100 Questions & Answers About Diabetes

Michael Bryer-Ash, MD
FRCP(Lond), FRCP(C)

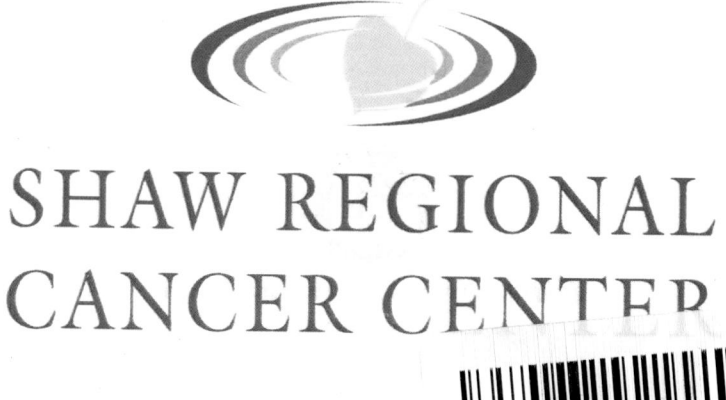

World Headquarters

Jones and Bartlett
  Publishers
40 Tall Pine Drive
Sudbury, MA 01776
978-443-5000
info@jbpub.com
www.jbpub.com

Jones and Bartlett
  Publishers Canada
6339 Ormindale Way
Mississauga, Ontario L5V 1J2
Canada

Jones and Bartlett
  Publishers International
Barb House, Barb Mews
London W6 7PA
United Kingdom

Jones and Bartlett's books and products are available through most bookstores and online book-sellers. To contact Jones and Bartlett Publishers directly, call 800-832-0034, fax 978-443-8000, or visit our website, www.jbpub.com.

Substantial discounts on bulk quantities of Jones and Bartlett's publications are available to corporations, professional associations, and other qualified organizations. For details and specific discount information, contact the special sales department at Jones and Bartlett via the above contact information or send an email to specialsales@jbpub.com

The authors, editor, and publisher have made every effort to provide accurate information. However, they are not responsible for errors, omissions, or for any outcomes related to the use of the contents of this book and take no responsibility for the use of the products and procedures described. Treatments and side effects described in this book may not be applicable to all people; likewise, some people may require a dose or experience a side effect that is not described herein. Drugs and medical devices are discussed that may have limited availability controlled by the Food and Drug Administration (FDA) for use only in a research study or clinical trial. Research, clinical practice, and government regulations often change the accepted standard in this field. When consideration is being given to use of any drug in the clinical setting, the health care provider or reader is responsible for determining FDA status of the drug, reading the package insert, and reviewing prescribing information for the most up-to-date recommendations on dose, precautions, and contraindications, and determining the appropriate usage for the product. This is especially important in the case of drugs that are new or seldom used.

Production Credits
Senior Acquisitions Editor: Alison Hankey
Senior Editorial Assistant: Jessica Acox
Associate Production Editor: Leah Corrigan
Senior Marketing Manager: Barb Bartoszek
Manufacturing and Inventory Supervisor: Amy Bacus
Composition: Glyph International
Cover Design: Carolyn Downer
Cover Images: © Lisa F. Young/Dreamstime.com, © Photos.com, © Bilderbuch/age fotostock
Printing and Binding: Malloy, Inc.
Cover Printing: Malloy, Inc.

Library of Congress Cataloging-in-Publication Data
Bryer-Ash, Michael.
    100 questions & answers about diabetes / Michael Bryer-Ash.
        p. cm.
    Includes index.
    ISBN 978-0-7637-5539-3 (alk. paper)
1. Diabetes--Miscellanea. 2. Diabetes--Popular works. I. Title. II. Title: One hundred questions and answers about diabetes.
    RC660.B79 2010
    616.4'62--dc22   2009038485

6048

Printed in the United States of America
13 12 11 10 09   10 9 8 7 6 5 4 3 2 1

This book is dedicated to the memory of the late Dr. Jonathan B. Jaspan (1947–1997), a consummate clinician and educator and a talented researcher, who gave much to the field of diabetes and touched the lives of many.

Contents

Part 5: Treatments for Diabetes 49

Questions 39–54 detail ways in which diabetes can be controlled, including exercise, diet, and medications:

- What should I eat and what should I avoid? Please be specific!
- Who should take pills and who should take insulin?
- Are there any medications prescribed for other conditions that can improve or worsen my diabetes?

Part 6: Monitoring and Living with Diabetes 73

Questions 55–69 offer help with the daily management of diabetes and how to live with the disease:

- What information should I bring to my doctor to help him or her manage my diabetes with me?
- How accurate are glucose monitors?
- How will my diabetes affect my work? Are there any jobs I cannot do?

Part 7: Diabetes and Special Situations 97

Questions 70–79 describe how to handle diabetes in special circumstances, such as pregnancy and travel:

- I have diabetes and want to get pregnant. What should I do?
- I will be traveling. How do I handle the time changes with my insulin shots?
- My child has diabetes and is about to start school. What steps should I take and how will the school help to ensure that things go well?

Part 8: Resources for People with Diabetes 111

Questions 80–89 provide useful sources for diabetes patients for information about the disease, diabetes research, advocacy, and more:

- I am interested in participating in research studies on new treatments for diabetes. How do I go about it?
- How can I find and join a diabetes support group in my area?
- How do I find out about the latest developments for treatment and monitoring of diabetes?

Part 9: When a Family Member or Loved One Has Diabetes 125

Questions 90–95 cover ways to help a loved one who has diabetes:

- What should a parent, spouse, partner, or caregiver know about diabetes in order to provide support to a loved one?
- My child has diabetes. What can I do when he or she is sick to help prevent the diabetes from going out of control?
- My spouse/partner has diabetes and we are planning a family. What is the risk that our children will develop diabetes?

Contents

Diabetes is a disease that is different from most other diseases for two important reasons. First, like hypertension, it can be a "silent killer." That is, there are few symptoms until late in the disease, at which time it is usually too late to reverse the damage. Because of this lack of symptoms, people with diabetes, and too often their physicians, do not give it a high priority. This is one of the reasons that diabetes is the leading cause of blindness in people less than 74 years of age, the leading cause of dialysis (using machines to replace kidney function), and the major reason for amputations of toes, feet, and legs. All of this need not happen if glucose levels in people with diabetes could be kept to near-normal levels.

Second, people with diabetes must be actively involved in its treatment. For almost all other diseases, doctors prescribe medicines and the only responsibility for the patient is to take them appropriately. Not so with diabetes. Patients must carefully watch their diet, exercise more often, measure their own glucoses in many cases, and keep appointments in which preventive tests (e.g., measurements of albumin leakage into the urine) and examinations (e.g., dilated eye exams by qualified ophthalmologists) are carried out—all of this when patients feel fine. Therefore, people with diabetes must know a lot about their disease to stay motivated and to be able to make appropriate decisions that would minimize bad outcomes from this disease.

Dr. Bryer-Ash's book, *100 Questions & Answers About Diabetes*, should be very helpful in that regard. In addition to basic information about diabetes, it discusses topics not usually covered by more basic books for the public. These topics include discussions of potential cures for diabetes, prevention of diabetes, important information for family members and caregivers of people with diabetes; hints for developing a professional career in diabetes, for volunteering in diabetes, for advocating for diabetes causes, for developing support groups; critical information for participating in sports, for smoothing the experience of children in their school environments, and for travel across time zones. The book is written for the sophisticated reader. This audience will benefit immeasurably from reading Dr. Bryer-Ash's book and certainly will not feel "talked down to." Instead, with this information, they will be important members, indeed the most important members, of the team that is caring for their diabetes.

Mayer B. Davidson, MD
Professor of Medicine
Charles Drew University &
David Geffen School of Medicine at UCLA
Past President, American Diabetes Association

Acknowledgments

I thank those who have given advice and assistance with this book, especially Dr. Mayer B. Davidson, who kindly reviewed the manuscript and gave many helpful suggestions, as he has done throughout my career. Jeffrey Hall, Janice Camino, and several of my patients contributed questions. Joann Jue provided administrative assistance. Michelle Dennison-Farris RD, CDE gave helpful advice on Questions 40 and 67 relating to nutrition and diet. I thank Dr. Keith G. Dawson for providing a superb clinical role model of a first-class diabetologist. Finally, I thank my family and loved ones for their patience and support. However, any omissions, oversights, or errors in this work are mine alone.

PART ONE

What Is Diabetes?

Why and how did I get diabetes?

What are the symptoms of diabetes?

Is there such a thing as borderline diabetes?
What is it?

More . . .

1. Why and how did I get diabetes?

Diabetes occurs for a number of reasons, but the ultimate cause of the high blood sugar that characterizes the disorder is either **deficiency** of the hormone **insulin** or a combination of insulin deficiency and resistance of the body tissues to its actions. In response to food intake, insulin is released by specialized cells in the **pancreas** and is necessary for adequate amounts of **glucose** and other nutrients from food to be absorbed into certain tissues of the body. When insulin is lacking or the body resists its actions, the level of glucose in the blood becomes excessively high and diabetes is diagnosed. The difference in the balance between the two characterizes the two major forms of diabetes—type 1 and type 2 (see Question 2). Whatever the form of diabetes, its basis is to some extent hereditary and to some extent environmental. The hereditary contribution is more or less constant throughout recent human evolution. It is the environmental component that has changed markedly over the last 100 years, leading to the dramatic rise in the frequency of diabetes in almost all societies. You developed diabetes because either you are strongly predisposed due to hereditary reasons or because there are factors in your lifestyle and environment (such as gaining weight, getting insufficient exercise, taking certain medications) that increase the likelihood of diabetes or, as is usually the case, a combination of both. This is not all bad, because the environment and lifestyle can often be changed, with dramatic improvement in the severity of the diabetes. For more on this, see Question 5.

2. What is the difference between type 1 and type 2 diabetes?

Type 1 diabetes is entirely due to an almost complete deficiency of insulin. The deficiency is the result of

Deficiency

A lack or shortage, especially of something essential to health.

Insulin

A hormone produced by the beta cells of the pancreas, which facilitates the entry of glucose and other substances into cells and which has several other functions.

Pancreas

A gland deep in the abdomen, behind the stomach, that produces hormones (insulin, glucagon) and digestive enzymes.

Glucose

A basic sugar used to fuel body cells.

Type 1 diabetes

Characterized by an almost complete deficiency of insulin due to the immune system erroneously attacking and destroying the insulin-producing cells in the pancreas.

the **immune system** erroneously attacking and destroying the insulin-producing cells in the pancreas. For the proper functioning of our bodies, it is necessary for insulin to be present at all times in the bloodstream and tissues, not only after we have eaten. Insulin is essential to maintain the structure of our tissues and prevent them from being broken down in an uncontrolled manner. Without any insulin present, our tissues literally melt away into simple compounds that leave our bodies when we urinate. Accordingly, people with type 1 diabetes have high levels of sugar and breakdown products of fat and protein in the bloodstream and urine and develop the typical symptoms described in Question 4.

Type 2 diabetes is due to a combination of our body tissues becoming resistant to the action of insulin (for the reasons described previously in Question 1) and the inability of the pancreas to make enough extra insulin to overcome it. Although this latter component of the problem is often viewed as a failure of the pancreas, it is not true in the strictest sense. While it is common for the insulin-producing capability of the pancreas to decline throughout later adult life, it was nevertheless sufficient throughout most of human evolution to prevent us from developing diabetes. It is only in recent times, when our lifestyle and environment have caused many of us to become very insulin resistant, that the insulin-producing capacity is unable to compensate. In the true sense, it fails because we impose an excessive load upon it. This is true, even for those of us who have a hereditary predisposition to becoming insulin resistant. The difference between the two forms of diabetes is illustrated in **Figure 1**.

Immune system

The body's system that protects it from foreign substances, cells, and tissues. The immune system includes the thymus, spleen, lymph nodes, lymphocytes, B-cells and T-cells, and antibodies.

Type 2 diabetes

Caused by a combination of body tissues becoming resistant to the action of insulin and the inability of the pancreas to make enough extra insulin to overcome it.

It is only in recent times, when our lifestyle and environment have caused many of us to become very insulin resistant, that the insulin-producing capacity is unable to compensate.

What Is Diabetes?

3

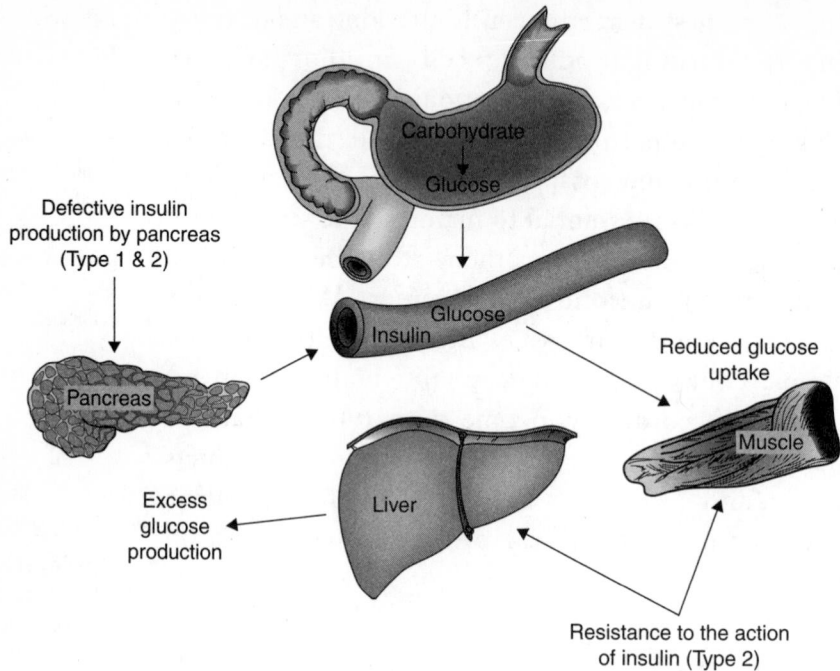

Figure 1   The cause of type 1 and type 2 diabetes.

3. What is the difference between diabetes mellitus and diabetes insipidus?

The word diabetes is an interesting one. Its origin is in the Greek language where it is derived from the word for a siphon or, more simply, a pipe or hose. This word was used to describe the disorder in ancient times (and diabetes was recognized in great antiquity) because those suffering from it produced such plentiful amounts of urine that they were reminiscent of a water pipe. The reason for the plentiful amounts of urine lies in the fact that when the sugar glucose reaches excessively high levels in our bloodstream, it is filtered into the kidney and enters the urine in large quantities. Due to its chemical and physical properties, when large amounts of glucose are filtered by our kidneys into the urine, it cannot be fully reabsorbed and retains a large amount of water with it, thus creating very large volumes of urine. The second part of the name, **mellitus**, is derived from the word meaning sweet, as in mellifluous music. Mellitus was added when it was discovered that the urine in a person with diabetes and very high blood sugar is sweet.

Diabetes insipidus is a disorder with an entirely different basis, but its sufferers share the siphon-like quality of very frequent and very high volume urination. Diabetes insipidus is due to failure of production or action of another vital hormone, known as **arginine vasopressin (AVP)**, also called **antidiuretic hormone (ADH)**, that is responsible for maintaining the normal volume and concentration of our urine. When AVP is deficient (usually due to damage or disease of the hypothalamus or pituitary gland) or fails to work (usually due to disease of or damage to the kidney), we are unable to concentrate our urine and it becomes excessively dilute. As such, it appears pale, almost colorless and watery—in a word insipid, hence *insipidus*. It is not sweet, as it has negligible amounts of sugar in it.

4. What are the symptoms of diabetes?

The typical symptoms of diabetes occur as a result of the high levels of glucose in the bloodstream and its passage into the urine and other tissues. These are frequent urination and thirst. Thirst arises as a result of the dehydration caused by the frequent urination. Dehydration and loss of nutrient calories in the urine lead to weight loss and hunger. Passage of glucose into the tissues of the eye can cause fluctuating

Diabetes mellitus

A condition characterized by inadequate production of insulin or resistance of the body's tissues to its actions, which results in excessive levels of glucose in the blood.

Diabetes insipidus

Increased urine production caused by inadequate secretion of vasopressin by the pituitary gland or by resistance of the kidney to its actions.

Arginine vasopressin (AVP)

A hormone that is responsible for maintaining the normal volume and concentration of our urine. Also called antidiuretic hormone (ADH).

Antidiuretic hormone (ADH)

A hormone that is responsible for maintaining the normal volume and concentration of our urine. Also called arginine vasopressin (AVP).

What Is Diabetes?

degrees of blurred vision. When these symptoms are prolonged and severe, as is typical with type 1 diabetes, serious changes occur in our blood chemistry due to the deficiency of insulin. Those changes, coupled with dehydration, result in dizziness, weakness, drowsiness, and ultimately coma, which if untreated can lead to death. Both type 1 and type 2 diabetes, when severe and inadequately treated, can be associated with coma and death. Although coma is less common in type 2 diabetes, it is more common for it to result in death, as people with type 2 diabetes tend to be older and to have more medical problems. Two other important points are worth noting. The first is that diabetes may not cause any symptoms. In fact, one of every four people believed to have diabetes is unaware of it and is undiagnosed. However, as diabetes of even moderate severity can lead to complications and shorten lifespan, it is important to make the diagnosis, even in people without symptoms. The second point is that the majority of people with diabetes may not have any symptoms from the elevated blood sugar, but it can still present with symptoms from its complications. Thus, people may be diagnosed with diabetes after presenting with symptoms of nerve damage (**neuropathy**—see Question 32) or a heart attack or stroke (see Question 35). In fact, one of every three people admitted with a sudden heart event is found to have diabetes or **prediabetes** (see Question 9) of which he or she or the doctor was unaware. Neuropathy is present in two of every five patients with type 2 diabetes at the time of diagnosis, while eye damage (**retinopathy**—see Question 33) is present in one of every five and kidney damage (**nephropathy**—see Question 34) is present in one in ten, indicating that the diabetes was ongoing for many months or even years before diagnosis.

One of every four people believed to have diabetes is unaware of it and is undiagnosed.

Neuropathy

Nerve damage.

Prediabetes

A condition in which abnormalities in plasma glucose levels lie in-between normal and standard accepted definitions of diabetes. "Borderline diabetes," "impaired fasting glucose," and "impaired glucose tolerance" are other terms used to describe types of this condition.

Retinopathy

Eye damage.

Nephropathy

Kidney damage.

5. Can diabetes be cured?

In general, we do not consider that diabetes can be cured once it has been diagnosed. People with type 2 diabetes can reverse the detectable abnormalities of diabetes by lifestyle adjustment without the use of medications (discussed in Question 28). However, the tendency to manifest high blood sugar again is always present if the patient is under significant metabolic stress, such as that caused by medications, severe illness, injury, regaining lost weight, cessation of exercise, aging, etc. Therefore we consider that diabetes can be under excellent control or in **remission**, but we do not usually use the word cured. Even people with type 1 diabetes who have undergone successful pancreas or islet transplantation and no longer require insulin therapy cannot be considered cured. There is a significant possibility that their diabetes will one day come back for a variety of reasons, including rejection of the transplant or a renewed attack on the transplanted **islet tissue** by the patient's immune system.

Perhaps the closest we have been able to come in the search for a true cure for diabetes is the effect of **bariatric surgery** ("weight loss surgery"), which either involves procedures to restrict the entry of food into the stomach or procedures to bypass the stomach and upper intestine, thus reducing food absorption. Procedures of the bypass type have shown prolonged remission of diabetes in up to 80% of cases for as long as 10 years. Remission for 10 years or more is approaching a definition of a true cure, and in the future this and other medications or procedures that provide a long-term reversal of obesity may come to be generally accepted as "curing" type 2 diabetes.

What Is Diabetes?

Remission
A temporary or permanent decrease of manifestations of a disease.

Islet tissue
Groups of cells found within the pancreas that produce and release insulin, glucagons, and other substances.

Bariatric surgery
Weight loss surgery.

6. Does diabetes affect all racial groups equally?

No, there are significant differences in the hereditary tendency to acquire diabetes (**Figure 2**). In general Caucasians (non-Hispanic whites) have a lower tendency to develop type 2 diabetes than other ethnic groups. The situation with regard to type 1 diabetes is the opposite, with the highest prevalence currently being in the regions in and near Finland, Sardinia, and Kuwait. Lifestyle does not appear to be more important than the hereditary tendency in determining the chance of a person to develop type 1 diabetes. However, in the case of type 2 diabetes it is an important factor. Thus, certain ethnic groups may have a very high tendency to develop type 2 diabetes under one set of environmental circumstances, but they may have a very low tendency under different environmental conditions. A case in point is the Pima tribe of Native Americans living in Arizona. Half of the Pima have type 2 diabetes, while their genetically related cousins living in the Chiapas region of Mexico pursuing a nonurban lifestyle have a low frequency of the disorder. The two most common and most important factors contributing to a high prevalence of type 2 diabetes in groups at high hereditary risk are weight gain and lack of physical exercise.

7. Are my brothers and sisters and my children at risk of diabetes?

If you have type 1 diabetes, your first-degree relatives (i.e. mother, father, brother, sister, and your children) are about ten times more likely than the general population to get type 1 diabetes. The frequency of type 1 diabetes in the general population is about half a percent (i.e., one in two hundred), so the risk in your first-degree relatives is about 10 × 1/2, or 5%. Fortunately, this is not particularly

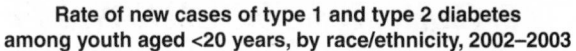

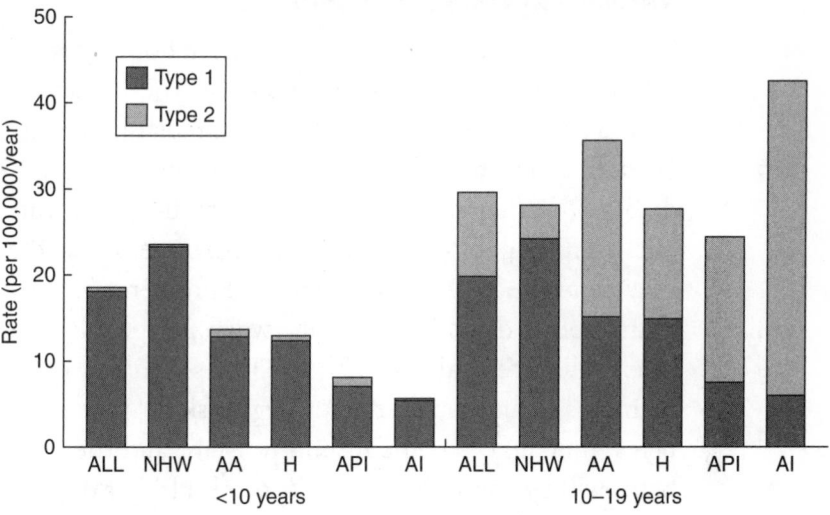

NHW = Non-Hispanic whites; AA = African Americans; H = Hispanics;
API = Asians/Pacific Islanders; AI = American Indians

Figure 2   Difference in frequency of occurrence of diabetes by race and ethnicity.

Source: Courtesy of SEARCH for diabetes in youth study.

high. Also, it is related to age. About 90% of cases of type 1 diabetes occur before age 35. Therefore, the parents of a person with type 1 diabetes are at considerably less, and ever decreasing, risk compared to his or her siblings and children. The risk of getting type 1 diabetes for an identical twin of a person with type 1 diabetes is 30–50%, indicating that environmental factors are very important, even though they are not well understood. In the case of type 2 diabetes, the risk is considerably higher. On average, one out of three of the children of an individual with type 2 diabetes will develop the disease. Two out of three of the children will develop diabetes when both parents have the disease. The risk of getting type 2 diabetes for an identical twin of a person with type 2 diabetes is 75–90%, indicating that genetic (hereditary) factors are very important.

What Is Diabetes?

8. Can a person have both type 1 and type 2 diabetes at the same time?

Generally speaking, we do not diagnose both disorders in the same individual. If people have type 1 diabetes, they are completely lacking effective circulating insulin. By definition, this is not the case in people with type 2 diabetes, so having the one disorder effectively rules out the other. However, people with type 1 diabetes may be prone to the same metabolic problems as those with type 2 diabetes. In other words, if people with type 1 diabetes gain weight, become sedentary, or are members of an ethnic group at high risk for type 2 diabetes, they may become insulin resistant and their diabetes will be more difficult to control. Higher doses of insulin will be required and they may develop the metabolic problems that tend to be associated with type 2 diabetes, such as cholesterol and related blood fat abnormalities, as well as high blood pressure. These will add to their risk of cardiovascular disease. Some people with apparent type 2 diabetes appear to have a partial form of type 1 diabetes, which has stopped short of complete destruction of their insulin-producing cells in the pancreas. This is known as LADA or *latent autoimmune diabetes of the adult*. They tend to require insulin treatment earlier in the course of their diabetes, but are not considered to have both diseases.

9. Is there such a thing as borderline diabetes? What is it?

The term **borderline diabetes** has now been replaced by the term *prediabetes*. Both terms indicate that a person has abnormalities in his or her plasma glucose levels that fall short of standard accepted definitions for frank diabetes. **Table 1** shows the normal ranges for both **fasting** plasma glucose and for plasma glucose after a

Borderline diabetes

A condition in which plasma glucose falls in between normal and standard accepted definitions for diabetes. "Prediabetes" is another term commonly used for the same condition.

Fasting

Abstaining from eating food, usually for nine hours or more.

Table 1 Definition of Diabetes & Prediabetes

Normal Blood Sugar	mg/dl	mmol/L
Fasting 2 hours after glucose*	60–99 less than 140	3.3–5.5 less than 7.8
Prediabetes: Fasting 2 hours after glucose	100–125 140–199	5.6–6.9 7.8–11.1
Diabetes: Fasting 2 hours after glucose Anytime	126 or above 200 or above 200 or above with symptoms**	7.0 or above 11.2 or above

*75 Grams of glucose by mouth.
**Such as thirst, frequent urination, weight loss or blurred vision.

glucose load by mouth. The reason that a standardized 75 gram (a little under 3 ounces) glucose load is used is to allow a direct comparison between different individuals under the same conditions. The table also shows the glucose levels above which diabetes is diagnosed. The range between the upper end of normal and diabetes itself is the prediabetic range. For fasting glucose, the range is 100 to 125 mg/dl and for glucose values 2 hours after a standard 75 gram glucose drink by mouth, it is 140 to 199 mg/dl. The former is termed *impaired fasting glucose*, or IFG, and the latter is termed *impaired glucose tolerance,* or IGT. When either is present, an individual is described as having prediabetes. There are at least two reasons why it is important to identify prediabetes. One reason is that people with prediabetes have a known increased risk of progression to frank type 2 diabetes and, second, prediabetes, especially of the IGT type, is associated with a significantly higher risk of cardiovascular disease and death. Therefore, knowledge that one has prediabetes necessitates regular follow-up and also permits early intervention to prevent progression to frank diabetes.

Knowledge that one has prediabetes necessitates regular follow-up and also permits early intervention to prevent progression to frank diabetes.

10. Why do some women get diabetes when they are pregnant? Is this dangerous for them or their baby?

Pregnancy is a situation in which insulin resistance (see Question 2) is a normal feature. This is because it is beneficial for the nutrients absorbed from a pregnant woman's meals to be channeled first to the growing fetus. The development of maternal insulin resistance in the second half of pregnancy assures that this will occur. At least part of the reason for the development of maternal insulin resistance is that the placenta produces substances that lead to insulin resistance and as the placenta grows, the insulin resistance increases. This is called physiologic (i.e., normal) insulin resistance. Indeed, a healthy pregnant woman may be more insulin resistant than the average patient with type 2 diabetes! However, the vast majority (>95%) of otherwise healthy pregnant women do not get diabetes in this situation because the pancreas is able to make enough insulin to overcome the insulin resistance and keep the glucose levels normal. A small minority of women cannot do so and their glucose levels rise. These women tend to be the same women who are destined to get type 2 diabetes later in life. The risk of developing type 2 diabetes is much higher in a woman who has had diabetes detected in pregnancy (**gestational diabetes mellitus** or GDM). GDM provides a unique opportunity to follow the natural history of type 2 diabetes in the years prior to its onset in women, since most GDM goes away very rapidly, often within hours, after the baby is delivered and reappears in later life as type 2 diabetes. If untreated, GDM can cause harm to both mother and baby, especially at or soon after delivery. Fortunately, outcomes of GDM are generally excellent in most developed countries.

A healthy pregnant woman may be more insulin resistant than the average patient with type 2 diabetes!

Gestational diabetes mellitus (GDM)

Diabetes detected in pregnancy.

PART TWO

Can Diabetes Be Prevented?

Does regular exercise help to prevent type 2 diabetes?

Is there a particular type of diet that will reduce my chance of type 2 diabetes?

Are there any natural herbs, minerals, or other remedies that prevent diabetes?

More . . .

11. How does my weight affect my risk of type 2 diabetes?

Body mass index (BMI)

A clinical means of relating weight to height by a formula. To calculate your own BMI, divide your weight in pounds by the square of your height in inches (i.e., your height multiplied by itself) and then multiply the answer by 703.

A BMI of 18 to almost 25 is considered to be healthy.

Weight and risk of type 2 diabetes are clearly linked. **Figure 3** shows the risk of development of type 2 diabetes, as it relates to body weight. For clinical purposes, weight is related to height by a formula known as **body mass index** or BMI. In our society, a BMI of 18 to almost 25 is considered to be healthy and from 25 to almost 30 is considered overweight. From 30 to 35 is considered to be obese and from 35 to 40 is severely obese. A BMI that is greater than 40 is considered morbidly obese, indicating that a person with this degree of obesity is at very serious risk of both immediate and long-term health problems. To calculate your own BMI, divide your weight in pounds by the square of your height in inches (i.e., your height multiplied by itself) and then multiply the answer

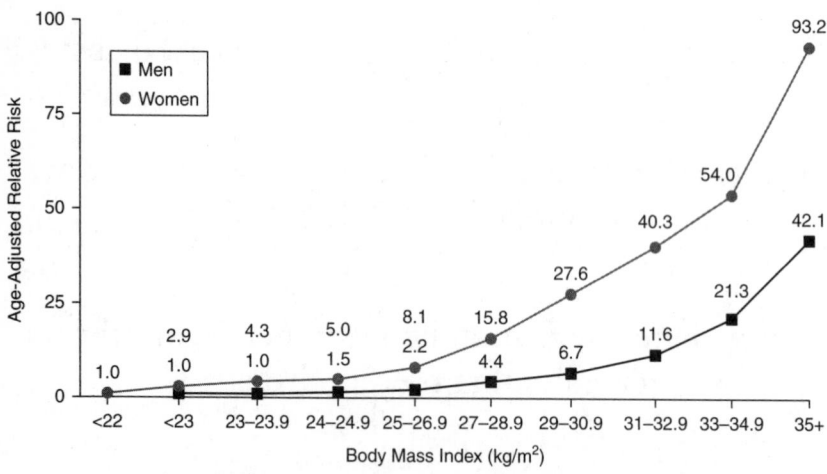

Figure 3   Relationship between weight risk of type 2 diabetes.

Source: Data from Chan JM et al. *Diabetes Care.* 1994;17:961–969; Colditz G et al. *Ann Intern Med.* 1995;122:481–486.

by 703. For example, if you are 5 feet 8 inches (68 inches) tall and weigh 148 pounds, your BMI will be 148 divided by 68 × 68, i.e., 148/4624 = 0.032 and then multiplied by 705, i.e., your BMI is 22.6. Congratulate yourself, as your weight is in the healthy range! Figure 3 shows the risk for development of type 2 diabetes according to weight for both men and women. The risk of having type 2 diabetes increases as weight increases, even within the normal range, especially for women. Severe and morbid obesity are associated with an almost 100 times greater chance of diabetes in women and almost 50 times for men. The reason for this is principally because the likelihood of having insulin resistance, a major causative factor for type 2 diabetes (see Question 2), increases as weight rises. Very physically active individuals who are overweight or obese by usual standards may be at little increased risk due to the protective effect of exercise (see Question 12).

12. Does regular exercise help to prevent type 2 diabetes?

Yes, regular exercise of at least moderate intensity provides some protection against the onset of type 2 diabetes. Exercise improves insulin resistance and thereby makes insulin more effective at removing glucose from the blood. In patients with prediabetes (see Question 9), exercise can prevent the progression of elevated glucose values toward the frankly diabetic range, or even restore them to normal. Exercise also consumes **calories** from those stored in the exercising muscle as starch (**glycogen**) and the need to replenish these stores draws glucose out of the bloodstream and thereby reduces the circulating levels. Exercise also helps to maintain a healthy body weight and avoid the weight gain that can lead to diabetes (see Question 11),

Regular exercise of at least moderate intensity provides some protection against the onset of type 2 diabetes.

Calorie

A unit used to express heat or energy value of food.

Glycogen

Starch, which comprises sugars linked together in a storage pattern.

although it is not as certain that exercise is as helpful in promoting weight reduction. Weight reduction is much more dependent on restriction of food intake. However, exercise is clearly important in maintaining weight loss. Finally, it is worth noting that exercise has beneficial effects on the other risk factors that combine with diabetes to cause vascular disease. For example, exercise increases the good (or **HDL**) cholesterol and improves levels of other blood fats, while lowering blood pressure and enhancing cardiovascular (i.e., heart and blood vessel) conditioning.

HDL

High-density lipoprotein; "good cholesterol."

13. Are there any medications I can take to help prevent diabetes?

Yes, there are a number of medications that will help to reduce the likelihood of a person developing type 2 diabetes, but not type 1 diabetes. These are shown in **Table 2**. None are labeled by the Food and Drug Administration for this indication. Our use of them is mainly confined to choosing a drug that will tend to slow progression to type 2 diabetes when the drug is needed for another condition. For example, when a patient at risk for diabetes needs treatment for high blood pressure, one would consider using a drug that has been shown to slow progression to diabetes in

Table 2   Medications That May Help to Prevent Diabetes

Medication	Approved Use
Ramipril	Blood pressure
Losartan	Blood pressure
Carvedilol	Blood pressure
Metformin	Type 2 diabetes
Acarbose	Type 2 diabetes
Hydroxychoroquine	Rheumatoid arthritis, malaria
Vitamin D	Vitamin supplementation
Aspirin	Pain and inflammation

those at high risk, as opposed to one that might actually accelerate it. Early use of drugs that are approved to treat type 2 diabetes in people at high risk of development of type 2 diabetes (mainly those with prediabetes—for definition see Question 9) has also been shown to prevent or delay the onset of the disease. Examples of this use are also shown in Table 2. Whether this represents prevention of diabetes or pretreatment of diabetes is not conclusively known. To be considered true prevention, the drug needs to modify the course and progression of the underlying factors leading to the disease and not merely lower the blood sugar. This means the rate at which those at risk progress to diabetes should be reduced in a sustained manner. It should be emphasized that one must be very cautious in advocating the use of oral antidiabetic drugs in this manner. The FDA and other authoritative bodies have not evaluated the ratio of risk to benefit sufficiently to recommend their use in prediabetes.

14. Is there a particular type of diet that will reduce my chance of type 2 diabetes?

The most important aspect of any diet to prevent type 2 diabetes is its calorie (i.e., energy) content. If calorie intake exceeds calorie usage, then the excess calories will, in the absence of other modifying factors, be directed toward the body's energy storage compartment, which is, of course, the fat tissue. Therefore, a diet that matches calorie consumption with output is the key to prevention of overweight and obesity and therefore diabetes. If one is already overweight, then the diet should provide fewer calories than are required, so that energy will be drawn from the body fat stores and gradual weight loss will occur. Even

The most important aspect of any diet to prevent type 2 diabetes is its calorie (i.e., energy) content.

modest weight loss can be very beneficial. The benefits can be shown very early, almost as soon as calorie intake drops below that required to maintain body weight and before significant weight loss actually occurs. The consumption side of this balance is, of course, food intake. The output side that we can control is exercise. Neither can operate successfully to regulate weight independent of the other. Very calorie-dense foods, such as those with a high fat content (e.g., cheese, ice cream, fried foods, and processed meats) are common components of diets that lead to weight gain, obesity, and ultimately diabetes. Although sugar itself does not cause diabetes, foods with a high content of refined sugar, such as sodas and candies, are also more likely to be associated with weight gain and diabetes than those with natural sugars. Natural sugars tend to be associated with **fiber**, which delays and limits their absorption. Thus, portion for portion, more sugar is consumed in foods high in refined sugar. The question of whether a specific diet composition can prevent diabetes, independent of its actual energy content, is not entirely known. Studies have shown that diets high in grain and fiber tend to be associated with a lower frequency of diabetes in the population. This may be related to the more gradual breakdown and absorption of the components of the meal, especially the **carbohydrates**, as discussed previously.

Since, in all parts of the world, the explosive rise in diabetes is clearly linked to weight gain (with some population groups being more susceptible than others) rather than to a specific type of diet, the dietary focus should remain on eating a healthy diet that provides the recommended amounts of important nutrients, in quantities necessary to maintain a healthy weight (see Question 11) and prevent undesirable weight gain.

Fiber

The structural part of plants and plant products that consists of carbohydrates that are wholly or partially indigestible.

Carbohydrates

Substances composed of long chains of oxygen, hydrogen, and carbon molecules. Carbohydrates in food (for example, sugar and starch) provide energy for the body and, if present in excess, are stored as fat.

For more information, visit http://www.diabetes.org/nutrition-and-recipes/nutrition/foodpyramid.jsp.

15. Does stress affect my risk of getting diabetes?

The perception of stress differs greatly among individuals. What one person may perceive as stressful, another may not. For this reason, stress is quite hard to measure in real-life situations. Artificial measures of accepted stress, such as electric shocks or deprivation of sleep, are very hard to apply to day-to-day life. However, people who report that they are more stressed, regardless of the actual nature of the stress itself, are more likely to suffer from diabetes. Furthermore, it has recently become apparent that measurable physical and psychological stress, such as that caused by sleep deprivation and social stress, is more likely to be associated with the presence of diabetes. This may in part explain the difference in the frequency of diabetes found in people of similar genetic background and measurable physical characteristics (body weight, amount of exercise, etc.) in different regions and societies. Exactly how perceived stress, whether physical, social, or psychological, leads to diabetes is not yet understood.

16. What other factors increase my risk of getting diabetes?

Besides excess weight, hereditary risk, and lack of exercise, another factor that can increase the risk of developing diabetes is the use of certain medications. Among these medications, the type associated most strongly with increased risk are the steroids (also called glucocorticoids), whose members include prednisone, methylprednisolone, hydrocortisone, and

Among these medications, the type associated most strongly with increased risk are the steroids (also called glucocorticoids).

dexamethasone. The steroids belong to a class of naturally occurring stress hormones known as **counterregulatory hormones**, which prepare the body to combat stress. They tend to raise blood sugar. Other stress hormones include the so-called *catecholamines* such as epinephrine (adrenaline) and norepinephrine (noradrenaline), which also raise the blood sugar. Synthetic versions of these compounds, which include some drugs used in weight loss medications, cold and allergy medications, asthma medications, and stimulants, can also cause a rise in blood sugar. Certain types of diuretic pills ("water pills") such as thiazides can also occasionally raise blood sugar, although these pills are commonly and appropriately used in people with diabetes. A certain type of cholesterol-modifying drug known as niacin can raise the blood sugar, sometimes quite markedly. The long-acting ("extended release") version of niacin is less likely to do this. Certain types of medications used to treat psychiatric conditions (the atypical antipsychotics) can lead to a higher frequency of diabetes, although this appears to be largely due to their tendency to cause weight gain. Certain classes of antiviral drugs, especially those used for the treatment of HIV/AIDS, can lead to diabetes.

Certain classes of antiviral drugs, especially those used for the treatment of HIV/AIDS, can lead to diabetes.

In the case of all these drugs, the prescribing physician needs to consider the potential benefit of the drug in question to the patient and weigh this against the known risks, including the risk of developing diabetes. In many cases, the potential benefit of using these drugs, which may be life-saving, is believed to outweigh the risks and the blood sugar should be monitored and treated appropriately if diabetes occurs. Once the drug in question is discontinued, the diabetes usually goes away and treatment can be discontinued.

17. Is there anything I can do to reduce my children's risk of getting diabetes?

There is presently little that can reliably be done to reduce a person's risk of type 1 diabetes, as discussed in Question 19. However, type 2 diabetes has undergone a dramatic increase in children and adolescents in recent years, and it is clear that this is driven, in the most part, by childhood and adolescent overweight and obesity as well as lack of regular exercise. Therefore, establishment of a healthy pattern of eating in childhood, without excess calorie intake, and encouragement of regular exercise can be the most effective means of preventing the development of diabetes. It is important not only to provide children with these elements, but to ensure that they understand how to make healthy choices for themselves and that they realize the lifelong benefits that maintenance of healthy body weight and regular exercise can bring. In this way, they are more likely to establish and attach importance to a healthy lifestyle in adulthood and thus reduce their likelihood of developing diabetes lifelong.

18. Are there any natural herbs, minerals, or other remedies that prevent diabetes?

While it would be premature to answer *yes* to this question, it does appear that certain compounds can favorably impact the blood sugar and may have the potential to delay or prevent diabetes. Those for whom there is at least some evidence include uncooked walnuts, gymnema sylvestre (also known as *gurmarbooti* or *gurmar*), green tea, and certain compounds of chromium, zinc, and vanadium. While it is not known how most of these compounds work, the metallic compounds may work by facilitating the body's mechanisms

Establishment of a healthy pattern of eating in childhood, without excess calorie intake, and encouragement of regular exercise can be the most effective means of preventing the development of diabetes.

for releasing insulin, or responding to insulin. Overall, the effect of most of these items is quite mild, and they may influence the blood sugar by a few points. However, occasional individuals have a fairly dramatic response. In addition, there is a known association between low levels of vitamin D and diabetes. It is possible that this may not result from the lack of vitamin D itself, but from other factors somehow related to low vitamin D levels. Replenishment of vitamin D has not been shown to prevent diabetes long term and it is too early to draw conclusions about this. Some of these compounds are shown in **Table 3**.

19. Can type 1 diabetes also be prevented?

At the present time, we do not think that type 1 diabetes can effectively be prevented. Part of the problem is that we do not know the exact environmental trigger(s), although there is provocative evidence for a number of factors, such as early exposure to cow's milk, certain viral strains, and lack of stimulation of the immune system at an early age by natural exposure to infective agents. The evidence is insufficient to make specific recommendations for avoidance of, or **immunization** against, specific potential triggering agents. A number of clinical trials of agents that

Immunization

The process of inducing immunity, usually through inoculation or vaccination.

Table 3   Herbs, Minerals, Etc. That May Help to Prevent Diabetes

Name
Chromium picolinate
Zinc
Walnuts
Bitter melon
Gymnema sylvestre
Tea
Flaxseed
Vitamin D

modify the immune system attack on the insulin-producing cells of the pancreas (see Question 2) are under way. In general, these agents cause a number of side effects. Trials are focused on patients with newly diagnosed diabetes, to determine whether very early diabetes can be reversed, before their use in people without symptoms who are at an increased risk of development of the disease can be justified. There is also a significant genetic (hereditary) component of risk for type 1 diabetes (see Question 7) that can presently not be modified. First, therapies based on genetic modification in general are still at a very early stage of development. Second, the exact gene or genes that require modification are not conclusively known.

20. Several members of my close family have diabetes. Will attempts at prevention still work for me?

Please refer to Question 19 regarding type 1 diabetes. Regarding type 2 diabetes, your success in preventing diabetes depends upon a combination of how successful you are at attaining the necessary goals and how susceptible your family is. Inherited susceptibility can range from modest to very high. The risk also depends very much on whether both sides of a person's family have a hereditary pattern of diabetes. If both the mother and the father's sides have a high frequency of diabetes, then their offspring will have a marked tendency to develop type 2 diabetes. The general degree of risk is described in Question 7. In spite of the importance of heredity, it is clear than environment and lifestyle play a major role. This is clearly the case because hereditary tendencies to disease change little over the course of a few generations, while environment and lifestyle can change very rapidly. The recent

If both the mother and the father's sides have a high frequency of diabetes, then their offspring will have a marked tendency to develop type 2 diabetes.

explosive rise in the frequency of type 2 diabetes in most regions of the world clearly implicates the latter as the most important factor. The most readily identifiable lifestyle factors that precipitate type 2 diabetes are weight gain and lack of exercise. Greater than 90% of type 2 diabetes in our society results from one, or usually both, of these factors. Depending on the severity of your inherited risk, a greater or lesser degree of adherence to a lifestyle that avoids overweight or obesity and engages you in regular exercise will effectively prevent you from developing type 2 diabetes.

PART THREE

How Do I Know I Have Diabetes?

How does my doctor confirm the diagnosis of diabetes?

My doctor says I have hypoglycemia. Isn't that the opposite of diabetes?

I have a strong family history of diabetes. How often should I be checked for it?

More . . .

21. What are the most common symptoms of diabetes?

The common and early symptoms of diabetes result from the effect of the high blood sugar entering the urine and drawing fluid from the body's tissues along with it. This leads to excess urine production with frequent urination. The loss of body fluid leads to thirst, in order to replace the fluid loss. As long as the person with diabetes is able to keep pace with his or her thirst by regular fluid intake, he or she will remain relatively well. However, without free access to fluid, which can occur for a variety of reasons, one will become dehydrated, which leads to dizziness upon standing upright drowsiness, confusion, and ultimately fainting and unconsciousness. Due to the wasting of calories as glucose in the urine, patients will complain of hunger and will usually lose weight if high blood sugar is very marked. However, it is important to note that only a minority of people with diabetes will experience these symptoms. Frequently, the degree of high blood sugar is more moderate, with little sugar entering the urine and causing no immediate symptoms. However, diabetes of even modest severity can cause considerable harm and lead to serious chronic complications. Therefore, it is important to detect diabetes that is **asymptomatic** (i.e., without symptoms), which is the reason that screening programs to detect diabetes in those at highest risk have been developed. If asymptomatic diabetes is not discovered for a sufficiently long period (many months or years), patients may actually present with long-term complications of the previously unrecognized diabetes, such as heart attack, stroke, heart failure, neuropathy (nerve damage), nephropathy (kidney damage), or retinopathy (eye damage). These are discussed in Questions 32 to 35.

Asymptomatic

Having no complaints or symptoms.

22. How does my doctor confirm the diagnosis of diabetes?

Your doctor will perform one of the standard measurements for the diagnosis of diabetes approved by the accepted authoritative body in whichever part of the world you live. In the United States, this is generally set by the American Diabetes Association (ADA) and is accepted by most practitioners, insurers, and health providers as valid. The most current ADA criteria for the diagnosis of diabetes are shown in Table 1 (see Question 9). Your doctor may or may not ask you to fast prior to measuring the blood glucose or he or she may perform a standard 2-hour test known as the oral glucose tolerance test. Unless they are clearly and indisputably abnormal, or accompanied by typical symptoms of diabetes (discussed in Question 4), the results should be confirmed on a different day, since the diagnosis of diabetes carries many implications and necessitates lifelong monitoring and treatment. Very soon, the test that measures the average blood glucose over the past 3 months (the Hemoglobin A1c or HbA1c test) is also likely to become a standard test for detection and diagnosis of diabetes.

Different diagnostic procedures are used for pregnant women, most of whom should be screened for the presence of diabetes of pregnancy ("gestational diabetes") during the 24th to 28th week of pregnancy or earlier if they are at high risk or had diabetes in a previous pregnancy. This involves an initial 1-hour screening test for which fasting is not required. If the screening test is positive, it is followed by a more detailed 3-hour test for which prior fasting is necessary.

23. Can I "feel" my high and low blood sugars reliably?

Although many people with diabetes confidently state that they can reliably detect both their high and low blood sugars without actual measurement, studies have shown that these beliefs are not usually accurate. It is generally easier to be aware of **hypoglycemia** ("low sugars") than high blood sugars. This is because the margin of safety between blood sugars in the lower part of the normal range and dangerously low blood sugars is quite narrow—only about 25 mg/dl—and the body has a vigorous and rapid response system, designed to ensure that a source of energy is rapidly found and consumed. Nevertheless, especially after longstanding diabetes or a period of very tight glucose control, symptoms of low blood sugar are often not detected by patients. If they are detected, they are perceived with insufficient time to take preventive action. Typical early symptoms of hypoglycemia are shakiness, sweatiness, hunger, abdominal discomfort, palpitations (i.e., a fluttering sensation in the chest), and headache. When blood sugar is very low, confusion and disorientation often occur together with sometimes bizarre behavior, but these features are generally noted by others rather than the affected person him- or herself. In the case of **hyperglycemia**, people with diabetes are usually quite unaware of the presence or severity of high sugars until secondary symptoms such as frequent urination and thirst occur. For the great majority of people, the only sure way to detect high blood sugar is to perform regular glucose monitoring.

Hypoglycemia

An abnormally low level of glucose in the blood; symptoms include shakiness, sweatiness, hunger, abdominal discomfort, palpitations, and confusion.

Hyperglycemia

An abnormally high level of glucose in the blood; secondary symptoms include frequent urination and thirst.

24. My doctor says I have hypoglycemia. Isn't that the opposite of diabetes?

Yes, hypoglycemia (low blood sugar) is the opposite of the hyperglycemia (high blood sugar) that characterizes diabetes. Certain treatments for diabetes and several conditions unrelated to diabetes can cause hypoglycemia. The most common form of hypoglycemia occurs in otherwise healthy young individuals, more commonly in women than men, and is quite benign, although it can be associated with distressing symptoms. Fortunately, it is usually treatable by adjustment of the composition and timing of meals. Sometimes, hypoglycemia can be caused by serious conditions and your doctor will be able to determine whether you are one of the small percentage of people who needs further investigation and specialist referral.

It is important to note that hypoglycemia can be an early feature of diabetes. This type of hypoglycemia occurs in people with prediabetes (see Question 9) who are resistant to the action of insulin and yet are still capable of mounting a vigorous insulin release from the pancreas to overcome it. In the later stages of absorption of calories from a meal, the insulin levels may remain high as the blood glucose level is falling quite rapidly. This may lead to a temporary but sometimes distressing period of low blood sugar that usually occurs about 3 to 5 hours after a meal. It tends to resolve if the prediabetes progresses to frank diabetes, but in some people, it may persist for some years. It is also often treatable by dietary adjustment or other means.

25. Could I have had diabetes for a long time and not known it?

Yes, indeed, you could have had diabetes for a considerable period of time, months or even years, and been unaware of it. However, it is unlikely that you could have had severe diabetes with very high blood sugars for a long time without having to seek medical attention, as you would have experienced complications. However, milder degrees of diabetes are often without obvious symptoms, although in retrospect patients will realize that all was not well when they start to feel the benefits of treatment. Studies have shown that, on average, type 2 diabetes has been present for several years by the time it is diagnosed. It is important that asymptomatic diabetes is detected and treated, because it can lead to serious health consequences, which may be irreversible when detected. About one of every three people has detectable neuropathy (nerve damage) at the time of diagnosis, indicating that longstanding diabetes has been present. Less commonly, eye damage (retinopathy) and/or kidney damage (nephropathy) are discovered at the time of diagnosis. These are serious consequences of diabetes and are the leading causes of blindness and kidney failure in working age adults in the United States, as well as much of the industrialized world. As serious, or even more serious than this, is the potential for undetected and untreated diabetes to lead to heart attacks, strokes, heart failure, or amputations. Indeed, almost 4 of every 10 patients admitted to hospital with a sudden serious cardiac event will be found to have previously unsuspected and undiagnosed diabetes or prediabetes. It is now clear that prediabetes is almost as serious a risk factor for such cardiac events and death from them as full-blown diabetes.

It is important that asymptomatic diabetes is detected and treated, because it can lead to serious health consequences, which may be irreversible when detected.

26. I have a strong family history of diabetes. How often should I be checked for it?

The frequency with which you should be checked for diabetes depends upon your degree of risk, your age, and lifestyle factors. Even if you have a strong family history of type 1 diabetes, your risk of developing it is still only about 5% and is much lower after the age of 35.

Furthermore, type 1 diabetes usually presents with obvious symptoms, such as those described in Question 21, and is unlikely to be missed. Since there is presently little that can be done to prevent type 1 diabetes, screening is usually not performed. If you have a strong family history of type 2 diabetes, the frequency with which you should be screened also depends on age and lifestyle factors. If you are young (younger than 30), physically active, and lean, then you are not at high risk and regular screening is not necessary. As you get older, especially if you get more sedentary and gain weight, as most of us do, then regular screening is advisable. Since screening for diabetes with a fasting or random blood glucose measurement is rapid and inexpensive, there is no reason not to perform it at least annually in individuals at high risk and every 2 to 3 years in those at lesser, but still significant, risk. In general, all pregnant women should be screened for gestational diabetes between 24 and 28 weeks of pregnancy. Some authorities exclude younger (younger than 25 years old) women, who are otherwise at low risk, from the need for screening.

27. I had diabetes during my last pregnancy. Am I at risk of diabetes in the future?

Yes, you are at high risk both of having type 2 diabetes in the future and of having diabetes again with your next pregnancy. The reason for this is that women destined to get type 2 diabetes in middle age or beyond tend to be the same women who will develop diabetes in pregnancy. Therefore, the presence of diabetes in pregnancy is an indicator of future risk for type 2 diabetes. Because type 2 diabetes is a disorder of aging, the diabetes in pregnancy tends to be more severe and requires more intensive treatment with each successive

If you are young (younger than 30), physically active, and lean, then you are not at high risk and regular screening is not necessary. As you get older, especially if you get more sedentary and gain weight, as most of us do, then regular screening is advisable.

pregnancy, unless steps are taken between pregnancies to reverse one or more risk factors, such as excess weight or lack of exercise.

28. Can diabetes sometimes be temporary and go away again?

Yes, this can and does occur, in the case of both types of diabetes. However, in the case of type 1 diabetes, the disappearance is very predictably temporary and the diabetes will almost inevitably return within months or a year or two. The reasons for it are complex and relate to the fact that type 1 diabetes is often diagnosed under conditions of physical stress. When the diabetes is treated and the stress to the body has resolved, there may be sufficient remaining insulin-producing capability in the pancreas to keep the blood sugar normal under most circumstances. Eventually, however, the pancreas fails and permanent diabetes supervenes.

In the case of type 2 diabetes, although the hereditary factors causing it cannot be reversed, the environmental and lifestyle factors can be changed. The latter are the cause of the explosive rise in the number of people affected with diabetes in recent years. Questions 1, 11, 12, 16, and 20 discuss some of these causative factors. Although we do not generally refer to type 2 diabetes as being cured once it has been diagnosed (see Question 5), it can certainly go into remission (cease to be an active medical problem) for long periods, depending on how successfully the causative factors are addressed. Because excess weight and sedentary lifestyle are the two most important and serious causative factors, weight reduction and adherence to an exercise program can often put type 2 diabetes into remission for as long as they are maintained. Sometimes, all medications, even insulin, can be stopped and all measures of diabetes, including blood glucose and hemoglobin A1c (HbA1c—the measure of your blood sugar control averaged over 3 months), will completely normalize. Other associated conditions, such as high blood pressure and cholesterol abnormalities, will also improve greatly. The possibility of stopping all medications is more likely to occur earlier in the course of diabetes and before long-term complications have developed. Unfortunately, many of us in modern society are unable to sustain weight reduction and exercise for long periods and the failure rate is high.

PART FOUR

What Are the Consequences of Diabetes?

What can happen if my diabetes is not properly treated and controlled?

What is diabetic neuropathy?

I hear a lot about footwear and foot care for diabetes. Why is this so important?

More . . .

29. What can happen if my diabetes is not properly treated and controlled?

Uncontrolled diabetes, which generally refers to glucose levels that are higher rather than lower than the target range, can lead to immediate short-term and longer-term consequences. The short-term consequences result from the very high blood glucose itself, which is described in Question 4. If severe enough or untreated for long enough, markedly high blood glucose levels can result in coma and ultimately death, due to the severe abnormalities of blood chemistry that occur. It is important to note that only a very small minority of patients with either form of diabetes will die in this way. Therefore, although immediate **decompensation** of diabetes is a serious and life-threatening condition, with a high death rate if detected and treated too late, the majority of people with diabetes should be more concerned about the damaging effects of diabetes that are not well controlled, yet not sufficiently poorly controlled to focus their attention.

The longer-term consequences of less than adequate diabetes control are the result of damage to the small (micro) and larger (macro) vessels of the circulation. The most common manifestations are diabetic eye disease (retinopathy), which is the leading cause of blindness in working-age adults in the United States; diabetic kidney disease (nephropathy), which is the leading cause of severe kidney failure necessitating dialysis or transplantation in working-age adults in the United States; and nerve damage (neuropathy), which is present in about 1 out of 3 people with diabetes at the time of diagnosis and in over 7 out of 10 by the time diabetes has been present for 10 years. Both retinopathy and nephropathy can be entirely without symptoms

Decompensation

A serious deterioration in a medical condition.

until they reach an advanced and irreversible stage, leading to blindness and the need for kidney dialysis or transplant. Diabetic neuropathy can cause very troublesome symptoms and lead to loss of sensation, mainly in the feet, which places the patient at high risk of trauma, infection, and amputations of the legs and feet.

Disease of the large blood vessels leads to a high rate of heart attack, stroke, heart failure, and amputation of the (usually lower) limbs. About two of every three patients with diabetes will die as a result of large vessel disease. Fortunately, studies have shown that good control of diabetes can prevent or delay the progression of many of these serious problems, but other contributing factors, such as blood pressure and cholesterol, must also be given careful attention.

However, we are only achieving target levels of diabetes control in about half of all people with diabetes in America today.

30. Does diabetes put me at risk of any other diseases or illnesses?

Aside from the direct consequences of high blood sugar itself, which are discussed in Question 29, people with diabetes are at risk of suffering from other associated diseases. In the case of type 1 diabetes, the diseases either result from the high blood sugar or from the root cause of the diabetes, which is a predisposition to destroy the hormone-producing tissues (called **autoimmunity**). Thus, a person with type 1 diabetes is more likely to suffer from adrenal gland damage (Addison's disease), thyroid gland damage (Graves' or, much more commonly, Hashimoto's disease), and several other disorders. Fortunately, except in the case of

Autoimmunity

A predisposition to produce autoantibodies.

thyroid disease, which affects about one in three people with type 1 diabetes, the likelihood of developing one of these other disorders is not high, but can be so in certain families. Most people with type 1 diabetes are screened annually for thyroid disease. In the case of type 2 diabetes, the other diseases appear to be independent, but related. In other words, they and the diabetes arise from a common soil in the affected person's metabolic makeup. These related diseases include cholesterol and other blood fat abnormalities (**dyslipidemia**), high blood pressure (**hypertension**), and gout. The first two are commonly seen in people with type 2 diabetes, while the third is less so.

Dyslipidemia
Cholesterol and other blood fat abnormalities.

Hypertension
High blood pressure.

31. What is diabetic coma?

Diabetic coma is loss of consciousness occurring as a result of very high blood sugar.

Diabetic coma is loss of consciousness occurring as a result of very high blood sugar. Its causes are similar in both type 1 and type 2 diabetes, but with the important difference that other abnormalities of the blood chemistry may contribute to the coma in type 1 diabetes. These other abnormalities occur as a result of the almost total lack of insulin that is present in type 1 diabetes. For this reason, while blood sugar is almost always very high in people with type 2 diabetes who are in diabetic coma, being several hundreds (of mg/dl) to 2000 or more, it can be less elevated in people with type 1 diabetes, sometimes as low as only 200 or 300. In the case of type 1 diabetes, diabetic coma can occur solely as a result of having insufficient insulin in the body (e.g., running out of or not taking one's insulin), while in the case of type 2 diabetes, there is almost always another stress to the body that precipitates the coma, such as infection, dehydration, etc. If the serious abnormalities of blood chemistry that led to diabetic coma are not corrected rapidly, death can occur. Although the derangements in blood chemistry are more complex and severe in type 1 diabetes than in type 2 diabetes, there is a higher mortality in type 2 diabetic coma because people suffering from it tend to be older, in less robust health, and with more cardiac risk factors. Also, additional symptoms of nausea, vomiting, and abdominal pain occur in the derangements of type 1 diabetes leading to coma and the diagnosis may be made earlier as a result. In the early stages of coma in type 2 diabetes, abnormalities of brain function and consciousness are more prominent due to the extreme degree of dehydration. Moreover, the illness that precipitated the coma may carry its own serious health risks. Although only a minority of patients with diabetes will succumb to coma, it remains an important medical emergency that requires immediate intervention.

32. What is diabetic neuropathy?

Diabetic neuropathy is the term used to describe the usually chronic damage to nerves that occurs as a result of untreated, or inadequately treated, high blood sugar. It results from a complex sequence of events that leads to damage and destruction of the minute blood vessels that nourish nerves along their course to the region of the body they serve after leaving the spinal canal. Each such nerve is a single cell. The longest nerves, much like long chains, are the most susceptible to damage. If a **peripheral nerve** (i.e., a nerve cell not contained in the brain or spinal column) emerging from the spinal column and traveling to the toes were the thickness of a piece of string, it would be 3 miles in length! At frequent intervals along its length, each peripheral nerve receives nourishment from tiny blood vessels. If any of these tiny blood vessels are irreversibly damaged, that part of the nerve dies and no signals are conducted in

Peripheral nerve
A nerve cell not contained in the brain or spinal column.

either direction along it, i.e., the chain fails at its weakest link. Although there are a vast number of individual nerve fibers serving any one area of the body, when a sufficiently large number get damaged, symptoms will result. Since the longest nerve fibers serve the parts of the body that are farthest from the spinal column, it is not surprising that they are the ones most frequently damaged. Therefore, diabetic neuropathy is most frequently a problem in the feet, hands, and male genitals. The symptoms represent a spectrum from those due to injury responses of the non-fatally injured nerves, such as pain, burning, and abnormal sensations such as bunched socks under the feet, to those due to loss of impulses, such as numbness and unperceived injury due to loss of **protective sensation**. This includes inability to perceive heat and sharp pain, leading to burns and puncture wounds. Although the typical form of diabetic neuropathy causes these symptoms, there are a number of other less common forms that can lead to sudden pain, weakness, and other unsuspected symptoms in almost every region of the body. Discussion of the whole range of these is beyond the scope of this book.

Diabetic neuropathy is most frequently a problem in the feet, hands, and male genitals.

Protective sensation

The perception of potential injury, such as awareness of sharp, rough, excessively hot or cold objects, or friction.

33. What is diabetic retinopathy?

Diabetic retinopathy is damage to the eye that results from chronically untreated or inadequately treated high blood sugar. In its more advanced form, it can result in severe visual loss or blindness if untreated, and this can occur suddenly without warning. It is the leading cause of blindness in working age adults in the United States and more than 20,000 people become blind as a result of diabetes each year. In order to prevent this, all people with diabetes should periodically be screened with an eye exam or photography of the inner lining of the eye (**retina**). Because it is often not possible to pinpoint precisely when type 2 diabetes actually develops, as it may be silent and unrecognized for months or even years, people with type 2 diabetes should be examined for retinopathy at the time of diagnosis, while those with type 1 diabetes should be examined between 3 and 5 years after the diagnosis has been made. The frequency with which follow-up visits is recommended will depend upon the findings and the measures taken to address them. For example, if no retinopathy is detected, follow-up examination in 2 years may be recommended, whereas in the case of serious findings requiring active treatment, follow-up in 3 months or fewer may be required.

Although it has clearly been shown that the rate of progression of diabetic retinopathy is related to the control of the blood sugar, there are several other factors involved. There is a hereditary tendency, so that if a close relative with diabetes developed retinopathy, you are more likely to do so. You should inform your eye doctor, who will be especially vigilant. Control of blood pressure has been shown to delay worsening of retinopathy and control of cholesterol abnormalities also plays a role in preventing progression. Quitting smoking can slow the progression of diabetic retinopathy. Therefore, all of these factors must be carefully addressed to prevent retinopathy successfully. Finally, it is important to note that retinopathy is not the only form of eye damage that can occur in diabetes. Other disorders, including **glaucoma** (increased pressure inside the eye) and **cataracts** (opacity of the lens of the eye), are more common in diabetes. Therefore, a comprehensive specialist eye exam is periodically needed and retinal photographs alone are not adequate.

Retina
The inner lining of the eye.

Glaucoma
Increased pressure inside the eye.

Cataracts
Opacity of the lens of the eye.

What Are the Consequences of Diabetes?

41

34. What is diabetic nephropathy?

Diabetic nephropathy is the term used to describe kidney damage that occurs in diabetes.

Diabetic nephropathy is the term used to describe kidney damage that occurs in diabetes, usually of long-standing. The damage to the kidney in diabetes can result from the high blood sugar itself, which leads to an expansion of certain types of material in the filtering mechanism of the kidney. This expansion damages the delicate cells responsible for filtering waste materials through the kidney. Eventually, there are abnormal pressures and changes in the important electrical balance in this complex structure. These changes lead to leakage of proteins that are usually either retained or reabsorbed by the kidney. The blood pressure can rise due to overload of fluid and constriction of small blood vessels. The rise in blood pressure further damages the kidney if not treated. If there is an excessive leak of protein, the body becomes protein deficient, which can lead to generalized puffiness and swelling. Eventually, the kidneys can fail and their functions must be replaced by the processes of either **hemodialysis** (blood filtering and removal of wastes through a machine) or **peritoneal dialysis** (a simpler process whereby wastes are exchanged into fluids introduced into the abdominal cavity), or a kidney transplant is required.

Hemodialysis

Blood filtering and removal of wastes through a machine.

Peritoneal dialysis

A process whereby wastes are exchanged into fluids introduced into the abdominal cavity.

Although complete kidney failure is not a common outcome in diabetes in percentage terms, diabetes is the most common cause of kidney failure in working age adults and occurs in more than 25,000 people each year in the United States. Kidney failure is extremely disruptive to the sufferer's life and is very expensive to treat. The tendency to get diabetic kidney damage has an inherited component, so that if a close relative with diabetes suffers from it, an individual is more likely to experience it. However, it can be delayed or even prevented. Good control of blood sugar and blood pressure, together with use of certain types of drugs known as *ACE-inhibitors* or *ARB*s, has been shown to markedly slow progression of diabetic kidney damage. Moreover, it can be detected very early by sensitive tests in common use.

35. Why is the risk of blood vessel diseases increased so much in diabetes?

There are several reasons why the risk of vascular diseases, such as heart attack, stroke, and diseases of the vessels in the limbs (**peripheral vascular disease**), is increased in both types of diabetes. The weight gain and lack of exercise common in people with type 2 diabetes lead to other conditions such as abnormal cholesterol levels and high blood pressure, which are potent causes of vascular disease. If all of these risk factors are not treated effectively, the probability of vascular disease remains high. High blood sugar over months and years leads to a chemical reaction of the sugar in the blood vessels, damaging them structurally. Perhaps most importantly, we now know that diabetes and obesity can be described as irritants to the body tissues, meaning that the body becomes generally inflamed. We know that this is so because we can measure high levels of compounds that indicate **inflammation** in the blood of many people with diabetes. It turns out that this inflammation, when maintained over time, extends to the lining of the blood vessels, which attracts inflammatory cells out of the bloodstream. Cholesterol also takes on an inflamed form, enters the lining of the blood vessels, and attracts still more inflammatory cells from the bloodstream, setting the stage for serious damage.

Peripheral vascular disease
Diseases of the vessels in the limbs.

Inflammation
Swelling, pain, tenderness, and disturbed function in an area of the body, usually as a result of injury.

Other contributors to vascular disease include the fact that high blood pressure results from nephropathy, which further damages blood vessels. This further damages the kidney and blood pressure rises still further, setting up a vicious cycle. Even short periods of high glucose, such as may occur after meals in people with diabetes and even prediabetes, can cause problems with the function of blood vessels, making them more sticky, inflamed, and less able to relax. Whether these repeated briefer periods of high blood sugar combine over time to cause permanent vascular damage is not known. However, it is known that the risk of vascular disease is already high in people with prediabetes.

36. Can my diabetes affect my sex life? If so, how and what can I do about it?

Diabetes can have a profound effect upon a person's sexual drive, functioning, and satisfaction. This is especially apparent in men, although there is some evidence that some women with diabetes can also experience adverse effects on their sexual responses. The reason for the significant effects on male sexual function arises from the complexity of the penile erection mechanism. This requires satisfactory nerve, blood vessel, and hormone function to be achieved and sustained. Diabetic nerve damage (see Question 32) can be of two main types. One form is damage to the system that serves conscious movement and sensation and the other is damage to the system that serves unconscious or automatic responses, such as bowel contraction and the heart beat. The erectile mechanism is served by the latter, while the sensation of pleasure in sexual performance is served by the former. Since the nerves to the genital area are relatively lengthy, they are prone to the damage described in

Question 32. Normal erectile function also depends on a healthy blood supply to the penis, as erection entails engorgement of the organ with blood. If the blood supply is compromised, the quality of the erection will be poor. As discussed in Question 35, vascular damage is commonly associated with diabetes and frequently affects the health of the vessels supplying the genitals. Finally, normal levels of the male hormone testosterone are necessary not only for sexual interest (**libido**), but also for perception of pleasurable sensations from sexual arousal. Low testosterone levels, already common in middle-aged and older men, are even more common in men with diabetes. Indeed, there is suggestive evidence that low testosterone levels may contribute to worsening of diabetes, thus creating a vicious cycle that further depresses hormone levels. In light of the three strikes of diabetic nerve damage, vascular damage, and diminished levels of male hormone, it is not surprising that poor sexual performance and diminished satisfaction are a frequent finding in men with diabetes. Indeed, more than half of all men with type 2 diabetes of five or more years' duration will complain of one or more symptoms of sexual dysfunction. Sometimes this is worsened by medications commonly used by people with diabetes, such as certain blood pressure-lowering drugs.

Libido
Sexual interest.

37. I feel as if my memory has gotten worse since I developed diabetes. Could I be right?

You may well be right. Studies have shown that memory, and other higher brain functions, can be negatively affected by diabetes. This pertains to both type 1 and type 2 diabetes and to both adults and children. A large part of this effect is related to blood sugar control. Children with repeated episodes of low blood sugar have been shown to have poor long-term memory performance. However, both high and low blood sugar levels are associated with poor memory performance. This affects recall of things previously remembered and memorization of new information. The effect of low blood sugar on memory appears to be the same whether a person is aware of the blood sugar or unaware of it. When memory problems are associated with high blood sugars, the good news is that they are often reversible with improved control of the diabetes, even in older people. Therefore, if you feel that your memory has deteriorated, a first step would be to ensure that your diabetes is under the best possible control, without unnecessary high or low blood sugars.

In addition to controlling blood sugars, it is important to remember that diabetes is a chronic disorder and that we age along with our diabetes. Memory function tends to decline with age, even in people without diabetes. Also, it is possible that some of the medications that you are taking may affect memory, independently of any effect on your blood sugar. This is particularly true of medications that may cause drowsiness (and therefore inattention to information that you may need to memorize) or low blood pressure. Medications given to treat the pain of neuropathy are the most likely to cause drowsiness. Finally, people with diabetes are at a significantly higher risk of diseases of the blood vessels, including those in the brain (see Question 35), and are at higher risk of brain injury. Such injury may not be noticed as a single severe event, but as a series of smaller unobserved events that ultimately lead to impaired brain functioning, including memory impairment.

38. I hear a lot about footwear and foot care for diabetes. Why is this so important?

Proper care and protection of the feet are extremely important for people with diabetes. This is due to the fact that the feet are frequently affected by diabetic nerve damage with a resultant loss of protective sensation. Protective sensation is the perception of potential injury, such as awareness of sharp, rough, or excessively hot or cold objects or friction, such as rubbing against the inside of shoes. When this is impaired, it is possible for the person with diabetes to sustain wounds, abrasions, burns, or freezing of which he or she may be unaware. Other types of injuries such as bites and blisters can similarly occur unnoticed. Even fractures to the bones of the foot can occur painlessly when more severe forms of diabetic nerve damage are present. The most serious consequence of unperceived injury is infection. Because the blood supply to the feet may also be impaired, the healing and immune response to both the injury and the infection can be compromised, so that a chronically infected wound results. The most dangerous consequences of chronically infected wounds are spread of infection to the deeper tissues, including the bones, and entry of infectious organisms into the bloodstream, which can lead to blood poisoning (**septicemia**) or spread by the bloodstream of infection to other body tissues. Both of these consequences can cause severe illness or even death. Local infection of the bones of the feet can require amputation, since infection in the bone (called "**osteomyelitis**") is very difficult to treat. Even powerful modern antibiotics given **intravenously** over several weeks may fail to completely eradicate infection in bone when its blood supply is poor.

Protective sensation is the perception of potential injury, such as awareness of sharp, rough, or excessively hot or cold objects or friction, such as rubbing against the inside of shoes.

Septicemia
Blood poisoning, due to infection, which is usually bacterial in origin.

Osteomyelitis
Infection in the bone.

Intravenously
Through a vein.

What Are the Consequences of Diabetes?

Diabetic nerve damage in the feet may lead to disturbance of the mechanics of the foot, such that pressure may occur on bony areas not designed to bear this. This can cause unusual prominences of the bones of the feet on all of their surfaces, which are more prone to injury than usual. Corns, calluses, cracks, fissures, and ulcers of the feet can all occur in people with diabetes in the absence of specific injury, but as a result of abnormal pressure distribution caused by nerve damage.

For all of these reasons, it is very important to protect the feet by wearing suitable footwear, not going barefoot, paying attention to the environment (i.e., removal or covering of protruding furniture legs etc. and hard, abrasive floor surfaces), performing daily inspection of the feet, foot hygiene, nail care, and prompt cleaning and dressing of minor injuries.

PART FIVE

Treatments for Diabetes

What should I eat and what should I avoid?
Please be specific!

Who should take pills and who should take insulin?

Are there any medications prescribed for
other conditions that can improve or worsen
my diabetes?

More . . .

39. Is diet and exercise management alone really effective for diabetes?

Diet and exercise are in fact the most effective treatments of all for most forms of type 2 diabetes, but are not primary measures for management of type 1 diabetes. In type 1 diabetes, profound insulin deficiency necessitates that insulin treatment is the principal form of treatment. Nevertheless, attention to diet and exercise can provide benefits in diabetes control and general health in patients with type 1 diabetes and should be included in the comprehensive treatment plan.

In the case of type 2 diabetes, the reason that diet and exercise are so effective is because lack of exercise and weight gain are the most significant causes of the disease and reversal of these issues can essentially reverse the problem of development of diabetes. Figure 3 (Question 11) shows the increasing likelihood of developing diabetes with increasing weight and this is discussed in Question 11. However, if one loses weight, one is able to travel back down the slope of diabetes to a large extent. Reduction in weight can reduce or even eliminate the need for medications in many patients, even those who have been on insulin injections for several years. The most striking example of this is bariatric surgery, which has been shown to reverse diabetes and to do so for several years, being effective as long as weight reduction is maintained. This is further discussed in Question 5.

Exercise works by making the body more sensitive to the actions of insulin and also by using up stored energy in the exercising muscles. The muscles then replace this energy by pulling in glucose and other sources of energy from the bloodstream. While this process can occur to some extent without insulin and in the absence of exercise, it occurs much more efficiently when the muscles are conditioned through regular exercise and normal levels of insulin are present. In addition, exercise helps to prevent recurrence of weight gain after successful attempts at reduction through diet. However, the longer diabetes has been present, the less effective diet and exercise are likely to be as treatment, although they are virtually always beneficial to some extent. Unfortunately, however, as we all know, there are many factors working against our ability to succeed in managing diabetes with diet and exercise in modern society. Longstanding success with diet and exercise alone is therefore the exception rather than the rule.

The longer diabetes has been present, the less effective diet and exercise are likely to be as treatment.

40. What should I eat and what should I avoid? Please be specific!

It depends. Nutrient needs are based on a number of different factors. Weight and coexisting conditions like high cholesterol and high blood pressure are important in determining an appropriate meal plan. Most people with type 2 diabetes need to treat all of these conditions.

Sugars and starches are primarily responsible for high blood sugar after a meal. These include fruit, juice, milk, soda, desserts, beans, peas, bread, pasta, rice, potatoes, and corn. A moderate restriction of these types of carbohydrates will help control after-meal blood sugar. However, restricting these foods too much may also be harmful, so it is important to seek professional guidance when choosing an appropriate carbohydrate amount. Avoiding fried foods and fatty meats (ground meat, sausage, bacon, bologna, hot dogs) and choosing healthier cooking oils, like canola and olive oil instead of shortening, lard, and butter, will help control your cholesterol levels and may assist with weight loss.

Treatments for Diabetes

51

If high blood pressure is a concern, then sodium restriction and weight loss may be helpful. Eliminating canned and jarred items (unless they are low sodium) and reducing added salt can help lower your blood pressure. Using fresh or frozen foods is a much better choice when reducing your sodium intake.

When attempting weight loss, smaller portions of high calorie density foods like processed meats, fats, and refined sugars are important. Increasing portions of low calorie foods like vegetables can make you feel full and therefore less likely to munch on foods that are not as healthy. As with any weight loss program it is recommended that you talk to your doctor before starting an exercise program.

An ideal meal for someone with typical type 2 diabetes who is accustomed to consuming about 2000 calories per day and who is interested in weight loss includes:

Fiber	>10 g/meal
Sodium	<650 mg
Carbohydrate	~45 g/meal
Fat	<20 g/meal
Saturated Fat	<5 g/meal
Cholesterol	<60 mg
Protein	35 g/meal
	(28 g = 1 oz)

Following these guidelines should produce the recommended 1-pound-per-week weight loss. Please note, however, that all dietary changes should be reviewed by your healthcare provider in regards to your particular health status. Those who have advanced kidney problems may need to decrease portions of protein.

To determine if you are meeting these recommendations you must look at the food label. All of this information can be found there.

41. What are the best and safest pills for diabetes?

There is really no best or safest pill for treatment of diabetes, because certain pills (usually called oral antidiabetic drugs or OADs) are appropriate for certain patients but not for others. Therefore, it is important for the prescribing physician to take a number of factors pertaining to the patient into account before recommending a specific OAD or combination of OADs. **Table 4** shows the currently available types of OAD and the main advantages and disadvantages of each. Although therapy must be individually selected for each patient, certain general statements can be made. The newer OADs sitagliptin and saxagliptin, which belong to a class of OADs known as DPP-IV inhibitors, appear to be especially safe, in that sitagliptin does not interact with other drugs (although saxagliptin alters plasma levels of some drugs and needs to be either not used or used with caution when taking these) and do not appear to have any serious side effects. Although a few patients may have experienced serious allergic reactions with sitagliptin, this is a very tiny minority of the many patients who have taken the drug. Which OAD could be considered the best (in the sense of most effective) is quite debatable, because several types of OAD have similar effectiveness and this varies according to the timing of their use in the course of the diabetes. One must also consider the fact that some OADs tend to fail after a certain time of use, while others have less of a tendency to do so. In addition, some OADs, such as pioglitazone, have other benefits in addition to their effect on blood sugar, such as improving the

Table 4 Pills for Diabetes Mellitus (Oral Antidiabetic Drugs—OADs)

Class	Name	Brand Name	Doses/Day	Potency	Benefits	Side Effects	Hypoglycemia	Effect on Weight	Cost
Biguanide	Metformin	Generic	2–3	+++		Diarrhea, nausea	–	↓	$
	Metformin ER	*Glucophage XR*®	1	+++	↓Side effects	Lactic acidosis*	–	↓	$$
Sulfonylurea	Glipizide	Generic	1–2	+++	Rapid onset	Occ. allergy	++	↑↑↑	$
	Glyburide	Generic	1–2	+++	Rapid onset	Occ. allergy	+++	↑↑↑	$
	Glimepiride	Generic	1	+++	Rapid onset	Occ. allergy	++	↑↑↑	$
Meglitinide	Repaglinide	*Prandin*®	3	+++	Short-acting		+	↑	$$
	Nateglinide	*Starlix*®	3	+++	Short-acting		+	↑	$$
TZD	Rosiglitazone	*Avandia*®	1–2	+++	↑HDL	CHF ↑MI slow onset	–	↑↑	$$$
	Pioglitazone	*Actos*®	1	+++	↑HDL ↓TG ↓MI	CHF slow onset	–	↑↑	$$$
DPP-IV I	Sitagliptin	*Januvia*®	1	++	Rhinitis§, URTI, HA, UTI	–		–	$$$
	Saxagliptin	*Onglyza*	1	++	URTI, HA, UTI			–	$$$
α-Glucosidase I	Acarbose	*Precose*®	3	+	↓CVD	Diarrhea, gas	–	–	$$
	Miglitol	*Starlix*®	3	+		Diarrhea, gas	–	–	$$
BABR	Colesevelam	*Welchol*®	3	+	↓Cholesterol	Bloating, gas		–	$$$

Abbreviations: ER: extended release; Occ: occasional; TZD: Thiazolidinedione (glitazone); HDL: high density lipoprotein (good cholesterol) CHF: congestive heart failure; MI: myocardial infarction (heart attack); TG: triglycerides; DPP-IV I: dipeptidyl peptidase IV inhibitor; URTI: upper respiratory tract infection (e.g., cold); HA: headache; UTI: urinary tract infection; α-glucosidase I: α-glucosidase inhibitor; CVD: cardiovascular disease; BABR: bile-acid binding resin;

Note: Many combination preparations of these medications are available. Combination use provides convenience and cost savings, but the properties of each of their component medications are unchanged.

*Lactic acidosis is a rare but serious side effect that can be prevented by not using this drug in persons with certain medical conditions.

§Rhinitis is nasal congestion, stuffiness, and runny nose.

cholesterol level and lowering blood pressure and perhaps even lowering the rate of heart attacks. Taken together, all this indicates that there is no single best drug for all patients with diabetes, but that for each patient there is one or more OADs that are safest and most effective for him or her.

42. Who should take pills and who should take insulin?

Presently, it is necessary for all patients with type 1 diabetes to take insulin by injection or pump. This is because they are profoundly deficient in insulin, which is essential for life. No other therapies can restore insulin in a person with type 1 diabetes apart from giving the hormone itself.

In the case of type 2 diabetes, the majority of patients can be controlled with one or more pills for their diabetes, usually for several years. The available types of oral medication for diabetes usually either improve the body's ability to make insulin, or make the body tissues more sensitive to it. Frequently, patients will take a combination of medicines that do both. A little over a decade ago, only one type of pill was available for diabetes in the United States but now there are at least six different classes of pills. Thus, by taking a combination of these, it is possible for people with diabetes to remain off insulin for longer, sometimes for many years. In addition to the blood glucose level, there are other factors that predict whether a person with type 2 diabetes will be likely to require insulin therapy earlier. People with type 2 diabetes who are not significantly overweight tend to require insulin treatment fairly early. About one out of every five people with type 2 diabetes actually seems to have a partial form of type 1 diabetes (the abbreviated name of which is LADA,

Treatments for Diabetes

short for "latent autoimmune diabetes of the adult"), based on clinical features, presence of related conditions or measurement of markers of immune attack against the insulin-producing cells of the pancreas (known as **autoantibodies**) in the blood. This partial form of type 1 diabetes appears to have become arrested before it became very severe. However, people with LADA usually respond better to insulin treatment than to pills.

Autoantibody

An antibody that an organism produces against any of its own tissues or cells.

In spite of the presence of indicators of LADA, the usual approach is to treat a patient with pills whenever it appears safe to do so. This means that certain people with a high blood sugar level who are being given a trial of pills will need to be followed very closely for the first few days or weeks to be sure that the blood sugar is responding. They will also need to check their own glucose and report these values to their physician or diabetes educator.

43. My doctor says that I need to start insulin. If I do, will I ever get off it?

People with type 1 diabetes usually cannot discontinue insulin use once they have started. This is because of the very severe deficiency of insulin in this disorder. However, there are a couple of exceptions to this general rule. First, there is often a brief period of improvement in pancreas function after the initial diagnosis of type 1 diabetes. This so-called "honeymoon period" can last for a few weeks to a couple of years. During this time, the amount of insulin needed to control the blood glucose is much lower and the occasional patient needs none at all. Second, people who have received either a pancreas transplant or a pancreatic islet cell transplant can sometimes stop using insulin. The latter procedure is still considered an experimental therapy. Although they can reduce or eliminate the need for insulin injections, these procedures should not be undertaken lightly, because they are associated with a lifelong need for powerful immunosuppressive (antirejection) drugs that can cause serious side effects.

In principle, it is possible for a person with type 2 diabetes to discontinue insulin once he or she has started it, if the lifestyle factors that led to the worsening of the diabetes can be reversed. Since the overwhelming majority of cases of type 2 diabetes are associated with overweight and lack of exercise, weight reduction and commencement of a regular exercise program will almost always result in significant improvement in glucose control and can lead a person on insulin being able to discontinue it. Unfortunately, in our society, it is very difficult for most people with type 2 diabetes to consistently pursue these goals and the majority will remain on insulin once it has been started. Also, it is a normal part of aging for the insulin-secreting cells of the pancreas (**beta cells**) to show declining function. The rate of this decline may be faster in people with type 2 diabetes. This leads to a need to intensify treatment over time and may explain in part why the majority of those who start insulin treatment will not be able to discontinue it without significant deterioration in control of their diabetes.

Beta cells

The insulin-producing cells of the pancreas.

44. I take several types of pills for my diabetes. How can I reduce the expense?

There are several ways in which the expense of your diabetes medications can be reduced. Many of them apply to medications in general. Whenever possible, you should try to use the medications that are on your insurance plan's preferred list or those that have the lowest co-pays. These are generally the generic med-ications. Your doctor should consider prescribing generic medications whenever possible, always weigh-ing in mind the benefits of saving money versus giving you the most effective and safe treatment for your individual condition. If brand-name medications are necessary, whenever possible your doctor will be will-ing to prescribe the specific brand that is preferred by your healthcare formulary with the lowest co-payment (first or second tier if more than one brand are available that have little difference between their efficacy and safety). Many plans will fill mail-in prescriptions for a 90-day supply with the same single co-pay as a 30-day supply at a retail pharmacy. Recently, some retail phar-macies have begun to offer the same programs. Also, some large national chain pharmacies, such as Wal-mart, have begun to maintain their own formularies with very low co-pays that discount further from those offered by your medical plan. Walmart, Target, and some Ralph's pharmacies, along with others, will pro-vide a 30-day supply of some generic antidiabetic, blood pressure, and cholesterol drugs for $4. They will honor these prices even if you do not have medical insurance coverage for your medications. Although the items on these formularies tend to be limited in num-ber and are usually generic, several of the medications commonly used by people with diabetes and related conditions can be found on them. Some plans cover only certain dosage strengths of medications at the lowest co-pay, so these should be prescribed by your doctor when there is a choice. Finally, a number of brand-name medications are available in a combina-tion formula with a generic medication (for example, pioglitazone with metformin and sitagliptin with met-formin) usually at the same price as the brand-name drug alone. In this case, the generic medication is free, as there is only one co-pay for a prescription. However, be sure that the combination preparation is not in a higher tier (co-pay level) than the individual preparations, as there may then be no saving.

Remember that one way *not* to save money is to ask your doctor to prescribe more medication than you are actually required to take on your prescription in order to make it last longer. This violates the terms of both the doctor's and your contract with your healthcare plan and the agreements between the healthcare plan and the pharmacy and could result in loss of coverage.

45. Why is it so important for people with diabetes to control their blood pressure and cholesterol as well?

It is very important for people to control their blood pressure and cholesterol because of the increased risk of vascular disease carried by people with diabetes (see Question 35). High blood pressure and abnormal levels of cholesterol and other blood fats are frequently found in people with diabetes and contribute additional risk for vascular disease. In some studies involving people with type 2 diabetes, control of cholesterol and blood pressure has been found to confer more protection against progression of small vessel (microvascular) disease than control of blood sugar itself! Not only is this the case, but the serious complications in the eyes, nerves, and kidneys caused by damage to the small blood vessels (discussed in Questions 32, 33, and 34) have been shown to be reduced by treatment of **cholesterol** and blood pressure. Some of the drugs used for these conditions may even provide a minor benefit in control of the blood sugar itself, while some may worsen it. When possible, your doctor will choose

In some studies involving people with type 2 diabetes, control of cholesterol and blood pressure has been found to confer more protection against progression of small vessel (microvascular) disease than control of blood sugar itself!

Cholesterol

A fatty substance normally present in blood.

those medications for blood pressure and cholesterol that will improve (or not worsen) control of your blood sugar and prevent or delay the progression of the complications of diabetes.

46. What is the difference between basal insulin and bolus insulin?

Basal insulin

The insulin required to control your blood sugar in the absence of food intake.

Basal insulin refers to the insulin required to control your blood sugar in the absence of food intake. A certain amount of insulin is always necessary to keep the blood sugar in the normal range, even in the absence of eating for prolonged periods. Without any insulin in the body, the starch, fat, and protein in the body will break down with severe health consequences, as occurs in people with type 1 diabetes. The amount of insulin that the body requires in the absence of food intake is known as the basal requirement and it is provided by the one or two injections of long-acting insulin that most patients give themselves each day. If a person is using an insulin pump, then it is covered by the basal setting on the pump. Modern insulin pumps offer several basal settings in each 24-hour period, as the basal insulin production in a healthy individual varies over the course of the day, being higher in the 2-to 3-hour period before arising in the morning, for example.

Bolus insulin

The insulin required to remove the energy derived from a meal from the bloodstream and into the tissues to replenish energy stores. Bolus insulin can also be given when the blood sugar is too high.

Bolus insulin refers to the insulin required to remove the energy derived from a meal from the bloodstream and into the tissues, to replenish energy stores. This is typically provided by the short-acting insulin injection given just prior to eating or by the bolus setting for patients on an insulin pump. Recently developed and marketed forms of insulin very closely match the pattern of insulin production from the pancreas itself in response to food. In this way, they are able to

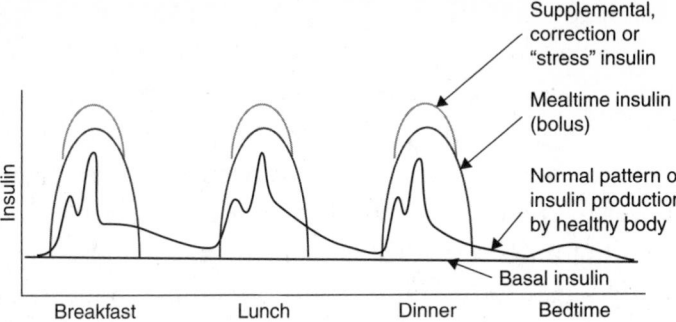

Figure 4   Basal, bolus, and stress/supplemental/correction insulin delivery.

prevent the blood sugar from rising excessively after a meal, while also preventing the occurrence of low blood sugar after the glucose from the meal has been cleared from the bloodstream. The latest insulin pumps offer different rates and patterns in which this bolus is given, in order to more effectively deal with rapidly or more slowly absorbed types of foods. **Figure 4** shows the normal pattern in which the body releases insulin and describes how basal, bolus, and supplemental insulin are given to mimic this as closely as possible.

Of course, once it has been delivered to the body, the insulin cannot distinguish between basal and meal-derived glucose and so different types of insulin preparation will overlap with each other in their action. Distinguishing between the two requires specialized knowledge and is beyond the scope of this book.

47. I am afraid that my diabetes treatment will cause me to gain weight. How can I prevent this?

Some types of medication for diabetes do tend to lead to weight gain. This is especially true of the classes of medications known as thiazolidinediones, sulfonylureas, meglitinides, and insulin itself. Members of each of these classes of medications have been described in Table 4 (see Question 41). These types of medications all have proven effectiveness in lowering blood sugar and controlling diabetes and have an important place in its management. However, weight gain is definitely an undesirable side effect associated with them. The ways in which weight gain can be minimized or prevented include using, whenever possible, medications that do not cause weight gain, such as the classes known as DPP-IV inhibitors or α-glucosidase inhibitors. Another option is to take medications that are actually known to cause weight reduction in many people who take them, such as the classes known as biguanides, incretin mimetics, or synthetic amylins (e.g., pramlintide). Some representatives of these classes can also be found in Table 4. If medications known to cause weight gain must be used, then your doctor will try to use them in the lowest effective dose, often by combining them with other types of medications.

Finally, it is important to remember that adhering to a diet and exercise plan is just as important when you are taking pills for diabetes as it was beforehand.

Finally, it is important to remember that adhering to a diet and exercise plan is just as important when you are taking pills for diabetes as it was beforehand. Many patients who are prescribed pills are told that they have failed diet and exercise. This is not entirely true. The diet and exercise may be making an important contribution to the control of the diabetes, but is not quite enough to control the blood sugar adequately. This important contribution will be lost if the program is not continued and some weight gain in people who start pills or injections for their diabetes is undoubtedly due to this.

48. I am afraid that I might forget I have taken my insulin and take it twice, or mistakenly take my long-acting dose for my short-acting and vice versa. What should I do if this happens?

If you think you have taken your insulin twice or taken more or less than you need at that particular point in time, you should not panic, but follow a plan designed to ensure that you do not experience serious consequences from this. First of all, it is surprising how often taking too much insulin does not actually lead to a seriously low level of blood glucose. Having said that, a careful response is needed if you suspect that you have taken too much insulin. In the case of too little insulin, it is often sufficient to monitor the glucose carefully—about every couple of hours is generally sufficient to detect any problems and address them—and be sure to take the right amount at the next scheduled dosage. A brief exposure to high glucose is usually not harmful (unless it is a repetitive event) and the glucose may take 24 hours or so to settle back to its usual pattern. If the reduced dosage is noted quickly, such as before eating the upcoming meal, then the remaining amount can be given. If the meal is underway already, then a slightly smaller meal or subsequent snack can be eaten. If the problem is noted later and the blood sugar is very high, then some additional (supplemental) insulin can be taken to bring it down. The best approach can vary among different patients and your doctor or diabetes educator will have a recommendation for a supplemental scale that may be right for you in these circumstances.

In the case of having taken too much insulin, the blood glucose should also be monitored every couple

It is surprising how often taking too much insulin does not actually lead to a seriously low level of blood glucose.

of hours and a snack should be kept with you until you feel comfortable that the danger of a serious low blood sugar has passed. You should probably not drive, work at heights, or operate heavy or dangerous machinery during this time. Many people with insulin-requiring diabetes keep a kit containing a syringe of glucagon, a hormone that counteracts the effects of insulin. If the blood sugar falls rapidly and oral glucose, sugar, or a snack is ineffective, glucagon can be given and will usually reverse the falling glucose within a few minutes. Your doctor can prescribe such a kit for you to keep on hand if you feel it is necessary and reassuring. If you recall that you have taken your insulin twice or taken too much fairly soon after having already done so, then you can take some additional carbohydrate at the meal or a larger-than-usual snack between meals.

49. I am on insulin for my diabetes and I am overweight. If I lose weight, will I be able to stop the insulin shots?

Encouragingly, the answer is yes. It is often a pleasant surprise to learn that you do not have to lose a dramatic amount of weight for this to occur. Even a loss of between 5% and 10% in your weight can have remarkable benefits on your blood sugars. Some patients often experience a significant reduction in the amount of insulin they need after only a modest weight reduction. Lowering the insulin dosage helps to control appetite and further helps efforts at weight reduction. Lowering the insulin dosage reduces appetite by reducing the likelihood of hypoglycemia, which must be treated by food intake, thus limiting the success of weight loss efforts. Unfortunately, even with such an incentive, the majority of people with diabetes who start insulin will need to remain on it, due to the difficulty of achieving

Some patients often experience a significant reduction in the amount of insulin they need after only a modest weight reduction.

and sustaining successful weight reduction and also to the fact that the body's own insulin production may by now be quite deficient (see Question 43). Available approved medications for weight reduction are also seldom helpful long term, due to limiting side effects and lack of effectiveness. However, patients who have undergone bariatric surgery (see Question 5) are often able to achieve sustained weight loss and discontinue insulin for the medium to long term. This approach is being increasingly used for people with severe degrees of obesity and serious health problems related to it, including diabetes.

50. Do any traditional or nonprescription remedies for diabetes really help control blood sugar? If so, which ones do you recommend?

There are a number of nonprescription remedies that are known to be effective at lowering blood sugar. In fact, one of the most frequently used and established treatments for diabetes, metformin, was derived from the traditional knowledge that the leaves of the French lilac plant reversed the symptoms of diabetes in some patients. This fact had been known to Europeans for more than 200 years before its eventual isolation and chemical modification to the medication that we now use. Other nonprescription remedies that have been found to be effective to varying degrees include cinnamon (it appears that the cinnamon stick itself must be used rather than powdered cinnamon alone), the herb gymnema sylvestre (gurmarbooti, gurmar), raw walnuts, bitter melon, and some compounds of the metals chromium and zinc. The beneficial effects of these are generally mild and can be more effective in some people with diabetes than in others, as is also the case for prescription medications. There is generally little down side to trying some of these supplements, as long as the glucose level is carefully

One of the most frequently used and established treatments for diabetes, metformin, was derived from the traditional knowledge that the leaves of the French lilac plant reversed the symptoms of diabetes in some patients.

monitored and conventional medications are also taken if they are needed. Since these remedies are not labeled or approved by the Food and Drug Administration for this use, there is no specific standardization for their formulation, which can therefore vary widely between manufacturers. Sometimes, exaggerated claims may be made for their effectiveness while at the same time a disclaimer is offered acknowledging that such compounds are not intended to diagnose or treat any disease!

51. Are there any medications prescribed for other conditions that can improve or worsen my diabetes?

Yes, there are a number of medications used to treat other conditions that can affect your blood sugar control. Most of these effects are small, but can be quite dramatic, such as the effect of certain types of steroid medications. Examples of various drugs and how they can affect your blood sugar are shown in **Table 5**.

Table 5 Examples of Medications in Common Use That Can Affect Blood Sugar

Medication	Usual Use	Effect on Sugar	Amount of Effect
Antiretroviral drugs (some)	HIV/AIDS	↑	++
Antidepressants (some)	Depression	↑	++ to +++
Carvedilol	Blood pressure	↓ or ↑	+
Estrogen	BCP, menopause	↑	+ to ++
Etanercept	RA, SLE, psoriasis	↓	++
Losartan	Blood pressure	↓	+
Niacin	Cholesterol	↑	+ to ++
Octreotide	Various	↑ or ↓	+
Pentamidine	Infection	↓ but later ↑	+ to ++
Pentoxifylline	Arterial disease	↓	+
Pseudoephedrine	Colds & allergies	↑	+
Ramipril	Blood pressure	↓	+
Steroids	Inflammation	↑	+++
Thiazides	Blood pressure	↑	+

Abbreviations: HIV: human immunodeficiency virus; AIDS: acquired immune deficiency syndrome; BCP: birth control pill; RA: rheumatoid arthritis; SLE: sytemic lupus erythematosus.

52. I hear that there are seven different types of pills for diabetes now. Is there a preferred order in which to try them and can they all be combined?

The various types of medications for diabetes are illustrated in Table 4 (Question 41). While there is no right or wrong order in which to try them, there are certain important principles that guide the use of diabetic medications. Important examples of these principles are effectiveness, safety, avoidance of weight gain, avoidance of low blood sugar, avoidance of side effects, long-lasting effectiveness, smallest number of pills required per day, lowest cost, and lack of interaction with other medications being taken by the patient. The overriding principle is that treatment must be tailored to the specific needs of each individual patient. Thus, while no medication can be said to be right for every patient, there is almost always a medication or combination of medications that can be used in each individual patient. Decision making is further complicated by the cost structure of your medical insurance company's drug formulary. Thus, while a certain pill may be more or less desirable from a medical perspective, the cost may factor significantly into the decision as to whether to use it and this can differ among various insurance plans.

Although many and complex factors must be taken into consideration, certain generally accepted patterns of practice have evolved among those caring for people with diabetes. Metformin is often the drug of first choice because it is inexpensive, does not cause weight gain (it may cause a modest weight loss), and does not cause low blood sugar. However, it has certain side effects and cannot be used in

Although many and complex factors must be taken into consideration, certain generally accepted patterns of practice have evolved among those caring for people with diabetes.

Treatments for Diabetes

patients who have various medical problems, such as liver and kidney disease or some forms of serious lung and heart problems. After metformin, the sulfonylureas are often used frequently, even though they can cause both low blood sugar and weight gain. However, they are generally very inexpensive. If this were not the case, sulfonylureas would probably be used much less often than they are and will probably be less and less used as the cost of safer alternative pills comes down over time. The newer class of pills known as DPP-IV inhibitors (e.g., sitagliptin) is very safe, convenient, and fairly effective, and does not cause weight gain or low blood sugar, but is more costly. The thiazolidinediones (TZDs or glitazones) are effective and do not cause low blood sugar, but they can be associated with weight gain and fluid retention and should not be used in people with, or at high risk for, heart failure. They are also expensive. The latter two types of pills therefore remain second line when cost is an issue. Other types of pills such as the meglitinides and the alpha-glucosidase inhibitors have their place in the management of diabetes, but are also usually not first-line drugs. **Table 6** shows an example of a common order in which diabetes pills can be used when considerations of cost are set aside.

These classes of pills can be used in most combinations. Not all of these combinations are specifically approved by the Food and Drug Administration, but many are. The only classes of medication that have been specifically shown to be no more effective when combined together than when used alone are the sulfonylureas and the meglitinides, since they both work through a similar mechanism to release insulin, although they activate it in different ways.

Table 6 Example of an Order in Which Oral Antidiabetic Drugs Can Be Tried

Medication	Choice	Reasons(s)
Metformin	1st	Potent, no weight gain, no hypoglycemia, inexpensive
DPP-IV-I	2nd	Mid-potent, no weight gain, no hypoglycemia, very few side effects, can be used with liver or kidney disease
Pioglitazone	3rd	Potent, durable effect, no hypoglycemia, cholesterol benefits, heart protective
Meglitinides	4th	Potent, rapid effect, less hypoglycemia
Sulfonylureas	5th	Potent, rapid effect, inexpensive
Acarbose	6th	No hypoglycemia, no weight gain
Colesevelam	7th	No hypoglycemia, no weight gain, cholesterol benefits

Note: This table does not take into account potential reasons why one or other drugs may not be suitable for a given patient. Treatment decisions must be tailored to the needs and for the safety of the patient. This is an example only.

53. How does the treatment based on "lizard spit" work?

The treatment based on lizard spit is exenatide (Byetta®), which is a synthetic version of a compound found in the saliva of a specific type of poisonous lizard that inhabits the southwestern United States and parts of Central America. The compound from the saliva is unrelated to the venom and is not poisonous. This compound (exendin-4) is a reptilian version of a compound that is released upon eating from cells lining the human intestine (glucagon-like peptide-1 or GLP-1). GLP-1 has several actions that favorably regulate glucose levels in the body. It travels in the bloodstream to the pancreas and increases the release of insulin, thereby lowering blood glucose. It also reduces the release of the hormone glucagon. This is useful because glucagon tends to raise blood glucose through an action on the liver. The remarkable feature of these actions of GLP-1 is that they only occur when the blood sugar is elevated above fasting levels. Thus, GLP-1 does not cause hypoglycemia. GLP-1 decreases the rate of emptying of the stomach, slowing delivery of calories to the intestine and making their absorption more gradual. This also serves to keep blood glucose levels lower. GLP-1 acts on the brain to increase the feeling of fullness after eating (known as *satiety*) and to reduce hunger, which helps to limit food intake.

Unfortunately, however, human GLP-1 is very rapidly broken down and inactivated by the body after release into the bloodstream, most being removed within a few minutes. This is where exenatide comes in. This derivative of the reptilian compound is resistant to the human mechanism for breaking it down and lasts in the bloodstream for several hours. This makes it approximately ten times as powerful as natural human GLP-1. For these reasons, exenatide, which must be taken by twice-daily injection, is effective at lowering blood sugar in people with diabetes and, in more than eight out of ten people who take it, it leads to weight loss, in part due to its appetite-suppressant properties. More than four out of ten people who start exenatide treatment will experience nausea and about one out of seven will experience at least one episode of vomiting. This often passes after a few uses, but some patients cannot tolerate this medication. To minimize this problem, it is given in a lower dose initially and the dosage is increased after the first month. It comes in prefilled pens containing one

- *Heloderma suspectum (Gila Monster)* and *Heloderma horridum (Beaded Lizard)* are the only venomous lizards in North America.
- Exendin-4 is *not* derived from nor related to the venom, but is produced in the salivary glands of the Gila monster.
- Exenatide is a synthetic version of the substance produced in the lizard's salivary glands. It is more potent than the equivalent human substance and more resistant to breakdown in the body.
- Exenatide must be given by injection. It lowers blood sugar and often leads to weight loss, although it can be effective even if the user does not lose weight.
- It often causes nausea initially and sometimes vomiting.
- Rarely, pancreatitis may occur.

Figure 5   Properties of exenatide.

month's treatment. **Figure 5** shows some of the properties of exenatide.

54. Many patients start on pills but end up on insulin. Why do pills tend to fail in the end and do they all fail at the same rate?

Pills for type 2 diabetes tend to fail after a period of time because the severity of the diabetes tends to progress. Diabetes is a disorder associated with aging, reduction in physical activity, and increasing body weight. Since all of these things tend to progress with time, it is not surprising that the severity of the diabetes tends to progress and the response to pills that were previously effective tends to be diminished. Not only this, but there appears to be a normal aging-related decline in the ability of the pancreas to make insulin that is steeper in those with diabetes. Since one is presently unable to prevent this or prevent aging from occurring, the only factors that are controllable to prevent progression of the diabetes are weight and exercise, and these are notoriously difficult to manage with consistent success. Therefore, it is not surprising that many people with type 2 diabetes tend to require more and higher doses of pills over time and that many eventually fail to be controlled on pills alone.

The pills do not all tend to fail at the same rate. The sulfonylurea drugs and metformin (see Questions 41 and 52 for a description) tend to fail at a rate of about 5% of patients who were previously controlled on them per year. Thus, after 10 years, half of the patients taking these drugs initially successfully will no longer be controlled on them. However, there is encouraging news from some of the newer types of pills for diabetes. It appears as if the medications of the TZD class and possibly the DPP-IV inhibitor class (see Questions 41 and 52 for a description) may actually modify the course of the diabetes itself and slow its progression. The TZD type of drugs acts to improve the body's response to the insulin it produces, while the DPP-IV inhibitor class may act to restore the health of the insulin-producing cells of the pancreas. Whether these types of drugs are able to achieve these improvements in a long-term manner, such that patients on them will not require insulin or other drugs by injection at all, remains to be shown by long-term studies.

PART SIX

Monitoring and Living with Diabetes

What information should I bring to my doctor to help him or her manage my diabetes with me?

How accurate are glucose monitors?

How will my diabetes affect my work? Are there any jobs I cannot do?

More . . .

55. How often do I need to check my blood sugar?

How often you need to check your blood sugar depends upon how the information that blood sugar testing provides will be used.

How often you need to check your blood sugar depends upon how the information that blood sugar testing provides will be used. All too often, people with diabetes are instructed to test their blood sugar frequently and yet neither they nor their physician or other caregivers make significant use of the information. Generally, when treatment (such as the amount of insulin to be taken before the next meal) is not being adjusted immediately or even day to day, there is little justification for very frequent testing. Except for people who cannot or will not test, all people with diabetes should be prepared to check their blood sugar frequently when they are sick, under severe physical stress, or taking medications that are known to markedly affect the blood sugar level, such as steroids. Examples of possible glucose monitoring schedules for various circumstances are shown in **Table 7**.

Table 7   Glucose Monitoring Strategies

Type of Diabetes	Testing Strategy
Type 1, 2, or GDM on intermittent insulin 2 to 4 times daily	Before meals, bedtime, occ. after meals, & during night
Type 1 or 2 on continuous insulin infusion (pump)	Before meals, bedtime, sometimes after meals, & during night
Type 2 on oral antidiabetic pills (OADs)	Before breakfast and supper alternating with before lunch and bedtime, 3 days/week
Type 2 or GDM on lifestyle intervention	As for type 2 on OADs, 1 to 3 days/week
All types, when sick or unstable	As needed to intervene effectively, q2-hours if needed

56. What is the target level for my blood sugar?

The target level for your blood sugar depends on who you are and on the other circumstances of your health. Various authoritative expert bodies have published blood sugar targets to aim at before and 2 hours after meals at various stages of life, including for children, adults, pregnant women, and the elderly. The various recommendations differ in certain respects, but are generally similar and those of the American Diabetes Association and the American Association of Clinical Endocrinologists are shown in **Table 8**. Wherever possible, otherwise healthy individuals with diabetes should aim to achieve blood sugar levels that are as close to normal as possible, as long as these can be reached without side effects that are either distressing or dangerous. This is a matter of judgment between you and your physician. The main side effects of the various pills for diabetes are shown in Table 4 (Question 41).

The target levels for blood sugar can either be described by blood sugar levels themselves or in overall terms, according to the Hemoglobin A1c

Table 8 Blood Sugar and A1c Targets for Diabetes

Time	ADA (mg/dl)	AACE (mg/dl)
Fasting	70–130	Less than 110
2 hours after eating	Less than 180	Less than 140
A1c	Less than 7.0% and as close to 6% as is safely achievable; less than 8% in young children, the elderly, and those at high risk of hypoglycemia	Less than 6.5%

Source: Data from ADA: American Diabetes Association; AACE: American Association of Clinical Endocrinologists.

(HbA1c or A1c), which is an average measure of blood sugar over the prior 3–4 months, approximately. For all people with diabetes, but especially those who do not need to perform frequent self-monitoring of blood sugar or who are unable to do so, the HbA1c is a very helpful measure and the American Diabetes Association recommends that it is performed at least twice per year. Recently, it has been recommended that the HbA1c should be reported in terms of the estimated average blood glucose (eAG) to which it corresponds, which may be more meaningful to most persons with diabetes. The corresponding values of each and the formula to make this calculation are shown in **Table 9**.

57. What information should I bring to my doctor to help him or her manage my diabetes with me?

The most important pieces of information that you can bring to your doctor are the results of your home

Table 9   The Relationship Between HbA1c and Estimated Average Glucose Level (eAG)

HbA1c (%)	eAG (mg/dl)
5	97
6	126
6.5	140
7	154
7.5	169
8	183
8.5	197
9	212
9.5	226
10	240
11	269
12	298

Formula used to calculate mean blood glucose (eAG) from A1c:
$eAG(mg/dl) = (28.7 \times HbA1c) - 46.7$.
Source: Data from American Diabetes Association (ADA).

glucose testing (and preferably your glucose monitor, also) and an updated list of the medications you are currently taking, not only for diabetes, but for other medical problems as well. The glucose testing results are important because they reflect the most current state of control of your blood sugar. Also, if you are taking your glucose tests at various times of day, your log will show where you are best controlled and where you are not so well controlled, which allows your doctor to recommend the most effective adjustment to your treatment, or to suggest factors that might be influencing your sugar levels. Generally speaking, the more complex your therapy and the longer you have had diabetes, the more important the home glucose test results become. For example, if you have developed diabetes relatively recently, are on one medication only, and your periodic HbA1c tests show that you are generally well controlled, the home glucose results are less critical than if you have had diabetes for several years, are on multiple pills and/or insulin, and have complications of your diabetes (see Part 4). The reason that it helps to bring your monitor is that the results may suggest a problem with it and it can be examined when you are seen. Also, the information in it can often be downloaded into the clinic computer and analyzed in a number of ways to show trends and patterns that can be very helpful. When you keep a record of your readings, it is much better to enter them into one of the commercially available logbooks designed for the purpose than to write them down one after the other on a sheet of paper, which often makes them quite hard to follow and understand.

The importance of the list of your current medications and dosages is that your doctor can only safely

If you are taking your glucose tests at various times of day, your log will show where you are best controlled and where you are not so well controlled.

Monitoring and Living with Diabetes

make adjustments to your medicines (for diabetes and other related conditions) in light of accurate knowledge of what you are presently taking. This includes herbs, supplements, and alternative medicines. This leads to one final important point, which is to remind you never to be hesitant to reveal to your doctor whether you are, or are not, taking your prescribed medicines correctly. Your doctor's aim is to serve your healthcare needs and to advise and assist you. He or she does not wish to judge or blame you. You have ownership and control of your medical problems and are free to make your own decisions as to whether to follow medical advice or not to do so. The only time a responsible physician will not agree to partner with you in such a decision is if it would be unethical or dangerous and his or her primary obligation not to harm you would be violated.

58. What tests should my doctor be doing on a regular basis to monitor my diabetes?

Some of the tests that your doctor will perform to monitor your diabetes and the status of any of its chronic complications are shown in **Table 10**. The main things that interest your doctor are monitoring the control of your blood sugar, the control of your cholesterol and blood pressure, and the presence or progress of any long-term complications of your diabetes (see Part 4 for discussion of these), and to check for the presence or absence of other related conditions. Tests in this context can refer to clinical examination, such as checking the condition of your feet and testing the sensation, laboratory blood tests, and special tests, as indicated, such as scans or other images. Many of these your doctor can do himself

Table 10   Items That May Be Checked Regularly in Persons with Diabetes

Item	Monitoring Tool
Glucose control	HbA1c, fructosamine, CBGs, eAG
Lipids	Fasting lipid panel ± special lipid tests
Blood pressure	BP cuff measurements
Large vessel health	EKG, carotid IMT
Small vessel health	
Feet	Inspection, microfilament, capillary refill, ABIs
Kidneys	Serum creatinine, estimated CCr, MACR
Eyes	Retinal imaging, dilated eye exam
Peripheral nerves	Monofilament, NCV testing, touch and vibration perception, proprioception*
Autonomic nerves	Postural BP, pulse, RR variation

Abbreviations: HbA1c: hemoglobin A1c; CBGs: capillary (fingerstick) blood glucoses; eAG: estimated average glucose; BP: blood pressure; EKG (ECG): electrocardiogram; IMT: intimal-medial thickness by ultrasound; ABIs: ankle-brachial indices; CCr: creatinine clearance; MACR: microalbumen-to-creatinine ratio; NCV: nerve conduction velocity; RR: R-wave to R-wave (on EKG). *Position sense.

and others may require referral to another specialist. A detailed eye examination is an example of the latter.

59. What is the best kind of glucose monitor?

Since insulin became available, probably nothing has more revolutionized the day-to-day management of diabetes, especially type 1 diabetes, than the arrival of the capillary glucose monitor. So successful has this technology been that this is a difficult question to answer specifically because there are up to 20 approved glucose monitors for use at any one time, with new or updated models appearing frequently. Also, different features are important to different individuals, depending on their needs. Probably the best way to answer this question is to discuss some of the available features. Size is one of the first that springs to mind. Monitors have been getting ever smaller since they first appeared more than 30 years ago. It is now possible to get a monitor that is about the same size as a standard lipstick (e.g., One Touch Ultra-Mini®) and is yet highly functional. Memory size is not as important as it might at first seem. A memory of about 100 readings is probably sufficient, although almost every monitor now has more. There is limited practical usefulness of going back too far, since treatment decisions should be based on recent information, rather than distant data. Sample size is sometimes important and most available meters now use much smaller blood samples than was previously the case. Microsample meters such as some Freestyle® and One Touch® models use samples less than 1/50th the size of an actual droplet of blood. Many monitors will permit sampling from sites other than the fingertip, such as the forearm (most) and palm, which is useful for those with sensitive fingers or for people who are heavily involved in manual or delicate work. The speed of obtaining the reading is now usually around 5 seconds after the blood sample is applied, although some models (such as the Prestige IQ®) can take up to 50 seconds. This is much shorter than models in the early days, which could take from 1 to 2 minutes. Most meters can now be linked by cable, Bluetooth, or broadband to a computer and their contents are downloadable, including to the Internet. Some meters have multistrip cassettes that dispense between 10 and 20 test strips, such as the Accuchek Compact Plus®, for added convenience. Other features include the ability to display results graphically (e.g., One Touch Ultrasmart®), to function at high altitude (e.g., Advocate Duo®), and to speak the results for those with limited vision (e.g., Prodigy Duo®). The features of 10 available glucose

Table 11 Features of 10 Available Capillary Glucose Monitors

Name	Vol	Site	Time	Mem	DL	Other
One Touch Ultra 2	1.0	F, A	5	500	+	
One Touch Ultrasmart	1.0	F, A	5	3000	+	Graphs
One Touch Ultramini	1.0	F, A	5	50	–	1.2 oz
Accuchek Compact+	1.5	F, A	5	300	+IR	Drum, no code
Accuchek Advantage	4.0	F	26	480	+	
Advance Microdraw	1.5	F, P	15	250	+	
Freestyle Flash	0.3	F, A	7	250	+IN	
Advocate Duo	0.7	F, A	7	450	+	To 10,742 ft
Prodigy Duo	0.6	F, A	6	450	+	Talks, 5 oz
Prestige IQ	4.0	F	50	365	+	WB/plasma

Vol: Sample vol in _L; F=finger; A=arm; P=palm; Time=time to results in seconds; Mem=memory capacity; DL=downloadable; IR=infrared; WB=whole blood.

monitors are shown in **Table 11** and an example of a typical data printout can be seen in **Figure 6**.

Finally, those with longstanding or complicated diabetes might want to consider the option of continuous glucose monitoring, which is discussed in Question 60. However, bear in mind that you will still require a conventional capillary glucose monitor.

Date	Breakfast					Lunch					Dinner					Night			Cmnt
	Bef	Aft	Meds	Carb	Other	Bef	Aft	Meds	Carb	Other	Bef	Aft	Meds	Carb	Other	Gluc	Meds	Carb	
12/08/02	68	131	20M	30							151		10M	60					
12/08/02											129								
12/07/02	172		20M	30		140			15		179		10M	45					
12/06/02	114		20M	30		88			15		144		10M	60		165		15	
12/05/02	264		20M	15		189	143		30				10M	120					
12/04/02		165	20M	30							303		4A	30					
12/04/02											223		5A						
Average	137	154				164	146				201	232				133			
In Target	40%	86%				43%	88%				27%	33%				71%			
# Results	15	7				14	8				11	3				7			

Figure 6 Example of a data printout from contemporary glucose monitor.

Source: Used with permission from LifeScan, Inc. © 2009

Monitoring and Living with Diabetes

60. Should I get one of the new continuous glucose monitors?

There are now three types of continuous glucose monitors available. They all transmit glucose results wirelessly from a small sensor placed just beneath the skin via a transmitter whose signal is received by the monitor placed anywhere from 5 to 10 feet away. Results are sent from every minute to every 5 minutes and the trend of the readings can be shown on graphs. One, the Medtronic Realtime System®, can transmit the results into the same unit that is used as the insulin pump. However, even though the same unit acts as both monitor and pump, it is still necessary for the wearer to program and set the amount of insulin to be delivered. Studies have shown that the additional information provided by the frequently delivered values and the graphed trends reduces high and low glucose events in the wearer by about half. It is important to note that all the current continuous glucose monitors are approved only for use with and alongside conventional glucose meters. This means that before acting on the information the continuous monitor provides, you should verify it by obtaining a reading with your regular monitor. Also, the two technologies provide similar but slightly different information. The conventional monitor measures blood glucose from the blood droplet resulting from the finger prick. The continuous meter does not use blood. Instead, it measures the glucose level in the fluid bathing the tissue under the skin. This is in fact derived from the blood plasma itself, but it takes several minutes to adjust to reflect the blood level. The available continuous meters need to be calibrated twice daily (Medtronic Guardian®, Dexcom 7®) with a conventional fingerstick reading, although the newer Abbott Freestyle Navigator® needs only four calibration readings in a 5-day period. Once introduced, the sensor/transmitter can be worn for 3 (Guardian), 5 (Navigator), or 7 (Dexcom-7) days before the sensor must be changed. Features of an available continuous monitor are shown in **Figure 7** and **Table 12**.

The decision as to whether to get one of these monitors depends on the value to the wearer of knowing his or her

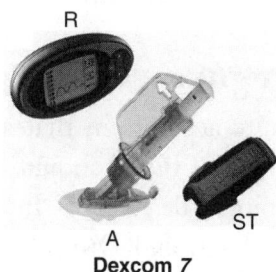

Dexcom *7*

A: Applicator; R: Receiver; ST: Sensor-Transmitter

Figure 7   A continuous glucose monitor.

Source: Dexcom.

Table 12   Features of Two Available Continuous Glucose Monitors

Feature	Dexcom *STS*	Medtronic *Guardian*
Sample site	Subcutaneous ISF	Subcutaneous ISF
Sensor life (days)	7	6
User age (years)	≥18	≥7
Set-up cost ($)	800	1339
Clark Error Grid A&B	95.4%	96.0%
Probe gauge	25	22
Battery	Rechargeable	Disposable AAA
Initialization (minutes)	120	140
Calibration (hours)	2, 8, then q12	0.5 × 2, then q12
Alarms	High and low	High and low
Integratable	No	Can transmit to *Paradigm* insulin pump
Transmitter range (feet)	5	6
Transmitter waterproof	Yes	Yes
Graphs trends (hours)	1, 3, and 9	3 and 24

readings on a minute-by-minute basis. For people early in the course of diabetes, on oral medications, and in good control, they are probably not necessary. For people on insulin, with a history of low and high readings, especially if they are hard to predict or explain, the information provided by continuous glucose sensing may be very valuable. However, approval for insurance coverage is often limited to specific circumstances, such as the frequent occurrence of very high or low blood sugars that cannot otherwise be prevented.

61. How accurate are glucose monitors?

Glucose monitors are quite accurate in that any given reading on the same sample of blood should only vary by a few percentage points (i.e., 5–10). In order to obtain approval from the Food and Drug Administration, such medical devices have to show that they are both precise and accurate. This means that they will obtain a similar result under similar conditions and that the result will be close to the real true value, as best as we are able to ascertain it, i.e., according to the accepted gold standard, which is glucose measured in the laboratory. Furthermore, when such a device is compared to the gold standard measurement in clinical trials, a specified number of readings have to fall very close to the readings obtained by the gold standard device. This value is more than 95%. The rules for approval of such devices have been published by the FDA and can be viewed at http://www.fda.gov/cdrh/oivd/guidance/1171.pdf. Although users are often surprised by the variation in results that they will see upon obtaining a reading within a very short space of time from a prior reading, it has to be acknowledged that the variation is seldom such that a different course of action would be taken. For example, insulin would be given or not given or a low blood sugar level would be treated or not treated. Actual numerical accuracy tends to be less when the glucose level is very low. However, since such a low value should always be treated, the accuracy of the actual reported number is not critical.

When a surprising glucose value that does not fit with the expected circumstances is obtained, it is always prudent to recheck that reading, on either the same or a different monitor. Also, it is advisable to check that the monitor is functioning well, by checking the low battery indicator, assuring that the correct coding has been entered and that the test strips are within date and inserted properly. Sometimes, variation in technique by the user accounts, at least partially, for variation in the result obtained. This can include liquid on the puncture site, contamination with glucose, excessive squeezing of the finger, and sweating.

62. How does stress affect my blood sugars?

Stress is a broad term that can have a number of meanings. For the purposes of this question, only emotional stress will be discussed. Emotional stress (whether its source is personal, professional, psychological, or social) can affect the blood sugar in a number of ways. The most frequent manifestation of stress is the result of the rise in the circulating level of stress hormones in the blood. The stress hormones, such as epinephrine or adrenaline and cortisol, release stored glucose into the blood, thus raising sugar levels. They also make the tissues resistant to insulin. The result is a rise in blood sugar levels, which often leads to a need for more insulin or other medication.

Stress can also affect blood sugar levels by its effect on eating behavior. When under stress, eating habits often change. This change may be predictable in a given

Stress can also affect blood sugar levels by its effect on eating behavior.

individual but is quite unpredictable in different individuals. It can vary from eating less and losing weight, to eating more or eating at different times, such as during the night. This can significantly alter one's pattern of blood sugar readings. Also, significant amounts of stress often interrupt established patterns of exercise and leisure sports, which can cause blood sugars to rise.

Furthermore, a person's adherence to a prescribed medical regimen often suffers during times of stress. The management of one's diabetes can consume a considerable amount of a person's time and attention and be a stress in itself. For this reason, people often reduce their frequency of glucose monitoring and sometimes the number of prescribed pills or injections that they actually take. Occasionally, this can have serious short-term consequences, but of significant concern is that people under prolonged stress who do not pay close attention to the management of their diabetes open themselves up to an increased risk of the serious long-term complications discussed in Part 4. Therefore, if you are a person with diabetes under stress, it is wise to focus on addressing and relieving that stress in the interests of your long-term health.

63. Is there a link between lack of sleep or disturbed sleep and my blood sugars?

There certainly can be. Studies have shown that sleep deprivation can have a negative effect on several aspects of metabolism, including blood sugar, blood pressure, and even cholesterol levels. Blood sugars can be increased by the stress of lack of sleep. What constitutes an adequate amount of sleep varies among individuals, so what may be a metabolic stress for one may not be so for another. The elevation in blood sugars will not necessarily occur upon awakening, but can occur anytime due to elevated levels of stress hormones throughout the day. As described in Question 62, stress hormones tend to push the blood sugar level up. Sometimes several days of deprived sleep are necessary to have a measurable effect on the blood sugars.

Several other factors are worth noting. If the lack of sleep is associated with restless behavior (e.g., tossing and turning or arising and pacing), the increased physical activity may actually lower the blood sugars. A condition known as obstructive sleep apnea, or OSA, can occur in people with obesity and type 2 diabetes. This can cause frequent awakening at night, with daytime sleepiness and napping. The net amount of sleep may be more or less than normal in people with OSA. Generally, a bed partner will notice snoring and a disturbed breathing pattern. This condition is treatable and sometimes constitutes medical justification for surgical intervention to control obesity. You should inform your doctor if you suspect you have this problem. Finally, shortened sleep tends to be associated with weight gain, so that restoration of a satisfactory sleep pattern can actually aid in efforts to reduce weight, which will generally help to control blood sugars.

64. How can I avoid getting bruises or swellings on my stomach from my insulin shots?

Bruises and swellings on the stomach (or more accurately the abdominal wall) due to insulin are caused by two distinct mechanisms and are not usually variations of the same thing. However, occasionally a bruise will be severe enough so as to cause an actual swelling.

Bruising is due to leakage of blood from small vessels penetrated at the time of the insulin injection. Some people are more likely to bruise than others, including the elderly and those on anticoagulant or antiplatelet medications (blood thinners) such as warfarin, heparin, clopidogrel, ticlopidine, and others. Some people on routine doses of aspirin for protection from stroke and heart attack will note an increased tendency to bruise with their insulin injections, while others do not. Injection tools or technique may also play a role. Those with relatively small amounts of body fat on their abdominal walls (or thighs or arms if you use them) need to be sure to lift and gently pinch the skin and insert the needle at an angle in the middle of the pinched tissue. Injecting the needle directly and to the hilt may lead to an inadvertent injection into the muscle. This will change the pattern of action of the insulin and lead to a bruise or sometimes a painful bleed into the muscle itself. Some types of needle are more prone to cause bruising in some individuals than others. If you bruise easily, use the smallest diameter (gauge) of needle you can find. Remember that the higher number of gauge means a smaller diameter.

Injecting the needle directly and to the hilt may lead to an inadvertent injection into the muscle.

Swellings, especially if they are chronic, are often due to a property of the insulin itself. Insulin is one of the hormones responsible for growth and maintenance of our tissues including muscle protein and fat stores. If insulin is injected repeatedly in the same area, additional fat can become laid down in that spot. This takes on the appearance of a painless fatty mound (**lipohypertrophy**), which can be somewhat disfiguring. Fortunately, these fatty mounds will disperse if the insulin is no longer injected there, although it may take several weeks or months to remodel. To avoid these, the insulin injection sites should be rotated. Keeping a simple map of your abdominal wall, divided into a grid of 20 or 30 boxes and checking off a box after you have used it, will allow you to avoid using

Lipohypertrophy

A painless, but potentially disfiguring, fatty mound.

the same spot repeatedly within a 3- or 4-week period. Rarely, the opposite of lipohypertrophy may occur, i.e., loss of body fat in a localized or more generalized way. This is known as *lipoatrophy*. This is sometimes preceded by a viral infection, but more often the underlying cause cannot be identified.

Red or itchy areas at the site of injection may indicate an allergic reaction to the insulin or a component of it. This is quite rare with modern insulins, but will necessitate a process known as desensitization, which needs to be performed under the supervision of a specialist. Larger red or discharging swellings, which are shiny and tender, indicate an abscess due to infection and you should seek medical attention promptly.

65. How will my diabetes affect my work? Are there any jobs I cannot do?

Whether your diabetes will affect your work depends upon the nature of your diabetes and the nature of your work. Thus, the impact can be almost negligible to highly significant and life-changing. People with early or well-controlled type 2 diabetes, especially if they are not taking medications known to cause hypoglycemia, should be able to perform satisfactorily in almost any type of work that they wish to do. In situations in which personal or public endangerment is a possibility (e.g., transportation and heavy equipment operation) glucose monitoring should be performed periodically, especially when feeling unwell, as high blood sugars can be associated with impaired mental functioning and increase the risk of dehydration and dizziness or drowsiness.

If you have type 1 diabetes or insulin-requiring type 2 diabetes, or have type 2 diabetes but are taking pills known to cause low blood sugar (for a list of these, see

Table 4 in Question 41), then the performance of certain occupations which could potentially endanger yourself or others places a special burden of care and attention upon you. With regards to motor transportation, motor vehicle departments have regulations, which may vary from state to state, as to licensure requirements. They may involve, for example, producing records from the memory of a glucose monitor to show that you have checked your blood sugar at regular intervals prior to and during driving and have had no significant low blood sugar readings while doing so. With regard to flying, there are federal regulations and states may have additional requirements. If you are considering a military career and have diabetes, you will have to inform your recruiter, who will advise you of your eligibility.

A number of occupations are not covered by specific regulations, but you will generally be held to the standard of reasonable behavior if you cause harm to people or property wholly or in part as a result of your diabetes. If you did not know what a reasonable person might be expected to know, or act on the knowledge that you have as a reasonable person might be expected to act, you could be judged to have recklessly endangered the lives of others or negligently damaged the property of others and could be subject to legal penalties. If in doubt, therefore, discuss your diabetes with your doctor and your employer and seek advice from experts on regulations that might apply to you.

66. I have heard that depression is more common in people with diabetes. Is this true?

Yes, it is true that people with diabetes (and with other long-term illnesses) can experience higher rates of depression. This can be due to factors relating to the diabetes itself, or it can be unrelated. There is no convincing evidence that the actual blood sugar level itself is reliably predictive of mood, even in those with a tendency to depression. The severity of the diabetes and its complications, as well as its impact upon a person's lifestyle and aspirations, can be an important predictor of depression. For some the impact may be major and for others much less so, even though the degree of severity of the diabetes is the same. It is important to remember that the vast majority of people in our society with treated diabetes (more than 15 million in the United States alone) are able to adjust to the disorder and have happy, productive, and rewarding lives. Some have even achieved astonishing things in all walks of life. Examples include the gold medal winning Olympic swimmer Gary Hall, the NBA basketball player Adam Morrison, and the actresses Halle Berry and Mary Tyler Moore and Supreme Court Justice Sonia Sotomayor, all of whom have lived with diabetes while achieving great success.

If you are experiencing unusual degrees of sadness, reduced enthusiasm or interest in life, or excessive stress that you perceive is related to your diabetes, your doctor or certified diabetes educator may be able to help you to identify resources that can help you cope. Some of these resources are discussed in Question 82. Many certified diabetes educators (CDEs) are trained to provide such psychosocial support. If you are truly suffering from depression, your diabetes may or may not be an underlying cause, even though it may seem that way. Your doctor or CDE will help you to identify whether expert professional psychological or psychiatric consultation is needed.

Monitoring and Living with Diabetes

67. How does the sugar in fruit drinks differ from the sugar in sodas?

Fructose

A simple sugar found in honey, many fruits, and some vegetables.

The sugar in fruit juices is predominantly **fructose**, which is a disaccharide, meaning that it contains two molecules of glucose joined together and must be broken down to glucose in order to be absorbed, which may cause a delayed or muted effect on the blood sugar. Fruit juices will also contain a moderate amount of some vitamins and minerals. Sodas do not contain significant amounts of vitamins or minerals. The sugar in regular non-diet sodas is glucose, which is very readily absorbed and sweeter tasting. The amount of sugar in a standard 12-ounce can of regular soda is equivalent to about 9 teaspoons of table sugar (which is neither glucose nor fructose, but sucrose, another disaccharide) and therefore provides a large amount of calories, which can raise the blood sugar level very quickly. This is helpful if a low blood sugar reaction is being treated, but not a recommended part of the diabetic diet, as it causes a very sharp rise in blood glucose to levels above those recommended. This rise is hard to prevent with either pills or insulin, without giving doses that will later lead to low blood sugar levels.

68. My doctor says I don't need to see a specialist for my diabetes. How do I know if my doctor is right?

At the time of writing, there are estimated to be about 16 million adults in the United States who are aware that they have diabetes. There are, however, only about 4000 certified adult diabetes specialists in clinical practice and not all of these are in full-time practice. Some, perhaps one in four, do not see patients with diabetes at all. This translates to one diabetes specialist for every 5000 people with diabetes. Those who are interested in learning more about the shortage of diabetes specialists in the United States can visit http://www.endo-society.org/advocacy/legislative/upload/A-Stewart-US-Endo-Workforce-A-Supply-Demand-Mismatch.pdf.

The average diabetes specialist carries a clinic census of several hundred active patients, each of whom he or she sees from two to several times per year. From these statistics, it is clear that the vast majority of people with diabetes will not be able to consult a specialist. However, not all people with diabetes need specialist input, and those who do will usually not require it for the majority of the course of the disease, especially in the case of type 2 diabetes. Much of the education necessary to effectively manage diabetes, especially that centering on glucose monitoring and diet and nutrition, is accessible by referral directly from your family doctor. Given its frequency, many family doctors see a considerable number of patients with diabetes and are competent in its routine management. They also generally make effective judgments as to when specialist consultation is advisable.

Some of the circumstances in which consultation with a diabetes specialist is often advisable are shown in **Table 13**.

69. I don't want my friends or co-workers to know I have diabetes. How can I manage it discreetly in public places?

It is sometimes surprising (and reassuring) to realize that, given the fact that about 1 in every 12 people in our society has diabetes, we encounter people with diabetes virtually every day in our daily lives and are quite unaware of it. This means that diabetes can

Table 13 Circumstances in Which Persons with Diabetes Might Benefit from Seeing a Specialist

1. Difficulty achieving target blood sugar control using routinely available medications with the best efforts of both the physician and the patient
2. Diabetes in which microvascular complications (such as eye, kidney, or nerve) have occurred or are progressing
3. Diabetes in which macrovascular complications (such as heart attack, heart failure, stroke, or other arterial disease) have occurred or are progressing
4. Frequent or unexplained high or low blood sugars
5. Pregnancy or planned pregnancy in a woman with diabetes
6. The use of multiple daily injections of insulin or a pump
7. Treatment of the diabetes complicated by other significant medical problems
8. During or following a hospital admission for decompensated diabetes or a diabetes complication, e.g., foot ulcer
9. When considering the decision to switch from pills to insulin
10. When considering pancreas or kidney transplantation
11. When a course of medium-or long-term oral steroid therapy is planned

indeed be managed discreetly and privately without undue attention and alarm by the vast majority of those who have it. A renowned diabetes specialist recently wrote that the most important contribution of the diabetes specialist is to help patients build diabetes into their lives rather than to build their lives around diabetes*. Thus, there are many ways in which management of diabetes can be built into our lives without unduly disrupting them.

Perhaps the two main challenges to discreet diabetes management are performing glucose monitoring and administering injectable medications, such as insulin, during the workday. The main challenge for many occurs in the middle of the day, when most people are at work and privacy is scarce. Many simply do not

---

*See Gale EAM. Who Needs the Diabetes Specialist Physician? *Diabetologia* 51:700–702, 2008.

check their blood sugar during the middle of the day and settle on a treatment regimen that avoids insulin shots during the day. Fortunately, some insulin treatment plans are designed to prevent this, as they entail use of one or two shots of longer-acting insulin and an injection of short-acting insulin before each main meal. Moreover, studies have shown that patients on insulin who do not check their blood sugar in the middle of the day achieve poorer control of their diabetes. Modern miniaturized glucose monitors and automated insulin pen devices are at least part of the answer for many people. Continuous glucose monitors (see Question 60) can offer a solution for others. Some glucose monitors, for example, the Lifescan One Touch Ultra Mini®, are little larger than a conventional tube of lipstick and will provide a reading within 5 seconds. Others, such as the Accuchek Compact Plus®, automatically produce a strip when switched on. While time is required to perform the finger (or arm) stick to obtain the drop of blood, the entire operation can be completed in about a minute, especially if the lancet was previously loaded into the spring-loaded autolancet device. Thus, this can be done at one's desk or in the restroom quite rapidly. Similarly, preloaded insulin pens can avoid the need to draw up insulin, or bring bottles and syringes. The dose can be dialed on the pen and given in seconds. Finally, continuous glucose monitors only require the wearer to check the readings they are displaying, much as we check our beepers and cell phones from time to time.

Remember that regular glucose monitoring during the day can help avoid unexpected low blood sugars, which can be the hardest to manage without attracting attention, especially if they are severe.

PART SEVEN

Diabetes and Special Situations

I have diabetes and want to get pregnant.
What should I do?

I will be traveling. How do I handle the time changes
with my insulin shots?

My child has diabetes and is about to start school.
What steps should I take and how will the school
help to ensure that things go well?

More . . .

70. I have diabetes and want to get pregnant. What should I do?

When a woman of childbearing age has diabetes, it is very important to plan the pregnancy ahead of time for a number of reasons. The first reason is that studies have shown that the risk of birth defects (called congenital malformations) is much higher if the diabetes is not well controlled at the time of becoming pregnant. Improving control of the diabetes as quickly as possible after discovering the pregnancy will not fully reverse this risk, which in some studies has been found to be as high as one in five. Therefore, it is important to establish and confirm that your diabetes is in the best possible control before proceeding with a plan to become pregnant.

The second issue is that women with longstanding diabetes who suffer from its microvascular complications (see Questions 32, 33, and 34 for discussion of these) are more likely to have a complicated pregnancy and will need to be reassessed prior to and during the pregnancy. Of particular importance are the possibility of progression of retinopathy and nephropathy during the course of pregnancy.

Finally, it may be necessary to change the type of treatment during the pregnancy, and this may require some forward planning. For example, pills are generally not used during pregnancy. Therefore, a woman with type 2 diabetes will almost always need to learn how to take insulin and it may be more convenient to do this as part of pre-pregnancy planning.

71. I am scheduled to have an operation. How do I prepare my diabetes for this?

The extent to which you and your physician prepare for your operation depends on the extent of the

Diabetes and Special Situations

operation, the severity of the condition that has led to it, and the treatment that you are taking for your diabetes. The fact that your operation is planned means that it is not urgent nor an emergency. However, many people with diabetes will experience surgical emergencies for which no preparation is possible. In general, the outcome will depend on the underlying emergency, with the overall management being made somewhat more complex by management of the diabetes during and after the operation. However, in recent years, studies have shown that very careful management of the blood sugar is very important in the days immediately following an operation. However, there is less convincing evidence that blood sugar management prior to and during an operation is quite as important.

In general, your surgeon will request assurance from the medical doctor caring for your diabetes that your blood sugar is under fair overall control, especially in the days and weeks running up to the operation. The severity of any large vessel complications, such as heart and other vascular disease, will need to be evaluated. Your blood pressure will need to be well controlled, as high blood pressure (hypertension) is a frequent accompaniment to diabetes and can lead to surgical complications if unregulated. Of the small vessel complications of diabetes, your kidney function will need to be evaluated and the result taken into account, as abnormal kidney function can affect blood pressure, lead to retention of intravenous fluids, and alter the rate of removal of certain medications from the body.

If you are taking pills and the operation is relatively minor and brief and your diabetes is under good

In general, your surgeon will request assurance from the medical doctor caring for your diabetes that your blood sugar is under fair overall control, especially in the days and weeks running up to the operation.

control, not taking your medication on the night prior to and/or the morning of the operation may be all that is needed and the medication can be resumed after surgery, with your first main meal. People who are taking insulin will generally be instructed to take a reduced dose of the longer-acting insulin the night prior to surgery and to take no set dose of short-acting insulin after the last meal has been eaten before surgery. Upon arrival at the hospital, the glucose will be monitored frequently by the hospital staff and insulin will be given if you need it. This is especially true for longer and more complicated operations. In all cases, you should monitor your blood sugar carefully at home in the days leading up to your operation.

72. Will having diabetes affect my ability to do my job?

The extent to which your diabetes will impact upon your job will depend on the nature of the job, the severity and complications of your diabetes, and the treatment you are taking for it. Many types of work will be affected only in a minor way, if at all, by the fact that you have diabetes. However, work that has implications for public safety, such as commercial operation of a vehicle (such as a bus, taxicab, train, or airplane), heavy machinery (such as a crane or a wrecker), or weapons (such as military weaponry) will be significantly impacted if you experience severe or unpredictable low blood sugar episodes. These are a significant risk if you take insulin or the type of pills known as sulfonylureas or meglitinides. Therefore, licensing authorities or your employer may be empowered (or even obliged) to limit your ability to perform these types of jobs, or set a strict set of criteria that must be satisfied (such as frequent verifiable glucose testing with a low frequency of low blood sugars) for you to do so.

Types of work where you are likely to place yourself, but not others, at higher risk are generally unregulated. Most involve a risk of falling from a height or self-injury with machinery. You should discuss with your doctor and/or diabetes educator the extent to which you are increasing your risk of injury and make an informed decision as to whether to pursue or continue this line of work. Examples of this type of job include roofing, commercial saw operation, and high-rise construction work.

73. I will be traveling. How do I handle the time changes with my insulin shots?

Traveling more than one or two time zones distant can temporarily throw off the timing of your injections and meals in relation to your previous injection pattern. This is further complicated by changes in your sleeping pattern, so that you may feel like eating at times other than set mealtimes or you may feel like sleeping when you would normally eat. Also, your daily pattern of hormonal changes (your diurnal rhythm), which can influence your blood sugars, may take several days to adjust to your new location. Moreover, travel these days can be quite stressful and your blood sugars can be affected by this, too. Therefore, some temporary disruption in your blood sugar control is to be expected, as many things are going on all at once.

If the journey is not too long and the stay will be relatively brief, some choose to adhere to their established meal and insulin injection pattern regardless of the time change and will take their shots and eat their meals correspondingly earlier or later. For most of us, this is not feasible as we need to be social with others at our destination. The key is to transition to a new pattern while trying to avoid a knock-on or stacking effect from the change in timing of insulin shots. When traveling west, your day will be longer, and will probably involve an additional meal or wider spacing in time between meals. When traveling east, a meal may be missed, but the next day's first meal will come earlier. In general, it is preferable to accept some higher blood sugars, which if moderate and short-lived, are not dangerous, versus low blood sugars, which may be more difficult to treat in an unfamiliar environment where access to food may be unpredictable. If taking a meal earlier in relation to the prior meal than is usual for you, you will probably eat less, and therefore a modest reduction in your short-acting insulin shot is probably wise. If taking a meal later, then a snack between meals may be more important than usual. Of course, checking your blood sugars regularly is very important, and including a correction factor for the unpredictable factors that may affect your blood sugar (e.g., stress, fatigue) is very helpful. Cycling the long-acting insulin shots into a new pattern can be the most challenging. If the next scheduled injection is much earlier than usual, based on the new time zone, it may be reasonable to delay it to some degree, especially if it is a relatively peakless insulin, such as glargine or detemir. A combination of dose reduction and a delay in timing can help to avoid hypoglycemia, with the goal of gradually moving it forward to fit into the new time zone. Conversely, if the injection needs to be delayed, this can often be managed with an additional injection of short-acting insulin, together with a snack, if needed to bridge the gap. It is recommended that you talk to your doctor about your travel plans and how to manage these. It is often helpful to keep your testing and meal schedule, when possible, on the time zone of the place from which you departed for the first 24 hours and then make adjustments when you are settled in the new location.

74. I will be getting a course of steroid treatment. I heard this could throw my diabetes out of control. What should I do?

Steroids are a type of medication based on compounds naturally produced by the body. Naturally occurring steroids are of several types, but one type, the glucocorticoids, have anti-inflammatory properties and are used to combat inflammation in a variety of conditions from asthma and allergic reactions to serious chronic diseases such as chronic bronchitis (COPD) and rheumatoid arthritis. Short courses of potent steroids, which can be given by mouth or injection, are generally effective and safe, but have the tendency to raise the blood sugar. Depending on the dosage, the potency of the steroid itself, and the underlying condition for which they are given, they can raise the blood sugar by a modest to a very marked degree. This will usually occur within a day of starting the course and will persist until the dosage is either lowered to levels normally produced by the body, or until a few days after discontinuing their use. In the case of a steroid injection given into an area of inflammation, such as the spine or a joint, the elevated blood sugars may persist for several days or even weeks, but are generally not as severe as when steroids are orally administered. In some people, administration of steroids may expose their tendency to diabetes for the first time.

Short courses of potent steroids, which can be given by mouth or injection, are generally effective and safe, but have the tendency to raise the blood sugar.

If you have diabetes and are either managed by pills or lifestyle adjustment alone, a course of high dose steroids may mean that you will need to take insulin for a period of time. This is because steroid-induced high blood sugars do not respond well to pills. Sometimes, when the course of steroids will be short, elevation of blood sugars, unless excessive, can be tolerated with the knowledge that it will resolve fairly rapidly when the medication is stopped. You should monitor your blood sugars regularly during a course of steroids and contact your doctor if the readings are climbing much above usual levels. Steroids taken in the morning often only have the tendency to raise the blood sugar in the afternoon and evening, with a return to your usual level by the next morning, so this is an expected pattern. If you already take insulin, you will probably need to raise your insulin dosage to combat rising blood sugars. Your doctor or diabetes educator can give you a strategy to do this, using supplemental insulin and possibly increasing your usual set doses, also.

75. How can I manage my blood sugar during sports and exercise activities?

Sports and exercise can affect the blood sugar in various ways. The use of energy by the body during the exercise will have the tendency to lower the blood sugar, as might be expected. If the exercise is vigorous, stressful to the body, or competitive, the release of stress hormones may occur, which will actually serve to raise the blood sugar. Also, so-called "**isometric**" exercise (meaning that tensing or rigidity of the muscle against forceful resistance is involved, such as in weight-lifting) tends to raise the blood sugar more than "**isotonic**" exercise (such as repeated movement against minimal resistance, such as jogging, swimming,

Steroid-induced high blood sugars do not respond well to pills.

Isometric exercise

Tensing or rigidity of the muscle against forceful resistance, such as in weight-lifting.

Isotonic exercise

Repeated movement against minimal resistance, such as jogging, swimming, or dancing.

or dancing), which will generally tend to lower it. Finally, the management of the blood sugar in the aftermath of exercise, meaning from hours to as much as half a day later, may be as important and challenging as during the period of activity itself. This is because the replenishment of depleted glycogen (starch) into the muscle requires drainage of glucose from the bloodstream into the muscle as the building blocks for the starch.

Exactly how best to manage your blood sugar during and after exercise is somewhat unique to each individual and becomes clearer after you have performed the same activity several times. It helps to plan ahead for the calorie consumption that may occur during anything other than brief exercise. Taking additional calories prior to, and sometimes during, exercise is preferable to cutting or stopping your diabetes medication during or prior to exercise, although sometimes it can be beneficial to reduce the insulin dosage modestly when exercise is planned ahead. This planning is helped by knowledge of your blood sugar levels leading up to the exercise and sometimes during it and certainly after it. Finally, account for the replenishment of glycogen stores over the hours following significant exercise by eating a sustaining meal later in the day afterward. It is not unusual for the blood sugar to be significantly lower, occasionally seriously so, the morning after exercise the previous evening if this is not factored into meal consumption.

76. What preparations should I make for traveling?

Questions 73 and 77 address the traveling-related issues of changing time zones and avoidance of low blood sugars when driving an automobile. General preparation for traveling may include some of the following considerations. Remember to take your glucose testing equipment and your diabetes medications. Take an extra supply of test strips and medication to allow for travel delays and changes in plans. Remember that not all of the medications that are available to you in your home town will be available to you in other countries if you should run out. It is a good idea to take your testing equipment and medications in your carry-on baggage when traveling by air, as your check-in baggage may get misdirected or lost. Most security and airport screening authorities recognize diabetes testing paraphernalia and insulin pens and syringes in industrialized countries, but cannot be relied on to do so in all parts of the world. It may be prudent to bring a note with you in the local language, if you do not speak it, that explains to authorities what these items are. If you are traveling to an exotic locale, where you are not sure of the local cuisine and your tolerance of it or your ability to accurately carbohydrate-count it, you may want to take a supply of familiar nonperishable food items with you to fall back on until you familiarize yourself with the local food or can locate a source of items that you recognize. If your diabetes is brittle or you have significant chronic complications, you may want to ask your physician or CDE for names of some local diabetes care providers that they can recommend in case you need them. This is especially valuable and important for students going away to college, who are likely to initially experience unpredictable lifestyle and diet adjustments and who will be away for lengthy periods. The farther away you are traveling, the less likely it is that your doctor or CDE will be able to identify resources for you at your destination. In this case, you may have to do your own homework. For the United States and Canada, the American Diabetes Association (ADA) directory of professional members (for this, go to http://www. diabetes.org) contains the names of physician and non-physician professional members throughout the United States, Canada, and the world. You may be able to contact them prior to your departure. Other ADA travel recommendations can be viewed at http://www. diabetes.org/pre-diabetes/travel/when-you-travel.jsp.

77. How can I prevent myself from having a low sugar reaction while driving?

If you are on the type of diabetes medication that has a significant risk of causing a low blood sugar (for details of these, see Question 41), you should check your fingerstick glucose before driving. If your blood sugar is low, you should treat the low blood sugar much as you treat a low blood sugar reaction in general, for example, by eating a snack providing a readily available source of calories and then rechecking your blood sugar 20–30 minutes later. If you cannot delay your trip, take a snack and an ongoing source of sugar, such as Life Savers or other type of hard candy, that you can consume over time. You should make sure that you have a snack with readily available sugar in the car at all times. When driving, it is strongly recommended that you stop every 2 hours and check your blood sugar and eat your normally scheduled meals and snacks. Do not use your glucose meter while you are driving! You need to pull over and do the test while parked.

Remember that your vehicle is a very heavy object traveling at high speed and, when out of control even for only short periods, can be highly dangerous not only to you, but others around you. Also recall that other factors that contribute to inattention and loss of control can be additive to the danger of low blood sugar while driving. These include fatigue and lack of sleep, alcohol and other drugs (prescription or recreational), physical illness, and mental stress.

78. I have heard that wounds heal more slowly in people with diabetes. Is this true and should I be worried when I go in for an operation?

In patients whose diabetes is under good control and who do not have complications from it, wound healing is generally fairly normal, especially in younger people. On the other hand, when diabetes is poorly controlled and when it is accompanied by chronic complications, wound healing can be significantly impaired. The long-term complications of diabetes (see Questions 32, 33, and 34 for detailed discussion of these) occur due to damage to the very small blood vessels nourishing the tissues and organs of the body. The skin is one of these organs and, although skin disorders due to diabetes are not common, they can and do occur. The body's ability to heal a wound depends upon a healthy blood supply, which is needed to deliver nutrients, on the cells that provide the protective defense against infection and those that cause inflammation. In this sense, inflammation is beneficial in that it leads to the mopping up and removal of dead and damaged tissue, which paves the way for its replacement by new healthy healing skin and underlying tissue. Second, short-term high blood sugar paralyzes these blood and tissue defenses, so that their infection-fighting and inflammatory actions are much weaker. Finally, insulin itself stimulates healing and regenerative actions in body tissues. If the diabetes is poorly controlled, this suggests that insulin is insufficient or ineffective, which can further impair healing.

For these reasons, your doctor will try to help you get your diabetes under the best possible control before you go in for a nonemergency operation. If you have chronic complications of your diabetes, special attention should be paid to measures that will help your surgical wound to heal, such as ensuring adequate blood supply by keeping the area warm and not placing excessive pressure on it, and meticulous attention to the avoidance of infection. Your blood glucose will also be carefully controlled during the period immediately following surgery, with insulin if necessary.

79. My child has diabetes and is about to start school. What steps should I take and how will the school help to ensure that things go well?

Nowadays, diabetes alone seldom prevents children from attending and participating fully in school activities, although special attention is required in certain circumstances. Fortunately, most children at the age of school entry have, by virtue of their age, not had diabetes for very long. Therefore, they rarely have chronic complications and their glucose control is more straightforward. The American Diabetes Association and other authoritative bodies recommend less stringent control of blood sugar in young children in order to avoid hypoglycemia, which is the overriding concern.

In general, it is important to remember that each person, young or old, experiences diabetes differently. This is challenging and humbling for those of us who see people with diabetes every day. For your child's teachers, whose primary role is education unrelated to diabetes, it can be a major challenge indeed. Therefore, preparation is the key. It is important to provide the school with a daily plan describing the way your child's diabetes is managed, so they know what to expect as routine. It is important to inform the school how things may present themselves when they go wrong. How does your child's diabetes respond when he or she is under the weather, under stress, or following strenuous sports activities? What behavior does he or she show when low blood sugar occurs? All these things should be written down and put in a folder for your child's school nurse and teacher. A meeting with the teacher prior to your child entering their class will help to smooth the way. There is also a document, known as a 504 plan, which is used to describe the expectations and roles of the parents and the school in the management of the diabetes and when things go wrong. Further details are beyond the scope of this book, but excellent sources of information, including sample 504 plans, can be found at various websites including those of the Juvenile Diabetes Research Foundation (go to http://kids.jdrf.org/index.cfm and click on *Your Life With Diabetes* and then select *To School*), American Diabetes Association (http://www.diabetes.org/for-parents-and kids/for-schools/diabetes-management.jsp), and the National Institutes of Health (http://ndep.nih.gov/diabetes/youth/youth.htm).

PART EIGHT

Resources for People with Diabetes

I am interested in participating in research studies on new treatments for diabetes. How do I go about it?

How can I find and join a diabetes support group in my area?

How do I find out about the latest developments for treatment and monitoring of diabetes?

More . . .

80. Whom can I contact when I have questions about my diabetes?

First and foremost, you can contact your family physician, internist, and, if you have one, your endocrinologist or diabetologist. You can also contact your certified diabetes educator (CDE) nurse educator, dietitian, or pharmacist for questions in their respective fields. All American Association of Diabetes Educators (AADE) certified diabetes educators, regardless of their underlying professional credentials, should have at least some knowledge in all the major areas of diabetes management. You can contact your local American Diabetes Association (ADA) or Juvenile Diabetes Research Foundation (JDRF) chapter. Contact information for the regional chapters (state and/or city) can be obtained through the website of the respective parent organizations. For ADA, go to http://www.diabetes.org, choose *Community Events and Local Programs*, and then select *What's Happening Locally* and enter your zip code or city. For JDRF, go to http://www.jdrf.org and select *JDRF in My Area* and enter your state. Many regional chapters will have affiliated support-type groups for people with either type 1 or type 2 diabetes. It is not usually necessary to become a member in order to attend and participate in these. There are a number of diabetes-related magazines and newspapers, both paper and online, that are published by these organizations. It is usually necessary to become a lay member in order to receive a subscription to these. There are also online and paper magazines that are independent. This is a changing and dynamic environment and the best way to find out which are currently available is to enter the term *diabetes magazine* into your favorite Internet search engine. The ADA website (see previous mention) will provide you with a link to its publications, many of which are directed at people with diabetes, and include informative books on diet, nutrition, and medications, among others. Finally, your friends, colleagues, and relatives with diabetes can often be a great resource for local information and tips about managing your diabetes, although issues that fall into the realm of medical advice should only be provided by a licensed practitioner.

81. I am interested in participating in research studies on new treatments for diabetes. How do I go about it?

There are two main routes through which one can volunteer to participate in research studies involving diabetes. The first is to contact your local ADA or JDF affiliate, or their national website. Additionally, you can go to the http://www.clinicalresearch.gov and choose *Where Can I Find Clinical Trials?* where various links will direct you to a list of NIH-sponsored research projects in which you can participate. For clinical trials organized and sponsored by the pharmaceutical industry, you can go to http://www.clinicalconnection.com and select *Find Clinical Trials*, then enter *diabetes* as a keyword and enter your zip code.

Alternatively, you can contact your local medical center, teaching hospital, or university department of medicine, or your doctor, and ask for information on approved projects in the field of diabetes. Remember that clinical research studies must be approved by the local or central body that governs ethical conduct of such research, the Institutional Review Board or "IRB." Clinical research staff can only discuss projects that have already been approved by the IRB, with a view to recruiting you. Other studies, even though they may be planned or pending, can only be discussed in general terms and no steps, such as qualifying blood tests, can be made at this stage. If you provide the clinical research contact person with your contact information and written permission, he or she will contact you if a suitable project becomes approved and available for enrollment.

No matter how ready, willing, and able you are to participate, it may well be the case that a study that is specifically tailored to your type of diabetes or type of treatment may not be available. Do not be discouraged, nor feel that your volunteerism is not appreciated. Clinical research investigators and their staff are always delighted to know of potential participants in clinical research and will certainly contact you if any appropriate study arises. Also, be sure to mention your interest in research participation to your doctor as well anytime you are considering a specific project. He or she can discuss with you whether it is advisable for you to participate, given your individual health issues.

Clinical research investigators and their staff are always delighted to know of potential participants in clinical research and will certainly contact you if any appropriate study arises.

82. How can I find and join a diabetes support group in my area?

A number of approved diabetes education programs have affiliated support groups for both type 1 and type 2 diabetes. The American Diabetes Association approves diabetes education programs and keeps a record of their locations and contact information. At http://www.diabetes.org/communityprograms-and-localevents/whatslocal.jsp you will be connected to the ADA site called *What's Happening Locally?* On this site there is a link to ADA-recognized education programs and a link to a message board on which you can post a question about local support groups or other activities, or you can call your local ADA affiliate. The staff of your local diabetes center or clinic will also probably know contact information for their affiliated support groups. You may find that other people whom you know with diabetes are a good resource for this kind of information, although this is a somewhat hit-and-miss resource, as the majority of people with diabetes are not members of a support group. Your diabetes educator (or the diabetes educator your doctor generally refers to) is often involved in some way with the local support groups or will be aware of their existence and be able to provide you with contact information. If you are in a rural or isolated area, there may well be no local support group available. However, there is nothing to stop you from starting your own, if you have identified that there is a need for one!

83. I want to be an advocate for diabetes. Where should I start?

Advocacy for diabetes can have several meanings, from fundraising to raising public awareness in the media or political arena or working in the healthcare field with and on behalf of those with, or at risk for, diabetes. To assure your effectiveness as an advocate, bring your available experience, talents, and skills to the table and consider your commitment in time very carefully. Using your skills and experience will help to ensure that, when possible, you are doing on behalf of diabetes advocacy what you do successfully in your professional life and at which you are good. While it is not always possible to seamlessly blend your professional abilities with your work on behalf of diabetes, it is often possible to blend them quite well and this is true for those in all walks of life. It is a good idea to give very careful consideration to the time commitment that you are able to make and how you are able to make it. If you are available in blocks of time intermittently, this might suit you for commitment to support individual events, whereas if you are available more or less continuously, you could take up a more permanent position in an organization. Do remember that, even though your commitment may be as a volunteer, the success of others around you may still depend on the performance of your assigned responsibility. Therefore, a smaller commitment in time that you can realistically and consistently provide is likely to be of more value than a commitment that you may not be able to fulfill reliably. It is also less likely to place a burden of stress upon your work and personal life and upon those around you and will, in the long run, be more sustainable and rewarding for you and for the cause you are supporting.

Advocacy can be done on an individual level, but is often more effective when combined with the efforts and energies of others.

Advocacy can be done on an individual level, but is often more effective when combined with the efforts and energies of others, especially as part of an established organization that has a track record of success in moving the cause of diabetes advocacy forward. Therefore, contacting your local chapter of such an organization is often a good place to start. Which organization you choose will depend on where your personal interest in the issue lies. You might be particularly interested in type 1 or type 2 diabetes, adults or children, prevention or cure, individual complications, availability of medications to those who need them, or pregnancy and healthcare coverage, just to name a few possibilities. The American Diabetes Association (http://www.diabetes.org) and the Juvenile Diabetes Foundation International (http://www.jdrf.org) are key organizations. Introduction through a friend who is already engaged in advocacy can often help to get you where you need to go, but almost always staff will welcome your interest and direct you to the right place.

84. Are there exercise programs for patients with diabetes covered by insurance or that are tax deductible?

Yes, although those that are tax deductible are not specifically aimed at diabetes and they are not government programs in themselves. Recently, in order to help to combat the growing amount of obesity and lack of exercise that now put Americans at risk of a number of diseases, including diabetes, the U.S. government has made provisions for a tax deduction on personal federal income tax for weight reduction programs when this is performed for specific medical indications. Losing a few pounds for your upcoming high school reunion (i.e., for your general appearance and overall health) is not included! Also, general gym or spa membership dues are not allowed under this credit. Although the program is specifically for weight reduction, exercise is an important component of weight maintenance and aids in weight reduction and is therefore included. The actual conditions of the program are contained in Internal Revenue Service (IRS) publication #502 that can be accessed at http://www.hsainsider.com/pdf/treasurypublications/TreasuryPub_23.pdf. Please see the information on pages 13 and 15 of this publication. It provides considerable detail on what is eligible for tax credit. This is a tax credit rather than a tax deduction, the important difference being that the entire cost of the program can be paid from your taxes. A very nice guide on how to actually prepare a submission to the IRS for the tax credit can be found at http://ezinearticles.com/?I.R.S.-Tax-Credit-for-Weight-Loss-and-Smoke-Cessation-Programs&id=345917. Of course, commonsense rules apply. The cost of a program of twice-weekly treadmill workouts or spinning sessions as part of a class at your local spa or health club is likely to be found to be acceptable, while the cost of membership in a darts or pool league at your favorite local bar is not. Whether the exercise involved can reasonably be expected to lead to weight loss or improved physical fitness is the issue that can determine its eligibility for a tax deduction. However, the IRS will not ask you to prove that you actually lost weight or expect you to produce copies of your split times on the stopwatch at your local track! In addition to the information available from the IRS link noted above, you can also get information from your qualified tax preparer.

Some health insurance programs will, with supporting documentation from your doctor, cover the costs of certain approved exercise or fitness interventions for certain categories of members. Details of these can be obtained from the administrator of your company health plan or from the healthcare provider staff themselves. There is also increasing awareness among employers that a healthy, physically active staff is a more productive staff who require fewer days off work for health-related reasons. Such enlightened employers sometimes provide incentives for their staff to join local healthcare facilities and occasionally provide such facilities themselves. They may sponsor some employees to participate in competitive athletic events or activities, sometimes to a high level of accomplishment. Programs such as this will be unique to each company and you will need to make inquiries about them from your human resources department.

There is also increasing awareness among employers that a healthy, physically active staff is a more productive staff who require fewer days off work for health-related reasons.

85. How do I access resources for people with diabetes from different cultures or creeds or who do not speak English?

Diabetes disproportionately affects those in our society who are non-Caucasian minorities and often it is harder to ensure that high quality care is provided. For example, only half as many Hispanic Americans with diabetes are currently achieving treatment goals for diabetes set by the American Diabetes Association as are achieved by Caucasian Americans. In some cases the reasons are cultural, in others economic, and in other cases they result from language and communication barriers. There is increasing interest in providing tools and resources to overcome these barriers and rectify these disparities. Many guides and booklets, such as diabetic recipe books, are also published in Spanish and other common languages. A number of diabetic cookbooks are available for different types of cuisine. Your local medical center will often provide translation services for visits with the doctor, nurse educator, or dietitian. These professionals often have materials in different languages to give you. Your local chapter of the American Diabetes Association or Juvenile Diabetes Foundation is generally a good place to start, as they often respond with commitment and energy to support the needs of particular groups who are represented in their local area. The website http://www. lacountyparks.org/cms1_033139.pdf also provides a listing of diabetes resources available for non-English-speaking people, while the Joslin Diabetes Center offers an innovative Chinese-English diabetes website at http://aadi.joslin.harvard.edu/.

Pharmaceutical representatives often provide tremendous support to the efforts of healthcare professionals in identifying resources to improve patients' access to care. Their commitment to patient care frequently extends beyond ensuring the availability of their companies' medications and they will usually go to great lengths to obtain helpful information. If you are taking a particular branded medication, it is not unreasonable to suggest to your doctor or diabetes educator that the representative of that company might help to find the information or resources that you need. They are often very happy to do so upon request.

86. How do I find out about the latest developments for treatment and monitoring of diabetes?

There are a number of resources that are available to inform people with diabetes and others who are interested about diabetes and the latest developments in treatment. These range from published magazines, periodicals, and newsletters to online e-zines and updates. It is important to ensure that the source of information is well informed and reliable. Therefore, it is advisable to start with a nationally or internationally recognized and respected organization. For diabetes in the United States, these include the American Diabetes Association (http://www.diabetes.org), the Juvenile Diabetes Foundation, and the International Diabetes Federation (IDF). Their websites all show links to helpful information on a variety of subjects. Each puts out publications for the lay person, such as *Diabetes Forecast* (ADA) and *Countdown* (JDRF). There are also a number of high quality independent newsletters, including *Diabetes-in-Control, DDN On Line, Diabetic LivingOnLine*, and *Diabetes Digest*. A listing of online diabetes publications for those with diabetes can be found at http://www.diabetesmonitor.com/journals.htm.

The local chapter of the ADA and JDF will be able to direct you to resources unique to your area. Their contact information can usually be found within the website of the parent national organization. Your local hospital, clinic, or doctor's office will generally have, or have access to, a diabetes education program, staffed by certified diabetes educators who are usually nurse practitioners, nurses, pharmacists, or registered dietitians. As a rule, CDEs are well informed on recent developments and on how to find out more about them and are happy to provide this information.

87. Where can I find out about interactive programs and games that make learning about diabetes fun for children and teenagers?

The American Diabetes Association recently unveiled a new interactive learning feature for young people with diabetes, which can be accessed at http://www. diabetes.org/for-parents-and-kids/resources.jsp and then by clicking on the link to *Youth Zone Games*. These are interactive short programs that hold children's attention by responding with an outcome to a specific set of choices relating to health and diabetes.

Pharmaceutical companies often provide educational resources. An example of a new interactive program for diabetes education is now offered by Merck Inc. It is called *Journey For Control* and uses a system of Conversation Maps for interactive education and decision making. The program and a video describing the conversation maps can be accessed at http://www. journeyforcontrol.com and then clicking on the link to the *Conversation Map Program*.

If sufficient resources were to be invested, very sophisticated interactive video games could be developed that could combine an educational message with a genuinely interesting and exciting adventure activity. However, since these types of programs are very expensive and unlikely to recoup their costs commercially, they will probably remain relatively short and simple until costs come down.

88. I am interested in a professional career in the field of diabetes. Where can I find out the various options and the prerequisites to apply?

Opportunities for a career in diabetes can be as diverse as the opportunities to be an advocate for diabetes (see Question 83), a caregiver in the diabetes medical field, or to work in the field of developing new technologies for diabetes care. However, building a career around your commitment to diabetes is complex, since you will almost certainly want and need to be paid for your work. Careers requiring higher professional qualifications, such as adult pediatric endocrinologists or diabetologists, physicians specializing in diabetic eye, kidney, or nerve diseases, diabetes nurse educators, and dietitians, generally require several years of planning and preparation to achieve and require a great deal of commitment due to the many demands placed upon them. Sometimes a person not previously involved in diabetes care may have skills, knowledge, or credentials that can be adapted to the field of diabetes, such as dietitians or nurses, who can take additional training, even in the middle of their careers, and specialize in the area of diabetes care. The same is true of qualified and experienced laboratory research professionals, who will use many of the same skills in the field of diabetes research that they used in other areas of medical or pharmaceutical research.

There are many other ways to develop a career committed to diabetes. Most medical institutions and industry or university research or clinical care organizations require the same administrative and technical support staff to ensure smooth and successful operations that other business organizations do. Even if you are working behind the scenes and do not have a job that allows direct interaction with patients or medical care, doing a job that helps to ensure smooth and successful running of an organization is a very important part of ensuring the overall success of the patient-related efforts. Therefore, it is recommended that you bring your skills to the table and contact organizations that you know are involved in some way with clinical care, education, research, or advocacy for diabetes and ask if they have openings for somebody with your skills. Be assured that sooner or later, doors will open!

89. What educational programs for diabetes are covered by Medicare and other governmental and private insurance plans? Who qualifies?

Medicare covers the cost of group diabetes education for eligible people with diabetes who fulfill certain criteria. Examples of these include people with newly diagnosed diabetes, poorly controlled diabetes, or the need to change from pills to insulin. Presently, Medicare will support up to 8 hours of diabetes, education performed in a center that is recognized as qualified. This means that their educational programs must be certified as meeting the required standard by the American Diabetes Association. A further hour of follow-up education can be provided in the first year to determine the success of the program. Unfortunately, most state medical care programs do not provide significant support for diabetes education, but provide a limited selection of medications and some support materials, such as a particular type of glucose testing meter.

Upon request, most private insurance providers will cover diabetes education upon the same, or similar, conditions. Also, most insurance companies will cover the cost of individual diabetes education by a certified diabetes educator. This includes dietary instruction, use of glucose meters, giving insulin injections, etc. As each healthcare plan varies, specific information on who qualifies is not realistic here, but it is recommended that you contact your healthcare plan to find out more details.

PART NINE

When a Family Member or Loved One Has Diabetes

What should a parent, spouse, partner, or caregiver know about diabetes in order to provide support to a loved one?

My child has diabetes. What can I do when he or she is sick to help prevent the diabetes from going out of control?

My spouse/partner has diabetes and we are planning a family. What is the risk that our children will develop diabetes?

More . . .

90. My partner/child/parent does not follow his or her doctor's advice on management of his or her diabetes. How can I help to improve things?

This is a very difficult question and is one that can be extended beyond diabetes to many aspects of a loved one's life where their behavior is apparently either endangering themselves or likely to lead to short- or long-term negative consequences. Sometimes it can be immensely frustrating for a caring parent/partner/friend or relative to experience lack of commitment to good healthcare practices on the part of someone they care about. Moreover, the knowledge that much of the burden of the consequences may fall on others can lead to anger and resentment.

There is no easy answer that can be applied universally, as everyone is different and their circumstances are unique. It is important to remember that, except in the case of a minor child, you must yield the control of the problem to the person who has it. For example, your spouse/partner owns his or her diabetes and must be empowered (except in very special circumstances) to make his or her own decisions on how to manage it. He or she is more likely to take advice if it is sought out than if it is given uninvited. They are likely to believe that they are giving as much attention to their diabetes as possible, whether or not it seems obvious to others that this is not the case. Frequent pressure to do more may engender a sense of failure and actually lead to doing less. Motivation through fear is generally not successful unless the object to be feared is immediately present. People with diabetes generally do not see or feel the consequences of the neglect of their diabetes on a day-to-day basis. When they finally do, it is too late to reverse them. For example, if you get too near the log fire in your living room, soon you realize that you do not want to get closer but should move away. There is no such warning before touching a hot iron or a burner on the stove. Thus, household cooktop and iron burns are much more common than burns from touching the blazing logs in the fireplace!

Perhaps the best that one can do is to help to ensure that our loved ones have access to high quality education about diabetes and its consequences, ensure that they are given the tools to do what is needed to take care of it, and to support them in that effort to the extent that they are willing to participate. After that, their autonomy must be respected, even though it may have some negative consequences for others. It is important to remember that you are not obliged to join your loved one in dangerous or destructive behaviors nor must you unquestioningly accept the consequences. Whether you choose to do so will depend on several factors, including your personal belief system.

> *It is important to remember that you are not obliged to join your loved one in dangerous or destructive behaviors nor must you unquestioningly accept the consequences.*

91. What should a parent, spouse, partner, or caregiver know about diabetes in order to provide support to a loved one?

The more informed a spouse, partner, or caregiver is about diabetes, the better source of support he or she can be to the affected person in their lives. Thus, the answer can be very open-ended. To be practical, let us focus on a few key issues that are especially important. If you are the main food preparer for the loved one in question, knowledge of diabetic diets and nutrition is very helpful (see Question 40 for more information). The appropriate type of diet for a person with diabetes is generally not complex, time-consuming, or expensive. Attending diabetes education with your loved one's dietitian is probably the most useful and important thing you can do. Getting to know as much as you can about diabetic meal preparation is very important, especially when there may be special requirements relating to kidney complications (nephropathy—see Question 34) or high blood pressure.

Knowing how to treat a low blood sugar reaction, whether moderate or severe, is very valuable. The mental alertness and coordination of the person with diabetes can be impaired with moderately severe low blood sugar reactions and he or she may not have insight into what is going on or how to treat it. In the case of severe low blood sugar, reactions, the affected loved one may be drowsy or unconscious and prompt action on your part is very important. Knowing how to check the blood sugar with their machine and how to treat a moderate low blood sugar, or how to use a glucagon kit to treat a severe low blood sugar, is very helpful indeed. This is addressed in detail in Question 92.

Finally, knowledge of how to manage sick days is very helpful. The body's response to illness can be somewhat unpredictable. In the case of an infection such as gastroenteritis or influenza, blood sugars may be high or low, depending on whether the body's stress reaction pushes the blood sugar higher or the failure to eat pushes it lower. Either way, during anything other than a minor illness, it is important to monitor the blood sugar frequently, and treat low or high sugars (the latter with insulin if necessary) and to ensure that your loved one is well hydrated, as dehydration will rapidly make the situation worse. Most important is to know when you are unable to keep pace, meaning that the blood sugar is rising in spite of your best efforts and your loved one is unable to take in fluids or is becoming drowsy. In this case, ensuring that he or she gets prompt medical attention is the most valuable thing you can do.

There are, of course, many other ways in which you can help by your knowledge of diabetes, but these are three of the most important.

92. How do I know when my relative with diabetes is having a low blood sugar reaction? What should I do to help?

The signs of a low blood sugar reaction can range from fairly obvious to quite subtle and hard to detect. The very young and the elderly are less likely to spontaneously complain of symptoms, but more often just slip into hypoglycemia. Those who have had diabetes for a long time, generally more than 10 years, may lose their ability to perceive hypoglycemia and fail to make complaints or take action to prevent seriously low blood sugar from occurring. This is much more common in longstanding type 1 diabetes than it is in type 2 diabetes. Those who are aware that something is wrong and who are able to voice their concerns will complain of a combination of hunger, headache, shakiness, sweating, palpitations (a sensation of fluttering in the chest), blurred vision, and inability to think straight or coordinate their actions, especially fine motor actions such as writing, typing, or dialing phone numbers. The very young, the elderly, or those with unawareness of low blood sugar will often exhibit confusion or bizarre behavior, shakiness, sweating, drowsiness, or restlessness in the earlier stages. Bizarre behavior can take many forms, from inappropriate laughing or crying, aggression, staring blankly, to making repetitive movements or inappropriate verbal responses to questions. Most people with diabetes will have their own individual pattern of behavior that tends to repeat itself each time their blood sugar is low. Therefore, familiarity is very helpful for recognition of low blood sugar in loved ones or colleagues.

If the low blood sugar is severe, loss of consciousness and seizures will occur. This is of course very worrisome to the observer and necessitates prompt action. Loss of consciousness can result from both very high and very low blood sugar. It comes on much more rapidly with low blood sugar than with high blood sugar and is usually more rapidly reversible if treated promptly and effectively. However, unless the circumstances unmistakably indicate high blood sugar, or a fingerstick glucose reading is available, the safest treatment is to administer sugar or glucose or use a glucagon injection kit. Additional glucose is unlikely to worsen in the short term the already serious situation of a coma due to high blood sugar, but could be lifesaving to a person with coma due to a very low blood sugar. Therefore, when in doubt, glucose or household sugar administration is the best route to take. Fortunately, the body has powerful mechanisms to prevent the blood sugar from becoming fatally low and these are generally intact in those with diabetes. For this reason, severely low blood sugar, while it is an emergency, is seldom fatal, considering how often it occurs.

93. My child has diabetes. What can I do when he or she is sick to help prevent the diabetes from going out of control?

Certain forms of illness are more likely to throw the diabetes out of control than others. Generally, those illnesses that provide quite intense stress to the body are more likely to cause the diabetes to go out of control than those that result in disability without general body stress. Illnesses associated with fever, infection, rapid heart rate, loss of appetite, and disordered bodily functions such as diarrhea, vomiting, breathlessness, etc. are often associated with loss of glucose control. It is important to remember that when a child is not eating due to a generalized illness, he or she may require as much or more insulin than he would take with a meal if he were eating. This is often very surprising to people with diabetes and their caregivers. When the body is under stress, it produces a variety of hormones that serve to counteract the stress, in part by raising the blood sugar. In those without diabetes, this response is generally beneficial. However, in those with diabetes it can be counterproductive. Therefore, the key to helping the sick child with diabetes from losing glucose control is to check the blood sugar frequently, such as every 2 hours, and to administer insulin according to the blood sugar level if the blood sugar level continues to rise and without regard to the intake of food. More insulin will be needed if the child is able to eat. Dehydration is a key contributor to worsening high blood sugar and therefore every attempt should be made to keep hydration up, with fluids that are not high in sugar (avoiding colas or juices, for example) as long as the blood sugar is high. Fluids that contain electrolytes, such as Pedialyte® or a similar product, are preferable to water alone in preventing dehydration. Remedies to reduce the severity of the illness, or the symptoms from it, can also help to keep glucose levels under control, such as sponging or antifever medications to lower a high temperature, antinauseants, or antidiarrheals to reduce intestinal disturbances. Reducing or minimizing psychological stress can also play a significant part, so this would not be the time to emphasize the homework that is not getting done or the test that might be missed!

It is important to remember that some illnesses are severe enough that they will throw the diabetes out of control in spite of a parent's best efforts to do everything to prevent it. Therefore, if the blood sugar is climbing in spite of frequent testing and administration of additional insulin or if is clear that dehydration is occurring, professional help should be sought without any sense of guilt or failure.

94. Can my child with diabetes participate in all sports in school or are there some that he or she should avoid?

If your child has type 2 diabetes, which is now not uncommon in children and has recently become more common in adolescent girls than type 1 diabetes, then participation in school sports is an excellent idea, as it will help to control weight and reverse insulin resistance. The only caveat would be concerning his or her medication and how it would be affected by exercise. Most children with type 2 diabetes do not require insulin, but some do take sulfonylureas (see Questions 41 and 52 for more details). Both of these therapies can cause low blood sugar in the face of energetic exercise, especially if prolonged. Therefore, the glucose should be checked prior to significant exercise and periodically during the exercise if greater than an hour or two at a stretch. If the glucose is well controlled before exercise, it is a good idea to provide calories prior to and sometimes during the event, in an amount designed to be readily available and commensurate with the amount of energy consumed during the sporting event. Your CDE can help with planning of calorie intake prior to, during, and after sporting events.

If your child has type 1 diabetes, the issues noted above also apply, but tend to be more critical, since children with type 1 diabetes are generally more susceptible to low glucose during physical activity and are on insulin therapy. Interestingly, competitive sports may actually result in increased glucose levels, even though the same amount, or more, of energy is expended as in non-competitive sports. This is because the levels of a number of hormones are raised in the heat of competition and these hormones tend to increase blood sugar levels. This is further discussed in Question 75.

95. My spouse/partner has diabetes and we are planning a family. What is the risk that our children will develop diabetes?

This depends on whether your spouse/partner has type 1 or type 2 diabetes. In the case of type 1 diabetes, in general the risk of type 1 diabetes is 10 times as great in a first-degree relative compared to the risk in the population at large. A first-degree relative is your parent, sibling, or child. The general population risk of type 1 diabetes is about one-third to one-half of 1%, i.e., about 1 in 200 to 250 people. In a first-degree relative of someone with type 1 diabetes, this increases to about 1 in 20 to 25 people or about a 4% or 5% chance. Most people consider that this is not a sufficiently high risk to deter them from having a family, but that is of course a personal and individual decision. The likelihood of developing type 1 diabetes declines with age, about 90% of cases being diagnosed younger than age 35.

In the case of type 2 diabetes, the risk is considerably higher and a general rule is that if both parents have type 2 diabetes, about two out of three of their children will develop it. If one parent has type 2 diabetes, about one out of three of their children will be affected. Decision making using these rough estimates is difficult. Most people destined to develop type 2 diabetes will not do so in their child-bearing years. Therefore, it is not really possible to estimate risk to the future children when it is as yet unknown whether the parents will get diabetes. Although type 2 diabetes is a highly inherited disorder, the risk of developing it can be very powerfully changed by an individual's lifestyle. Even people with a high hereditary risk may not get type 2 diabetes if they maintain a healthy weight and exercise regularly. However, if your spouse/partner has type 2 diabetes, you can factor in your own parents' health history in the risk to your future children. If either of your parents has type 2 diabetes, this increases the risk to your child to more than one in three. Of course, in contrast to type 1 diabetes, type 2 diabetes tends to develop later in life, so children at risk are still most likely to have a healthy childhood and diabetes-free youth.

PART TEN

What Does the Future Hold for People with Diabetes?

What is the likelihood of a cure for type 2 diabetes?
What form will it take and when will it be available?

When and how will we be able to prevent
type 1 diabetes?

How can we stop the dramatic increase in diabetes
presently occurring throughout the world?

More . . .

96. What is the likelihood of a cure for type 1 diabetes? What form will it take and when will it be available?

A true cure is likely to be some years off. Although pancreas transplants and islet transplants can lead to independence from insulin treatment and have resulted in dramatic improvement in quality of life for some, they remain a limited proposition for most, in view of the need for risky and expensive antirejection drugs and the late failure that tends to occur. In addition, donor tissues are in short supply. Manipulation of stem cells (early forms of cells that have the potential to develop into an array of different cell types) into pancreatic islet cells that produce insulin has a great deal of potential, but there are a number of operational issues that need to be addressed before this will become an accepted clinical therapy.

Even in a person with established type 1 diabetes, the use of an efficient closed-loop pump system would revolutionize management of the diabetes. Closed-loop means that detecting the blood glucose level and responding to it by injecting the right amount of insulin are both handled by the pump automatically, without the need for decision-making input from the patient. While this is actually more of a management tool than a cure, it would so effectively relieve the patient of the burden of their diabetes that it is for practical purposes almost as good. A number of companies are, as you might expect, actively working on this approach.

Since type 1 diabetes is an immunologic disorder, effective cure may result from manipulation of the immune system, especially if performed early in the course of the disease. An immunologic disorder in this case means one in which a person's own immune system attacks his or her tissues in error. Type 1 diabetes results from an attack of the immune system on the insulin-producing cells of the pancreas, ultimately destroying most of them. Therapies aimed at slowing, halting, or reversing this attack are currently in clinical trials. They are limited by the fact that the diabetes needs to be in an early stage for the treatment to be effective, that manipulating the immune system can cause a number of undesirable side effects, and that it tends to be a lengthy and complicated form of treatment, requiring admission to the hospital.

The latter approach in some form or another is likely to offer the best chance of cure for type 1 diabetes, as it addresses the root cause. Although the fact that clinical trials are ongoing is certainly encouraging, this option remains some way off.

While type 1 diabetes is a lifelong disorder that requires continuous attention and work by those affected, it is important to keep in mind that any cure must be safer and more effective than currently available treatments, which are continually improving and already allow the majority of people with type 1 diabetes to lead healthy and productive lives with few limitations.

97. What is the likelihood of a cure for type 2 diabetes? What form will it take and when will it be available?

The likelihood of a cure for type 2 diabetes arising from a single drug or therapy is quite small. Many factors are involved in the development of the disorder and it can almost be considered to arise from the body being under a generalized form of environmental and genetic stress—the stress being, in this case, the environmental stress of being overweight, lacking exercise, and other less well-recognized and understood factors. Most type 2 diabetes are predicated to some degree or another on being overweight (although this varies considerably from ethnic group to ethnic group) and therefore a medication or intervention that reverses or prevents obesity and overweight would be expected to have the additional benefit of preventing or curing type 2 diabetes. Indeed this has been conclusively shown to be true for bariatric surgery, which is a type of surgical operation that leads to weight reduction by either restricting the intake of food into the intestine, or leading to it being poorly absorbed from the intestine. Certain types of bariatric surgical procedures may lead to up to 90% reversal (we do not yet use the word *cure* here) of established type 2 diabetes and effective prevention of progression from prediabetes to frank diabetes. Surgical intervention of this kind is at present reserved for those at highest risk and is not feasible for everyone. There are some risks due to complications of the procedures themselves. Fortunately these are quite uncommon. There are also some subsequent side effects, such as a risk of inadequate balanced nutrition or vitamin deficiency with the bypass type of procedure as well as low blood sugar and diarrhea. However, this means of achieving effective weight loss can prevent or cure type 2 diabetes and a medication that leads to safe, durable, and effective weight reduction could achieve the same result. Possibly environmental adjustment on a social level to promote healthier lifestyles may achieve similar benefits for society as a whole, but this is notoriously difficult!

98. When and how will we be able to prevent type 1 diabetes?

There are a number of approaches that might reasonably lead to the prevention of type 1 diabetes in the foreseeable future. Although hereditary factors are involved in a person's risk of getting type 1 diabetes, it is clear that there is an important trigger in the environment. For example, if one of a pair of identical twins has type 1 diabetes, the chance of the other twin getting the disease is smaller than 50%. Definite identification of a major risk factor (such as an infectious agent, nutrient, or other chemical) could lead to effective protection against exposure or immunization against it. Whatever the trigger may be, the process that ultimately leads to type 1 diabetes is caused by the body's immune system, which activates a destructive attack on the insulin-producing cells of the pancreas. There are a number of ways in which this destructive process can be slowed or suppressed. Earlier efforts were either ineffective or led to a general suppression of the body's immune system, increasing the risk of infections. However, clinical trials of drugs that specifically target the self-destructive process in the pancreas are presently underway. These treatments require prolonged administration into the blood vessels over several days and often have unpleasant side effects. Also, to be truly preventive, they must be given when early evidence of future diabetes is discovered, but before the actual onset of diabetes, by which time intense and often irreversible destruction of the insulin-producing cells has already occurred. It is probable that it will be several years before any of these drugs is readily available. There is a great deal of investigation currently ongoing into the development of stem cells for use as replacements for lost insulin-producing cells. Stem cells are a small proportion of cells in tissues and organs that have not yet developed into final form. As such, when treated in a certain way, they can be persuaded to commit themselves to developing into one specific desired type of cell. There are a lot of questions remaining to be answered regarding the safety, effectiveness, and durability of stem cell treatments and there remains the issue that the immune system problem that destroyed the original insulin-producing cells might also destroy their replacements. However, clinical trials are underway in other diseases which, if successful, could accelerate interest in the use of stem cells for type 1 diabetes.

99. When and how will we be able to prevent type 2 diabetes?

The prevention of type 2 diabetes in global terms depends upon the prevention of overweight and obesity and the performance of healthy amounts of exercise. These two factors are responsible for the overwhelming majority of cases of type 2 diabetes in the world today, especially those in younger people. However, it is not clear that this can be achieved by individual education. Most adults who are overweight are aware that they overeat and take insufficient exercise, yet few are able to address these issues successfully in a long-term way. This is not because they are lazy or weak-minded, but because humans, and other species, have been conditioned throughout their evolution to defend themselves against starvation and backbreaking labor, both of which are injurious to survival. It is not surprising therefore that strong drives exist within us to take in as much food energy as we can to protect us against impending famine, and to seek a life of ease to protect us from injury and environmental exposure. It is only within the past century or two that sufficient food to lead to overweight has been available year-round for all but a fortunate few. Not surprisingly, therefore, human conditioning has not yet been able to adjust to this very recent change.

It is likely that significant reductions in weight and increases in exercise will come from social changes that build these into our environment and lifestyles. Some of these are already beginning to occur. Many states and school districts are increasing the amount of exercise in the core school curriculum and removing ready access to snacks and sweetened beverages on campus. Urban planners are considering new ways to make walking to school, work, and local shops appealing and limiting the access of automobiles to the inner city. Restaurant chains are attempting, with some success, to offer alternatives to calorie-dense high fat food items. It is important than such alternatives are appealing in taste and satisfying to hunger, or they will not be chosen.

Of course, modern medicine has a role to play in the prevention of type 2 diabetes, by developing safe and effective medications to suppress appetite or prevent weight gain. Also, drugs that can be taken by people at high risk to prevent early abnormalities in blood sugar from developing into full-blown diabetes will be valuable. However, since type 2 diabetes is largely a disease of the industrialized urban world, the healthiest and most generally effective way to prevent it will be to make the environment of the future less conducive to those habits that lead to its occurrence.

100. How can we stop the dramatic increase in diabetes presently occurring throughout the world?

Although both type 1 and type 2 diabetes are increasing in frequency throughout the world, it is type 2 diabetes that has shown the explosive rise in occurrence in the past couple of decades. Since this rise is most clearly associated with weight gain and lack of exercise brought on by our current lifestyle, this trend will probably only be stopped, or reversed, by addressing these two factors, as discussed in Question 99. While individual counseling and education are worthwhile and effective in some cases, a broader approach will be necessary to impact favorably upon weight and exercise in population terms. Interventions such as increasing the amount of exercise in the core school curriculum, provision of healthy school meals, and improved policies on the access of snack food vendors to school premises are among measures that are already taking hold and will hopefully have a favorable impact on our youth. The engineering of the workplace and social areas to encourage physical activity, such as removing automobile access to the inner city, providing convenient and pleasant walkways and bicycle paths through frequently traveled areas of town, and probably financial disincentives from excessive automobile use should help to mobilize us. Countries with emerging economies are particularly affected by the switch to urban industrialized living, in terms of rising numbers of people with diabetes, yet they have perhaps the best opportunity to effect change. They are in the planning and growth stages and can make social and environmental decisions to improve the future before diabetes becomes an overwhelming problem.

While individual counseling and education are worthwhile and effective in some cases, a broader approach will be necessary to impact favorably upon weight and exercise in population terms.

Glossary

Antidiuretic hormone (ADH): A hormone that is responsible for maintaining the normal volume and concentration of our urine. Also called arginine vasopressin (AVP).

Arginine vasopressin (AVP): A hormone that is responsible for maintaining the normal volume and concentration of our urine. Also called antidiuretic hormone (ADH).

Asymptomatic: Having no complaints or symptoms.

Autoantibody: An antibody that an organism produces against any of its own tissues or cells.

Autoimmunity: A predisposition to produce autoantibodies.

Bariatric surgery: Weight loss surgery.

Basal insulin: The insulin required to control your blood sugar in the absence of food intake.

Beta cells: The insulin-producing cells of the pancreas.

Body mass index (BMI): A clinical means of relating weight to height by a formula. To calculate your own BMI, divide your weight in pounds by the square of your height in inches (i.e., your height multiplied by itself) and then multiply the answer by 703.

Bolus insulin: The insulin required to remove the energy derived from a meal from the bloodstream and into the tissues to replenish energy stores. Bolus insulin can also be given when the blood sugar is too high.

Borderline diabetes: A condition in which plasma glucose falls in-between normal and standard accepted definitions for diabetes. "Prediabetes" is another term commonly used for the same condition.

Calorie: A unit used to express heat or energy value of food.

Carbohydrates: Substances composed of long chains of oxygen, hydrogen, and carbon molecules. Carbohydrates in food (for example, sugar and starch) provide energy for the body and, if present in excess, are stored as fat.

Cataracts: Opacity of the lens of the eye.

Cholesterol: A fatty substance normally present in blood.

Counterregulatory hormones: Naturally occurring hormones that prepare the body to combat stress.

Decompensation: A serious deterioration in a medical condition.

Deficiency: A lack or shortage, especially of something essential to health.

Diabetes insipidus: Increased urine production caused by inadequate secretion of vasopressin by the pituitary gland or by resistance of the kidney to its actions.

Diabetes mellitus: A condition characterized by inadequate production of insulin or resistance of the body's tissues to its actions, which results in excessive levels of glucose in the blood.

Dyslipidemia: Cholesterol and other blood fat abnormalities.

Fasting: Abstaining from eating food, usually for nine hours or more.

Fiber: The structural part of plants and plant products that consists of carbohydrates that are wholly or partially indigestible.

Fructose: A simple sugar found in honey, many fruits, and some vegetables.

Gestational diabetes mellitus (GDM): Diabetes detected in pregnancy.

Glaucoma: Increased pressure inside the eye.

Glucose: A basic sugar used to fuel body cells.

Glycogen: Starch, which comprises sugars linked together in a storage pattern.

HDL: High-density lipoprotein; "good cholesterol."

Hemodialysis: Blood filtering and removal of wastes through a machine.

Hyperglycemia: An abnormally high level of glucose in the blood; secondary symptoms include frequent urination and thirst.

Hypertension: High blood pressure.

Hypoglycemia: An abnormally low level of glucose in the blood; symptoms include shakiness, sweatiness, hunger, abdominal discomfort, palpitations, and confusion.

Immune system: The body's system that protects it from foreign substances, cells, and tissues. The immune system includes the thymus, spleen, lymph nodes, lymphocytes, B-cells and T-cells, and antibodies.

Immunization: The process of inducing immunity, usually through inoculation or vaccination.

Inflammation: Swelling, pain, tenderness, and disturbed function in an area of the body, usually as a result of injury.

Insulin: A hormone produced by the beta cells of the pancreas, which facilitates the entry of glucose and other substances into cells and which has several other functions.

Intravenously: Through a vein.

Islet tissue: Groups of cells found within the pancreas that produce and release insulin, glucagons, and other substances.

Isometric exercise: Tensing or rigidity of the muscle against forceful resistance, such as in weight-lifting.

Isotonic exercise: Repeated movement against minimal resistance, such as jogging, swimming, or dancing.

Libido: Sexual interest.

Lipohypertrophy: A painless, but potentially disfiguring, fatty mound.

Nephropathy: Kidney damage.

Neuropathy: Nerve damage.

Osteomyelitis: Infection in the bone.

Pancreas: A gland deep in the abdomen, behind the stomach, that produces hormones (insulin, glucagon) and digestive enzymes.

Peripheral nerve: A nerve cell not contained in the brain or spinal column.

Peripheral vascular disease: Diseases of the vessels in the limbs.

Peritoneal dialysis: A process whereby wastes are exchanged into fluids introduced into the abdominal cavity.

Prediabetes: A condition in which abnormalities in plasma glucose levels lie in-between normal and standard accepted definitions of diabetes.

"Borderline diabetes," "impaired fasting glucose," and "impaired glucose tolerance" are other terms used to describe types of this condition.

Protective sensation: The perception of potential injury, such as awareness of sharp, rough, excessively hot or cold objects, or friction.

Remission: A temporary or permanent decrease of manifestations of a disease.

Retina: The inner lining of the eye.

Retinopathy: Eye damage.

Septicemia: Blood poisoning, due to infection, which is usually bacterial in origin.

Type 1 diabetes: Characterized by an almost complete deficiency of insulin due to the immune system erroneously attacking and destroying the insulin-producing cells in the pancreas.

Type 2 diabetes: Caused by a combination of body tissues becoming resistant to the action of insulin and the inability of the pancreas to make enough extra insulin to overcome it.

Vasopressin: Also called antidiuretic hormone (ADH) or arginine vasopressin (AVP) hormone. A hormone that is responsible for maintaining the normal volume and concentration of our urine.

Index

Index

LIPPINCOTT'S
Nursing
Drug Guide

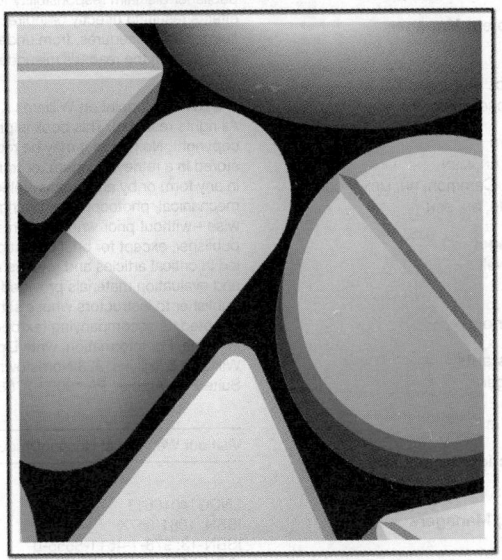

Amy M. Karch, RN, MS

Associate Professor of Clinical Nursing
University of Rochester School of Nursing
Rochester, New York

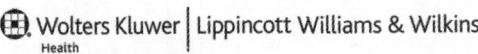

Wolters Kluwer | Lippincott Williams & Wilkins
Health
Philadelphia · Baltimore · New York · London
Buenos Aires · Hong Kong · Sydney · Tokyo

Staff

Publisher
Jay Abramovitz

Chief Nurse
Judith A. Schilling McCann, RN, MSN

Product Director
David Moreau

Art Director
Elaine Kasmer

Electronic Project Manager
John Macalino

Clinical Project Manager
Beverly Ann Tscheschlog, RN, MS

Clinical Editors
Anita Lockhart, RN, MSN
Shari A. Regina-Cammon, RN, MSN, PCCN
Leigh Ann Trujillo, RN, BSN

Product Manager
Rosanne Hallowell

Editor
Karen C. Comerford

Editorial Assistants
Megan L. Aldinger
Jeri O'Shea
Linda K. Ruhf

Senior Production Project Manager
Cynthia Rudy

Manufacturing Managers
Beth J. Welsh
Kathleen Brown

Production Services
Aptara, Inc.

The clinical procedures described and recommended in this publication are based on research and consultation with nursing, medical, pharmaceutical, and legal authorities. To the best of our knowledge, these procedures reflect currently accepted practice; nevertheless, they can't be considered absolute and universal recommendations. For individual application, all recommendations must be considered in light of the patient's clinical condition and, before the administration of new or infrequently used drugs, in light of the latest package-insert information. The authors and publisher disclaim responsibility for adverse effects resulting directly or indirectly from the suggested procedures, from undetected errors, or from the reader's misunderstanding of the text.

Visit our Web site at NursingDrugGuide.com

LNDG14010613
ISSN: 1081-857X
ISBN-13: 978-1-4511-8655-0
ISBN-10: 1-4511-8655-X
ISBN-13: 978-1-4698-2074-3 (Canada)
ISBN-10: 1-4698-2074-9 (Canada)

Contents

A quick-access full-color photoguide to pills and capsules
is found between pages 750 and 751.

Consultants

Lawrence Carey, PharmD
Director, Physician Assistant Program
Philadelphia University
Philadelphia, Pennsylvania

Catherine A. Cashmore, MS, PharmD, ANP, FASCP
Associate Dean
Idaho State University College of Pharmacy
Pocatello, Idaho

Glen E. Farr, PharmD
Professor of Clinical Pharmacy and Associate Dean
University of Tennessee College of Pharmacy
Knoxville, Tennessee

Jennifer Faulkner, PharmD, BCPP
Director of Education, Pharmacy
Central Texas Veterans Health Care System
Temple, Texas

Tatyana Gurvich, PharmD, CGP
Clinical Pharmacist
University of Southern California School of Pharmacy
Los Angeles, California

Toshal Hallowell, BS, PharmD
Pharmacist
Edward M. Kennedy Community Health Center
Worcester, Massachusetts

Mary Kate Kelly, RPh, PharmD
Pharmacy Manager
QOL Meds
Pottstown, Pennsylvania

Bruce H. Livengood, PharmD
Associate Professor
Duquesne University
Mylan School of Pharmacy
Pittsburgh, Pennsylvania

Hannah J. Livengood, PharmD
Resident
MedStar Washington Hospital Center
Washington, DC

Kristy H. Lucas, PharmD
Professor and Interim Chair
Department of Pharmacy Practice
University of Charleston School of Pharmacy
Charleston, West Virginia

Michael A. Mancano, PharmD
Clinical Professor of Pharmacy
Interim Chair, Department of Pharmacy Practice
Temple University School of Pharmacy
Philadelphia, Pennsylvania

Chijioke Okafor, PharmD
Neuroscience Medical Science Liaison
Bristol-Myers Squibb Company
Plainsboro, New Jersey

Maha Saad, PharmD, CGP, BCPS
Assistant Clinical Professor
St. John's University College of Pharmacy and Health Sciences
Queens, New York

Michele F. Shepherd, MS, PharmD, BCPS, FASHP
Clinical Specialist
Abbott Northwestern Hospital
Minneapolis, Minnesota

Suzzanne Tairu, PharmD
Medical Science Liaison
Collegeville, Pennsylvania

Preface

The number of clinically important drugs increases every year, as does the nurse's responsibility for drug therapy. No nurse can memorize all the drug information needed to provide safe and efficacious drug therapy. The *2014 Lippincott's Nursing Drug Guide* provides the drug information nurses need in a concise, ready-access format. This edition was completely updated and then it was reviewed by independent clinical reviewers, including pharmacists and nurses, to ensure that nurses will have the most up-to-date and accurate information possible.

This book presents nursing considerations related to drug therapy in the format of the nursing process, a framework for applying basic pharmacologic information to patient care. It is intended for the student nurse who is just learning how to apply pharmacologic data in the clinical situation, as well as for the busy practicing professional nurse who needs a quick, easy-to-use guide to the clinical use of drugs.

This book provides broad coverage of the drugs commonly encountered by nurses and of drugs whose use commonly involves significant nursing intervention. *Anatomy of a monograph,* found inside the front cover, explains how the information in each monograph can be used to implement the nursing process. Commonly used medical abbreviations are used throughout the book and are defined in the *Guide to abbreviations,* which follows this Preface.

Before the drug monographs, you will see shaded pages that begin with **Nursing Process Guidelines**, a concise review of the nursing process and its application to pharmacologic situations. This section includes concise examples of how to use the drug guide to apply the nursing process and to make a patient teaching guide. Next is a section on **Patient Safety and Medication Administration**, which covers the seven rights of drug administration, and provides guidelines for ensuring patient safety and avoiding medication errors. Safety Net charts cover common dangerous abbreviations to avoid; patient teaching to prevent medication errors; and medication disposal guidelines. Following this section is **Pharmacologic Classes**, a review of selected drug classifications, which provides a convenient, complete summary of the drug information pertinent to drugs in each class.

Complete drug monographs

Drug information is presented in monograph form, with the monographs arranged alphabetically by generic name. Each page of the book contains guide words at the top, much like a dictionary, to facilitate easy access to any drug. The right-hand edge of the book contains letter guides, again to facilitate finding a drug as quickly as possible.

Each drug monograph is complete in itself—that is, it includes all of the clinically important information that a nurse needs to know to administer the drug safely and effectively. Every monograph begins with the drug's generic (nonproprietary) name; any alternate names follow in parentheses; an alphabetical list of the most common brand names, including common brand names found only in Canada (noted by the designation CAN); the drug's pregnancy category classification, and its schedule, if it is a controlled substance. The names of drugs that are described in Appendix R, *Less commonly used drugs,* appear alphabetically in the text and are cross referenced to the index.

Preventing medication errors is a critical component of patient care. Clinical practice has revealed that some drugs are especially dangerous when involved in a medication error. The monographs for these drugs are marked with the "dangerous drug" logo to alert the nurse to use exceptional care during administration. TALL man lettering, approved by the Food and Drug Administration (FDA) to help decrease medication errors and confusion, will appear with those drugs on the list.

Each monograph provides a commonly accepted pronunciation (after *USAN* and the *USP Dictionary of Drug Names, 2012*) to help the nurse feel more comfortable discussing the drug with other members of the health care team. After the pronunciation, each monograph gives you these features:

- The clinically important drug classes of each drug are indicated to put the drug in appropriate context.

- The therapeutically useful actions of the drug are described, including, where known, the mechanism(s) by which these therapeutic effects are produced; no attempt is made to list *all* of the drug's known actions here.
- Clinical indications for the drug are listed, including important unlabeled indications not approved by the FDA, as well as orphan drug uses where appropriate. New indications for a drug are emphasized by the "New indication" logo.
- Contraindications to drug use and cautions that should be considered when using the drug are listed.
- The pharmacokinetic profile of the drug is given in table form to allow easy access to such information as half-life, peak levels, distribution, and so on, offering a quick reference on how the drug is handled by the body.
- Dosage information is listed next, including dosages for adults, pediatric patients, and geriatric patients, and dosages for indications when these differ. A listing of the available forms of each drug serves as a guide for prescribing or suggesting alternate routes of administration. Details of drug administration that must not be overlooked for the safe administration of the drug (eg, "Dilute before infusing" or "Infuse slowly over 30 min") are included in the dosage section, but other aspects of drug administration (eg, directions for reconstituting a powder for injection) are presented under *Interventions* in the next section of the monograph. If there is a treatment for the overdose of this drug, that information is indicated in *Interventions*.
- The *IV Facts* section, with a prominent logo, gives concise, important information that is needed for drugs given IV—dilution, flow rate, compatibilities—making it unnecessary to have a separate IV handbook.
- Commonly encountered adverse effects are listed by body system, with the most commonly encountered adverse effects appearing in *italics* to make it easier to assess the patient for adverse effects and to teach the patient about what to expect. Potentially life-threatening adverse effects are in **bold** for easy access. Adverse effects that have been reported, but appear less commonly or rarely, are also listed to make the drug information as complete as possible.
- Clinically important interactions are listed separately for easy access: drug-drug, drug-food, drug-lab test, drug-alternative therapy—for interferences to consider when using the drug and any nursing action that is necessary because of this interaction.
- The "Dangerous drug" heading indicates those drugs proved more likely to be involved in serious patient reactions.
- Drugs that cannot be cut, crushed, or chewed have a "Do Not Crush"(⬛) logo to immediately alert you about this caution.
- A "Black box" warning logo highlights FDA Black Box warnings regarding safe use of the drug.
- The "Warning" logo highlights important facts and potential safety issues; warnings appear in antibiotic monographs for those antibiotics with a higher incidence of the development of multidrug-resistant organisms (MDRO); warnings appear in proton pump inhibitor monographs regarding the increased risk of *Clostridium difficile* infection.

Clinically focused nursing considerations

The remainder of each monograph is concerned with nursing considerations, which are presented in the format of the nursing process. The steps of the nursing process are given slightly different names by different authorities; this handbook includes: assessment (history and physical examination), interventions, and teaching points for each of the drugs presented.

"Clinical alert" provides important information about reported name confusions that have occurred with a given drug to help prevent potential medication errors.

- **Assessment:** Outlines the information that should be collected before administering the drug. This section is further divided into two subsections:
  –History: Includes a list of those underlying conditions that constitute contraindications and cautions for use of the drug.
  –Physical: Provides data, by organ system, that should be collected before beginning drug therapy, both to allow detection of conditions that are contraindications or cautions to the use of the drug and to provide baseline data for detecting adverse reactions to the drug and monitoring for therapeutic response.

- **Interventions:** Lists, in chronologic order, those nursing activities that should be undertaken in the course of caring for a patient who is receiving the drug. This section includes interventions related to drug preparation and administration, the provision of comfort and safety measures, and drug levels to monitor, as appropriate.
- **Teaching points:** Includes specific information that is needed for teaching the patient who is receiving this drug. Proved "what to say" advice can be transferred directly to patient teaching printouts and used as a written reminder.

Evaluation

Evaluation is usually the last step of the nursing process. In all drug therapy, the patient should be evaluated for the desired effect of the drug as listed in the *Indications* section; the occurrence of adverse effects, as listed in the *Adverse effects* section; and learning following patient teaching, as described in the *Teaching points* section. These points are essential. In some cases, evaluation includes monitoring specific therapeutic serum drug levels; these cases are specifically mentioned in the *Interventions* section. The *Nursing process guidelines* chapter gives an example of how the drug monograph can be used to establish a nursing care plan, to develop a patient teaching printout, and to incorporate the nursing process into drug therapy.

Appendices

The appendices contain information that is useful to nursing practice but may not lend itself to the monograph format—alternative and complementary therapies; important drug-related dietary guidelines for patient teaching; a list of drugs that interact with grapefruit juice; recommended routes of administration; formulas for pediatric dosage calculations; schedules of controlled substances (for U.S. and Canadian drugs); pregnancy categories (for U.S. drugs); cardiovascular guidelines—including standards for lipid levels and blood pressure monitoring; normal laboratory values; Canadian drug information, including mini-monographs of drugs that are used in Canada but not in the United States; topical drugs and corticosteroids; ophthalmic drugs; laxatives; detailed combination drug references; information about hormonal contraceptives; commonly used biologics; less commonly used drugs; 50 common disorders and the drugs used to treat them; and a quick guide to reputable Internet sites. A bibliography follows the appendices.

Index

An extensive index provides a ready reference to drug information. The **generic** name of each drug is highlighted in bold. If the generic name of a drug is not known, the drug may be found quickly by using whatever name is known. *Brand names* are listed in italics, commonly used chemical names and any commonly used "jargon" name (such as IDU for idoxuridine) are listed alphabetically in plain font. In addition, the index lists drugs by clinically important classes— pharmacologic and therapeutic. If you know a patient is taking an antianginal drug and don't remember the name, reviewing the list of drugs under *Antianginals* may well help you recall the name. Chlorpromazine, for example, is listed by its generic name, by all of its brand names, and by classes as an antipsychotic (a therapeutic classification), as a phenothiazine (the pharmacologic class), and as a dopaminergic blocking drug (a classification by postulated mechanism of action). The comprehensive index helps to avoid cross-referencing from within the text, which is time consuming and often confusing.

2014 Quick-access photoguide

The full-color quick-access photoguide located in the center of the book presents more than 400 pills and capsules, representing the most commonly prescribed generic and brand drugs. Photos of certain brands were provided by the following companies: Forest Pharmaceuticals, Inc. (Campral); Novartis Pharmaceuticals (Enablex); Sepracor, Inc. (Lunesta); Teva Pharmaceuticals (Azilect); and Pfizer (Sutent). Photos of the following drugs were provided by Jeff Sigler, © SFI Medical Publishing, Inc.: Aciphex, Actos, Aricept, Clozaril, Dexilant, Diovan HCT, Effient, Flomax, Lyrica, Nexium, Plavix, Pristiq, Seroquel, Topamax, TriCor, Valtrex, Vytorin, and Zyprexa.

What's new

The new features in the book include:

- More than 45 new drugs
- More than 1,200 updates
- More "Warning" logos that highlight potential complications
- More FDA-issued Black Box Warnings, to improve patient safety.

Web site

Through the NursingDrugGuide.com Web site you will be able to access patient-teaching print-outs for more than 200 of the most commonly prescribed drugs, which you can use to prepare your own study aids, develop nursing care plans, and customize patient and staff teaching tools. You'll also find tips for avoiding common drug errors, information on toxic drug-drug interactions, and many other patient safety resources. Pharmacology information, therapeutic guidelines, and tools such as a dosage calculator, pronunciation guide, and Spanish-English resources are also provided on the Web site.

Added benefit

With this guide comes access to free monthly drug updates available to you throughout the year via the NursingDrugGuide.com Web site. Get the most recent drug information available, including the latest FDA drug approvals and advances in clinical pharmacology. In addition, you will be able to access new continuing education tests via the Web site and earn contact hours.

This 19th edition incorporates many of the suggestions and requests that have been made by the users of earlier editions of this book. It is hoped that the overall organization and concise, straight-forward presentation of the material in the *2014 Lippincott's Nursing Drug Guide* will make it a readily used and clinically useful reference for the nurse who needs easily accessible information to facilitate the provision of drug therapy within the framework of the nursing process. It is further hoped that the thoroughness of the additional sections of the book will make it an invaluable resource that will replace the need for several additional references.

Amy M. Karch, RN, MS

Guide to abbreviations

ACE	angiotensin-converting enzyme	CML	chronic myelogenous leukemia
ACT	activated clotting time	CNS	central nervous system
ACTH	adrenocorticotropic hormone	COPD	chronic obstructive pulmonary disease
ADH	antidiuretic hormone	CPR	cardiopulmonary resuscitation
ADHD	attention-deficit hyperactivity disorder	CR	controlled release
ADLs	activities of daily living	CrCl	creatinine clearance
AIDS	acquired immunodeficiency syndrome	CSF	cerebrospinal fluid
		CTZ	chemoreceptor trigger zone
ALL	acute lymphocytic leukemia	CV	cardiovascular
ALT	alanine transaminase (formerly called SGPT)	CVP	central venous pressure
		CYP450	cytochrome P-450
AML	acute myelogenous leukemia	D_5W	dextrose 5% in water
ANA	anti-nuclear antibodies	DEA	Drug Enforcement Administration
ANC	absolute neutrophil count	DIC	disseminated intravascular coagulopathy
aPTT	activated partial thromboplastin time	dL	deciliter (100 mL)
ARB	angiotensin II receptor blocker	DNA	deoxyribonucleic acid
ARC	AIDS-related complex	DR	delayed release
ASA	acetylsalicylic acid	DTP	diphtheria-tetanus-pertussis (vaccine)
AST	aspartate transaminase (formerly called SGOT)	DVT	deep vein thrombosis
AV	atrioventricular	ECG	electrocardiogram
bid	twice a day *(bis in die)*	ECT	electroconvulsive therapy
BP	blood pressure	ED	erectile dysfunction
BPH	benign prostatic hypertrophy	EEG	electroencephalogram
BUN	blood urea nitrogen	EENT	eye, ear, nose, and throat
C	centigrade, Celsius	ER	extended release
CAD	coronary artery disease	EST	electroshock therapy
cAMP	cyclic adenosine monophosphate	F	Fahrenheit
CBC	complete blood count	FDA	Food and Drug Administration
CDC	Centers for Disease Control and Prevention	5-FU	fluorouracil
CK	creatine kinase	5-HIAA	5-hydroxyindole acetic acid

FSH	follicle-stimulating hormone	L	liter
g	gram	lb	pound
GABA	gamma-aminobutyric acid	LDH	lactic dehydrogenase
GERD	gastroesophageal reflux disease	LDL	low-density lipoproteins
GFR	glomerular filtration rate	LFT	liver function test
GGTP	gamma-glutamyl transpeptidase	LH	luteinizing hormone
GI	gastrointestinal	LHRH	luteinizing hormone-releasing hormone
G6PD	glucose-6-phosphate dehydroge-nase	m	meter
GU	genitourinary	MAO	monoamine oxidase
HCG	human chorionic gonadotropin	MAOI	monoamine oxidase inhibitor
Hct	hematocrit	mcg	microgram
HDL	high-density lipoproteins	MDRO	multidrug-resistant organisms
HF	heart failure	mg	milligram
Hg	mercury	MI	myocardial infarction
Hgb	hemoglobin	min	minute
Hib	*Haemophilus influenzae* type b	mL	milliliter
HIV	human immunodeficiency virus	mo	month
HMG-CoA	3-hydroxy-3-methylglutaryl coenzyme A	MS	multiple sclerosis
HPA	hypothalamic–pituitary axis	ng	nanogram
hr	hour	NMS	neuroleptic malignant syndrome
HR	heart rate	NPO	nothing by mouth *(nihil per os)*
HSV	herpes simplex virus	NSAID	nonsteroidal anti-inflammatory drug
IBS	irritable bowel syndrome	OCD	obsessive compulsive disorder
IHSS	idiopathic hypertrophic subaortic stenosis	OTC	over-the-counter
I & O	intake and output	P	pulse
IM	intramuscular	PABA	para-aminobenzoic acid
INR	international normalized ratio	PAT	paroxysmal atrial tachycardia
IOP	intraocular pressure	PBI	protein-bound iodine
IPPB	intermittent (or inspiratory) positive pressure breathing	PCWP	pulmonary capillary wedge pressure
IUD	intrauterine device	PDA	patent ductus arteriosus
IV	intravenous	PE	pulmonary embolus
JVP	jugular venous pressure	PFT	pulmonary function test
kg	kilogram	PG	prostaglandin
		pH	hydrogen ion concentration

PID	pelvic inflammatory disease
PMDD	premenstrual dysphoric disorder
PMS	premenstrual syndrome
PO	orally, by mouth *(per os)*
PRN	when required *(pro re nata)*
PSA	prostate-specific antigen
PT	prothrombin time
PTSD	post-traumatic stress disorder
PTT	partial thromboplastin time
PVCs	premature ventricular contractions
qid	four times a day *(quarter in die)*
R	respiratory rate
RAS	reticular-activating system
RBC	red blood cell
RDA	recommended dietary allowance
RDS	respiratory distress syndrome
REM	rapid eye movement
RNA	ribonucleic acid
RSV	respiratory syncytial virus
SA	sinoatrial
SBE	subacute bacterial endocarditis
sec	seconds
SIADH	syndrome of inappropriate anti-diuretic hormone secretion
SLE	systemic lupus erythematosus
SMA-12	sequential multiple analysis-12

SR	sustained release
SSRI	selective serotonin reuptake inhibitor
STD	sexually transmitted disease
Subcut.	subcutaneous
SWSD	shift-work sleep disorder
T	temperature
$T_{1/2}$	half-life
T_3	triiodothyronine
T_4	thyroxine (tetraiodothyronine)
TB	tuberculosis
TCA	tricyclic antidepressant
TIA	transient ischemic attack
tid	three times a day *(ter in die)*
URI	upper respiratory (tract) infection
US	United States
USP	United States Pharmacopeia
UTI	urinary tract infection
UV	ultraviolet
VLDL	very–low-density lipoproteins
VMA	vanillylmandelic acid
VRE	vancomycin-resistant enterococcus
WBC	white blood cell
WBCT	whole blood clotting time
wk	week
yr	year

Author's acknowledgments

I would like to thank the many people who have had an impact on making this book possible. Students and practicing nurses, patients and patients' families, past and present, who have helped me learn how to make pharmacology clinically useful; the many users of past editions of the book who have taken the time to offer suggestions and provide valuable comments; Judy McCann, Chief Nurse at the Ambler office of Lippincott Williams & Wilkins; Beverly Tscheschlog, my go-to person, trusted ally, and fellow dog-lover; Rosanne Hallowell, my new ally; Joan Robinson, who has been so patient, supportive, and helpful; Linda Ruhf, who secures the reviewers; and Karen Comerford, who makes it all come together.

A special thanks to those people who continue to inspire and teach and amaze me: Dr. Todd Wihlen, Dr. Michael Koch, Dr. Kent Burgesser, Dr. Paul Black, and the amazing staff of the MVA and VSES, who exhibit so much professionalism, compassion, empathy, and amazing support; to Jen Bidwell and Dr. Simon Kirk for keeping the dream alive and well; to Dr. Patrick Hopkins and Dr. Rebecca Tucker, my allies and co-conspirators; and to Tim, Jyoti, Mark, Tracey, Cortney, Bryan, and Kathryn for their unwavering support; Vikas, Nisha, Zara, Logan, Connor, and Jack for bringing the sunshine back into our lives and for reviving the joy of learning; and to Dixie and Brodie, my harshest critics and most joyous supporters, who keep everything in perspective.

Amy M. Karch, RN, MS

Nursing Process Guidelines

The delivery of medical care is in a constant state of change and sometimes in crisis. The population is aging, resulting in more chronic disease and more complex care issues. The population is transient, resulting in unstable support systems and fewer at-home care providers and helpers. At the same time, medicine is undergoing a technological and pharmacological boom. Patients are being discharged earlier from the acute-care facility or not being admitted at all for procedures that used to be done in the hospital with follow-up support and monitoring. Patients are becoming more responsible for their own care and for following complicated medical regimens at home.

Nursing is a unique and complex science and a nurturing and caring art. Traditionally, nurses minister to and soothe the sick; currently, nursing also requires using more technical and scientific skills. Nurses have had to assume increasing responsibilities involved not only with nurturing and caring, but also with assessing, diagnosing, and intervening with patients to treat, prevent, and educate to help people cope with various health states.

The nurse deals with the whole person—the physical, emotional, intellectual, and spiritual aspects—considering the ways that a person responds to disease and treatment, and the change in lifestyle that may be required by both. The nurse is the key health care provider in a position to assess the patient (physical, social, and emotional aspects), administer therapy and medications, teach the patient how best to cope with the therapy to ensure the most effectiveness, and evaluate the effectiveness of therapy. This role requires a broad base of knowledge in the basic sciences (anatomy, physiology, nutrition, chemistry, pharmacology), the social sciences (sociology, psychology), and education (learning approaches, evaluation).

Although all nursing theorists do not completely agree on the process that defines the practice of nursing, most include certain key elements in the nursing process. These elements are the basic components of the decision-making or problem-solving process:

assessment (gathering of information), diagnosis (defining that information to arrive at some conclusions), planning (developing a plan of care), intervention (eg, administration, education, comfort measures), and evaluation (determining the effects of the interventions that were performed). Using this process each time a situation arises ensures a method of coping with the overwhelming scientific and technical information. However, the unique emotional, social, and physical aspects that each patient brings to the situation can confound matters. Using the nursing process format in each instance of drug therapy will ensure that the patient receives the best, most efficient, scientifically based holistic care.

Assessment

The first step of the nursing process is the systematic, organized collection of data about the patient. Because the nurse is responsible for holistic care, these data must include information about physical, intellectual, emotional, social, and environmental factors. They will provide the nurse with information needed to plan discharge, plan educational programs, arrange for appropriate consultations, and monitor physical response to treatment or to disease. In actual clinical practice, this process never ends. The patient is not in a steady state but is dynamic, adjusting to physical, emotional, and environmental influences. Each nurse develops a unique approach to the organization of the assessment, an approach that is functional, useful, and appropriate in the clinical setting and that makes sense to that nurse and that clinical situation.

Drug therapy is a complex, integral, and important part of health care today, and the principles of drug therapy need to be incorporated into every patient assessment plan. The particular information that is needed and that should be assessed will vary with each drug, but the concepts involved are similar and are based on the principles of drug therapy. Two important areas that need to be assessed are history and physical presentation.

History

Past experiences and past illnesses and surgeries impact the actual effect of a drug.

Chronic conditions: These may be contraindications to the use of a drug or may require that caution be used or that drug dosage be adjusted.

Drug use: Prescription drugs, over-the-counter (OTC) drugs, herbs and alternative therapies, street drugs, alcohol, nicotine, and caffeine all may have an impact on the effect of a drug. Patients often neglect to mention OTC drugs, herbal and alternative therapies, vitamin and mineral supplements, and contraceptives, not considering them actual drugs, and should be asked specifically about the use of OTC drugs, herbals, supplements, contraceptives, or any drug that might be taken on a long-term basis and not mentioned.

Allergies: Past exposure to a drug or other allergen can predict a future reaction or need to use certain drugs, food, or animal products cautiously.

Level of education: This information will help to provide a basis for patient education programs and level of explanation.

Level of understanding of disease and therapy: This information also will direct the development of educational information.

Social supports: Patients are being discharged earlier than ever before and often need assistance at home to provide care and institute and monitor drug therapy.

Financial supports: The financial impact of health care and the high cost of medications need to be considered when prescribing drugs. These factors may impact a patient's ability to follow through with drug therapy.

Pattern of health care: The way that a patient seeks health care will give the nurse valuable information to include in educational information. Does this patient routinely seek physical examinations and follow-up care or wait for emergency situations?

Physical assessment

Weight: Weight is an important factor when determining if the recommended dosage of a drug is appropriate. The recommended dosage is based on the 150-lb adult male. Patients who are much lighter or much heavier will need a dosage adjustment.

Age: Patients at the extremes of the age spectrum—pediatric and geriatric—often require dosage adjustments based on the functional level of the liver and kidneys and the responsiveness of other organs.

Physical parameters related to the disease state or known drug effects: Assessment of these factors before beginning drug therapy will give a baseline level with which future assessments can be compared to determine the effects of drug therapy. The specific parameters that need to be assessed will depend on the disease process being treated and on the expected therapeutic and adverse effects of the drug therapy. Because the nurse has the greatest direct and continual contact with the patient, the nurse has the best opportunity to detect the minute changes that will determine the course of drug therapy and therapeutic success or the need for discontinuation because of adverse or unacceptable responses.

The monographs in this book include the specific parameters that need to be assessed in relation to the particular drug being discussed (see the sample monograph in the preface). This assessment provides not only the baseline information needed before giving that drug, but the data needed to evaluate the effects of that drug on the patient. The information given in this area should supplement the overall nursing assessment of the patient, which will include social, intellectual, financial, environmental, and other physical data.

Nursing diagnosis

Once data have been collected, the nurse must organize and analyze that information to arrive at a nursing diagnosis. A nursing diagnosis is simply a statement of the patient's status from a nursing perspective. This statement directs appropriate nursing interventions. A nursing diagnosis will show actual or potential alteration in patient function based on the assessment of the clinical situation. Because drug therapy is only a small part of the overall patient situation, the nursing diagnoses that are related to drug therapy must be incorporated into a total picture of the patient. In many cases the drug therapy will not present a new nursing diagnosis, but the desired effects and adverse effects related to each drug given should be considered in the identified nursing diagnoses for each patient. NANDA International (NANDA-I) produces a coded list of accepted nursing diagnoses that are updated every 3 years.

Interventions

The assessment and diagnosis of the patient's situation will direct specific nursing interventions. Four types of interventions are frequently involved in drug therapy: Drug administration, provision of comfort measures, monitoring the effects of drug therapy, and patient and family teaching.

Drug administration

Drug: Ensuring that the drug being administered is the correct dose of the correct drug at the correct time, and is being given to the correct patient, is standard nursing practice.

Storage: Some drugs require specific storage environments (eg, refrigeration, protection from light).

Route: Determining the best route of administration is often determined by the prescription of the drug. Nurses can often have an impact on modifying the prescribed route to determine the most efficient route and the most comfortable one for the patient based on his or her specific situation. When establishing the prescribed route, it is important to check the proper method of administering a drug by that route.

Dosage: Drug dosage may need to be calculated based on available drug form, patient body weight or surface area, or kidney function.

Preparation: Some drugs require specific preparation before administration. Oral drugs may need to be shaken or crushed; parenteral drugs may need to be reconstituted or diluted with specific solutions; topical drugs may require specific handling before administration.

Timing: Actual administration of a drug may require coordination with the administration of other drugs, foods, or physical parameters. The nurse, as the caregiver most frequently involved in administering a drug, must be aware of and juggle all of these factors and educate the patient to do this on his or her own.

Documentation: Once the nurse has assessed the patient, made the appropriate nursing diagnoses, and delivered the correct drug by the correct route, in the correct dose, and at the correct time, that information needs to be recorded in accordance with the local requirements for documenting medication administration.

Each monograph in this book contains pertinent guidelines for storage, dosage, preparation, and administration of the drug being discussed.

Comfort measures

Nurses are in the unique position to help the patient cope with the effects of drug therapy. **Placebo effect:** The anticipation that a drug will be helpful (placebo effect) has been proved to have tremendous impact on the actual success of drug therapy, so the nurse's attitude and support can be a critical part of drug therapy. A back rub, a kind word, and a positive approach may be as beneficial as the drug itself. **Side effects:** These interventions can be directed at decreasing the impact of the anticipated side effects of the drug and promoting patient safety. Such interventions include environmental control (eg, temperature, lighting), safety measures (eg, avoiding driving, avoiding the sun, using side rails), physical comfort (eg, skin care, laxatives, frequent meals).

Lifestyle adjustment: Some drug effects will require that a patient change his or her lifestyle to cope effectively. Diuretic users may have to rearrange the day to be near toilet facilities when the drug works. MAOI users have to adjust their diet to prevent serious drug effects.

Each monograph in this book will include a list of pertinent comfort measures appropriate to that particular drug.

Education

With patients becoming more responsible for their own care, it is essential that they have all of the information necessary to ensure safe and effective drug therapy at home. Many states now require that the patient be given written information. Key elements that need to be included in any drug education include the following:

- Name, dose, and action of drug: With many people seeing more than one health care provider, this information is important for ensuring safe and effective drug therapy.

- Timing of administration: Patients need to know specifically when to take the drug with regard to frequency, other drugs, and meals.

- Special storage and preparation instructions: Some drugs require particular handling that the patient will need to have spelled out.

- Specific OTC drugs, vitamin and mineral supplements, or alternative therapies to avoid: Many people do not consider these to be actual drugs and may inadvertently take them and cause unwanted or even dangerous drug interactions. Explaining problems will help the patient avoid these potential situations.

- Special comfort or safety measures that need to be considered: Alerting the patient to ways to cope with anticipated side effects will prevent a great deal of anxiety and noncompliance with drug therapy. The patient also may need to be alerted to the need to return for follow-up tests or evaluation.

- Safety measures: All patients need to be alerted to keep drugs out of the reach of children. They also need to be reminded to tell any health care provider whom they see that they are taking this drug. This can prevent drug-drug interactions, polypharmacy, and misdiagnosing based on drug effects.
- Specific points about drug toxicity: Warning signs of drug toxicity that the patient should be aware of should be listed. He or she can be advised to notify the health care provider if any of these effects occur.
- Specific warnings about drug discontinuation: Some drugs with a small margin of safety and drugs with particular systemic effects cannot be stopped abruptly without dangerous effects. Patients taking these drugs need to be alerted to the problem and encouraged to call immediately if they cannot take their medication for any reason (eg, illness, financial).

Each drug monograph in this book lists specific teaching points that relate to that particular drug. An example of a compact, written drug card developed from the information in the monograph is shown on page 5.

Evaluation

Evaluation is part of the continual process of patient care that leads to changes in assessment, diagnosis, and intervention. The patient is continually evaluated for therapeutic response, the occurrence of drug side effects, and the occurrence of drug-drug, drug-food, drug-laboratory test, or drug-alternative therapy interactions.

The efficacy of the nursing interventions and the education program must be evaluated. In some situations, the nurse will evaluate the patient simply by reapplying the beginning steps of the nursing process and analyzing for change. In some cases of drug therapy, particular therapeutic drug levels need to be evaluated as well.

Monographs in this book list only specific evaluation criteria, such as therapeutic serum levels, as they apply to each drug. Regular evaluation of drug effects, side effects, and the efficacy of comfort measures and education programs will not be specifically listed but can be deduced from information in the monograph regarding therapeutic effects and adverse effects. See *Nursing care plan: Patient receiving oral linezolid,* page 6. *Anatomy of a monograph,* in the preface, provides additional guidelines for using each section of a monograph as it applies to the nursing process.

Patient Drug Sheet: Oral Linezolid

Patient's Name: Mr. Kors
Prescriber's Name: J. Smith, ANP
Phone Number: 555-555-5555

Instructions:

1. The name of your drug is *linezolid*; the brand name is *Zyvox*. This drug is an antibiotic that is being used to treat your *pneumonia*. This drug is very specific in its action and is only indicated for your particular infection. Take the full course of your drug. Do not share this drug with other people or save tablets for future use.
2. The dose of the drug that has been prescribed for you is: *600 mg (1 tablet)*.
3. The drug should be taken *once every 12 hours*. The best time for you to take this drug will be *8:00 in the morning and 8:00 in the evening*. Do not skip any doses. Do not take two doses at once if you forget a dose. If you miss a dose, take the dose as soon as you remember and then again in 12 hours.
4. The drug can be taken with food if GI upset is a problem. Avoid foods that are rich in tyramine (list is below) while you are taking this drug.
5. The following side effects may occur:
   Nausea, vomiting, abdominal pain (taking the drug with food and eating frequent small meals may help).
   Diarrhea (ensure ready access to bathroom facilities). Notify your health care provider if this becomes severe.
6. Do not take this drug with over-the-counter drugs or herbal remedies without first checking with your health care provider. Many of these agents can cause problems with your drug.
7. Tell any nurse, physician, or dentist who is taking care of you that you are on this drug.
8. Keep this and all medications out of the reach of children.

Notify your health care provider if any of the following occur:
   Rash, severe GI problems, bloody or excessive diarrhea, weakness, tremors, increased bleeding or bruising, anxiety.

> Foods high in tyramine to avoid: Aged cheeses, avocados, bananas, beer, bologna, caffeinated beverages, chocolate, liver, over-ripe fruit, pepperoni, pickled fish, red wine, salami, smoked fish, yeast, yogurt.

Nursing care plan: Patient receiving oral linezolid

Assessment	Nursing diagnoses	Interventions	Evaluation
History (contraindications and cautions) Hypertension Hyperthyroidism Blood dyscrasias Hepatic dysfunction Pheochromocytoma Phenylketonuria Carcinoid syndrome Pregnancy Lactation Known allergy to linezolid	Imbalanced nutrition, less than body requirements, related to GI effects Acute pain related to GI effects, headache Ineffective tissue perfusion related to bone marrow effects Deficient knowledge related to drug therapy	Safe and appropriate administration of drug: Culture infection site to ensure appropriate use of drug Provision of safety and comfort measures: • Monitor BP periodically • Monitor platelet counts before and periodically during therapy • Alleviation of GI upset • Ready access to bathroom facilities • Nutritional consult • Safety provisions if dizziness and CNS effects occur • Avoidance of tyramine-rich foods	Monitor patient for therapeutic effects of drug: Resolution of infection. If resolution does not occur, reculture site. Monitor patient for adverse effects of drug: • GI upset—nausea, vomiting, diarrhea • Liver function changes • Pseudomembranous colitis • Blood dyscrasias— changes in platelet counts • Fever • Rash • Sweating • Photosensitivity • Acute hypersensitivity reactions
Medication History (possible drug-drug interactions) Pseudoephedrine SSRIs MAOIs Antiplatelet drugs			
Diet History (possible drug-food interactions) Foods high in tyramine		Patient teaching regarding: • Drug • Side effects to anticipate • Warnings • Reactions to report	Evaluate effectiveness of patient teaching program: Patient can name drug, dose of drug, use of drug, adverse effects to expect, reactions to report.
Physical Assessment (screen for contraindications and to establish a baseline for evaluating effects and adverse effects) **CNS:** Affect, reflexes, orientation **CV:** P, BP, peripheral perfusion **GI:** Bowel sounds, liver evaluation **Hematologic:** CBC with differential, liver function tests **Local:** Culture site of infection **Skin:** Color, lesions		Support and encouragement to cope with disease, high cost of therapy, and side effects Provision of emergency and life-support measures in cases of acute hypersensitivity	Monitor patient for drug-drug, drug-food interactions as appropriate. Evaluate effectiveness of life-support measures if needed.

Patient Safety and Medication Administration

Growing numbers of patients—and drugs—bring increased risk of medication errors. Compounding this risk are the tremendous upsurge in the use of over-the-counter (OTC) drugs and herbal remedies and the overwhelming impact of the Internet and direct-to-consumer advertising in influencing patient compliance and decision making. There have always been checkpoints in ensuring medication safety. There have traditionally been three levels of checks protecting the patient—the prescriber who chooses and orders a drug, the pharmacist who fills the prescription and, finally, the nurse who actually administers the drug to the patient. Each serves as a check within the system to catch errors—the wrong drug, the wrong patient, the wrong dose, the wrong route, or the wrong time.

Back in the 1950s and 1960s, most drugs were given in a hospital or institutional setting and these checks were effective in catching wrong drugs, wrong doses, and so forth. But in today's world, with skyrocketing health care costs and the push for early discharge, more people are being treated outside the hospital than in the hospital. National studies published in 2008 predicted that, with so many patients managing their own drug regimens at home, over 5 million preventable medication errors can occur each year with an estimated annual cost of $350 billion and untold personal suffering. The usual checks are still in place, but the patient is now responsible for administering the drug and the nurse is the person with the responsibility for discharging patients to home with the knowledge and tools they will need to manage a potentially complicated drug regimen.

The rights of medication administration

In the clinical setting, the monumental task of ensuring medication safety can be managed by consistently using the seven rights of drug administration: right drug, right route, right dose, right time, right patient, right response, and right documentation.

Right drug

- Always review a drug order before administering the drug.
- Do not assume that a computer system is always right and will protect the patient. Always double-check.
- Make sure the drug name is correct. Ask for a brand name and a generic name. Because many drug names look and sound alike (note the Clinical Alerts throughout the monographs), the chance of reading the name incorrectly is greatly reduced if both generic and brand names are used.
- Avoid taking verbal or telephone orders whenever possible. If you must, have a second person listen in to verify and clarify the order.
- Abbreviations can be confusing between and even within health care facilities. Do not be afraid or embarrassed to ask the meaning of an abbreviation, even a common one. For instance, many people use "hs" to mean "hour of sleep"; others may read it as "every hour." As much as possible, spell out abbreviations for clarification.
- Consider whether the drug makes sense for the patient's diagnosis. If you do not know or you have questions, look up the drug and ask the patient what it is being used for.

Right route

- Review the available forms of a drug to make sure the drug can be given according to the order.
- Check the routes available and the appropriateness of the route for this patient. Be familiar with the appropriate and safe technique for administration by the ordered route.
- Make sure the patient is able to take the drug by the route indicated. If you know that the patient has trouble swallowing, for example, you also know that a liquid form of the drug may be better than a tablet or capsule.
- Do not use abbreviations for routes because the danger of confusion is too great. For example, "SC" is often used to mean "subcutaneous," but it has been misinterpreted to

mean "sublingual" among other misinterpretations. Also, "IV" can be misinterpreted to mean "IU," or international units.

Right dose

- Make sure the dose about to be delivered is the dose the prescriber ordered.
- There should always be a 0 to the left of a decimal point, and there should never be a 0 to the right of a decimal point. For example, "0.5" is correct (not ".5," which can be easily mistaken for "5") and "5" is correct (not "5.0," which can be easily mistaken for "50"). If you see an ordered dose that starts with a decimal point, question it. And if a dose seems much too big, question that.
- Double-check drug calculations. If a dose has to be calculated for pediatric or other use, always have someone double-check the math, even if a computer did the calculations. This is especially important with drugs that have small margins of safety, such as digoxin and insulin.
- Check the measuring devices used for liquid drugs. Advise patients not to use kitchen teaspoons or tablespoons to measure drug doses.
- Do not cut tablets in half to get the correct dose without checking the warnings that come with the drug. Many drugs cannot be cut, crushed, or chewed because of the matrix systems that have been developed to prepare the drugs.

Right time

- Increased workloads, decreased nursing staffs, and constant interruptions can interfere with the delivery of medications at the right times. Even at home, patients are busy, have tight schedules, and may fail to follow a precise schedule. Ensure the timely delivery of the patient's drugs by scheduling dosage with other drugs, meals, or other consistent events to maintain the serum level.
- Teach patients the importance of timing critical drugs. Keep in mind that patients tend to take all of their daily drugs at once, in the morning, to reduce the risk of forgetting them. But with critical drugs, such as those with a small margin of safety, those that interact, and those that need meticu-

lous spacing, you will need to stress the importance of accurate timing. As needed, make detailed medication schedules and prepare pill boxes.

Right patient

- Check the patient's identification even if you think you know who the patient is. Ask for the patient's full name, and check the patient's identification band if available.
- Review the patient's diagnosis, and verify that the drug matches the diagnosis. If a drug does not make sense for the patient's diagnosis, look it up and, if necessary, consult the prescriber.
- Make sure all allergies have been checked before giving a drug. Serious adverse reactions can be avoided if allergies are known.
- Ask patients specifically about OTC drugs, vitamin and mineral supplements, herbal remedies, and routine drugs that they may not think to mention, such as oral contraceptives, thyroid hormones, and insulin. Serious overdoses, adverse reactions, and drug interactions can be avoided if this information is acquired early.
- Review the patient's drug regimen to prevent potential interactions between the drug you are about to give and drugs the patient already takes. If you are not sure about potential interactions, consult a drug reference.

The bottom line in avoiding medication errors is simple: "If in doubt, check it out." A strange abbreviation, a drug or dosage that is new to you, and a confusing name are all examples that signal a need for follow-up. Look up the drug in your drug guide or call the prescriber or the pharmacy to double-check. Never give a drug until you have satisfied yourself that it is the right drug, given by the right route, at the right dose, at the right time, and to the right patient.

Right Response

Monitor the patient's response to the drug administered to make sure that the response is what is anticipated. A response that is not anticipated could indicate that the wrong drug is being used or that this particular patient has a unique reaction that needs to be addressed.

Right Documentation

Document according to facility policy. Include the drug name, dose, route, and time of administration. Note special circumstances, such as the patient having difficulty swallowing or the site of the injection. Include the patient's response to the drug and any special nursing interventions that were used. Remember, "if it isn't written, it didn't happen." Accurate documentation provides continuity of care and helps prevent medication errors.

Preventing miscommunication

As with so many things in the world, miscommunication can be the source of many safety issues in medicine and nursing. Working to prevent miscommunication is a complicated task for the entire health care team.

Although abbreviations can save time, they also raise the risk of misinterpretation, which can lead to potentially disastrous consequences, especially when dealing with drug administration. To help reduce the risk of being misunderstood, always take the time to write legibly and to spell out anything that could be misread. This caution extends to how you write numbers as well as drug names and other drug-related instructions. The Joint Commission is enforcing a growing list of abbreviations that should not be used in medical records to help alleviate this problem. It is important to be familiar with the abbreviations used in your clinical area and to avoid the use of any other abbreviations. (See *Common dangerous abbreviations,* page 10.)

Dosages

When writing a drug dosage, never add a zero after a decimal point and always add a zero before a decimal point. If you see "1.0 mg" instead of the correct "1 mg," the dosage easily could be misread as "10 mg." Likewise, if you see ".5 mg" instead of the correct "0.5 mg," the dosage could be misread as "5 mg."

Drug names

Be careful with drug names. For instance, if you write "$MgSO_4$" as shorthand for "magnesium sulfate," it could be misread as meaning "morphine sulfate." The opposite is also true; if you write "MS" or "MSO_4," meaning "morphine sulfate," it could be misread as meaning "magnesium sulfate." Instead, make sure to clearly write out all drug names, particularly those that could be dangerous if confused or that could be easily confused.

Patient and family teaching

In today's world, once the right drug, right dose, right route, right time, and right patient have been established, the patient is usually left to manage on his or her own. The most important safety check after all is said and done is the patient—the patient is the only person in the system who has all the pertinent information to prevent medication errors, both inside and outside the health care facility. Only the patient actually knows what health care providers he or she is seeing; what prescription drugs, OTC drugs, and herbal remedies are actually being used; and how they are being used. Today's patient needs to be educated about all drugs being taken and empowered to speak up and protect himself or herself against medication errors.

Medication errors present a constant risk, particularly for patients who take multiple drugs prescribed by multiple health care providers. (See *Patient teaching to prevent medication errors,* pages 11 and 12.)

Elderly patients

The elderly population is the most rapidly growing group in our country. Frequently, these patients have chronic diseases, are on multiple drugs, and have increasing health problems that can be a challenge to following a drug regimen. They are also more likely to suffer adverse reactions to drugs and drug combinations. Advise them to keep a medication list with them to share with all health care providers and to post a list somewhere in their home (on the refrigerator, on the back of the front door) for easy access by emergency personnel. It is frequently helpful to prepare drug boxes for the week, draw up injectables (if stable) for the week, and provide daily reminders to take their medications. Elderly patients need strong patient advocates to ensure drug safety.

SAFETY NET

Common dangerous abbreviations

Try to avoid these common—and dangerous—abbreviations, especially those that appear in color.

Abbreviation	Intended use	Potential misreading	Preferred use
BT	bedtime	May be read as "bid" or twice daily	Spell out "bedtime."
cc	cubic centimeters	May be read as "u" or units	Use "milliliters," abbreviated as "mL" or "ml."
D/C	discharge or discontinue	May lead to premature discontinuation of drug therapy or premature discharge	Spell out "discharge" or "discontinue."
hs	at bedtime	May be read as "half-strength"	Spell out "at bedtime."
HS	half-strength	May be read as "at bedtime"	Spell out "half-strength."
IJ	injection	May be read as "IV"	Spell out "injection."
IN	intranasal	May be read as "IM" or "IV"	Spell out "intranasal" or use "NAS."
IU	international unit	May be read as "IV" or "10"	Spell out "international unit."
µg	microgram	May be read as "mg"	Use "mcg."
o.d. or O.D.	once daily	May be read as "right eye"	Spell out "once daily."
per os	by mouth	May be read as "left eye"	Use "PO" or spell out "orally."
q.d. or QD	daily	May be read as "qid"	Spell out "daily."
q1d	once daily	May be read as "qid"	Spell out "once daily."
qhs	every bedtime	May be read as "qhr" (every hour)	Spell out "nightly" or "at bedtime."
qn	every night	May be read as "qh" (every hour)	Spell out "nightly" or "at bedtime."
q.o.d. or QOD	every other day	May be read as "q.d." (daily) or "q.i.d." (four times daily)	Spell out "every other day."
SC, SQ	subcutaneous	May be read as "SL" (sublingual) or "5 every"	Spell out "subcutaneous" or use "subcut."
U or u	unit	May be read as "0" (100 instead of 10U)	Spell out "unit."
×7d	for 7 days	May be read as "for seven doses"	Spell out "for 7 days."
°	hour	May be read as a zero	Spell out "hour" or use "hr."

SAFETY NET

Patient teaching to prevent medication errors

When being prescribed medications, patients should learn these key points to reduce the risk of medication errors.

- Keep a list: Keep a written list of all the drugs you take, including over-the-counter drugs, herbal products, and other supplements. Make sure the list includes brand names, generic names, the amount you take, and how often you take each product. Then make sure to carry this list with you and show it to all your health care providers, including dentists and emergency personnel.

- Watch for problems: Drugs can be lost in luggage, or other problems can occur. Drugs may have different brand names in other countries, and the brand name you are used to may belong to a very different drug. For instance, *Ambien* (zolpidem) in the United States is used as a sleeping aid, and in the United Kingdom *Ambyn* (amiodarone) is a very potent antiarrhythmic. When asking for a replacement for *Ambien,* for example, when in another country, make sure that you are not getting a very different and potentially dangerous drug.

- Know your drugs: Make sure you know why you take each of your drugs. If you know why you are taking each drug, you will have a better understanding of what to report, what to watch for, and when to report to your health care provider if the drug is not working.

- Follow the directions: Carefully read the label of each of your drugs, and follow the directions for taking it safely. Do not stop taking a drug without first consulting the prescriber. It is easy to make up your own schedule or to take everything all at once in the morning. Always check the labels to see if there are specific times you should be taking your drugs. Make a calendar if you take drugs on alternating days. Using a weekly pillbox may also help to keep things straight.

- Store carefully: Always store drugs in a dry place, safely out of the reach of children and pets. Storing drugs in the bathroom, where it is often hot and steamy, can cause them to break down faster and become ineffective. Also, make sure to keep all drugs in their original, labeled containers.

- Speak up: You, the patient, are the most important member of your health care team. You have very important information to share that impacts your health and your drug regimen. Tell your health care providers about your health history, allergies (especially drug allergies), medications (including over-the-counter drugs and herbal remedies), and current health problems. *Never be afraid to ask questions* about your health or your treatments.

Keep children safe

Children present unique challenges related to medication errors. Children frequently cannot speak for themselves and rely on a caregiver or caregivers to manage their drug regimen. Because their bodies are still developing, they respond differently than adults to many drugs; the risk of serious adverse reactions is greater in children. The margin of safety with many drugs is very small when dealing with children. When teaching parents about their children's drug regimens, be sure to include the following instructions

If you are a parent or a child's caregiver, take these steps to prevent medication errors.

- Keep a list of all medications you are giving your child, including prescription, over-the-counter, and herbal medications. Share this list with any health care provider who cares for your child. Never assume that a health care provider already knows what your child is taking.

- Never use adult medications to treat a child. The body organs and systems of children, primarily their liver and kidneys, are very different from those of an adult. As a result, children respond differently to drugs.

- Read all labels before giving your child a drug. Many over-the-counter drugs contain the same ingredients, and you could accidentally overdose your child if you are not careful. In addition, some over-the-counter drugs are not to be used in children younger than a certain age. Dosages also may differ for children.

(continued)

> **Patient teaching to prevent medication errors** (continued)
>
> - Measure liquid medications using appropriate measuring devices. Never use your flatware teaspoon or tablespoon to measure your child's drugs. Always use a measured dosing device or the spoon from a measuring set.
> - Call your health care provider immediately if your child seems to get worse or seems to be having trouble with a drug. Do not hesitate; many drugs can cause serious or life-threatening problems in children, and you should act immediately.
> - When in doubt, do not hesitate to ask questions. You are your child's best advocate.

Women of childbearing age

As a general rule, it is best to avoid taking any drugs while pregnant. Advise women who may be pregnant of Pregnancy Category X drugs (statins, hormones) that could cause serious harm to the fetus. Advise any woman who is pregnant to avoid all OTC drugs and herbal therapies until she has checked with her obstetrician for safety. Also advise her to question all prescription drugs and check carefully to make sure that they are safe for the fetus. A woman who is breast-feeding should always check for safety of prescribed drugs, OTC drugs, or herbal therapies she is considering using to make sure that the drug or therapy will not adversely affect the baby.

Medication disposal

The White House Office of National Drug Control Policy, the Department of Health and Human Services, and the Environmental Protection Agency have established guidelines for the proper disposal of unused, unneeded, or expired medications to promote consumer safety, block access to them by potential abusers, and protect the water supply and the environment from possible contamination. (See *Medication disposal guidelines,* page 13.)

Error reporting

In recent years, the incidence of medication errors has become a frequent media headline. As the population ages and more people are taking multiple medications—and as more drugs become available—the possibilities for medication errors seem to be increasing.

Institutions have adopted policies for reporting errors, which protect patients and staff and identify the need for educational programs within the institution, but it is also important to submit information about errors to national programs. These national programs, coordinated by the US Pharmacopeia (USP), help to gather and disseminate information about errors, to prevent their recurrence at other sites and by other providers. These reports might prompt the issuing of prescriber warnings to alert health care providers about potential or actual medication errors and to prevent these same errors from recurring. The reporting of actual or potential errors results in alerts and publicity about sound-alike drug names, problems with abbreviations, the need for clear writing of dosages and times, incorrect calculations, and transcribing issues.

The strongest warning that the Food and Drug Administration (FDA) can give about potential drug problems is called a "black box warning." This warning may be part of the initial drug prescribing information, if a drug is found to have potentially serious adverse effects before approval, or the warning may be added as a result of postmarketing reports of adverse effects or serious errors involving the drug. The black box warning alerts the health care provider and patient about screening to be done, adverse effects to watch for, and other drugs to avoid. The monographs in this book highlight black box warnings to help bring attention to these reported effects and to help decrease medication errors and promote patient safety.

SAFETY NET
Medical disposal guidelines

It is important to know how to safely dispose of medications. When disposing of medications, follow these guidelines:

Disposing in trash
- Take unused, unneeded, or expired medications out of their original containers.
- Mix the medication with an undesirable substance, such as coffee grounds or used kitty litter, and place it in an impermeable, nondescript container, such as an empty can or a sealable storage bag. These steps help keep the medication from being diverted for illicit use or being accidentally ingested by children or animals.
- Place the closed container in your household trash.

Disposing in toilet
- Flush prescription drugs down the toilet only if the accompanying patient information specifically instructs you to do so.

Disposing at a hospital or government-sponsored site
- You may be able to return unused, unneeded, or expired prescription drugs to a pharmaceutical take-back location that offers safe disposal. Check with your local hospital, health department, or local government for a site near you.

Witnessing an error

If you witness or participate in an actual or potential medication error, it is important to report that error to the national clearinghouse to ultimately help other professionals avoid similar errors. To help streamline the process of reporting and make it as easy as possible for professionals to participate, the USP maintains one central reporting center, from which it disseminates information to the FDA, drug manufacturers, and the Institute for Safe Medication Practices (ISMP). You can report an actual error or potential error by calling 1-800-23-ERROR, the USP Medication Errors Reporting Program. Their office will send you a mailer to fill out and return to them. Or, you can log on to www.usp.org to report an error online or to print out the form to mail or fax back to the USP. You may request to remain anonymous to all institutions to which the report is subsequently disseminated if you feel uncomfortable sharing this information. If you are not sure about what you want to report, you may report errors to the USP through the ISMP website at www.ismp.org, which also offers a discussion forum on medication errors.

What kinds of errors should be reported?

Errors (or potential errors) to report include administration of the wrong drug, strength, or dose of a drug; incorrect routes of administration; miscalculations; misuse of medical equipment; mistakes in prescribing or transcribing (misunderstanding of verbal orders); and errors resulting from sound-alike or look-alike names.

In your report, you will be asked to include the following:
1. A description of the error or preventable adverse drug reaction. What went wrong?
2. Was this an actual medication accident (reached the patient) or are you expressing concern about a potential error or writing about an error that was discovered before it reached the patient?
3. Patient outcome. Did the patient suffer any adverse effects?
4. Type of practice site (eg, hospital, private office, retail pharmacy, drug company, long-term care facility)
5. Generic name (International Nonproprietary Name [INN] or official name) of all products involved

6. Brand name of all products involved
7. Dosage form, concentration or strength, and so forth
8. Where the error was based on a communication problem, is a sample of the order available? Are package label samples or pictures available if requested?
9. Your recommendations for error prevention. You will also be asked to provide your name, title, facility address, and e-mail, fax, or phone number if someone wants to contact you about details. You can remain anonymous and no one will contact your employer to discuss the report. The ISMP publishes case studies and publicizes warnings and alerts based on clinician reports of medication errors. Their efforts have helped to increase recognition of the many types of errors, such as those involving sound-alike names, look-alike names and packaging, instructions on equipment and delivery devices, and others.

Pharmacologic Classes

PREGNANCY CATEGORY D

Therapeutic actions

Alkylating drugs are cytotoxic: They alkylate cellular DNA, interfering with the replication of susceptible cells and causing cell death. Their action is most evident in rapidly dividing cells.

Indications

- Palliative treatment of chronic lymphocytic leukemia; malignant lymphomas, including lymphosarcoma, giant follicular lymphoma; brain tumors; Hodgkin's lymphoma; multiple myelomas; testicular cancers; pancreatic cancer; ovarian and breast cancers
- Used as part of multiple-drug regimens

Contraindications and cautions

- Contraindicated with hypersensitivity to the drugs, concurrent radiation therapy, hematopoietic suppression, pregnancy, lactation.

Adverse effects

- **CNS:** *Tremors, muscular twitching, confusion,* agitation, ataxia, flaccid paresis, hallucinations, seizures
- **Dermatologic:** *Skin rash, urticaria, alopecia,* keratitis
- **GI:** Nausea, vomiting, anorexia, **hepatotoxicity**
- **GU:** Sterility
- **Hematologic:** *Bone marrow depression,* hyperuricemia
- **Respiratory:** Bronchopulmonary dysplasia, **pulmonary fibrosis**
- **Other:** *Cancer, acute leukemia*

■ Nursing considerations

Assessment

- **History:** Hypersensitivity to drug, radiation therapy, hematopoietic depression, pregnancy, lactation
- **Physical:** T; weight; skin color, lesions; R, adventitious sounds; liver evaluation; CBC, differential, Hgb, uric acid, LFTs, renal function tests

Interventions

⊗ **Black box warning** Arrange for blood tests to evaluate hematopoietic function prior to and weekly during therapy; severe bone marrow suppression is possible.

- Restrict dosage within 4 wk after a full course of radiation therapy or chemotherapy because of risk of severe bone marrow suppression.
- Ensure that patient is well hydrated before treatment.
- Arrange for frequent small meals and dietary consultation to maintain nutrition if GI upset occurs.
- Arrange for skin care for rashes.

⊗ **Black box warning** Suggest use of contraception; serious fetal abnormalities or death is possible.

Teaching points

- You may experience these side effects: Nausea, vomiting, loss of appetite (dividing dose may help; frequent small meals may help; maintain fluid intake and nutrition; drink at least 10–12 glasses of fluid each day); infertility (potentially irreversible and irregular menses to amenorrhea and aspermia; discuss feelings with your health care provider); these drugs can cause severe birth defects; use birth control methods while on these drugs.
- Report unusual bleeding or bruising; fever, chills, sore throat; cough, shortness of breath; yellowing of the skin or eyes; flank or stomach pain.

Representative drugs

altretamine
bendamustine
busulfan
carboplatin
carmustine
chlorambucil
cisplatin
cyclophosphamide
dacarbazine
estramustine

ifosfamide
lomustine
mechlorethamine
melphalan
oxaliplatin
procarbazine
streptozocin
thiotepa

Alpha₁-adrenergic Blockers

PREGNANCY CATEGORY C

Therapeutic actions

Alpha₁-adrenergic blockers selectively block postsynaptic alpha₁-adrenergic receptors, decreasing sympathetic tone on the vasculature, dilating arterioles and veins, and lowering both supine and standing BP; unlike conventional alpha-adrenergic blockers (phentolamine), they do not also block alpha₂ presynaptic receptors, so they do not cause reflex tachycardia. They also relax smooth muscle of bladder and prostate.

Indications

- Treatment of hypertension (alone or with other drugs)
- Treatment of BPH (alfuzosin, doxazosin, terazosin, tamsulosin)
- Unlabeled uses: Symptomatic treatment of chronic abacterial prostatitis (terazosin)

Contraindications and cautions

- Contraindicated with hypersensitivity to any alpha₁-adrenergic blocker, lactation.
- Use cautiously with heart failure, renal failure, pregnancy.

Adverse effects

- **CNS:** *Dizziness, headache, drowsiness, lack of energy, weakness,* nervousness, vertigo, depression, paresthesias
- **CV:** *Palpitations,* sodium and water retention, increased plasma volume, edema, dyspnea, syncope, tachycardia, orthostatic hypotension
- **Dermatologic:** Rash, pruritus, lichen planus
- **EENT:** Blurred vision, reddened sclera, epistaxis, tinnitus, dry mouth, nasal congestion

- **GI:** *Nausea,* vomiting, diarrhea, constipation, abdominal discomfort or pain
- **GU:** Urinary frequency, incontinence, impotence
- **Other:** Diaphoresis

Interactions

✳ **Drug-drug** • Severity and duration of hypotension following first dose of drug may be greater in patients receiving beta-adrenergic blockers (propranolol), verapamil • Risk of severe hypotension if combined with sildenafil, tadalafil, vardenafil • Increased risk of hypotension if combined with alcohol

■ Nursing considerations
Assessment

- **History:** Hypersensitivity to any alpha₁-adrenergic blocker, heart failure, renal failure, lactation
- **Physical:** Weight; skin color, lesions; orientation, affect, reflexes; ophthalmologic examination; P, BP, orthostatic BP, supine BP, perfusion, edema, auscultation; R, adventitious sounds, status of nasal mucous membranes; bowel sounds, normal output; voiding pattern, normal output; renal function tests, urinalysis

Interventions

- Administer, or have patient take, first dose at night to lessen likelihood of first-dose syncope believed to be caused by excessive orthostatic hypotension.
- Have patient lie down, and treat supportively if syncope occurs; condition is self-limiting.
- Monitor patient for orthostatic hypotension: most marked in the morning, accentuated by hot weather, alcohol, exercise.
- Monitor edema, weight in patients with incipient cardiac decompensation; arrange to add a thiazide diuretic to the drug regimen if sodium and fluid retention, signs of impending heart failure occur.
- Provide frequent small meals, frequent mouth care if GI effects occur.
- Establish safety precautions if CNS, hypotensive changes occur (side rails, accompany patient).
- Arrange for analgesic for patients experiencing headache.

Teaching points

- Take these drugs exactly as prescribed. Take the first dose at bedtime. Do not drive a car

or operate machinery for 4 hours after the first dose.
- Avoid over-the-counter drugs (nose drops, cold remedies) while taking these drugs. If you feel you need one of these preparations, consult your health care provider.
- You may experience these side effects: Dizziness, weakness may occur when changing position, in the early morning, after exercise, in hot weather, and after consuming alcohol; tolerance may occur after taking these drugs for a while, but avoid driving or engaging in tasks that require alertness while experiencing these symptoms; change position slowly, and use caution in climbing stairs; lie down if dizziness persists; GI upset (frequent small meals may help); dry mouth (sucking on sugarless candies, ice chips may help); stuffy nose. Most of these effects will stop with continued therapy.
- Report frequent dizziness or faintness.

Representative drugs
alfuzosin
doxazosin
prazosin
silodosin
tamsulosin
terazosin

Aminoglycosides

PREGNANCY CATEGORY D

Therapeutic actions
Aminoglycosides are antibiotics that are bactericidal. They inhibit protein synthesis in susceptible strains of gram-negative bacteria and appear to disrupt the functional integrity of bacterial cell membrane, causing cell death. Oral aminoglycosides are very poorly absorbed and are used for the suppression of GI bacterial flora.

Indications
- Short-term treatment of serious infections caused by susceptible strains of *Pseudomonas* species, *Escherichia coli*, indole-positive *Proteus* species, *Providencia* species, *Klebsiella-Enterobacter-Serratia* species, *Acinetobacter* species
- Suspected gram-negative infections before results of susceptibility studies are known

- Initial treatment of staphylococcal infections when penicillin is contraindicated or when infection may be caused by mixed organisms
- Neonatal sepsis when other antibiotics cannot be used (used in combination with penicillin-type drug)
- Unlabeled uses: As part of a multidrug regimen for treatment of *Mycobacterium avium* complex (a common infection in AIDS patients) and orally for the treatment of intestinal amebiasis; adjunctive treatment of hepatic coma and for suppression of intestinal bacteria for surgery

Contraindications and cautions
- Contraindicated with allergy to any aminoglycosides, renal disease, hepatic disease, preexisting hearing loss, myasthenia gravis, parkinsonism, infant botulism, lactation.
- Use cautiously in elderly patients; patients with diminished hearing; patients with decreased renal function, dehydration, neuromuscular disorders, pregnancy.

Adverse effects
- **CNS:** *Ototoxicity,* confusion, disorientation, depression, lethargy, nystagmus, visual disturbances, headache, fever, numbness, tingling, tremor, paresthesias, muscle twitching, seizures, muscular weakness, neuromuscular blockade, apnea
- **CV:** Palpitations, hypotension, hypertension
- **GI:** Nausea, vomiting, anorexia, diarrhea, weight loss, stomatitis, increased salivation, splenomegaly
- **GU:** *Nephrotoxicity*
- **Hematologic:** Leukemoid reaction, agranulocytosis, granulocytosis, leukopenia, leukocytosis, thrombocytopenia, eosinophilia, pancytopenia, anemia, hemolytic anemia, increased or decreased reticulocyte count, electrolyte disturbances
- **Hepatic:** Hepatic toxicity, hepatomegaly
- **Hypersensitivity:** Purpura, rash, urticaria, exfoliative dermatitis, itching
- **Other:** *Superinfections, pain and irritation at IM injection sites*

Interactions
✳ **Drug-drug** • Increased ototoxic and nephrotoxic effects if taken with potent diuretics and similarly toxic drugs (cephalosporins) • Increased likelihood of neuromuscular blockade if given shortly after general anesthetics,

depolarizing and nondepolarizing neuromuscular junction blockers

■ **Nursing considerations**

Assessment

- **History:** Allergy to any aminoglycosides, renal disease, hepatic disease, preexisting hearing loss, myasthenia gravis, parkinsonism, infant botulism, lactation, diminished hearing, decreased renal function, dehydration, neuromuscular disorders
- **Physical:** Arrange culture and sensitivity tests of infection prior to therapy; renal function tests before, during, and after therapy; eighth cranial nerve function, and state of hydration, during and after therapy; LFTs, CBC; skin color, lesions; orientation, affect; reflexes, bilateral grip strength; body weight; bowel sounds

Interventions

⊗ **Black box warning** Monitor patient carefully for severe renal toxicity and ototoxicity; discontinue drug or adjust dosage at first indication of either.

- Arrange for culture and sensitivity testing of infected area prior to treatment.
- Monitor duration of treatment: Usual duration is 7–10 days. If no clinical response within 3–5 days, stop therapy. Prolonged treatment leads to increased risk of toxicity. If drug is used longer than 10 days, monitor auditory and renal function daily.
- Give IM dosage by deep injection.
- Ensure that patient is well hydrated before and during therapy.
- Establish safety measures if CNS, vestibular nerve effects occur (use of side rails, assistance with ambulation).
- Provide frequent small meals if nausea, anorexia occur.
- Provide comfort measures and medication for superinfections.
- Monitor drug levels periodically if used for prolonged periods.

Teaching points

- Take full course of oral neomycin, drink plenty of fluids.
- You may experience these side effects: Ringing in the ears, headache, dizziness (reversible; safety measures need to be taken if severe); nausea, vomiting, loss of appetite (frequent small meals, frequent mouth care may help).

- Report pain at injection site, severe headache, dizziness, loss of hearing, changes in urine pattern, difficulty breathing, rash or skin lesions.

Representative drugs

amikacin
gentamicin
neomycin
streptomycin
tobramycin

Angiotensin-converting Enzyme (ACE) Inhibitors

PREGNANCY CATEGORY C
(FIRST TRIMESTER)

PREGNANCY CATEGORY D
(SECOND AND THIRD TRIMESTERS)

Therapeutic actions

ACE inhibitors block ACE in the lungs from converting angiotensin I, activated when renin is released from the kidneys, to angiotensin II, a powerful vasoconstrictor. Blocking this conversion leads to decreased BP, decreased aldosterone secretion, a small increase in serum potassium levels, and sodium and fluid loss; increased prostaglandin synthesis also may be involved in the antihypertensive action.

Indications

- Treatment of hypertension (alone or with thiazide-type diuretics)
- Treatment of heart failure (used with diuretics and digitalis)
- Treatment of stable patients within 24 hr of acute MI to improve survival (lisinopril)
- Reduction in risk of MI, stroke, and death from CV causes (ramipril)
- Treatment of left ventricular dysfunction post-MI (captopril, trandolapril)
- Treatment of asymptomatic left ventricular dysfunction (enalapril)
- Treatment of diabetic nephropathy (captopril)
- Unlabeled uses: Renovascular hypertension, nondiabetic nephropathy, migraine prophylaxis, stroke prevention, heart failure, high risk of CAD, diabetes, chronic renal disease, scleroderma renal crisis

Adverse effects in *italics* are most common; those in **bold** are life-threatening. ⊂▭⊃ Do not crush.

Contraindications and cautions

- Contraindicated with allergy to the drug, impaired renal function, heart failure, salt or volume depletion, lactation, pregnancy, history of angioedema, bilateral renal artery stenosis.

Adverse effects

- **CNS:** Dizziness, headache, fatigue
- **CV:** Tachycardia, angina pectoris, **MI,** Raynaud's syndrome, heart failure, hypotension in salt- or volume-depleted patients
- **Dermatologic:** *Rash,* pruritus, alopecia, pemphigoid-like reaction, scalded mouth sensation, exfoliative dermatitis, photosensitivity
- **GI:** *Gastric irritation, aphthous ulcers,* peptic ulcers, dysgeusia, cholestatic jaundice, hepatocellular injury, anorexia, constipation
- **GU:** Proteinuria, renal insufficiency, **renal failure,** polyuria, oliguria, urinary frequency
- **Hematologic:** Neutropenia, agranulocytosis, thrombocytopenia, hemolytic anemia, **pancytopenia,** hyperkalemia
- **Other:** *Cough,* malaise, dry mouth, lymphadenopathy, angioedema

Interactions

✴ **Drug-drug** ● Increased risk of hypersensitivity reactions with allopurinol ● Decreased antihypertensive effects with indomethacin ● Increased risk of hyperkalemia if combined with aldosterone blockers, potassium-sparing diuretics, aliskiren, cyclosporine, potassium supplements
✴ **Drug-food** ● Decreased absorption of selected drugs if taken with food
✴ **Drug-lab test** ● False-positive test for urine acetone

■ Nursing considerations
Assessment

- **History:** Allergy to ACE inhibitors, impaired renal function, heart failure, salt or volume depletion, pregnancy, lactation
- **Physical:** Skin color, lesions, turgor; T, P, BP, peripheral perfusion; mucous membranes; bowel sounds; liver evaluation; urinalysis, LFTs, renal function tests, CBC and differential, potassium levels

Interventions

⊗ **Black box warning** Ensure that patient is not pregnant before beginning therapy; serious fetal effects can occur.

- Administer 1 hr before or 2 hr after meals; is affected by food in GI tract (captopril, moexipril).
- Alert surgeon and mark patient's chart that ACE inhibitor is being taken; angiotensin II formation subsequent to compensatory renin release during surgery will be blocked; hypotension may be reversed with volume expansion.
- Monitor patient closely in situations that may lead to a fall in BP due to reduction in fluid volume (excessive perspiration and dehydration, vomiting, diarrhea) because excessive hypotension may occur.
- Arrange for reduced dosage in patients with impaired renal function.
- Arrange for bowel program if constipation occurs.
- Provide frequent small meals if GI upset is severe.
- Provide frequent mouth care and oral hygiene if mouth sores, alteration in taste occur.
- Caution patient to change position slowly if orthostatic changes occur.
- Provide skin care as needed.

Teaching points

- Take these drugs 1 hour before or 2 hours after meals; do not take with food (captopril, moexipril).
- Do not stop taking the medication without consulting your health care provider.
- Be careful with any conditions that may lead to a drop in blood pressure (such as diarrhea, sweating, vomiting, dehydration); if light-headedness or dizziness occurs, consult your health care provider.
- Avoid over-the-counter drugs, especially cough, cold, allergy medications. If you need one of these, consult your health care provider.
- You may experience these side effects: GI upset, loss of appetite, change in taste perception (limited effects; if they persist or become a problem, consult your health care provider); mouth sores (frequent mouth care may help); rash; fast heart rate; dizziness, light-headedness (passes after a few days of therapy; if it occurs, change position slowly and limit activities requiring alertness and precision); cough.
- Report mouth sores; sore throat, fever, chills; swelling of the hands, feet; irregular heartbeat, chest pains; swelling of the face, eyes, lips, tongue; difficulty breathing.

Representative drugs
benazepril
captopril
enalapril
enalaprilat
fosinopril
lisinopril
moexipril
perindopril
quinapril
ramipril
trandolapril

Angiotensin II Receptor Blockers (ARBs)

PREGNANCY CATEGORY C
(FIRST TRIMESTER)

PREGNANCY CATEGORY D
(SECOND AND THIRD TRIMESTERS)

Therapeutic actions
ARBs selectively block the binding of angiotensin II to specific tissue receptors found in the vascular smooth muscle and adrenal gland. This action blocks the vasoconstriction effect of the renin-angiotensin system as well as the release of aldosterone leading to decreased BP; may block vessel remodeling that occurs in hypertension and contributes to the development of atherosclerosis.

Indications
- Treatment of hypertension, alone or in combination with other antihypertensives
- Nephropathy in type 2 diabetes (losartan, irbesartan)
- Treatment of heart failure in patients resistant to ACE inhibitors (valsartan)
- Reduction in the risk of stroke in patients with hypertension and left ventricular hypertrophy (losartan)

Contraindications and cautions
- Contraindicated with hypersensitivity to any ARB, pregnancy (use during the second or third trimester can cause injury or even death to the fetus), lactation.
- Use cautiously with renal impairment, hypovolemia.

Adverse effects
- **CNS:** Headache, dizziness, syncope, muscle weakness, *fatigue, depression*
- **CV:** Hypotension
- **Dermatologic:** Rash, inflammation, urticaria, pruritus, alopecia, dry skin
- **GI:** Diarrhea, *abdominal pain,* nausea, constipation
- **Respiratory:** *URI symptoms,* cough, sinus disorders
- **Other:** Cancer in preclinical studies, UTIs, pain

Interactions
✳ **Drug-drug** ● Decreased effectiveness if combined with phenobarbital ● Risk of increased lithium levels ● Risk of hyperkalemia if combined with potassium-sparing diuretics, potassium supplements, salt substitutes, aliskiren

■ Nursing considerations
Assessment
- **History:** Hypersensitivity to any ARB, pregnancy, lactation, renal impairment, hypovolemia
- **Physical:** Skin lesions, turgor; body T; reflexes, affect; BP; R, respiratory auscultation; renal function tests

Interventions
- Administer without regard to meals.
- ⊗ **Black box warning** Ensure that patient is not pregnant before beginning therapy; suggest the use of barrier contraception; fetal injury and deaths have been reported.
- Find an alternative method of feeding infant if ARBs are given to a nursing mother. Depression of the renin-angiotensin system in infants is potentially very dangerous.
- Alert surgeon and mark on patient's chart that an ARB is being taken. The blockage of the renin-angiotensin system after surgery can produce problems. Hypotension may be reversed with volume expansion.
- If BP control does not reach desired levels, diuretics or other antihypertensives may be added to the drug regimen. Monitor patient's BP carefully.
- Monitor patient closely in situations that may cause a decrease in BP secondary to reduction in fluid volume—excessive perspiration, dehydration, vomiting, diarrhea—excessive hypotension can occur.

Adverse effects in *italics* are most common; those in **bold** are life-threatening. ⊂⊃ Do not crush.

Teaching points

- Take these drugs without regard to meals. Do not stop taking these drugs without consulting your health care provider.
- Use a barrier method of birth control while using these drugs; if you become pregnant or desire to become pregnant, consult your physician.
- You may experience these side effects: Dizziness (avoid driving a car or performing hazardous tasks); nausea, abdominal pain (proper nutrition is important; consult a dietitian to maintain nutrition); symptoms of upper respiratory tract or urinary tract infection, cough (do not self-medicate, consult your health care provider if this becomes uncomfortable).
- Report fever, chills, dizziness, pregnancy.

Representative drugs

azilsartan
candesartan
eprosartan
irbesartan
losartan
olmesartan
telmisartan
valsartan

Antiarrhythmics

PREGNANCY CATEGORY C

Therapeutic actions

Antiarrhythmics act at specific sites to alter the action potential of cardiac cells and interfere with the electrical excitability of the heart. Most of these drugs may cause new or worsened arrhythmias (proarrhythmic effect) and must be used with caution and with continual cardiac monitoring and patient evaluation.

Indications

- Treatment of tachycardia when rapid but short-term control of ventricular rate is desirable (patients with atrial fibrillation, atrial flutter, in both perioperative and postoperative situations)
- Treatment of noncompensatory tachycardia when heart rate requires specific intervention
- Treatment of atrial arrhythmias

Contraindications and cautions

- There are no contraindications; reserve for emergency situations.
- Use cautiously during pregnancy or lactation.

Adverse effects

- **CNS:** *Light-headedness, speech disorder, midscapular pain, weakness, rigors,* somnolence, confusion
- **CV:** *Hypotension,* pallor, arrhythmias
- **GI:** *Taste perversion*
- **GU:** *Urine retention*
- **Local:** *Inflammation,* induration, edema, erythema, burning at the site of infusion
- **Other:** Fever, rhonchi, flushing

Interactions

✳ **Drug-drug** ● Increased risk of drug interactions with antiarrhythmic use; monitor patients

■ Nursing considerations

Assessment

- **History:** Cardiac disease, cerebrovascular disease
- **Physical:** P, BP, ECG; orientation, reflexes; R, adventitious sounds; urinary output

Interventions

- Ensure that more toxic drug is not used in chronic settings when transfer to another drug is anticipated.
- Monitor BP, heart rate, and rhythm closely.
- Provide comfort measures for pain, rigors, fever, flushing, if patient is awake.
- Provide supportive measures appropriate to condition being treated.
- Provide support and encouragement to deal with drug effects and discomfort of IV lines.
- Monitor drug levels for procainamide and amiodarone, as indicated.

Teaching points

- Reserved for emergency use. Incorporate information about these drugs into the overall teaching program for patient. Patients maintained on oral drugs will need specific teaching.

Representative drugs

Type IA

disopyramide
quinidine

Type IB
lidocaine
mexiletine
phenytoin
Type IC
flecainide
propafenone
Type II
acebutolol
esmolol
propranolol
Type III
amiodarone
dofetilide
ibutilide
sotalol
Type IV
diltiazem
verapamil
Other
adenosine
digoxin
dronedarone

Anticoagulants

DANGEROUS DRUG

PREGNANCY CATEGORY C
(HEPARIN, DABIGATRAN,
RIVAROXABAN), X (WARFARIN), B
(LOW–MOLECULAR-WEIGHT HEPARINS)

Therapeutic actions

Oral anticoagulants interfere with the hepatic synthesis of vitamin K–dependent clotting factors (factors II, prothrombin, VII, IX, and X), resulting in their eventual depletion and prolongation of clotting times; parenteral anticoagulants interfere with the conversion of prothrombin to thrombin, blocking the final step in clot formation but leaving the circulating levels of clotting factors unaffected.

Indications

- Treatment and prevention of pulmonary embolism and venous thrombosis and its extension
- Treatment of atrial fibrillation with embolization
- Prevention of DVT
- Prophylaxis of systemic embolization after acute MI

- Prevention of thrombi following specific surgical procedures and prolonged bedrest (low–molecular-weight heparins)
- Unlabeled uses: Prevention of recurrent TIAs and MI

Contraindications and cautions

- Contraindicated with allergy to the drug; SBE; hemorrhagic disorders; TB; hepatic diseases; GI ulcers; renal disease; indwelling catheters, spinal puncture; aneurysm; diabetes; visceral carcinoma; uncontrolled hypertension; severe trauma (including recent or contemplated CNS, eye surgery, recent placement of IUD); threatened abortion, menometrorrhagia; pregnancy (oral drugs cause fetal damage and death); or lactation (heparin if anticoagulation is required).
- Use cautiously with heart failure, diarrhea, fever, thyrotoxicosis; patients with dementia, psychosis, depression.

Adverse effects

- **Bleeding:** *Hemorrhage;* GI or urinary tract bleeding (hematuria, dark stools; paralytic ileus; intestinal obstruction from hemorrhage into GI tract); petechiae and purpura, bleeding from mucous membranes; hemorrhagic infarction, vasculitis, skin necrosis of female breast; adrenal hemorrhage and resultant adrenal insufficiency; compressive neuropathy secondary to hemorrhage near a nerve
- **Dermatologic:** *Alopecia, urticaria, dermatitis*
- **GI:** *Nausea,* vomiting, anorexia, abdominal cramping, diarrhea, retroperitoneal hematoma, hepatitis, jaundice, mouth ulcers
- **GU:** Priapism, nephropathy, red-orange urine
- **Hematologic:** Granulocytosis, leukopenia, eosinophilia
- **Other:** Fever, "purple toes" syndrome

Interactions

✳ **Drug-drug** • Increased bleeding tendencies with salicylates, chloral hydrate, phenylbutazone, disulfiram, chloramphenicol, metronidazole, cimetidine, ranitidine, cotrimoxazole, sulfinpyrazone, quinidine, thyroid drugs, glucagon, erythromycin, androgens, amiodarone, cefoxitin, ceftriaxone, mefenamic acid, famotidine, nizatidine, nalidixic acid, fluoroquinolones
• Possible decreased anticoagulation effect with barbiturates, rifampin, phenytoin, carbamazepine, vitamin K, vitamin E, cholestyramine

Adverse effects in *italics* are most common; those in **bold** are life-threatening. ▭ Do not crush.

• Altered effects of warfarin with methimazole, propylthiouracil • Increased activity and toxicity of phenytoin with oral anticoagulants

✳ **Drug-alternative therapy** • Increased risk of bleeding with chamomile, garlic, ginger, ginkgo, ginseng therapy, turmeric, horse chestnut, green tea leaf, grape seed extract, feverfew, dong quai

✳ **Drug-lab test** • Red-orange discoloration of alkaline urine may interfere with some lab tests

■ Nursing considerations

Assessment

• **History:** Allergy to the drug; SBE; hemorrhagic disorders; tuberculosis; hepatic diseases; GI ulcers; renal diseases; indwelling catheters, spinal puncture; aneurysm; diabetes; visceral carcinoma; uncontrolled hypertension; severe trauma; threatened abortion; menometrorrhagia; pregnancy; lactation; heart failure, diarrhea, fever; thyrotoxicosis; senile, psychotic, or depressed patients

• **Physical:** Skin lesions, color, T, orientation, reflexes, affect; P, BP, peripheral perfusion, baseline ECG; R, adventitious sounds; liver evaluation, bowel sounds, normal output; CBC, urinalysis, guaiac stools, PT, INR, LFTs, renal function tests, WBCT, aPTT

Interventions

• Monitor INR (warfarin) or aPTT (heparin) to adjust dosage.

• Do not change brand names once stabilized; bioavailability problems can occur.

• Evaluate patient for signs of blood loss (petechiae, bleeding gums, bruises, dark stools, dark urine).

• Establish safety measures to protect patient from injury.

⊗ **Black box warning** Do not give to patients receiving epidural/spinal anesthesia; risk of epidural/spinal hematoma with neurologic impairment.

• Do not give patient IM injections. Monitor sites of invasive procedures; ensure prolonged compression of bleeding vessels.

• Double-check other drugs that are ordered for potential interaction: Dosages of both drugs may need to be adjusted.

• Use caution when discontinuing other medications; dosage of warfarin may need to be adjusted; carefully monitor PT and INR values.

• Keep vitamin K available in case of overdose of oral drugs; keep protamine sulfate available for parenteral drug.

• Arrange for frequent follow-up, including blood tests to evaluate drug effects.

• Evaluate for therapeutic effects: PT, 1.5–2.5 times the control value; INR, 2–3 (2.5–3.5 with prosthetic valve in place); aPTT, 1.5–2 times the control.

Teaching points

• Many factors may change your body's response to these drugs—fever, change of diet, change of environment, other medications. The dosage of the drug may have to be changed. Be sure to write down all changes prescribed.

• Do not change any medication that you are taking (adding or stopping another drug) without consulting your health care provider. Other drugs affect the way anticoagulants work; starting or stopping another drug can cause excessive bleeding or interfere with the desired effects of these drugs.

• Carry or wear a medical alert tag stating that you are using one of these drugs. This will alert medical personnel in an emergency that you are taking an anticoagulant.

• Avoid situations in which you could be easily injured—contact sports, shaving with a straight razor.

• Arrange periodic blood tests to check on the action of the drug. It is very important that you have these tests.

• Use contraceptive measures while taking these drugs; it is important that you do not become pregnant.

• You may experience these side effects: Stomach bloating, cramps (passes with time; if it becomes too uncomfortable, contact your health care provider); loss of hair, skin rash (this is a frustrating and upsetting effect; if it becomes a problem, discuss it with your health care provider); orange-red discoloration to the urine (this may be mistaken for blood; add vinegar to urine, the color should disappear).

• Report unusual bleeding (when brushing your teeth, excessive bleeding from injuries, excessive bruising), black or bloody stools, cloudy or dark urine, sore throat, fever, chills, severe headaches, dizziness, suspected pregnancy.

Representative drugs
Oral
dabigatran
rivaroxaban
warfarin sodium
Parenteral
argatroban
bivalirudin
desirudin
fondaparinux
heparin
lepirudin
Low–molecular-weight heparins
dalteparin
enoxaparin
tinzaparin

Antidiabetics

PREGNANCY CATEGORY C, B
(GLYBURIDE, METFORMIN)

Therapeutic actions
Oral antidiabetics include several drug types. One type, called the sulfonylureas, stimulates insulin release from functioning beta cells in the pancreas and may either improve binding between insulin and insulin receptors or increase the number of insulin receptors. Second-generation sulfonylureas (glipizide and glyburide) are thought to be more potent than first-generation sulfonylureas. Other types include drugs that increase insulin receptor sensitivity (thiazolidinediones); drugs that delay or alter glucose absorption (acarbose, miglitol); drugs that increase the stimulus for insulin release (DPP-4 inhibitors, incretin mimetics); and insulin, which is used for replacement therapy.

Indications
- Adjuncts to diet and exercise to lower blood glucose in patients with type 2 (non–insulin-dependent) diabetes mellitus
- Adjuncts to insulin therapy in the stabilization of certain cases of insulin-dependent maturity-onset diabetes, reducing the insulin requirement and decreasing the chance of hypoglycemic reactions
- Replacement therapy in type 1 (insulin-dependent) diabetes mellitus and when oral

drugs cannot control glucose levels in type 2 diabetes

Contraindications and cautions
- Contraindicated with allergy to sulfonylureas; diabetes complicated by fever, severe infections, severe trauma, major surgery, ketosis, acidosis, coma (insulin is indicated); type 1 diabetes, serious hepatic impairment, serious renal impairment, uremia, thyroid or endocrine impairment, glycosuria, hyperglycemia associated with primary renal disease; labor and delivery (if glipizide is used during pregnancy, discontinue drug at least 1 mo before delivery); lactation, safety not established.

Adverse effects
- **CV:** Increased risk of CV mortality
- **Endocrine:** *Hypoglycemia*
- **GI:** *Anorexia, nausea,* vomiting, *epigastric discomfort, heartburn, diarrhea*
- **Hematologic:** Leukopenia, thrombocytopenia, anemia
- **Hypersensitivity:** *Allergic skin reactions,* eczema, pruritus, erythema, urticaria, photosensitivity, fever, eosinophilia, jaundice

Interactions
✳ **Drug-drug** • Increased risk of hypoglycemia with sulfonamides, chloramphenicol, salicylates • Decreased effectiveness of both sulfonylurea and diazoxide if taken concurrently • Increased risk of hyperglycemia with rifampin, thiazides • Risk of hypoglycemia and hyperglycemia with ethanol; "disulfiram reaction" has also been reported

✳ **Drug-alternative therapy** • Increased risk of hypoglycemia with juniper berries, ginseng, garlic, fenugreek, coriander, dandelion root, celery

■ Nursing considerations
Assessment
- **History:** Allergy to sulfonylureas; diabetes complicated by fever, severe infections, severe trauma, major surgery, ketosis, acidosis, coma (insulin is indicated); type 1 diabetes, serious hepatic impairment, serious renal impairment, uremia, thyroid or endocrine impairment, glycosuria, hyperglycemia associated with primary renal disease
- **Physical:** Skin color, lesions; T; orientation, reflexes, peripheral sensation; R,

adventitious sounds; liver evaluation, bowel sounds; urinalysis, BUN, serum creatinine, LFTs, blood glucose, CBC

Interventions
- Administer in appropriate relationship to meals, based on drug.
- Monitor urine or serum glucose levels to determine effectiveness of drug and dosage.
- Arrange for transfer to insulin therapy during high stress (infections, surgery, trauma).
- Arrange for use of IV glucose if severe hypoglycemia occurs as a result of overdose.
- Arrange consultation with dietitian to establish weight loss program and dietary control as appropriate.
- Arrange thorough diabetic teaching program to include disease, dietary control, exercise, signs and symptoms of hypoglycemia and hyperglycemia, avoidance of infection, hygiene.
- Provide skin care to prevent breakdown.
- Ensure access to bathroom facilities if diarrhea occurs.
- Establish safety precautions if CNS effects occur.

Teaching points
- Do not stop taking these drugs without consulting your health care provider.
- Monitor urine or blood for glucose and ketones.
- Learn to recognize symptoms of low blood sugar and have a source of glucose readily available.
- Do not use these drugs during pregnancy (except insulin).
- Avoid alcohol while on these drugs.
- Report fever, sore throat, unusual bleeding or bruising, skin rash, dark urine, light-colored stools, hypoglycemia, or hyperglycemic reactions.

Representative drugs
acarbose
chlorpropamide
exenatide
glimepiride
glipizide
glyburide
insulin
linagliptin
liraglutide
metformin
miglitol
nateglinide
pioglitazone
pramlintide
repaglinide
rosiglitazone
saxagliptin
sitagliptin
tolazamide
tolbutamide

Antifungals

PREGNANCY CATEGORY C

Therapeutic actions
Antifungals bind to or impair sterols of fungal cell membranes, allowing increased permeability and leakage of cellular components and causing the death of the fungal cell.

Indications
- Systemic fungal infections: Candidiasis, chronic mucocutaneous candidiasis, oral thrush, candiduria, blastomycosis, coccidioidomycosis, histoplasmosis, chromomycosis, paracoccidioidomycosis, dermatophytosis, ringworm infections of the skin
- Treatment of onychomycosis, pityriasis versicolor, vaginal candidiasis; topical treatment of tinea corporis and tinea cruris caused by *Trichophyton rubrum, Trichophyton mentagrophytes,* and *Epidermophyton floccosum;* treatment of tinea versicolor caused by *Malassezia furfur* (topical); and reduction of scaling due to dandruff (shampoo)

Contraindications and cautions
- Contraindicated with allergy to any antifungal, fungal meningitis, pregnancy, lactation.
- Use cautiously with hepatocellular failure (increased risk of hepatocellular necrosis).

Adverse effects
- **CNS:** Headache, dizziness, somnolence, photophobia
- **GI: Hepatotoxicity,** *nausea, vomiting,* abdominal pain
- **GU:** Impotence, oligospermia (with very high doses), **nephrotoxicity**
- **Hematologic:** Thrombocytopenia, leukopenia, hemolytic anemia
- **Hypersensitivity:** Urticaria to anaphylaxis

- **Local:** *Severe irritation, pruritus, stinging* with topical application
- **Other:** *Pruritus,* fever, chills, gynecomastia, electrolyte abnormalities (amphotericin B)

Interactions

✳ **Drug-drug** • Decreased blood levels with rifampin • Increased blood levels of cyclosporine and risk of toxicity with antifungals • Increased duration of adrenal suppression when methylprednisolone, corticosteroids are taken with antifungals

■ Nursing considerations

Assessment

- **History:** Allergy to antifungals, fungal meningitis, hepatocellular failure, pregnancy, lactation
- **Physical:** Skin color, lesions; orientation, reflexes, affect; bowel sounds, liver evaluation, LFTs; CBC and differential; culture of area involved

Interventions

⊗ **Black box warning** Reserve systemic antifungals for patients with progressive and potentially fatal infections because of severe toxicity.

- Arrange for culture before beginning therapy; treatment should begin prior to lab results.
- Maintain epinephrine on standby in case of severe anaphylaxis after first dose.
- Administer oral drug with food to decrease GI upset.
- Administer until infection is eradicated: candidiasis, 1–2 wk; other systemic mycoses, 6 mo; chronic mucocutaneous candidiasis often requires maintenance therapy; tinea versicolor, 2 wk of topical application.
- Discontinue treatment and consult physician about diagnosis if no improvement within 2 wk of topical application.
- Discontinue topical applications if sensitivity or chemical reaction occurs.
- Administer shampoo as follows: Moisten hair and scalp thoroughly with water; apply sufficient shampoo to produce a lather; gently massage for 1 min; rinse hair with warm water; repeat, leaving on hair for 3 min.
- Provide hygiene measures to control sources of infection or reinfection.

- Provide frequent small meals if GI upset occurs.
- Provide comfort measures appropriate to site of fungal infection.
- Arrange hepatic function tests prior to therapy and at least monthly during treatment.
- Establish safety precautions if CNS effects occur (side rails, assistance with ambulation).

Teaching points

- Take the full course of therapy. Long-term use of the drug will be needed; beneficial effects may not be seen for several weeks. Take oral drugs with meals to decrease GI upset. Apply topical drugs to affected area and surrounding area. Shampoo—moisten hair and scalp thoroughly with water; apply to produce a lather; gently massage for 1 minute; rinse with warm water; repeat, leaving on for 3 minutes. Shampoo twice a week for 4 weeks with at least 3 days between shampooing.
- Use hygiene measures to prevent reinfection or spread of infection.
- You may experience these side effects: Nausea, vomiting, diarrhea (take drug with food); sedation, dizziness, confusion (avoid driving or performing tasks that require alertness); stinging, irritation (local application).
- Report skin rash, severe nausea, vomiting, diarrhea, fever, sore throat, unusual bleeding or bruising, yellowing of skin or eyes, dark urine or pale stools, severe irritation (local applications).

Representative drugs

amphotericin B
anidulafungin
butenafine
butoconazole
caspofungin
ciclopirox
clotrimazole
econazole
fluconazole
flucytosine
griseofulvin
itraconazole
ketoconazole
micafungin
miconazole
naftifine
nystatin

oxiconazole
posaconazole
sertaconazole
terbinafine
tolnaftate
voriconazole

Antihistamines

PREGNANCY CATEGORY B OR C

Therapeutic actions
Antihistamines competitively block the effects of histamine at peripheral H_1 receptor sites, have anticholinergic (atropine-like) and antipruritic effects.

Indications
- Relief of symptoms associated with perennial and seasonal allergic rhinitis, vasomotor rhinitis, allergic conjunctivitis, mild, uncomplicated urticaria and angioedema
- Amelioration of allergic reactions to blood or plasma
- Treatment of dermatographism
- Management of tremor in early parkinsonian syndrome and drug-induced extrapyramidal reactions
- Control of nausea, vomiting, and dizziness from motion sickness (buclizine, cyclizine, diphenhydramine, meclizine)
- Adjunctive therapy in anaphylactic reactions
- Unlabeled uses: Relief of lower respiratory conditions, such as histamine-induced bronchoconstriction in asthmatics and exercise- and hyperventilation-induced bronchospasm

Contraindications and cautions
- Contraindicated with allergy to antihistamines, pregnancy, or lactation.
- Use cautiously with narrow-angle glaucoma, stenosing peptic ulcer, symptomatic prostatic hypertrophy, asthmatic attack, bladder neck obstruction, pyloroduodenal obstruction.

Adverse effects
- **CNS:** *Depression,* nightmares, sedation
- **CV:** Arrhythmia, increase in QTc intervals
- **Dermatologic:** Alopecia, angioedema, skin eruption and itching
- **GI:** *Dry mouth, GI upset,* anorexia, increased appetite, nausea, vomiting, diarrhea, constipation

- **GU:** Galactorrhea, menstrual disorders, dysuria, hesitancy
- **Respiratory:** *Bronchospasm, cough, thickening of secretions*
- **Other:** Musculoskeletal pain, mild to moderate transaminase elevations

Interactions
✳ **Drug-drug** • Altered antihistamine metabolism with ketoconazole, troleandomycin • Increased antihistaminic anticholinergic effects with MAOIs • Additive CNS depressant effects with alcohol, CNS depressants

■ Nursing considerations
Assessment
- **History:** Allergy to any antihistamines, narrow-angle glaucoma, stenosing peptic ulcer, symptomatic prostatic hypertrophy, asthmatic attack, bladder neck obstruction, pyloroduodenal obstruction, pregnancy, lactation
- **Physical:** Skin color, lesions, texture; orientation, reflexes, affect; vision examination; R, adventitious sounds; prostate palpation; serum transaminase levels

Interventions
- Administer with food if GI upset occurs.
- Provide mouth care, sugarless candies for dry mouth.
- Arrange for humidifier if thickening of secretions, nasal dryness become bothersome; encourage intake of fluids.
- Provide skin care for dermatologic effects.

Teaching points
- Avoid excessive dosage.
- Take with food if GI upset occurs.
- Avoid alcohol; serious sedation could occur.
- You may experience these side effects: Dizziness, sedation, drowsiness (use caution driving or performing tasks that require alertness); dry mouth (mouth care, sucking sugarless candies may help); thickening of bronchial secretions, dryness of nasal mucosa (use a humidifier); menstrual irregularities.
- Report difficulty breathing, hallucinations, tremors, loss of coordination, unusual bleeding or bruising, visual disturbances, irregular heartbeat.

Representative drugs

azelastine (nasal spray only)
brompheniramine
cetirizine
chlorpheniramine
clemastine
cyclizine
cyproheptadine
desloratadine
dexchlorpheniramine
dimenhydrinate
diphenhydramine
fexofenadine
hydroxyzine
levocetirizine
loratadine
meclizine
promethazine

Antimetabolites

DANGEROUS DRUG

PREGNANCY CATEGORY D

Therapeutic actions

Antimetabolites are antineoplastic drugs that inhibit DNA polymerase. They are cell-cycle-phase–specific to S phase (stage of DNA synthesis), causing cell death for cells in the S phase; they also block progression of cells from G_1 to S in the cell cycle.

Indications

• Induction and maintenance of remission in acute myelocytic leukemia (higher response rate in children than in adults), chronic lymphocytic leukemia
• Treatment of acute lymphocytic leukemia, chronic myelocytic leukemia and erythroleukemia, meningeal leukemia, psoriasis and rheumatoid arthritis (methotrexate)
• Palliative treatment of GI adenocarcinoma, carcinomas of the colon, rectum, breast, stomach, pancreas
• Part of combination therapy for treatment of non-Hodgkin's lymphoma in children

Contraindications and cautions

• Contraindicated with allergy to the drug, pregnancy, lactation, premature infants.
• Use cautiously with hematopoietic depression secondary to radiation or chemotherapy; impaired liver function.

Adverse effects

• **CNS:** Neuritis, neural toxicity
• **Dermatologic:** Fever, rash, urticaria, freckling, skin ulceration, pruritus, conjunctivitis, alopecia
• **GI:** *Anorexia, nausea, vomiting, diarrhea, oral and anal inflammation or ulceration;* esophageal ulcerations, esophagitis, abdominal pain, *hepatic impairment* (jaundice), acute pancreatitis
• **GU:** Renal impairment, urine retention
• **Hematologic:** Bone marrow depression, hyperuricemia
• **Local:** Thrombophlebitis, cellulitis at injection site
• **Other:** *Fever, rash*

Interactions

✳ **Drug-drug** • Decreased therapeutic action of digoxin with cytarabine • Enhanced toxicity of 5-FU with leucovorin • Potentially fatal reactions if methotrexate is taken with various NSAIDs

■ Nursing considerations

Assessment

• **History:** Allergy to drug, hematopoietic depression, impaired hepatic function, lactation
• **Physical:** Weight; T; skin lesions, color; hair; orientation, reflexes; R, adventitious sounds; mucous membranes, liver evaluation, abdominal examination; CBC, differential; LFTs; renal function tests; urinalysis

Interventions

⊗ **Black box warning** Arrange for tests to evaluate hematopoietic status prior to and during therapy; serious to fatal bone marrow suppression can occur.

• Arrange for discontinuation of drug therapy if platelet count is lower than 50,000/mm³ or polymorphonuclear granulocyte count is lower than 1,000/mm³; consult physician for dosage adjustment.
• Monitor injection site for signs of thrombophlebitis, inflammation.
• Provide mouth care for mouth sores.
• Provide frequent small meals and dietary consultation to maintain nutrition when GI effects are severe.
• Establish safety measures if dizziness, CNS effects occur.

- Arrange for patient to obtain a wig or some other suitable head covering if alopecia occurs; ensure that head is covered in extremes of temperature.
- Protect patient from exposure to infections.
- Provide skin care.
- Arrange for comfort measures if anal inflammation, headache, or other pain associated with cytarabine syndrome occurs.
- Arrange for treatment of fever if it occurs.

Teaching points

- Keep the prepared calendar of treatment days available for your reference.
- Use birth control; these drugs may cause birth defects or miscarriages.
- Arrange to have frequent, regular medical follow-up, including frequent blood tests.
- You may experience these side effects: Nausea, vomiting, loss of appetite (medication may be ordered; frequent small meals may help; it is important to maintain nutrition); malaise, weakness, lethargy (these are all effects of the drug; consult your health care provider and avoid driving or operating dangerous machinery); mouth sores (frequent mouth care will be needed); diarrhea; loss of hair (you may wish to obtain a wig or other suitable head covering; keep the head covered in extremes of temperature); anal inflammation (consult with your health care provider; comfort measures can be ordered).
- Report black, tarry stools; fever, chills; sore throat; unusual bleeding or bruising; shortness of breath; chest pain; difficulty swallowing.

Representative drugs

capecitabine
cladribine
clofarabine
cytarabine
floxuridine
fludarabine
5-FU (fluorouracil)
gemcitabine
mercaptopurine
methotrexate
pemetrexed
pentostatin
rasburicase
thioguanine

Antimigraine Drugs (Triptans)

PREGNANCY CATEGORY C

Therapeutic actions

Triptans bind to serotonin receptors to cause vascular constrictive effects on cranial blood vessels, causing the relief of migraine in selective patients.

Indications

- Treatment of acute migraine attacks with or without aura
- Treatment of cluster headaches (sumatriptan injection)

Contraindications and cautions

- Contraindicated with allergy to any triptan, active coronary artery disease, uncontrolled hypertension, hemiplegic migraine, pregnancy.
- Use cautiously in the elderly; with lactation.

Adverse effects

- **CNS:** *Dizziness, vertigo,* headache, anxiety, malaise or fatigue, *weakness, myalgia*
- **CV:** *BP alterations, tightness or pressure in chest,* **MI**
- **GI:** Abdominal discomfort, dysphagia
- **Local:** *Injection site discomfort*
- **Other:** *Tingling, warm or hot sensations, burning sensation, feeling of heaviness, pressure sensation, numbness, feeling of tightness,* feeling strange, cold sensation

Interactions

✳ **Drug-drug** • Prolonged vasoactive reactions when taken concurrently with ergot-containing drugs, MAOIs, other triptans • Risk of increased blood levels and prolonged effects with hormonal contraceptives; monitor patient very closely if this combination must be used • Risk of serious serotonin syndrome if combined with SSRIs

✳ **Drug-alternative therapy** • Increased risk of severe reaction if combined with St. John's Wort

■ Nursing considerations
Assessment

- **History:** Allergy to any triptan, active coronary artery disease, uncontrolled hypertension, hemiplegic migraine, pregnancy, lactation

- **Physical:** Skin color and lesions; orientation, reflexes, peripheral sensation; P, BP; LFTs, renal function tests

Interventions

- Administer to relieve acute migraine, not as a prophylactic measure.
- Administer as prescribed—by inhalation, injection, or orally.
- Establish safety measures if CNS, visual disturbances occur.
- Provide appropriate analgesics as needed for pains related to therapy.
- Monitor injection sites—pain and redness are common—for signs of infection or irritation.
- Control environment as appropriate to help relieve migraine (eg, lighting, temperature).
- Monitor BP of patients with possible coronary artery disease; discontinue triptan at any sign of angina, prolonged high BP.

Teaching points

- Learn to use the autoinjector; injection may be repeated in no less than 1 hour if relief is not obtained; do not administer more than two injections in 24 hours (if appropriate).
- These drugs should not be taken during pregnancy; if you suspect that you are pregnant, contact your health care provider and refrain from using the drug.
- Continue to do anything that usually helps you feel better during a migraine—control lighting, noise.
- Take these drugs at first sign of a migraine.
- Contact your health care provider immediately if you experience chest pain or pressure that is severe or does not go away.
- You may experience these side effects: Dizziness, drowsiness (avoid driving or operating dangerous machinery while using these drugs); numbness, tingling, feelings of tightness or pressure.
- Report feelings of heat, flushing, tiredness, sickness, swelling of lips or eyelids.

Representative drugs

almotriptan
eletriptan
frovatriptan
naratriptan
rizatriptan
sumatriptan
zolmitriptan

Antivirals

PREGNANCY CATEGORY B or C

Therapeutic actions

Antiviral drugs inhibit viral DNA or RNA replication in the virus, preventing replication and leading to viral death.

Indications

- Initial and recurrent mucosal and cutaneous HSV-1 and HSV-2 infections in immuno-compromised patients, encephalitis, herpes zoster
- HIV infections (part of combination therapy)
- Cytomegalovirus (CMV) retinitis in patients with AIDS
- Severe initial and recurrent genital herpes infections
- Treatment and prevention of influenza A respiratory tract illness
- Prevention of CMV infection in patients receiving kidney, heart, or pancreas transplant who are considered at high risk for CMV infection
- Treatment of initial HSV genital infections and limited mucocutaneous HSV infections in immunocompromised patients (ointment)
- Unlabeled uses: Treatment of herpes zoster, CMV and HSV infection following transplant, herpes simplex infections, infectious mononucleosis, varicella pneumonia, and varicella zoster in immunocompromised patients

Contraindications and cautions

- Contraindicated with allergy to drug, seizures, heart failure, renal disease, lactation.

Adverse effects

Systemic administration

- **CNS:** Headache, vertigo, depression, tremors, encephalopathic changes, fatigue
- **Dermatologic:** *Inflammation or phlebitis at injection sites,* rash, hair loss, sweating
- **GI:** *Nausea, vomiting,* diarrhea, anorexia, taste perversion
- **GU:** Crystalluria with rapid IV administration, hematuria
- **Metabolic:** Hyperglycemia, dyslipidemia

Topical administration

- **Skin:** *Transient burning at the site of application*

Adverse effects in *italics* are most common; those in **bold** are life-threatening. Do not crush.

Interactions

✳ **Drug-drug** • Increased drug effects with probenecid • Increased nephrotoxicity with other nephrotoxic drugs

✳ **Drug-alternative therapy** • Decreased effectiveness if combined with St. John's Wort

■ Nursing considerations

Assessment

- **History:** Allergy to drug, seizures, heart failure, renal disease, lactation
- **Physical:** Skin color, lesions; orientation; BP, P, auscultation, perfusion, edema; R, adventitious sounds; urinary output; BUN, creatinine clearance

Interventions

Systemic administration

- Ensure that the patient is well hydrated with IV or PO fluids.
- Provide support and encouragement to deal with disease.
- Provide frequent small meals if systemic therapy causes GI upset.
- Provide skin care, analgesics if needed for rash.

Topical administration

- Start treatment as soon as possible after onset of signs and symptoms.
- Wear a rubber glove or finger cot when applying drug.

Teaching points

Systemic administration

- Complete the full course of oral therapy, and do not exceed the prescribed dose.
- These drugs are not a cure for your disease but they should make you feel better.
- Avoid sexual intercourse if lesions are visible.
- You may experience these side effects: Nausea, vomiting, loss of appetite, diarrhea, headache, dizziness.
- Report difficulty urinating, skin rash, increased severity or frequency of recurrences.

Topical administration

- Wear rubber gloves or finger cots to apply the drug to prevent autoinoculation of other sites and transmission of the disease.
- These drugs do not cure the disease; applying the drug during symptom-free periods will not prevent recurrences.

- Avoid sexual intercourse while visible lesions are present.
- These drugs may cause burning, stinging, itching, rash; notify your health care provider if these are pronounced.

Representative drugs

abacavir
acyclovir
acyclovir sodium
adefovir
amantadine
atazanavir
boceprevir
cidofovir
darunavir
delavirdine
didanosine
docosanol
efavirenz
emtricitabine
entecavir
etravirine
famciclovir
fosamprenavir
foscarnet
ganciclovir
imiquimod
indinavir
lamivudine
lopinavir
maraviroc
nelfinavir
nevirapine
oseltamivir
penciclovir
peramivir
raltegravir
ribavirin
rilpivirine
rimantadine
ritonavir
saquinavir
sinecatechins
stavudine
telaprevir
telbivudine
tenofovir
tipranavir
trifluridine
valacyclovir
valganciclovir
zanamivir
zidovudine

Barbiturates

PREGNANCY CATEGORY D

CONTROLLED SUBSTANCE C-II

Therapeutic actions

Barbiturates act as sedatives, hypnotics, and antiepileptics. They are general CNS depressants. Barbiturates inhibit impulse conduction in the ascending reticular activating system, depress the cerebral cortex, alter cerebellar function, depress motor output, and can produce excitation, sedation, hypnosis, anesthesia, and deep coma; at anesthetic doses, they have anticonvulsant activity.

Indications

- Sedatives or hypnotics for short-term treatment of insomnia
- Preanesthetic medications
- Antiepileptics, in anesthetic doses, for emergency control of certain acute seizure episodes (eg, status epilepticus, eclampsia, meningitis, tetanus, toxic reactions to strychnine or local anesthetics)

Contraindications and cautions

- Contraindicated with hypersensitivity to barbiturates, manifest or latent porphyria, marked hepatic impairment, nephritis, severe respiratory distress, respiratory disease with dyspnea, obstruction, or cor pulmonale, previous addiction to sedative-hypnotic drugs, pregnancy (causes fetal damage, neonatal withdrawal syndrome), or lactation.
- Use cautiously with acute or chronic pain (paradoxical excitement or masking of important symptoms could result), seizure disorders (abrupt discontinuation of daily doses of drug can result in status epilepticus), fever, hyperthyroidism, diabetes mellitus, severe anemia, pulmonary or cardiac disease, status asthmaticus, shock, uremia.

Adverse effects

- **CNS:** *Somnolence, agitation, confusion, hyperkinesia, ataxia, vertigo, CNS depression, nightmares, lethargy, residual sedation (hangover), paradoxical excitement, nervousness, psychiatric disturbance, hallucinations, insomnia, anxiety, dizziness, abnormal thinking*

- **CV:** *Bradycardia, hypotension, syncope*
- **GI:** *Nausea, vomiting, constipation, diarrhea, epigastric pain*
- **Hypersensitivity:** Skin rashes, angioneurotic edema, serum sickness, morbilliform rash, urticaria; rarely, exfoliative dermatitis, **Stevens-Johnson syndrome**
- **Local:** *Pain, tissue necrosis at injection site,* gangrene; arterial spasm with inadvertent intra-arterial injection; thrombophlebitis; permanent neurologic deficit if injected near a nerve
- **Respiratory:** *Hypoventilation, apnea, respiratory depression,* **laryngospasm, bronchospasm,** circulatory collapse
- **Other:** Tolerance, psychological and physical dependence; **withdrawal syndrome**

Interactions

✴ **Drug-drug** • Increased CNS depression with alcohol • Decreased effects of the following drugs given with barbiturates: oral anticoagulants, corticosteroids, oral contraceptives and estrogens, beta-adrenergic blockers (especially propranolol, metoprolol), theophylline, metronidazole, doxycycline, phenylbutazones, quinidine

■ Nursing considerations

Assessment

- **History:** Hypersensitivity to barbiturates; manifest or latent porphyria; marked hepatic impairment; nephritis; severe respiratory distress; respiratory disease with dyspnea, obstruction, or cor pulmonale; previous addiction to sedative-hypnotic drugs; acute or chronic pain; seizure disorders; pregnancy; lactation; fever, hyperthyroidism; diabetes mellitus; severe anemia; pulmonary or cardiac disease; status asthmaticus; shock; uremia
- **Physical:** Weight; T; skin color, lesions, injection site; orientation, affect, reflexes; P, BP, orthostatic BP; R, adventitious sounds; bowel sounds, normal output, liver evaluation; LFTs, renal function tests, blood and urine glucose, BUN

Interventions

- Do not administer intra-arterially; may produce arteriospasm, thrombosis, gangrene.
- Administer IV doses slowly.
- Administer IM doses deep in a muscle mass.

Adverse effects in *italics* are most common; those in **bold** are life-threatening. ⊂⊃ Do not crush.

- Do not use parenteral dosage forms if solution is discolored or contains a precipitate.
- Monitor injection sites carefully for irritation, extravasation (IV); solutions are alkaline and very irritating to the tissues.
- Monitor P, BP, R carefully during IV administration.
- Keep resuscitative facilities available in case of respiratory depression, hypersensitivity reaction.
- Provide frequent small meals, frequent mouth care if GI effects occur.
- Use safety precautions if CNS changes occur (use side rails, accompany patient).
- Provide skin care if dermatologic effects occur.
- Provide comfort measures, reassurance for patients receiving pentobarbital for tetanus, toxic seizures.
- Offer support and encouragement to patients receiving this drug for preanesthetic medication.
- Taper dosage gradually after repeated use, especially in patients with epilepsy.

Teaching points

When giving these drugs as preanesthetic, incorporate teaching about the drug into general teaching about the procedure. Include these points:

- This drug will make you drowsy and less anxious.
- Do not try to get up after you have received this drug (request assistance if you must sit up or move about for any reason).

Outpatients

- Take these drugs exactly as prescribed. These drugs are habit forming; the drug's effectiveness in facilitating sleep disappears after a short time. Do not take these drugs longer than 2 weeks (for insomnia), and do not increase the dosage without consulting your health care provider. If the drug appears to be ineffective, consult your health care provider.
- Avoid becoming pregnant while taking these drugs. The use of hormonal contraceptives while taking these drugs is not recommended as the contraceptives lose their effectiveness.
- You may experience these side effects: Drowsiness, dizziness, hangover, impaired thinking (these effects may become less pronounced after a few days; avoid driving a car or engaging in activities that require

alertness); GI upset (taking the drug with food may help); dreams, nightmares, difficulty concentrating, fatigue, nervousness (these are effects of the drug that will go away when the drug is discontinued; consult your health care provider if these become bothersome).

- Report severe dizziness, weakness, drowsiness that persists, rash or skin lesions, pregnancy.

Representative drugs

amobarbital
methohexital
pentobarbital
pentobarbital sodium
phenobarbital
primidone
secobarbital
thiopental

Benzodiazepines

PREGNANCY CATEGORY D OR X

CONTROLLED SUBSTANCE C-IV

Therapeutic actions

Benzodiazepines are anxiolytics, antiepileptics, muscle relaxants, and sedative-hypnotics. Their exact mechanisms of action are not understood, but it is known that benzodiazepines potentiate the effects of GABA, an inhibitory neurotransmitter.

Indications

- Management of anxiety disorders, short-term relief of symptoms of anxiety
- Short-term treatment of insomnia
- Alone or as adjunct in treatment of Lennox-Gastaut syndrome (petit mal variant), akinetic and myoclonic seizures
- May be useful in patients with absence (petit mal) seizures who have not responded to succinimides; up to 30% of patients show loss of effectiveness of drug within 3 mo of therapy (may respond to dosage adjustment)
- Unlabeled use: Treatment of panic attacks, treatment of IBS, acute alcohol withdrawal syndrome, chemotherapy-induced nausea and vomiting, psychogenic catatonic depression, PMS

Contraindications and cautions

- Contraindicated with hypersensitivity to benzodiazepines, psychoses, acute narrow-angle glaucoma, shock, coma, acute alcoholic intoxication with depression of vital signs, pregnancy (risk of congenital malformations, neonatal withdrawal syndrome), labor and delivery ("floppy infant" syndrome reported), or lactation (infants become lethargic and lose weight).
- Use cautiously with impaired hepatic or renal function, debilitation.

Adverse effects

- **CNS:** *Transient, mild drowsiness initially; sedation, depression, lethargy, apathy, fatigue, light-headedness, disorientation, anger, hostility,* episodes of mania and hypomania, *restlessness, confusion, crying,* delirium, *headache,* slurred speech, dysarthria, stupor, rigidity, tremor, dystonia, vertigo, euphoria, nervousness, difficulty in concentration, vivid dreams, psychomotor retardation, extrapyramidal symptoms; mild paradoxical excitatory reactions during first 2 wk of treatment
- **CV:** Bradycardia, tachycardia, CV collapse, hypertension and hypotension, palpitations, edema
- **Dermatologic:** Urticaria, pruritus, skin rash, dermatitis
- **EENT:** Visual and auditory disturbances, diplopia, nystagmus, depressed hearing, nasal congestion
- **GI:** *Constipation, diarrhea, dry mouth,* salivation, *nausea,* anorexia, vomiting, difficulty in swallowing, gastric disorders, hepatic impairment, encopresis
- **GU:** Incontinence, urine retention, changes in libido, menstrual irregularities
- **Hematologic:** Elevations of blood enzymes—LDH, alkaline phosphatase, AST, ALT; blood dyscrasias—agranulocytosis, leukopenia
- **Other:** Hiccups, fever, diaphoresis, paresthesias, muscular disturbances, gynecomastia; *drug dependence with withdrawal syndrome when drug is discontinued; more common with abrupt discontinuation of higher dosage used for longer than 4 mo*

Interactions

✳ **Drug-drug** • Increased CNS depression with alcohol • Increased effect with cimetidine, disulfiram, omeprazole, hormonal contraceptives
- Decreased effect with theophylline

■ Nursing considerations

Assessment

- **History:** Hypersensitivity to benzodiazepines, psychoses, acute narrow-angle glaucoma, shock, coma, acute alcoholic intoxication with depression of vital signs, pregnancy, lactation, impaired hepatic or renal function, debilitation
- **Physical:** Skin color, lesions; T; orientation, reflexes, affect, ophthalmologic examination; P, BP; R, adventitious sounds; liver evaluation, abdominal examination, bowel sounds, normal output; CBC, LFTs, renal function tests

Interventions

- Keep addiction-prone patients under careful surveillance.
- Monitor liver function, blood counts in patients on long-term therapy.
- Ensure ready access to bathroom if GI effects occur; establish bowel program if constipation occurs.
- Provide frequent small meals, frequent mouth care if GI effects occur.
- Provide measures appropriate to care of urinary problems (protective clothing, bed changing).
- Establish safety precautions if CNS changes occur (eg, side rails, accompany patient).
- Taper dosage gradually after long-term therapy, especially in patients with epilepsy; arrange to substitute another antiepileptic.
- Monitor patient for therapeutic drug levels; levels vary with drug being used.
- Arrange for patient to wear medical alert identification indicating epilepsy and drug therapy.

Teaching points

- Take drug exactly as prescribed; do not stop taking these drugs (long-term therapy) without consulting your health care provider.
- Avoid alcohol, sleep-inducing drugs, or over-the-counter drugs.
- You may experience these side effects: Drowsiness, dizziness (may become less pronounced after a few days; avoid driving or engaging in other dangerous activities); GI upset (take drug with food); fatigue; depression; dreams;

crying; nervousness; depression, emotional changes; bed wetting, urinary incontinence.
• Report severe dizziness, weakness, drowsiness that persists, rash or skin lesions, difficulty voiding, palpitations, swelling in the extremities.

Representative drugs
alprazolam
chlordiazepoxide
clobazam
clonazepam
clorazepate
diazepam
estazolam
flurazepam
lorazepam
midazolam
nitrazepam (CAN)
oxazepam
quazepam
temazepam
triazolam

Beta-adrenergic Blockers (β-blockers)

PREGNANCY CATEGORY C (MOST), D (ATENOLOL), B (ACEBUTOLOL, PINDOLOL, SOTALOL)

Therapeutic actions
Beta-adrenergic blockers are antianginals, antiarrhythmics, and antihypertensives. These drugs competitively block beta-adrenergic receptors in the heart and juxtaglomerular apparatus. They decrease the influence of the sympathetic nervous system on these tissues, the excitability of the heart, cardiac workload, oxygen consumption, and the release of renin; they lower BP. They have membrane-stabilizing (local anesthetic) effects that contribute to their antiarrhythmic action. They also act in the CNS to reduce sympathetic outflow and vasoconstrictor tone.

Indications
• Hypertension (alone or with other drugs, especially diuretics)
• Angina pectoris caused by coronary atherosclerosis
• Hypertrophic subaortic stenosis, to manage associated stress-induced angina, palpitations, and syncope; cardiac arrhythmias, especially supraventricular tachycardia, and ventricular tachycardias induced by digoxin or catecholamines; essential tremor, familial or hereditary
• Prevention of reinfarction in clinically stable patients when started 1–4 wk after MI
• Adjunctive therapy for pheochromocytoma after treatment with an alpha-adrenergic blocker, to manage tachycardia before or during surgery or if the pheochromocytoma is inoperable
• Prophylaxis for migraine headache (propranolol)
• Management of acute situational stress reaction (stage fright); essential tremor (propranolol)
• Unlabeled uses: Treatment of recurrent GI bleeding in cirrhotic patients, schizophrenia, tardive dyskinesia, acute panic symptoms, vaginal contraceptive, acute alcohol withdrawal

Contraindications and cautions
• Contraindicated with allergy to beta-adrenergic blockers, sinus bradycardia, second- or third-degree heart block, cardiogenic shock, heart failure, bronchial asthma, bronchospasm, COPD, pregnancy (neonatal bradycardia, hypoglycemia, and apnea have occurred in infants whose mothers received propranolol; low birth weight occurs with chronic maternal use during pregnancy), or lactation.
• Use cautiously with hypoglycemia and diabetes, thyrotoxicosis, hepatic impairment.

Adverse effects
• **Allergic reactions:** Pharyngitis, erythematous rash, fever, sore throat, laryngospasm, respiratory distress
• **CV:** *Bradycardia, heart failure, cardiac arrhythmias, sinoatrial or AV nodal block, tachycardia,* peripheral vascular insufficiency, claudication, **stroke,** pulmonary edema, hypotension
• **Dermatologic:** Rash, pruritus, sweating, dry skin
• **EENT:** Eye irritation, dry eyes, conjunctivitis, blurred vision
• **GI:** *Gastric pain, flatulence, constipation, diarrhea, nausea, vomiting,* anorexia, ischemic colitis, renal and mesenteric

arterial thrombosis, retroperitoneal fibrosis, hepatomegaly, acute pancreatitis
- **GU:** *Impotence, decreased libido,* Peyronie's disease, dysuria, nocturia, frequency
- **Musculoskeletal:** Joint pain, arthralgia, muscle cramps
- **Neurologic:** Dizziness, vertigo, tinnitus, *fatigue,* emotional depression, paresthesias, sleep disturbances, hallucinations, disorientation, memory loss, slurred speech
- **Respiratory:** Bronchospasm, dyspnea, cough, bronchial obstruction, nasal stuffiness, rhinitis, pharyngitis
- **Other:** *Decreased exercise tolerance, development of antinuclear antibodies,* hyperglycemia or hypoglycemia, elevated serum transaminase, alkaline phosphatase, and LDH

Interactions
✳ Drug-drug • Increased effects with verapamil, diltiazem • Decreased effects with indomethacin, ibuprofen, piroxicam, sulindac, barbiturates • Prolonged hypoglycemic effects of insulin with beta-adrenergic blockers • Peripheral ischemia possible if combined with ergot alkaloids • Initial hypertensive episode followed by bradycardia with epinephrine • Increased "first-dose response" to prazosin with beta-adrenergic blockers • Increased serum levels and toxic effects with lidocaine, cimetidine • Increased serum levels of beta-adrenergic blockers and phenothiazines, hydralazine if the two drugs are taken concurrently • Paradoxical hypertension when clonidine is given with beta-adrenergic blockers; increased rebound hypertension when clonidine is discontinued • Decreased serum levels and therapeutic effects if taken with methimazole, propylthiouracil • Decreased bronchodilator effects of theophyllines • Decreased antihypertensive effects with NSAIDs (eg, ibuprofen, indomethacin, piroxicam, sulindac), rifampin
✳ Drug-lab test • Interference with glucose or insulin tolerance tests, glaucoma screening tests

■ Nursing considerations
Assessment
- **History:** Allergy to beta-adrenergic blockers, sinus bradycardia, second- or third-degree heart block, cardiogenic shock, heart failure, bronchial asthma, bronchospasm, COPD, hypoglycemia and diabetes, thyrotoxicosis, hepatic impairment, pregnancy, lactation
- **Physical:** Weight, skin color, lesions, edema, T; reflexes, affect, vision, hearing, orientation; BP, P, ECG, peripheral perfusion; R, auscultation; bowel sounds, normal output, liver evaluation; bladder palpation; LFTs, thyroid function test, blood and urine glucose

Interventions
- Do not stop drug abruptly after long-term therapy (hypersensitivity to catecholamines may have developed, causing exacerbation of angina, MI, and ventricular arrhythmias). Taper drug gradually over 2 wk with monitoring.
- Consult physician about withdrawing drug if patient is to undergo surgery (controversial).
- Give oral drug with food to facilitate absorption.
- Provide side rails and assistance with walking if CNS, vision changes occur.
- Position patient to decrease effects of edema, respiratory obstruction.
- Space activities, and provide rest periods.
- Provide frequent small meals if GI effects occur.
- Provide comfort measures to help patient cope with eye, GI, joint, CNS, dermatologic effects.

Teaching points
- Take these drugs with meals. Do not stop taking these drugs abruptly; this can worsen the disorder being treated.
- If you have diabetes, the normal signs of hypoglycemia (tremor, tachycardia) may be blocked by these drugs; monitor your blood or urine glucose carefully; be sure to eat regular meals, and take your diabetic medication regularly.
- You may experience these side effects: Dizziness, drowsiness, light-headedness, blurred vision (avoid driving or performing hazardous tasks); nausea, loss of appetite (frequent small meals may help); nightmares, depression (notify your health care provider, who may be able to change your medication); sexual impotence (you may want to discuss this with your health care provider).

Adverse effects in italics *are most common; those in* **bold** *are life-threatening.* ⬛ *Do not crush.*

- Report difficulty breathing, night cough, swelling of extremities, slow pulse, confusion, depression, rash, fever, sore throat.

Representative drugs
acebutolol
atenolol
betaxolol
bisoprolol
carvedilol
esmolol
labetalol
levobunolol
metipranolol
metoprolol
nadolol
nebivolol
penbutolol
pindolol
propranolol
sotalol
timolol

Bisphosphonates

PREGNANCY CATEGORY D
(PARENTERAL), C (ORAL)

Therapeutic actions
Bisphosphonates inhibit bone resorption, possibly by inhibiting osteoclast activity and promoting osteoclast cell apoptosis; this action leads to decreased release of calcium from bone and decreased serum calcium level.

Indications
- Treatment of Paget's disease of bone (oral)
- Treatment of osteoporosis (oral) (postmenopausal and in males)
- Treatment of heterotopic ossification (oral)
- Treatment of hypercalcemia of malignancy in patients inadequately managed by diet or oral hydration (parenteral)
- Treatment of hypercalcemia of malignancy, which persists after adequate hydration has been restored (parenteral)
- Prevention of new clinical fractures in patients with low-trauma hip fractures (parenteral)

Contraindications and cautions
- Contraindicated with allergy to bisphosphonates, hypocalcemia, pregnancy, lactation, severe renal impairment.

- Use cautiously in the presence of renal impairment, upper GI disease.

Adverse effects
- **CNS:** *Headache,* dizziness
- **CV:** Hypertension, chest pain
- **GI:** *Nausea, diarrhea,* altered taste, metallic taste, *abdominal pain,* anorexia, esophageal erosion
- **Hematologic:** Elevated BUN, serum creatinine, hypophosphatemia, hypokalemia, hypomagnesemia, hypocalcemia
- **Respiratory:** Dyspnea, coughing, pleural effusion
- **Skeletal:** *Increased or recurrent bone pain* (Paget's disease), focal osteomalacia, *arthralgia*
- **Other:** *Infections* (UTI, candidiasis), *fever,* progression of cancer

Interactions
✳ **Drug-drug** ● Increased risk of GI distress if taken with aspirin ● Decreased absorption if oral form is taken with antacids, calcium, iron, multivalent cations; separate dosing by at least 30 min ● Possible increased risk of hypocalcemia if parenteral form is given with aminoglycosides, loop diuretics; if this combination is used, monitor serum calcium levels closely
✳ **Drug-food** ● Significantly decreased absorption and serum levels if oral form is taken with any food; administer on an empty stomach, 30 min before meals

■ Nursing considerations
Assessment
- **History:** Allergy to bisphosphonates, renal failure, upper GI disease, lactation, pregnancy
- **Physical:** Muscle tone, bone pain, bowel sounds, urinalysis, serum calcium, renal function tests

Interventions
- Administer oral drug with a full glass of water, 30 min to 1 hr before meals or any other medication; make sure that patient stays upright for at least 30 min after administration.
- Make sure that patient is well hydrated before and during therapy with parenteral agents.
- Monitor serum calcium levels before, during, and after therapy.

- Ensure a 3-mo rest period after treatment for Paget's disease if retreatment is required; allow 7 days between treatments for hypercalcemia of malignancy.
- Ensure adequate vitamin D and calcium intake.
- Provide comfort measures if bone pain returns.

Teaching points
- Take these drugs with a full glass of water 30 to 60 minutes before meals or any other medication; stay upright for at least 30 minutes after taking these drugs.
- Periodic blood tests may be required to monitor your calcium levels.
- You may experience these side effects: Nausea, diarrhea, bone pain, headache (analgesics may help).
- Report twitching, muscle spasms, dark-colored urine, severe diarrhea, GI distress, epigastric pain.

Representative drugs
alendronate
etidronate
ibandronate
pamidronate
risedronate
tiludronate
zoledronic acid

> ### Calcium Channel Blockers

PREGNANCY CATEGORY C

Therapeutic actions
Calcium channel blockers are antianginal and antihypertensive. They inhibit the movement of calcium ions across the membranes of cardiac and arterial muscle cells. This inhibition of transmembrane calcium flow results in the depression of impulse formation in specialized cardiac pacemaker cells, slowing of the velocity of conduction of the cardiac impulse, depression of myocardial contractility, and dilation of coronary arteries and arterioles and peripheral arterioles. These effects lead to decreased cardiac work, decreased cardiac energy consumption, and increased delivery of oxygen to myocardial cells.

Indications
- Treatment of angina pectoris caused by coronary artery spasm (Prinzmetal's variant angina), chronic stable angina (effort-associated angina), hypertension, arrhythmias (supraventricular, those related to digoxin [verapamil]), subarachnoid hemorrhage (nimodipine)
- Orphan drug use in the treatment of interstitial cystitis, hypertensive emergencies, migraines, Raynaud's syndrome
- Unlabeled uses: Treatment of preterm labor, Raynaud's phenomenon, acute ischemic stroke, vascular headaches, hypertensive emergencies

Contraindications and cautions
- Contraindicated with heart block, allergy to calcium channel blockers, sick sinus syndrome, ventricular dysfunction, pregnancy.
- Use cautiously during lactation.

Adverse effects
- **CNS:** *Dizziness, light-headedness, headache, asthenia,* fatigue, *nervousness,* sleep disturbances, blurred vision
- **CV:** *Peripheral edema, angina,* hypotension, arrhythmias, bradycardia, *AV block,* asystole
- **Dermatologic:** *Flushing, rash,* dermatitis, pruritus, urticaria
- **GI:** *Nausea, diarrhea, constipation,* flatulence, cramps, hepatic injury
- **Other:** *Nasal congestion, cough,* fever, chills, shortness of breath, muscle cramps, joint stiffness, sexual difficulties

Interactions
✳ **Drug-drug** • Increased effects with cimetidine, ranitidine • Increased toxicity of cyclosporine
✳ **Drug-food** • Increased serum levels when combined with grapefruit juice

■ Nursing considerations
Assessment
- **History:** Allergy to calcium channel blockers, sick sinus syndrome, heart block, ventricular dysfunction; pregnancy; lactation
- **Physical:** Skin lesions, color, edema; orientation, reflexes; P, BP, baseline ECG, peripheral perfusion, auscultation; R,

adventitious sounds; liver evaluation, normal GI output; LFTs

Interventions

- Monitor patient carefully (BP, cardiac rhythm, and output) while drug is being titrated to therapeutic dose; the dosage may be increased more rapidly in hospitalized patients under close supervision.
- Ensure that patients do not chew or divide sustained-release tablets.
- Taper dosage of beta-adrenergic blockers before beginning calcium channel blocker therapy.
- Protect drug from light and moisture.
- Ensure ready access to bathroom.
- Provide comfort measures for skin rash, headache, nervousness.
- Establish safety precautions if CNS changes occur.
- Position patient to alleviate peripheral edema.
- Provide frequent small meals if GI upset occurs.

Teaching points

- Do not chew or divide sustained-release tablets. Swallow whole.
- Avoid grapefruit juice while taking this drug.
- You may experience these side effects: Nausea, vomiting (frequent small meals may help); dizziness, light-headedness, vertigo (avoid driving, operating hazardous machinery; avoid falling); muscle cramps, joint stiffness, sweating, sexual difficulties (should stop when the drug therapy is stopped; discuss with your health care provider if these become too uncomfortable).
- Report irregular heartbeat, shortness of breath, swelling of the hands or feet, pronounced dizziness, constipation.

Representative drugs

amlodipine
clevidipine
diltiazem
felodipine
isradipine
nicardipine
nifedipine
nimodipine
nisoldipine
verapamil

Cephalosporins

PREGNANCY CATEGORY B

Therapeutic actions

Cephalosporins are antibiotics. They are bactericidal, inhibiting synthesis of bacterial cell wall, causing cell death in susceptible bacteria.

Indications

- Treatment of pharyngitis, tonsillitis caused by *Streptococcus pyogenes*; otitis media caused by *Streptococcus pneumoniae, Haemophilus influenzae, Moraxella catarrhalis, S. pyogenes;* respiratory infections caused by *S. pneumoniae, Haemophilus parainfluenzae, Staphylococcus aureus, Escherichia coli, Klebsiella, H. influenzae, S. pyogenes;* UTIs caused by *E. coli, Klebsiella pneumoniae;* dermatologic infections caused by *S. aureus, S. pyogenes, E. coli, Klebsiella, Enterobacter;* uncomplicated and disseminated gonorrhea caused by *Neisseria gonorrhea;* septicemia caused by *S. pneumoniae, S. aureus, E. coli, Klebsiella, H. influenzae;* meningitis caused by *S. pneumoniae, H. influenzae, S. aureus, Neisseria meningitidis;* bone and joint infections caused by *S. aureus*
- Perioperative prophylaxis

Contraindications and cautions

- Contraindicated with allergy to cephalosporins or penicillins, renal failure, or lactation.

Adverse effects

- **CNS:** Headache, dizziness, lethargy, paresthesias, seizures
- **GI:** *Nausea, vomiting, diarrhea, anorexia, abdominal pain, flatulence,* pseudomembranous colitis, hepatotoxicity
- **GU:** Nephrotoxicity
- **Hematologic:** Bone marrow depression; decreased WBC, platelets, Hct
- **Hypersensitivity:** Ranging from *rash, fever* to **anaphylaxis;** serum sickness reaction
- **Local:** *Pain,* abscess at injection site, *phlebitis,* inflammation at IV site
- **Other:** *Superinfections, disulfiram-like reaction with alcohol*

Interactions
✳ **Drug-drug** • Increased nephrotoxicity with aminoglycosides • Increased bleeding effects with oral anticoagulants • Disulfiram-like reaction may occur if alcohol is taken within 72 hr after cephalosporin administration

✳ **Drug-lab test** • Possibility of false results on tests of urine glucose using Benedict's solution, Fehling's solution, Clinitest tablets; urinary 17-ketosteroids; direct Coombs' test

■ Nursing considerations
Assessment
• **History:** Allergy to any cephalosporin, hepatic and renal impairment, lactation, pregnancy
• **Physical:** Skin status, LFTs, renal function tests, culture of affected area, sensitivity tests

Interventions
• Culture infected area and arrange for sensitivity tests before beginning drug therapy and during therapy if expected response is not seen.
• Administer oral drug with food to decrease GI upset and enhance absorption.
• Administer liquid drug to children who cannot swallow tablets; crushing the drug results in a bitter, unpleasant taste.
• Have vitamin K available in case hypoprothrombinemia occurs.
• Discontinue drug if hypersensitivity reaction occurs.
• Ensure ready access to bathroom and provide frequent small meals if GI complications occur.
• Arrange for treatment of superinfections.

Teaching points
Oral drug
• Take full course of therapy.
• These drugs are specific to an infection and should not be used to self-treat other problems.
• Swallow tablets or capsules whole; do not crush.
• Take the drug with food.
• Avoid drinking alcoholic beverages while taking and for 3 days after stopping this drug because severe reactions often occur (even with parenteral forms).

• You may experience these side effects: Stomach upset or diarrhea.
• Report severe diarrhea with blood, pus, or mucus; rash; difficulty breathing; unusual tiredness, fatigue; unusual bleeding or bruising; unusual itching or irritation, pain at injection site.

Representative drugs
First generation
cefadroxil
cefazolin
cephalexin

Second generation
cefaclor
cefoxitin
cefprozil
cefuroxime

Third generation
cefdinir
cefotaxime
cefpodoxime
ceftazidime
ceftibuten
ceftriaxone

Fourth generation
cefditoren
cefepime
ceftaroline

Corticosteroids

PREGNANCY CATEGORY C

Therapeutic actions
Corticosteroids enter target cells and bind to cytoplasmic receptors, initiating many complex reactions that are responsible for anti-inflammatory, immunosuppressive (glucocorticoid), and salt-retaining (mineralocorticoid) actions. Some of these actions are considered undesirable, depending on the indication for which the drug is being used.

Indications
Systemic administration
• Replacement therapy in adrenal cortical insufficiency
• Treatment of hypercalcemia associated with cancer
• Short-term management of inflammatory and allergic disorders such as rheumatoid

arthritis, collagen diseases (eg, SLE), dermatologic diseases (eg, pemphigus), status asthmaticus, and autoimmune disorders
- Management of hematologic disorders—thrombocytopenic purpura, erythroblastopenia
- Treatment of trichinosis with neurologic or myocardial involvement
- Treatment of ulcerative colitis, acute exacerbations of MS, and palliation in some leukemias and lymphomas

Inhalation
- Treatment of asthma

Intra-articular or soft-tissue administration
- Treatment of arthritis, psoriatic plaques

Retention enema
- For ulcerative colitis, proctitis

Dermatologic preparations
- Relief of inflammatory and pruritic manifestations of dermatoses that are steroid-responsive

Anorectal cream, suppositories
- Relief of discomfort from hemorrhoids and perianal itching or irritation

Contraindications and cautions

- *Systemic administration:* Infections, especially tuberculosis, fungal infections, amebiasis, hepatitis B, vaccinia, or varicella, and antibiotic-resistant infections; kidney disease (predisposes to edema); liver disease, cirrhosis, hypothyroidism; ulcerative colitis with impending perforation; diverticulitis; recent GI surgery; active or latent peptic ulcer; inflammatory bowel disease (drug may cause exacerbations or bowel perforation); hypertension, heart failure; thromboembolitic tendencies, thrombophlebitis, osteoporosis, convulsive disorders, metastatic carcinoma, diabetes mellitus; lactation.
- *Retention enemas, intrarectal foam:* Systemic fungal infections; recent intestinal surgery; extensive fistulas.
- *Topical dermatologic administration:* Fungal, tubercular, herpes simplex skin infections; vaccinia, varicella; ear application when eardrum is perforated; lactation.

Adverse effects
Systemic administration
- **CNS:** *Vertigo, headache,* paresthesias, insomnia, seizures, psychosis

- **CV:** *Hypotension, shock,* hypertension and CHF secondary to fluid retention, thromboembolism, thrombophlebitis, fat embolism, cardiac arrhythmias secondary to electrolyte disturbances
- **Dermatologic:** *Thin, fragile skin; petechiae, ecchymoses,* purpura, striae, subcutaneous fat atrophy
- **Endocrine:** *Amenorrhea, irregular menses,* growth retardation, decreased carbohydrate tolerance and diabetes mellitus, cushingoid state (long-term therapy), hypothalamic-pituitary-adrenal (HPA) suppression systemic with therapy longer than 5 days
- **Eye:** Cataracts, glaucoma (long-term therapy), increased IOP
- **GI:** *Peptic or esophageal ulcer, pancreatitis,* abdominal distention, nausea, vomiting, increased appetite and weight gain (long-term therapy)
- **Hematologic:** *Sodium and fluid retention, hypokalemia,* hypocalcemia, increased blood sugar, increased serum cholesterol, decreased serum T_3 and T_4 levels
- **Hypersensitivity:** Anaphylactoid or hypersensitivity reactions
- **Musculoskeletal:** *Muscle weakness,* steroid myopathy and loss of muscle mass, osteoporosis, spontaneous fractures (long-term therapy)
- **Other:** *Immunosuppression, aggravation or masking of infections, impaired wound healing*

The following effects are related to specific routes of administration:

IM repository injections
Atrophy at injection site

Retention enema
Local pain, burning; rectal bleeding; systemic absorption and adverse effects (see above)

Inhalation
Cough, throat irritation, oral thrush

Intra-articular
Osteonecrosis, tendon rupture, infection

Intraspinal
Meningitis, adhesive arachnoiditis, conus medullaris syndrome

Intralesional therapy—head and neck
Blindness (rare)

Intrathecal administration
Arachnoiditis

Topical forms

Local burning, irritation, acneiform lesions, striae, skin atrophy

Systemic absorption can lead to HPA suppression (see above), growth retardation in children, and other systemic adverse effects. Children may be at special risk of systemic absorption because of their larger skin surface area-to-body weight ratio.

Interactions

✳ Drug-drug • Increased steroid blood levels if taken with hormonal contraceptives, troleandomycin • Decreased steroid blood levels if taken with phenytoin, phenobarbital, rifampin, cholestyramine • Decreased serum level of salicylates if taken with corticosteroids • Decreased effectiveness of anticholinesterases (ambenonium, edrophonium, neostigmine, pyridostigmine) if taken with corticosteroids

✳ Drug-lab test • False-negative nitrobluetetrazolium test for bacterial infection (with systemic absorption) • Suppression of skin test reactions

■ Nursing considerations

Assessment

- **History:** Infections, especially TB, fungal infections, amebiasis, hepatitis B, vaccinia, varicella, and antibiotic-resistant infections; kidney disease; liver disease, cirrhosis, hypothyroidism; ulcerative colitis with impending perforation; diverticulitis; recent GI surgery; active or latent peptic ulcer; inflammatory bowel disease; hypertension, heart failure; thromboembolitic tendencies, thrombophlebitis, osteoporosis, seizure disorders, metastatic carcinoma, diabetes mellitus; lactation

  Retention enemas, intrarectal foam: Systemic fungal infections; recent intestinal surgery, extensive fistulas

  Topical dermatologic administration: Fungal, tubercular, herpes simplex skin infections; vaccinia, varicella; ear application when eardrum is perforated

- **Physical:** *Systemic administration:* Body weight, T; reflexes, affect, bilateral grip strength, ophthalmologic examination; BP, P, auscultation, peripheral perfusion, discoloration, pain or prominence of superficial vessels; R, adventitious sounds, chest X-ray; upper GI X-ray (history or symptoms of peptic ulcer), liver palpation; CBC, serum electrolytes, 2-hr postprandial blood glucose, urinalysis, thyroid function tests, serum cholesterol

  Topical, dermatologic preparations: Affected area, integrity of skin

Interventions

Systemic administration

- Administer once a day before 9 AM to mimic normal peak diurnal corticosteroid levels and minimize HPA suppression.
- Space multiple doses evenly throughout the day.
- Do not give IM injections if patient has thrombocytopenia purpura.
- Rotate sites of IM repository injections to avoid local atrophy.
- Use minimal doses for shortest duration of time to minimize adverse effects.
- ⊗ **Black box warning** Arrange to taper doses when discontinuing high-dose or long-term therapy or when transferring from systemic to inhaled corticosteroids. Monitor for signs and symptoms of adrenal insufficiency.
- Arrange for increased dosage when patient is subject to unusual stress.
- Use alternate-day maintenance therapy with short-acting corticosteroids when possible.
- Do not give live-virus vaccines with immunosuppressive doses of glucocorticoids.
- Provide skin care if patient is bedridden.
- Provide frequent small meals to minimize GI distress.
- Provide antacids between meals to help avoid peptic ulcer.
- Arrange for bed rails, other safety precautions if CNS, musculoskeletal effects occur.
- Avoid exposing patient to infection.

Inhalation

- Teach patient the proper technique for using the delivery device prescribed.

Topical dermatologic administration

- Use caution with occlusive dressings, tight or plastic diapers over affected area; these can increase systemic absorption.
- Avoid prolonged use, especially near eyes, in genital and rectal areas, on face and in skin creases.
- Provide careful wound care if lesions are present.
- Provide measures to deal with pain, discomfort on administration.

Teaching points
Systemic administration
- Take these drugs exactly as prescribed. Do not stop taking these drugs without notifying your health care provider; drug dosage must be slowly tapered to avoid problems.
- Take with meals or snacks if GI upset occurs.
- Take single daily or alternate-day doses before 9 AM; mark a calendar or use other measure as a reminder of treatment days.
- Arrange for frequent follow-up visits to your health care provider so that your response to the drug may be determined and the dosage adjusted if necessary.
- Wear a medical identification tag (if you are on long-term therapy) so that any emergency medical personnel will know that you are taking one of these drugs.
- With dosage reductions, you may experience signs of adrenal insufficiency; report fatigue, muscle and joint pains, anorexia, nausea, vomiting, diarrhea, weight loss, weakness, dizziness, low blood sugar (if you monitor blood sugar).
- You may experience these side effects: Increase in appetite, weight gain (some of the weight gain may be from fluid retention; watching calories may help); heartburn, indigestion (eat frequent small meals; use antacids between meals); increased susceptibility to infection (avoid crowded areas during peak cold or flu seasons and avoid contact with anyone with a known infection); poor wound healing (if you have an injury or wound, consult your health care provider); muscle weakness, fatigue (frequent rest periods may help).
- Report unusual weight gain, swelling of lower extremities, muscle weakness, black or tarry stools, vomiting of blood, epigastric burning, puffing of face, menstrual irregularities, fever, prolonged sore throat, cold or other infection, worsening of symptoms.

Inhalation
- Follow directions you have been given regarding proper use of the drug delivery device.
- Brush your teeth or rinse your mouth after each use.

Intra-articular, intralesional administration
- Do not overuse the injected joint even if the pain is gone. Follow directions you have been given for proper rest and exercise.

Topical dermatologic administration
- Apply sparingly and rub in lightly.
- Avoid eye contact.
- Report burning, irritation, or infection of the site, worsening of the condition.
- Avoid prolonged use.

Anorectal preparations
- Maintain normal bowel function by proper diet, adequate fluid intake, and regular exercise.
- Use stool softeners or bulk laxatives if needed.
- Notify your health care provider if symptoms do not improve in 7 days, or if bleeding, protrusion, or seepage occurs.

Representative drugs
alclometasone
amcinonide
beclomethasone
betamethasone
budesonide
ciclesonide
clobetasol
clocortolone
cortisone
desonide
desoximetasone
dexamethasone
diflorasone
difluprednate
fludrocortisone
flunisolide
fluocinolone
fluocinonide
fluoromethalone
flurandrenolide
fluticasone
halcinonide
halobetasol
hydrocortisone
methylprednisolone
mometasone
prednicarbate
prednisolone
prednisone
rimexolone
triamcinolone

Diuretics

PREGNANCY CATEGORY B OR C

Therapeutic actions

Diuretics are divided into several subgroups. Thiazide and thiazide-related diuretics inhibit reabsorption of sodium and chloride in the distal renal tubule, increasing the excretion of sodium, chloride, and water by the kidneys. Loop diuretics inhibit the reabsorption of sodium and chloride in the loop of Henle and in the distal renal tubule; because of this added effect, loop diuretics are more potent. Potassium-sparing diuretics block the effect of aldosterone on the renal tubule, leading to a loss of sodium and water and the retention of potassium; their overall effect is much weaker. Osmotic diuretics pull fluid out of the tissues with a hypertonic effect. Overall effect of diuretics is a loss of water and electrolytes from the body.

Indications

- Adjunctive therapy in edema associated with heart failure, cirrhosis, corticosteroid and estrogen therapy, renal impairment
- Treatment of hypertension, alone or in combination with other antihypertensives
- Reduction of intracranial pressure before and during neurosurgery
- Reduction of intraocular pressure in acute episodes of glaucoma when other therapies are not successful
- Unlabeled uses: Treatment of diabetes insipidus, especially nephrogenic diabetes insipidus, reduction of incidence of osteoporosis in postmenopausal women

Contraindications and cautions

- Contraindicated with fluid or electrolyte imbalances, renal or hepatic disease, gout, SLE, glucose tolerance abnormalities, hyperparathyroidism, manic-depressive disorders, or lactation.

Adverse effects

- **CNS:** *Dizziness, vertigo,* paresthesias, weakness, headache, drowsiness, fatigue
- **CV:** Orthostatic hypotension, venous thrombosis, volume depletion, cardiac arrhythmias, chest pain

- **Dermatologic:** Photosensitivity, rash, purpura, exfoliative dermatitis
- **GI:** *Nausea, anorexia, vomiting, dry mouth, diarrhea, constipation,* jaundice, hepatitis, pancreatitis
- **GU:** *Polyuria, nocturia, impotence,* loss of libido
- **Hematologic:** Leukopenia, thrombocytopenia, agranulocytosis, aplastic anemia, neutropenia, fluid and electrolyte imbalances
- **Other:** Muscle cramps and muscle spasms, fever, hives, gouty attacks, flushing, weight loss, rhinorrhea, electrolyte imbalance

Interactions

✴ **Drug-drug** • Increased thiazide effects and possible acute hyperglycemia with diazoxide • Decreased absorption with cholestyramine, colestipol • Increased risk of cardiac glycoside toxicity if hypokalemia occurs • Increased risk of lithium toxicity • Increased dosage of antidiabetics may be needed • Risk of hyperkalemia if potassium-sparing diuretics are given with potassium preparations or ACE inhibitors • Increased risk of ototoxicity if loop diuretics are taken with aminoglycosides or cisplatin

✴ **Drug-lab test** • Monitor for decreased PBI levels without clinical signs of thyroid disturbances

■ Nursing considerations

Assessment

- **History:** Fluid or electrolyte imbalances, renal or liver disease, gout, SLE, glucose tolerance abnormalities, hyperparathyroidism, bipolar disorders, lactation
- **Physical:** Orientation, reflexes, muscle strength; pulses, BP, orthostatic BP, perfusion, edema, baseline ECG; R, adventitious sounds; liver evaluation, bowel sounds; CBC, serum electrolytes, blood glucose; LFTs, renal function tests; serum uric acid, urinalysis

Interventions

- Administer with food or milk if GI upset occurs.
- Administer early in the day so increased urination will not disturb sleep.
- Ensure ready access to bathroom.
- Establish safety precautions if CNS effects, orthostatic hypotension occur.

- Measure and record regular body weights to monitor fluid changes.
- Provide mouth care and frequent small meals as needed.
- Monitor IV sites for any sign of extravasation.
- Monitor electrolytes frequently with parenteral use, periodically with chronic use.

Teaching points
- Take these drugs early in the day so sleep will not be disturbed by increased urination.
- Weigh yourself daily and record weights.
- Protect your skin from exposure to the sun or bright lights.
- If taking a potassium-sparing diuretic, avoid foods high in potassium and avoid using salt substitutes.
- Take prescribed potassium replacement, and eat foods high in potassium if taking a thiazide or loop diuretic.
- Increased urination will occur (stay close to bathroom facilities).
- Use caution if dizziness, drowsiness, or faintness occurs.
- Report rapid weight gain or loss, swelling in ankles or fingers, unusual bleeding or bruising, muscle cramps.

Representative drugs
Carbonic anhydrase inhibitors
acetazolamide
methazolamide
Thiazide and related diuretics
chlorothiazide
chlorthalidone
hydrochlorothiazide
indapamide
methyclothiazide
metolazone
Loop diuretics
bumetanide
ethacrynic acid
furosemide
torsemide
Potassium-sparing diuretics
amiloride
spironolactone
triamterene
Osmotic diuretic
mannitol

Fluoroquinolones

PREGNANCY CATEGORY C

Therapeutic actions
Fluoroquinolones are antibacterial. They interfere with DNA replication in susceptible gram-negative bacteria, preventing cell reproduction and leading to death of bacteria.

Indications
- Treatment of infections caused by susceptible gram-negative bacteria, including *Escherichia coli, Proteus mirabilis, Klebsiella pneumoniae, Enterobacter cloacae, Proteus vulgaris, Providencia rettgeri, Morganella morganii, Pseudomonas aeruginosa, Citrobacter freundii, Staphylococcus aureus, S. epidermidis,* group D streptococci, *Streptococcus pneumoniae*
- Unlabeled use: Treatment of patients with cystic fibrosis who have pulmonary exacerbations

Contraindications and cautions
- Contraindicated with allergy to any fluoroquinolone, pregnancy, lactation, history of myasthenia gravis.
- Use cautiously with renal impairment, seizures.

Adverse effects
- **CNS:** *Headache,* dizziness, insomnia, fatigue, somnolence, depression, blurred vision
- **GI:** *Nausea,* vomiting, dry mouth, *diarrhea,* abdominal pain
- **Hematologic:** Elevated BUN, AST, ALT, serum creatinine and alkaline phosphatase; decreased WBC, neutrophil count, Hct
- **Other:** Fever, rash, **photosensitivity,** QT-interval prolongation, tendinitis, tendon rupture

Interactions
✳ **Drug-drug** • Decreased therapeutic effect with iron salts, sucralfate • Decreased absorption with antacids • Increased serum levels and toxic effects of theophyllines with fluoroquinolones • Risk of prolonged QT interval if combined with other drugs that prolong QT interval

✳ **Drug-alternative therapy** • Increased photosensitivity reactions with St. John's Wort

■ Nursing considerations

Assessment

- **History:** Allergy to fluoroquinolones, renal impairment, seizures, lactation
- **Physical:** Skin color, lesions; T; orientation, reflexes, affect; mucous membranes, bowel sounds; LFTs, renal function tests

Interventions

⊗ **Black box warning** Drug increases risk of tendinitis and tendon rupture, especially in older patients, patients with organ transplants, and patients on corticosteroids; may exacerbate weakness in patients with myasthenia gravis. Avoid use in these patients.

- Arrange for culture and sensitivity tests before beginning therapy.
- Continue therapy for 2 days after the signs and symptoms of infection have disappeared.
- Administer oral drug 1 hr before or 2 hr after meals with a glass of water.
- Ensure that patient is well hydrated during course of drug therapy.
- Administer antacids, if needed, at least 2 hr after dosing.
- Monitor clinical response; if no improvement is seen or a relapse occurs, repeat culture and sensitivity.
- Ensure ready access to bathroom if diarrhea occurs.
- Arrange for appropriate bowel training program if constipation occurs.
- Provide frequent small meals if GI upset occurs.
- Arrange for monitoring of environment (noise, temperature) and analgesics, for headache.
- Establish safety precautions if CNS, visual changes occur.
- Encourage patient to complete full course of therapy.

Teaching points

- Take oral drugs on an empty stomach, 1 hour before or 2 hours after meals. If you need an antacid, do not take it within 2 hours of ciprofloxacin dose.
- Drink plenty of fluids.
- You may experience these side effects: Nausea, vomiting, abdominal pain (frequent small meals may help); diarrhea or constipation (consult your health care provider); drowsiness, blurring of vision,

dizziness (observe caution if driving or using hazardous equipment).
- Report rash, visual changes, severe GI problems, weakness, tremors.

Representative drugs

ciprofloxacin
gemifloxacin
levofloxacin
moxifloxacin
norfloxacin
ofloxacin

Histamine$_2$ (H$_2$) Antagonists

PREGNANCY CATEGORY B

Therapeutic actions

H$_2$ antagonists inhibit the action of histamine at the H$_2$ receptors of the stomach, inhibiting gastric acid secretion and reducing total pepsin output; the resultant decrease in acid allows healing of ulcerated areas.

Indications

- Short-term and maintenance treatment of active duodenal ulcer and benign gastric ulcer
- Treatment of pathologic hypersecretory conditions (Zollinger-Ellison syndrome) and erosive GERD
- Prophylaxis of stress-induced ulcers and acute upper GI bleed in critically ill patients
- Treatment of GERD, heartburn, acid indigestion, sour stomach

Contraindications and cautions

- Contraindicated with allergy to H$_2$ antagonists, impaired renal or hepatic function, or lactation.

Adverse effects

- **CNS:** Dizziness, somnolence, headache, confusion, hallucinations, peripheral neuropathy, symptoms of brain stem dysfunction (dysarthria, ataxia, diplopia)
- **CV:** Cardiac arrhythmias, arrest; hypotension (IV use)
- **GI:** *Diarrhea*
- **Hematologic:** Increases in plasma creatinine, serum transaminase

- **Other:** Impotence (reversible with drug withdrawal), gynecomastia (long-term treatment), rash, vasculitis, pain at IM injection site

Interactions
❋ **Drug-drug** • Increased risk of decreased white blood cell counts with antimetabolites, alkylating agents, other drugs known to cause neutropenia • Increased serum levels and risk of toxicity of warfarin-type anticoagulants, phenytoin, beta-adrenergic blockers, alcohol, quinidine, lidocaine, theophylline, chloroquine, certain benzodiazepines (alprazolam, chlordiazepoxide, diazepam, flurazepam, triazolam), nifedipine, pentoxifylline, tricyclic antidepressants, procainamide, carbamazepine when taken with H$_2$ antagonists

■ Nursing considerations
Assessment
- **History:** Allergy to H$_2$ antagonists, impaired renal or hepatic function, lactation
- **Physical:** Skin lesions; orientation, affect; pulse, baseline ECG (continuous with IV use); liver evaluation, abdominal examination, normal output; CBC, LFTs, renal function tests

Interventions
- Administer drug with food and at bedtime.
- Decrease doses in renal and hepatic impairment.
- Administer IM dose undiluted, deep into large muscle group.
- Ensure ready access to bathroom.
- Provide comfort measures for rash, headache.
- Establish safety measures if CNS changes occur (side rails, accompany patient).
- Arrange for regular follow-up, including liver and renal function tests, to evaluate effects.

Teaching points
- Take these drugs with food and at bedtime; therapy may continue for 4–6 weeks or longer.
- Take antacids exactly as prescribed; be careful of the time.
- Inform your health care provider about your cigarette smoking habits. Cigarette smoking decreases the effectiveness of these drugs.
- Have regular medical follow-up while on this drug to evaluate your response.
- Report sore throat, fever, unusual bruising or bleeding, tarry stools, confusion, hallucinations, dizziness, muscle or joint pain.

Representative drugs
cimetidine
famotidine
nizatidine
ranitidine

HMG-CoA Inhibitors

PREGNANCY CATEGORY X

Therapeutic actions
HMG-CoA inhibitors are antihyperlipidemic. They are a fungal metabolite that inhibits the enzyme that catalyzes the first step in the cholesterol synthesis pathway in humans, resulting in a decrease in serum cholesterol and serum LDLs (associated with increased risk of CAD); either an increase or no change in serum HDLs (associated with decreased risk of CAD); and a decrease in triglycerides.

Indications
- Adjunct to diet in the treatment of elevated total and LDL cholesterol in patients with primary hypercholesterolemia (types IIa and IIb) whose response to dietary restriction of saturated fat and cholesterol and other nonpharmacologic measures has not been adequate
- Primary prevention of coronary events (lovastatin, pravastatin)
- Secondary prevention of CV events (fluvastatin, lovastatin, pravastatin, simvastatin)

Contraindications and cautions
- Contraindicated with allergy to HMG-CoA inhibitors, fungal byproducts, pregnancy, or lactation, concurrent gemfibrozil therapy.
- Use cautiously with impaired hepatic function, cataracts.

Adverse effects
- **CNS:** *Headache, blurred vision,* dizziness, insomnia, fatigue, muscle cramps, cataracts
- **GI:** *Flatulence, abdominal pain, cramps, constipation, nausea, vomiting,* heartburn, elevations of CK, alkaline phosphatase, and transaminases
- **Musculoskeletal: Rhabdomyolysis with possible renal failure**

Interactions

✱ **Drug-drug** • Monitor patients receiving HMG-CoA inhibitors for possible severe myopathy or rhabdomyolysis if taken with cyclosporine, erythromycin, gemfibrozil, niacin, azole antifungals

✱ **Drug-food** • Risk of increased serum levels if combined with grapefruit juice

■ **Nursing considerations**

Assessment

- **History:** Allergy to HMG-CoA inhibitors, fungal byproducts; impaired hepatic function; cataracts; pregnancy; lactation
- **Physical:** Orientation, affect, ophthalmologic examination; liver evaluation; lipid studies, LFTs

Interventions

- Administer drug at bedtime; highest rates of cholesterol synthesis are between midnight and 5 AM.
- Consult with dietitian about low-cholesterol diets.
- Arrange for diet and exercise consultation.
- Arrange for regular follow-up during long-term therapy.
- Provide comfort measures to deal with headache, muscle cramps, nausea.
- Arrange for periodic ophthalmologic examination to check for cataract development.
- Offer support and encouragement to deal with disease, diet, drug therapy, and follow-up.

Teaching points

- Take these drugs at bedtime.
- Institute appropriate diet changes.
- Use contraceptive measures to avoid pregnancy while using these drugs.
- Avoid grapefruit juice while taking these drugs.
- You may experience these side effects: Nausea (eat frequent small meals); headache, muscle and joint aches and pains (may lessen with time).
- Have periodic ophthalmic examinations while you are using these drugs.
- Report severe GI upset, changes in vision, unusual bleeding or bruising, dark urine or light-colored stools; muscle pain, weakness.

Representative drugs

atorvastatin
fluvastatin
lovastatin
pitavastatin
pravastatin
rosuvastatin
simvastatin

Macrolide Antibiotics

PREGNANCY CATEGORY B OR C

Therapeutic actions

Macrolides are antibiotics. They are bacteriostatic or bactericidal in susceptible bacteria; they bind to cell membranes and cause changes in protein function, leading to bacterial cell death.

Indications

- Treatment of acute infections caused by sensitive strains of *Streptococcus pneumoniae, Mycoplasma pneumoniae, Listeria monocytogenes, Legionella pneumophila;* URIs, lower respiratory tract infections, skin and soft-tissue infections caused by group A beta-hemolytic streptococci when oral treatment is preferred to injectable benzathine penicillin; PID caused by *Neisseria gonorrhoeae* in patients allergic to penicillin; intestinal amebiasis caused by *Entamoeba histolytica;* infections in the newborn and in pregnancy that are caused by *Chlamydia trachomatis* and in adult chlamydial infections when tetracycline cannot be used; primary syphilis (*Treponema pallidum*) in penicillin-allergic patients; eliminating *Bordetella pertussis* organisms from the nasopharynx of infected individuals and as prophylaxis in exposed and susceptible individuals; superficial ocular infections caused by susceptible strains of microorganisms; prophylaxis of ophthalmia neonatorum caused by *N. gonorrhoeae* or *C. trachomatis*
- In conjunction with sulfonamides to treat URIs caused by *Haemophilus influenzae*
- Adjunct to antitoxin in infections caused by *Corynebacterium diphtheriae* and *Corynebacterium minutissimum*
- Prophylaxis against alpha-hemolytic streptococcal endocarditis before dental or other procedures in patients allergic to penicillin who have valvular heart disease and against infection in minor skin abrasions

- Unlabeled uses: Treatment of severe diarrhea associated with *Campylobacter* enteritis or enterocolitis; treatment of genital, inguinal, or anorectal lymphogranuloma venereum infection; treatment of *Haemophilus ducreyi* (chancroid); treatment of acne vulgaris and skin infections caused by sensitive microorganisms

Contraindications and cautions
- Contraindicated with allergy to any macrolide antibiotic.
- Use cautiously with hepatic impairment or lactation (secreted and may be concentrated in breast milk; may modify bowel flora of breast-fed infant and interfere with fever workups).

Adverse effects
- **CNS:** Reversible hearing loss, confusion, uncontrollable emotions, abnormal thinking, headache
- **Dermatologic:** Edema, urticaria, dermatitis, angioneurotic edema
- **GI:** *Abdominal cramping, anorexia, diarrhea, vomiting,* pseudomembranous colitis, hepatotoxicity
- **Hypersensitivity:** Allergic reactions ranging from rash to **anaphylaxis**
- **Local:** *Irritation, burning, itching* at site of application
- **Other:** *Superinfections*

Interactions
✱ **Drug-drug** • Increased serum levels of digoxin • Increased effects of oral anticoagulants, theophyllines, carbamazepine • Increased therapeutic and toxic effects of corticosteroids • Increased levels of cyclosporine and risk of renal toxicity • Increased irritant effects with peeling, desquamating, or abrasive agents used with dermatologic preparations • Risk of prolonged QT interval if combined with other drugs that prolong QT interval

✱ **Drug-lab test** • Interferes with fluorometric determination of urinary catecholamines • Decreased urinary estriol levels caused by inhibition of hydrolysis of steroids in the gut

■ Nursing considerations
Assessment
- **History:** Allergy to macrolides, hepatic impairment, lactation, viral, fungal, myco-

bacterial infections of the eye (ophthalmologic)
- **Physical:** Site of infection, skin color, lesions; orientation, affect, hearing tests; R, adventitious sounds; GI output, bowel sounds, liver evaluation; culture and sensitivity tests of infection, urinalysis, LFTs

Interventions
- Culture site of infection before therapy.
- Administer oral erythromycin base or stearate on an empty stomach, 1 hr before or 2–3 hr after meals, with a full glass of water (oral erythromycin estolate, ethylsuccinate, and certain enteric-coated tablets; see manufacturer's instructions; may be given without regard to meals).
- Administer drug around the clock to maximize therapeutic effect; scheduling may have to be adjusted to minimize sleep disruption.
- ⊗ **Black box warning** Monitor liver function in patients on prolonged therapy; serious toxicity can occur.
- Institute hygiene measures and treatment if superinfections occur.
- If GI upset occurs with oral therapy, some preparations (see previous) may be given with meals, or it may be possible to substitute one of these preparations.
- Provide frequent small meals if GI problems occur.
- Establish safety measures (accompany patient, side rails) if CNS changes occur.
- Give patient support and encouragement to continue with therapy.
- Wash affected area, rinse well, and dry before topical application.

Teaching points
- Take oral drugs on an empty stomach, 1 hr before or 2–3 hrs after meals, with a full glass of water, or, as appropriate, drug may be taken without regard to meals. These drugs should be taken around the clock; schedule to minimize sleep disruption. It is important that you finish the *full course* of the drug therapy.
- Wash and rinse area and pat it dry before applying topical solutions; use fingertips or an applicator; wash hands thoroughly after application.

- You may experience these side effects: Stomach cramping, discomfort (taking the drug with meals, if appropriate, may alleviate this problem); uncontrollable emotions, crying, laughing, abnormal thinking (will end when the drug is stopped).
- Report severe or watery diarrhea, severe nausea or vomiting, dark urine, yellowing of the skin or eyes, loss of hearing, skin rash or itching.

Representative drugs
  azithromycin
  clarithromycin
  erythromycin
  fidaxomicin

Nitrates

PREGNANCY CATEGORY C

Therapeutic actions
Nitrates are antianginals. They relax vascular smooth muscle with a resultant decrease in venous return and decrease in arterial blood pressure, which reduces left ventricular workload and decreases myocardial oxygen consumption, relieving the pain of angina.

Indications
- Treatment of acute angina (sublingual, translingual, inhalant preparations)
- Prophylaxis of angina (oral sustained release, sublingual, topical, transdermal, translingual, transmucosal preparations)
- Treatment of angina unresponsive to recommended doses of organic nitrates or betablockers (IV preparations)
- Management of perioperative hypertension, heart failure associated with acute MI (IV preparations)
- Produce controlled hypotension during surgery (IV preparations)
- Unlabeled uses: Reduction of cardiac workload in acute MI and in heart failure (sublingual, topical); diffuse esophageal spasm without reflux

Contraindications and cautions
- Contraindicated with allergy to nitrates, angle-closure glaucoma, severe anemia, early MI, head trauma, cerebral hemorrhage, cardiomyopathy, concommitant use with phosphodiesterase type 5 (PDE5) inhibitors, pregnancy, or lactation.
- Use cautiously with hepatic or renal disease, hypotension or hypovolemia, increased intracranial pressure, constrictive pericarditis, pericardial tamponade, low ventricular filling pressure or low pulmonary capillary wedge pressure (PCWP).

Adverse effects
- **CNS:** *Headache,* apprehension, restlessness, weakness, vertigo, dizziness, faintness
- **CV:** Tachycardia, retrosternal discomfort, palpitations, **hypotension,** syncope, collapse, orthostatic hypotension, angina
- **Dermatologic:** Rash, exfoliative dermatitis, cutaneous vasodilation with flushing, pallor, perspiration, cold sweat, contact dermatitis (transdermal preparations), topical allergic reactions (topical nitroglycerin ointment)
- **GI:** Nausea, vomiting, incontinence of urine and feces, abdominal pain
- **Local:** Local burning sensation at the point of dissolution (sublingual)
- **Other:** Ethanol intoxication with high dose IV use (alcohol in diluent)

Interactions
✳ **Drug-drug** ● Increased risk of hypertension and decreased antianginal effect with ergot alkaloids ● Decreased pharmacologic effects of heparin ● Risk of orthostatic hypotension with calcium channel blockers ● Profound hypotension with PDE5 inhibitors
✳ **Drug-lab test** ● False report of decreased serum cholesterol if done by the Zlatkis-Zak color reaction

■ Nursing considerations
Assessment
- **History:** Allergy to nitrates, severe anemia, early MI, head trauma, cerebral hemorrhage, hypertrophic cardiomyopathy, hepatic or renal disease, hypotension or hypovolemia, increased intracranial pressure, constrictive pericarditis, pericardial tamponade, low ventricular filling pressure or low PCWP, pregnancy, lactation
- **Physical:** Skin color, T, lesions; orientation, reflexes, affect; P, BP, orthostatic BP, baseline ECG, peripheral perfusion; R, adventitious sounds; liver evaluation, normal output; LFTs (IV); renal function tests (IV); CBC, Hgb

Interventions
- Administer sublingual preparations under the tongue or in the buccal pouch. Encourage the patient not to swallow. Ask patient if the tablet "fizzles" or burns. Check the expiration date on the bottle; store at room temperature, protected from light. Discard unused drug 6 mo after bottle is opened (conventional tablets); stabilized tablets (*Nitrostat*) are less subject to loss of potency.
- Administer sustained-release preparations with water; tell the patient not to chew the tablets or capsules; do not crush these preparations.
- Administer topical ointment by applying it over a $6'' \times 6''$ area in a thin, uniform layer using the applicator. Cover area with plastic wrap held in place by adhesive tape. Rotate sites of application to decrease the chance of inflammation and sensitization; close tube tightly when finished.
- Administer transdermal systems to skin site free of hair and not subject to much movement. Shave areas that have a lot of hair. Do not apply to distal extremities. Change sites slightly to decrease the chance of local irritation and sensitization. Remove transdermal system before attempting defibrillation or cardioversion. Remove old system before applying new system.
- Administer transmucosal tablets by placing them between the lip and gum above the incisors or between the cheek and gum. Encourage patient not to swallow and not to chew the tablet.
- Administer the translingual spray directly onto the oral mucosa; preparation is not to be inhaled.
- Withdraw drug gradually; 4–6 wk recommended period for the transdermal preparations.
- Establish safety measures if CNS effects, hypotension occur.
- Keep environment cool, dim, and quiet.
- Provide periodic rest periods for patient.
- Provide comfort measures and arrange for analgesics if headache occurs.
- Maintain life support equipment on standby if overdose occurs or cardiac condition worsens.
- Provide support and encouragement to deal with disease, therapy, and needed lifestyle changes.

Teaching points
- Place sublingual tablets under your tongue or in your cheek; do not chew or swallow the tablet; the tablet should burn or "fizzle" under the tongue. Take nitroglycerin before chest pain begins, when you anticipate that your activities or situation may precipitate an attack. Do not buy large quantities; these drugs do not store well. Keep these drugs in a dark, dry place, in a dark-colored glass bottle with a tight lid; do not combine with other drugs. You may repeat your dose every 5 minutes for a total of three tablets; if the pain is still not relieved, go to an emergency room.
- Do not chew or crush the timed-release preparations; take on an empty stomach.
- Spread a thin layer of topical ointment on the skin using the applicator. Do not rub or massage the area. Cover with plastic wrap held in place with adhesive tape. Wash your hands after application. Keep the tube tightly closed. Rotate the sites frequently to prevent local irritation.
- To use transdermal systems, you may need to shave an area for application. Apply to a slightly different area each day. Use care if changing brands; each system has a different concentration. Remove the old system before applying a new one.
- Place transmucosal tablets between the lip and gum or between the gum and cheek. Do not chew; try not to swallow.
- Spray translingual spray directly onto oral mucous membranes; do not inhale. Use 5–10 minutes before activities that you anticipate will precipitate an attack.
- Take these drugs exactly as directed; do not exceed recommended dosage.
- Do not take erectile dysfunction drugs while you are using a nitrate.
- You may experience these side effects: Dizziness, light-headedness (this may pass as you adjust to the drug; change positions slowly); headache (lying down in a cool environment and resting may help; over-the-counter preparations may not help); flushing of the neck or face (this usually passes as the drug's effects pass).
- Report blurred vision, persistent or severe headache, skin rash, more frequent or more severe angina attacks, fainting.

Representative drugs

isosorbide dinitrate
isosorbide mononitrate
nitroglycerin

Nondepolarizing Neuromuscular Junction Blockers (NMJ Blockers)

DANGEROUS DRUG

PREGNANCY CATEGORY C

Therapeutic actions

NMJ blockers interfere with neuromuscular transmission and cause flaccid paralysis by blocking acetylcholine receptors at the skeletal neuromuscular junction.

Indications

- Adjuncts to general anesthetics to facilitate endotracheal intubation and relax skeletal muscle; to relax skeletal muscle to facilitate mechanical ventilation

Contraindications and cautions

- Contraindicated with hypersensitivity to NMJ blockers and the bromide ion.
- Use cautiously with myasthenia gravis; pregnancy (teratogenic in preclinical studies; may be used in cesarean section, but reversal may be difficult if patient has received magnesium sulfate to manage preeclampsia); renal or hepatic disease, respiratory depression, altered fluid or electrolyte balance; patients in whom an increase in heart rate may be dangerous.

Adverse effects

- **CV:** *Increased heart rate*
- **Hypersensitivity:** Hypersensitivity reactions, especially rash
- **Musculoskeletal:** Profound and prolonged muscle paralysis
- **Respiratory:** *Depressed respiration, apnea,* bronchospasm

Interactions

＊ **Drug-drug** ● Increased intensity and duration of neuromuscular block with some anesthetics (isoflurane, enflurane, halothane, diethyl ether), some parenteral antibiotics (aminogly-

cosides, clindamycin, lincomycin, bacitracin, polymyxin B), ketamine, quinine, quinidine, calcium channel-blocking drugs (eg, verapamil), Mg^{2+} salts, and in hypokalemia (from K^+-depleting diuretics) ● Decreased intensity of neuromuscular block with acetylcholine, cholinesterase inhibitors, K^+ salts, theophyllines, phenytoins, azathioprine, mercaptopurine, carbamazepine

■ Nursing considerations

Assessment

- **History:** Hypersensitivity to NMJ blockers and the bromide ion, myasthenia gravis, pregnancy, renal or hepatic disease, respiratory depression, altered fluid or electrolyte balance
- **Physical:** Weight, T, skin condition, hydration, reflexes, bilateral grip strength, pulse, BP, R and adventitious sounds, LFTs, renal function tests, serum electrolytes

Interventions

⊗ **Black box warning** Drug should be given only by trained personnel (anesthesiologists); intubation will be necessary.

- Arrange to have facilities on standby to maintain airway and provide mechanical ventilation.
- Provide neostigmine, pyridostigmine, or edrophonium (cholinesterase inhibitors) on standby to overcome excessive neuromuscular block.
- Provide atropine or glycopyrrolate on standby to prevent parasympathomimetic effects of cholinesterase inhibitors.
- Provide a peripheral nerve stimulator on standby to assess degree of neuromuscular block, as needed.
- Change patient's position frequently, and provide skin care to prevent decubitus ulcer formation when drug is used for other than brief periods.
- Monitor conscious patient for pain or distress that he may not be able to communicate.
- Reassure conscious patients frequently.

Teaching points

- Teaching points about what these drugs do and how the patient will feel should be incorporated into the overall teaching program about the procedure.

Representative drugs

atracurium
cisatracurium
pancuronium
rocuronium
vecuronium

Nonsteroidal Anti-inflammatory Drugs (NSAIDs)

PREGNANCY CATEGORY B OR C
(FIRST AND SECOND TRIMESTERS)
PREGNANCY CATEGORY D
(THIRD TRIMESTER)

Therapeutic actions

NSAIDs have anti-inflammatory, analgesic, and antipyretic activities largely related to inhibition of prostaglandin synthesis; exact mechanisms of action are not known.

Indications

- Relief of signs and symptoms of rheumatoid arthritis, osteoarthritis, and juvenile arthritis
- Relief of mild to moderate pain
- Treatment of primary dysmenorrhea
- Fever reduction
- Reduction of number of adenomatous colorectal polyps in adults with familial adenomatous polyposis

Contraindications and cautions

- Contraindicated with allergy to salicylates or other NSAIDs (more common in patients with rhinitis, asthma, chronic urticaria, nasal polyps); CV dysfunction, hypertension; peptic ulceration, GI bleeding; pregnancy or lactation.
- Use cautiously with impaired hepatic function, impaired renal function, heart failure.

Adverse effects

- **CNS:** *Headache, dizziness, somnolence, insomnia,* fatigue, tiredness, tinnitus, ophthalmologic effects
- **Dermatologic:** *Rash,* pruritus, sweating, dry mucous membranes, stomatitis
- **GI:** *Nausea, dyspepsia, GI pain,* diarrhea, vomiting, constipation, flatulence
- **GU:** Dysuria, renal impairment

- **Hematologic:** Bleeding, platelet inhibition with higher doses, neutropenia, eosinophilia, leukopenia, pancytopenia, thrombocytopenia, agranulocytosis, granulocytopenia, aplastic anemia, decreased Hgb or Hct, bone marrow depression, menorrhagia
- **Respiratory:** Dyspnea, hemoptysis, pharyngitis, bronchospasm, rhinitis
- **Other:** Peripheral edema, anaphylactoid reactions to **anaphylactic shock**

Interactions

✳ **Drug-drug** • Increased toxic effects of lithium with NSAIDs • Decreased diuretic effect with loop diuretics: bumetanide, furosemide, ethacrynic acid • Potential decrease in antihypertensive effect of beta-adrenergic blockers

■ Nursing considerations

Assessment

- **History:** Allergy to salicylates or other NSAIDs; CV dysfunction, hypertension; peptic ulceration, GI bleeding; impaired hepatic function; impaired renal function; pregnancy; lactation
- **Physical:** Skin color, lesions; T; orientation, reflexes, ophthalmologic evaluation, audiometric evaluation, peripheral sensation; P, BP, edema; R, adventitious sounds; liver evaluation, bowel sounds; CBC, clotting times, urinalysis, LFTs, renal function tests, serum electrolytes, stool guaiac

Interventions

⊗ *Black box warning* Monitor patient for CV events, GI bleed; risk may be increased.

- Administer drug with food or after meals if GI upset occurs.
- Establish safety measures if CNS, visual disturbances occur.
- Arrange for periodic ophthalmologic examination during long-term therapy.
- Arrange for discontinuation of drug if eye changes, symptoms of hepatic impairment, renal impairment occur.
- Institute emergency procedures if overdose occurs (gastric lavage, induction of emesis, supportive therapy).
- Provide comfort measures to reduce pain and to reduce inflammation.
- Provide frequent small meals if GI upset is severe.

Teaching points

- Use these drugs only as suggested. Do not exceed the prescribed dosage. Take these drugs with food or after meals if GI upset occurs.
- Avoid over-the-counter drugs while taking these drugs. Many of these drugs contain similar medications; serious overdosage can occur. If you feel you need one of these preparations, consult your health care provider.
- Avoid alcohol while taking these drugs.
- You may experience these side effects: Nausea, GI upset, dyspepsia (take with food); diarrhea or constipation; drowsiness, dizziness, vertigo, insomnia (use caution when driving or operating dangerous machinery).
- Report sore throat, fever, rash, itching, weight gain, swelling in ankles or fingers, changes in vision, black or tarry stools.

Representative drugs

celecoxib
diclofenac
diflunisal
etodolac
fenoprofen
flurbiprofen
ibuprofen
indomethacin
ketoprofen
ketorolac
mefenamic acid
meloxicam
nabumetone
naproxen
oxaprozin
piroxicam
sulindac
tolmetin

Opioids

PREGNANCY CATEGORY B OR C
CONTROLLED SUBSTANCE C-II, C-III

Therapeutic actions

Opioids act as agonists at specific opioid receptors in the CNS to produce analgesia, euphoria, sedation; the receptors mediating these effects are thought to be the same as those mediating the effects of endogenous opioids (enkephalins, endorphins).

Indications

- Relief of moderate to severe acute and chronic pain
- Preoperative medication to sedate and allay apprehension, facilitate induction of anesthesia, and reduce anesthetic dosage
- Analgesic adjunct during anesthesia
- Intraspinal use with microinfusion devices for the relief of intractable pain
- Unlabeled use: Relief of dyspnea associated with acute left ventricular failure and pulmonary edema

Contraindications and cautions

- Contraindicated with hypersensitivity to opioids, diarrhea caused by poisoning until toxins are eliminated, during labor or delivery of a preterm infant (may cross immature blood–brain barrier more readily), after biliary tract surgery or following surgical anastomosis, pregnancy, or labor (can cause respiratory depression of neonate; may prolong labor).
- Use cautiously with head injury and increased intracranial pressure; acute asthma, COPD, cor pulmonale, preexisting respiratory depression, hypoxia, hypercapnia (may decrease respiratory drive and increase airway resistance); lactation (may be safer to wait 4–6 hr after administration to nurse the baby); acute abdominal conditions; CV disease, supraventricular tachycardias; myxedema; seizure disorders; acute alcoholism, delirium tremens; cerebral arteriosclerosis; ulcerative colitis; fever; kyphoscoliosis; Addison's disease; prostatic hypertrophy, urethral stricture; recent GI or GU surgery; toxic psychosis; renal or hepatic impairment.

Adverse effects

- **CNS:** *Light-headedness, dizziness, sedation,* euphoria, dysphoria, delirium, insomnia, agitation, anxiety, fear, hallucinations, disorientation, drowsiness, lethargy, impaired mental and physical performance, coma, mood changes, weakness, headache, tremor, seizures, miosis, visual disturbances, suppression of cough reflex
- **CV:** Facial flushing, peripheral circulatory collapse, tachycardia, *bradycardia,* arrhythmia, palpitations, chest wall rigidity, hypertension, hypotension, orthostatic hypotension, syncope

Adverse effects in *italics* are most common; those in **bold** are life-threatening. ⬛ Do not crush.

- **Dermatologic:** Pruritus, urticaria, laryngospasm, bronchospasm, edema
- **GI:** *Nausea, vomiting,* dry mouth, anorexia, *constipation,* biliary tract spasm; increased colonic motility in patients with chronic ulcerative colitis
- **GU:** Ureteral spasm, spasm of vesical sphincters, urinary retention or hesitancy, oliguria, antidiuretic effect, reduced libido or potency
- **Local:** Tissue irritation and induration (subcutaneous injection)
- **Major hazards: Respiratory depression, apnea, circulatory depression, respiratory arrest, shock, cardiac arrest**
- **Other:** *Sweating,* physical tolerance and dependence, psychological dependence

Interactions

☀ **Drug-drug** • Increased likelihood of respiratory depression, hypotension, profound sedation, or coma in patients receiving barbiturate general anesthetics

☀ **Drug-lab test** • Elevated biliary tract pressure (an effect of opioids) may cause increases in plasma amylase, lipase; determinations of these levels may be unreliable for 24 hr

■ Nursing considerations
Assessment

- **History:** Hypersensitivity to opioids; diarrhea caused by poisoning; labor or delivery of a premature infant; biliary tract surgery or surgical anastomosis; head injury and increased intracranial pressure; acute asthma, COPD, cor pulmonale, preexisting respiratory depression, hypoxia, hypercapnia; acute abdominal conditions; CV disease, supraventricular tachycardias; myxedema; seizure disorders; acute alcoholism, delirium tremens; cerebral arteriosclerosis; ulcerative colitis; fever; kyphoscoliosis; Addison's disease; prostatic hypertrophy; urethral stricture; recent GI or GU surgery; toxic psychosis; renal or hepatic impairment; pregnancy; lactation
- **Physical:** T; skin color, texture, lesions; orientation, reflexes, bilateral grip strength, affect; P, auscultation, BP, orthostatic BP, perfusion; R, adventitious sounds; bowel sounds, normal output; urinary frequency, voiding pattern, normal output; ECG; EEG; LFTs, thyroid and renal function tests

Interventions

- Caution patient not to chew or crush controlled-release preparations.
- Dilute and administer IV slowly to minimize likelihood of adverse effects.
- Direct patient to lie down during IV administration.
- Keep opioid antagonist and equipment for assisted or controlled respiration readily available during IV administration.
- Use caution when injecting IM or subcutaneously into chilled areas or in patients with hypotension or in shock; impaired perfusion may delay absorption; with repeated doses, an excessive amount may be absorbed when circulation is restored.
- Monitor injection sites for irritation, extravasation.
- Instruct postoperative patients in pulmonary toilet; drug suppresses cough reflex.
- Monitor bowel function and arrange for anthraquinone laxatives for severe constipation.
- Institute safety precautions (use side rails, assist with walking) if CNS, vision effects occur.
- Provide frequent small meals if GI upset occurs.
- Control environment if sweating, visual difficulties occur.
- Provide back rubs, positioning, and other nondrug measures to alleviate pain.
- Reassure patient about addiction liability; most patients who receive opioids for medical reasons do not develop dependence syndromes.

Teaching points

When these drugs are used as a preoperative medication, teach the patient about the drug when explaining the procedure.

- Take these drugs exactly as prescribed. Avoid alcohol, antihistamines, sedatives, tranquilizers, and over-the-counter drugs.
- Do not take any leftover medication for other disorders, and do not let anyone else take your prescription.
- You may experience these side effects: Nausea, loss of appetite (take the drug with food and lie quietly); constipation (notify your health care provider if this is severe; a laxative may help); dizziness, sedation, drowsiness, impaired visual acuity (avoid driving or performing other tasks requiring alertness, visual acuity).

- Report severe nausea, vomiting, constipation, shortness of breath or difficulty breathing, skin rash.

Representative drugs
alfentanil
buprenorphine
butorphanol
codeine
fentanyl
hydrocodone
hydromorphone
levorphanol
meperidine
methadone
morphine sulfate
nalbuphine
opium
oxycodone
oxymorphone
pentazocine
sufentanil
tapentadol
tramadol

Penicillins

PREGNANCY CATEGORY B

Therapeutic actions
Penicillins are antibiotics. They are bactericidal, inhibiting the synthesis of cell wall of sensitive organisms, causing cell death in susceptible organisms.

Indications
- Treatment of moderate to severe infections caused by sensitive organisms: streptococci, pneumococci, staphylococci, *Neisseria gonorrhoeae, Treponema pallidum,* meningococci, *Actinomyces israelii, Clostridium perfringens, Clostridium tetani, Leptotrichia buccalis* (Vincent's disease), *Spirillum minus* or *Streptobacillus moniliformis, Listeria monocytogenes, Pasteurella multocida, Erysipelothrix insidiosa, Escherichia coli, Enterobacter aerogenes, Alcaligenes faecalis, Salmonella, Shigella, Proteus mirabilis, Corynebacterium diphtheriae, Bacillus anthracis*
- Treatment of syphilis, gonococcal infections
- Unlabeled use: Treatment of Lyme disease

Contraindications and cautions
- Contraindicated with allergy to penicillins, cephalosporins, other allergens.
- Use cautiously with renal disease, pregnancy, lactation (may cause diarrhea or candidiasis in the infant).

Adverse effects
- **CNS:** Lethargy, hallucinations, seizures
- **GI:** *Glossitis, stomatitis, gastritis, sore mouth,* furry tongue, black "hairy" tongue, *nausea, vomiting, diarrhea,* abdominal pain, bloody diarrhea, enterocolitis, pseudomembranous colitis, nonspecific hepatitis
- **GU:** Nephritis-oliguria, proteinuria, hematuria, casts, azotemia, pyuria
- **Hematologic:** Anemia, thrombocytopenia, leukopenia, neutropenia, prolonged bleeding time
- **Hypersensitivity:** *Rash, fever, wheezing,* **anaphylaxis**
- **Local:** *Pain, phlebitis,* thrombosis at injection site, Jarisch-Herxheimer reaction when used to treat syphilis
- **Other:** *Superinfections,* sodium overload, leading to heart failure

Interactions
✳ **Drug-drug** ● Decreased effectiveness with tetracyclines ● Inactivation of parenteral aminoglycosides (amikacin, gentamicin, kanamycin, neomycin, streptomycin, tobramycin) if mixed in the same solution ● Risk of increased serum levels if combined with aspirin, indomethacin, diuretics, sulfonamides
✳ **Drug-lab test** ● False-positive Coombs' test (IV)

■ Nursing considerations
Assessment
- **History:** Allergy to penicillins, cephalosporins, other allergens, renal disease, lactation
- **Physical:** Culture infected area; skin rashes, lesions; R, adventitious sounds; bowel sounds, normal output; CBC, LFTs, renal function tests, serum electrolytes, Hct, urinalysis; skin test with benzylpenicilloyl-polylysine if hypersensitivity reactions have occurred

Interventions

- Culture infected area before beginning treatment; reculture area if response is not as expected.
- Use the smallest dose possible for IM injection to avoid pain and discomfort.
- Arrange to continue treatment for 48–72 hr after the patient becomes asymptomatic.
- Monitor serum electrolytes and cardiac status if penicillin G is given by IV infusion. Na or K preparations have been associated with severe electrolyte imbalances.
- Check IV site carefully for signs of thrombosis or local drug reaction.
- Do not give IM injections repeatedly in the same site; atrophy can occur. Monitor injection sites.
- Explain the reason for parenteral routes of administration; offer support and encouragement to deal with therapy.
- Provide frequent small meals if GI upset occurs.
- Arrange for comfort and treatment measures for superinfections.
- Provide for frequent mouth care if GI effects occur.
- Ensure that bathroom facilities are readily available if diarrhea occurs.
- Keep epinephrine, IV fluids, vasopressors, bronchodilators, oxygen, and emergency equipment readily available in case of serious hypersensitivity reaction.
- Arrange for the use of corticosteroids, antihistamines for skin reactions.

Teaching points

- You may experience these side effects: Upset stomach, nausea, vomiting (eat frequent small meals); sore mouth (provide frequent mouth care); diarrhea; pain or discomfort at the injection site (report if very uncomfortable).
- Report unusual bleeding, sore throat, rash, hives, fever, severe diarrhea, difficulty breathing.

Representative drugs

amoxicillin
ampicillin
oxacillin
penicillin G benzathine
penicillin G potassium
penicillin G procaine
penicillin V
piperacillin

Phenothiazines

PREGNANCY CATEGORY C

Therapeutic actions

Mechanism of action of phenothiazines is not fully understood. Antipsychotic drugs block postsynaptic dopamine receptors in the brain, but this may not be necessary and sufficient for antipsychotic activity; depresses the RAS, including the parts of the brain involved with wakefulness and emesis; anticholinergic, antihistaminic (H_1), and alpha-adrenergic blocking activity also may contribute to some of its therapeutic (and adverse) actions.

Indications

- Management of manifestations of psychotic disorders
- Control of severe nausea and vomiting, intractable hiccups

Contraindications and cautions

- Contraindicated with coma or severe CNS depression, bone marrow depression, blood dyscrasia, circulatory collapse, subcortical brain damage, Parkinson's disease, liver damage, cerebral arteriosclerosis, coronary disease, severe hypotension or hypertension, prolonged QTc interval.
- Use cautiously with respiratory disorders ("silent pneumonia" may develop); glaucoma, prostatic hypertrophy; epilepsy or history of epilepsy; breast cancer; thyrotoxicosis; peptic ulcer, decreased renal function; myelography within previous 24 hr or scheduled within 48 hr; exposure to heat or phosphorous insecticides; pregnancy; lactation; children younger than 12 yr, especially those with chickenpox, CNS infections (children are especially susceptible to dystonias that may confound the diagnosis of Reye's syndrome).

Adverse effects

- **Autonomic:** Dry mouth, salivation, nasal congestion, nausea, vomiting, anorexia, fever, pallor, flushed facies, sweating, constipation, paralytic ileus, urine retention, incontinence, polyuria, enuresis, priapism, ejaculation inhibition, male impotence

- **CNS:** *Drowsiness,* insomnia, vertigo, headache, weakness, tremor, ataxia, slurring, cerebral edema, seizures, exacerbation of psychotic symptoms, extrapyramidal syndromes—*pseudoparkinsonism; dystonias; akathisia,* tardive dyskinesias, potentially irreversible (no known treatment) **neuroleptic malignant syndrome**
- **CV:** Hypotension, orthostatic hypotension, hypertension, tachycardia, bradycardia, cardiac arrest, heart failure, cardiomegaly, **refractory arrhythmias,** pulmonary edema, **prolonged QTc interval**
- **EENT:** Glaucoma, *photophobia, blurred vision,* miosis, mydriasis, deposits in the cornea and lens (opacities), pigmentary retinopathy
- **Endocrine:** Lactation, breast engorgement in females, galactorrhea; syndrome of inappropriate ADH secretion; amenorrhea, menstrual irregularities; gynecomastia in males; changes in libido; hyperglycemia or hypoglycemia; glycosuria; hyponatremia; pituitary tumor with hyperprolactinemia; inhibition of ovulation, infertility, pseudopregnancy; reduced urinary levels of gonadotropins, estrogens, progestins
- **Hematologic:** Eosinophilia, leukopenia, leukocytosis, anemia; aplastic anemia; hemolytic anemia; thrombocytopenic or nonthrombocytopenic purpura; pancytopenia
- **Hypersensitivity:** Jaundice, urticaria, angioneurotic edema, laryngeal edema, photosensitivity, eczema, asthma, anaphylactoid reactions, exfoliative dermatitis
- **Respiratory:** Bronchospasm, laryngospasm, dyspnea; suppression of cough reflex and potential for aspiration (**sudden death related to asphyxia** or cardiac arrest has been reported)
- **Other:** *Urine discolored pink to red-brown*

Interactions

✳ **Drug-drug** • Additive CNS depression with alcohol • Additive anticholinergic effects and possibly decreased antipsychotic efficacy with anticholinergic drugs • Increased likelihood of seizures with metrizamide (contrast agent used in myelography) • Increased chance of severe neuromuscular excitation and hypotension if given to patients receiving barbiturate anesthetics (methohexital, phenobarbital, thiopen-

tal) • Increased risk of cardiac arrhythmias and serious adverse effects if combined with drugs that prolong the QTc interval

✳ **Drug-lab test** • False-positive pregnancy tests (less likely if serum test is used) • Increase in protein-bound iodine, not attributable to an increase in thyroxine

■ Nursing considerations
Assessment

- **History:** Coma or severe CNS depression; bone marrow depression; blood dyscrasia; circulatory collapse; subcortical brain damage; Parkinson's disease; liver damage; cerebral arteriosclerosis; coronary disease; severe hypotension or hypertension; respiratory disorders; glaucoma, prostatic hypertrophy; epilepsy or history of epilepsy; breast cancer; thyrotoxicosis; peptic ulcer, decreased renal function; myelography within previous 24 hr or myelography scheduled within 48 hr; exposure to heat or phosphorous insecticides; pregnancy; children younger than 12 yr, especially those with chickenpox, CNS infections
- **Physical:** Weight; T; reflexes, orientation, IOP; P, BP, orthostatic BP; R, adventitious sounds; bowel sounds and normal output, liver evaluation; urinary output, prostate size; CBC, urinalysis, thyroid, LFTs, renal function tests, ECG analysis

Interventions

- Obtain baseline ECG with QTc interval noted.
- Dilute oral concentrate *only* with water, saline, *7-Up,* homogenized milk, carbonated orange drink, and pineapple, apricot, prune, orange, *V-8,* tomato, or grapefruit juices; use 60 mL of diluent for each 16 mg (5 mL) of concentrate.
- Do *not* mix with beverages that contain caffeine (coffee, cola), tannics (tea), or pectinates (apple juice); physical incompatibility may result.
- Give IM injections only to seated or recumbent patients, and observe for adverse effects for a brief period afterward.
- Monitor pulse and BP continuously during IV administration.
- Do not change long-term therapy dosage more often than weekly; it takes 4–7 days to achieve steady-state plasma levels of drug.

- Avoid skin contact with oral solution; contact dermatitis has occurred.
- Arrange for discontinuation of drug if serum creatinine, BUN become abnormal or if WBC count is depressed.
- Monitor bowel function, arrange therapy for severe constipation; adynamic ileus with fatal complications has occurred.
- Monitor elderly patients for dehydration and institute remedial measures promptly; sedation and decreased sensation of thirst related to CNS effects of drug can lead to severe dehydration.
- Consult physician regarding warning of patient or patient's guardian about tardive dyskinesias.
- Consult physician about reducing dosage, using anticholinergic antiparkinsonians (controversial) if extrapyramidal effects occur.
- Provide safety measures (side rails, assist) if sedation, ataxia, vertigo, orthostatic hypotension, vision changes occur.
- Provide positioning to relieve discomfort of dystonias.
- Provide reassurance to deal with extrapyramidal effect, sexual dysfunction.

Teaching points

- Take these drugs exactly as prescribed. The full effect may require 6 weeks–6 months of therapy.
- Avoid skin contact with drug solutions.
- Avoid driving or engaging in activities requiring alertness if CNS, vision changes occur.
- Avoid prolonged exposure to sun or use a sunscreen or covering garments.
- Maintain fluid intake, and use precautions against heatstroke in hot weather.
- Report sore throat, fever, unusual bleeding or bruising, rash, weakness, tremors, impaired vision, dark urine (pink or reddish brown urine is to be expected), pale stools, yellowing of the skin or eyes.

Representative drugs

chlorpromazine
fluphenazine
perphenazine
prochlorperazine
thioridazine

Phosphodiesterase Type 5 Inhibitors

PREGNANCY CATEGORY B

Therapeutic actions

Selectively inhibits cGMP-specific phosphodiesterase type 5. The mechanism of penile erection involves the release of nitric oxide into the corpus cavernosum of the penis during sexual stimulation. Nitrous oxide activates cGMP, which causes smooth muscle relaxation allowing the flow of blood into the corpus cavernosum. Phosphodiesterase type 5 inhibitors prevent the breakdown of cGMP by phosphodiesterase, leading to increased cGMP levels and prolonged smooth muscle relaxation promoting the flow of blood into the corpus cavernosum.

Indications

- Treatment of erectile dysfunction in the presence of sexual stimulation
- Treatment of pulmonary arterial hypertension

Contraindications and cautions

- Contraindicated with allergy to any component of the drugs, for women or children; concurrent use of nitrates or alpha blockers.
- Use cautiously with hepatic or renal impairment; with anatomical deformation of the penis; with known cardiac disease (effects of sexual activity need to be evaluated); congenital prolonged QT interval; unstable angina; hypotension (systolic lower than 90); uncontrolled hypertension (higher than 170/110); severe hepatic impairment; end-stage renal disease with dialysis; hereditary degenerative retinal disorders.

Adverse effects

- **CNS:** *Headache,* abnormal vision, changes in color vision, fatigue, hearing loss
- **CV:** *Flushing,* angina, chest pain, hypertension, hypotension, **MI,** palpitations, orthostatic hypotension, tachycardia
- **GI:** *Dyspepsia,* diarrhea, abdominal pain, dry mouth, esophagitis, gastritis, GERD, nausea, abnormal LFT
- **GU:** Abnormal erection, spontaneous erection, priapism
- **Respiratory:** Rhinitis, sinusitis, dyspnea, epistaxis, pharyngitis, nasal congestion

- **Other:** Flulike symptoms, edema, pain, rash, sweating, myalgia

Interactions

❋ **Drug-drug** • Possible severe hypotension and serious cardiac events if combined with nitrates, alpha blockers; this combination is contraindicated • Possible increased levels and effects if taken with ketoconazole, itraconazole, erythromycin; monitor patient and reduce dosage as needed • Increased serum levels if combined with indinavir, ritonavir; if these drugs are being used, limit dosage • Reduced levels and effectiveness if combined with rifampin • Risk for increased cardiac effects, decreased BP, flushing if combined with alcohol; warn patient of this possibility if alcohol is used

❋ **Drug-food** • Possible increased levels if taken with grapefruit juice

■ Nursing considerations

Assessment

- **History:** Allergy to any component of the tablet, concurrent use of nitrates or alpha blockers; unstable angina; hypotension; uncontrolled hypertension; severe hepatic impairment; end-stage renal disease with dialysis; hereditary degenerative retinal disorders; anatomical deformation of the penis, cardiac disease, congenital prolonged QT interval
- **Physical:** Orientation, affect; skin color, lesions; R, adventitious sounds; P, BP, ECG, LFTs, renal function tests

Interventions

- Assure diagnosis of erectile dysfunction and determine underlying causes and other appropriate treatment.
- Advise patient that drug does not work in the absence of sexual stimulation. Limit use to once per day.
- Remind patient that drug does not protect against STDs and that appropriate measures should be taken.
- ⊗ **Black box warning** Advise patient to never take this drug with nitrates or alpha blockers; serious and even fatal complications can occur.
- Warn patient of the risk of lowered BP and dizziness if taken with alcohol.

Teaching points

- Take these drugs before anticipated sexual activity; the drug will stay in your body for up to 4 hours (sildenafil, vardenafil), or up to 36 hours (tadalafil). The drug will have no effect in the absence of sexual stimulation.
- These drugs will not protect you from sexually transmitted diseases; use appropriate precautions.
- Do not take these drugs if you are taking any nitrates or alpha blockers or other drugs for treating erectile dysfunction; serious side effects and even death can occur.
- Many drugs may interact with these drugs; consult your health care provider before taking any drug, including over-the-counter drugs and herbal therapies; dosage adjustments may be needed.
- Know that combining these drugs with alcohol could cause dizziness, loss of blood pressure, increased flushing.
- You may experience these side effects: Headache, dizziness, upset stomach, runny nose, muscle pains; these side effects should go away within a couple of hours. If side effects persist, consult your health care provider.
- Report difficult or painful urination, vision changes, hearing loss, fainting, erection that persists for longer than 4 hours (if this occurs, seek medical assistance as soon as possible).

Representative drugs

avanafil
sildenafil
tadalafil
vardenafil

Selective Serotonin Reuptake Inhibitors (SSRIs)

PREGNANCY CATEGORY C

Therapeutic actions

The SSRIs act as antidepressants by inhibiting CNS neuronal uptake of serotonin with little or no effect on norepinephrine; they are also thought to antagonize muscarinic, histaminergic, and alpha$_1$-adrenergic receptors. The increase in serotonin levels at neuroreceptors is thought to act as a stimulant, counteracting depression and increasing motivation.

Indications

- Treatment of depression; most effective in patients with major depressive disorder

- Treatment of OCD, PTSD, social anxiety, generalized anxiety disorder, panic disorder, PMDD
- Unlabeled uses: Treatment of bulimia

Contraindications and cautions

- Contraindicated with hypersensitivity to any SSRI; pregnancy.
- Use cautiously with impaired hepatic or renal function, diabetes mellitus, lactation.

Adverse effects

- **CNS:** *Headache, nervousness, insomnia, drowsiness, anxiety, tremor, dizziness, light-headedness,* agitation, sedation, abnormal gait, seizures
- **CV:** Hot flashes, palpitations
- **Dermatologic:** *Sweating, rash, pruritus,* acne, alopecia, contact dermatitis
- **GI:** *Nausea, vomiting, diarrhea, dry mouth, anorexia, dyspepsia, constipation, taste changes,* flatulence, gastroenteritis, dysphagia, gingivitis
- **GU:** *Painful menstruation, sexual dysfunction,* frequency, cystitis, impotence, urgency, vaginitis
- **Respiratory:** *URIs, pharyngitis,* cough, dyspnea, bronchitis, rhinitis
- **Other:** *Weight loss, asthenia, fever*

Interactions

✴ **Drug-drug** • Increased therapeutic and toxic effects of TCAs with SSRIs • Decreased therapeutic effects with cyproheptadine • Risk for severe to fatal hypertensive crisis with MAOIs; avoid this combination

✴ **Drug-alternative therapy** • Increased risk of severe reaction with St. John's Wort

■ Nursing considerations
Assessment

- **History:** Hypersensitivity to any SSRI; impaired hepatic or renal function; diabetes mellitus; lactation; pregnancy
- **Physical:** Weight; T; rash, lesions; reflexes, affect; bowel sounds, liver evaluation; P, peripheral perfusion; urinary output; LFTs, renal function tests, CBC

Interventions

- Arrange for lower dose or less frequent administration in elderly patients and patients with hepatic or renal impairment.

- Establish suicide precautions for severely depressed patients. Dispense only a small number of capsules at a time to these patients.
- ⊗ ***Black box warning*** Monitor children, adolescents, and young adults for suicidal thoughts and behavior, especially when changing dosage.
- Administer drug in the morning. If dose of more than 20 mg/day is needed, administer in divided doses.
- Monitor patient response for up to 4 wk before increasing dose because of lack of therapeutic effect. It frequently takes several weeks to see the desired effect.
- Provide frequent small meals if GI upset or anorexia occurs. Monitor weight loss; a nutritional consultation may be needed.
- Provide sugarless candies, frequent mouth care if dry mouth is a problem.
- Ensure ready access to bathroom facilities if diarrhea occurs. Establish bowel program if constipation is a problem.
- Establish safety precautions (use side rails, appropriate lighting; accompany patient) if CNS effects occur.
- Provide appropriate comfort measures if CNS effects, insomnia, rash, sweating occur.
- Encourage patient to maintain therapy for treatment of underlying cause of depression.

Teaching points

- It may take up to 4 weeks to get a full antidepressant effect from these drugs. These drugs should be taken in the morning (or in divided doses if necessary).
- Do not take these drugs during pregnancy. If you think that you are pregnant or you wish to become pregnant, consult your health care provider.
- You may experience these side effects: Dizziness, drowsiness, nervousness, insomnia (avoid driving or performing hazardous tasks); nausea, vomiting, weight loss (frequent small meals may help; monitor your weight loss—if it becomes marked, consult your health care provider); sexual dysfunction (drug effect); flulike symptoms (if severe, consult your health care provider for appropriate treatment); photosensitivity (avoid exposure to sunlight).
- Report rash, mania, seizures, severe weight loss.

Representative drugs
citalopram
desvenlafaxine
escitalopram
fluoxetine
fluvoxamine
paroxetine
sertraline
venlafaxine
vilazodone

Sulfonamides

PREGNANCY CATEGORY C

PREGNANCY CATEGORY D (AT TERM)

Therapeutic actions
Sulfonamides are antibiotics. They are bacteriostatic; competitively antagonize para-aminobenzoic acid, an essential component of folic acid synthesis, in susceptible gram-negative and gram-positive bacteria, causing cell death.

Indications
- Treatment of ulcerative colitis, otitis media, inclusion conjunctivitis, meningitis, nocardiosis, toxoplasmosis, trachoma, UTIs
- Management of rheumatoid arthritis, collagenous colitis, Crohn's disease

Contraindications and cautions
- Contraindicated with allergy to sulfonamides, sulfonylureas, thiazides; pregnancy (teratogenic in preclinical studies; at term, may bump fetal bilirubin from plasma protein–binding sites and cause kernicterus); or lactation (risk of kernicterus, diarrhea, rash).
- Use cautiously with impaired renal or hepatic function, G6PD deficiency, porphyria.

Adverse effects
- **CNS:** Headache, peripheral neuropathy, *mental depression*, seizures, ataxia, hallucinations, tinnitus, vertigo, insomnia, hearing loss, drowsiness, transient lesions of posterior spinal column, transverse myelitis
- **Dermatologic:** Photosensitivity, cyanosis, petechiae, alopecia
- **GI:** *Nausea, emesis, abdominal pains, diarrhea,* bloody diarrhea, anorexia, pancreatitis, stomatitis, impaired folic acid absorption, hepatitis, hepatocellular necrosis
- **GU:** Crystalluria, hematuria, proteinuria, nephrotic syndrome, toxic nephrosis with oliguria and anuria, oligospermia, infertility
- **Hematologic: Agranulocytosis, aplastic anemia,** thrombocytopenia, leukopenia, hemolytic anemia, hypoprothrombinemia, methemoglobinemia, megaloblastic anemia
- **Hypersensitivity: Stevens-Johnson syndrome,** generalized skin eruptions, epidermal necrolysis, urticaria, serum sickness, pruritus, **exfoliative dermatitis, anaphylactoid reactions,** periorbital edema, conjunctival and scleral redness, photosensitization, arthralgia, allergic myocarditis, transient pulmonary changes with eosinophilia, decreased pulmonary function
- **Other:** Drug fever, chills, periarteritis nodosum

Interactions
❋ **Drug-drug** ● Increased risk of hypoglycemia when tolbutamide, tolazamide, glyburide, glipizide, chlorpropamide are taken concurrently ● Increased risk of folate deficiency if taking sulfonamides; monitor patients receiving folic acid carefully for signs of folate deficiency

❋ **Drug-lab test** ● Possible false-positive urinary glucose tests using Benedict's method

■ Nursing considerations
Assessment
- **History:** Allergy to sulfonamides, sulfonylureas, thiazides; pregnancy; lactation; impaired renal or hepatic function; G6PD deficiency; porphyria
- **Physical:** T; skin color, lesions; culture of infected site; orientation, reflexes, affect, peripheral sensation; R, adventitious sounds; mucous membranes, bowel sounds, liver evaluation; LFTs, renal function tests, CBC and differential, urinalysis

Interventions
- Arrange for culture and sensitivity tests of infected area prior to therapy; repeat cultures if response is not as expected.
- Administer drug after meals or with food to prevent GI upset. Administer the drug around the clock.

- Ensure adequate fluid intake.
- Discontinue drug immediately if hypersensitivity reaction occurs.
- Establish safety precautions if CNS effects occur (side rails, assistance, environmental control).
- Protect patient from exposure to light (use sunscreen, protective clothing) if photosensitivity occurs.
- Provide frequent small meals if GI upset occurs.
- Provide mouth care for stomatitis.
- Offer support and encouragement to deal with side effects of drug therapy, including changes in sexual function.

Teaching points

- Complete the full course of therapy.
- Take these drugs with food or meals to decrease GI upset.
- Drink eight glasses of water per day.
- These drugs are specific to the disease being treated; do not use to self-treat any other infection.
- You may experience these side effects: Sensitivity to sunlight (use sunscreens; wear protective clothing); dizziness, drowsiness, difficulty walking, loss of sensation (avoid driving or performing tasks that require alertness); nausea, vomiting, diarrhea (ensure ready access to bathroom); loss of fertility; yellow-orange urine.
- Report blood in the urine, rash, ringing in the ears, difficulty breathing, fever, sore throat, chills.

Representative drugs
    balsalazide
    sulfadiazine
    sulfamethoxazole (always used in combination with trimethoprim)
    sulfasalazine
    sulfisoxazole

Tetracyclines

PREGNANCY CATEGORY D

Therapeutic actions
Tetracyclines are antibiotics. They are bacteriostatic; inhibit protein synthesis of susceptible bacteria, preventing cell replication.

Indications

- Treatment of infections caused by rickettsiae; *Mycoplasma pneumoniae;* agents of psittacosis, ornithosis, lymphogranuloma venereum, and granuloma inguinale; *Borrelia recurrentis, Haemophilus ducreyi, Pasteurella pestis, Pasteurella tularensis, Bartonella bacilliformis, Bacteroides, Vibrio comma, Vibrio fetus, Brucella, Escherichia coli, Escherichia aerogenes, Shigella, Acinetobacter calcoaceticus, Haemophilus influenzae, Staphylococcus aureus, Diplococcus pneumoniae, Klebsiella;* when penicillin is contraindicated, infections caused by *Neisseria gonorrhoeae, Listeria monocytogenes, Treponema pallidum, Treponema pertenue, Clostridium, Bacillus anthracis, Actinomyces, Fusobacterium fusiforme, Neisseria meningitidis*
- Adjunct to amebicides in acute intestinal amebiasis
- Treatment of malaria
- Treatment of anthrax
- Treatment of acne
- Treatment of complicated urethral, endocervical, or rectal infections in adults caused by *Chlamydia trachomatis*
- Treatment of superficial ocular infections caused by susceptible strains of microorganisms
- Prophylaxis of ophthalmia neonatorum caused by *N. gonorrhoeae* or *C. trachomatis*
- Unlabeled uses: Lyme disease, endocarditis, facial nerve paralysis, arthritis, early syphilis, chlamydial infection, PID, epididymitis, prophylaxis after sexual assault

Contraindications and cautions

- Contraindicated with allergy to any tetracyclines, allergy to tartrazine (in 250-mg tetracycline capsules marketed under brand name *Sumycin*), pregnancy (toxic to fetus), lactation (causes damage to the teeth of infants).
- Use cautiously with hepatic or renal impairment; ocular viral, mycobacterial, or fungal infections.

Adverse effects

- **Dermatologic:** *Phototoxic reactions, rash,* **exfoliative dermatitis**
- **GI:** *Discoloring and inadequate calcification of primary teeth of fetus if used by pregnant women, discoloring and inadequate calcification of permanent teeth if*

*used during period of dental develop-
ment,* fatty liver, hepatic failure, *anorexia,
nausea, vomiting, diarrhea, glossitis, dysphagia,* enterocolitis, esophageal ulcers
- **Hematologic:** Hemolytic anemia, thrombocytopenia, neutropenia, eosinophilia,
leukocytosis, leukopenia
- **Hypersensitivity:** Reactions from urticaria to **anaphylaxis,** including intracranial hypertension
- **Local:** *Transient irritation, stinging, itching,* angioneurotic edema, urticaria, dermatitis, superinfections with ophthalmic or
dermatologic use
- **Other:** *Superinfections,* local irritation at
parenteral injection sites

Interactions

✳ **Drug-drug** ● Decreased absorption with
calcium salts, magnesium salts, zinc salts,
aluminum salts, bismuth salts, iron, urine alkalinizers, food, dairy products, charcoal ● Increased digoxin toxicity ● Decreased effectiveness of hormonal contraceptives (rare) with a
risk of breakthrough bleeding or pregnancy
● Decreased activity of penicillins

■ Nursing considerations
Assessment

- **History:** Allergy to any of the tetracyclines;
allergy to tartrazine; hepatic or renal impairment, pregnancy, lactation; ocular viral, mycobacterial, or fungal infections
- **Physical:** Site of infection, skin color, lesions; R, adventitious sounds; bowel sounds,
output, liver evaluation; urinalysis, BUN,
LFTs, renal function tests

Interventions

- Administer oral medication on an empty
stomach, 1 hr before or 2–3 hr after meals.
Do not give with antacids. If antacids must
be used, give them 3 hr after the dose of tetracycline.
- Culture infected area prior to drug therapy.
- Do not use outdated drugs; degraded drug
is highly nephrotoxic and should not be
used.
- Do not give oral drug with meals, antacids,
or food.
- Provide frequent hygiene measures if superinfections occur.
- Protect patient from sunlight and bright
lights if photosensitivity occurs.

- Arrange for regular renal function tests if
long-term therapy is used.
- Use topical preparations of this drug only
when clearly indicated. Sensitization from
the topical use of this drug may preclude its
later use in serious infections. Topical preparations containing antibiotics that are not
ordinarily given systemically are preferable.

Teaching points
Systemic administration

- Take these drugs throughout the day for best
results. These drugs should be taken on an
empty stomach, 1 hour before or 2–3 hours
after meals, with a full glass of water. Do not
take these drugs with food, dairy products,
iron preparations, or antacids.
- Take the full course of therapy prescribed;
if any drug is left, discard it immediately.
Never take an outdated product.
- Pregnancy may occur when taking tetracycline with hormonal contraceptives. To be
sure of avoiding pregnancy, use an additional type of contraceptive while using this
drug.
- Report severe cramps, watery diarrhea, rash
or itching, difficulty breathing, dark urine or
light-colored stools, yellowing of the skin or
eyes.

Eyedrop administration

- To give eyedrops: Lie down or tilt your head
backward and look at the ceiling. Drop suspension drug inside your lower eyelid while
looking up. Close your eye, and apply gentle pressure to the inner corner of the eye for
1 minute.
- Apply ointment inside the lower eyelid; close
your eyes, and roll your eyeball in all directions.
- These drugs may cause temporary blurring
of vision or stinging after application.
- Notify your health care provider if stinging
or itching becomes severe.
- Take the full course of therapy prescribed;
discard any leftover medication.
- Apply dermatologic solution until skin is
wet; avoid eyes, nose, and mouth.

Topical administration

- You may experience transient stinging or
burning; this will subside quickly; skin in
the treated area may become yellow; this
will wash off.
- Use cosmetics as you usually do.

Adverse effects in *italics* are most common; those in **bold** are life-threatening. ▣ Do not crush.

- Wash area before applying (unless contraindicated); this drug may stain clothing.
- You may experience these side effects: Stomach upset, nausea; superinfections in the mouth, vagina (frequent washing may help; if it becomes severe, medication may help); sensitivity of the skin to sunlight (use protective clothing and sunscreen).
- Report worsening of condition, rash, irritation.

Representative drugs
demeclocycline
doxycycline
minocycline
tetracycline

Tricyclic Antidepressants (TCAs)

PREGNANCY CATEGORY C OR D
(AMITRIPTYLINE, IMIPRAMINE, NORTRIPTYLINE)

Therapeutic actions
Mechanism of action is unknown. The TCAs are structurally related to the phenothiazine antipsychotic drugs (eg, chlorpromazine), but in contrast to them, TCAs inhibit the presynaptic reuptake of the neurotransmitters norepinephrine and serotonin; anticholinergic at CNS and peripheral receptors; the relation of these effects to clinical efficacy is unknown.

Indications
- Relief of symptoms of major depressive disorders
- Treatment of OCDs
- Unlabeled uses: Treatment of obstructive sleep apnea, panic disorder, eating disorders, PMS, migraine, ADHD, insomnia associated with depression, fibromyalgia, neuropathic pain, adult enuresis

Contraindications and cautions
- Contraindicated with hypersensitivity to any tricyclic drug, concomitant therapy with an MAOI, recent MI, myelography within previous 24 hr or scheduled within 48 hr, pregnancy (limb reduction abnormalities reported), or lactation.
- Use cautiously with EST; preexisting CV disorders (severe coronary heart disease, progressive heart failure, angina pectoris, paroxysmal tachycardia); angle-closure glaucoma, increased IOP, urine retention, ureteral or urethral spasm; seizure disorders (lower seizure threshold); hyperthyroidism (predisposes to CVS toxicity, including cardiac arrhythmias); impaired hepatic, renal function; psychiatric patients; schizophrenic or paranoid may exhibit a worsening of psychosis; manic-depressive disorder may shift to hypomanic or manic phase; elective surgery (discontinue as long as possible before surgery).

Adverse effects
- **CNS:** *Sedation and anticholinergic (atropine-like) effects* (dry mouth, blurred vision, disturbance of accommodation for near vision, mydriasis, increased IOP), *confusion* (especially in elderly), *disturbed concentration,* hallucinations, disorientation, decreased memory, feelings of unreality, delusions, anxiety, nervousness, restlessness, agitation, panic, insomnia, nightmares, hypomania, mania, exacerbation of psychosis, drowsiness, weakness, fatigue, headache, numbness, tingling, paresthesia of extremities, incoordination, motor hyperactivity, akathisia, ataxia, tremors, peripheral neuropathy, extrapyramidal symptoms, *seizures,* speech blockage, dysarthria, tinnitus, altered EEG
- **CV:** *Orthostatic hypotension,* hypertension, syncope, tachycardia, palpitations, MI, arrhythmias, heart block, precipitation of heart failure, **stroke**
- **Endocrine:** Elevated or depressed blood sugar; elevated prolactin levels; inappropriate ADH secretion
- **GI:** *Dry mouth, constipation,* paralytic ileus, *nausea,* vomiting, anorexia, epigastric distress, diarrhea, flatulence, dysphagia, peculiar taste, increased salivation, stomatitis, glossitis, parotid swelling, abdominal cramps, black "hairy" tongue
- **GU:** Urine retention, delayed micturition, dilation of the urinary tract, gynecomastia, testicular swelling; breast enlargement, menstrual irregularity, and galactorrhea; change in libido; impotence

- **Hematologic:** Bone marrow depression, including agranulocytosis; eosinophilia; purpura; thrombocytopenia; leukopenia
- **Hypersensitivity:** Skin rash, pruritus, vasculitis, petechiae, photosensitization, edema (generalized, face and tongue), drug fever
- **Withdrawal:** Symptoms with abrupt discontinuation of prolonged therapy; nausea, headache, vertigo, nightmares, malaise
- **Other:** Nasal congestion, excessive appetite, weight change; sweating, alopecia, lacrimation, hyperthermia, flushing, chills

Interactions

✳ Drug-drug ● Increased TCA levels and pharmacologic effects with cimetidine, fluoxetine, ranitidine ● Altered response, including arrhythmias and hypertension, with sympathomimetics ● Risk of severe hypertension with clonidine ● Hyperpyretic crises, severe seizures, hypertensive episodes, and death with MAOIs

■ Nursing considerations
Assessment

- **History:** Hypersensitivity to any tricyclic drug; concomitant therapy with an MAOI; recent MI; myelography within previous 24 hr or scheduled within 48 hr; pregnancy; lactation; preexisting disorders; angle-closure glaucoma, increased IOP; urinary retention, ureteral or urethral spasm; seizure disorders; hyperthyroidism; impaired hepatic, renal function; psychiatric, manic-depressive disorder; elective surgery
- **Physical:** Weight; T; skin color, lesions; orientation, affect, reflexes, vision and hearing; P, BP, orthostatic BP, perfusion; bowel sounds, normal output, liver evaluation; urine flow, normal output; usual sexual function, frequency of menses, breast and scrotal examination; LFTs, urinalysis, CBC, ECG

Interventions

- Ensure that depressed and potentially suicidal patients have limited access to drug.
- Reduce dosage if minor side effects develop; discontinue drug if serious side effects occur.
- Arrange for CBC if patient develops fever, sore throat, or other sign of infection.
- Ensure ready access to bathroom if GI effects occur; establish bowel program for constipation.

- Provide frequent small meals, frequent mouth care if GI effects occur; provide sugarless candies for dry mouth.
- Establish safety precautions if CNS changes occur (side rails, assist walking).

Teaching points
- Take these drugs exactly as prescribed; do not stop taking these drugs abruptly or without consulting your health care provider.
- Avoid alcohol, sleep-inducing drugs, over-the-counter drugs.
- Avoid prolonged exposure to sunlight or sunlamps; use a sunscreen or protective garments if unavoidable.
- You may experience these side effects: Headache, dizziness, drowsiness, weakness, blurred vision (reversible; safety measures may be needed if severe; avoid driving or performing tasks requiring alertness); nausea, vomiting, loss of appetite, dry mouth (frequent small meals, mouth care, and sucking sugarless candies may help); nightmares, inability to concentrate, confusion; changes in sexual function.
- Report dry mouth, difficulty in urination, excessive sedation.

Representative drugs
amitriptyline
amoxapine
clomipramine
desipramine
doxepin
imipramine
nortriptyline
protriptyline
trimipramine

▷**abacavir sulfate**
(ah **bak'** ah veer)

Ziagen

PREGNANCY CATEGORY C

Drug classes
Antiviral
Nucleoside reverse transcriptase inhibitor

Therapeutic actions
Nucleoside reverse transcriptase inhibitor; obstructs RNA and DNA synthesis and inhibits viral reproduction. Used in combination with other anti-HIV drugs to reduce the viral load as low as possible and decrease the chance of further viral mutation. Thought to cross the blood–brain barrier and be effective in the treatment of HIV-related dementia. There are no long-term studies on the effectiveness of this drug.

Indications
- Treatment of HIV-1 infection in combination with other antiretrovirals

Contraindications and cautions
- Contraindicated with life-threatening allergy or hypersensitivity to any component, moderate to severe hepatic impairment, lactation.
- Use cautiously with mild hepatic impairment, lactic acidosis, pregnancy.

Available forms
Tablets—300 mg; oral solution—20 mg/mL

Dosages
Adults
300 mg PO bid or 600 mg PO once daily.
Adults with mild hepatic impairment
200 mg PO bid (solution).
Pediatric patients 3 mo–16 yr
8 mg/kg PO bid; do not exceed 300 mg/dose.
Pediatric patients younger than 3 mo
Not recommended.

Pharmacokinetics

Route	Onset	Peak
Oral	Rapid	2–4 hr

Metabolism: Hepatic; $T_{1/2}$: 1–2 hr
Distribution: Crosses placenta; may enter breast milk
Excretion: Urine, feces

Adverse effects
- **CNS:** *Headache, weakness, malaise, fatigue, insomnia,* dizziness, anxiety, depression
- **Dermatologic:** *Rash*
- **GI:** *Diarrhea, nausea,* anorexia, *vomiting,* dyspepsia, liver enzyme elevations, liver enlargement, **risk of severe to fatal hepatomegaly**
- **Other: Severe hypersensitivity reactions** (fever, malaise, nausea, vomiting, rash), **severe to fatal lactic acidosis,** fat redistribution, increased lipid levels, **MI**

Interactions
✳ **Drug-drug** ● Risk of severe toxic effects if combined with alcohol

■ **Nursing considerations**
Assessment
- **History:** Life-threatening allergy to any component, impaired hepatic or renal function, lactic acidosis, pregnancy, lactation
- **Physical:** T; affect, reflexes, peripheral sensation; R, adventitious sounds; bowel sounds, liver evaluation; LFTs, renal function tests

Interventions
- Administer with meals or a light snack if GI upset occurs.

⊗ *Black box warning* Monitor patient for signs of potentially fatal hypersensitivity reaction; give patient hypersensitivity reaction warning card provided by manufacturer. Advise patient to stop drug at first sign of reaction. Do not try the drug again if patient has a hypersensitivity reaction.

⊗ *Black box warning* Monitor patient for lactic acidosis and severe hepatomegaly; increased risk with other antivirals.

⊗ *Black box warning* Patients with HLA-B*5701 allele are at high risk for hypersensitivity reactions. Screening for HLA-B*5701 allele is recommended.

- Administer the drug concurrently with other anti-HIV drugs.
- Recommend the use of barrier contraceptives while on this drug.

Teaching points

- Take drug exactly as prescribed; take missed doses as soon as possible and return to normal schedule; do not double skipped doses; take with meals or a light snack if GI upset occurs.
- This drug is not a cure for AIDS or AIDS-related complex; opportunistic infections may occur and regular medical follow-up is needed.
- Long-term effects of this drug are unknown.
- Treatment does not reduce the risk of transmission of HIV by sexual contact or blood contamination; use precautions.
- Do not drink alcohol while taking this drug.
- Use barrier contraceptives; hormonal contraceptives may not be effective.
- This drug has been connected with severe hypersensitivity reactions, which usually occur early in the use of the drug. Keep your hypersensitivity list readily available, and stop the drug if any of these effects occur.
- You may experience these side effects: Nausea, loss of appetite, diarrhea (eat frequent small meals; medication is available to control the diarrhea); dizziness, loss of feeling (take appropriate precautions).
- Report extreme fatigue, lethargy, severe headache, severe nausea, vomiting, difficulty breathing, rash, fever.

▽abatacept

See Appendix R, *Less commonly used drugs*.

▽abciximab
*(ab **six'** ab mab)*

ReoPro

PREGNANCY CATEGORY C

Drug classes
Antiplatelet
Glycoprotein IIb/IIIa inhibitor

Therapeutic actions
Interferes with platelet membrane function by inhibiting fibrinogen binding and platelet–platelet interactions; inhibits platelet aggregation and prolongs bleeding time; effect is irreversible for life of the platelet.

Indications

- Adjunct to percutaneous coronary intervention (PCI) for the prevention of cardiac ischemic complications in patients undergoing PCI and with unstable angina not responding to conventional therapy when PCI is planned within 24 hr; intended to be used with heparin and aspirin therapy
- Unlabeled uses: Early treatment of acute MI or acute ischemic stroke

Contraindications and cautions

- Contraindicated with allergy to abciximab; neutropenia; thrombocytopenia (fewer than 100,000 cells/mcL); hemostatic disorders; bleeding ulcer; intracranial bleeding; major trauma; vasculitis; recent major surgery; aneurysm; use of IV dextran (before or during PCI); pregnancy; severe, uncontrolled hypertension; active internal bleeding; recent (within 6 wk) GI or GU bleeding; history of stroke within 2 yr; administration of oral anticoagulants within 7 days (unless PT is 1.2 times control or less).
- Use cautiously during lactation and with concurrent use of anticoagulants, thrombolytics, or antiplatelet drugs.

Available forms
Injection—2 mg/mL

Dosages
Efficacy of abciximab has only been studied in combination with heparin and aspirin.
Adults
- *Adjunct to PCI:* 0.25 mg/kg by IV bolus 10–60 min prior to procedure, followed by continuous infusion of 0.125 mcg/kg/min (maximum dose 10 mcg/min) for 12 hr.
- *Unstable angina not responding to conventional medical therapy when PCI is planned within 24 hr:* 0.25 mg/kg by IV bolus over at least 1 min; then 10 mcg/min by IV infusion for 18–24 hr, concluding 1 hr after PCI.
Pediatric patients
Safety and efficacy not established.

Pharmacokinetics

Route	Onset	Peak
IV	Rapid	30 min

Metabolism: Cellular; $T_{1/2}$: less than 10 min, then 30 min

Adverse effects in *italics* are most common; those in **bold** are life-threatening. ⬛ Do not crush.

Distribution: Crosses placenta; may enter breast milk

Excretion: Unknown

▼ IV FACTS

Preparation: Withdraw the necessary amount through a 0.2- or 0.5-micron filter for bolus injection. Prepare infusion by withdrawing necessary amount through filter into syringe; inject into 250 mL 0.9% sterile saline or 5% dextrose; an 0.2- or 0.22-micron filter should be used for continuous infusion. Do not use any solution that contains visibly opaque particles; discard solution after 12 hr. Do not shake; refrigerate solution.

Infusion (as adjunct to PCI): 10–60 min before procedure give bolus of 0.25 mg/kg over at least 1 min; give continuous infusion at rate of 0.125 mcg/kg/min (to a maximum dose of 10 mcg/min) for 12 hr.

Incompatibilities: Do not mix in solution with any other medication; give through a separate IV line.

Adverse effects

- **CNS:** Dizziness, confusion, anxiety
- **CV:** Bradycardia, *hypotension,* arrhythmias, edema
- **GI:** *Nausea, vomiting*
- **Hematologic: Thrombocytopenia, bleeding**
- **Local:** Pain, *edema*
- **Respiratory:** Pneumonia, pleural effusion

Interactions

✳ **Drug-drug** • Risk of increased bleeding if combined with anticoagulants, antiplatelets, or thrombolytics; monitor patient accordingly.

■ Nursing considerations

Assessment

- **History:** Allergy to abciximab, neutropenia, thrombocytopenia, hemostatic disorders, bleeding ulcer, intracranial bleeding, severe liver disease, lactation, renal disorders, pregnancy, recent trauma or surgery
- **Physical:** Skin color, lesions; orientation; bowel sounds, normal output; CBC, LFTs, renal function tests

Interventions

- Monitor CBC count before use and frequently while initiating therapy.

- Monitor patient for signs and symptoms of bleeding.
- Arrange for concomitant aspirin and heparin therapy.
- Establish safety precautions to prevent injury and bleeding (such as using electric razor, not playing contact sports).
- Provide increased precautions against bleeding during invasive procedures—bleeding will be prolonged.
- Mark chart of any patient receiving abciximab to alert medical personnel to potential for increased bleeding in surgery or dental surgery.

Teaching points

- It may take longer than normal to stop bleeding while on this drug; avoid playing contact sports, use electrical razors, and take other precautions. Apply pressure for extended periods to bleeding sites.
- You may experience these side effects: Upset stomach, nausea.
- Report fever, chills, sore throat, rash, bruising, bleeding, dark stools or urine.

▷ abiraterone

See Appendix R, *Less commonly used drugs.*

▷ acamprosate calcium

(a kam pro' sate)

Campral

PREGNANCY CATEGORY C

Drug classes

Antialcoholic drug

GABA analogue

Therapeutic actions

Exact mechanism of action not understood; acts with glutamate and GABA neurotransmitter systems in the CNS to restore balance between neuronal excitation and inhibition that may be altered by chronic alcohol exposure.

Indications

- Maintenance of abstinence from alcohol in patients with alcohol dependence who are abstinent at treatment initiation as part of a comprehensive management program that includes psychosocial support

Contraindications and cautions

- Contraindicated with allergy to any component of the drug or severe renal impairment (creatinine clearance 30 mL/min or less).
- Use cautiously with pregnancy, lactation, moderate renal impairment, history of depression and suicidal thoughts.

Available forms

DR tablets—333 mg

Dosages

Adults

666 mg (two 333-mg tablets) PO tid; may be taken with meals to aid compliance. Dosage should begin as soon as possible after period of alcohol withdrawal when the patient has achieved abstinence, and should be maintained if patient relapses. Should be part of a comprehensive psychosocial treatment program.

Pediatric patients

Safety and efficacy not established.

Patients with renal impairment

Moderate impairment (creatinine clearance 30–50 mL/min): 333 mg PO tid; severe renal impairment (creatinine clearance 30 mL/min or less): do not use acamprosate.

Pharmacokinetics

Route	Onset	Peak
Oral	Slow	3–8 hr

Metabolism: Not metabolized; $T_{1/2}$: 20–30 hr
Distribution: May cross placenta; may pass into breast milk
Excretion: Urine, unchanged

Adverse effects

- **CNS:** Anxiety, depression, dizziness, impaired judgment, insomnia, paresthesia, asthenia, insomnia, **suicidal thoughts**
- **GI:** Anorexia, *diarrhea,* dry mouth, flatulence, nausea
- **Respiratory:** Bronchitis, cough, dyspnea, pharyngitis, rhinitis
- **Skin:** Increased sweating, pruritus
- **Other:** Back pain, flulike symptoms, impotence, muscle aches and pains, weight gain

■ Nursing considerations

Assessment

- **History:** Allergy to any component of the drug, renal impairment, pregnancy, lactation, history of depression and suicidal thoughts, alcohol intake
- **Physical:** Skin, lesions; orientation, reflexes, affect; abdominal examination

Interventions

- Ensure that patient is abstaining from alcohol intake when treatment is initiated.
- Ensure that patient is participating in a comprehensive program, including psychological and social support, to manage abstinence from alcohol.
- Give drug three times a day with meals— timing may be helpful in aiding compliance to the regimen when the patient is managing the drug regimen at home. However, drug may be given without regard to meals.
- Instruct patient to continue to take the drug even if a relapse to alcohol consumption occurs; encourage patient to notify health care provider if a relapse occurs.
- Encourage use of barrier contraceptives during treatment with this drug; fetal abnormalities are possible.

Teaching points

- This drug is given as part of a comprehensive program to support your abstinence from alcohol; it is important that you continue that program while taking this drug.
- Take this drug three times a day; taking the drug with meals may be a helpful reminder.
- If you forget a dose, take it as soon as you remember and return to your usual regimen. Do not make up doses and do not take more than three doses in 24 hours.
- Continue to take the drug even if you relapse and drink alcohol. Notify your health care provider to discuss the renewed drinking.
- You may experience impaired judgment, impaired thinking, or impaired motor skills. You should not drive or operate hazardous machinery or sign important documents or make important decisions until you are certain that *Campral* has not affected your ability to engage in these activities safely.

Adverse effects in *italics* are most common; those in **bold** are life-threatening. ▣ Do not crush.

- You should not take this drug during pregnancy; if you suspect that you are pregnant, or wish to become pregnant, consult your health care provider.
- You should find another method of feeding the infant if you are breast-feeding; it is not known if this drug crosses into breast milk.
- You may experience these side effects: Flatulence, diarrhea, abdominal discomfort; depression; thoughts of suicide (if this occurs, consult with your health care provider); muscle or joint aches and pains (consult your health care provider, an analgesic may be helpful).
- Report depression or thoughts of suicide, numbness or tingling, fever, severe diarrhea.

▽ **acarbose**
(a kar' boz)

Prandase (CAN), Precose

PREGNANCY CATEGORY B

Drug classes
Alpha-glucosidase inhibitor
Antidiabetic

Therapeutic actions
Alpha-glucosidase inhibitor obtained from the fermentation process of a microorganism; delays the digestion of ingested carbohydrates, leading to a smaller increase in blood glucose following meals and a decrease in glycosylated Hgb; does not enhance insulin secretion, so its effects are additive to those of the sulfonylureas in controlling blood glucose.

Indications
- Monotherapy or adjunct to diet to lower blood glucose in those patients with type 2 diabetes mellitus whose hyperglycemia cannot be managed by diet alone
- Combination therapy with a sulfonylurea, metformin, or insulin to enhance glycemic control in patients who do not receive adequate control with diet and either drug alone

Contraindications and cautions
- Contraindicated with hypersensitivity to drug; diabetic ketoacidosis; cirrhosis; inflammatory bowel disease; conditions that deteriorate with increased gas in the bowel; type 1 diabetes; existence of or predisposition to intestinal obstruction; colonic ulceration.
- Use cautiously with renal impairment, pregnancy, lactation.

Available forms
Tablets—25, 50, 100 mg

Dosages
Adults
- *Monotherapy:* Initially, 25 mg PO tid with first bite of each meal. May start with 25 mg/day and gradually increase to tid if GI side effects are a problem. Increase as needed every 4–8 wk as indicated by 1-hr postprandial glucose levels or glycosylated Hgb level and tolerance. For patient 60 kg or less, maximum dosage 50 mg tid; for patient more than 60 kg, maximum dosage 100 mg tid.
- *Combination with sulfonylurea or insulin:* Blood glucose may be much lower; monitor closely and adjust dosages of each drug accordingly.

Pediatric patients
Safety and efficacy not established.

Pharmacokinetics

Route	Onset	Peak
Oral	Rapid	1 hr

Metabolism: Intestinal; $T_{1/2}$: 2 hr
Distribution: Very little
Excretion: Feces, urine

Adverse effects
- **Endocrine:** *Hypoglycemia*
- **GI:** *Abdominal pain, flatulence, diarrhea,* anorexia, nausea, vomiting

Interactions
✳ **Drug-drug** • Possible decrease in digoxin levels if combined; monitor patients closely if this combination is used • Decreased effects of acarbose if taken with digestive enzymes or charcoal; avoid these combinations • Increased risk of hypoglycemia when given with other antidiabetic drugs

✳ **Drug-alternative therapy** • Increased risk of hypoglycemia if taken with juniper berries, ginseng, garlic, fenugreek, coriander, dandelion root, celery

■ **Nursing considerations**

Assessment

- **History:** Hypersensitivity to drug; diabetic ketoacidosis; cirrhosis; inflammatory bowel disease; existence of or predisposition to intestinal obstruction; type 1 diabetes; conditions that would deteriorate with increased gas in bowel; renal impairment; pregnancy; lactation
- **Physical:** Skin color, lesions; T; orientation, reflexes, peripheral sensation; R, adventitious sounds; liver evaluation, bowel sounds; urinalysis, BUN, blood glucose, CBC

Interventions

- Give drug tid with the first bite of each meal.
- Monitor serum glucose levels frequently to determine drug effectiveness and dosage; monitor LFTs every 3 mo for 1 year, then periodically. Oral glucose should be given if hypoglycemia occurs; sucrose absorption will be inhibited.
- Inform patient of likelihood of abdominal pain and flatulence.
- Consult dietitian to establish weight loss program and dietary control.
- Arrange for thorough diabetic teaching program, including disease, dietary control, exercise, signs and symptoms of hypoglycemia and hyperglycemia, avoidance of infection, hygiene.

Teaching points

- Do not discontinue this drug without consulting health care provider.
- Take drug three times a day with first bite of each meal.
- Monitor blood for glucose as prescribed.
- Continue diet and exercise program established for control of diabetes.
- You may experience these side effects: Abdominal pain, flatulence, bloating.
- Report fever, sore throat, unusual bleeding or bruising, severe abdominal pain.

▽**acebutolol hydrochloride**

(a se byoo' toe lole)

Apo-Acebutolol (CAN), Gen-Acebutolol (CAN), Rhotral (CAN), Sectral

PREGNANCY CATEGORY B

Drug classes

Antiarrhythmic
Antihypertensive
Beta$_1$-selective adrenergic blocker

Therapeutic actions

Blocks beta-adrenergic receptors of the sympathetic nervous system in the heart and juxtaglomerular apparatus (kidney); decreases excitability of the heart, cardiac output and oxygen consumption, and release of renin from the kidneys; and lowers BP.

Indications

- Hypertension, alone or with other antihypertensive drugs, especially diuretics
- Management of ventricular premature beats
- Unlabeled uses: Ventricular tachycardia, thyrotoxicosis, essential tremor

Contraindications and cautions

- Contraindicated with bradycardia (HR lower than 45 beats per min), second- or third-degree heart block (PR interval greater than 0.24 sec), cardiogenic shock, heart failure, asthma, COPD, lactation.
- Use cautiously with diabetes or thyrotoxicosis, hepatic impairment, renal failure, pregnancy, bronchospastic disease, peripheral vascular disease, anesthesia, major surgery.

Available forms

Capsules—200, 400 mg

Dosages

Adults

- *Hypertension:* Initially 400 mg/day in one or two doses PO; usual maintenance dosage range is 200 mg/day, up to 1,200 mg/day given in two divided doses.
- *Ventricular arrhythmias:* 200 mg bid PO; increase dosage gradually until optimum response is achieved (usually at 600–1,200 mg/day); discontinue gradually over 2 wk.

Pediatric patients

Safety and efficacy not established.

Geriatric patients

Because bioavailability doubles, lower doses may be required; maintain at 800 mg/day or less.

Patients with impaired renal or hepatic function
Reduce daily dose by 50% when creatinine clearance is less than 50 mL/min; reduce by 75% when creatinine clearance is less than 25 mL/min; use caution with hepatic impairment.

Pharmacokinetics

Route	Onset	Peak	Duration
Oral	Varies	3–4 hr	6–8 hr

Metabolism: Hepatic; $T_{1/2}$: 3–4 hr
Distribution: Crosses placenta; enters breast milk
Excretion: Bile, feces, urine

Adverse effects

- **Allergic reactions:** Pharyngitis, erythematous rash, fever, sore throat, *laryngospasm, respiratory distress*
- **CNS:** Dizziness, vertigo, tinnitus, *fatigue,* emotional depression, paresthesias, sleep disturbances, vision changes, hallucinations, disorientation, memory loss, slurred speech (because acebutolol is less lipid soluble than propranolol, it is less likely to penetrate the blood–brain barrier and cause CNS effects)
- **CV:** *Bradycardia, heart failure, cardiac arrhythmias, sinoatrial or AV nodal block, tachycardia,* peripheral vascular insufficiency, claudication, **stroke,** pulmonary edema, hypotension
- **Dermatologic:** Rash, pruritus, sweating, dry skin
- **EENT:** Eye irritation, dry eyes, conjunctivitis, blurred vision
- **GI:** *Gastric pain, flatulence, constipation, diarrhea, nausea, vomiting,* anorexia
- **GU:** *Impotence, decreased libido,* Peyronie's disease, dysuria, nocturia, frequent urination
- **Musculoskeletal:** Joint pain, arthralgia, muscle cramp
- **Respiratory: Bronchospasm,** dyspnea, cough, bronchial obstruction, nasal stuffiness, rhinitis
- **Other:** *Decreased exercise tolerance, development of antinuclear antibodies,* hyperglycemia or hypoglycemia, elevated serum transaminase

Interactions

✳ **Drug-drug** • Increased effects of both drugs if combined with calcium channel blockers • Increased risk of orthostatic hypotension with beta blockers, alpha blockers, prazosin • Possible increased BP-lowering effects with aspirin, bismuth subsalicylate, magnesium salicylate • Decreased antihypertensive effects with NSAIDs, clonidine • Possible increased hypoglycemic effect of insulin

■ Nursing considerations
Assessment

- **History:** Sinus bradycardia, second- or third-degree heart block, cardiogenic shock, heart failure, asthma, COPD, pregnancy, lactation, diabetes, or thyrotoxicosis
- **Physical:** Weight, skin condition, neurologic status, P, BP, ECG, respiratory status, renal and thyroid function tests, blood glucose

Interventions

- Give with meals if needed.
- Do not discontinue drug abruptly after long-term therapy. Taper drug gradually over 2 wk with monitoring (abrupt withdrawal may cause serious beta-adrenergic rebound effects).
- ⊗ **Warning** Monitor apical pulse; do not administer if P is less than 50.
- Consult physician about withdrawing drug if patient is to undergo surgery (withdrawal is controversial).
- Provide comfort measures for coping with drug effects.
- Provide safety precautions if CNS effects occur.

Teaching points

- Take drug with meals.
- Do not stop taking unless so instructed by your health care provider; drug must be slowly withdrawn.
- Avoid driving or dangerous activities if dizziness or weakness occurs.
- You may experience these side effects: Dizziness, light-headedness, loss of appetite, nightmares, depression, sexual impotence.
- Report difficulty breathing, night cough, swelling of extremities, slow pulse, confusion, depression, rash, fever, sore throat.

▷acetaminophen (N-acetyl-p-aminophenol)

(a seet a min' a fen)

Suppositories: Acephen

Oral: Aminofen, Anacin Aspirin Free, APAP, Apo-Acetaminophen (CAN), Atasol (CAN), Cetafen, Feverall, Genapap, Mapap Arthritis Pain⬛, Masophen, Q-Pap, Silapap, Tylenol, UN-Aspirin, Valorin

Injection: Ofirmev

PREGNANCY CATEGORY B

Drug classes
Analgesic (nonopioid)
Antipyretic

Therapeutic actions
Antipyretic: Reduces fever by acting directly on the hypothalamic heat-regulating center to cause vasodilation and sweating, which helps dissipate heat.
Analgesic: Site and mechanism of action unclear.

Indications
• Temporary reduction of fever; temporary relief of minor aches and pains caused by common cold and influenza, headache, sore throat, toothache (patients 2 yr and older), backache, menstrual cramps, minor arthritis pain, and muscle aches (patients older than 12 yr)
• Unlabeled use: Prophylaxis in children and patients at risk for seizures who are receiving DTP vaccination to reduce incidence of fever and pain

Contraindications and cautions
• Contraindicated with allergy to acetaminophen.
• Use cautiously with impaired hepatic function, chronic alcoholism, pregnancy, lactation.

Available forms
Suppositories—80, 120, 325, 650 mg; chewable tablets—80, 160, 500 mg; tablets—325, 500 mg; ER tablets⬛—650 mg; disintegrating tablets—80, 160 mg; rapid-release tablets—500 mg; capsules—500 mg; elixir—160 mg/5 mL; liquid—160 mg/5 mL, 166.6 mg/5 mL, 500 mg/5 mL; solution—80 mg/mL, 100 mg/mL, 160 mg/5 mL; suspension—160 mg/5 mL solution for injection—10 mg/mL.

Dosages
Adults and children older than 12 yr
PO or rectal suppositories
By suppository, 325–650 mg every 4–6 hr PO, or 1,300 mg ER tablets every 8 hr. Do not exceed 4,000 mg/day.
Adults and children 13 yr and older, weighing 50 kg or more
1,000 mg every 6 hr or 650 mg every 4 hr IV; maximum dose, 1,000 mg/dose or 4,000 mg/day.
Pediatric patients
PO or rectal doses may be repeated 4–5 times/day; do not exceed five doses in 24 hr or 10 mg/kg.
PO

Age	Dosage (mg)
0–3 mo	40
4–11 mo	80
12–23 mo	120
2–3 yr	160
4–5 yr	240
6–8 yr	320
9–10 yr	400
11 yr	480

Rectal suppositories

Age	Dosage
3–11 mo	80 mg every 6 hr
12–36 mo	80 mg every 4 hr
3–6 yr	120 mg every 4–6 hr
6–12 yr	325 mg every 4–6 hr

13 yr, weighing less than 50 kg: 15 mg/kg every 6 hr or 12.5 mg/kg every 4 hr IV; maximum dose, 3,750 mg or 75 mg/kg/day.
2–12 yr: 15 mg/kg every 6 hr or 12 mg/kg every 4 hr IV; maximum dose, 75 mg/kg/day.

▼ **IV FACTS**

Preparation: Use as prepared. For small, pediatric doses, draw solution into a syringe and administer using a syringe pump. Do not refrigerate. Use within 6 hr of breaking vacuum seal on vial.
Infusion: Infuse over 15 min.
Incompatibilities: Do not add other medications to vial or infusion device. Physically

incompatible with diazepam and chlorpromazine; do not administer simultaneously.

Pharmacokinetics

Route	Onset	Peak	Duration
Oral	Varies	0.5–2 hr	4–6 hr

Metabolism: Hepatic; $T_{1/2}$: 1–3 hr
Distribution: Crosses placenta; enters breast milk
Excretion: Urine

Adverse effects

- **CNS:** Headache
- **CV:** Chest pain, dyspnea, **myocardial damage** when doses of 5–8 g/day are ingested daily for several weeks or when doses of 4 g/day are ingested for 1 yr
- **GI: Hepatic toxicity and failure,** jaundice
- **GU:** Acute renal failure, renal tubular necrosis
- **Hematologic:** Methemoglobinemia—cyanosis; hemolytic anemia—hematuria, anuria; neutropenia, leukopenia, pancytopenia, thrombocytopenia, hypoglycemia
- **Hypersensitivity:** Rash, fever

Interactions

✳ **Drug-drug** ● Increased toxicity with long-term, excessive ethanol ingestion ● Increased hypoprothrombinemic effect of oral anticoagulants ● Increased risk of hepatotoxicity and possible decreased therapeutic effects with barbiturates, carbamazepine, hydantoins, rifampin, sulfinpyrazone ● Possible delayed or decreased effectiveness with anticholinergics ● Possible reduced absorption of acetaminophen with activated charcoal ● Possible decreased effectiveness of zidovudine

✳ **Drug-lab test** ● Interference with *Chemstrip G, Dextrostix,* and *Visidex II* home blood glucose measurement systems; effects vary

■ Nursing considerations
Assessment

- **History:** Allergy to acetaminophen, impaired hepatic function, chronic alcoholism, pregnancy, lactation
- **Physical:** Skin color, lesions; T; liver evaluation; CBC, LFTs, renal function tests

Interventions

- Do not exceed the recommended dosage.

- Consult physician if needed for children younger than 3 yr; if needed for longer than 10 days; if continued fever, severe or recurrent pain occurs (possible serious illness).
- Reduce dosage with hepatic impairment.
- Avoid using multiple preparations containing acetaminophen. Carefully check all OTC products.
- Give drug with food if GI upset occurs.
- Discontinue drug if hypersensitivity reactions occur.
- Treatment of overdose: Monitor serum levels regularly, *N*-acetylcysteine should be available as a specific antidote; basic life support measures may be necessary.

Teaching points

- Do not exceed recommended dose; do not take for longer than 10 days unless directed by prescriber.
- Chew the chewable tablets before swallowing; dissolve dispersable tablets in mouth before swallowing; shake liquid forms well before using; do not cut, crush, or chew extended-relief forms.
- Take the drug only for complaints indicated; it is not an anti-inflammatory agent.
- Avoid the use of other over-the-counter or prescription preparations containing acetaminophen. Serious overdose can occur. If you need an over-the-counter preparation, consult your health care provider.
- Report rash, unusual bleeding or bruising, yellowing of skin or eyes, changes in voiding patterns.

▷ **acetaZOLAMIDE**
(ah set a zole' ah mide)

Apo-Acetazolamide (CAN),
Diamox Sequels

PREGNANCY CATEGORY C

Drug classes
Antiepileptic
Antiglaucoma drug
Carbonic anhydrase inhibitor
Diuretic
Sulfonamide (nonbacteriostatic)

Therapeutic actions

Inhibits the enzyme carbonic anhydrase. This action decreases aqueous humor formation in the eye, IOP, and hydrogen ion secretion by renal tubule cells, and increases sodium, potassium, bicarbonate, and water excretion by the kidney, causing a diuretic effect. In epilepsy, carbonic anhydrase inhibition seems to retard abnormal, excessive discharge from CNS neurons.

Indications

- Adjunctive treatment of chronic open-angle glaucoma, secondary glaucoma
- Preoperative use in acute angle-closure glaucoma when delay of surgery is desired to lower IOP
- Edema caused by heart failure, drug-induced edema
- Centrencephalic epilepsy (absence, unlocalized seizures)
- Prophylaxis and treatment of acute mountain sickness
- Unlabeled uses: Malignant glaucoma, migraine prevention, familial periodic paralysis, cystine or uric acid renal calculi prevention, tardive dyskinesia

Contraindications and cautions

- Contraindicated with allergy to acetazolamide, antibacterial sulfonamides, or thiazides; chronic noncongestive angle-closure glaucoma; cirrhosis.
- Use cautiously with fluid or electrolyte imbalance (specifically decreased Na$^+$, decreased K$^+$, hyperchloremic acidosis), renal disease, hepatic disease (risk of hepatic coma if acetazolamide is given), adrenocortical insufficiency, respiratory acidosis, COPD, lactation.

Available forms

Tablets—125, 250 mg; ER capsules—500 mg; powder for injection—500 mg/vial

Dosages
Adults
- *Open-angle glaucoma:* 250 mg–1 g/day PO, usually in divided doses or ER capsules–1 capsule bid (morning and evening). Do not exceed 1 g/day.
- *Acute congestive angle-closure glaucoma:* 500 mg PO bid (ER capsules) or 250 mg PO q4h; may use a leading dose of 500 mg followed by 125–250 mg every 4 hr.

- *Secondary glaucoma and preoperatively:* 250 mg every 4 hr or 250 mg bid PO or 500 mg PO bid (ER capsules), or 500 mg followed by 125–250 mg every 4 hr. May be given IV for rapid relief of increased IOP—500 mg IV, then 125–250 mg PO every 4 hr.
- *Diuresis in heart failure:* 250–375 mg (5 mg/kg) daily in the morning. Most effective if given on alternate days or for 2 days alternating with a day of rest.
- *Drug-induced edema:* 250–375 mg once every day or for 1 or 2 days alternating with a day of rest.
- *Epilepsy:* 8–30 mg/kg/day in divided doses. When given in combination with other antiepileptics, starting dose is 250 mg daily. SR preparation is not recommended for this use. Range of dosing: 375–1,000 mg/day.
- *Acute mountain sickness:* 500 mg–1 g/day PO in divided doses of tablets or ER capsules. For rapid ascent, the 1-g dose is recommended. When possible, begin dosing 24–48 hr before ascent and continue for 48 hr or longer as needed while at high altitude.

Pediatric patients 12 yr and older
- *Acute mountain sickness:* 500–1,000 mg/day PO in divided doses.

Pediatric patients 11 yr and younger
- Safety and efficacy not established.

Pharmacokinetics

Route	Onset	Peak	Duration
Oral	1 hr	4 hr	8–12 hr
SR	2 hr	3–6 hr	18–24 hr
IV	1–2 min	15–18 min	4–5 hr

Metabolism: T$_{1/2}$: 5–6 hr
Distribution: Crosses placenta; enters breast milk
Excretion: Urine, unchanged

▼ IV FACTS

Preparation: Reconstitute 500-mg vial with 5 mL of sterile water for injection; stable for 3 days if refrigerated, but use within 12 hr is recommended.
Infusion: Give over 1 min for single injection, over 4–8 hr in solution.
Incompatibilities: Do not mix with diltiazem or in multivitamin infusion.

Adverse effects
- **CNS:** Weakness, fatigue, nervousness, sedation, drowsiness, dizziness, depression,

tremor, ataxia, headache, paresthesias, seizures, flaccid paralysis, transient myopia
- **Dermatologic:** Urticaria, pruritus, photosensitivity, rash, erythema multiforme (Stevens-Johnson syndrome)
- **GI:** Anorexia, nausea, vomiting, constipation, melena, hepatic insufficiency
- **GU:** Hematuria, glycosuria, *urinary frequency,* renal colic, renal calculi, crystalluria, polyuria
- **Hematologic:** Bone marrow depression
- **Other:** Weight loss, fever, acidosis, changes in blood glucose levels

Interactions

✳ **Drug-drug** • Decreased renal excretion of quinidine, amphetamine, procainamide, TCAs • Increased excretion of salicylates, lithium • Increased risk of salicylate toxicity due to metabolic acidosis with acetazolamide

✳ **Drug-lab test** • False-positive results of tests for urinary protein

■ Nursing considerations

CLINICAL ALERT!
Name confusion has occurred between *Diamox* (acetazolamide) and *Trimox* (ampicillin); use caution.

Assessment

- **History:** Allergy to acetazolamide, antibacterial sulfonamides, or thiazides; chronic noncongestive angle-closure glaucoma; fluid or electrolyte imbalance; renal or hepatic disease; adrenocortical insufficiency; respiratory acidosis; COPD; lactation
- **Physical:** Skin color, lesions; edema, weight, orientation, reflexes, muscle strength, IOP; R, pattern, adventitious sounds; liver evaluation, bowel sounds, urinary output patterns; CBC, serum electrolytes, LFTs, renal function tests, urinalysis

Interventions

⊗ **Black box warning** Fatalities have occurred due to severe reactions, including Stevens-Johnson syndrome, toxic epidermal necrolysis, fulminant hepatic necrosis, and blood dyscrasias. Discontinue immediately at any sign of serious reactions.

⊗ **Black box warning** Use caution if patient is receiving high-dose aspirin; anorexia,

tachypnea, lethargy, coma, and death have been reported.
- Administer by direct IV if parenteral use is necessary; IM use is painful.
- Give with food or milk if GI upset occurs.
- Use caution if giving with other drugs with excretion inhibited by urine alkalinization.
- Make oral liquid form by crushing tablets and suspending in cherry, chocolate, raspberry, or other sweet syrup, or one tablet may be submerged in 10 mL of hot water with 1 mL of honey or syrup; do not use alcohol or glycerin as a vehicle.
- Establish safety precautions if CNS effects occur; protect patient from sun or bright lights if photophobia occurs.
- Obtain regular weight to monitor fluid changes.
- Monitor serum electrolytes and acid–base balance during course of drug therapy.

Teaching points

- Take drug with meals if GI upset occurs.
- Arrange to have intraocular pressure checked periodically.
- Weigh yourself on a regular basis, at the same time of the day and in the same clothing. Record weight on calendar.
- You may experience these side effects: Increased volume and frequency of urination; dizziness, feeling faint on arising, drowsiness, fatigue (do not engage in hazardous activities like driving a car); sensitivity to sunlight (use sunglasses; wear protective clothing or use a sunscreen when outdoors); GI upset (taking the drug with meals, eat frequent small meals).
- Report weight change of more than 3 pounds in 1 day, unusual bleeding or bruising, sore throat, dizziness, trembling, numbness, fatigue, muscle weakness or cramps, flank or loin pain, rash.

▽acetylcysteine (*N*-acetylcysteine)
*(a se teel **sis'** tay een)*

Acetadote

PREGNANCY CATEGORY B

Drug classes
Antidote
Mucolytic

Therapeutic actions

Mucolytic activity: Splits links in the muco-proteins contained in respiratory mucus secretions, decreasing the viscosity of the mucus. Antidote to acetaminophen hepato-toxicity: Protects liver cells by maintaining cell function and detoxifying acetaminophen metabolites.

Indications

- Mucolytic adjuvant therapy for abnormal, viscid, or inspissated mucus secretions in acute and chronic bronchopulmonary disease (emphysema with bronchitis, asthmatic bronchitis, tuberculosis, pneumonia, primary bronchiectasis, lung amyloidosis), in pulmonary complications of cystic fibrosis, and in tracheostomy care; pulmonary complications associated with surgery, anesthesia, post-traumatic chest conditions; diagnostic bronchial studies (oral solution only)
- To prevent or lessen hepatic injury that may occur after ingestion of a potentially hepatotoxic dose of acetaminophen; treatment must start as soon as possible; most effective if administered within 8–10 hr of ingestion, but can be given within 24 hr after ingestion; IV use approved for this indication
- Unlabeled uses: As ophthalmic solution to treat keratoconjunctivitis sicca (dry eye); as an enema to treat bowel obstruction due to meconium ileus or its equivalent; prevention of radiocontrast-induced nephrotoxicity; chronic blepharitis

Contraindications and cautions
Mucolytic use
- Contraindicated with hypersensitivity to acetylcysteine; use caution and discontinue immediately if bronchospasm occurs.
Antidotal use
- No contraindications; use caution with esophageal varices, peptic ulcer.

Available forms
Solution—10%, 20%; injection—200 mg/mL

Dosages
Adult and pediatric patients
Mucolytic use
- Nebulization with face mask, mouthpiece, tracheostomy: 3–5 mL of the 20% solution or 6–10 mL of the 10% solution tid or qid.

- Nebulization with tent, croupette: Very large volumes are required, occasionally up to 300 mL, during a treatment period. The dose is the volume or solution that will maintain a very heavy mist in the tent or croupette for the desired period. Administration for intermittent or continuous prolonged periods, including overnight, may be desirable.

Instillation
- Direct or by tracheostomy: 1–2 mL of a 10%–20% solution every 1–4 hr; may be introduced into a particular segment of the bronchopulmonary tree by way of a plastic catheter (inserted under local anesthesia and with direct visualization). Instill 2–5 mL of the 20% solution by a syringe connected to the catheter.
- Percutaneous intratracheal catheter: 1–2 mL of the 20% solution or 2–4 mL of the 10% solution every 1–4 hr by a syringe connected to the catheter.
- Diagnostic bronchogram: Before the procedure, give two to three administrations of 1–2 mL of the 20% solution or 2–4 mL of the 10% solution by nebulization or intratracheal instillation.

Antidotal use
- For acetaminophen overdose, oral: Administer acetylcysteine immediately if 8 hr or less have elapsed since acetaminophen ingestion, using the following protocol: ● If activated charcoal has been administered by lavage, charcoal may adsorb acetylcysteine and reduce its effectiveness. ● Draw blood for acetaminophen plasma assay and for baseline AST, ALT, bilirubin, PT, creatinine, BUN, blood sugar, and electrolytes; if acetaminophen assay cannot be obtained or dose is clearly in the toxic range, give full course of acetylcysteine therapy; monitor hepatic and renal function, fluid and electrolyte balance.
● Administer acetylcysteine PO 140 mg/kg loading dose. ● See manufacturer's directions for preparation of oral dose using 10% or 20% solution and cola or other soft drink as diluent. ● Administer 17 maintenance doses of 70 mg/kg every 4 hr, starting 4 hr after loading dose; administer full course of doses unless acetaminophen assay shows nontoxic level. ● If patient vomits loading or maintenance dose within 1 hr of administration, repeat that dose; if patient is persistently unable to retain oral dosing, may administer by duodenal intubation.

Adverse effects in *italics* are most common; those in **bold** are life-threatening. ▣ Do not crush.

• *IV:* Dilute in 5% dextrose. Loading dose—150 mg/kg in 200 mL given IV over 60 min; then first maintenance dose 50 mg/kg in 500 mL IV over 4 hr followed by a second maintenance dose 100 mg/kg in 1,000 mL given IV over 16 hr. Total IV dose is 300 mg/kg over 21 hr. • Children less than 40 kg and patients who need fluid restriction should receive lowest infusion volume possible. See prescribing information for details. • Repeat blood chemistry assays as described above daily if acetaminophen plasma level is in toxic range.

Pharmacokinetics

Route	Onset	Peak	Duration
Oral	30–60 min	1–2 hr	Not known
Instillation, Inhalation	1 min	5–10 min	2–3 hr
IV	Immediate	5 min	2–3 hr

Metabolism: Hepatic; $T_{1/2}$: 5.6–6.25 hr
Excretion: Urine (30%)

▼ IV FACTS

Preparation: Dilute in 5% dextrose only. Solution may change from colorless to pink or purple when the stopper is punctured. Reconstituted solution is stable 24 hr at room temperature. Discard any unused portion of the vial. Solution is preservative-free.

Infusion: Infuse loading dose over 15 min, first maintenance dose over 4 hr, second maintenance dose over 16 hr.

Incompatibilities: Do not mix with other drugs. Avoid solution contact with rubber and metals, particularly iron, copper, nickel.

Adverse effects
Mucolytic use
• **GI:** Nausea, stomatitis
• **Hypersensitivity:** Urticaria
• **Respiratory: Bronchospasm,** especially in patients with asthma
• **Other:** *Rhinorrhea*
Antidotal use
• **Dermatologic:** Rash
• **GI:** *Nausea, vomiting, other GI symptoms*
• **Other: Anaphylactoid reactions**

■ Nursing considerations
Assessment
• **History:** Mucolytic use: Hypersensitivity to acetylcysteine, asthma. Antidotal use: Esophageal varices, peptic ulcer
• **Physical:** Weight, T, skin color, lesions; BP, P; R, adventitious sounds, bowel sounds, liver palpation

Interventions
Mucolytic use
• Dilute the 20% acetylcysteine solution with either normal saline or sterile water for injection; use the 10% solution undiluted. Refrigerate unused, undiluted solution, and use within 96 hr. Drug solution in the opened bottle may change color, but this does not alter safety or efficacy.
• Administer the following drugs separately, because they are incompatible with acetylcysteine solutions: Tetracyclines, erythromycin lactobionate, amphotericin B, iodized oil chymotrypsin, trypsin, hydrogen peroxide.
• Use water to remove residual drug solution on the patient's face after administration by face mask.
• Inform patient that nebulization may produce an initial disagreeable odor, but the odor will soon disappear.
• Monitor nebulizer for buildup of drug from evaporation; dilute with sterile water for injection to prevent concentrate from impeding nebulization and drug delivery.
• Establish routine for pulmonary toilet; have suction equipment on standby.
Antidotal use
• Dilute the 20% acetylcysteine solution with cola drinks or other soft drinks to a final concentration of 5%; if administered by gastric tube or Miller-Abbott tube, water may be used as diluent. Dilution minimizes the risk of vomiting.
• Prepare fresh solutions, and use within 1 hr; undiluted solution in opened vials may be kept for 96 hr.
• Treat fluid and electrolyte imbalance, hypoglycemia.
• Give vitamin K_1 if prothrombin ratio exceeds 1.5; give fresh-frozen plasma if prothrombin ratio exceeds 3.
• Do not administer diuretics.
• Monitor timing of IV doses.
• Follow acetaminophen assays carefully to determine appropriate dosage.

Teaching points
- You may experience these side effects: Increased productive cough, nausea, GI upset.
- Report difficulty breathing or nausea.

▷ **acitretin**

See Appendix R, *Less commonly used drugs*.

▷ **aclidinium bromide**
(a clih din' ee um)

Tudorza Pressair

PREGNANCY CATEGORY C

Drug classes
Anticholinergic
Bronchodilator

Therapeutic actions
Long-acting anticholinergic that blocks acetylcholine at muscarinic receptors, leading to bronchodilation; effect of inhaled drug is predominantly site specific, with less generalized parasympatholytic activity than systemic agents.

Indications
- Long-term maintenance treatment of bronchospasm associated with COPD, including chronic bronchitis and emphysema

Contraindications and cautions
- Contraindicated with history of serious hypersensitivity reactions to components of the drug; acute bronchospasm.
- Use cautiously with bladder outlet obstruction, BPH, glaucoma, pregnancy, lactation, known milk protein hypersensitivity.

Available forms
Dry powder inhaler—400 mcg/actuation

Dosages
Adults
400 mcg bid by oral inhalation using multidose inhalation device.
Pediatric patients
Safety and efficacy not established

Pharmacokinetics

Route	Onset	Peak
Inhalation	Rapid	10 min

Metabolism: Hepatic; $T_{1/2}$: 5-8 hr
Distribution: May cross placenta; may enter breast milk
Excretion: Urine

Adverse effects
- **CNS:** *Headache*, worsening glaucoma
- **GI:** Nausea, diarrhea, vomiting, dry mouth
- **GU:** Urine retention
- **Respiratory:** *Nasopharyngitis*, rhinitis, cough, paradoxical bronchospasm
- **Other:** Toothache, hypersensitivity reactions

Interactions
✳ **Drug-drug** • Risk of additive anticholinergic effects if combined with other anticholinergics; avoid this combination

■ Nursing considerations
Assessment
- **History:** Allergy to components of the drug, lactation, BPH, bladder outlet obstruction, pregnancy, glaucoma, acute bronchospasm, milk protein hypersensitivity
- **Physical:** P, BP; R, adventitious sounds; bladder exam; IOP measurement

Interventions
- Ensure diagnosis of chronic bronchospasm associated with COPD; drug is not for use with acute bronchospasm.
- Administer using the *Tudorza Pressair* inhaler; review proper use with patient.
- Monitor patient for acute hypersensitivity reaction (difficulty breathing, swelling of face or tongue, rash, hives), which is more common with patients who have milk protein sensitivity. Stop drug and provide supportive care if these signs and symptoms occur.
- Discontinue drug and arrange for other therapy if paradoxical bronchospasm occurs.
- Assess patient for possible urine retention and BPH before beginning therapy; monitor for worsening of condition. Have patient void before each dose if this is a problem.
- Assess patients with narrow-angle glaucoma before and periodically during treatment; monitor for worsening of condition.

A

Teaching points

- This drug must be inhaled. Review the proper use of the *Tudorza Pressair* inhaler; use the inhaler twice a day. Do not clean the inhaler; it may be wiped off with a dry paper towel. Discard the inhaler and start a new one when the dose indicator is in the red zone or shows a zero.
- If you miss a dose, begin taking the drug again with the next scheduled dose. Do not take more than two doses a day.
- This drug is taken daily; it is not a rescue drug for acute problems. Do not increase the dose if your symptoms are worsening. You should discuss a rescue treatment with your health care provider.
- It is not known how this drug could affect a developing fetus; if you are pregnant or are thinking about becoming pregnant while taking this drug, discuss the risks with your health care provider.
- It is not known how this drug could affect a breast-feeding infant; if you are breast-feeding, discuss the risks with your health care provider.
- You may experience these side effects: Headache, worsening of glaucoma (if you have glaucoma, report changes in vision, eye pain, nausea, or vomiting), urine retention (this is more likely if you have an enlarged prostate or preexisting urine retention; empty your bladder before each dose and report increased difficulty emptying your bladder); hypersensitivity reaction (immediately report swelling of the face or tongue, rash, hives, difficulty breathing).
- Report difficulty urinating, rash, difficulty breathing, worsening of symptoms, blurred vision.

▽acyclovir (acycloguanosine)

(ay sye' kloe ver)

Apo-Acyclovir (CAN), Gen-Acyclovir (CAN), ratio-Acyclovir (CAN), Zovirax

PREGNANCY CATEGORY B

Drug classes

Antiviral
Purine nucleoside analogue

Therapeutic actions

Antiviral activity; inhibits viral DNA replication.

Indications

- Initial and recurrent mucosal and cutaneous HSV-1 and HSV-2 and varicella zoster infections in immunocompromised patients
- Severe initial and recurrent genital herpes infections in immunocompromised patients
- Herpes simplex encephalitis
- Treatment of neonatal HSV infections
- Acute treatment of herpes zoster (shingles) and chickenpox (varicella)
- Ointment: Initial herpes genital infections; limited mucocutaneous HSV infections in immunocompromised patients
- Cream: Recurrent herpes labialis (cold sores) in patients 12 yr or older
- Unlabeled uses: Cytomegalovirus and HSV infection following transplant, ocular and other herpes simplex infections, varicella pneumonia, disseminated primary eczema herpeticum

Contraindications and cautions

- Contraindicated with allergy to acyclovir, renal disease, lactation.
- Use cautiously with pregnancy.

Available forms

Tablets—400, 800 mg; capsules—200 mg; suspension—200 mg/5 mL; powder for injection—500 mg/vial, 1,000 mg/vial; injection—50 mg/mL; ointment—50 mg/g; cream—50 mg/g

Dosages

Adults

Parenteral

- *Herpes genitalis:* 5 mg/kg IV infused over 1 hr every 8 hr for 5 days.
- *Herpes encephalitis:* 10 mg/kg IV infused over 1 hr every 8 hr for 10 days.
- *Herpes simplex, immunocompromised patients:* 5 mg/kg IV infused over 1 hr every 8 hr for 7 days.
- *Varicella zoster, immunocompromised patients:* 10 mg/kg IV infused over 1 hr every 8 hr for 7 days.

Oral

- *Initial genital herpes:* 200 mg every 4 hr five times daily (1,000 mg/day) for 10 days.

- *Long-term suppressive therapy:* 400 mg bid for up to 12 mo.
- *Recurrent therapy:* 200 mg every 4 hr five times daily for 5 days.
- *Acute herpes zoster:* 800 mg every 4 hr five times daily while awake for 7–10 days.
- *Chickenpox:* 800 mg qid for 5 days.

Pediatric patients
Parenteral

- *HSV infections in patients younger than 12 yr:* 10 mg/kg infused IV over 1 hr every 8 hr for 7 days.
- *Varicella zoster infection in patients younger than 12 yr:* 20 mg/kg IV over 1 hr every 8 hr for 7 days.
- *Shingles, HSV encephalitis in patients 3 mo to 12 yr:* 20 mg/kg IV over 1 hr every 8 hr for 14–21 days.
- *Neonatal HSV:* 10 mg/kg infused over 1 hr every 8 hr for 10 days.

Oral
Younger than 2 yr: Safety not established.
2 yr or older and 40 kg or less: 20 mg/kg per dose qid (80 mg/kg/day) for 5 days.
More than 40 kg: Use adult dosage.
12 yr or older: Use adult dosage.

Geriatric patients or patients with renal impairment
Oral

For creatinine clearance less than 10 mL/min, 200 mg every 12 hr. If usual regimen was 200 mg every 4 hr or 400 mg every 12 hr; if normal dose is 800 mg every 4 hr, give 800 mg every 12 hr. If on hemodialysis, an additional dose should be given after each dialysis session.

IV

CrCl (mL/min)	100% of usual dose at dosing interval (IV)
More than 50	Every 8 hr
25–50	Every 12 hr
10–25	Daily
0–10	50% of dose every 24 hr

Topical

Ointment (all ages): Apply sufficient quantity to cover all lesions 6 times/day (every 3 hr) for 7 days; 1.25-cm (0.5-in) ribbon of ointment covers 2.5 cm^2 (4 in^2) surface area.
Cream (12 yr and older): Apply enough to cover all lesions 5 times/day for 4 days.

Pharmacokinetics

Route	Onset	Peak	Duration
Oral	Varies	1.5–2 hr	Not known
IV	Immediate	1 hr	8 hr
Topical	Absorption is minimal		

Metabolism: $T_{1/2}$: 2.5–5 hr
Distribution: Crosses placenta; enters breast milk
Excretion: Unchanged in urine

▼ IV FACTS

Preparation: Reconstitute 500-mg vial in 10 mL sterile water for injection; do not use bacteriostatic water for injection containing benzyl alcohol, 1,000-mg vial in 20 mL; concentration will be 50 mg/mL. Do not dilute drug with bacteriostatic water containing parabens. Use reconstituted solution within 12 hr; dilute IV solution to concentration of 7 mg/mL or less. Do not use biologic or colloidal fluids such as blood products or protein solutions. Warm drug to room temperature to dissolve precipitates formed during refrigeration.

Infusion: Administer by slow IV infusion of parenteral solutions; avoid bolus or rapid injection. Infuse over at least 1 hr to avoid renal damage.

Incompatibilities: Do not mix with diltiazem, dobutamine, dopamine, fludarabine, foscarnet, idarubicin, meperidine, morphine, ondansetron, piperacillin, sargramostim, vinorelbine.

Adverse effects
Systemic administration

- **CNS:** Headache, vertigo, depression, tremors, encephalopathic changes
- **Dermatologic:** *Inflammation or phlebitis at injection sites,* rash, hair loss
- **GI:** *Nausea, vomiting,* diarrhea, anorexia
- **GU:** Crystalluria with rapid IV administration, hematuria, increased BUN.

Topical administration

- **Dermatologic:** Transient burning at site of application

Interactions
Systemic administration

✳ **Drug-drug** • Increased effects with probenecid • Increased nephrotoxicity with other nephrotoxic drugs • Extreme drowsiness with zidovudine

■ Nursing considerations
Assessment
- **History:** Allergy to acyclovir, renal disease, lactation, pregnancy
- **Physical:** Skin color, lesions; orientation; BP, P, auscultation, perfusion, edema; R, adventitious sounds; urinary output; BUN, creatinine clearance

Interventions
Systemic administration
- Ensure that the patient is well hydrated.

Topical administration
- Start treatment as soon as possible after onset of signs and symptoms.
- Wear a rubber glove or finger cot when applying drug.

Teaching points
Systemic administration
- Complete the full course of oral therapy, and do not exceed the prescribed dose.
- Oral acyclovir is not a cure for your disease but should make you feel better.
- Avoid sexual intercourse while visible lesions are present.
- You may experience these side effects: Nausea, vomiting, loss of appetite, diarrhea; headache, dizziness.
- Report difficulty urinating, rash, increased severity or frequency of recurrences.

Topical administration
- Wear rubber gloves or finger cots when applying the drug to prevent autoinoculation of other sites and transmission to others.
- This drug does not cure the disease; application during symptom-free periods will not prevent recurrences.
- Avoid sexual intercourse while visible lesions are present.
- This drug may cause burning, stinging, itching, rash; notify your health care provider if these are pronounced.

▽**adalimumab**

See Appendix R, *Less commonly used drugs*.

▽**adefovir dipivoxil**
*(ah **def'** o veer dye pih **vocks'** ill)*

Hepsera

PREGNANCY CATEGORY C

Drug classes
Antiviral
Reverse transcriptase inhibitor

Therapeutic actions
Antiviral activity; nucleotide analogue of adenosine that inhibits hepatitis B virus reverse transcriptase and causes DNA chain termination and blocked viral replication.

Indications
- Treatment of chronic hepatitis B in adults and children 12 yr and older with evidence of active viral replication and either evidence of persistent elevations in ALT or AST or histologically active disease

Contraindications and cautions
- Contraindicated with allergy to adefovir or any components of the product, lactation.
- Use cautiously with pregnancy, renal impairment, signs of lactic acidosis, risk factors for severe liver disease, the elderly.

Available forms
Tablets—10 mg

Dosages
Adults and children 12 yr and older
10 mg/day PO.
Pediatric patients
Safety and efficacy not established.
Patients with renal impairment
For creatinine clearance 30–49 mL/min, 10 mg every 48 hr; for creatinine clearance 10–29 mL/min, 10 mg every 72 hr. For hemodialysis patients, 10 mg every 7 days following dialysis. Drug not recommended for creatinine clearance less than 10 mL/min if patient is not on dialysis.

Pharmacokinetics

Route	Onset	Peak
Oral	Rapid	0.6–4 hr

Metabolism: Hepatic; $T_{1/2}$: 7.5 hr

Distribution: May cross placenta; may enter breast milk
Excretion: Urine

Adverse effects

- **CNS:** Headache, *asthenia*
- **GI:** Nausea, diarrhea, abdominal pain, flatulence, dyspepsia, **severe hepatomegaly with steatosis, sometimes fatal; exacerbation of hepatitis if therapy is discontinued,** *elevated liver enzymes*
- **GU: Nephrotoxicity,** hematuria, glycosuria
- **Metabolic: Lactic acidosis, sometimes severe,** elevated CK, elevated amylase levels
- **Other:** HIV resistance if used to treat patients with unrecognized HIV infection

Interactions

✳ **Drug-drug** • Increased risk of nephrotoxicity if combined with other drugs that cause nephrotoxicity; if this combination is used, monitor renal function closely and evaluate risks versus benefits of continuing the combination

■ Nursing considerations
Assessment

- **History:** Allergy to adefovir or any component of the drug, renal or hepatic impairment, lactic acidosis, pregnancy, lactation
- **Physical:** T; orientation, reflexes; abdominal examination, LFTs, renal function tests

Interventions

- Ensure that HIV antibody testing has been done before initiating therapy to reduce risk of emergence of HIV resistance.

⊗ *Black box warning* Caution patient not to run out of this drug; patients who stop taking it may develop worsened or severe hepatitis.

⊗ *Black box warning* Monitor patients regularly to evaluate renal function and liver enzymes; severe nephrotoxicity and hepatotoxicity can occur.

⊗ *Black box warning* Withdraw drug and monitor patient if patient develops signs of lactic acidosis or hepatotoxicity, including hepatomegaly and steatosis.

⊗ *Black box warning* HIV resistance may occur in unrecognized or untreated HIV

infection; test patients for HIV infection before beginning therapy.

- Encourage women of childbearing age to use barrier contraceptives while on this drug as the effects of the drug on the fetus are not known.
- Advise women who are breast-feeding to find another method of feeding the infant.
- Advise patient that this drug does not cure the disease and there is still a risk of transmitting the disease to others; advise the use of barrier contraceptives.

Teaching points

- Take this drug once a day.
- Take the full course of therapy as prescribed; if you miss a dose, take it as soon as you remember and then take the next dose at the usual time the next day. Do not double any doses.
- You will be asked to have an HIV antibody test if your HIV status is not known; some people with HIV who are treated with this drug develop resistant strains of HIV.
- This drug does not cure chronic hepatitis B infection; long-term effects are not yet known; continue to take precautions as the risk of transmission is not reduced by this drug.
- Do not stop taking this drug; you may experience very serious or worsening hepatitis B if the drug is stopped after you have been taking it. Consult your health care provider if your prescription is getting low and make sure that you do not skip any doses.
- You may experience these side effects: Nausea, diarrhea, abdominal pain, headache; try to maintain nutrition and fluid intake as much as possible—eat frequent small meals.
- Report severe weakness, muscle pain, trouble breathing, dizziness, cold feelings in your arms or legs, palpitations.

▽ adenosine

See Appendix R, *Less commonly used drugs*.

▽ aflibercept

See Appendix R, *Less commonly used drugs*.

▽ agalsidase beta

See Appendix R, *Less commonly used drugs*.

Adverse effects in *italics* are most common; those in **bold** are life-threatening. ▭▭ Do not crush.

▷albumin, human (normal serum albumin)
(al byoo' min)

5%: Albuminar-5, Albutein 5%
Normal Serum Albumin 5%
Solution, Plasbumin-5
20%: Plasbumin-20
25%: Albuminar-25, Albutein 25%,
Buminate 25%, Human Albumin Grifols,
Normal Serum Albumin 25%
Solution, Plasbumin-25

PREGNANCY CATEGORY C

Drug classes
Blood product
Plasma protein

Therapeutic actions
Normal blood protein; maintains plasma osmotic pressure and is important in maintaining normal blood volume.

Indications
- Emergency treatment of shock due to burns, trauma, surgery, and infections (20% or 25%); 5% for use in nonemergency cases
- Burns: Albumin 5% used to prevent hemoconcentration and water and protein losses in conjunction with adequate infusions of crystalloid. 20% or 25% used beyond 24 hr.
- Hypoproteinemia in postoperative patients, patients with sepsis, or intensive care patients (20%, 25%)
- Adult respiratory distress syndrome: Albumin 20% or 25% with a diuretic may be helpful
- Cardiopulmonary bypass: Preoperative blood dilution with 20% or 25% albumin. 5% may be used as adjunct therapy.
- Acute liver failure (20% or 25%)
- Sequestration of protein-rich fluids (20%, 25%)
- Erythrocyte resuspension: Albumin 20% or 25% may be added to the isotonic suspension of washed red cells immediately before transfusion
- Acute nephrosis: Albumin 20% or 25% and loop diuretic may help to control edema repeated daily for 7–10 days
- Renal dialysis: Albumin 20% or 25% may be useful in treatment of shock and hypotension. 5% solution may be used as adjunct in hemodialysis.
- Hyperbilirubinemia and erythroblastosis fetalis: Adjunct in exchange transfusions
- Neonatal hemolytic disease: 20%–25% solution

Contraindications and cautions
- Contraindicated with allergy to albumin; severe anemia, cardiac failure, normal or increased intravascular volume, current use of cardiopulmonary bypass.
- Use cautiously with hepatic or renal failure.

Available forms
Injection—5%, 20%, 25%

Dosages
Administer by IV infusion only; contains 130–160 mEq sodium/L.
Adults
- *Hypovolemic shock:* 5% albumin: Initial dose of 500 mL is given as rapidly as possible; additional 500 mL may be given in 15–30 min. Base therapy on clinical response if more than 1,000 mL is required; consider the need for whole blood. In patients with low blood volume, administer at rate of 1–2 mL/min. 20% or 25% albumin: Base therapy on clinical response. Administer as rapidly as tolerated; 1 mL/min may be given to patients with low blood volume.
- *Erythrocyte resuspension:* 25 g of albumin per liter of erythrocytes, add to isotonic suspension of washed RBCs before transfusion.
- *Hypoproteinemia:* 5% albumin may be given for acute replacement of protein; use 20% or 25% albumin 50–75 g/day. Do not exceed 2 mL/min. Adjust the rate of infusion based on patient response.
- *Burns:* 20% or 25% albumin can be helpful in maintaining colloid osmotic pressure; goal is to maintain plasma albumin concentration at 2.5 ± 0.5 g/100 mL with a plasma oncotic pressure of 20 mm Hg.
- *Hepatic cirrhosis:* 25% may be effective in temporary restoration of plasma protein levels.
- *Nephrosis:* Initial dose of 100 mL of 25% albumin may be repeated daily for 7–10 days, with a loop diuretic; effects are not sustained because of the underlying problem.
Pediatric patients
- Use of albumin 5% has not been evaluated.

- Usual rate of administration is 1/4 to 1/2 adult rate, or dosage may be calculated on basis of 0.6–1 g/kg.
- *Hypoproteinemia:* 25 g/day of 20% or 25% albumin.
- *Hyperbilirubinemia and erythroblasto-sis fetalis:* 1 g/kg 1 hr before transfusion.

Pharmacokinetics

Route	Onset	Peak
IV	Immediate	End of infusion

Metabolism: Tissue; $T_{1/2}$: Unknown
Distribution: Crosses placenta; enters breast milk
Excretion: Urine

▼ IV FACTS

Preparation: Swab stopper top with antiseptic immediately before removing seal and entering the vial. Use a 16-gauge needle or dispensing pin with vials 20 mL or larger. Inspect for particulate matter and discoloration. Store at room temperature; do not freeze. Do not dilute 5% albumin; 25% albumin may be undiluted or diluted in normal saline; if sodium restriction is required, may dilute 25% albumin with D_5W.

Infusion: Give by IV infusion slowly enough to prevent rapid plasma volume expansion 1–2 mL/min for adults, 0.25–1 mL/min for children. Give in combination with or through the same administration set as solutions of saline or carbohydrates.

Incompatibilities: Do not use with solutions containing alcohol or protein hydrolysates— precipitates may form.

Adverse effects

- **CV:** Hypotension, heart failure, pulmonary edema after rapid infusion
- **Hypersensitivity:** Fever, chills, *changes in blood pressure,* flushing, nausea, vomiting, changes in respiration, rashes

■ Nursing considerations
Assessment

- **History:** Allergy to albumin, severe anemia, heart failure, current use of cardiopulmonary bypass, hepatic failure, renal failure
- **Physical:** Skin color, lesions; T; P, BP, peripheral perfusion; R, adventitious sounds;

LFTs, renal function tests, Hct, serum electrolytes

Interventions

- Give to all blood groups or types.
- Consider using whole blood; infusion provides only symptomatic relief of hypoproteinemia.
- Monitor BP; discontinue infusion if hypotension occurs.
- Stop infusion if headache, flushing, fever, changes in BP occur; treat reaction with antihistamines. If a plasma protein is still needed, try material from a different lot number.
- Monitor patient's clinical response, and adjust infusion rate accordingly.

Teaching points

- Report headache, nausea, vomiting, difficulty breathing, back pain.

▷ albuterol sulfate
(al byoo' ter ole)

AccuNeb, ProAir HFA, Proventil HFA, Ventolin Diskus (CAN), Ventolin HFA, Ventolin Oral Liquid (CAN), VoSpire ER ⓒⓝⓒ

PREGNANCY CATEGORY C

Drug classes
Antiasthmatic
Beta$_2$-selective adrenergic agonist
Bronchodilator
Sympathomimetic

Therapeutic actions

In low doses, acts relatively selectively at beta$_2$-adrenergic receptors to cause bronchodilation and vasodilation; at higher doses, beta$_2$ selectivity is lost, and the drug acts at beta$_2$ receptors to cause typical sympathomimetic cardiac effects.

Indications

- Relief and prevention of bronchospasm in patients with reversible obstructive airway disease or COPD
- Inhalation: Treatment of acute attacks of bronchospasm; prevention of exercise-induced bronchospasm

• Unlabeled use, inhalation: Adjunct in treating moderate to severe hyperkalemia in dialysis patients; seems to lower potassium concentrations when inhaled by patients on hemodialysis

Contraindications and cautions

• Contraindicated with hypersensitivity to albuterol; tachyarrhythmias, tachycardia caused by digitalis glycoside intoxication; general anesthesia with halogenated hydrocarbons or cyclopropane (these sensitize the myocardium to catecholamines); unstable vasomotor system disorders; hypertension; coronary insufficiency, CAD; history of stroke; COPD patients with degenerative heart disease.

• Use cautiously with diabetes mellitus (large IV doses can aggravate diabetes and ketoacidosis); hyperthyroidism; history of seizure disorders; psychoneurotic individuals; labor and delivery (oral use has delayed second stage of labor; parenteral use of beta$_2$-adrenergic agonists can accelerate fetal heart beat and cause hypoglycemia, hypokalemia, pulmonary edema in the mother and hypoglycemia in the neonate); lactation; the elderly (more sensitive to CNS effects).

Available forms

Tablets—2, 4 mg; ER tablets ◖ONE◗—4, 8 mg; syrup—2 mg/5 mL; aerosol—90 mcg/actuation; solution for inhalation—0.021%, 0.042%, 0.083%, 0.5%.

Dosages
Adults
Oral
Initially, 2 or 4 mg (1–2 tsp syrup) tid–qid PO; may cautiously increase dosage if necessary to 4 or 8 mg qid, not to exceed 32 mg/day. ER tablets, 4–8 mg q 12 hr. Limit use of doses over 4 mg/qid; increase dose only if patient fails to respond.
Inhalation
• *Asthma, bronchospasm:* 1 to 2 inhalations every 4 to 6 hr, maximum dose, 12 inhalations every 24 hr.
• *Prevention of exercise-induced bronchospasm:* 2 inhalations 15 to 30 min prior to exercise.
Solution for inhalation
2.5 mg tid to qid by nebulization.

Pediatric patients
Oral, tablets
6–12 yr: 2 mg tid–qid. May be increased if needed, but do not exceed 24 mg/day. ER tablets, 4 mg q 12 hr.
12 yr and older: Use adult dosage.
Oral, syrup
Younger than 2 yr: Safety and efficacy not established.
2–5 yr: Initially 0.1 mg/kg tid, not to exceed 2 mg (1 tsp) tid; if necessary, cautiously increase stepwise to 0.2 mg/kg tid. Do not exceed 4 mg (2 tsp) tid.
6–14 yr: 2 mg (1 tsp) tid–qid; if necessary, cautiously increase dosage. Do not exceed 24 mg/day in divided doses.
Older than 14 yr: Use adult dosage.
Inhalation solution
2–12 yr: For child less than 15 kg, use 0.5% solution (2.5 mg/0.5 mL) tid to qid by nebulization over 5–15 min; for child more than 15 kg, use 2.5 mg bid or tid by nebulization.
12 yr and older: Use adult dosage.
AccuNeb for patients 2–12 yr: Usual starting dose, 1.25 mg or 0.63 mg tid or qid as needed by nebulization over 5–15 min. More frequent administration is not recommended.
Geriatric patients or patients sensitive to beta-adrenergic stimulation
Restrict initial dose to 2 mg tid or qid; individualize dosage thereafter to as much as 8 mg tid–qid. Patients older than 60 yr are more likely to develop adverse effects.

Pharmacokinetics

Route	Onset	Peak	Duration
Oral	30 min	2–2.5 hr	4–8 hr
Inhalation	5 min	1.5–2 hr	3–8 hr

Metabolism: Hepatic; T$_{1/2}$: 2–4 hr
Distribution: Crosses placenta; enters breast milk
Excretion: Urine

Adverse effects

• **CNS:** *Restlessness, apprehension, anxiety, fear, CNS stimulation,* hyperkinesia, insomnia, tremor, drowsiness, irritability, weakness, vertigo, headache
• **CV: Cardiac arrhythmias,** tachycardia, palpitations, PVCs (rare), anginal pain

- **Dermatologic:** *Sweating, pallor, flushing*
- **GI:** *Nausea,* vomiting, heartburn, unusual or bad taste in mouth
- **GU:** Increased incidence of leiomyomas of uterus when given in higher than human doses in preclinical studies
- **Respiratory:** Respiratory difficulties, pulmonary edema, coughing, **bronchospasm;** paradoxical airway resistance with repeated, excessive use of inhalation preparations

Interactions

✳ **Drug-drug** • Increased sympathomimetic effects with other sympathomimetic drugs • Increased risk of toxicity, especially cardiac, when used with theophylline, aminophylline • Decreased bronchodilating effects with beta-adrenergic blockers (eg, propranolol) • Decreased effectiveness of insulin, oral hypoglycemic drugs • Decreased serum levels and therapeutic effects of digoxin • Increased risk of QT-interval prolongation when combined with other drugs that prolong QT interval • Risk of severe toxicity if combined with or used within 2 wk of linezolid

■ Nursing considerations

Assessment

- **History:** Hypersensitivity to albuterol; tachyarrhythmias, tachycardia caused by digitalis intoxication; general anesthesia with halogenated hydrocarbons or cyclopropane; unstable vasomotor system disorders; hypertension; coronary insufficiency, CAD; history of stroke; COPD patients who have developed degenerative heart disease; diabetes mellitus; hyperthyroidism; history of seizure disorders; psychoneurotic individuals; lactation
- **Physical:** Weight; skin color, T, turgor; orientation, reflexes, affect; P, BP; R, adventitious sounds; blood and urine glucose, serum electrolytes, thyroid function tests, ECG

Interventions

- Use minimal doses for minimal periods; drug tolerance can occur with prolonged use.
- Maintain a beta-adrenergic blocker (cardioselective beta-blocker, such as atenolol, should be used with respiratory distress) on standby in case cardiac arrhythmias occur.

- Prepare solution for inhalation by diluting 0.5 mL 0.5% solution with 2.5 mL normal saline; deliver over 5–15 min by nebulization.
- Do not exceed recommended dosage; administer pressurized inhalation drug forms during second half of inspiration, because the airways are open wider and the aerosol distribution is more extensive.

Teaching points

- Do not exceed recommended dosage; adverse effects or loss of effectiveness may result. Read the instructions that come with respiratory inhalant.
- Do not cut, crush, or chew ER tablets; swallow them whole.
- You may experience these side effects: Dizziness, drowsiness, fatigue, headache (use caution if driving or performing tasks that require alertness); nausea, vomiting, change in taste (eat frequent small meals); rapid heart rate, anxiety, sweating, flushing, insomnia.
- Report chest pain, dizziness, insomnia, weakness, tremors or irregular heartbeat, difficulty breathing, productive cough, failure to respond to usual dosage.

▽aldesleukin

See Appendix R, *Less commonly used drugs*.

▽alendronate sodium

(ah len' dro nate)

Binosto, Co-Alendronate (CAN), Fosamax, Novo-Alendronate (CAN), PMS-Alendronate (CAN), ratio-Alendronate (CAN)

PREGNANCY CATEGORY C

Drug classes

Bisphosphonate
Calcium regulator

Therapeutic actions

Slows normal and abnormal bone resorption without inhibiting bone formation and mineralization.

Indications

- Treatment and prevention of osteoporosis in postmenopausal women
- Treatment of men with osteoporosis
- Treatment of glucocorticoid-induced osteoporosis
- Treatment of Paget's disease of bone in patients with alkaline phosphatase at least two times upper limit of normal, those who are symptomatic, those at risk for future complications
- Unlabeled uses: Osteoporosis with spinal cord injury, vitamin D intoxication, hypercalcemia of malignancy; postoperative knee arthroplasty, osteogenesis imperfecta

Contraindications and cautions

- Contraindicated with allergy to bisphosphonates, hypocalcemia, esophageal abnormalities, inability to stay upright for at least 30 min, and in those at risk for aspiration (oral solution).
- Use cautiously with renal impairment, upper GI disease, pregnancy, lactation.

Available forms

Tablets—5, 10, 35, 40, 70 mg; effervescent tablet—70 mg

Dosages
Adults

- *Postmenopausal osteoporosis:* 10 mg/day PO in AM with full glass of water, at least 30 min before the first beverage, food, or medication of the day, or 70 mg PO once a wk or one bottle of 70 mg oral solution once a wk. Avoid lying down for 30 min after taking drug.
- *Men with osteoporosis:* 10 mg/day PO or 70 mg tablet or effervescent tablet once a wk.
- *Prevention of osteoporosis:* 5 mg/day PO or 35 mg PO once a wk.
- *Paget's disease:* 40 mg/day PO in AM with full glass of water, at least 30 min before the first beverage, food, or medication of the day for 6 mo; may retreat after 6-mo treatment-free period.
- *Glucocorticoid-induced osteoporosis:* 5 mg/day PO with calcium and vitamin D (for men and women); 10 mg/day PO for postmenopausal women not on estrogen.

Pediatric patients
Safety and efficacy not established.

Patients with renal impairment
Dosage adjustment not necessary for creatinine clearance 35–60 mL/min; not recommended if creatinine clearance less than 35 mL/min.

Pharmacokinetics

Route	Onset	Duration
Oral	Slow	Days

Metabolism: Not metabolized; $T_{1/2}$: More than 10 yr
Distribution: Crosses placenta; may enter breast milk
Excretion: Urine

Adverse effects

- **CNS:** *Headache*
- **GI:** *Nausea, diarrhea, GI irritation, pain, esophageal erosion*
- **Skeletal:** *Increased or recurrent bone pain,* focal osteomalacia, osteonecrosis of the jaw

Interactions

❋ **Drug-drug** • Increased risk of GI distress with aspirin and NSAIDs • Decreased absorption if taken with antacids, calcium, iron, multivalent cations; separate dosing by at least 30 min • Increased risk of toxicity if combined with ranitidine; if this combination is used, alendronate dosage may need to be reduced
❋ **Drug-food** • Significantly decreased absorption and serum levels if taken with food; separate dosing from food and beverage by at least 30 min

■ Nursing considerations

CLINICAL ALERT!
Name confusion has occurred between *Fosamax* (alendronate) and *Flomax* (tamsulosin); use caution.

Assessment

- **History:** Allergy to bisphosphonates, renal failure, upper GI disease, lactation, pregnancy
- **Physical:** Muscle tone, bone pain; bowel sounds; urinalysis, serum calcium

Interventions

⊗ *Warning* Give in AM with full glass of water at least 30 min before the first beverage, food, or medication of the day. Patient must stay upright for 30 min to decrease risk of potentially serious esophageal erosion.

• Monitor serum calcium levels before, during, and after therapy.

• Ensure 6-mo rest period after treatment for Paget's disease if retreatment is required.

• Ensure adequate vitamin D and calcium intake.

• Provide comfort measures if bone pain returns.

Teaching points

• Take drug in the morning with a full glass of plain water (not mineral water), at least 30 minutes before any beverage, food, or medication, and stay upright for 30 minutes and until after the first food of the day; mark calendar for once-weekly dosing.

• You must maintain adequate intake of calcium and vitamin D.

• You may experience these side effects: Nausea, diarrhea; bone pain, headache (analgesic may help).

• Report twitching, muscle spasms, dark-colored urine, severe diarrhea, difficulty swallowing.

▷ **alfuzosin hydrochloride**

(al foo zow' sin)

Uroxatral ⊙ⓝⓖ

PREGNANCY CATEGORY B

Drug classes
Alpha adrenergic blocker
BPH drug

Therapeutic actions
Blocks the smooth muscle alpha-1 adrenergic receptors in the prostate, prostatic capsule, prostatic urethra, and bladder neck, leading to the relaxation of the bladder and prostate and improving the flow of urine and improvement in symptoms in patients with BPH.

Indications
• Treatment of the signs and symptoms of BPH

Contraindications and cautions
• Contraindicated with allergy to any component of the product; hepatic insufficiency, pregnancy, lactation.
• Use cautiously with hypotension, renal insufficiency, prolonged QTc interval, CAD.

Available forms
ER tablets ⓝⓖ—10 mg

Dosages
Adults
10 mg/day PO after the same meal each day.
Pediatric patients
Safety and efficacy not established.

Pharmacokinetics

Route	Onset	Peak
Oral	Varies	8 hr

Metabolism: Hepatic; $T_{1/2}$: 10 hr
Distribution: Crosses placenta; may enter breast milk
Excretion: Feces, urine

Adverse effects
• **CNS:** Dizziness, headache
• **CV:** Orthostatic hypotension, syncope, tachycardia, chest pain
• **GI:** Abdominal pain, dyspepsia, constipation, nausea
• **GU:** Impotence, priapism
• **Respiratory:** Cough, bronchitis, sinusitis, pharyngitis, URI
• **Other:** Fatigue, pain

Interactions
✳ **Drug-drug** • Increased serum levels and risk of adverse effects of alfuzosin if combined with CYP3A4 inhibitors, ketoconazole, itraconazole, ritonavir; use of these combinations is contraindicated • Increased risk of orthostatic hypotension and syncope if combined with antihypertensive medications; monitor patient closely and adjust antihypertensive dosage accordingly • Increased risk of adverse effects if combined with other adrenergic blockers; monitor patients closely and adjust dosages as needed • Risk of serious adverse effects if combined

---

with protease inhibitors; this combination is contraindicated

■ **Nursing considerations**
Assessment
- **History:** Allergy to alfuzosin, hepatic or renal impairment, CAD, prolonged QTc interval, pregnancy, lactation
- **Physical:** Body weight; skin color, lesions; orientation, affect, reflexes; P, BP, orthostatic BP; R, adventitious sounds; PSA level; voiding pattern, normal output, urinalysis

Interventions
- Ensure that patient does not have prostatic cancer before beginning treatment; check for normal PSA levels.
- Administer once a day, after the same meal each day.
- Ensure that patient does not crush, chew, or cut tablet. Tablet should be swallowed whole.
- Store tablets in a dry place, protected from light.

⊗ **Warning** Monitor patient carefully for orthostatic hypotension; chance of orthostatic hypotension, dizziness, and syncope are greatest with the first dose. Establish safety precautions as appropriate.

Teaching points
- Take this drug exactly as prescribed, once a day. Do not chew, crush, or cut tablets; tablets must be swallowed whole. Use care when beginning therapy; dizziness and syncope are most likely at the beginning of therapy. Change position slowly to avoid increased dizziness. Take the drug after the same meal each day. Do not take the drug on an empty stomach.
- You may experience these side effects: Dizziness, weakness (these are more likely to occur when you change position, in the early morning, after exercise, in hot weather, and when you have consumed alcohol; some tolerance may occur after you have taken the drug for a while. Avoid driving a car or engaging in tasks that require alertness while you are experiencing these symptoms; remember to change position slowly, use caution when climbing stairs, lie down for a while if dizziness persists); GI upset (eat frequent small meals); impotence (you may wish to discuss this with your health care provider); fatigue.

- Report frequent dizziness or fainting, worsening of symptoms, chest pain.

▽ **alglucosidase alfa**

See Appendix R, *Less commonly used drugs*.

▽ **aliskiren**
*(ah liss **kye**' ren)*

Tekturna

PREGNANCY CATEGORY C
(FIRST TRIMESTER)

PREGNANCY CATEGORY D
(SECOND AND THIRD TRIMESTERS)

Drug classes
Antihypertensive
Renin inhibitor

Therapeutic actions
Directly inhibits renin, which decreases plasma renin activity and inhibits conversion of angiotensinogen to angiotensin I. Inhibition of the renin-angiotensin-aldosterone system leads to decreased blood pressure, decreased aldosterone release, and decreased sodium resorption.

Indications
- Treatment of hypertension, alone or with other antihypertensives

Contraindications and cautions
- Contraindicated with known hypersensitivity to any component of the drug, second or third trimester of pregnancy, lactation.
- Use cautiously with history of impaired renal function, hyperkalemia.

Available forms
Tablets—150, 300 mg

Dosages
Adults
150 mg/day PO. May be increased to 300 mg/day PO if needed to control BP.
Pediatric patients
Safety and efficacy not established.

Patients with severe renal impairment

No dosage adjustment needed with mild to moderate renal dysfunction; caution should be used with severe dysfunction because clinical experience is limited.

Pharmacokinetics

Route	Onset	Peak
Oral	Slow	1–3 hr

Metabolism: Hepatic; $T_{1/2}$: 24 hr
Distribution: Crosses placenta; may enter breast milk
Excretion: Urine

Adverse effects

- **CNS:** Dizziness, fatigue, headache, seizures
- **CV:** Edema, hypotension
- **GI:** Diarrhea, abdominal pain, dyspepsia, GERD
- **Respiratory:** Cough, URI, **angioedema with respiratory symptoms**
- **Other:** Back pain

Interactions

✳ **Drug-drug** • Risk of decreased effectiveness of furosemide if combined with aliskiren; monitor patient closely • Risk of increased serum levels and effects of aliskiren if combined with atorvastatin, ketoconazole; monitor patient closely • Risk of increased uric acid levels if combined with thiazides; monitor patient • Risk of hyperkalemia if combined with ACE inhibitors, other drugs that alter potassium levels; monitor potassium level periodically • Decreased serum aliskiren level if combined with irbesartan; monitor blood pressure carefully • Risk of renal impairment, hypotension, hyperkalemia if combined with ACE inhibitors or ARBs in patients with renal impairment or diabetes; avoid these combinations in these patients.

✳ **Drug-food** • Substantial decrease in absorption if taken with high-fat foods; do not give with high-fat meals

■ Nursing considerations

⊗ **Black box warning** Use during second and third trimesters of pregnancy can cause fetal injury or death; if pregnancy occurs, discontinue drug as soon as possible.

Assessment

- **History:** Hypersensitivity to any component of the drug, second or third trimester of pregnancy, lactation, history of impaired renal function, hyperkalemia
- **Physical:** Orientation, affect; BP; R, lung sounds; abdominal examination; renal function tests, electrolytes

Interventions

- Ensure that patient is not pregnant before starting drug; suggest use of contraceptive measures.
- Monitor serum potassium level periodically.
- Monitor patients also receiving furosemide for possible loss of diuretic effects.
- Continue other antihypertensive drugs as needed to control blood pressure.

Teaching points

- Take this drug once a day, at about the same time each day. If you miss a dose, take it as soon as you remember; then resume your usual schedule the next day. Do not make up missed doses. Do not take more than one dose each day.
- Store this drug at room temperature in a dry place (not in the bathroom or near the kitchen sink). Do not share this drug with any other people; keep it out of the reach of children.
- You may also be taking other drugs to control your blood pressure; check with your health care provider, and follow your drug regimen as directed.
- This drug should not be taken during pregnancy; use of contraceptive measures is advised. If you wish to become pregnant, discuss this with your health care provider. If you become pregnant while taking *Tekturna,* stop the drug and consult your health care provider about a different treatment for your hypertension.
- It is not known how this drug could affect a breast-feeding infant. Because of the potential for serious adverse effects in the infant, another method of feeding should be used while you are taking this drug.
- Your health care provider will monitor your blood pressure regularly while you are taking this drug.
- You may experience low blood pressure if you are also taking diuretics, if you become

dehydrated, or if you have dialysis treatments. If you feel faint or dizzy, lie down and call your health care provider right away.

• Report difficulty breathing; swelling of the face, lips, or tongue; dizziness or lightheadedness; pregnancy.

▽allopurinol
*(al ob **pure'** i nole)*

Aloprim, Apo-Allopurinol (CAN), Zyloprim

PREGNANCY CATEGORY C

Drug classes
Antigout drug
Purine analogue

Therapeutic actions
Inhibits the enzyme responsible for the conversion of purines to uric acid, thus reducing the production of uric acid with a decrease in serum and sometimes in urinary uric acid levels, relieving the signs and symptoms of gout.

Indications
• Management of the signs and symptoms of primary and secondary gout
• Management of patients with leukemia, lymphoma, and malignancies who are undergoing chemotherapy expected to result in elevations of serum and urinary uric acid
• Management of patients with recurrent calcium oxalate calculi whose daily uric acid excretion exceeds 800 mg/day (males) or 750 mg/day (females)
• Orphan drug use: Treatment of Chagas' disease; cutaneous and visceral leishmaniasis
• Unlabeled uses: Amelioration of granulocyte suppression with 5-FU; as a mouthwash to prevent 5-FU–induced stomatitis; prevention of ischemic reperfusion tissue damage; reduction of perioperative mortality and postoperative arrhythmias in CABG surgery; reduction of relapse of *Helicobacter pylori*–induced duodenal ulcers; treatment of hematemesis from NSAID–induced erosive gastritis; alleviation of pain of acute pancreatitis; vivo preservation and function of organs for liver and kidney transplantation; reduction of rejection in adult cadaver

renal transplant recipients; epileptic seizures

Contraindications and cautions
• Contraindicated with allergy to allopurinol, blood dyscrasias.
• Use cautiously with liver disease, renal failure, lactation, pregnancy.

Available forms
Tablets—100, 300 mg; powder for injection—500 mg

Dosages
Adults
• *Gout and hyperuricemia:* 100–800 mg/day PO in divided doses, depending on the severity of the disease (200–300 mg/day is usual dose). *Maintenance:* Establish dose that maintains serum uric acid levels within normal limits.
• *Hyperuricosuria:* 200–300 mg/day PO; adjust dose based on 24-hr urinary urate levels.
• *Prevention of acute gouty attacks:* 100 mg/day PO; increase the dose by 100 mg at weekly intervals until uric acid levels are 6 mg/dL or less.
• *Prevention of uric acid nephropathy in certain malignancies:* 600–800 mg/day PO for 2–3 days with a high fluid intake; maintenance dose should then be established as above.
• *Recurrent calcium oxalate stones:* 200–300 mg/day PO; adjust dose based on 24-hr urinary urate determinations.
• *Parenteral:* 200–400 mg/m^2/day IV to maximum of 600 mg/day as continuous infusion or at 6-, 8-, 12-hr intervals.

Pediatric patients
• *Secondary hyperuricemia associated with various malignancies:*
  6–10 yr: 300 mg/day PO.
  Younger than 6 yr: 150 mg/day; adjust dosage after 48 hr of treatment based on serum uric acid levels.
• *Parenteral:* 200 mg/m^2/day IV as continuous infusion or at 6-, 8-, 12-hr intervals.

Geriatric patients or patients with renal impairment
For geriatric patients or for patients with creatinine clearance 10–20 mL/min, 200 mg/day; for creatinine clearance less than 10 mL/min,

100 mg/day; for creatinine clearance less than 3 mL/min, extend intervals between doses based on patient's serum uric acid levels.

Pharmacokinetics

Route	Onset	Peak
Oral	Slow	1–2 hr
IV	10–15 min	30 min

Metabolism: Hepatic; $T_{1/2}$: 1–1.5 hr, then 23–24 hr
Distribution: Crosses placenta; may enter breast milk
Excretion: Urine

▼ IV FACTS

Preparation: Dissolve contents of each vial with 25 mL of sterile water for injection. Further dilute with NSS or D_5W to final concentration of 6 mg/mL or less. Administer within 10 hr of reconstitution.
Infusion: Administer as a continuous infusion or infused every 6, 8, or 12 hr with rate dependent on volume used.
Incompatibilities: Incompatible with many other drugs and solutions containing sodium bicarbonate. Do not mix with any other drug in same solution.

Adverse effects

- **CNS:** *Headache, drowsiness,* peripheral neuropathy, neuritis, paresthesias
- **Dermatologic: Rashes—maculopapular, scaly or exfoliative—sometimes fatal**
- **GI:** *Nausea, vomiting, diarrhea,* abdominal pain, gastritis, hepatomegaly, hyperbilirubinemia, cholestatic jaundice
- **GU:** Exacerbation of gout and renal calculi, renal failure
- **Hematologic:** Anemia, leukopenia, agranulocytosis, thrombocytopenia, aplastic anemia, bone marrow depression

Interactions

✳ **Drug-drug** ● Increased risk of hypersensitivity reaction with ACE inhibitors ● Increased toxicity with thiazide diuretics ● Increased risk of rash with ampicillin or amoxicillin ● Increased risk of bone marrow suppression with cyclophosphamide, other cytotoxic agents ● Increased half-life of oral anticoagulants ● Increased serum levels of theophylline ● Increased risk of toxic effects with thiopurines,

6-MP (azathioprine dose and dose of 6-MP should be reduced to one-third to one-fourth the usual dose)

■ Nursing considerations

Assessment

- **History:** Allergy to allopurinol, blood dyscrasias, liver disease, renal failure, lactation
- **Physical:** Skin lesions, color; orientation, reflexes; liver evaluation, normal urinary output; normal output; CBC, LFTs, renal function tests, urinalysis

Interventions

- Administer drug following meals.
- Encourage patient to drink 2.5–3 L/day to decrease the risk of renal stone development.
- Check urine alkalinity—urates crystallize in acid urine; sodium bicarbonate or potassium citrate may be ordered to alkalinize urine.
- ⊗ *Warning* Discontinue drug at first sign of skin rash; severe to fatal skin reactions have occurred.
- Arrange for regular medical follow-up and blood tests.

Teaching points

- Take the drug after meals.
- Avoid over-the-counter medications. Many of these preparations contain vitamin C or other agents that might increase the likelihood of kidney stone formation. If you need an over-the-counter preparation, check with your health care provider.
- You may experience these side effects: Exacerbation of gouty attack or renal stones (drink 2.5–3 liters of fluids per day while on this drug); nausea, vomiting, loss of appetite (take after meals or eat frequent small meals); drowsiness (use caution while driving or performing hazardous tasks).
- Report rash; unusual bleeding or bruising; fever, chills; gout attack; numbness or tingling; flank pain, rash.

▷**almotriptan malate**
(*al moh **trip**' tan **mah**' layt*)

Axert

PREGNANCY CATEGORY C

Drug classes
Antimigraine
Serotonin selective agonist
Triptan

Therapeutic actions
Binds to serotonin receptors to cause vascular constrictive effects on cranial blood vessels, causing the relief of migraine in selective patients.

Indications
• Treatment of acute migraines with or without aura

Contraindications and cautions
• Contraindicated with allergy to almotriptan, active coronary artery disease, Prinzmetal's angina, peripheral or cerebrovascular syndromes, uncontrolled hypertension, use of an ergot compound or other triptan within 24 hours, pregnancy.
• Use cautiously with hepatic or renal impairment, risk factors for CAD, lactation.

Available forms
Tablets—6.25, 12.5 mg

Dosages
Adults
6.25–12.5 mg PO as a single dose at first sign of migraine; if headache returns, may be repeated after 2 hr; do not use more than 2 doses/24 hr. Maximum daily dose, 25 mg.
Pediatric patients
12–17 yr: 6.25–12.5 mg PO; may be repeated after 2 hr. Maximum daily dosage, 25 mg. Safety and efficacy not established for patients younger than 12 yr.
Patients with hepatic or renal impairment
Starting dose—6.25 mg; do not exceed 12.5 mg/24 hr.

Pharmacokinetics

Route	Onset	Peak
Oral	Varies	1–3 hr

Metabolism: Hepatic; $T_{1/2}$: 3–4 hr
Distribution: Crosses placenta; may enter breast milk
Excretion: Feces, urine

Adverse effects
• **CNS:** *Dizziness,* headache, anxiety, malaise or fatigue, weakness, myalgia, somnolence
• **CV:** *BP alterations, tightness or pressure in chest,* arrhythmias, **MI**
• **GI:** *Nausea, dry mouth,* abdominal discomfort, dysphagia
• **Other:** Tingling; cold, warm, or hot sensations; burning sensation; feeling of heaviness; pressure sensation; numbness; feeling of tightness; feeling strange

Interactions
✳ **Drug-drug** • Prolonged vasoactive reactions when taken concurrently with ergot-containing drugs, other triptans • Risk of severe effects if taken with or within 2 wk of discontinuation of an MAOI • Increased effects and possible toxicity if taken with ketoconazole and other antifungals, nefazodone, macrolide antibiotics, antivirals; monitor patient closely if this combination is used • Risk of serotonin syndrome when combined with SSRIs, other antidepressants; monitor patient carefully if combination cannot be avoided

■ Nursing considerations
Assessment
• **History:** Allergy to almotriptan, active coronary artery disease, Prinzmetal's angina, pregnancy, lactation, peripheral vascular syndromes, uncontrolled hypertension, use of an ergot compound or other triptan within 24 hr, risk factors for CAD
• **Physical:** Skin color and lesions; orientation, reflexes, peripheral sensation; P, BP; LFTs, renal function tests

Interventions
• Administer to relieve acute migraine, not as a prophylactic measure.
⊗ **Warning** Ensure that the patient has not taken an ergot-containing compound or other triptan within 24 hr; risk of potentially serious vasospastic events.
• Do not administer more than 2 doses in a 24-hr period.

- Establish safety measures if CNS, visual disturbances occur.
- Control environment as appropriate to help relieve migraine (lighting, temperature, noise).
- Monitor BP of patients with possible coronary artery disease; discontinue at any sign of angina, prolonged high BP, and so forth.

Teaching points
- Take drug exactly as prescribed, at the onset of headache or aura. Do not take this drug to prevent a migraine; it is only used to treat migraines that are occurring. If the headache persists after you take this drug, you may repeat the dose after 2 hours have passed.
- Do not take more than 2 doses in a 24-hour period. Do not take any other migraine medication while you are taking this drug. If the headache is not relieved, call your health care provider.
- This drug should not be taken during pregnancy; if you suspect that you are pregnant, contact your health care provider and refrain from using drug.
- Continue to do anything that usually helps you feel better during a migraine (such as controlling lighting and reducing noise).
- Contact your health care provider immediately if you experience chest pain or pressure that is severe or does not go away.
- You may experience these side effects: Dizziness, drowsiness (avoid driving or the use of dangerous machinery while on this drug), numbness, tingling, feelings of tightness or pressure.
- Report feeling hot, tired, or sick; flushing; swelling of lips or eyelids.

▽alosetron hydrochloride
*(ah **loss' e** tron)*

Lotronex

PREGNANCY CATEGORY B

Drug classes
5-HT$_3$ (serotonin) antagonist
IBS drug

Therapeutic actions
Blocks 5-HT$_3$ (serotonin) receptors in the enteric nervous system of the GI tract; interacting with these receptors blocks visceral sensitivity, increases colonic transit time, decreases GI motility, may also decrease the perception of abdominal pain and discomfort.

Indications
- Treatment of severe diarrhea-predominant IBS in women who have chronic IBS (longer than 6 mo), have no anatomic or biochemical abnormalities of the GI tract, and who have failed to respond to conventional therapy

Contraindications and cautions
- Contraindicated with hypersensitivity to the drug, history of chronic or severe constipation or sequelae from constipation; history of intestinal obstruction, stricture, toxic megacolon, GI perforation or adhesions; history of ischemic colitis, impaired intestinal circulation, thrombophlebitis, or hypercoagulable state; history of or current Crohn's disease, ulcerative colitis, diverticulitis; severe hepatic impairment; inability to understand or comply with the Physician–Patient Agreement.
- Use cautiously with pregnancy, lactation, elderly patients, hepatic impairment.

Available forms
Tablets—0.5, 1 mg

Dosages
Adults
0.5 mg PO bid for 4 wk; may be continued if drug is tolerated and symptoms of IBS are under adequate control. Dose may be increased up to 1 mg bid PO after 4 wk if well tolerated and needed.
Pediatric patients
Safety and efficacy not established for patients younger than 18 yr.
Geriatric patients or patients with mild to moderate hepatic impairment
These patients may be at increased risk for complications from constipation; monitor very closely.

Pharmacokinetics

Route	Onset	Peak
Oral	Rapid	1 hr

Metabolism: Hepatic; $T_{1/2}$: 1.5 hr
Distribution: Crosses placenta; enters into breast milk
Excretion: Bile, urine, feces

Adverse effects

• **CNS:** Anxiety, tremors, dreams, headache
• **Dermatologic:** Sweating, urticaria
• **GI:** Abdominal pain, nausea, *constipation, ischemic colitis*
• **Other:** Malaise, fatigue, pain

Interactions

✴ **Drug-drug** • Increased risk of constipation if taken with other drugs that cause decreased GI motility; if this combination cannot be avoided, monitor patient very carefully and discontinue drug at first sign of constipation or ischemic colitis • Contraindicated for use with fluvoxamine • Avoid use with fluoroquinolones, cimetidine because of risk of adverse effects • Risk of increased alosetron serum levels if combined with clarithromycin, itraconazole, ketoconazole, protease inhibitors, telithromycin, voriconazole; use caution

■ Nursing considerations

Assessment

• **History:** Hypersensitivity to the drug, history of chronic or severe constipation or sequelae from constipation; history of intestinal obstruction, stricture, toxic megacolon, GI perforation or adhesions; history of ischemic colitis, impaired intestinal circulation, thrombophlebitis, or hypercoagulable state; history of Crohn's disease, ulcerative colitis, diverticulitis; inability to understand or comply with the Physician–Patient Agreement, pregnancy, lactation, elderly patients, hepatic impairment
• **Physical:** Skin lesions; T; reflexes, affect; urinary output, abdominal examination; bowel patterns

Interventions

⊗ **Black box warning** Ensure that the patient has read and understands the Physician–Patient Agreement, which outlines the risks associated with the use of the drug, including risk for ischemic colitis, and warning

signs to report. Drug is only indicated for women with severe diarrhea-dominant IBS who have failed to respond to conventional therapy.
⊗ **Black box warning** Discontinue drug immediately if patient develops constipation or signs and symptoms of ischemic colitis. Do not restart drug if ischemic colitis has occurred.
• Ensure that the Physician–Patient Agreement is in the patient's permanent record.
• Administer drug without regard to food.
• Arrange for further evaluation of patient after 4 wk of therapy to determine effectiveness of drug; discontinue drug if symptoms are not controlled at 1 mg bid.
• Encourage the use of barrier contraceptives to prevent pregnancy while patient is using this drug.
• Maintain supportive treatment as appropriate for underlying problem.
• Provide additional comfort measures to alleviate discomfort from GI effects, headache.
• Monitor patient for any signs of constipation; discontinue drug at first sign of constipation or ischemic colitis and alert the prescribing physician.

Teaching points

• Read and sign the Physician–Patient Agreement, which outlines the risks and benefits of therapy with this drug.
• Arrange to have regular medical follow-up while you are on this drug.
• Use barrier contraceptives while on this drug; serious adverse effects could occur during pregnancy; if you become or wish to become pregnant, consult your health care provider.
• Maintain all of the usual activities and restrictions that apply to your condition. If this becomes difficult, consult your health care provider.
• You may experience these side effects: Headache (consult your health care provider if these become bothersome, medications may be available to help); nausea, vomiting (proper nutrition is important, consult a dietitian to maintain nutrition).
• Report constipation, signs of ischemic colitis—worsening abdominal pain, bloody diarrhea, blood in the stool; continuation of IBS symptoms without relief.

▷ alpha₁-proteinase inhibitor

See Appendix R, *Less commonly used drugs.*

▷ alprazolam

*(al **prah**' zoe lam)*

Alprazolam Extended Relief ⚫, Alprazolam Intensol, Apo-Alpraz (CAN), Apo-Alpraz TS (CAN), Gen-Alprazolam (CAN), Niravam, Novo-Alprazol (CAN), Xanax, Xanax TS (CAN), Xanax XR ⚫

PREGNANCY CATEGORY D

CONTROLLED SUBSTANCE C-IV

Drug classes
Anxiolytic
Benzodiazepine

Therapeutic actions
Exact mechanisms of action not understood; main sites of action may be the limbic system and reticular formation; increases the effects of GABA, an inhibitory neurotransmitter; anxiety blocking effects occur at doses well below those necessary to cause sedation, ataxia.

Indications
- Management of anxiety disorders, short-term relief of symptoms of anxiety; anxiety associated with depression
- Treatment of panic attacks with or without agoraphobia (*Niravam, Xanax, Xanax XR*)

Contraindications and cautions
- Contraindicated with hypersensitivity to benzodiazepines, psychoses, acute narrow-angle glaucoma, shock, coma, acute alcoholic intoxication with depression of vital signs, pregnancy (crosses the placenta; risk of congenital malformations, neonatal withdrawal syndrome), labor and delivery ("floppy infant" syndrome), lactation (secreted in breast milk; infants become lethargic and lose weight).
- Use cautiously with impaired liver or renal function, debilitation.

Available forms
Tablets—0.25, 0.5, 1, 2 mg; ER tablets ⚫—0.5, 1, 2, 3 mg; oral solution—1 mg/mL; rapidly disintegrating tablets—0.25, 0.5, 1, 2 mg

Dosages
Individualize dosage; increase dosage gradually to avoid adverse effects; decrease dosage gradually (no more than 0.5 mg q 3 days) when discontinuing drug.

Adults
- *Anxiety disorders:* Initially, 0.25–0.5 mg PO tid; adjust to maximum daily dose of 4 mg/day in divided doses at intervals of 3–4 days or extended-release form once per day in the AM once dosage is established (immediate release, intensol solution).
- *Panic disorder:* Initially, 0.5 mg PO tid; increase dose at 3- to 4-day intervals in increments of no more than 1 mg/day; ranges of 1–10 mg/day have been needed. ER tablets—Initially, 0.5–1 mg/day; dosage range, 3–6 mg/day.

Geriatric patients or patients with advanced hepatic or debilitating disease
Initially, 0.25 mg bid–tid PO; gradually increase if needed and tolerated; ER tablets—0.5 mg PO once each day; gradually increase if needed and tolerated.

Pharmacokinetics

Route	Onset	Peak	Duration
Oral	30 min	1–2 hr	4–6 hr

Metabolism: Hepatic; $T_{1/2}$: 6.3–26.9 hr
Distribution: Crosses placenta; enters breast milk
Excretion: Urine

Adverse effects
- **CNS:** *Transient, mild drowsiness initially; sedation, depression, lethargy, apathy, fatigue, light-headedness, disorientation, anger, hostility,* episodes of mania and hypomania, *restlessness, confusion, crying,* delirium, *headache,* slurred speech, dysarthria, stupor, rigidity, tremor, dystonia, vertigo, euphoria, nervousness, difficulty in concentration, vivid dreams, psychomotor retardation, extrapyramidal symptoms; *mild paradoxical excitatory reactions during first 2 wk of treatment*

- **CV:** Bradycardia, tachycardia, **CV collapse,** hypertension, hypotension, palpitations, edema
- **Dermatologic:** Urticaria, pruritus, rash, dermatitis
- **EENT:** Visual and auditory disturbances, diplopia, nystagmus, depressed hearing, nasal congestion
- **GI:** *Constipation, diarrhea, dry mouth,* salivation, *nausea,* anorexia, vomiting, difficulty in swallowing, gastric disorders, hepatic impairment
- **GU:** Incontinence, changes in libido, urine retention, menstrual irregularities
- **Hematologic:** Elevations of liver enzymes—LDH, alkaline phosphatase, AST, ALT; blood dyscrasias—agranulocytosis, leukopenia
- **Other:** Hiccups, fever, diaphoresis, paresthesias, muscular disturbances, gynecomastia. *Drug dependence with withdrawal syndrome when drug is discontinued; more common with abrupt discontinuation of higher dosage used for longer than 4 mo*

Interactions
✴ **Drug-drug** ● Increased CNS depression with alcohol, other CNS depressants, propoxyphene ● Increased effect with cimetidine, disulfiram, omeprazole, isoniazid, hormonal contraceptives, valproic acid ● Decreased effect with carbamazepine, rifampin, theophylline ● Possible increased risk of digitalis toxicity with digoxin ● Decreased antiparkinson effectiveness of levodopa with benzodiazepines ● Contraindicated with ketoconazole, itraconazole; serious toxicity can occur

✴ **Drug-food** ● Decreased metabolism and risk of toxic effects if combined with grapefruit juice; avoid this combination

✴ **Drug-alternative therapy** ● Risk of coma if combined with kava therapy ● Additive sedative effects with valerian root

■ **Nursing considerations**

★ CLINICAL ALERT!
Name confusion has occurred among *Xanax* (alprazolam), *Celexa* (citalopram), and *Cerebyx* (fosphenytoin), and between alprazolam and lorazepam; use caution.

Assessment
- **History:** Hypersensitivity to benzodiazepines; psychoses; acute narrow-angle glaucoma; shock; coma; acute alcoholic intoxication with depression of vital signs; labor and delivery; lactation; impaired liver or renal function; debilitation; pregnancy
- **Physical:** Skin color, lesions; T; orientation, reflexes, affect, ophthalmologic examination; P, BP; liver evaluation, abdominal examination, bowel sounds, normal output; CBC, LFTs, renal function tests

Interventions
- Arrange to taper dosage gradually after long-term therapy, especially in epileptic patients.
- Do not administer with grapefruit juice or within 48 hr of grapefruit juice.
- Taper drug slowly, decrease by no more than 0.5 mg every 3 days.

Teaching points
- Take this drug exactly as prescribed; take extended-release form once a day in the morning; do not cut, crush, or chew extended-release tablets. Place the rapidly disintegrating tablet on top of your tongue, where it will disintegrate and can be swallowed with saliva.
- Do not drink grapefruit juice while on this drug.
- Do not stop taking drug (in long-term therapy) without consulting health care provider; drug should not be stopped suddenly.
- Avoid alcohol, sleep-inducing, or over-the-counter drugs.
- You may experience these side effects: Drowsiness, dizziness (these effects will be less pronounced after a few days, avoid driving a car or engaging in other dangerous activities if these occur); GI upset (take drug with food); fatigue; depression; dreams; crying; nervousness.
- Report severe dizziness, weakness, drowsiness that persists, rash or skin lesions, difficulty voiding, palpitations, swelling in the extremities.

▽ alprostadil

(al pross' ta dil)

IV: Prostin VR Pediatric
Intracavernous: Caverject, Caverject Impulse, Edex, Muse

PREGNANCY CATEGORY
(NOT APPLICABLE)

Drug class
Prostaglandin

Therapeutic actions
Relaxes vascular smooth muscle; the smooth muscle of the ductus arteriosus is especially sensitive to this action and will relax and stay open; this is beneficial in infants who have congenital defects that restrict pulmonary or systemic blood flow and who depend on a patent ductus arteriosus for adequate blood oxygenation and lower body perfusion. Treatment of erectile dysfunction due to neurogenic, vasculogenic, psychogenic, or mixed etiology.

Indications
- Palliative therapy to temporarily maintain the patency of the ductus arteriosus until corrective or palliative surgery can be performed in neonates with congenital heart defects who depend on a patent ductus (eg, pulmonary atresia or stenosis, tetralogy of Fallot, coarctation of the aorta), men for whom sexual activity is unadvisable
- Treatment of erectile dysfunction (intracavernous injection)
- Unlabeled use: Raynaud's disease

Contraindications and cautions
- Contraindicated with respiratory distress syndrome (IV), conditions that might predispose to priapism, deformation of the penis, penile implants (intracavernous injection), known hypersensitivity, urethral strictures, severe hypospadias and curvature, acute or chronic urethritis, tendency for thromboembolism (urogenital).
- Use cautiously with patients with bleeding tendencies (drug inhibits platelet aggregation), hypotension, dizziness.

Available forms
Powder for injection—10, 20, 40 mcg/mL; 10, 20 mcg/0.5 mL; injection (IV)—10, 20 mcg/mL; 40 mcg/2 mL (penile); 500 mcg/mL; pellets—125, 250, 500, 1,000 mcg

Dosages
Adults
Intracavernous injection
0.2–60 mcg by intracavernous injection using 0.5-in 27–30 gauge needle; may be repeated up to three times weekly with at least 24 hr between doses. Self-injection over 6-mo period has been successful. Reduce dose if erection lasts more than 1 hr.
Urogenital
Initially, 125–250 mcg; maximum dosage, 2 systems per 24 hr.
Pellet
125, 250, 500, or 1,000 mcg based on patient response. Maximum dosage, two systems in 24 hr administered intraurethrally.
Pediatric patients
Preferred administration is through a continuous IV infusion into a large vein; may be administered through an umbilical artery catheter placed at the ductal opening. Begin infusion with 0.05–0.1 mcg/kg/min. After an increase in partial pressure of oxygen (pO_2) or in systemic BP and blood pH is achieved, reduce infusion to the lowest possible dosage that maintains the response (often achieved by reducing dosage from 0.1–0.05 to 0.025–0.01 mcg/kg/min). Up to 0.4 mcg/kg/min may be used for maintenance if required; higher dosage rates are not more effective.

Pharmacokinetics

Route	Onset	Peak
IV	5–25 min	End of infusion
Intracavernous	10 min	30–60 min
Pellet	5–10 min	30–60 min

Metabolism: Lungs, local metabolism in GU tract; $T_{1/2}$: 5–10 min
Excretion: Urine

▼ IV FACTS

Preparation: Prepare solution by diluting 500 mcg alprostadil with sodium chloride injection or dextrose injection; dilute to volumes required for pump delivery system. Discard and prepare fresh infusion solutions every 24 hr; refrigerate drug ampules.

Infusion:

Add 500 mg Alprostadil to	Approximate Concentration of Resulting Solution	Infusion Rate (mL/kg/min)
250 mL	2 mcg/mL	0.05
100 mL	5 mcg/mL	0.02
50 mL	10 mcg/mL	0.01
25 mL	20 mcg/mL	0.005

Adverse effects

- **CNS:** *Seizures,* cerebral bleeding, hypothermia, jitteriness, lethargy, stiffness
- **CV:** *Bradycardia, flushing, tachycardia, hypotension,* **cardiac arrest,** heart block
- **GI:** Diarrhea, gastric outlet obstruction (neonates)
- **GU (with intracavernous injection):** Penile pain, rash, **fibrosis,** erection, priapism, urethral burning or bleeding
- **Hematologic:** Inhibited platelet aggregation, bleeding, anemia, DIC, hypokalemia
- **Respiratory:** *Apnea,* respiratory distress
- **Other:** Cortical proliferation of the long bones (with prolonged use; regresses after treatment is stopped), sepsis

■ Nursing considerations

CLINICAL ALERT!
Confusion has been reported with *Prostin VR Pediatric* (alprostadil), *Prostin F₂* (dinoprost—available outside United States), *Prostin E₂* (dinoprostone), *Prostin 15M* (carboprost in Europe); use extreme caution.

Assessment

- **History:** Respiratory distress, bleeding tendencies
- **Physical:** T; cyanosis; skeletal development, reflexes, state of agitation, arterial pressure (using auscultation or Doppler), P, auscultation, peripheral perfusion; R, adventitious sounds, bleeding times, arterial blood gases, blood pH

Interventions
IV

- Constantly monitor arterial pressure; decrease infusion rate immediately if any fall in arterial pressure occurs.

- Regularly monitor arterial blood gases to determine efficacy of alprostadil (pO_2 in infants with restricted pulmonary flow; pH and systemic BP in infants with restricted systemic flow).

⊗ ***Black box warning*** Apnea occurs within first hr of drug infusion in 10%–12% of neonates treated with alprostadil, particularly those weighing less than 2 kg. Monitor respiratory status continuously, have ventilatory assistance readily available, and move the neonate often during first hr of infusion.

Intracavernous

- Reconstitute vial with 1 mL diluent. 1 mL of solution will contain 5.4–41.1 mcg of alprostadil.
- Use solution immediately after reconstitution; do not store or freeze.
- Inject along the dorsal-lateral aspect of the proximal third of the penis using sterile technique.

Intraurethral

- Teach patient proper technique for intraurethral insertion.
- Store foil packets for pellets in the refrigerator and do not open them until ready to use.

Teaching points
IV

- Teaching about this drug should be incorporated into a total teaching program for the parents of the infant with a cyanotic congenital heart defect; specifics that they will need to know include the following:
  - Your infant will be continually monitored and have frequent blood tests to follow the effects of the drug.
  - Your infant may look better, breathe easier, become fussy, and so forth, but the drug treatment is only a temporary solution, and the baby will require corrective surgery.

Intracavernous

- Learn and repeat self-injection technique. Plan for the first injection in the physician's office under supervision. Do not self-inject more than three times per week; wait at least 24 hours between injections.
- Return for regular medical follow-up and evaluation.
- You may experience these side effects: Penile pain, swelling, rash.
- Report prolonged erection, swelling, or severe pain.

Intraurethral

- If you are prescribed the pellet form for intraurethral insertion, you will need to learn proper administration technique.
- Store foil packets for pellets in the refrigerator and do not open them until ready to use.
- Do not use more than two systems in a 24-hour period.

DANGEROUS DRUG

▽alteplase, recombinant (recombinant tissue-type plasminogen activator, rt-PA)
(al ti plaze')

Activase, Cathflo Activase

PREGNANCY CATEGORY C

Drug classes
Thrombolytic enzyme
Tissue plasminogen activator (TPA)

Therapeutic actions
Human tissue enzyme produced by recombinant DNA techniques; converts plasminogen to the enzyme plasmin (fibrinolysin), which degrades fibrin clots; lyses thrombi and emboli; is most active at the site of the clot and causes little systemic fibrinolysis.

Indications
- Treatment of coronary artery thrombosis associated with acute MI; improvement of ventricular function following MI; reduction of the incidence of heart failure and mortality associated with MI *(Activase)*
- Treatment of acute, massive pulmonary embolism in adults *(Activase)*
- Treatment of acute ischemic stroke *(Activase)*
- Restoration of function to central venous access devices occluded as assessed by the ability to withdraw blood *(Cathflo Activase)*
- Unlabeled uses: Treatment of unstable angina, frostbite, pleural effusion

Contraindications and cautions
- Contraindicated with allergy to TPA; active internal bleeding; recent (within 2 mo) stroke; intracranial or intraspinal surgery or neoplasm; recent major surgery, obstetric delivery, organ biopsy, or rupture of a noncompressible blood vessel; recent serious GI bleed; recent serious trauma, including CPR; SBE; hemostatic defects; cerebrovascular disease; early-onset, insulin-dependent diabetes; septic thrombosis; severe uncontrolled hypertension; subarachnoid hemorrhage; concurrent use of anticoagulants; low platelet count; administration of heparin within 48 hr.
- Use cautiously with hepatic disease in elderly (more than 75 yr—risk of bleeding may be increased), pregnancy, lactation.

Available forms
Powder for injection—50, 100 mg; single use powder for injection *(Cathflo Activase)*—2 mg

Dosages
Careful patient assessment and evaluation are needed to determine the appropriate dose of this drug. Because experience is limited with this drug, careful monitoring is essential.
Adults
- *Acute MI:* For patients weighing more than 67 kg, 100 mg as a 15-mg IV bolus followed by 50 mg infused over 30 min. Then 35 mg over the next 60 min. For patients weighing 67 kg or less, 15-mg IV bolus followed by 0.75 mg/kg infused over 30 min (not to exceed 50 mg). Then 0.5 mg/kg over the next 60 min (not to exceed 35 mg). For a 3-hr infusion, 60 mg in first hr (6–10 mg as a bolus); 20 mg over second hr; 20 mg over third hr. Patients weighing less than 65 kg should receive 1.25 mg/kg over 3 hr.
⊗ *Warning* Do not use a total dose of 150 mg because of the increased risk of intracranial bleeding.
- *Pulmonary embolism:* 100 mg administered by IV infusion over 2 hr, followed immediately by heparin therapy when PTT or thrombin time returns to twice normal or less.
- *Acute ischemic stroke:* 0.9 mg/kg (not to exceed 90 mg total dose) infused over 60 min with 10% given as an IV bolus over the first 1 min.
- *Restoration of function of central venous access devices (Cathflo Activase):* 2 mg in 2 mL of sterile water for injection from single-use vial injected into device; may repeat after 2 hr if necessary for patient weighing 30 kg (66 lb) or more. For patients

weighing 10 kg to less than 30 kg, use 110% of internal lumen volume of catheter, not to exceed 2 mg in 2 mL.

Pharmacokinetics

Route	Onset	Peak	Duration
IV	Immediate	5–10 min	2.5–3 hr

Metabolism: Hepatic; $T_{1/2}$: 26 min
Distribution: Crosses placenta
Excretion: Liver

▼ IV FACTS

Preparation: Do not use if vacuum is not present; add volume of the sterile water for injection provided with vial using a large bore needle and directing stream into the cake; slight foaming may occur but will dissipate after standing undisturbed for several min; reconstitute immediately before use. Do not shake. Refrigerate reconstituted solution and use within 8 hr. Do not use bacteriostatic water for injection. Reconstituted solution should be colorless or pale yellow and transparent; contains 1 mg/mL with a pH of 7.3.

Infusion: Administer as reconstituted or further dilute with an equal volume of 0.9% sodium chloride injection or 5% dextrose injection to yield 0.5 mg/mL; stable for up to 8 hr in these solutions. Avoid excessive agitation; mix by gentle swirling or slow inversion. Discard unused solution.

Incompatibilities: Do not add other medications to infusion solution; use 0.9% sodium chloride injection or 5% dextrose injection and no other solutions.

Y-site compatibility: Lidocaine.

Y-site incompatibilities: Dobutamine, dopamine, heparin, nitroglycerin.

Adverse effects

- **CV: Cardiac arrhythmias with coronary reperfusion,** hypotension
- **Hematologic:** *Bleeding*—particularly at venous or arterial access sites, GI bleeding, **intracranial hemorrhage**
- **Other:** Urticaria, nausea, vomiting, fever

Interactions

✳ **Drug-drug** • Increased risk of hemorrhage if used with heparin or oral anticoagulants, aspirin, dipyridamole

■ Nursing considerations

✯ CLINICAL ALERT!
Confusion has been reported between alteplase and *Altace* (ramipril); use caution.

Assessment

- **History:** Allergy to TPA; active internal bleeding; recent (within 2 mo) obstetric delivery, organ biopsy, or rupture of a noncompressible blood vessel; recent serious GI bleed; recent serious trauma, including CPR; SBE; hemostatic defects; cerebrovascular disease; type 1 diabetes; septic thrombosis; severe uncontrolled hypertension; liver disease
- **Physical:** Skin color, T, lesions; orientation, reflexes; P, BP, peripheral perfusion, baseline ECG; R, adventitious sounds; liver evaluation, Hct, platelet count, thrombin time, aPTT, PT

Interventions

- Discontinue heparin and alteplase if serious bleeding occurs.
- Monitor coagulation studies; PT or aPTT should be less than two times control.
- Apply pressure or pressure dressings to control superficial bleeding (at invaded or disturbed areas).
- Avoid arterial invasive procedures.
- Type and cross-match blood in case serious blood loss occurs and whole-blood transfusions are required.
- Institute treatment within 6 hr of onset of symptoms for evolving MI, within 3 hr of onset of stroke.

Teaching points

- This drug can only be given IV. You will be closely monitored during drug treatment.
- Report difficulty breathing, dizziness, disorientation, headache, numbness, tingling.

▽ altretamine

See Appendix R, *Less commonly used drugs.*

▷aluminum hydroxide gel

(a loo' mi num)

AlternaGEL, Amphojel

PREGNANCY CATEGORY
UNDETERMINED

Drug class
Antacid

Therapeutic actions
Neutralizes or reduces gastric acidity, resulting in an increase in the pH of the stomach and duodenal bulb and inhibiting the proteolytic activity of pepsin, which protects the lining of the stomach and duodenum; binds with phosphate ions in the intestine to form insoluble aluminum–phosphate complexes, lowering phosphate in hyperphosphatemia and chronic renal failure; may cause hypophosphatemia in other states.

Indications
- Symptomatic relief of upset stomach associated with hyperacidity
- Hyperacidity associated with uncomplicated peptic ulcer, gastritis, peptic esophagitis, gastric hyperacidity, hiatal hernia
- Unlabeled uses: Prophylaxis of GI bleeding, stress ulcer; reduction of phosphate absorption in hyperphosphatemia in patients with chronic renal failure; suspected GERD laryngitis (adults)

Contraindications and cautions
- Contraindicated with allergy to aluminum products, gastric outlet destruction, hypophosphatemia, lactation.
- Use cautiously with pregnancy, renal impairment, hyperphosphatemia, constipation.

Available forms
Tablets—600 mg; capsules—500 mg; suspension—320 mg/5 mL, 450 mg/5 mL, 675 mg/5 mL; liquid—600 mg/5 mL

Dosages
Adults
Tablets and capsules: 500–1,500 mg 3–6 times/day PO between meals and at bedtime.
Liquid: 5–10 mL between meals, at bedtime, or as directed.
Pediatric patients
- *General guidelines:* 5–15 mL PO every 3–6 hr or 1–3 hr after meals and at bedtime.
- *Hyperphosphatemia:* 50–150 mg/kg every 24 hr PO in divided doses every 4–6 hr; adjust dosage to normal serum phosphorus.
- *Prophylaxis of GI bleeding in critically ill infants:* 2–5 mL/dose every 1–2 hr PO.
- *Prophylaxis of GI bleeding in critically ill children:* 5–15 mL/dose every 1–2 hr PO.

Pharmacokinetics

Route	Onset
Oral	Varies

Metabolism: Hepatic
Distribution: Long-term use, small amounts may be absorbed systemically and cross the placenta and enter breast milk
Excretion: Feces

Adverse effects
- **GI:** *Constipation;* intestinal obstruction; decreased absorption of fluoride; accumulation of aluminum in serum, bone, and CNS; rebound hyperacidity
- **Musculoskeletal:** Osteomalacia and chronic phosphate deficiency with bone pain, malaise, muscular weakness

Interactions
✳ **Drug-drug** ● Do not administer other oral drugs within 1–2 hr of antacid; change in gastric pH may interfere with absorption of oral drugs ● Decreased pharmacologic effect of corticosteroids, diflunisal, digoxin, fluoroquinolones, iron, isoniazid, penicillamine, phenothiazines, ranitidine, tetracyclines ● Increased pharmacologic effect of benzodiazepines

■ Nursing considerations
Assessment
- **History:** Allergy to aluminum products; gastric outlet obstruction; hypertension, heart failure; hypophosphatemia; lactation
- **Physical:** Bone strength, muscle strength; P, auscultation, BP, peripheral edema; abdominal examination, bowel sounds; serum phosphorous, serum fluoride; bone X-ray is appropriate

Interventions

- Give hourly for first 2 wk when used for acute peptic ulcer; during the healing stage, give 1–3 hr after meals and at bedtime.

⊗ **Warning** Do not administer oral drugs within 1–2 hr of antacid administration.

- Have patient chew tablets thoroughly; follow with a glass of water.
- Monitor serum phosphorus levels periodically during long-term therapy.

Teaching points

- Take this drug between meals and at bedtime; ulcer patients need to strictly follow prescribed dosage pattern. If tablets are being used, chew thoroughly before swallowing, and follow with a glass of water.
- Do not take maximum dosage of antacids for longer than 2 weeks except under medical supervision.
- Do not take this drug with any other oral medications; absorption of those medications can be inhibited. Take other oral medications at least 1–2 hours after aluminum salt. Consult with your health care provider before using other drugs.
- Constipation may occur.
- Report constipation; bone pain, muscle weakness; coffee ground vomitus, black tarry stools; no relief from symptoms being treated.

▽ **alvimopan**

See Appendix R, *Less commonly used drugs.*

▽ **amantadine hydrochloride**

(a man' ta deen)

Endantadine (CAN), Gen-Amantadine (CAN), Symmetrel

PREGNANCY CATEGORY C

Drug classes

Antiviral
Antiparkinsonian

Therapeutic actions

May inhibit penetration of influenza A virus into the host cell; may increase dopamine release in the nigrostriatal pathway of patients with Parkinson's disease, relieving their symptoms.

Indications

- Prevention and treatment of influenza A virus respiratory infection, especially in high-risk patients
- Adjunct to late vaccination against influenza A virus, to provide interim coverage; supplement to vaccination in immunodeficient patients; prophylaxis when vaccination is contraindicated
- Treatment of Parkinson's disease and drug-induced extrapyramidal reactions

Contraindications and cautions

- Contraindicated with allergy to drug product, psychoses, lactation.
- Use cautiously with renal or hepatic disease, seizures, heart failure, pregnancy, eczematoid rash.

Available forms

Tablets—100 mg; capsules—100 mg; syrup—50 mg/5 mL

Dosages

Adults

- *Influenza A virus prophylaxis:* 200 mg/day PO or 100 mg bid PO for 10 days after exposure, for the duration of known influenza A in the community if vaccination is impossible and exposure is repeated. If used in conjunction with influenza vaccine, administer for 2–4 wk after vaccine has been given.
- *Uncomplicated influenza A virus treatment:* Same dose as above; start treatment as soon after exposure as possible, continuing for 24–48 hr after symptoms are gone.
- *Parkinsonism treatment:* 100 mg bid (up to 400 mg/day) PO when used alone; reduce in patients receiving other antiparkinsonian drugs. Use initial dose of 100 mg/day in patients with severe associated medical illnesses.
- *Drug-induced extrapyramidal reactions:* 100 mg bid PO, up to 300 mg/day in divided doses has been used.

Patients with seizure disorders
Observe patient closely for increased seizure activity.

Patients with renal disease

For patients on hemodialysis, 200 mg PO every 7 days. For patients with reduced creatinine clearance, use dosage as outlined below:

CrCl (mL/min)	Dosage
Less than 15	200 mg PO every 7 days
15–29	200 mg PO first day, then 100 mg on alternate days
30–50	200 mg PO first day, then 100 mg/day

Pediatric patients

Not recommended for children younger than 1 yr.

- *Influenza A virus prophylaxis:*
  1–9 yr: 4.4–8.8 mg/kg/day PO in one or two divided doses, not to exceed 150 mg/day.
  9–12 yr: 100 mg PO bid.
- *Influenza A virus treatment:* As above; start as soon after exposure as possible, continuing for 24-48 hr after symptoms are gone.

Geriatric patients

- *Influenza A prophylaxis treatment:* For patients older than 65 yr with no recognized renal disease, 100 mg once daily PO.
- *Parkinsonism:* 100 mg/day for patients with serious associated medical illnesses or who are using other parkinsonism drugs. May increase to 100 mg bid if necessary after 1 wk or longer.

Pharmacokinetics

Route	Onset	Peak
Oral	36–48 hr	1.5–8 hr

Metabolism: $T_{1/2}$: 10–25 hr
Distribution: Crosses placenta; enters breast milk
Excretion: Unchanged in the urine

Adverse effects

- **CNS:** *Light-headedness, dizziness, insomnia,* confusion, irritability, ataxia, psychosis, depression, hallucinations, headache, somnolence, suicidal ideation
- **CV:** HF, orthostatic hypotension, dyspnea
- **GI:** *Nausea,* anorexia, constipation, dry mouth, diarrhea
- **GU:** Urine retention, fatigue

Interactions

❊ **Drug-drug** • Increased atropine-like side effects with anticholinergic drugs • Increased amantadine effects with hydrochlorothiazide, triamterene • Increased risk of QT-interval prolongation if combined with other drugs that prolong QT interval

■ Nursing considerations

Assessment

- **History:** Allergy to drug product, seizures, hepatic disease, eczematoid rash, psychoses, HF, renal disease, lactation
- **Physical:** Orientation, vision, speech, reflexes; BP, orthostatic BP, P, auscultation, perfusion, edema; R, adventitious sounds; urinary output; BUN, creatinine clearance

Interventions

- Do not discontinue abruptly when treating parkinsonism syndrome; parkinsonian crisis may occur.
- Be aware that the smallest amount possible should be prescribed; deaths have been reported from overdose.

Teaching points

- Mark your calendar if you are on alternating dosage schedules; it is very important to take the full course of the drug.
- You may experience these side effects: Drowsiness, blurred vision (use caution when driving or using dangerous equipment); dizziness, light-headedness (avoid sudden position changes); irritability or mood changes (common effect; if severe, drug may be changed).
- Report swelling of the fingers or ankles; shortness of breath; difficulty urinating, walking; tremors, slurred speech; thoughts of suicide.

▷ **ambenonium chloride**

*(am be **noe'** nee um)*

Mytelase

PREGNANCY CATEGORY C

Drug classes

Antimyasthenic
Cholinesterase inhibitor
Parasympathomimetic (indirectly acting)

Therapeutic actions

Increases the concentration of acetylcholine at the sites of cholinergic transmission (parasympathetic neurons and skeletal muscles) and prolongs and exaggerates the effects of acetylcholine by inhibiting the enzyme acetylcholinesterase; this causes parasympathomimetic effects and facilitates transmission at the skeletal neuromuscular junction. Also has direct stimulating effects on skeletal muscle and has a longer duration of effect and fewer side effects than other agents.

Indications
• Treatment of myasthenia gravis

Contraindications and cautions
• Contraindicated with hypersensitivity to anticholinesterases, intestinal or urogenital tract obstruction, peritonitis, lactation, concurrent use of atropine.
• Use cautiously with asthma, peptic ulcer, bradycardia, cardiac arrhythmias, recent coronary occlusion, vagotonia, hyperthyroidism, epilepsy, pregnancy.

Available forms
Tablets—10 mg

Dosages
Adults
5–25 mg PO tid–qid (5–75 mg per dose has been used). Start dosage with 5 mg, and gradually increase to determine optimum dosage based on optimal muscle strength and no GI disturbances; increase dose every 1–2 days. Dosage above 200 mg/day requires close supervision to avoid overdose.
Pediatric patients
Safety and efficacy not established.

Pharmacokinetics

Route	Onset	Duration
Oral	20–30 min	3–8 hr

Metabolism: $T_{1/2}$: Unknown
Distribution: Crosses placenta; enters breast milk
Excretion: Unknown

Adverse effects
Parasympathomimetic effects
• **CNS:** Seizures, dysarthria, dysphonia, drowsiness, dizziness, headache, loss of consciousness
• **CV:** *Bradycardia,* **cardiac arrhythmias,** AV block and nodal rhythm, **cardiac**

arrest, decreased cardiac output, leading to hypotension, syncope
• **Dermatologic:** Diaphoresis, flushing
• **EENT:** *Lacrimation, miosis,* spasm of accommodation, diplopia, conjunctival hyperemia
• **GI:** *Salivation, dysphagia, nausea, vomiting, increased peristalsis, abdominal cramps,* flatulence, diarrhea
• **GU:** *Urinary frequency and incontinence,* urinary urgency
• **Respiratory:** *Increased pharyngeal and tracheobronchial secretions,* **laryngospasm, bronchospasm,** bronchiolar constriction, dyspnea
Skeletal muscle effects
• **Peripheral:** Skeletal muscle weakness, fasciculations, muscle cramps, arthralgia
• **Respiratory:** Respiratory muscle paralysis, **central respiratory paralysis**

Interactions
✳ **Drug-drug** • Decreased neuromuscular blockade of succinylcholine • Decreased effects of ambenonium and possible muscular depression with corticosteroids • Risk of severe toxicity with atropine; combination is contraindicated • Risk of toxicity if given with other anticholinesterases, antiarrhythmics, local and general anesthetics

■ Nursing considerations
Assessment
• **History:** Hypersensitivity to anticholinesterases, intestinal or urogenital tract obstruction, peritonitis, asthma, peptic ulcer, bradycardia, cardiac arrhythmias, recent coronary occlusion, vagotonia, hyperthyroidism, epilepsy, lactation
• **Physical:** Skin color, texture, lesions; reflexes, bilateral grip strength; P, auscultation; BP; R, adventitious sounds; salivation, bowel sounds, normal output; frequency, voiding pattern, normal urinary output; EEG, thyroid function tests

Interventions
• Overdose can cause muscle weakness (cholinergic crisis) that is difficult to differentiate from myasthenic weakness (use of edrophonium for differential diagnosis is recommended). The administration of atropine may mask the parasympathetic

effects of anticholinesterase overdose and further confound the diagnosis.

⊗ **Warning** Keep atropine sulfate readily available as an antidote and antagonist in case of cholinergic crisis or hypersensitivity reaction.

- Use edrophonium (2 mg IV given 1 hr after last ambenonium dose) to evaluate adequacy of dose. Transient increase in strength occurring in 30 sec and lasting 3–5 min indicates inadequate dose; adequate maintenance dose will reflect no change, or transient decrease in strength will occur.
- Monitor patient response carefully if increasing dosage.
- Discontinue drug and consult physician if excessive salivation, emesis, frequent urination, or diarrhea occurs.
- Arrange for decreased dosage of drug if excessive sweating, nausea, or GI upset occurs.

Teaching points

- Take this drug exactly as prescribed; does not need to be taken at night. You and your home caregiver need to know about the effects of the drug, the signs and symptoms of myasthenia gravis, the fact that muscle weakness may be related to drug overdose and to exacerbation of the disease, and that it is important to report muscle weakness promptly to your health care provider so that proper evaluation can be made.
- You may experience these side effects: Blurred vision, difficulty with far vision, difficulty with dark adaptation (use caution while driving, especially at night, or performing hazardous tasks in reduced light); increased urinary frequency, abdominal cramps (if these become a problem, notify your health care provider); sweating (avoid hot or excessively humid environments).
- Report muscle weakness, nausea, vomiting, diarrhea, severe abdominal pain, excessive sweating, excessive salivation, frequent urination, urinary urgency, irregular heartbeat, difficulty breathing.

▽ **ambrisentan**

See Appendix R, *Less commonly used drugs*.

▽ **amifostine**

See Appendix R, *Less commonly used drugs*.

▽ **amikacin sulfate**
*(am i **kay'** sin)*

Amikin

PREGNANCY CATEGORY D

Drug class
Aminoglycoside

Therapeutic actions
Bactericidal: Inhibits protein synthesis in susceptible strains of gram-negative bacteria, and the functional integrity of bacterial cell membrane appears to be disrupted, causing cell death.

Indications

- Short-term treatment of serious infections caused by susceptible strains of *Pseudomonas* species, *Escherichia coli*, indole-positive and indole-negative *Proteus* species, *Providencia* species, *Klebsiella*, *Enterobacter*, and *Serratia* species, *Acinetobacter* species
- Suspected gram-negative infections before results of susceptibility studies are known (effective in infections caused by gentamicin- or tobramycin-resistant strains of gram-negative organisms)
- Initial treatment of staphylococcal infections when penicillin is contraindicated or infection may be caused by mixed organisms
- Treatment of serious infections such as bacterial septicemia (including neonatal sepsis); infections of the respiratory tract, bones, joints, CNS, skin and soft tissues; intra-abdominal infections; postoperative infections; recurrent and complicated UTIs
- Unlabeled uses: Intrathecal or intraventricular administration at 8 mg/24 hr; part of a multidrug regimen for treatment of *Mycobacterium avium* complex, a common infection in AIDS patients; aerosolized for the treatment of pneumonia or cystic fibrosis; second-line therapy for drug-resistant tuberculosis

Contraindications and cautions

- Contraindicated with allergy to any aminoglycosides, renal or hepatic disease, preexisting hearing loss, myasthenia gravis, parkinsonism, infant botulism, lactation.
- Use cautiously with elderly patients, any patient with diminished hearing, decreased renal function, dehydration, neuromuscular disorders, pregnancy.

Available forms

Injection—50 mg/mL, 250 mg/mL

Dosages

Adults and pediatric patients

15 mg/kg/day IM or IV divided into two to three equal doses at equal intervals, not to exceed 1.5 g/day. Usual course of treatment is 7–10 days. Uncomplicated infections should respond in 24–48 hr. If no clinical response is seen in 3–5 days, reevaluate therapy.

- *UTIs:* 250 mg bid IM or IV; treatment is usually required for 7–10 days. If treatment is required for longer, carefully monitor serum levels and renal and neurologic function.

Neonatal patients

Loading dose of 10 mg/kg IM or IV; then 7.5 mg/kg every 12 hr.

Geriatric patients or patients with renal failure

Reduce dosage, and carefully monitor serum drug levels and renal function tests throughout treatment; regulate dosage based on these values. If creatinine clearance is not available and patient condition is stable, calculate a dosage interval in hours for the normal dose by multiplying patient's serum creatinine by 9. Dosage guide if creatinine clearance is known: Maintenance dose every 12 hr = observed creatinine clearance ÷ normal creatinine clearance × calculated loading dose (mg). For patients on dialysis, approximately one-half of the normal dose can be administered after hemodialysis. Before peritoneal dialysis, 7.5 mg/kg is given, then drug is instilled in peritoneal dialysis at the desired concentration.

Pharmacokinetics

Route	Onset	Peak
IV	Immediate	30–90 min
IM	Varies	45–120 min

Metabolism: $T_{1/2}$: 2–3 hr
Distribution: Crosses placenta; enters breast milk
Excretion: Urine, unchanged

▼ IV FACTS

Preparation: Prepare IV solution by adding the contents of a 500-mg vial to 100 or 200 mL of sterile diluent. Do not physically mix with other drugs. Administer amikacin separately. Prepared solution is stable in concentrations of 0.25 and 5 mg/mL for 24 hr at room temperature.
Infusion: Administer to adults or pediatric patients over 30–60 min; infuse to infants over 1–2 hr.
Compatibilities: Amikacin is stable in 5% dextrose injection; 5% dextrose and 0.2%, 0.45%, or 0.9% sodium chloride injection; lactated Ringer's injection; *Normosol M* in 5% dextrose injection; *Normosol R* in 5% dextrose injection; *Plasma-Lyte* 56 or 148 injection in D_5W.
Y-site compatibilities: May be given with enalaprilat, furosemide, magnesium sulfate, morphine, ondansetron.
Y-site incompatibility: Do not give with hetastarch.

Adverse effects

- **CNS:** *Ototoxicity,* confusion, disorientation, depression, lethargy, nystagmus, visual disturbances, headache, fever, numbness, tingling, tremor, paresthesias, muscle twitching, seizures, muscular weakness, neuromuscular blockade, apnea
- **CV:** Palpitations, hypotension, hypertension
- **GI:** *Nausea, vomiting, anorexia, diarrhea,* weight loss, stomatitis, increased salivation, splenomegaly
- **GU: Nephrotoxicity**
- **Hematologic:** Leukemoid reaction, agranulocytosis, granulocytosis, leukopenia, leukocytosis, thrombocytopenia, eosinophilia, pancytopenia, anemia, hemolytic anemia, increased or decreased reticulocyte count, electrolyte disturbances
- **Hypersensitivity:** Purpura, rash, urticaria, exfoliative dermatitis, itching
- **Other:** *Superinfections, pain, and irritation at IM injection sites*

Interactions

✳ **Drug-drug** • Increased ototoxic and nephrotoxic effects with potent diuretics and other similarly toxic drugs (eg, cephalosporins) • Risk of inactivation if mixed parenterally with penicillins • Increased likelihood of neuromuscular blockade if given shortly after general anesthetics, depolarizing and nondepolarizing neuromuscular junction blockers

■ Nursing considerations

CLINICAL ALERT!
Name confusion has occurred between amikacin and anakinra; use caution.

Assessment

• **History:** Allergy to any aminoglycosides, renal or hepatic disease, preexisting hearing loss, myasthenia gravis, parkinsonism, infant botulism, lactation, diminished hearing, decreased renal function, dehydration, neuromuscular disorders
• **Physical:** Arrange culture and sensitivity tests on infection prior to therapy; eighth cranial nerve function and state of hydration prior to, during, and after therapy; LFTs, renal function tests, CBC, skin color and lesions, orientation and affect, reflexes, bilateral grip strength, weight, bowel sounds

Interventions

⊗ **Black box warning** Monitor patient for nephrotoxicity, ototoxicity with baseline and periodic renal function and neurologic examinations; risk for serious toxicity, including neuromuscular blockade and respiratory paralysis.
• Arrange for culture and sensitivity testing of infected area before treatment.
⊗ **Warning** Monitor duration of treatment: Usually 7–10 days. If clinical response does not occur within 3–5 days, stop therapy. Prolonged treatment leads to increased risk of toxicity. If drug is used longer than 10 days, monitor auditory and renal function daily.
• Give IM dosage by deep injection.
• Ensure that patient is well hydrated before and during therapy.

Teaching points

• This drug is only available for IM or IV use.
• You may experience these side effects: Ringing in the ears, headache, dizziness (reversible; safety measures may need to be taken if severe); nausea, vomiting, loss of appetite (eat frequent small meals, frequent mouth care may help).
• Report pain at injection site, severe headache, dizziness, loss of hearing, changes in urine pattern, difficulty breathing, rash or skin lesions.

▽amiloride hydrochloride

(a mill' oh ride)

Midamor

PREGNANCY CATEGORY B

Drug class

Potassium-sparing diuretic

Therapeutic actions

Inhibits sodium reabsorption in the renal distal tubule, causing loss of sodium and water and retention of potassium.

Indications

• Adjunctive therapy with thiazide or loop diuretics in heart failure and in hypertension to treat hypokalemia or to prevent hypokalemia in patients who would be at high risk if hypokalemia occurred (digitalized patients, patients with cardiac arrhythmias)
• Unlabeled uses: Inhalation in the treatment of cystic fibrosis; reduction of lithium-induced polyuria without increasing lithium levels

Contraindications and cautions

• Contraindicated with allergy to amiloride, hyperkalemia, severe renal disease, diabetic nephropathy, potassium-rich diet.
• Use cautiously with renal or hepatic disease, diabetes mellitus, metabolic or respiratory acidosis, lactation, pregnancy.

Available forms

Tablets—5 mg

Dosages
Adults
- *Adjunctive therapy:* Add 5 mg/day PO to usual antihypertensive or dosage of kaliuretic diuretic; if necessary, increase dose to 10 mg/day or to 15–20 mg/day with careful monitoring of electrolytes.
- *Single-drug therapy:* Start with 5 mg/day PO; if necessary, increase to 10 mg/day or to 15–20 mg/day with careful monitoring of electrolytes.

Pediatric patients
Safety and efficacy not established.

Pharmacokinetics

Route	Onset	Peak	Duration
Oral	2 hr	6–10 hr	24 hr

Metabolism: Hepatic; $T_{1/2}$: 6–9 hr
Distribution: Crosses placenta; enters breast milk
Excretion: Urine, unchanged

Adverse effects
- **CNS:** *Headache,* dizziness, drowsiness, fatigue, paresthesias, tremors, confusion, encephalopathy
- **GI:** *Nausea, anorexia, vomiting, diarrhea,* dry mouth, constipation, jaundice, gas pain, GI bleeding
- **GU:** Polyuria, dysuria, *impotence,* decreased libido
- **Musculoskeletal:** *Weakness, fatigue, muscle cramps* and muscle spasms, joint pain
- **Respiratory:** Cough, dyspnea
- **Other:** Rash, pruritus, itching, alopecia, *hyperkalemia*

Interactions
＊**Drug-drug** ● Increased hyperkalemia with triamterene, spironolactone, potassium supplements, diets rich in potassium, ACE inhibitors ● Reduced effectiveness of digoxin with amiloride

■ Nursing considerations
Assessment
- **History:** Allergy to amiloride, hyperkalemia, renal or liver disease, diabetes mellitus, metabolic or respiratory acidosis, lactation
- **Physical:** Skin color, lesions, edema; orientation, reflexes, muscle strength; pulses, baseline ECG, BP; R, pattern, adventitious sounds; liver evaluation, bowel sounds, urinary output patterns; CBC, serum electrolytes, blood sugar, LFTs, renal function tests, urinalysis

Interventions
⊗ **Black box warning** Monitor patient for hyperkalemia (serum potassium level greater than 5.5 mEq/L).
- Administer with food or milk to prevent GI upset.
- Administer early in the day so increased urination does not disturb sleep.
- Measure and record weight regularly to monitor mobilization of edema fluid.
- Avoid foods and salt substitutes high in potassium. See Appendix B for listing of high-potassium foods.
- Provide frequent mouth care and sugarless candies to suck.
- Arrange for regular evaluation of serum electrolytes.

Teaching points
- Take single dose early in the day so increased urination will not disturb sleep.
- Take the drug with food or meals to prevent GI upset.
- Avoid foods that are high in potassium and any flavoring that contains potassium (such as a salt substitute).
- Weigh yourself on a regular basis at the same time and in the same clothing, and record the weight on your calendar.
- You may experience these side effects: Increased volume and frequency of urination; dizziness, feeling faint on arising, drowsiness (avoid rapid position changes, hazardous activities like driving, and the use of alcohol which may intensify these problems); decrease in sexual function; increased thirst (sucking on sugarless candies may help; frequent mouth care also may help); avoid foods that are rich in potassium (eg, fruits, *Sanka*).
- Report loss or gain of more than 3 pounds in 1 day; swelling in your ankles or fingers; dizziness, trembling, numbness, fatigue; muscle weakness or cramps.

▽amino acids
(a mee' noe)

Aminosyn, FreAmine, HepatAmine,
Novamine, Primene (CAN),
ProcalAmine, Travasol, TrophAmine

PREGNANCY CATEGORY C

Drug classes
Caloric agent
Protein substrate

Therapeutic actions
Essential and nonessential amino acids provided in various combinations to supply calories and proteins and provide a protein-building and a protein-sparing effect for the body (a positive nitrogen balance).

Indications
• Provide nutrition to patients who are in a negative nitrogen balance when GI tract cannot absorb protein; when protein needs exceed the ability to absorb protein (with burns, trauma, infections); when bowel rest is needed; when tube feeding cannot supply adequate nutrition; when health can be improved or restored by replacing lost amino acids
• Treatment of hepatic encephalopathy in patients with cirrhosis or hepatitis (*HepatAmine*)
• Nutritional support of uremic patients when oral nutrition is not feasible or is impractical or insufficient

Contraindications and cautions
• Contraindicated with hypersensitivity to any component of the solution; severe electrolyte or acid–base imbalance; inborn errors in amino acid metabolism; decreased circulating blood volume; severe renal or hepatic disease; hyperammonemia; bleeding abnormalities.
• Use cautiously with hepatic or renal impairment, diabetes mellitus, heart failure, hypertension, decreased circulating blood volume.

Available forms
Many forms available for IV injections.

Dosages
Dosage must be individualized with careful observation of cardiac status and BUN and evaluation of metabolic needs. Recommended protein dietary allowances are 0.9 g/kg/day for healthy adults, 1.4–2.2 g/kg/day in healthy infants and children. Requirements increase with trauma or in those who are malnourished.
• *Hepatic encephalopathy:* 80–120 g amino acid/day; 500 mL *HepatAmine* with 500 mL 50% dextrose and electrolyte solution over 8–12 hr per day.

Adults
1–1.5 g/kg/day amino acid injection IV into a peripheral vein; 250–500 mL/day amino acid injection IV mixed with appropriate dextrose, vitamins, and electrolytes as part of a total parenteral nutrition (TPN) solution.

Pediatric patients
• *Renal failure:* 0.5–1 g/kg/day amino acid IV mixed with dextrose as appropriate; more than 1 g/kg/day not recommended.
• *Allowances of protein in infant nutrition:* 2–4 g/protein/kg/day
• *Amino acids:*
16 yr and older: 1.5 g/kg/day
13–15 yr: 1.7 g/kg/day
4–12 yr: 2 g/kg/day
1–3 yr: 2–2.5 g/kg/day

Pharmacokinetics

Route	Onset
IV	Immediate

Metabolism: Part of normal anabolic processes
Distribution: Crosses placenta; enters breast milk
Excretion: Urine

▼ IV FACTS
Preparation: Strict aseptic technique is required in mixing solution; use of a laminar flow hood in the pharmacy is recommended. A 0.22-micron filter should be used to block any particulate matter and bacteria. Use mixed solution immediately. If not used within 1 hr, refrigerate solution. Mixed solutions must be used within 24 hr. Use strict aseptic technique when changing bottles, catheter tubing, and so forth. Replace all IV apparatus every 24 hr. Change dressing every 24 hr to assess insertion site.

A

Infusion: Use a volumetric infusion pump. Infuse only if solution is absolutely clear and without particulate matter. Infuse slowly. If infusion falls behind, do not try to speed up infusion rate; serious overload could occur. Infusion rates of 20–30 mL/hr up to a maximum of 60–100 mL/hr have been used.

Incompatibilities: Do not mix with amphotericin B, ampicillin, gentamicin, metronidazole, tetracycline, ticarcillin.

Adverse effects

- **CNS:** *Headache, dizziness,* mental confusion, loss of consciousness
- **CV:** Hypertension, heart failure, **pulmonary edema,** tachycardia, *generalized flushing*
- **Endocrine:** Hypoglycemia, hyperglycemia, fatty acid deficiency, azotemia, hyperammonemia
- **GI:** *Nausea, vomiting,* abdominal pain, liver impairment, fatty liver
- **Hypersensitivity:** Fever, chills, rash, papular eruptions
- **Local:** *Pain, infection,* phlebitis, venous thrombosis, tissue sloughing at injection site

Interactions

✴ **Drug-drug** • Reduced protein-sparing effects of amino acids if taken with tetracyclines

■ Nursing considerations

Assessment

- **History:** Hypersensitivity to any component of the solution; severe electrolyte or acid–base imbalance; inborn errors in amino acid metabolism; decreased circulating blood volume; hepatic or renal disease; hyperammonemia; bleeding abnormalities; diabetes mellitus; heart failure; hypertension
- **Physical:** T, weight, height; orientation, reflexes; P, BP, edema; R, lung auscultation; abdominal examination; urinary output; CBC, platelet count, PT, electrolytes, BUN, blood glucose, uric acid, bilirubin, creatinine, plasma proteins, LFTs, renal function tests; urine glucose, osmolarity

Interventions

- Assess nutritional status before and frequently during treatment; weigh patient

daily to monitor fluid load and nutritional status.

- Monitor vital signs often during infusion; monitor I&O continually during treatment.
- Observe infusion site at least daily for infection, phlebitis; change dressing using strict aseptic technique at least every 24 hr.
- Arrange to give D₅W or D₁₀W for injection by a peripheral line to avoid hypoglycemia rebound if TPN infusion needs to be stopped.
- Monitor urine glucose, acetone, and specific gravity every 6 hr during initial infusion period, at least bid when the infusion has stabilized; stop solution at any sign of renal failure.
- Monitor patient for vascular overload or hepatic impairment; decrease rate of infusion or discontinue.

Teaching points

- This drug can be given only through an intravenous or central line.
- This drug helps you to build new proteins and regain strength and healing power.
- You may experience these side effects: Headache, dizziness (medication may be ordered to help); nausea, vomiting; pain at infusion site.
- Report fever, chills, severe pain at infusion site, changes in color of urine or stool, severe headache, rash.

▷ **aminocaproic acid**
*(a mee noe ka **proe'** ik)*

Amicar

PREGNANCY CATEGORY C

Drug class

Systemic hemostatic drug

Therapeutic actions

Inhibits fibrinolysis by inhibiting plasminogen activator substances and by antiplasmin activity; this action prevents the breakdown of clots.

Indications

- Treatment of excessive bleeding resulting from systemic hyperfibrinolysis and urinary fibrinolysis

- Unlabeled uses: Prevention of recurrence of subarachnoid hemorrhage; management of amegakaryocytic thrombocytopenia; to decrease the need for platelet administration; to abort and treat attacks of hereditary angioneurotic edema; to reduce postoperative bleeding complications in cardiac and orthopedic procedures; acute promyelocytic leukemia with coagulopathy associated with low levels of alpha-2-plasmin inhibitor

Contraindications and cautions

- Contraindicated with allergy to aminocaproic acid, active intravascular clotting, cardiac disease, renal impairment, hematuria of upper urinary tract origin, hepatic impairment, lactation.
- Use cautiously with hyperfibrinolysis, pregnancy.

Available forms

Tablets—500, 1,000 mg; injection—250 mg/mL; oral solution—250 mg/mL

Dosages
Adults

- *Treatment of excessive bleeding:* Initial dose of 5 g PO or IV followed by 1–1.25 g every hr to produce and sustain plasma levels of 0.13 mg/mL; do not administer more than 30 g/day.
- *Acute bleeding:* 4–5 g IV in 250 mL of diluent during the first hour of infusion; then continuous infusion of 1 g/hr in 50 mL of diluent. Continue for 8 hr or until bleeding stops.
- *Prevention of recurrence of subarachnoid hemorrhage:* 36 g/day in six divided doses, PO or IV.

Pediatric patients
Safety and efficacy not established.

Pharmacokinetics

Route	Onset	Peak	Duration
Oral	Rapid	2 hr	Not known
IV	Immediate	Minutes	2–3 hr

Metabolism: $T_{1/2}$: 2 hr
Distribution: Crosses placenta; may enter breast milk
Excretion: Urine, unchanged

▼ IV FACTS

Preparation: Dilute in compatible IV fluid. Rapid IV infusion undiluted is not recommended. Dilute 4 mL (1 g) of solution with 50 mL of diluent. For acute bleed, dilute 4–5 g in 250 mL diluent and give over 1 hr; then a continuous infusion of 1 g/hr given in 50 mL diluent. Store at room temperature.
Infusion: Infuse at 4–5 g the first hour of treatment, then 1 g/hr by continuous infusion; administer slowly to avoid hypotension, bradycardia, arrhythmias. Continue infusion for 8 hr or until bleeding is controlled. Undiluted, rapid injection is not recommended.
Compatibilities: Compatible with sterile water for injection, normal saline, 5% dextrose, Ringer's solution.

Adverse effects

- **CNS:** *Dizziness, tinnitus, headache,* delirium, hallucinations, psychotic reactions, weakness, conjunctival suffusion, nasal stuffiness
- **CV:** Hypotension, cardiac myopathy, bradycardia
- **GI:** *Nausea, cramps, diarrhea,* vomiting
- **GU:** Intrarenal obstruction, renal failure, *fertility problems*
- **Hematologic:** *Elevated serum CPK,* aldolase, AST, elevated serum potassium
- **Musculoskeletal:** *Malaise,* myopathy, symptomatic weakness, fatigue
- **Respiratory:** Dyspnea, **pulmonary embolism**
- **Other:** Rash, thrombophlebitis

Interactions

✳ **Drug-drug** • Risk of hypercoagulable state with hormonal contraceptives, estrogens
✳ **Drug-lab test** • Elevation of serum K+ levels, especially with impaired renal function

■ Nursing considerations
Assessment

- **History:** Allergy to aminocaproic acid, DIC, cardiac disease, renal impairment; hematuria of upper urinary tract origin, hepatic impairment, lactation, hyperfibrinolysis
- **Physical:** Skin color, lesions; muscular strength; orientation, reflexes, affect; BP, P, baseline ECG, peripheral perfusion; liver

evaluation, bowel sounds, output; clotting studies, CPK, urinalysis, LFTs, renal function tests

Interventions
- Patient on oral therapy may need up to 10 tablets the first hour of treatment and tablets around the clock during treatment.
- Orient patient and offer support if hallucinations, delirium, or psychoses occur.
- Monitor patient for signs of clotting.

Teaching points
- You may experience these side effects: Dizziness, weakness, headache, hallucinations (avoid driving or the use of dangerous machinery; take special precautions to avoid injury); nausea, diarrhea, cramps (eat frequent small meals); infertility problems (menstrual irregularities, dry ejaculation—should go away when the drug is stopped); weakness, malaise (plan activities, take rest periods as needed).
- Report severe headache, restlessness, muscle pain and weakness, blood in the urine.

▷ aminolevulinic acid hydrochloride

See Appendix R, *Less commonly used drugs.*

▷ aminophylline (theophylline ethylenediamine)
(am in off′ i lin)

PREGNANCY CATEGORY C

Drug classes
Bronchodilator
Xanthine

Therapeutic actions
Relaxes bronchial smooth muscle, causing bronchodilation and increasing vital capacity, which has been impaired by bronchospasm and air trapping; in higher concentrations, it also inhibits the release of slow-reacting substance of anaphylaxis (SRS-A) and histamine and suppresses the response of airways to stimuli.

Indications
- Symptomatic relief or prevention of bronchial asthma and reversible bronchospasm associated with chronic bronchitis and emphysema
- As adjunct to inhaled beta$_2$ selective adrenergic agonists and systemic corticosteroids for the treatment of acute exacerbations of the symptoms and reversible airflow obstruction associated with asthma and other obstructive lung diseases
- Unlabeled uses: Respiratory stimulant in Cheyne-Stokes respiration; treatment of apnea and bradycardia in premature babies

Contraindications and cautions
- Contraindicated with hypersensitivity to any xanthine or to ethylenediamine, peptic ulcer, active gastritis.
- Use cautiously with cardiac arrhythmias, acute myocardial injury, heart failure, cor pulmonale, severe hypertension, severe hypoxemia, renal or hepatic disease, hyperthyroidism, alcoholism, labor, lactation, pregnancy.

Available forms
Injection—25 mg/mL

Dosages
Individualize dosage. Because of poor distribution of drug in body fat, dosing should be calculated based on ideal body weight. Base dosage adjustments on clinical response. Monitor serum theophylline levels and maintain a therapeutic range of 10–20 mcg/mL. Aminophylline is approximately 79% anhydrous theophylline by weight. To convert a theophylline dose to aminophylline, divide the theophylline dose by 0.8.
Adults and pediatric patients

▼ IV FACTS
Loading dose is 5.7 mg/kg (aminophylline) calculated on ideal body weight. Administer over 30 min. This should produce a peak serum level of 6–16 mcg/mL. Determine serum levels 30 min after administering dose. If patient has had theophylline within 24 hr, monitor levels before administering loading dose and adjust dosage accordingly.

Initial theophylline infusion rates after loading dose to target 10 mcg/mL serum level. (Divide theophylline dose by 0.8 to arrive at aminophylline dose.)

Age	Initial infusion rate
Neonates 24 days or younger	1 mg/kg every 12 hr
Neonates older than 24 days	1.5 mg/kg every 12 hr
Infants 6–52 wk	mg/kg/hr = 0.008 × age in weeks + 0.21
Children 1–9 yr	0.8 mg/kg/hr
Children 9–12 yr and adolescent smokers	0.7 mg/kg/hr
Nonsmoking adolescents 12–16 yr	0.5 mg/kg/hr; do not exceed 900 mg theophylline/day
Healthy, nonsmoking adults	0.4 mg/kg/hr; do not exceed 900 mg theophylline/day
Adults older than 60 yr	0.3 mg/kg/hr; do not exceed 400 mg theophylline/day
Adults with cardiac decompensation, cor pulmonale, hepatic impairment, sepsis with multiorgan failure, shock	0.2 mg/kg/hr; do not exceed 400 mg theophylline/day; do not exceed 17 mg/hr

Infusion dosage should be adjusted based on serum theophylline levels as noted under oral dosing.

Compatibilities: Aminophylline is compatible with most IV solutions, but do not mix in solution with other drugs, including vitamins.

Y-site incompatibilities: Dobutamine, hydralazine, ondansetron.

Patients with impaired renal function No dosage adjustment needed in adults or children older than 3 mo. Frequent monitoring and dosage reduction are needed for neonates with renal impairment.

Pharmacokinetics

Route	Onset	Peak
Oral	Rapid	1–2 hr

Metabolism: Hepatic; $T_{1/2}$: 6–23 hr
Distribution: May cross placenta; may enter breast milk
Excretion: Urine

Adverse effects

- **Serum theophylline levels less than 20 mcg/mL:** Adverse effects uncommon
- **Serum theophylline levels more than 20–25 mcg/mL:** Nausea, vomiting, diarrhea, headache, insomnia, irritability (75% of patients)
- **Serum theophylline levels more than 30–35 mcg/mL:** Hyperglycemia, hypotension, cardiac arrhythmias, **seizures,** tachycardia (more than 10 mcg/mL in premature newborns), **brain damage**
- **CNS:** Irritability (especially in children); restlessness, dizziness, muscle twitching, seizures, severe depression, stammering speech; abnormal behavior characterized by withdrawal, mutism, and unresponsiveness alternating with hyperactive periods
- **CV:** Palpitations, sinus tachycardia, ventricular tachycardia, life-threatening ventricular arrhythmias, **circulatory failure**
- **GI:** Loss of appetite, hematemesis, epigastric pain, gastroesophageal reflux during sleep, increased AST
- **GU:** Proteinuria, increased excretion of renal tubular cells and RBCs; diuresis (dehydration), urine retention in men with prostate enlargement
- **Respiratory:** Tachypnea, **respiratory arrest**
- **Other:** Fever, flushing, hyperglycemia, SIADH, rash

Interactions

✳ **Drug-drug** • Increased effects with acyclovir, allopurinol, cimetidine, erythromycin, troleandomycin, clindamycin, lincomycin, methotrexate, diltiazem, disulfiram, enoxacin, fluvoxamine, inteferon alfa-2a, mexiletine, pentoxifylline, ticlopidine, verapamil, zileuton, influenza virus vaccine, fluoroquinolones, hormonal contraceptives • Possibly increased effects with allopurinol • Increased cardiac toxicity with halothane; increased likelihood of seizures when given with ketamine; increased likelihood of adverse GI effects when given with tetracyclines • Increased or decreased effects with furosemide, levothyroxine, liothyronine, liotrix, thyroglobulin, thyroid hormones • Decreased effects in patients who are cigarette smokers (1–2 packs per day); theophylline dosage may need to be increased 50%–100% • Decreased effects with phenobarbital, carbamazepine, isoproterenol, rifamycins • Increased effects, toxicity of sympathomimetics (especially ephedrine) with theophylline preparations • Decreased effects of phenytoin and theophylline preparations when given concomitantly • Decreased effects of lithium carbonate, nondepolarizing neuromuscular blockers given with theophylline preparations • Mutually antagonistic effects of beta-blockers and theophylline preparations

✴ **Drug-food** • Elimination is increased by a low-carbohydrate, high-protein diet and by charcoal-broiled beef • Elimination is decreased by a high-carbohydrate, low-protein diet • Food may alter bioavailability and absorption of timed-release theophylline preparations, causing toxicity; these forms should be taken on an empty stomach

✴ **Drug-lab test** • Interference with spectrophotometric determinations of serum theophylline levels by furosemide, phenylbutazone, probenecid, theobromine; coffee, tea, cola beverages, chocolate, acetaminophen cause falsely high values • Alteration in assays of uric acid, urinary catecholamines, plasma free fatty acids by theophylline preparations

■ **Nursing considerations**
Assessment
- **History:** Hypersensitivity to any xanthine or to ethylenediamine, peptic ulcer, active gastritis, cardiac arrhythmias, acute myocardial injury, heart failure, cor pulmonale, severe hypertension, severe hypoxemia, renal or hepatic disease, hyperthyroidism, alcoholism, labor, lactation
- **Physical:** Bowel sounds, normal output; P, auscultation, BP, perfusion, ECG; R, adventitious sounds; frequency of urination, voiding, normal output pattern, urinalysis, LFTs, renal function tests; liver palpation; thyroid function tests; skin color, texture, lesions; reflexes, bilateral grip strength, affect, EEG

Interventions
- Administer to pregnant patients only when clearly needed—neonatal tachycardia, jitteriness, and withdrawal apnea observed when mothers received xanthines up until delivery.
- Give tablets, liquid dosage forms with food if GI effects occur.
- Maintain adequate hydration.

- Monitor results of serum theophylline levels carefully, and arrange for reduced dosage if serum levels exceed therapeutic range of 10–20 mcg/mL.
- Take serum samples to determine peak theophylline concentration drawn 15–30 min after an IV loading dose.
- Monitor for clinical signs of adverse effects, particularly if serum theophylline levels are not available.
- Ensure that diazepam and/or phenobarbital are readily available to treat seizures.

Teaching points
- This drug will be given IV.
- This drug may be given continuously around the clock for adequate control of asthma attacks.
- Avoid excessive intake of coffee, tea, cocoa, cola beverages, and chocolate.
- Smoking cigarettes or other tobacco products impacts the drug's effectiveness. Try not to smoke. Notify your health care provider if smoking habits change while taking this drug.
- Frequent blood tests may be necessary to monitor the effect of this drug and to ensure safe and effective dosage; keep all appointments for blood tests and other monitoring.
- You may experience these side effects: Nausea, loss of appetite; difficulty sleeping, depression, emotional lability (reversible).
- Report nausea, vomiting, severe GI pain, restlessness, seizures, irregular heartbeat.

DANGEROUS DRUG

▽**amiodarone hydrochloride**
(a mee o' da rone)

Apo-Amiodarone (CAN), Cordarone, Gen-Amiodarone (CAN), Nexterone, Novo-Amiodarone (CAN), Pacerone, PMS-Amiodarone (CAN), ratio-Amiodarone (CAN)

PREGNANCY CATEGORY D

Drug classes
Adrenergic blocker (not used as sympatholytic drug)
Antiarrhythmic

Therapeutic actions

Type III antiarrhythmic: Acts directly on cardiac cell membrane; prolongs repolarization and refractory period; increases ventricular fibrillation threshold; acts on peripheral smooth muscle to decrease peripheral resistance.

Indications

- Only for treatment of the following documented life-threatening recurrent ventricular arrhythmias that do not respond to documented adequate doses of other antiarrhythmics or when alternative agents are not tolerated: Recurrent ventricular fibrillation, recurrent hemodynamically unstable ventricular tachycardia. Serious and even fatal toxicity has been reported with this drug; use alternative agents first; very closely monitor patient receiving this drug
- Unlabeled uses: Treatment of refractory sustained or paroxysmal atrial fibrillation and paroxysmal supraventricular tachycardia; postoperative conversion of atrial fibrillation, atrial flutter

Contraindications and cautions

- Contraindicated with hypersensitivity to amiodarone; sinus node dysfunction, heart block, cardiogenic shock, severe bradycardia; hypokalemia; lactation; sensitivity to iodine.
- Use cautiously with thyroid dysfunction, pregnancy.

Available forms

Tablets—100, 200, 400 mg; injection—1.5 mg/mL, 1.8 mg/mL, 50 mg/mL

Dosages

Careful patient assessment and evaluation with continual monitoring of cardiac response are necessary for titrating the dosage. Therapy should begin in the hospital with continual monitoring and emergency equipment on standby. The following is a guide to usual dosage.

Adults

Oral

Loading dose, 800–1,600 mg/day PO in divided doses for doses of 1,000 mg or more or with GI intolerance, for 1–3 wk; reduce dose to 600–800 mg/day in divided doses for 1 mo; if rhythm is stable, reduce dose to 400 mg/day in one to two divided doses for maintenance dose. Adjust to the lowest possible dose to limit side effects.

IV

1,000 mg IV over 24 hr—150 mg loading dose over 10 min (15 mg/min), followed by 360 mg over 6 hr at rate of 1 mg/min, then 540 mg at 0.5 mg/min over the next 18 hr. After the first 24 hr, a maintenance infusion of 0.5 mg/min (720 mg/24 hr) or less can be cautiously continued for 2–3 wk. Switch to oral form as soon as possible.

Converting from IV to PO

IV dose of 720 mg/day at 0.5 mg/min: Convert to PO dose based on duration of IV therapy. Less than 1 wk—initial oral dose 800–1,600 mg; 1–3 wk—initial oral dose 600–800 mg; more than 3 wk—initial oral dose 400 mg.

Pediatric patients

Safety and efficacy not established.

Pharmacokinetics

Route	Onset	Peak	Duration
Oral	2–3 days	3–7 hr	6–8 hr
IV	Immediate	20 min	Infusion

Metabolism: Hepatic; $T_{1/2}$: 10 days, then 40–55 days
Distribution: Crosses placenta; enters breast milk
Excretion: Bile, feces

▼ IV FACTS

Preparation: Do not use PVC container if infusion is to exceed 2 hr; use glass or polyolefin instead. Dilute 150 mg in 100 mL D_5W for rapid loading dose (1.5 mg/mL). Dilute 900 mg in 500 mL D_5W for slow infusions (1.8 mg/mL). Administer via PVC tubing using an in-line filter. Concentrations of more than 2 mg/mL should be given via central venous catheter. *Nexterone* is available as premixed injection in dextrose; no further preparation is needed. Store at room temperature and use within 24 hr.

Infusion: Infuse loading dose over 10 min. Immediately follow with slow infusion of 1 mg/min or 33.3 mL/hr. Maintenance infusion of 0.5 mg/min or 16.6 mL/hr can be continued up to 96 hr. Use of an infusion pump is advised.

Adverse effects in *italics* are most common; those in **bold** are life-threatening. ⊜⊜ Do not crush.

Incompatibilities: Do not mix with aminophylline, cefazolin, heparin, sodium bicarbonate; do not mix in solution with other drugs.

Adverse effects

- **CNS:** *Malaise, fatigue, dizziness, tremors, ataxia,* paresthesias, lack of coordination
- **CV: Cardiac arrhythmias,** heart failure, **cardiac arrest,** *hypotension,* bradycardia
- **EENT:** *Corneal microdeposits* (photophobia, dry eyes, halos, blurred vision); ophthalmic abnormalities including permanent blindness
- **Endocrine:** *Hypothyroidism or hyperthyroidism*
- **GI:** *Nausea, vomiting, anorexia, constipation, abnormal LFT,* **hepatotoxicity**
- **Respiratory: Pulmonary toxicity**— pneumonitis, infiltrates (shortness of breath, cough, rales, wheezes)
- **Other:** *Photosensitivity,* angioedema, fever

Interactions

✳ **Drug-drug** • Increased digitalis toxicity with digoxin • Increased risk of rhabdomyolysis if combined with simvastatin; limit simvastatin to less than 20 mg/dose • Increased quinidine toxicity with quinidine • Increased flecainide toxicity with amiodarone • Increased risk of arrhythmias with azole antifungals, fluoroquinolones, macrolide antibiotics, ranolazine, trazodone, thioridazine, vardenafil, ziprasidone • Increased phenytoin toxicity with phenytoin, ethotoin • Increased bleeding tendencies with warfarin • Potential sinus arrest and heart block with beta-blockers, calcium channel blockers

✳ **Drug-lab test** • Increased T_4 levels, increased serum reverse T_3 levels

✳ **Drug-food** • Increased risk of toxicity if oral form combined with grapefruit juice; avoid this combination

■ Nursing considerations

CLINICAL ALERT!
Name confusion has occurred with amrinone (name has now been changed to inamrinone, but confusion may still occur); use caution.

Assessment

- **History:** Hypersensitivity to amiodarone, sinus node dysfunction, heart block, severe bradycardia, hypokalemia, lactation, thyroid dysfunction, pregnancy
- **Physical:** Skin color, lesions; reflexes, gait, eye examination; P, BP, auscultation, continuous ECG monitoring; R, adventitious sounds, baseline chest X-ray; liver evaluation; LFTs, serum electrolytes, T_4, and T_3

Interventions

⊗ **Black box warning** Reserve use for life-threatening arrhythmias; serious toxicity, including arrhythmias, pulmonary toxicity can occur.

- Monitor cardiac rhythm continuously.
- Monitor for an extended period when dosage adjustments are made.

⊗ **Warning** Monitor for safe and effective serum levels (0.5–2.5 mcg/mL).

⊗ **Warning** Doses of digoxin, quinidine, phenytoin, and warfarin may need to be reduced one-third to one-half when amiodarone is started.

- Give drug with meals to decrease GI problems.
- Arrange for ophthalmologic examinations; reevaluate at any sign of optic neuropathy.
- Arrange for periodic chest X-ray to evaluate pulmonary status (every 3–6 mo).
- Arrange for regular periodic blood tests for liver enzymes, thyroid hormone levels.

Teaching points

- Drug dosage will be changed in relation to response of arrhythmias; you will need to be hospitalized during initiation of drug therapy; you will be closely monitored when dosage is changed.
- Avoid grapefruit juice while on this drug.
- Have regular medical follow-up, monitoring of cardiac rhythm, chest X-ray, eye examination, blood tests.
- You should avoid pregnancy while taking this drug. If you are breast-feeding, you should use another method of feeding the infant.
- You may experience these side effects: Changes in vision (halos, dry eyes, sensitivity to light; wear sunglasses, monitor light exposure); nausea, vomiting, loss of appetite (take with meals; eat frequent small meals); sensitivity to the sun (use a sunscreen or protective clothing when outdoors); constipation (a laxative may be ordered); tremors, twitching, dizziness, loss of coordination (do not drive, operate dangerous machinery, or

undertake tasks that require coordination until drug effects stabilize and your body adjusts to it).

- Report unusual bleeding or bruising; fever, chills; intolerance to heat or cold; shortness of breath, difficulty breathing, cough; swelling of ankles or fingers; palpitations; difficulty with vision.

▷ **amitriptyline hydrochloride**
*(a mee **trip'** ti leen)*

Apo-Amitriptyline (CAN)

PREGNANCY CATEGORY D

Drug classes
Antidepressant
TCA; tertiary amine

Therapeutic actions
Mechanism of action unknown; TCAs inhibit the reuptake of the neurotransmitters norepinephrine and serotonin, leading to an increase in their effects; anticholinergic at CNS and peripheral receptors; sedative.

Indications
- Relief of symptoms of depression (endogenous most responsive); sedative effects may help when depression is associated with anxiety and sleep disturbance
- Unlabeled uses: Control of chronic pain (eg, intractable pain of cancer, central pain syndromes, peripheral neuropathies, postherpetic neuralgia, tic douloureux); prevention of onset of cluster and migraine headaches; treatment of pathologic weeping and laughing secondary to forebrain disease (due to MS); insomnia; fibromyalgia; adult enuresis; bulimia nervosa

Contraindications and cautions
- Contraindicated with hypersensitivity to any tricyclic drug; concomitant therapy with an MAOI; recent MI; myelography within previous 24 hr or scheduled within 48 hr; lactation.
- Use cautiously with electroshock therapy; preexisting CV disorders (severe heart disease, progressive heart failure, angina pectoris, paroxysmal tachycardia); angle-closure glaucoma, increased IOP, urinary retention,

ureteral or urethral spasm; seizure disorders; hyperthyroidism; impaired hepatic, renal function; psychiatric patients (schizophrenic or paranoid patients may exhibit a worsening of psychosis with TCA therapy); patients with bipolar disorder; elective surgery (discontinue as long as possible before surgery).

Available forms
Tablets—10, 25, 50, 75, 100, 150 mg

Dosages
Adults
- *Depression, hospitalized patients:* Initially, 100 mg/day PO in divided doses; gradually increase to 200–300 mg/day as required.
- *Depression, outpatients:* Initially, 75 mg/day PO, in divided doses; may increase to 150 mg/day. Increases should be made in late afternoon or at bedtime. Total daily dosage may be administered at bedtime. Initiate single daily dose therapy with 50–100 mg at bedtime; increase by 25–50 mg as necessary to a total of 150 mg/day. Maintenance dose, 40–100 mg/day, which may be given as a single bedtime dose. After satisfactory response, reduce to lowest effective dosage. Continue therapy for 3 mo or longer to lessen possibility of relapse.
- *Chronic pain:* 75–150 mg/day PO.

Pediatric patients 12 yr and older
10 mg tid PO and then 20 mg at bedtime.

Pediatric patients younger than 12 yr
Not recommended.

Geriatric patients
10 mg tid PO and then 20 mg at bedtime.

Pharmacokinetics

Route	Onset	Peak	Duration
Oral	Varies	2–4 hr	2–4 wk

Metabolism: Hepatic; $T_{1/2}$: 10–50 hr
Distribution: Crosses placenta; enters breast milk
Excretion: Urine

Adverse effects
- **CNS:** *Disturbed concentration, sedation and anticholinergic (atropine-like) effects, confusion* (especially in elderly), hallucinations, disorientation, decreased memory, feelings of unreality, delusions, anxiety, nervousness, restlessness, agitation, panic, insomnia, nightmares, hypomania, mania,

Adverse effects in *italics* are most common; those in **bold** are life-threatening. ⊂⊃ Do not crush.

exacerbation of psychosis, drowsiness, weakness, fatigue, headache, numbness, tingling, paresthesias of extremities, incoordination, motor hyperactivity, akathisia, ataxia, tremors, peripheral neuropathy, extrapyramidal symptoms, seizures, speech blockage, dysarthria, tinnitus, altered EEG

- **CV:** *Orthostatic hypotension,* hypertension, syncope, tachycardia, palpitations, **MI,** arrhythmias, heart block, precipitation of heart failure, **stroke**
- **Endocrine:** Elevated or depressed blood sugar, elevated prolactin levels, inappropriate ADH secretion
- **GI:** *Dry mouth, constipation,* paralytic ileus, *nausea,* vomiting, anorexia, epigastric distress, diarrhea, flatulence, dysphagia, peculiar taste, increased salivation, stomatitis, glossitis, parotid swelling, abdominal cramps, black tongue, hepatitis, jaundice (rare), elevated transaminase, altered alkaline phosphatase
- **GU:** Urinary retention, delayed micturition, dilation of the urinary tract, gynecomastia, testicular swelling; breast enlargement, menstrual irregularity and galactorrhea; increased or decreased libido; impotence
- **Hematologic:** Bone marrow depression, including agranulocytosis; eosinophilia, purpura, thrombocytopenia, leukopenia
- **Hypersensitivity:** Rash, pruritus, vasculitis, petechiae, photosensitization, edema (generalized, face, tongue), drug fever
- **Withdrawal:** Symptoms on abrupt discontinuation of prolonged therapy: Nausea, headache, vertigo, nightmares, malaise
- **Other:** Nasal congestion, excessive appetite, weight change; sweating, alopecia, lacrimation, hyperthermia, flushing, chills

Interactions

✳ **Drug-drug •** Increased TCA levels and pharmacologic (especially anticholinergic) effects with cimetidine, fluoxetine • Increased TCA levels with methylphenidate, phenothiazines, hormonal contraceptives, disulfiram • Hyperpyretic crises, severe seizures, hypertensive episodes and deaths with MAOIs, furazolidone • Increased antidepressant response and cardiac arrhythmias with thyroid medication • Increased or decreased effects with estrogens • Delirium with disulfiram • Sympathetic hyperactivity, sinus tachycardia, hypertension, agitation with levodopa • Increased biotransformation of TCAs

in patients who smoke cigarettes • Increased sympathomimetic (especially beta-adrenergic) effects of direct-acting sympathomimetic drugs (norepinephrine, epinephrine) • Increased anticholinergic effects of anticholinergics (including anticholinergic antiparkinsonians) • Increased response (especially CNS depression) to barbiturates • Decreased antihypertensive effect of clonidine, other antihypertensives • Decreased effects of indirect-acting sympathomimetic drugs (ephedrine) • Increased risk of QT-interval prolongation if combined with other drugs that prolong QT interval

▪ Nursing considerations
Assessment

- **History:** Hypersensitivity to any tricyclic drug; concomitant therapy with an MAOI; recent MI; myelography within previous 24 hr or scheduled within 48 hr; lactation; EST; preexisting CV disorders; angle-closure glaucoma, increased IOP, urinary retention, ureteral or urethral spasm; seizure disorders; hyperthyroidism; impaired hepatic, renal function; psychiatric patients; manic-depressive patients; elective surgery
- **Physical:** Weight; T; skin color, lesions; orientation, affect, reflexes, vision and hearing; P, BP, orthostatic BP, perfusion; bowel sounds, normal output, liver evaluation; urine flow, normal output; usual sexual function, frequency of menses, breast and scrotal examination; LFTs, urinalysis, CBC, ECG

Interventions

⊗ **Black box warning** Children, adolescents, and young adults have increased risk of suicidality; monitor patient carefully.

- Restrict drug access for depressed and potentially suicidal patients.
- Administer major portion of dose at bedtime if drowsiness, severe anticholinergic effects occur (note that the elderly may not tolerate single-daily-dose therapy).
- Reduce dosage if minor side effects develop; discontinue if serious side effects occur.
- Arrange for CBC if patient develops fever, sore throat, or other sign of infection.
- Be aware that drug's sedative effects may be apparent before the antidepressant effect is seen.

Teaching points

- Take drug exactly as prescribed; do not stop abruptly or without consulting your health care provider.
- Drug's sedative effects may be apparent before the antidepressant effect is seen.
- Avoid using alcohol, other sleep-inducing drugs, over-the-counter drugs.
- Avoid prolonged exposure to sunlight or sunlamps; use sunscreen or protective garments.
- You may experience these side effects: Headache, dizziness, drowsiness, weakness, blurred vision (reversible; if severe, avoid driving and tasks requiring alertness while these persist); nausea, vomiting, loss of appetite, dry mouth (eat frequent small meals; use frequent mouth care and suck on sugarless candies); nightmares, inability to concentrate, confusion; changes in sexual function.
- Report dry mouth, difficulty in urination, excessive sedation, thoughts of suicide.

▷**amlodipine besylate**
(am loe' di peen beh' sah layt)

Norvasc

PREGNANCY CATEGORY C

Drug classes

Antianginal
Antihypertensive
Calcium channel blocker

Therapeutic actions

Inhibits the movement of calcium ions across the membranes of cardiac and arterial muscle cells; inhibits transmembrane calcium flow, which results in the depression of impulse formation in specialized cardiac pacemaker cells, slowing of the velocity of conduction of the cardiac impulse, depression of myocardial contractility, and dilation of coronary arteries and arterioles and peripheral arterioles; these effects lead to decreased cardiac work, decreased cardiac oxygen consumption, and in patients with vasospastic (Prinzmetal's) angina, increased delivery of oxygen to cardiac cells.

Indications

- Angina pectoris due to coronary artery spasm (Prinzmetal's variant angina)
- Chronic stable angina, alone or in combination with other drugs
- To reduce the risk of hospitalization due to angina and to reduce the need for coronary revascularization procedures in patients with angiographically documented CAD without heart failure or ejection fraction less than 40%
- Essential hypertension, alone or in combination with other antihypertensives

Contraindications and cautions

- Contraindicated with allergy to amlodipine, impaired hepatic function, sick sinus syndrome, heart block (second or third degree), lactation.
- Use cautiously with HF, pregnancy.

Available forms

Tablets—2.5, 5, 10 mg

Dosages

Adults
Initially, 5 mg PO daily; dosage may be gradually increased over 7–14 days to a maximum dose of 10 mg PO daily.
Pediatric patients 6–17 yr
- *Hypertension:* 2.5–5 mg/day PO.
Geriatric patients or patients with hepatic impairment
Initially, 2.5–5 mg PO daily; dosage may be gradually adjusted over 7–14 days based on clinical assessment.

Pharmacokinetics

Route	Onset	Peak
Oral	Unknown	6–12 hr

Metabolism: Hepatic; T$_{1/2}$: 30–50 hr
Distribution: Crosses placenta; may enter breast milk
Excretion: Urine

Adverse effects

- **CNS:** *Dizziness, light-headedness, headache,* asthenia, *fatigue, lethargy*
- **CV:** *Peripheral edema,* arrhythmias
- **Dermatologic:** *Flushing,* rash
- **GI:** *Nausea,* abdominal discomfort

Adverse effects in *italics* are most common; those in **bold** are life-threatening. ⬚ Do not crush.

■ **Nursing considerations**

CLINICAL ALERT!
Name confusion has been reported between *Norvasc* (amlodipine) and *Navane* (thiothixene); use caution.

Assessment
- **History:** Allergy to amlodipine, impaired hepatic function, sick sinus syndrome, heart block, lactation, heart failure
- **Physical:** Skin lesions, color, edema; P, BP, baseline ECG, peripheral perfusion, auscultation; R, adventitious sounds; liver evaluation, GI normal output; LFTs, renal function tests, urinalysis

Interventions
⊗ *Warning* Monitor patient carefully (BP, cardiac rhythm, and output) while adjusting drug to therapeutic dose; use special caution if patient has heart failure.
- Monitor BP very carefully if patient is also on nitrates.
- Monitor cardiac rhythm regularly during stabilization of dosage and periodically during long-term therapy.
- Administer drug without regard to meals.

Teaching points
- Take with meals if upset stomach occurs.
- You may experience these side effects: Nausea, vomiting (eat frequent small meals); headache (adjust lighting, noise, and temperature; medication may be ordered).
- Report irregular heartbeat, shortness of breath, swelling of the hands or feet, pronounced dizziness, constipation.

▽ **ammonium chloride**
(ah mo' nee um)

PREGNANCY CATEGORY C

Drug classes
Electrolyte
Urinary acidifier

Therapeutic actions
Converted to urea in the liver; liberated hydrogen and chloride ions in blood and extracellular fluid lower the pH and correct alkalosis; lowers the urinary pH, producing an acidic urine that changes the excretion rate of many metabolites and drugs.

Indications
- Treatment of hypochloremic states and metabolic alkalosis
- Acidification of urine

Contraindications and cautions
- Contraindicated with renal function impairment; hepatic impairment; metabolic alkalosis due to vomiting of hydrochloric acid when it is accompanied by loss of sodium bicarbonate in the urine.
- Use cautiously with pregnancy, primary respiratory acidosis, high total CO_2 and buffer base, lactation.

Available forms
Injection—26.75% (5 mEq/mL)

Dosages
An oral dosage form of the drug is no longer commercially available.
Adults
Dosage is determined by patient's condition and tolerance; monitor dosage rate and amount by repeated serum bicarbonate determinations. IV infusion should not exceed a concentration of 1%–2% of ammonium chloride.
Pediatric patients
Safety and efficacy for injection in children have not been established.

Pharmacokinetics

Route	Onset	Peak
IV	Rapid	1–3 hr

Metabolism: Hepatic
Distribution: Crosses placenta; enters breast milk
Excretion: Urine

▼ IV FACTS
Preparation: Add contents of one or two vials (100–200 mEq) to 500 or 1,000 mL isotonic (0.9%) sodium chloride injection. Concentration should not exceed 1%–2% ammonium chloride. Avoid excessive heat; protect from freezing. If crystals do appear, warm the solution to room temperature in a water bath prior to use.

Infusion: Do not exceed rate of 5 mL/min in adults (1,000 mL infused over 3 hr). Infuse slowly. Reduce rate in infants and children.
Incompatibilities: Do not mix with levorphanol, norepinephrine, dobutamine.

Adverse effects
- **GI:** Severe hepatic impairment
- **Local:** *Pain or irritation at injection site,* fever, venous thrombosis, phlebitis, extravasation
- **Metabolic:** Metabolic acidosis, hypervolemia, **ammonia toxicity**—pallor, sweating, irregular breathing, retching, bradycardia, arrhythmias, twitching, seizures, coma; hypokalemia

Interactions
✳ **Drug-drug** ● Decreased therapeutic levels due to increased elimination of amphetamine, methamphetamine, dextroamphetamine, ephedrine, flecainide, pseudoephedrine, methadone, mexiletine when taken with ammonium chloride ● Increased effects of chlorpropamide with ammonium chloride

■ Nursing considerations
Assessment
- **History:** Renal or hepatic impairment; metabolic alkalosis due to vomiting of hydrochloric acid when it is accompanied by loss of sodium, respiratory acidosis
- **Physical:** P, BP; skin color, texture; T; injection site evaluation; LFTs, renal function tests, serum bicarbonate, urinalysis

Interventions
- Infuse IV slowly to avoid irritation; check infusion site frequently to monitor for reaction.
- Monitor IV doses for possible fluid overload.
- Monitor for acidosis (increased R, restlessness, sweating, increased blood pH); decrease infusion as appropriate. Ensure that sodium bicarbonate or sodium lactate is readily available in case of overdose.

Teaching points
- Frequent monitoring of blood tests is needed when receiving IV drugs to determine dosage and rate of drug.
- Report pain or irritation at IV site; confusion, restlessness, sweating, headache; severe GI upset, fever, chills.

▽ amoxapine
(a mox' a peen)

PREGNANCY CATEGORY C

Drug classes
Anxiolytic
TCA

Therapeutic actions
Mechanism of action unknown; TCAs inhibit the reuptake of the neurotransmitters norepinephrine and serotonin, leading to an increase in their effects; anticholinergic at CNS and peripheral receptors; sedative.

Indications
- Relief of symptoms of depression in patients with neurotic or reactive depressive disorders and in those with endogenous and psychotic depression (endogenous depression most responsive)
- Treatment of depression accompanied with anxiety or agitation

Contraindications and cautions
- Contraindicated with hypersensitivity to tricyclic drugs; concomitant use with an MAOI; recent MI; myelography within previous 24 hr or scheduled within 48 hr; lactation.
- Use cautiously with EST; preexisting CV disorders (severe coronary heart disease, progressive heart failure, angina pectoris, paroxysmal tachycardia); angle-closure glaucoma, increased IOP, urinary retention, ureteral or urethral spasm; seizure disorders; hyperthyroidism; psychiatric patients (schizophrenic or paranoid patients may exhibit a worsening of psychosis); patients with bipolar disorder; elective surgery (discontinue as soon as possible before surgery), pregnancy.

Available forms
Tablets—25, 50, 100, 150 mg

Dosages
Adults
Initially, 50 mg PO bid–tid; gradually increase to 100 mg bid–tid by end of first wk if tolerated; increase above 300 mg/day only if this dosage ineffective for at least 2 wk. Hospitalized patients refractory to antidepressant

therapy and with no history of seizures may be given up to 600 mg/day in divided doses; after effective dosage is established, drug may be given in a single dose at bedtime (maximum, 300 mg). Usual effective dose is 200–300 mg/day.

Pediatric patients

Not recommended for patients younger than 16 yr.

Geriatric patients

Initially, 25 mg bid–tid; if tolerated, dosage may be increased by end of first week to 50 mg bid–tid. For many elderly patients, 100–150 mg/day may be adequate; some may require up to 300 mg/day. Once effective dose is established, give as single dose at bedtime, not to exceed 300 mg.

Pharmacokinetics

Route	Onset	Peak	Duration
Oral	Varies	90 min	2–4 wk

Metabolism: Hepatic; $T_{1/2}$: 8–30 hr
Distribution: Crosses placenta; enters breast milk
Excretion: Urine

Adverse effects

- **CNS:** *Disturbed concentration, sedation and anticholinergic (atropine-like) effects, confusion* (especially in elderly), hallucinations, disorientation, decreased memory, feelings of unreality, delusions, anxiety, nervousness, restlessness, agitation, panic, insomnia, nightmares, hypomania, mania, exacerbation of psychosis, drowsiness, weakness, fatigue, headache, numbness, tingling, paresthesias of extremities, incoordination, motor hyperactivity, akathisia, ataxia, tremors, peripheral neuropathy, extrapyramidal symptoms, seizures, speech blockage, dysarthria, tinnitus, altered EEG, **neuroleptic malignant syndrome**
- **CV:** *Orthostatic hypotension,* hypertension, syncope, tachycardia, palpitations, **MI,** arrhythmias, heart block, precipitation of heart failure, **stroke**
- **Endocrine:** Elevated or depressed blood sugar, elevated prolactin levels, inappropriate ADH secretion
- **GI:** *Dry mouth, constipation,* paralytic ileus, *nausea,* vomiting, anorexia, epigastric distress, diarrhea, flatulence, dysphagia, peculiar taste, increased salivation, stomatitis, glossitis, parotid swelling, abdominal cramps, black tongue, hepatitis, jaundice (rare); elevated transaminase, altered alkaline phosphatase
- **GU:** Urinary retention, delayed micturition, dilation of the urinary tract, gynecomastia, testicular swelling in men; breast enlargement, menstrual irregularity, and galactorrhea in women; changes in libido; impotence
- **Hematologic:** Bone marrow depression
- **Hypersensitivity:** Rash, pruritus, vasculitis, petechiae, photosensitization, edema (generalized, facial, tongue), drug fever
- **Withdrawal:** Symptoms on abrupt discontinuation of prolonged therapy: Nausea, headache, vertigo, nightmares, malaise
- **Other:** Nasal congestion, excessive appetite, weight gain or loss, sweating, alopecia, lacrimation, hyperthermia, flushing, chills

Interactions

✳ Drug-drug ● Increased TCA levels and pharmacologic (especially anticholinergic) effects with cimetidine, fluoxetine ● Increased TCA levels with methylphenidate, phenothiazines, hormonal contraceptives, disulfiram, cimetidine, ranitidine ● Hyperpyretic crises, severe seizures, hypertensive episodes, and deaths with MAOIs, furazolidone ● Increased antidepressant response and cardiac arrhythmias with thyroid medication ● Increased or decreased effects with estrogens ● Delirium with disulfiram ● Sympathetic hyperactivity, sinus tachycardia, hypertension, agitation with levodopa ● Increased biotransformation of TCAs in patients who smoke cigarettes ● Increased sympathomimetic (especially alpha-adrenergic) effects of direct-acting sympathomimetic drugs (norepinephrine, epinephrine) ● Increased anticholinergic effects of anticholinergic drugs (including anticholinergic antiparkinsonians) ● Increased response (especially CNS depression) to barbiturates ● Decreased antihypertensive effect of clonidine, other antihypertensives

■ Nursing considerations
Assessment

- **History:** Hypersensitivity to any tricyclic drug; concomitant therapy with an MAOI; recent MI; myelography within previous 24 hr or scheduled within 48 hr; lactation;

EST; preexisting CV disorders; angle-closure glaucoma, increased IOP; urinary retention, ureteral or urethral spasm; seizure disorders; hyperthyroidism; psychiatric disorders; manic-depression; elective surgery

- **Physical:** Weight; T; skin color, lesions; orientation, affect, reflexes, vision and hearing; P, BP, orthostatic BP, perfusion; bowel sounds, normal output, liver evaluation; urine flow, normal output; usual sexual function, frequency of menses, breast and scrotal examination; LFTs, urinalysis, CBC, ECG

Interventions

- Restrict drug access for depressed and potentially suicidal patients.
- ⊗ **Black box warning** Children, adolescents, and young adults have increased risk of suicidality; monitor patient carefully.
- Give most of dose at bedtime if drowsiness, severe anticholinergic effects occur (elderly patients may not tolerate single daily dose).
- Reduce dosage if minor side effects develop; discontinue if serious side effects occur.
- Arrange for CBC if patient develops fever, sore throat, or other sign of infection.
- Encourage elderly men or men with prostate problems to void before taking drug.

Teaching points

- Do not stop taking this drug abruptly or without consulting your health care provider.
- Avoid using alcohol, other sleep-inducing drugs, and over-the-counter drugs.
- Avoid prolonged exposure to sunlight or sunlamps; use a sunscreen or protective garments.
- You may experience these side effects: Headache, dizziness, drowsiness, weakness, blurred vision (reversible; safety measures may need to be taken if severe; avoid driving or tasks requiring alertness); nausea, vomiting, loss of appetite, dry mouth (eat frequent small meals, frequent mouth care, and sucking sugarless candies may help); nightmares, inability to concentrate, confusion; changes in sexual function.
- Report dry mouth, difficulty in urination, excessive sedation, thoughts of suicide.

▷ **amoxicillin trihydrate**
*(a mox i **sill'** in try **high'** drayt)*

Amoxil, Apo-Amoxi (CAN), DisperMox, Gen-Amoxicillin (CAN), Moxatag ⊙, Novamoxin (CAN), Nu-Amoxi (CAN), Trimox

PREGNANCY CATEGORY B

Drug class
Antibiotic (penicillin–ampicillin type)

Therapeutic actions
Bactericidal: Inhibits synthesis of cell wall of sensitive organisms, causing cell death.

Indications

- Treatment of tonsillitis and pharyngitis caused by *Streptococcus pyogenes* (ER tablet)
- Infections due to susceptible strains of *Haemophilus influenzae, Escherichia coli, Proteus mirabilis, Neisseria gonorrhoeae, Streptococcus pneumoniae, Enterococcus faecalis,* streptococci, non–penicillinase-producing staphylococci
- *Helicobacter pylori* infection in combination with other agents
- Postexposure prophylaxis against *Bacillus anthracis*
- Unlabeled uses: *Chlamydia trachomatis* in pregnancy, mild to moderate otitis media in children, Lyme disease

Contraindications and cautions

- Contraindicated with allergies to penicillins, cephalosporins, or other allergens.
- Use cautiously with renal disorders, lactation.

Available forms
Chewable tablets—125, 250 mg; tablets—500, 875 mg; capsules—250, 500 mg; powder for oral suspension—125 mg/5 mL, 200 mg/5 mL, 250 mg/5 mL; tablets for oral suspension—200, 400 mg; ER tablets ⊙—775 mg
Available in oral preparations only.

Dosages
Adults and pediatric patients weighing more than 40 kg

- *URIs, GU infections, skin and soft-tissue infections:* Mild to moderate—250 mg PO

Adverse effects in *italics* are most common; those in **bold** are life-threatening. ⊙ Do not crush.

every 8 hr—500 mg PO every 12 hr; severe infection—500 mg every 8 hr or 875 mg every 12 hr.

• *Postexposure anthrax prophylaxis:* 500 mg PO tid to complete a 60-day course after 14–21 days of a fluoroquinolone or doxycycline.

• *Lower respiratory infections:* 500 mg PO every 8 hr or 875 mg PO bid.

• *Uncomplicated gonococcal infections:* 3 g amoxicillin PO as a single dose.

• C. trachomatis *in pregnancy:* 500 mg PO tid for 7 days or 875 mg PO bid.

• *Tonsillitis or pharyngitis:* 775 mg/day PO for 10 days with food (ER tablet).

• H. pylori *infections:* 1 g bid with clarithromycin 500 mg bid and lansoprazole 30 mg bid for 14 days.

Pediatric patients 3 mo and older weighing less than 40 kg

• *URIs, GU infections, skin and soft-tissue infections:* Mild to moderate infection— 20 mg/kg/day PO in divided doses every 8 hr or 25 mg/kg/day PO in divided doses every 12 hr. Severe infection—40 mg/kg/day in divided doses every 8 hr or 45 mg/kg/day PO in divided doses every 12 hr.

• *Postexposure anthrax prophylaxis:* 80 mg/kg/day PO divided into 3 doses to complete a 60-day course after 14–21 days of fluoroquinolone or doxycycline therapy.

Pediatric patients 3 mo and older

• *Mild to moderate URIs, GU infections, and skin infections:* 20 mg/kg daily in divided doses every 8 hr or 25 mg/kg in divided doses every 12 hr.

• *Acute otitis media:* 80–90 mg/kg/day PO for 10 days (severe cases) or for 5–7 days (moderate cases).

• *Gonorrhea in prepubertal children:* 50 mg/kg PO with 25 mg/kg probenecid as a single dose (probenecid contraindicated in children younger than 2 yr).

• *For lower respiratory infections, or severe URIs, GU, or skin infections:* 40 mg/kg daily in divided doses every 8 hr or 45 mg/kg daily in divided doses every 12 hr.

Pediatric patients up to 12 wk

Up to 30 mg/kg daily in divided doses every 12 hr.

Patients with renal impairment

Do not use 875-mg tablet if GFR is less than 30 mL/min. For GFR of 10–30 mL/min, 250–500 mg every 12 hr; for GFR less than 10 mL/min, 250–500 mg every 24 hr; for hemodialysis patients, 250–500 mg every 24 hr with additional doses during and after dialysis.

Pharmacokinetics

Route	Onset	Peak	Duration
Oral	Varies	1 hr	6–8 hr

Metabolism: $T_{1/2}$: 1–1.4 hr
Distribution: Crosses placenta; enters breast milk
Excretion: Urine, unchanged

Adverse effects

• **CNS:** Lethargy, hallucinations, seizures
• **GI:** *Glossitis, stomatitis, gastritis, sore mouth,* furry tongue, black "hairy" tongue, *nausea, vomiting, diarrhea, abdominal pain,* bloody diarrhea, enterocolitis, pseudomembranous colitis, nonspecific hepatitis
• **GU:** Nephritis
• **Hematologic:** Anemia, thrombocytopenia, leukopenia, neutropenia, prolonged bleeding time
• **Hypersensitivity:** *Rash, fever, wheezing,* **anaphylaxis**
• **Other:** *Superinfections*—oral and rectal moniliasis, vaginitis

Interactions

✴ **Drug-drug** • Increased effect with probenecid • Decreased effectiveness with tetracyclines, chloramphenicol • Decreased efficacy of hormonal contraceptives
✴ **Drug-food** • Delayed or reduced GI absorption with food

■ Nursing considerations

Assessment

• **History:** Allergies to penicillins, cephalosporins, or other allergens; renal disorders; lactation
• **Physical:** Culture infected area; skin color, lesion; R, adventitious sounds; bowel sounds; CBC, LFTs, renal function tests, serum electrolytes, Hct, urinalysis

Interventions

• Culture infected area prior to treatment; reculture area if response is not as expected.
• Give in oral preparations only; amoxicillin is not affected by food. Ensure that patient does not cut, crush, or chew ER tablets.

- Continue therapy for at least 2 days after signs of infection have disappeared; continuation for 10 full days is recommended.
- Use corticosteroids or antihistamines for skin reactions.

Teaching points
- Take this drug around-the-clock.
- Take the full course of therapy; do not stop because you feel better. Do not cut, crush, or chew ER tablets (*Moxatag*).
- This antibiotic is specific for this problem and should not be used to self-treat other infections.
- Be aware that oral contraceptives may lose effectiveness while you are taking this drug; you should use a second form of contraception.
- You may experience these side effects: Nausea, vomiting, GI upset (eat frequent small meals); diarrhea; sore mouth (frequent mouth care may help).
- Report unusual bleeding or bruising, sore throat, fever, rash, hives, severe diarrhea, difficulty breathing.

DANGEROUS DRUG

▽amphotericin B
(am foe ter' i sin)

amphotericin B cholesteryl sulfate

amphotericin B, liposome
Abelcet, AmBisome, Amphotec

PREGNANCY CATEGORY B

Drug class
Antifungal

Therapeutic actions
Binds to sterols in the fungal cell membrane with a resultant change in membrane permeability, an effect that can destroy fungal cells and prevent their reproduction; fungicidal or fungistatic depending on concentration and organism.

Indications
- Reserve use for patients with progressive, potentially fatal infections: Cryptococcosis; North American blastomycosis; systemic candidiasis; disseminated moniliasis; coccidioidomycosis and histoplasmosis; mucormycosis caused by species of *Mucor, Rhizopus, Absidia, Conidiobolus, Basidiobolus;* sporotrichosis; aspergillosis. Not for use in treating noninvasive fungal infections
- Adjunct treatment of American mucocutaneous leishmaniasis (not choice in primary therapy)
- Treatment of aspergillosis in patients refractory to conventional therapy (*Abelcet, Amphotec*)
- Treatment of cryptococcal meningitis in HIV-infected patients (*AmBisome*)
- Treatment of invasive aspergillosis where renal toxicity precludes use of conventional amphotericin B (*Amphotec*)
- Treatment of presumed fungal infections in febrile, neutropenic patients (*AmBisome*)
- Treatment of *Aspergillis, Candida,* or *Cryptococcus* infections in patients intolerant to or refractory to conventional amphotericin B (*AmBisome*)
- Treatment of visceral leishmaniasis (*AmBisome*)
- Treatment of any type of progressive fungal infection that does not respond to conventional therapy
- Unlabeled uses: Prophylactic to prevent fungal infections in bone marrow transplants, bladder irrigation for candidal cystitis, primary treatment of amoebic meningoencephalitis, ocular aspergillosis, treatment of severe meningitis in patients unresponsive to IV therapy (intrathecal administration)

Contraindications and cautions
- Contraindicated with allergy to amphotericin B, renal impairment, lactation (except when life-threatening and treatable only with this drug).
- Use cautiously with pregnancy.

Available forms
Injection—50 mg; suspension for injection—5 mg/mL; powder for injection—50, 100 mg/vial

Dosages
Adults and pediatric patients
Abelcet
Consider test dose; if tolerated, may proceed to regular dosing regimen.

- *Fungal infections, systemic:* 5 mg/kg/day given as a single infusion at 2.5 mg/kg/hr.

Amphotec
Use test dose (10 mL of final preparation infused over 15–30 min).

- *Aspergillosis:* Initially, 3–4 mg/kg/day IV. Infuse at 1 mg/kg/hr.

AmBisome
Consider test dose; if tolerated, may proceed to regular dosing regimen.

- *Presumed fungal infection in febrile neutropenic patients:* 3 mg/kg/day IV.
- *Cryptococcal meningitis in HIV:* 6 mg/kg/day IV.
- *Aspergillosis:* 3 mg/kg/day IV, give over more than 2 hr.
- *Leishmaniasis:* 3 mg/kg/day IV, days 1–5, 14, and 21 for immunocompetent patients; 4 mg/kg/day IV, days 1–5, 10, 17, 24, 31, and 38 for immunocompromised patients.

Pharmacokinetics

Route	Onset	Peak	Duration
IV	20–30 min	1–2 hr	20–24 hr

Metabolism: $T_{1/2}$: 24 hr initially and then 15 days; 173.4 hr *(Abelcet)*
Distribution: Crosses placenta; may enter breast milk
Excretion: Urine

▼ IV FACTS

Abelcet: Shake vial gently until no yellow sediment is seen. Withdraw dose, replace needle with a 5-micron filter needle. Inject into bag containing 5% dextrose injection to a concentration of 1 mg/mL. May be further diluted. Store vials in refrigerator; stable for 48 hr once prepared if refrigerated, for 6 hr at room temperature.
Amphotec: Reconstitute with sterile water for injection. 10 mL to 50 mg/vial or 20 mL to 100 mg/vial. Dilute to 0.6 mg/mL. Refrigerate after reconstitution; use within 24 hr.
AmBisome: Add 12 mL sterile water to each vial to yield 4 mg/mL; immediately shake vial for 30 sec until yellow translucent suspension formed; draw up dose via syringe, attach 5 micron filter, and inject into appropriate volume at 5% dextrose to final concentration of 1–2 mg/mL (0.2–0.5 mg/mL for infants/small children).

Infusion: *Amphotericin B:* Protect from exposure to light if not infused within 8 hr of preparation. Infuse slowly over 6 hr.
Abelcet: Infuse at rate of 2.5 mg/kg/hr. If infusion takes more than 2 hr, remix bag by shaking.
Amphotec: Infuse at 1 mg/kg/hr over at least 2 hr; do not use an in-line filter.
AmBisome: Flush line with D_5W prior to infusion. Infuse over more than 2 hr if tolerated; stop immediately at any sign of anaphylactic reaction.

Incompatibilities: Do not mix with saline-containing solution, parenteral nutrional solutions, aminoglycosides, penicillins, phenothiazines, calcium preparations, cimetidine, methyldopa, polymyxin, potassium chloride, ranitidine, verapamil, clindamycin, cotrimoxazole, dopamine, dobutamine, tetracycline, vitamins, lidocaine, procaine, or heparin. **If line must be flushed, do not use heparin or saline; use D_5W.**
Y-site incompatibilities: Foscarnet, ondansetron.

Adverse effects
Systemic administration

- **CNS:** Fever (often with shaking chills), headache, malaise, generalized pain
- **GI:** *Nausea, vomiting, dyspepsia, diarrhea,* cramping, epigastric pain, anorexia
- **GU:** Hypokalemia, azotemia, hyposthenuria, renal tubular acidosis, nephrocalcinosis
- **Hematologic:** Normochromic, normocytic anemia
- **Local:** *Pain at the injection site* with phlebitis and thrombophlebitis
- **Other:** Weight loss

Interactions
✱ Drug-drug ● Do not administer with corticosteroids unless these are needed to control symptoms ● Increased risk of nephrotoxicity with other nephrotoxic antibiotics, antineoplastics, zidovudine ● Increased effects and risk of toxicity of digitalis, skeletal muscle relaxants, flucytosine ● Increased nephrotoxic effects with cyclosporine ● Increased risk of hypokalemia with thiazide diuretics

■ Nursing considerations

CLINICAL ALERT!

Dosages between the amphotericin products are not the same and are not interchangeable. Ensure correct drug is ordered and given.

Assessment

- **History:** Allergy to amphotericin B, renal impairment, lactation
- **Physical:** Skin color, lesions; T; weight; injection site; orientation, reflexes, affect; bowel sounds, liver evaluation; LFTs, renal function tests; CBC and differential; culture of area involved

Interventions

⊗ **Black box warning** Reserve use for progressive or potentially fatal infections; not for use in noninvasive disease; toxicity can be severe.

- Arrange for immediate culture of infection but begin treatment before lab results are returned.
- Monitor injection sites and veins for signs of phlebitis.
- Provide aspirin, antihistamines, and antiemetics, and maintain sodium balance to ease drug discomfort. Minimal use of IV corticosteroids may decrease febrile reactions. Meperidine has been used to relieve chills and fever.
- Amphotericin B products may cause severe electrolyte abnormalities, such as magnesium wasting. Monitor electrolytes often.
- Monitor renal function tests weekly; discontinue or decrease dosage of drug at any sign of increased renal toxicity.

Teaching points

- Long-term use of this drug will be needed; beneficial effects may not be seen for several weeks; the drug can only be given IV.
- Use good hygiene to prevent reinfection or spread of infection.
- You may experience these side effects: Nausea, vomiting, diarrhea (eat frequent small meals); discoloring, drying of the skin, staining of fabric with topical forms (washing with soap and water or cleaning fabric with standard cleaning fluid should remove stain); stinging, irritation with local application; fever, chills, muscle aches and pains, headache (medications may be ordered to help you to deal with these discomforts of the drug).
- Report pain, irritation at injection site; GI upset, nausea, loss of appetite; difficulty breathing; local irritation, burning (topical application).

▽ **ampicillin**
(am pi sill' in)

ampicillin sodium

Oral: Novo-Ampicillin (CAN), Principen

PREGNANCY CATEGORY B

Drug classes
Antibiotic
Penicillin

Therapeutic actions
Bactericidal action against sensitive organisms; inhibits synthesis of bacterial cell wall, causing cell death.

Indications

- Treatment of infections caused by susceptible strains of *Shigella, Salmonella, S. typhosa, Escherichia coli, Haemophilus influenzae, Proteus mirabilis, Neisseria gonorrhoeae,* enterococci, gram-positive organisms (penicillin G–sensitive staphylococci, streptococci, pneumococci)
- Meningitis caused by *Neisseria meningitidis*
- Prevention of bacterial endocarditis following dental, oral, or respiratory procedures in very high-risk patients
- Unlabeled use: Prophylaxis in cesarean section in certain high-risk patients

Contraindications and cautions

- Contraindicated with allergies to penicillins, cephalosporins, or other allergens.
- Use cautiously with renal disorders.

Available forms
Capsules—250, 500 mg; powder for oral suspension—125 mg/5 mL, 250 mg/5 mL; powder for injection—125, 250, 500 mg, 1, 2 g

Dosages

Maximum recommended dosage, 8–14 g/day (reserve 14 g for serious infections, such as meningitis, septicemia); may be given IV, IM, or PO. Use parenteral routes for severe infections; switch to oral route as soon as possible.

Adults

- *Prevention of bacterial endocarditis for dental, oral, or upper respiratory procedures in patients at high risk:* 2 g ampicillin IM or IV within 30 min of procedure.
- *GU infections:* 500 mg every 6 hr.
- *Respiratory tract infections:* 250 mg every 6 hr.
- *Digestive system infections:* 500 mg PO every 6 hr for 48–72 hr after patient becomes asymptomatic or eradication is evident.
- *STDs in patients allergic to tetracycline:* 3.5 g ampicillin PO with 1 g probenecid.

Pediatric patients

- *Prevention of bacterial endocarditis for GI or GU surgery or instrumentation:* 50 mg/kg ampicillin IM or IV within 30 minutes of procedure. Six hours later, give 25 mg/kg ampicillin IM or IV or 25 mg/kg amoxicillin PO.
- *Prevention of bacterial endocarditis for dental, oral, or upper respiratory procedures in patients at high risk:* 50 mg/kg ampicillin IM or IV within 30 min of procedure.

Adults and pediatric patients

- *Respiratory and soft-tissue infections:*
  40 kg or more: 250–500 mg IV or IM every 6 hr.
  Less than 40 kg: 25–50 mg/kg/day IM or IV in equally divided doses at 6- to 8-hr intervals.
  20 kg or more: 250 mg PO every 6 hr.
  Less than 20 kg: 50 mg/kg/day PO in equally divided doses every 6–8 hr.
- *GI and GU infections, including women with* N. gonorrhoeae:
  More than 40 kg: 500 mg IM or IV every 6 hr.
  40 kg or less: 50 mg/kg/day IM or IV in equally divided doses every 6–8 hr.
  20 kg or more: 500 mg PO every 6 hr.
  Less than 20 kg: 100 mg/kg/day PO in equally divided doses every 6–8 hr.
- *Bacterial meningitis:* 150–200 mg/kg/day by continuous IV drip and then IM injections in equally divided doses every 3–4 hr.
- *Septicemia:* 150–200 mg/kg/day IV for at least 3 days, then IM every 3–4 hr.

Patients with renal impairment

If creatinine clearance is 10–50 mL/min, give dose every 6–12 hr. If clearance is less than 10 mL/min, give dose every 12–16 hr.

Pharmacokinetics

Route	Onset	Peak	Duration
Oral	30 min	2 hr	6–8 hr
IM	15 min	1 hr	6–8 hr
IV	Immediate	5 min	6–8 hr

Metabolism: $T_{1/2}$: 1–2 hr
Distribution: Crosses placenta; enters breast milk
Excretion: Urine, unchanged

▼ IV FACTS

Preparation: Reconstitute with sterile or bacteriostatic water for injection; piggyback vials may be reconstituted with sodium chloride injection; use reconstituted solution within 1 hr. Do not mix in the same IV solution as other antibiotics. Use within 1 hr after preparation because potency may decrease significantly after that.

Infusion: 125-, 250-, or 500-mg dose given over 3–5 min; 1- or 2-g dose given over 10–15 min.

IV piggyback: Administer alone or further dilute with compatible solution.

Compatibilities: Ampicillin is compatible with 0.9% sodium chloride, D_5W, or 0.45% sodium chloride solution, 10% invert sugar water, M/6 sodium lactate solution, lactated Ringer's solution, sterile water for injection. Diluted solutions are stable for 2–8 hr; check manufacturer's inserts for specifics. Discard solution after allotted time period.

Incompatibilities: Do not mix with lidocaine, verapamil, other antibiotics, dextrose solutions.

Y-site incompatibilities: Do not give with epinephrine, hydralazine, or ondansetron.

Adverse effects

- **CNS:** Lethargy, hallucinations, seizures
- **CV:** Heart failure
- **GI:** *Glossitis, stomatitis, gastritis, sore mouth,* furry tongue, black "hairy" tongue, *nausea, vomiting, diarrhea,* abdominal pain, bloody diarrhea, enterocolitis, pseudomembranous colitis, nonspecific hepatitis
- **GU: Nephritis**

- **Hematologic:** Anemia, thrombocytopenia, leukopenia, neutropenia, prolonged bleeding time
- **Hypersensitivity:** *Rash, fever, wheezing,* anaphylaxis
- **Local:** *Pain, phlebitis,* thrombosis at injection site (parenteral)
- **Other:** *Superinfections*—oral and rectal moniliasis, vaginitis

Interactions

✳ **Drug-drug** • Increased ampicillin effect with probenecid • Increased risk of rash with allopurinol • Decreased effectiveness with tetracyclines, chloramphenicol • Decreased efficacy of hormonal contraceptives, atenolol with ampicillin
✳ **Drug-food** • Oral ampicillin may be less effective with food; take on an empty stomach
✳ **Drug-lab test** • False-positive Coombs' test if given IV • Decrease in plasma estrogen concentrations in pregnant women • False-positive urine glucose tests if Clinitest, Benedict's solution, or Fehling's solution is used; enzymatic glucose oxidase methods (*Clinistix, Tes-Tape*) should be used to check urine glucose

■ Nursing considerations
Assessment

- **History:** Allergies to penicillins, cephalosporins, or other allergens; renal disorders; lactation
- **Physical:** Culture infected area; skin color, lesion; R, adventitious sounds; bowel sounds; CBC, LFTs, renal function tests, serum electrolytes, Hct, urinalysis

Interventions

- Culture infected area before treatment; reculture area if response is not as expected.
- Check IV site carefully for signs of thrombosis or drug reaction.
- Do not give IM injections in the same site; atrophy can occur. Monitor injection sites.
- Administer oral drug on an empty stomach, 1 hr before or 2 hr after meals with a full glass of water; do not give with fruit juice or soft drinks.

Teaching points

- Take this drug around the clock.
- Take the full course of therapy; do not stop taking the drug if you feel better.

- Take the oral drug on an empty stomach, 1 hour before or 2 hours after meals; do not take with fruit juice or soft drinks; the oral solution is stable for 7 days at room temperature or 14 days refrigerated.
- This antibiotic is specific to your problem and should not be used to self-treat other infections.
- If you are a woman and you use a hormonal contraceptive, you should use a second form of birth control for 1–2 weeks while taking this drug.
- You may experience these side effects: Nausea, vomiting, GI upset (eat frequent small meals), diarrhea.
- Report pain or discomfort at sites, unusual bleeding or bruising, mouth sores, rash, hives, fever, itching, severe diarrhea, difficulty breathing.

▷ **anagrelide hydrochloride**
*(an **agh' rah** lide)*

Agrylin

PREGNANCY CATEGORY C

Drug class
Antiplatelet drug

Therapeutic actions
Thought to reduce platelet production by decreasing megakaryocyte hypermaturation; inhibits cyclic AMP and ADP collagen-induced platelet aggregation. At therapeutic doses has no effect on WBC counts or coagulation parameters; may affect RBC parameters.

Indications

- Treatment of essential thrombocythemia secondary to myeloproliferative disorders to reduce elevated platelet count and the risk of thrombosis and to improve associated symptoms, including thrombohemorrhagic events

Contraindications and cautions

- Contraindicated with known allergy to anagrelide or severe hepatic or renal impairment.

Adverse effects in *italics* are most common; those in **bold** are life-threatening. ⬤▭⬤ Do not crush.

- Use cautiously with renal or hepatic disorders, pregnancy, lactation, known heart disease, thrombocytopenia.

Available forms
Capsules—0.5, 1 mg

Dosages
Adults
Initially, 0.5 mg PO qid or 1 mg PO bid. After 1 wk, reevaluate and adjust the dosage as needed. Dosage is based on platelet counts; goal is less than 600,000 mm³. Do not increase by more than 0.5 mg/day each week. Maximum dose, 10 mg/day or 2.5 mg as a single dose.
Pediatric patients
Initially, 0.5 mg/day–0.5 mg qid. Adjust to lowest effective dose to keep platelet count below 600,000/mm³. Do not increase by more than 0.5 mg/day each week. Maximum dose, 10 mg/day or 2.5 mg in a single dose.
Patients with moderate hepatic impairment
Initially, 0.5 mg/day for at least 1 wk. Monitor patient closely. Do not increase dose by more than 0.5 mg/day in 1 wk.

Pharmacokinetics

Route	Onset	Peak
Oral	Rapid	1 hr

Metabolism: Hepatic; T$_{1/2}$: 1.3 hr
Distribution: Crosses placenta; may enter breast milk
Excretion: Feces, urine

Adverse effects
- **CNS:** Dizziness, *headaches, asthenia,* paresthesias
- **CV: Heart failure,** tachycardia, **MI, complete heart block,** atrial fibrillation, hypotension, *palpitations,* **stroke**
- **GI:** *Diarrhea, nausea, vomiting, abdominal pain,* flatulence, dyspepsia, anorexia, **pancreatitis,** ulcer
- **Hematologic:** *Thrombocytopenia,* anemia
- **Other:** Rash, purpura, edema

Interactions
✳ **Drug-food** • Risk of increased toxicity with grapefruit juice; avoid this combination

■ Nursing considerations

◆ CLINICAL ALERT!
Confusion has been reported with *Agrylin* and *Aggrastat* (tirofiban); use caution.

Assessment
- **History:** Allergy to anagrelide, thrombocytopenia, hemostatic disorders, bleeding ulcer, intracranial bleeding, severe liver disease, lactation, renal disorders, pregnancy, known heart disease
- **Physical:** Skin color, lesions; orientation; bowel sounds, normal output; CBC, LFTs, renal function tests

Interventions
- Perform platelet counts every 2 days during the first week of therapy and at least weekly thereafter; if thrombocytopenia occurs, decrease dosage of drug and arrange for supportive therapy. During first 2 wk, also monitor CBC, LFTs, serum creatinine, BUN.
- Administer drug on an empty stomach if at all tolerated.
- Establish safety precautions to prevent injury and bleeding (eg, use an electric razor, avoid contact sports).
- Monitor BP before and periodically during therapy.
- Advise patient to use barrier contraceptives while receiving this drug; it may harm the fetus.
- Monitor patient for any sign of excessive bleeding—eg, bruises, dark stools—and monitor bleeding times.
- Mark chart of any patient receiving anagrelide to alert medical personnel of potential for increased bleeding in cases of surgery or dental surgery, invasive procedures.

Teaching points
- Take drug on an empty stomach.
- Do not drink grapefruit juice while on this drug.
- You will need frequent and regular blood tests to monitor your response to this drug.
- It may take longer than normal to stop bleeding while taking this drug, so avoid contact sports, use electric razors, and take other precautions to avoid bleeding. Apply pressure for extended periods to bleeding sites.

- Avoid pregnancy while taking this drug because it could harm the fetus. Using barrier contraceptives is suggested.
- Notify any dentist or surgeon that you are taking this drug before invasive procedures.
- You may experience these side effects: Upset stomach, nausea, diarrhea, loss of appetite (eat frequent small meals).
- Report fever, chills, sore throat, rash, bruising, bleeding, dark stools or urine, palpitations, chest pain.

▽ **anakinra**

(ann ack' in rah)

Kineret

PREGNANCY CATEGORY B

Drug classes
Antiarthritic
Interleukin-1 receptor antagonist

Therapeutic actions
A recombinant human interleukin-1 receptor antagonist; blocks the activity of interleukin 1 that is elevated in response to inflammatory and immune stimulation and is responsible for the degradation of cartilage due to the rapid loss of proteoglycans in rheumatoid arthritis.

Indications
- Reduction of the signs and symptoms and slowing of progression of moderately to severely active rheumatoid arthritis in patients 18 yr and older who have failed on one or more disease-modifying antirheumatic drugs (methotrexate, sulfasalazine, hydroxychloroquine, gold, penicillamine, leflunomide, azathioprine); used alone or with disease-modifying anti-rheumatic drugs other than tumor necrosis factor blocking agents
- Unlabeled use: Juvenile idiopathic arthritis

Contraindications and cautions
- Contraindicated with allergy to anakinra or proteins produced by *Escherichia coli.*
- Use cautiously with immunosuppression, active infection, pregnancy, lactation, renal impairment.

Available forms
Prefilled glass syringes—100 mg/0.67 mL

Dosages
Adults
- 100 mg/day subcutaneously at approximately the same time each day.
Pediatric patients
- Safety and efficacy not established.
Patients with renal impairment
For patients with end-stage renal disease or creatinine clearance less than 30 mL/min, 100 mg every other day.

Pharmacokinetics

Route	Onset	Peak
Subcut.	Slow	3–7 hr

Metabolism: Tissue; $T_{1/2}$: 4–6 hr
Distribution: May cross placenta; may enter breast milk
Excretion: Urine

Adverse effects
- **CNS:** Headache
- **GI:** Nausea, diarrhea, abdominal pain
- **Hematologic:** Neutropenia, thrombocytopenia
- **Respiratory:** *URI, sinusitis*
- **Other:** *Injection-site reactions, infections,* flulike symptoms

Interactions
✳ **Drug-drug** ⊗ *Warning* Increased risk of serious infections and neutropenia if combined with etanercept or other tumor necrosis factor blocking drugs; avoid this combination (if no alternative is available; use extreme caution and monitor patient closely)
- Immunizations given while on anakinra may be less effective

■ **Nursing considerations**

CLINICAL ALERT!
Name confusion has occurred between anakinra and amikacin; use caution.

Assessment
- **History:** Allergy to anakinra or proteins produced by *E. coli,* immunosuppression, renal impairment, pregnancy, lactation
- **Physical:** T, body weight, P, BP, R, adventitious sounds, CBC, renal function tests

Adverse effects in *italics* are most common; those in **bold** are life-threatening. ⊞ Do not crush.

Interventions

- Make sure that patient does not have an active infection before administering.
- Store the drug in the refrigerator, protected from light; use by expiration date because solution contains no preservatives.
- Administer the subcutaneous injection at about the same time each day.
- Inspect solution before injection. Do not use solution if it is discolored or contains particulate matter.
- Discard any unused portion of the drug; do not store for later use.
- Provide analgesics if headache or muscle pain are a problem.
- Monitor injection sites for erythema, ecchymosis, inflammation, and pain. Rotating sites may help to decrease severe reactions.
- Advise women of childbearing age to use a barrier form of contraception while taking this drug.
- Monitor CBC before and periodically during therapy; drug should not be given during active infections.

Teaching points

- This drug must be injected subcutaneously once each day at approximately the same time each day.
- The drug must be stored in the refrigerator, protected from light. Use the drug by the expiration date on the box; the drug contains no preservatives and will not be effective after that date. Do not use any drug that is discolored or contains particulate matter.
- You and a family member or significant other should learn the proper way to administer a subcutaneous injection, including the proper disposal of needles and syringes. Prepare a chart of injection sites to ensure that you rotate the sites. Dispose of syringes in appropriate container.
- Avoid infection while you are taking this drug; avoid crowded areas or people with known infections.
- This drug does not cure your rheumatoid arthritis, and appropriate therapies to deal with the disease should be followed.
- You may experience these side effects: Reactions at the injection site (rotating sites and applying heat may help); headache, pain (use of an analgesic may help; consult your health care provider); increased risk of infection (contact your health care provider at any sign of infection [fever, muscular aches and pains, respiratory problems] because it may be necessary to stop the drug during the infection).
- Report fever, chills, difficulty breathing, severe discomfort at injection site.

DANGEROUS DRUG

▽ anastrozole
(an **abs**' troh zol)

Arimidex

PREGNANCY CATEGORY X

Drug classes

Antiestrogen
Aromatase inhibitor

Therapeutic actions

Selective nonsteroidal aromatase inhibitor that significantly reduces serum estradiol levels with no significant effect on adrenocortical steroids or aldosterone.

Indications

- Treatment of advanced breast cancer in postmenopausal women with disease progression following tamoxifen therapy
- First-line treatment of postmenopausal women with hormone receptor positive or hormone receptor unknown locally advanced or metastatic breast cancer
- Adjuvant treatment of postmenopausal women with hormone receptor positive early breast cancer
- Unlabeled uses: Male infertility, breast cancer prevention

Contraindications and cautions

- Contraindicated with allergy to anastrozole, pregnancy, lactation.
- Use cautiously with hepatic or renal impairment, high cholesterol states.

Available forms

Tablets—1 mg

Dosages

Adults
1 mg PO daily.
Pediatric patients
Not recommended.

Pharmacokinetics

Route	Onset	Peak
Oral	Varies	2 hr

Metabolism: Hepatic; T$_{1/2}$: 50 hr
Distribution: Crosses placenta; enters breast milk
Excretion: Feces, urine

Adverse effects

- **CNS:** Depression, light-headedness, dizziness, *asthenia, headache,* **insomnia**
- **CV:** Vasodilation, hypertension, ischemic CV events
- **Dermatologic:** *Hot flashes, rash*
- **GI:** *Nausea, vomiting,* food distaste, dry mouth, *pharyngitis,* constipation
- **GU:** Vaginal bleeding, vaginal pain, UTIs
- **Other:** *Peripheral edema, bone pain, back pain; decreased bone density;* increased HDL, LDL levels; *fractures*

Interactions

✻ Drug-drug • Loss of effectiveness with estrogens; combination is not recommended
• Decreased effectiveness with tamoxifen; avoid this combination

■ Nursing considerations

Assessment

- **History:** Allergy to anastrozole, hepatic or renal impairment, pregnancy, lactation, treatment profile for breast cancer, hypercholesterolemia
- **Physical:** Skin lesions, color, turgor; pelvic examination; orientation, affect, reflexes; peripheral pulses, edema; LFTs, renal function tests

Interventions

- Administer once daily without regard to meals.
- Arrange for periodic lipid profiles during therapy.
- Arrange for appropriate analgesic measures if pain and discomfort become severe.

Teaching points

- Take the drug once a day without regard to meals.
- You may experience these side effects: Bone pain; hot flashes (staying in cool temperatures may help); nausea, vomiting (eat frequent small meals); dizziness, headache,

light-headedness (use caution if driving or performing tasks that require alertness); birth defects (avoid pregnancy; use of barrier contraceptives is advised).
- Report changes in color of stool or urine, severe vomiting, or inability to eat.

▷ **anidulafungin**
(an ah doo' lah fun gin)

Eraxis

PREGNANCY CATEGORY C

Drug classes

Antifungal
Echinocandin

Therapeutic actions

Inhibits glucan synthesis, an enzyme present in fungal cells but not human cells; this inhibition prevents the fungal cell wall from forming and results in cell death.

Indications

- Treatment of candidemia and other forms of *Candida* infections (intra-abdominal abscess, peritonitis)
- Treatment of esophageal candidiasis
- Unlabeled use: Catheter-related bloodstream infections

Contraindications and cautions

- Contraindicated with hypersensitivity to anidulafungin or any other echinocandin, or to any component of the drug.
- Use cautiously with liver impairment, pregnancy, lactation.

Available forms

Single-use vials—50, 100 mg with diluent vial

Dosages

Adults

- Treatment of candidemia and other forms *Candida* infections: 200 mg by IV infusion on day 1, then 100 mg/day by IV infusion; generally continued for at least 14 days after the last positive culture.
- Esophageal candidiasis: 100 mg by IV infusion on day 1, then 50 mg/day by IV infusion

---

for a minimum of 14 days and for at least 7 days following resolution of symptoms.

Pediatric patients
Safety and efficacy not established.

Pharmacokinetics

Route	Onset	Peak
IV infusion	Rapid	End of infusion

Metabolism: Degradation; $T_{1/2}$: 40–50 hr
Distribution: May cross placenta; may enter breast milk
Excretion: Feces

▼ IV FACTS

Preparation: Reconstitute with the diluent provided, giving a concentration of 3.33 mg/mL; then dilute with 5% dextrose injection or 0.9% sodium chloride injection to a concentration of 0.5 mg/mL. Store prepared solution at room temperature; must be used within 24 hr after dilution. Inspect solution for particulate matter or discoloration, and discard if observed.
Infusion: Infuse at no more than 1.1 mg/min.
Incompatibilities: Do not combine with any other drug or with any solution other than those listed.

Adverse effects

- **CNS:** Headache
- **CV:** Hypotension
- **GI:** Nausea, abdominal pain, vomiting, dyspepsia, elevated liver enzymes
- **Hematologic:** Leukopenia, neutropenia
- **Other:** Rash, urticaria, flushing, pruritus

■ Nursing considerations

Assessment

- **History:** Hypersensitivity to anidulafungin or any other echinocandin or to any component of the drug, hepatic impairment, pregnancy, lactation
- **Physical:** Skin, BP, abdominal examination, LFTs, culture of infected area

Interventions

- Culture infected area prior to starting drug; drug can be started before results are known, but appropriate adjustments in treatment should be made when culture results are evaluated.

- Periodically monitor LFTs to make sure hepatotoxicity does not occur.
- Suggest the use of contraceptive measures while using this drug; the potential effects on a fetus are not known.
- Advise breast-feeding mothers that another method of feeding the infant will need to be used while on this drug.
- Provide supportive measures if histamine reaction occurs; symptoms include hypotension, flushing, rash. A reaction is less likely if infusion rate does not exceed 1.1 mg/min.

Teaching points

- This drug must be given by a daily IV infusion.
- It is very important to maintain your fluid and food intake, which will help healing. Notify your health care provider if nausea or vomiting prevents this.
- You may need blood tests to evaluate the effects of the drug on your body.
- It is not known how this drug could affect a fetus, if you are pregnant or decide to become pregnant while on this drug, consult your health care provider.
- It is not known how this drug could affect a breast-feeding infant. If you are breast-feeding, another method of feeding the baby should be selected.
- You may experience these side effects: Headache, nausea (consult your health care provider, medications may be available that could help).
- Report changes in the color of urine or stool, rash, yellowing of the skin or eyes, extreme fatigue, shortness of breath, tightness in the chest.

▽ antihemophilic factor (AHF, Factor VIII)

(an tee hee moe fill' ik fack' tur)

Advate, Alphanate, Helixate FS, Hemofil M, Humate-P, Koate-DVI, Kogenate FS, Monoclate-P, Recombinate, ReFacto, Wilate, Xyntha

PREGNANCY CATEGORY C

Drug class
Antihemophilic

Therapeutic actions

A normal plasma protein that is needed for the transformation of prothrombin to thrombin, the final step of the intrinsic clotting pathway.

Indications

- Treatment of classical hemophilia (hemophilia A), in which there is a demonstrated deficiency of factor VIII; provides a temporary replacement of clotting factors to correct or prevent bleeding episodes or to allow necessary surgery
- Short-term prophylaxis (*ReFacto*) to reduce frequency of spontaneous bleeding
- Surgical and/or invasive procedures in patients with von Willebrand disease in whom desmopressin is ineffective or contraindicated to control bleeding; not for major surgery (*Advate, Alphanate, Xyntha*)
- ■■ **NEW INDICATION:** Routine prophylaxis to prevent or reduce the frequency of bleeding episodes in patients with hemophilia A (*Advate*)

Contraindications and cautions

- Contraindicated with antibodies to mouse, hamster, or bovine proteins or to porcine or murine factor.
- Use cautiously with pregnancy.

Available forms

IV injection—250, 500, 1,000, 1,500, 2,000, 3,000 international units/vial in numerous preparations; 450, 900 units (*Wilate*)

Dosages

Adult and pediatric patients

Administer IV using a plastic syringe; dose depends on weight, severity of deficiency, and severity of bleeding. Follow treatment carefully with factor VIII level assays.

Formulas used as a guide for dosage are:

$$\text{(\% of normal)} = \frac{\text{Expected Factor VIII increase}}{\text{weight in kg}}$$

$$\text{AHF/IU required} = \text{weight (kg)} \times \text{desired factor VIII increase (\% of normal)} \times 0.5$$

- *Prophylaxis of spontaneous hemorrhage:* Level of factor VIII required to prevent spontaneous hemorrhage is 5% of normal; 30%

of normal is the minimum required for hemostasis following trauma or surgery; smaller doses may be needed if treated early. *ReFacto* is given at least two times per wk for short-term prevention or to decrease the frequency of spontaneous musculoskeletal hemorrhage in patients with hemophilia.

- *Prevention of bleeding episodes:* 20–40 international units/kg every other day (three to four times per wk) IV; or give dose every third day. Base dose on patient response to maintain factor VIII through levels at 1% or more (*Advate*).
- *Mild hemorrhage:* Do not repeat therapy unless further bleeding occurs.
- *Moderate hemorrhage or minor surgery:* 30%–50% of normal is desired for factor VIII levels; initial dose of 15–25 AHF/international units/kg with maintenance dose of 10–15 AHF/international units/kg every 8–12 hr is usually sufficient. (*Koate-DVI*)
- *Severe hemorrhage:* Factor VIII level of 80%–100% normal is desired; initial dose of 40–50 AHF/international units/kg and a maintenance dose of 20–25 AHF/international units/kg is given every 8–12 hr (*Monoclate-P, Koate-DVI*).
- *Major surgery:* Dose of AHF to achieve factor VIII levels of 80%–100% of normal given as a preoperative dose of 50 units/kg an hour before surgery; repeat infusions may be necessary every 6–12 hr initially. Maintain factor VIII levels at least 30% normal for a healing period of 10–14 days (*Koate-DVI*).
- *Surgery/invasive procedures:* Preoperative dose 60 international units/kg; infusion of 40–60 international units/kg at 8- to 12-hr intervals. *Children:* 75 international units/kg preoperatively; then 50–75 international units/kg infused at 8- to 12-hr intervals (*Alphanate*).
- *Dental extraction:* Factor VIII level of 60%–80% is recommended; administer 1 hr before procedure in combination with antifibrinolytic therapy (*Hemofil M*).

Pharmacokinetics

Route	Onset
IV	Immediate

Metabolism: $T_{1/2}$: 12 hr
Distribution: Does not readily cross placenta

Adverse effects in *italics* are most common; those in **bold** are life-threatening. ◉■◉ Do not crush.

Excretion: Cleared from the body by normal metabolism

▼ IV FACTS

Preparation: Reconstitute using solution provided. Refrigerate unreconstituted preparations. Before reconstitution, warm diluent and dried concentrate to room temperature. Add diluent and rotate or shake vial until completely dissolved. Do not refrigerate reconstituted preparations; give within 3 hr of reconstitution.

Infusion: Give by IV only; use a plastic syringe; solutions may stick to glass. Give preparations at a rate of 2 mL/min; can be given at up to 10 mL/min; administration of entire dose in 5–10 min is generally well tolerated.

Adverse effects

- **Allergic reactions:** Erythema, hives, fever, backache, **bronchospasm,** urticaria, chills, nausea, *stinging at the infusion site,* vomiting, headache
- **Hematologic:** Hemolysis with large or frequently repeated doses
- **Other: Hepatitis, AIDS** (risks associated with repeated use of blood products)

■ Nursing considerations
Assessment

- **History:** Antibodies to mouse, hamster, or bovine protein; porcine or murine factor; von Willebrand disease; pregnancy
- **Physical:** Skin color, lesions; P, peripheral perfusion; R, adventitious sounds; factor VIII levels, Hct, direct Coombs' test, HIV screening, hepatitis screening

Interventions

- Monitor pulse during administration; if a significant increase occurs, reduce the rate or discontinue and consult physician.
- Monitor patient's clinical response and factor VIII levels regularly; if no response is noted with large doses, consider the presence of factor VIII inhibitors and need for anti-inhibitor complex therapy.

Teaching points

- Dosage is highly variable. All known safety precautions are taken to ensure that this blood product is pure and the risk of AIDS and hepatitis is as minimal as possible.

- Wear or carry a medical alert ID tag to alert medical emergency personnel that you require this treatment.
- Report headache; rash, itching; backache; difficulty breathing.

▷ antithrombin, recombinant

See Appendix R, *Less commonly used drugs.*

▷ antithrombin III

See Appendix R, *Less commonly used drugs.*

▷ apomorphine

See Appendix R, *Less commonly used drugs.*

▷ aprepitant
(ah pre' pit ant)
Emend

fosaprepitant
Emend for Injection

PREGNANCY CATEGORY B

Drug classes
Antiemetic
Substance P and neurokinin 1 receptor antagonist

Therapeutic actions
Selectively blocks human substance P and neurokinin 1 (NK1) receptors in the CNS, blocking the nausea and vomiting caused by highly emetogenic chemotherapeutic agents. Does not affect serotonin, dopamine, or corticosteroid receptors.

Indications

- In combination with other antiemetics for prevention of acute and delayed nausea and vomiting associated with initial and repeat courses of moderately or highly emetogenic cancer chemotherapy, including high-dose cisplatin
- Prevention of postoperative nausea and vomiting (oral only)

Contraindications and cautions

- Contraindicated with hypersensitivity to any component of aprepitant, concurrent use of pimozide, lactation.
- Use cautiously with concomitant use of any CYP3A4 inhibitors (docetaxel, vinblastine, vincristine, ifosfamide, irinotecen, imatinib, vinorelbine, paclitaxel, etoposide), warfarin and with pregnancy, severe hepatic impairment.

Available forms

Capsules—40, 80, 125 mg; powder for injection—150 mg (fosaprepitant)

Dosages

Adults

- *Highly emetogenic cancer chemotherapy:* 150 mg IV (fosaprepitant) over 20–30 min, starting 30 min prior to chemotherapy or 125 mg PO 1 hr prior to chemotherapy (day 1) and 80 mg PO once daily in the morning on days 2 and 3; given in combination with 12 mg dexamethasone PO 30 min before chemotherapy on day 1 and 8 mg dexamethasone PO days 2 to 4 and 32 mg ondansetron IV on day 1 only.
- *Moderately emetogenic cancer chemotherapy:* 115 mg IV (fosaprepitant) over 15 min, starting 30 min prior to chemotherapy or 125 mg PO 1 hr before chemotherapy on day 1 with 12 mg dexamethasone PO and two 8-mg doses ondansetron PO (the first given 1 hr before, the second 8 hr after chemotherapy); 80 mg PO on days 2 and 3 in the morning.
- *Postopereative nausea and vomiting:* 40 mg PO within 3 hr before induction of anesthesia.

Pediatric patients

Safety and efficacy not established.

- *Parenteral administration (fosaprepitant):* 115 mg IV 30 min before chemotherapy on day 1 of antiemetic regimen; infuse over 15 min. Use oral form on days 2 and 3.

Pharmacokinetics

Route	Onset	Peak
Oral	Rapid	4 hr

Metabolism: Hepatic; $T_{1/2}$: 9–13 hr
Distribution: Crosses placenta; enters breast milk
Excretion: Feces, urine

▼ IV FACTS

Preparation: Inject 5 mL 0.9% sodium chloride along vial wall to prevent foaming. Swirl vial gently. Add to infusion bag containing 110 mL saline; gently invert bag two to three times. Drug is stable for 24 hr at room temperature.
Infusion: Infuse over 15–30 min.
Incompatibilities: Do not mix with other solutions; do not mix with divalent cations such as lactated Ringer's solution or Hartmann's solution.

Adverse effects

- **CNS:** Dizziness, *anorexia,* neuropathy, tinnitus, headache, insomnia, asthenia
- **GI:** *Constipation, diarrhea,* epigastric discomfort, gastritis, heartburn, *nausea,* vomiting, elevated ALT or AST, abdominal pain, stomatitis
- **Respiratory:** Hiccups
- **Other:** *Fatigue,* dehydration, fever, neutropenia

Interactions

✳ **Drug-drug** • Risk of increased serum levels and toxic effects of aprepitant and pimozide if combined; do not use this combination • Possible increased serum levels of docetaxel, paclitaxel, etoposide, irinotecan, ifosfamide, imatinib, vinorelbine, vinblastine, vincristine, paclitaxel; monitor patient very closely if this combination is used • Increased risk of decreased effectiveness of warfarin if combined with aprepitant; monitor patient closely and adjust warfarin dose as needed • Risk of decreased effectiveness of hormonal contraceptives if combined with aprepitant; suggest using barrier contraceptives while aprepitant is being used • Risk of altered response when aprepitant is combined with any drug that inhibits CYP3A4; use caution when adding any drug to a regimen that contains aprepitant

■ Nursing considerations

Assessment

- **History:** Hypersensitivity to any component of aprepitant, concurrent use of pimozide; lactation, concomitant use of any CYP3A4 inhibitors; pregnancy
- **Physical:** T, orientation, reflexes, affect; bowel sounds; LFT, CBC

Interventions

- Administer first oral dose along with dexamethasone 1 hr before beginning of chemotherapy. Give IV 15–30 min before chemotherapy.
- Administer additional doses of dexamethasone as well as ondansetron as indicated as part of antiemetic regimen.
- Administer within 3 hr before induction of anesthesia if used to prevent postoperative nausea and vomiting.
- Establish safety precautions (eg, side rails, assistance with ambulation, proper lighting) if CNS, visual effects occur.
- Provide appropriate analgesics for headache if needed.
- Suggest the use of barrier contraceptives to women of childbearing age.

Teaching points

- When giving drug to prevent postoperative nausea and vomiting, incorporate teaching into overall teaching plan.
- This drug is given as part of a drug regimen to alleviate the nausea and vomiting associated with your chemotherapy drug; take the first dose 1 hour before your chemotherapy and then again in the morning of days 2 and 3; you will also be taking dexamethasone and, possibly, ondansetron with this drug.
- If you miss a dose, take the drug as soon as you think of it. If you miss an entire day, consult your health care provider. Do not take two doses in the same day.
- You should avoid getting pregnant while receiving chemotherapy. Using barrier contraceptives is advised; hormonal contraceptives may be ineffective while you are taking *Emend.*
- If you are breast-feeding, another method of feeding the infant should be used.
- Tell any health care provider who is taking care of you that you are taking this drug— it may react with many other drugs; you should not add or remove any drugs from your medical regimen without checking with your health care provider.
- You may experience these side effects: Dizziness, drowsiness (if these occur, use caution if driving or performing tasks that require alertness); constipation; headache (appropriate medication will be arranged to alleviate this problem).

- Report changes in color of urine or stool, severe constipation or diarrhea, severe headache.

▽ arformoterol tartrate

*(ar for **mob**' ter ol)*

Brovana

PREGNANCY CATEGORY C

Drug classes

Beta$_2$-adrenergic agonist, long-acting
Bronchodilator

Therapeutic actions

Long-acting agonist that binds to beta$_2$-adrenergic receptors in the lungs, causing bronchodilation; also inhibits release of inflammatory mediators in the lungs, blocking swelling and inflammation.

Indications

- Long-term maintenance treatment of bronchoconstriction in patients with COPD, including chronic bronchitis and emphysema

Contraindications and cautions

- Contraindicated with allergy to any component of the drug, acutely deteriorating COPD, acute bronchospasm, asthma without the use of a long-term control medication.
- Use cautiously with CV disease, convulsive disorders, thyrotoxicosis, pregnancy, lactation.

Available forms

Inhalation solution—7.5 mcg/mL

Dosages

Adults
15 mcg bid (morning and evening) by nebulization. Do not exceed total daily dose of 30 mcg.
Pediatric patients
Safety and efficacy not established.

Pharmacokinetics

Route	Onset	Peak
Inhalation	Rapid	30–60 min

Metabolism: Direct conjugation; T$_{1/2}$: 26 hr
Distribution: Crosses placenta; may pass into breast milk
Excretion: Urine

Adverse effects

- **CV:** Hypertension, prolonged QT interval, tachycardia, chest pain, peripheral edema
- **GI:** Diarrhea
- **Musculoskeletal:** Leg cramps
- **Respiratory: Paradoxical broncho-spasm,** dyspnea, chest congestion, sinusi-tis, **increase in asthma-related deaths**
- **Skin:** Rash
- **Other:** Pain, flulike symptoms

Interactions

✳ Drug-drug • Potential for increased toxicity if combined with MAOIs, TCAs, drugs that prolong the QT interval; use caution • Risk for decreased therapeutic effects and severe bronchospasm if combined with beta-adrenergic blockers; avoid this combination if at all possible; use a beta-specific blocker if combination must be used • Increased risk of hypokalemia if combined with non–potassium-sparing diuretics

■ Nursing considerations
Assessment

- **History:** Allergy to any component of the drug, acutely deteriorating COPD, acute bron-chospasm, CV disease, convulsive disorders, thyrotoxicosis, pregnancy, lactation
- **Physical:** Skin color, lesions; R, adventitious sounds; P, BP, baseline ECG

Interventions

⊗ **Black box warning** Long-lasting beta agonists may increase risk of asthma-related death; alert patient accordingly. Contraindicated for use in asthma without use of a long-term control med-ication.

- Ensure that drug is not used to treat acute attacks or worsening or deteriorating COPD.
- Instruct patient in the proper use of nebuliz-er; instruct patient not to swallow or inject solution.
- Ensure that patient continues with appropri-ate use of other drugs to manage COPD as in-structed.
- Store foil pouches in the refrigerator; use im-mediately after opening.
- Arrange for periodic evaluation of respirato-ry condition while on this drug.

Teaching points

- This drug is not for use during an acute at-tack, use your rescue medication if you are having an acute problem.

- You should take this drug through your neb-ulizer in the morning and in the evening.
- You should be aware that this type of drug is associated with an increased risk of asthma-related deaths; you should discuss this with your health care provider.
- Use this drug in your nebulizer only; do not swallow or inject this solution.
- The foil pouches should be stored in the re-frigerator and protected from heat and light. Do not use after the expiration date. Use im-mediately after opening the foil pouch.
- Do not use any solution that is discolored or contains particles.
- Arrange for periodic evaluation of your res-piratory problem while on this drug.
- It is not known if this drug could affect a fe-tus. If you are pregnant, or are thinking about becoming pregnant, consult your health care provider.
- It is not known how this drug could affect a breast-feeding infant; discuss the use of this drug during lactation with your health care provider.
- You should continue to use other medications prescribed for the treatment of your COPD as directed by your health care provider.
- Report palpitations, worsening of your COPD, tremors, nervousness.

▽ argatroban

See Appendix R, *Less commonly used drugs.*

▽ aripiprazole
*(air eh **pip'** rah zole)*

Abilify, Abilify Discmelt

PREGNANCY CATEGORY C

Drug classes

Atypical antipsychotic
Dopamine, serotonin agonist and antagonist
Psychotropic drug

Therapeutic actions

Acts as an agonist at dopamine and serotonin sites and antagonist at other serotonin recep-tor sites.

Indications

- Treatment of schizophrenia in patients 13 yr and older

Adverse effects in *italics* are most common; those in **bold** are life-threatening. ⬛ Do not crush.

A

- Treatment of major depressive disorder as adjunct to antidepressant therapy
- Treatment and maintenance of acute manic and mixed episodes associated with bipolar disorders in patients 10 yr and older
- Adjunct to lithium or valproate for acute treatment and maintenance of manic or mixed episodes associated with bipolar disorder in patients 10 yr and older
- Irritability associated with autistic disorder in children 6–17 yr
- Treatment of agitation associated with schizophrenia or bipolar disorder, manic or mixed (injection)
- Unlabeled uses: Restless leg syndrome, cocaine dependence, Tourette syndrome

Contraindications and cautions

- Contraindicated with allergy to aripiprazole, lactation.
- Use cautiously with suicidal ideation, pregnancy, cerebral vascular disease or other conditions causing hypotension, known CV disease, seizure disorders, exposure to extreme heat, Alzheimer's disease, dysphagia (risk for aspiration pneumonia), parkinsonism, elderly patients with dementia-related psychosis.

Available forms

Tablets—2, 5, 10, 15, 20, 30 mg; oral solution—1 mg/mL; orally disintegrating tablets—10, 15 mg; injection—7.5 mg/mL

Dosages
Adults
- *Schizophrenia:* 10–15 mg/day PO. Increase dose every 2 wk to maximum of 30 mg/day. Oral solution may be substituted on a mg-to-mg basis up to 25 mg of tablet. Patients taking 30-mg tablets should receive 25 mg if switched to solution.
- *Bipolar disorder:* 15 mg/day PO as one dose; maintenance dosage, 15–30 mg/day PO. Oral solution may be substituted on a mg-to-mg basis to 25 mg. Patients taking 30-mg tablets should take 25 mg if switched to solution.
- *Major depressive disorder:* Initial dose, 2–5 mg/day PO; maintenance dose, 2–15 mg/day as adjunct therapy. Dose adjustments up to 5 mg/day should occur at intervals of 1 wk or longer.

- *Agitation:* 5.25–15 mg IM; usual dose, 9.75 mg IM. Cumulative doses of up to 30 mg/day may be given.
Pediatric patients 13–17 yr
- *Schizophrenia:* Initially, 2 mg/day PO. Adjust to 5 mg/day after 2 days then to target dosage of 10 mg/day. Maximum, 30 mg/day.
Pediatric patients 10–17 yr
- *Bipolar disorder:* Initially, 2 mg/day PO; titrate to 5 mg/day after 2 days, then to 10 mg/day after another 2 days. Target dose, 10 mg/day; maximum dose, 30 mg/day.
Pediatric patients 6–17 yr
- *Irritability associated with autistic disorder:* 2 mg/day PO; titrate to maintenance dosage of 5–15 mg/day.

Pharmacokinetics

Route	Onset	Peak
Oral	Slow	3–5 hr
IM	Rapid	1–3 hr

Metabolism: Hepatic; $T_{1/2}$: 75 hr for extensive metabolizers, 146 hr for poor metabolizers
Distribution: May cross placenta; may enter breast milk
Excretion: Urine and feces

Adverse effects

- **CNS:** Headache, anxiety, insomnia, lightheadedness, somnolence, tremor, asthenia, tardive dyskinesia, blurred vision, **seizures (potentially life-threatening),** akathisia, dizziness, restlessness
- **CV:** Orthostatic hypotension
- **Dermatologic:** Rash
- **GI:** Nausea, vomiting, constipation, diarrhea, abdominal pain, esophageal dysmotility
- **Respiratory:** Rhinitis, cough
- **Other:** Fever, **neuroleptic malignant syndrome, increased suicide risk,** development of diabetes mellitus

Interactions

✳ **Drug-drug** • Risk of serious toxic effects if combined with strong inhibitors of the CYP3A4 system (such as ketoconazole), if any of these drug are being used, initiate treatment with one-half the usual dose of aripiprazole and monitor patient closely • Potential for increased serum levels and toxicity if taken with potential CYP2D6 inhibitors—quinidine, fluoxetine, paroxetine; reduce the dose of aripiprazole to one-half the normal dose • Decreased serum levels and loss of effectiveness if combined with CYP3A4 inducers such as carbamazepine—dosage of aripiprazole should be doubled and the patient monitored closely Risk of severe sedation, orthostatic hypotension if IM aripiprazole is combined with lorazepam injection • Risk of increased CNS depression and impairment if combined with alcohol or other CNS depressants

■ Nursing considerations

> ★ **CLINICAL ALERT!**
> Confusion between aripiprazole and proton pump inhibitors has occurred; use extreme caution.

Assessment

- **History:** Allergy to aripiprazole, lactation, suicidal ideation, pregnancy, hypotension or known CV disease, seizure disorders, exposure to extreme heat, patients with Alzheimer's disease, dysphagia, parkinsonism
- **Physical:** T, orientation, reflexes, vision; BP; R; abdominal examination

Interventions

⊗ *Black box warning* Elderly patients with dementia-related psychosis have an increased risk of death if given atypical antipsychotics; these drugs are not approved for treating patients with dementia-related psychosis.

⊗ *Black box warning* Risk of suicidal ideation increases with antidepressant drug use, especially in children, adolescents, and young adults. Observe and monitor patient accordingly.

- Dispense the least amount of drug possible to patients with suicidal ideation.
- Have patient place orally disintegrating tablet on tongue, allow to dissolve, then swallow.
- Protect patient from extremes of heat; monitor BP if overheating occurs.
- Administer drug once a day without regard to food.
- Establish baseline orientation and affect before beginning therapy.
- Ensure that patient is well hydrated while taking this drug.
- Monitor patient regularly for signs and symptoms of diabetes mellitus.

- Establish appropriate safety precautions if patient experiences adverse CNS effects.
- If a breast-feeding patient is taking this drug, suggest another method of feeding the infant.
- Advise women of childbearing age to use contraceptives while taking this drug.
- Consider switching to oral solution for patients who have difficulty swallowing.

Teaching points

- Take this drug once a day as prescribed. If you forget a dose, take the next dose as soon as you remember and then resume taking the drug the next day. Do not take more than one dose in any 24-hour period.
- If taking orally disintegrating tablet, place the tablet on your tongue, allow to dissolve, and then swallow. It is recommended that you use no liquid to take the tablet; if you do use liquid, use the smallest amount possible.
- This drug may interact with many other medications and with alcohol. Alert any health care provider caring for you that you are taking this drug.
- This drug should not be taken during pregnancy or when breast-feeding; using barrier contraceptives is suggested.
- Make sure that you are well hydrated while taking this drug.
- You may experience these side effects: Dizziness, impaired thinking and motor coordination (use caution and avoid driving a car or performing other tasks that require alertness if you experience these effects); inability to cool body effectively (avoid extremes of heat, heavy exercise, dehydration while using this drug).
- Report severe dizziness, trembling, lightheadedness, suicidal thoughts, blurred vision.

▷ **armodafinil**
*(are moe **daff'** ih nill)*

Nuvigil

PREGNANCY CATEGORY C

CONTROLLED SUBSTANCE C-IV

Drug classes

CNS stimulant
Narcolepsy drug

Therapeutic actions

A CNS stimulant that helps to improve vigilance and decrease excessive daytime sleepiness associated with narcolepsy and other sleep disorders. May act through dopaminergic mechanisms; exact mechanism of action is not known. Not associated with the cardiac and other systemic stimulatory effects of amphetamines.

Indications

- To improve wakefulness in patients with excessive sleepiness associated with obstructive sleep apnea/hypopnea syndrome, narcolepsy, and shift work sleep disorder

Contraindications and cautions

- Contraindicated with known hypersensitivity to any component of the drug or to modafinil.
- Use cautiously with a history of psychosis, depression, mania; pregnancy, lactation; history of drug abuse or dependence; hepatic impairment, LV hyertrophy, mitral valve prolapse, history of severe rash, Tourette syndrome.

Available forms

Tablets—50, 150, 250 mg

Dosages

Adults

- Obstructive sleep apnea/hypopnea syndrome, narcolepsy: 150–250 mg/day PO as a single dose in the morning.
- Shift work sleep disorder: 150 mg/day PO taken 1 hr before start of work shift.

Patients with severe hepatic impairment, elderly patients
Consider use of a lower dose.

Pharmacokinetics

Route	Onset	Peak
Oral	Rapid	2 hr

Metabolism: Hepatic; $T_{1/2}$: 15 hr
Distribution: May cross placenta; may enter breast milk
Excretion: Urine

Adverse effects

- **CNS:** *Headache, dizziness, insomnia,* disturbance in attention, tremor, paresthesia, anxiety, depression, agitation, nervousness
- **CV:** Tachycardia, chest pain, palpitations
- **Dermatologic:** Dermatitis, **Stevens-Johnson syndrome,** rash
- **GI:** *Nausea,* diarrhea, dry mouth, dyspepsia, constipation, vomiting, anorexia
- **GU:** Polyuria
- **Respiratory:** Dyspnea
- **Other:** Fatigue, pyrexia, flulike symptoms, dependence

Interactions

❊ **Drug-drug** • Possible decreased effectiveness of hormonal contraceptives during and up to 1 month after treatment; suggest use of barrier contraceptive • Risk of increased levels and effects of warfarin, phenytoin, omeprazole, TCAs; dosage adjustment may be needed • Risk of decreased levels and effectiveness of cyclosporine, ethinyl estradiol, midazolam, triazolam; dosage adjustment may be needed

■ Nursing considerations

Assessment

- **History:** Hypersensitivity to any component of the drug or to modafinil, history of drug abuse or dependence, psychosis, depression, pregnancy, lactation, hepatic impairment
- **Physical:** T; skin color, lesions; orientation, affect, reflexes; bowel sounds; LFTs

Interventions

- Ensure proper diagnosis before administering drug to rule out underlying medical problems.
- Drug therapy should be part of a comprehensive program to include measures to improve sleep patterns.
- Administer once a day in the morning for narcolepsy or sleep apnea disorders; for shift work sleep disorders, have patient take tablet approximately 1 hour before shift begins.
- Establish safety precautions if CNS changes occur (dizziness, changes in thought process).

Teaching points

- This drug is a controlled substance with abuse potential; keep it in a secure place. It is illegal to sell or give this drug to other people.
- This drug should be part of an overall plan, including measures to improve your sleep habits. It is not a substitute for sleep.
- Your health care provider will run tests to accurately diagnose your sleep disorder.

- Take only your prescribed dose. Do not change your dosage or the time of day you are taking the drug without consulting your health care provider.
- Take your dose once each day in the morning if you have sleep apnea or narcolepsy. If you have shift work sleep disorder, take it 1 hour before your shift begins.
- Avoid drinking alcohol while you are taking this drug.
- This drug can decrease the effectiveness of hormonal contraceptives. The use of a barrier contraceptive is advised while you are taking this drug and for 1 month after you have stopped the drug.
- It is not known how this drug could affect a developing fetus. If you are pregnant or you wish to become pregnant, discuss this with your health care provider.
- It is not known how this drug could affect a breast-feeding infant. If you are breast-feeding, consult with your health care provider.
- You may experience these side effects: dizziness, insomnia, nervousness, impaired thinking (do not drive a car or engage in activities that require alertness if these effects occur); headache (consult with your health care provider for possible medication to relieve this).
- Report rash; hives; peeling skin blisters; swelling of the face, eyes, lips, tongue, or throat; trouble swallowing or breathing; hoarse voice; chest pain or palpitations; thoughts of suicide; hallucinations; depression; or anxiety.

▷ arsenic trioxide

See Appendix R, *Less commonly used drugs*.

▷ asenapine

(ah sin' ah peen)

Saphris

PREGNANCY CATEGORY C

Drug classes
Atypical antipsychotic
Dopamine/serotonin antagonist

Therapeutic actions
Mechanism of action not fully understood; blocks dopamine and serotonin receptors in the brain and depresses the reticular activating system. Suppresses many of the negative aspects of schizophrenia, including blunted affect, social withdrawal, lack of motivation, and anger.

Indications
- Acute treatment of schizophrenia in adults
- Acute treatment of manic or mixed episodes associated with bipolar I disorder in adults
- Adjunctive therapy with lithium or valproate for acute treatment of manic or mixed episodes associated with bipolar I disorder in adults

Contraindications and cautions
- Contraindicated with known hypersensitivity to any component of drug, pregnancy, lactation.
- Use cautiously in prolonged QT interval, history of seizures, diabetes, suicidal ideation, bone marrow suppression, neuroleptic malignant syndrome, history of CV events.

Available forms
Sublingual tablets—5, 10 mg

Dosages
Adults
Schizophrenia: 5–10 mg sublingually bid
Bipolar disorder: 5–10 mg sublingually bid; may be decreased to 5 mg/bid if needed
Pediatric patients
Safety and efficacy not established
Patients with hepatic impairment
Not recommended for patients with severe hepatic impairment, Child-Pugh C

Pharmacokinetics

Route	Onset	Peak
Sublingual	Rapid	30–90 min

Metabolism: Hepatic; $T_{1/2}$: 24 hr
Distribution: May cross placenta; may enter breast milk
Excretion: Urine and feces

Adverse effects
- **CNS:** *Dizziness, somnolence, extrapyramidal disorders, akathisia,* tremor, lethargy, blurred vision, altered thinking
- **CV:** Orthostatic hypotension, hypertension, tachycardia, prolonged QT interval, peripheral edema

Adverse effects in *italics* are most common; those in **bold** are life-threatening. ▭ Do not crush.

- **GI:** *Nausea,* diarrhea, dry mouth, abdominal discomfort
- **GU:** Priapism, ejaculation failure
- **Respiratory:** URI, nasal pharyngitis
- **Other:** Fatigue, lethargy, bone marrow suppression, **neuroleptic malignant syndrome (NMS),** hyperglycemia, *weight gain,* gynecomastia, galactorrhea

Interactions

✳ **Drug-drug** • Increased risk of serious cardiac arrhythmias if taken with other drugs that prolong QT interval; avoid this combination. If combination must be used, monitor patient carefully • Risk of increased effectiveness of antihypertensives if used in combination; monitor patient closely and adjust antihypertensive dosage as needed • Risk of increased CNS effects if combined with centrally acting drugs or alcohol; use caution if this combination is used • Increased risk of toxic effects of both drugs if combined with fluvoxamine; use caution • Risk of paroxetine toxicity if combined with asenapine; monitor patient closely

■ Nursing considerations

Assessment

- **History:** Hypersensitivity to any component of drug; pregnancy, lactation; prolonged QT interval; history of seizures; diabetes; suicidal ideation
- **Physical:** Weight; orientation, affect, reflexes; BP, P; abdominal exam; liver evaluation (LFTs); ECG, CBC, blood glucose level

Interventions

⊗ **Black box warning** Risk of death increases if used in elderly patients with dementia-related psychosis. Do not use for these patients; drug not approved for this use.

- Obtain baseline ECG to rule out prolonged QT interval; monitor patient periodically throughout therapy.
- Place tablet under the tongue and allow to dissolve completely, which should occur within seconds. Tell patient not to swallow tablet. Ensure that patient avoids eating and drinking for 10 minutes after administration.
- Monitor patient regularly for signs and symptoms of increased blood glucose level.
- Provide safety measures, especially early in treatment, if orthostatic hypotension occurs.

- Be aware of risk of extrapyramidal effects in newborns if drug is taken in last trimester.
- Advise patient who is breast-feeding to select another method of feeding the infant.
- Monitor patient for signs and symptoms of NMS (high fever, muscle rigidity, altered mental status, high or low blood pressure, diaphoresis, tachycardia); discontinue drug and support patient if these occur. Carefully consider reintroduction of drug because NMS recurrence is likely.
- Provide safety measures as needed if patient develops extrapyramidal effects or orthostatic hypotension.
- Be aware that patient may experience changes in cognitive and motor function.
- Because of risk of suicidal ideation with treatment, limit amount of drug dispensed to the smallest effective amount, to decrease chances of overdose.
- Continue other measures being used to deal with schizophrenia or bipolar disorder.

Teaching points

- Take this drug once a day, exactly as prescribed.
- If you miss a dose, take the next dose as soon as you remember. Do not take more than the prescribed amount each day.
- Avoid alcohol while taking this drug. Tell your health care provider about any other drugs, over-the-counter drugs, or herbal therapies that you are using; serious drug interactions are possible.
- If you are diabetic, monitor your blood glucose level very carefully and adjust treatment as ordered.
- It is not known how this drug could affect a fetus. If you should become pregnant while taking this drug, consult your health care provider. If drug is taken in last trimester, infant may exhibit abnormal movements (tremors, shaking).
- It is not known how this drug could affect a breast-feeding infant. Because of the potential for serious adverse effects in an infant, you should use another method of feeding the infant while you are taking this drug.
- This drug may cause your blood pressure to fall when you stand up; this is called orthostatic hypotension.
- Use care when standing or changing positions, especially when starting the drug and when changing dosage.

- You may experience the following side effects: dizziness, changes in motor performance and impaired thinking (do not drive a car or engage in activities that require alertness if these effects occur), nausea, dry mouth (small frequent meals may help; sucking sugarless candies may also be helpful).
- Report fever accompanied by sweating, changes in mental status, muscle rigidity; heart palpitations; feeling faint; loss of consciousness; thoughts of suicide.

▷**asparaginase *Erwinia chrysantheni***

See Appendix R, *Less commonly used drugs.*

▷**aspirin**

(ass' pir in)

Bayer, Bayer Advanced Aspirin, Easprin, Ecotrin, Empirin, Genprin, Halfprin 81, Heartline, Norwich, St. Joseph, ZORprin ⊙

Buffered aspirin products:
Adprin-B, Alka-Seltzer, Ascriptin, Bufferin, Buffex

PREGNANCY CATEGORY D

Drug classes
Analgesic (nonopioid)
Anti-inflammatory
Antiplatelet
Antipyretic
Antirheumatic
NSAID
Salicylate

Therapeutic actions
Analgesic and antirheumatic effects are attributable to aspirin's ability to inhibit the synthesis of prostaglandins by inhibiting cyclooxygenase 1 and 2, important mediators of inflammation. Antipyretic effects are not fully understood, but aspirin probably acts in the thermoregulatory center of the hypothalamus to block effects of endogenous pyrogen by inhibiting synthesis of the prostaglandin intermediary. Inhibition of platelet aggregation is attributable to the inhibition of platelet synthesis of thromboxane A_2, a potent vasoconstrictor and inducer of platelet aggregation. This effect occurs at low doses and lasts for the life of the platelet (8 days). Higher doses inhibit the synthesis of prostacyclin, a potent vasodilator and inhibitor of platelet aggregation.

Indications
- Mild to moderate pain
- Fever
- Inflammatory conditions—rheumatic fever, rheumatoid arthritis, osteoarthritis, juvenile rheumatoid arthritis, spondyloarthropathies
- Reduction of risk of recurrent TIAs or stroke in patients with history of TIA due to fibrin platelet emboli or ischemic stroke
- Reduction of risk of death or nonfatal MI in patients with history of infarction or unstable angina pectoris or suspected acute MI
- Patients who have undergone revascularization procedures (eg, coronary artery bypass graft [CABG], percutaneous transluminal coronary angioplasty [PTCA], endarterectomy)
- Unlabeled uses: Prophylaxis against cataract formation with long-term use; prosthetic valve thromboprophylaxis, Kawasaki disease, antithrombotic therapy in children with Blalock-Taussing shunt and after Fontan procedure

Contraindications and cautions
- Contraindicated with allergy to salicylates or NSAIDs (more common with nasal polyps, asthma, chronic urticaria); allergy to tartrazine (cross-sensitivity to aspirin is common); hemophilia, bleeding ulcers, hemorrhagic states, blood coagulation defects, hypoprothrombinemia, vitamin K deficiency (increased risk of bleeding); Reye syndrome.
- Use cautiously with impaired renal function; chickenpox, influenza (risk of Reye syndrome in children and teenagers); children with fever accompanied by dehydration; surgery scheduled within 1 wk; peptic ulcer disease; gout; pregnancy (maternal anemia, antepartal and postpartal hemorrhage, prolonged gestation, and prolonged labor have been reported; readily crosses the placenta; possibly teratogenic; maternal

ingestion of aspirin during late pregnancy has been associated with the following adverse fetal effects: low birth weight, increased intracranial hemorrhage, stillbirths, neonatal death); lactation.

Available forms
Tablets—81, 165, 325, 500, 650, 975 mg; SR tablets ⓒᴀɴ—650, 800 mg; suppositories—120, 200, 300, 600 mg; rapidly dissolving tablets—325, 500 mg

Dosages
Available in oral and suppository forms. Also available as chewable tablets, gum; enteric coated, SR, and buffered preparations (SR aspirin is not recommended for antipyresis, short-term analgesia, or children younger than 12 yr).

Adults
- *Ischemic stroke, TIA:* 50–325 mg/day.
- *Angina, recurrent MI prevention:* 75–325 mg/day.
- *Suspected MI:* 160–325 mg as soon as possible; continue daily for 30 days.
- *CABG:* 325 mg 6 hr after procedure, then daily for 1 yr.
- *PTCA:* 325 mg 2 hr before procedure, then 160–325 mg/day.
- *Carotid endarterectomy:* 80 mg/day–650 mg bid started before the procedure and then continued after the procedure.
- *Spondyloarthritis:* Up to 4 g/day in divided doses.
- *Osteoarthritis:* Up to 3 g/day in divided doses.
- *Analgesic and antipyretic:* Tablets—325–1,000 mg, every 4–6 hr; maximum dosage, 4,000 mg/day; SR tablets—1,300 mg, then 650–1,300 mg every 8 hr; maximum dosage, 3,900 mg/day. Suppositories—1 rectally every 4 hr.
- *Arthritis and rheumatic conditions:* 3 g/day in divided doses.
- *Acute rheumatic fever:* 5–8 g/day; modify to maintain serum salicylate level of 15–30 mg/dL.

Pediatric patients
- *Analgesic and antipyretic:* 10–15 mg/kg/dose every 4 hr, up to 60–80 mg/kg/day. Do not administer to patients with chickenpox or influenza symptoms.

Age (yr)	Dosage (mg every 4 hr)
2–3	162
4–5	243
6–8	324
9–10	405
11	486
12 or older	648 (or 1 suppository, rectally)

- *Juvenile rheumatoid arthritis:* 90–130 mg/kg per 24 hr in divided doses at 6- to 8-hr intervals. Maintain a serum level of 150–300 mcg/mL.
- *Acute rheumatic fever:* Initially, 100 mg/kg/day, then decrease to 75 mg/kg/day for 4–6 wk. Therapeutic serum salicylate level is 150–300 mcg/mL.
- *Kawasaki disease:* 80–100 mg/kg/day divided every 6 hr; after fever resolves; 1–5 mg/kg/day once daily.

Pharmacokinetics

Route	Onset	Peak	Duration
Oral	5–30 min	15–120 min	3–6 hr
Rectal	1–2 hr	4–5 hr	6–8 hr

Metabolism: Hepatic (salicylate); $T_{1/2}$: 15 min–12 hr
Distribution: Crosses placenta; enters breast milk
Excretion: Urine

Adverse effects
- **Acute aspirin toxicity:** Respiratory alkalosis, hyperpnea, tachypnea, hemorrhage, excitement, confusion, asterixis, pulmonary edema, seizures, tetany, metabolic acidosis, fever, coma, CV collapse, renal and respiratory failure (dose related, 20–25 g in adults, 4 g in children)
- **Aspirin intolerance:** Exacerbation of bronchospasm, rhinitis (with nasal polyps, asthma)
- **Dermatologic:** rash, hives, urticaria
- **GI:** *Nausea, dyspepsia, heartburn, epigastric discomfort,* anorexia, hepatotoxicity
- **Hematologic:** *Occult blood loss, hemostatic defects, bleeding, anemia*
- **Hypersensitivity:** Anaphylactoid reactions to anaphylactic shock
- **Salicylism:** *Dizziness, tinnitus, difficulty hearing, nausea,* vomiting, diarrhea, mental confusion, lassitude (dose related)

Interactions

❋ **Drug-drug** • Increased risk of bleeding with oral anticoagulants, heparin • Increased risk of GI ulceration with steroids, alcohol, NSAIDs • Increased serum salicylate levels due to decreased salicylate excretion with urine acidifiers (ammonium chloride, ascorbic acid, methionine) • Increased risk of salicylate toxicity with carbonic anhydrase inhibitors, furosemide • Decreased serum salicylate levels with corticosteroids • Decreased serum salicylate levels due to increased renal excretion of salicylates with acetazolamide, methazolamide, certain antacids, alkalinizers • Decreased absorption of aspirin with nonabsorbable antacids • Increased methotrexate levels and toxicity with aspirin • Increased effects of valproic acid secondary to displacement from plasma protein sites • Greater glucose lowering effect of sulfonylureas, insulin with large doses (more than 2 g/day) of aspirin • Decreased antihypertensive effect of captopril, beta-adrenergic blockers with salicylates; consider discontinuation of aspirin • Decreased uricosuric effect of probenecid • Possible decreased diuretic effects of spironolactone, furosemide (in patients with compromised renal function) • Unexpected hypotension may occur with nitroglycerin

❋ **Drug-lab test** • Decreased serum protein bound iodine (PBI) due to competition for binding sites • False-negative readings for urine glucose by glucose oxidase method and copper reduction method with moderate to large doses of aspirin • Interference with urine 5-HIAA determinations by fluorescent methods but not by nitrosonaphthol colorimetric method • Interference with urinary ketone determination by the ferric chloride method • Falsely elevated urine VMA levels with most tests; a false decrease in VMA using the Pisano method

■ Nursing considerations

Assessment

• **History:** Allergy to salicylates or NSAIDs; allergy to tartrazine; hemophilia, bleeding ulcers, hemorrhagic states, blood coagulation defects, hypoprothrombinemia, vitamin K deficiency; impaired hepatic function; impaired renal function; chickenpox; influenza; children with fever accompanied by dehydration; surgery scheduled within 1 wk; pregnancy; lactation

• **Physical:** Skin color, lesions; T; eighth cranial nerve function, orientation, reflexes, affect; P, BP, perfusion; R, adventitious sounds; liver evaluation, bowel sounds; CBC, clotting times, urinalysis, stool guaiac, LFTs, renal function tests

Interventions

⊗ **Warning** Do not use in children and teenagers to treat chickenpox or flu symptoms without review for Reye syndrome, a rare but fatal disorder associated with aspirin use.

• Give drug with food or after meals if GI upset occurs.

• Give drug with full glass of water to reduce risk of tablet or capsule lodging in the esophagus.

• Do not crush, and ensure that patient does not chew SR preparations.

• Do not use aspirin that has a strong vinegar-like odor.

⊗ **Warning** Institute emergency procedures if overdose occurs: Gastric lavage, induction of emesis, activated charcoal, supportive therapy.

Teaching points

• Take extra precautions to keep this drug out of the reach of children; this drug can be very dangerous for children.

• Use the drug only as suggested; avoid overdose. Avoid the use of other over-the-counter drugs while taking this drug. Many of these drugs contain aspirin, and serious overdose can occur.

• Take the drug with food or after meals if GI upset occurs.

• Do not cut, crush, or chew sustained-release products.

• Over-the-counter aspirins are equivalent. Price does not reflect effectiveness. Do not use aspirin that has a strong vinegar odor.

• You may experience these side effects: Nausea, GI upset, heartburn (take drug with food); easy bruising, gum bleeding (related to aspirin's effects on blood clotting).

• Report ringing in the ears; dizziness, confusion; abdominal pain; rapid or difficult breathing; nausea, vomiting, bloody stools.

▷ atazanavir sulfate
*(ah **taz'** ah nah veer)*

Reyataz

PREGNANCY CATEGORY B

Drug classes
Anti-HIV drug
Antiretroviral
Protease inhibitor

Therapeutic actions
HIV-1 protease inhibitor; selectively inhibits processing of viral proteins in HIV-infected cells, preventing the formation of mature viruses.

Indications
- In combination with other antiretrovirals for the treatment of HIV-1 infection

Contraindications and cautions
- Contraindicated with allergy to any components of the product, lactation (HIV-infected mothers are discouraged from breast-feeding).
- Use cautiously with pregnancy; hepatic impairment; signs of lactic acidosis; risk factors for lactic acidosis, including female gender and obesity; hemophilia.

Available forms
Capsules—100, 150, 200, 300 mg

Dosages
Adults
Therapy-naïve patients: 300 mg/day PO with 100 mg ritonavir once daily; if unable to tolerate ritonavir, 400 mg PO once daily can be used. Taken with food. If taken with didanosine, give atazanavir with food 2 hr before or 1 hr after the didanosine. If taken with efavirenz, 400 mg/day PO atazanavir, and 100 mg ritonavir with food and 600 mg efavirenz as a single daily dose on an empty stomach, preferably at bedtime. Atazanavir should not be used with efavirenz without ritonavir. If taken with tenofovir, 300 mg tenofovir PO with 300 mg atazanavir PO and 100 mg ritonavir PO once daily with food.
Therapy-experienced patients: 300 mg/day PO with 100 mg ritonavir PO taken with food.

Concomitant therapy: With histamine-2 (H_2) receptor antagonists, do not exceed equivalent of 40 mg famotidine bid (for therapy-naïve patients) or 20 mg famotidine bid (for therapy-experienced patients); administer 300 mg atazanavir with 100 mg ritonavir simultaneously with first dose of H_2-receptor antagonist. Administer second dose of H_2-receptor antagonist 10 hr later. With proton pump inhibitors, do not exceed equivalent of 20 mg omeprazole. Administer 12 hr prior to atazanavir for therapy-naïve patients. Do not use proton pump inhibitors in therapy-experienced patients.

Pediatric patients 6 yr to under 18 yr
Do not exceed recommended adult doses.

Patient type	Body weight (kg)	Atazanavir dose (mg)	Ritonavir dose (mg)
Therapy naïve	15 to less than 25	150	80
	25 to less than 32	200	100
	32 to less than 39	250	100
	39 or more	300	100
Therapy experienced	25 to less than 32	200	100
	32 to less than 39	250	100
	39 or more	300	100

Patients with hepatic impairment
300 mg/day PO with moderate impairment (Child-Pugh class B); do not use with severe hepatic impairment or hepatic insufficiency (Child-Pugh class C).

Patients with renal impairment
No dosage adjustment needed if patient is not on dialysis. Do not use in treatment-experienced patients with end-stage renal disease who are on hemodialysis. Treatment-naïve patients on dialysis should receive 300 mg with ritonavir 100 mg.

Pharmacokinetics

Route	Onset	Peak
Oral	Rapid	2–2.5 hr

Metabolism: Hepatic; T$_{1/2}$: 6.5–7.9 hr
Distribution: May cross placenta; may enter breast milk
Excretion: Feces, urine

Adverse effects

- **CNS:** *Headache,* depression, insomnia, dizziness, peripheral neurologic symptoms
- **CV:** Prolonged PR interval
- **GI:** *Nausea,* diarrhea, abdominal pain, vomiting, jaundice, **severe hepatomegaly with steatosis, sometimes fatal;** *elevated liver enzymes and bilirubin, lipase elevations*
- **Metabolic:** Lactic acidosis, sometimes severe; hyperglycemia, increased triglycerides
- **Respiratory:** Cough
- **Other:** *Rash,* arthralgia, fever, fatigue, pain, fat redistribution, back pain, increased CK

Interactions

✳ **Drug-drug** • Increased risk of severe toxicity if combined with other drugs that are metabolized via the CYP450 pathway—midazolam, triazolam, ergot derivatives, pimozide; the use of these drugs with atazanavir is contraindicated • Risk of increased toxicity of lovastatin, simvastatin, indinavir, proton pump inhibitors, irinotecan; coadministration of atazanavir with these drugs is not recommended • Increased risk of serious adverse effects if taken with sildenafil; encourage patient to report any adverse effects to the health care provider • Risk of decreased therapeutic effects of rifampin if combined with atazanavir; this combination is not recommended • Decreased absorption of atazanavir if taken with antacids or buffered medications; if this combination is used, administer atazanavir 1 hr before or 2 hr after these drugs • Potential for increased bleeding if combined with warfarin; if this combination is used, monitor INR carefully and adjust warfarin dosage accordingly • Risk of serious adverse effects if taken with bosentan without ritonavir; ensure that patients on bosentan taking atazanavir are also receiving ritonavir

✳ **Drug-alternative therapy** • Decreased concentrations of atazanavir and loss of therapeutic effects if combined with St. John's Wort; this combination is not recommended

■ Nursing considerations

Assessment

- **History:** Allergy to any components of the product, lactation, pregnancy, hepatic impairment, signs of lactic acidosis, obesity, hemophilia
- **Physical:** T; orientation, reflexes; R, adventitious sounds; abdominal examination, LFTs, cholesterol levels

Interventions

- Ensure that HIV antibody testing has been done before initiating therapy to reduce risk of emergence of HIV resistance.
- Ensure that patient is taking this drug in combination with other antiretroviral drugs.
- Monitor patients regularly to evaluate hepatic function; establish baseline ECG to monitor P-R interval.
- Administer this drug with food.
- ⊗ **Warning** Withdraw drug and monitor patient if patient develops signs of lactic acidosis or hepatotoxicity, including hepatomegaly and steatosis.
- Encourage women of childbearing age to use barrier contraceptives while taking this drug because the effects of the drug on the fetus are not known. If drug is used in pregnancy, patient should be registered with the antiretroviral pregnancy registry.
- Advise women who are breast-feeding to find another method of feeding the infant; HIV-infected women are advised to not breast-feed.
- Advise patient that this drug does not cure the disease and there is still a risk of transmitting the disease to others.

Teaching points

- Take this drug once a day with food and in combination with your other antiviral drugs.
- Take the drug every day; if you miss a dose, take it as soon as you remember and then take the next dose at the usual time the next day. Do not double any doses.
- Tell any other health care provider that you see that you are taking this drug; the drug interacts with many other drugs and caution may be needed; the drug also changes your ECG reading and that may be important.
- Avoid the use of St. John's Wort while taking this drug; the effectiveness of this drug can be blocked.

Adverse effects in *italics* are most common; those in **bold** are life-threatening. ⊂⊃ Do not crush.

- If you use *Viagra* or *Revatio,* you could experience serious adverse effects with this drug; report any adverse effects to your health care provider.
- This drug does not cure your HIV infection and you will still be able to pass it to others; using condoms is advised. Women of childbearing age are discouraged from becoming pregnant while taking this drug; using barrier contraceptives is recommended.
- With some antiviral drugs, there is a redistribution of body fat—a "buffalo hump" may develop—and fat is distributed around the trunk while fat is lost in the limbs; the long-term effects of this redistribution are not known.
- You may experience these side effects: Nausea, diarrhea, abdominal pain, headache (try to maintain nutrition and fluid intake as much as possible; eat frequent small meals; and always take the drug with food).
- Report severe weakness, muscle pain, trouble breathing, dizziness, cold feelings in your arms or legs, palpitations, yellowing of the eyes or skin.

▽atenolol
(a ten' o lole)

Apo-Atenolol (CAN), Gen-Atenolol (CAN), Novo-Atenol (CAN), ratio-Atenolol (CAN), Tenormin

PREGNANCY CATEGORY D

Drug classes
Antianginal
Antihypertensive
Beta₁-selective adrenergic blocker

Therapeutic actions
Blocks beta-adrenergic receptors of the sympathetic nervous system in the heart and juxtaglomerular apparatus (kidney), thus decreasing the excitability of the heart, decreasing cardiac output and oxygen consumption, decreasing the release of renin from the kidney, and lowering BP.

Indications
- Treatment of angina pectoris due to coronary atherosclerosis

- Hypertension, alone or with other drugs, especially diuretics
- Treatment of MI in hemodynamically stable patients
- Unlabeled uses: Prevention of migraine headaches; treatment of ventricular and supraventricular arrhythmias; prevention of variceal bleeding; unstable angina

Contraindications and cautions
- Contraindicated with sinus bradycardia, second- or third-degree heart block, cardiogenic shock, pregnancy, hypersensitivity to any component of the drug.
- Use cautiously with renal failure, diabetes or thyrotoxicosis (atenolol can mask the usual cardiac signs of hypoglycemia and thyrotoxicosis), lactation, respiratory disease (including bronchospastic disease), heart failure (controlled by digoxin or diuretics).

Available forms
Tablets—25, 50, 100 mg

Dosages
Adults
- *Hypertension:* Initially, 50 mg PO once a day; after 1–2 wk, dose may be increased to 100 mg/day.
- *Angina pectoris:* Initially, 50 mg PO daily. If optimal response is not achieved in 1 wk, increase to 100 mg daily; up to 200 mg/day may be needed.
- *Acute MI:* 100 mg PO daily or 50 mg PO bid for 6–9 days or until discharge from the hospital.

Pediatric patients
Safety and efficacy not established.

Geriatric patients or patients with renal impairment
Dosage reduction is required because atenolol is excreted through the kidneys. For elderly patients, use initial dose of 25 mg/day PO. The following dosage is suggested for patients with renal impairment:

CrCl (mL/min)	Half-life (hr)	Maximum Dosage
15–35	16–27	50 mg/day
Less than 15	More than 27	25 mg/day

For patients on hemodialysis, give 25–50 mg after each dialysis; give only in hospital setting; severe hypotension can occur.

Pharmacokinetics

Route	Onset	Peak	Duration
Oral	Varies	2–4 hr	24 hr

Metabolism: $T_{1/2}$: 6–7 hr
Distribution: Crosses placenta; enters breast milk
Excretion: Bile, feces, urine

Adverse effects

- **Allergic reactions:** Pharyngitis, erythematous rash, fever, sore throat, **laryngospasm,** respiratory distress
- **CNS:** Dizziness, vertigo, tinnitus, fatigue, emotional depression, paresthesias, sleep disturbances, hallucinations, disorientation, memory loss, slurred speech
- **CV:** *Bradycardia, HF, cardiac arrhythmias, sinoatrial or AV nodal block, tachycardia,* peripheral vascular insufficiency, claudication, **stroke,** pulmonary edema, hypotension, cold extremities
- **Dermatologic:** Rash, pruritus, sweating, dry skin
- **EENT:** Eye irritation, dry eyes, conjunctivitis, blurred vision
- **GI:** *Gastric pain, flatulence, constipation, diarrhea, nausea, vomiting,* anorexia, ischemic colitis, renal and mesenteric arterial thrombosis, retroperitoneal fibrosis, hepatomegaly, acute pancreatitis
- **GU:** *Impotence, decreased libido,* Peyronie's disease, dysuria, nocturia, frequent urination
- **Musculoskeletal:** Joint pain, arthralgia, muscle cramps
- **Respiratory: Bronchospasm,** dyspnea, cough, bronchial obstruction, nasal stuffiness, rhinitis, pharyngitis (less likely than with propranolol)
- **Other:** *Decreased exercise tolerance, development of antinuclear antibodies,* hyperglycemia or hypoglycemia, elevated serum transaminase, alkaline phosphatase, and LDH

Interactions

✳ **Drug-drug** • Increased effects with verapamil, anticholinergics, quinidine • Increased risk of orthostatic hypotension with prazosin • Increased risk of lidocaine toxicity with atenolol • Possible increased BP-lowering effects with aspirin, bismuth subsalicylate, magnesium salicylate, hormonal contraceptives • Decreased antihypertensive effects with NSAIDs, clonidine • Decreased antihypertensive and antianginal effects of atenolol with ampicillin, calcium salts • Possible masked hypoglycemic effect of insulin
✳ **Drug-lab test** • Possible false results with glucose or insulin tolerance tests

■ Nursing considerations
Assessment

- **History:** Sinus bradycardia, second- or third-degree heart block, cardiogenic shock, heart failure, renal failure, diabetes or thyrotoxicosis, lactation, pregnancy
- **Physical:** Baseline weight, skin condition, neurologic status, P, BP, ECG, respiratory status, renal and thyroid function tests, blood and urine glucose, cholesterol, triglycerides

Interventions

⊗ **Black box warning** Do not discontinue drug abruptly after long-term therapy (hypersensitivity to catecholamines may have developed, causing exacerbation of angina, MI, and ventricular arrhythmias). Taper drug gradually over 2 wk with monitoring.

- Consult physician about withdrawing drug if patient is to undergo surgery (withdrawal is controversial).

Teaching points

- Take drug with meals if GI upset occurs.
- Do not stop taking this drug unless told to do so by a health care provider.
- Avoid driving or dangerous activities if dizziness or weakness occurs.
- You may experience these side effects: Dizziness, light-headedness, loss of appetite, nightmares, depression, sexual impotence.
- Report difficulty breathing, night cough, swelling of extremities, slow pulse, confusion, depression, rash, fever, sore throat.

▽ **atomoxetine hydrochloride**
*(at oh **mox'** ah teen)*

Strattera

PREGNANCY CATEGORY C

Drug class
Selective norepinephrine reuptake inhibitor

Adverse effects in *italics* are most common; those in **bold** are life-threatening. ▣ Do not crush.

Therapeutic actions

Selectively blocks the reuptake of norepinephrine at the neuronal synapse. The mechanism by which this action has a therapeutic effect in ADHD is not understood.

Indications

• Treatment of ADHD as part of a total treatment program
• Unlabeled uses: Treatment of obesity, binge eating disorder, nocturnal enuresis

Contraindications and cautions

• Contraindicated with hypersensitivity to atomoxetine or constituents of *Strattera;* use of MAOIs within the past 14 days; narrow-angle glaucoma; pheochromocytoma.
• Use cautiously with hypertension, tachycardia, CV or cerebrovascular disease, pregnancy, lactation, severe hepatic impairment.

Available forms

Capsules—10, 18, 25, 40, 60, 80, 100 mg

Dosages
Adults and children weighing more than 70 kg
40 mg/day PO, increase after a minimum of 3 days to a target total daily dose of 80 mg PO given as a single dose in the morning or two evenly divided doses, in the morning and late afternoon or early evening; after 2–4 additional wk, total dosage may be increase to a maximum of 100 mg/day if needed.
Pediatric patients 6 yr and older weighing 70 kg or less
Initially, 0.5 mg/kg/day PO; increase after a minimum of 3 days to a target total daily dose of approximately 1.2 mg/kg/day PO as a single daily dose in the morning; may be given in two evenly divided doses in the morning and late afternoon or early evening. Do not exceed 1.4 mg/kg or 100 mg/day, whichever is less.
Patients with hepatic impairment
For moderate hepatic impairment (Child-Pugh class B), reduce dose to 50% of the normal dose; for severe hepatic impairment (Child-Pugh class C), reduce dose to 25% of the normal dose.

Pharmacokinetics

Route	Onset	Peak
Oral	Rapid	1–2 hr

Metabolism: Hepatic; $T_{1/2}$: 5 hr
Distribution: May cross placenta; may enter breast milk
Excretion: Feces, urine

Adverse effects

• **CNS:** Aggression, irritability, somnolence, dizziness, *headache,* mood swings, *insomnia,* **possible suicidal ideation in children, adolescents, and young adults**
• **CV:** Palpitations, **sudden CV death**
• **Dermatologic:** Dermatitis, increased sweating
• **GI:** *Dry mouth, nausea,* dyspepsia, flatulence, *decreased appetite, constipation, upper abdominal pain, vomiting*
• **GU:** Urinary hesitation, urinary retention, dysmenorrhea, erectile problems
• **Respiratory:** *Cough,* rhinorrhea, sinusitis
• **Other:** Fever, rigors, sinusitis, weight loss, myalgia, fatigue

Interactions

✳ **Drug-drug** • Possible increased serum levels if combined with potent CYP2D6 inhibitors—paroxetine, fluoxetine, quinidine, or CYP3A4 substrates; dosage adjustment may be necessary
• Risk of neuroleptic malignant syndrome if combined with MAOIs; do not combine with an MAOI and do not give atomoxetine within 14 days of using an MAOI; do not start MAOI within 2 wk after discontinuing atomoxetine

■ Nursing considerations
Assessment

• **History:** Hypersensitivity to atomoxetine or constituents of *Strattera;* use of MAOIs within the past 14 days; narrow-angle glaucoma, hypertension, tachycardia, CV or cerebrovascular disease, pregnancy, lactation
• **Physical:** Height, weight, T; skin color, lesions; orientation, affect; P, BP, auscultation; R, adventitious sounds; bowel sounds, normal output

Interventions

⊗ *Black box warning* Adolescents and children have an increased risk of suicidality when treated with atomoxetine. Monitor patient closely, and alert caregivers of risk.

• Ensure proper diagnosis before administering to children for behavioral syndromes; drug should not be used until other causes and concomitants of abnormal behavior (learning disability, EEG abnormalities, neurologic deficits) are ruled out.

- Be aware that patient may be at increased risk for sudden CV death; evaluate use carefully and monitor patient.
- Ensure that drug is being used as part of an overall treatment program including education and psychosocial interventions.
- Be aware of an increased risk of inappropriate and aggressive behavior; monitor patient accordingly and include this information in teaching program.
- Arrange to interrupt drug dosage periodically in children being treated for behavioral disorders to determine if symptoms recur at an intensity that warrants continued drug therapy.
- Monitor growth and weight of children on long-term atomoxetine therapy.
- Administer drug before 6 PM to prevent insomnia if that is a problem.
- Monitor BP early in treatment, particularly with adult patients.
- Arrange for consult with school nurse for school-age patients receiving this drug.
- For women of childbearing age who are using this drug, suggest using contraceptives.

Teaching points

- Take this drug exactly as prescribed. It can be taken once a day in the morning; if adverse effects are a problem, the drug can be taken in two evenly divided doses in the morning and in the late afternoon or early evening.
- Do not open capsule; swallow it whole.
- Take drug before 6 PM to avoid nighttime sleep disturbance.
- Avoid the use of alcohol and over-the-counter drugs, including nose drops, cold remedies, and herbal therapies while taking this drug; some of these products cause dangerous effects. If you think that you need one of these preparations, consult your health care provider.
- The effects of this drug on a fetus are not known; women of childbearing age are advised to use contraceptives.
- You may experience these side effects: Dizziness, insomnia, moodiness (these effects may become less pronounced after a few days; avoid driving a car or engaging in activities that require alertness if these occur; notify your health care provider if these are

pronounced or bothersome); headache (analgesics may be available to help) loss of appetite, dry mouth (eat frequent small meals and suck on sugarless candies); thoughts of suicide (if you are a minor, report this to your parents or health care provider); changes in behavior.

- Report palpitations, dizziness, weight loss, severe dry mouth and difficulty swallowing, pregnancy, thoughts of suicide, aggressive or inappropriate behavior.

▷ **atorvastatin calcium**
*(ah **tor'** va stah tin)*

Lipitor

PREGNANCY CATEGORY X

Drug classes
Antihyperlipidemic
HMG-CoA reductase inhibitor

Therapeutic actions
Inhibits HMG-CoA reductase, the enzyme that catalyzes the first step in the cholesterol synthesis pathway, resulting in a decrease in serum cholesterol, serum LDLs (associated with increased risk of CAD), and increases serum HDLs (associated with decreased risk of CAD); increases hepatic LDL recapture sites, enhances reuptake and catabolism of LDL; lowers triglyceride levels.

Indications
- Adjunct to diet in treatment of elevated total cholesterol, serum triglycerides, and LDL cholesterol and to increase HDL-C in patients with primary hypercholesterolemia (types IIa and IIb) and mixed dyslipidemia and primary dysbetalipoproteinemia, whose response to dietary restriction of saturated fat and cholesterol and other nonpharmacologic measures has not been adequate
- To reduce total cholesterol and LDL-C in patients with homozygous familial hypercholesterolemia as adjunct to lipid-lowering treatments
- Reduction of risk of MI and stroke in patients with type 2 diabetes and in those with multiple risk factors for CAD (such as age 55 or older, smoking, hypertension, low

HDL-C, family history of early CAD) but no clinical evidence of CAD
- Adjunct to diet to treat elevated serum triglyceride levels (Fredrickson Type IV)
- Adjunct to diet in treatment of boys and postmenarchal girls ages 10–17 with heterozygous familial cholesterolemia if diet alone is not adequate to control lipid levels and LDL-C levels are 190 mg/dL or greater or if LDL-C level is 160 mg/dL or greater and there is a family history of premature CV disease or the child has two or more risk factors for the development of coronary disease
- Reduction of risk of MI, fatal and nonfatal stroke, revascularization procedures, heart failure, hospitalization, and angina in patients with clinically evident CAD
- Prevention of CV disease in adults without clinically evident coronary disease but with multiple risk factors for CAD; to reduce the risk of MI and risk for revascularization procedures and angina

Contraindications and cautions
- Contraindicated with allergy to atorvastatin, fungal byproducts, active hepatic disease, or unexplained and persistent elevations of transaminase levels, pregnancy, lactation.
- Use cautiously with impaired endocrine function, history of liver disease, alcoholism.

Available forms
Tablets—10, 20, 40, 80 mg

Dosages
Adults
Initially, 10–20 mg PO once daily without regard to meals; if more than 45% reduction in LDL is needed, may start with 40 mg daily; for maintenance, 10–80 mg PO daily. May be combined with bile acid–binding resin. Check lipid levels initially and with dosage adjustments, which may be made every 2–4 wk; adjust dose as needed.
Pediatric patients 10–17 yr
Initially, 10 mg PO daily. Maximum, 20 mg/day; do not change dose at intervals less than 4 wk.

Pharmacokinetics

Route	Onset	Peak
Oral	Slow	1–2 hr

Metabolism: Hepatic and cellular; $T_{1/2}$: 14 hr
Distribution: Crosses placenta; enters breast milk
Excretion: Bile

Adverse effects
- **CNS:** *Headache,* asthenia, cataracts
- **GI:** *Flatulence, abdominal pain, cramps, constipation, nausea,* dyspepsia, heartburn, **liver failure,** diarrhea, transaminase elevations
- **Respiratory:** Sinusitis, pharyngitis
- **Other: Rhabdomyolysis with acute renal failure,** arthralgia, myalgia, infections

Interactions
✴ **Drug-drug** • Possible severe myopathy or rhabdomyolysis with erythromycin, cyclosporine, nefazodone, tacrolimus, niacin, fibric acid derivatives, antifungals, clarithromycin, diltiazem, cimetidine, protease inhibitors, other HMG-CoA reductase inhibitors; limit dose to 10 mg/day with cyclosporine; limit dose to 20 mg/day with clarithromycin or protease inhibitors • Increased digoxin levels with possible toxicity if taken together; monitor digoxin levels • Increased estrogen levels with hormonal contraceptives; monitor patients on this combination
✴ **Drug-food** • Decreased metabolism and risk of toxic effects if combined with grapefruit juice; avoid this combination

■ Nursing considerations

> **CLINICAL ALERT!**
> Name confusion has been reported between written orders for *Lipitor* (atorvastatin) and *Zyrtec* (cetirizine). Use extreme caution.

Assessment
- **History:** Allergy to atorvastatin, fungal byproducts; active hepatic disease; acute serious illness; pregnancy; lactation
- **Physical:** Orientation, affect, muscle strength; liver evaluation, abdominal examination; lipid studies, LFTs, renal function tests

Interventions
- Obtain LFTs as a baseline and periodically during therapy; discontinue drug if AST or ALT levels increase to 3 times normal levels.

⊗ **Warning** Withhold atorvastatin in any acute, serious condition (severe infection, hypotension, major surgery, trauma, severe metabolic or endocrine disorder, seizures) that may suggest myopathy or serve as risk factor for development of renal failure.

- Ensure that patient has tried cholesterol-lowering diet regimen for 3–6 mo before beginning therapy.
- Administer drug without regard to food, but at same time each day.
- Atorvastatin may be combined with a bile acid-binding agent. Do not combine with other HMG-CoA reductase inhibitors or fibrates.
- Consult dietitian about low-cholesterol diets.

⊗ **Warning** Ensure that patient is not pregnant and has appropriate contraceptives available during therapy; serious fetal damage has been associated with this drug.

Teaching points

- Take this drug once a day, at about the same time each day, preferably in the evening; may be taken with food. Do not drink grapefruit juice while taking this drug.
- Institute appropriate dietary changes.
- Arrange to have periodic blood tests while you are taking this drug.
- Alert any health care provider that you are taking this drug; it will need to be discontinued if acute injury or illness occurs.
- Do not become pregnant while you are taking this drug; use barrier contraceptives. If you wish to become pregnant or think you are pregnant, consult your health care provider.
- You may experience these side effects: Nausea (eat frequent small meals); headache, muscle and joint aches and pains (may lessen over time).
- Report muscle pain, weakness, tenderness; malaise; fever; changes in color of urine or stool; swelling.

▽ **atovaquone**

(*a **toe'** va kwon*)

Mepron

PREGNANCY CATEGORY C

Drug class
Antiprotozoal

Therapeutic actions
Directly inhibits enzymes required for nucleic acid and ATP synthesis in protozoa; effective against *Pneumocystis carinii,* now called *Pneumocystis jiroveci.*

Indications

- Prevention and acute oral treatment of mild to moderate *P. jiroveci* pneumonia in patients who are intolerant to trimethoprim-sulfamethoxazole

Contraindications and cautions

- Contraindicated with development or history of potentially life-threatening allergic reactions to any of the components of the drug.
- Use cautiously with severe *P. Jiroveci* infections, the elderly, lactation, hepatic impairment.

Available forms
Suspension—750 mg/5 mL

Dosages
Adults and patients 13–16 yr

- *Prevention of* P. jiroveci *pneumonia:* 1,500 mg PO daily with a meal.
- *Treatment of* P. jiroveci *pneumonia:* 750 mg PO bid with food for 21 days.

Pediatric patients younger than 13 yr
Safety and efficacy not established.
Geriatric patients
Use caution, and evaluate patient response regularly.

Pharmacokinetics

Route	Onset	Peak	Duration
Oral	Varies	1–8 hr	3–5 days

Metabolism: $T_{1/2}$: 2.2–2.9 days
Distribution: Crosses placenta; may enter breast milk
Excretion: Feces

Adverse effects

- **CNS:** Dizziness, *insomnia, headache, depression*
- **Dermatologic:** *Rash,* pruritus, sweating, dry skin
- **GI:** Constipation, *diarrhea, nausea, vomiting,* anorexia, abdominal pain, oral monilia infections

- **Other:** *Fever,* elevated liver enzymes, hyponatremia, increased cough, dyspnea, flulike syndrome, sweating

Interactions
✳ **Drug-drug** • Decreased effects if taken with rifamycins
✳ **Drug-food** • Markedly increased absorption of atovaquone when taken with food

■ Nursing considerations
Assessment
- **History:** History of potentially life-threatening allergic reactions to any components of the drug, severe *P. jiroveci* pneumonia, elderly, lactation
- **Physical:** T, skin condition, neurologic status, abdominal evaluation, serum electrolytes, LFTs

Interventions
- Give drug with meals.
- Ensure that this drug is taken for 21 days as treatment.

Teaching points
- Take drug with food; food increases the absorption of the drug. Complete the full course of therapy.
- You may experience these side effects: Dizziness, insomnia, headache (medication may be ordered); nausea, vomiting (eat frequent small meals); diarrhea or constipation (consult your health care provider for appropriate treatment); superinfections (therapy may be ordered); rash (good skin care may help).
- Report fever, mouth infection, severe headache, severe nausea or vomiting, rash.

▽**atropine sulfate**
(a' troe peen)

Parenteral and oral preparations: AtroPen
Ophthalmic solution: Atropine Sulfate Ophthalmic, Isopto Atropine Ophthalmic

PREGNANCY CATEGORY C

Drug classes
Anticholinergic
Antidote

Antimuscarinic
Antiparkinsonian
Belladonna alkaloid
Diagnostic agent (ophthalmic preparations)
Parasympatholytic

Therapeutic actions
Competitively blocks the effects of acetylcholine at muscarinic cholinergic receptors that mediate the effects of parasympathetic postganglionic impulses, depressing salivary and bronchial secretions, dilating the bronchi, inhibiting vagal influences on the heart, relaxing the GI and GU tracts, inhibiting gastric acid secretion (high doses), relaxing the pupil of the eye (mydriatic effect), and preventing accommodation for near vision (cycloplegic effect); also blocks the effects of acetylcholine in the CNS.

Indications
Systemic administration
- Antisialagogue for preanesthetic medication to prevent or reduce respiratory tract secretions
- Treatment of parkinsonism; relieves tremor and rigidity (injection)
- Restoration of cardiac rate and arterial pressure during anesthesia when vagal stimulation produced by intra-abdominal traction causes a decrease in pulse rate, lessening the degree of AV block when increased vagal tone is a factor (eg, some cases due to cardiac glycosides)
- Relief of bradycardia and syncope due to hyperactive carotid sinus reflex
- Relief of pylorospasm, hypertonicity of the small intestine, and hypermotility of the colon
- Relaxation of the spasm of biliary and ureteral colic and bronchospasm
- Relaxation of the tone of the detrusor muscle of the urinary bladder in the treatment of urinary tract disorders
- Control of crying and laughing episodes in patients with brain lesions (injection)
- Treatment of closed head injuries that cause acetylcholine release into CSF, EEG abnormalities, stupor, neurologic signs
- Relaxation of uterine hypertonicity
- Management of peptic ulcer (injection)
- Control of rhinorrhea of acute rhinitis or hay fever

- Antidote (with external cardiac massage) for CV collapse from overdose of parasympathomimetic (cholinergic) drugs (choline esters, pilocarpine), or cholinesterase inhibitors (eg, physostigmine, isoflurophate, organophosphorus insecticides)
- Antidote for poisoning by certain species of mushroom (eg, *Amanita muscaria*) (injection)
- Initial treatment of muscarinic symptoms of insecticide or nerve agent poisoning

Ophthalmic preparations

- Diagnostically to produce mydriasis and cycloplegia-pupillary dilation in acute inflammatory conditions of the iris and uveal tract

Contraindications and cautions

- Contraindicated with hypersensitivity to anticholinergic drugs.

Systemic administration

- Contraindicated with glaucoma, adhesions between iris and lens; stenosing peptic ulcer; pyloroduodenal obstruction; paralytic ileus; intestinal atony; severe ulcerative colitis; toxic megacolon; symptomatic prostatic hypertrophy; bladder neck obstruction; bronchial asthma; COPD; cardiac arrhythmias; tachycardia; myocardial ischemia; impaired metabolic, hepatic, or renal function; myasthenia gravis.
- Use cautiously with Down syndrome, brain damage, spasticity, hypertension, hyperthyroidism, pregnancy, lactation.

Ophthalmic solution

- Contraindicated with glaucoma or tendency to glaucoma.

Available forms

Tablets—0.4 mg; injection—0.05, 0.1, 0.3, 0.4, 0.5, 0.8, 1, 2 mg/mL; ophthalmic ointment—1%; ophthalmic solution—0.5%, 1%, 2%; auto-injector—0.25, 0.5, 1, 2 mg

Dosages
Adults

Systemic administration
0.4–0.6 mg PO, IM, IV, or subcutaneously.

- *Hypotonic radiography:* 1 mg IM.
- *Surgery:* 0.5 mg (0.4–0.6 mg) IM (or subcutaneously or IV) prior to induction of anesthesia; during surgery, give IV; reduce dose

to less than 0.4 mg with cyclopropane anesthesia.

- *Bradyarrhythmias:* 0.4–1 mg (up to 2 mg) IV every 1–2 hr as needed.
- *Antispasmodic:* 0.4 mg every 4–6 hr as needed.
- *Secretion reduction:* 0.4 mg every 4–6 hr as needed.
- *Antidote:* For poisoning due to cholinesterase inhibitor insecticides, give large doses of at least 2–3 mg parenterally, and repeat until signs of atropine intoxication appear; for rapid type of mushroom poisoning, give in doses sufficient to control parasympathetic signs before coma and CV collapse intervene. Auto-injector provides rapid administration.

Ophthalmic solution

- *For refraction:* Instill 1–2 drops into eye 1 hr before refracting.
- *For uveitis:* Instill 1–2 drops into eye tid.

Pediatric patients

Systemic administration
Refer to the following table:

Weight	Dose (mg)
7–16 lb (3.2–7.3 kg)	0.1
16–24 lb (7.3–10.9 kg)	0.15
24–40 lb (10.9–18.1 kg)	0.2
40–65 lb (18.1–29.5 kg)	0.3
65–90 lb (29.5–40.8 kg)	0.4
> 90 lb (> 40.8 kg)	0.4–0.6

- *Surgery:* For infants weighing less than 5 kg, 0.04 mg/kg; infants weighing more than 5 kg, 0.03 mg/kg. Repeat every 4–6 hr as needed. For children, 0.01 mg/kg to a maximum of 4 mg; repeat every 4–6 hr.
- *Bradyarrhythmias:* 0.01–0.03 mg/kg IV.

Autoinjection

- *Antidote:*
  90 lb or more: 2 mg auto-injector.
  40–90 lb: 1-mg auto-injector.
  15–40 lb: 0.5 mg auto-injector.
  Less than 15 lb: Do not treat with auto-injector—inject IM as individual doses at 0.05 mg/kg.

Geriatric patients
More likely to cause serious adverse reactions, especially CNS reactions, in elderly patients; use with caution.

Adverse effects in *italics* are most common; those in **bold** are life-threatening. ▣ Do not crush.

Pharmacokinetics

Route	Onset	Peak	Duration
IM	10–15 min	30 min	4 hr
IV	Immediate	2–4 min	4 hr
Subcut.	Varies	1–2 hr	4 hr
Topical	5–10 min	30–40 min	7–14 days

Metabolism: Hepatic; $T_{1/2}$: 2.5 hr
Distribution: Crosses placenta; enters breast milk
Excretion: Urine

▼ IV FACTS

Preparation: Give undiluted or dilute in 10 mL sterile water.
Infusion: Give direct IV; administer 1 mg or less over 1 min.

Adverse effects
Systemic administration

- **CNS:** Blurred vision, mydriasis, cycloplegia, photophobia, increased IOP, headache, flushing, nervousness, weakness, dizziness, insomnia, mental confusion or excitement (after even small doses in the elderly), nasal congestion
- **CV:** *Palpitations, bradycardia* (low doses), *tachycardia* (higher doses)
- **GI:** *Dry mouth, altered taste perception, nausea,* vomiting, dysphagia, heartburn, constipation, bloated feeling, **paralytic ileus,** gastroesophageal reflux
- **GU:** *Urinary hesitancy and retention;* impotence
- **Other:** *Decreased sweating and predisposition to heat prostration,* suppression of lactation

Ophthalmic preparations
- **Local:** Transient stinging
- **Systemic:** Systemic adverse effects, depending on amount absorbed

Interactions

✳ **Drug-drug** • Increased anticholinergic effects with other drugs that have anticholinergic activity—certain antihistamines, certain antiparkinsonians, TCAs, MAOIs • Decreased antipsychotic effectiveness of haloperidol with atropine • Decreased effectiveness of phenothiazines, but increased incidence of paralytic ileus • If cholinesterase inhibitors and atropine are given together, opposing effects will render both drugs ineffective

■ Nursing considerations
Assessment

- **History:** Hypersensitivity to anticholinergics; glaucoma; adhesions between iris and lens; stenosing peptic ulcer, pyloroduodenal obstruction, paralytic ileus, intestinal atony, severe ulcerative colitis, toxic megacolon, symptomatic prostatic hypertrophy, bladder neck obstruction, bronchial asthma, COPD, cardiac arrhythmias, myocardial ischemia, impaired metabolic, liver, or renal function, myasthenia gravis, Down syndrome, brain damage, spasticity, hypertension, hyperthyroidism, lactation
- **Physical:** Skin color, lesions, texture; T; orientation, reflexes, bilateral grip strength; affect; ophthalmic examination; P, BP; R, adventitious sounds; bowel sounds, normal GI output; normal urinary output; prostate palpation; LFTs, renal function tests, ECG

Interventions

- Ensure adequate hydration; provide environmental control (temperature) to prevent hyperpyrexia.
- Have patient void before taking medication if urinary retention is a problem.
- Monitor heart rate.

Teaching points

When used preoperatively or in other acute situations, incorporate teaching about the drug with teaching about the procedure; the ophthalmic solution is mainly used acutely and will not be self-administered by the patient; the following apply to oral medication for outpatients:

- Take as prescribed, 30 minutes before meals; avoid excessive dosage.
- Avoid hot environments; you will be heat intolerant, and dangerous reactions may occur.
- You may experience these side effects: Dizziness, confusion (use caution driving or performing hazardous tasks); constipation (ensure adequate fluid intake, proper diet); dry mouth (sugarless candies, frequent mouth care may help; may be transient); blurred vision, sensitivity to light (reversible; avoid tasks that require acute vision; wear sunglasses in bright light); impotence (reversible); difficulty in urination (empty the bladder prior to taking drug).
- Report rash; flushing; eye pain; difficulty breathing; tremors, loss of coordination;

irregular heartbeat, palpitations; headache; abdominal distention; hallucinations; severe or persistent dry mouth; difficulty swallowing; difficulty in urination; constipation; sensitivity to light.

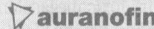

▷ auranofin

See Appendix R, *Less commonly used drugs*.

▷ avanafil
(ah van' ah fil)

Stendra

PREGNANCY CATEGORY C

Drug classes
Impotence drug
Phosphodiesterase-5 inhibitor

Therapeutic actions
Selectively inhibits cyclic guanosine monophosphate (cGMP)–specific phosphodiesterase type 5. The mechanism of penile erection involves the release of nitric oxide into the corpus cavernosum of the penis during sexual simulation. Nitric oxide activates cGMP, causing smooth muscle relaxation and allowing the flow of blood into the corpus cavernosum. Phosphodiesterase type 5 is responsible for the deactivation of cGMP; preventing its deactivation leads to prolonged smooth muscle relaxation and increased blood flow. There is no effect in the absence of sexual stimulation.

Indications
• Treatment of ED

Contraindications and cautions
• Contraindicated with history of serious hypersensitivity reactions to components of the drug; concurrent use of organic nitrates. Not for use in women or children.
• Use cautiously with alpha blockers or other antihypertensives, CV conditions limiting sexual activity.

Available forms
Tablets—50, 100, 200 mg

Dosages
Adults
100 mg PO approximately 30 min before sexual activity; no more than one dose/day. May be increased to 200 mg or decreased to 50 mg as needed.
Patients with severe renal or hepatic impairment
Not recommended.

Pharmacokinetics

Route	Onset	Peak
Oral	Rapid	30–45 min

Metabolism: Hepatic; $T_{1/2}$: 5 hr
Distribution: May cross placenta; may enter breast milk
Excretion: Feces

Adverse effects
• **CNS:** *Headache*, abnormal vision, fatigue, sudden hearing loss
• **CV:** Hypotension, *flushing*, **MI**, palpitations, tachycardia
• **GI:** *Dyspepsia*, abdominal pain, dry mouth
• **GU:** Abnormal erection, priapism, hematuria, UTI
• **Respiratory:** *Nasal congestion, nasopharyngitis*
• **Other:** Back pain

Interactions
✳ **Drug-drug** • Risk of severe hypotension with organic nitrates; this combination is contraindicated • Risk of severe hypotension with alpha blockers, other antihypertensives, alcohol; if this combination must be used, monitor patient closely • Potential for increased effects and toxicity if combined with strong CYP3A4 inhibitors (itraconazole, ketoconazole, ritonavir); these combinations are not recommended • Risk of toxic effects with amprenavir, aprepitant, diltiazem, erythromycin, fluconazole, fosamprenavir, verapamil; limit avanafil dose to 50 mg/day if this combination is used

✳ **Drug-food** • Possible increased levels and toxicity if combined with grapefruit juice; limit this combination

■ Nursing considerations
Assessment
- **History:** Allergy to components of the drug; concurrent use of interacting drugs; severe hepatic or renal impairment; CV disorders
- **Physical:** P, BP; orientation; LFTs, renal function

Interventions
- Ensure diagnosis of ED and rule out underlying medical issues requiring treatment.
- Ensure that sexual activity is advisable for patient based on medical condition.
- Advise patient that drug does not work in the absence of sexual stimulation.
- Remind patient that drug does not protect from sexually transmitted diseases and appropriate precautions should be taken.

⊗ **Warning** Advise patient never to use nitrates or alpha blockers with this drug; fatal complications have occurred.

- Advise patient to stop drug and seek medical assistance if sudden vision or hearing loss or erection lasting longer than 4 hours occurs.

Teaching points
- Take this drug approximately 30 min before sexual activity; use this drug only once in a 24-hour period.
- Know that sexual stimulation is required to see drug's effects. This drug does not protect you from sexually transmitted diseases; take appropriate precautions.
- Do not take this drug if you are using nitrates for chest pain or if you are taking antihypertensive medications; serious adverse effects could occur.
- Do not drink alcohol while taking this drug; serious low blood pressure could occur.
- Do not drink large amounts of grapefruit juice while taking this drug.
- Stop the drug immediately and seek medical assistance if you experience sudden vision or hearing loss or an erection lasting 4 hours or longer.
- You may experience these side effects: Dizziness, headache, upset stomach (these symptoms usually pass quickly; consult your health care provider if they persist).
- Report difficulty urinating, dizziness, fainting, loss of vision or hearing, erection lasting longer than 4 hours.

▽ **axitinib**

See Appendix R, *Less commonly used drugs.*

▽ **azacitidine**

See Appendix R, *Less commonly used drugs.*

▽ **azathioprine**
(ay za thye' oh preen)

Azasan, Imuran

PREGNANCY CATEGORY D

Drug class
Immunosuppressant

Therapeutic actions
Suppresses cell-mediated hypersensitivities and alters antibody production; exact mechanisms of action in increasing homograft survival and affecting autoimmune diseases not clearly understood.

Indications
- Renal homotransplantation: Adjunct for prevention of rejection
- Rheumatoid arthritis: Use only with adults meeting criteria for classic rheumatoid arthritis and not responding to conventional management
- Unlabeled uses: Treatment of chronic ulcerative colitis, myasthenia gravis, Behçet's syndrome, Crohn's disease, clinically definite MS (alone or in combination with other drugs), psoriasis

Contraindications and cautions
- Contraindicated with allergy to azathioprine; rheumatoid arthritis patients previously treated with alkylating agents, increasing their risk for neoplasia; pregnancy.
- Use cautiously with bone marrow suppression, hepatic impairment, lactation, serious infection.

Available forms
Tablets—50, 75, 100 mg; injection—100 mg/vial

Dosages

Adults

- *Renal homotransplantation:* Initially, 3–5 mg/kg/day PO or IV as a single dose on the day of transplant; for maintenance, use 1–3 mg/kg/day PO. Do not increase dose to decrease risk of rejection.
- *Rheumatoid arthritis:* Usually given daily; initial dose is 1 mg/kg PO given as a single dose or bid. Dose may be increased at 6–8 wk and thereafter by steps at 4-wk intervals. Dose increments should be 0.5 mg/kg/day up to a maximum dose of 2.5 mg/kg/day. Once patient is stabilized, dose should be decreased to lowest effective dose; decrease in 0.5-mg/kg increments. Patients who do not respond in 12 wk are probably refractory.

Pediatric patients

Safety and efficacy not established.

Geriatric patients or patients with renal impairment

Lower doses may be required because of decreased rate of excretion and increased sensitivity to the drug.

Pharmacokinetics

Route	Onset	Peak
Oral	Varies	1–2 hr
IV	Immediate	30–45 min

Metabolism: Hepatic; $T_{1/2}$: 5 hr
Distribution: Crosses placenta; may enter breast milk
Excretion: Urine

▼ IV FACTS

Preparation: Add 10 mL sterile water for injection and swirl until a clear solution results; use within 24 hr. Further dilution into sterile saline or dextrose is usually made for infusion.
Infusion: Infuse over 30–60 min; can range from 5 min–8 hr for the daily dose.

Adverse effects

- **GI:** *Nausea, vomiting,* hepatotoxicity (especially in homograft patients)
- **Hematologic:** *Leukopenia, thrombocytopenia, macrocytic anemia*
- **Other: Serious infections** (fungal, bacterial, protozoal infections secondary to immunosuppression), *carcinogenesis* (increased risk of neoplasia, especially in homograft patients)

Interactions

* **Drug-drug** • Increased effects with allopurinol; reduce azathioprine to one-third to one-fourth the usual dose • Reversal of the neuromuscular blockade of nondepolarizing neuromuscular junction blockers (atracurium, pancuronium, tubocurarine, vecuronium) with azathioprine

■ Nursing considerations

Assessment

- **History:** Allergy to azathioprine; rheumatoid arthritis patients previously treated with alkylating agents; pregnancy or male partners of women trying to become pregnant; lactation
- **Physical:** T; skin color, lesions; liver evaluation, bowel sounds; LFTs, renal function tests, CBC

Interventions

- Give drug IV if oral administration is not possible; switch to oral route as soon as possible.
- Administer in divided daily doses or with food if GI upset occurs.

⊗ **Black box warning** Monitor blood counts regularly; severe hematologic effects may require the discontinuation of therapy; increases risk of neoplasia. Alert patient accordingly.

Teaching points

- Take drug in divided doses with food if GI upset occurs.
- You will need to have regular blood tests to check the effects of this drug on your body.
- Avoid infections; avoid crowds or people who have infections. Notify your physician at once if you are injured.
- Notify your health care provider if you think you are pregnant or wish to become pregnant, or if you are a man whose sex partner wishes to become pregnant.
- You may experience these side effects: Nausea, vomiting (take drug in divided doses or with food), diarrhea, rash.
- Report unusual bleeding or bruising, fever, sore throat, mouth sores, signs of infection, abdominal pain, severe diarrhea, darkened urine or pale stools, severe nausea and vomiting.

Adverse effects in *italics* are most common; those in **bold** are life-threatening. ▭▭ Do not crush.

A

▽azilsartan medoxomil
(ay' zil sar' tan)

Edarbi

PREGNANCY CATEGORY C
(FIRST TRIMESTER)

PREGNANCY CATEGORY D
(SECOND AND THIRD
TRIMESTERS)

Drug classes
Angiotensin II receptor blocker
Antihypertensive

Therapeutic actions
Selectively blocks the binding of angiotensin II to specific tissue receptors found in vascular smooth muscle and the adrenal gland; this action blocks the vasoconstrictive effect of the renin-angiotensin system as well as the release of aldosterone, leading to a decrease in BP.

Indications
• Treatment of hypertension, alone or with other antihypertensives

Contraindications and cautions
• Contraindicated with hypersensitivity to components of the drug, pregnancy (use during second or third trimester can cause fetal injury or even death), lactation.
• Use cautiously with renal impairment, volume or salt depletion.

Available forms
Tablets—40, 80 mg

Dosages
Adults
80 mg/day PO; for patients on high dose of diuretics or who are volume-depleted, consider a starting dose of 40 mg/day and titrate if tolerated.
Pediatric patients younger than 18 yr
Safety and efficacy not established.

Pharmacokinetics

Route	Onset	Peak
Oral	Rapid	1.5–3 hr

Metabolism: Hepatic; $T_{1/2}$: 11 hr
Distribution: Crosses placenta; enters breast milk
Excretion: Urine, feces

Adverse effects
• **CNS:** Headache, dizziness, asthenia, fatigue
• **CV:** Hypotension, orthostatic hypotension
• **GI:** *Diarrhea,* nausea, constipation, dry mouth, abdominal pain
• **Other:** Rash, pruritus

Interactions
✳ **Drug-drug** • Increased risk of renal damage, including renal failure, if combined with NSAIDs in patients with renal dysfunction, elderly patients, and volume-depleted patients; if this combination is used, monitor renal function carefully • Increased risk of hypotension if combined with NSAIDs; if this combination is used, monitor BP regularly

■ Nursing considerations
Assessment
• **History:** Known hypersensitivity to components of the drug, lactation, pregnancy, renal dysfunction, hypovolemia
• **Physical:** Skin lesions, turgor; reflexes, affect; GI exam; renal function tests

Interventions
⊗ **Black box warning** Ensure patient is not pregnant before start of therapy; suggest the use of barrier contraceptives during therapy; fetal injury and death have been reported. When pregnancy is detected, discontinue drug as soon as possible.
• Administer without regard to meals.
• If the patient is breast-feeding, help her find an alternative method of feeding the infant; depression of the renin-angiotensin system in infants is potentially very dangerous.
⊗ **Warning** Alert surgeon and mark patient's chart with notice that patient is taking azilsartan; blockage of the renin-angiotensin system after surgery can produce problems. Hypotension may need to be reversed with volume expansion.
• Be aware that patient may need additional antihypertensives if BP control is not achieved.
• Monitor patient closely in situations that may lead to a decrease in BP secondary to reduction in fluid volume (such as

excessive perspiration, vomiting, diarrhea); excessive hypotension may occur.

Teaching points

- Take this drug without regard to meals. Do not stop taking this drug without consulting your health care provider.
- You need to be careful in situations that could result in loss of fluid (such as excess perspiration, diarrhea, and vomiting) because your blood pressure could become very low. Try to maintain fluid intake at all times.
- Do not take this drug if you are pregnant; the drug can have serious effects on the fetus and can even cause fetal death. Use of a barrier contraceptive is advised. If you should become pregnant, consult your health care provider immediately.
- If you are breast-feeding, you should use another method of feeding the baby while you are on this drug. This drug could cause serious adverse effects in the baby.
- You may experience these side effects: Dizziness (use caution when moving about, change position slowly, and avoid driving a car or using dangerous machinery if dizziness occurs); nausea and diarrhea (small, frequent meals may help; medication may be available to relieve these symptoms).
- Report severe diarrhea, pregnancy, dizziness with position changes.

▷ azithromycin
(ay zi thro my' sin)

AzaSite, Zithromax, Zmax

PREGNANCY CATEGORY B

Drug class
Macrolide antibiotic

Therapeutic actions
Bacteriostatic or bactericidal in susceptible bacteria; interferes with protein synthesis.

Indications
- Treatment of lower respiratory infections: Acute bacterial exacerbations of COPD due to *Haemophilus influenzae, Moraxella catarrhalis, Streptococcus pneumoniae;* community-acquired pneumonia due to *S. pneumoniae, H. influenzae, Mycoplasma pneumoniae; Chlamydophilia pneumoniae*
- Treatment of lower respiratory infections: Streptococcal pharyngitis and tonsillitis due to *Streptococcus pyogenes* in those who cannot take penicillins
- Treatment of genital ulcer disease caused by *Haemophilus ducreyi* (chancroid) in men
- Treatment of uncomplicated skin infections due to *Staphylococcus aureus, S. pyogenes, Streptococcus agalactiae*
- Treatment of nongonococcal urethritis and cervicitis due to *Chlamydia trachomatis;* treatment of PID
- Treatment of otitis media caused by *H. influenzae, M. catarrhalis, S. pneumoniae* in children older than 6 mo
- Treatment of pharyngitis and tonsillitis caused by *S. pyogenes* in children older than 2 yr who cannot use first-line therapy
- Prevention and treatment of disseminated *Mycobacterium avium* complex (MAC) in patients with advanced HIV infection
- Treatment of patients with mild to moderate acute bacterial sinusitis caused by *H. influenzae, M. catarrhalis, S. pneumoniae* (*Zmax*)
- Treatment of mild to moderate community-acquired pneumonia caused by *C. pneumoniae, H. influenzae, M. pneumoniae, S. pneumoniae* (*Zmax*)
- Treatment of bacterial conjunctivitis (*AzaSite*)
- Unlabeled uses: Uncomplicated gonococcal infections caused by *N. gonorrhoeae,* gonococcal pharyngitis caused by *N. gonorrhoeae,* chlamydial infections caused by *C. trachomatis,* prophylaxis after sexual attack, babesiosis, early Lyme disease, granuloma inguinale, treatment of cholera in adults

Contraindications and cautions
- Contraindicated with hypersensitivity to azithromycin, erythromycin, or any macrolide antibiotic, mild to moderate pneumonia, cystic fibrosis, bacteremia, immunocompromised patients, elderly patients.
- Use cautiously with gonorrhea or syphilis, pseudomembranous colitis, hepatic or renal impairment, lactation.

Available forms
Tablets—250, 500, 600 mg; powder for injection—500 mg; injection—2.5 g; powder for

oral suspension–100 mg/5 mL, 200 mg/5 mL, 1 g/packet; bottles for oral suspension—2 g to be reconstituted with 60 mL water (*Zmax*); ophthalmic solution—1%

Dosages
Adults

- *Mild to moderate acute bacterial exacerbations of COPD, pneumonia, pharyngitis and tonsillitis (as second-line), uncomplicated skin and skin structure infections:* 500 mg PO single dose on first day, followed by 250 mg PO daily on days 2–5 for a total dose of 1.5 g or 500 mg/day PO for 3 days.
- *Nongonococcal urethritis, genital ulcer disease, and cervicitis due to* C. trachomatis: A single 1-g PO dose.
- *Gonococcal urethritis and cervicitis:* A single dose of 2 g PO.
- *Disseminated MAC infections:* For prevention, 1,200 mg PO taken once weekly. For treatment, 600 mg/day PO with etambutol.
- *Acute sinusitis:* 500 mg/day PO for 3 days or a single 2-g dose of *Zmax*.
- *Mild to moderate acute bacterial sinusitis, community acquired pneumonia:* 2 g PO as a single dose (*Zmax*).
- *Community-acquired pneumonia (patients 16 yr and older):* 500 mg IV daily for at least 2 days; then 500 mg PO for a total of 7–10 days.
- *Mild community-acquired pneumonia:* 500 mg PO on day 1, then 250 mg PO for 4 days.
- *PID:* 500 mg IV daily for 1–2 days; then 250 mg/day PO for a total of 7 days.

Pediatric patients 6 mo and older

- *Otitis media:* Initially, 10 mg/kg PO as a single dose, then 5 mg/kg on days 2–5 or 30 mg/kg PO as a single dose; or 10 mg/kg/day PO for 3 days.
- *Community-acquired pneumonia (patients 6 mo–15 yr):* 10 mg/kg PO as a single dose on first day, then 5 mg/kg PO on days 2–5, or 60 mg/kg *Zmax* as a single dose; children weighing more than 34 kg (75 lb) should receive adult dosage.
- *Pharyngitis or tonsillitis (patients 2 yr and older):* 12 mg/kg/day PO on days 1–5 (maximum of 500 mg/day). Safety and efficacy for children younger than 2 yr have not been established.
- *Acute sinusitis:* 10 mg/kg/day PO for 3 days.

Ophthalmic solution

- *Patients 1 yr and older:* 1 drop to affected eye(s) bid for 2 days, then 1 drop/day for 5 days.

Pharmacokinetics

Route	Onset	Peak	Duration
Oral	Varies	2.5–3.2 hr	24 hr

Metabolism: $T_{1/2}$: 11–48 hr
Distribution: Crosses placenta; enters breast milk
Excretion: Bile, urine—unchanged

▼ IV FACTS

Preparation: Add 4.8 mL sterile water for injection to 500-mg vial. Shake until drug is dissolved; may be further diluted in 0.9% normal saline; 0.45% normal saline, D_5W in water, 5% dextrose in lactated Ringer's solution, 1/2 or 1/3 normal saline, lactated Ringer's solution, *Normosol-M or Normosol-R* in 5% dextrose. Drug is stable for 24 hr at room temperature or for 7 days refrigerated.
Infusion: Infuse over 60 minutes or longer.
Guidelines: 1 mg/mL solution over 3 hr; 2 mg/mL over 1 hr.

Adverse effects

- **CNS:** Dizziness, headache, vertigo, somnolence, fatigue
- **CV:** QT-interval, prolongation
- **GI:** *Diarrhea, abdominal pain, nausea,* dyspepsia, flatulence, vomiting, melena, pseudomembranous colitis, *Clostridium difficile* diarrhea
- **Other:** *Superinfections,* **angioedema,** rash, photosensitivity, vaginitis

Interactions

✳ **Drug-drug** • Decreased serum levels and effectiveness of azithromycin with aluminum and magnesium-containing antacids • Possible increased effects of theophylline • Possible increased anticoagulant effects of warfarin • Increased risk of QT prolongation if combined with other drugs that prolong QT interval.

✳ **Drug-food** • Food greatly decreases the absorption of azithromycin

■ Nursing considerations

Assessment

- **History:** Hypersensitivity to azithromycin, erythromycin, or any macrolide antibiotic; gonorrhea or syphilis, pseudomembranous colitis, hepatic or renal impairment, lactation
- **Physical:** Site of infection; skin color, lesions; orientation, GI output, bowel sounds, liver evaluation; culture and sensitivity tests of infection, urinalysis, LFTs, renal function tests; tests for syphilis, gonorrhea as appropriate

Interventions

- Culture site of infection before therapy.
- Administer *Zmax* on an empty stomach 1 hr before or 2–3 hr after meals. Food affects the absorption of this drug. Patients may take all other forms without regard to food.
- Prepare *Zmax* by adding 60 mL water to bottle, shake well.
- Counsel patients being treated for STDs about appropriate precautions and additional therapy.

Teaching points

- Take the full course prescribed. Do not take with antacids. Tablets and oral suspension can be taken with or without food.
- Prepare *Zmax* by adding 60 mL (¼ cup) water to bottle, shake well, drink all at once.
- You may experience these side effects: Stomach cramping, discomfort, diarrhea; fatigue, headache (medication may help); additional infections in the mouth or vagina (consult your health care provider for treatment).
- Report severe or watery diarrhea, severe nausea or vomiting, rash or itching, mouth sores, vaginal sores.

▽**aztreonam**
(az' tree oh nam)

Azactam, Cayston

PREGNANCY CATEGORY B

Drug class

Monobactam antibiotic

Therapeutic actions

Bactericidal: Interferes with bacterial cell wall synthesis, causing cell death in susceptible gram-negative bacteria, ineffective against gram-positive and anaerobic bacteria.

Indications

- Treatment of UTIs, lower respiratory infections, skin and skin-structure infections, septicemia, intra-abdominal infections and gynecologic infections caused by susceptible strains of *Escherichia coli, Enterobacter, Serratia, Proteus, Salmonella, Providencia, Pseudomonas, Citrobacter, Haemophilus, Neisseria, Klebsiella*
- Adjunct to surgery in managing infections caused by susceptible organisms (especially gram-negative aerobic pathogens)
- Improvement of respiratory symptoms in cystic fibrosis patients with *Pseudomonas aeruginosa* infections (inhalation)
- Unlabeled use: 1 g IM for treatment of acute uncomplicated gonorrhea as alternative to spectinomycin in penicillin-resistant gonococci

Contraindications and cautions

- Contraindicated with allergy to aztreonam.
- Use cautiously with immediate hypersensitivity reaction to penicillins or cephalosporins, renal and hepatic disorders, lactation.

Available forms

Powder for injection—500 mg, 1 g, 2 g; single-use vial for inhalation—75 mg

Dosages

Available for IV and IM use and inhalation; maximum recommended dose, 8 g/day.

Adults
- *UTIs:* 500 mg–1 g IM or IV every 8–12 hr.
- *Moderately severe systemic infection:* 1–2 g IM or IV every 8–12 hr.
- *Severe systemic infection:* 2 g IM or IV every 6–8 hr.

Pediatric patients 9 mo and older
- *Mild to moderate infections:* 30 mg/kg IM or IV every 8 hr.
- *Moderate to severe infections:* 30 mg/kg IM or IV every 6–8 hr.

Maximum recommended dose, 120 mg/kg/day.

Adults and children 7 yr and older
Cystic fibrosis patients with P. aeruginosa *infections:* 75 mg inhalation using *Altera Nebulizer System* tid for 28 days; space doses at least 4 hr apart. Follow with 28 days off aztreonam.

Patients with renal impairment
Reduce dosage by one-half in patients who have estimated creatinine clearances between 10 and 30 mL/min/1.73m² after an initial loading dose

A

of 1 or 2 g. For creatinine clearance less than 10 mL/min; reduce dosage by 25%. For patients on hemodialysis, give 500 mg, 1 g, or 2 g initially; maintenance dose should be one-fourth the usual initial dose at fixed intervals of 6, 8, or 12 hr. In serious or life-threatening infections, give an additional one-eighth of the initial dose after each hemodialysis session.

Pharmacokinetics

Route	Onset	Peak	Duration
IM	Varies	60–90 min	6–8 hr
IV	Immediate	30 min	6–8 hr
Inhalation	Immediate	10 min	6–8 hr

Metabolism: $T_{1/2}$: 1.5–2 hr
Distribution: Crosses placenta; enters breast milk
Excretion: Urine

▼ IV FACTS

Preparation: After adding diluent to container, shake immediately and vigorously. Constituted solutions are not for multiple-dose use; discard any unused solution. Solution should be colorless to light straw yellow, or it may be slightly pink.
IV injection: Reconstitute contents of 15-mL vial with 6–10 mL sterile water for injection. Inject slowly over 3–5 min directly into vein or into IV tubing of compatible IV infusion.
IV infusion: Reconstitute contents of 100-mL bottle to make a final concentration of 20 mg/mL or less (add at least 50 mL of one of the following solutions per gram of aztreonam): 0.9% sodium chloride injection, Ringer's injection, lactated Ringer's injection, 5% or 10% dextrose injection, 5% dextrose and 0.2%, 0.45%, or 0.09% sodium chloride, sodium lactate injection, *Ionosol B with 5% Dextrose, Isolyte E, Isolyte E with 5% Dextrose, Isolyte M with 5% Dextrose, Normosol-R, Normosol-R and 5% Dextrose, Normosol-M and 5% Dextrose,* 5% and 10% mannitol injection, lactated Ringer's and 5% dextrose injection, *Plasma-Lyte M and 5% Dextrose, 10% Travert Injection, 10% Travert and Electrolyte no. 1, 2, or 3 Injection.* Use reconstituted solutions promptly after preparation; those prepared with sterile water for injection or sodium chloride injection should be used within 48 hr if stored at room temperature and within 7 days if refrigerated. Administer over 20–60 min. If giving into IV tub-

ing that is used to administer other drugs, flush tubing with delivery solution before and after aztreonam administration.
Incompatibilities: Do not mix with nafcillin sodium or metronidazole; other admixtures are not recommended because data are not available.
Y-site incompatibility: Vancomycin.

Adverse effects

- **Dermatologic:** *Rash, pruritus*
- **GI:** *Nausea, vomiting, diarrhea,* transient elevation of AST, ALT, LDH
- **Hypersensitivity: Anaphylaxis**
- **Local:** *Local phlebitis or thrombophlebitis* at IV injection site, swelling or discomfort at IM injection site
- **Respiratory:** Bronchospasm, cough, congestion, sore throat, wheezing (inhaled form)
- **Other:** Superinfections

■ Nursing considerations
Assessment

- **History:** Allergy to aztreonam, immediate hypersensitivity reaction to penicillins or cephalosporins, renal and hepatic disorders, lactation
- **Physical:** Skin color, lesions; injection sites; T; GI mucous membranes, bowel sounds, liver evaluation; GU mucous membranes; culture and sensitivity tests of infected area; LFTs, renal function tests

Interventions

- Arrange for culture and sensitivity tests of infected area before therapy. In acutely ill patients, therapy may begin before test results are known. If therapeutic effects are not noted, reculture area.
- For IM administration, reconstitute contents of 15-mL vial with at least 3 mL of diluent per gram of aztreonam. Appropriate diluents are sterile water for injection, bacteriostatic water for injection, 0.9% sodium chloride injection, bacteriostatic sodium chloride injection. Inject deeply into a large muscle mass. Do not mix with any local anesthetic.
- ⊗ **Warning** Discontinue drug and provide supportive measures if hypersensitivity reaction or anaphylaxis occurs.
- Monitor injection sites and provide comfort measures.

- Prepare inhaled form immediately before use. Administer using *Altera Nebulizer System*; each dose should take 2–3 min. Space doses at least 4 hr apart.
- Administer a bronchodilator before giving inhaled form: If bronchodilator is short-acting, give 15 min to 4 hr before each dose; if long-acting, give 30 min to 12 hr before each dose. If patient is on multiple inhaled therapies, use the following order—bronchodilator, mucolytic, aztreonam.
- Provide treatment and comfort measures if superinfections occur.
- Monitor patient's nutritional status, and provide small, frequent meals and mouth care if GI effects or superinfections interfere with nutrition.

Teaching points

- This drug can be given IM or IV or by inhalation.
- If you are using the inhaled form, it may be stored at room temperature for up to 28 days. Do not use after expiration date. The powder must be diluted with the saline provided. Use immediately after you have prepared the drug. Do not mix with other solutions. Use only with the *Altera Nebulizer System*. Space your daily treatments at least 4 hr apart. Use this drug for the full 28 days. If you are using other inhaled drugs, take them in the following order—bronchodilators, mucolytics, then this drug.
- You may experience these side effects: Nausea, vomiting, diarrhea.
- Report pain, soreness at injection site; difficulty breathing; mouth sores; facial swelling.

▽ bacitracin
*(bass i **tray**' sin)*

Powder for injection: Baci-IM, BaciJect (CAN)
Topical ointment: Baciguent (CAN)

PREGNANCY CATEGORY C

Drug class
Antibiotic

Therapeutic actions
Antibacterial; inhibits cell wall synthesis of susceptible bacteria, primarily staphylococci, causing cell death.

Indications
- IM: Pneumonia and empyema caused by susceptible strains of staphylococci in infants
- Ophthalmic preparations: Superficial ocular infections involving the conjuctiva or cornea caused by susceptible strains of staphylococci
- Topical ointment: Prophylaxis of minor skin abrasions; treatment of superficial infections of the skin caused by susceptible staphylococci

Contraindications and cautions
- Contraindicated with allergy to bacitracin, renal disease (IM use), lactation.
- Use cautiously with pregnancy, dehydration.

Available forms
Powder for injection—50,000 units; ophthalmic ointment—500 units/g; topical ointment—500 units/g

Dosages
Adults and pediatric patients
Ophthalmic
Administration and dosage vary depending on the product used. See the product's package insert.
Topical
Apply to affected area one to three times per day; cover with sterile bandage if needed. Do not use longer than 1 wk.
IM
Infants weighing less than 2.5 kg: 900 units/kg/day IM in two to three divided doses.
Infants weighing more than 2.5 kg: 1,000 units/kg/day IM in two to three divided doses.

Pharmacokinetics

Route	Onset	Peak	Duration
IM	Rapid	1–2 hr	12–14 hr

Metabolism: Hepatic; $T_{1/2}$: 6 hr
Distribution: Crosses placenta; enters breast milk
Excretion: Urine

Adverse effects
- **GI:** Nausea, vomiting
- **GU:** *Nephrotoxicity*
- **Local:** *Pain at injection site* (IM); *contact dermatitis* (topical ointment); *irritation, burning, stinging, itching, blurring of vision* (ophthalmic preparations)
- **Other:** Superinfections

Interactions
✴ **Drug-drug** • Increased neuromuscular blockade and muscular paralysis with anesthetics, nondepolarizing neuromuscular blocking drugs, drugs with neuromuscular blocking activity • Increased risk of respiratory paralysis and renal failure with aminoglycosides

■ Nursing considerations
Assessment
- **History:** Allergy to bacitracin, renal disease, lactation
- **Physical:** Site of infection; skin color, lesions; normal urinary output; urinalysis, serum creatinine, renal function tests

Interventions
- For IM use, reconstitute 50,000-unit vial with 9.8 mL 0.9% sodium chloride injection with 2% procaine hydrochloride; reconstitute the 10,000-unit vial with 2 mL of diluent (resulting concentration of 5,000 units/mL). Do not use diluents containing parabens; precipitates can form. Refrigerate unreconstituted vials. Reconstituted solutions are stable for 1 wk, refrigerated.
- For topical application, cleanse the area before applying new ointment.
- Culture infected area before therapy.
- Ensure adequate hydration to prevent renal toxicity.

⊗ **Black box warning** During IM therapy, monitor renal function tests daily; risk of serious renal toxicity.

Teaching points
- Give ophthalmic preparation as follows: Tilt head back; place medication inside the eyelid and close eyes; gently hold the inner corner of the eye for 1 minute. Do not touch tube to eye. For topical application, cleanse area being treated before applying

new ointment; cover with sterile bandage (if possible).
- You may experience these side effects: Superinfections (frequent hygiene measures, medications may help); transient burning, stinging, or blurring of vision (ophthalmic).
- Report rash or skin lesions; change in urinary voiding patterns; changes in vision, severe stinging, or itching (ophthalmic).

▽baclofen
(bak' loe fen)

Apo-Baclofen (CAN), Gablofen, Gen-Baclofen, (CAN), Kemstro, Lioresal, Lioresal Intrathecal, PMS-Baclofen (CAN), ratio-Baclofen (CAN)

PREGNANCY CATEGORY C

Drug class
Centrally acting skeletal muscle relaxant

Therapeutic actions
Precise mechanism not known; GABA analogue but does not appear to produce clinical effects by actions on GABA-minergic systems; inhibits both monosynaptic and polysynaptic spinal reflexes; CNS depressant.

Indications
- Alleviation of signs and symptoms of spasticity resulting from MS, particularly for the relief of flexor spasms and concomitant pain, clonus, muscular rigidity (for patients with reversible spasticity to aid in restoring residual function); treatment of severe spasticity (intrathecal route)
- Spinal cord injuries and other spinal cord diseases—may be of some value (oral)
- Unlabeled uses: Trigeminal neuralgia (tic douloureux); may be beneficial in reducing spasticity in cerebral palsy in children (intrathecal use); intractable hiccups unresponsive to other therapies, alcohol and opiate withdrawal (oral), GERD, migraine prevention

Contraindications and cautions

- Contraindicated with hypersensitivity to baclofen; skeletal muscle spasm resulting from rheumatic disorders.
- Use cautiously with stroke, cerebral palsy, Parkinson's disease, seizure disorders, lactation, pregnancy.

Available forms

Tablets—10, 20 mg; intrathecal—0.05 mg/mL, 0.5 mg/mL, 2 mg/mL, 10 mg/20 mL, 10 mg/5 mL; oral disintegrating tablets—10, 20 mg

Dosages
Adults
Oral

Individualize dosage; start at low dosage and increase gradually until optimum effect is achieved (usually 40–80 mg/day). The following dosage schedule is suggested: 5 mg PO tid for 3 days; 10 mg tid for 3 days; 15 mg tid for 3 days; 20 mg tid for 3 days. Thereafter, additional increases may be needed, but do not exceed 80 mg/day (20 mg qid); use lowest effective dose. If benefits are not evident after a reasonable trial period, gradually withdraw the drug.

Intrathecal

Refer to manufacturer's instructions on pump implantation and initiation of long-term infusion. Testing is usually done with 50 mcg/mL injected into intrathecal space over 1 min. Patient is observed for 4–8 hr, then dose of 75 mcg/1.5 mL is given; patient is observed for 4–8 hr; a final screening bolus of 100 mcg/2 mL is given 24 hr later if the response is still not adequate. Patients who do not respond to this dose are not candidates for the implant. Maintenance dose is determined by monitoring patient response. Maintenance dose for spasticity of cerebral origin ranges from 22–1,400 mcg/day. Maintenance dose for spasticity of spinal cord origin ranges from 12–2,003 mcg/day; usual range is 300–800 mcg/day. Smallest dose possible to achieve muscle tone without adverse effects is desired.

Pediatric patients

Safety for use in children younger than 12 yr not established; orphan drug use to decrease spasticity in children with cerebral palsy is being studied.

Geriatric patients or patients with renal impairment

Dosage reduction may be necessary; monitor closely (drug is excreted largely unchanged by the kidneys).

Pharmacokinetics

Route	Onset	Peak	Duration
Oral	1 hr	2 hr	4–8 hr
Intrathecal	30–60 min	4 hr	4–8 hr

Metabolism: Hepatic; $T_{1/2}$: 3–4 hr
Distribution: Crosses placenta; enters breast milk
Excretion: Urine

Adverse effects

- **CNS:** *Transient drowsiness, dizziness, weakness, fatigue, confusion, headache, insomnia*
- **CV:** *Hypotension,* palpitations
- **GI:** Nausea, constipation
- **GU:** *Urinary frequency,* dysuria, enuresis, impotence
- **Other:** Rash, pruritus, ankle edema, excessive perspiration, weight gain, nasal congestion, increased AST, elevated alkaline phosphatase, elevated blood sugar, weakness

Interactions

✳ **Drug-drug** • Increased CNS depression with alcohol, other CNS depressants

■ Nursing considerations
Assessment

- **History:** Hypersensitivity to baclofen, skeletal muscle spasm resulting from rheumatic disorders, stroke, cerebral palsy, Parkinson's disease, seizure disorders, lactation, pregnancy
- **Physical:** Weight; T; skin color, lesions; orientation, affect, reflexes, bilateral grip strength, visual examination; P, BP; bowel sounds, normal GI output, liver evaluation; normal urinary output; LFTs, renal function tests, blood and urine glucose

Interventions

- Patients given implantable device for intrathecal delivery need to learn about the programmable delivery system, frequent checks; how to adjust dose and programming.

Adverse effects in *italics* are most common; those in **bold** are life-threatening. ⬚ Do not crush.

B

• Give with caution to patients whose spasticity contributes to upright posture or balance in locomotion or whenever spasticity is used to increase function.

⊗ **Black box warning** Taper dosage gradually to prevent rebound spasticity, hallucinations, possible psychosis, rhabdomyolysis, or other serious effects; abrupt discontinuation can cause serious reactions.

Teaching points
• Take this drug exactly as prescribed. Do not stop taking this drug without consulting your health care provider; abrupt discontinuation may cause hallucinations or other serious effects.
• Avoid alcohol, sleep-inducing, or over-the-counter drugs because these could cause dangerous effects.
• Do not take this drug during pregnancy. If you decide to become pregnant or find that you are pregnant, consult your health care provider.
• You may experience these side effects: Drowsiness, dizziness, confusion (avoid driving or engaging in activities that require alertness); nausea (eat frequent small meals); insomnia, headache, painful or frequent urination (effects reversible; will go away when the drug is discontinued).
• Report frequent or painful urination, constipation, nausea, headache, insomnia, or confusion that persists or is severe.

⮞**balsalazide disodium**
(bal sal' a zyde)

Colazal

PREGNANCY CATEGORY B

Drug class
Anti-inflammatory

Therapeutic actions
Mechanism of action is unknown; thought to be direct, delivered intact to the colon; a local anti-inflammatory effect occurs in the colon where balsalazide is converted to mesalamine (5-ASA), which blocks cyclooxygenase and inhibits prostaglandin production in the colon.

Indications
• Treatment of mildly to moderately active ulcerative colitis

Contraindications and cautions
• Contraindicated with hypersensitivity to salicylates or mesalamine.
• Use cautiously with renal impairment, pregnancy, lactation.

Available forms
Capsules—750 mg

Dosages
Adults
Three 750-mg capsules PO tid for a total daily dose of 6.75 g. Continue for up to 12 wk.
Pediatric patients 5–17 yr
Three 750-mg capsules PO tid (6.75 g/day) with or without food for 8 wk, or one 750 mg capsule PO tid (2.25 g/day) with or without food for up to 8 wk.

Pharmacokinetics
Route	Onset	Peak
Oral	Varies	1–2 hr

Metabolism: Hepatic; $T_{1/2}$: Unknown
Distribution: Crosses placenta; may enter breast milk
Excretion: Feces and urine

Adverse effects
• **CNS:** *Headache, fatigue, malaise, depression,* dizziness, asthenia, insomnia
• **GI:** *Abdominal pain, cramps, vomiting, discomfort; gas; flatulence; nausea; diarrhea, dyspepsia,* bloating, hemorrhoids, rectal pain, constipation, diarrhea, dry mouth
• **Other:** *Flulike symptoms, rash,* fever, cold, back pain, peripheral edema, *arthralgia*

■ Nursing considerations

★ **CLINICAL ALERT!**
Name confusion has occurred between *Colazal* (balsalazide) and *Clozaril* (clozapine). Serious effects have occurred; use extreme caution.

Assessment
• **History:** Hypersensitivity to salicylates; renal impairment; pregnancy, lactation

- **Physical:** T, hair status; reflexes; affect; abdominal examination, rectal examination; urinary output, renal function tests

Interventions
- May be given for up to 12 wk (8 wk for children 5–17 yr).
- Monitor patients with renal impairment for possible adverse effects.
- Observe for possible worsening of ulcerative colitis.
- Ensure ready access to bathroom facilities if diarrhea occurs.
- Offer support and encouragement to deal with GI discomfort, CNS effects.
- Arrange for appropriate measures to deal with headache, arthralgia, GI problems.
- Provide small, frequent meals if GI upset is severe.
- Maintain all therapy (such as dietary restrictions, reduced stress) necessary to support remission of the ulcerative colitis.

Teaching points
- Take the drug without regard to meals in evenly divided doses. You can swallow the capsule whole, or you can open it and sprinkle the contents on applesauce.
- Maintain all of the usual restrictions and therapy that apply to your colitis. If this becomes difficult, consult your health care provider.
- You may experience these side effects: Abdominal cramping, discomfort, pain, diarrhea (ensure ready access to bathroom facilities, taking the drug with meals may help), headache, fatigue, fever, flulike symptoms (consult health care provider if these become bothersome, medications may be available to help); rash, itching (skin care may help; consult your health care provider if this becomes a problem).
- Report severe diarrhea, malaise, fatigue, fever, blood in the stool.

▷basiliximab

See Appendix R, *Less commonly used drugs*.

▷BCG intravesical

See Appendix R, *Less commonly used drugs*.

▷beclomethasone dipropionate
*(be kloe **meth*** a sone)*

Apo-Beclomethasone (CAN), Gen-Beclo AQ (CAN), Propaderm (CAN), QNASL, QVAR, ratio-Beclomethasone AQ (CAN)

beclomethasone dipropionate monohydrate
Beconase AQ

PREGNANCY CATEGORY C

Drug classes
Corticosteroid
Glucocorticoid
Hormone

Therapeutic actions
Anti-inflammatory effects; local administration into lower respiratory tract or nasal passages maximizes beneficial effects on these tissues while decreasing the likelihood of adverse corticosteroid effects from systemic absorption.

Indications
- Maintenance and prophylactic treatment of asthma in patients 5 yr and older
- Respiratory inhalant use: Control of bronchial asthma that requires corticosteroids along with other therapy
- Intranasal use: Relief of symptoms of seasonal or perennial and nonallergic rhinitis that respond poorly to other treatments; prevention of recurrence of nasal polyps following surgical removal

Contraindications and cautions
- Respiratory inhalant therapy: Contraindicated with acute asthmatic attack, status asthmaticus. Use caution with systemic fungal infections (may cause exacerbations), allergy to any ingredient, status asthmaticus, lactation.
- Intranasal therapy: Use caution with untreated local infections (may cause exacerbations); nasal septal ulcers, recurrent epistaxis, nasal surgery or trauma (interferes with healing); lactation.

Adverse effects in *italics* are most common; those in **bold** are life-threatening. ⊝ Do not crush.

Available forms

Inhalation aerosol—40 mcg/actuation, 80 mcg/actuation; nasal spray—0.042% (42 mcg/inhalation); nasal aerosol—80 mcg/actuation

Dosages
Respiratory inhalant use
Adults and children 12 yr and older
40–160 mcg bid. Do not exceed 320 mcg/bid. Titrate to response. "Low" dose: 80–240 mcg/day; "medium" dose: 240–480 mcg/day; "high" dose: more than 480 mcg/day.
Pediatric patients 5–11 yr
40 mcg bid. Do not exceed 80 mcg bid.
Pediatric patients younger than 5 yr
Do not use.
Intranasal therapy
Each actuation delivers 42 mcg or 80 mcg (*QNASL*). Discontinue therapy after 3 wk if no significant symptomatic improvement.
Adults and children 12 yr and older
One to two inhalations (42–84 mcg) in each nostril bid (total dose 168–336 mcg/day). For *QNASL*, give a total of four nasal aerosol sprays per day.
Pediatric patients 6–12 yr
One inhalation in each nostril bid. Total dose 168 mcg. With more severe symptoms, may increase to two inhalations in each nostril bid (336 mcg).

Pharmacokinetics

Route	Onset	Peak
Inhalation	1–2 wk	Rapid

Metabolism: Lungs, GI, and liver; $T_{1/2}$: 3–15 hr
Distribution: Crosses placenta; may enter breast milk
Excretion: Feces

Adverse effects
Respiratory inhalant use
- **Endocrine:** Cushing's syndrome with overdose, suppression of HPA function due to systemic absorption
- **Local:** *Oral, laryngeal, pharyngeal irritation,* fungal infections
Intranasal use
- **Local:** Nasal irritation, fungal infections
- **Respiratory:** *Epistaxis, rebound congestion,* perforation of the nasal septum, anosmia

- **Other:** *Headache, nausea,* urticaria

■ Nursing considerations
Assessment
- **History:** Acute asthmatic attack, status asthmaticus; systemic fungal infections; allergy to any ingredient; lactation; untreated local infections, nasal septal ulcers, recurrent epistaxis, nasal surgery or trauma
- **Physical:** Weight; T; P, BP, auscultation; R, adventitious sounds; chest radiograph before respiratory inhalant therapy; examination of nares before intranasal therapy

Interventions
⊗ *Warning* Taper systemic steroids carefully during transfer to inhalation steroids; deaths resulting from adrenal insufficiency have occurred during and after transfer from systemic to aerosol steroids.
- Use decongestant nose drops to facilitate penetration of intranasal steroids if edema or excessive secretions are present.

Teaching points
- This respiratory inhalant has been prescribed to prevent asthmatic attacks, not for use during an attack.
- Allow at least 1 minute between puffs (respiratory inhalant); if you also are using an inhalational bronchodilator (albuterol, levalbuterol, metaproterenol, epinephrine), use it several minutes before using the steroid aerosol.
- Rinse your mouth after using the respiratory inhalant aerosol.
- Use a decongestant before the intranasal steroid, and clear your nose of all secretions if nasal passages are blocked; intranasal steroids may take several days to produce full benefit.
- Use this product exactly as prescribed; do not take more than prescribed, and do not stop taking the drug without consulting your health care provider. The drug must not be stopped abruptly but must be slowly tapered.
- You may experience these side effects: Local irritation (use the device correctly), headache (consult your health care provider for treatment).
- Report sore throat or sore mouth.

▷ belatacept
(bel at' ab sept)

Nulogix

PREGNANCY CATEGORY C

Drug class
T-cell costimulation blocker

Therapeutic actions
Inhibits cytokine production by T cells required for antigen-specific antibody production by B cells, leading to a decrease in mean immunoglobulin concentrations.

Indications
• Prophylaxis of organ rejection in adults receiving kidney transplant (used with basiliximab induction, mycophenolate, corticosteroids)

Contraindications and cautions
• Contraindicated with history of serious hypersensitivity to belatacept; Epstein-Barr seronegative or unknown status Epstein-Barr serostatus, pregnancy, lactation, transplants of other organs.
• Use cautiously with infections, tuberculosis.

Available forms
Powder for injection—250 mg/vial

Dosages
Adults
Day of transplant—10 mg/kg IV over 30 min; repeat on day 5, end of week 2, 4, 8 and 12 after transplant. Maintenance—beginning end of wk 16, 5 mg/kg IV over 30 min every 4 wk.
Pediatric patients
Safety and efficacy not established.

Pharmacokinetics

Route	Onset	Peak
IV	Slow	8 wk

Metabolism: $T_{1/2}$: 10–13 days
Distribution: May cross placenta; may enter breast milk
Excretion: Tissue

▼ IV FACTS

Preparation: Reconstitute using only the silicone-free disposable syringe provided. Re-

constitute each vial with 10.5 mL of diluent using an 18G–21G needle. Reconstitute with sterile water for injection, 0.9% sodium chloride, or D_5W; rotate vial with gentle swirling motion. Vial will contain 25 mg/mL and should be clear to slightly opalescent and colorless to pale yellow; do not use if particles, discoloration appear. Further dilute correct dose with solution used for reconstitution. Withdraw volume of infusion fluid equal to volume of drug to be given and, using the silicone-free syringe, withdraw the drug solution from the vial and inject into the infusion container; gently rotate to mix.
Administration: Infuse over 30 min using a 0.2–1.2 micron filter.
Incompatibilities: Do not mix in solution with other drugs or add to solutions containing other drugs.

Adverse effects
• **CNS:** *Headache,* **progressive multifocal encephalopathy (PML), posttransplant lymphoproliferative disorder,** dizziness, insomnia, anxiety
• **CV:** *Hypertension, hypotension, edema*
• **GI:** *Constipation, diarrhea, nausea, vomiting, abdominal pain*
• **GU:** *UTI, hematuria, proteinuria*
• **Hematologic:** *Anemia, leukopenia*
• **Metabolic:** *Hypokalemia, hyperkalemia, hyperglycemia, hypoglycemia, dyslipidemia*
• **Respiratory:** *Cough*
• **Other: Serious to fatal infections, cancers,** *fever,* pain, *graft dysfunction*

Interactions
✳ **Drug-drug** • Live-virus vaccines should not be given to patient taking belatacept • Increased serum levels of mycophenolate when given with belatacept; monitor patient accordingly

■ Nursing considerations
Assessment
• **History:** Hypersensitivity to components of the drug; Epstein-Barr exposure status, pregnancy, lactation, infections
• **Physical:** T, BP, R; GI exam, neurologic status, renal function tests, CBC, serum electrolytes, lipid profile, Epstein-Barr serosensitivity, TB testing

Interventions

⊗ **Black box warning** Increased risk of post-transplant lymphoproliferative disorder, more likely in patients without Epstein-Barr exposure. Check Epstein-Barr serosensitivity before beginning treatment; monitor neurologic function closely.

⊗ **Black box warning** Increased risk of serious to fatal infections and malignancies related to immune suppression; only physicians experienced in immunosuppressive therapy should prescribe this drug.

• Use approved only for kidney transplants, not for other transplants.
• Check Epstein-Barr serostatus and do TB testing before beginning therapy.
• Regularly monitor neurologic function; consider lowering dosage or discontinuing drug if evidence of PML occurs.
• Protect patient from exposure to infection; monitor for signs of infection.
• Encourage regular cancer screening.
• Suggest another method of feeding the baby if drug is used by breast-feeding women.
• Patient should avoid sun exposure; use of sunscreen and protective clothing is suggested.

Teaching points

• This drug must be given IV; you should prepare a calendar of infusion dates.
• This drug will be given with other drugs to prevent rejection of your transplanted kidney.
• It is not known how this drug could affect a fetus. If you are pregnant or thinking about becoming pregnant, discuss this with your health care provider.
• This drug is not recommended for use while breast-feeding. If you are breast-feeding, you should use another method of feeding your baby.
• You will be at increased risk for infections and cancer development while taking this drug because your immune system will be depressed. Avoid exposure to infections and arrange for regular cancer screening.
• Avoid sun exposure; use of sunscreens and protective clothing is recommended.
• Do not get immunizations while taking this drug; consult your health care provider.
• Report signs of infection (fever, swelling, flu-like symptoms), changes in mood or behavior, tremor, visual disturbances.

▽ belimumab

See Appendix R, *Less commonly used drugs.*

▽ benazepril hydrochloride
(ben a' za pril)

Lotensin

PREGNANCY CATEGORY C (FIRST TRIMESTER)

PREGNANCY CATEGORY D (SECOND AND THIRD TRIMESTERS)

Drug classes

ACE inhibitor
Antihypertensive

Therapeutic actions

Blocks ACE from converting angiotensin I to angiotensin II, a potent vasoconstrictor, leading to decreased BP, decreased aldosterone secretion, a small increase in serum potassium levels, and sodium and fluid loss; increased prostaglandin synthesis also may be involved in the antihypertensive action.

Indications

• Treatment of hypertension alone or in combination with thiazide diuretics
• Unlabeled uses: Nondiabetic neuropathy, HF, post MI, diabetes, chronic kidney disease, recurrent stroke prevention

Contraindications and cautions

• Contraindicated with allergy to benazepril or other ACE inhibitors, pregnancy, history of angioedema.
• Use cautiously with impaired renal function, immunosuppression, hypotension, heart failure, salt or volume depletion, lactation, first trimester of pregnancy, hyperkalemia.

Available forms

Tablets—5, 10, 20, 40 mg

Dosages
Adults

Initial dose, 10 mg PO daily. Maintenance dose, 20–40 mg/day PO, single or two divided doses. Patients using diuretics should discontinue them 2–3 days prior to benazepril therapy.

If BP is not controlled, add diuretic slowly. If diuretic cannot be discontinued, begin benazepril therapy with 5 mg. Maximum dose, 80 mg.

Pediatric patients (6 yr and older)
0.1–0.6 mg/kg/day. Starting dose for monotherapy—0.2 mg/kg/day. Do not exceed 0.6 mg/kg/day (40 mg daily).

Patients with renal impairment
For creatinine clearance less than 30 mL/min (serum creatinine greater than 3 mg/dL), 5 mg PO daily. Dosage may be gradually increased until BP is controlled, up to a maximum of 40 mg/day. Not recommended for children with renal impairment.

Pharmacokinetics

Route	Onset	Peak	Duration
Oral	0.5–1 hr	3–4 hr	24 hr

Metabolism: Hepatic; $T_{1/2}$: 10–11 hr
Distribution: Crosses placenta; enters breast milk
Excretion: Urine

Adverse effects

• **CNS:** Dizziness, fatigue, headache, somnolence
• **CV:** Angina pectoris, hypotension in salt- or volume-depleted patients, palpitations
• **Dermatologic:** Rash, pruritus, diaphoresis, flushing, **Stevens-Johnson syndrome**
• **GI:** *Nausea,* abdominal pain, vomiting, constipation
• **Respiratory:** *Cough,* asthma, bronchitis, dyspnea, sinusitis
• **Other:** Angioedema, impotence, decreased libido, asthenia, myalgia, arthralgia

Interactions

✷ **Drug-drug** • Increased risk of hypersensitivity reactions with allopurinol • Increased coughing with capsaicin • Decreased antihypertensive effects with indomethacin and other NSAIDs • Increased lithium levels and neurotoxicity may occur if combine • Increased risk of hyperkalemia with potassium-sparing diuretics or potassium supplements

■ Nursing considerations
Assessment

• **History:** Allergy to benazepril or other ACE inhibitors, impaired renal function, heart failure, salt or volume depletion, lactation, pregnancy
• **Physical:** Skin color, lesions, turgor; T; P; BP, peripheral perfusion; mucous membranes, bowel sounds, liver evaluation; urinalysis, LFTs, renal function tests, CBC and differential

Interventions

⊗ **Warning** Alert surgeon: Note use of benazepril on patient's chart; the angiotensin II formation subsequent to compensatory renin release during surgery will be blocked; hypotension may be reversed with volume expansion.
• Monitor patient for possible drop in BP secondary to reduction in fluid volume (excessive perspiration and dehydration, vomiting, diarrhea) because excessive hypotension may occur.

⊗ **Black box warning** Ensure that patient is not pregnant; fetal abnormalities and death have occurred if used during second or third trimester. Encourage use of contraceptive measures.
• Reduce dosage in patients with impaired renal function.

Teaching points

• Do not stop taking the medication without consulting your health care provider.
• Be careful with any conditions that may lead to a drop in blood pressure (such as diarrhea, sweating, vomiting, dehydration); if light-headedness or dizziness occurs, consult your health care provider.
• You should not become pregnant while on this drug. Serious fetal abnormalities could occur; use of contraceptives is advised.
• You may experience these side effects: GI upset, loss of appetite (transient effects; if persistent, consult health care provider); light-headedness (transient; change position slowly, and limit activities to those that do not require alertness and precision); dry cough (irritating but not harmful; consult your health care provider).
• Report mouth sores; sore throat, fever, chills; swelling of the hands, feet; irregular heartbeat, chest pains; swelling of the face, eyes, lips, tongue, difficulty breathing, persistent cough.

Adverse effects in *italics* are most common; those in **bold** are life-threatening. ▨ Do not crush.

DANGEROUS DRUG

▽**bendamustine hydrochloride**
(*ben' dah moos' teen*)

Treanda

PREGNANCY CATEGORY D

Drug classes
Alkylating agent
Antineoplastic

Therapeutic actions
Cytotoxic; alkylates DNA and RNA and inhibits several enzymatic processes, leading to cell death.

Indications
- Treatment of chronic lymphocytic leukemia (CLL)
- Treatment of indolent B-cell non-Hodgkin lymphoma that has progressed during or within 6 mo of rituximab therapy or a rituximab-containing regimen

Contraindications and cautions
- Contraindicated with known hypersensitivity to bendamustine or mannitol, pregnancy, lactation, moderate or severe hepatic impairment, severe renal impairment.
- Use cautiously in patients with moderate renal impairment, mild hepatic impairment.

Available forms
Single-use vials—25, 100 mg

Dosages
Adults
- *CLL:* 100 mg/m^2 IV over 30 min on days 1 and 2 of a 28-day cycle for up to 6 cycles; dosage may need to be lowered based on patient response and drug toxicity.
- *Non-Hodgkin lymphoma:* 120 mg/m^2 IV over 60 min on days 1 and 2 of a 21-day cycle for up to 8 cycles; dosage may need to be adjusted based on patient response.
Pediatric patients
Safety and efficacy not established.
Patients with hepatic or renal impairment
Use caution with mild dysfunction; do not use with moderate to severe hepatic dysfunction and severe renal dysfunction.

Pharmacokinetics

Route	Onset	Peak
IV	Rapid	End of infusion

Metabolism: Hepatic; $T_{1/2}$: 3 hr
Distribution: Crosses placenta; may enter breast milk
Excretion: Feces

▼ IV FACTS
Preparation: Reconstitute 100-mg vial with 20 mL sterile water for injection; solution should be clear yellow with concentration of 5 mg/mL. Withdraw desired dose and transfer immediately to 500 mL 0.9% sodium chloride injection or 500 mL 2.5% dextrose/0.45% sodium chloride injection within 30 min of reconstitution; thoroughly mix bag. Drug is stable for 24 hr if refrigerated, 3 hr at room temperature.
Infusion: Administer complete infusion over 30 min (CLL) or 60 min for non-Hodgkin lymphoma.
Incompatibilities: Do not mix in solution with any other medications. Administer only with sterile water for injection diluent and 0.9% sodium chloride injection or 2.5% dextrose/0.45% sodium chloride injection.

Adverse effects
- **Dermatologic:** Rash to **toxic skin reactions,** pruritus
- **GI:** *Diarrhea, nausea, vomiting*
- **Hematologic:** *Myelosuppression,* hyperuricemia
- **Respiratory:** Nasopharyngitis, cough
- **Other:** *Infusion reaction,* tumor lysis syndrome, *infections, fever, fatigue,* chills, weight loss

Interactions
✳ **Drug-drug •** Concurrent use of CYP1A2 inhibitors (fluvoxamine, ciprofloxacin) or inducers (omeprazole, nicotine) can lead to treatment failure or increased toxicity; an alternative treatment should be considered

■ Nursing considerations
Assessment
- **History:** Hypersensitivity to mannitol or bendamustine, pregnancy, lactation, hepatic or renal impairment

- **Physical:** T; skin color, lesions; R, adventitious sounds; GI exam, renal function tests, LFTs

Interventions

- Monitor hematopoietic function before therapy and weekly during therapy to monitor patient response and ensure dosage is reduced when needed.

- Review safety precautions for bone marrow suppression with patient, such as avoiding infections and injuries and arranging rest periods throughout the day.

- Monitor patient carefully during infusion; severe infusion reactions have been reported. Antihistamines, antipyretics and corticosteroids may be needed if reactions do occur. Consider discontinuing drug if severe reactions occur.

- Monitor patient for tumor lysis syndrome, especially during the first cycle; provide appropriate fluid volume, monitor electrolytes, and consider prophylactic allopurinol for high-risk patients.

- Assess skin regularly. If skin reactions occur and become severe or progressive, drug may need to be stopped.

Teaching points

- Mark your calendar with the days you will need to have IV infusions.

- You will need to have regular blood tests, including tests right before your infusion, to monitor the drug's effects on your body and determine the dose you will need.

- You may feel tired because your red blood cell count is decreased. Plan rest periods during the day.

- You may experience increased bruising and bleeding because your platelet count is decreased. Try to avoid activities that could lead to injury.

- You are susceptible to infection because your white blood cell count is decreased. Avoid crowded places, people with known infections, and digging in the dirt (unless you are wearing gloves).

- This drug could harm a fetus. You should use contraceptive measures while you are on this drug. If you become pregnant, notify your health care provider immediately.

- It is not known how this drug could affect a breast-feeding infant. Because of the po-

tential for serious adverse effects, another method of feeding the infant should be used while you are on this drug.

- You may experience these side effects: Nausea, vomiting (small, frequent meals may help; medication may be available to relieve these symptoms), diarrhea (medications may also help this symptom), rash, fever.

- Report rash of any kind, any signs of infection (fever, fatigue, muscle aches and pains), significant bleeding, shortness of breath, swelling of the face, persistent or severe nausea, vomiting, or diarrhea.

▷ benzonatate
(ben zoe' na tate)

Benzonatate Softgels⬚, Tessalon⬚, Tessalon Perles⬚, Zonatuss

PREGNANCY CATEGORY C

Drug class
Antitussive (nonopioid)

Therapeutic actions
Related to the local anesthetic tetracaine; anesthetizes the stretch receptors in the respiratory passages, lungs, and pleura, hampering their activity and reducing the cough reflex at its source.

Indications
- Symptomatic relief of nonproductive cough
- Unlabeled use: To reduce cough reflex during procedures (ie, endoscopy)

Contraindications and cautions
- Contraindicated with allergy to benzonatate or related compounds (tetracaine); lactation.
- Use cautiously with pregnancy.

Available forms
Capsules⬚—100, 150, 200 mg

Dosages
Adults and pediatric patients 10 yr and older
100–200 mg PO tid; up to 600 mg/day may be used.

Pharmacokinetics

Route	Onset	Duration
Oral	15–20 min	3–8 hr

Metabolism: Hepatic; $T_{1/2}$: 2–4 hr
Distribution: Crosses placenta; may enter breast milk
Excretion: Urine

Adverse effects

- **CNS:** *Sedation, headache, mild dizziness,* hallucinations, nasal congestion, sensation of burning in the eyes
- **Dermatologic:** Pruritus, skin eruptions
- **GI:** *Constipation, nausea,* GI upset
- **Other:** Vague "chilly" feeling, numbness in the chest

■ Nursing considerations

Assessment

- **History:** Allergy to benzonatate or related compounds (tetracaine); lactation, pregnancy
- **Physical:** Nasal mucous membranes; skin color, lesions; orientation, affect; adventitious sounds

Interventions

⊗ *Warning* Administer orally; caution patient not to chew or break capsules but to swallow them whole; choking could occur if drug is released in the mouth.

Teaching points

- Swallow the capsules whole; do not chew or break capsules because numbness of the throat and mouth could occur, and swallowing could become difficult.
- You may experience these side effects: Rash, itching (skin care may help); constipation, nausea, GI upset; sedation, dizziness (avoid driving or tasks that require alertness).
- Report restlessness, tremor, difficulty breathing, constipation, rash, bizarre behavior.

▽ **benztropine mesylate**
(benz' troe peen)

Apo-Benztropine (CAN), Cogentin

PREGNANCY CATEGORY C

Drug class

Antiparkinsonian (anticholinergic type)

Therapeutic actions

Has anticholinergic activity in the CNS that is believed to help normalize the hypothesized imbalance of cholinergic and dopaminergic neurotransmission in the basal ganglia of the brain of a parkinsonism patient. Reduces severity of rigidity and, to a lesser extent, akinesia and tremor; less effective overall than levodopa; peripheral anticholinergic effects suppress secondary symptoms of parkinsonism, such as drooling.

Indications

- Adjunct in the therapy of parkinsonism (postencephalitic, arteriosclerotic, and idiopathic types)
- Control of extrapyramidal disorders (except tardive dyskinesia) due to neuroleptic drugs (phenothiazines)

Contraindications and cautions

- Contraindicated with hypersensitivity to benztropine; glaucoma, especially angle-closure glaucoma; pyloric or duodenal obstruction, stenosing peptic ulcers, achalasia (megaesophagus); prostatic hypertrophy or bladder neck obstructions; myasthenia gravis, megacolon.
- Use cautiously with tachycardia, cardiac arrhythmias, hypertension, hypotension, hepatic or renal impairment, alcoholism, chronic illness, work in hot environments; hot weather; lactation, Alzheimer's disease, thin patients, pregnancy.

Available forms

Tablets—0.5, 1, 2 mg; injection—1 mg/mL

Dosages

Adults

- *Parkinsonism:* Initially, 0.5–1 mg PO at bedtime; a total daily dose of 0.5–6 mg given at bedtime or in two to four divided doses is usual. Increase initial dose in 0.5-mg increments at 5- to 6-day intervals to the smallest amount necessary for optimal relief. Maximum daily dose, 6 mg. May be given IM or IV in same dosage as oral. When used with other drugs, gradually substitute benztropine for all or part of them and gradually reduce dosage of the other drug.
- *Drug-induced extrapyramidal symptoms:* For acute dystonic reactions, initially,

1–2 mg IM (preferred) or IV to control condition; may repeat if parkinsonian effect begins to return. After that, 1–4 mg PO daily or bid to prevent recurrences. Some patients may require higher doses.

• *Extrapyramidal disorders occurring early in neuroleptic treatment:* 1–2 mg PO bid to tid. Withdraw drug after 1 or 2 wk to determine its continued need; reinstitute if disorder reappears.

Pediatric patients
Safety and efficacy not established.

Geriatric patients
Strict dosage regulation may be necessary; patients older than 60 yr often develop increased sensitivity to the CNS effects of anticholinergic drugs.

Pharmacokinetics

Route	Onset	Duration
Oral	1 hr	6–10 hr
IM, IV	15 min	6–10 hr

Metabolism: Hepatic; $T_{1/2}$: Unknown
Distribution: Crosses placenta; enters breast milk
Excretion: Unknown

▼ IV FACTS

Preparation: Give undiluted. Store in tightly covered, light-resistant container. Store at room temperature.
Injection: Administer direct IV at a rate of 1 mg over 1 min.

Adverse effects
Peripheral anticholinergic effects

• **CV:** Tachycardia, palpitations, hypotension, orthostatic hypotension
• **Dermatologic:** Rash, urticaria, other dermatoses
• **EENT:** *Blurred vision,* mydriasis, diplopia, increased intraocular tension, angle-closure glaucoma
• **GI:** *Dry mouth, constipation,* dilation of the colon, paralytic ileus, *nausea,* vomiting, epigastric distress
• **GU:** *Urinary retention, urinary hesitancy,* dysuria, difficulty achieving or maintaining an erection
• **Other:** Flushing, decreased sweating, elevated temperature

CNS effects, characteristic of centrally acting anticholinergic drugs

• **CNS:** Disorientation, confusion, memory loss, hallucinations, psychoses, agitation, nervousness, delusions, delirium, paranoia, euphoria, excitement, light-headedness, dizziness, depression, drowsiness, weakness, giddiness, paresthesia, heaviness of the limbs
• **Other:** Muscular weakness, muscular cramping; inability to move certain muscle groups (high doses), numbness of fingers

Interactions

✳ **Drug-drug** • Paralytic ileus, hyperthermia, heat stroke, sometimes fatal, when given with other anticholinergic drugs, or drugs that have anticholinergic properties (phenothiazines, TCAs) • Additive adverse CNS effects (toxic psychosis) with other drugs that have CNS anticholinergic properties (TCAs, phenothiazines) • Possible masking of the development of persistent extrapyramidal symptoms, tardive dyskinesia, in patients on long-term therapy with antipsychotic drugs (phenothiazines, haloperidol) • Decreased therapeutic efficacy of antipsychotic drugs (phenothiazines, haloperidol), possibly due to central antagonism

■ Nursing considerations
Assessment

• **History:** Hypersensitivity to benztropine; glaucoma; pyloric or duodenal obstruction, stenosing peptic ulcers, achalasia; prostatic hypertrophy or bladder neck obstructions; myasthenia gravis; cardiac arrhythmias, hypertension, hypotension; hepatic or renal impairment; alcoholism, chronic illness, people who work in hot environments; other anticholinergics; lactation, pregnancy
• **Physical:** Weight; T; skin color, lesions; orientation, affect, reflexes, bilateral grip strength, visual examination including tonometry; P, BP, orthostatic BP; adventitious sounds; bowel sounds, normal output, liver evaluation; normal urinary output, voiding pattern, prostate palpation; LFTs, renal function tests

Interventions

• Decrease dosage or discontinue temporarily if dry mouth makes swallowing or speaking difficult.

- Do not give to patients on cholinesterase inhibitors. Benztropine directly counteracts the effects of these drugs.

⊗ **Warning** Give with caution and reduce dosage in hot weather. Drug interferes with sweating and body's ability to maintain heat equilibrium; provide sugarless candies or ice chips to suck for dry mouth.
- Give with meals if GI upset occurs; give before meals for dry mouth; give after meals if drooling or nausea occurs.
- Ensure patient voids before receiving each dose if urinary retention is a problem.

Teaching points
- Take this drug exactly as prescribed.
- Avoid alcohol, sedatives, and over-the-counter drugs (could cause dangerous effects).
- You may experience these side effects: Drowsiness, dizziness, confusion, blurred vision (avoid driving or engaging in activities that require alertness and visual acuity); nausea (eat frequent small meals); dry mouth (suck sugarless candies or ice chips); painful or difficult urination (empty bladder immediately before each dose); constipation (maintain adequate fluid intake and exercise regularly); use caution in hot weather (you are susceptible to heat prostration).
- Report difficult or painful urination, constipation, rapid or pounding heartbeat, confusion, eye pain, or rash.

▽**beractant (natural lung surfactant)**
(*ber ak' tant*)

Survanta

PREGNANCY CATEGORY
UNKNOWN

Drug class
Lung surfactant

Therapeutic actions
A natural bovine compound containing lipids and apoproteins that reduce surface tension and allow expansion of the alveoli; replaces the surfactant missing in the lungs of neonates suffering from respiratory distress syndrome (RDS).

Indications
- Prophylactic treatment of infants at risk of developing RDS; infants with birth weights less than 1,250 g or infants with birth weights more than 1,250 g who have evidence of pulmonary immaturity
- Rescue treatment of premature infants who have developed RDS

Contraindications and cautions
- Because beractant is used as an emergency drug in acute respiratory situations, the benefits usually outweigh any possible risks.

Available forms
Suspension—25 mg/mL suspended in 0.9% sodium chloride injection

Dosages
Pediatric patients
Accurate determination of birth weight is essential for correct dosage. Beractant is instilled into the trachea using a catheter inserted into the endotracheal tube.
- *Prophylactic treatment:* Give first dose of 100 mg phospholipids/kg birth weight (4 mL/kg) soon after birth, preferably within 15 min. After determining the needed dose, inject one-quarter of the dose into the endotracheal tube over 2–3 sec. Remove the catheter and ventilate the baby. Repeat the procedure to give the remaining one-quarter dose. A repeat dose may be given no sooner than 6 hr after previous dose if infant remains intubated and requires at least 30% inspired oxygen to maintain a partial pressure of arterial oxygen of 80 mm Hg or less. Four doses can be administered in the first 48 hr of life.
- *Rescue treatment:* Administer 100 mg phospholipids/kg birth weight (4 mL/kg) intratracheally. Administer the first dose as soon as possible within 8 hr of birth after the diagnosis of RDS is made and patient is on the ventilator. Repeat doses can be given based on clinical improvement and blood gases. Administer subsequent doses no sooner than every 6 hr. Mechanically ventilate after each dose.

Pharmacokinetics

Route	Onset	Peak
Intratracheal	Immediate	Hours

Metabolism: Normal surfactant metabolic pathways; $T_{1/2}$: Unknown
Distribution: Lung tissue

Adverse effects

- **CNS:** Seizures
- **CV:** *Patent ductus arteriosus,* **intraventricular hemorrhage, hypotension, bradycardia**
- **Respiratory: Pulmonary hemorrhage,** oxygen desaturation
- **Other:** *Sepsis, nonpulmonary infections*

■ Nursing considerations
Assessment

- **History:** Time of birth, exact birth weight
- **Physical:** Skin T, color; R, adventitious sounds, oximeter, endotracheal tube position and patency, chest movement; ECG, P, BP, peripheral perfusion, arterial pressure (desirable); oxygen saturation, blood gases, CBC; muscular activity, facial expression, reflexes

Interventions

- Monitor ECG and transcutaneous oxygen saturation continually during administration.
- Ensure that endotracheal tube is in the correct position, with bilateral chest movement and lung sounds.
- Have staff view manufacturer's teaching video before regular use to cover all the technical aspects of administration.
- Suction the infant immediately before administration, but do not suction for 1 hr after administration unless clinically necessary.
- Inspect vial for discoloration. Vial should contain off-white to brown liquid. Gently mix. Warm to room temperature before using—20 min standing or 8 min warmed by hand. Do not use other warming methods.
- Store drug in refrigerator. Protect from light. Enter drug vial only once. Discard remaining drug after use. Unopened, unused vials warmed to room temperature may be returned to refrigerator within 8 hr of warming.
- Insert 5 French catheter into the endotracheal tube; do not instill into the mainstem bronchus.
- Instill dose slowly; inject one-fourth dose over 2–3 sec; remove catheter and reattach infant to ventilator for at least 30 sec or until stable; repeat procedure administering one-fourth dose at a time. Keep accurate records of doses and timing.

- Do not suction infant for 1 hr after completion of full dose; do not flush catheter.
- Continually monitor patient's color, lung sounds, ECG, oximeter, and blood gas readings during administration and for at least 30 min after.

Teaching points

- Details of drug effects and administration are best incorporated into parents' comprehensive teaching program.

▷ **betamethasone**
*(bay ta **meth**' a sone)*

betamethasone
Topical dermatologic ointment, cream, lotion, gel

betamethasone dipropionate
*(dye proh **py**' oh nayt)*

Topical dermatologic ointment, cream, lotion, aerosol: Diprolene, Diprolene AF, Maxivate, Taro-Sone (CAN)

betamethasone sodium phosphate and acetate
Systemic, IM, and local intra-articular, intralesional, intra-dermal injection: Celestone Soluspan

betamethasone valerate
*(val **ayr**' ayt)*

Topical dermatologic ointment, cream, lotion, foam:
Betaderm (CAN),
Beta-Val, Luxiq, Prevex B (CAN),
Psorion Cream, Valisone

PREGNANCY CATEGORY D
(FIRST TRIMESTER)

PREGNANCY CATEGORY C
(SECOND AND THIRD TRIMESTERS)

Drug classes

Corticosteroid (long-acting)
Glucocorticoid
Hormone

B

Therapeutic actions

Binds to intracellular corticosteroid receptors, thereby initiating many natural complex reactions that are responsible for its anti-inflammatory and immunosuppressive effects.

Indications
Systemic administration

- Treatment of primary or secondary adreno-corticoid insufficiency
- Hypercalcemia associated with cancer
- Short-term management of inflammatory and allergic disorders, such as rheumatoid arthritis, collagen diseases (eg, SLE), dermatologic diseases (eg, pemphigus), status asthmaticus, and autoimmune disorders
- Hematologic disorders: Thrombocytopenia purpura, erythroblastopenia
- Ulcerative colitis, acute exacerbations of MS, and palliation in some leukemias and lymphomas
- Trichinosis with neurologic or myocardial involvement

Intra-articular or soft-tissue administration

- Arthritis, psoriatic plaques, and so forth

Dermatologic preparations

- Relief of inflammatory and pruritic manifestations of steroid-responsive dermatoses

Contraindications and cautions
Systemic (oral and parenteral) administration

- Contraindicated with infections, especially tuberculosis, fungal infections, amebiasis, vaccinia and varicella, and antibiotic-resistant infections, lactation.

All forms

- Use cautiously with kidney or liver disease, hypothyroidism, ulcerative colitis with impending perforation, diverticulitis, active or latent peptic ulcer, inflammatory bowel disease, heart failure, hypertension, thrombo-embolic disorders, osteoporosis, seizure disorders, diabetes mellitus, active infections.

Available forms

Syrup—0.6 mg/5 mL; injection—3 mg betamethasone sodium phosphate with 3 mg betamethasone acetate; ointment—0.1%, 0.05%; cream—0.01%, 0.05%, 0.1%; lotion—0.1%, 0.05%; gel—0.05%

Dosages
Adults
Systemic administration

Individualize dosage, based on severity and response. Give daily dose before 9 AM to minimize adrenal suppression. Reduce initial dosage in small increments until the lowest dose that maintains satisfactory clinical response is reached. If long-term therapy is needed, alternate-day therapy with a short-acting corticosteroid should be considered. After long-term therapy, withdraw drug slowly to prevent adrenal insufficiency.

- *Oral (betamethasone):* Initial dosage, 0.6–7.2 mg/day.
- *IM (betamethasone sodium phosphate; betamethasone sodium phosphate and acetate):* Initial dosage, 0.5–9 mg/day. Dosage range is one-third to one-half oral dose given every 12 hr. In life-threatening situations, dose can be in multiples of the oral dose.

Intrabursal, intra-articular, intradermal, intralesional (betamethasone sodium phosphate and acetate)

1.5–12 mg intra-articular, depending on joint size; 0.2 mL/cm^3 intradermally, not to exceed 1 mL/wk; 0.25–1 mL at 3- to 7-day intervals for disorders of the foot.

Topical dermatologic cream, ointment (betamethasone dipropionate)

Apply sparingly to affected area daily or bid.

Pediatric patients
Systemic administration

Individualize dosage on the basis of severity and response rather than by formulas that correct adult doses for age or weight. Carefully observe growth and development in infants and children on prolonged therapy.

Pharmacokinetics

Route	Onset	Duration
Systemic	Varies	3 days

Metabolism: Hepatic; $T_{1/2}$: 36–54 hr
Distribution: Crosses placenta; enters breast milk
Excretion: Urine, unchanged

Adverse effects

- **CNS:** *Vertigo, headache,* paresthesias, insomnia, seizures, psychosis, cataracts, increased IOP, glaucoma (in long-term therapy)

- **CV:** Hypotension, shock, hypertension, and heart failure secondary to fluid retention, thromboembolism, thrombophlebitis, fat embolism, cardiac arrhythmias
- **Electrolyte imbalance:** *Na⁺ and fluid retention,* hypokalemia, hypocalcemia
- **Endocrine:** Amenorrhea, irregular menses, growth retardation, decreased carbohydrate tolerance, diabetes mellitus, cushingoid state (long-term effect), increased blood sugar, increased serum cholesterol, decreased T_3 and T_4 levels, HPA suppression with systemic therapy longer than 5 days
- **GI:** Peptic or esophageal ulcer, pancreatitis, abdominal distention, nausea, vomiting, *increased appetite, weight gain (long-term therapy)*
- **Musculoskeletal:** Muscle weakness, steroid myopathy, loss of muscle mass, osteoporosis, spontaneous fractures (long-term therapy)
- **Other:** *Immunosuppression, aggravation, or masking of infections; impaired wound healing;* thin, fragile skin; petechiae, ecchymoses, purpura, striae; subcutaneous fat atrophy; hypersensitivity or anaphylactoid reactions

Effects related to various local routes of steroid administration

- **Intra-articular:** Osteonecrosis, tendon rupture, infection
- **Intralesional therapy:** Blindness when applied to face and head
- **Topical dermatologic ointments, creams, sprays:** *Local burning, irritation,* acneiform lesions, striae, skin atrophy, skin infections

Interactions

❋ **Drug-drug** • Risk of severe deterioration of muscle strength in myasthenia gravis patients receiving ambenonium, edrophonium, neostigmine, pyridostigmine • Decreased steroid blood levels with barbiturates, phenytoin, rifampin • Decreased effectiveness of salicylates with betamethasone

❋ **Drug-lab test** • False-negative nitrobluetetrazolium test for bacterial infection • Suppression of skin test reactions

■ Nursing considerations
Assessment

- **History:** (systemic administration): Infections, fungal infections, amebiasis, vaccinia and varicella, and antibiotic-resistant infections; kidney or liver disease; hypothyroidism; ulcerative colitis with impending perforation; diverticulitis; active or latent peptic ulcer; inflammatory bowel disease; heart failure; hypertension; thromboembolic disorders; osteoporosis; seizure disorders; diabetes mellitus; lactation
- **Physical:** Baseline weight, T, reflexes and grip strength, affect and orientation, P, BP, peripheral perfusion, prominence of superficial veins, R and adventitious sounds, serum electrolytes, blood glucose

Interventions
Systemic use

- Give daily dose before 9 AM to mimic normal peak corticosteroid blood levels.
- Increase dosage when patient is subject to stress.
- Taper doses when discontinuing high-dose or long-term therapy.
- Do not give live-virus vaccines with immunosuppressive doses of corticosteroids.

Topical dermatologic preparations

- Examine area for infections and skin integrity before application.
- Administer cautiously to pregnant patients; topical corticosteroids have caused teratogenic effects and can be absorbed from systemic site.

⊗ **Warning** Use caution when occlusive dressings or tight diapers cover affected area; these can increase systemic absorption of the drug.

- Avoid prolonged use near eyes, in genital and rectal areas, and in skin creases.

Teaching points
Systemic use

- Do not stop taking the oral drug without consulting your health care provider.
- Take single dose or alternate-day doses before 9 AM.
- Avoid exposure to infections; ability to fight infections is reduced.
- Wear a medical alert tag so emergency care providers will know that you are on this medication.

Adverse effects in *italics* are most common; those in **bold** are life-threatening. ⬚ Do not crush.

- You may experience these side effects: Increase in appetite, weight gain (counting calories may help); heartburn, indigestion (eat frequent small meals; take antacids); poor wound healing (consult your health care provider); muscle weakness, fatigue (frequent rest periods will help).
- Report unusual weight gain, swelling of the extremities, muscle weakness, black or tarry stools, fever, prolonged sore throat, colds or other infections, worsening of original disorder.

Intrabursal, intra-articular therapy

- Do not overuse joint after therapy, even if pain is gone.

Topical dermatologic preparations

- Apply sparingly; do not cover with tight dressings.
- Avoid contact with the eyes.
- Report irritation or infection at the site of application.

▽ betaxolol hydrochloride

(beh tax' oh lol)

Ophthalmic: Betoptic S
Oral: Kerlone

PREGNANCY CATEGORY C

Drug classes

Antiglaucoma drug
Antihypertensive
Beta$_1$-selective adrenergic blocker

Therapeutic actions

Blocks beta-adrenergic receptors of the sympathetic nervous system in the heart and juxtaglomerular apparatus (kidneys), decreasing the excitability of the heart, decreasing cardiac output and oxygen consumption, decreasing the release of renin from the kidneys, and lowering BP. Decreases IOP by decreasing the secretion of aqueous humor.

Indications

- Oral: Hypertension, used alone or with other antihypertensive agents, particularly thiazide-type diuretics

- Ophthalmic: Treatment of ocular hypertension and open-angle glaucoma alone or in combination with other antiglaucoma drugs

Contraindications and cautions

- Contraindicated with sinus bradycardia, second- or third-degree heart block, cardiogenic shock, heart failure.
- Use cautiously with renal failure, diabetes, or thyrotoxicosis (betaxolol masks the cardiac signs of hypoglycemia and thyrotoxicosis), lactation, pregnancy.

Available forms

Tablets—10, 20 mg; ophthalmic solution (0.5%)—5.6 mg/mL; ophthalmic suspension (0.25%)—2.8 mg/mL

Dosages
Adults
Oral
Initially, 10 mg PO daily, alone or added to diuretic therapy. Full antihypertensive effect is usually seen in 7–14 days. If desired response is not achieved, dose may be doubled.
Ophthalmic
One or two drops bid to affected eye or eyes.
Pediatric patients
Safety and efficacy not established.
Geriatric patients or patients with severe renal impairment; patients undergoing dialysis
Oral
Consider reducing initial dose to 5 mg PO daily.

Pharmacokinetics

Route	Onset	Peak	Duration
Oral	30–60 min	2 hr	12–15 hr
Ophthalmic	≤ 30 min	2 hr	12 hr

Metabolism: Hepatic; $T_{1/2}$: 14–22 hr
Distribution: Crosses placenta; enters breast milk
Excretion: Urine

Adverse effects
Oral form
- **Allergic reactions:** Pharyngitis, erythematous rash, fever, sore throat, laryngospasm, respiratory distress
- **CNS:** Dizziness, vertigo, tinnitus, fatigue, emotional depression, paresthesias, sleep disturbances, hallucinations, disorientation, memory loss, slurred speech

- **CV:** *Bradycardia, heart failure, cardiac arrhythmias, sinoatrial or AV nodal block, tachycardia,* peripheral vascular insufficiency, claudication, stroke, **pulmonary edema,** hypotension
- **Dermatologic:** Rash, pruritus, sweating, dry skin
- **EENT:** Eye irritation, dry eyes, conjunctivitis, blurred vision
- **GI:** Gastric pain, flatulence, constipation, *diarrhea, nausea, vomiting,* anorexia, ischemic colitis, renal and mesenteric arterial thrombosis, retroperitoneal fibrosis, hepatomegaly, acute pancreatitis
- **GU:** Impotence, decreased libido, Peyronie's disease, dysuria, nocturia, frequent urination
- **Musculoskeletal:** Joint pain, arthralgia, muscle cramp
- **Respiratory: Bronchospasm,** dyspnea, cough, bronchial obstruction, nasal stuffiness, rhinitis, pharyngitis (less likely than with propranolol)
- **Other:** *Decreased exercise tolerance, development of ANA,* hyperglycemia or hypoglycemia, elevated serum transaminase, alkaline phosphatase, and LDH

Betaxolol ophthalmic solution

- **CNS:** Insomnia, depressive neurosis
- **Local:** *Brief ocular discomfort, occasional tearing, itching, decreased corneal sensitivity,* corneal staining, keratitis, photophobia, blurred vision, dry eyes

Interactions

✳ **Drug-drug** • Increased effects with verapamil, anticholinergics • Increased risk of orthostatic hypotension with prazosin • Possible increased antihypertensive effects with aspirin, bismuth subsalicylate, magnesium salicylate, hormonal contraceptives • Decreased antihypertensive effects with NSAIDs • Possible masked hypoglycemic effect of insulin with betaxolol
✳ **Drug-lab test** • Possible false results with glucose or insulin tolerance tests

■ Nursing considerations

Assessment
- **History:** Sinus bradycardia, second- or third-degree heart block, cardiogenic shock, heart failure, renal failure, diabetes or thyrotoxicosis, lactation, pregnancy
- **Physical:** Baseline weight, skin condition, neurologic status, P, BP, ECG, R, renal and thyroid function tests, blood and urine glucose

Interventions

⊗ **Warning** Do not discontinue drug abruptly after long-term therapy (hypersensitivity to catecholamines may develop, exacerbating angina, MI, and ventricular arrhythmias). Taper drug gradually over 2 wk with monitoring.
- Consult physician about withdrawing drug if patient is to undergo surgery (withdrawal is controversial).
- With ophthalmic use, protect eye from injury if corneal sensitivity is lost.

Teaching points
- Administer eyedrops as instructed to minimize systemic absorption of the drug.
- Take oral drug as prescribed.
- Do not stop taking unless told to do so by a health care provider.
- Avoid driving or dangerous activities if dizziness or weakness occurs.
- You may experience these side effects: Dizziness, light-headedness, loss of appetite, nightmares, depression, sexual impotence.
- Report difficulty breathing, night cough, swelling of extremities, slow pulse, confusion, depression, rash, fever, sore throat; eye pain or irritation (ophthalmic).

▽ **bethanechol chloride**
*(beh **than' e** kole)*

PMS-Bethanechol (CAN), Urecholine

PREGNANCY CATEGORY C

Drug classes
Cholinergic
Parasympathomimetic

Therapeutic actions
Acts at cholinergic receptors in the urinary bladder (and GI tract) to mimic the effects of acetylcholine and parasympathetic stimulation; increases the tone of the detrusor muscle and causes the emptying of the urinary bladder; not destroyed by the enzyme cholinesterase, so effects are more prolonged than those of acetylcholine.

Indications
- Acute postoperative and postpartum nonobstructive urinary retention and neurogenic atony of the urinary bladder with retention

- Unlabeled uses: Reflux esophagitis, gastro-esophageal reflux (pediatric use)

Contraindications and cautions

- Contraindicated with unusual sensitivity to bethanechol or tartrazine, hyperthyroidism, peptic ulcer, latent or active asthma, bradycardia, vasomotor instability, coronary artery disease, epilepsy, parkinsonism, hypotension, obstructive uropathies or intestinal obstruction, recent surgery on GI tract or bladder.
- Use cautiously with lactation, pregnancy.

Available forms

Tablets—5, 10, 25, 50 mg

Dosages

Determine and use the minimum effective dose; larger doses may increase side effects.
Adults
10–50 mg PO three or four times a day. Initial dose of 5–10 mg with gradual increases hourly until desired effect is seen; or until 50 mg has been given.
Pediatric patients
Safety and efficacy not established.

Pharmacokinetics

Route	Onset	Peak	Duration
Oral	30–90 min	60–90 min	1–6 hr

Metabolism: Unknown
Distribution: Crosses placenta; may enter breast milk
Excretion: Unknown

Adverse effects

- **CV:** Transient heart block, **cardiac arrest,** orthostatic hypotension (with large doses)
- **GI:** *Abdominal discomfort, salivation, nausea, vomiting,* involuntary defecation, abdominal cramps, diarrhea, belching
- **GU:** Urinary urgency
- **Respiratory:** Dyspnea
- **Other:** Malaise, headache, *sweating, flushing,* lacrimation, diaphoresis

Interactions

* **Drug-drug** • Increased cholinergic effects with other cholinergic drugs, cholinesterase in-

hibitors • Critical drop in BP may occur if taken with ganglionic blockers

■ Nursing considerations
Assessment

- **History:** Unusual sensitivity to bethanechol or tartrazine, hyperthyroidism, peptic ulcer, latent or active asthma, bradycardia, vasomotor instability, CAD, epilepsy, parkinsonism, hypotension, obstructive uropathies or intestinal obstruction, recent surgery on GI tract or bladder, lactation, pregnancy
- **Physical:** Skin color, lesions; T; P, rhythm, BP; bowel sounds, urinary bladder palpation; bladder tone evaluation, urinalysis

Interventions

- Administer on an empty stomach (1 hr before or 2 hr after meals) to avoid nausea and vomiting.
- Monitor response to establish minimum effective dose.
- ⊗ *Warning* Keep atropine readily available to reverse overdose or severe response.
- Monitor bowel function, especially in elderly patients who may become impacted or develop serious intestinal problems.

Teaching points

- Take this drug on an empty stomach (1 hour before or 2 hours after meals) to avoid nausea and vomiting.
- Dizziness, light-headedness, or fainting may occur when getting up from sitting or lying down.
- You may experience these side effects: Increased salivation, sweating, flushing, abdominal discomfort.
- Report diarrhea, headache, belching, substernal pressure or pain, dizziness.

▷ **bevacizumab**

See Appendix R, *Less commonly used drugs.*

▷ **bexarotene**

See Appendix R, *Less commonly used drugs.*

▷ **bicalutamide**

See Appendix R, *Less commonly used drugs.*

▽ bismuth subsalicylate

(**bis'** mith sub sah **lih'** sih late)

Bismatrol, Kao-Tin, Kaopectate, Kaopectate Maximum Strength, Maalox Total Stomach Relief, Peptic Relief, Pepto-Bismol, Pepto-Bismol Maximum Strength, Pink Bismuth

PREGNANCY CATEGORY C
(FIRST AND SECOND TRIMESTERS)

PREGNANCY CATEGORY D
(THIRD TRIMESTER)

Drug class
Antidiarrheal

Therapeutic actions
Adsorbent actions remove irritants from the intestine; forms a protective coating over the mucosa and soothes the irritated bowel lining. Antimicrobial and antisecretory effects.

Indications
- To control diarrhea, gas, upset stomach, indigestion, heartburn, nausea
- To reduce the number of bowel movements and help firm stool
- To control traveler's diarrhea
- Unlabeled uses: Prevention of traveler's diarrhea; treatment of chronic infantile diarrhea

Contraindications and cautions
- Contraindicated with allergy to any components or to aspirin or other salicylates; chickenpox or influenza (risk of Reye's syndrome).
- Use cautiously with pregnancy, lactation.

Available forms
Caplets—262 mg; chewable tablets—262 mg; liquid—87 mg/5 mL, 130 mg/15 mL, 262 mg/15 mL, 524 mg/15 mL; suspension—525 mg/15 mL; tablets—262 mg

Dosages
Adults and children 12 yr and older
2 tablets or 30 mL (524 mg) PO, repeat every 30 min–1 hr as needed, up to eight doses per 24 hr.
- *Traveler's diarrhea:* 1 ounce (524 mg) every 30 min for a total of 8 doses.
Pediatric patients 9–11 yr
One tablet or 15 mL (1 tablespoon) PO.
Pediatric patients 6–8 yr
Two-thirds tablet or 10 mL (2 teaspoons) PO.
Pediatric patients 3–5 yr
One-third tablet or 5 mL (1 teaspoon) PO.
Pediatric patients younger than 3 yr
Dosage not established.

Pharmacokinetics

Route	Onset
Oral	Varies

Metabolism: Hepatic; $T_{1/2}$: Unknown
Distribution: Crosses placenta
Excretion: Urine

Adverse effects
- **GI:** *Darkening of the stool,* impaction in infants or debilitated patients
- **Salicylate toxicity:** Ringing in the ears, rapid respirations

Interactions
✳ **Drug-drug** • Increased risk of salicylate toxicity with aspirin-containing products • Increased toxic effects of methotrexate, valproic acid if taken with salicylates • Use caution with drugs used for diabetes • Decreased effectiveness with corticosteroids • Decreased absorption of oral tetracyclines • Decreased effectiveness of sulfinpyrazone with salicylates
✳ **Drug-lab test** • May interfere with radiologic examinations of GI tract; bismuth is radiopaque

■ Nursing considerations
Assessment
- **History:** Allergy to any components
- **Physical:** T; orientation, reflexes; R and depth of respirations; abdominal examination, bowel sounds; serum electrolytes; acid–base levels

Interventions
- Shake liquid well before administration; have patient chew tablets thoroughly or dissolve in mouth; do not swallow whole.

- Discontinue drug if any sign of salicylate toxicity (ringing in the ears) occurs.

Teaching points
- Take this drug as prescribed; do not exceed prescribed dosage. Shake liquid well before using. Chew tablets thoroughly or let them dissolve in your mouth; do not swallow whole.
- Darkened stools may occur.
- Do not take this drug with other drugs containing aspirin or aspirin products; serious overdose can occur.
- Report fever or diarrhea that does not stop after 2 days, ringing in the ears, rapid respirations.

▽bisoprolol fumarate
*(bis **ob'** pro lole **few'** mah rate)*

Apo-Bisoprolol (CAN), Zebeta

PREGNANCY CATEGORY C

Drug classes
Antihypertensive
Beta$_1$-selective adrenergic blocker

Therapeutic actions
Blocks beta-adrenergic receptors (primarily beta$_1$) of the sympathetic nervous system in the heart and juxtaglomerular apparatus (kidney), thus decreasing the excitability of the heart, decreasing cardiac output and oxygen consumption, decreasing the release of renin from the kidneys, and lowering BP.

Indications
- Management of hypertension, used alone or with other antihypertensives

Contraindications and cautions
- Contraindicated with sinus bradycardia, second- or third-degree heart block, cardiogenic shock.
- Use cautiously with renal failure, diabetes or thyrotoxicosis (bisoprolol can mask the usual cardiac signs of hypoglycemia and thyrotoxicosis), pregnancy, lactation, and in those with bronchospastic disease, heart failure.

Available forms
Tablets—5, 10 mg

Dosages
Adults
Initially, 5 mg PO daily, alone or added to diuretic therapy; 2.5 mg may be appropriate; up to 20 mg PO daily has been used.
Pediatric patients
Safety and efficacy not established.
Patients with renal or hepatic impairment
Initially, 2.5 mg PO; adjust, and use extreme caution in dose titration.

Pharmacokinetics

Route	Onset	Peak	Duration
Oral	30–60 min	2 hr	12–15 hr

Metabolism: Hepatic; T$_{1/2}$: 9–12 hr
Distribution: Crosses placenta; may enter breast milk
Excretion: Urine

Adverse effects
- **Allergic reactions:** Pharyngitis, erythematous rash, fever, sore throat, **laryngospasm,** respiratory distress
- **CNS:** Dizziness, vertigo, tinnitus, *fatigue,* emotional depression, paresthesia, sleep disturbances, hallucinations, disorientation, memory loss, slurred speech, *headache*
- **CV:** *Bradycardia, heart failure, cardiac arrhythmias, sinoatrial or AV nodal block, tachycardia,* peripheral vascular insufficiency, claudication, stroke, **pulmonary edema,** hypotension
- **Dermatologic:** Rash, pruritus, sweating, dry skin
- **EENT:** Eye irritation, dry eyes, conjunctivitis, blurred vision
- **GI:** *Gastric pain, flatulence, constipation, diarrhea, nausea, vomiting,* anorexia, ischemic colitis, renal and mesenteric arterial thrombosis, retroperitoneal fibrosis, hepatomegaly, acute pancreatitis
- **GU:** *Impotence, decreased libido,* Peyronie's disease, dysuria, nocturia, frequent urination
- **Musculoskeletal:** Joint pain, arthralgia, muscle cramp

- **Respiratory: Bronchospasm,** dyspnea, cough, bronchial obstruction, nasal stuffiness, rhinitis, pharyngitis (less likely than with propranolol)
- **Other:** *Decreased exercise tolerance, development of antinuclear antibodies,* hyperglycemia or hypoglycemia, elevated serum transaminase, alkaline phosphatase, and LDH

Interactions

❋ **Drug-drug** • Increased effects with verapamil, anticholinergics • Increased risk of orthostatic hypotension with prazosin • Possible increased BP-lowering effects with aspirin, bismuth subsalicylate, magnesium salicylate, sulfinpyrazone, hormonal contraceptives • Decreased antihypertensive effects with NSAIDs • Possible masked hypoglycemic effect of insulin • Possible masking of hypoglycemic symptoms in patients with diabetes

❋ **Drug-lab test** • Possible false results with glucose or insulin tolerance tests

■ Nursing considerations

> **CLINICAL ALERT!**
> Name confusion has occurred between *Zebeta* (bisoprolol) and *DiaBeta* (glyburide); use caution.

Assessment

- **History:** Sinus bradycardia, cardiac arrhythmias, cardiogenic shock, heart failure, renal failure, diabetes or thyrotoxicosis, pregnancy, lactation
- **Physical:** Baseline weight, skin condition, neurologic status, P, BP, ECG, R, LFTs, renal function tests, blood and urine glucose

Interventions

⊗ *Warning* Do not discontinue drug abruptly after long-term therapy (hypersensitivity to catecholamines may have developed, causing exacerbation of angina, MI, and ventricular arrhythmias). Taper drug gradually over 2 wk with monitoring.

- Be aware that half-life can be up to 21 hr in patients with cirrhosis and 36 hr in patients with creatinine clearance less than 40 mL/min.
- Consult with physician about withdrawing drug if patient is to undergo surgery (withdrawal is controversial).

Teaching points

- Do not stop taking this drug unless instructed to do so by a health care provider.
- Avoid over-the-counter medications.
- Avoid driving or dangerous activities if dizziness or weakness occurs.
- If you are diabetic, monitor your blood glucose regularly because this drug may mask the signs of hypoglycemia.
- You may experience these side effects: Dizziness, light-headedness, loss of appetite, nightmares, depression, sexual impotence.
- Report difficulty breathing, night cough, swelling of extremities, slow pulse, confusion, depression, rash, fever, sore throat.

▽ **bivalirudin**

See Appendix R, *Less commonly used drugs.*

DANGEROUS DRUG

▽ **bleomycin sulfate**
(blee oh mye' sin)

BLM

PREGNANCY CATEGORY D

Drug classes
Antibiotic
Antineoplastic

Therapeutic actions
Inhibits DNA, RNA, and protein synthesis in susceptible cells, preventing cell division; cell cycle phase-specific agent with major effects in G2 and M phases.

Indications

- Palliative treatment of squamous cell carcinoma, lymphomas, testicular carcinoma, alone or with other drugs
- Treatment of malignant pleural effusion and prevention of recurrent pleural effusions
- Unlabeled uses: Mycosis fungoides, osteosarcoma, AIDS-related Kaposi sarcoma, germ cell tumors, sclerosis of pleural effusions, palliative treatment of children with lymphomas, malignant pericardial effusion, malignant peritoneal effusion, warts (intralesional)

Adverse effects in *italics* are most common; those in **bold** are life-threatening. ⊕ Do not crush.

Contraindications and cautions

- Contraindicated with allergy to bleomycin sulfate; lactation, pregnancy.
- Use cautiously with pulmonary disease; hepatic or renal impairment.

Available forms

Powder for injection—15, 30 units

Dosages

Adults

Treat lymphoma patients with 2 units or less for the first two doses; if no acute anaphylactoid reaction occurs, use the regular dosage schedule:

- *Squamous cell carcinoma, non-Hodgkin's lymphoma, testicular carcinoma:* 0.25–0.5 unit/kg IV, IM, or subcutaneously, once or twice weekly.
- *Hodgkin's lymphoma:* 0.25–0.5 unit/kg IV, IM, or subcutaneously once or twice weekly. After a 50% response, give maintenance dose of 1 unit/day or 5 units/wk, IV or IM. Response should be seen within 2 wk (Hodgkin's lymphoma, testicular tumors) or 3 wk (squamous cell cancers). If no improvement is seen by then, it is unlikely to occur.
- *Malignant pleural effusion:* 60 units dissolved in 50–100 mL 0.9% saline solution, given via thoracostomy tube.

Pediatric patients

Safety and efficacy not established.

Patients with renal impairment

CrCl (mL/min)	% of Initial Dosage
50 or more	100
40–50	70
30–40	60
20–30	55
10–20	45
5–10	40

Pharmacokinetics

Route	Onset	Peak
IV	Immediate	10–20 min
IM, Subcut.	15–20 min	30–60 min

Metabolism: Hepatic; $T_{1/2}$: 2 hr
Distribution: May cross placenta; may enter breast milk
Excretion: Urine

▼ IV FACTS

Preparation: Dissolve contents of 15-unit vial with 1–5 mL or 30-unit vial with 2–10 mL physiologic saline, sterile water for injection, or bacteriostatic water for injection. Do not use D_5W or dextrose-containing diluents; stable for 24 hr at room temperature in saline solution. Powder should be refrigerated.
Infusion: Infuse slowly over 10 min.
Incompatibilities: Incompatible in solution with aminophylline, ascorbic acid, carbenicillin, diazepam, hydrocortisone, methotrexate, mitomycin, nafcillin, penicillin G, terbutaline.

Adverse effects

- **Dermatologic:** *Rash, striae, vesiculation, hyperpigmentation, skin tenderness, hyperkeratosis, nail changes, alopecia, pruritus*
- **GI:** Hepatic toxicity, *stomatitis, vomiting,* anorexia, weight loss
- **GU:** Renal toxicity
- **Hypersensitivity:** Idiosyncratic reaction similar to anaphylaxis: Hypotension, mental confusion, fever, chills, wheezing (lymphoma patients, 1% occurrence)
- **Respiratory:** *Dyspnea, rales, pneumonitis,* **pulmonary fibrosis**
- **Other:** *Fever, chills*

Interactions

✳ **Drug-drug** • Decreased serum levels and effectiveness of digoxin and phenytoin • Increased risk of pulmonary toxicity if combined with oxygen use

■ Nursing considerations

Assessment

- **History:** Allergy to bleomycin sulfate, pregnancy, lactation, pulmonary disease, hepatic or renal impairment
- **Physical:** T; skin color, lesions; weight; R, adventitious sounds; liver evaluation, abdominal status; PFTs, urinalysis, LFTs, renal function tests, chest radiograph

Interventions

- Reconstitute for IM or subcutaneous use by dissolving contents of 15-unit vial in 1–5 mL, 30-unit vial with 2–10 mL of sterile water for injection, sodium chloride for injection, bacteriostatic water for injection.

- Label drug solution with date and hour of preparation; check label before use. Stable at room temperature for 24 hr in 0.9% sodium chloride; discard after that time.

⊗ *Black box warning* Monitor pulmonary function regularly and chest radiograph weekly or biweekly to monitor onset of pulmonary toxicity; consult physician immediately if changes occur. Risk is markedly increased with doses over 400 units/day.

- Arrange for periodic monitoring of LFTs and renal function tests.
- Advise women of childbearing age to avoid pregnancy while on this drug.

⊗ *Black box warning* Be alert for rare, severe idiosyncratic reaction including fever, chills, hypertension in lymphoma patients.

⊗ *Black box warning* Only physicians experienced in chemotherapy should administer this drug.

Teaching points

- This drug has to be given by injection. Mark calendar with dates for injection.
- This drug may cause fetal harm; using a barrier contraceptive is advised.
- You may experience these side effects: Rash, skin lesions, loss of hair, changes in nails (you may want to invest in a wig, skin care may help); loss of appetite, nausea, mouth sores (try frequent mouth care, eat frequent small meals; maintain good nutrition).
- Report difficulty breathing, cough, yellowing of skin or eyes, severe GI upset, fever, chills.

▽**boceprevir**

(*boe* **seb'** *preh veer*)

Victrelis

PREGNANCY CATEGORY B

PREGNANCY CATEGORY X

(IF TAKEN WITH PEGINTERFERON, RIBAVIRIN)

Drug classes
Antiviral
Protease inhibitor

Therapeutic actions
Antiviral; inhibits hepatitis C virus–specific protease, which inhibits viral replication in the hepatitis C–infected cell.

Indications
- Treatment of chronic hepatitis C virus, genotype-1 infection, in adults with compensated liver disease who are previously untreated or have failed on interferon and ribavirin therapy; must be given with peginterferon alfa and ribavirin

Contraindications and cautions
- Contraindicated with history of serious hypersensitivity reactions to boceprevir, concurrent use of CYP3A4/5 inducers or inhibitors, pregnancy, lactation.
- Use cautiously with co-infection with HIV, hepatitis B; elderly patients.

Available forms
Capsules—200 mg

Dosages
Adults
800 mg PO tid (every 7–9 hr) with food for 28–48 wk. Patient should receive 4 wk of ribavirin and peginterferon alfa before beginning therapy; these drugs must continue during boceprevir therapy.
Pediatric patients
Safety and efficacy not established.

Pharmacokinetics

Route	Onset	Peak
Oral	Rapid	2 hr

Metabolism: Hepatic; $T_{1/2}$: 3.4 hr
Distribution: May cross placenta; may enter breast milk
Excretion: Feces

Adverse effects
- **CNS:** *Headache, dizziness, insomnia, irritability*
- **GI:** *Nausea, dysgeusia, vomiting, decreased appetite*
- **Hematologic:** *Anemia,* neutropenia
- **Other:** *Fatigue, alopecia, dry skin, chills,* **thrombotic events**

Interactions
❋ **Drug-drug** • Increased toxicity if combined with alfuzosin, carbamazepine, cisapride, drospirenone, ergot derivatives, lovastatin, midazolam, pimozide, phenobarbital, phenytoin, rifampin, sildenafil, simvastatin, tadalafil, triazolam; use of these drugs with

---

Adverse effects in *italics* are most common; those in **bold** are life-threatening. ⬛ Do not crush.

boceprevir is contraindicated • Increased digoxin levels if combined; monitor patient closely • Increased colchicine levels; dosage must be reduced; combination should not be used in patients with renal or hepatic impairment • Possible decreased effectiveness of atazanavir, boceprevir, darunavir, lopinavir/ritonavir with combined use, leading to increased HIV and hepatitis C infections; avoid these combinations

✳ **Drug-alternative therapy** • Loss of effectiveness if taken with St. John's Wort; avoid this combination

■ **Nursing considerations**
Assessment

• **History:** Hypersensitivity to components of the drug, pregnancy, lactation, concurrent infection with HIV, hepatitis B
• **Physical:** Neurologic exam; skin evaluation; GI exam; CBC; HIV, hepatitis B testing

Interventions

• Drug must be given with peginterferon alfa and ribavirin; consider all cautions and contraindications for those drugs.
• Rule out HIV and hepatitis B infection before beginning therapy.
• Ensure patient has received 4 wk of peginterferon alfa and ribavirin before start of therapy.
• Administer tid with food, with 7–9 hr between doses.
• Encourage small, frequent meals and comfort measures if GI upset, taste changes are severe.
• Ensure that patient is not pregnant; this combination of drugs can cause severe fetal abnormalities. Men on this combination should not father a child. Two forms of contraception should be used; routine, monthly pregnancy tests should be performed.
• Patient should be advised that transmission of hepatitis C may still occur and to take appropriate precautions.

Teaching points

• This drug must be taken with peginterferon alfa and ribavirin.
• Take boceprevir three times a day with food; allow 7 to 9 hours between doses. If you miss a dose and it is less than 2 hours before the next dose is due, skip that dose. If you miss a dose and it is more than 2 hours before the next dose is due, take the missed dose with food and resume the normal dosing schedule.
• Tell your health care provider about all drugs, OTC products, and herbs you might be taking; boceprevir interacts with many other drugs and dosage adjustment may be needed. Do not use St. John's Wort while taking this drug.
• This combination of drugs can cause serious fetal abnormalities. Use two forms of contraception to ensure that pregnancy does not occur; a routine, monthly pregnancy test will be done. Men should not father a child while taking these drugs and should suggest the use of two forms of contraception to their partner.
• These drugs may appear in breast milk; if you are breast-feeding, you should use a different method of feeding your baby.
• Transmission of hepatitis C may still occur while you are taking boceprevir; take precautions to prevent transmission.
• You may be more susceptible to infection while taking these drugs; avoid exposure to infection.
• You may experience these side effects: GI upset, taste changes, nausea (small, frequent meals may help), fatigue, anemia (spacing activities throughout the day may help); headache (consult your health care provider for an appropriate pain medication).
• Report fever, muscle or calf pain, chest pain, difficulty breathing, signs of infection.

▽**bortezomib**

See Appendix R, *Less commonly used drugs.*

DANGEROUS DRUG

▽**bosentan**
(bow sen' tan)

Tracleer

PREGNANCY CATEGORY X

Drug classes
Endothelin receptor antagonist
Pulmonary antihypertensive
Vasodilator

Therapeutic actions

Specifically blocks receptor sites for endothelin ET_A and ET_B in the endothelium and vascular smooth muscles; these endothelins are elevated in plasma and lung tissue of patients with pulmonary arterial hypertension.

Indications

- Treatment of pulmonary arterial hypertension in patients with World Health Organization class II to class IV symptoms, to improve exercise ability and to decrease the rate of clinical worsening
- Unlabeled uses: Prevention of Raynaud's phenomenon; prevention of digital ulcers in systemic sclerosis

Contraindications and cautions

- Contraindicated with allergy to bosentan, severe liver impairment, pregnancy, lactation.
- Use cautiously with hepatic impairment, anemia.

Available forms

Tablets—62.5, 125 mg

Dosages

Adults and children older than 12 yr

62.5 mg PO bid for 4 wk. Then, for patients weighing 40 kg or more, maintenance dose is 125 mg PO bid. For patients weighing less than 40 kg, but older than 12 yr, maintenance dose is 62.5 mg PO bid. Administer in the morning and evening. Discontinue 36 hr before initiating ritonavir therapy; if patient is on ritonavir, initiate bosentan at 62.5 mg/day PO or once every other day.

Pediatric patients

Safety and efficacy not established.

Patients with hepatic impairment

Avoid use in moderate to severe hepatic impairment; reduce dosage and monitor patients closely with mild hepatic impairment. If ALT/AST is more than 3 to 5 or less times the upper limit of normal (ULN), reduce dose to 62.5 mg PO bid or interrupt treatment. Restart treatment only if liver enzyme levels return to pretreatment levels. Stop treatment if ALT/AST is more than 5 to 8 times ULN.

Pharmacokinetics

Route	Onset	Peak
Oral	Varies	3–5 hr

Metabolism: Hepatic; $T_{1/2}$: 5 hr
Distribution: Crosses placenta; may enter breast milk
Excretion: Feces

Adverse effects

- **CNS:** *Headache,* fatigue
- **CV:** *Flushing, edema, hypotension,* palpitations
- **EENT:** *Nasopharyngitis*
- **GI: Liver injury,** dyspepsia
- **Hematologic:** Decreased Hgb level, decreased Hct
- **Skin:** Pruritus
- **Other:** Spermatogenesis inhibition

Interactions

* **Drug-drug** • Potential for decreased effectiveness of hormonal contraceptives; advise using barrier contraceptives • Bosentan serum concentrations increased with cyclosporine A, and cyclosporine A concentrations decrease by 50% with bosentan; avoid this combination • Decreased serum levels of statins if combined with bosentan; if the combination is used, patients should have serum cholesterol levels monitored regularly • Increased risk of liver damage if combined with glyburide; avoid this combination • Increased bosentan concentrations with ketoconazole and tacrolimus; monitor patients for adverse effects • Risk of serious toxicity if taken with atazanavir without ritonavir; always administer atazanavir with ritonavir if bosentan is needed. Give bosentan at 62.5 mg every other day, starting 10 days after starting ritonavir. If patient on bosentan is to be started on ritonavir, stop bosentan 3 days befor starting ritonavir; resume bosentan 10 days after starting ritonavir.

■ Nursing considerations

Assessment

- **History:** Allergy to bosentan, severe liver impairment, anemia, pregnancy, lactation
- **Physical:** Skin color and lesions, orientation, BP, LFTs, CBC, Hgb level, pregnancy test

B

Interventions

⊗ **Black box warning** Make sure that the patient is not pregnant before initiating therapy and that patient will conform to use of two forms of contraception during therapy and for 1 mo after stopping drug. Verify pregnancy status monthly.

⊗ **Black box warning** Obtain baseline and then monthly liver enzyme levels; dosage reduction or drug withdrawal is indicated at signs of elevated liver enzymes. Liver failure is possible.

⊗ **Warning** Obtain baseline Hgb level and then repeat at 1 and 3 mo, then every 3 mo. If Hgb drops, the situation should be evaluated and appropriate action taken.

- Do not administer to any patient taking cyclosporine or glyburide.
- Administer in the morning and in the evening with or without food.

⊗ **Warning** Monitor patients who are discontinuing bosentan; dose may need to be tapered to avoid sudden worsening of disease.

- Provide analgesics as appropriate for patients who develop headache.
- Monitor patient's functional level to note improvement in exercise tolerance.
- Maintain other measures used to treat pulmonary arterial hypertension.
- Be aware that drug can only be prescribed and dispensed through a restricted distribution program because of risks associated with use.

Teaching points

- This drug is only available through the Tracleer Access Program. You will need to be enrolled in the program before beginning therapy.
- Take drug exactly as prescribed, in the morning and the evening.
- This drug should not be taken during pregnancy; serious fetal abnormalities have occurred. A negative pregnancy test will be required before the drug is started. The use of two reliable forms of contraception during therapy and for 1 month after stopping bosentan is required.
- Keep a chart of your exercise tolerance to help monitor improvement in your condition.
- Continue your usual procedures for treating your pulmonary arterial hypertension.

- You will need frequent blood tests to evaluate the effect of this drug on your liver and your hemoglobin.
- You may experience these side effects: Headache (analgesics may be available that will help); stomach upset (taking the drug with food may help).
- Report swelling, changes in color of urine or stool, yellowing of the eyes or skin.

▷ **botulinum toxin type A (onabotulinumtoxinA)**

(*bot' yoo lin um*)

Botox, Botox Cosmetic, Dysport, Xeomin

PREGNANCY CATEGORY C

Drug class
Neurotoxin

Therapeutic actions

Blocks neuromuscular transmission by binding to receptor sites on the motor nerve terminals and inhibiting the release of acetylcholine; this blocking results in localized muscle denervation, which causes local muscle paralysis; this denervation can lead to muscle atrophy and reinnervation if the muscle develops new acetylcholine receptors.

Indications

- Temporary improvement in the appearance of moderate to severe glabellar lines—associated with corrugator or procerus muscle activity in adults 65 yr and younger (*Botox Cosmetic, Dysport, Xeomin*)
- Treatment of cervical dystonia in adults to decrease severity of abnormal head position and neck pain (*Botox, Dysport, Xeomin*)
- Treatment of severe primary axillary hyperhidrosis that is not adequately managed with topical agents (*Botox* only)
- Treatment of strabismus and blepharospasm associated with dystonia in patients 12 yr and older (*Botox* only)
- Treatment of spasticity of the elbow, wrist, and fingers in adults following stroke, traumatic brain injury, progression of multiple sclerosis (*Botox* only)

- Prophylaxis of headaches in adults with chronic migraines (at least 15 days/month lasting 4 hr a day or longer) (*Botox* only)
- Treatment of blepharospasm in adults previously treated with *Botox* (*Xeomin* only)
- ■ **NEW INDICATION:** Treatment of urinary incontinence in patients with neurological conditions, such as spinal cord injury or MS, who have overactive bladder (*Botox*)
- Unlabeled uses: Achalasia, cosmetic improvement of facial lines and wrinkles, gustatory sweating, hand dystonia, tension headache, palmar hyperhidrosis, sialorrhea

Contraindications and cautions

- Contraindicated with hypersensitivity to any component of the drug, active infection at the injection site area.
- Use cautiously with peripheral neuropathic diseases (amyotrophic lateral sclerosis [ALS], motor neuropathies); neuromuscular disorders such as myasthenia gravis; inflammation in the injection area; compromised respiratory function, bronchitis, or URIs when used for limb spasticity; lactation, pregnancy; known CV disease.

Available forms

Powder for injection—50, 100, 200, 300, 500 units/vial

Dosages
Adults

- *Glabellar lines:* Total of 20 units (0.5 mL solution) injected as divided doses of 0.1 mL into each of five sites—two in each corrugator muscle, and one in the procerus muscle; injections usually need to be repeated every 3–4 mo to maintain effect (*Botox*). Or, 50 units in five equal injections every 4 mo (*Dysport*).
- *Cervical dystonia:* 236 units (range 198–300 units) divided among affected muscles and injected into each muscle in patients with known tolerance. In patients without prior use, 100 units or less, then adjust dosage based on patient response (*Botox*). 120 units IM (*Xeomin*) or 250–1,000 units IM every 12 wk (*Dysport*).
- *Primary axillary hyperhidrosis:* 50 units per axilla injected intradermally 0.1–0.2 mL aliquots at multiple sites (10–15), approximately 1–2 cm apart. Repeat as needed.

- *Blepharospasm associated with dystonia:* 1.25–2.5 units injected into the medial and lateral pretarsal orbicularis oculi of the lower lid and upper lid. Repeat approximately every 3 mo.
- *Strabismus associated with dystonia:* 1.25–50 units in any one muscle.
- *Upper limb spasticity:* Base dosage on muscles affected and severity of activity; electromyographic guidance is recommended. Use no more than 50 units per site.
- *Chronic migraine:* 155 units IM as 0.1 mL (5 units) at each site; divide into seven head/neck muscle areas (*Botox*).
- *Blepharospasm in previously treated adults:* 35 units per eye (*Xeomin*).
- *Bladder overactivity with neurological conditions:* 200 units as 1-mL injections across 30 sites into the detrusor muscle.

Pharmacokinetics
Not absorbed systemically

Adverse effects

- **CNS:** *Headache,* blepharoptosis, transient ptosis, *dizziness,* dyphonia
- **CV:** Arrhythmias, **MI** (patients with preexisting disease), hypertension
- **GI:** Nausea, difficulty swallowing, dyspepsia, tooth disorder
- **Respiratory:** Pneumonia, bronchitis, sinusitis, pharyngitis, URI, breathing difficulty
- **Other:** Redness, edema, and pain at injection site, *flulike symptoms,* paralysis of facial muscles, facial pain, infection, skin tightness, ecchymosis, **anaphylactic reactions, spread of toxin effects that can lead to death,** urine retention when injected into detrusor muscle

Interactions
✳ **Drug-drug** • Risk for additive effects if combined with aminoglycosides or other drugs that interfere with neuromuscular transmission—neuromuscular junction blockers, lincosamides, quinidine, magnesium sulfate, anticholinesterases, succinylcholine, polymyxin; use extreme caution if this combination is used

■ Nursing considerations
Assessment
- **History:** Hypersensitivity to any component of the drug; active infection in the

injection site area, pregnancy, peripheral neuropathic diseases (ALS, motor neuropathies), neuromuscular disorders such as myasthenia gravis, inflammation in the injection area, lactation, known CV disease, lactose allergy (*Dysport*)

• **Physical:** T; reflexes; R, respiratory auscultation, assessment of injection site and muscle function

Interventions

⊗ *Black box warning* Drug is not for the treatment of muscle spasticity; toxin may spread from injection area and cause signs and symptoms of botulism (CNS alterations, trouble speaking and swallowing, loss of bladder conrol). Use only for approved indications.

• Store vials in the refrigerator before reconstitution.
• Reconstitute with 0.9% sterile, preservative-free saline as indicated for each use using a 21-gauge needle. Inject saline into vial; gently rotate vial to reconstitute and label vial with time and date of reconstitution. Reconstituted solution may be refrigerated but must be used within 4 hr. Discard after that time.
• Inspect vial for particulate matter or discoloration before use.
• Check manufacturer's guidelines for appropriate needle-gauge for each use.
• Be aware that *Dysport* contains lactose.

⊗ *Warning* Ensure that epinephrine is readily available in case of anaphylactic reaction to the drug.

• Inform the patient that the effect of the drug may not be seen for 1 or 2 days, with the full effect taking up to a week. The effect usually lasts 3–4 mo. Do not administer the drug more often than every 3–4 mo.
• Advise patient not to become pregnant while this drug is being used; advise using contraceptives.

Teaching points

• This drug will be injected into your muscles to block the contraction of particular muscles.
• The effects of the drug may not be apparent for 1–2 days and may not be fully apparent for a week. The effects of the drug persist for 3–4 months.
• Avoid pregnancy while using this drug; the effects on the fetus are not known. If you

become pregnant or desire to become pregnant, consult your health care provider. Using contraceptives is advised.
• You may experience these side effects: Pain, redness at injection site, and headache (analgesics may be helpful), drooping of the eyelid (this is usually transient), nausea, flu-like symptoms.
• Report difficulty swallowing, facial paralysis; difficulty speaking; difficulty breathing; persistent pain, redness, or swelling at injection site.

▽ botulinum toxin type B

See Appendix R, *Less commonly used drugs*.

▽ brentuximab vedotin

See Appendix R, *Less commonly used drugs*.

▽ bromocriptine mesylate

*(broe moe **krip'** teen **mess'** ah late)*

Apo-Bromocriptine (CAN), Cycloset, Parlodel, Parlodel SnapTabs

PREGNANCY CATEGORY B

Drug classes

Antidiabetic
Antiparkinsonian
Dopamine receptor agonist
Semisynthetic ergot derivative

Therapeutic actions

Parkinsonism: Acts as an agonist directly on postsynaptic dopamine receptors of neurons in the brain, mimicking the effects of the neurotransmitter dopamine, which is deficient in parkinsonism. Unlike levodopa, bromocriptine does not require biotransformation by the nigral neurons that are deficient in parkinsonism patients; thus, bromocriptine may be effective when levodopa has begun to lose its efficacy.

Hyperprolactinemia: Acts directly on postsynaptic dopamine receptors of the prolactin-secreting cells in the anterior pituitary, mimicking the effects of prolactin inhibitory factor, inhibiting the release of prolactin and galactorrhea. Also restores normal ovulatory menstrual cycles in patients with amenorrhea or galactorrhea, and inhibits the release of growth hormone in patients with acromegaly. Diabetes: Stimulates CNS dopamine activity, which indirectly improves glycemic control; exact mechanism of action not known, but these patients may have decreased dopamine activity as part of their metabolic syndrome.

Indications

- Treatment of postencephalitic or idiopathic Parkinson's disease; may provide additional benefit in patients currently maintained on optimal dosages of levodopa with or without carbidopa, beginning to deteriorate or develop tolerance to levodopa, and experiencing "end of dose failure" on levodopa therapy; may allow reduction of levodopa dosage and decrease the dyskinesias and "on-off" phenomenon associated with long-term levodopa therapy
- Short-term treatment of amenorrhea or galactorrhea associated with hyperprolactinemia due to various etiologies, excluding demonstrable pituitary tumors
- Treatment of hyperprolactinemia associated with pituitary adenomas to reduce elevated prolactin levels, cause shrinkage of macroprolactinomas; may be used to reduce the tumor mass before surgery
- Female infertility associated with hyperprolactinemia in the absence of a demonstrable pituitary tumor
- Acromegaly; used alone or with pituitary irradiation or surgery to reduce serum growth hormone level
- Treatment of type 2 diabetes as monotherapy or in combination with other antidiabetics (*Cycloset* only)
- Unlabeled uses: Hepatic encephalopathy, traumatic brain injury

Contraindications and cautions

- Contraindicated with hypersensitivity to bromocriptine or any ergot alkaloid; severe ischemic heart disease or peripheral vascular disease; uncontrolled hypertension; pregnancy, lactation.
- Use cautiously with history of MI with residual arrhythmias (atrial, nodal, or ventricular); renal or hepatic disease, history of peptic ulcer (fatal bleeding ulcers have oc-

curred in patients with acromegaly treated with bromocriptine).

Available forms

Capsules—5 mg; tablets—0.8, 2.5 mg

Dosages

Adults and pediatric patients 15 yr and older

Give drug with food; individualize dosage; increase dosage gradually to minimize side effects; adjust dosage carefully to optimize benefits and minimize side effects.

- *Hyperprolactinemia:* Initially, 1.25–2.5 mg PO daily; an additional 2.5-mg tablet may be added as tolerated every 2–7 days until optimal response is achieved; therapeutic dosage range is 2.5–15 mg/day.
- *Acromegaly:* Initially, 1.25–2.5 mg PO for 3 days at bedtime; add 1.25–2.5 mg as tolerated every 3–7 days until optimal response is achieved. Evaluate patient monthly, and adjust dosage based on growth hormone levels. Usual dosage range is 20–30 mg/day; do not exceed 100 mg/day; withdraw patients treated with pituitary irradiation for a yearly 4- to 8-wk reassessment period.
- *Parkinson's disease:* 1.25 mg PO bid; assess every 2 wk, and adjust dosage carefully to ensure lowest dosage producing optimal response. If needed, increase dosage by increments of 2.5 mg/day every 14–28 days; do not exceed 100 mg/day.
- *Type 2 diabetes:* 0.8 mg/day PO in the morning within 2 hr of waking; increase by 1 tablet per wk to maximum daily dose of 6 tablets (4.8 mg) or until maximum tolerated dose between 2 and 6 tablets/day (*Cycloset*).

Pediatric patients

Safety for use in patients younger than 16 yr not established.

Pharmacokinetics

Route	Onset	Peak	Duration
Oral	Varies	1–3 hr	14 hr

Metabolism: Hepatic; $T_{1/2}$: 3 hr (initial phase), 45–50 hr (terminal phase)
Excretion: Bile

Adverse effects
Hyperprolactinemic indications
- **CNS:** *Dizziness, fatigue,* light-headedness, nasal congestion, drowsiness, headache, CSF rhinorrhea in patients who have had trans-sphenoidal surgery, pituitary radiation
- **CV:** *Hypotension*
- **GI:** *Constipation, diarrhea, nausea, vomiting, abdominal cramps*

Physiologic lactation
- **CNS:** Headache, dizziness, nausea, vomiting, fatigue, syncope
- **CV:** Hypotension
- **GI:** Diarrhea, cramps

Acromegaly
- **CNS:** Nasal congestion, digital vasospasm, drowsiness
- **CV:** Exacerbation of Raynaud's syndrome, *orthostatic hypotension*
- **GI:** *Nausea, constipation, anorexia,* indigestion, dry mouth, vomiting, GI bleeding

Parkinson's disease
- **CNS:** Abnormal involuntary movements, hallucinations, confusion, "on-off" phenomenon, dizziness, drowsiness, faintness, asthenia, visual disturbance, ataxia, insomnia, depression, vertigo
- **CV:** *Hypotension, shortness of breath*
- **GI:** *Nausea, vomiting, abdominal discomfort, constipation*

Interactions
✳ **Drug-drug** • Increased serum bromocriptine levels and increased pharmacologic and toxic effects with erythromycin • Decreased effectiveness with phenothiazines for treatment of prolactin-secreting tumors • Increased bromocriptine adverse effects if combined with sympathomimetics

■ Nursing considerations
Assessment
- **History:** Hypersensitivity to bromocriptine or any ergot alkaloid; severe ischemic heart disease or peripheral vascular disease; pregnancy; history of MI with residual arrhythmias; hepatic, renal disease; history of peptic ulcer, lactation
- **Physical:** Skin T (especially fingers), color, lesions; nasal mucous membranes; orientation, affect, reflexes, bilateral grip

strength, vision examination, including visual fields; P, BP, orthostatic BP, auscultation; R, depth, adventitious sounds; bowel sounds, normal output, liver evaluation; LFTs, renal function tests, CBC with differential

Interventions
- Evaluate patients with amenorrhea or galactorrhea before drug therapy begins; syndrome may result from pituitary adenoma that requires surgical or radiation procedures.
- Arrange to administer drug with food.
- Taper dosage in patients with Parkinson's disease if drug must be discontinued.
- Monitor hepatic, renal, and hematopoietic function periodically during therapy.
- Ensure that patients with type 2 diabetes continue diet and exercise program and any other medications associated with maintaining glycemic control.

Teaching points
- Take drug exactly as prescribed with food; take the first dose at bedtime while lying down.
- If taking this drug for diabetes, take once a day in the morning. Continue diet and exercise program. You may also be taking other antidiabetic drugs.
- Do not discontinue drug without consulting health care provider (patients with macroadenoma may experience rapid growth of tumor and recurrence of original symptoms).
- Use barrier contraceptives while taking this drug (amenorrhea or galactorrhea); pregnancy may occur before menses, and the drug is contraindicated in pregnancy (estrogen contraceptives may stimulate a prolactinoma).
- You may experience these side effects: Drowsiness, dizziness, confusion (avoid driving or engaging in activities that require alertness); nausea (take the drug with meals, eat frequent small meals); dizziness or faintness when getting up (change position slowly, be careful climbing stairs); headache, nasal stuffiness (medication may help).
- Report fainting; light-headedness; dizziness; uncontrollable movements of the face, eyelids, mouth, tongue, neck, arms, hands, or legs; mental changes; irregular heartbeat or palpitations; severe or persistent nausea or

vomiting; coffee-ground vomitus; black tarry stools; vision changes (macroadenoma); any persistent watery nasal discharge (hyperprolactinemic).

▷brompheniramine maleate (parabromdylamine maleate)

(brome fen ir' a meen mal' ee ate)

BroveX, BroveX CT, J-Tan, Lodrane 12 hr, Lodrane 24 hr, Lodrane XR, LoHist 12 Hour ⓞⓣⓒ, P-Tex, Respa BR, VaZol

PREGNANCY CATEGORY C

Drug class
Antihistamine (alkylamine type)

Therapeutic actions
Competitively blocks the effects of histamine at H_1-receptor sites; has anticholinergic (atropine-like), antipruritic, and sedative effects.

Indications
- Symptomatic relief of symptoms associated with perennial and seasonal allergic rhinitis—runny nose, sneezing, itching nose and throat, watery eyes
- Temporary relief of sneezing and runny nose due to common cold; treatment of allergic and nonallergic pruritic symptoms; mild urticaria and angioedema; amelioration of allergic reactions to blood or plasma; adjunctive therapy in anaphylactic reactions (*VaZol*)

Contraindications and cautions
- Contraindicated with allergy to any antihistamines, allergy to tartrazine (*BroveX CT*), third trimester of pregnancy (newborn or preterm infants may have severe reactions); patients receiving MAOIs, alcohol.
- Use cautiously with lactation, narrow-angle glaucoma, stenosing peptic ulcer, symptomatic prostatic hypertrophy, asthma attack, bladder neck obstruction, pyloroduodenal obstruction. Use cautiously in the elderly (this population is extremely sensitive to anticholinergic side effects of this drug).

Available forms
Chewable tablets—12 mg; ER tablets ⓞⓣⓒ—6 mg; ER capsules ⓞⓣⓒ—12 mg; drops—1 mg; liquid—1 mg/mL, 2 mg/5 mL; oral suspension—4 mg/5 mL, 8 mg/5 mL, 10 mg/5 mL, 12 mg/5 mL

Dosages
Adults and pediatric patients 12 yr and older
Products vary widely. Check manufacturer's instructions before use. ER tablets: 6–12 mg PO every 12 hr. Chewable tablets: 12–24 mg PO every 12 hr, maximum 48 mg/day. ER capsules: 12–24 mg/day PO. Oral suspension (*BroveX*): 5–10 mL (12–24 mg) PO every 12 hr; maximum 48 mg/day. Oral liquid: 10 mL (4 mg) PO 4 times/day. Oral suspension (*Lodrane XR*): 5 mL PO every 12 hr; do not exceed 2 doses/day.
Pediatric patients 6–12 yr
ER tablets: 6 mg PO every 12 hr. Chewable tablets: 6–12 mg PO every 12 hr, maximum 24 mg/day. ER capsules: 12 mg/day PO. Oral liquid: 5 mL (2 mg) PO 4 times/day. Oral suspension (*BroveX*): 5 mL (12 mg) PO every 12 hr; maximum 24 mg/day. Oral suspension (*Lodrane XR*): 2.5 mL PO every 12 hr; up to 5 mL/day.
Pediatric patients 2–6 yr
Chewable tablets: 6 mg PO every 12 hr; maximum 12 mg/day. Oral liquid: 2.5 mL (1 mg) PO 4 times/day. Oral suspension (*BroveX*): 2.5 mL (6 mg) PO every 12 hr up to 12 mg/day. Oral suspension (*Lodrane XR*): 1.25 mL PO every 12 hr; maximum 2.5 mg/day.
Pediatric patients 12 mo–2 yr
Oral suspension: 1.25 mL (3 mg) PO every 12 hr up to 2.5 mL (6 mg)/day. Oral liquid: Titrate dose based on 0.5 mg/kg/day PO in equally divided doses four times/day.
Geriatric patients
More likely to cause dizziness, sedation, syncope, toxic confusional states, and hypotension in elderly patients; use with caution.

Pharmacokinetics

Route	Onset	Peak	Duration
Oral	15–30 min	1–2 hr	4–6 hr

Metabolism: Hepatic; $T_{1/2}$: 12–35 hr
Distribution: Crosses placenta; enters breast milk
Excretion: Urine

Adverse effects

- **CNS:** *Drowsiness, sedation, dizziness, faintness, disturbed coordination,* fatigue, confusion, restlessness, excitation, nervousness, tremor, headache, blurred vision, diplopia, vertigo, tinnitus, acute labyrinthitis, hysteria, tingling, heaviness and weakness of the hands
- **CV:** Hypotension, palpitations, bradycardia, tachycardia, extrasystoles
- **GI:** Epigastric distress, anorexia, increased appetite and weight gain, nausea, vomiting, diarrhea or constipation
- **GU:** Urinary frequency, dysuria, urinary retention, early menses, decreased libido, impotence
- **Hematologic:** Hemolytic anemia, hypoplastic anemia, thrombocytopenia, leukopenia, agranulocytosis, pancytopenia
- **Hypersensitivity:** Urticaria, rash, **anaphylactic shock,** photosensitivity
- **Respiratory:** *Thickening of bronchial secretions,* chest tightness, wheezing, nasal stuffiness, dry mouth, dry nose, dry throat, sore throat

Interactions

✳ **Drug-drug** • Increased sedation with alcohol, other CNS depressants • Increased and prolonged anticholinergic (drying) effects with MAOIs

■ Nursing considerations
Assessment

- **History:** Allergy to any antihistamines, tartrazine, narrow-angle glaucoma, stenosing peptic ulcer, symptomatic prostatic hypertrophy, asthmatic attack, bladder neck obstruction, pyloroduodenal obstruction, third trimester of pregnancy, lactation
- **Physical:** Skin color, lesions, texture; orientation, reflexes, affect; vision examination; P, BP; R, adventitious sounds; bowel sounds; prostate palpation; CBC with differential

Interventions

- Give orally with food if GI upset occurs.
- Ensure that patient does not cut, crush, or chew ER forms.
- Double-check all dosages before use; products vary widely.

Teaching points

- Take as prescribed; avoid excessive dosage; take with food if GI upset occurs. Swallow extended-release forms whole; do not cut, crush, or chew them.
- Avoid alcohol while on this drug; serious sedation could occur.
- Oral liquid and oral suspensions differ in strength; do not use interchangeably.
- You may experience these side effects: Dizziness, sedation, drowsiness (use caution if driving or performing tasks that require alertness); epigastric distress, diarrhea or constipation (take with meals); dry mouth (frequent mouth care, sucking sugarless candies may help); thickening of bronchial secretions, dryness of nasal mucosa (try a humidifier).
- Report difficulty breathing, hallucinations, tremors, loss of coordination, unusual bleeding or bruising, visual disturbances, irregular heartbeat.

▷ budesonide
*(byoo **des'** oh nide)*

Inhalation: Entocort (CAN), Pulmicort Flexhaler, Pulmicort Respules, Rhinocort Aqua, Rhinocort Turbuhaler (CAN)
Oral: Entocort EC

PREGNANCY CATEGORY B (INHALATION), C (CAPSULE)

Drug class
Corticosteroid

Therapeutic actions
Anti-inflammatory effect; local administration into nasal passages maximizes beneficial effects on these tissues, while decreasing the likelihood of adverse effects from systemic absorption.

Indications
- *Rhinocort Aqua:* Management of symptoms of seasonal or perennial allergic rhinitis in adults and children 6 yr and older
- *Respules/Flexhaler:* Maintenance treatment of asthma as prophylactic therapy in adults

and children age 6 yr and older and for patients requiring corticosteroids for asthma
- Inhalation suspension: Maintenance treatment and prophylaxis therapy of asthma in children 12 mo–8 yr
- Oral: Treatment and maintenance of clinical remission for up to 3 mo of mild to moderate active Crohn's disease involving the ileum or ascending colon
- Unlabeled use: Eosinophilic esophagitis in children

Contraindications and cautions
Inhalation
- Contraindicated with hypersensitivity to drug or for relief of acute asthma or bronchospasm.
- Use cautiously with TB, systemic infections, lactation.
Oral
- Contraindicated with hypersensitivity to drug, lactation.
- Use cautiously with TB, hypertension, diabetes mellitus, osteoporosis, peptic ulcer disease, glaucoma, cataracts, family history of diabetes or glaucoma, other conditions in which glucocorticosteroids may have unwanted effects.
Nasal
- Contraindicated with hypersensitivity to drug, nasal infections, nasal trauma, nasal septal ulcers, recent nasal surgery.
- Use cautiously with lactation, TB, systemic infection.

Available forms
Spray—32 mcg/actuation; dry powder for inhalation (*Pulmicort Flexhaler*)—90 mcg (delivers 80 mcg), 180 mcg (delivers 160 mcg); inhalation suspension—0.25 mg/2 mL, 0.5 mg/2 mL, 1 mg/2 mL; capsules ⊙ᴿ—3 mg

Dosages
Nasal inhalation
Adults and patients 6 yr and older
Initial dose, 64 mcg/day given as 1 spray (32 mcg) in each nostril once daily. After desired clinical effect is achieved, reduce dosage to the smallest dose possible to maintain the control of symptoms. Maximum daily dose for patients older than 12 yr is 256 mcg/day given as 4 sprays per nostril once daily. Patients 6 to younger than 12 yr should not exceed 128 mcg/day (given as 2 sprays per nostril once daily). Generally takes approximately 2 wk to achieve maximum clinical effect.

Pulmicort Flexhaler
Adults and children 12 yr and older
360 mcg bid; maximum dose, 720 mcg bid. "Low" dose: 180–600 mcg/day; "medium" dose: 600–1,200 mcg/day; "high" dose: more than 1,200 mcg/day.
Pediatric patients 5–11 yr
180 mcg bid; maximum dose, 360 mcg bid. "Low" dose: 180–400 mcg/day; "medium" dose: 400–800 mcg/day; "high" dose: more than 800 mcg/day.

Pulmicort Respules
Pediatric patients 0–11 yr
0.5–1 mg once daily or in two divided doses using jet nebulizer. Maximum dose, 1 mg/day. "Low" dose: 0.25–0.5 mg/day (0–4 yr), 0.5 mg/day (5–11 yr); "medium" dose: 0.5–1 mg/day (0–4 yr), 1 mg/day (5–11 yr); "high" dose: more than 1 mg/day (0–4 yr), 2 mg/day (5–11 yr).

Oral
Adults
9 mg/day PO taken in the morning for up to 8 wk. Recurrent episodes may be retreated for 8-wk periods. Maintenance treatment, 6 mg/day PO for up to 3 mo, then taper until cessation is complete.
Pediatric patients younger than 6 yr
Safety and efficacy not established.
Patients with hepatic impairment
Monitor patients very closely for signs of hypercorticism; reduced dosage should be considered with these patients.

Pharmacokinetics

Route	Onset	Peak	Duration
Intranasal, inhaled	Immediate	Rapid	8–12 hr
Oral	Slow	0.5–10 hr	Unknown

Metabolism: Hepatic; $T_{1/2}$: 2–3.6 hr (oral); $T_{1/2}$: 2.8 hr (inhalation)
Distribution: Crosses placenta; may enter breast milk
Excretion: Urine

Adverse effects
- **CNS:** *Headache, dizziness,* lethargy, *fatigue,* paresthesias, nervousness

- **Dermatologic:** Rash, edema, pruritus, alopecia
- **Endocrine:** HPA suppression, Cushing's syndrome with overdosage and systemic absorption
- **GI:** Nausea, dyspepsia, dry mouth
- **Local:** *Nasal irritation,* fungal infection
- **Respiratory:** Epistaxis, rebound congestion, *pharyngitis, cough*
- **Other:** Chest pain, asthenia, moon face, acne, bruising, *back pain*

Interactions
Oral use

✳ **Drug-drug** • Increased risk of corticosteroid toxic effects if combined with ketoconazole, itraconazole, ritonavir, indinavir, saquinavir, erythromycin, or other known CYP3A4 inhibitors; if drugs must be used together, decrease dosage of budesonide and monitor patient closely

✳ **Drug-food** • Risk of increased toxic effects if combined with grapefruit juice; avoid this combination

■ Nursing considerations
Assessment

- **History:** Untreated local nasal infections, nasal trauma, septal ulcers, recent nasal surgery, lactation
- **Physical:** BP, P, auscultation; R, adventitious sounds; examination of nares

Interventions
Inhalation

⊗ **Warning** Taper systemic steroids carefully during transfer to inhalational steroids; deaths from adrenal insufficiency have occurred.

- Arrange for use of decongestant nose drops to facilitate penetration if edema, excessive secretions are present.
- Use spray within 6 mo of opening. Shake well before each use.
- Store *Pulmicort Respules* upright and protected from light; gently shake before use; open envelopes should be discarded after 2 wk.
- Store *Flexhaler* tightly closed at room temperature. Do not remove or twist mouthpiece. Do not immerse in water or use liquid to clean *Flexhaler.*

Nasal inhalation

- Prime pump eight times before first use. If not used for 2 consecutive days, reprime with

1 spray or until fine mist appears. If not used for more than 14 days, rinse applicator and reprime with 2 sprays or until fine mist appears.

Oral

- Make sure patient does not cut, crush, or chew capsules; they must be swallowed whole.
- Administer the drug once each day, in the morning; have patient avoid drinking grapefruit juice.
- Encourage patient to complete full 8 wk of drug therapy.

⊗ **Warning** Monitor patient for signs of hypercorticism—acne, bruising, moon face, swollen ankles, hirsutism, skin striae, buffalo hump—which could indicate need to decrease dosage.

Teaching points
Inhalation

- Do not use more often than prescribed; do not stop without consulting your health care provider.
- It may take several days to achieve good effects; do not stop if effects are not immediate.
- Use decongestant nose drops first if nasal passages are blocked.
- Store *Pulmicort Respules* upright, protect from light; discard open envelopes after 2 weeks; gently shake before use.
- Store *Flexhaler* at room temperature. Keep tightly closed. Do not immerse in water and do not use liquid to clean the device. Do not twist or remove mouthpiece. Rinse mouth after using oral inhaler.
- You may experience these side effects: Local irritation (use your device correctly), dry mouth (suck sugarless candies).
- Prime the pump eight times before its first use. If it is not used for 2 consecutive days, reprime it with 1 spray or until a fine mist appears. If it is not used for more than 14 days, rinse the applicator off and reprime it with 2 sprays or until fine mist appears.
- Report sore mouth, sore throat, worsening of symptoms, severe sneezing, exposure to chickenpox or measles, eye infections.

Oral

- Take the drug once a day in the morning. Do not cut, crush, or chew the capsules, they must be swallowed whole.

- If you miss a day, take the capsules as soon as you remember them. Take the next day's capsules at the regular time. Do not take more than three capsules in a day.
- Take the full course of the drug therapy (8 weeks in most cases).
- Do not take this drug with grapefruit juice; avoid grapefruit juice entirely while using this drug.
- You may experience these side effects: Dizziness, headache (avoid driving or operating dangerous machinery if these effects occur); nausea, flatulence (small, frequent meals may help; try to maintain your fluid and food intake).
- Report chest pain, ankle swelling, respiratory infections, increased bruising.

▷ bumetanide

See Appendix R, *Less commonly used drugs*.

DANGEROUS DRUG

▷ buprenorphine hydrochloride
*(byoo pre **nor' feen**)*

Buprenex, Butrans Transdermal System

PREGNANCY CATEGORY C

CONTROLLED SUBSTANCE C-III

Drug class
Opioid agonist-antagonist analgesic

Therapeutic actions
Acts as an agonist at specific mu opioid receptors in the CNS to produce analgesia; also acts as an opioid antagonist; exact mechanism of action not understood.

Indications
- Parenteral: Relief of moderate to severe pain
- Oral: Treatment of opioid dependence, preferably used as induction treatment
- Transdermal system: Management of moderate to severe chronic pain in patients requiring a continuous, around-the-clock opioid analgesic for an extended period of time

Contraindications and cautions
- Contraindicated with hypersensitivity to buprenorphine.
- Use cautiously with physical dependence on opioid analgesics (withdrawal syndrome may occur); compromised respiratory function; increased intracranial pressure (buprenorphine may elevate CSF pressure; may cause miosis and coma, which could interfere with patient evaluation), myxedema, Addison's disease, toxic psychosis, prostatic hypertrophy or urethral stricture, acute alcoholism, delirium tremens, kyphoscoliosis, biliary tract dysfunction (may cause spasm of the sphincter of Oddi), hepatic or renal impairment; respiratory depression, paralytic ileus, severe bronchial asthma; lactation, pregnancy.

Available forms
Injection—0.324 mg/mL (equivalent to 0.3 mg); sublingual tablets—2, 8 mg; transdermal patches—5, 10, 20 mcg/hr

Dosages
Adults
Transdermal system: Initially, 5 mcg/hr, intended to be worn for 7 days; if needed, dosage may be increased after wearing system for 72 hr. Maximum dose, 20 mcg/hr.
Adults and pediatric patients older than 13 yr
Parenteral
- *Relief of pain:* 0.3 mg IM or by slow (over 2 min) IV injection. May repeat once, 30–60 min after first dose; repeat every 6 hr as needed. If necessary, nonrisk patients may be given up to 0.6 mg by deep IM injection.
Adults and pediatric patients 16 yr and older
Oral
- *Opioid dependence:* Initially, 8 mg on day 1, 16 mg on day 2 and subsequent induction days (can be 3–4 days); use buprenorphine/naloxone combination (*Suboxone*) for maintenance. Maintenance dose, 12–16 mg/day sublingually (*Suboxone*).
Pediatric patients (2–12 yr)
2–6 mcg/kg of body weight IM or slow IV injection every 4–6 hr.
Geriatric or debilitated patients
Reduce dosage to one-half usual adult dose.

Adverse effects in *italics* are most common; those in **bold** are life-threatening. ⬛ Do not crush.

Pharmacokinetics

Route	Onset	Peak	Duration
Oral	15 min	1 hr	6 hr
Patch	Slow	3 days	7 days
IV	10 min	30–45 min	6 hr

Metabolism: Hepatic; $T_{1/2}$: 2–3 hr (patch, 26 hr)
Distribution: Crosses placenta; may enter breast milk
Excretion: Feces

▼ IV FACTS

Preparation: May be diluted with isotonic saline, lactated Ringer's solution, 5% dextrose and 0.9% saline, 5% dextrose. Protect from light and excessive heat.
Injection: Administer slowly over 2 min.
Compatibilities: Compatible IV with scopolamine HBr, haloperidol, glycopyrrolate, droperidol and hydroxyzine HCl.
Incompatibilities: Do not mix with diazepam and lorazepam.

Adverse effects

- **CNS:** *Sedation, dizziness or vertigo, headache,* confusion, dreaming, psychosis, euphoria, weakness, fatigue, nervousness, slurred speech, paresthesia, depression, malaise, hallucinations, depersonalization, coma, tremor, dysphoria, agitation, seizures, tinnitus
- **CV:** *Hypotension,* hypertension, tachycardia, bradycardia, Wenckebach's block
- **Dermatologic:** *Sweating,* pruritus, rash, pallor, urticaria
- **EENT:** *Miosis,* blurred vision, diplopia, conjunctivitis, visual abnormalities, amblyopia
- **GI:** *Nausea, vomiting,* dry mouth, constipation, flatulence
- **Local:** Injection-site reaction
- **Respiratory:** *Hypoventilation,* dyspnea, cyanosis, apnea

Interactions

✳ **Drug-drug** • Potentiation of effects of buprenorphine with other opioid analgesics, phenothiazines, tranquilizers, barbiturates, general anesthetics, benzodiazepines

■ Nursing considerations
Assessment

- **History:** Hypersensitivity to buprenorphine, physical dependence on opioid analgesics,

timing of last heroin dose, compromised respiratory function, increased intracranial pressure, myxedema, Addison's disease, toxic psychosis, prostatic hypertrophy or urethral stricture, acute alcoholism, delirium tremens, kyphoscoliosis, biliary tract dysfunction, hepatic or renal impairment, lactation, pregnancy
- **Physical:** Skin color, texture, lesions; orientation, reflexes, bilateral grip strength, affect; pupil size, vision; pulse, auscultation, BP; R, adventitious sounds; bowel sounds, normal output, liver palpation; prostate palpation, normal urine output; LFTs, renal, thyroid, adrenal function tests

Interventions

⊗ *Warning* Keep opioid antagonist and facilities for assisted or controlled respiration readily available in case respiratory depression occurs.

- Have the patient hold sublingual tablets beneath the tongue until they dissolve; these tablets should not be swallowed. Place all tablets for a single dose under patient's tongue at once; if not possible, place two tablets at a time. If using the transdermal patch, apply patch to clean, dry area; leave in place for 7 days. Remove old patch before applying new one.
- Apply transdermal system for 7 days. Remove old system before applying a new system. Allow a minimum of 3 wk before applying new system to the same site.
- Instruct patient being treated for opioid dependence that CNS depression and death can occur with overdose of these drugs, or if this drug is combined with sedatives, alcohol, tranquilizers, antidepressants, or benzodiazepines.
- Manage overdose by providing ventilation and support.
- If discontinuing, taper dosage as part of a comprehensive treatment plan.

Teaching points

- Hold sublingual tablets under the tongue until they dissolve. Do not swallow these tablets. If possible, place all tablets for a single dose under the tongue at once; if not possible, place two tablets at a time. If using the transdermal system, apply patch to clean, dry area; leave patch in place for 7 days.

Remove old patch before applying new one; do not apply a new patch to any area you have already used for at least 3 wk.

• Inform all health care or emergency workers that you are opioid dependent and using this drug for maintenance; serious effects could occur if certain drugs are used with this drug.

• Avoid combining sublingual tablets with any alcohol, antidepressants, sedatives, benzodiazepines, or tranquilizers; serious CNS depression could occur. Do not crush and inject these tablets.

• Overdose with sublingual tablets can result in coma and death; use this drug exactly as prescribed.

• Do not stop this drug suddenly; the drug should be tapered within your treatment program.

• This drug is not recommended for use in pregnancy or while breast-feeding.

• You may experience these side effects: Dizziness, sedation, drowsiness, impaired visual acuity (avoid driving, performing other tasks that require alertness); nausea, loss of appetite (lie quietly, eat frequent small meals).

• Report severe nausea, vomiting, palpitations, shortness of breath or difficulty breathing, urinary difficulty.

▷ **buPROPion**
(byoo proe' pee on)

buPROPion hydrobromide
Aplenzin ⊕

buPROPion hydrochloride
Wellbutrin, Wellbutrin SR ⊕,
Wellbutrin XL ⊕, Zyban

PREGNANCY CATEGORY C

Drug classes
Antidepressant
Smoking deterrent

Therapeutic actions
The neurochemical mechanism of the antidepressant effect of bupropion is not understood; it is chemically unrelated to other antidepressant agents; it is a weak blocker of neuronal uptake of serotonin and norepinephrine and inhibits the reuptake of dopamine to some extent.

Indications
• Treatment of major depressive disorder
• Aid to smoking cessation treatment (*Zyban*)
• Prevention of major depressive episodes in patients with seasonal affective disorder (*Wellbutrin XL*)
■ **NEW INDICATION:** Treatment of seasonal affective disorder (*Aplenza*)
• Unlabeled uses: Treatment of neuropathic pain, ADHD, weight loss, aphthous ulcers, migraine prevention, PMDD

Contraindications and cautions
• Contraindicated with hypersensitivity to bupropion; history of seizure disorder, bulimia or anorexia, head trauma, CNS tumor (increased risk of seizures); treatment with MAOIs; lactation.
• Use cautiously with renal or liver disease; heart disease, history of MI, pregnancy.

Available forms
Tablets—75, 100 mg; SR tablets ⊕—100, 150, 200 mg; ER tablets ⊕—150, 200, 300 mg; 174, 348, 522 mg (*Aplenzin*)

Dosages
Adults
• *Depression:* 300 mg PO given as 100 mg tid; begin treatment with 100 mg PO bid; if clinical response warrants, increase to 300 mg/day (given as 100 mg tid) 3 days after beginning treatment. If 4 wk after treatment, no clinical improvement is seen, dose may be increased to 150 mg PO tid (450 mg/day). Do not exceed 150 mg in any one dose. Discontinue drug if no improvement occurs at the 450-mg/day level. *SR:* 150 mg PO bid; allow at least 8 hr between doses. *ER:* Initially, 150 mg/day PO as a once-a-day dose. May increase as early as day 4; range 300–450 mg/day. *ER (Aplenzin):* 174–348 mg/day PO. Maximum dose, 522 mg/day.
• *Smoking cessation:* 150 mg (*Zyban*) PO daily for 3 days, then increase to 300 mg/day

in two divided doses at least 8 hr apart. Treat for 7–12 wk.

- *Seasonal affective disorder:* 150 mg (*Wellbutrin XL*) PO daily in the morning; may increase after 1 wk to 300 mg/day PO. Begin in autumn and taper off (150 mg/day for 2 wk before discontinuation) in early spring.

Pediatric patients

Safety and efficacy in patients younger than 18 yr not established.

Patients with impaired renal function

Bupropion is excreted through the kidneys; use with caution, and monitor patients carefully.

Patients with impaired hepatic function

Consider reduced dose or frequency in patients with mild or moderate impairment. For those with severe impairment, do not exceed 75 mg/day (*Wellbutrin*), 100 mg/day or 150 mg every other day (*Wellbutrin SR*), 150 mg every other day (*Wellbutrin XL* and *Zyban*), or 174 mg/48 hr (*Aplenzin*).

Pharmacokinetics

Route	Onset	Peak	Duration
Oral	Varies	2 hr	8–12 hr
SR Oral	Varies	3 hr	16–20 hr
ER Oral	Varies	5 hr	15–25 hr

Metabolism: Hepatic; $T_{1/2}$: 14 hr; 21 hr (*Wellbutrin SR*)

Distribution: May cross placenta; may enter breast milk

Excretion: Feces, urine

Adverse effects

- **CNS:** *Agitation,* dizziness, *insomnia, headache, migraine, tremor,* ataxia, incoordination, *seizures,* mania, alterations in libido, hallucinations, visual disturbances
- **CV:** *Tachycardia,* edema, ECG abnormalities, chest pain, shortness of breath
- **Dermatologic:** Rash, alopecia, dry skin
- **GI:** *Dry mouth, constipation,* nausea, vomiting, stomatitis
- **GU:** Nocturia, vaginal irritation, testicular swelling
- **Other:** *Weight loss,* flulike symptoms

Interactions

✳ **Drug-drug** • Increased risk of adverse effects with levodopa, amantadine, fluvoxamine, paroxetine, cyclophosphamide, sertraline • Increased risk of toxicity with MAOIs • Increased risk of seizures with drugs that lower seizure threshold, including alcohol

■ Nursing considerations

Assessment

- **History:** Hypersensitivity to bupropion, history of seizure disorder, bulimia or anorexia, head trauma, CNS tumor, treatment with MAOI, renal or hepatic disease, heart disease, lactation
- **Physical:** Skin, weight; orientation, affect, vision, coordination; P, rhythm, auscultation; R, adventitious sounds; bowel sounds, condition of mouth

Interventions

- Check dosages and drugs carefully; products vary widely.
- Avoid use in patients with a history of seizure disorders.
- Give drug three times a day for depression; do not administer more than 150 mg in any one dose. Administer SR forms twice a day with at least 8 hr between doses. Administer ER forms once a day. Caution patient not to cut, crush, or chew ER or SR forms.
- Increase dosage slowly to reduce the risk of seizures.
- Administer 100-mg immediate-release tablets four times a day for depression, with at least 6 hr between doses, if patient is receiving more than 300 mg/day; use combinations of 75-mg tablets to avoid giving more than 150 mg in any single dose.
- Arrange for patient evaluation after 6 wk.
- Discontinue MAOI therapy for at least 14 days before beginning bupropion.
- Monitor hepatic and renal function tests in patients with a history of hepatic or renal impairment.
- Have patient quit smoking within first 2 wk of treatment for smoking cessation; may be used with transdermal nicotine.

⊗ **Black box warning** Monitor response and behavior; suicide is a risk in depressed patients, children, adolescents, and young adults. Serious mental health events, including changes in behavior, depression, and hostility, have been reported.

⊗ **Black box warning** Be aware the *Aplenzin, Wellbutrin, Wellbutrin SR,* and *Wellbutrin XL* are not indicated for smoking cessation; risk of serious neuropsychiatric events, including suicide, when used for this purpose.

Teaching points

- Take this drug in equally divided doses three to four times a day as prescribed for depression. Take sustained-release forms twice a day, at least 8 hours apart. Do not combine doses or make up missed doses. Take once a day, or divided into two doses at least 8 hours apart for smoking cessation. Do not cut, crush, or chew ER or SR forms.
- Avoid or limit the use of alcohol while on this drug. Seizures can occur if these are combined.
- May be used with transdermal nicotine; most effective for smoking cessation if combined with behavioral support program.
- You may experience these side effects: Dizziness, lack of coordination, tremor (avoid driving or performing tasks that require alertness); dry mouth (use frequent mouth care, suck sugarless candies); headache, insomnia (consult your health care provider if these become a problem; do not self-medicate); nausea, vomiting, weight loss (eat frequent small meals).
- Report dark urine, light-colored stools; rapid or irregular heartbeat; hallucinations; severe headache or insomnia; thoughts of suicide; fever, chills, sore throat.

▽ **busPIRone**

See Appendix R, *Less commonly used drugs.*

DANGEROUS DRUG

▽ **busulfan**
(byoo sul' fan)

Busulfex, Myleran

PREGNANCY CATEGORY D

Drug classes
Alkylating drug
Antineoplastic

Therapeutic actions
Cytotoxic: Interacts with normal function of DNA, causing cell death; cell cycle nonspecific.

Indications

- Tablets: Palliative treatment of chronic myelogenous leukemia; less effective in patients without the Philadelphia chromosome (Ph1); ineffective in the blastic stage
- Injection: In combination with cyclophosphamide as conditioning regimen prior to allogenic hematopoietic progenitor cell transplant for CML
- Oral: Other myeloproliferative disorders, including severe thrombocytosis and polycythemia vera, myelofibrosis; bone marrow transplantation

Contraindications and cautions

- Contraindicated with allergy to busulfan, history of resistance to busulfan, chronic lymphocytic leukemia, acute leukemia, blastic phase of chronic myelogenous leukemia, hematopoietic depression, pregnancy, lactation.
- Use cautiously with bone marrow suppression, history of seizure disorders, hepatic impairment.

Available forms
Tablets—2 mg; injection—6 mg/mL

Dosages
Adults
Oral

- *Remission induction:* 4–8 mg or 60 mcg/kg (WBC count more likely to drop with doses above 4 mg/day) total dose PO daily.

Adverse effects in *italics* are most common; those in **bold** are life-threatening. ⏣ Do not crush.

Continue until WBC has dropped to 15,000/mm³; WBC may continue to fall for 1 mo after drug is discontinued. Normal WBC count is usually achieved in approximately 12–20 wk in most cases.

- *Maintenance therapy:* Resume treatment with induction dosage when WBC count reaches 50,000/mm³. If remission is shorter than 3 mo, maintenance therapy of 1–3 mg PO daily is advised to keep hematologic status under control.

Parenteral
- *Conditioning regimen:* 0.8 mg/kg of ideal body weight or actual body weight, whichever is lower, as a 2-hr infusion every 6 hr for 4 consecutive days (16 doses) via central venous catheter.

Pediatric patients
Oral
Children may be dosed at 60–120 mcg/kg/day *or* 1.8–4.6 mg/m²/day (body surface) for remission induction.

Patients with hepatic impairment
Monitor patient closely; dosage adjustment may be needed.

Pharmacokinetics

Route	Onset	Peak	Duration
Oral, IV	30 min–2 hr	2–3 hr	4 hr

Metabolism: Hepatic; T₁/₂: 2.5 hr
$$T_{1/2}$$
Metabolism: Hepatic; $T_{1/2}$: 2.5 hr
Distribution: Crosses placenta; enters breast milk
Excretion: Urine

▼ IV FACTS

Preparation: Dilute to 10 times the busulfan volume using 0.9% sodium chloride injection or D₅W. Use enclosed 5-micron filter when withdrawing drug from ampule. Final concentration should be greater than or equal to 0.5 mg/mL. Use strict aseptic technique. Always add busulfan to the diluent. Mix by inverting bag several times. Stable at room temperature for 8 hr (infusion must be completed within that timeframe), then discard.

Infusion: Use an infusion pump to deliver total dose over 2 hr. Flush catheter with 5 mL D₅W or 0.9% sodium chloride before and after

each dose. Infusion must be completed within 8 hr.
Incompatibilities: Do not infuse with any other solution or drugs.

Adverse effects
- **CNS:** Seizures
- **CV:** Hypertension, tachycardia, thrombosis
- **Dermatologic:** *Hyperpigmentation,* urticaria, **Stevens-Johnson syndrome,** erythema nodosum, alopecia, porphyria cutanea tarda, excessive dryness and fragility of the skin with anhidrosis
- **EENT:** Cataracts (with prolonged use)
- **Endocrine:** *Amenorrhea, ovarian suppression, menopausal symptoms,* interference with spermatogenesis, testicular atrophy, syndrome resembling adrenal insufficiency (weakness, fatigue, anorexia, weight loss, nausea, vomiting, melanoderma)
- **GI:** Dryness of the oral mucous membranes and cheilosis; *nausea, vomiting,* abdominal pain, anorexia
- **GU:** Hyperuricemia
- **Hematologic:** *Leukopenia, thrombocytopenia, anemia,* **pancytopenia** (prolonged)
- **Respiratory: Pulmonary dysplasia**
- **Other:** Cancer

■ Nursing considerations
Assessment
- **History:** Allergy to or history of resistance to busulfan, chronic lymphocytic leukemia, acute leukemia, blastic phase of chronic myelogenous leukemia, hematopoietic depression, pregnancy, lactation, hepatic impairment, seizure disorders
- **Physical:** Weight; skin color, lesions, turgor; earlobe tophi; eye examination; bilateral hand grip; R, adventitious sounds; mucous membranes; CBC, differential; urinalysis; serum uric acid; PFTs; bone marrow examination if indicated

Interventions
⊗ Black box warning Arrange for blood tests to evaluate bone marrow function prior to therapy as well as weekly during and

for at least 3 wk after therapy has ended. Severe bone marrow suppression is possible.

⊗ *Warning* Arrange for respiratory function tests before beginning therapy, periodically during therapy, and periodically after busulfan therapy has ended, to monitor for pulmonary dysplasia.

• Reduce dosage in cases of bone marrow depression.
• Give at the same time each day.
• Suggest barrier contraceptive use during therapy.

⊗ *Warning* Ensure patient is hydrated before and during therapy; alkalinization of the urine or allopurinol may be needed to prevent adverse effects of hyperuricemia.

• Monitor patient for cataracts.
• Administer IV busulfan through a central venous catheter.
• Premedicate patient receiving IV busulfan with phenytoin to decrease occurrence of seizures.
• Medicate patient receiving IV busulfan with antiemetics prior to the first dose and on a fixed schedule through the administration regimen.

Teaching points
Oral drug
• Take drug at the same time each day.
• Drink 10–12 glasses of fluid each day.
• Have regular medical follow-up, including blood tests, to monitor effects of the drug.
• Consider using barrier contraceptives. This drug has been known to cause fetal damage.
• You may experience these side effects: Darkening of the skin, rash, dry and fragile skin (skin care suggestions will be outlined for you to help to prevent skin breakdown); weakness, fatigue (consult with health care provider if pronounced); loss of appetite, nausea, vomiting, weight loss (eat frequent small meals); amenorrhea in women, change in sperm production in men (may affect fertility).
• Report unusual bleeding or bruising; fever, chills, sore throat; stomach, flank, or joint pain; cough, shortness of breath.

DANGEROUS DRUG

▷**butorphanol tartrate**
(byoo **tor'** *fa nole)*

Stadol

PREGNANCY CATEGORY C
(DURING PREGNANCY)

PREGNANCY CATEGORY D
(DURING LABOR AND DELIVERY)

CONTROLLED SUBSTANCE C-IV

Drug class
Opioid agonist-antagonist analgesic

Therapeutic actions
Acts as an agonist at opioid receptors in the CNS to produce analgesia, sedation (therapeutic effects), but also acts to cause hallucinations (adverse effect); has low abuse potential.

Indications
• Relief of moderate to severe pain when use of an opioid analgesic is appropriate
• For preoperative or preanesthetic medication, to supplement balanced anesthesia, and to relieve prepartum pain (parenteral)
• Nasal spray: Relief of moderate to severe pain

Contraindications and cautions
• Contraindicated with hypersensitivity to butorphanol or benzethonium chloride preservative, physical dependence on an opioid analgesic, pregnancy, lactation.
• Use cautiously with bronchial asthma, COPD, respiratory depression, anoxia, increased intracranial pressure, acute MI, ventricular failure, coronary insufficiency, hypertension, biliary tract surgery, renal or hepatic impairment, geriatric patients.

Available forms
Injection—1 mg/mL, 2 mg/mL; nasal spray—10 mg/mL

Dosages
Adults
IM
Usual single dose is 2 mg every 3–4 hr; patient must be able to remain recumbant.

Dosage range is 1–4 mg every 3–4 hr; single doses should not exceed 4 mg.
- *Preoperative:* 2 mg IM, 60–90 min before surgery.

IV

Usual single dose is 1 mg every 3–4 hr. Dosage range is 0.5–2 mg every 3–4 hr.
- *Balanced anesthesia:* 2 mg IV shortly before induction or 0.5–1 mg IV in increments during anesthesia.

IV or IM

- *Labor:* 1–2 mg IV or IM at full term during early labor; repeat every 4 hr. Use alternative analgesia for pain associated with delivery or if delivery is expected within 4 hr.

Nasal

- *Relief of pain:* 1 mg (1 spray per nostril). May repeat in 60–90 min if adequate relief is not achieved. May repeat two-dose sequence every 3–4 hr.

Pediatric patients

Not recommended for patients younger than 18 yr.

Geriatric patients or patients with renal or hepatic impairment

Parenteral

Use one-half the usual dose at least 6 hr apart. Monitor patient response.

Nasal

Initially, 1 mg. Allow 90–120 min to elapse before a second dose is given. Repeat dose sequence based on patient response. There are generally at least 6-hr intervals between dose sequences.

Pharmacokinetics

Route	Onset	Peak	Duration
IV	Rapid	0.5–1 hr	3–4 hr
IM	10–15 min	0.5–1 hr	3–4 hr
Nasal	15 min	1–2 hr	4–5 hr

Metabolism: Hepatic; $T_{1/2}$: 2.1–9.2 hr
Distribution: Crosses placenta; enters breast milk
Excretion: Feces, urine

▼ IV FACTS

Preparation: May be given undiluted. Store at room temperature. Protect from light.
Injection: Administer direct IV over 3–5 min.

Compatibilities: Do not mix in solution with dimenhydrinate or pentobarbital.
Y-site compatibility: Enalaprilat.

Adverse effects

- **CNS:** Sedation, clamminess, sweating, headache, vertigo, floating feeling, dizziness, lethargy, confusion, light-headedness, nervousness, unusual dreams, agitation, euphoria, hallucinations
- **CV:** Palpitation, increase or decrease in BP
- **Dermatologic:** Rash, hives, pruritus, flushing, warmth, sensitivity to cold
- **EENT:** Diplopia, blurred vision
- **GI:** *Nausea,* dry mouth
- **Respiratory:** Slow, shallow respiration

Interactions

* **Drug-drug** • Potentiation of effects of butorphanol when given with barbiturate anesthetics

■ Nursing considerations
Assessment

- **History:** Hypersensitivity to butorphanol, physical dependence on a narcotic analgesic, pregnancy, lactation, bronchial asthma, COPD, increased intracranial pressure, acute MI, ventricular failure, coronary insufficiency, hypertension, biliary tract surgery, renal or hepatic impairment
- **Physical:** Orientation, reflexes, bilateral grip strength, affect; pupil size, vision; pulse, auscultation, BP; R, adventitious sounds; bowel sounds, normal output; LFTs, renal function tests

Interventions

- Ensure that opioid antagonist facilities for assisted or controlled respiration is readily available during parenteral administration.

Teaching points

- You may experience these side effects: Dizziness, sedation, drowsiness, impaired visual acuity (avoid driving, performing other tasks that require alertness); nausea, loss of appetite (lie quietly, eat frequent small meals).

- Report severe nausea, vomiting, palpitations, shortness of breath or difficulty breathing, nasal lesions or discomfort (nasal spray).

▷C1-Inhibitor (human)

See Appendix R, *Less commonly used drugs*.

▷cabazitaxel

See Appendix R, *Less commonly used drugs*.

▷caffeine
(kaf een')

Caffedrine, Enerjets, Fastlene, Keep Alert, Keep Going, Molie, NoDoz, Overtime, Stay Awake, Valentine, Vivarin

caffeine citrate
Cafcit

PREGNANCY CATEGORY C

Drug classes
Analeptic
CNS stimulant
Xanthine

Therapeutic actions
Increases calcium permeability in sarcoplasmic reticulum, promotes the accumulation of cAMP, and blocks adenosine receptors; stimulates the CNS, cardiac activity, gastric acid secretion, and diuresis.

Indications
- An aid in staying awake and restoring mental awareness
- Adjunct to analgesic formulations
- IM: Possibly an analeptic in conjunction with supportive measures to treat respiratory depression associated with overdose with CNS depressants
- Caffeine citrate: Short-term treatment of apnea of prematurity in infants between 28 and 33 wk gestation
- Unlabeled uses: Headache, obesity, alcohol intoxication, postprandial hypotension

Contraindications and cautions
- Contraindicated with duodenal ulcers, diabetes mellitus, lactation.
- Use cautiously with pregnancy, renal or hepatic impairment, depression, CV disease.

Available forms
Tablets—200 mg; capsules—200 mg; lozenges—75 mg; injection—250 mg/mL; caffeine citrate injection and oral solution—20 mg/mL

Dosages
20 mg caffeine citrate = 10 mg caffeine base; use caution.
Adults
100–200 mg PO every 3–4 hr as needed.
- *Respiratory depression:* 500 mg–1 g caffeine and sodium benzoate (250–500 mg caffeine) IM; do not exceed 2.5 g/day; may be given IV in severe emergency situation.
Pediatric patients
- *Neonatal apnea:* 20 mg/kg IV over 30 min followed 24 hours later by 5 mg/kg/day IV over 10 min or PO as maintenance *(CAFCIT)*.

Pharmacokinetics

Route	Onset	Peak
Oral	15 min	15–45 min
IV	Immediate	End of infusion

Metabolism: Hepatic; $T_{1/2}$: 3–7.5 hr, 100 hr (neonates)
Distribution: Crosses placenta; enters breast milk
Excretion: Urine

▼ IV FACTS
Preparation: Dissolve 10 g caffeine citrate powder in 250 mL sterile water for injection USP to 500 mL; filter and autoclave. Final concentration is 10 mg/mL caffeine base (20 mg/mL caffeine citrate). Stable for 3 mo. Or dissolve 10 mg caffeine powder and 10.9 g citric acid powder in bacteriostatic water for injection, USP to 1 L. Sterilize by filtration. *CAFCIT:* 60 mg/3 mL vial may be diluted to achieve desired dose.
Infusion: IV single dose of 500 mg caffeine may be given slowly over 2 min in emergency situations; not recommended. *CAFCIT:* Give 20 mg/kg as a single dose over 30 min; maintain with infusion of 5 mg/kg/day.

Adverse effects in *italics* are most common; those in **bold** are life-threatening. ▢▢▢ Do not crush.

Adverse effects

- **CNS:** *Insomnia, restlessness, excitement,* nervousness, tinnitus, muscular tremor, headaches, light-headedness
- **CV:** *Tachycardia,* hypertension, extrasystoles, palpitations
- **GI:** Nausea, vomiting, diarrhea, stomach pain
- **GU:** *Diuresis*
- **Other:** Withdrawal syndrome: Headache, anxiety, muscle tension

Interactions

✳ **Drug-drug** • Increased CNS effects of caffeine with cimetidine, hormonal contraceptives, disulfiram, ciprofloxacin, mexiletine • Decreased effects of caffeine while smoking • Increased serum levels of theophylline, clozapine with caffeine

✳ **Drug-alternative therapy** • Avoid concomitant administration with guarana, ma huang, or ephedra; may cause additive effects

✳ **Drug-lab test** • Possible false elevations of serum urate, urine VMA, resulting in false-positive diagnosis of pheochromocytoma or neuroblastoma

■ Nursing considerations

Assessment

- **History:** Depression, duodenal ulcer, diabetes mellitus, lactation, pregnancy
- **Physical:** Neurologic status, P, BP, ECG, normal urinary output, abdominal examination, blood glucose

Interventions

⊗ *Warning* Do not stop the drug abruptly after long-term use to avoid withdrawal reactions.

- Monitor diet for caffeine-containing foods that may contribute to overdose.
- Parents of infants being treated with caffeine citrate for apnea should have drug information incorporated into the overall teaching plan.

Teaching points

- Do not stop taking this drug abruptly; withdrawal symptoms may occur.
- Avoid foods high in caffeine (coffee, tea, cola, chocolate), which may cause symptoms of overdose.
- Avoid driving or dangerous activities if dizziness, tremors, or restlessness occur.
- Consult your health care provider if fatigue continues.

- You may experience these side effects: Diuresis, restlessness, insomnia, muscular tremors, light-headedness; nausea, abdominal pain.
- Report abnormal heart rate, dizziness, palpitations.

▽ **calcitonin**
*(kal si **toe'** nin)*

calcitonin, salmon
Apo-Calcitonin (CAN), Calcimar, Caltine (CAN), Fortical, Miacalcin, Miacalcin Nasal Spray, Osteocalcin, Salmonine

PREGNANCY CATEGORY C

Drug classes
Hormone
Calcium regulator

Therapeutic actions
The calcitonins are polypeptide hormones secreted by the thyroid; salmon calcitonin appears to be a chemically identical polypeptide to human calcitonin but with greater potency per milligram and longer duration; inhibits bone resorption; lowers elevated serum calcium in children and patients with Paget disease; increases the excretion of filtered phosphate, calcium, and sodium by the kidneys.

Indications
- Treatment of Paget disease
- Treatment of postmenopausal osteoporosis in conjunction with adequate calcium and vitamin D intake to prevent loss of bone mass
- Treatment of hypercalcemia, emergency treatment (injection only)

Contraindications and cautions
- Contraindicated with allergy to salmon calcitonin or fish products, lactation.
- Use cautiously with renal insufficiency, osteoporosis, pernicious anemia.

Available forms
Injection—200 units/mL; nasal spray—200 units/actuation

Dosages
Adults
Calcitonin, salmon
- *Skin testing:* 0.1 mL of a 10 units/mL solution injected subcutaneously.
- *Paget disease:* Initial dose, 100 units/day IM or subcutaneously. For maintenance, 50 units/day or every other day. Actual dose should be determined by patient response.
- *Postmenopausal osteoporosis:* 100 units every other day IM or subcutaneously, with supplemental calcium (calcium carbonate, 1.5 g/day) and vitamin D (400 units/day) or 200 units intranasally daily, alternating nostrils daily.
- *Hypercalcemia:* Initial dose, 4 units/kg every 12 hr IM or subcutaneously. If response is not satisfactory after 1–2 days, increase to 8 units/kg every 12 hr; if response remains unsatisfactory after 2 more days, increase to 8 units/kg every 6 hr.

Pediatric patients
Safety and efficacy not established.

Pharmacokinetics

Route	Onset	Peak	Duration
IM, Subcut.	15 min	16–25 min	8–24 hr
Nasal	Rapid	31–39 min	8–24 hr

Metabolism: Renal; $T_{1/2}$: 43 min (salmon), 1 hr (human)
Distribution: May enter breast milk
Excretion: Urine

Adverse effects
- **Dermatologic:** *Flushing of face or hands, rash*
- **GI:** *Nausea, vomiting*
- **GU:** *Urinary frequency*
- **Local:** *Local inflammatory reactions at injection site,* nasal irritation (nasal spray)

■ Nursing considerations
Assessment
- **History:** Allergy to salmon calcitonin or fish products, lactation, osteoporosis, pernicious anemia, renal disease
- **Physical:** Skin lesions, color, T; muscle tone; urinalysis, serum calcium, serum alkaline phosphatase and urinary hydroxyproline excretion

Interventions
⊗ **Warning** Give skin test to patients with any history of allergies; salmon calcitonin is a protein, and risk of allergy is significant. Prepare solution for skin test as follows: Withdraw 0.05 mL of the 200 units/mL solution into a tuberculin syringe. Fill to 1 mL with sodium chloride injection. Mix well. Discard 0.9 mL, and inject 0.1 mL (about 1 unit) subcutaneously into the inner aspect of the forearm. Observe after 15 min; the presence of a wheal or more than mild erythema indicates a positive response.
- Ensure that parenteral calcium is readily available in case hypocalcemic tetany develops.
- Monitor serum alkaline phosphatase and urinary hydroxyproline excretion prior to therapy and during first 3 mo and every 3–6 mo during long-term therapy.
- Periodically examine urine sediment for casts in patients on chronic therapy.
⊗ **Warning** Inject doses of more than 2 mL IM, not subcutaneously; use multiple injection sites.
- Refrigerate nasal spray until activated, then store at room temperature.

Teaching points
- This drug is given IM or subcutaneously; you or a significant other must learn how to do this at home. Refrigerate the drug vials. Dispose of needles and syringes in an appropriate container.
- For intranasal use, alternate nostrils daily; notify health care provider if significant nasal irritation occurs.
- Before first use, activate spray by holding bottle upright and depressing the two white side arms toward bottle six times, until a faint spray appears.
- You may experience these side effects: Nausea, vomiting (this passes); irritation at injection site (rotate sites); flushing of the face or hands, rash.
- Report twitching, muscle spasms, dark urine, hives, rash, difficulty breathing.

▷calcium salts
(kal si' uhm)

calcium carbonate
Apo-Cal (CAN), Calcite 500 (CAN), Caltrate, Chooz, Equilet, Os-Cal, Oyst-Cal, PMS-Calcium (CAN), Surpass, Tums

calcium chloride

calcium glubionate
Calcionate, Calciquid

calcium gluconate
Cal-G

calcium lactate
Cal-Lac

PREGNANCY CATEGORY C

Drug classes
Antacid
Electrolyte

Therapeutic actions
Essential element of the body; helps maintain the functional integrity of the nervous and muscular systems; helps maintain cardiac function, blood coagulation; is an enzyme cofactor and affects the secretory activity of endocrine and exocrine glands; neutralizes or reduces gastric acidity (oral use).

Indications
• Dietary supplement when calcium intake is inadequate
• Treatment of calcium deficiency in tetany of the newborn, acute and chronic hypoparathyroidism, pseudohypoparathyroidism, postmenopausal and senile osteoporosis, rickets, osteomalacia
• Prevention of hypocalcemia during exchange transfusions
• Adjunctive therapy for insect bites or stings, such as black widow spider bites; sensitivity reactions, particularly when characterized by urticaria; depression due to overdose of magnesium sulfate; acute symptoms of lead colic
• Calcium chloride: Combats the effects of hyperkalemia as measured by ECG, pending correction of increased potassium in the extracellular fluid
• Improves weak or ineffective myocardial contractions when epinephrine fails in cardiac resuscitation, particularly after open heart surgery
• Calcium carbonate: Symptomatic relief of upset stomach associated with hyperacidity; hyperacidity associated with peptic ulcer, gastritis, peptic esophagitis, gastric hyperacidity, hiatal hernia
• Calcium carbonate: Prophylaxis of GI bleeding, stress ulcers, and aspiration pneumonia; possibly useful
• Unlabeled uses: Treatment of hypertension in some patients with indices suggesting calcium "deficiency"; treatment of premenstrual syndrome (calcium glubionate); treatment of calcium channel–blocker, beta-blocker overdose

Contraindications and cautions
• Contraindicated with allergy to calcium, renal calculi, hypercalcemia, ventricular fibrillation during cardiac resuscitation and patients with the risk of existing digitalis toxicity.
• Use cautiously with renal impairment, pregnancy, lactation.

Available forms
Tablets—250, 300, 500, 650, 975 mg, 1 g, 1.25 g, 1.5 g; powder—2,400 mg; injection—10%, 1.1 g/5 mL; syrup—1.8 g/5 mL; chewable tablets—400, 420, 500, 750, 1,000, 1,177, 1,250 mg; gum—300, 400, 500 mg

Dosages
Adults
Calcium carbonate or lactate
• *RDA:*
14–18 yr: 1,300 mg/day
19–50 yr: 1,000 mg/day
Older than 50 yr: 1,200 mg/day
Pregnant or lactating
14–18 yr: 1,300 mg/day
19–50 yr: 1,000 mg/day
• *Dietary supplement:* 500 mg–2 g PO, bid–qid.
• *Antacid:* 0.5–2 g PO calcium carbonate as needed.
Calcium chloride
For IV use only. 1 g contains 273 mg (13.6 mEq) calcium.

- *Hypocalcemic disorders:* 500 mg–1 g IV at intervals of 1–3 days; response may dictate more frequent injections.
- *Magnesium intoxication:* 500 mg IV promptly. Observe patient for signs of recovery before giving another dose.
- *Hyperkalemic ECG disturbances of cardiac function:* Adjust dosage according to ECG response.
- *Cardiac resuscitation:* 500 mg–1 g IV or 200–800 mg into the ventricular cavity.

Calcium gluconate

IV infusion preferred. 1 g contains 93 mg (4.65 mEq) calcium. 0.5–2 g IV as required; daily dose 1–15 g.

Pediatric patients

Calcium carbonate or lactate

- *RDA:*
  0–6 mo: 210 mg/day
  7–12 mo: 270 mg/day
  1–3 yr: 500 mg/day
  4–8 yr: 800 mg/day
  9–13 yr: 1,300 mg/day

Calcium chloride

2.7–5 mg/kg IV or 0.027–0.05 mL/kg IV every 4–6 hr.

Calcium gluconate

200–500 mg/day IV (2–5 mL of 10% solution); for infants, no more than 200 mg IV (2 mL of 10% solution) given in divided doses.

Pharmacokinetics

Route	Onset	Peak
Oral	3–5 min	N/A
IV	Immediate	3–5 min

Metabolism: Hepatic; $T_{1/2}$: 1–3 hr
Distribution: Crosses placenta; enters breast milk
Excretion: Feces, urine

▼ IV FACTS

Preparation: Warm solutions to body temperature; use a small needle inserted into a large vein to decrease irritation.
Infusion: Infuse slowly, 0.5–2 mL/min. Stop infusion if patient complains of discomfort; resume when symptoms disappear. Repeated injections are often necessary.
Incompatibilities: Avoid mixing calcium salts with carbonates, phosphates, sulfates, tartrates, amphotericin, cefazolin, clindamycin, dobutamine, prednisolone.

Adverse effects

- **CV:** *Slowed heart rate, tingling, "heat waves"* (rapid IV administration); *peripheral vasodilation, local burning, drop in BP* (calcium chloride injection)
- **Local:** *Local irritation,* severe necrosis, sloughing and abscess formation (IM, subcutaneous use of calcium chloride)
- **Metabolic:** Hypercalcemia (*anorexia, nausea, vomiting, constipation,* abdominal pain, dry mouth, thirst, polyuria), *rebound hyperacidity* and milk-alkali syndrome (hypercalcemia, alkalosis, renal damage with calcium carbonate used as an antacid)

Interactions

✳ **Drug-drug** ● Decreased serum levels of oral tetracyclines, oral fluoroquinolones, salicylates, iron salts with oral calcium salts; give these drugs at least 1 hr apart ● Increased serum levels of quinidine and possible toxicity with calcium salts ● Antagonism of effects of verapamil with calcium ● Decreased effect of thyroid hormone replacement; space doses 2 hr apart if this combination is used

✳ **Drug-food** ● Decreased absorption of oral calcium when taken concurrently with oxalic acid (found in rhubarb and spinach), phytic acid (bran and whole-grain cereals), phosphorus (milk and dairy products)

✳ **Drug-lab test** ● False-negative values for serum and urinary magnesium

■ **Nursing considerations**

Assessment

- **History:** Allergy to calcium; renal calculi; hypercalcemia; ventricular fibrillation during cardiac resuscitation; digitalis toxicity, renal impairment, pregnancy, lactation
- **Physical:** Injection site; P, auscultation, BP, peripheral perfusion, ECG; abdominal examination, bowel sounds, mucous membranes; serum electrolytes, urinalysis

Interventions

- Give drug hourly for first 2 wk when treating acute peptic ulcer. During healing stage, administer 1–3 hr after meals and at bedtime.
- Do not administer oral drugs within 1–2 hr of antacid administration.

- Have patient chew antacid tablets thoroughly before swallowing; follow with a glass of water or milk.
- Give calcium carbonate antacid 1 and 3 hr after meals and at bedtime.

⊗ **Warning** Avoid extravasation of IV injection; it irritates the tissues and can cause necrosis and sloughing. Use a small needle in a large vein.

- Have patient remain recumbent for a short time after IV injection.
- Administer into ventricular cavity during cardiac resuscitation, not into myocardium.
- Warm calcium gluconate if crystallization has occurred.
- Monitor serum phosphorus levels periodically during long-term oral therapy.
- Monitor cardiac response closely during parenteral treatment with calcium.

Teaching points
Parenteral
- Report any pain or discomfort at the injection site as soon as possible.

Oral
- Take drug between meals and at bedtime. Ulcer patients must take drug as prescribed. Chew tablets thoroughly before swallowing, and follow with a glass of water or milk.
- Do not take with other oral drugs. Absorption of those medications can be blocked; take other oral medications at least 1–2 hours after calcium carbonate.
- You may experience these side effects: Constipation (can be medicated), nausea, GI upset, loss of appetite (special dietary consultation may be necessary).
- Report loss of appetite, nausea, vomiting, abdominal pain, constipation, dry mouth, thirst, increased voiding.

▽**calfactant (DDPC, natural lung surfactant)**
(*cal fak' tant*)

Infasurf

Drug class
Lung surfactant

Therapeutic actions
A natural bovine compound containing lipids and apoproteins that reduce surface tension, allowing expansion of the alveoli; replaces the surfactant missing in the lungs of neonates suffering from RDS.

Indications
- Prophylactic treatment of infants at risk of developing RDS; infants less than 29 wk gestation
- Rescue treatment of premature infants up to 72 hr of age who have developed RDS and require endotracheal intubation; best if started within 30 min after birth

Contraindications and cautions
- Because calfactant is used as an emergency drug in acute respiratory situations, the benefits usually outweigh any possible risks.

Available forms
Intratracheal suspension—35 mg/mL

Dosages
Infants
Accurate determination of birth weight is essential for determining appropriate dosage. Calfactant is instilled into the trachea using a catheter inserted into the endotracheal tube.
- *Prophylactic and rescue treatment:* Instill 3 mL/kg of birth weight in two doses of 1.5 mL/kg each. Repeat doses of 3 mL/kg of birth weight up to a total of three doses 12 hr apart.

Pharmacokinetics

Route	Onset	Peak
Intratracheal	Immediate	Hours

Metabolism: Normal surfactant metabolic pathways; $T_{1/2}$: less than 24 hr
Distribution: Lung tissue
Excretion: Unknown

Adverse effects
- **CNS: Seizures, intracranial hemorrhage**
- **CV: Patent ductus arteriosus, intraventricular hemorrhage,** *hypotension, bradycardia*
- **Hematologic:** *Hyperbilirubinemia, thrombocytopenia*
- **Respiratory: Pneumothorax,** *pulmonary air leak,* **pulmonary hemorrhage** (more often seen with infants weighing less than 700 g), *apnea,* pneumomediastinum, emphysema
- **Other:** *Sepsis, nonpulmonary infections*

■ Nursing considerations
Assessment
- **History:** Time of birth, exact birth weight
- **Physical:** T, color; R, adventitious sounds, oximeter, endotracheal tube position and patency, chest movement; ECG, P, BP, peripheral perfusion, arterial pressure (desirable); oxygen saturation, blood gases, CBC; muscular activity, facial expression, reflexes

Interventions
- Arrange for appropriate assessment and monitoring of critically ill infant.
- Monitor ECG and transcutaneous oxygen saturation continually during administration.
- Ensure that endotracheal tube is in the correct position, with bilateral chest movement and lung sounds.
- Do not dilute or mix calfactant with any other drugs or solutions. Administer as provided. Warm unopened vials to room temperature. Gently swirl to mix contents.
- Suction the infant immediately before administration; but do not suction for 2 hr after administration unless clinically necessary.
- Store drug in refrigerator. Protect from light. Enter drug vial only once. Discard remaining drug after use. Avoid repeated warmings to room temperature.
- Administer through a side-port adapter into the endotracheal tube or insert 5 French feeding catheter into the endotracheal tube; do not instill into the mainstream bronchus.
- Two attendants, one to instill drug and one to monitor, are needed. Administer total dose in two aliquots of 1.5 mL/kg each. After each instillation, position infant on either right or left side dependent. Administer while continuing ventilation over 20–30 breaths for each aliquot, with small bursts timed during inspiration cycles. A pause followed by evaluation of respiratory status and repositioning should separate the two aliquots. May repeat doses of 3 mL/kg up to a total of three doses 12 hr apart.
- Endotracheal suctioning and/or reintubation is sometimes needed if signs of airway obstruction occur after surfactant.

⊗ **Warning** Continually monitor patient color, lung sounds, ECG, oximeter and blood gas readings during administration and for at least 30 min following administration.
- Maintain appropriate interventions for critically ill infant.
- Offer support and encouragement to parents.

Teaching points
- Parents of the critically ill infant will need a comprehensive teaching and support program. Details of drug effects and administration are best incorporated into the comprehensive program.

▽ canakinumab

See Appendix R, *Less commonly used drugs*.

▽ candesartan cilexetil
*(can dah **sar'** tan)*

Atacand

PREGNANCY CATEGORY C (FIRST TRIMESTER)

PREGNANCY CATEGORY D (SECOND AND THIRD TRIMESTERS)

Drug classes
Angiotensin II receptor antagonist
Antihypertensive

Therapeutic actions
Selectively blocks the binding of angiotensin II to specific tissue receptors found in vascular smooth muscle and adrenal gland; this action blocks the vasoconstriction effect of the renin–angiotensin system as well as the release of aldosterone leading to decreased BP.

Indications
- Treatment of hypertension, alone or in combination with other antihypertensives
- Treatment of heart failure (New York Heart Association classes II–IV, ejection fraction 40% or less) to reduce risk of CV death and to reduce hospitalization for heart failure; may be combined with an ACE inhibitor
- ■ **NEW INDICATION:** Unlabeled use: Prevention of migraines

Contraindications and cautions

- Contraindicated with hypersensitivity to candesartan, pregnancy (use during the second or third trimester can cause injury or even death to the fetus), lactation.
- Use cautiously with renal impairment, hypovolemia.

Available forms

Tablets—4, 8, 16, 32 mg

Dosages
Adults

- *Hypertension:* Usual starting dose, 16 mg PO daily. Can be administered in divided doses bid with a total daily dose of 32 mg/day. Dose range: 8–32 mg a day.
- *Heart failure:* 4 mg/day PO; may be doubled at 2 wk intervals to achieve target dose of 32 mg/day PO as a single dose.

Pediatric patients 6 to younger than 17 yr
- *Hypertension*

More than 50 kg: 8–16 mg/day PO; range, 4–32 mg/day PO once daily or in divided doses. *Less than 50 kg:* 4–8 mg/day PO; range, 2–16 mg/day PO.

Pediatric patients 1 to younger than 6 yr
- *Hypertension*

Initially, 0.20 mg/kg/day oral suspension; range, 0.05–0.4 mg/kg/day oral suspension once daily or in divided doses.

Patients with volume depletion
Consider using lower dose; keep patient under close medical supervision.

Pharmacokinetics

Route	Onset	Peak
Oral	Rapid	3–4 hr

Metabolism: Hepatic; $T_{1/2}$: 9 hr
Distribution: Crosses placenta; enters breast milk
Excretion: Feces, urine

Adverse effects

- **CNS:** *Headache, dizziness,* syncope, muscle weakness
- **CV:** Hypotension
- **Dermatologic:** Rash, inflammation, urticaria, pruritus, alopecia, dry skin
- **GI:** *Diarrhea, abdominal pain, nausea,* constipation, dry mouth, dental pain

- **Respiratory:** *URI symptoms,* cough, sinus disorders
- **Other:** Cancer in preclinical studies, back pain, fever, gout, hyperkalemia, changes in renal function

■ Nursing considerations
Assessment

- **History:** Hypersensitivity to candesartan, pregnancy, lactation, renal impairment, hypovolemia
- **Physical:** Skin lesions, turgor; T; reflexes, affect; BP; R, respiratory auscultation; renal function tests

Interventions

- Administer without regard to meals.
- Have pharmacist prepare oral suspension for children 1–6 yr. Do not administer to children younger than 1 yr.

⊗ **Black box warning** Ensure that patient is not pregnant before beginning therapy, suggest the use of barrier birth control while using candesartan; fetal injury and deaths have been reported. When pregnancy is detected, discontinue candesartan as soon as possible.

- Find an alternate method of feeding the infant for a breast-feeding mother. Depression of the renin-angiotensin system in infants is potentially very dangerous.

⊗ **Warning** Alert surgeon and mark patient's chart with notice that candesartan is being taken. The blockage of the renin-angiotensin system following surgery can produce problems. Hypotension may be reversed with volume expansion.

- If BP control does not reach desired levels, diuretics or other antihypertensives may be added to candesartan. Monitor patient's BP carefully.
- Monitor patient closely in any situation that may lead to a decrease in BP secondary to reduction in fluid volume—excessive perspiration, dehydration, vomiting, diarrhea—excessive hypotension can occur.

Teaching points

- Take this drug without regard to meals. Do not stop taking this drug without consulting your health care provider.
- Use a barrier method of birth control while on this drug; if you become pregnant or desire to become pregnant, consult your health care provider.

- Maintain your fluid intake, especially in situations that could cause loss of fluids, such as diarrhea, vomiting, or excessive sweating.
- You may experience these side effects: Dizziness (avoid driving a car or performing hazardous tasks); headache (medications may be available to help); nausea, vomiting, diarrhea (proper nutrition is important, consult with your dietitian to maintain nutrition); symptoms of URI, cough (do not self-medicate, consult your health care provider if this becomes uncomfortable).
- Report fever, chills, dizziness, pregnancy.

DANGEROUS DRUG

▽ capecitabine
*(kap ah **seat'** ah been)*

Xeloda

PREGNANCY CATEGORY D

Drug classes
Antimetabolite
Antineoplastic

Therapeutic actions
A prodrug of 5-fluorouridine that is readily converted to 5-FU; inhibits thymidylate synthetase, leading to inhibition of DNA and RNA synthesis and cell death.

Indications
- Treatment of breast cancer in patients with metastatic breast cancer resistant to both paclitaxel and doxorubicin or doxorubicin-equivalent chemotherapy
- Treatment of breast cancer in combination with docetaxel in patients with metastatic disease after failure with anthracycline chemotherapy
- Treatment of metastatic colorectal cancer as first-time treatment when treatment with fluoropyrimidine therapy is preferred
- Adjuvant post-surgery treatment of patients with Dukes C colon cancer who have undergone complete resection of the primary tumor who are candidates for single oral agent chemotherapy
- Unlabeled uses: Adjunct treatment of pancreatic cancer; with lopatinib for treatment of advanced or metastatic breast cancer in women with HER 2-overexpressing tumors previously treated with anthracycline and trastuzumab; with ixabepilone for advanced or metastatic breast cancer in women treated with anthracycline and ataxane

Contraindications and cautions
- Contraindicated with allergy to 5-FU; pregnancy; lactation; severe renal impairment, concomitant warfarin therapy.
- Use cautiously with renal or hepatic impairment, severe diarrhea or intestinal disease, coronary artery disease, bleeding disorders (adverse cardiac effects are more common).

Available forms
Tablets—150, 500 mg

Dosages
Adults
- *Breast and colorectal cancers:* Starting dose, 2,500 mg/m^2/day PO in two divided doses 12 hr apart within 30 min after a meal for 2 wk followed by a 1-wk rest period; given in 3-wk cycles.
- *Adjuvant post-surgery Dukes C colon cancer:* 1,250 mg/m^2 PO twice daily, morning and evening within 30 min after a meal, for 2 wk, followed by 1 wk rest, given as 3-wk cycles for a total of 8 cycles (24 wk).

Pediatric patients
Safety and efficacy not established.

Geriatric patients or patients with hepatic impairment
These patients may be more sensitive to the toxic effects of the drug. Monitor closely and decrease dosage as needed to avoid toxicity.

Patients with renal impairment
For creatinine clearance 51–80 mL/min, no adjustment recommended, but monitor carefully; for creatinine clearance 30–50 mL/min, give 75% of normal starting dose; for creatinine clearance less than 30 mL/min, use is contraindicated.

Patients on concurrent therapy with docetaxel
Severe toxicity may result, as manifested by NCIC grade 2–4 toxicity criteria; monitor and adjust doses of both drugs as needed.

Pharmacokinetics

Route	Onset	Peak
Oral	Rapid	1.5 hr

Metabolism: Hepatic and cellular; $T_{1/2}$: 45 min
Distribution: Crosses placenta; may enter breast milk
Excretion: Lungs, urine

Adverse effects

- **CNS:** Fatigue, paresthesias, headache, dizziness, insomnia
- **CV: MI,** angina, arrhythmias, ECG changes
- **Dermatologic:** *Hand-and-foot syndrome* (numbness, dysesthesias, tingling, pain, swelling, blisters, pain), *dermatitis,* nail disorders
- **GI: Diarrhea,** *anorexia, nausea, vomiting, cramps, constipation, stomatitis*
- **Hematologic:** *Leukopenia, thrombocytopenia,* anemia
- **Other:** Fever, edema, myalgia

Interactions

✳ Drug-drug ⊗ *Warning* Increased capecitabine levels and toxicity, with possibility of death, when combined with leucovorin; avoid this combination.

⊗ **Black box warning** Increased risk of excessive bleeding and even death if combined with warfarin anticoagulants; avoid this combination. If the combination must be used, INR and prothrombin levels should be monitored very closely and anticoagulant dose adjusted as needed.

- Increased capecitabine levels when taken with antacids ● Increased phenytoin levels if taken together; consider reduction of phenytoin dose

■ Nursing considerations
Assessment

- **History:** Allergy to 5-FU; impaired hepatic or renal function; pregnancy; lactation; diarrhea, intestinal disease, coronary disease, warfarin therapy
- **Physical:** Weight; T; skin lesions, color; orientation, reflexes, affect, sensation; P, BP, cardiac rhythm, peripheral perfusion; mucous membranes, liver evaluation, abdominal examination; CBC, differential; LFTs, renal function tests

Interventions

- Evaluate renal function before starting therapy to ensure accurate dosage.
- Always administer drug with water, within 30 min of a meal. Have patient swallow drug with water.
- Monitor for toxicities, especially if used with docetaxel; dosage may need to be adjusted based on toxicity.

⊗ *Warning* Arrange for discontinuation of drug therapy if any sign of toxicity occurs— severe nausea, vomiting, diarrhea, hand-and-foot syndrome, stomatitis.

- Monitor nutritional status and fluid and electrolyte balance when GI effects occur; provide supportive care and fluids as needed; loperamide may be helpful for severe diarrhea.
- Provide frequent mouth care for stomatitis or mouth sores.

⊗ *Warning* Arrange for frequent small meals and dietary consultation to maintain nutrition when GI effects are severe.

- Protect patient from exposure to infection; monitor temperature and CBC regularly.
- Suggest use of barrier contraceptives while patient is using this drug; serious birth defects can occur.
- Monitor for toxicities, especially if used with docetaxel; dosage may need to be adjusted, based on toxicity.

Teaching points

- Take this drug every 12 hours, within 30 minutes of a meal; always take the drug after you have eaten and have food in your stomach. Swallow the tablets with water.
- Prepare a calendar of treatment days to follow. The drug is given in 3-week cycles.
- Arrange to have frequent, regular medical follow-up, including frequent blood tests to follow the effects of the drug on your body.
- Avoid pregnancy while taking this drug; using barrier contraceptives is advised. This drug can cause serious birth defects if taken during pregnancy.
- You may experience these side effects: Nausea, vomiting, loss of appetite (medication may be ordered to help; eat frequent small meals; it is very important to maintain your nutrition while you are taking this drug); mouth sores (frequent mouth care will be needed); diarrhea (have ready access to bathroom facilities if this occurs).

- Report fever, chills, sore throat; chest pain; mouth sores; pain or tingling in hands or feet; severe nausea, vomiting or diarrhea (more than five episodes of any of these per day); dizziness.

▽ **capreomycin**

(kap ree oh mye' sin)

Capastat Sulfate

PREGNANCY CATEGORY C

Drug classes
Antibiotic
Antituberculotic ("third line")

Therapeutic actions
Polypeptide antibiotic; mechanism of action against *Mycobacterium tuberculosis* unknown.

Indications
- Treatment of pulmonary tuberculosis that is not responsive to first-line antituberculosis agents but is sensitive to capreomycin in conjunction with other antituberculosis agents

Contraindications and cautions
- Contraindicated with allergy to capreomycin; preexisting auditory impairment.
- Use cautiously with lactation, renal impairment, pregnancy.

Available forms
Solution for injection—1 g/10 mL

Dosages
Always give in combination with other antituberculotics.

Adults
1 g daily (not to exceed 20 mg/kg/day) IM or IV for 60–120 days, followed by 1 g IM two to three times weekly for 12–24 mo. Can also give IV infusion after further dilution in 100 mL 0.9% sodium chloride and infuse over 60 min.

Pediatric patients
Safety and efficacy have not been established.

Geriatric patients or patients with renal impairment

CrCl (mL/min)	Dose (mg/kg) at These Intervals		
	24 hr	48 hr	72 hr
0–9	1.29	2.58	3.87
10	2.43	4.87	7.3
20	3.58	7.16	10.7
30	4.72	9.45	14.2
40	5.87	11.7	–
50	7.01	14	–
60	8.16	–	–
80	10.4	–	–
100	12.7	–	–
110	13.9	–	–

Pharmacokinetics

Route	Onset	Peak	Duration
IM	20–30 min	1–2 hr	8–12 hr

Metabolism: $T_{1/2}$: 4–6 hr
Distribution: Crosses placenta; may enter breast milk
Excretion: Urine

▼ IV FACTS
Preparation: Dissolve vial contents in 2 mL 0.9% sodium chloride or sterile water and allow 3 min for full dissolution. Further dilute in 100 mL 0.9% sodium chloride.
Infusion: Infuse over 60 min.

Adverse effects
- **CNS:** *Ototoxicity*
- **GI:** Hepatic impairment
- **GU:** *Nephrotoxicity*
- **Hematologic:** Leukocytosis, leukopenia, eosinophilia, hypokalemia
- **Hypersensitivity:** Urticaria, rashes, fever
- **Local:** Pain, induration at injection sites, sterile abscesses

Interactions
✳ **Drug-drug** • Increased nephrotoxicity and ototoxicity if used with similarly toxic drugs
• Increased risk of peripheral neuromuscular blocking action with nondepolarizing muscle relaxants (atracurium, pancuronium, tubocurarine, vecuronium)

Adverse effects in italics *are most common; those in* **bold** *are life-threatening.* � Do not crush.

■ **Nursing considerations**
Assessment

- **History:** Allergy to capreomycin; renal insufficiency; auditory impairment; lactation, pregnancy
- **Physical:** Skin color, lesions; T; orientation, reflexes, affect, audiometric measurement, vestibular function tests; liver evaluation; LFTs, renal function tests, CBC, serum K+

Interventions

- Arrange for culture and sensitivity studies before use.
- Administer this drug only when other forms of therapy have failed.
- Administer only in conjunction with other antituberculotics to which the mycobacteria are susceptible.
- Prepare solution by dissolving in 2 mL of 0.9% sodium chloride injection or sterile water for injection; allow 2–3 min for dissolution. To administer 1 g, use entire vial—if less than 1 g is needed, see the manufacturer's instructions for dilution. Reconstituted solution may be stored for 24 hr refrigerated. Solution may acquire a straw color and darken with time; this is not associated with loss of potency. Can also give IV infusion after further dilution in 100 mL 0.9% sodium chloride and infuse over 60 min.
- Administer by deep IM injection into a large muscle mass.

⊗ **Black box warning** Arrange for audiometric testing and assessment of vestibular function, renal function tests, and serum potassium before and at regular intervals during therapy; risk of renal failure, auditory damage is severe.

⊗ **Black box warning** Be aware that safety of drug has not been established in children or pregnant women.

Teaching points

- This drug can be given by IM injection or IV infusion.
- Take this drug regularly; avoid missing doses. You must not discontinue this drug without first consulting your health care provider.
- Arrange to have regular, periodic medical checkups, including blood tests.
- You may experience these side effects: Loss of hearing, dizziness, vertigo (avoid injury).

- Report rash, loss of hearing, decreased urine output, palpitations.

▽ **captopril**
(*kap' toe pril*)

Apo-Capto (CAN), Capoten, Gen-Captopril (CAN), PMS-Captopril (CAN)

PREGNANCY CATEGORY C
(FIRST TRIMESTER)

PREGNANCY CATEGORY D
(SECOND AND THIRD TRIMESTERS)

Drug classes
ACE inhibitor
Antihypertensive

Therapeutic actions
Blocks ACE from converting angiotensin I to angiotensin II, a powerful vasoconstrictor, leading to decreased BP, decreased aldosterone secretion, a small increase in serum potassium levels, and sodium and fluid loss; increased prostaglandin synthesis also may be involved in the antihypertensive action.

Indications

- Treatment of hypertension alone or in combination with thiazide-type diuretics
- Treatment of heart failure in patients unresponsive to conventional therapy; used with diuretics and cardiac glycosides
- Treatment of diabetic nephropathy
- Treatment of left ventricular dysfunction after MI
- Unlabeled uses: Management of hypertensive crises; treatment of rheumatoid arthritis; diagnosis of anatomic renal artery stenosis, hypertension related to scleroderma renal crisis; diagnosis of primary aldosteronism, idiopathic edema; Bartter syndrome; Raynaud syndrome

Contraindications and cautions

- Contraindicated with allergy to captopril, history of angioedema, second or third trimester of pregnancy.
- Use cautiously with renal impairment, heart failure, salt or volume depletion, history of renal artery stenosis, lactation.

Available forms
Tablets—12.5, 25, 50, 100 mg

Dosages
Adults
- *Hypertension:* 25 mg PO bid or tid; if satisfactory response is not noted within 1–2 wk, increase dosage to 50 mg bid–tid; usual range is 25–150 mg bid–tid PO with a mild thiazide diuretic. Do not exceed 450 mg/day.
- *Heart failure:* Initially, 6.25–12.5 mg PO tid in patients who may be salt or volume depleted. Usual initial dose, 25 mg PO tid; maintenance dose, 50–100 mg PO tid. Do not exceed 450 mg/day. Use in conjunction with diuretic and cardiac glycoside therapy.
- *Left ventricular dysfunction after MI:* Initially, 6.25 mg PO, then 12.5 mg PO tid; increase slowly to 50 mg PO tid starting as early as 3 days post MI.
- *Diabetic nephropathy:* Reduce dosage; suggested dose is 25 mg PO tid.

Pediatric patients
Safety and efficacy not established.

Geriatric patients and patients with renal impairment
Excretion is reduced in renal failure; use smaller initial dose; adjust at smaller doses with 1- to 2-wk intervals between increases; slowly adjust to smallest effective dose. Use a loop diuretic with renal impairment.

Pharmacokinetics

Route	Onset	Peak
Oral	15 min	30–90 min

Metabolism: $T_{1/2}$: 2 hr
Distribution: Crosses placenta; enters breast milk
Excretion: Urine

Adverse effects
- **CV:** *Tachycardia,* angina pectoris, **heart failure, MI,** Raynaud syndrome, hypotension in salt- or volume-depleted patients
- **Dermatologic:** Alopecia, *rash, pruritus,* scalded mouth sensation, pemphigoid-like reaction, exfoliative dermatitis, photosensitivity
- **GI:** *Gastric irritation, aphthous ulcers, peptic ulcers, dysgeusia,* cholestatic jaundice, hepatocellular injury, anorexia, constipation

- **GU:** *Proteinuria,* renal insufficiency, renal failure, polyuria, oliguria, urinary frequency
- **Hematologic:** Neutropenia, **agranulocytosis,** thrombocytopenia, hemolytic anemia, **pancytopenia**
- **Other:** *Cough,* malaise, dry mouth, lymphadenopathy

Interactions
✳ **Drug-drug** • Increased risk of hypersensitivity reactions with allopurinol • Decreased antihypertensive effects with indomethacin • Increased captopril effects with probenecid
✳ **Drug-food** • Decreased absorption of captopril with food
✳ **Drug-lab test** • False-positive test for urine acetone

■ Nursing considerations
Assessment
- **History:** Allergy to captopril, history of angioedema, impaired renal function, heart failure, salt or volume depletion, pregnancy, lactation
- **Physical:** Skin color, lesions, turgor; T; P, BP, peripheral perfusion; mucous membranes, bowel sounds, liver evaluation; urinalysis, LFTs, renal function tests, CBC and differential

Interventions
- Administer 1 hr before meals.
- ⊗ **Black box warning** Ensure that patient is not pregnant before beginning treatment. Encourage use of contraceptives; if pregnancy is detected, stop drug.
- ⊗ **Warning** Alert surgeon and mark patient's chart with notice that captopril is being taken; the angiotensin II formation subsequent to compensatory renin release during surgery will be blocked; hypotension may be reversed with volume expansion.
- Monitor patient for drop in BP secondary to reduction in fluid volume (due to excessive perspiration, dehydration, vomiting, or diarrhea); excessive hypotension may occur.
- Reduce dosage in patients with impaired renal function.

Teaching points
- Take drug 1 hour before meals; do not take with food. Do not stop taking drug without consulting your health care provider.

- Watch for drop in blood pressure (occurs most often with diarrhea, sweating, vomiting, or dehydration); if light-headedness or dizziness occurs, consult your health care provider.
- Severe fetal damage can occur if captopril is taken during pregnancy. Use of contraceptives is advised; if pregnancy should occur, stop drug and notify health care provider.
- Avoid over-the-counter medications, especially cough, cold, or allergy medications that may contain ingredients that will interact with ACE inhibitors. Consult your health care provider.
- You may experience these side effects: cough, GI upset, loss of appetite, change in taste perception (limited effects, will pass); mouth sores (frequent mouth care may help); rash; fast heart rate; dizziness, light-headedness (usually passes after the first few days; change position slowly, and limit activities to those that do not require alertness and precision).
- Report mouth sores; sore throat; fever; chills; swelling of the hands or feet; irregular heartbeat; chest pains; swelling of the face, eyes, lips, or tongue; difficulty breathing.

▷ carbamazepine
(kar ba maz' e peen)

Apo-Carbamazepine (CAN),
Carbatrol ⓐ, Epitol, Equetro ⓐ,
Gen-Carbamazepine CR (CAN) ⓐ,
PMS-Carbamazepine (CAN),
Tegretol, Tegretol-XR ⓐ

PREGNANCY CATEGORY D

Drug class
Antiepileptic

Therapeutic actions
Mechanism of action not understood; antiepileptic activity may be related to its ability to inhibit polysynaptic responses and block post-tetanic potentiation. Drug is chemically related to the TCAs.

Indications
- Refractory seizure disorders: Partial seizures with complex symptoms (psychomotor, temporal lobe epilepsy), generalized tonic-clonic (grand mal) seizures, mixed seizure patterns or other partial or generalized seizures. Reserve for patients unresponsive to other agents with seizures difficult to control or who are experiencing marked side effects, such as excessive sedation
- Trigeminal neuralgia (tic douloureux): Treatment of pain associated with true trigeminal neuralgia; also beneficial in glossopharyngeal neuralgia
- Treatment of acute manic and mixed episodes associated with bipolar 1 disorder (*Equetro*)
- Unlabeled uses: Certain psychiatric disorders, including schizoaffective illness, resistant schizophrenia, and dyscontrol syndrome associated with limbic system dysfunction; alcohol withdrawal (800–1,000 mg/day); restless leg syndrome (100–300 mg/day at bedtime); non-neuritic pain syndrome (600–1,400 mg/day)

Contraindications and cautions
- Contraindicated with hypersensitivity to carbamazepine or TCAs, history of bone marrow depression, concomitant use of MAOIs, lactation, pregnancy.
- Use cautiously with history of adverse hematologic reaction to any drug (increased risk of severe hematologic toxicity), glaucoma or increased IOP; history of cardiac, hepatic, or renal damage; psychiatric patients (may activate latent psychosis).

Available forms
Tablets—200 mg; chewable tablets—100 mg; ER tablets ⓐ—100, 200, 400 mg; ER capsules ⓐ—100, 200, 300 mg; suspension—100 mg/5 mL

Dosages
Individualize dosage; a low initial dosage with gradual increase is advised.
Adults
- *Epilepsy:* Initial dose, 200 mg PO bid on the first day; increase gradually by up to 200 mg/day in divided doses every 6–8 hr, until best response is achieved. *Suspension:* 100 mg PO qid. Do not exceed 1,200 mg/day in patients older than age 15; doses up to 1,600 mg/day have been used in adults (rare). For maintenance, adjust to minimum effective level, usually 800–1,200 mg/day.

- *Trigeminal neuralgia:* Initial dose, 100 mg PO bid on the first day; may increase by up to 200 mg/day, using 100-mg increments every 12 hr as needed. Do not exceed 1,200 mg/day. For maintenance, control of pain can usually be maintained with 400–800 mg/day (range 200–1,200 mg/day). Attempt to reduce the dose to the minimum effective level or to discontinue the drug at least once every 3 mo. *Suspension:* Start at 50 mg PO qid; increase by 50 mg PO qid as needed to maximum dose.
- *Combination therapy:* When added to existing antiepileptic therapy, do so gradually while other antiepileptics are maintained or discontinued.
- *Bipolar 1 disorder:* 400 mg/day PO in divided doses; may be increased in 200 mg/day increments. Do not exceed 1,600 mg/day (*Equetro*).

Pediatric patients older than 12 yr
Use adult dosage. Do not exceed 1,000 mg/day in patients 12–15 yr; 1,200 mg/day in patients older than 15 yr.

Pediatric patients 6–12 yr
Initial dose, 100 mg PO bid on the first day. Increase gradually by adding 100 mg/day at 6- to 8-hr intervals until best response is achieved. Do not exceed 1,000 mg/day. Dosage also may be calculated on the basis of 20–30 mg/kg/day in divided doses tid–qid.

Pediatric patients younger than 6 yr
Optimal daily dose, less than 35 mg/kg/day.

Geriatric patients
Use caution; may cause confusion, agitation.

Pharmacokinetics

Route	Onset	Peak
Oral	Slow	4–5 hr
ER oral	Slow	3–12 hr

Metabolism: Hepatic; $T_{1/2}$: 25–65 hr, then 12–17 hr
Distribution: Crosses placenta; enters breast milk
Excretion: Feces, urine

Adverse effects

- **CNS:** *Dizziness, drowsiness, unsteadiness,* disturbance of coordination, confusion, headache, fatigue, visual hallucinations, depression with agitation, behavioral changes in children, talkativeness, speech distur-

bances, abnormal involuntary movements, paralysis and other symptoms of cerebral arterial insufficiency, peripheral neuritis and paresthesias, tinnitus, hyperacusis, blurred vision, transient diplopia and oculomotor disturbances, nystagmus, scattered punctate cortical lens opacities, conjunctivitis, ophthalmoplegia, fever, chills; SIADH, suicidal ideation
- **CV: Heart failure,** increased hypertension, hypotension, syncope and collapse, edema, primary thrombophlebitis, thrombophlebitis reccurence, aggravation of CAD, arrhythmias and AV block; **CV complications**
- **Dermatologic:** Pruritic and erythematous rashes, urticaria, **Stevens-Johnson syndrome,** photosensitivity reactions, alterations in pigmentation, exfoliative dermatitis, alopecia, diaphoresis, erythema multiforme and nodosum, purpura, aggravation of lupus erythematosus
- **GI:** *Nausea, vomiting,* gastric distress, abdominal pain, diarrhea, constipation, anorexia, dryness of mouth or pharynx, glossitis, stomatitis; abnormal LFT, cholestatic and hepatocellular jaundice, **hepatitis, massive hepatic cellular necrosis with total loss of intact liver tissue**
- **GU:** Urinary frequency, acute urinary retention, oliguria with hypertension, renal failure, azotemia, impotence, proteinuria, glycosuria, elevated BUN, microscopic deposits in urine
- **Hematologic: Hematologic disorders** (severe bone marrow suppression)
- **Respiratory:** Pulmonary hypersensitivity characterized by fever, dyspnea, pneumonitis or pneumonia

Interactions

✴ **Drug-drug** • Increased serum levels and manifestations of toxicity with erythromycin, cimetidine, danazol, isoniazid, verapamil; dosage of carbamazepine may need to be reduced (reductions of about 50% recommended with erythromycin) • Increased CNS toxicity with lithium • Increased risk of hepatotoxicity with isoniazid (MAOI qualities); because of the chemical similarity of carbamazepine to the TCAs and because of the serious adverse interaction of TCAs and MAOIs, discontinue MAOIs for minimum of 14 days before carbamazepine administration • Decreased absorption with charcoal • Decreased serum levels and decreased effects of carbamazepine with barbiturates • Increased metabolism but no loss of seizure control with phenytoin, primidone • Increased metabolism of phenytoin, valproic acid • Decreased anticoagulant effect of warfarin, oral anticoagulants; dosage of warfarin may need to be increased during concomitant therapy but decreased if carbamazepine is withdrawn • Decreased effects of nondepolarizing muscle relaxants, haloperidol • Decreased antimicrobial effects of doxycycline

■ Nursing considerations
Assessment
• History: Hypersensitivity to carbamazepine or TCAs; history of bone marrow depression; concomitant use of MAOIs; history of adverse hematologic reaction to any drug; glaucoma or increased IOP; history of cardiac, hepatic, or renal damage; psychiatric history; lactation; pregnancy
• Physical: Weight; T; skin color, lesions; palpation of lymph glands; orientation, affect, reflexes; ophthalmologic examination (including tonometry, funduscopy, slit lamp examination); P, BP, perfusion; auscultation; peripheral vascular examination; R, adventitious sounds; bowel sounds, normal output; oral mucous membranes; normal urinary output, voiding pattern; CBC including platelet, reticulocyte counts and serum iron; LFTs, urinalysis, BUN, thyroid function tests, EEG

Interventions
• Use only for classifications listed. Do not use as a general analgesic. Use only for epileptic seizures that are refractory to other safer agents.
• Give drug with food to prevent GI upset.
• Do not mix suspension with other medications or elements—precipitation may occur.
⊗ Warning Reduce dosage, discontinue, or substitute other antiepileptic medication gradually. Abrupt discontinuation of all antiepileptic medication may precipitate status epilepticus.
⊗ Warning There is an increased risk of suicidal ideation with antiepileptic administration. Caution patient and monitor accordingly.
• Suspension will produce higher peak levels than tablets—start with a lower dose given more frequently.

• Ensure that patient swallows ER tablets whole—do not cut, crush, or chew. Equetro capsules may be opened and contents sprinkled over soft food, such as 1 tsp applesauce.
• Arrange for frequent LFTs; discontinue drug immediately if hepatic impairment occurs.
⊗ Black box warning There is a risk of aplastic anemia and agranulocytosis. Arrange for patient to have CBC, including platelet, reticulocyte counts, and serum iron determination, before initiating therapy; repeat weekly for the first 3 mo of therapy and monthly thereafter for at least 2–3 yr. Discontinue drug if there is evidence of marrow suppression, as follows:
⊗ Black box warning Serious to fatal dermatologic reactions, including Stevens-Johnson syndrome, have been reported. Risk increases with Asian patients with HLA-B*1502 allele. Patients testing positive for this allele should not be treated with carbamazepine.

Erythrocytes	Less than 4 million/mm³
Hct	Less than 32%
Hgb	Less than 11 gm/dL
Leukocytes	Less than 4,000/mm³
Platelets	Less than 100,000/mm³
Reticulocytes	Less than 0.3% (20,000/mm²)
Serum iron	Less than 150 g/100 mL

• Arrange for frequent eye examinations, urinalysis, and BUN determinations.
• Arrange for frequent monitoring of serum levels of carbamazepine and other antiepileptics given concomitantly, especially during the first few weeks of therapy. Adjust dosage on basis of data and clinical response.
• Counsel women who wish to become pregnant; advise the use of barrier contraceptives.
• Evaluate for therapeutic serum levels (usually 4–12 mcg/mL).

Teaching points
• Take drug with food as prescribed. Swallow extended-release tablets whole; do not cut, crush, or chew them. If using Equetro capsules, they may be opened and contents sprinkled over soft food, such as 1 teaspoon of applesauce.
• Do not discontinue this drug abruptly or change dosage, except on the advice of your physician.

- Avoid alcohol, sleep-inducing, or over-the-counter drugs; these could cause dangerous effects.
- Arrange for frequent checkups, including blood tests, to monitor your response to this drug. Keep all appointments for checkups.
- Use contraceptives at all times; if you wish to become pregnant, you should consult your physician.
- Wear a medical alert tag at all times so that any emergency medical personnel will know that you have epilepsy and are taking antiepileptic medication.
- You may experience these side effects: Drowsiness, dizziness, blurred vision (avoid driving or performing other tasks requiring alertness or visual acuity); GI upset (take the drug with food or milk, eat frequent small meals).
- Report bruising, unusual bleeding, abdominal pain, yellowing of the skin or eyes, pale feces, darkened urine, impotence, central nervous system disturbances, edema, fever, chills, sore throat, mouth ulcers, rash, pregnancy, thoughts of suicide.

DANGEROUS DRUG

▷**carboplatin**

(*kar' boe pla tin*)

PREGNANCY CATEGORY D

Drug classes

Alkylating drug
Antineoplastic

Therapeutic actions

Cytotoxic: Heavy metal that produces cross-links within and between strands of DNA, thus preventing cell replication; cell cycle nonspecific.

Indications

- Initial treatment of advanced ovarian carcinoma in combination with other antineoplastics
- Palliative treatment of patients with ovarian carcinoma recurrent after prior chemotherapy, including patients who have been treated with cisplatin
- Unlabeled uses: Alone or with other agents to treat small-cell lung cancer, squamous cell cancer of the head and neck, endometrial cancer, relapsed or refractory acute leukemia, seminoma of testicular cancer

Contraindications and cautions

- Contraindicated with history of severe allergic reactions to carboplatin, cisplatin, platinum compounds, mannitol; severe bone marrow depression; lactation.
- Use cautiously in renal impairment, pregnancy, history of neuropathic disorders.

Available forms

Powder for injection—150 mg; injection—10 mg/mL

Dosages

Adults

- *As a single agent:* 360 mg/m^2 IV on day 1 every 4 wk. Do not repeat single doses of carboplatin until the neutrophil count is at least 2,000/mm^3 and the platelet count is at least 100,000/mm^3. These adjustments of dosage can be used: For platelets more than 100,000 and neutrophils more than 2,000, use dosage 125% of prior course; for platelets 50,000–100,000 and neutrophils 500–2,000, no adjustment in dosage; for platelets less than 50,000 and neutrophils less than 500—dosage 75% of previous course. Doses of more than 125% are not recommended. May also be given at 300 mg/m^2 in combination with cyclophosphamide.

Pediatric patients

Safety and efficacy not established.

Geriatric patients and patients with renal impairment

Increased risk of bone marrow depression with renal impairment. Use caution.

CrCl (mL/min)	Dose (mg/m^2 on Day 1)
41–59	250
16–40	200
15 or less	No data available

Pharmacokinetics

Route	Onset	Duration
IV	Rapid	48–96 hr

Metabolism: T$_{1/2}$: 1.2–2 hr, then 2.6–5.9 hr
Distribution: Crosses placenta; may enter breast milk
Excretion: Urine

C

▼ IV FACTS

Preparation: Immediately before use, reconstitute the contents of each powder vial with sterile water for injection, D_5W, or sodium chloride injection. For a concentration of 10 mg/mL, combine 150-mg vial with 15 mL of diluent. Carboplatin can be further diluted using D_5W or sodium chloride injection. Store unopened vials at room temperature. Protect from exposure to light. Reconstituted solution is stable for 8 hr at room temperature. Discard after 8 hr. Do not use needles of IV administration sets that contain aluminum; carboplatin can precipitate and lose effectiveness when in contact with aluminum.

Infusion: Administer by slow infusion lasting at least 15 min.

Adverse effects

- **CNS:** *Peripheral neuropathies,* ototoxicity, visual disturbances, change in taste perception
- **GI:** *Vomiting, nausea, abdominal pain, diarrhea, constipation*
- **GU:** *Increased BUN or serum creatinine*
- **Hematologic: Bone marrow depression;** *decreased serum sodium, magnesium, calcium, potassium*
- **Hypersensitivity:** *Anaphylactic-like reaction,* rash, urticaria, erythema, pruritus, **bronchospasm**
- **Other:** *Pain, alopecia, asthenia,* **cancer**

Interactions

✳ **Drug-drug** • Decreased potency of carboplatin and precipitate formation in solution using needles or administration sets containing aluminum

■ Nursing considerations

Assessment

- **History:** Severe allergic reactions to carboplatin, cisplatin, platinum compounds, mannitol; severe bone marrow depression; renal impairment; pregnancy, lactation
- **Physical:** Weight, skin, and hair evaluation; eighth cranial nerve evaluation; reflexes; sensation; CBC, differential; renal function tests; serum electrolytes; serum uric acid; audiogram

Interventions

⊗ **Black box warning** Evaluate bone marrow function before and periodically during therapy. Do not give next dose if bone marrow depression is marked. Consult physician for dosage.

⊗ **Black box warning** Ensure that epinephrine, corticosteroids, and antihistamines are readily available in case of anaphylactic-like reactions, which may occur within minutes of administration.

- Arrange for an antiemetic if nausea and vomiting are severe.

Teaching points

- This drug can only be given IV. Prepare a calendar of treatment days.
- Use contraceptives while taking this drug. This drug may cause birth defects or miscarriages.
- Have frequent, regular medical follow-up, including frequent blood tests to monitor drug effects.
- You may experience these side effects: Nausea, vomiting (medication may be ordered; eat frequent small meals); numbness, tingling, loss of taste, ringing in ears, dizziness, loss of hearing; rash, loss of hair (you can use a wig or scarves).
- Report loss of hearing, dizziness; unusual bleeding or bruising; fever, chills, sore throat; leg cramps, muscle twitching; changes in voiding patterns; difficulty breathing.

▽ carboprost tromethamine

(kar' boe prost)

Hemabate

PREGNANCY CATEGORY C

Drug classes

Abortifacient
Prostaglandin

Therapeutic actions

Stimulates the myometrium of the gravid uterus to contract in a manner that is similar to the contractions of the uterus during labor, thus evacuating the contents of the gravid uterus.

Indications

- Termination of pregnancy 13–20 wk from the first day of the last menstrual period

- Evacuation of the uterus in instance of missed abortion or intrauterine fetal death in the second trimester
- Postpartum hemorrhage due to uterine atony unresponsive to conventional methods

Contraindications and cautions

- Contraindicated with allergy to prostaglandin preparations; acute PID; active cardiac, hepatic, pulmonary, renal disease.
- Use cautiously with history of asthma; hypotension; hypertension; CV, adrenal, renal, or hepatic disease; anemia; jaundice; diabetes; epilepsy; scarred uterus; cervicitis, infected endocervical lesions; acute vaginitis.

Available forms

Injection—250 mcg/mL

Dosages
Adults

- *Abortion:* Initially, 250 mcg (1 mL) IM; give 250 mcg IM at 1.5- to 3.5-hr intervals, depending on uterine response; may be increased to 500 mcg if uterine contractility is inadequate after several 250-mcg doses; do not exceed 12 mg total dose or continuous administration over 2 days.
- *Refractory postpartum uterine bleeding:* 250 mcg IM as one dose; in some cases, multiple doses at 15- to 90-min intervals may be used; do not exceed a total dose of 2 mg (8 doses).

Pharmacokinetics

Route	Onset	Peak
IM	15 min	2 hr

Metabolism: Hepatic and lung; $T_{1/2}$: 8 hr
Distribution: Crosses placenta; may enter breast milk
Excretion: Urine

Adverse effects

- **CNS:** Headache, paresthesias, *flushing,* anxiety, weakness, syncope, dizziness
- **CV:** *Hypotension,* arrhythmias, chest pain
- **GI:** Vomiting, diarrhea, *nausea*
- **GU:** Endometritis, **perforated uterus, uterine rupture,** uterine or vaginal pain, incomplete abortion
- **Respiratory:** Coughing, dyspnea
- **Other:** Chills, diaphoresis, backache, breast tenderness, eye pain, skin rash, pyrexia

■ Nursing considerations
Assessment

- **History:** Allergy to prostaglandin preparations; acute PID; active cardiac, hepatic, pulmonary, renal disease; history of asthma; hypotension; hypertension; anemia; jaundice; diabetes; epilepsy; scarred uterus; cervicitis, infected endocervical lesions; acute vaginitis
- **Physical:** T; BP, P, auscultation; R, adventitious sounds; bowel sounds, liver evaluation; vaginal discharge, pelvic examination, uterine tone; LFTs, renal function tests, WBC, urinalysis, CBC

Interventions

- Refrigerate unopened vials.
- Administer a test dose of 100 mcg (0.4 mL) prior to abortion if indicated.
- Administer by deep IM injection.
- Arrange for pretreatment or concurrent treatment with antiemetics and antidiarrheals to decrease the incidence of GI side effects.

⊗ **Warning** Ensure that abortion is complete or that other measures are used to complete the abortion if drug effects are not sufficient.

- Monitor T, using care to differentiate prostaglandin-induced pyrexia from postabortion endometritis pyrexia.
- Monitor uterine tone and vaginal discharge during procedure and several days after to assess drug effects and recovery.
- Ensure adequate hydration throughout procedure.

Teaching points

- Several IM injections may be required to achieve desired effect.
- You may experience these side effects: Nausea, vomiting, diarrhea, uterine or vaginal pain, fever, headache, weakness, dizziness.
- Report severe pain, difficulty breathing, palpitations, eye pain, rash.

▽ carfilzomib

See Appendix R, *Less commonly used drugs.*

▽ carglumic acid

See Appendix R, *Less commonly used drugs.*

Adverse effects in *italics* are most common; those in **bold** are life-threatening. ▭ Do not crush.

▽ **carisoprodol (isomeprobamate)**

(kar eye soe proe' dol)

Soma

PREGNANCY CATEGORY C

Drug class
Centrally acting skeletal muscle relaxant

Therapeutic actions
Precise mechanism not known; chemically related to meprobamate, an anxiolytic; has sedative properties; also found in animal studies to inhibit interneuronal activity in descending reticular formation and spinal cord; does not directly relax tense skeletal muscles.

Indications
• Relief of discomfort associated with acute, painful musculoskeletal conditions as an adjunct to rest, physical therapy, and other measures

Contraindications and cautions
• Contraindicated with allergic or idiosyncratic reactions to carisoprodol, meprobamate (reported cross-reactions with meprobamate); acute intermittent porphyria, suspected porphyria, lactation.
• Use cautiously with renal or hepatic impairment, pregnancy.

Available forms
Tablets—250, 350 mg

Dosages
Adults and children older than 16 yr
250–350 mg PO tid–qid; take last dose at bedtime for a maximum of 2–3 wk.
Pediatric patients
Not recommended for children younger than 16 yr.
Patients with hepatic or renal impairment
Dosage reduction may be necessary; monitor closely.

Pharmacokinetics

Route	Onset	Peak	Duration
Oral	30 min	1–2 hr	4–6 hr

Metabolism: Hepatic; $T_{1/2}$: 8 hr
Distribution: May cross placenta; enters breast milk
Excretion: Urine

Adverse effects
• **CNS:** *Dizziness, drowsiness, vertigo, ataxia, tremor, agitation, irritability*
• **CV:** Tachycardia, orthostatic hypotension, facial flushing
• **GI:** Nausea, vomiting, hiccups, epigastric distress
• **Hypersensitivity: Allergic or idiosyncratic reactions** (seen with first to fourth dose in patients new to drug)—rash, erythema multiforme, pruritus, eosinophilia, fixed drug eruption; asthmatic episodes, fever, weakness, dizziness, angioneurotic edema, smarting eyes, hypotension, **anaphylactoid shock**

■ Nursing considerations
Assessment
• **History:** Allergic or idiosyncratic reactions to carisoprodol, meprobamate; acute intermittent porphyria, suspected porphyria; lactation
• **Physical:** T; skin color, lesions; orientation, affect; P, BP, orthostatic BP; bowel sounds, liver evaluation; LFTs, renal function tests, CBC

Interventions
⊗ *Warning* Monitor patient for potentially serious idiosyncratic reactions—most likely with first few doses.
• Reduce dose with hepatic impairment.
• Provide safety measures if CNS effects occur.
• Drug may be habit forming. Monitor patient.

Teaching points
• Take this drug exactly as prescribed; do not take a higher dosage; take with food if GI upset occurs.
• Avoid alcohol, sleep-inducing, or over-the-counter drugs; these could cause dangerous effects; if you feel you need one of these preparations, consult your health care provider.
• You may experience these side effects: Drowsiness, dizziness, vertigo (avoid driving or activities that require alertness); dizziness when you get up or climb stairs (avoid sudden changes in position, use caution climbing stairs); nausea (take drug with

food, eat frequent small meals); insomnia, headache, depression (transient effects).
- Report rash, severe nausea, dizziness, insomnia, fever, difficulty breathing.

DANGEROUS DRUG

▽ **carmustine (BCNU)**
(car mus' teen)

BiCNU, Gliadel

PREGNANCY CATEGORY D

Drug classes
Alkylating agent
Nitrosourea
Antineoplastic

Therapeutic actions
Cytotoxic: Alkylates DNA and RNA and inhibits several enzymatic processes, leading to cell death.

Indications
- Palliative therapy alone or with other agents (injection) for brain tumors: Glioblastomas, brainstem glioma, medullablastoma, astrocytoma, ependymoma, metastatic brain tumors
- Hodgkin lymphoma and non-Hodgkin lymphomas (as secondary therapy)
- Multiple myeloma (with prednisone)
- Adjunct to surgery for the treatment of recurrent glioblastoma as implantable wafer after removal of tumor (wafer)
- Treatment of newly diagnosed high-grade malignant glioma as adjunct to surgery and radiation (wafer)
- Unlabeled uses: Treatment of mycosis fungoides (topical), cutaneous T-cell lymphoma, hematopoietic stem-cell transplantation, colorectal carcinoma, malignant melanoma

Contraindications and cautions
- Contraindicated with allergy to carmustine.
- Use cautiously with radiation therapy, chemotherapy, hematopoietic depression, impaired renal or hepatic function, pregnancy (teratogenic and embryotoxic), lactation.

Available forms
Powder for injection—100 mg; wafer (*Gliadel*)—7.7 mg

Dosages
⊗ **Black box warning** Do not give doses more often than every 6 wk because of delayed bone marrow toxicity.

Adults and pediatric patients
IV
As single agent in untreated patients, 150–200 mg/m² IV every 6 wk as a single dose or in divided daily injections (75–100 mg/m² on 2 successive days). Do not repeat dose until platelets exceed 100,000/mm³, leukocytes exceed 4,000/mm³. Adjust dosage after initial dose based on hematologic response, as follows:

Leukocytes	Platelets	Percentage of Prior Dose to Give
More than 4,000	More than 100,000	100%
3,000–3,999	75,000–99,999	100%
2,000–2,999	25,000–74,999	70%
Less than 2,000	Less than 25,000	50%

Wafer
Implanted in resection cavity as part of a surgical procedure; up to 8 wafers at a time.

Pharmacokinetics

Route	Onset	Peak
IV	Immediate	15 min
Wafer	Absorbed locally	Unknown

Metabolism: Hepatic; T$_{1/2}$: 15–30 min
Distribution: Crosses placenta; may enter breast milk
Excretion: Lungs, urine

▼**IV FACTS**

Preparation: Reconstitute with 3 mL of supplied sterile diluent, then add 27 mL of sterile water for injection to the alcohol solution; resulting solution contains 3.3 mg/mL of carmustine in 10% ethanol, pH is 5.6–6; may be further diluted with 5% dextrose injection. Refrigerate unopened vials. Protect reconstituted solution from light; lacking preservatives, solution decomposes with time, but is stable for 8 hr at room temperature. Check vials before use for absence of oil film residue; if present, discard vial.

Infusion: Administer reconstituted solution by IV drip over 1–2 hr; shorter infusion time may cause intense pain and burning. Stability

of dextrose-diluted solutions at a concentration
of 0.2 mg/mL is 8 hr at room temperature.
Incompatibility: Do not add to sodium bicarbonate.

Adverse effects

- **CNS:** Ocular toxicity—nerve fiber-layer in-
farcts, retinal hemorrhage
- **GI:** *Nausea, vomiting, stomatitis, hepatotoxicity*
- **GU:** Renal toxicity—decreased renal size,
azotemia, **renal failure**
- **Hematologic:** *Myelosuppression, leukopenia, thrombocytopenia, anemia* (delayed for 4–6 wk)
- **Respiratory:** *Pulmonary infiltrates,* **pulmonary fibrosis**
- **Other:** *Local burning at site of injection;* intense flushing of the skin, suffusion of the conjunctiva with rapid IV infusion; **cancer**

Interactions

✳ Drug-drug • Increased toxicity and myelosuppression with cimetidine • Decreased serum
levels of digoxin, phenytoin • Risk of corneal
and epithelial damage with mitomycin

■ Nursing considerations
Assessment

- **History:** Allergy to carmustine; radiation
therapy; chemotherapy; hematopoietic depression; impaired renal or hepatic function;
pregnancy; lactation
- **Physical:** T; weight; ophthamologic examination; R, adventitious sounds; mucous
membranes, liver evaluation; CBC, differential; urinalysis, LFTs, renal function tests; PFTs

Interventions

⊗ **Black box warning** Evaluate hematopoietic function before therapy and weekly during and for at least 6 wk after therapy to monitor for bone marrow suppression.
- Do not give full dosage within 2–3 wk after
a full course of radiation therapy or chemotherapy because of the risk of severe bone
marrow depression; reduced dosage may be
needed.
⊗ **Black box warning** Monitor patient
for pulmonary toxicity and delayed toxicity,
which can occur years after therapy; even death
can occur. Cumulative doses of 1,400 mg/m^2
increase the risk.

- Unopened foil pouches of wafer may be kept
at ambient room temperature for a maximum of 6 hr.
- Reduce dosage in patients with depressed
bone marrow function.
- Arrange for pretherapy medicating with
antiemetic to decrease the severity of nausea and vomiting.
- Monitor injection site for any adverse reaction; accidental contact of carmustine with
the skin can cause burning and hyperpigmentation of the area.
- Monitor ophthalmologic status.
- Monitor urine output for volume and any
sign of renal failure.
- Monitor LFTs, renal function tests, and
PFTs.

Teaching points

- This drug can only be given IV or implanted during surgery.
- Maintain your fluid intake and nutrition.
- Use contraceptives; this drug can cause severe birth defects.
- You may experience these side effects: Nausea, vomiting, loss of appetite (an antiemetic may be ordered; eat frequent small meals);
increased susceptibility to infection (avoid
exposure to infection by avoiding crowded
places; avoid injury).
- Report unusual bleeding or bruising, fever,
chills, sore throat, stomach or flank pain,
changes in vision, difficulty breathing, shortness of breath, burning or pain at IV injection site.

▽ **carvedilol**
(kar vah' da lol)

Apo-Carvedilol (CAN), Coreg,
Coreg CR ⊙ⅅⅭ, PMS-Carvedilol (CAN),
ratio-Carvedilol (CAN)

PREGNANCY CATEGORY C

Drug classes

Alpha- and beta-adrenergic blocker
Antihypertensive

Therapeutic actions

Competitively blocks alpha-, beta-, and beta$_2$-
adrenergic receptors and has some sympathomimetic activity at beta$_2$-receptors. Both

alpha- and beta-blocking actions contribute to the BP-lowering effect; beta blockade prevents the reflex tachycardia seen with most alpha-blocking drugs and decreases plasma renin activity. Significantly reduces plasma renin activity.

Indications

- Hypertension, alone or with other oral drugs, especially diuretics
- Treatment of mild to severe heart failure of ischemic or cardiomyopathic origin with digitalis, diuretics, ACE inhibitors
- Left ventricular dysfunction (LVD) after MI
- Unlabeled uses: Angina (25–50 mg bid), hiccups, idiopathic cardiomyopathy

Contraindications and cautions

- Contraindicated with decompensated heart failure, bronchial asthma, heart block, cardiogenic shock, hypersensitivity to carvedilol, pregnancy, lactation.
- Use cautiously with hepatic impairment, peripheral vascular disease, thyrotoxicosis, diabetes, anesthesia, major surgery.

Available forms

Tablets—3.125, 6.25, 12.5, 25 mg; CR capsules ⊙⊞⊙—10, 20, 40, 80 mg

Dosages
Adults

- *Hypertension:* 6.25 mg PO bid; maintain for 7–14 days, then increase to 12.5 mg PO bid if needed to control BP. Do not exceed 50 mg/day.
- *Heart failure:* Monitor patient very closely, individualize dose based on patient response. Initial dose, 3.125 mg PO bid for 2 wk, may then be increased to 6.25 mg PO bid. Do not increase doses at intervals shorter than 2 wk. Maximum dose, 25 mg PO bid in patients weighing less than 85 kg or 50 mg PO bid in patients weighing more than 85 kg.
- *LVD following MI:* 6.25 mg PO bid; increase after 3–10 days to target dose of 25 mg bid. For conversion from tablets to CR capsules, follow these instructions. For dosage of 6.25 mg daily (3.125 mg bid), give 10 mg CR capsules once daily. For 12.5 mg (6.25 mg bid), give 20 mg CR capsules once daily. For 25 mg (12.5 mg bid), give 40 mg CR capsules once daily. For 50 mg (25 mg bid), give 80 mg CR capsules once daily.

Pediatric patients
Safety and efficacy not established.
Patients with hepatic impairment
Do not administer to any patient with severe hepatic impairment.

Pharmacokinetics

Route	Onset	Peak	Duration
Oral	Rapid	30 min	8–10 hr

Metabolism: Hepatic; $T_{1/2}$: 7–10 hr
Distribution: Crosses placenta; may enter breast milk
Excretion: Bile, feces

Adverse effects

- **CNS:** *Dizziness, vertigo, tinnitus, fatigue,* emotional depression, paresthesias, sleep disturbances
- **CV:** *Bradycardia,* orthostatic hypertension, **heart failure,** cardiac arrhythmias, pulmonary edema, *hypotension*
- **GI:** *Gastric pain, flatulence, constipation, diarrhea,* **hepatic failure**
- **Respiratory:** *Rhinitis,* pharyngitis, dyspnea
- **Other:** *Fatigue,* back pain, infections

Interactions

✳ **Drug-drug** • Increased effectiveness of antidiabetics; monitor blood glucose and adjust dosages appropriately • Increased effectiveness of clonidine; monitor patient for potential severe bradycardia and hypotension • Increased serum levels of digoxin; monitor serum levels and adjust dosage accordingly • Increased plasma levels of carvedilol with rifampin • Potential for dangerous conduction system disturbances with verapamil or diltiazem; if this combination is used, closely monitor ECG and BP

✳ **Drug-food** • Slowed rate of absorption but not decreased effectiveness with food

■ Nursing considerations
Assessment

- **History:** Heart failure, bronchial asthma, heart block, cardiogenic shock, hypersensitivity to carvedilol, pregnancy, lactation, hepatic impairment, peripheral vascular disease, thyrotoxicosis, diabetes, anesthesia or major surgery
- **Physical:** Baseline weight, skin condition, neurologic status, P, BP, ECG, respiratory

---

Adverse effects in *italics* are most common; those in **bold** are life-threatening. ⊙⊞⊙ Do not crush.

status, LFTs, renal and thyroid function tests, blood and urine glucose

Interventions

⊗ **Warning** Do not discontinue drug abruptly after chronic therapy (hypersensitivity to catecholamines may have developed, causing exacerbation of angina, MI, and ventricular arrhythmias); taper drug gradually over 2 wk with monitoring.

- Consult with physician about withdrawing drug if patient is to undergo surgery (withdrawal is controversial).
- Give with food to decrease orthostatic hypotension and adverse effects.
- Ensure that patient swallows controlled-release capsules whole; do not cut, crush, or allow patient to chew capsules.
- Monitor for orthostatic hypotension and provide safety precautions.
- Monitor diabetic patient closely; drug may mask hypoglycemia or worsen hyperglycemia.

⊗ **Warning** Monitor patient for any sign of hepatic impairment (pruritus, dark urine or stools, anorexia, jaundice, pain); arrange for LFTs and discontinue drug if tests indicate liver injury. Do not restart carvedilol.

Teaching points

- Take drug with meals.
- Do not cut, crush, or chew controlled-release capsules; swallow capsules whole.
- Do not stop taking drug unless instructed to do so by a health care provider.
- Avoid use of over-the-counter medications.
- If you are diabetic, promptly report changes in glucose level.
- You may experience these side effects: Depression, dizziness, light-headedness (avoid driving or performing dangerous activities; getting up and changing positions slowly may help ease dizziness), decreased tears with contact lenses.
- Report difficulty breathing, swelling of extremities, changes in color of stool or urine, very slow heart rate, continued dizziness.

▽ **caspofungin acetate**

See Appendix R, *Less commonly used drugs*.

▽ **cefaclor**
(sef' a klor)

Apo-Cefaclor (CAN), Ceclor, Ceclor Pulvules, Cefaclor⊙⊙⊙, Raniclor

PREGNANCY CATEGORY B

Drug classes
Antibiotic
Cephalosporin (second generation)

Therapeutic actions
Bactericidal: Inhibits synthesis of bacterial cell wall, causing cell death.

Indications

- Lower respiratory infections caused by *Streptococcus pneumoniae, Haemophilus influenzae, Streptococcus pyogenes*
- URIs caused by *S. pyogenes*
- Dermatologic infections caused by *Staphylococcus aureus*
- UTIs caused by *Escherichia coli, Proteus mirabilis, Klebsiella,* coagulase-negative staphylococci
- Otitis media caused by *S. pneumoniae, H. influenzae, S. pyogenes,* staphylococci
- ER tablets: Acute exacerbations of chronic bronchitis, secondary infections of acute bronchitis, pharyngitis, and tonsillitis due to *S. pyogenes;* uncomplicated skin infections
- Unlabeled use: Acute uncomplicated UTI in select patients, single 2-g dose

Contraindications and cautions

- Contraindicated with allergy to cephalosporins or penicillins.
- Use cautiously with renal failure, lactation, pregnancy.

Available forms
Capsules—250, 500 mg; ER tablets⊙⊙⊙—375, 500 mg; powder for oral suspension—125 mg/5 mL, 187 mg/5 mL, 250 mg/5 mL, 375 mg/5 mL

Dosages
Adults
250 mg PO every 8 hr or 375–500 mg PO every 12 hr for 7–10 days; dosage may be doubled in severe cases. **Do not exceed 4 g/day.**

Pediatric patients

20 mg/kg per day PO in divided doses every 8 hr; in severe cases 40 mg/kg/day PO may be given. **Do not exceed 1 g/day.**

- *Otitis media and pharyngitis:* Total daily dosage may be divided and administered every 12 hr.

Pharmacokinetics

Route	Peak	Duration
Oral	30–60 min	8–10 hr

Metabolism: $T_{1/2}$: 30–60 min
Distribution: Crosses the placenta; enters breast milk
Excretion: Urine, unchanged

Adverse effects

- **CNS:** Headache, dizziness, lethargy, paresthesias
- **GI:** *Nausea, vomiting, diarrhea, anorexia, abdominal pain, flatulence,* **pseudomembranous colitis,** hepatotoxicity
- **GU:** Nephrotoxicity
- **Hematologic:** Bone marrow depression
- **Hypersensitivity:** *Ranging from rash to fever* to **anaphylaxis;** serum sickness reaction
- **Other:** *Superinfections*

Interactions

＊ **Drug-drug** ● Increased nephrotoxicity with aminoglycosides ● Increased bleeding effects with oral anticoagulants ● Decreased serum level of ER form if taken with antacids; separate by at least 2 hr

＊ **Drug-lab test** ● Possibility of false results on tests of urine glucose using Benedict solution, Fehling solution, Clinitest tablets; urinary 17-ketosteroids; direct Coombs test

■ Nursing considerations

Assessment

- **History:** Penicillin or cephalosporin allergy, pregnancy or lactation
- **Physical:** Renal function tests, respiratory status, skin status, culture and sensitivity tests of infected area

Interventions

- Culture infection site before drug therapy.
- Give drug with meals or food to decrease GI discomfort. Ensure that patient swallows ER

tablets whole; do not cut, crush, or allow patient to chew them.

- Refrigerate suspension after reconstitution, and discard after 14 days.
- Discontinue drug if hypersensitivity reaction occurs.
- Evaluate patient for *Clostridium difficile* infection if diarrhea occurs.
- Give patient yogurt or buttermilk in case of diarrhea.
- Arrange for oral vancomycin for serious colitis that fails to respond to discontinuation of drug.

Teaching points

- Take this drug with meals or food.
- Complete the full course of this drug, even if you feel better.
- Do not cut, crush, or chew ER form; swallow tablets whole.
- This drug is prescribed for this particular infection; do not self-treat any other infection.
- You may experience these side effects: Stomach upset, loss of appetite, nausea (take drug with food); diarrhea; headache, dizziness.
- Report severe diarrhea with blood, pus, or mucus; rash or hives; difficulty breathing; unusual tiredness or fatigue; unusual bleeding or bruising.

▷ **cefadroxil**

*(sef a **drox'** ill)*

Apo-Cefadroxil (CAN)

PREGNANCY CATEGORY B

Drug classes

Antibiotic
Cephalosporin (first generation)

Therapeutic actions

Bactericidal: Inhibits the formation of bacterial cell wall, causing the cell's death.

Indications

- UTIs caused by *Escherichia coli, Proteus mirabilis, Klebsiella* species
- Pharyngitis, tonsillitis caused by group A beta-hemolytic streptococci
- Skin and skin structure infections caused by staphylococci, streptococci

Contraindications and cautions

- Contraindicated with allergy to cephalosporins or penicillins.
- Use cautiously with renal failure, lactation, pregnancy.

Available forms

Capsules—500 mg; tablets—1,000 mg; powder for oral suspension—125 mg/5 mL, 250 mg/5 mL, 500 mg/5 mL

Dosages

Adults

- *UTIs:* 1–2 g/day PO in single dose or two divided doses for uncomplicated lower UTIs. For all other UTIs, 2 g/day in two divided doses.
- *Skin and skin-structure infections:* 1 g/day PO in single dose or two divided doses.
- *Pharyngitis, tonsillitis caused by group A beta-hemolytic streptococci:* 1 g/day PO in single dose or two divided doses for 10 days.

Pediatric patients

- *UTIs, dermatologic infections:* 30 mg/kg per day PO in divided doses every 12 hr.
- *Pharyngitis, tonsillitis caused by group A beta-hemolytic streptococci:* 30 mg/kg/day in single or two divided doses every 12 hr, continue for 10 days.

Geriatric patients or patients with impaired renal function

1 g PO loading dose, followed by 500 mg PO at these intervals:

CrCl (mL/min)	Interval (hr)
25–50	12
10–25	24
0–10	36

Pharmacokinetics

Route	Peak	Duration
Oral	1.5–2 hr	20–22 hr

Metabolism: $T_{1/2}$: 78–96 min
Distribution: Crosses the placenta; enters breast milk
Excretion: Urine

Adverse effects

- **CNS:** Headache, dizziness, lethargy, paresthesias
- **GI:** *Nausea, vomiting, diarrhea, anorexia, abdominal pain, flatulence,* **pseudomembranous colitis,** hepatotoxicity
- **GU:** Nephrotoxicity
- **Hematologic: Bone marrow depression**
- **Hypersensitivity:** Ranging from *rash* to *fever* to **anaphylaxis;** serum sickness reaction
- **Other:** *Superinfections*

Interactions

✳ **Drug-drug** • Decreased bactericidal activity if used with bacteriostatic agents • Increased serum levels of cephalosporins if used with probenecid • Increased nephrotoxicity with aminoglycosides

✳ **Drug-lab test** • False-positive urine glucose using Benedict solution, Fehling solution, Clinitest tablets • False-positive direct Coombs test • Falsely elevated urinary 17-ketosteroids

■ Nursing considerations

Assessment

- **History:** Penicillin or cephalosporin allergy, pregnancy or lactation, renal failure
- **Physical:** Renal function tests, respiratory status, skin status, culture and sensitivity tests of infected area

Interventions

- Culture infection site before drug therapy.
- Give drug with meals or food to decrease GI discomfort.
- Refrigerate suspension after reconstitution, and discard after 14 days; shake refrigerated suspension well before using.
- Discontinue if hypersensitivity reaction occurs.
- Evaluate patient for *Clostridium difficile* infection of diarrhea occurs.
- Give the patient yogurt or buttermilk in case of diarrhea.

⊗ *Warning* Arrange for oral vancomycin for serious colitis that fails to respond to discontinuation of drug.

Teaching points

- Take this drug only for this infection; do not use to treat other problems; complete the full course of therapy, even if you feel better.
- Refrigerate the suspension, and discard unused portion after 14 days; shake suspension well before each use.
- You may experience these side effects: Stomach upset, loss of appetite, nausea (take drug with food), diarrhea, headache, dizziness.

- Report severe diarrhea with blood, pus, or mucus; rash; difficulty breathing; unusual tiredness, fatigue; unusual bleeding or bruising.

▷**cefdinir**

(sef' din er)

Omnicef

PREGNANCY CATEGORY B

Drug classes

Antibiotic
Cephalosporin (third generation)

Therapeutic actions

Bactericidal: Inhibits synthesis of bacterial cell wall, causing cell death.

Indications

Adults and adolescents

- Community-acquired pneumonia caused by *Haemophilus influenzae, Haemophilus parainfluenzae, Streptococcus pneumoniae, Moraxella catarrhalis*
- Acute exacerbations of chronic bronchitis caused by *H. influenzae, H. parainfluenzae, S. pneumoniae, M. catarrhalis*
- Acute maxillary sinusitis caused by *H. influenzae, S. pneumoniae, M. catarrhalis*
- Pharyngitis and tonsillitis caused by *Streptococcus pyogenes*
- Uncomplicated skin and skin structure infections caused by *Staphylococcus aureus, S. pyogenes*

Pediatric patients

- Acute bacterial otitis media caused by *H. influenzae, S. pneumoniae, M. catarrhalis*
- Pharyngitis and tonsillitis caused by *S. pyogenes*
- Uncomplicated skin and skin-structure infections caused by *S. aureus, S. pyogenes*

Contraindications and cautions

- Contraindicated with allergy to cephalosporins or penicillins.
- Use cautiously with renal failure, lactation, pregnancy.

Available forms

Capsules—300 mg; oral suspension—125 mg/5 mL; 250 mg/5 mL

Dosages

Adults and adolescent patients

- *Community-acquired pneumonia, uncomplicated skin or skin-structure infections:* 300 mg PO every 12 hr for 10 days.
- *Acute exacerbation of chronic bronchitis, acute maxillary sinusitis, pharyngitis, or tonsillitis:* 300 mg every 12 hr PO for 5–10 days or 600 mg every 24 hr PO for 10 days.

Pediatric patients 6 mo–12 yr

- *Otitis media, acute maxillary sinusitis, pharyngitis, tonsillitis:* 7 mg/kg every 12 hr PO or 14 mg/kg every 24 hr PO for 5–10 days up to maximum dose of 600 mg/day.
- *Skin and skin-structure infections:* 7 mg/kg PO every 12 hr for 10 days.

Patients with renal impairment

For adults with creatinine clearance less than 30 mL/min, 300 mg PO daily. For patients on dialysis, 300 mg PO every other day; start with 300 mg PO at the end of dialysis and then every other day.

Pediatric patients with renal impairment

For creatinine clearance less than 30 mL/min, 7 mg/kg (up to 300 mg) once daily. On dialysis—7 mg/kg every other day; give a supplemental dose of 300 mg or 7 mg/kg at the end of each dialysis period.

Pharmacokinetics

Route	Peak	Duration
Oral	60 min	8–10 hr

Metabolism: $T_{1/2}$: 100 min
Distribution: Crosses the placenta, enters breast milk
Excretion: Urine, unchanged

Adverse effects

- **CNS:** Headache, dizziness, lethargy, paresthesias
- **GI:** *Nausea, vomiting, diarrhea, anorexia, abdominal pain, flatulence,* **pseudomembranous colitis,** hepatotoxicity
- **GU:** Nephrotoxicity
- **Hematologic:** Bone marrow depression
- **Hypersensitivity:** Ranging from *rash* to *fever* to **anaphylaxis;** serum sickness reaction
- **Other:** *Superinfections*

Adverse effects in *italics* are most common; those in **bold** are life-threatening. ⬛ Do not crush.

Interactions

❋ **Drug-drug** • Increased nephrotoxicity with aminoglycosides • Increased bleeding effects if taken with oral anticoagulants • Interferes with absorption of cefdinir if taken with antacids containing magnesium or aluminum or with iron supplements; separate by at least 2 hr

❋ **Drug-lab test** • Possibility of false results on tests of urine glucose using Benedict solution, Fehling solution, Clinitest tablets; urinary 17-ketosteroids; direct Coombs test

■ Nursing considerations

Assessment

- **History:** Penicillin or cephalosporin allergy; pregnancy or lactation, renal failure
- **Physical:** Renal function tests, respiratory status, skin status; culture and sensitivity tests of infected area

Interventions

- Arrange for culture and sensitivity tests of infected area before beginning drug therapy and during therapy if infection does not resolve.
- Reconstitute oral suspension by adding 38 mL water to the 60 mL bottle, 63 mL water to the 100 mL bottle; shake well before each use. Store at room temperature. Discard after 10 days.
- Give drug with meals; arrange for small, frequent meals if GI complications occur. Separate antacids or iron supplements by 2 hr from the cefdinir dose.
- Arrange for treatment of superinfections if they occur.
- Evaluate patient for *Clostridium difficile* infection if diarrhea occurs.

Teaching points

- Take this drug with meals or food. Store suspension at room temperature, shake well before each use; discard any drug after 10 days.
- Complete the full course of this drug, even if you feel better before the course of treatment is over.
- This drug is prescribed for this particular infection; do not self-treat any other infection with this drug.
- You may experience these side effects: Stomach upset, loss of appetite, nausea (taking the drug with food may help); diarrhea (stay near bathroom facilities); headache, dizziness.
- Report severe diarrhea with blood, pus, or mucus; rash or hives; difficulty breathing; unusual tiredness, fatigue; unusual bleeding or bruising.

▽ **cefditoren pivoxil**
(sef' di tore en)

Spectracef

PREGNANCY CATEGORY B

Drug classes
Antibiotic
Cephalosporin

Therapeutic actions

Bactericidal. Inhibits synthesis of susceptible gram-negative and gram-positive bacterial cell wall, causing cell death. Effective in the presence of beta-lactamases, including penicillinases and cephalosporinases.

Indications

- Acute exacerbations of chronic bronchitis caused by *Haemophilus influenzae, Haemophilus parainfluenzae, Streptococcus pneumoniae, Moraxella catarrhalis*
- Community-acquired pneumonia caused by *H. influenzae, H. parainfluenzae, S. pneumoniae, M. catarrhalis*
- Pharyngitis and tonsillitis caused by *Streptococcus pyogenes*
- Uncomplicated skin and skin-structure infections caused by *Staphylococcus aureus, S. pyogenes*

Contraindications and cautions

- Contraindicated with allergy to cephalosporins or penicillins, carnitine deficiencies, milk protein hypersensitivities, renal failure, lactation.
- Use cautiously with renal or hepatic impairment, pregnancy.

Available forms
Tablets—200, 400 mg

Dosages
Adults and patients older than 12 yr
- *Uncomplicated skin or skin-structure infections; pharyngitis or tonsillitis:* 200 mg PO bid for 10 days.

- *Acute exacerbation of chronic bronchitis, community-acquired pneumonia:* 400 mg PO bid for 10 days (chronic bronchitis) or 14 days (pneumonia).

Patients with renal impairment
For creatinine clearance 30–49 mL/min, 200 mg PO bid; creatinine clearance less than 30 mL/min, 200 mg PO daily.

Pharmacokinetics

Route	Peak	Duration
Oral	1.5–3 hr	8–10 hr

Metabolism: $T_{1/2}$: 100–115 min
Distribution: Crosses the placenta; enters breast milk
Excretion: Urine, primarily unchanged

Adverse effects

- **CNS:** Headache, dizziness, lethargy, paresthesias, nervousness
- **GI:** *Nausea, vomiting, diarrhea,* anorexia, *abdominal pain,* **pseudomembranous colitis, hepatotoxicity**
- **GU:** Nephrotoxicity, vaginitis, urinary frequency
- **Hematologic:** Bone marrow depression, carnitine deficiency with long-term use
- **Hypersensitivity:** Ranging from *rash* to *fever* to **anaphylaxis;** serum sickness reaction
- **Other:** *Superinfections*

Interactions

✳ **Drug-drug** • Increased bleeding effects if taken with oral anticoagulants • Interference with absorption of cefditoren if taken with antacids containing magnesium or aluminum or with histamine₂-receptor antagonists; separate by at least 2 hr if concomitant use is necessary

✳ **Drug-lab test** • Possibility of false results on tests of urine glucose using Benedict solution, Fehling solution, Clinitest tablets; urinary 17-ketosteroids; direct Coombs test

■ Nursing considerations
Assessment

- **History:** Penicillin or cephalosporin allergy, carnitine deficiency, milk protein hypersensitivity, renal or hepatic impairment, pregnancy, lactation
- **Physical:** Renal function tests, respiratory status, skin status, culture and sensitivity tests of infected area, GI function, orientation, affect

Interventions

- Arrange for culture and sensitivity tests of infected area before therapy and during therapy if infection does not resolve.
- Do not administer for longer than 10 days; risk of carnitine deficiency with prolonged use.
- ⊗ **Warning** Do not administer drug to patients with hypersensitivity to sodium caseinate or milk protein; this is not lactose intolerance.
- Give drug with meals; arrange for small, frequent meals if GI complications occur. Separate antacids or histamine₂-receptor antagonists by 2 hr from the cefditoren dose.
- Arrange for treatment of superinfections if they occur.
- Evaluate patient for *Clostridium difficile* infection if diarrhea occurs.

Teaching points

- Take this drug with meals or food.
- Complete the full course of this drug, even if you feel better before the course of treatment is over.
- This drug is prescribed for this particular infection; do not self-treat any other infection with this drug.
- Do not take this drug with antacids or histamine₂-receptor antagonists because they decrease absorption.
- You may experience these side effects: Stomach upset, loss of appetite, nausea (taking the drug with food may help); diarrhea (stay near bathroom facilities); headache, dizziness.
- Report severe diarrhea with blood, pus, or mucus; rash or hives; difficulty breathing; unusual tiredness, fatigue; unusual bleeding or bruising.

▽ **cefepime hydrochloride**
(sef' ah peem)

PREGNANCY CATEGORY B

Drug classes
Antibiotic
Cephalosporin (third generation)

Therapeutic actions
Bactericidal: Inhibits synthesis of bacterial cell wall, causing cell death.

CrCl (mL/min)	Recommended Maintenance Schedule			
More than 60 (Normal recommended schedule)	500 mg every 12 hr	1 g every 12 hr	2 g every 12 hr	2 g every 8 hr
30–60	500 mg every 24 hr	1 g every 24 hr	2 g every 24 hr	2 g every 12 hr
11–29	500 mg every 24 hr	500 mg every 24 hr	1 g every 24 hr	2 g every 24 hr
Less than 11	250 mg every 24 hr	250 mg every 24 hr	500 mg every 24 hr	1 g every 24 hr
CAPD	500 mg every 48 hr	1 g every 48 hr	2 g every 48 hr	2 g every 48 hr
Hemodialysis*	1 g on day 1, then 500 mg every 24 hr thereafter			1 g every 24 hr

*On hemodialysis days, cefepime should be administered following hemodialysis. Whenever possible, cefepime should be administered at the same time each day.

Indications
- UTIs caused by *Escherichia coli, Proteus mirabilis, Klebsiella* species, including *Klebsiella pneumoniae*
- Pneumonia caused by *Streptococcus pneumoniae, Pseudomonas aeruginosa, K. pneumoniae, Enterobacter*
- Uncomplicated skin and skin-structure infections caused by *Staphylococcus aureus* group or *Streptococcus pyogenes*
- Empiric therapy for febrile neutropenic patients
- Complicated intra-abdominal infections in combination with metronidazole
- Unlabeled use: catheter-related bloodstream infections

Contraindications and cautions
- Contraindicated with allergy to cephalosporins or penicillins.
- Use cautiously with renal failure, lactation, pregnancy.

Available forms
Powder for injection—500 mg; 1, 2 g

Dosages
Adults
0.5–2 g IV or IM every 8–12 hr.
- *Mild to moderate UTI:* 0.5–1 g IM or IV every 12 hr for 7–10 days.
- *Severe UTI:* 2 g IV every 12 hr for 10 days.
- *Moderate to severe pneumonia:* 1–2 g IV every 12 hr for 10 days.
- *Moderate to severe skin infections:* 2 g IV every 12 hr for 10 days.
- *Empiric therapy for febrile neutropenic patients:* 2 g IV every 8 hr for 7 days.
- *Complicated intra-abdominal infections:* 2 g IV every 12 hr for 7–10 days.

Pediatric patients older than 2 mo, weighing less than 40 kg
50 mg/kg IV or IM every 12 hr for 7–10 days depending on severity of infection. Consider IM route for mild to moderate infections when IM route is considered more appropriate. If treating febrile neutropenia, give every 8 hr (maximum dose, 2 g/day).

Geriatric patients or patients with impaired renal function
Use recommended adult starting dose and then maintenance dose as shown in the table above.

Pharmacokinetics

Route	Onset	Peak	Duration
IM	30 min	1.5–2 hr	10–12 hr
IV	Immediate	5 min	10–12 hr

Metabolism: $T_{1/2}$: 102–138 min
Distribution: Crosses placenta; enters breast milk
Excretion: Urine, unchanged

▼ IV FACTS
Preparation: Dilute with 50–100 mL 0.9% sodium chloride, 5% and 10% dextrose injection, M/6 sodium lactate injection, 5% dextrose and 0.9% sodium chloride injection, lactated Ringer and 5% dextrose injection, *Normosol-R, Normosol-M and D₅W* injection. Diluted solution is stable for 24 hr at room temperature or up to 7 days if refrigerated. Protect from light.
Infusion: Infuse slowly over 30 min.
Incompatibilities: Do not mix with ampicillin, metronidazole, vancomycin, gentamicin, tobramycin, or aminophylline. If concurrent therapy is needed, administer each drug separately. If possible, do not give any other drug in same solution as cefepime.

Adverse effects

- **CNS:** Headache, dizziness, lethargy, paresthesias, nonconvulsive status epilepticus (more common with renal impairment)
- **GI:** *Nausea, vomiting, diarrhea, anorexia, abdominal pain, flatulence,* **pseudomembranous colitis, hepatotoxicity**
- **GU:** Nephrotoxicity
- **Hematologic:** Bone marrow depression
- **Hypersensitivity:** Ranging from *rash* to *fever* to **anaphylaxis;** serum sickness reaction
- **Other:** *Superinfections, pain,* abscess (redness, tenderness, heat, tissue sloughing), inflammation at injection site, *phlebitis, disulfiram-like reaction with alcohol*

Interactions

✳ **Drug-drug** • Increased nephrotoxicity with aminoglycosides; monitor renal function tests • Increased bleeding effects with oral anticoagulants; reduced dosage may be needed • Increased toxicity if combined with alcohol; avoid this combination during and for 3 days after completing therapy

✳ **Drug-lab test** • False reports of urine glucose using Benedict solution, Fehling solution, Clinitest tablets; urinary 17-ketosteroids; direct Coombs test

■ Nursing considerations

Assessment

- **History:** Penicillin or cephalosporin allergy; pregnancy, lactation
- **Physical:** Renal function tests, respiratory status, skin status; culture and sensitivity tests of infection area, injection site

Interventions

- Culture infected area and arrange for sensitivity tests before beginning therapy.
- Reconstitute for IM use with 0.9% sodium chloride, 5% dextrose injection, 0.5% or 1% lidocaine HCl or bacteriostatic water with parabens or benzyl alcohol. Reserve IM use for mild to moderate UTIs due to *E. coli.*
- Adjust dose in patients with renal impairment because of increased risk of nonconvulsive status epilepticus. If this condition occurs, it may clear on its own or with hemodialysis.
- Have vitamin K available in case hypoprothrombinemia occurs.

- Evaluate patient for *Clostridium difficile* infection if diarrhea occurs.

Teaching points

- Do not drink alcohol while taking this drug and for 3 days after drug has been stopped; severe reactions may occur.
- You may experience these side effects: Stomach upset, loss of appetite, nausea (take drug with food); diarrhea (stay near bathroom); headache, dizziness.
- Report severe diarrhea, difficulty breathing, unusual tiredness or fatigue, pain at injection site.

▽ **cefotaxime sodium**
(sef oh **taks'** *eem)*

Claforan

PREGNANCY CATEGORY B

Drug classes

Antibiotic
Cephalosporin (third generation)

Therapeutic actions

Bactericidal: Inhibits synthesis of bacterial cell wall, causing cell death.

Indications

- Lower respiratory infections caused by *Streptococcus pneumoniae, Staphylococcus aureus, Klebsiella* species, *Haemophilus influenzae, Escherichia coli, Proteus mirabilis, Enterobacter* species, *Serratia marcescens, Streptococcus pyogenes,* indole-positive *Proteus* and *Pseudomonas* species
- UTIs caused by *Enterococcus* species, *S. epidermidis, S. aureus, Citrobacter* species, *Enterobacter* species, *E. coli, Klebsiella* species, *P. mirabilis, Proteus* species, *S. marcescens, Pseudomonas* species
- Gynecologic infections caused by *S. epidermidis, Enterococcus* species, *E. coli, P. mirabilis, Bacteroides* species, *Clostridium* species, *Peptococcus* species, *Peptostreptococcus* species, streptococci*;* and uncomplicated gonorrhea caused by *N. gonorrhoeae*
- Dermatologic infections caused by *S. aureus, E. coli, Serratia* species, *Proteus* species, *Klebsiella* species, *Enterobacter* species, *Pseudomonas, S. marcescens,*

Bacteroides species, *Peptococcus* species, *Peptostreptococcus* species, *P. mirabilis, S. epidermidis, S. pyogenes, Enterococcus* species

- Septicemia caused by *E. coli, Klebsiella* species, *S. marcescens*
- Peritonitis and intra-abdominal infections caused by *E. coli, Peptostreptococcus* species, *Bacteroides* species, *Peptococcus* species, *Klebsiella* species
- CNS infections caused by *E. coli, H. influenzae, Neisseria meningitidis, S. pneumoniae, K. pneumoniae*
- Bone and joint infections caused by *S. aureus, Streptococcus* species, *Pseudomonas* species, *P. mirabilis*
- Perioperative prophylaxis

Contraindications and cautions

- Contraindicated with allergy to cephalosporins or penicillins.
- Use cautiously with renal failure, lactation, pregnancy.

Available forms

Powder for injection—500 mg, 1, 2 g; injection—1, 2 g

Dosages
Adults

2–8 g/day IM or IV in equally divided doses every 6–8 hr. Do not exceed 12 g/day.
- *Gonorrhea:* 0.5–1 g IM in a single injection.
- *Disseminated infection:* 1–2 g IV every 8 hr.
- *Life-threatening infections:* 2 g IV every 4 hr, up to 12 g/day.
- *Perioperative prophylaxis:* 1 g IV or IM 30–90 min before surgery.
- *Cesarean section:* 1 g IV after cord is clamped and then 1 g IV or IM at 6 and 12 hr.

Pediatric patients 1 mo–12 yr weighing less than 50 kg

50–180 mg/kg/day IV or IM in four to six divided doses.

Pediatric patients 1–4 wk

50 mg/kg IV every 8 hr.

Pediatric patients 0–1 wk

50 mg/kg IV every 12 hr.

Geriatric patients or patients with reduced renal function

For creatinine clearance less than 20 mL/min, reduce dosage by half.

Pharmacokinetics

Route	Onset	Peak	Duration
IV	Immediate	5 min	18–24 hr
IM	5–10 min	30 min	18–24 hr

Metabolism: $T_{1/2}$: 1 hr
Distribution: Crosses the placenta; enters breast milk
Excretion: Urine

▼ IV FACTS

Preparation: Reconstitute for intermittent IV injection with 1 or 2 g with 10 mL sterile water for injection. Reconstitute vials for IV infusion with 10 mL of sterile water for injection. Reconstitute infusion bottles with 50 or 100 mL of 0.9% sodium chloride injection or 5% dextrose injection. Drug solution may be further diluted with 50–100 mL of 5% or 10% dextrose injection; 5% dextrose and 0.2%, 0.45%, or 0.9% sodium chloride injection; lactated Ringer solution; 0.9% sodium chloride injection; sodium lactate injection (M/6); 10% invert sugar. Reconstituted solution is stable for 24 hr at room temperature or 5 days if refrigerated. Powder and reconstituted solution darken with storage.

Infusion: Inject slowly into vein over 3–5 min or over a longer time through IV tubing; give intermittent IV infusions over 20–30 min. If administered with aminoglycosides, administer at different sites.

Incompatibilities: Do not mix in solutions with aminoglycoside solutions.

Y-site incompatibility: Hetastarch.

Adverse effects

- **CNS:** Headache, dizziness, lethargy, paresthesias
- **GI:** *Nausea, vomiting, diarrhea, anorexia, abdominal pain, flatulence,* **pseudomembranous colitis, hepatotoxicity**
- **GU:** Nephrotoxicity
- **Hematologic: Bone marrow depression**—decreased WBC count, decreased platelets, decreased Hct
- **Hypersensitivity:** *Ranging from rash* to *fever* to **anaphylaxis;** serum sickness reaction
- **Local:** *Pain,* abscess at injection site, *phlebitis,* inflammation at IV site
- **Other:** *Superinfections, disulfiram-like reaction with alcohol*

Interactions

❋ Drug-drug • Increased nephrotoxicity with aminoglycosides • Increased bleeding effects with oral anticoagulants • Risk of severe toxicity if combined with alcohol; avoid this combination during and for 3 days after completing therapy

❋ Drug-lab test • Possibility of false results on tests of urine glucose using Benedict solution, Fehling solution, Clinitest tablets; urinary 17-ketosteroids; direct Coombs test

■ Nursing considerations

Assessment

- **History:** Hepatic and renal impairment, lactation, pregnancy
- **Physical:** Skin status, LFTs, renal function tests, culture of affected area, sensitivity tests

Interventions

- Culture infection site, and arrange for sensitivity tests before and during therapy if expected response is not seen.
- Reconstitution of drug varies by size of package; see manufacturer's directions for details.
- Reconstitute drug for IM use with sterile water or bacteriostatic water for injection; divide doses of 2 g and administer at two different sites by deep IM injection.
- Discontinue if hypersensitivity reaction occurs.
- Evaluate patient for *Clostridium difficile* infection if diarrhea occurs.

Teaching points

- Avoid alcohol while taking this drug and for 3 days after because severe reactions often occur.
- You may experience these side effects: Stomach upset, diarrhea.
- Report severe diarrhea, difficulty breathing, unusual tiredness or fatigue, pain at injection site.

▽ cefoxitin sodium
(se ***fox'*** *i tin)*

PREGNANCY CATEGORY B

Drug classes

Antibiotic
Cephalosporin (second generation)

Therapeutic actions

Bactericidal: Inhibits synthesis of bacterial cell wall, causing cell death.

Indications

- Lower respiratory infections caused by *Streptococcus pneumoniae, Staphylococcus aureus,* streptococci, *Escherichia coli, Klebsiella, Haemophilus influenzae, Bacteroides*
- Skin and skin structure infections caused by *S. aureus, Staphylococcus epidermidis,* streptococci, *E. coli, Proteus mirabilis, Klebsiella, Bacteroides, Clostridium, Peptococcus, Peptostreptococcus*
- UTIs caused by *E. coli, P. mirabilis, Klebsiella, Morganella morganii, Proteus rettgeri, Proteus vulgaris, Providencia*
- Uncomplicated gonorrhea caused by *Neisseria gonorrhoeae*
- Intra-abdominal infections caused by *E. coli, Klebsiella, Bacteroides, Clostridium*
- Gynecologic infections caused by *E. coli, N. gonorrhoeae, Bacteroides, Clostridium, Peptococcus, Peptostreptococcus,* group B streptococci
- Septicemia caused by *S. pneumoniae, S. aureus, E. coli, Klebsiella, Bacteroides*
- Bone and joint infections caused by *S. aureus*
- Perioperative prophylaxis

Contraindications and cautions

- Contraindicated with allergy to cephalosporins or penicillins.
- Use cautiously with renal failure, lactation, pregnancy.

Available forms

Powder for injection—1, 2 g; injection— 1 g/50 mL, 2 g/50 mL in D$_5$W

Dosages

Adults

1–2 g IM or IV every 6–8 hr, depending on the severity of the infection.

- *Uncomplicated gonorrhea:* 2 g IM with 1 g oral probenecid.
- *Uncomplicated lower respiratory infections, UTIs, skin infections:* 1 g every 6–8 hr IV.
- *Moderate to severe infections:* 1 g every 4 hr IV to 2 g every 6–8 hr IV.
- *Severe infections:* 2 g every 4 hr IV or 3 g every 6 hr IV.

- *Perioperative prophylaxis:* 2 g IV or IM 30–60 min prior to initial incision and every 6 hr for 24 hr after surgery.
- *Cesarean section:* 2 g IV as soon as the umbilical cord is clamped, followed by 2 g IM or IV at 4 and 8 hr, then every 6 hr for up to 24 hr.
- *Transurethral prostatectomy:* 1 g prior to surgery and then 1 g every 8 hr for up to 5 days.

Pediatric patients 3 mo or older
80–160 mg/kg/day IM or IV in divided doses every 4–6 hr. Do not exceed 12 g/day.

- *Prophylactic use:* 30–40 mg/kg per dose IV or IM every 6 hr.

Geriatric patients or patients with impaired renal function
IV loading dose of 1–2 g. If patient is on hemodialysis, give loading dose after session. Maintenance dosages are as follows:

CrCl (mL/min)	Maintenance Dosage
30–50	1–2 g every 8–12 hr
10–29	1–2 g every 12–24 hr
5–9	0.5–1 g every 12–24 hr
Less than 5	0.5–1 g every 24–48 hr

Pharmacokinetics

Route	Onset	Peak	Duration
IV	Immediate	5 min	6–8 hr
IM	5–10 min	20–30 min	6–8 hr

Metabolism: $T_{1/2}$: 45–60 min
Distribution: Crosses the placenta; enters breast milk
Excretion: Urine

▼ **IV FACTS**

Preparation: For IV intermittent administration, reconstitute 1 or 2 g with 10–20 mL sterile water for injection. For continuous IV infusion, add reconstituted solution to 5% dextrose injection, 0.9% sodium chloride injection, 5% dextrose and 0.9% sodium chloride injection, or 5% dextrose injection with 0.02% sodium bicarbonate solution. Store dry powder in cool, dry area. Powder and reconstituted solution darken with storage. Infusion bottles stable for 24 hr at room temperature; reconstituted vials stable for 6 hr at room temperature.
Infusion: For intermittent administration, slowly inject over 3–5 min, or give over longer time through IV tubing; discontinue other so-

lutions temporarily. If given with aminoglycosides, give each at a different site.
Incompatibilities: Do not mix aminoglycosides and cefoxitin in the same IV solution.
Y-site incompatibility: Hetastarch.

Adverse effects

- **CNS:** Headache, dizziness, lethargy, paresthesias
- **GI:** *Nausea, vomiting, diarrhea, anorexia, abdominal pain, flatulence,* **pseudomembranous colitis, hepatotoxicity**
- **GU:** Nephrotoxicity
- **Hematologic: Bone marrow depression**—decreased WBC count, decreased platelets, decreased Hct
- **Hypersensitivity:** Ranging from *rash* to *fever* to **anaphylaxis,** serum sickness reaction
- **Local:** *Pain,* abscess at injection site, *phlebitis,* inflammation at IV site
- **Other:** *Superinfections, disulfiram-like reaction with alcohol*

Interactions

✳ **Drug-drug** • Increased nephrotoxicity with aminoglycosides • Increased bleeding effects with oral anticoagulants • Disulfiram-like reaction may occur if alcohol is taken during or within 72 hr after cefoxitin administration

✳ **Drug-lab test** • Possibility of false results on tests of urine glucose using Benedict solution, Fehling solution, Clinitest tablets; urinary 17-ketosteroids; direct Coombs test

■ Nursing considerations
Assessment

- **History:** Hepatic and renal impairment, lactation, pregnancy
- **Physical:** Skin status, LFTs, renal function tests, culture of affected area, sensitivity tests

Interventions

- Culture infection site, and arrange for sensitivity tests before and during therapy if expected response is not seen.
- Reconstitute each gram for IM use with 2 mL sterile water for injection or with 2 mL of 0.5% lidocaine HCl solution (without epinephrine) to decrease pain at injection site. Inject deeply into large muscle group.
- Dry powder and reconstituted solutions darken slightly at room temperature.

- Have vitamin K available in case hypoprothrombinemia occurs.
- Discontinue if hypersensitivity reaction occurs.
- Evaluate patient for *Clostridium difficile* infection if diarrhea occurs.

Teaching points
- Avoid alcohol while taking this drug and for 3 days after because severe reactions often occur.
- You may experience these side effects: Stomach upset, diarrhea.
- Report severe diarrhea, difficulty breathing, unusual tiredness or fatigue, pain at injection site.

▽cefpodoxime proxetil
(sef poe docks' eem)

Vantin

PREGNANCY CATEGORY B

Drug classes
Antibiotic
Cephalosporin (third generation)

Therapeutic actions
Bactericidal: Inhibits synthesis of bacterial cell wall, causing cell death.

Indications
- Lower respiratory infections, including community-acquired pneumonia, caused by *Streptococcus pneumoniae, Haemophilus influenzae*
- URIs, including acute maxillary sinusitis, caused by *Streptococcus pyogenes, H. influenzae, Moraxella catarrhalis*
- Uncomplicated skin and skin structure infections caused by *Staphylococcus aureus, S. pyogenes*
- UTIs caused by *Escherichia coli, Proteus mirabilis, Klebsiella, Staphylococcus saprophyticus*
- Otitis media caused by *S. pneumoniae, H. influenzae, M. catarrhalis*
- STD caused by *Neisseria gonorrhoeae*

Contraindications and cautions
- Contraindicated with allergy to cephalosporins or penicillins.
- Use cautiously with renal failure, lactation, pregnancy.

Available forms
Tablets—100, 200 mg; oral suspension—50 mg/5 mL, 100 mg/5mL

Dosages
Adults
100–400 mg every 12 hr PO depending on severity of infection; continue for 5–14 days.
Pediatric patients
5 mg/kg per dose PO every 12 hr; do not exceed 100–200 mg per dose; continue for 10 days.
- *Acute otitis media:* 10 mg/kg/day PO divided every 12 hr; do not exceed 400 mg/day; continue for 5 days.
Geriatric patients or patients with renal impairment
For creatinine clearance less than 30 mL/min, increase dosing interval to every 24 hr. For patient on hemodialysis, give dose three times weekly after session.

Pharmacokinetics

Route	Peak	Duration
Oral	30–60 min	16–18 hr

Metabolism: $T_{1/2}$: 120–180 min
Distribution: Crosses the placenta; enters breast milk
Excretion: Renal, unchanged

Adverse effects
- **CNS:** Headache, dizziness, lethargy, paresthesias
- **GI:** *Nausea, vomiting, diarrhea, anorexia, abdominal pain, flatulence,* **pseudomembranous colitis, hepatotoxicity**
- **GU:** Nephrotoxicity
- **Hematologic: Bone marrow depression**
- **Hypersensitivity:** *Ranging from rash to fever to* **anaphylaxis;** serum sickness reaction
- **Other:** *Superinfections*

Interactions
✳ **Drug-drug** • Increased nephrotoxicity with aminoglycosides • Increased bleeding effects with oral anticoagulants
✳ **Drug-food** • Increased absorption and increased effects of cefpodoxime if taken with food
✳ **Drug-lab test** • Possibility of false results on tests of urine glucose using Benedict

solution, Fehling solution, Clinitest tablets; urinary 17-ketosteroids; direct Coombs test

■ **Nursing considerations**
Assessment
- **History:** Penicillin or cephalosporin allergy, pregnancy or lactation, renal failure
- **Physical:** Renal function tests, respiratory status, skin status; culture and sensitivity tests of infected area

Interventions
- Culture infection site before drug therapy.
- Give drug with meals or food to enhance absorption.
- Store solution in refrigerator. Shake well before using; use within 14 days, then discard.
- Discontinue drug if hypersensitivity reaction occurs.
- Evaluate patient for *Clostridium difficile* infection if diarrhea occurs.
- Give the patient yogurt or buttermilk in case of diarrhea.
- Arrange for oral vancomycin for serious colitis that fails to respond to discontinuation.

Teaching points
- Take this drug with food.
- Complete the full course of this drug even if you feel better.
- If using suspension, store in refrigerator and shake well before each use. Discard after 14 days.
- This drug is prescribed for this particular infection; do not self-treat any other infection.
- You may experience these side effects: Stomach upset, loss of appetite, nausea (take drug with food); diarrhea; headache, dizziness.
- Report severe diarrhea with blood, pus, or mucus; rash or hives; difficulty breathing; unusual tiredness, fatigue; unusual bleeding or bruising.

▽ **cefprozil**
(sef pro' zil)

PREGNANCY CATEGORY B

Drug classes
Antibiotic
Cephalosporin (second generation)

Therapeutic actions
Bactericidal: Inhibits synthesis of bacterial cell wall, causing cell death.

Indications
- Pharyngitis or tonsillitis caused by *Streptococcus pyogenes*
- Secondary bacterial infection of acute bronchitis and exacerbation of chronic bronchitis caused by *Streptococcus pneumoniae, Haemophilus influenzae, Moraxella catarrhalis*
- Dermatologic infections caused by *Staphylococcus aureus, S. pyogenes*
- Otitis media caused by *S. pneumoniae, H. influenzae, M. catarrhalis*
- Acute sinusitis caused by *S. pneumoniae, S. aureus, H. influenzae, M. catarrhalis*

Contraindications and cautions
- Contraindicated with allergy to cephalosporins or penicillins.
- Use cautiously with renal failure, lactation, pregnancy.

Available forms
Tablets—250, 500 mg; powder for suspension—125 mg/5 mL, 250 mg/5 mL

Dosages
Adults
250–500 mg PO every 12–24 hr. Continue treatment for 10 days.
Pediatric patients
Acute sinusitis, otitis media
- *6 mo–12 yr:* 7.5–15 mg/kg PO every 12 hr for 10 days.
Pharyngitis, tonsillitis
- *2–12 yr:* 7.5 mg/kg PO every 12 hr; continue treatment for 10 days.
Skin and skin structure infection
- *2–12 yr:* 20 mg/kg PO once daily; continue treatment for 10 days.
Geriatric patients or patients with renal impairment
For creatinine clearance of 30–120 mL/min, use standard dose; for creatinine clearance of 0–29 mL/min, use 50% of standard dose; if patient is on hemodialysis, give dose after dialysis period.

Pharmacokinetics

Route	Peak	Duration
Oral	6–10 hr	24–28 hr

Metabolism: $T_{1/2}$: 78 min
Distribution: Crosses the placenta, enters breast milk
Excretion: Urine, unchanged

Adverse effects

- **CNS:** Headache, dizziness, lethargy, paresthesias
- **GI:** *Nausea, vomiting, diarrhea, anorexia, abdominal pain, flatulence,* **pseudomembranous colitis, hepatotoxicity**
- **GU:** Nephrotoxicity
- **Hematologic: Bone marrow depression**
- **Hypersensitivity:** Ranging from *rash* to *fever* to **anaphylaxis;** serum sickness reaction
- **Other:** *Superinfections*

Interactions

✳ **Drug-drug** • Increased nephrotoxicity with aminoglycosides • Increased bleeding effects if taken with oral anticoagulants

✳ **Drug-lab test** • Possibility of false results on tests of urine glucose using Benedict solution, Fehling solution, Clinitest tablets; urinary 17-ketosteroids; direct Coombs test

■ Nursing considerations
Assessment

- **History:** Penicillin or cephalosporin allergy, pregnancy or lactation, renal failure
- **Physical:** Renal function tests, respiratory status, skin status, culture and sensitivity tests of infected area

Interventions

- Culture infection site before drug therapy.
- Give drug with food to decrease GI discomfort.
- Refrigerate suspension after reconstitution, and discard after 14 days.
- Discontinue if hypersensitivity reaction occurs.
- Evaluate patient for *Clostridium difficile* infection if diarrhea occurs.
- Give the patient yogurt or buttermilk in case of diarrhea.
- Arrange for oral vancomycin or metronidazole for serious colitis that fails to respond to discontinuation.

Teaching points

- Take this drug with food.
- Complete the full course of this drug, even if you feel better.
- This drug is prescribed for this particular infection; do not use it to self-treat any other infection.
- You may experience these side effects: Stomach upset, loss of appetite, nausea (take drug with food); diarrhea; headache, dizziness.
- Report severe diarrhea with blood, pus, or mucus; rash or hives; difficulty breathing; unusual tiredness, fatigue; unusual bleeding or bruising.

▷ **ceftaroline fosamil**
*(sef **tar'** oh leen)*

Teflaro

PREGNANCY CATEGORY B

Drug class
Cephalosporin

Therapeutic actions
Bactericidal; inhibits synthesis of bacterial cell wall, causing cell death.

Indications

- Treatment of acute bacterial skin and skin-structure infections caused by susceptible bacteria: *Staphylococcus aureus* (including methicillin-susceptible and methicillin-resistant strains), *Streptococcus pyogenes, Streptococcus agalactiae, Escherichia coli, Klebsiella pneumoniae, Klebsiella oxytoca*
- Treatment of community-acquired bacterial pneumonia caused by susceptible bacteria: *Streptococcus pneumoniae, S. aureus* (methicillin-susceptible only), *Haemophilus influenzae, K. pneumoniae, K. oxytoca, E. coli*

Contraindications and cautions

- Contraindicated with history of serious hypersensitivity reactions to cephalosporins.
- Use cautiously with renal dysfunction, pregnancy, lactation.

Available forms
Powder for injection—400, 600 mg/vial

Dosages

Adults

600 mg every 12 hr by IV infusion over 1 hr for 5–14 days (skin and skin-structure infections) or 5–7 days (community-acquired pneumonia).

Pediatric patients

Safety and efficacy not established.

Patients with renal impairment

For creatinine clearance of more than 30 and up to 50 mL/min, 400 mg IV over 1 hr every 12 hr; if clearance is more than 15 and up to 30 mL/min, 300 mg IV over 1 hr every 12 hr; for end-stage renal disease and patients on hemodialysis, 200 mg IV over 1 hr every 12 hr. (Administer after dialysis on dialysis days.)

Pharmacokinetics

Route	Onset	Peak
IV	Rapid	1 hr

Metabolism: Hepatic; $T_{1/2}$: 1.6 hr
Distribution: May cross placenta; may enter breast milk
Excretion: Urine

▼ **IV FACTS**

Preparation: Reconstitute vial with 20 mL sterile water for injection; mix gently to ensure that contents have dissolved. Further dilute with at least 250 mL of 0.9% sodium chloride injection, 5% dextrose injection, 2.5% dextrose injection, 0.45% sodium chloride injection, or lactated Ringer injection. Solution should be clear with no particulates and light to dark yellow. Use within 6 hr of reconstitution if stored at room temperature, within 24 hr if refrigerated.

Administration: Infuse slowly over 1 hr.

Incompatibilities: Do not mix in solution with other drugs or add to solutions containing other drugs.

Adverse effects

- **CNS:** Dizziness
- **CV:** Bradycardia, palpitations
- **GI:** Nausea, diarrhea, vomiting, constipation, abdominal pain, *Clostridium difficile* diarrhea
- **Hematological:** Hemolytic anemia
- **Renal: Renal failure**
- **Other:** Urticaria, hyperglycemia, hyperkalemia, injection-site reactions, fever, rash, **hypersensitivity reactions**

■ Nursing considerations

Assessment

- **History:** Hypersensitivity to components of ceftaroline or to other cephalosporins, renal dysfunction, pregnancy, lactation
- **Physical:** T, P, GI exam, skin status, renal function tests, culture of affected area, sensitivity tests

Interventions

- Culture infected site and arrange for sensitivity tests before beginning therapy and during therapy if results are not as expected.
- Monitor injection site for possible reactions.
- Monitor blood counts before and periodically during therapy; if anemia occurs, obtain work-up for potential hemolytic anemia.
- Monitor patient for *C. difficile* diarrhea if diarrhea occurs.
- Encourage small, frequent meals and comfort measures if GI upset is severe.

Teaching points

- This drug is specific to your infection. It must be given by IV infusion over 1 hour each day.
- You may experience GI upset, diarrhea, or nausea; small frequent meals may help. Notify your health care provider if these symptoms become severe.
- It is not known how this drug affects a fetus. If you are pregnant or thinking about becoming pregnant, discuss this with your health care provider.
- It is not known if this drug enters breast milk or how this could affect a breast-feeding infant; if you are breast-feeding, discuss this with your health care provider.
- Report severe or persistent diarrhea, pain at the injection site, difficulty breathing, rash.

▽ **ceftazidime**

(sef taz' i deem)

Ceptaz, Fortaz, Tazicef, Tazidime

PREGNANCY CATEGORY B

Drug classes

Antibiotic
Cephalosporin (third generation)

Therapeutic actions
Bactericidal: Inhibits synthesis of bacterial cell wall, causing cell death.

Indications
- Lower respiratory infections caused by *Pseudomonas aeruginosa*, other *Pseudomonas, Streptococcus pneumoniae, Staphylococcus aureus, Klebsiella, Haemophilus influenzae, Proteus mirabilis, Escherichia coli, Enterobacter, Serratia, Citrobacter*
- UTIs caused by *P. aeruginosa, Enterobacter, E. coli, Klebsiella, P. mirabilis, Proteus*
- Gynecologic infections caused by *E. coli*
- Skin and skin structure infections caused by *P. aeruginosa, S. aureus, E. coli, Serratia, Proteus, Klebsiella, Enterobacter, Streptococcus pyogenes*
- Septicemia caused by *P. aeruginosa, E. coli, Klebsiella, H. influenzae, Serratia, S. pneumoniae, S. aureus*
- Intra-abdominal infections caused by *E. coli, S. aureus, Bacteroides, Klebsiella*
- CNS infections caused by *H. influenzae, Neisseria meningitidis*
- Bone and joint infections caused by *P. aeruginosa, Klebsiella, Enterobacter, S. aureus*
- Unlabeled use: Catheter-related bloodstream infections in children and adolescents

Contraindications and cautions
- Contraindicated with allergy to cephalosporins or penicillins.
- Use cautiously with renal failure, lactation, pregnancy.

Available forms
Powder for injection—500 mg, 1, 2 g; injection—1, 2 g

Dosages
Adults
Usual dose, 1 g (range 250 mg–2 g) every 8–12 hr IM or IV. Do not exceed 6 g/day. Dosage will vary with infection.
- *UTI:* 250–500 mg IV or IM every 8–12 hr.
- *Pneumonia, skin and skin structure infections:* 500 mg–1 g IV or IM every 8 hr.
- *Bone and joint infections:* 2 g IV every 12 hr.
- *Gynecologic, intra-abdominal, life-threatening infections, meningitis:* 2 g IV every 8 hr.

Pediatric patients 1 mo–12 yr
30–50 mg/kg IV every 8 hr. Do not exceed 6 g/day.
Pediatric patients 0–4 wk
30 mg/kg IV every 12 hr.
Geriatric patients or patients with reduced renal function
Loading dose of 1 g IV, followed by:

CrCl (mL/min)	Dosage
31–50	1 g every 12 hr
16–30	1 g every 24 hr
6–15	500 mg every 24 hr
5 or less	500 mg every 48 hr

Pharmacokinetics

Route	Onset	Peak	Duration
IV	Rapid	1 hr	24–28 hr
IM	30 min	1 hr	24–28 hr

Metabolism: $T_{1/2}$: 114–120 min
Distribution: Crosses the placenta; enters breast milk
Excretion: Urine

▼ IV FACTS

Preparation: Reconstitute drug for direct IV injection with sterile water for injection. Reconstituted solution is stable for 24 hr at room temperature for *Fortaz* and *Tazidime*, or 18 hr at room temperature for *Ceptaz* and *Tazicef* or 7 days if refrigerated. For 500-mg vial, mix with 5 mL diluent; resulting concentration, 11 mg/mL. For 1-g vial, mix with 5 (10) mL diluent; resulting concentration, 180 (100) mg/mL. For 2-g vial, mix with 10 mL diluent; resulting concentration, 170–180 mg/mL.

Infusion: For IV, reconstitute 1- or 2-g infusion pack with 100 mL sterile water for injection; infuse slowly. For direct injection, slowly over 3–5 min. For infusion, over 30 min. If patient is also receiving aminoglycosides, administer at separate sites.

Incompatibilities: Do not mix with sodium bicarbonate injection or aminoglycoside solutions.

Adverse effects
- **CNS:** Headache, dizziness, lethargy, paresthesias
- **GI:** *Nausea, vomiting, diarrhea, anorexia, abdominal pain, flatulence,* **pseudomembranous colitis, hepatotoxicity**

Adverse effects in *italics* are most common; those in **bold** are life-threatening. ▣ Do not crush.

- **GU:** Nephrotoxicity
- **Hematologic: Bone marrow depression**—decreased WBC count, decreased platelets, decreased Hct
- **Hypersensitivity:** Ranging from *rash* to *fever* to **anaphylaxis; serum sickness reaction**
- **Local:** *Pain,* abscess at injection site; *phlebitis,* inflammation at IV site
- **Other:** *Superinfections, disulfiram-like reaction with alcohol*

Interactions

✳ **Drug-drug** • Increased nephrotoxicity with aminoglycosides • Increased bleeding effects with oral anticoagulants • Disulfiram-like reaction if combined with alcohol during or for 3 days after completion of therapy

✳ **Drug-lab test** • Possibility of false results on tests of urine glucose using Benedict solution, Fehling solution, Clinitest tablets; urinary 17-ketosteroids; direct Coombs test

■ Nursing considerations
Assessment
- **History:** Hepatic and renal impairment, lactation, pregnancy
- **Physical:** Skin status, LFTs, renal function tests, culture of affected area, sensitivity tests

Interventions
- Culture infection site, and arrange for sensitivity tests before and during therapy if expected response is not seen.
- Reconstitute drug for IM use with sterile water or bacteriostatic water for injection or with 0.5% or 1% lidocaine HCl injection to reduce pain; inject deeply into large muscle group.
- ⊗ **Warning** Do not mix with aminoglycoside solutions. Administer these drugs separately.
- Powder and reconstituted solution darken with storage.
- Have vitamin K available in case hypoprothrombinemia occurs.
- Discontinue if hypersensitivity reaction occurs.
- Evaluate patient for *Clostridium difficile* infection if diarrhea occurs.

Teaching points
- Avoid alcohol while taking this drug and for 3 days after because severe reactions often occur.
- You may experience these side effects: Stomach upset or diarrhea.

- Report severe diarrhea, difficulty breathing, unusual tiredness or fatigue, pain at injection site.

▷ **ceftibuten**
*(sef ta **byoo' ten**)*
Cedax

PREGNANCY CATEGORY B

Drug classes
Antibiotic
Cephalosporin (third generation)

Therapeutic actions
Bactericidal: Inhibits synthesis of bacterial cell wall, causing cell death.

Indications
- Acute bacterial exacerbations of chronic bronchitis due to *Haemophilus influenzae, Moraxella catarrhalis, Streptococcus pneumoniae*
- Acute bacterial otitis media due to *H. influenzae, M. catarrhalis, Streptococcus pyogenes*
- Pharyngitis and tonsillitis due to *S. pyogenes*

Contraindications and cautions
- Contraindicated with allergy to cephalosporins or penicillins.
- Use cautiously with renal failure; lactation, pregnancy.

Available forms
Capsules—400 mg; oral suspension—90 mg/5 mL, 180 mg/5 mL

Dosages
Adults
400 mg PO daily for 10 days.
Pediatric patients
9 mg/kg/day PO for 10 days to a maximum daily dose of 400 mg/day.
Patients with renal impairment

CrCl (mL/min)	Dose
More than 50	9 mg/kg or 400 mg PO every 24 hr
30–49	4.5 mg/kg or 200 mg PO every 24 hr
5–29	2.25 mg/kg or 100 mg PO every 24 hr

Pharmacokinetics

Route	Peak	Duration
Oral	30–60 min	8–10 hr

Metabolism: $T_{1/2}$: 30–60 min
Distribution: Crosses placenta; enters breast milk
Excretion: Urine, unchanged

Adverse effects

- **CNS:** Headache, dizziness, lethargy, paresthesias
- **GI:** *Nausea, vomiting, diarrhea, anorexia, abdominal pain, flatulence,* **pseudomembranous colitis, hepatotoxicity**
- **GU:** Nephrotoxicity
- **Hematologic: Bone marrow depression**
- **Hypersensitivity:** Ranging from *rash* to *fever* to **anaphylaxis;** serum sickness reaction
- **Other:** *Superinfections*

Interactions

✴ **Drug-drug** • Increased nephrotoxicity with aminoglycosides • Increased bleeding effects with oral anticoagulants • Disulfiram-like reaction may occur if alcohol is taken within 72 hr after administration

✴ **Drug-lab test** • Possibility of false results on tests of urine glucose using Benedict solution, Fehling, Clinitest tablets; urinary 17-ketosteroids; direct Coombs test

■ Nursing considerations
Assessment

- **History:** Allergy to penicillin or cephalosporin; pregnancy, lactation, renal failure
- **Physical:** Renal function tests, respiratory status, skin status; culture and sensitivity tests of infection

Interventions

- Culture infection site before beginning drug therapy.
- Give capsules with meals to decrease GI discomfort; suspension must be given on an empty stomach at least 2 hr before or 1 hr after meals.
- Refrigerate suspension after reconstitution; shake vigorously before use and discard after 14 days.
- Discontinue drug if hypersensitivity reaction occurs.
- Evaluate patient for *Clostridium difficile* infection if diarrhea occurs.
- Give patient yogurt or buttermilk in case of diarrhea.
- Arrange for treatment of superinfections.
- Reculture infection if patient fails to respond.

Teaching points

- Take capsules with meals or food; suspension must be taken on an empty stomach, at least 2 hours before or 1 hour after meals.
- Refrigerate suspension; shake vigorously after use and discard after 14 days.
- Complete the full course of this drug, even if you feel better before the course of treatment is over.
- Avoid alcohol while taking this drug and for 3 days after completion of therapy; serious reactions can occur.
- This drug is prescribed for this particular infection; do not use it to self-treat any other infection.
- You may experience these side effects: Stomach upset, loss of appetite, nausea (take drug with food); diarrhea (yogurt and buttermilk are often helpful if this is a problem); headache, dizziness.
- Report severe diarrhea with blood, pus, or mucus; rash or hives; difficulty breathing; unusual tiredness, fatigue; unusual bleeding or bruising.

▷ **ceftriaxone sodium**
(sef try ax' ohn)

Rocephin

PREGNANCY CATEGORY B

Drug classes
Antibiotic
Cephalosporin (third generation)

Therapeutic actions
Bactericidal: Inhibits synthesis of bacterial cell wall, causing cell death.

Indications

- Lower respiratory infections caused by *Streptococcus pneumoniae, Staphylococcus aureus, Klebsiella, Haemophilus influenzae, Escherichia coli, Proteus mirabilis, Enterobacter aerogenes,*

Serratia marcescens, Haemophilus para-influenzae, Streptococcus (excluding enterococci)

- Acute bacterial otitis media caused by *S. pneumoniae, H. influenzae, Moraxella catarrhalis*
- UTIs caused by *E. coli, Klebsiella, Proteus vulgaris, Proteus mirabilis, Morganella morganii*
- Gonorrhea caused by *Neisseria gonorrhoeae*
- Intra-abdominal infections caused by *E. coli, Klebsiella pneumoniae*
- PID caused by *N. gonorrhoeae*
- Skin and skin structure infections caused by *S. aureus, Klebsiella, Enterobacter cloacae, P. mirabilis, Staphylococcus epidermidis, Pseudomona aeruginosa, Streptococcus* (excluding enterococci)
- Septicemia caused by *E. coli, S. pneumoniae, H. influenzae, S. aureus, K. pneumoniae*
- Bone and joint infections caused by *S. aureus, Streptococcus* (excluding enterococci), *P. mirabilis, S. pneumoniae, E. coli, K. pneumoniae, Enterobacter*
- Meningitis caused by *H. influenzae, S. pneumoniae, Neisseria meningitidis*
- Perioperative prophylaxis for patients undergoing coronary artery bypass surgery and in contaminated or potentially contaminated surgical procedures (eg, vaginal or abdominal hysterectomy)
- Unlabeled uses: Treatment of Lyme disease in doses of 2 g IV daily for 14–28 days, epididymitis, proctitis, proctocolitis, enteritis, gonococcal meningitis, endocarditis

Contraindications and cautions

- Contraindicated with allergy to cephalosporins or penicillins.
- Use cautiously with renal failure, lactation, pregnancy.

Available forms

Powder for injection—250 mg, 500 mg, 1 g, 2 g; injection—1, 2 g

Dosages
Adults

1–2 g/day IM or IV once a day or in equal divided doses bid. Do not exceed 4 g/day.
- *Gonorrhea:* Single 250-mg IM dose.

- *Meningitis:* 1–2 g IM or IV once a day or in equal divided doses bid for 4–14 days. Longer therapy may be required. Do not exceed 4 g/day.
- *Perioperative prophylaxis:* Give 1 g IV 30–120 min before surgery.

Pediatric patients

50–75 mg/kg/day IV or IM in divided doses every 12 hr. Do not exceed 2 g/day.
- *Meningitis:* 100 mg/kg/day IV or IM in divided doses every 12 hr for 7–14 days. Do not exceed 4 g/day. Loading dose of 100 mg/kg may be used.

Pharmacokinetics

Route	Onset	Peak	Duration
IV	Rapid	Immediate	15–18 hr
IM	30 min	1.5–4 hr	15–18 hr

Metabolism: $T_{1/2}$: 5–10 hr
Distribution: Crosses the placenta; enters breast milk
Excretion: Bile, urine

▼ IV FACTS

Preparation: Dilute reconstituted solution for IV infusion with 50–100 mL of 5% or 10% dextrose injection, 5% dextrose and 0.45% or 0.9% sodium chloride injection, 0.9% sodium chloride injection, 10% invert sugar, 5% sodium bicarbonate, *FreAmine 111, Normosol-M in 5% Dextrose, Ionosol-B in 5% Dextrose,* 5% or 10% mannitol, sodium lactate.

Package Size	Diluent to Add	Resulting Concentration
250-mg vial	2.4 mL	100 mg/mL
500-mg vial	4.8 mL	100 mg/mL
1-g vial	9.6 mL	100 mg/mL
2-g vial	19.2 mL	100 mg/mL
Piggyback 1 g	10 mL	
Piggyback 2 g	20 mL	

Stability of reconstituted and diluted solution depends on diluent, concentration and type of container (eg, glass, PVC); check manufacturer's inserts for specific details. Protect drug from light.

Infusion: Administer by intermittent infusion over 15–30 min. Do not mix ceftriaxone with any other antimicrobial drug.

Incompatibilities: Do not mix aminoglycosides and ceftriaxone in the same IV solution.

Adverse effects

- **CNS:** Headache, dizziness, lethargy, paresthesias
- **GI:** *Nausea, vomiting, diarrhea, anorexia, abdominal pain, flatulence,* **pseudomembranous colitis, hepatotoxicity**
- **GU:** Nephrotoxicity
- **Hematologic: Bone marrow depression**—decreased WBC count, decreased platelets, decreased Hct
- **Hypersensitivity:** *Ranging from rash to fever to* **anaphylaxis;** serum sickness reaction
- **Local:** *Pain,* abscess at injection site; *phlebitis,* inflammation at IV site
- **Other:** *Superinfections, disulfiram-like reaction with alcohol*

Interactions

✳ **Drug-drug** • Increased nephrotoxicity with aminoglycosides • Increased bleeding effects with oral anticoagulants • Disulfiram-like reaction may occur if alcohol is taken within 72 hr after ceftriaxone administration

✳ **Drug-lab test** • Possibility of false results on tests of urine glucose using Benedict solution, Fehling solution, Clinitest tablets; urinary 17-ketosteroids; direct Coombs test

■ Nursing considerations

Assessment

- **History:** Hepatic and renal impairment, lactation, pregnancy
- **Physical:** Skin status, LFTs, renal function tests, culture of affected area, sensitivity tests

Interventions

- Culture infection site, and arrange for sensitivity tests before and during therapy if expected response is not seen.
- Reconstitute for IM use with sterile water for injection, 0.9% sodium chloride solution, 5% dextrose solution, bacteriostatic water with 0.9% benzyl alcohol, or 1% lidocaine solution (without epinephrine); inject deeply into a large muscle group.
- Check manufacturer's inserts for specific details. Stability of reconstituted and diluted solution depends on diluent, concentration and type of container (eg, glass, PVC).
- Protect drug from light.
- ⊗ *Warning* Do not mix ceftriaxone with any other antimicrobial drug.

- Monitor ceftriaxone blood levels in patients with severe renal impairment and in patients with renal and hepatic impairment.
- Have vitamin K available in case hypoprothrombinemia occurs.
- Discontinue if hypersensitivity reaction occurs.
- Evaluate patient for *Clostridium difficile* infection if diarrhea occurs.

Teaching points

- Avoid alcohol while taking this drug and for 3 days after because severe reactions often occur.
- You may experience these side effects: Stomach upset or diarrhea.
- Report severe diarrhea, difficulty breathing, unusual tiredness or fatigue, pain at injection site.

▷ **cefuroxime**
(se fyoor ox' eem)

cefuroxime axetil
Ceftin ᴄᴀɴ

cefuroxime sodium
Zinacef

PREGNANCY CATEGORY B

Drug classes

Antibiotic
Cephalosporin (second generation)

Therapeutic actions

Bactericidal: Inhibits synthesis of bacterial cell wall, causing cell death.

Indications

Oral (cefuroxime axetil)

- Pharyngitis, tonsillitis caused by *Streptococcus pyogenes*
- Otitis media caused by *Streptococcus pneumoniae, S. pyogenes, Haemophilus influenzae, Moraxella catarrhalis*
- Acute bacterial maxillary sinusitis caused by *S. pneumoniae, H. influenzae*
- Lower respiratory infections caused by *S. pneumoniae, Haemophilus parainfluenzae, H. influenzae*
- UTIs caused by *Escherichia coli, Klebsiella pneumoniae*

Adverse effects in *italics* are most common; those in **bold** are life-threatening. ᴄᴀɴ Do not crush.

- Uncomplicated gonorrhea (urethral and endocervical)
- Skin and skin structure infections, including impetigo caused by *Streptococcus aureus, S. pyogenes*
- Treatment of early Lyme disease

Parenteral (cefuroxime sodium)
- Lower respiratory infections caused by *S. pneumoniae, S. aureus, E. coli, Klebsiella pneuemoniae, H. influenzae, S. pyogenes*
- Dermatologic infections caused by *S. aureus, S. pyogenes, E. coli, K. pneuemoniae, Enterobacter*
- UTIs caused by *E. coli, K. pneumoniae*
- Uncomplicated and disseminated gonorrhea caused by *N. gonorrhoeae*
- Septicemia caused by *S. pneumoniae, S. aureus, E. coli, K. pneumoniae, H. influenzae*
- Meningitis caused by *S. pneumoniae, H. influenzae, S. aureus, N. meningitidis*
- Bone and joint infections due to *S. aureus*
- Perioperative prophylaxis
- Treatment of acute bacterial maxillary sinusitis in patients 3 mo–12 yr

Contraindications and cautions
- Contraindicated with allergy to cephalosporins or penicillins.
- Use cautiously with renal failure, lactation, pregnancy.

Available forms
Tablets—125, 250, 500 mg; suspension—125 mg/5 mL, 250 mg/5 mL; powder for injection—750 mg, 1.5 g; injection—750 mg, 1.5 g

Dosages
Oral
Adults and patients 12 yr and older
250 mg bid. For severe infections, may be increased to 500 mg bid. Treat for up to 10 days.
- *Uncomplicated UTIs:* 250 mg bid. Treat for 7–10 days.
- *Uncomplicated gonorrhea:* 1,000 mg once as a single dose.
Pediatric patients younger than 12 yr
125 mg bid.
- *Acute otitis media:*
  3 mo–12 yr: 250 mg PO bid for 10 days in children who can swallow tablets whole. Or,

30 mg/kg/day (maximum, 1 g/day) in two divided doses for 10 days (oral solution).
- *Pharyngitis or tonsillitis:*
  3 mo–12 yr: 125 mg PO every 12 hr for 10 days in children who can swallow tablets whole. Or, 20 mg/kg/day (maximum, 500 mg/day) in two divided doses for 10 days (oral solution).
- *Acute sinusitis:*
  3 mo–12 yr: 250 mg PO bid for 10 days in children who can swallow tablets whole. Or, 30 mg/kg/day (maximum, 1 g/day) in two divided doses for 10 days (oral solution).
- *Impetigo:*
  3 mo–12 yr: 30 mg/kg/day PO (maximum, 1 g/day) in two divided doses for 10 days (oral suspension).

Parenteral
Adults
750 mg–1.5 g IM or IV every 8 hr, depending on severity of infection, for 5–10 days.
- *Uncomplicated gonorrhea:* 1.5 g IM (at two different sites) with 1 g of oral probenecid.
- *Perioperative prophylaxis:* 1.5 g IV 30–60 min prior to initial incision; then 750 mg IV or IM every 8 hr for 24 hr after surgery.
Pediatric patients older than 3 mo
50–100 mg/kg/day IM or IV in divided doses every 6–8 hr.
- *Bacterial meningitis:* 200–240 mg/kg/day IV in divided doses every 6–8 hr.
Pediatric patients with impaired renal function
Adjust adult dosage for renal impairment by weight or age of child.
Geriatric patients or adults with impaired renal function

CrCl (mL/min)	Dosage
More than 20	750 mg–1.5 g every 8 hr
10–20	750 mg every 12 hr
Less than 10	750 mg every 24 hr

Pharmacokinetics

Route	Onset	Peak	Duration
IV	Rapid	Immediate	18–24 hr
IM	20 min	30 min	18–24 hr
Oral	Varies	2 hr	18–24 hr

Metabolism: $T_{1/2}$: 1–2 hr
Distribution: Crosses the placenta; enters breast milk
Excretion: Urine

▼ IV FACTS

Preparation: Preparation of parenteral drug solutions and suspensions differs for different starting preparations and different brand names; check the manufacturer's directions carefully. Reconstitute parenteral drug with sterile water for injection, D_5W, 0.9% sodium chloride, or any of the following, which also may be used for further dilution: 0.9% sodium chloride, 5% or 10% dextrose injection, 5% dextrose and 0.45% or 0.9% sodium chloride injection, or 1/6 M sodium lactate injection. Stability of solutions depends on diluent and concentration: Check manufacturer's specifications.

⊗ **Warning** Do not mix with IV solutions containing aminoglycosides. Powder form, solutions, and suspensions darken during storage.

Infusion: Inject slowly over 3–5 min directly into vein for IV administration, or infuse over 30 min; may be given by continuous infusion. Give aminoglycosides and cefuroxime at different sites.

Incompatibilities: Do not mix aminoglycosides and cefuroxime in the same IV solution.

Adverse effects

- **CNS:** Headache, dizziness, lethargy, paresthesias
- **GI:** *Nausea, vomiting, diarrhea, anorexia, abdominal pain, flatulence,* **pseudomembranous colitis, hepatotoxicity**
- **GU:** Nephrotoxicity
- **Hematologic: Bone marrow depression** (decreased WBC, decreased platelets, decreased Hct)
- **Hypersensitivity:** *Ranging from rash* to *fever* to **anaphylaxis;** serum sickness reaction
- **Local:** *Pain,* abscess at injection site, *phlebitis,* inflammation at IV site
- **Other:** *Superinfections, disulfiram-like reaction with alcohol*

Interactions

✳ **Drug-drug** • Increased nephrotoxicity with aminoglycosides • Increased bleeding effects with oral anticoagulants • Risk of disulfiram-like reaction with alcohol; avoid this combination during and for 3 days after completion of therapy

✳ **Drug-lab test** • Possibility of false results on tests of urine glucose using Benedict solution, Fehling solution, Clinitest tablets; urinary 17-ketosteroids; direct Coombs test

■ Nursing considerations

Assessment

- **History:** Hepatic and renal impairment, lactation, pregnancy
- **Physical:** Skin status, LFTs, renal function tests, culture of affected area, sensitivity tests

Interventions

- Culture infection site, and arrange for sensitivity tests before and during therapy if expected response is not seen.
- Give oral drug with food to decrease GI upset and enhance absorption.
- Give oral tablets to children who can swallow tablets; crushing the drug results in a bitter, unpleasant taste. Use solution for children who cannot swallow tablets.
- Have vitamin K available in case hypoprothrombinemia occurs.
- Discontinue if hypersensitivity reaction occurs.
- Evaluate patient for *Clostridium difficile* infection if diarrhea occurs.

Teaching points

Oral drug

- Take full course of therapy even if you are feeling better.
- This drug is specific for this infection and should not be used to self-treat other problems.
- Swallow tablets whole; do not crush them. Take the drug with food.
- Store solution in the refrigerator. Shake well before each use.
- You may experience these side effects: Stomach upset or diarrhea.
- Report severe diarrhea with blood, pus, or mucus; rash; difficulty breathing; unusual tiredness, fatigue; unusual bleeding or bruising; unusual itching or irritation.

Parenteral drug

- Avoid alcohol while taking this drug and for 3 days after because severe reactions often occur.
- You may experience these side effects: Stomach upset or diarrhea.
- Report severe diarrhea, difficulty breathing, unusual tiredness or fatigue, pain at injection site.

▽**celecoxib**

*(sell ah **cocks**' ib)*

Celebrex

PREGNANCY CATEGORY C
(FIRST AND SECOND TRIMESTER)

PREGNANCY CATEGORY D
(THIRD TRIMESTER)

Drug classes

Analgesic (nonopioid)
NSAID
Specific COX-2 enzyme inhibitor

Therapeutic actions

Analgesic and anti-inflammatory activities related to inhibition of the COX-2 enzyme, which is activated in inflammation to cause the signs and symptoms associated with inflammation; does not affect the COX-1 enzyme, which protects the lining of the GI tract and has blood clotting and renal functions.

Indications

- Acute and long-term treatment of signs and symptoms of rheumatoid arthritis and osteoarthritis
- Management of acute pain
- Treatment of primary dysmenorrhea
- Relief of signs and symptoms of ankylosing spondylitis
- Relief of signs and symptoms of juvenile rheumatoid arthritis
- Unlabeled uses: Treatment of preterm labor; prevention of colorectal cancer; adjunctive therapy in schizophrenia

Contraindications and cautions

- Contraindicated with allergies to sulfonamides, celecoxib, NSAIDs, or aspirin; significant renal impairment; perioperative pain post CABG surgery; pregnancy (third trimester); lactation.
- Use cautiously with impaired hearing, hepatic and CV conditions.

Available forms

Capsules—50, 100, 200, 400 mg

Dosages

Adults

Initially, 100 mg PO bid; may increase to 200 mg/day PO bid as needed.

- *Acute pain, dysmenorrhea:* 400 mg, then 200 mg PO bid.
- *Osteoarthritis:* 200 mg/day PO.
- *Rheumatoid arthritis:* 100–200 mg PO bid.
- *Ankylosing spondylitis:* 200 mg/day PO; after 6 wk, a trial of 400 mg/day may be tried for 6 wk; if no effect is seen, suggest another therapy.

Pediatric patients 2 yr and older

- *Juvenile rheumatoid arthritis: 10 kg to 25 kg or less:* 50 mg capsule PO bid.
More than 25 kg: 100 mg capsule PO bid.

Patients with moderate hepatic impairment

Reduce dosage by 50%.

Patients with renal impairment or severe hepatic impairment

Not recommended.

Pharmacokinetics

Route	Onset	Peak
Oral	Slow	3 hr

Metabolism: Hepatic; $T_{1/2}$: 11 hr
Distribution: Crosses placenta; may enter breast milk
Excretion: Bile, urine

Adverse effects

- **CNS:** *Headache, dizziness, somnolence, insomnia,* fatigue, tiredness, dizziness, tinnitus, ophthalmologic effects
- **CV: MI, stroke**
- **Dermatologic:** *Rash,* pruritus, sweating, dry mucous membranes, stomatitis
- **GI:** Nausea, abdominal pain, *dyspepsia,* flatulence, GI bleed
- **Hematologic:** Neutropenia, eosinophilia, leukopenia, pancytopenia, thrombocytopenia, **agranulocytosis,** granulocytopenia, aplastic anemia, decreased Hgb or Hct, bone marrow depression, menorrhagia
- **Other:** Peripheral edema, **anaphylactoid reactions** to **anaphylactic shock**

Interactions

✱ **Drug-drug** • Increased risk of bleeding if taken concurrently with warfarin. Monitor patient closely and reduce warfarin dose as appropriate ● Increased lithium levels and toxicity ● Increased risk of GI bleeding with long-term alcohol use, smoking

■ **Nursing considerations**

CLINICAL ALERT!
Name confusion has occurred between *Celebrex* (celecoxib), *Celexa* (citalopram), *Xanax* (alprazolam), and *Cerebyx* (fosphenytoin); use caution.

Assessment
● **History:** Renal impairment, impaired hearing, allergies, hepatic and CV conditions, lactation, pregnancy
● **Physical:** Skin color and lesions; orientation, reflexes, ophthalmologic and audiometric evaluation; peripheral sensation; P, edema; R, adventitious sounds; liver evaluation; CBC, LFTs, renal function tests; serum electrolytes

Interventions
⊗ **Black box warning** Be aware that patient may be at increased risk for CV events, GI bleeding; monitor accordingly.
● Administer drug with food or after meals if GI upset occurs.
● Establish safety measures if CNS or visual disturbances occur.
● Arrange for periodic ophthalmologic examination during long-term therapy.
⊗ **Warning** If overdose occurs, institute emergency procedures—gastric lavage, induction of emesis, supportive therapy.
● Provide further comfort measures to reduce pain (eg, positioning, environmental control) and to reduce inflammation (eg, warmth, positioning, rest).

Teaching points
● Take drug with food or meals if GI upset occurs.
● Take only the prescribed dosage; do not increase dosage.
● You may experience these side effects: Dizziness, drowsiness (avoid driving or the use of dangerous machinery while taking this drug).
● Report sore throat, fever, rash, itching, weight gain, swelling in ankles or fingers; changes in vision; chest pain, shortness of breath, slurred speech.

▽ **cellulose sodium phosphate (CSP)**

See Appendix R, *Less commonly used drugs.*

▽ **cephalexin**
*(sef a **lex'** in)*

Apo-Cephalex (CAN), Keflex, Novo-Lexin (CAN), Nu-Cephalex (CAN)

PREGNANCY CATEGORY B

Drug classes
Antibiotic
Cephalosporin (first generation)

Therapeutic actions
Bactericidal: Inhibits synthesis of bacterial cell wall, causing cell death.

Indications
● Respiratory tract infections caused by *Streptococcus pneumoniae,* group A beta-hemolytic streptococci
● Skin and skin-structure infections caused by staphylococcus, streptococcus
● Otitis media caused by *S. pneumoniae, Haemophilus influenzae,* streptococcus, staphylococcus, *Moraxella catarrhalis*
● Bone infections caused by staphylococcus, *Proteus mirabilis*
● GU infections caused by *Escherichia coli, P. mirabilis, Klebsiella*

Contraindications and cautions
● Contraindicated with allergy to cephalosporins or penicillins.
● Use cautiously with renal failure, lactation, pregnancy.

Available forms
Capsules—250, 500, 750 mg; tablets—250, 500 mg; oral suspension—125 mg/5 mL, 250 mg/5 mL

Dosages
Adults
1–4 g/day in divided doses; 250 mg PO every 6 hr usual dose.

Adverse effects in *italics* are most common; those in **bold** are life-threatening. ⊂⊃ Do not crush.

- *Skin and skin-structure infections, strep-tococcal pharyngitis, uncomplicated cystitis:* 500 mg PO every 12 hr. Larger doses may be needed in severe cases; do not exceed 4 g/day.

Pediatric patients
25–50 mg/kg/day PO in divided doses.

- *Skin and skin-structure infections:* Divide total daily dose, and give every 12 hr. Dosage may be doubled in severe cases.
- *Otitis media:* 75–100 mg/kg/day PO in four divided doses.

Pharmacokinetics

Route	Peak	Duration
Oral	60 min	8–10 hr

Metabolism: $T_{1/2}$: 50–80 min
Distribution: Crosses the placenta, enters breast milk
Excretion: Urine

Adverse effects

- **CNS:** Headache, dizziness, lethargy, paresthesias
- **GI:** *Nausea, vomiting, diarrhea, anorexia, abdominal pain, flatulence,* **pseudomembranous colitis, hepatotoxicity**
- **GU:** Nephrotoxicity
- **Hematologic: Bone marrow depression**
- **Hypersensitivity:** *Ranging from rash* to *fever* to **anaphylaxis;** serum sickness reaction
- **Other:** *Superinfections*

Interactions

✲ **Drug-drug** • Increased nephrotoxicity with aminoglycosides • Increased bleeding effects with oral anticoagulants • Disulfiram-like reaction may occur if alcohol is taken within 72 hr after cephalexin administration

✲ **Drug-lab test** • Possibility of false results on tests of urine glucose using Benedict solution, Fehling solution, Clinitest tablets; urinary 17-ketosteroids; direct Coombs test

■ Nursing considerations
Assessment

- **History:** Penicillin or cephalosporin allergy, pregnancy, or lactation
- **Physical:** Renal function tests, respiratory status, skin status; culture and sensitivity tests of infected area

Interventions

- Arrange for culture and sensitivity tests of infection before and during therapy if infection does not resolve.
- Give drug with meals; arrange for small, frequent meals if GI complications occur.
- Refrigerate suspension, discard after 14 days.
- Evaluate patient for *Clostridium difficile* infection if diarrhea occurs.

Teaching points

- Take this drug with food. Refrigerate suspension; discard any drug after 14 days.
- Complete the full course of this drug even if you feel better.
- This drug is prescribed for this particular infection; do not self-treat any other infection.
- You may experience these side effects: Stomach upset, loss of appetite, nausea (take drug with food); diarrhea; headache, dizziness.
- Avoid alcohol while taking cephalexin and for 3 days after completion of therapy.
- Report severe diarrhea with blood, pus, or mucus; rash or hives; difficulty breathing; unusual tiredness, fatigue; unusual bleeding or bruising.

▷ **certolizumab**

See Appendix R, *Less commonly used drugs.*

▷ **cetirizine hydrochloride**
(se teer' i zeen)

Reactine (CAN), Zyrtec, Zyrtec Allergy, Zyrtec Children's Allergy, Zyrtec Children's Hives Relief, Zyrtec Hives Relief

PREGNANCY CATEGORY B

Drug class
Antihistamine

Therapeutic actions
Potent specific histamine (H_1) receptor antagonist; inhibits histamine release and eosinophil chemotaxis during inflammation, leading to reduced swelling and decreased inflammatory response.

Indications

- Management of seasonal and perennial allergic rhinitis, allergies, hay fever
- Treatment of chronic, idiopathic urticaria
- Unlabeled uses: To decrease wheal response and pruritus of mosquito bites; possible use in allergic asthma

Contraindications and cautions

- Contraindicated with allergy to any antihistamines, hydroxyzine.
- Use cautiously with narrow-angle glaucoma, stenosing peptic ulcer, symptomatic prostatic hypertrophy, asthmatic attack, bladder neck obstruction, pyloroduodenal obstruction (avoid use or use with caution as condition may be exacerbated by drug effects); lactation.

Available forms

Tablets—5, 10 mg; chewable tablets—5, 10 mg; capsules—10 mg; syrup—1 mg/mL

Dosages

Adults and children 6 yr and older
10 mg/day PO or 5 mg PO bid; maximum dose 10 mg/day.
Pediatric patients 6–11 yr
5 or 10 mg PO daily.
Pediatric patients 2–6 yr
2.5 mg PO once daily to a maximum 5 mg/day.
Patients with hepatic or renal impairment, elderly patients
Dosage adjustment necessary; suggested dose, 5 mg PO daily.

Pharmacokinetics

Route	Onset	Peak	Duration
Oral	Rapid	1 hr	24 hr

Metabolism: Hepatic; $T_{1/2}$: 7–10 hr
Distribution: Crosses placenta; enters breast milk
Excretion: Feces, urine

Adverse effects

- **CNS:** *Somnolence, sedation*
- **CV:** Palpitation, edema, dizziness
- **GI:** Nausea, diarrhea, abdominal pain, constipation, dry mouth
- **Respiratory: Bronchospasm,** pharyngitis
- **Other:** Fever, photosensitivity, rash, myalgia, arthralgia, angioedema, fatigue

■ Nursing considerations

 CLINICAL ALERT!
Name confusion has occurred between *Zyrtec* (cetirizine) and *Zyprexa* (olanzapine) and between *Zyrtec* (cetirizine) and *Zantac* (ranitidine); use caution.

Assessment

- **History:** Allergy to any antihistamines, hydroxyzine; narrow-angle glaucoma, stenosing peptic ulcer, symptomatic prostatic hypertrophy, asthmatic attack, bladder neck obstruction, pyloroduodenal obstruction; lactation
- **Physical:** Skin color, lesions, texture; orientation, reflexes, affect; vision examination; R, adventitious sounds; prostate palpation; renal and hepatic function tests

Interventions

- Give without regard to meals.
- Provide syrup form or chewable tablets for pediatric use if needed.
- Arrange for use of humidifier if thickening of secretions, nasal dryness become bothersome; encourage adequate intake of fluids.
- Provide skin care for urticaria.

Teaching points

- Take this drug without regard to meals.
- You may experience these side effects: Dizziness, sedation, drowsiness (use caution if driving or performing tasks that require alertness); thickening of bronchial secretions, dry nasal mucosa (humidifier may help).
- Report difficulty breathing, hallucinations, tremors, loss of coordination, irregular heartbeat.

▷ cetrorelix acetate

See Appendix R, *Less commonly used drugs.*

▷ cetuximab

See Appendix R, *Less commonly used drugs.*

▷ cevimeline hydrochloride

See Appendix R, *Less commonly used drugs.*

Adverse effects in *italics* are most common; those in **bold** are life-threatening. ▨ Do not crush.

▷charcoal, activated
(char' kole)

OTC: Actidose-Aqua, Actidose with Sorbitol, CharcoAid, CharcoAid 2000, Liqui-Char

PREGNANCY CATEGORY UNDETERMINED

Drug class
Antidote

Therapeutic actions
Adsorbs toxic substances swallowed into the GI tract, inhibiting GI absorption; maximum amount of toxin absorbed is 100–1,000 mg/g charcoal.

Indications
• Emergency treatment in poisoning by most drugs and chemicals

Contraindications and cautions
• Contraindicated with poisoning or overdosage of cyanide, mineral acids, alkalies.
• Use cautiously; not effective with ethanol, methanol, and iron salts.

Available forms
Powder—15, 30, 40, 120, 240 g; liquid—208 mg/mL, 12.5 g/60 mL, 15 g/75 mL, 15 g/120 mL, 25 g/120 mL, 30 g/120 mL, 50 g/240 mL; suspension—15, 30 g; granules—15 g

Dosages
Adults
50–60 g or 1 g/kg PO or approximately 8–10 times by volume the amount of poison ingested, as an oral suspension; administer as soon as possible after poisoning.
• *Gastric dialysis:* 20–40 g every 6 hr for 1–2 days for severe poisonings; for optimum effect, administer within 30 min of poisoning.
Pediatric patients 1–12 yr
Weighing more than 32 kg: 50–60 g.
Weighing 16–32 kg: 25–30 g.
Weighing less than 16 kg and younger than 1 yr: Not recommended.

Pharmacokinetics
Not absorbed systemically
Excretion: Feces

Adverse effects
• **GI:** *Vomiting* (related to rapid ingestion of high doses), *constipation, diarrhea,* black stools

Interactions
✳ **Drug-drug** • Adsorption and inactivation of laxatives with activated charcoal • Decreased effectiveness of other medications because of adsorption by activated charcoal
✳ **Drug-food** • Decreased adsorptive capacity if taken with milk, ice cream, or sherbet

■ Nursing considerations

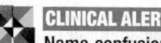 **CLINICAL ALERT!**
Name confusion can occur between *Actidose* (charcoal) and *Actos* (pioglitazone); use caution.

Assessment
• **History:** Poisoning or overdosage of cyanide, mineral acids, alkalies, ethanol, methanol, and iron salts
• **Physical:** Stools, bowel sounds

Interventions
• Repeat dose if patient vomits shortly after administration.
• Give drug to conscious patients only.
• Take measures to prevent aspiration of charcoal powder; fatalities have occurred.
• Give drug as soon after poisoning as possible; most effective results are seen if given within 30 min.
• Prepare suspension of powder in 6–8 oz of water; taste may be gritty and disagreeable. Sorbitol is added to some preparations to improve taste; diarrhea more likely with these preparations.
• Store in closed containers; activated charcoal adsorbs gases from the air and will lose its effectiveness with prolonged exposure to air.
• Ensure that life-support equipment is readily available for poisoning and overdose.

Teaching points
• Drink 6–8 glasses of liquid per day to avoid constipation.
• You may experience these side effects: Black stools, diarrhea, constipation.

▷chenodiol

See Appendix R, *Less commonly used drugs.*

DANGEROUS DRUG

▷chloral hydrate

(klor al hye' drate)

Chloral Hydrate-Odan (CAN),
Somnote⊕

PREGNANCY CATEGORY C

CONTROLLED SUBSTANCE C-IV

Drug class
Sedative-hypnotic (nonbarbiturate)

Therapeutic actions
Mechanism by which CNS is affected is not known; hypnotic dosage produces mild cerebral depression and quiet, deep sleep; does not depress REM sleep, produces less hangover than most barbiturates and benzodiazepines.

Indications
- Nocturnal sedation
- Preoperative sedation to lessen anxiety and induce sleep without depressing respiration or cough reflex
- Adjunct to opiates and analgesics in postoperative care and control of pain

Contraindications and cautions
- Contraindicated with hypersensitivity to chloral derivatives, severe cardiac disease, gastritis, gastric or duodenal ulcers; hepatic or renal impairment, lactation.
- Use cautiously with acute intermittent porphyria (may precipitate attacks).

Available forms
Capsules⊕—500 mg; syrup—250 mg/5 mL, 500 mg/5 mL

Dosages
Adults
Single doses or daily dose should not exceed 2 g.
- *Hypnotic:* 500 mg–1 g PO 15–30 min before bedtime or 30 min before surgery. It is not usually considered safe practice to give oral medication to patients who are NPO for anesthesia or surgery.
- *Sedative:* 250 mg PO tid after meals.

Pediatric patients
- *Hypnotic:* 50 mg/kg/day PO up to 1 g per single dose; may be given in divided doses.
- *Sedative:* 25 mg/kg/day PO up to 500 mg per single dose; may be given in divided doses.

Pharmacokinetics

Route	Onset	Peak	Duration
Oral, rectal	30–60 min	1–3 hr	4–8 hr

Metabolism: Hepatic; $T_{1/2}$: 7–10 hr
Distribution: Crosses placenta; enters breast milk
Excretion: Bile, urine

Adverse effects
- **CNS:** *Somnambulism, disorientation, incoherence, paranoid behavior,* excitement, delirium, drowsiness, staggering gait, ataxia, light-headedness, vertigo, nightmares, malaise, mental confusion, headache, hallucinations
- **Dermatologic:** *Skin irritation;* allergic rashes including hives, erythema, eczematoid dermatitis, urticaria
- **GI:** Gastric irritation, nausea, vomiting, **gastric necrosis** (following intoxicating doses), flatulence, diarrhea, unpleasant taste
- **Hematologic:** Leukopenia, eosinophilia
- **Other:** Physical, psychological dependence; tolerance; withdrawal reaction; hangover

Interactions
✳ **Drug-drug** • Additive CNS depression with alcohol, other CNS depressants • Mutual inhibition of metabolism with alcohol • Complex effects on oral (warfarin) anticoagulants given with chloral hydrate; monitor prothrombin levels and adjust warfarin dosage whenever chloral hydrate is instituted or withdrawn from drug regimen
✳ **Drug-lab test** • Interference with the copper sulfate test for glycosuria, fluorometric tests for urine catecholamines, and urinary 17-hydroxycorticosteroid determinations (when using the Reddy, Jenkins, and Thorn procedure)

■ Nursing considerations
Assessment
- **History:** Hypersensitivity to chloral derivatives, severe cardiac disease, gastritis,

hepatic or renal impairment, acute intermittent porphyria, lactation
• **Physical:** Skin color, lesions; orientation, affect, reflexes; P, BP, perfusion; bowel sounds, normal output, liver evaluation; LFTs, renal function tests, CBC and differential, stool guaiac test

Interventions
• Give capsules with a full glass of liquid; ensure that patient swallows capsules whole; give syrup in half glass of water, fruit juice, or ginger ale.
• Supervise dose and amount of drug prescribed for patients who are addiction prone or alcoholic; give least amount feasible to patients who are depressed or suicidal.
• Withdraw gradually over 2 wk if patient has been maintained on high doses for weeks or months; if patient has built up high tolerance, withdrawal should occur in a hospital, using supportive therapy similar to that for barbiturate withdrawal; fatal withdrawal reactions have occurred.
• Reevaluate patients with prolonged insomnia; therapy for the underlying cause (eg, pain, depression) is preferable to prolonged use of sedative-hypnotic drugs.

Teaching points
• Take this drug exactly as prescribed: Swallow capsules whole with a full glass of liquid (take syrup in half glass of water, fruit juice, or ginger ale).
• Do not discontinue the drug abruptly. Consult your health care provider if you wish to discontinue the drug.
• Avoid alcohol, sleep-inducing, or over-the-counter drugs; these could cause dangerous effects.
• You may experience these side effects: Drowsiness, dizziness, light-headedness (avoid driving or performing tasks requiring alertness); GI upset (eat frequent small meals); sleep-walking, nightmares, confusion (use caution: close doors, keep medications out of reach so inadvertent overdose does not occur while confused).
• Report rash, coffee ground vomitus, black or tarry stools, severe GI upset, fever, sore throat.

DANGEROUS DRUG

▽**chlorambucil**
(klor am' byoo sil)

Leukeran

PREGNANCY CATEGORY D

Drug classes
Alkylating drug
Nitrogen mustard derivative
Antineoplastic

Therapeutic actions
Cytotoxic: Alkylates cellular DNA, interfering with the replication of susceptible cells.

Indications
• Palliative treatment of chronic lymphocytic leukemia; malignant lymphomas, including lymphosarcoma; giant follicular lymphoma; and Hodgkin lymphoma
• Unlabeled uses: Ovarian and testicular carcinomas, Waldenström macroglobulinemia, non-Hodgkin lymphoma, polycythemia vera

Contraindications and cautions
• Contraindicated with allergy to chlorambucil; cross-sensitization with melphalan, pregnancy.
• Use cautiously with radiation therapy, chemotherapy, myelosuppression, lactation.

Available forms
Tablets—2 mg

Dosages
Individualize dosage based on hematologic profile and response.
Adults
• *Initial dose and short-course therapy:* 0.1–0.2 mg/kg per day PO for 3–6 wk; single daily dose may be given.
• *Chronic lymphocytic leukemia (alternate regimen):* 0.4 mg/kg PO every 2 wk, increasing by 0.1 mg/kg with each dose until therapeutic or toxic effect occurs.
• *Maintenance dose:* 0.03–0.1 mg/kg/day PO. Do not exceed 0.1 mg/kg/day. Short courses of therapy are safer than continuous maintenance therapy; base dosage and duration on patient response and bone marrow status.
Pediatric patients
Safety and efficacy not established.

Patients with renal impairment

CrCl (mL/min)	% of Usual Dose
More than 50	100%
10–50	75%
Less than 10	50%
Dialysis	50%, no supplemental dose needed

Pharmacokinetics

Route	Onset	Peak	Duration
Oral	Varies	1 hr	15–20 hr

Metabolism: Hepatic; $T_{1/2}$: 60–90 min
Distribution: Crosses placenta; enters breast milk
Excretion: Urine

Adverse effects

• **CNS:** Tremors, muscular twitching, confusion, agitation, ataxia, flaccid paresis, hallucinations, seizures
• **Dermatologic:** Rash, urticaria, *alopecia,* keratitis, **Stevens-Johnson syndrome, erythema multiforme**
• **GI:** *Nausea, vomiting, stomatitis,* anorexia, **hepatotoxicity,** jaundice (rare)
• **GU:** *Sterility* (especially in prepubertal or pubertal males and adult men; amenorrhea can occur in females)
• **Hematologic: Bone marrow depression,** hyperuricemia
• **Respiratory:** Bronchopulmonary dysplasia, pulmonary fibrosis
• **Other:** Cancer, **acute leukemia**

■ Nursing considerations

CLINICAL ALERT!
Name confusion has occurred between *Leukeran* (chlorambucil), *Myleran* (busulfan), *Alkeran* (melphalan), and leucovorin; use caution.

Assessment

• **History:** Allergy to chlorambucil, cross-sensitization with melphalan (rash), radiation therapy, chemotherapy, hematopoietic depression, pregnancy, lactation
• **Physical:** T; weight; skin color, lesions; R, adventitious sounds; liver evaluation; CBC, differential, Hgb, uric acid, LFTs

Interventions

⊗ *Black box warning* Arrange for blood tests to evaluate hematopoietic function before and weekly during therapy. Severe bone marrow suppression can occur.
⊗ *Black box warning* This drug is carcinogenic. Monitor patient regularly.
• Do not give full dosage within 4 wk after a full course of radiation therapy or chemotherapy because of risk of severe bone marrow depression.
• Ensure that patient is well hydrated before treatment.
⊗ *Black box warning* Ensure that patient is not pregnant before beginning therapy; encourage use of barrier contraceptives because this drug is teratogenic. This drug may also cause infertility.
⊗ *Warning* Monitor uric acid levels; ensure adequate fluid intake, and prepare for appropriate treatment of hyperuricemia if it occurs.
• Divide single daily dose if nausea and vomiting occur with large single dose.

Teaching points

• Take this drug once a day and take it with food. If nausea and vomiting occur, consult health care provider about dividing the dose.
• You may experience these side effects: Nausea, vomiting, loss of appetite (dividing dose, eat frequent small meals; maintain your fluid intake and nutrition; drink at least 10–12 glasses of fluid each day); infertility (from irregular menses to complete amenorrhea; men may stop producing sperm—may be irreversible; discuss with your health care provider); severe birth defects—use barrier contraceptives; cancer—follow all suggested screening protocols.
• Report unusual bleeding or bruising, fever, chills, sore throat; cough, shortness of breath, yellow skin or eyes, flank or stomach pain.

▷ **chloramphenicol**
(klor am fen' i kole)

chloramphenicol sodium succinate

PREGNANCY CATEGORY C

Drug class
Antibiotic

Therapeutic actions
Bacteriostatic effect against susceptible bacteria; prevents cell replication.

Indications
Systemic
- Serious infections for which no other antibiotic is effective
- Acute infections caused by *Salmonella typhi*
- Serious infections caused by *Salmonella, Haemophilus influenzae*, rickettsiae, lymphogranuloma—psittacosis group
- Cystic fibrosis regimen

Contraindications and cautions
- Contraindicated with allergy to chloramphenicol.
- Use cautiously with renal failure, hepatic failure, G6PD deficiency, intermittent porphyria, pregnancy (may cause gray syndrome in premature infants and newborns), lactation.

Available forms
Powder for injection—1 g/vial

Dosages
⊗ **Black box warning** Severe and sometimes fatal blood dyscrasias (in adults) and severe and sometimes fatal gray syndrome (in newborns and premature infants) may occur. Use should be restricted to situations in which no other antibiotic is effective. Serum levels should be monitored at least weekly to minimize risk of toxicity (therapeutic concentrations: peak, 10–20 mcg/mL; trough, 5–10 mcg/mL).
Adults
50 mg/kg/day IV in divided doses every 6 hr up to 100 mg/kg/day in severe cases.
Pediatric patients
50–100 mg/kg/day IV in divided doses every 6 hr.
- *Meningitis:* 50–100 mg/kg/day IV in divided doses every 6 hr.
- *Neonates:* Usual dose, 25 mg/kg/day IV; individualize doses at 6-hr intervals. Dosage adjustment—after first 2 wk of life, full-term neonates may receive up to 50 mg/kg/day in divided doses at 6-hr intervals.
- *Infants and children with immature metabolic processes:* 25 mg/kg/day IV (monitor serum concentration carefully).

Geriatric patients or patients with renal or hepatic failure
Use serum concentration of the drug to adjust dosage.

Pharmacokinetics
Route	Onset	Peak	Duration
IV	20–30 min	1 hr	48–72 hr

Metabolism: Hepatic; $T_{1/2}$: 1.5–4 hr
Distribution: Crosses placenta; enters breast milk
Excretion: Urine

▼ IV FACTS
Preparation: Dilute with 10 mL of sterile water for injection, or 5% dextrose injection.
Infusion: Administer as a 10% solution over 3–5 min, single-dose infusion over 30–60 min.

Adverse effects
Systemic
- **CNS:** Headache, mild depression, mental confusion, delirium
- **GI:** Nausea, vomiting, glossitis, stomatitis, diarrhea
- **Hematologic: Blood dyscrasias**
- **Other:** Fever, macular rashes, urticaria, **anaphylaxis; gray baby syndrome** (seen in neonates and premature infants—abdominal distention, pallid cyanosis, vasomotor collapse, irregular respirations), **superinfections**

Interactions
✳ **Drug-drug** • Increased serum levels and drug effects of warfarin, phenytoins, tolbutamide, glipizide, glyburide, tolazamide with chloramphenicol • Decreased hematologic response to iron salts, vitamin B_{12} with chloramphenicol • Risk of increased bone marrow suppression if taken with other drugs that suppress bone marrow

■ Nursing considerations
Assessment
- **History:** Allergy to chloramphenicol, renal or hepatic failure, G6PD deficiency, intermittent porphyria, pregnancy, lactation
- **Physical:** Culture infection; orientation, reflexes, sensation; R, adventitious sounds; bowel sounds, output, liver evaluation; urinalysis, BUN, CBC, LFTs, renal function tests

Interventions
Systemic administration
- Culture infection site before beginning therapy. Use only in situations in which a less dangerous antibiotic is ineffective or contraindicated.
- ⊗ **Warning** Do not give this drug IM because it is ineffective.
- ⊗ **Black box warning** Monitor hematologic data carefully, especially with long-term therapy by any route of administration. Serious and fatal blood dyscrasias have occurred.
- Reduce dosage in patients with renal or hepatic disease.
- Monitor serum levels periodically as indicated in dosage section.
- Change to another antibiotic as soon as possible.

Teaching points
- This drug can only be given IV.
- You may experience these side effects: Nausea, vomiting; diarrhea (reversible); headache (request medication); confusion (avoid driving or operating machinery); superinfections (good hygiene may help; medications are available if severe).
- Report sore throat, tiredness, unusual bleeding or bruising (even as late as several weeks after you finish the drug), numbness, tingling, pain in the extremities, pregnancy; discomfort at IV site.

▽ **chlordiazepoxide**
(metaminodiazepoxide hydrochloride)

(klor dye az e pox' ide)

Apo-Chlordiazepoxide (CAN), Librium

PREGNANCY CATEGORY D

CONTROLLED SUBSTANCE C-IV

Drug classes
Anxiolytic
Benzodiazepine

Therapeutic actions
Exact mechanisms of action not understood; acts mainly at subcortical levels of the CNS; main sites of action may be the limbic system and reticular formation; potentiates the effects of GABA.

Indications
- Management of anxiety disorders or for short-term relief of symptoms of anxiety
- Acute alcohol withdrawal; may be useful in symptomatic relief of acute agitation, tremor, delirium tremens, hallucinosis
- Preoperative relief of anxiety and tension

Contraindications and cautions
- Contraindicated with hypersensitivity to benzodiazepines, psychoses, acute narrow-angle glaucoma, shock, coma, acute alcoholic intoxication with depression of vital signs, pregnancy (increased risk of congenital malformations, neonatal withdrawal syndrome), labor and delivery ("floppy infant" syndrome reported), lactation (infants may become lethargic and lose weight).
- Use cautiously with hepatic or renal impairment, debilitation and in geriatric patients who are at increased risk for mental status changes.

Available forms
Capsules—5, 10, 25 mg

Dosages
Adults
Individualize dosage; increase dosage cautiously to avoid adverse effects.
- *Anxiety disorders:* 5 or 10 mg PO, up to 20 or 25 mg, tid–qid, depending on severity of symptoms.
- *Preoperative apprehension:* 5–10 mg PO tid–qid on days preceding surgery.
- *Alcohol withdrawal:* Initial dose is 50–100 mg PO, followed by repeated doses as needed up to 300 mg/day; then reduce to maintenance levels.
Pediatric patients
Younger than 6 yr: Not recommended.
Older than 6 yr: Initially, 5 mg PO bid–qid; may be increased in some children to 10 mg bid–tid.
Geriatric patients or patients with debilitating disease
5 mg PO bid–qid

Adverse effects in *italics* are most common; those in **bold** are life-threatening. ⬛ Do not crush.

Pharmacokinetics

Route	Onset	Peak	Duration
Oral	Varies	1–4 hr	48–72 hr
IM	10–15 min	15–30 min	48–72 hr

Metabolism: Hepatic; $T_{1/2}$: 24–48 hr
Distribution: Crosses placenta; enters breast milk
Excretion: Urine

Adverse effects

- **CNS:** *Transient, mild drowsiness initially; sedation, depression, lethargy, apathy, fatigue, light-headedness, disorientation, restlessness, confusion,* crying, delirium, headache, slurred speech, dysarthria, stupor, rigidity, tremor, psychomotor retardation, extrapyramidal symptoms; *mild paradoxical excitatory reactions during first 2 wk of treatment* (especially in psychiatric patients, aggressive children, and those with high dosage), visual and auditory disturbances, diplopia, nystagmus, depressed hearing, nasal congestion
- **CV:** Bradycardia, tachycardia, **CV collapse,** hypertension and hypotension, palpitations, edema
- **Dependence:** *Drug dependence with withdrawal syndrome* when drug is discontinued (more common with abrupt discontinuation of higher dosage used for longer than 4 mo)
- **Dermatologic:** Urticaria, pruritus, skin rash, dermatitis
- **GI:** *Constipation, diarrhea,* dry mouth, salivation, nausea, anorexia, vomiting, difficulty in swallowing, gastric disorders, hepatic impairment, jaundice
- **GU:** *Incontinence, urinary retention, changes in libido,* menstrual irregularities
- **Hematologic:** Decreased Hct, blood dyscrasias
- **Other:** Hiccups, fever, diaphoresis, paresthesias, muscular disturbances, gynecomastia

Interactions

✳ **Drug-drug** • Increased CNS depression with alcohol, omeprazole • Increased pharmacologic effects with cimetidine, disulfiram, hormonal contraceptives • Decreased sedative effects with theophylline, aminophylline, dyphylline, smoking

✳ **Drug-alternative therapy** • Risk of increased CNS effects with kava

■ Nursing considerations

Assessment

- **History:** Hypersensitivity to benzodiazepines; psychoses; acute narrow-angle glaucoma; shock; coma; acute alcoholic intoxication; pregnancy; lactation; impaired hepatic or renal function
- **Physical:** Skin color, lesions; T; orientation, reflexes, affect, ophthalmologic examination; P, BP; R, adventitious sounds; liver evaluation, abdominal examination, bowel sounds, normal output; CBC, LFTs, renal function tests

Interventions

- Monitor LFTs, renal function tests, and CBC at intervals during long-term therapy.
- ⊗ **Warning** Taper dosage gradually after long-term therapy, especially in epileptic patients.
- Advise use of barrier contraceptives; serious fetal abnormalities have been reported.

Teaching points

- Take drug exactly as prescribed.
- Do not stop taking this drug (long-term therapy) without consulting your health care provider. Avoid alcohol and sleep-inducing or over-the-counter drugs.
- Avoid becoming pregnant while taking this drug; serious adverse effects could occur. Using barrier contraceptives is suggested.
- You may experience these side effects: Drowsiness, dizziness (transient; avoid driving or engaging in other dangerous activities); GI upset (take drug with water); depression, dreams, emotional upset, crying.
- Report severe dizziness, weakness, drowsiness that persists, rash or skin lesions, palpitations, swelling of the extremities, visual changes, difficulty voiding, smoking (can decrease effectiveness).

▷ **chloroquine phosphate**

(klo' ro kwin)

Aralen Phosphate

PREGNANCY CATEGORY C

Drug classes

4-aminoquinoline
Amebicide
Antimalarial

Therapeutic actions

Inhibits protozoal reproduction and protein synthesis. Mechanism of anti-inflammatory action in rheumatoid arthritis is not known.

Indications

- Treatment of extraintestinal amebiasis
- Prophylaxis and treatment of acute attacks of malaria caused by susceptible strains of *Plasmodia*
- Unlabeled use: Treatment of rheumatoid arthritis (150 mg PO daily)

Contraindications and cautions

- Contraindicated with allergy to chloroquine and other 4-aminoquinolines; retinal or visual field changes.
- Use cautiously with porphyria, psoriasis, retinal disease, hepatic disease, G6PD deficiency, alcoholism, lactation, pregnancy.

Available forms

Tablets—250, 500 mg

Dosages

⊗ *Warning* Dosage is often expressed as chloroquine base.

Adults

- *Amebiasis:* 1 g (600 mg base)/day PO for 2 days; then 500 mg (300 mg base)/day for 2–3 wk.
- *Malaria:* For suppression, 300 mg base (500 mg) PO once a week on the same day for 2 wk before exposure and continuing until 8 wk after exposure. For acute attack, initially 600 mg base (1 g) PO; then 300 mg base (500 mg) 6–8 hr, 24 hr, 48 hr after the initial dose for a total dose of 1.5 g base (2.5 g) in 3 days.

Pediatric patients

- *Amebiasis:* Not recommended.
- *Malaria:* For suppression, 5 mg base/kg PO once a week on the same day for 2 wk before exposure and continuing for 8 wk after leaving endemic area. For acute attack, 10 mg base/kg PO initially (do not exceed single dose of 600 mg base); then 5 mg base/kg (do not exceed single dose of 300 mg base) 6 hr later; then third dose 18 hr later; then last dose 24 hr after third dose.

Pharmacokinetics

Route	Onset	Peak	Duration
Oral	Varies	1–2 hr	1 wk

Metabolism: Hepatic; $T_{1/2}$: 70–120 hr
Distribution: May cross placenta; enters breast milk
Excretion: Urine

Adverse effects

- **CNS:** *Visual disturbances,* possibly permanent retinal changes (blurring of vision, difficulty in focusing), ototoxicity, muscle weakness
- **CV:** Hypotension, ECG changes
- **Dermatologic:** Skin eruptions, pruritus, hair loss
- **GI:** *Nausea, vomiting, diarrhea,* loss of appetite, abdominal pain
- **Hematologic:** Blood dyscrasias, hemolysis in patients with G6PD deficiency

Interactions

＊**Drug-drug** • Increased effects of chloroquine with cimetidine

■ Nursing considerations

Assessment

- **History:** Allergy to chloroquine and other 4-aminoquinolines, porphyria, psoriasis, retinal disease, hepatic disease, G6PD deficiency, alcoholism, lactation, pregnancy
- **Physical:** Reflexes, muscle strength, auditory and ophthalmologic screening; BP, ECG; liver palpation; CBC, G6PD in deficient patients, LFTs

Interventions

- Administer with meals if GI upset occurs.
- Schedule weekly, same-day therapy on a calendar.
- ⊗ *Warning* Double check pediatric doses; children are very susceptible to overdosage.
- Arrange for ophthalmologic examinations during long-term therapy.

Teaching points

- Take full course of drug therapy. Take drug with meals if GI upset occurs. Mark your calendar with the days you should take your drug for malarial prophylaxis.
- Arrange to have regular ophthalmologic examinations if long-term use is indicated.

Adverse effects in *italics* are most common; those in **bold** are life-threatening. ⊂▣⊃ Do not crush.

- You may experience these side effects: Stomach pain, loss of appetite, nausea, vomiting, or diarrhea.
- Report blurring of vision, loss of hearing, ringing in the ears, muscle weakness, fever.

▽ **chlorothiazide**

*(klor oh **thye'** a zide)*

Diuril

chlorothiazide sodium

PREGNANCY CATEGORY C

Drug class
Thiazide diuretic

Therapeutic actions
Inhibits reabsorption of sodium and chloride in distal renal tubule, increasing the excretion of sodium, chloride, and water by the kidneys.

Indications
- Adjunctive therapy in edema associated with heart failure, cirrhosis, corticosteroid, and estrogen therapy, renal impairment
- Treatment of hypertension, alone or with other antihypertensives
- Unlabeled uses: Treatment of diabetes insipidus, especially nephrogenic diabetes insipidus; reduction of incidence of osteoporosis in postmenopausal women, calcium nephrolithiasis

Contraindications and cautions
- Contraindicated with anuria, renal failure, allergy to thiazide diuretics or other sulfonamide drugs, hepatic coma.
- Use cautiously with fluid or electrolyte imbalances, renal or liver disease, gout, SLE, glucose tolerance abnormalities, hyperparathyroidism, bipolar disorder, lactation, pregnancy.

Available forms
Tablets—250, 500 mg; oral suspension—250 mg/5 mL; powder for injection—500 mg

Dosages
Note: Dosage should be individualized according to patient response, and the lowest possible dose should be used.

Adults
- *Edema:* 0.5–2 g daily PO or IV (if patient unable to take PO), daily in one or two doses.
- *Hypertension:* 0.5–2 g/day PO as a single or divided dose; adjust dosage to BP response, giving up to 2 g/day in divided doses. IV use is not recommended.

Pediatric patients
10–20 mg/kg/day PO in a single dose or two doses.

Pediatric patients 2–12 yr
375 mg–1 g PO in two divided doses.

Pediatric patients 2 yr or younger
125–375 mg PO in two divided doses.

Pediatric patients younger than 6 mo
Up to 30 mg/kg per day PO in two doses. IV use not recommended.

Pharmacokinetics

Route	Onset	Peak	Duration
Oral	2 hr	3–6 hr	6–12 hr
IV	15 min	30 min	2 hr

Metabolism: $T_{1/2}$: 45–120 min
Distribution: Crosses placenta; enters breast milk
Excretion: Urine

▼ IV FACTS

Preparation: Dilute vial for parenteral solution with 18 mL sterile water for injection. Never add less than 18 mL. Discard diluted solution after 24 hr.
Infusion: Administer slowly. Switch to oral drug as soon as possible.
Compatibilities: Compatible with dextrose and sodium chloride solutions.
Incompatibilities: Do not give parenteral solution with whole blood or blood products.

Adverse effects
- **CNS:** *Dizziness, vertigo,* paresthesias, weakness, headache, drowsiness, fatigue
- **CV:** Orthostatic hypotension, venous thrombosis, volume depletion, cardiac arrhythmias, chest pain
- **Dermatologic:** Photosensitivity, rash, purpura, exfoliative dermatitis
- **GI:** *Nausea, anorexia, vomiting, dry mouth, diarrhea, constipation,* jaundice, hepatitis, pancreatitis

- **GU:** *Polyuria, nocturia, impotence,* loss of libido, renal failure
- **Hematologic:** Leukopenia, thrombocytopenia, **agranulocytosis, aplastic anemia,** neutropenia, fluid and electrolyte imbalances
- **Other:** Muscle cramps and muscle spasms, fever, hives, gouty attacks, flushing, weight loss, rhinorrhea, electrolyte imbalances

Interactions
✳ **Drug-drug** • Increased thiazide effects and chance of acute hyperglycemia with diazoxide • Decreased absorption with cholestyramine • Increased risk of cardiac glycoside toxicity if hypokalemia occurs • Increased risk of lithium toxicity • Increased dosage of antidiabetics may be needed • Possible potentiation of hypotension with alcohol, opioids • Potentiation of hypokalemia with corticosteroids
✳ **Drug-lab test** • Monitor for decreased PBI levels without clinical signs of thyroid disturbances

■ Nursing considerations
Assessment
- **History:** Fluid or electrolyte imbalances, renal or liver disease, gout, SLE, glucose tolerance abnormalities, hyperparathyroidism, manic-depressive disorders, lactation
- **Physical:** Orientation, reflexes, muscle strength; pulses, BP, orthostatic BP, perfusion, edema, baseline ECG; R, adventitious sounds; liver evaluation, bowel sounds; CBC, serum electrolytes, blood glucose, LFTs, renal function tests, serum uric acid, urinalysis

Interventions
- Administer with food or milk if GI upset occurs.
- Do not administer drug IM or subcutaneously.
- Administer early in the day, so increased urination will not disturb sleep.
- Measure and record weight to monitor fluid changes.

Teaching points
- Take drug early in the day, so your sleep will not be disturbed by increased urination.
- Weigh yourself daily, and record weights.
- Protect skin from exposure to the sun or bright lights.
- Increased urination will occur; you may want to plan activities accordingly.

- You may experience these side effects: Dizziness, drowsiness, or feeling faint (use caution).
- Report rapid weight change of more than 3 pounds a day, swelling in ankles or fingers, unusual bleeding or bruising, muscle cramps.

▽ **chlorpheniramine maleate**
(klor fen ir' a meen mal' ee ate)

Aller-Chlor; Allergy; Allergy Relief; Chlo-Amine; Chlor-Trimeton Allergy 8 hr, and 12 hr; ED-CHLOR-TAN ⓄⓉⒸ; Efidac 24 ⓄⓉⒸ; QDALL-AR ⓄⓉⒸ

PREGNANCY CATEGORY C

Drug class
Antihistamine (alkylamine type)

Therapeutic actions
Competitively blocks the effects of histamine at H_1-receptor sites; has atropine-like, antipruritic, and sedative effects.

Indications
- Symptomatic relief of symptoms associated with perennial and seasonal allergic rhinitis; vasomotor rhinitis; common cold; allergic conjunctivitis

Contraindications and cautions
- Contraindicated with allergy to any antihistamines, narrow-angle glaucoma, stenosing peptic ulcer, symptomatic prostatic hypertrophy, asthmatic attack, bladder neck obstruction, pyloroduodenal obstruction, third trimester of pregnancy, lactation.
- Use cautiously in pregnancy, geriatric patients.

Available forms
Chewable tablets—2 mg; tablets—4 mg; ER tablets ⓄⓉⒸ—8, 12, 16 mg; syrup—2 mg/5 mL; SR capsules ⓄⓉⒸ—8, 12 mg; ER capsules ⓄⓉⒸ—12 mg; caplets—8 mg

Dosages
Adults and children older than 12 yr
Tablets or syrup
4 mg PO every 4–6 hr; do not exceed 24 mg in 24 hr.

SR
8–12 mg PO at bedtime or every 8–12 hr during the day; do not exceed 24 mg in 24 hr.
ER (Efidac 24)
16 mg with liquid PO every 24 hr.
ER capsules
12 mg/day PO; do not exceed 24 mg/day.
Caplets
8–12 mg/day PO every 12 hr.
Pediatric patients
Tablets or syrup
Younger than 6 yr: Consult health care provider.
6–12 yr: 2 mg every 4–6 hr PO; do not exceed 12 mg in 24 hr.
SR
Younger than 6 yr: Not recommended.
6–12 yr: 8 mg PO at bedtime or during the day.
Geriatric patients
More likely to cause dizziness, sedation, syncope, toxic confusional states, and hypotension in elderly patients; use with caution.

Pharmacokinetics

Route	Onset	Peak
Oral	0.5–6 hr	2–6 hr

Metabolism: Hepatic; $T_{1/2}$: 12–15 hr
Distribution: Crosses placenta; may enter breast milk
Excretion: Urine

Adverse effects
- **CNS:** *Drowsiness, sedation, dizziness, disturbed coordination,* fatigue, confusion, restlessness, excitation, nervousness, tremor, headache, blurred vision, diplopia, vertigo, tinnitus, acute labyrinthitis, hysteria, tingling, heaviness and weakness of the hands
- **CV:** Hypotension, palpitations, bradycardia, tachycardia, extrasystoles
- **GI:** *Epigastric distress,* anorexia, increased appetite and weight gain, nausea, vomiting, diarrhea, or constipation
- **GU:** Urinary frequency, dysuria, urinary retention, early menses, decreased libido, impotence
- **Hematologic:** Hemolytic anemia, **aplastic anemia,** thrombocytopenia, leukopenia, **agranulocytosis,** pancytopenia
- **Respiratory:** *Thickening of bronchial secretions,* chest tightness, wheezing, nasal

stuffiness, dry mouth, dry nose, dry throat, sore throat
- **Other:** Urticaria, rash, **anaphylactic shock,** photosensitivity, excessive perspiration, chills

Interactions
✳ **Drug-drug** • Increased depressant effects with alcohol, other CNS depressants

■ **Nursing considerations**
Assessment
- **History:** Allergy to any antihistamines; narrow-angle glaucoma, stenosing peptic ulcer, symptomatic prostatic hypertrophy, asthmatic attack, bladder neck obstruction, pyloroduodenal obstruction, pregnancy, lactation
- **Physical:** Skin color, lesions, texture; orientation, reflexes, affect; vision examination; P, BP; R, adventitious sounds; bowel sounds; prostate palpation; CBC with differential

Interventions
- Administer with food if GI upset occurs.
- Caution patient not to crush or chew SR or ER preparations.
- Arrange for periodic blood tests during prolonged therapy.

Teaching points
- Take as prescribed; avoid excessive dosage. Take with food if GI upset occurs; do not cut, crush, or chew the sustained-release or extended-release preparations.
- Avoid over-the-counter drugs; many contain ingredients that could cause serious reactions if taken with this antihistamine.
- Avoid alcohol; serious sedation may occur.
- You may experience these side effects: Dizziness, sedation, drowsiness (use caution driving or performing tasks that require alertness); epigastric distress, diarrhea, or constipation (take with meals; consult your health care provider if severe); dry mouth (frequent mouth care, sucking sugarless candies may help); thickening of bronchial secretions, dryness of nasal mucosa (use a humidifier).
- Report difficulty breathing; hallucinations, tremors, loss of coordination; unusual bleeding or bruising; visual disturbances; irregular heartbeat.

▷ chlorproMAZINE hydrochloride

(klor proe' ma zeen)

Novo-Chlorpromazine (CAN)

PREGNANCY CATEGORY C

Drug classes
Antiemetic
Antipsychotic
Anxiolytic
Dopaminergic blocker
Phenothiazine

Therapeutic actions
Mechanism not fully understood; antipsychotic drugs block postsynaptic dopamine receptors in the brain; depress those parts of the brain involved with wakefulness and emesis; anticholinergic, antihistaminic (H_1), and alpha-adrenergic blocking.

Indications
- Management of manifestations of psychotic disorders; control of manic phase of manic-depressive illness; treatment of schizophrenia
- Relief of preoperative restlessness and apprehension
- Adjunct in treatment of tetanus
- Acute intermittent porphyria therapy
- Severe behavioral problems in children
- Therapy for combativeness, hyperactivity
- Control of nausea and vomiting, intractable hiccups

Contraindications and cautions
- Contraindicated with allergy to chlorpromazine, comatose or severely depressed states, bone marrow depression, circulatory collapse, subcortical brain damage, Parkinson disease, liver damage, cerebral or coronary arteriosclerosis, severe hypotension or hypertension.
- Use cautiously with respiratory disorders; glaucoma; epilepsy or history of epilepsy; peptic ulcer or history of peptic ulcer; decreased renal function; prostate hypertrophy; breast cancer; thyrotoxicosis; myelography within 24 hr or scheduled within 48 hr; lactation; exposure to heat, phosphorous insecticides; children with chickenpox, CNS infections (makes children more susceptible to dystonias, confounding the diagnosis of

Reye syndrome or other encephalopathy; antiemetic effects of drug may mask symptoms of Reye syndrome, encephalopathies); pregnancy, lactation.

Available forms
Tablets—10, 25, 50, 100, 200 mg; injection—25 mg/mL

Dosages
Full clinical antipsychotic effects may require 6 wk to 6 mo of therapy.

Adults
- *Excessive anxiety, agitation in psychiatric patients, schizophrenia:* 25 mg IM; may repeat in 1 hr with 25–50 mg IM. Increase dosage gradually in inpatients, up to 400 mg every 4–6 hr. Switch to oral dosage as soon as possible, 25–50 mg PO tid for outpatients; up to 2,000 mg/day PO for inpatients. Initial oral dosage, 10 mg tid–qid PO or 25 mg PO bid–tid; increase daily dosage by 20–50 mg semiweekly until optimum dosage is reached (maximum response may require months); doses of 200–800 mg/day PO are not uncommon in discharged mental patients.
- *Surgery:* Preoperatively, 25–50 mg PO 2–3 hr before surgery or 12.5–25 mg IM 1–2 hr before surgery; intraoperatively, 12.5 mg IM, repeated in 30 min or 2 mg IV repeated every 2 min up to 25 mg total to control vomiting (if no hypotension occurs); postoperatively, 10–25 mg PO every 4–6 hr or 12.5–25 mg IM repeated in 1 hr (if no hypotension occurs).
- *Acute intermittent porphyria:* 25–50 mg PO or 25 mg IM tid–qid until patient can take oral therapy.
- *Tetanus:* 25–50 mg IM tid–qid, usually with barbiturates, or 25–50 mg IV diluted and infused at rate of 1 mg/min.
- *Antiemetic:* 10–25 mg PO every 4–6 hr; 25 mg IM as a single dose. If no hypotension, give 25–50 mg every 3–4 hr. Switch to oral dose when vomiting ends.
- *Intractable hiccups:* 25–50 mg PO tid–qid. If symptoms persist for 2–3 days, give 25–50 mg IM; if inadequate response, give 25–50 mg IV in 500–1,000 mL of saline with BP monitoring and administer to patient flat in bed.

Pediatric patients 6 mo–12 yr
Generally not used in children younger than 6 mo.

Adverse effects in *italics* are most common; those in **bold** are life-threatening. ⬛ Do not crush.

C

- *Psychiatric outpatients:* 0.55 mg/kg PO every 4–6 hr; 0.55 mg/kg IM every 6–8 hr, not to exceed 40 mg/day (up to 5 yr) or 75 mg/day (5–12 yr).
- *Surgery:* Preoperatively, 0.55 mg/kg PO 2–3 hr before surgery or 0.55 mg/kg IM 1–2 hr before surgery; intraoperatively, 0.25 mg/kg IM or 1 mg (diluted) IV, repeated at 2-min intervals up to total IM dose; postoperatively, 0.55 mg/kg PO every 4–6 hr or 0.55 mg/kg IM, repeated in 1 hr if no hypotension.
- *Psychiatric inpatients:* 50–100 mg/day PO; maximum of 40 mg/day IM for children up to 5 yr; maximum of 75 mg/day IM for children 5–12 yr.
- *Tetanus:* 0.55 mg/kg IM every 6–8 hr or 0.5 mg/min IV, not to exceed 40 mg/day for children up to 23 kg; 75 mg/day for children 23–45 kg.
- *Antiemetic:* 0.55 mg/kg PO every 4–6 hr; or 0.55 mg/kg IM every 6–8 hr. Maximum IM dosage, 40 mg/day for children up to 5 yr or 75 mg/day for children 5–12 yr.

Geriatric patients
Start dosage at lower doses than those given in younger adults and increase more gradually.

Pharmacokinetics

Route	Onset	Peak	Duration
Oral	30–60 min	2–4 hr	4–6 hr
IM	10–15 min	15–20 min	4–6 hr

Metabolism: Hepatic, $T_{1/2}$: 2 hr, then 30 hr
Distribution: Crosses placenta; enters breast milk
Excretion: Urine

▼ IV FACTS

Preparation: Dilute drug for IV injection to a concentration of 1 mg/mL or less.
Injection: Reserve IV injections for hiccups, tetanus, or use during surgery. Administer at a rate of 1 mg/min for adults, 0.5 mg/min for children.
Incompatibilities: Precipitate or discoloration may occur when mixed with morphine, meperidine, cresols.

Adverse effects

- **CNS:** *Drowsiness,* insomnia, *vertigo,* headache, weakness, tremors, ataxia, slurring, cerebral edema, seizures, exacerbation of psychotic symptoms, *extrapyramidal syn-*dromes, **neuroleptic malignant syndrome,** tardive dyskinesia
- **CV:** *Hypotension, orthostatic hypotension,* hypertension, tachycardia, bradycardia, **cardiac arrest, heart failure, cardiomegaly,** refractory arrhythmias, **pulmonary edema**
- **EENT:** Nasal congestion, glaucoma, *photophobia, blurred vision,* miosis, mydriasis, deposits in the cornea and lens, pigmentary retinopathy
- **Endocrine:** Lactation; breast engorgement in females; galactorrhea; SIADH; amenorrhea; menstrual irregularities; gynecomastia; changes in libido; hyperglycemia; inhibition of ovulation; infertility; pseudopregnancy; reduced urinary levels of gonadotropins, estrogens, and progestins
- **GI:** *Dry mouth, salivation, nausea, vomiting, anorexia, constipation,* paralytic ileus, incontinence
- **GU:** *Urinary retention,* polyuria, incontinence, priapism, ejaculation inhibition, male impotence, urine discolored pink to red-brown
- **Hematologic:** Eosinophilia, leukopenia, leukocytosis, anemia, **aplastic anemia,** hemolytic anemia, thrombocytopenic or nonthrombocytopenic purpura, pancytopenia, elevated serum cholesterol
- **Hypersensitivity:** Jaundice, *urticaria,* angioneurotic edema, laryngeal edema, photosensitivity, eczema, asthma, **anaphylactoid reactions,** exfoliative dermatitis, contact dermatitis
- **Respiratory: Bronchospasm, laryngospasm,** dyspnea, suppression of cough reflex and potential aspiration
- **Other:** Fever, heatstroke, pallor, flushed facies, sweating, *photosensitivity*

Interactions

✳ **Drug-drug** • Additive anticholinergic effects and possibly decreased antipsychotic efficacy with anticholinergic drugs • Additive CNS depression, hypotension if given preoperatively with barbiturate anesthetics, alcohol, meperidine • Additive effects of both drugs if taken concurrently with beta blockers • Increased risk of tachycardia, hypotension with epinephrine, norepinephrine

✳ **Drug-lab test** • False-positive pregnancy tests (less likely if serum test is used) • Increase in protein-bound iodine, not attributable to an increase in thyroxine • False positive on PKU test

■ Nursing considerations

CLINICAL ALERT!
Name confusion has occurred between chlorpromazine, chlorpropamide, and clomipramine; use caution.

Assessment

• **History:** Allergy to chlorpromazine; comatose or severely depressed states; bone marrow depression; circulatory collapse; subcortical brain damage, Parkinson disease; liver damage; cerebral or coronary arteriosclerosis; severe hypotension or hypertension; respiratory disorders; glaucoma; epilepsy or history of epilepsy; peptic ulcer or history of peptic ulcer; decreased renal function; prostate hypertrophy; breast cancer; thyrotoxicosis; myelography within 24 hr or scheduled within 48 hr; lactation; exposure to heat, phosphorous insecticides; children with chickenpox; CNS infections; pregnancy, lactation.

• **Physical:** T; weight; skin color, turgor; reflexes, orientation, IOP, ophthalmologic examination; P, BP, orthostatic BP, ECG; R, adventitious sounds; bowel sounds, normal output, liver evaluation; prostate palpation, normal urine output; CBC; urinalysis; thyroid, LFTs, renal function tests; EEG

Interventions

⊗ *Black box warning* Increased risk of mortality in elderly patients with dementia-related psychosis; not approved for treatment of elderly patients with dementia-related psychosis.

• Do not give by subcutaneous injection; give slowly by deep IM injection into upper outer quadrant of buttock.

• Keep patient recumbent for 30 min after injection to avoid orthostatic hypotension.

• If giving drug via continuous infusion for intractable hiccups, keep patient flat in bed during infusion and monitor BP.

• Avoid skin contact with parenteral drug solutions due to possible contact dermatitis.

• Patient or the patient's guardian should be advised about the possibility of tardive dyskinesias.

⊗ *Warning* Be alert to potential for aspiration because of suppressed cough reflex.

• Monitor renal function tests; discontinue if serum creatinine or BUN becomes abnormal.

• Monitor CBC; discontinue if WBC count is depressed.

• Consult with physician about dosage reduction or use of anticholinergic antiparkinsonian drugs (controversial) if extrapyramidal effects occur.

• Withdraw drug gradually after high-dose therapy; possible gastritis, nausea, dizziness, headache, tachycardia, insomnia after abrupt withdrawal.

• Monitor elderly patients for dehydration; sedation and decreased sensation of thirst; CNS effects can lead to dehydration, hemoconcentration, and reduced pulmonary ventilation; promptly institute remedial measures.

• Avoid epinephrine as vasopressor if drug-induced hypotension occurs.

Teaching points

• Take drug exactly as prescribed. Avoid over-the-counter drugs and alcohol unless you have consulted your health care provider.

• Use caution in hot weather; risk of heatstroke; keep up fluid intake, and do not overexercise in a hot climate.

• You may experience these side effects: Drowsiness (avoid driving or operating dangerous machinery; avoid alcohol, which increases drowsiness); sensitivity to the sun (avoid prolonged sun exposure, wear protective garments or use a sunscreen); pink or reddish brown urine (expected effect); faintness, dizziness (change position slowly; use caution climbing stairs; usually transient).

• Report sore throat, fever, unusual bleeding or bruising, rash, weakness, tremors, impaired vision, dark urine, pale stools, yellowing of the skin and eyes.

▽ **chlorproPAMIDE**

See Appendix R, *Less commonly used drugs.*

▽ **chlorthalidone**
(klor thal' i done)

Apo-Chlorthalidone (CAN), Thalitone

PREGNANCY CATEGORY B

Drug class
Thiazide-like diuretic

Adverse effects in *italics* are most common; those in **bold** are life-threatening. ⬛ Do not crush.

Therapeutic actions

Inhibits reabsorption of sodium and chloride in distal renal tubule, increasing excretion of sodium, chloride, and water by the kidneys.

Indications

- Adjunctive therapy in edema associated with heart failure, cirrhosis, corticosteroid and estrogen therapy, renal impairment
- Hypertension, alone or with other antihypertensives
- Unlabeled use: Pediatric hypertension

Contraindications and cautions

- Contraindicated with anuria, renal failure, allergy to any thiazides or sulfonamides, hepatic coma.
- Use cautiously with fluid or electrolyte imbalances, renal or hepatic disease, gout, SLE, glucose tolerance abnormalities, hyperparathyroidism, manic-depressive disorders, lactation, pregnancy.

Available forms

Tablets—15, 25, 50, 100 mg

Dosages
Adults

- *Edema:* 50–100 mg/day PO or 100 mg PO every other day; up to 200 mg/day. Or 30–60 mg/day PO or 60 mg PO every other day, up to 120 mg/day. (*Thalitone*)
- *Hypertension:* Initiate with 25 mg/day; if response is insufficient, increase to 50 mg/day. If additional control is needed, increase to 100 mg/day or add a second antihypertensive. Increases in serum uric acid and decreases in serum potassium are dose-related over the 25–100 mg/day range. Or 15 mg/day PO, may be increased to 30, 45, or 50 mg/day as a single dose (*Thalitone*); if control is still not achieved, add a second antihypertensive.

Pediatric patients
Safety and efficacy not established.

Pharmacokinetics

Route	Onset	Peak	Duration
Oral	2–3 hr	2–6 hr	24–72 hr

Metabolism: Eliminated primarily as unchanged drug; $T_{1/2}$: 40–60 hr
Distribution: Crosses placenta; enters breast milk
Excretion: Urine

Adverse effects

- **CNS:** *Dizziness, vertigo,* paresthesias, weakness, headache, drowsiness, fatigue
- **CV:** Orthostatic hypotension, venous thrombosis, volume depletion, cardiac arrhythmias, chest pain
- **Dermatologic:** Photosensitivity, rash, purpura, exfoliative dermatitis
- **GI:** *Nausea, anorexia, vomiting, dry mouth, diarrhea, constipation,* jaundice, hepatitis, pancreatitis
- **GU:** *Polyuria, nocturia, impotence,* loss of libido
- **Hematologic:** Leukopenia, thrombocytopenia, **agranulocytosis, aplastic anemia,** neutropenia, fluid and electrolyte imbalances
- **Other:** Muscle cramps and muscle spasms, fever, hives, gouty attacks, flushing, weight loss

Interactions

⁑ **Drug-drug** • Increased thiazide effects and chance of acute hyperglycemia with diazoxide • Decreased absorption with cholestyramine, colestipol • Increased risk of cardiac glycoside toxicity if hypokalemia occurs • Increased risk of lithium toxicity • Increased dosage of antidiabetics may be needed

⁑ **Drug-lab test** • Decreased PBI levels without clinical signs of thyroid disturbances

■ Nursing considerations
Assessment

- **History:** Fluid or electrolyte imbalances, renal or hepatic disease, gout, SLE, glucose tolerance abnormalities, hyperparathyroidism, bipolar disorder, lactation, allergy to thiazides or sulfonamides, pregnancy
- **Physical:** Skin color and lesions; orientation, reflexes, muscle strength; pulses, BP, orthostatic BP, perfusion, edema, baseline ECG; R, adventitious sounds; liver evaluation, bowel sounds; CBC, serum electrolytes, blood glucose, LFTs, renal function tests, serum uric acid, urinalysis

Interventions

⊗ *Warning* Differentiate between *Thalitone* and other preparations; dosage varies.
- Give with food or milk if GI upset occurs.
- Administer early in the day, so increased urination will not disturb sleep.
- Mark calendars or other reminders of drug days for outpatients on every other day or 3- to 5-day/wk therapy.

- Measure and record weight to monitor fluid changes.

Teaching points
- Take drug early in the day, so your sleep will not be disturbed by increased urination.
- Weigh yourself daily, and record weights.
- Protect skin from exposure to the sun or bright lights.
- Increased urination will occur.
- You may experience these side effects: Dizziness, drowsiness, feeling faint (use caution).
- Report rapid weight change, swelling in ankles or fingers, unusual bleeding or bruising, muscle cramps.

▷ chlorzoxazone
(klor zox' a zone)

Paraflex, Parafon Forte DSC, Remular-S

PREGNANCY CATEGORY C

Drug class
Skeletal muscle relaxant (centrally acting)

Therapeutic actions
Precise mechanism not known; has sedative properties; acts at spinal and supraspinal levels of the CNS to depress reflex arcs involved in producing and maintaining skeletal muscle spasm.

Indications
- Relief of discomfort associated with acute, painful musculoskeletal conditions, adjunct to rest, physical therapy, and other measures

Contraindications and cautions
- Contraindicated with allergic or idiosyncratic reactions to chlorzoxazone.
- Use cautiously with history of allergies or allergic drug reactions, lactation, pregnancy.

Available forms
Tablets—250, 375, 500, 750 mg

Dosages
Adults
Usual dose, 250 mg PO tid–qid; painful conditions may require 500 mg PO tid–qid; may increase to 750 mg tid–qid; reduce dosage as improvement occurs.

Pediatric patients
Safety and efficacy not established.

Pharmacokinetics

Route	Onset	Peak	Duration
Oral	30–60 min	1–2 hr	3–4 hr

Metabolism: Hepatic; $T_{1/2}$: 60 min
Distribution: Crosses placenta; may enter breast milk
Excretion: Urine

Adverse effects
- **CNS:** *Dizziness, light-headedness, drowsiness,* malaise, overstimulation
- **GI:** *GI disturbances,* GI bleeding (rare)
- **GU:** Urine discoloration (orange to purple-red)
- **Hypersensitivity:** Rashes, petechiae, ecchymoses, angioneurotic edema, **anaphylaxis** (rare)

Interactions
✳ **Drug-drug** • Additive CNS effects with alcohol, other CNS depressants

■ Nursing considerations
Assessment
- **History:** Allergic or idiosyncratic reactions to chlorzoxazone; history of allergies or allergic drug reactions; lactation, pregnancy
- **Physical:** Skin color, lesions; orientation; liver evaluation; LFTs

Interventions
⊗ *Warning* Discontinue if signs or symptoms of hepatic impairment or allergic reaction (urticaria, redness, or itching) occur.
- Institute rest, physical therapy, and other measures to relieve discomfort.

Teaching points
- Take this drug exactly as prescribed; do not take a higher dosage.
- Avoid alcohol and sleep-inducing or over-the-counter drugs; these could cause dangerous effects.
- You may experience these side effects: Drowsiness, dizziness, light-headedness (avoid driving or engaging in activities that require alertness); nausea (take with food and eat frequent small meals); discolored urine (expected effect).

Adverse effects in *italics* are most common; those in **bold** are life-threatening. ▣ Do not crush.

- Report rash, severe nausea, coffee-ground vomitus, black or tarry stools, pale stools, yellow skin or eyes, difficulty breathing.

▽cholestyramine
(koe less' tir a meen)

Cholestyramine Light,
PMS-Cholestyramine (CAN), Prevalite,
Questran, Questran Light

PREGNANCY CATEGORY C

Drug classes
Antihyperlipidemic
Bile acid sequestrant

Therapeutic actions
Binds bile acids in the intestine, allowing excretion in the feces; as a result, cholesterol is oxidized in the liver to replace the bile acids lost; serum cholesterol and LDL are lowered.

Indications
- Adjunctive therapy: Reduction of elevated serum cholesterol in patients with primary hypercholesterolemia (elevated LDL)
- Pruritus associated with partial biliary obstruction
- Unlabeled uses: Antibiotic-induced pseudomembranous colitis, treatment of thyroid hormone overdose, treatment of digitalis toxicity, treatment of certain diarrheas including *Clostridium difficile* (binds to toxins in the intestine), hyperoxaluria

Contraindications and cautions
- Contraindicated with allergy to bile acid sequestrants, tartrazine (tartrazine sensitivity occurs often with allergies to aspirin); complete biliary obstruction.
- Use cautiously with abnormal intestinal function, pregnancy, lactation.

Available forms
Powder for suspension—4 g per packet or scoopful

Dosages
Adults
Initially, 4 g one to two times per day PO. In patients with constipation, start with 4 g once/day. Individualize dose based on response. For maintenance, 8–16 g/day divided into two doses. Increase dose gradually with periodic assessment of lipid/lipoprotein levels at intervals of at least 4 wk. Maximum dose 6 packets or scoopfuls. May be administered 1–6 doses/day. Maximum dose, 24 g/day.
Pediatric patients
240 mg/kg/day in 2–3 divided doses, not to exceed 8 g/day. Dose is based on anhydrous cholestyramine resin. Optimal dose schedule has not been established.

Pharmacokinetics
Not absorbed systemically
Excretion: Feces

Adverse effects
- **CNS:** Headache, anxiety, vertigo, dizziness, fatigue, syncope, drowsiness
- **Dermatologic:** Rash and irritation of skin, tongue, perianal area
- **GI:** *Constipation* to *fecal impaction, exacerbation of hemorrhoids,* abdominal cramps, pain, flatulence, anorexia, heartburn, nausea, vomiting, steatorrhea
- **GU:** Hematuria, dysuria, diuresis
- **Hematologic:** *Increased bleeding tendencies related to vitamin K malabsorption,* vitamins A and D deficiencies, reduced serum and red cell folate, hyperchloremic acidosis
- **Other:** Osteoporosis, backache, muscle and joint pain, arthritis, fever

Interactions
✳ **Drug-drug** ● Decreased or delayed absorption with warfarin, thiazide diuretics, digitalis preparations, thyroid, corticosteroids ● Malabsorption of fat-soluble vitamins with cholestyramine

■ Nursing considerations
Assessment
- **History:** Allergy to bile acid sequestrants, tartrazine; complete biliary obstruction; abnormal intestinal function; lactation, pregnancy
- **Physical:** Skin lesions, color, T; orientation, affect, reflexes; P, auscultation, baseline ECG, peripheral perfusion; liver evaluation, bowel sounds; lipid studies, LFTs, clotting profile

Interventions

- Mix contents of one packet or one level scoop of powder with 2–6 fluid oz of beverage (water, milk, fruit juices, noncarbonates), highly fluid soup, pulpy fruits (applesauce, pineapple); do not give drug in dry form.
- Administer drug before meals.

⊗ *Warning* Monitor intake of other oral drugs due to risk of binding in the intestine and delayed or decreased absorption; give oral medications 1 hr before or 4–6 hr after the cholestyramine.

- Alert patient about potentially high cost of drug.

Teaching points

- Take drug before meals; do not take the powder in the dry form; mix one packet or one scoop with 2–6 ounces of fluid—water, milk, juice, noncarbonated drinks, highly fluid soups, cereals, pulpy fruits such as applesauce or pineapple.
- Take other medications 1 hour before or 4–6 hours after cholestyramine.
- You may experience these side effects: Constipation (ask about measures that may help); nausea, heartburn, loss of appetite (eat frequent small meals); dizziness, drowsiness, vertigo, fainting (avoid driving and operating dangerous machinery); headache, muscle and joint aches and pains (may lessen with time).
- Report unusual bleeding or bruising, severe constipation, severe GI upset, chest pain, difficulty breathing, rash, fever.

▷ **choline magnesium trisalicylate**

See Appendix R, *Less commonly used drugs*.

▷ **chorionic gonadotropin (human chorionic gonadotropin, HCG)**

*(kor e **awn** ick goe **nad'** oh troe pin)*

Novarel, Pregnyl

PREGNANCY CATEGORY X

Drug class

Hormone

Therapeutic actions

A human placental hormone with actions identical to pituitary LH; stimulates production of testosterone and progesterone.

Indications

- Prepubertal cryptorchidism not due to anatomic obstruction
- Treatment of selected cases of hypogonadotropic hypogonadism in males
- Induction of ovulation in the anovulatory, infertile woman in whom the cause of anovulation is secondary and not due to primary ovarian failure and who has been pretreated with human menotropins

Contraindications and cautions

- Contraindicated with known sensitivity to chorionic gonadotropin, precocious puberty, prostatic carcinoma or androgen-dependent neoplasm, pregnancy.
- Use cautiously with epilepsy, migraine, asthma, cardiac or renal disease, lactation.

Available forms

Powder for injection—5,000, 10,000, 20,000 units/vial with 10 mL diluent

Dosages
Patients older than 4 yr
For IM use only; individualize dosage; the following dosage regimens are suggested:

- *Prepubertal cryptorchidism not due to anatomic obstruction:* 4,000 USP units IM, three times per week for 3 wk; 5,000 USP units IM, every second day for 4 injections; 15 injections of 500–1,000 USP units over 6 wk; 500 USP units three times per week for 4–6 wk; if not successful, start another course 1 mo later, giving 1,000 USP units/injection.
- *Hypogonadotropic hypogonadism in males:* 500–1,000 USP units, IM three times per week for 3 wk; followed by the same dose twice a week for 3 wk; 1,000–2,000 USP units IM three times per week; 4,000 USP units three times per week for 6–9 mo; reduce dosage to 2,000 USP units three times per week for an additional 3 mo.
- *Induction of ovulation and pregnancy:* 5,000–10,000 units IM, 1 day following the last dose of menotropins.

Pediatric patients
Safety and efficacy in children younger than 4 yr have not been established.

Adverse effects in *italics* are most common; those in **bold** are life-threatening. ▭ Do not crush.

Pharmacokinetics

Route	Onset	Peak
IM	2 hr	6 hr

Metabolism: Hepatic; T$_{1/2}$: 23 hr
Distribution: Crosses placenta; may enter breast milk
Excretion: Urine

Adverse effects

- **CNS:** *Headache, irritability, restlessness,* depression, fatigue
- **CV:** Edema, arterial thromboembolism
- **Endocrine:** *Precocious puberty, gynecomastia,* ovarian hyperstimulation (sudden ovarian enlargement, ascites, rupture of ovarian cysts, multiple births)
- **Other:** *Pain at injection site,* **ovarian malignancy**

■ Nursing considerations

Assessment

- **History:** Sensitivity to chorionic gonadotropin, precocious puberty, prostatic carcinoma or androgen-dependent neoplasm, epilepsy, migraine, asthma, cardiac or renal disease, lactation, pregnancy
- **Physical:** Skin texture, edema; prostate examination; injection site; sexual development; orientation, affect, reflexes; R, adventitious sounds; P, auscultation, BP, peripheral edema; liver evaluation; renal function tests

Interventions

⊗ **Black box warning** Be aware that this drug has no known effect on fat metabolism and is not for treatment of obesity.

- Prepare solution for injection using manufacturer's instructions; brand and concentrations vary.

⊗ **Warning** Discontinue at any sign of ovarian overstimulation, and have patient admitted to the hospital for observation and supportive measures.

- Provide comfort measures for CNS effects, pain at injection site.

Teaching points

- This drug can only be given IM. Prepare a calendar with a treatment schedule. If you will be giving the drug at home, learn proper administration and disposal of needles and syringes.

- You may experience these side effects: Headache, irritability, restlessness, depression, fatigue (reversible; if uncomfortable, consult your health care provider).
- Report pain at injection site, severe headache, restlessness, swelling of ankles or fingers, difficulty breathing, severe abdominal pain.

▽ chorionic gonadotropin alfa

See Appendix R, *Less commonly used drugs.*

▽ cidofovir

See Appendix R, *Less commonly used drugs.*

▽ cilostazol

*(sill **abs'** tah zoll)*

Pletal

PREGNANCY CATEGORY C

Drug class

Antiplatelet

Therapeutic actions

Reversibly inhibits platelet aggregation induced by a variety of stimuli including ADP, thrombin, collagen, shear stress, epinephrine, and arachidonic acid by inhibiting cAMP phosphodiesterase III; produces vascular dilation in vascular beds with a specificity for femoral beds; seems to have no effect on renal arteries.

Indications

- Reduction of symptoms of intermittent claudication allowing increased walking distance

Contraindications and cautions

- Contraindicated with allergy to cilostazol, heart failure of any severity (decreased survival rates have occurred), active bleeding, hemostatic disorders.
- Use cautiously with pregnancy, lactation, renal dysfunction.

Available forms

Tablets—50, 100 mg

Dosages
Adults
100 mg PO bid taken at least 30 min before or 2 hr after breakfast and dinner. Response may not be noted for 2–4 wk and may take up to 12 wk.
Pediatric patients
Safety and efficacy not established.

Pharmacokinetics

Route	Onset	Peak
Oral	Gradual	4–6 hr

Metabolism: Hepatic; $T_{1/2}$: 11–13 hr
Distribution: Crosses placenta; may enter breast milk
Excretion: Urine

Adverse effects
- **CNS:** *Dizziness, headaches*
- **CV: Heart failure,** tachycardia, *palpitations*
- **GI:** *Diarrhea, nausea, flatulence, dyspepsia*
- **Respiratory:** Cough, pharyngitis, *rhinitis*
- **Other:** Peripheral edema, infection, back pain

Interactions
✳ **Drug-drug** • Increased serum levels and risk of toxic effects of cilostazol if combined with macrolide antibiotics, diltiazem, azole antifungals (itraconazole, ketoconazole), or omeprazole; if this combination is used, consider decreasing cilostazol dose to 50 mg bid and monitor patient closely • Smoking decreased cilostazol exposure by 20%

✳ **Drug-food** • Increased absorption if taken with high-fat meal; administer drug at least 30 min before or 2 hr after meals • Increased serum levels and risk of adverse effects if combined with grapefruit juice; avoid grapefruit juice if taking this drug

■ Nursing considerations
Assessment
- **History:** Allergy to cilostazol, heart failure, lactation, CV disorders, pregnancy
- **Physical:** Skin color, lesions; orientation; bowel sounds, normal output; P, BP; R, adventitious sounds; CBC, LFTs, renal function tests

Interventions
⊗ **Black box warning** Do not administer to patients with heart failure; decreased survival has been reported.

- Administer drug on an empty stomach, at least 30 min before or 2 hr after breakfast and dinner.
- Encourage patient to avoid the use of grapefruit juice.
- Establish baseline walking distance to monitor drug effectiveness.
- ⊗ **Warning** Establish safety precautions to prevent injury and bleeding (eg, tell patient to use an electric razor, avoid contact sports).
- Advise patient to use barrier contraceptives while receiving this drug; potentially, it could harm the fetus.
- Encourage patient to continue therapy; results may not be seen for 2–4 wk and in some cases may take up to 12 wk.
- Advise patient that the CV risks associated with this drug are not known; potentially serious CV effects have occurred in laboratory animals but drug has been successfully used in patients with CAD.

Teaching points
- Take drug on an empty stomach at least 30 minutes before or 2 hours after breakfast and dinner.
- Avoid drinking grapefruit juice while you are taking this drug.
- The therapeutic effects of this drug may not be seen for 2–4 weeks and may take up to 12 weeks.
- Avoid pregnancy while taking this drug; it could potentially harm the fetus. Use barrier contraceptives; notify your health care provider immediately if you think you are pregnant.
- You may experience these side effects: Upset stomach, nausea, diarrhea, loss of appetite (eat frequent small meals).
- Report fever, chills, sore throat, palpitations, chest pain, edema or swelling, difficulty breathing, fatigue, bleeding, or bruising.

▽ **cimetidine**
*(sye **met**' i deen)*

Apo-Cimetidine (CAN), Gen-Cimetidine (CAN), Nu-Cimet (CAN), Tagamet, Tagamet HB, Tagamet HB Suspension

PREGNANCY CATEGORY B

Adverse effects in *italics* are most common; those in **bold** are life-threatening. ⊞ Do not crush.

Drug class
Histamine$_2$ (H$_2$) antagonist

Therapeutic actions
Inhibits the action of histamine at the H$_2$ receptors of the stomach, inhibiting gastric acid secretion and reducing total pepsin output.

Indications
- Short-term treatment and maintenance of active duodenal ulcer
- Short-term treatment of benign gastric ulcer
- Treatment of pathologic hypersecretory conditions (Zollinger-Ellison syndrome)
- Prophylaxis of stress-induced ulcers and acute upper GI bleeding in critical patients
- Treatment of erosive GERD
- OTC use: Relief of symptoms of heartburn, acid indigestion, sour stomach
- Unlabeled uses: Part of multidrug regimen for *Helicobacter pylori;* urticaria, warts, interstitial cystitis

Contraindications and cautions
- Contraindicated with allergy to cimetidine.
- Use cautiously with impaired renal or hepatic function, lactation, pregnancy.

Available forms
Tablets—200, 300, 400, 800 mg; liquid—300 mg/5 mL; injection—150 mg/mL; injection premixed—300 mg/50 mL

Dosages
Adults
- *Active duodenal ulcer:* 800 mg PO at bedtime or 300 mg PO qid with meals and at bedtime or 400 mg PO bid; continue for 4–6 wk unless healing is demonstrated by endoscopy. For intractable ulcers, 300 mg IM or IV every 6–8 hr.
- *Maintenance therapy for duodenal ulcer:* 400 mg PO at bedtime.
- *Active benign gastric ulcer:* 300 mg PO qid with meals and at bedtime or 800 mg at bedtime. Treat for 8 wk.
- *Pathologic hypersecretory syndrome:* 300 mg PO qid with meals and at bedtime, or 300 mg IV or IM every 6 hr. Individualize doses as needed; do not exceed 2,400 mg/day.
- *Erosive GERD:* 1,600 mg PO in divided doses bid–qid for 12 wk.

- *Prevention of upper GI bleeding:* Continuous IV infusion of 50 mg/hr. Do not treat beyond 7 days.
- *Heartburn, acid indigestion:* 200 mg as symptoms occur; up to 400 mg/24 hr. Do not take maximum dose for more than 2 wk.

Pediatric patients
Not recommended for children younger than 12 yr.

Geriatric patients or patients with impaired renal function
Accumulation may occur. Use lowest dose possible, 300 mg PO or IV every 12 hr; may be increased to every 8 hr if patient tolerates it and levels are monitored; if creatinine clearance is less than 30 mL/min, give half the recommended dose IV for prevention of upper GI bleed. Consider further dose reduction if concurrent hepatic impairment exists.

Pharmacokinetics

Route	Onset	Peak
Oral	Varies	1–1.5 hr
IV, IM	Rapid	1–1.5 hr

Metabolism: Hepatic; T$_{1/2}$: 2 hr
Distribution: Crosses placenta; enters breast milk
Excretion: Urine

▼ IV FACTS

Preparation: For IV injections, dilute in 0.9% sodium chloride injection, 5% or 10% dextrose injection, lactated Ringer solution, 5% sodium bicarbonate injection to a volume of 20 mL. Solution is stable for 48 hr at room temperature. For IV infusions, dilute 300 mg in at least 50 mL of 5% dextrose injection or one of above listed solutions.

Infusion: Inject by direct injection over not less than 5 min; by infusion, slowly over 15–20 min.

Incompatibilities: Incompatible with aminophylline, barbiturate in IV solutions; pentobarbital sodium and pentobarbital sodium and atropine in the same syringe.

Adverse effects
- **CNS:** *Dizziness, somnolence, headache, confusion, hallucinations,* peripheral neuropathy; symptoms of brain stem dysfunction (dysarthria, ataxia, diplopia)
- **CV:** Cardiac arrhythmias, **cardiac arrest,** hypotension (IV use)

- **GI:** *Diarrhea*
- **Hematologic:** Increases in plasma creatinine, serum transaminase
- **Other:** *Impotence* (reversible), gynecomastia (in long-term treatment), rash, vasculitis, pain at IM injection site

Interactions

✳ **Drug-drug** • Increased risk of decreased white blood cell counts with antimetabolites, alkylating agents, other drugs known to cause neutropenia • Increased serum levels and risk of toxicity of warfarin-type anticoagulants, phenytoin, beta-adrenergic blocking agents, alcohol, quinidine, lidocaine, theophylline, chloroquine, certain benzodiazepines (alprazolam, chlordiazepoxide, diazepam, flurazepam, triazolam), nifedipine, pentoxifylline, TCAs, carbamazepine when taken with cimetidine

■ Nursing considerations

Assessment

- **History:** Allergy to cimetidine, impaired renal or hepatic function, lactation
- **Physical:** Skin lesions; orientation, affect; pulse, baseline ECG (continuous with IV use); liver evaluation, abdominal examination, normal output; CBC, LFTs, renal function tests

Interventions

- Give drug with meals and at bedtime.
- Decrease doses in patients with renal and hepatic impairment.
- Administer IM dose undiluted deep into large muscle group.
- Arrange for regular follow-up, including blood tests to evaluate effects.

Teaching points

- Take drug with meals and at bedtime; therapy may continue for 4–6 weeks or longer.
- Take antacids as prescribed and at recommended times.
- Inform your health care provider about your cigarette smoking habits. Cigarette smoking decreases the drug's effectiveness.
- Have regular medical follow-up care to evaluate your response to drug.
- Tell your health care providers about all medications, over-the-counter drugs, or herbs you take; this drug may interact with many of these.

- Report sore throat, fever, unusual bruising or bleeding, tarry stools, confusion, hallucinations, dizziness, muscle or joint pain.

▷ **cinacalcet hydrochloride**
(sin ah kal' set)

Sensipar ⓞⓣⓒ

PREGNANCY CATEGORY C

Drug classes

Calcimimetic
Calcium-lowering drug

Therapeutic actions

Increases the sensitivity to extracellular calcium of the calcium-sensing receptors on the surface of the chief cell of the parathyroid gland, resulting in a decrease in parathyroid hormone secretion. The drop in parathyroid hormone level leads to a decrease in serum calcium levels.

Indications

- Secondary hyperparathyroidism in patients receiving dialysis for chronic renal disease
- Treatment of hypercalcemia in patients with parathyroid carcinoma
- Treatment of severe hypercalcemia in patients with primary hyperparathyroidism unable to have parathyroidectomy.

Contraindications and cautions

- Contraindicated with allergy to any component of the drug, lactation, hypocalcemia.
- Use cautiously with a history of seizure disorders, moderate to severe hepatic impairment, pregnancy.

Available forms

Tablets ⓞⓣⓒ—30, 60, 90 mg

Dosages

Adults

- *Secondary hyperparathyroidism:* 30 mg/day PO; monitor serum calcium and phosphorous levels within 1 wk after starting therapy and intact parathyroid hormone levels within 1–4 wk of starting therapy to adjust dosage to therapeutic level. May increase dose 30 mg every 2–4 wk to a maximum dose of 180 mg/day. Titrate to target intact parathyroid hormone levels of 150–300 pg/mL. May be combined with vitamin D and phosphate binders.

- *Hypercalcemia associated with parathyroid carcinoma or severe hypercalcemia in patients with primary hyperparathyroidism:* Initially 30 mg PO bid to maintain calcium levels within a normal range; may adjust dosage every 2–4 wk in sequential dosages of 60 mg bid, then 90 mg bid to a maximum dosage of 90 mg tid to qid.

Pediatric patients
Safety and efficacy not established.

Pharmacokinetics

Route	Onset	Peak
Oral	Slow	2–6 hr

Metabolism: Hepatic; $T_{1/2}$: 30–40 hr
Distribution: May cross placenta; may pass into breast milk
Excretion: Urine

Adverse effects

- **CNS:** Asthenia, *dizziness,* **seizures**
- **CV:** Chest pain, hypertension
- **GI:** Anorexia, diarrhea, *nausea, vomiting*
- **Other:** Adynamic bone disease, hypocalcemia, *myalgia*

Interactions

✳ **Drug-drug** ● Risk of increased amitriptyline levels if used concomitantly; monitor patient ● Risk of increased serum levels of flecainide, vinblastine, thioridazine, TCAs; if this combination is used, monitor patient and adjust dosage accordingly ● Risk of increased serum levels of cinacalcet and resulting hypocalcemia if combined with ketoconazole, erythromycin, itraconazole; monitor serum calcium levels carefully and adjust dosage accordingly

■ Nursing considerations
Assessment

- **History:** Allergy to any component of the drug, pregnancy, lactation, history of seizure disorders, moderate to severe hepatic impairment
- **Physical:** Orientation, reflexes; BP; abdominal examination; LFTs, renal function tests; serum calcium, phosphorous levels, intact parathyroid hormone levels

Interventions

- Monitor serum calcium levels before and regularly during therapy.

- Administer with food or shortly after a meal; ensure that patient does not cut, crush or chew the tablet.
- Suggest alternative method of feeding the infant if patient is breast-feeding; it is not known if this drug passes into breast milk, but it does cross in animal studies.
- Monitor patient's nutritional status as nausea, vomiting, and diarrhea are common.

Teaching points

- Take this drug with food or shortly after a meal.
- Do not cut, crush, or chew this tablet; it must be swallowed whole.
- If you miss a dose, take the dose as soon as you remember. Take the next dose the next day; do not make up or double doses.
- If you are taking this drug with hemodialysis, you will also be taking vitamin D and phosphate binders.
- If you are breast-feeding, choose a different method of feeding the baby while you are on this drug.
- You will need to have regular follow-ups, including blood tests to monitor your calcium levels while you are on this drug.
- You may experience these side effects: Dizziness, drowsiness (avoid driving or use of dangerous machinery while on this drug); nausea, vomiting, loss of appetite (it is important to try to maintain your nutrition and fluid intake; if this becomes a problem, consult your health care provider); confusion, hallucinations (it might help to know that this is a drug effect; consult your health care provider if this becomes a problem).
- Report muscle cramping, tingling, pain; fever, flulike symptoms, seizure activity.

▷ **ciprofloxacin**

(si proe flox' a sin)

Apo-Ciprofloxacin (CAN), Ciloxan, Cipro, Cipro HC Otic, Cipro I.V., Co Ciprofloxacin (CAN), Gen-Ciprofloxacin (CAN), PMS-Ciprofloxacin (CAN), Proquin XR ⓞⓡ, ratio-Ciprofloxacin (CAN)

PREGNANCY CATEGORY C

Drug classes
Antibacterial
Fluoroquinolone

Therapeutic actions
Bactericidal; interferes with DNA replication in susceptible bacteria preventing cell reproduction.

Indications
- For the treatment of infections caused by susceptible gram-negative bacteria, including *Escherichia coli, Proteus mirabilis, Klebsiella pneumoniae, Enterobacter cloacae, Proteus vulgaris, Proteus rettgeri, Morganella morganii, Pseudomonas aeruginosa, Citrobacter freundii, Staphylococcus aureus, Staphylococcus epidermidis,* group D streptococci, *Serratia marcescens* (such as chancroid, granuloma inguinale, infective endocarditis, plague, tularemia, multi-drug-resistant tuberculosis, disseminated gonorrhea); surgical, urologic, gynecologic procedure prophylaxis
- Treatment of uncomplicated UTIs caused by *E. coli, K. pneumoniae* as a one-time dose in patients at low risk of nausea, diarrhea (*Proquin XR*)
- Treatment of acute otitis externa (otic)
- Treatment of chronic bacterial prostatitis
- Treatment of nosocomial pneumonia caused by *Haemophilus influenzae, K. pneumoniae* (IV)
- Typhoid fever (oral)
- STDs caused by *Neisseria gonorrheae* (oral)
- Prevention of anthrax following exposure to anthrax bacillus (prophylactic use in regions suspected of using germ warfare)
- Acute sinusitis: Caused by *H. influenzae, Streptococcus pneumoniae,* or *Moraxella catarrhalis*
- Lower respiratory tract infections: Caused by *E. coli, Klebsiella, Enterobacter* species, *P. mirabilis, P. aeruginosa, H. influenzae, Haemophilus parainfluenzae, S. pneumoniae*
- Unlabeled uses: Cystic fibrosis in patients who have pulmonary exacerbations, gastroenteritis in children, mycobacterial infection, traveler's diarrhea

Contraindications and cautions
- Contraindicated with allergy to ciprofloxacin, norfloxacin or other fluoroquinolones, pregnancy, lactation.
- Use cautiously with renal impairment, seizures, tendinitis or tendon rupture associated with fluoroquinolone use.

Available forms
Tablets—100, 250, 500, 750 mg; ER tablets ⊙⊙⊙—500, 1,000 mg; injection—200, 400 mg; microcapsules for suspension—250, 500 mg; ophthalmic ointment—3.33 mg/g; ophthalmic solution—3.5 mg/mL; otic suspension—2 mg/mL; otic single-use container—0.25 mL

Dosages
Adults
- *Uncomplicated UTIs:* 250 mg PO every 12 hr for 3 days or 500 mg PO daily (ER tablets) for 3 days. *Proquin XR*—500 mg PO once a day for 3 days.
- *Mild to moderate UTIs:* 250 mg every 12 hr PO for 7–14 days or 200 mg IV every 12 hr for 7–14 days.
- *Complicated UTIs:* 500 mg every 12 hr PO for 7–14 days or 400 mg IV every 12 hr or 1,000 mg (ER tablets) PO daily every 7–14 days.
- *Chronic bacterial prostatitis:* 500 mg PO every 12 hr for 28 days or 400 mg IV every 12 hr for 28 days.
- *Infectious diarrhea:* 500 mg every 12 hr PO for 5–7 days.
- *Anthrax postexposure:* 500 mg PO every 12 hr for 60 days or 400 mg IV every 12 hr for 60 days.
- *Respiratory infections:* 500–750 mg PO every 12 hr or 400 mg IV every 8–12 hr for 7–14 days.
- *Acute sinusitis:* 500 mg PO every 12 hr or 400 mg IV every 12 hr for 10 days.
- *Acute uncomplicated pyelonephritis:* 1,000 mg ER tablets PO daily every 7–14 days.
- *Bone, joint, skin infections:* 500–750 mg PO every 12 hr or 400 mg IV every 8–12 hr for 4–6 wk.
- *Nosocomial pneumonia:* 400 mg IV every 8 hr for 10–14 days.
- *Ophthalmic infections caused by susceptible organisms not responsive to other therapy:* 1 or 2 drops every 2 hr while awake

for 2 days or every 4 hr for 5 days, or ½ inch ribbon of ointment into conjunctival sac tid on first 2 days, then apply ½ inch ribbon bid for next 5 days.

• *Acute otitis externa:* 4 drops in infected ear, tid–qid, or 1 single-use container (0.25 mL) in infected ear bid for 7 days.

Pediatric patients

⊗ *Warning* There is increased incidence of adverse reactions in children, including reactions to the joints and/or surrounding tissue.

⊗ *Warning* Safety and efficacy of ER tablets have not been established in children younger than 18 yr.

Inhalational anthrax: 15 mg/kg/dose PO every 12 hr for 60 days or 10 mg/kg/dose IV every 12 hr for 60 days; do not exceed 500 mg/dose PO or 400 mg/dose IV.

Patients with impaired renal function

For creatinine clearance of 30–50 mL/min, give 250–500 mg PO every 12 hr. For creatinine clearance of 5–29 mL/min, give 250–500 mg PO every 18 hr or 200–400 mg IV every 18–24 hr. For patients on peritoneal or hemodialysis, give 250–500 mg every 24 hr, after dialysis.

Pharmacokinetics

Route	Onset	Peak	Duration
Oral	Varies	60–90 min	4–5 hr
IV	10 min	30 min	4–5 hr

Metabolism: Hepatic; $T_{1/2}$: 3.5–4 hr
Distribution: Crosses placenta; enters breast milk
Excretion: Bile, urine

▼ IV FACTS

Preparation: Dilute to a final concentration of 1–2 mg/mL with 0.9% sodium chloride injection or 5% dextrose injection. Stable up to 14 days refrigerated or at room temperature.
Infusion: Administer slowly over 60 min.
Incompatibilities: Discontinue the administration of any other solutions during ciprofloxacin infusion. Incompatible with aminophylline, amoxicillin, clindamycin, heparin in solution.

Adverse effects

• **CNS:** *Headache,* dizziness, insomnia, fatigue, somnolence, depression, blurred vision, hallucinations, ataxia, nightmares

• **CV:** Arrhythmias, hypotension, angina
• **EENT:** Dry eye, eye pain, keratopathy
• **GI:** *Nausea,* vomiting, dry mouth, *diarrhea,* abdominal pain
• **GU:** Renal failure
• **Hematologic:** Elevated BUN, AST, ALT, serum creatinine and alkaline phosphatase; decreased WBC count, neutrophil count, Hct
• **Other:** Fever, rash

Interactions

✳ **Drug-drug** • Decreased therapeutic effect with iron salts, sucralfate • Decreased absorption with antacids, didanosine • Increased serum levels and toxic effects of theophyllines if taken concurrently with ciprofloxacin • Increased effects of coumarin or its derivatives • Increased risk of seizures with foscarnet

✳ **Drug-alternative therapy** • Increased risk of severe photosensitivity reactions if combined with St. John's Wort

■ Nursing considerations
Assessment

• **History:** Allergy to ciprofloxacin, norfloxacin or other quinolones; renal impairment; seizures; lactation
• **Physical:** Skin color, lesions; T; orientation, reflexes, affect; mucous membranes, bowel sounds; LFTs, renal function tests

Interventions

⊗ *Black box warning* Risk of tendinitis and tendon rupture exists; risk is higher in patients older than 60 yr; those on steroids; and those with renal, heart, or lung transplant.

⊗ *Black box warning* Avoid use in patients with a history of myasthenia gravis because drug may exacerbate weakness.

• Arrange for culture and sensitivity tests before beginning therapy.
• Continue therapy for 2 days after signs and symptoms of infection are gone.
• Be aware that *Proquin XR* is not interchangeable with other forms.
• Ensure that patient swallows ER tablets whole; do not cut, crush, or chew.
• Ensure that patient is well hydrated.
• Give antacids at least 2 hr after dosing.
• Monitor clinical response; if no improvement is seen or a relapse occurs, repeat culture and sensitivity.
• Encourage patient to complete full course of therapy.

Teaching points

- If an antacid is needed, take it at least 2 hours before or after dose. Swallow ER tablets whole; do not cut, crush, or chew them.
- Take *Proquin XR* with the main meal of the day, preferably the evening meal.
- Do not touch tip of eye ointment or solution as this may contaminate the product.
- Drink plenty of fluids while you are taking this drug.
- You may experience these side effects: Nausea, vomiting, abdominal pain (eat frequent small meals); diarrhea or constipation; drowsiness, blurring of vision, dizziness (use caution if driving or using dangerous equipment).
- Report rash, visual changes, severe GI problems, weakness, tremors.

DANGEROUS DRUG

▷ **cisplatin (CDDP)**

(sis' pla tin)

PREGNANCY CATEGORY D

Drug classes
Alkylating drug
Antineoplastic
Platinum agent

Therapeutic actions
Cytotoxic: Heavy metal that inhibits cell replication by alkylating DNA; cell cycle nonspecific.

Indications
- Metastatic testicular tumors: Combination therapy with bleomycin sulfate and vinblastine sulfate after surgery or radiotherapy
- Metastatic ovarian tumors: As single therapy in resistant patients or in combination therapy with doxorubicin or cyclophosphamide after surgery or radiotherapy
- Advanced bladder cancer: Single agent for transitional cell bladder cancer no longer amenable to surgery or radiotherapy
- Unlabeled uses: Lung cancer; endometrial cancer; osteogenic sarcoma; liver cancer; breast cancer; squamous cell carcinoma of the head, neck, cervix; brain tumor; esophageal cancer; carcinoma of adrenal cortex

Contraindications and cautions
- Contraindicated with allergy to cisplatin, platinum-containing products; hematopoi-etic depression; impaired renal function; hearing impairment; pregnancy; lactation.
- Use cautiously with hepatic impairment, peripheral vascular disease.

Available forms
Injection—1 mg/mL

Dosages
Dose is often given in combination with another chemotherapeutic drug.

Adults
- *Metastatic testicular tumors:*
  Remission induction: Cisplatin, 20 mg/m^2 per day IV for 5 consecutive days (days 1–5) every 3 wk for three courses of therapy; bleomycin, 30 units IV weekly (day 2 of each wk) for 12 consecutive doses; vinblastine, 0.15–0.2 mg/kg IV twice weekly (days 1 and 2) every 3 wk for four courses.
  Maintenance: Vinblastine, 0.3 mg/kg IV every 4 wk for 2 yr.
- *Metastatic ovarian tumors:* 75–100 mg/m^2 IV once every 4 wk. For combination therapy, administer sequentially: Cisplatin, 75–100 mg/m^2 IV once every 3–4 wk; cyclophosphamide, 600 mg/m^2 IV once every 4 wk. Single dose: 100 mg/m^2 IV once every 4 wk.
- *Advanced bladder cancer:* 50–70 mg/m^2 IV once every 3–4 wk; in heavily pretreated (radiotherapy or chemotherapy) patients, give an initial dose of 50 mg/m^2 repeated every 4 wk. Do not give repeated courses until serum creatinine is lower than 1.5 mg/dL or BUN is lower than 25 mg/dL or until platelets exceed 100,000/mm^3 and WBCs exceed 4,000/mm^3. Do not give subsequent doses until audiometry indicates hearing is within normal range.

Patients with renal impairment
Creatinine clearance of 10–50 mL/min, give 75% normal dose; creatinine clearance of less than 10 mL/min, give 50% normal dose but consider not using this drug; creatinine clearance of 0–9 mL/min, do not give.

Pharmacokinetics

Route	Onset	Peak	Duration
IV	8–10 hr	18–23 days	30–35 days

Metabolism: Hepatic; T$_{1/2}$: 25–49 min, then 58–73 hr
Distribution: Crosses placenta; enters breast milk
Excretion: Urine

Adverse effects in *italics* are most common; those in **bold** are life-threatening. ⊝ Do not crush.

▼ IV FACTS

Preparation: Available solution contains 1 mg/mL cisplatin; stable for 28 days protected from light or 7 days under room light at room temperature—do not refrigerate. Dilute drug in 1–2 L of 5% dextrose in one-half or one-third normal saline containing 37.5 g mannitol.

Infusion: Hydrate patient with 1–2 L of fluid infused for 8–12 hr before drug therapy; infuse dilute drug over 6–8 hr.

Adverse effects

- **CNS:** *Ototoxicity,* peripheral neuropathies, seizures, loss of taste
- **GI:** *Nausea, vomiting, anorexia,* liver impairment
- **GU:** *Nephrotoxicity,* dose limiting
- **Hematologic:** *Leukopenia, thrombocytopenia, anemia,* hypomagnesemia, hypocalcemia, hypokalemia, hypophosphatemia, hyperuricemia
- **Hypersensitivity: Anaphylactic-like reactions,** facial edema, bronchoconstriction, tachycardia, hypotension (treat with epinephrine, corticosteroids, antihistamines)

Interactions

✳ **Drug-drug** • Additive ototoxicity with furosemide, bumetanide, ethacrynic acid • Decreased serum levels of phenytoins with cisplatin • Additive nephrotoxicity with aminoglycosides

■ **Nursing considerations**
Assessment

- **History:** Allergy to cisplatin, platinum-containing products; hematopoietic depression; impaired renal function; hearing impairment; pregnancy, lactation
- **Physical:** Weight; eighth cranial nerve evaluation; reflexes; sensation; CBC, differential; renal function tests; serum electrolytes; serum uric acid; audiogram

Interventions

⊗ *Black box warning* Arrange for audiometric testing before beginning therapy and prior to subsequent doses. Do not give dose if audiometric acuity is outside normal limits.

⊗ *Black box warning* Monitor renal function; severe toxicity related to dose is possible.

⊗ *Black box warning* Have epinephrine and corticosteroids available in case the patient has anaphylaxis-like reactions.

⊗ *Warning* Do not use needles of IV sets containing aluminum parts; can cause precipitate and loss of drug potency. Use gloves while preparing drug to prevent contact with the skin or mucosa; contact can cause skin reactions. If contact occurs, wash area immediately with soap and water.

- Maintain adequate hydration and urinary output for the 24 hr following drug therapy.
- Use of prophylactic antiemetics is required (ondansetron).
- Monitor uric acid levels; if markedly increased, allopurinol may be ordered.
- Monitor electrolytes and maintain by supplements.

Teaching points

- This drug can only be given IV. Prepare a calendar of treatment days.
- Use contraceptives; drug may cause birth defects or miscarriages.
- Have frequent, regular medical follow-up care, including frequent blood tests, to monitor drug effects.
- You may experience these side effects: Nausea, vomiting (medication may be ordered; eat frequent small meals); numbness, tingling, loss of taste, ringing in the ears, dizziness, loss of hearing (reversible).
- Report loss of hearing, dizziness; unusual bleeding or bruising, fever, chills, sore throat, leg cramps, muscle twitching, changes in voiding patterns.

▽ **citalopram hydrobromide**

*(si **tal**' oh pram hi dro **broh**' myde)*

Apo-Citalopram (CAN)⬛, Celexa⬛, Co Citalopram (CAN)⬛, Gen-Citalopram (CAN)⬛, PMS-Citalopram (CAN)⬛, ratio-Citalopram (CAN)⬛

PREGNANCY CATEGORY C

Drug classes
Antidepressant
SSRI

Therapeutic actions
Potentiates serotonergic activity in the CNS by inhibiting neuronal reuptake of serotonin, resulting in antidepressant effect, with little

effect on norepinephrine or dopamine reuptake.

Indications

- Treatment of depression, particularly effective in major depressive disorders
- Unlabeled uses: OCD, panic disorder, PMDD, social phobia, trichotillomania, PTSD, alcoholism, binge eating, third-line treatment of diabetic neuropathy, impulsive-aggressive behavior, irritable bowel syndrome, gambling, stuttering

Contraindications and cautions

- Contraindicated with MAOI use; allergy to drug or any component of the drug or other SSRIs; concomitant use of pimozide.
- Use cautiously with renal or hepatic impairment, pregnancy, and lactation, patients with prolonged QT interval, patients predisposed to low potassium or low magnesium levels, and in patients who are elderly or suicidal.

Available forms

Tablets ⊙⊙—10, 20, 40 mg; oral solution—2 mg/mL

Dosages

Adults
Initially, 20 mg/day PO as a single daily dose. If needed, after at least 1 wk, may be increased to 40 mg/day. Maximum daily dose, 40 mg/day (20 mg/day if also taking cimetidine or other CYP2C19 inhibitors).

Pediatric patients
Safety and efficacy not established.

Geriatric patients or patients with renal or hepatic impairment
20 mg/day PO as a single dose; increase to 40 mg/day only if clearly needed and patient is not responding.

Pharmacokinetics

Route	Onset	Peak
Oral	Slow	2–4 hr

Metabolism: Hepatic; $T_{1/2}$: 35 hr
Distribution: Crosses placenta; enters breast milk
Excretion: Urine

Adverse effects

- **CNS:** *Somnolence, dizziness, insomnia, tremor,* nervousness, headache, anxiety, paresthesia, blurred vision
- **CV:** Palpitations, vasodilation, orthostatic hypotension, hypertension, prolonged QT interval
- **Dermatologic:** *Sweating,* rash, redness
- **GI:** *Nausea, dry mouth,* constipation, diarrhea, anorexia, flatulence, vomiting
- **GU:** *Ejaculatory disorders*
- **Respiratory:** Sinusitis, URI, cough, rhinitis

Interactions

✳ **Drug-drug** • Increased citalopram levels and toxicity if taken with MAOIs; ensure that patient has been off the MAOI for at least 14 days before administering citalopram • Increased citalopram levels with azole antifungals, macrolides • Possible severe adverse effects if combined with TCAs, erythromycin; use caution • Possible increased effects of beta blockers; monitor patient and reduce beta-blocker dose as needed • Possible increased bleeding with warfarin; monitor patient carefully • Risk of prolonged QT interval and potentially fatal cardiac arrhythmias if combined with pimozide; avoid this combination • Risk of serotonin syndrome with linezolid • Increased citalopram levels with cimetidine and other CYP2C19 inhibitors

✳ **Drug-alternative therapy** • Increased risk of severe reaction if combined with St. John's Wort

■ Nursing considerations

CLINICAL ALERT!
Name confusion has occurred between *Celexa* (citalopram), *Celebrex* (celecoxib), *Xanax* (alprazolam), and *Cerebyx* (fosphenytoin); use caution.

Assessment

- **History:** MAOI use; allergy to drug or any component of the drug; renal or hepatic impairment, the elderly, pregnancy, lactation, suicidal tendencies
- **Physical:** Orientation, reflexes; P, BP, perfusion; bowel sounds, normal output; urinary output; liver evaluation; LFTs, renal function tests

Interventions

⊗ **Black box warning** Be aware of increased risk of suicidality in children, adolescents, and young adults; monitor accordingly.

⊗ **Warning** Do not use doses over 40 mg; increased risk of prolonged QT interval and potentially fatal arrhythmias at higher doses.

- Administer once a day, in the morning; may be taken with food if desired.
- Encourage patient to continue use for 4–6 wk, as directed, to ensure adequate levels to affect depression.
- Limit amount of drug given in prescription to potentially suicidal patients.
- Establish appropriate safety precautions if patient experiences adverse CNS effects.
- Institute appropriate therapy for patient suffering from depression.

Teaching points

- Take this drug exactly as directed, and as long as directed; it may take a few weeks to realize the benefits of the drug. The drug may be taken with food if desired. Do not cut, crush, or chew tablets.
- This drug should not be taken during pregnancy or when breast-feeding; use of barrier contraceptives is suggested.
- You may experience these side effects: Drowsiness, dizziness, tremor (use caution and avoid driving a car or performing other tasks that require alertness if you experience daytime drowsiness); GI upset (eat frequent small meals, perform frequent mouth care); alterations in sexual function (it may help to know that this is a drug effect, and will pass when drug therapy is ended).
- Report severe nausea, vomiting; palpitations; blurred vision; excessive sweating; thoughts of suicide.

DANGEROUS DRUG

▽ **cladribine (CdA, 2-chlorodeoxyadenosine)**

(kla′ dri been)

Leustatin

PREGNANCY CATEGORY D

Drug classes

Antimetabolite
Antineoplastic
Purine analogue

Therapeutic actions

Blocks DNA synthesis and repair, causing cell death in active and resting lymphocytes and monocytes.

Indications

- Treatment of active hairy cell leukemia
- Unlabeled uses: Chronic lymphocytic leukemia, non-Hodgkin lymphomas, acute myeloid leukemia, Waldenström macroglobulinemia

Contraindications and cautions

- Contraindicated with hypersensitivity to cladribine or any components, pregnancy, lactation.
- Use cautiously with active infection, myelosuppression, debilitating illness, renal or hepatic impairment.

Available forms

IV solution—1 mg/mL

Dosages

Adults

Single course given by continuous IV infusion of 0.09–0.1 mg/kg/day for 7 days.

Pediatric patients

Safety and efficacy not established.

Pharmacokinetics

Route	Onset	Peak
IV	Rapid	8–10 hr

Metabolism: Hepatic; $T_{1/2}$: 5.4 hr
Distribution: Crosses placenta; may enter breast milk
Excretion: Urine

▼ **IV FACTS**

Preparation: Prepare daily dose by adding calculated dose to 500-mL bag of 0.9% sodium chloride injection. Stable for 24 hr at room temperature. Prepare 7-day infusion using aseptic technique, and add calculated dose to 100 mL bacteriostatic, 0.9% sodium chloride injection (0.9% benzyl alcohol preserved) through a sterile 0.22-micron filter. Store unopened vials in refrigerator; protect from light. Vials are single-use only; discard after use.

Infusion: Infuse daily dose slowly over 24 hr. 7-day dose should be infused continuously over the 7-day period. Stable for 7 days in CADD medication cassettes.

Incompatibilities: Do not mix with any other solutions, drugs, or additives. Do not infuse through IV line with any other drug or additive.

Adverse effects

- **CNS:** *Fatigue, headache,* dizziness, insomnia, **neurotoxicity**
- **CV:** Tachycardia, edema
- **Dermatologic:** *Rash,* pruritus, pain, erythema, petechiae, purpura
- **GI:** *Nausea, anorexia, vomiting, diarrhea, constipation,* abdominal pain
- **GU: Nephrotoxicity**
- **Hematologic:** *Neutropenia,* **myelosuppression,** anemia, thrombocytopenia, *lymphopenia*
- **Local:** *Injection site redness, swelling, pain;* thrombosis, phlebitis
- **Respiratory:** *Cough, abnormal breath sounds,* shortness of breath
- **Other:** *Fever, chills,* asthenia, diaphoresis, myalgia, arthralgia, **infection,** cancer

■ Nursing considerations
Assessment

- **History:** Allergy to cladribine or any component, renal or hepatic impairment, myelosuppression, infection, pregnancy, lactation
- **Physical:** Weight, skin condition, neurologic status, abdominal examination, P, respiratory status, LFTs, renal function tests, CBC, uric acid levels

Interventions

⊗ *Warning* Use disposable gloves and protective garments when handling cladribine. If drug contacts skin or mucous membranes, wash immediately with copious amounts of water.

- Ensure continuous infusion of drug over 7 days.
- Alert patients of childbearing age to drug's severe effects on fetus; advise using birth control during and for several weeks after treatment.

⊗ **Black box warning** Monitor complete hematologic profile and LFTs and renal function tests before and frequently during treatment. Consult with physician at first sign

of toxicity; consider delaying or discontinuing dose if neurotoxicity or renal toxicity occurs.

Teaching points

- This drug must be given continuously for 7 days.
- Frequent monitoring of blood tests is needed during the treatment and for several weeks thereafter to assess the drug's effect.
- Using barrier contraceptives is advised during therapy and for several weeks following therapy.
- You may experience these side effects: Fever, headache, rash, nausea, vomiting, fatigue, pain at injection site.
- Report numbness or tingling, severe headache, nausea, rash, extreme fatigue, edema, pain or swelling at injection site.

▽ **clarithromycin**
*(klar **ith'** ro my sin)*

Biaxin, Biaxin XL ⬛

PREGNANCY CATEGORY C

Drug class
Macrolide antibiotic

Therapeutic actions
Inhibits protein synthesis in susceptible bacteria, causing cell death.

Indications

- Treatment of URIs caused by *Streptococcus pyogenes, Streptococcus pneumoniae*
- Treatment of lower respiratory infections caused by *Mycoplasma pneumoniae, S. pneumoniae, Haemophilus influenzae, Moraxella catarrhalis, Haemophilus parainfluenzae*
- Treatment of skin and skin structure infections caused by *Staphylococcus aureus, S. pyogenes*
- Treatment and prevention of disseminated mycobacterial infections due to *Mycobacterium avium* and *Mycobacterium intracellulare*
- Treatment of active duodenal ulcer associated with *Helicobacter pylori* in combination with proton pump inhibitor

---

- Treatment of acute otitis media, acute maxillary sinusitis due to *H. influenzae, M. catarrhalis, S. pneumoniae*
- Treatment of mild to moderate community-acquired pneumonia

Contraindications and cautions

- Contraindicated with hypersensitivity to clarithromycin, erythromycin, or any macrolide antibiotic.
- Use cautiously with colitis, hepatic or renal impairment, pregnancy, lactation.

Available forms

Tablets—250, 500 mg; granules for suspension—125, 250 mg/5 mL; ER tablets ⓄⓇⒸ—500 mg

Dosages

Adults

- *Pharyngitis, tonsillitis; pneumonia due to* S. pneumoniae, M. pneumoniae; *skin or skin structure infections; lower respiratory infections due to* S. pneumoniae, M. catarrhalis: 250 mg PO every 12 hr for 7–14 days.
- *Acute maxillary sinusitis, acute otitis media, lower respiratory infections caused by* H. influenzae, M. catarrhalis, S. pneumoniae: 500 mg PO every 12 hr for 14 days or 1,000 mg ER tablets PO every 24 hr.
- *Mycobacterial infections:* 500 mg PO bid.
- *Duodenal ulcers:* 500 mg PO tid plus omeprazole 40 mg PO every AM for 14 days, then omeprazole 20 mg PO every AM for 14 days.
- *Community-acquired pneumonia:* 250 mg PO every 12 hr for 7–14 days or 1,000 mg PO of ER tablets every 24 hr for 7 days.

Pediatric patients

Usual dosage, 15 mg/kg/day PO divided every 12 hr for 10 days.

- *Mycobacterial infections:* 7.5 mg/kg PO bid, up to 500 mg PO bid.

Geriatric patients or patients with impaired renal function

Decrease dosage or prolong dosing intervals as appropriate. If creatinine clearance is less than 30 mL/min, halve the dose or double the interval.

Pharmacokinetics

Route	Onset	Peak
Oral	Varies	2 hr

Metabolism: Hepatic; $T_{1/2}$: 3–7 hr
Distribution: Crosses placenta; enters breast milk
Excretion: Urine

Adverse effects

- **CNS:** Dizziness, headache, vertigo, somnolence, fatigue
- **GI:** *Diarrhea, abdominal pain, nausea,* dyspepsia, flatulence, vomiting, melena, pseudomembranous colitis, abnormal taste
- **Other:** *Superinfections,* increased PT, decreased WBC count

Interactions

✳ **Drug-drug** • Increased serum levels and effects of carbamazepine, theophylline, lovastatin, phenytoin
✳ **Drug-food** • Food decreases the rate of absorption of clarithromycin but does not alter effectiveness • Decreased metabolism and risk of toxic effects if combined with grapefruit juice; avoid this combination

■ Nursing considerations

Assessment

- **History:** Hypersensitivity to clarithromycin, erythromycin, or any macrolide antibiotic; pseudomembranous colitis, hepatic or renal impairment, lactation, pregnancy
- **Physical:** Site of infection; skin color, lesions; orientation, GI output, bowel sounds, liver evaluation; culture and sensitivity tests of infection, urinalysis, LFTs, renal function tests

Interventions

- Culture infection site before therapy.
- Do not cut or crush, and ensure that patient does not chew ER tablets.
- Monitor patient for anticipated response.
- Administer without regard to meals; administer with food if GI effects occur.

Teaching points

- Take drug with food if GI effects occur. Take the full course of therapy. Do not drink grapefruit juice while taking this drug.
- Shake suspension before use; do not refrigerate; do not cut, crush, or chew extended-release tablets; swallow them whole.
- You may experience these side effects: Stomach cramping, discomfort, diarrhea; fatigue, headache (medication may be ordered);

additional infections in the mouth or vagina (consult your health care provider for treatment).

• Report severe or watery diarrhea, severe nausea or vomiting, rash or itching, mouth sores, vaginal sores.

▷ **clemastine fumarate**
(klem' as teen)

Dayhist-1, Tavist Allergy

PREGNANCY CATEGORY B

Drug class
Antihistamine

Therapeutic actions
Blocks the effects of histamine at H_1-receptor sites; has atropine-like, antipruritic, and sedative effects.

Indications
• Symptomatic relief of symptoms associated with perennial and seasonal allergic rhinitis; vasomotor rhinitis; allergic conjunctivitis
• Mild, uncomplicated urticaria and angioedema

Contraindications and cautions
• Contraindicated with allergy to any antihistamines, third trimester of pregnancy, lactation.
• Use cautiously with narrow-angle glaucoma, stenosing peptic ulcer, symptomatic prostatic hypertrophy, asthmatic attack, bladder neck obstruction, pyloroduodenal obstruction.

Available forms
Tablets—1.34, 2.68 mg; syrup—0.67 mg/5 mL

Dosages
Adults and children older than 12 yr
• *Allergic rhinitis:* 1.34 mg PO bid. Do not exceed 8.04 mg/day (syrup); 2.68 mg/day (tablets).
• *Urticaria or angioedema:* 2.68 mg PO daily–tid. Do not exceed 8.04 mg/day.
Pediatric patients 6–12 yr
• *Allergic rhinitis (syrup only):* 0.67 mg PO as syrup bid. Do not exceed 4.02 mg/day.

• *Urticaria or angioedema (syrup only):* 1.34 mg PO as syrup bid. Do not exceed 4.02 mg/day.
Pediatric patients younger than 6 yr
Safety and efficacy not established.
Geriatric patients
More likely to cause dizziness, sedation, syncope, toxic confusional states, and hypotension in elderly patients; use with caution.

Pharmacokinetics

Route	Onset	Peak	Duration
Oral	15–30 min	1–2 hr	12 hr

Metabolism: Hepatic; $T_{1/2}$: 3–4 hr
Distribution: Crosses placenta; enters breast milk
Excretion: Urine

Adverse effects
• **CNS:** *Drowsiness, sedation, dizziness, disturbed coordination,* fatigue, confusion, restlessness, excitation, nervousness, tremor, headache, blurred vision, diplopia, vertigo, tinnitus, acute labyrinthitis, hysteria, tingling, heaviness and weakness of the hands
• **CV:** Hypotension, palpitations, bradycardia, tachycardia, extrasystoles
• **GI:** *Epigastric distress,* anorexia, increased appetite and weight gain, nausea, vomiting, diarrhea or constipation
• **GU:** Urinary frequency, dysuria, urinary retention, early menses, decreased libido, impotence
• **Hematologic:** Hemolytic anemia, aplastic anemia, thrombocytopenia, leukopenia, **agranulocytosis,** pancytopenia
• **Respiratory:** *Thickening of bronchial secretions,* chest tightness, wheezing, nasal stuffiness, dry mouth, dry nose, dry throat, sore throat
• **Other:** Urticaria, rash, **anaphylactic shock,** photosensitivity, excessive perspiration, chills

Interactions
✳ **Drug-drug** • Increased depressant effects with alcohol, other CNS depressants • Increased and prolonged anticholinergic (drying) effects with MAOIs; avoid this combination

Adverse effects in *italics* are most common; those in **bold** are life-threatening. ▭ Do not crush.

■ Nursing considerations
Assessment
- **History:** Allergy to any antihistamines; narrow-angle glaucoma, stenosing peptic ulcer, symptomatic prostatic hypertrophy, asthmatic attack, bladder neck obstruction, pyloroduodenal obstruction; lactation, pregnancy
- **Physical:** Skin color, lesions, texture; orientation, reflexes, affect; vision examination; P, BP; R, adventitious sounds; bowel sounds; prostate palpation; CBC with differential

Interventions
- Administer with food if GI upset occurs.
- Administer syrup form if patient is unable to take tablets; children 6–12 yr should receive only syrup form.
- Encourage patient to drink plenty of fluids (unless contraindicated); use a humidifier if dry mucosa is an issue.
- Monitor patient response, adjust to lowest possible effective dose.

Teaching points
- Take drug as prescribed; avoid excessive dosage.
- Take with food if GI upset occurs.
- Avoid alcohol; serious sedation could occur.
- You may experience these side effects: Dizziness, sedation, drowsiness (use caution if driving or performing tasks that require alertness); epigastric distress, diarrhea, or constipation (take with meals; consult your health care provider as needed); dry mouth (frequent mouth care, sucking sugarless candies may help); thickening of bronchial secretions, dryness of nasal mucosa (use a humidifier).
- Report difficulty breathing, hallucinations, tremors, loss of coordination, unusual bleeding or bruising, visual disturbances, irregular heartbeat.

▽clevidipine butyrate
*(klev **id'** ib peen)*

Cleviprex

PREGNANCY CATEGORY C

Drug classes
Antihypertensive
Calcium channel blocker

Therapeutic actions
Blocks the influx of calcium in the arterial smooth muscle, leading to arterial muscle relaxation and decreased vascular resistance, which lowers BP; does not affect preload or cardiac filling pressure, showing no effect on venous vessels.

Indications
- BP reduction when oral therapy is not possible or is not desirable

Contraindications and cautions
- Contraindicated with known hypersensitivity to any component of the drug, soy, or egg products; defective lipid metabolism; acute pancreatitis; severe aortic stenosis.
- Use cautiously with heart failure, pregnancy, lactation.

Available forms
Single-use vials—0.5 mg/mL

Dosages
Adults
- Initially, give IV infusion of 1–2 mg/hr; titrate quickly by doubling the dose every 90 sec to achieve desired BP. Maintenance dose is usually 4–6 mg/hr. Maximum dose, 21 mg/hr per 24-hr period.

Pediatric patients
- Safety and efficacy not established.

Pharmacokinetics

Route	Onset	Peak
IV	Rapid	End of infusion

Metabolism: Blood and tissues; $T_{1/2}$: 15 min
Distribution: May cross placenta; may enter breast milk
Excretion: Blood and tissues

▼IV·FACTS
Preparation: Maintain strict sterile technique; product contains phospholipids, which can support microbial growth. Administer within 12 hr of puncturing the stopper; discard any unused drug. Invert vial several times to dispense drug. Drug should appear milky; inspect for any particulate matter, which indicates a contaminated product. Do not dilute. May be administered with water for injection, sodium chloride (0.9%) injection, 5% dextrose

injection, 5% dextrose in 0.9% sodium chloride, 5% dextrose in lactated Ringer solution, lactated Ringer injection, 10% amino acids.

Infusion: Monitor patient's BP and cardiac status continuously. Infuse using a controlled infusing device that allows for calibrated titration.

Incompatibilities: Do not administer in the same line as any other medications.

Adverse effects
- **CNS:** *Headache*
- **CV:** Hypotension, reflex tachycardia, hypertension, **heart failure**
- **GI:** *Nausea, vomiting*

■ Nursing considerations

Assessment
- **History:** Known hypersensitivity to any component of the drug, soy, or egg products; defective lipid metabolism; acute pancreatitis; severe aortic stenosis; heart failure; pregnancy; lactation
- **Physical:** Orientation, affect; BP, P, peripheral perfusion, auscultation

Interventions
- Continuously monitor BP and cardiac status during administration; titrate drug accordingly to achieve desired BP.
- Be aware that drug does not protect from rebound affect of beta-blocker discontinuation; if patient has been maintained on a beta blocker, drug should be tapered to avoid rebound tachycardia and hypertension.
- Patient should be switched to an oral antihypertensive as appropriate to maintain BP control. If patient is not started on an oral antihypertensive, be prepared for effects of rebound hypertension for at least 8 hr after discontinuation of clevidipine.
- Be aware that drug should be handled using strict sterile technique because drug contains phospholipids that can support microbial growth.
- Use drug within 4 hr of puncturing the stopper.

Teaching points
- This drug must be given IV to regulate your high blood pressure. You will be continuously monitored and the dosage will be adjusted to achieve the desired blood pressure.

- You will need to have regular medical follow-up appointments with your health care provider to monitor your hypertension. Oral medications may be ordered to maintain a safe blood pressure.
- You may experience these side effects: Headache (medications may be available to help); nausea and vomiting (frequent small meals may help, medication may be available to relieve these symptoms).
- Report changes in vision, swelling of the ankles or legs, changes in orientation or alertness, difficulty breathing, fast heart rate.

▽**clindamycin**
*(klin da **mye**' sin)*

clindamycin hydrochloride
Oral: Cleocin, Dalacin C (CAN)

clindamycin palmitate hydrochloride
Oral: Cleocin Pediatric, Dalacin C Flavored Granules (CAN)

clindamycin phosphate
Oral, parenteral, topical dermatologic solution for acne, vaginal preparation: Cleocin Phosphate, Cleocin Phosphate IV, Cleocin T, Cleocin Vaginal Ovules, Clinda-Derm (CAN), Clindagel, ClindaMax, Clindesse, Dalacin C Phosphate (CAN), Dalacin Vaginal Cream (CAN), Dalacin T (CAN), Evoclin

PREGNANCY CATEGORY B

Drug class
Lincosamide antibiotic

Therapeutic actions
Inhibits protein synthesis in susceptible bacteria, causing cell death.

Indications
- Systemic administration: Serious infections caused by susceptible strains of anaerobes, streptococci, staphylococci, pneumococci; reserve use for penicillin-allergic patients or

---

when penicillin is inappropriate; less toxic antibiotics (erythromycin) should be considered
- Parenteral: Treatment of septicemia caused by staphylococci, streptococci; acute hematogenous osteomyelitis; adjunct to surgical treatment of chronic bone and joint infections due to susceptible organisms; do not use to treat meningitis; does not cross the blood–brain barrier.
- Topical dermatologic solution: Treatment of acne vulgaris
- Vaginal preparation: Treatment of bacterial vaginosis

Contraindications and cautions
Systemic administration
- Contraindicated with allergy to clindamycin, lactation.
- Use cautiously in newborns and infants due to benzyl alcohol content (associated with gasping syndrome) and in patients with tartrazine sensitivity or hepatic or renal impairment.

Topical dermatologic solution, vaginal preparation
- Contraindicated with allergy to clindamycin or lincomycin.
- Use caution with history of regional enteritis or ulcerative colitis; history of antibiotic-associated colitis.

Available forms
Capsules—75, 150, 300 mg; granules for oral solution—75 mg/5 mL; injection—150 mg/mL, 300 mg/2 mL, 600 mg/4 mL, 900 mg/6 mL; 300, 600, 900 mg/50 mL; topical gel—1%; topical lotion—1%; topical suspension—1%; vaginal cream—2%; vaginal suppository—100 mg

Dosages
Adults
Oral
150–300 mg every 6 hr, up to 300–450 mg every 6 hr in more severe infections.
Parenteral
600–2,700 mg/day in two to four equal doses; up to 4.8 g/day IV or IM may be used for life-threatening situations.
Vaginal
One applicator (100 mg clindamycin phosphate) intravaginally, preferably at bedtime for 7 consecutive days in pregnant women and 3 or 7 days in nonpregnant women; or insert vaginal suppository, preferably at bedtime for 3 days for *Cleocin Vaginal Ovules.*
Topical
Apply a thin film to affected area bid.
Pediatric patients
Oral
For clindamycin hydrochloride, 8–16 mg/kg/day (serious infections) or 16–20 mg/kg/day (more serious infections) in three or four equal doses. For clindamycin palmitate hydrochloride, 8–25 mg/kg/day in three or four equal doses; for children weighing less than 10 kg, use 37.5 mg tid as the minimum dose.
Parenteral
Neonates: 15–20 mg/kg/day in three or four equal doses.
Older than 1 mo: 20–40 mg/kg/day in three or four equal doses or 350 mg/m²/day to 450 mg/m²/day.
Patients with renal failure
Reduce dose, and monitor patient carefully.

Pharmacokinetics

Route	Onset	Peak	Duration
Oral	Varies	1–2 hr	8–12 hr
IM	20–30 min	1–3 hr	8–12 hr
IV	Immediate	Minutes	8–12 hr

Metabolism: Hepatic; $T_{1/2}$: 2–3 hr
Distribution: Crosses placenta; enters breast milk
Excretion: Feces, urine
Topical: Minimal systemic absorption

▼ IV FACTS

Preparation: Store unreconstituted product at room temperature. Reconstitute by adding 75 mL of water to 100-mL bottle of palmitate in two portions. Shake well; do not refrigerate reconstituted solution. Reconstituted solution is stable for 2 wk at room temperature. Dilute reconstituted solution to a concentration of 300 mg/50 mL or more of diluent using 0.9% sodium chloride injection, 5% dextrose injection, or lactated Ringer solution. Do not exceed 18 mg/mL. Solution is stable for 16 days at room temperature.

Infusion: ⊗ *Warning* Do not administer more than 1,200 mg in a single 1-hr infusion. Infusion rates: 300 mg in 50 mL diluent, 10 min; 600 mg in 50 mL diluent, 20 min; 900 mg in 50–100 mL diluent, 30 min; 1,200 mg in 100 mL diluent, 40 min. Do not infuse faster than

30 mg/min; rapid infusion can cause cardiac arrest.

Incompatibilities: Do not mix with calcium gluconate, ampicillin, phenytoin, barbiturates, aminophylline, and magnesium sulfate. May be mixed with sodium chloride, dextrose, calcium, potassium, vitamin B complex, kanamycin, gentamicin, penicillin. Incompatible in syringe with tobramycin.

Adverse effects
Systemic administration
- **CV:** Hypotension, **cardiac arrest** (with rapid IV infusion)
- **GI:** Severe colitis, including **pseudomembranous colitis,** *nausea, vomiting, diarrhea, abdominal pain, esophagitis, anorexia,* jaundice, hepatic function changes
- **Hematologic:** Neutropenia, leukopenia, **agranulocytosis,** eosinophilia
- **Hypersensitivity:** *Rashes,* urticaria to **anaphylactoid** reactions
- **Local:** *Pain following injection,* induration and sterile abscess after IM injection, thrombophlebitis after IV use

Topical dermatologic solution
- **CNS:** Fatigue, headache
- **Dermatologic:** *Contact dermatitis, dryness,* gram-negative folliculitis
- **GI:** Pseudomembranous colitis, diarrhea, bloody diarrhea; abdominal pain, sore throat
- **GU:** Urinary frequency

Vaginal preparation
- **GU:** Cervicitis, vaginitis, vulvar irritation

Interactions
Systemic administration
✳ **Drug-drug** • Increased neuromuscular blockade with neuromuscular blocking agents
- Decreased GI absorption with kaolin, aluminum salts

■ Nursing considerations
Assessment
- **History:** Allergy to clindamycin, history of asthma or other allergies, allergy to tartrazine (in 75- and 150-mg capsules); hepatic or renal impairment; lactation; history of regional enteritis or ulcerative colitis; history of antibiotic-associated colitis
- **Physical:** Site of infection or acne; skin color, lesions; BP; R, adventitious sounds; bowel sounds, output, liver evaluation; complete blood count, LFTs, renal function tests

Interventions
Systemic administration
- Culture infection site before therapy.
- Administer oral drug with a full glass of water or with food to prevent esophageal irritation.
- Do not give IM injections of more than 600 mg; inject deep into large muscle to avoid serious problems.
- Do not use for minor bacterial or viral infections.
- ⊗ **Black box warning** Be aware that serious to fatal colitis, including *Clostridium difficile*–associated diarrhea, can occur up to several wk after completion of therapy; reserve use, and monitor patient closely.
- Monitor LFTs and renal function tests, and blood counts with prolonged therapy.

Topical dermatologic administration
- Keep solution away from eyes, mouth, and abraded skin or mucous membranes; alcohol base will cause stinging. Shake well before use.
- Keep cool tap water available to bathe eye, mucous membranes, abraded skin inadvertently contacted by drug solution.

Vaginal preparation
- Give intravaginally, preferably at bedtime.

Teaching points
Systemic administration
- Take oral drug with a full glass of water or with food.
- Take full prescribed course of oral drug. Do not stop taking without notifying your health care provider.
- You may experience these side effects: Nausea, vomiting (eat frequent small meals); superinfections in the mouth, vagina (use frequent hygiene measures, request treatment if severe).
- Report severe or watery diarrhea, abdominal pain, inflamed mouth or vagina, skin rash or lesions.

Topical dermatologic administration
- Apply thin film of acne solution to affected area twice daily, being careful to avoid eyes, mucous membranes, abraded skin; if solution contacts one of these areas, flush with lots of cool water.
- Report abdominal pain, diarrhea.

Vaginal preparation

- Use vaginal preparation for 7 or 3 consecutive days, preferably at bedtime. Refrain from sexual intercourse during treatment with this product.
- Report vaginal irritation, itching; diarrhea, no improvement in complaint being treated.

▷clobazam
(kloe' bah zam)

Onfi

PREGNANCY CATEGORY C

Drug classes
Antiepileptic
Benzodiazepine

Therapeutic actions
Potentiates GABA action by binding to GABA receptor sites. GABA is an inhibitory neurotransmitter; the exact action causing the clinical effects is not understood.

Indications
- Adjunct treatment of seizures associated with Lennox-Gastaut syndrome in patients 2 yr and older

Contraindications and cautions
- Contraindicated with history of serious hypersensitivity reactions to clobazam.
- Use cautiously with concurrent use of other CNS depressants, pregnancy, lactation.

Available forms
Tablets—5, 10, 20 mg

Dosages
Adults and children 2 yr and older
30 kg or less: Initially, 5 mg/day PO. Increase to 5 mg PO bid starting on day 7; increase to 10 mg PO bid starting on day 14. *Over 30 kg:* Initially, 5 mg PO bid. Increase to 10 mg PO bid starting on day 7; increase to 20 mg PO bid staring on day 14.
Geriatric patients, poor CYP2C19 metabolizers, patients with mild to moderate hepatic impairment
Initially, 5 mg/day PO. Titrate according to weight at half the usual dose to a maximum

of 20–40 mg/day based on weight, starting on day 21, if tolerated.

Pharmacokinetics

Route	Onset	Peak
Oral	Rapid	0.5–4 hr

Metabolism: Hepatic; $T_{1/2}$: 38–42 hr, then 71–82 hr
Distribution: May cross placenta; enters breast milk
Excretion: Urine

Adverse effects
- **CNS:** *Sedation, somnolence, insomnia, fatigue, aggression, drooling,* ataxia, **suicidality**
- **GI:** *Constipation,* vomiting
- **Respiratory:** Cough, URI
- **Renal:** UTI
- **Other:** *Dysarthria, withdrawal with rapid dose reduction,* physical dependence, *fever*

Interactions
✳ **Drug-drug** • Increased toxicity if combined with alcohol • Potential loss of effectiveness of hormonal contraceptives; suggest use of alternative form of contraception • Potential for altered effectiveness if combined with fluconazole, fluvoxamine, ticlopidine, omeprazole; if these combinations are used, monitor patient response closely

■ Nursing considerations
Assessment
- **History:** Hypersensitivity to components of the drug, pregnancy, lactation
- **Physical:** T, R, adventitious sounds; orientation, affect, reflexes

Interventions
- Arrange to taper gradually after long-term use; risk of withdrawal reaction with rapid dose reduction.
- Limit amount of drug dispensed and follow patient closely if there is a history of substance abuse; physical dependence is possible.
- Be aware of risk of suicidality; monitor patient accordingly.
- Administer whole or crushed and mixed in applesauce.
- Advise women of childbearing age to avoid pregnancy; fetal harm has been reported.

Teaching points

- Take this drug twice a day. Swallow the tablet whole, or you can crush it and mix it in applesauce.
- Do not stop taking this drug suddenly. Make sure you have a supply on hand; suddenly stopping the drug can cause serious effects;
- This drug could cause harm to the fetus if taken while you are pregnant. This drug may make hormonal contraceptives ineffective; use of barrier contraceptives is advised. If you are pregnant or thinking about becoming pregnant, discuss this with your health care provider.
- This drug appears in breast milk. If you are breast-feeding, you will need to find another method of feeding the baby.
- This drug is a controlled substance and can lead to addiction or dependence; make sure you secure the drug to prevent abuse or misuse by others.
- Do not drink alcohol while taking this drug; increased sedation and dizziness may occur.
- This drug can lead to increased thoughts of suicide; report thoughts of suicide or worsening depression.
- You may experience these side effects: Dizziness, sleepiness, slowed thinking (do not drive or operate hazardous machinery if these effects occur); constipation (medication may be available to help).
- Report fever, thoughts of suicide, worsening of seizure activity.

<hr>

▷ clofarabine

See Appendix R, *Less commonly used drugs*.

<hr>

▷ clomiPHENE citrate
(kloe' mi feen)

Clomid, Milophene, Serophene

PREGNANCY CATEGORY X

Drug classes

Fertility drug
Hormone

Therapeutic actions

Binds to estrogen receptors, decreasing the number of available estrogen receptors, which gives the hypothalamus and pituitary the false signal to increase FSH and LH secretion, resulting in ovarian stimulation.

Indications

- Treatment of ovulatory failure in patients with normal liver function and normal endogenous estrogen levels, whose partners are fertile and potent
- Unlabeled use: Treatment of male infertility

Contraindications and cautions

- Contraindicated with known sensitivity to clomiphene, liver disease, uterine fibroids, abnormal vaginal bleeding of undetermined origin, ovarian cyst, uncontrolled thyroid or adrenal dysfunction, organic intracranial lesions, pregnancy.
- Use cautiously with lactation.

Available forms

Tablets—50 mg

Dosages
Adults

- *Treatment of ovulatory failure:*
  Initial therapy: 50 mg/day PO for 5 days started anytime there has been no recent uterine bleeding or about the fifth day of the cycle if uterine bleeding does occur.
  Second course: If ovulation does not occur after the first course, administer 100 mg/day PO for 5 days; start this course as early as 30 days after the previous one.
  Third course: Repeat second course regimen; if patient does not respond to three courses of treatment, further treatment is not recommended.

Pharmacokinetics

Route	Onset	Duration
Oral	5–8 days	6 wk

Metabolism: Hepatic; $T_{1/2}$: 5 days
Distribution: Crosses placenta
Excretion: Feces

Adverse effects

- **CNS:** Visual symptoms (blurring, spots, flashes), nervousness, insomnia, dizziness, light-headedness, photophobia, diplopia
- **CV:** *Vasomotor flushing*
- **GI:** *Abdominal discomfort, distention, bloating, nausea, vomiting*

- **GU:** Uterine bleeding, *ovarian enlargement*, **ovarian overstimulation**, birth defects in resulting pregnancies
- **Other:** *Breast tenderness*

Interactions

✳ Drug-lab test • Increased levels of serum thyroxine, thyroxine-binding globulin

■ Nursing considerations

⬥ CLINICAL ALERT!
Name confusion has occurred between *Serophene* (clomiphene) and *Sarafem* (fluoxetine); use caution.

Assessment

- **History:** Sensitivity to clomiphene, liver disease, uterine fibroids, abnormal vaginal bleeding of undetermined origin, ovarian cyst, pregnancy, thyroid or adrenal dysfunction, intracranial lesions
- **Physical:** Skin color, T; affect, orientation, ophthalmologic examination; abdominal examination, pelvic examination, liver evaluation; urinary estrogens and estriol levels (women); LFTs

Interventions

- Complete a pelvic examination before each treatment to rule out ovarian enlargement, pregnancy, and other uterine difficulties.
- Check urine estrogen and estriol levels before therapy; normal levels indicate appropriate patient selection.
- Refer patient for complete ophthalmic examination; if visual symptoms occur, discontinue drug.
- ⊗ *Warning* Discontinue drug at any sign of ovarian overstimulation, admit patient to hospital for observation and supportive measures.
- Provide women with calendar of treatment days and explanations about signs of estrogen and progesterone activity; caution patient that 24-hr urine collections will be needed periodically; timing of intercourse is important for achieving pregnancy.
- Alert patient to risks and hazards of multiple births.
- Explain failure to respond after three courses of therapy probably means drug will not help, and treatment will be discontinued.

Teaching points

- Prepare a calendar showing the treatment schedule, plotting ovulation.
- There is an increased incidence of multiple births in women using this drug.
- You may experience these side effects: Abdominal distention; flushing; breast tenderness; dizziness, drowsiness, light-headedness, visual disturbances (use caution driving or performing tasks that require alertness).
- Report bloating, stomach pain, blurred vision, yellow skin or eyes, unusual bleeding or bruising, fever, chills, visual changes.

▷ clomiPRAMINE hydrochloride

*(kloe **mi'** pra meen)*

Anafranil, Apo-Clomipramine (CAN), Co Clomipramine (CAN), Gen-Clomipramine (CAN)

PREGNANCY CATEGORY C

Drug class

TCA (tertiary amine)

Therapeutic actions

Mechanism unknown; inhibits the presynaptic reuptake of the neurotransmitters norepinephrine and serotonin; anticholinergic at CNS and peripheral receptors.

Indications

- Treatment of obsessions and compulsions in patients with OCD, whose obsessions or compulsions cause marked distress, are time-consuming, or interfere with social or occupational functioning
- Unlabeled uses: Panic disorders, PMS, prevention of migraine, stuttering

Contraindications and cautions

- Contraindicated with hypersensitivity to any tricyclic drug, concomitant therapy with an MAOI, patients in the acute recovery phase following MI, myelography within previous 24 hr or scheduled within 48 hr, lactation.
- Use cautiously with allergy to dibenzazepines, ECT, preexisting CV disorders (eg, severe coronary heart disease, progressive heart failure, angina pectoris, paroxysmal

tachycardia); angle-closure glaucoma, increased IOP, urinary retention, ureteral or urethral spasm; seizure disorders; hyperthyroidism; impaired hepatic, renal function; psychiatric patients (schizophrenic or paranoid patients may exhibit a worsening of psychosis with TCA therapy); patients with bipolar disorder; elective surgery; pregnancy; lactation.

Available forms
Capsules—25, 50, 75 mg

Dosages
Adults
- *Initial treatment:* 25 mg PO daily; gradually increase as tolerated to approximately 100 mg during the first 2 wk. Then increase gradually over the next several weeks to a maximum dose of 250 mg/day. At maximum dose, give once a day at bedtime to minimize sedation.
- *Maintenance therapy:* Adjust to maintain the lowest effective dosage, and periodically assess need for treatment. Effectiveness after 10 wk has not been documented.

Pediatric patients
- *Initial treatment:* 25 mg PO daily; gradually increase as tolerated during the first 2 wk to a maximum of 3 mg/kg or 100 mg, whichever is smaller. Administer in divided doses with meals to reduce GI side effects. Then increase dosage to a daily maximum of 3 mg/kg or 200 mg, whichever is smaller. At maximum, give once a day at bedtime to minimize sedation.
- *Maintenance therapy:* Adjust dosage to maintain lowest effective dosage, and periodically assess patient to determine the need for treatment. Effectiveness after 10 wk has not been documented.

Pharmacokinetics

Route	Onset	Duration
Oral	Slow	1–6 wk

Metabolism: Hepatic; $T_{1/2}$: 19–37 hr
Distribution: Crosses placenta; enters breast milk
Excretion: Bile, feces, urine

Adverse effects
- **CNS:** *Sedation and anticholinergic (atropine-like) effects; confusion* (espe-

cially in elderly), *disturbed concentration, dizziness, tremor,* hallucinations, disorientation, decreased memory, feelings of unreality, delusions, anxiety, nervousness, restlessness, agitation, panic, insomnia, nightmares, hypomania, mania, *asthenia,* aggressive reaction
- **CV:** *Orthostatic hypotension,* hypertension, syncope, tachycardia, palpitations, **MI,** arrhythmias, heart block, **precipitation of heart failure, stroke**
- **Endocrine:** Hyperglycemia or hypoglycemia; elevated prolactin levels; inappropriate ADH secretion
- **GI:** *Dry mouth, constipation,* paralytic ileus, *nausea,* vomiting, anorexia, epigastric distress, diarrhea, flatulence, dysphagia, peculiar taste, increased salivation, stomatitis, parotid swelling, abdominal cramps, black tongue, *eructation*
- **GU:** Urinary retention, delayed or frequent micturition, dilation of the urinary tract, gynecomastia, testicular swelling; breast enlargement, *menstrual irregularity* and galactorrhea in women; increased or decreased libido; *impotence,* painful ejaculation
- **Hematologic:** Bone marrow depression, including **agranulocytosis;** eosinophilia, purpura, thrombocytopenia, leukopenia, anemia
- **Hypersensitivity:** Skin rash, pruritus, vasculitis, petechiae, photosensitization, edema (generalized, facial, tongue), drug fever
- **Withdrawal:** Symptoms on abrupt discontinuation of prolonged therapy—nausea, headache, vertigo, nightmares, malaise
- **Other:** *Nasal congestion, laryngitis,* excessive appetite, weight change; sweating hyperthermia, flushing, chills

Interactions
✳ **Drug-drug** • Increased TCA levels and pharmacologic effects with cimetidine • Increased TCA levels with fluoxetine, methylphenidate, phenothiazines, hormonal contraceptives, disulfiram • Hyperpyretic crises, severe seizures, hypertensive episodes and deaths when MAOIs, furazolidone, clonidine are given with TCAs; don't give within 14 days before or after an MAOI • Increased antidepressant response and cardiac arrhythmias when given with thyroid medication • Increased anticholinergic effects of anticholinergic drugs when given with TCAs

• Increased response to alcohol, barbiturates, benzodiazepines, other CNS depressants with TCAs • Decreased effects of indirect-acting sympathomimetic drugs (ephedrine) with TCAs • Risk of arrhythmias if combined with fluoroquinolones • Decreased levels with drugs that induce CYP450 (such as rifampin, phenytoin)
* Drug-alternative therapy • Clomipramine levels reduced with St. John's Wort

■ **Nursing considerations**

CLINICAL ALERT!
Name confusion has occurred between clomipramine and chlorpromazine; use caution.

Assessment

• **History:** Hypersensitivity to any tricyclic drug; concomitant therapy with an MAOI; myelography within previous 24 hr or scheduled within 48 hr; lactation; ECT; preexisting CV disorders; angle-closure glaucoma, increased IOP, urinary retention, ureteral or urethral spasm; seizure disorders; hyperthyroidism, impaired hepatic, renal function; psychiatric patients; elective surgery, pregnancy
• **Physical:** Weight; T; skin color, lesions; orientation, affect, reflexes, vision and hearing; P, BP, orthostatic BP, perfusion; bowel sounds, normal output, liver evaluation; urine flow, normal output; usual sexual function, frequency of menses; breast and scrotal examination; LFTs, urinalysis, CBC, ECG

Interventions

⊗ **Black box warning** Increased risk of suicidal thinking and behavior in children, adolescents, and young adults; use caution, and monitor patient accordingly.

• Limit depressed and potentially suicidal patients' access to drug.
• Administer in divided doses with meals to reduce GI side effects while increasing dosage to therapeutic levels.
• Give maintenance dose once daily at bedtime to decrease daytime sedation.
• Reduce dose if minor side effects develop; discontinue drug if serious side effects occur.
• Arrange for CBC if patient develops fever, sore throat, or other signs of infection.

Teaching points

• Take this drug as prescribed; do not stop taking abruptly or without consulting your health care provider.
• Avoid alcohol, sleep-inducing drugs, and over-the-counter drugs.
• Avoid prolonged exposure to sun or sunlamps; use a sunscreen or protective garments if exposure to sun is unavoidable.
• You may experience these side effects: Headache, dizziness, drowsiness, weakness, blurred vision (reversible; take safety measures if severe; avoid driving or performing tasks that require alertness); nausea, vomiting, loss of appetite, dry mouth (eat frequent small meals; practice frequent mouth care; and suck sugarless candies); nightmares, inability to concentrate, confusion; changes in sexual function.
• Report dry mouth, difficulty urinating, excessive sedation.

▽**clonazepam**
(kloe na' ze pam)

Apo-Clonazepam (CAN),
CO Clonazepam (CAN), Gen-
Clonazepam (CAN), Klonopin,
PMS-Clonazepam (CAN), ratio-
Clonazepam (CAN), Rivotril (CAN)

PREGNANCY CATEGORY D

CONTROLLED SUBSTANCE C-IV

Drug classes
Antiepileptic
Benzodiazepine

Therapeutic actions
Exact mechanisms not understood; benzodiazepines potentiate the effects of GABA, an inhibitory neurotransmitter.

Indications
• Used alone or as adjunct in treatment of Lennox-Gastaut syndrome (petit mal variant), akinetic and myoclonic seizures; may be useful in patients with absence (petit mal) seizures who have not responded to succinimides; up to 30% of patients show loss of anticonvulsant activity of drug, often within 3 mo of therapy (may respond to dosage adjustment)

- Treatment of panic disorder with or without agoraphobia
- Unlabeled uses: Periodic leg movements during sleep; hypokinetic dysarthria; acute manic episodes; multifocal tic disorders; neuralgias; adjunct in managing schizophrenia

Contraindications and cautions

- Contraindicated with hypersensitivity to benzodiazepines, psychoses, acute narrow-angle glaucoma, shock, coma, acute alcoholic intoxication with depression of vital signs; pregnancy (risk of congenital malformations, neonatal withdrawal syndrome), labor and delivery ("floppy infant" syndrome), lactation (infants become lethargic and lose weight).
- Use cautiously with hepatic or renal impairment, debilitation; elderly patients.

Available forms

Tablets—0.5, 1, 2 mg; orally disintegrating tablets—0.125, 0.25, 0.5, 1, 2 mg

Dosages

Individualize dosage; increase dosage gradually to avoid adverse effects; drug is available only in oral dosage forms.

Adults

Seizure disorders: Initial dose should not exceed 1.5 mg/day PO divided into three doses; increase in increments of 0.5–1 mg PO every 3 days until seizures are adequately controlled or until side effects preclude further increases. Maximum recommended dosage is 20 mg/day.

Panic disorders: Initial dose 0.25 mg PO bid; gradually increase to a target dose of 1 mg/day. Do not exceed 4 mg/day.

Pediatric patients at least 10 yr or 30 kg

Initially, 0.01–0.03 mg/kg/day PO; do not exceed 0.05 mg/kg/day PO, given in two or three doses. Increase dosage by not more than 0.25–0.5 mg every third day until a daily maintenance dose of 0.1–0.2 mg/kg has been reached, unless seizures are controlled by lower dosage or side effects preclude increases. Whenever possible, divide daily dose into three equal doses, or give largest dose at bedtime.

Pharmacokinetics

Route	Onset	Peak	Duration
Oral	Varies	1–2 hr	Weeks

Metabolism: Hepatic; $T_{1/2}$: 18–50 hr
Distribution: Crosses placenta; enters breast milk
Excretion: Urine

Adverse effects

- **CNS:** *Transient, mild drowsiness initially; sedation, depression, lethargy, apathy, fatigue, light-headedness, disorientation, anger, hostility,* episodes of mania and hypomania, restlessness, confusion, crying, delirium, suicidal ideation, headache, slurred speech, dysarthria, stupor, rigidity, tremor, dystonia, vertigo, euphoria, nervousness, difficulty in concentration, vivid dreams, psychomotor retardation, extrapyramidal symptoms; *mild paradoxical excitatory reactions during first 2 wk of treatment*
- **CV:** Bradycardia, tachycardia, **CV collapse,** hypertension and hypotension, palpitations, edema
- **Dermatologic:** Urticaria, pruritus, rash, dermatitis
- **EENT:** Visual and auditory disturbances, diplopia, nystagmus, depressed hearing, nasal congestion
- **GI:** *Constipation, diarrhea, dry mouth,* salivation, *nausea,* anorexia, vomiting, difficulty in swallowing, gastric disorders, encoporesis
- **GU:** Incontinence, urinary retention, changes in libido, menstrual irregularities
- **Hematologic:** Elevations of blood enzymes—LDH, alkaline phosphatase, AST, ALT; blood dyscrasias: **agranulocytosis,** leukopenia
- **Other:** Hiccups, fever, diaphoresis, paresthesias, muscular disturbances, gynecomastia. Drug dependence with withdrawal syndrome when drug is discontinued; more common with abrupt discontinuation of higher dosage used for longer than 4 mo

Interactions

✳ **Drug-drug** • Increased CNS depression with alcohol and other CNS depressants • Increased effect with cimetidine, disulfiram, omeprazole, hormonal contraceptives • Decreased effect with theophylline • Risk of increased digoxin levels and toxicity; monitor patient carefully

■ Nursing considerations

 CLINICAL ALERT!

Name confusion has occurred between *Klonopin* (clonazepam) and clonidine; use caution.

Assessment

- **History:** Hypersensitivity to benzodiazepines; psychoses; acute narrow-angle glaucoma; shock; coma; acute alcoholic intoxication; pregnancy; lactation; hepatic or renal impairment, debilitation
- **Physical:** Skin color, lesions; T; orientation, reflexes, affect, ophthalmologic examination; P, BP; R, adventitious sounds; liver evaluation, abdominal examination, bowel sounds, normal output; CBC, LFTs, renal function tests

Interventions

- Monitor addiction-prone patients carefully because of their predisposition to habituation and drug dependence.
- Monitor patient for suicidal ideation.
- Monitor liver function and blood counts periodically in patients on long-term therapy.
- ⊗ *Warning* Taper dosage gradually after long-term therapy, especially in patients with epilepsy; substitute another antiepileptic.
- Monitor patient for therapeutic drug levels: 20–80 nanograms/mL.
- If patient has epilepsy, arrange for patient to wear medical alert identification indicating patient has epilepsy and is receiving drug therapy.

Teaching points

- Take drug exactly as prescribed; do not stop taking drug (long-term therapy) without consulting your health care provider.
- Avoid alcohol and sleep-inducing or over-the-counter drugs.
- Avoid pregnancy; serious adverse effects can occur. Using barrier contraceptives is advised while taking this drug.
- It is advisable to wear or carry a medical alert identification indicating your diagnosis and drug therapy.
- You may experience these side effects: Drowsiness, dizziness (may become less pronounced; avoid driving or engaging in other dangerous activities); GI upset (take drug with food); fatigue; dreams; crying; nervousness; depression, emotional changes; bed-wetting, urinary incontinence.
- Report severe dizziness, weakness, drowsiness that persists, rash or skin lesions, difficulty voiding, palpitations, swelling in the extremities, thoughts of suicide.

▽ **clonidine hydrochloride**

(kloe' ni deen)

Oral: Apo-Clonidine (CAN), Catapres, Kapvay⊙ᴿ, Nexiclon XR
Transdermal preparations:
Catapres-TTS-1, Catapres-TTS-2, Catapres-TTS-3, Dixarit (CAN), Duraclon
Analgesic: Duraclon

PREGNANCY CATEGORY C

Drug classes

Antihypertensive
Central analgesic
Sympatholytic (centrally acting)

Therapeutic actions

Stimulates CNS alpha₂-adrenergic receptors, inhibits sympathetic cardioaccelerator and vasoconstrictor centers, and decreases sympathetic outflow from the CNS.

Indications

- Hypertension, used alone or as part of combination therapy
- Treatment of severe pain in cancer patients in combination with opiates; epidural more effective with neuropathic pain (*Duraclon*)
- Treatment of ADHD in children 6–17 yr, as monotherapy or in combination with stimulants (*Kapvay*)
- Unlabeled uses: Tourette syndrome; migraine, decreases severity and frequency; menopausal flushing, decreases severity and frequency of episodes; chronic methadone detoxification; rapid opiate detoxification (in doses up to 17 mcg/kg/day); alcohol and benzodiazepine withdrawal treatment; management of hypertensive "urgencies" (oral clonidine "loading" is used; initial dose of 0.2 mg then 0.1 mg every hour until a dose of 0.7 mg is reached or until BP is controlled); atrial fibrillation; post-herpetic

neuralgia, smoking cessation (transdermal), hot flashes, hyperhidrosis, ulcerative colitis, diabetic diarrhea

Contraindications and cautions

• Contraindicated with hypersensitivity to clonidine or any adhesive layer components of the transdermal system.
• Use cautiously with severe coronary insufficiency, recent MI, cerebrovascular disease; chronic renal failure; pregnancy, lactation.

Available forms

Tablets—0.1, 0.2, 0.3 mg; ER tablets ⓒⒻⓒ— 0.1, 0.2 mg; modified-release tablets—0.1 mg; ER suspension—0.09 mg/mL; transdermal— 0.1, 0.2, 0.3 mg/24 hr; epidural injection— 100 mcg/mL, 500 mcg/mL

Dosages

Adults

Oral therapy

Individualize dosage. Initial dose is 0.1 mg bid; for maintenance dosage, increase in increments of 0.1 or 0.2 mg to reach desired response. Common range is 0.2–0.6 mg/day, in divided doses or once daily if using extended-release form; maximum dose is 2.4 mg/day. Minimize sedation by slowly increasing daily dosage; giving majority of daily dose at bedtime. Modified-release tablets use same dosage, but are not interchangeable with other forms; dosage adjustment may be needed if switching between forms.

Transdermal system

Apply to a hairless area of intact skin of upper arm or torso once every 7 days. Change skin site for each application. If system loosens while wearing, apply adhesive overlay directly over the system to ensure adhesion. Start with the 0.1-mg system (releases 0.1 mg/24 hr); if, after 1–2 wk, desired BP reduction is not achieved, add another 0.1-mg system, or use a larger system. Dosage of more than two 0.3-mg systems does not improve efficacy. Antihypertensive effect may only begin 2–3 days after application; therefore, when substituting transdermal systems, a gradual reduction of prior dosage is advised. Remove old system before applying new one. Previous antihypertensive medication may have to be continued, particularly with severe hypertension.

Epidural

• *Pain management:* 30 mcg/hr by continuous epidural infusion.

Pediatric patients 6–17 yr

• *ADHD:* Initially, 0.1 mg PO at bedtime; titrate at 0.1 mg/wk to a total of 0.2 mg, with 0.1 mg in AM and 0.1 mg in PM, then 0.1 mg in AM and 0.2 mg in PM. Maintenance dose, 0.2 mg in AM and 0.2 mg in PM. If discontinuing, taper in increments of no more than 0.1 mg every 7 day (*Kapvay* only).

Pharmacokinetics

Route	Onset	Peak	Duration
Oral	30–60 min	3–5 hr	24 hr
Transdermal	Slow	2–3 days	7 days
Epidural	Rapid	19 min	Variable

Metabolism: Hepatic; $T_{1/2}$: 12–16 hr, 19 hr (transdermal system); 48 hr (epidural)
Distribution: Crosses placenta; enters breast milk
Excretion: Urine

Adverse effects

• **CNS:** *Drowsiness, sedation, dizziness,* headache, fatigue that tend to diminish within 4–6 wk, dreams, nightmares, insomnia, hallucinations, delirium, nervousness, restlessness, anxiety, depression, retinal degeneration
• **CV:** Heart failure, orthostatic hypotension, palpitations, tachycardia, bradycardia, Raynaud phenomenon, ECG abnormalities manifested as Wenckebach period or ventricular trigeminy
• **Dermatologic:** Rash, angioneurotic edema, hives, urticaria, hair thinning and alopecia, pruritus, dryness, itching or burning of the eyes, pallor
• **GI:** *Dry mouth, constipation,* anorexia, malaise, nausea, vomiting, parotid pain, parotitis, mild transient abnormalities in LFTs
• **GU:** Impotence, sexual dysfunction, nocturia, difficulty in micturition, urinary retention
• **Other:** Weight gain, transient hyperglycemia or elevated serum creatine phosphokinase level, gynecomastia, weakness, muscle or joint pain, cramps of the lower limbs, dryness of the nasal mucosa, fever

Transdermal system

• **CNS:** Drowsiness, fatigue, headache, lethargy, sedation, insomnia, nervousness
• **GI:** *Dry mouth,* constipation, nausea, change in taste, dry throat

- **GU:** Impotence, sexual dysfunction
- **Local:** *Transient localized skin reactions,* pruritus, erythema, allergic contact sensitization and contact dermatitis, localized vesiculation, hyperpigmentation, edema, excoriation, burning, papules, throbbing, blanching, generalized macular rash

Interactions

❋ **Drug-drug** ● Decreased antihypertensive effects with TCAs (imipramine) ● Paradoxical hypertension with propranolol; also greater withdrawal hypertension when abruptly discontinued and patient is taking beta-adrenergic blocking agents ● Additive sedation with CNS depressants, alcohol

■ Nursing considerations

 CLINICAL ALERT!
Name confusion has occurred between clonidine and *Klonopin* (clonazepam); use caution.

Assessment

- **History:** Hypersensitivity to clonidine or adhesive layer components of the transdermal system; severe coronary insufficiency, recent MI, cerebrovascular disease; chronic renal failure; lactation, pregnancy
- **Physical:** Body weight; T; skin color, lesions, T; mucous membranes color, lesions; breast examination; orientation, affect, reflexes; ophthalmologic examination; P, BP, orthostatic BP, perfusion, edema, auscultation; bowel sounds, normal output, liver evaluation; palpation of salivary glands; normal urinary output, voiding pattern; LFTs, ECG

Interventions

⊗ **Warning** Do not discontinue use abruptly; discontinue therapy by reducing the dosage gradually over 2–4 days to avoid rebound hypertension, tachycardia, flushing, nausea, vomiting, cardiac arrhythmias (hypertensive encephalopathy and death have occurred after abrupt cessation of clonidine).
- Do not discontinue transdermal therapy prior to surgery; monitor BP carefully during surgery; have other BP-controlling drugs readily available.
- Continue oral clonidine therapy to within 4 hr of surgery then resume as soon as possible thereafter.

- Be alert that *Kapvay,* used to treat ADHD, is not interchangeable with any other clonidine product. *Kapvay* cannot be cut, crushed, or chewed.

⊗ **Black box warning** Epidural route is not recommended for obstetric, postpartum, or perioperative pain because of the risk of hemodynamic instability.
- Store epidural injection at room temperature; discard any unused portions.
- Reevaluate therapy if clonidine tolerance occurs; giving concomitant diuretic increases the antihypertensive efficacy of clonidine.
- Monitor BP carefully when discontinuing clonidine; hypertension usually returns within 48 hr.

⊗ **Warning** Remove transdermal patch before defibrillation to prevent arcing. Remove system if patient is having an MRI.
- Assess compliance with drug regimen in a supportive manner with pill counts, or other methods.

Teaching points

- Take this drug exactly as prescribed. Do not miss doses. Do not discontinue the drug unless instructed by your health care provider. Do not discontinue abruptly; life-threatening adverse effects may occur. If you travel, take an adequate supply of drug. If using *Kapvay* for ADHD, swallow tablet whole; do not cut, crush, or chew tablet.
- Use the transdermal system as prescribed; refer to directions in package insert, or contact your health care provider with questions. Be sure to remove old systems before applying new ones. System must be removed if you are going to have an MRI; inform technician that you are using this system.
- Attempt lifestyle changes that will reduce your blood pressure: Stop smoking and using alcohol; lose weight; restrict intake of salt; exercise regularly.
- Use caution with alcohol. Your sensitivity may increase while using this drug.
- You may experience these side effects: Drowsiness, dizziness, light-headedness, headache, weakness (often transient; observe caution driving or performing other tasks that require alertness or physical dexterity); dry mouth (sucking on sugarless candies or ice chips may help); GI upset (eat frequent small meals); dreams, nightmares (reversible); dizziness, light-headedness when you change

position (get up slowly; use caution climbing stairs); impotence, other sexual dysfunction, decreased libido (discuss with your health care provider); breast enlargement, sore breasts; palpitations.

- Report urinary retention, changes in vision, blanching of fingers, rash.

▷ clopidogrel bisulfate
(cloe *pid'* oh grel)

Plavix

PREGNANCY CATEGORY B

Drug classes
Adenosine diphosphate (ADP) receptor antagonist
Antiplatelet

Therapeutic actions
Inhibits platelet aggregation by blocking ADP receptors on platelets, preventing clumping of platelets.

Indications
- Treatment of patients at risk for ischemic events—recent MI, recent ischemic stroke, peripheral artery disease
- Treatment of patients with acute coronary syndrome
- Unlabeled use: As loading dose with aspirin to prevent adverse cardiac events in coronary stent implantation

Contraindications and cautions
- Contraindicated with allergy to clopidogrel, active pathologic bleeding such as peptic ulcer or intracranial hemorrhage, lactation.
- Use cautiously with bleeding disorders, recent surgery, hepatic impairment, pregnancy.

Available forms
Tablets—75, 300 mg

Dosages
Adults
- *Recent MI, stroke, or established peripheral arterial disease:* 75 mg PO daily.
- *Acute coronary syndrome:* 300 mg PO loading dose, then 75 mg/day PO with aspirin, given at a dose from 75–325 mg once daily.

Pharmacokinetics

Route	Onset	Peak	Duration
Oral	Varies	1 hr	2 hr

Metabolism: Hepatic; $T_{1/2}$: 8 hr
Distribution: Crosses placenta; enters breast milk
Excretion: Bile, feces, urine

Adverse effects
- **CNS:** *Headache, dizziness,* weakness, syncope, flushing
- **CV:** Hypertension, edema
- **Dermatologic:** *Rash,* pruritus
- **GI:** Nausea, GI distress, constipation, diarrhea, **GI bleed**
- **Other:** Increased bleeding risk

Interactions
* **Drug-drug** • Increased risk of GI bleeding with NSAIDs, monitor patient carefully • Increased risk of bleeding with warfarin; monitor carefully

■ Nursing considerations
Assessment
- **History:** Allergy to clopidogrel, pregnancy, lactation, bleeding disorders, recent surgery, hepatic impairment, peptic ulcer
- **Physical:** Skin color, T, lesions; orientation, reflexes, affect; P, BP, orthostatic BP, baseline ECG, peripheral perfusion; R, adventitious sounds

Interventions
⊗ **Black box warning** Slow or poor metabolizers may experience less effects, as drug is activated in the liver by CYP2C19. Genotype testing for poor metabolizers is suggested before beginning drug.
- Provide frequent small meals if GI upset occurs (not as common as with aspirin).
- Provide comfort measures and arrange for analgesics if headache occurs.
- Monitor patient for increased bleeding; limit invasive procedures.

Teaching points
- Take daily as prescribed. May be taken with meals. You may also be taking aspirin.
- You may experience these side effects: Dizziness, light-headedness (this may pass as you adjust to the drug); headache (lie down in a cool environment and rest;

Adverse effects in *italics* are most common; those in **bold** are life-threatening. ⬛ Do not crush.

over-the-counter preparations may help); nausea, gastric distress (eat frequent small meals); prolonged bleeding (alert dentists and health care providers of this drug use).
- Report rash, chest pain, fainting, severe headache, abnormal bleeding or bruising.

▷**clorazepate dipotassium**
(klor az' e pate)

Apo-Clorazepate (CAN), Tranxene-T-tab

PREGNANCY CATEGORY D

CONTROLLED SUBSTANCE C-IV

Drug classes
Antiepileptic
Anxiolytic
Benzodiazepine

Therapeutic actions
Exact mechanisms not understood; benzodiazepines potentiate the effects of GABA, an inhibitory neurotransmitter; anxiolytic effects occur at doses well below those necessary to cause sedation, ataxia.

Indications
- Management of anxiety disorders or for short-term relief of symptoms of anxiety
- Symptomatic relief of acute alcohol withdrawal
- Adjunctive therapy for partial seizures

Contraindications and cautions
- Contraindicated with hypersensitivity to benzodiazepines; psychoses; acute narrow-angle glaucoma; shock; coma; acute alcoholic intoxication with depression of vital signs; pregnancy (risk of congenital malformations, neonatal withdrawal syndrome); labor and delivery ("floppy infant" syndrome); lactation (infants tend to become lethargic and lose weight).
- Use cautiously with impaired liver or renal function, debilitation; elderly patients.

Available forms
Tablets—3.75, 7.5, 15 mg

Dosages
Individualize dosage; increase dosage gradually to avoid adverse effects. Drug is available only in oral forms.
Adults
- *Anxiety:* Usual dose is 30 mg/day PO in divided doses tid; adjust gradually within the range of 15–60 mg/day; also may be given as a single daily dose at bedtime with a maximum starting dose of 15 mg. For maintenance, give the 22.5-mg PO tablet in a single daily dose as an alternate form for patients stabilized on 7.5 mg PO tid; do not use to initiate therapy.
- *Adjunct to antiepileptic medication:* Maximum initial dose is 7.5 mg PO tid. Increase dosage by no more than 7.5 mg every wk, do not exceed 90 mg/day.
- *Acute alcohol withdrawal:* Day 1: 30 mg PO initially, then 30–60 mg in divided doses. Day 2: 45–90 mg PO in divided doses. Day 3: 22.5–45 mg PO in divided doses. Day 4: 15–30 mg PO in divided doses. Thereafter, gradually reduce dose to 7.5–15 mg/day PO, and stop as soon as condition is stable.
Pediatric patients
- *Adjunct to antiepileptic medication:* Older than 12 yr: Use adult dosage. 9–12 yr: Maximum initial dose is 7.5 mg PO bid; increase dosage by no more than 7.5 mg every wk, and do not exceed 60 mg/day. Younger than 9 yr: Not recommended.
Geriatric patients or patients with debilitating disease
- *Anxiety:* Initially, 7.5–15 mg/day PO in divided doses. Adjust as needed and tolerated.

Pharmacokinetics

Route	Onset	Peak	Duration
Oral	Fast	1–2 hr	Days

Metabolism: Hepatic; $T_{1/2}$: 40–50 hr
Distribution: Crosses placenta; enters breast milk
Excretion: Urine

Adverse effects
- **CNS:** *Transient, mild drowsiness initially; sedation, depression, lethargy, apathy, fatigue, light-headedness, disorientation, anger, hostility,* episodes of mania and hypomania, restlessness, confusion, crying, delirium, *headache,* slurred speech, dysarthria, stupor, rigidity, tremor, dystonia,

vertigo, euphoria, nervousness, difficulty in concentration, vivid dreams, psychomotor retardation, extrapyramidal symptoms; *mild paradoxical excitatory reactions during first 2 wk of treatment*
- **CV:** Bradycardia, tachycardia, **CV collapse,** hypertension and hypotension, palpitations, edema
- **Dermatologic:** Urticaria, pruritus, rash, dermatitis
- **EENT:** Visual and auditory disturbances, diplopia, nystagmus, depressed hearing, nasal congestion
- **GI:** *Constipation, diarrhea, dry mouth,* salivation, *nausea,* anorexia, vomiting, difficulty in swallowing, gastric disorders, hepatic impairment, encopresis
- **GU:** Incontinence, urinary retention, changes in libido, menstrual irregularities
- **Hematologic:** Elevations of blood enzymes—LDH, alkaline phosphatase, AST, ALT; blood dyscrasias—**agranulocytosis,** leukopenia
- **Other:** Hiccups, fever, diaphoresis, paresthesias, muscular disturbances, gynecomastia; drug dependence with withdrawal syndrome is common with abrupt discontinuation of higher dosage used for longer than 4 mo

Interactions
✳ **Drug-drug** ● Increased CNS depression with alcohol and other CNS depressants ● Increased effect with cimetidine, disulfiram, omeprazole, hormonal contraceptives ● Decreased effect with theophylline ● Risk of increased digoxin levels and toxicity; monitor patient carefully
✳ **Drug-alternative therapy** ● Increased CNS effects with kava

■ Nursing considerations

CLINICAL ALERT!
Name confusion has occurred between clorazepate and clofibrate; use caution.

Assessment
- **History:** Hypersensitivity to benzodiazepines; psychoses; acute narrow-angle glaucoma; shock; coma; acute alcoholic intoxication; pregnancy; lactation; renal or hepatic impairment; debilitation
- **Physical:** Skin color, lesions; T; orientation, reflexes, affect, ophthalmologic examination; P, BP; R, adventitious sounds; liver evalua-

tion, abdominal examination, bowel sounds, normal output; CBC, LFTs, renal function tests

Interventions
⊗ **Warning** Taper dosage gradually after long-term therapy, especially in epileptics.
- Arrange for patients with epilepsy to wear medical alert identification, indicating disease and medication usage.
- Because of increased risk of suicide, monitor patient for suicidal ideation.

Teaching points
- Take drug exactly as prescribed; do not stop taking drug (long-term therapy) without consulting your health care provider.
- Avoid alcohol and sleep-inducing or over-the-counter drugs.
- Avoid pregnancy while taking this drug; use of barrier contraceptives is advised. If you become pregnant, do not stop the drug; contact your health care provider.
- You may experience these side effects: Drowsiness, dizziness (may be transient; avoid driving a car or engaging in other dangerous activities); GI upset (take with food); fatigue; depression; dreams; crying; nervousness; depression, emotional changes; bed-wetting, urinary incontinence.
- Report severe dizziness, weakness, drowsiness that persists, rash or skin lesions, difficulty voiding, palpitations, swelling in the extremities, thoughts of suicide.

▽ clotrimazole
*(kloe **trim' a** zole)*

Oral, Topical use only: Mycelex Troche
Vaginal preparations: Canesten Vaginal (CAN), Gyne-Lotrimin 3, Gyne-Lotrimin 3 Combination Pack, Mycelex-7, Mycelex-7 Combination Pack
Topical preparations: Canesten Topical (CAN), Clotrimaderm (CAN), Cruex, Desenex, Fungoid, Lotrimin AF, Lotrimin Ultra

PREGNANCY CATEGORY B
(TOPICAL, VAGINAL FORMS)

PREGNANCY CATEGORY C
(ORAL TROCHE)

Drug class
Antifungal

Therapeutic actions
Fungicidal and fungistatic: Binds to fungal cell membrane with a resultant change in membrane permeability, allowing leakage of intracellular components, causing cell death.

Indications
- Troche: Treatment of oropharyngeal candidiasis; prevention of oropharyngeal candidiasis in immunocompromised patients receiving radiation, chemotherapy, or steroid therapy
- Vaginal preparations: Local treatment of vulvovaginal candidiasis (moniliasis)
- Topical preparations: Topical treatment of tinea pedia, tinea cruris, tinea corporis due to *Trichophyton rubrum, Trichophyton mentagrophytes, Epidermophyton floccosum, Microsporum canis;* candidiasis due to *Candida albicans;* tinea versicolor due to *Malassezia furfur*

Contraindications and cautions
- Contraindicated with allergy to clotrimazole or components used in preparation. Vaginal products contraindicated in girls younger than 12 yr.
- Use vaginal and topical preparations cautiously with pregnancy, lactation.
- Use oral troche only when benefits to mother outweigh risk to fetus.

Available forms
Vaginal suppositories—100, 200 mg; vaginal cream, solution, lotion—1%, 2%; topical cream, solution, lotion—1%; oral troche—10 mg

Dosages
Oral troche, patients 2 yr and older
For treatment, dissolve slowly in the mouth five times daily for 14 days. For prevention, tid for the duration of chemotherapy or radiation therapy or until steroids are reduced to maintenance levels.
Topical, patients 2 yr and older
Gently massage into affected and surrounding skin areas bid in the morning and evening for 14 days. Relief is usually noted during first week of therapy; therapy 2–4 wk.

Vaginal suppository, patients 12 yr and older
100-mg suppository intravaginally at bedtime for 7 consecutive nights; 200-mg suppository for 3 consecutive nights.
Vaginal preparation, cream, patients 12 yr and older
One applicator (5 g/day), preferably at bedtime for 3–7 consecutive days.

Pharmacokinetics
Action is primarily local; pharmacokinetics are not known.

Adverse effects
Troche
- **GI:** *Nausea, vomiting, abnormal LFTs*
Vaginal
- **Dermatologic:** Rash
- **GI:** *Lower abdominal cramps,* bloating (elevated AST), unpleasant mouth sensations
- **GU:** *Slight urinary frequency; burning or irritation in the sex partner*
Topical
- **Local:** Erythema, stinging, blistering, peeling, edema, pruritus, urticaria, general skin irritation

■ Nursing considerations

 CLINICAL ALERT!
Name confusion has occurred between clotrimazole and co-trimoxazole; use caution.

Assessment
- **History:** Allergy to clotrimazole or components used in preparation, pregnancy, lactation
- **Physical:** Skin color, lesions, area around lesions; bowel sounds; culture of area involved, LFTs

Interventions
- Culture fungus involved before therapy.
- Have patient dissolve troche slowly in mouth.
- Insert vaginal suppository into vagina at bedtime for 3–7 consecutive nights. Provide sanitary napkin to protect clothing from stains.
- Administer vaginal cream high into vagina using the applicator supplied with the product. Administer for 3–7 consecutive

nights, even during menstrual period. During pregnancy, use of vaginal applicator may be contraindicated.

- Cleanse affected area before topical application. Do not apply to eyes or near eyes.
- Monitor response to drug therapy. If no response is noted, arrange for more cultures to determine causative organism.
- Ensure that patient receives full course of therapy to eradicate the fungus and prevent recurrence.
- Discontinue topical or vaginal administration if rash or sensitivity occurs.
- Supervise children younger than 12 yr using topical products.

Teaching points
- Take the full course of drug therapy, even if symptoms improve. Continue during menstrual period if vaginal route is being used. Long-term use of the drug may be needed; beneficial effects may not be seen for several weeks. Vaginal creams should be inserted high into the vagina. Troche preparation should be allowed to dissolve slowly in the mouth. Apply topical preparation by gently massaging into the affected area.
- Use hygiene measures to prevent reinfection or spread of infection.
- With vaginal use, refrain from sexual intercourse, or advise partner to use a condom to avoid reinfection. Use a sanitary napkin to prevent staining of clothing.
- You may experience these side effects: Nausea, vomiting, diarrhea (oral use); irritation, burning, stinging (local).
- Report worsening of the condition being treated, local irritation, burning (topical), rash, irritation, pelvic pain (vaginal), nausea, GI distress (oral administration).

▽clozapine
(kloe' za peen)

Apo-Clozapine (CAN), Clozaril, FazaClo, Gen-Clozapine (CAN)

PREGNANCY CATEGORY B

Drug classes
Antipsychotic
Dopaminergic blocker

Therapeutic actions
Mechanism not fully understood: Blocks dopamine receptors in the brain, depresses the RAS; anticholinergic, antihistaminic (H_1), and alpha-adrenergic blocking activity may contribute to some of its therapeutic (and adverse) actions. Clozapine produces fewer extrapyramidal effects than other antipsychotics.

Indications
- Management of severely ill schizophrenics who are unresponsive to standard antipsychotic drugs
- Reduction of the risk of recurrent suicidal behavior in patients with schizophrenia or schizoaffective disorder (not orally disintegrating tablet)

Contraindications and cautions
- Contraindicated with allergy to clozapine, myeloproliferative disorders, history of clozapine-induced agranulocytosis or severe granulocytopenia, severe CNS depression, comatose states, history of seizure disorders, lactation, therapy with other drugs that cause bone marrow suppression.
- Use cautiously with CV disease, narrow-angle glaucoma, pregnancy.

Available forms
Tablets—12.5, 25, 50, 100, 200 mg; orally disintegrating tablets—12.5, 25, 100, 150, 200 mg

Dosages
Adults
- *Initial therapy:* 12.5 mg PO once or twice daily. Continue to 25 mg PO daily or bid; then gradually increase with daily increments of 25–50 mg/day, if tolerated, to a dose of 300–450 mg/day by the end of second week. Adjust later dosage no more often than twice weekly in increments of less than 100 mg. Do not exceed 900 mg/day.
- *Maintenance:* Maintain at the lowest effective dose for remission of symptoms.
- *Discontinuation of therapy:* Gradual reduction over a 1- to 2-wk period is preferred. If abrupt discontinuation is required, carefully monitor patient for signs of acute psychotic symptoms.
- *Reinitiation of treatment:* Follow initial dosage guidelines, use extreme care; increased risk of severe adverse effects with re-exposure.

Pediatric patients
Safety and efficacy in patients younger than 16 yr not established.

Pharmacokinetics

Route	Onset	Peak	Duration
Oral	Varies	1–6 hr	Weeks

Metabolism: Hepatic; $T_{1/2}$: 4–12 hr
Distribution: Crosses placenta; enters breast milk
Excretion: Feces, urine

Adverse effects

- **CNS:** *Drowsiness, sedation,* **seizures**, *dizziness, syncope, headache,* tremor, disturbed sleep, nightmares, restlessness, agitation, increased salivation, sweating, tardive dyskinesia, neuroleptic malignant syndrome
- **CV:** *Tachycardia, hypotension,* hypertension, ECG changes, **potentially fatal myocarditis**
- **GI:** *Nausea, vomiting, constipation,* abdominal discomfort, dry mouth
- **GU:** Urinary abnormalities
- **Hematologic:** Leukopenia, **agranulocytosis**
- **Other:** *Fever,* weight gain, rash, development of diabetes mellitus

Interactions

✻ Drug-drug • Increased therapeutic and toxic effects with cimetidine, caffeine, other CYP450 inhibitors • Decreased therapeutic effect with phenytoin, ethotoin, other CYP450 inducers

■ Nursing considerations

CLINICAL ALERT!
Name confusion has occurred with *Clozaril* (clozapine) and *Colazal* (balsalazide); dangerous effects could occur. Use caution.

Assessment

- **History:** Allergy to clozapine, myeloproliferative disorders, history of clozapine-induced agranulocytosis or severe granulocytopenia, severe CNS depression, comatose states, history of seizure disorders, CV disease, narrow-angle glaucoma, lactation, pregnancy
- **Physical:** T, weight; reflexes, orientation, IOP, ophthalmologic examination; P, BP, orthostatic BP, ECG; R, adventitious sounds; bowel sounds, normal output, liver evaluation; prostate palpation, normal urine output; CBC, urinalysis, LFTs, renal function tests, EEG

Interventions

⊗ **Black box warning** Use only when unresponsive to conventional antipsychotic drugs; risk of serious CV and respiratory effects, including myocarditis.

- Obtain clozapine through the *Clozaril* Patient Assistance Program. For more information, call 1-800-448-5938.
- Dispense only 1 wk supply at a time.
- Monitor WBC count carefully prior to first dose.

⊗ **Black box warning** Monitor WBC count weekly during treatment and for 4 wk thereafter. Dosage must be adjusted based on WBC count. Potentially fatal agranulocytosis has been reported.

⊗ **Black box warning** Elderly patients with dementia-related psychosis are at increased risk for death; drug is not approved for these patients.

- Monitor T. If fever occurs, rule out underlying infection, and consult physician for comfort measures.

⊗ **Black box warning** Monitor for seizures; with history of seizures, risk of seizures increases as dose increases.

- Monitor elderly patients for dehydration. Institute remedial measures promptly; sedation and decreased thirst related to CNS effects can lead to dehydration.
- Monitor patient regularly for signs and symptoms of diabetes mellitus.
- Encourage voiding before taking drug to decrease anticholinergic effects of urinary retention.
- Follow guidelines for discontinuation or reinstitution of the drug.
- Educate patient on seriousness of potential agranulocytosis.

Teaching points

- Weekly blood tests will be taken to determine safe dosage; dosage will be increased gradually to achieve most effective dose. Only 1 week of medication can be dispensed at a time and will depend on your white blood cell count. Do not take more than your prescribed dosage. Do not make up missed doses; instead contact your health care provider. Do not stop taking this drug suddenly; gradual reduction of dosage is needed to prevent side effects.

- If you think you are pregnant or wish to become pregnant, contact your health care provider.
- You may experience these side effects: Drowsiness, dizziness, sedation, seizures (avoid driving or performing tasks that require concentration); dizziness, faintness on arising (change positions slowly); increased salivation (reversible); constipation (consult your health care provider for correctives); fast heart rate (rest, take your time).
- Report lethargy, weakness, fever, sore throat, malaise, mouth ulcers, and flulike symptoms.

▷ coagulation factor VIIa (recombinant)

See Appendix R, *Less commonly used drugs*.

DANGEROUS DRUG

▷ codeine phosphate
(koe' deen)

PREGNANCY CATEGORY C
(DURING PREGNANCY)

PREGNANCY CATEGORY D
(DURING LABOR)

CONTROLLED SUBSTANCE C-II

Drug classes
Antitussive
Opioid agonist analgesic

Therapeutic actions
Acts at opioid receptors in the CNS to produce analgesia, euphoria, sedation; acts in the medullary cough center to depress cough reflex.

Indications
- Relief of mild to moderate pain in adults and children
- Suppression of coughing induced by chemical or mechanical irritation of the respiratory system

Contraindications and cautions
- Contraindicated with hypersensitivity to opioids, physical dependence on an opioid analgesic (drug may precipitate withdrawal).
- Use cautiously with pregnancy, labor, lactation, bronchial asthma, COPD, respiratory depression, anoxia, increased intracranial pressure, acute MI, ventricular failure, coronary insufficiency, hypertension, biliary tract surgery, renal or hepatic impairment.

Available forms
Tablets—15, 30, 60 mg; injection—15, 30 mg/mL

Dosages
Adults
Analgesic
15–60 mg PO, IM, IV or subcutaneously every 4–6 hr; do not exceed 360 mg/24 hr.
Antitussive
10–20 mg PO every 4–6 hr; do not exceed 120 mg/24 hr.
Pediatric patients
Contraindicated in premature infants.
Analgesic
1 yr and older: 0.5 mg/kg or 15 mg/m^2 IM or subcutaneously every 4 hr.
Antitussive
2–6 yr: 2.5–5 mg PO every 4–6 hr; do not exceed 12–18 mg/day based on age.
6–12 yr: 5–10 mg PO every 4–6 hr; do not exceed 60 mg/24 hr.
Geriatric patients or impaired adults
Use caution; respiratory depression may occur in elderly, the very ill, or those with respiratory problems. Reduced dosage may be necessary.

Pharmacokinetics

Route	Onset	Peak	Duration
Oral, IM, IV	10–30 min	30–60 min	4–6 hr

Metabolism: Hepatic; $T_{1/2}$: 3 hr
Distribution: Crosses placenta; enters breast milk
Excretion: Urine

▼ IV FACTS
Preparation: Protect vials from light.
Infusion: Administer slowly over 5 min by direct injection or into running IV tubing.

Adverse effects
- **CNS:** *Sedation, clamminess, sweating, headache, vertigo, floating feeling, dizziness, lethargy, confusion, light-headedness,* nervousness, unusual dreams, agitation,

euphoria, hallucinations, delirium, insomnia, anxiety, fear, disorientation, impaired mental and physical performance, coma, mood changes, weakness, tremor, seizures

- **CV:** Palpitation, increase or decrease in BP, circulatory depression, **cardiac arrest, shock,** tachycardia, bradycardia, arrhythmia
- **Dermatologic:** Rash, hives, pruritus, flushing, warmth, sensitivity to cold
- **EENT:** Diplopia, blurred vision
- **GI:** *Nausea, vomiting,* dry mouth, anorexia, *constipation,* biliary tract spasm
- **GU:** Ureteral spasm, spasm of vesical sphincters, urinary retention or hesitancy, oliguria, antidiuretic effect, reduced libido or potency
- **Local:** Phlebitis following IV injection; pain at injection site; tissue irritation and induration (subcutaneous injection)
- **Respiratory:** Slow, shallow respiration; apnea; suppression of cough reflex; **laryngospasm; bronchospasm**
- **Other:** Physical tolerance and dependence, psychological dependence

Interactions
✴ **Drug-drug** • Additive CNS effects when given with CNS depressants • Potentiation of effects of codeine with barbiturate anesthetics; decrease dose of codeine when coadministering
✴ **Drug-lab test** • Elevated biliary tract pressure may increase plasma amylase, lipase; determinations of these levels may be unreliable for 24 hr after administration of opioids

■ Nursing considerations

CLINICAL ALERT!
Name confusion has occurred between codeine and *Cardene* (nicardipine); use caution.

Assessment
- **History:** Hypersensitivity to codeine, physical dependence on an opioid analgesic, pregnancy, labor, lactation, bronchial asthma, COPD, increased intracranial pressure, acute MI, ventricular failure, coronary insufficiency, hypertension, biliary tract surgery, renal or hepatic impairment
- **Physical:** Orientation, reflexes, bilateral grip strength, affect; pupil size, vision; pulse, auscultation, BP; R, adventitious sounds; bowel sounds, normal output; LFTs, renal function tests

Interventions
- Give to breast-feeding women 4–6 hr before scheduled feeding to minimize drug in milk.
- Use the smallest effective dose for the shortest period.
⊗ **Warning** Breast-feeding mothers should monitor infants for evidence of overdose (increased sleepiness, difficulty breathing, limpness) and seek medical help immediately if it occurs.
⊗ **Warning** During parenteral administration, ensure that opioid antagonist and facilities for assisted or controlled respirations are readily available.
- Use caution when injecting subcutaneously into chilled body areas or in patients with hypotension or in shock; impaired perfusion may delay absorption; with repeated doses, an excessive amount may be absorbed when circulation is restored.
⊗ **Warning** Do not use IV in children.
- Instruct postoperative patients in pulmonary toilet; drug suppresses cough reflex.
- Monitor bowel function, arrange for stimulant laxatives to be given regularly, and initiate bowel training program if severe constipation occurs.

Teaching points
- Take drug exactly as prescribed.
- Do not take any leftover drug for other disorders, and do not let anyone else take it.
- If you are breast-feeding, take drug 4 to 6 hours before scheduled feeding. Monitor baby for increased sleepiness or difficulty breathing.
- You may experience these side effects: Dizziness, sedation, drowsiness, impaired visual acuity (avoid driving and performing other tasks that require alertness); nausea, loss of appetite (lie quietly, eat frequent small meals); constipation (use a laxative).
- Report severe nausea, vomiting, palpitations, constipation, shortness of breath or difficulty breathing.

 colchicine
(kol' chih seen)

Colcrys

PREGNANCY CATEGORY C

Drug class
Antigout drug

Therapeutic actions

Exact mechanism of action unknown; decreases deposition of uric acid, inhibits kinin formation and phagocytosis, and decreases inflammatory reaction to urate crystal deposition.

Indications

- Prophylaxis and treatment of acute gout flares in adults
- Treatment of familial Mediterranean fever in adults and children 4 yr and older
- Unlabeled uses: Behçet syndrome, hepatic cirrhosis, pericarditis

Contraindications and cautions

- Contraindicated with hypersensitivity to colchicine, concurrent use of cyclosporine, ranolazine, or strong to moderate CYP3A4 inhibitors in presence of hepatic or renal impairment.
- Use cautiously with hepatic or renal impairment, pregnancy, lactation, and in elderly patients.

Available forms

Tablets—0.6 mg

Dosages

Adults

Acute gout flares: 1.2 mg PO at first sign of gout flare, followed by 0.6 mg 1 hour later. Maximum recommended dosage is 1.8 mg over a 1-hour period.

Prophylaxis of gout flares in patients 16 yr and older: 0.6 mg PO once or twice a day; maximum dose, 1.2 mg/day.

Familial Mediterranean fever: 1.2–2.4 mg/day PO in one or two divided doses; increase or decrease in 0.3-mg increments as needed.

Pediatric patients

Treatment and prophylaxis of acute gout flares: Safety and efficacy not established.

Familial Mediterranean fever: 4–6 yr: 0.3–1.8 mg/day PO; 6–12 yr: 0.9–1.8 mg/day PO; older than 12 yr: use adult dosage. May be given as one dose or in two divided doses.

Patients with hepatic impairment

Acute gout flares: For mild to moderate impairment, no dosage adjustment is needed. For severe impairment, dosage should be the same but should not be repeated more often than once every 2 wk. Prophylaxis not recommended.

Familial Mediterranean fever: Monitor patient closely. Consider dosage reduction with careful monitoring.

Patients with renal impairment

Acute gout flares: For mild to moderate impairment, no dosage adjustment is needed. For severe impairment (CrCl less than 30 mL/min), dosage adjustment is not needed, but do not repeat more than once every 2 wk. For patient on dialysis, give 0.6 mg as a single dose; do not repeat more than once every 2 wk.

Prophylaxis of gout flares: Mild to moderate impairment, no dosage adjustment needed, but follow patient closely. Severe renal impairment, 0.3 mg/day PO. On dialysis, 0.3 mg PO twice a week.

Familial Mediterranean fever: For mild to moderate impairment, consider dosage reduction; monitor patient closely. For severe impairment, start with 0.3 mg/day and increase with careful monitoring. Patients on dialysis, starting dose of 0.3 mg/day; dose may then be increased with close monitoring.

Pharmacokinetics

Route	Onset	Peak
Oral	Slow	1–2 hr

Metabolism: Hepatic; $T_{1/2}$: 26–31 hr
Distribution: Crosses placenta; may enter breast milk
Excretion: Urine, bile

Adverse effects

- **CNS:** Peripheral neuropathy
- **Dermatologic:** Alopecia, rash, purpura, dermatoses
- **GI:** *Nausea, diarrhea, vomiting, abdominal pain,* dyspepsia
- **GU:** Azoospermia, oligospermia
- **Hematologic: Bone marrow suppression,** elevated AST and ALT, aplastic anemia
- **Other:** Myopathy, muscle pain, weakness, **rhabdomyolysis**

Interactions

✳ **Drug-drug** • Increased risk of serious toxic effects, including fatalities if combined with cyclosporine, ranolazine; this combination is contraindicated but if combination must be used, monitor patient closely and limit dose to maximum of 0.6 mg/day • Significant increase in serum colchicine level and toxicity if combined with atazanavir, clarithromycin, indinavir, itracona-zole, ketoconazole, nefazodone, nelfinavir, riton-avir, saquinavir, telithromycin; this combination is contraindicated but if combination must be used, monitor patient closely and limit dose to 0.6 mg followed by 0.3 mg in 1 hour (for gout), repeat no earlier than every 3 days; 0.6 mg/day (for familial Mediterranean fever); avoid this com-bination in patients with renal or hepatic im-pairment • Risk of significant increase in colchicine plasma level and toxicity with amprenavir, aprepi-tant, diltiazem, erythromycin, fluconazole, fos-amprenavir, verapamil; these combinations are contraindicated, but if combination must be used, limit dose to 1.2 mg (for gout), repeat no earlier than every 3 days; 1.2 mg/day (for familial Mediter-ranean fever) • Risk of altered pharmacokinetics or pharmacodynamics if combined with atorvas-tatin, digoxin, fibrates, fluvastatin, gemfibrozil, pravastatin, simvastatin; weigh benefit versus risk in use of these combinations and carefully mon-itor patient for muscle pain or weakness

✳ **Drug-food** • Risk of serious adverse effects if combined with grapefruit juice; avoid this combination

■ Nursing considerations
Assessment
- **History:** Hypersensitivity to components of drug; blood dyscrasias; serious GI, hepatic or renal disorders; pregnancy; lactation
- **Physical:** T; skin color, lesions; orientation, reflexes; P, BP; liver evaluation; normal bow-el output; normal urine output; CBC, LFTs, renal function tests, urinalysis

Interventions
- Obtain baseline and periodic liver and renal function tests, serum uric acid levels, CBC.
- Administer drug as prescribed. Do not make up missed doses.
- Encourage patient to avoid grapefruit juice.
- Check patient's complete drug list and en-sure that interacting drugs are not being used, and that appropriate dosage adjust-ments have been considered.
- Monitor patient for relief of pain and signs and symptoms of acute gout flare. Begin therapy at first sign of acute flare for best therapeutic effect.
- Monitor GI effects; antidiarrheal medica-tion may be needed.
- Fatal overdoses have occurred; keep out of reach of children.

Teaching points
- Take this drug exactly as prescribed. If tak-ing this drug for acute gout, take it at the first sign of an acute flare; then take the sec-ond dose 1 hour later.
- If you are taking this drug for familial Mediterranean fever and forget a dose, take the next dose at the regular time. Do not at-tempt to make up or double doses.
- Do not drink grapefruit juice while you are tak-ing drug; serious adverse effects could occur.
- Continue to take this drug as prescribed; do not discontinue this drug without consult-ing your health care provider. Keep drug out of the reach of children.
- Keep a record of all drugs, herbs, and over-the-counter medications you are taking and review it with your health care provider. This drug interacts with many of these drugs and serious complications could occur. Your health care provider may need to adjust the dosages of these drugs for your safety.
- This drug can suppress the activity of your bone marrow, resulting in lower than nor-mal red blood cells (you may feel fatigued), platelets (you may bleed more than nor-mal), and white blood cells (you may have increased susceptibility to infections).
- You may experience these side effects: Nau-sea, vomiting, diarrhea, abdominal pain (small, frequent meals may help; consult your health care provider if abdominal pain becomes too uncomfortable), loss of hair (which is reversible), rash
- You will need periodic medical examina-tions and blood tests to evaluate the effects of this drug.
- Report severe diarrhea, muscle pain or weak-ness, tingling or numbness in the fingers or toes, persistent gout attacks, extreme fatigue, unusual bleeding or bruising, fever and chills, signs of infection.

▽ colesevelam hydrochloride
*(koe leh **seve'** eh lam)*

WelChol

PREGNANCY CATEGORY B

Drug classes
Antihyperlipidemic
Bile acid sequestrant

Therapeutic actions

Binds bile acids in the intestine allowing excretion in the feces; as a result, cholesterol is oxidized in the liver to replace the bile acids lost; serum cholesterol and LDLs are lowered.

Indications

- Reduction of elevated LDLs as adjunct to diet and exercise in patients with primary hypercholesterolemia; used alone or in conjunction with an HMG-CoA reductase inhibitor
- As adjunct to diet and exercise to improve glycemic control in adults with type 2 diabetes
- Adjunct to diet and exercise to reduce LDL in boys and postmenarchal girls ages 10–17 yr with familial hypercholesterolemia not responsive to diet alone

Contraindications and cautions

- Contraindicated with allergy to bile acid sequestrants; complete biliary obstruction; intestinal obstruction; lactation.
- Use cautiously with difficulty swallowing; GI motility disorders; major GI tract surgery; patients susceptible to fat-soluble vitamin deficiency, pregnancy.

Available forms

Tablets—625 mg; oral powder packets—3.75-g packets

Dosages
Adults

- *Monotherapy for hyperlipidemia:* 3 tablets bid PO with meals or 6 tablets daily PO with a meal; do not exceed 7 tablets/day. Can also give 3.75 g/day of powder.
- *Combination therapy with an HMG-CoA inhibitor:* 3 tablets PO bid with meals or 6 tablets once a day PO with a meal; do not exceed 6 tablets/day. Can also give 3.75 g/day of powder.
- *Type 2 diabetes:* 6 tablets/day PO or 3 tablets PO bid.

Pediatric patients 10–17 yr

- *Familial hypercholesterolemia:* 3.75 g/day PO oral powder. Tablets are not recommended for use in children.

Pharmacokinetics

Not absorbed systemically
Excretion: Feces

Adverse effects

- **CNS:** Headache, anxiety, vertigo, dizziness, fatigue, syncope, drowsiness
- **GI:** *Constipation to fecal impaction,* exacerbation of hemorrhoids, abdominal cramps, pain, flatulence, nausea, vomiting, diarrhea, heartburn
- **GU:** Hematuria, dysuria, diuresis
- **Hematologic:** Increased bleeding tendencies related to vitamin K malabsorption, vitamins A and D deficiencies, reduced serum and red cell folate, hyperchloremic acidosis
- **Other:** Osteoporosis, backache, muscle and joint pain, arthritis, fever, pharyngitis

Interactions

✳ **Drug-drug** • Malabsorption of fat-soluble vitamins if taken concurrently with cholestyramine • Decreased absorption of oral drugs; take other oral drugs 1 hr before or 4–6 hr after colesevelam • Decreased bioavailability of SR verapamil

■ Nursing considerations
Assessment

- **History:** Allergy to bile acid sequestrants; complete biliary obstruction; intestinal obstruction; pregnancy; lactation; difficulty swallowing, GI motility disorders; major GI tract surgery; susceptibility to fat-soluble vitamin deficiency
- **Physical:** Skin lesions, color, T; orientation, affect, reflexes; P, auscultation, baseline ECG, peripheral perfusion; liver evaluation, bowel sounds; lipid studies, LFTs, clotting profile

Interventions

- Monitor serum cholesterol, LDLs, triglycerides, and serum glucose before starting treatment and periodically during treatment.
- For hyperlipidemia, administer drug with meals. For type 2 diabetes, administer once or twice a day.
- Store at room temperature; protect from moisture.
- Mix oral suspension packet with 4–8 oz of water; do not use dry. Administer with meals.
- Establish bowel program to deal with constipation.
- Monitor nutritional status and arrange for consults if needed.
- Consult with dietitian regarding low-cholesterol diets and provide information regarding exercise programs.

- Ensure that patients with type 2 diabetes follow diet and exercise regimen.
- Arrange for regular follow-up during long-term therapy.

Teaching points

- If this drug was prescribed for hyperlipidemia, take drug with meals. If drug was prescribed for type 2 diabetes, take drug once or twice per day without regard to meals.
- Take this drug at least 1 hour before or 4–6 hours after other drugs.
- Continue to follow your low-fat or diabetic diet and participate in an exercise program.
- If using the oral solution, mix entire content of packet with 4–8 ounces of water, fruit juice, or diet soft drink. Take with meals. Do not use dry.
- Plan to return for periodic blood tests to evaluate the effectiveness of this drug.
- You may experience these side effects: Constipation (this may resolve, or other measures may need to be taken to alleviate this problem); nausea, heartburn, loss of appetite (eat frequent small meals); dizziness, drowsiness, vertigo, fainting (avoid driving and operating dangerous machinery until you know how this drug affects you); headache, muscle and joint aches and pains (this may decrease over time; if it becomes bothersome, consult your health care provider).
- Report unusual bleeding or bruising, severe constipation, severe GI upset, chest pain, difficulty breathing, rash, fever.

▽colestipol hydrochloride

(koe les' ti pole)

Colestid

PREGNANCY CATEGORY C

Drug classes

Antihyperlipidemic
Bile acid sequestrant

Therapeutic actions

Binds bile acids in the intestine to form a complex that is excreted in the feces; as a result, cholesterol is lost, oxidized in the liver, and serum cholesterol and LDL are lowered.

Indications

- Adjunctive therapy: Reduction of elevated serum cholesterol in patients with primary hypercholesterolemia (elevated LDL)
- Unlabeled uses: Digitalis toxicity, hyperoxaluria, relief of pruritus associated with biliary obstruction, adjunctive treatment of hyperthyroidism, binding of *Clostridium difficile* toxin

Contraindications and cautions

- Contraindicated with allergy to bile acid sequestrants, complete biliary obstruction.
- Use cautiously with abnormal intestinal function, pregnancy, lactation.

Available forms

Tablets—1 g; granules—5-g powder/dose

Dosages

Adults

- For suspension, 5–30 g/day PO once or in divided doses two to four times/day. Start with 5 g daily or bid PO, and increase in 5-g/day increments at 1- to 2-mo intervals. For tablets, 2–16 g/day PO in 1–2 divided doses; initially, 2 g once or twice daily; increasing in 2-g increments at 1- to 2-mo intervals.

Pediatric patients

Safety and efficacy not established.

Pharmacokinetics

Not absorbed systemically
Excretion: Feces

Adverse effects

- **CNS:** *Headache,* anxiety, vertigo, dizziness, fatigue, syncope, drowsiness
- **Dermatologic:** Rash and irritation of skin, tongue, perianal area
- **GI:** *Constipation* to fecal impaction, *exacerbation of hemorrhoids,* abdominal cramps, *abdominal pain,* flatulence, anorexia, heartburn, nausea, vomiting, steatorrhea
- **GU:** Hematuria, dysuria, diuresis
- **Hematologic:** Increased bleeding tendencies related to vitamin K malabsorption, vitamins A and D deficiencies, hyperchloremic acidosis
- **Other:** Osteoporosis, chest pain, backache, muscle and joint pain, arthritis, fever

Interactions

✳ **Drug-drug** • Decreased serum levels or delayed absorption of thiazide diuretics, digitalis preparations • Malabsorption of fat-soluble vitamins • Decreased absorption of oral drugs; administer 1 hr before or 4–6 hr after colestipol

■ Nursing considerations

Assessment

• **History:** Allergy to bile acid sequestrant, complete biliary obstruction, abnormal intestinal function, pregnancy, lactation
• **Physical:** Skin lesions, color, T; orientation, affect, reflexes; P, auscultation, baseline ECG, peripheral perfusion; liver evaluation, bowel sounds; lipid studies, LFTs, clotting profile

Interventions

• Do not administer drug in dry form. Mix in liquids, soups, cereals, or pulpy fruits; add the prescribed amount to a glassful (90 mL) of liquid; stir until completely mixed. The granules will not dissolve. May be mixed with carbonated beverages, slowly stirred in a large glass. Rinse the glass with a small amount of additional beverage to ensure that the entire dose has been taken.
• Make sure that patient swallows tablets whole; do not cut, crush, or chew them. Tablets should be taken with plenty of fluids.
• Administer drug before meals.
⊗ **Warning** Monitor administration of other oral drugs for binding in the intestine and delayed or decreased absorption. Give them 1 hr before or 4–6 hr after the colestipol.
• Arrange for regular follow-up care during long-term therapy.
• Alert patient and concerned others about the high cost of drug.

Teaching points

• Take drug before meals. Do not take the powder in the dry form. Mix in liquids, soups, cereals, or pulpy fruit; add the prescribed amount to a glassful of the liquid; stir until completely mixed. The granules will not dissolve; rinse the glass with a small amount of additional liquid to ensure that you receive the entire dose of the drug. Or, carbonated beverages may be used; mix by slowly stirring in a large glass. If taking tablet form, swallow tablet whole with plenty of fluids; do not cut, crush, or chew it.

• This drug may interfere with the absorption of other oral medications. Take other oral medications 1 hour before or 4–6 hours after colestipol.
• You may experience these side effects: Constipation (transient, if it persists, request correctives); nausea, heartburn, loss of appetite (eat frequent small meals); dizziness, drowsiness, vertigo, fainting (avoid driving and operating dangerous machinery); headache, muscle and joint aches and pains (may decrease with time).
• Report unusual bleeding or bruising, severe constipation, severe GI upset, chest pain, difficulty breathing, rash, fever.

▽ collagenase clostridium histolyticum

See Appendix R, *Less commonly used drugs*.

▽ corticotropin (ACTH, adrenocorticotropin, corticotrophin)

*(kor ti koe **troe'** pin)*

Repository injection: H.P. Acthar Gel

PREGNANCY CATEGORY C

Drug classes

Anterior pituitary hormone
Diagnostic agent

Therapeutic actions

Stimulates the adrenal cortex to synthesize and secrete adrenocortical hormones.

Indications

• Allergic states unresponsive to conventional treatments
• Therapy of some glucocorticoid-sensitive disorders
• Nonsuppurative thyroiditis
• Hypercalcemia associated with cancer
• Acute exacerbations of MS
• Tuberculous meningitis with subarachnoid block
• Trichinosis with neurologic or myocardial involvement

Adverse effects in *italics* are most common; those in **bold** are life-threatening. ⊂▣⊃ Do not crush.

- Rheumatic, collagen, dermatologic, allergic, ophthalmologic, respiratory, hematologic, edematous, and GI diseases
- Palliative management of leukemias, lymphomas
- Unlabeled use: Treatment of infantile spasms

Contraindications and cautions

- Contraindicated with adrenocortical insufficiency or hyperfunction; infections, especially systemic fungal infections, ocular herpes simplex; scleroderma, osteoporosis; recent surgery; heart failure, hypertension; allergy to pork or pork products (corticotropin is isolated from porcine pituitaries); liver disease; ulcerative colitis with impending perforation; recent GI surgery; active or latent peptic ulcer; inflammatory bowel disease; hypothyroidism; pregnancy, lactation.
- Use cautiously with mental disturbances, diabetes, diverticulitis, renal impairment, myasthenia gravis.

Available forms

Repository injection—80 units/mL

Dosages

Adults

- *Therapy:* 40–80 units IM or subcutaneously every 24–72 hr; when indicated, gradually reduce dosage by increasing intervals between injections or decreasing the dose injected, or both.
- *Acute exacerbations of MS:* 80–120 units/day IM for 2–3 wk.

Pediatric patients

Use only if necessary, and only intermittently and with careful observation. Prolonged use will inhibit skeletal growth.

Pharmacokinetics

Route	Onset	Peak	Duration
IM, Subcut.	Rapid	1 hr	2–4 hr

Metabolism: $T_{1/2}$: 15 min
Distribution: Does not cross placenta; may enter breast milk

Adverse effects

- **CNS:** Seizures, vertigo, *headaches,* pseudotumor cerebri, *euphoria, insomnia, mood swings, depression,* psychosis, intracerebral hemorrhage, reversible cerebral atrophy in infants, cataracts, increased IOP, glaucoma

- **CV:** *Hypertension,* heart failure, necrotizing angiitis
- **Endocrine:** Growth retardation, decreased carbohydrate tolerance, diabetes mellitus, cushingoid state, *secondary adrenocortical and pituitary unresponsiveness*
- **GI:** Peptic or esophageal ulcer, pancreatitis, abdominal distention
- **GU:** *Amenorrhea, irregular menses*
- **Hematologic:** *Fluid and electrolyte disturbances,* negative nitrogen balance
- **Hypersensitivity: Anaphylactoid reaction** or hypersensitivity reactions
- **Musculoskeletal:** *Muscle weakness,* steroid myopathy, loss of muscle mass, osteoporosis, spontaneous fractures
- **Other:** *Impaired wound healing, petechiae, ecchymoses, increased sweating, thin and fragile skin, acne, immunosuppression and masking of signs of infection,* activation of latent infections, including tuberculosis, fungal, and viral eye infections, pneumonia, abscess, septic infection, GI and GU infections

Interactions

✳ **Drug-drug** ● Decreased effects with barbiturates ● Decreased effects of anticholinesterases with corticotropin; profound muscular depression is possible ● Decreased effectiveness of insulin, antidiabetics; monitor patient closely and increase dosage as needed

✳ **Drug-lab test** ● Suppression of skin test reactions

■ Nursing considerations

Assessment

- **History:** Adrenocortical insufficiency or hyperfunction; infections, ocular herpes simplex; scleroderma, osteoporosis; recent surgery; heart failure, hypertension; allergy to pork or pork products; liver disease: cirrhosis; ulcerative colitis; diverticulitis; active or latent peptic ulcer; inflammatory bowel disease, lactation; diabetes mellitus; hypothyroidism; pregnancy
- **Physical:** Weight, T; skin color, integrity; reflexes, bilateral grip strength, ophthalmologic examination, affect, orientation; P, BP, auscultation, peripheral perfusion, status of veins; R, adventitious sounds, chest X-ray; upper GI X-ray (peptic ulcer symptoms), liver palpation; CBC, serum electrolytes, 2-hr postprandial blood glucose, thyroid function tests, urinalysis

Interventions

- Verify adrenal responsiveness (increased urinary and plasma corticosteroid levels) to corticotropin before therapy; use the administrative route proposed for treatment.
- Administer only by IM or subcutaneous injection.
- Use minimal doses for minimal duration to minimize adverse effects.
- Taper doses when discontinuing high-dose or long-term therapy.
- Administer a rapidly acting corticosteroid before, during, and after stress when patients are on long-term therapy.
- Do not give patients receiving corticotropins live virus vaccines.

Teaching points

- Avoid immunizations with live vaccines.
- Diabetics may require an increased dosage of insulin or oral hypoglycemic drug; consult your health care provider.
- Take antacids between meals to reduce heartburn.
- Avoid exposure to people with contagious diseases. This drug masks signs of infection and decreases resistance to infection; wash hands carefully after touching contaminated surfaces.
- Report unusual weight gain, swelling of lower extremities, muscle weakness, abdominal pain, seizures, headache, fever, prolonged sore throat, cold or other infection, worsening of symptoms for which drug is being taken.

▷ cosyntropin

See Appendix R, *Less commonly used drugs*.

▷ cromolyn sodium

See Appendix R, *Less commonly used drugs*.

▷ cyanocobalamin, intranasal

*(sigh' an oh cob **ball**' a min)*

Nascobal

PREGNANCY CATEGORY C

Drug class

Synthetic vitamin

Therapeutic actions

Intranasal gel that allows absorption of vitamin B_{12}, which is essential to cell growth and reproduction, hematopoiesis, and nucleoprotein and myelin synthesis, and has been associated with fat and carbohydrate metabolism and protein synthesis.

Indications

- Maintenance of patients in hematologic remission after IM vitamin B_{12} therapy for pernicious anemia, inadequate secretion of intrinsic factor, dietary deficiency, malabsorption, competition by intestinal bacteria or parasites, or inadequate utilization of vitamin B_{12}
- Maintenance of effective therapeutic levels of vitamin B_{12} in patients with HIV, AIDS, MS, and Crohn disease

Contraindications and cautions

- Contraindicated with hypersensitivity to cobalt, vitamin B_{12}, or any component of drug.
- Use cautiously with pregnancy or lactation, Leber disease, nasal lesions, or URIs.

Available forms

Spray—500 mcg/0.1 mL

Dosages

Adults
One spray (500 mcg) in one nostril, once per wk.
Pediatric patients
Safety and efficacy not established.

Pharmacokinetics

Route	Onset	Peak
Nasal	Slow	1–2 hr

Metabolism: $T_{1/2}$: Unknown
Distribution: May cross placenta, may enter breast milk
Excretion: Urine

Adverse effects

- **CNS:** *Headache*
- **Hematologic:** Bone marrow suppression
- **Local:** *Rhinitis, nasal congestion*
- **Other:** Fever, pain, local irritation

Interactions

✳ **Drug-drug** • Decreased effectiveness may be seen with antibiotics, methotrexate, colchicine, para-aminosalicylic acid, excessive alcohol use

■ Nursing considerations

Assessment

- **History:** Pregnancy or lactation, Leber disease, nasal lesions or URIs; history of pernicious anemia, vitamin B_{12} deficiency, dates of IM cyanocobalamin therapy
- **Physical:** State of nasal mucous membranes; serum vitamin B_{12} levels, CBC, potassium level

Interventions

- Confirm diagnosis before administering; ensure that patient is hemodynamically stable after IM therapy.
- Monitor serum vitamin B_{12} levels before starting, 1 mo after starting, and every 3–6 mo during therapy.
- Do not administer if nasal congestion, rhinitis, or URI is present.
- Evaluate patient response and consider need for folate or iron replacement.

Teaching points

- Take drug as prescribed, one spray in one nostril once a week.
- Periodic blood tests will be needed to monitor your response to this drug.
- Take drug 1 hour before or 1 hour after ingestion of hot foods or liquids because hot foods can cause nasal secretions and interfere with absorption.
- Do not administer if you have nasal congestion, rhinitis, or upper respiratory tract infection; consult your health care provider.
- You may experience these side effects: Headache (analgesics may help), nausea (eat frequent small meals).
- Report nasal pain, nasal sores, fatigue, weakness, easy bruising.

▽**cyclizine**

(sye' kli zeen)

Marezine

PREGNANCY CATEGORY B

Drug classes

Anticholinergic
Antiemetic
Antihistamine
Anti–motion-sickness drug

Therapeutic actions

Reduces sensitivity of the labyrinthine apparatus; peripheral anticholinergic effects may contribute to efficacy.

Indications

- Prevention and treatment of nausea, vomiting, dizziness associated with motion sickness

Contraindications and cautions

- Contraindicated with allergy to cyclizine.
- Use cautiously with pregnancy, lactation, narrow-angle glaucoma, stenosing peptic ulcer, symptomatic prostatic hypertrophy, bronchial asthma, bladder neck obstruction, pyloroduodenal obstruction, cardiac arrhythmias; postoperative patients (hypotensive effects may be confusing and dangerous).

Available forms

Tablets—25, 50 mg

Dosages

Adults

50 mg PO 30 min before exposure to motion; repeat every 4–6 hr. Do not exceed 200 mg in 24 hr.

Pediatric patients 6–12 yr

25 mg PO up to three times a day; maximum dose, 75 mg/day.

Geriatric patients

More likely to cause dizziness, sedation, syncope, toxic confusional states, and hypotension in elderly patients; use with caution.

Pharmacokinetics

Route	Onset	Peak	Duration
Oral	30–60 min	60–90 min	4–6 hr

Metabolism: Hepatic; $T_{1/2}$: 2–3 hr
Distribution: Crosses placenta; enters breast milk
Excretion: Unknown

Adverse effects

- **CNS:** *Drowsiness, confusion,* euphoria, nervousness, restlessness, insomnia and excitement, seizures, vertigo, tinnitus, blurred vision, diplopia, auditory and visual hallucinations
- **CV:** Hypotension, palpitations, tachycardia

- **Dermatologic:** Urticaria, drug rash
- **GI:** *Dry mouth, anorexia, nausea,* vomiting, diarrhea or constipation, cholestatic jaundice
- **GU:** *Urinary frequency, difficult urination,* urinary retention
- **Respiratory:** Respiratory depression, dry nose and throat

Interactions
✳ Drug-drug • Increased depressant effects with alcohol, other CNS depressants

■ Nursing considerations
Assessment
- **History:** Allergy to cyclizine, narrow-angle glaucoma, stenosing peptic ulcer, symptomatic prostatic hypertrophy, bronchial asthma, bladder neck obstruction, pyloroduodenal obstruction, cardiac arrhythmias, recent surgery, lactation
- **Physical:** Skin color, lesions, texture; orientation; reflexes, affect; vision examination; P, BP; R, adventitious sounds; bowel sounds; prostate palpation; CBC

Interventions
- Monitor elderly patients carefully for adverse effects.

Teaching points
- Take drug as prescribed; avoid excessive dosage.
- Use before motion sickness occurs; antimotion sickness drugs work best if used prophylactically.
- Avoid alcohol; serious sedation could occur.
- You may experience these side effects: Dizziness, sedation, drowsiness (use caution driving or performing tasks that require alertness); epigastric distress, diarrhea or constipation (take drug with food); dry mouth (practice frequent mouth care, suck sugarless candies); thickening of bronchial secretions, dryness of nasal mucosa (consider another type of motion sickness remedy).
- Report difficulty breathing, hallucinations, tremors, loss of coordination, unusual bleeding or bruising, visual disturbances, irregular heartbeat.

▽ **cyclobenzaprine hydrochloride**
*(sye kloe **ben'** za preen)*

Amrix, Apo-Cyclobenzaprine (CAN), Flexeril, Gen-Cyclobenzaprine (CAN), PMS-Cyclobenzaprine (CAN), ratio-Cyclobenzaprine (CAN)

PREGNANCY CATEGORY B

Drug class
Skeletal muscle relaxant (centrally acting)

Therapeutic actions
Precise mechanism not known; does not directly relax tense skeletal muscles but appears to act mainly at brain stem levels or in the spinal cord.

Indications
- Relief of discomfort associated with acute, painful musculoskeletal conditions, as adjunct to rest, physical therapy
- Unlabeled use: Adjunct in the management of fibrositis syndrome

Contraindications and cautions
- Contraindicated with hypersensitivity to cyclobenzaprine, acute recovery phase of MI, arrhythmias, heart block or conduction disturbances, heart failure, hyperthyroidism.
- Use cautiously with urinary retention, angle-closure glaucoma, increased IOP, lactation, mild hepatic impairment.

Available forms
Tablets—5, 7.5, 10 mg; ER capsules—15, 30 mg

Dosages
Adults
5 mg PO tid, up to 10 mg PO tid. Do not exceed 30 mg/day; do not use longer than 2 or 3 wk. For ER capsules, 15 mg once/day; some patients need 30 mg/day.
Pediatric patients
Safety and efficacy in patients younger than 15 yr not established.
Geriatric patients
Initiate at 5 mg/day PO; titrate slowly while monitoring patient. Do not use capsules.

Patients with hepatic impairment
For muscle spasms in patients with mild impairment, initial dose is 5 mg with slow titration. For moderate to severe impairment, do not use.

Pharmacokinetics

Route	Onset	Peak	Duration
Oral	1 hr	4–6 hr	12–24 hr

Metabolism: Hepatic; $T_{1/2}$: 1–3 days, 18 hr (range 8–37 hr)
Distribution: Crosses placenta; may enter breast milk
Excretion: Urine

Adverse effects
- **CNS:** *Drowsiness, dizziness,* fatigue, asthenia, blurred vision, headache, nervousness, confusion
- **CV:** Arrhythmias, **MI**
- **GI:** *Dry mouth,* nausea, constipation, dyspepsia, unpleasant taste, liver toxicity
- **GU:** Frequency, urinary retention

Interactions
✳ **Drug-drug** • Additive CNS effects with alcohol, barbiturates, other CNS depressants, MAOIs, TCAs; avoid concomitant use • Risk of hyperpyretic crisis and seizures if given within 14 days of MAOIs • Increased risk of seizures with tramadol

■ Nursing considerations
Assessment
- **History:** Hypersensitivity to cyclobenzaprine, acute recovery phase of MI, arrhythmias, heart failure, hyperthyroidism, urinary retention, angle-closure glaucoma, increased IOP, lactation
- **Physical:** Orientation, affect, ophthalmic examination (tonometry); bowel sounds, normal GI output; prostate palpation, normal voiding pattern; thyroid function tests

Interventions
- Arrange for analgesics if headache occurs.
- Monitor elderly patients closely; they are at increased risk for adverse effects.

Teaching points
- Take this drug exactly as prescribed. Do not take a higher dosage.

- Avoid alcohol and sleep-inducing or over-the-counter drugs; these may cause dangerous effects.
- You may experience these side effects: Drowsiness, dizziness, blurred vision (avoid driving or engaging in activities that require alertness); dyspepsia (take drug with food, eat frequent small meals); dry mouth (suck sugarless candies or ice chips).
- Report urinary retention or difficulty voiding, pale stools, yellow skin or eyes.

DANGEROUS DRUG

▷ **cyclophosphamide**
*(sye kloe **foss'** fa mide)*

Procytox (CAN)

PREGNANCY CATEGORY D

Drug classes
Alkylating drug
Antineoplastic
Nitrogen mustard derivative

Therapeutic actions
Cytotoxic: Interferes with the replication of susceptible cells. Not specific to cell cycle.
Immunosuppressive: Lymphocytes are especially sensitive to drug effects.

Indications
- Treatment of malignant lymphomas, multiple myeloma, leukemias, mycosis fungoides, neuroblastoma, adenocarcinoma of the ovary, retinoblastoma, carcinoma of the breast; used concurrently or sequentially with other antineoplastic drugs
- Treatment of minimal change nephrotic syndrome in children
- Unlabeled uses: Severe rheumatologic conditions, Wegener granulomatosis, steroid-resistant vasculitis, SLE, numerous other cancers

Contraindications and cautions
- Contraindicated with allergy to cyclophosphamide, pregnancy, lactation.
- Use cautiously with radiation therapy; tumor cell infiltration of the bone marrow; adrenalectomy with steroid therapy; infections, especially varicella-zoster; hematopoietic depression, impaired hepatic or renal function.

Available forms

Tablets—25, 50 mg; injection—500 mg, 1 g, 2 g

Dosages

Consult current chemotherapeutic reference for appropriate protocol, and individualize dosage based on hematologic profile and response.

Adults

- **Induction therapy:** 40–50 mg/kg IV given in divided doses over 2–5 days or 1–5 mg/kg/day PO.
- **Alternative dosing:** 1–5 mg/kg/day PO, 10–15 mg/kg IV every 7–10 days, or 3–5 mg/kg IV twice weekly.

Pediatric patients

- **Minimal change nephrotic syndrome:** 2.5–3 mg/day PO for 60–90 days.

Patients with renal impairment

Creatinine clearance less than 10 mL/min, reduce dose to 75% of usual dose.

Patients with hepatic impairment

Bilirubin 3.1–5 mg/dL or AST more than 180 mg/dL, give 75% of dose. Bilirubin more than 5 mg/dL, do not give.

Pharmacokinetics

Route	Onset	Peak
Oral	Varies	1 hr
IV	Rapid	15–30 min

Metabolism: Hepatic; $T_{1/2}$: 3–12 hr
Distribution: Crosses placenta; enters breast milk
Excretion: Urine

▼ IV FACTS

Preparation: Add sterile water for injection or bacteriostatic water for injection to the vial, and shake gently. Use 25 mL for 500-mg vial, 50 mL for 1-g vial, 100 mL for 2-g vial. Prepared solutions may be injected IV, IM, intraperitoneally, intrapleurally. Use within 24 hr if stored at room temperature or within 6 days if refrigerated. If bacteriostatic water for injection is not used, use within 6 hr.

Infusion: Infuse in 5% dextrose injection, 5% dextrose and 0.9% sodium chloride injection; infuse over 15 min or longer (infusion can be painful).

Adverse effects

- **CV:** Cardiotoxicity

- **Dermatologic:** *Alopecia,* darkening of skin and fingernails
- **GI:** *Anorexia, nausea, vomiting, diarrhea, stomatitis*
- **GU:** Bladder fibrosis, hematuria to potentially **fatal hemorrhagic cystitis,** increased uric acid levels, infertility
- **Hematologic:** *Leukopenia,* thrombocytopenia, anemia
- **Respiratory: Interstitial pulmonary fibrosis**
- **Other:** SIADH, immunosuppression secondary to malignancy

Interactions

✴ Drug-drug • Prolonged apnea with succinylcholine: Metabolism is inhibited by cyclophosphamide • Decreased serum levels and therapeutic activity of digoxin • Myelosuppressive effects are enhanced with coadministration of allopurinol • Increased anticoagulant effects with anticoagulants • Increased cardiac effects with doxorubicin • Reduced activity of cyclophosphamide with chloramphenicol

✴ Drug-food • Decreased metabolism and risk of toxic effects if combined with grapefruit juice; avoid this combination

■ Nursing considerations

Assessment

- **History:** Allergy to cyclophosphamide, radiation therapy, chemotherapy, tumor cell infiltration of the bone marrow, adrenalectomy with steroid therapy, infections, hematopoietic depression, impaired hepatic or renal function, pregnancy, lactation
- **Physical:** T; weight; skin color, lesions; hair; P, auscultation, baseline ECG; R, adventitious sounds; mucous membranes, liver evaluation; CBC, differential; urinalysis; LFTs, renal function tests

Interventions

- Arrange for blood tests to evaluate hematopoietic function before therapy and weekly during therapy.
- ⊗ *Warning* Do not give full dosage within 4 wk after a full course of radiation therapy due to the risk of severe bone marrow depression; reduced dosage may be needed.
- Arrange for reduced dosage in patients with impaired renal or hepatic function.
- ⊗ *Warning* Ensure that patient is well hydrated before treatment to reduce risk of cystitis.

Adverse effects in *italics* are most common; those in **bold** are life-threatening. ⊞ Do not crush.

- Prepare oral solution by dissolving injectable cyclophosphamide in aromatic elixir. Refrigerate in a glass container and use within 14 days.
- Give tablets on an empty stomach. If severe GI upset occurs, tablet may be given with food. Use protective gloves when handling drug.
- Counsel male patients not to father a child during or immediately after therapy; infant cardiac and limb abnormalities have occurred.
- Make sure that antiemetics have been ordered before each dose.

Teaching points
- Take drug on an empty stomach. If severe GI upset occurs, the tablet may be taken with food. Do not drink grapefruit juice while taking this drug. Wear protective gloves when handling drug.
- Try to maintain your fluid intake and nutrition (drink at least 10–12 glasses of fluid each day).
- Both men and women should use birth control during and after drug use; this drug can cause severe birth defects.
- You may experience these side effects: Nausea, vomiting, loss of appetite (take drug with food, eat frequent small meals); darkening of the skin and fingernails; loss of hair (obtain a wig or other head covering prior to hair loss; head must be covered in extremes of temperature).
- Report unusual bleeding or bruising, fever, chills, sore throat, cough, shortness of breath, blood in the urine, painful urination, rapid heartbeat, swelling of the feet or hands, stomach or flank pain.

▷ cycloSERINE
(sye kloe ser' een)

Seromycin Pulvules

PREGNANCY CATEGORY C

Drug classes
Antibiotic
Antituberculotic (third line)

Therapeutic actions
Inhibits cell wall synthesis in susceptible strains of gram-positive and gram-negative bacteria and in *Mycobacterium tuberculosis,* causing cell death.

Indications
- Treatment of active pulmonary and extrapulmonary (including renal) TB that is not responsive to first-line antituberculotics in conjunction with other antituberculotics
- UTIs caused by susceptible bacteria

Contraindications and cautions
- Contraindicated with allergy to cycloserine, epilepsy, depression, severe anxiety or psychosis, severe renal insufficiency, excessive concurrent use of alcohol, lactation.
- Use cautiously with pregnancy.

Available forms
Capsules—250 mg

Dosages
Adults
Initial dose, 250 mg bid PO at 12-hr intervals for first 2 wk; monitor serum levels (above 30 mcg/mL is generally toxic). Maintenance dose, 500 mg–1 g/day PO in divided doses monitored by blood levels. Do not exceed 1 g/day.
Pediatric patients
Safety and efficacy not established.

Pharmacokinetics

Route	Onset	Peak	Duration
Oral	Varies	4–8 hr	48–72 hr

Metabolism: $T_{1/2}$: 10 hr
Distribution: Crosses placenta; enters breast milk
Excretion: Feces, urine

Adverse effects
- **CNS:** *Drowsiness, somnolence, headache, tremor, vertigo, confusion,* disorientation, loss of memory, psychoses (possibly with suicidal tendencies), hyperirritability, aggression, paresis, hyperreflexia, paresthesias, seizures, coma
- **Dermatologic:** Rash
- **Hematologic:** Elevated serum transaminase levels

■ Nursing considerations
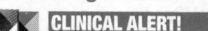 **CLINICAL ALERT!**
Name confusion has occurred among cycloserine, cyclosporine, and cyclophosphamide; use caution.

Assessment

- **History:** Allergy to cycloserine, epilepsy, depression, severe anxiety or psychosis, severe renal insufficiency, excessive concurrent use of alcohol, lactation, pregnancy
- **Physical:** Skin color, lesions; orientation, reflexes, affect, EEG; liver evaluation; LFTs

Interventions

- Arrange for culture and sensitivity studies before use.
- Give this drug only when other therapy has failed, and only in conjunction with other antituberculotics, when treating TB.
- Arrange for follow-up of LFTs, renal function tests, hematologic tests, and serum drug levels.
- Consult with physician regarding the use of antiepileptics, sedatives, or pyridoxine if CNS effects become severe.
- Discontinue drug, and notify physician if rash or severe CNS reactions occur.

Teaching points

- Avoid excessive alcohol consumption while on this drug.
- Take this drug regularly; avoid missing doses. Do not discontinue this drug without first consulting your health care provider.
- Avoid taking with a high-fat meal.
- Have regular, periodic medical checkups, including blood tests to evaluate the drug's effects.
- You may experience these side effects: Drowsiness, tremor, disorientation (use caution operating a car or dangerous machinery); depression, personality change, numbness, tingling.
- If you experience trouble breathing or if signs or symptoms of heart failure occur, notify your health care provider immediately, especially if you are receiving more than 1 to 1.5 g per day.
- Report rash, headache, tremors, shaking, confusion, dizziness.

▽ **cycloSPORINE**
(cyclosporin A)
(sye' kloe spor een)

Gengraf, Neoral, Sandimmune

PREGNANCY CATEGORY C

Drug class

Immunosuppressant

Therapeutic actions

Exact mechanism of immunosuppressant is not known; specifically and reversibly inhibits immunocompetent lymphocytes in the G0 or G1 phase of the cell cycle; inhibits T-helper and T-suppressor cells, lymphokine production, and release of interleukin-2 and T-cell growth factor.

Indications

- Prophylaxis for organ rejection in kidney, liver, and heart transplants in conjunction with adrenal corticosteroids
- Treatment of chronic rejection in patients previously treated with other immunosuppressive agents (*Sandimmune*)
- *Neoral, Gengraf:* Alone, or in combination with methotrexate for treatment of patients with severe active rheumatoid arthritis
- *Neoral, Gengraf:* Treatment of recalcitrant, plaque psoriasis in non–immune-compromised adults
- Unlabeled uses: Aplastic anemia; resistant leukemias; other procedures, including pancreas, bone marrow, lung transplants; Crohn disease, SLE, MS

Contraindications and cautions

- Contraindicated with allergy to cyclosporine or polyoxyethylated castor oil, lactation.
- Use cautiously with impaired renal function, malabsorption, pregnancy, uncontrolled hypertension.

Available forms

Capsules—25, 100 mg; soft gel capsules for microemulsion—25, 100 mg; oral solution—100 mg/mL; IV solution—50 mg/mL

Dosages

Adults and pediatric patients
Neoral, Gengraf, and *Sandimmune* are not bioequivalent—do not interchange. Concentrations should be monitored when switching because of variable bioavailability.
Oral

- *Organ rejection:* 15 mg/kg/day PO (*Sandimmune*) initially given 4–12 hr prior to transplantation; continue dose postoperatively for 1–2 wk, then taper by 5% per wk to a maintenance level of 5–10 mg/kg/day.

- *Rheumatoid arthritis:* 2.5 mg/kg/day (*Neoral, Gengraf*) PO in divided doses bid; may increase up to 4 mg/kg/day. If no benefit after 16 wks, discontinue drug.
- *Psoriasis:* 2.5 mg/kg/day (*Neoral, Gengraf*) PO divided bid for 4 wk, then may increase up to 4 mg/kg/day. If no satisfactory response after 6 wk at 4 mg/kg/day, discontinue drug.

Parenteral
Patients unable to take oral solution preoperatively or postoperatively may be given IV infusion (*Sandimmune*) at one-third the oral dose (ie, 5–6 mg/kg/day given 4–12 hr prior to transplantation, administered as a slow infusion over 2–6 hr). Continue this daily dose postoperatively. Switch to oral drug as soon as possible.

Pharmacokinetics

Route	Onset	Peak
Oral	Varies	3.5 hr
IV	Rapid	1–2 hr

Metabolism: Hepatic; $T_{1/2}$: 10–27 hr (*Sandimmune*), 5–18 hr (*Neoral, Gengraf*)
Distribution: Crosses placenta; enters breast milk
Excretion: Bile, urine

▼ IV FACTS

Preparation: Dilute IV solution immediately before use. Dilute 1 mL concentrate in 20–100 mL of 0.9% sodium chloride injection or 5% dextrose injection. Discard unused infusion solutions after 24 hr.
Infusion: Give in a slow IV infusion over 2–6 hr.
Incompatibility: Do not mix with magnesium sulfate.

Adverse effects

- **CNS:** *Tremor,* seizures, headache, paresthesias
- **CV:** *Hypertension*
- **GI: Hepatotoxicity,** *gum hyperplasia, diarrhea,* nausea, vomiting, anorexia
- **GU:** *Renal impairment,* nephrotoxicity
- **Hematologic:** Leukopenia, *hyperkalemia, hypomagnesemia,* hyperuricemia
- **Other:** *Hirsutism, acne,* lymphomas, infections, elevated serum creatinine and BUN

Interactions

✳ **Drug-drug** • Increased risk of nephrotoxicity with other nephrotoxic agents (aminoglycosides, amphotericin B, acyclovir) • Increased risk of digoxin toxicity • Risk of severe myopathy or rhabdomyolysis with HMG-CoA reductase inhibitors • Increased risk of toxicity if taken with SSRIs, diltiazem, metoclopramide, nicardipine, amiodarone, androgens, azole antifungals, colchicine, hormonal contraceptives, foscarnet, macrolides, metoclopramide • Increased plasma concentration of cyclosporine with ketoconazole • Decreased therapeutic effect with hydantoins, rifampin, phenobarbital, carbamazepine, orlistat

✳ **Drug-food** • Increased serum levels and adverse effects if combined with grapefruit juice • Decreased absorption of *Neoral* if taken with a high-fat meal

✳ **Drug-alternate therapy** • Decreased cyclosporine levels with use of St. John's Wort

■ Nursing considerations

CLINICAL ALERT!
Name confusion has been associated with cyclosporine, cycloserine, and cyclophosphamide; use caution.

Assessment

- **History:** Allergy to cyclosporine or polyoxyethylated castor oil, impaired renal function, malabsorption, lactation
- **Physical:** T; skin color, lesions; BP, peripheral perfusion; liver evaluation, bowel sounds; gum evaluation; LFTs, renal function tests, CBC

Interventions

- Mix oral solution with milk, chocolate milk, or orange juice at room temperature. Stir well, and administer at once. Do not allow mixture to stand before drinking. Use a glass container, and rinse with more diluent to ensure that the total dose is taken.
- Use parenteral administration only if patient is unable to take the oral solution; transfer to oral solution as soon as possible. *Sandimmune* must be taken with corticosteroids.
- Do not refrigerate oral solution; store at room temperature and use within 2 mo after opening.

⊗ *Black box warning* Monitor patient for infections, malignancies; risks are increased.

⊗ **Black box warning** Monitor LFTs and renal function tests prior to and during therapy; marked decreases in function may require dosage adjustment or discontinuation.

⊗ **Black box warning** Monitor BP; heart transplant patients may require concomitant antihypertensive therapy.

Teaching points

- Dilute solution with milk, chocolate milk, or orange juice at room temperature; drink immediately after mixing. Rinse the glass with the solution to ensure that all of the dose is taken. Store solution at room temperature. Use solution within 2 months of opening the bottle.
- Do not drink grapefruit juice while taking this drug.
- Do not take with high-fat meals or within 30 minutes of high-fat meals.
- Do not use St. John's Wort while taking this drug.
- Avoid infection; avoid crowds or people who have infections. Notify your health care provider at once if you injure yourself.
- This drug should not be taken during pregnancy. Use of barrier contraceptives is advised. If you think that you are pregnant or you want to become pregnant, discuss this with your health care provider.
- This drug interacts with many drugs. Make sure you report all drugs, OTC products, or herbal supplements you are using; dosage adjustments may be needed.
- Have periodic blood tests to monitor your response to drug effects.
- Do not discontinue this medication without your health care provider's advice.
- You may experience these side effects: Nausea, vomiting (take the drug with food); diarrhea; rash; mouth sores (practice frequent mouth care).
- Report unusual bleeding or bruising, fever, sore throat, mouth sores, tiredness.

▷ **cyproheptadine hydrochloride**

(si proe **hep'** ta deen)

PREGNANCY CATEGORY B

Drug class
Antihistamine (piperidine type)

Therapeutic actions
Blocks the effects of histamine at H_1 receptor sites; has atropine-like, antiserotonin, antipruritic, sedative, and appetite-stimulating effects.

Indications
- Relief of symptoms associated with perennial and seasonal allergic rhinitis; vasomotor rhinitis; allergic conjunctivitis; mild, uncomplicated urticaria and angioedema; amelioraton of allergic reactions to blood or plasma; dermatographism; adjunctive therapy in anaphylactic reactions
- Treatment of cold urticaria
- Unlabeled uses: Treatment of vascular cluster headaches, appetite stimulation, treatment of nightmares associated with PTSD, prevention of vascular headaches such as migraines

Contraindications and cautions
- Contraindicated with allergy to any antihistamines, third trimester of pregnancy, newborns, preterm infants, elderly patients.
- Use cautiously with narrow-angle glaucoma, stenosing peptic ulcer, symptomatic prostatic hypertrophy, asthmatic attack, bladder neck obstruction, pyloroduodenal obstruction, lactation.

Available forms
Tablets—4 mg; syrup—2 mg/5 mL

Dosages
Adults
For initial therapy, 4 mg tid PO. For maintenance therapy, 4–20 mg/day in three divided doses PO; do not exceed 0.5 mg/kg/day.
Pediatric patients 2–6 yr
2 mg PO bid or tid; do not exceed 12 mg/day.
Pediatric patients 7–14 yr
4 mg PO bid or tid; do not exceed 16 mg/day.
Geriatric patients
More likely to cause dizziness, sedation, syncope, toxic confusional states, and hypotension in elderly patients.

Pharmacokinetics

Route	Onset	Peak	Duration
Oral	15–30 min	1–2 hr	4–6 hr

Metabolism: Hepatic; $T_{1/2}$: 3–4 hr
Distribution: Crosses placenta; enters breast milk
Excretion: Urine

Adverse effects in *italics* are most common; those in **bold** are life-threatening. ⊗ Do not crush.

Adverse effects

- **CNS:** *Drowsiness, sedation, dizziness, disturbed coordination,* fatigue, confusion, restlessness, excitation, nervousness, tremor, headache, blurred vision, diplopia, vertigo, tinnitus, acute labyrinthitis, hysteria, tingling, heaviness and weakness of the hands
- **CV:** Hypotension, palpitations, bradycardia, tachycardia, extrasystoles
- **GI:** *Epigastric distress,* anorexia, increased appetite and weight gain, nausea, vomiting, diarrhea or constipation
- **GU:** Urinary frequency, dysuria, urinary retention, early menses, decreased libido, impotence
- **Hematologic:** Hemolytic anemia, hypoplastic anemia, thrombocytopenia, leukopenia, **agranulocytosis, pancytopenia**
- **Respiratory:** *Thickening of bronchial secretions,* chest tightness, wheezing, nasal stuffiness, dry mouth, dry nose, dry throat, sore throat
- **Other:** Urticaria, rash, **anaphylactic shock,** photosensitivity, excessive perspiration, chills

Interactions

✷ **Drug-drug** ● Subnormal pituitary-adrenal response to metyrapone ● Decreased effects of fluoxetine ● Increased and prolonged anticholinergic (drying) effects if taken with MAOIs ● Increased sedation with alcohol, CNS depressants

■ Nursing considerations
Assessment

- **History:** Allergy to any antihistamines; narrow-angle glaucoma, stenosing peptic ulcer, symptomatic prostatic hypertrophy, asthmatic attack, bladder neck obstruction, pyloroduodenal obstruction; lactation, pregnancy
- **Physical:** Skin color, lesions, texture; orientation, reflexes, affect; vision examination; P, BP; R, adventitious sounds; bowel sounds; prostate palpation; CBC with differential

Interventions

- Administer with food if GI upset occurs.
- Give syrup form if unable to take tablets.
- Monitor patient response, and adjust dosage to lowest possible effective dose.

Teaching points

- Take as prescribed; avoid excessive dosage.
- Take drug with food if GI upset occurs.
- Avoid alcohol; serious sedation could occur.
- You may experience these side effects: Dizziness, sedation, drowsiness (use caution if driving or performing tasks that require alertness); epigastric distress, diarrhea, or constipation (take drug with meals); dry mouth (practice frequent mouth care, suck sugarless candies); thickening of bronchial secretions, dryness of nasal mucosa (use humidifier).
- Report difficulty breathing, hallucinations, tremors, loss of coordination, unusual bleeding or bruising, visual disturbances, irregular heartbeat.

DANGEROUS DRUG

▷**cytarabine
(cytosine arabinoside)**
*(sye **tare**' a been)*

DepoCyt, Tarabine PFS

PREGNANCY CATEGORY D

Drug classes

Antimetabolite
Antineoplastic

Therapeutic actions

Inhibits DNA polymerase; cell cycle phase specific—S phase (stage of DNA synthesis); also blocks progression of cells from G1 to S.

Indications

- Induction and maintenance of remission in AML (higher response rate in children than in adults)
- Treatment of acute lymphocytic leukemia in adults and children; treatment of chronic myelocytic leukemia and erythroleukemia
- Intrathecal use: Treatment of meningeal leukemia
- Liposomal: Treatment of lymphomatous meningitis
- In combination therapy: Treatment of non-Hodgkin lymphoma in children
- Unlabeled uses: Hodgkin lymphoma, bone marrow transplantation

Contraindications and cautions

- Contraindicated with allergy to cytarabine, active meningeal infection (liposomal).
- Use cautiously with hematopoietic depression secondary to radiation or chemotherapy; hepatic impairment, pregnancy, lactation, premature infants.

Available forms

Powder for injection—100, 500 mg, 1, 2 g; injection—20 mg/mL, 100 mg/mL, 10 mg/mL (liposomal)

Dosages

Doses vary based on protocol; consult a current chemotherapy reference.

Adults

- *AML induction of remission:* 100 mg/m^2/day by continuous IV infusion (days 1–7) or 100 mg/m^2 IV every 12 hr (days 1–7). Individualize dosage based on hematologic response.
- *Maintenance of AML:* Use same dosage and schedule as induction; often a longer rest period is allowed.
- *ALL:* Dosage similar to AML.
- *Meningeal leukemia:* 5 mg/m^2 to 75 mg/m^2 once daily for 4 days or once every 4 days. Most common dose is 30 mg/m^2 every 4 days until CSF is normal, followed by one more treatment.
- *Treatment of lymphomatous meningitis:* 50 mg liposomal cytarabine intrathecal every 14 days for two doses; then every 14 days for three doses; repeat every 28 days for four doses.

Pediatric patients

- *Remission induction and maintenance of AML:* Calculate dose by body weight or surface area.
- *ALL:* Same dosage as AML.

Combination therapies

For persistent leukemias, give at 2- to 4-wk intervals.
Cytarabine: 100 mg/m^2/day by continuous IV infusion, days 1–10. *Doxorubicin:* 30 g/m^2/day by IV infusion over 30 min, days 1–3.
Cytarabine: 100 mg/m^2/day by IV infusion over 30 min every 12 hr, days 1–7. *Thioguanine:* 100 mg/m^2 PO every 12 hr, days 1–7. *Daunorubicin:* 60 mg/m^2/day by IV infusion, days 5–7.
Cytarabine: 100 mg/m^2/day by continuous infusion, days 1–7. *Doxorubicin:* 30 mg/m^2/day

by IV infusion, days 1–3. *Vincristine:* 1.5 mg/m^2/day by IV infusion, days 1 and 5.
Prednisone: 40 mg/m^2/day by IV infusion every 12 hr, days 1–5.
Cytarabine: 100 mg/m^2/day by continuous infusion, days 1–7.
Daunorubicin: 45 mg/m^2/day by IV push, days 1–3.

Pharmacokinetics

Route	Onset	Peak	Duration
IV	Rapid	20–60 min	12–18 hr

Metabolism: Hepatic; T$_{1/2}$ in plasma: 1–3 hr; T$_{1/2}$ in CSF: 2 hr.
Distribution: Crosses placenta; may enter breast milk
Excretion: Urine

▼ IV FACTS

Preparation: Reconstitute 100-mg vial with 5 mL of bacteriostatic water for injection with benzyl alcohol 0.9%; resultant solution contains 20 mg/mL cytarabine. Reconstitute 500-mg vial with 10 mL of the above; resultant solution contains 50 mg/mL cytarabine. Reconstitute 1-g vial and 2-g vial with 10 mL, 20 mL of the above respectively; resultant solution contains 100 mg/mL cytarabine. Store at room temperature for up to 48 hr. Discard solution if a slight haze appears. Can be further diluted with water for injection, D$_5$W, or sodium chloride injection; stable for 8 days.

Infusion: Administer by IV infusion over at least 30 min, IV injection over 1–3 min for each 100 mg, or subcutaneously; patients can usually tolerate higher doses when given by rapid IV injection. There is no clinical advantage to any particular route.

Incompatibilities: Do not mix with insulin, heparin, penicillin G, oxacillin, nafcillin, 5-FU.

Adverse effects

- **CNS:** Neuritis, neural toxicity
- **Dermatologic:** Fever, rash, urticaria, freckling, skin ulceration, pruritus, conjunctivitis, alopecia
- **GI:** *Anorexia, nausea, vomiting, diarrhea, oral and anal inflammation or ulceration;* esophageal ulcerations, esophagitis, abdominal pain, hepatic impairment (jaundice), acute pancreatitis

---

Adverse effects in *italics* are most common; those in **bold** are life-threatening. ⬛ Do not crush.

- **GU:** Renal impairment, urine retention
- **Hematologic:** Bone marrow depression, hyperuricemia, *leukopenia, thrombocytopenia,* anemia
- **Local:** *Thrombophlebitis,* cellulitis at injection site
- **Other:** Cytarabine syndrome (fever, myalgia, bone pain, occasional chest pain, maculopapular rash, conjunctivitis, malaise, which is sometimes responsive to corticosteroids), *fever, rash,* arachnoiditis (liposomal preparation)

Interactions

✷ **Drug-drug** • Decreased therapeutic action of digoxin if taken with cytarabine

■ Nursing considerations

Assessment

- **History:** Allergy to cytarabine, hematopoietic depression, impaired liver function, lactation, pregnancy
- **Physical:** Weight; T; skin lesions, color; hair; orientation, reflexes; R, adventitious sounds; mucous membranes, liver evaluation, abdominal exam; CBC, differential; LFTs, renal function tests; urinalysis

Interventions

- Evaluate hematopoietic status before and frequently during therapy.

⊗ *Warning* Discontinue drug therapy if platelet count is less than 50,000/mm³ or neutrophil count is less than 1,000/mm³; consult physician for dosage adjustment.

- Use Elliott's B solution for diluent, similar to CSF, for intrathecal use. Administer within 4 hr after withdrawal from vial; contains no preservatives. Do not use in-line filters; inject directly into CSF.
- Use caution to avoid skin contact with liposomal form; use liposomal form within 4 hr of withdrawing from vial.
- Make sure antiemetics are ordered before each dose.
- Give comfort measures for anal inflammation, headache, other pain associated with cytarabine syndrome.

Teaching points

- Prepare a calendar of treatment days. Drug must be given IV, subcutaneously, or intrathecally.

- Use contraceptives; this drug may cause birth defects or miscarriages.
- Have frequent, regular medical follow-up care, including blood tests to assess drug's effects.
- You may experience these side effects: Nausea, vomiting, loss of appetite (medication may be ordered; eat frequent small meals; maintain nutrition); malaise, weakness, lethargy (reversible; avoid driving or operating dangerous machinery); mouth sores (practice frequent mouth care); diarrhea; loss of hair (obtain a wig or other head covering; keep the head covered in extreme temperatures); anal inflammation (use comfort measures).
- Report black, tarry stools; fever; chills; sore throat; unusual bleeding or bruising; shortness of breath; chest pain; difficulty swallowing.

▽ dabigatran etexilate mesylate

(da bye gah' tron)

Pradaxa 🆑

PREGNANCY CATEGORY C

Drug class

Direct thrombin inhibitor

Therapeutic actions

Competitive, direct thrombin inhibitor; thrombin enables the conversion of fibrinogen to fibrin fibers during the clotting cascade. Inhibiting this process prevents clot development. Dabigatran inhibits free and clot-bound thrombin and thrombin-induced platelet aggregation.

Indications

- Reduction of the risk of stroke and systemic embolism in patients with nonvalvular atrial fibrillation

Contraindications and cautions

- Contraindicated with history of serious hypersensitivity reactions to dabigatran; active pathologic bleeding.
- Use cautiously with invasive procedures, surgery, pregnancy, lactation.

Available forms

Capsules 🆑—75, 150 mg

Dosages

Adults

150 mg PO bid. If converting from warfarin to dabigatran, stop warfarin and begin dabigatran when INR is less than 2. If converting from a parenteral anticoagulant, start dabigatran 0–2 hr before next dose of parenteral drug would have been given, or at time of discontinuation of continuous infusion of parenteral anticoagulant. If patient is taking dabigatran and needs to be started on a parenteral anticoagulant, wait 12 hr (if creatinine clearance is 30 mL/min or more) or 24 hr (if creatinine clearance is less than 30 mL/min) after last dose of dabigatran before beginning parenteral drug.

Pediatric patients

Safety and efficacy not established.

Patients with renal impairment

If creatinine clearance is 15–30 mL/min, give 75 mg PO bid.

Pharmacokinetics

Route	Onset	Peak
Oral	Rapid	1–4 hr

Metabolism: Hepatic; $T_{1/2}$: 12–17 hr
Distribution: May cross placenta; may enter breast milk
Excretion: Urine

Adverse effects

- **GI:** *Dyspepsia, gastritis-like symptoms, gastritis,* **gastric hemorrhage,** gastric ulcer
- **Other: Bleeding, serious hypersensitivity reactions**

Interactions

✳ **Drug-drug** • Potential for decreased effectiveness if combined with P-gp inducers (such as rifampin); avoid this combination
• Increased risk of bleeding if combined with other drugs that increase bleeding, NSAIDs, aspirin, platelet inhibitors, warfarin; if these combinations are used, monitor patient closely for potential bleeding problems

■ Nursing considerations

Assessment

- **History:** History of serious hypersensitivity reactions to dabigatran; pathologic bleeding, planned invasive procedures, pregnancy, lactation

- **Physical:** Abdominal exam, renal function tests, aPPT

Interventions

- Assess renal function before and periodically during therapy. Discontinue if acute renal failure develops.
- If possible, discontinue drug, 1–2 days (if CrCl is 50 mL/min or more) or 3–5 days (if CrCl is less than 50 mL/min) before surgery or invasive procedure.
- Ensure that patient swallows capsules whole; capsules should not be cut, crushed, or chewed.
- Administer at approximately the same time each day; do not double up any missed doses.
- Provide safety measures if bleeding becomes an issue.
- Provide small, frequent meals if GI upset is severe.
- Do not interrupt drug unless absolutely necessary (surgery, bleeding); risk of stroke increases when dabigatran is stopped.
- Be aware that a reversal agent is not available; drug is dialyzable. Use of concentrated platelets can also be considered if severe bleeding occurs.

Teaching points

- Take this drug once a day at approximately the same time each day. Store at room temperature protected from moisture and in the original container or blister pack; do not store in any other container (such as a pill organizer). Remove one capsule at a time and immediately tightly close the bottle. Once opened, the bottle must be used within 60 days; mark the bottle to expire in 60 days so you remember.
- If you forget a dose, take it as soon as you remember, then begin your usual dosage the next day. Do not make up skipped doses and do not take more than one dose each day.
- Do not stop taking this drug without consulting your health care provider.
- Tell your health care provider about any over-the-counter drugs, herbs, or other drugs you may be taking that might affect bleeding and that could require a dosage change while you are taking this drug.
- Swallow the capsules whole, and do not cut, crush, or chew them; do not open the capsule to take granules separately.

Adverse effects in italics *are most common; those in* **bold** *are life-threatening.* ▣ *Do not crush.*

- It is not known how this drug affects a fetus. If you are pregnant or thinking about becoming pregnant, discuss this with your health care provider.
- This drug may enter breast milk, but it is not known how this could affect a breast-feeding infant. If you are breast-feeding, you should find another method of feeding the baby.
- This drug will increase your risk of bleeding; tell all health care professionals who are taking care of you that you are on this drug. This is especially important before any procedure that could cause bleeding, such as dental work or surgery.
- Report the use of other prescription drugs, OTC drugs, or herbal supplements; dosage adjustment may be needed.
- You may experience these side effects: GI upset, nausea, abdominal discomfort (small, frequent meals may help; consult your health care provider if this becomes an issue); increased risk of bleeding (use a soft-bristled toothbrush and an electric razor; avoid contact sports).
- Report unusual bruising, pink or brown urine, red or black stool, coughing up blood, vomiting blood, nose bleeds, bleeding that takes a long time to stop, heavier than normal menstrual flow, headache, dizziness, weakness.

DANGEROUS DRUG

▽**dacarbazine**
(DTIC, imidazole carboxamide)

(da kar' ba zeen)

DTIC-Dome

PREGNANCY CATEGORY C

Drug classes
Alkylating agent
Antineoplastic

Therapeutic actions
Cytotoxic: Exact mechanism of action unknown; inhibits DNA and RNA synthesis, causing cell death; cell cycle nonspecific.

Indications
- Metastatic malignant melanoma
- Hodgkin disease—second-line therapy in combination with other drugs

- Unlabeled uses: Malignant pheochromocytoma with cyclophosphamide and vincristine; metastatic soft tissue sarcoma; alone or in combination therapy for Kaposi sarcoma; alone or in combination for the treatment of neuroblastomas, fibrosarcoma, rhabdomyosarcoma, islet-cell carcinoma, medullary carcinoma of the thyroid

Contraindications and cautions
- Contraindicated with allergy to dacarbazine, lactation.
- Use cautiously with impaired hepatic function, bone marrow depression, pregnancy, lactation; choose another method of feeding a baby.

Available forms
Powder for injection—100, 200, 500 mg

Dosages
- *Adult and pediatric malignant melanoma:* 2–4.5 mg/kg/day IV for 10 days, repeated at 4-wk intervals or 250 mg/m² per day IV for 5 days, repeated every 3 wk.
- *Adult Hodgkin disease:* 150 mg/m² per day for 5 days in combination with other drugs, repeated every 4 wk or 375 mg/m² on day 1 in combination with other drugs, repeated every 15 days.

Pharmacokinetics

Route	Onset	Duration
IV	15–20 min	6–8 hr

Metabolism: Hepatic; $T_{1/2}$: 19 min then 5 hr
Distribution: Crosses placenta; enters breast milk
Excretion: Urine

IV FACTS

Preparation: Reconstitute 100-mg vials with 9.9 mL and the 200-mg vials with 19.7 mL of sterile water for injection; the resulting solution contains 10 mg/mL of dacarbazine. Reconstituted solution may be further diluted with 5% dextrose injection or 0.9% sodium chloride injection and administered as an IV infusion. Reconstituted solution is stable for 72 hr if refrigerated, 8 hr at room temperature. If further diluted, solution is stable for 24 hr if refrigerated or 8 hr at room temperature. Protect reconstituted solution from light.

Infusion: Infuse slowly over 30–60 min; avoid extravasation.
Incompatibility: Do not combine with hydrocortisone sodium succinate.

Adverse effects

- **Dermatologic:** *Photosensitivity,* erythematous and urticarial rashes, alopecia
- **GI:** *Anorexia, nausea, vomiting,* hepatotoxicity, **hepatic necrosis**
- **Hematologic: Leukopenia, thrombocytopenia**
- **Hypersensitivity: Anaphylaxis**
- **Local:** *Local tissue damage and pain if extravasation occurs*
- **Other:** Facial flushing and paresthesias, flulike symptoms, cancer

■ Nursing considerations
Assessment

- **History:** Allergy to dacarbazine, impaired hepatic function, bone marrow depression, lactation, pregnancy
- **Physical:** Weight; T; skin color, lesions; hair; mucous membranes, liver evaluation; CBC, LFTs, renal function tests

Interventions

⊗ **Black box warning** Arrange for lab tests (liver function; WBC, RBC, platelet counts) before and frequently during therapy; serious bone marrow suppression, hepatotoxicity may occur.

⊗ **Black box warning** Drug is carcinogenic in animals; monitor patient accordingly.

⊗ **Warning** Give IV only; avoid extravasation into the subcutaneous tissues during administration because tissue damage and severe pain may occur.

- Apply hot packs to relieve pain locally if extravasation occurs.
- Restrict oral intake of fluid and foods for 4–6 hr before therapy to alleviate nausea and vomiting.
- Consult with physician for antiemetic if severe nausea and vomiting occur. Phenobarbital and prochlorperazine may be used. Assure patient that nausea usually subsides after 1–2 days.

Teaching points

- Prepare a calendar for treatment days and additional therapy.

- Have regular blood tests to monitor drug's effects.
- You may experience these side effects: Loss of appetite, nausea, vomiting (frequent mouth care, eat frequent small meals; maintain good nutrition; consult a dietitian; antiemetic available); rash; loss of hair (reversible; keep head covered in extreme temperature); sensitivity to UV light (use a sunscreen and protective clothing); increased risk of infection (avoid crowded areas, people with known infections).
- Report fever, chills, sore throat, unusual bleeding or bruising, yellow skin or eyes, light-colored stools, dark urine, pain or burning at IV injection site.

DANGEROUS DRUG

▷ **dactinomycin (actinomycin D, ACT)**
(dak ti noe mye' sin)

Cosmegen

PREGNANCY CATEGORY D

Drug classes
Antibiotic
Antineoplastic

Therapeutic actions
Cytotoxic: Inhibits synthesis of messenger RNA, causing cell death; cell cycle nonspecific.

Indications

- Wilms tumor, rhabdomyosarcoma, Ewing sarcoma, in combination therapy
- Testicular cancer (metastatic nonseminomatous) in combination
- Gestational trophoblastic neoplasia, as monotherapy or in combination
- Palliative treatment or adjunct to tumor resection via isolation-perfusion technique for solid malignancies
- Unlabeled uses: Osteosarcoma, malignant melanoma, Paget disease

Contraindications and cautions

- Contraindicated with allergy to dactinomycin; chickenpox, herpes zoster (severe, generalized disease and death could result); pregnancy; lactation.

Adverse effects in *italics* are most common; those in **bold** are life-threatening. ⬚ Do not crush.

- Use cautiously with bone marrow suppression, radiation therapy, and patients with reduced renal and hepatic function.

Available forms
Powder for injection—500 mcg

Dosages
⊗ *Warning* Individualize dosage. Toxic reactions are frequent, limiting the amount of the drug that can be given. Give drug in short courses.

Adults
Do not exceed 15 mcg/kg/day or 400–600 mcg/m² per day for 5 days. Calculate dosage for obese or edematous patients on the basis of surface area as an attempt to relate dosage to lean body mass.
- *Nonseminomatous testicular carcinoma:* 1,000 mcg/m² IV on day 1 of a combination regimen.
- *Gestational trophoblastic neoplasia:* 12 mcg/kg/day IV for 5 days when used as monotherapy. When used as part of a combination regimen, can give 500 mcg IV on days 1 and 2.
- *Isolation-perfusion technique:* 50 mcg/kg for lower extremity or pelvis; 35 mcg/kg for upper extremity. Use lower dose for obese patients or when previous chemotherapy or radiation therapy has been used.

Pediatric patients
Do not give to children younger than 6 mo. 15 mcg/kg/day IV for 5 days; do not exceed 15 mcg/kg/day or 400–600 mcg/m²/day for 5 days.

Pharmacokinetics
Route	Onset	Duration
IV	Rapid	9 days

Metabolism: Hepatic; T₁/₂: 36 hr
Distribution: Crosses placenta; may enter breast milk
Excretion: Feces, urine

▼ IV FACTS
Preparation: Reconstitute by adding 1.1 mL of sterile water for injection (without preservatives) to vial, creating a 500 mcg/mL concentration solution. Discard any unused portion. Highly toxic—handle and administer cautiously. Avoid inhalation of dust or vapors and contact with mucous membranes, especially the eyes. Protective equipment should be worn when handling.
Infusion: Add to IV infusions of 5% dextrose or to sodium chloride, or inject into IV tubing of a running IV infusion. Direct drug injection without infusion requires two needles, one sterile needle to remove drug from vial and another for the direct IV injection. Do not inject into IV lines with cellulose ester membrane filters; drug may be partially removed by filter. Inject over 2–3 min; infuse slowly over 20–30 min. Protect from light.

Adverse effects
- **Dermatologic:** *Alopecia, skin eruptions,* acne, erythema, increased pigmentation of previously irradiated skin
- **GI:** *Cheilitis, dysphagia, esophagitis,* ulcerative stomatitis, pharyngitis, *anorexia, abdominal pain, diarrhea,* GI ulceration, proctitis, nausea, vomiting, **hepatotoxicity**
- **GU:** Renal abnormalities
- **Hematologic:** *Anemia,* **aplastic anemia, agranulocytosis, leukopenia, thrombocytopenia, pancytopenia, reticulopenia**
- **Local:** *Tissue necrosis at sites of extravasation*
- **Other:** *Malaise, fever, fatigue, lethargy, myalgia,* hypocalcemia, **death,** increased incidence of second primary tumors with radiation

Interactions
✷ **Drug-lab test** • Inaccurate bioassay procedure results for determination of antibacterial drug levels

■ Nursing considerations

CLINICAL ALERT!
Name confusion has been reported between dactinomycin and daptomycin. Use extreme caution.

Assessment
- **History:** Allergy to dactinomycin; chickenpox, herpes zoster; bone marrow suppression, prior chemotherapy, radiation therapy; pregnancy, lactation
- **Physical:** T; skin color, lesions; weight; hair; local injection site; mucous membranes,

abdominal examination; CBC, LFTs, renal function tests, urinalysis

Interventions

⊗ **Black box warning** Use strict handling procedures; drug is extremely toxic to skin and eyes.

• Do not give IM or subcutaneously; severe local reaction and tissue necrosis occur; IV use only.

⊗ **Black box warning** Monitor injection site for extravasation, burning, or stinging. Discontinue infusion immediately, apply cold compresses to the area, and restart in another vein. Local infiltration with injectable corticosteroid and flushing with saline may lessen reaction.

• Monitor response, including CBC, often at start of therapy; adverse effects may require a decrease in dose or discontinuation of the drug; consult physician.

• Adverse effects may not occur immediately, may be worst 1–2 wk after therapy.

Teaching points

• Prepare a calendar for therapy days.

• Have regular medical follow-up, including blood tests to monitor the drug's effects.

• Adverse effects of the drug may not occur immediately; may be 1 week after therapy before maximal effects.

• You may experience these side effects: Rash, skin lesions, loss of hair (obtain a wig; use skin care); loss of appetite, nausea, mouth sores (frequent mouth care, eat frequent small meals; maintain good nutrition; consult a dietitian; antiemetic may be ordered).

• Report severe GI upset, diarrhea, vomiting, fever, burning or pain at injection site, unusual bleeding or bruising, severe mouth sores, sore throat, GI lesions.

▽ **dalfampridine**

See Appendix R, *Less commonly used drugs.*

DANGEROUS DRUG

▽ **dalteparin sodium**
(dahl' tep ah rin)

Fragmin

PREGNANCY CATEGORY B

Drug classes

Anticoagulant
Antithrombotic
Low–molecular-weight heparin

Therapeutic actions

Low–molecular-weight heparin that inhibits thrombus and clot formation by blocking factor Xa, factor IIa, preventing the formation of clots.

Indications

• Treatment of unstable angina and non–Q-wave MI for the prevention of complications in patients on aspirin or standard therapy

• Prevention of DVT, which may lead to pulmonary embolism, following abdominal or hip replacement surgery

• Extended treatment of symptomatic venous thromboembolism, DVT, or pulmonary embolism to reduce the recurrence of venous thromboembolism in patients with cancer

• Unlabeled uses: Systemic anticoagulation in venous and arterial thromboembolic complications; prophylaxis of DVT in situations that may lead to PE

Contraindications and cautions

• Contraindicated with hypersensitivity to dalteparin, heparin, pork products, or benzyl alcohol; severe thrombocytopenia; uncontrolled bleeding; use of unstable angina dosage in patients undergoing regional anesthesia; pregnancy.

• Use cautiously with lactation; history of GI bleed; severe hepatic or renal impairment; recent childbirth or surgery; history of heparin-induced thrombocytopenia; severe and uncontrolled hypertension; spinal tap; spinal/epidural anesthesia.

Available forms

Injection (prefilled syringes)—2,500 international units/0.2 mL, 5,000 international units/0.2 mL, 7,500 international units/0.3 mL, 10,000 international units/mL, 10,000 international units/0.4 mL, 12,500 international units/0.5 mL, 15,000 international units/0.6 mL, 18,000 international units/0.72 mL, 95,000 international units/3.8 or 9.5 mL.

Dosages

Adults

• *Unstable angina:* 120 international units/kg subcutaneously every 12 hr with aspirin

Adverse effects in *italics* are most common; those in **bold** are life-threatening. ⊙ Do not crush.

therapy for 5–8 days; not to exceed 10,000 international units every 12 hr.

• *DVT prophylaxis, abdominal surgery:* 2,500 international units subcutaneously given 1–2 hr before surgery and repeated once daily for 5–10 days after surgery; high-risk patients, 5,000 international units subcutaneously starting the evening before surgery; then daily for 5–10 days.

• *Hip replacement surgery:* 5,000 international units subcutaneously the evening before surgery *or* 2,500 international units within 2 hr before surgery *or* 2,500 international units 4–8 hr after surgery; then, 5,000 international units subcutaneously each day for 5–10 days or up to 14 days.

• *Extended treatment of venous thromboembolism:*
Month 1: 200 international units/kg/day subcutaneously; do not exceed 18,000 international units/day
Months 2–6: 150 international units/kg/day subcutaneously; do not exceed 18,000 international units/day.

Pediatric patients
Safety and efficacy not established.
Patients with thrombocytopenia on extended treatment
Reduce daily dose by 2,500 international units until platelet count exceeds 100,000/mm3. If platelet count is less than 50,000/mm3, discontinue drug until platelet count recovers above 50,000/mm3.
Patients with renal insufficiency on extended treatment
If creatinine clearance is less than 30 mL/min, target anti-Xa range is 0.5–1.5 international units/mL; after at least 3–4 doses have been given, draw blood 4–6 hr after dose

Pharmacokinetics

Route	Onset	Peak	Duration
Subcut.	20–60 min	3–5 hr	2–12 hr

Metabolism: T₁/₂: 4.5 hr
Distribution: May cross placenta, may enter breast milk
Excretion: Urine

Adverse effects
• **Hematologic: Hemorrhage,** *bruising,* thrombocytopenia
• **Hepatic:** Elevated concentrations of AST, ALT

• **Hypersensitivity:** Chills, fever, urticaria, asthma
• **Other:** Fever; pain; local irritation, hematoma, erythema at site of injection; risk of spinal or epidural hematoma if used with spinal/epidural anesthesia or spinal tap, skin necrosis

Interactions
✳ **Drug-drug** • Increased bleeding tendencies with oral anticoagulants or platelet inhibitors; clopidogrel, ticlopidine, salicylates
• Risk of severe bleeding with heparin; avoid this combination
✳ **Drug-lab test** • Increased AST, ALT levels
✳ **Drug-alternative therapy** • Increased risk of bleeding if combined with chamomile, garlic, ginger, ginkgo biloba, and ginseng therapy, high-dose vitamin E

■ Nursing considerations
Assessment
• **History:** Recent surgery or injury; sensitivity to heparin, pork products, either low–molecular-weight heparins or enoxaparin, tinzaparin, benzyl alcohol; lactation, pregnancy; history of GI bleed; renal or hepatic impairment
• **Physical:** Peripheral perfusion, R, stool guaiac test, PTT or other tests of blood coagulation, platelet count, LFTs, renal function tests

Interventions
⊗ **Black box warning** Carefully monitor patients with spinal epidural anesthesia for signs of neurologic impairment; risk of spinal hematoma and paralysis.
• Give 1–2 hr before abdominal surgery.
• Do not give dalteparin by IM injection.
• Administer by deep subcutaneous injection; patient should be lying down; alternate administration between the left and right anterolateral and left and right posterolateral abdominal wall. Introduce the whole length of the needle into a skin fold at a 45 to 90 degree angle held between the thumb and forefinger; hold the skin fold throughout the injection.
• Cannot be used interchangeably (unit for unit) with other low–molecular-weight heparin or unfractionated heparin.

- Apply pressure to all injection sites after needle is withdrawn; inspect injection sites for signs of hematoma.
- Do not massage injection sites.
- Do not mix with other injections or infusions.
- Store at room temperature; fluid should be clear, colorless to pale yellow.
- Alert all health care providers that patient is on dalteparin.
- If thromboembolic episode should occur despite therapy, discontinue and initiate appropriate therapy.

⊗ **Warning** Keep protamine sulfate (dalteparin antidote) readily available in case of overdose.

- Treatment of overdose: Protamine sulfate (1% solution). Administer 1 mg of protamine per 100 antifactor Xa international units of dalteparin. Give very slowly IV over 10 min.

Teaching points

- This drug must be given by a parenteral route (not orally). You or your caregiver need to learn to administer the drug subcutaneously, and to safely dispose of needles and syringes.
- Periodic blood tests are needed to monitor response.
- Avoid injury while using this drug—use an electric razor, avoid potentially injurious activities.
- Report nose bleed, bleeding of the gums, unusual bruising, black or tarry stools, cloudy or dark urine, abdominal or lower back pain, severe headache, light-headedness, or dizziness.

▽ **dantrolene sodium**

(*dan' troe leen*)

Dantrium, Dantrium Intravenous

PREGNANCY CATEGORY C

Drug class
Skeletal muscle relaxant (direct acting)

Therapeutic actions
Relaxes skeletal muscle within the skeletal muscle fiber, probably by interfering with the release of calcium from the sarcoplasmic retic-

ulum; does not interfere with neuromuscular transmission or affect the surface membrane of skeletal muscle.

Indications

- Oral: Control of clinical spasticity resulting from upper motor neuron disorders, such as spinal cord injury, stroke, cerebral palsy, or MS; not indicated for relief of skeletal muscle spasm resulting from rheumatic disorders; continued long-term administration is justified if use significantly reduces painful or disabling spasticity (clonus); significantly reduces the intensity or degree of nursing care required; rids the patient of problematic manifestation of spasticity
- Oral: Preoperatively to prevent or attenuate the development of malignant hyperthermia in susceptible patients who must undergo surgery or anesthesia; after a malignant hyperthermia crisis to prevent recurrence
- Parenteral (IV): Management of the fulminant hypermetabolism of skeletal muscle characteristic of malignant hyperthermia crisis; preoperative prevention of malignant hyperthermia
- Unlabeled uses: Exercise-induced muscle pain, neuroleptic malignant syndrome

Contraindications and cautions

- Contraindicated with active hepatic disease; spasticity used to sustain upright posture, balance in locomotion or to gain or retain increased function; lactation.
- Use cautiously with female patients and patients older than 35 yr (increased risk for potentially fatal, hepatocellular disease); impaired pulmonary function; severely impaired cardiac function due to myocardial disease; history of previous liver disease or impairment.
- Malignant hyperthermia is a medical emergency that would override contraindications and cautions.

Available forms
Capsules—25, 50, 100 mg; powder for injection—20 mg/vial

Dosages
Adults
Oral

- *Chronic spasticity:* Titrate and individualize dosage; establish a therapeutic goal before therapy, and increase dosage until maximum performance compatible with the dysfunction is achieved. Initially, 25 mg daily; increase to 25 mg tid for 7 days; then increase to 50 mg tid and to 100 mg tid if necessary. Most patients will respond to 400 mg/day or less; maintain each dosage level for 7 days to evaluate response. Discontinue drug after 45 days if benefits are not evident.

• *Preoperative prophylaxis of malignant hyperthermia:* 4–8 mg/kg/day PO in three to four divided doses for 1–2 days prior to surgery; give last dose about 3–4 hr before scheduled surgery with a minimum of water. Adjust dosage to the recommended range to prevent incapacitation due to drowsiness and excessive GI irritation.

• *Postcrisis follow-up:* 4–8 mg/kg/day PO in four divided doses for 1–3 days to prevent recurrence.

Parenteral
• *Treatment of malignant hyperthermia:* Discontinue all anesthetics as soon as problem is recognized. Give dantrolene by continuous rapid IV push beginning at a minimum dose of 1 mg/kg and continuing until symptoms subside or a maximum cumulative dose of 10 mg/kg has been given. If physiologic and metabolic abnormalities reappear, repeat regimen. Give continuously until symptoms subside.

• *Preoperative prophylaxis of malignant hyperthermia:* 2.5 mg/kg IV 1¼ hr before surgery infused over 1 hr.

Pediatric patients
Safety for use in children younger than 5 yr not established. Since adverse effects may appear only after many years, weigh benefits and risks of long-term use carefully.

Oral
• *Chronic spasticity:* Use an approach similar to that for the adult. Initially, 0.5 mg/kg PO once daily for 7 days, followed by 0.5 mg/kg PO tid for 7 days; then 1 mg/kg tid for 7 days; then 2 mg/kg tid if necessary. Do not exceed dosage of 100 mg qid.

• *Malignant hyperthermia:* Dosage orally and IV is same as adult.

Pharmacokinetics

Route	Onset	Peak	Duration
Oral	Slow	4–6 hr	8–10 hr
IV	Rapid	5 hr	6–8 hr

Metabolism: Hepatic; $T_{1/2}$: 9 hr (oral), 4–8 hr (IV)
Distribution: Crosses placenta; enters breast milk
Excretion: Urine

▼ **IV FACTS**
Preparation: Add 60 mL of sterile water for injection (without bacteriostatics) to each vial; shake until solution is clear. Use within 6 hr; store at room temperature and protect from light.
Infusion: Administer by rapid continuous IV push. Administer continuously until symptoms subside; prophylactic doses infused over 1 hr.
Incompatibilities: Dantrolene sodium is not compatible with 5% dextrose or 0.9% sodium chloride or bacteriostatic water for injection.

Adverse effects
Oral
• **CNS:** *Drowsiness, dizziness, weakness, general malaise, fatigue,* speech disturbance, seizure, headache, light-headedness, visual disturbance, diplopia, alteration of taste, insomnia, mental depression, mental confusion, increased nervousness
• **CV:** Tachycardia, erratic BP, phlebitis, **heart failure**
• **Dermatologic:** Abnormal hair growth, acnelike rash, pruritus, urticaria, eczematoid eruption, sweating, photosensitivity
• **GI:** *Diarrhea,* constipation, GI bleeding, anorexia, dysphagia, gastric irritation, abdominal cramps, **hepatitis**
• **GU:** Increased urinary frequency, hematuria, crystalluria, difficult erection, urinary incontinence, nocturia, dysuria, urinary retention
• **Hematologic: Aplastic anemia,** leukopenia, thrombocytopenia
• **Other:** Myalgia, backache, chills and fever, feeling of suffocation, respiratory depression

Parenteral
• None of the above reactions with short-term IV therapy for malignant hyperthermia

Interactions
✳ **Drug-drug** • Risk of hyperkalemia, myocardial depression if combined with verapamil

■ Nursing considerations
Assessment
- **History:** Active hepatic disease; spasticity used to sustain upright posture and balance in locomotion or to gain and retain increased function; female patient and patients older than 35 yr; impaired pulmonary function; severely impaired cardiac function; history of previous liver disease; lactation, pregnancy
- **Physical:** T; skin color, lesions; orientation, affect, reflexes, bilateral grip strength, vision; P, BP, auscultation; adventitious sounds; bowel sounds, normal GI output; prostate palpation, normal output, voiding pattern; urinalysis, LFTs

Interventions
⊗ *Warning* Monitor IV injection sites, and ensure that extravasation does not occur—drug is very alkaline and irritating to tissues.

⊗ *Warning* Ensure that all appropriate measures are used to treat malignant hyperthermia: Discontinue triggering drugs, monitor and provide for increased oxygen requirements, manage metabolic acidosis and electrolyte imbalance, use cooling measures if necessary.

- Establish a therapeutic goal before beginning long-term oral therapy to gain or enhance ability to engage in therapeutic exercise program, use of braces, transfer maneuvers.
- Withdraw oral drug for 2–4 days to confirm therapeutic benefits; clinical impression of exacerbation of spasticity would justify use of this potentially dangerous drug.
- Discontinue if diarrhea is severe; it may be possible to reinstitute drug at a lower dose.

⊗ **Black box warning** Have liver function tests done periodically; arrange to discontinue at first sign of abnormality; early detection of liver abnormalities may permit reversion to normal function. Hepatotoxicity is possible.

Teaching points
Preoperative prophylaxis of malignant hyperthermia
- Call for assistance if you wish to get up; do not move about alone; this drug can cause drowsiness.
- Report GI upset; a dosage change is possible; eat frequent small meals.

Long-term oral therapy for spasticity
- Take this drug exactly as prescribed; do not take a higher dosage.
- Avoid alcohol and sleep-inducing or over-the-counter drugs; these could cause dangerous effects.
- You may experience these side effects: Drowsiness, dizziness, blurred vision (avoid driving or engaging in activities that require alertness); diarrhea; nausea (take with food, eat frequent small meals); difficulty urinating, increased urinary frequency, urinary incontinence (empty bladder just before taking medication); headache, malaise (an analgesic may be allowed); photosensitivity (avoid sun and ultraviolet light or use sunscreens, protective clothing).
- Report rash, itching, bloody or black tarry stools, pale stools, yellowish discoloration of the skin or eyes, severe diarrhea.

▷dapsone

See Appendix R, *Less commonly used drugs*.

▷daptomycin
*(dap toe **mye**' sin)*

Cubicin

PREGNANCY CATEGORY B

Drug class
Cyclic lipopeptide antibiotic

Therapeutic actions
Binds to bacterial cell membranes, causing a rapid depolarization of membrane potential. The loss of membrane potential leads to the inhibition of protein, DNA, and RNA synthesis, which results in bacterial cell death.

Indications
- Treatment of complicated skin and skin-structure infections caused by susceptible strains of the following gram-positive bacteria: *Staphylococcus aureus* (including methicillin-resistant strains), *Streptococcus pyogenes, Streptococcus agalactiae, Streptococcus dysgalactiae,* and *Enterococcus faecalis* (vancomycin-susceptible strains only)

- Treatment of *S. aureus* bloodstream infections, including right-sided endocarditis caused by methicillin-susceptible and methicillin-resistant *S. aureus*
- ◢■ **NEW INDICATION:** Unlabeled use: Treatment of vancomycin-resistant *Enterococcus faecium*

Contraindications and cautions

- Contraindicated with known allergy to daptomycin.
- Use cautiously with pregnancy, lactation, renal impairment.

Available forms

Powder for injection—500 mg/vial

Dosages

Adults

Skin and skin-structure infections: 4 mg/kg IV given over 30 min or as an IV injection over 2 min in 0.9% sodium chloride injection every 24 hr for 7–14 days.
Bacteremia: 6 mg/kg/day IV over 30 min or as an IV injection over 2 min for 2–6 wk or longer.

Pediatric patients

Safety and efficacy not established.

Patients with renal impairment

For patients with creatinine clearance less than 30 mL/min or for those on dialysis, give 4 mg/kg IV once every 48 hr (6 mg/kg for *S. aureus* bloodstream infections).

Pharmacokinetics

Route	Onset	Peak
IV	Rapid	30 min

Metabolism: Hepatic; $T_{1/2}$: 8–9 hr
Distribution: May cross placenta; may enter breast milk
Excretion: Urine

▼ IV FACTS

Preparation: Reconstitute with 10 mL (500-mg vial) 0.9% sodium chloride injection; further dilute with 0.9% sodium chloride injection for infusion. Final concentration should not exceed 20 mg/mL. Reconstituted and diluted solution is stable for 12 hr at room temperature, up to 48 hr if refrigerated; date bag to ensure that solution is discarded after that

time; solution should be clear and free of particulate matter.
Infusion: Infuse over 30 min.
Injection: Inject reconstituted drug over 2 min.
Compatibilities: Compatible with 0.9% sodium chloride injection, lactated Ringer solution.
Incompatibilities: Do not mix with dextrose solutions; do not mix in solution with any other drugs, if a line is used for several drugs, flush the line with compatible fluids between drugs.

Adverse effects

- **CNS:** *Headache, insomnia,* dizziness, peripheral neuropathy
- **CV:** Hypotension, hypertension
- **GI:** *Constipation, nausea, diarrhea, vomiting,* dyspepsia, **pseudomembranous colitis,** *Clostridium difficile* diarrhea
- **Respiratory:** Dyspnea, eosinophilic pneumonia
- **Other:** *Injection site reactions,* fever, *rash,* pruritus, arthralgia, limb pain, **myopathy,** *superinfections,* anemia

Interactions

✳ **Drug-drug** • Potential for increased effects of oral anticoagulants if combined; monitor patient closely and adjust dosage as needed • Risk of altered effects of both drugs if combined with tobramycin; if this combination is used, monitor patient very closely • Increased risk of myopathy if combined with HMG-CoA inhibitors; consider discontinuing the HMG-CoA inhibitor while daptomycin is being used

■ Nursing considerations

✖ CLINICAL ALERT!

Name confusion has been reported between dactinomycin and daptomycin. Use extreme caution.

Assessment

- **History:** Allergy to daptomycin, renal impairment, pregnancy, lactation
- **Physical:** Site of infection, skin color, lesions; orientation, affect; R, adventitious sounds; GI output, bowel sounds; orientation, affect; culture and sensitivity tests of infection, renal function tests

D

Interventions

- Culture site of infection before beginning therapy.
- Monitor CPK levels weekly to assess for myopathy.
- ⊗ *Warning* Discontinue drug and provide supportive care for any patient developing signs of pseudomembranous colitis.
- ⊗ *Warning* Discontinue drug with any unexplained signs of myopathy (muscle pain or weakness) or with increasing levels of CK. Consider discontinuing any other drugs that are associated with myopathy (HMG-CoA inhibitors) while daptomycin is being used.
- ⊗ *Warning* Discontinue drug and provide medical support for signs and symptoms of eosinophilic pneumonia.
- Monitor renal function in patients before beginning therapy.
- Institute appropriate hygiene measures and arrange treatment if superinfections occur.
- If GI upset occurs, provide small, frequent meals; encourage patient to maintain fluid intake and nutrition.
- Establish safety measures (eg, accompany patient, use side rails) if CNS changes occur.

Teaching points

- This drug will be given IV over 30 minutes or by IV injection over 2 minutes once a day for 7–14 days or longer.
- You may experience these side effects: Nausea, diarrhea, discomfort (eat frequent small meals); headache (analgesics may be available to help; consult your health care provider); dizziness (ask for help when you are walking); reaction at the injection site (if this becomes painful, notify your health care provider).
- Report severe or watery diarrhea, rash, muscle pain or weakness, difficulty breathing.

▽**darbepoetin alfa**

(dar bah poe e' tin)

Aranesp

PREGNANCY CATEGORY C

Drug class

Erythropoiesis-stimulating hormone

Therapeutic actions

An erythropoietin-like glycoprotein hormone produced by recombinant DNA technology; stimulates RBC production in the bone marrow in the same manner as naturally occurring erythropoietin, a hormone released into the bloodstream in response to renal hypoxia.

Indications

- Treatment of anemia associated with chronic renal failure, including during dialysis
- Treatment of chemotherapy-induced anemia in patients with nonmyeloid malignancies
- Unlabeled use: Anemia associated with malignancy

Contraindications and cautions

- Contraindicated with uncontrolled hypertension or hypersensitivity to any component of the drug.
- Use cautiously with hypertension, pregnancy, lactation.

Available forms

Polysorbate solution for injection—25, 40, 60, 100, 200, 300, 500 mcg/mL; 25 mcg/0.42 mL, 40 mcg/0.4 mL; 60 mcg/0.3 mL; 100 mcg/0.5 mL; 150 mcg/0.3 or 0.75 mL; 200 mcg/0.4 mL; 300 mcg/0.6 mL

Dosages

Adults

Chronic renal disease

- *Starting dose:* 0.45 mcg/kg IV or subcutaneously once per wk or 0.75 mcg IV or subcutaneously once every 2 wk. Dosage may be adjusted no more frequently than once per mo. Target Hgb level is 12 g/dL. Adjust dosage by 25% at a time to achieve that level. Avoid rapid increase in Hgb.
- *Switching from epoetin alfa:*

Epoetin Alfa Dose in Units/wk	Darbepoetin Alfa Dose in mcg/wk (adult)	Darbepoetin Alfa Dose in mcg/wk (pediatric)
1,500–2,499	6.25	6.25
2,500–4,999	12.5	10
5,000–10,999	25	20
11,000–17,999	40	40
18,000–33,999	60	60
34,000–89,999	100	100
90,000 or more	200	200

Adverse effects in *italics* are most common; those in **bold** are life-threatening. ⊞ Do not crush.

Patients who were receiving epoetin two to three times per week should receive darbepoetin once per wk. Patients who were receiving epoetin once per wk should receive darbepoetin once every 2 wk.

- *Chemotherapy-induced anemia:* 2.25 mcg/kg subcutaneously once per wk; adjust to maintain acceptable Hgb levels. Or 500 mcg by subcutaneous injection once every 3 wk; adjust dosage to maintain Hgb level at 12 g/dL.
- *Anemia of chronic renal failure:* Start with single subcutaneous injection every 2 wk. Dosage should start slowly and be increased based on Hgb levels; check Hgb levels weekly until stable, then monthly.

Pediatric patients

Safety and efficacy in children with cancer have not been established.

Pharmacokinetics

Route	Peak	Duration
Subcut.	34 hr	24–72 hr
IV	14 hr	24–72 hr

Metabolism: Serum; $T_{1/2}$: 21 hr (IV), 49 hr (subcutaneously)
Distribution: May cross placenta; enters breast milk
Excretion: Urine

▼ IV FACTS

Preparation: Administer as provided; no additional preparation needed. Enter vial only once; discard any unused solution. Refrigerate. Do not shake vial. Inspect for any discoloring or precipitates before use.
Infusion: Administer by direct IV injection or into tubing of running IV.
Incompatibilities: Do not mix with any other drug solution.

Adverse effects

- **CNS:** *Headache, fatigue, asthenia,* dizziness, **seizure,** TIA, **stroke**
- **CV:** *Hypertension, edema, hypotension,* chest pain, arrhythmias, chest pain, **MI**
- **GI:** *Nausea, vomiting, diarrhea, abdominal pain*
- **Respiratory:** *URI, dyspnea, cough*
- **Other:** *Arthralgias, myalgias,* limb pain, clotting of access line, pain at injection site, **development of anti-erythropoietin antibodies with subsequent pure red cell aplasia and extreme anemia; tumor progression with cancer**

■ Nursing considerations
Assessment

- **History:** Hypertension; hypersensitivity to any component of product, pregnancy, lactation
- **Physical:** Reflexes, affect, BP, P, R, adventitious sounds, urinary output, renal function tests, CBC, hemoglobin, Hct, iron levels, electrolytes

Interventions

⊗ *Warning* Ensure chronic, renal nature of anemia or response to chemotherapy. Darbepoetin is not intended as a treatment of severe anemia and is not a substitute for emergency transfusion.

⊗ *Black box warning* Risk of death and serious CV events increases if hemoglobin target exceeds 12 g/dL. Use lowest level of any drug needed to increase hemoglobin to lowest level needed to avoid transfusion.

⊗ *Black box warning* Risk of DVT is higher in patients who receive erythropoietin-stimulating agents preoperatively to decrease need for transfusion; note that darbepoetin is not approved for this use.

⊗ *Black box warning* Risk of death or tumor progression increases when drug is used in cancer patients with Hgb target range exceeding 12 g/dL. Monitor Hgb closely in these patients.

- Prepare solution by gently mixing. Do not shake; shaking may denature the glycoprotein. Use only one dose per vial; do not reenter the vial. Discard unused portions.
- Patients with chronic renal failure on hemodialysis should receive this drug IV, not by subcutaneous injection, to decrease the risk of developing anti-erythropoietin antibodies.
- Do not administer with any other drug solution.
- Administer dose once weekly. If administered independent of dialysis, administer into venous access line. If patient is not on dialysis, administer IV or subcutaneously.
- Evaluate chemotherapy patients for once-every-3-wk treatment program.
- Monitor access lines for signs of clotting.

- Arrange for Hct or Hgb reading before administration of each dose to determine appropriate dosage. Do not exceed Hgb target of 12 g/dL. If patient fails to respond within 4 wk of therapy, evaluate patient for other causes of the problem.
- Evaluate iron stores before and periodically during therapy. Supplemental iron may be needed.
- Monitor patient for sudden loss of response and severe anemia with low reticulocyte count; hold drug and check patient for anti-erythropoetin antibodies. If antibodies are present, discontinue drug permanently and do not switch to any other erythropoetic agent; cross-sensitivity can occur.
- Monitor diet and assess nutrition; arrange for nutritional consult as necessary.
- Establish safety precautions (eg, siderails, environmental control, lighting) if CNS effects occur.
- Maintain seizure precautions during administration.
- Provide additional comfort measures, as necessary, to alleviate discomfort from GI effects, headache.
- Offer support and encouragement to deal with chronic disease and need for prolonged therapy and testing.

Teaching points

- The drug will need to be given once a week or once every 3 wk, as prescribed, and can only be given IV or subcutaneously or into a dialysis access line. Prepare a schedule of administration dates. You and a significant other should learn to administer subcutaneous injections. Dispose of needles and syringes properly.
- Keep appointments for blood tests; frequent blood tests will be needed to determine the effects of the drug on your blood count and to determine the appropriate dosage needed.
- Maintain all of the usual activities and restrictions that apply to your chronic renal failure. If this becomes difficult, consult your health care provider.
- You may experience these side effects: Dizziness (avoid driving a car or performing hazardous tasks); headache, fatigue, joint pain (consult your health care provider if these become bothersome; medications may be available to help); nausea, vomiting, diarrhea (proper nutrition is important; consult with your dietitian to maintain nutrition and ensure ready access to bathroom facilities); upper respiratory infection, cough (consult your health care provider if this occurs).
- Report difficulty breathing, numbness or tingling, chest pain, seizures, severe headache.

▷ **darifenacin hydrobromide**

(da ree fen' ah sin high droh broh' myde)

Enablex ⒪ⓜⓡ

PREGNANCY CATEGORY C

Drug classes
Muscarinic receptor antagonist
Urinary antispasmodic

Therapeutic actions
Counteracts smooth muscle spasm of the urinary tract by relaxing the detrusor and other smooth muscles through action at the muscarinic parasympathetic receptors.

Indications

- Treatment of overactive bladder with symptoms of urge urinary incontinence, urgency and urinary frequency

Contraindications and cautions

- Contraindicated with allergy to drug or any component of the drug, urinary retention, gastric retention, uncontrolled narrow-angle glaucoma.
- Use cautiously with bladder outflow obstruction, GI obstructive disorders, decreased GI motility, controlled narrow-angle glaucoma, reduced hepatic function, pregnancy, lactation.

Available forms
ER tablets ⒪ⓜⓡ—7.5, 15 mg

Dosages
Adults

7.5 mg/day PO taken with liquid and swallowed whole. May be increased to 15 mg/day PO as early as week 2, if needed for patient response.

Adverse effects in *italics* are most common; those in **bold** are life-threatening. ⒪ⓜⓡ Do not crush.

Pediatric patients
Safety and efficacy not established.
Patients with moderate hepatic impairment
Do not exceed 7.5 mg/day PO.
Patients with severe hepatic impairment
Not recommended.

Pharmacokinetics

Route	Onset	Peak
Oral	Slow	6.5–7.5 hr

Metabolism: Hepatic; $T_{1/2}$: 13–19 hr
Distribution: May cross placenta; may enter breast milk
Excretion: Feces, urine

Adverse effects

- **CNS:** Dizziness, asthenia, headache, confusion
- **EENT:** Dry eyes, blurred vision
- **GI:** *Dry mouth, constipation,* nausea, dyspepsia, abdominal pain, diarrhea
- **GU:** UTI, urinary retention
- **Other:** Flulike symptoms

Interactions

✳ **Drug-drug** • Risk of increased serum levels and toxic effects if combined with clarithromycin, ketoconazole, itraconazole, ritonavir, nelfinavir, clarithromycin, nefazodone; if this combination is used, monitor patient and do not exceed 7.5 mg/day darifenacin • Risk of increased toxic effects of flecainide, thioridazine, TCAs; monitor patient closely and use caution if this combination is used • Risk of increased anticholinergic adverse effects (dry mouth, constipation, blurred vision) if combined with anticholinergic drugs; monitor patient carefully if this combination is used

■ Nursing considerations
Assessment

- **History:** Allergy to drug or any component of the drug; urinary retention, gastric retention, uncontrolled narrow-angle glaucoma, bladder outflow obstruction, GI obstructive disorders, decreased GI motility, reduced renal or hepatic function, pregnancy, lactation
- **Physical:** Orientation, affect, reflexes, ophthalmic examination, ocular pressure measurement; P; bowel sounds, oral mucous membranes; LFTs

Interventions

- Arrange for definitive treatment of underlying medical conditions that may be causing overactive bladder.
- Ensure that patient swallows tablet whole; do not cut, crush, or allow patient to chew tablet.
- Provide sugarless candies for patient to suck and frequent mouth care if dry mouth is a serious problem.
- Provide small, frequent meals if GI upset occurs.
- Establish bowel program if constipation is a problem.
- Arrange for ophthalmic examination before beginning therapy and periodically during therapy.
- Establish safety precautions if CNS effects occur.

Teaching points

- Take drug once a day with water. Swallow whole, do not cut, crush, or chew tablet. Take with or without food.
- Be aware that this drug is meant to relieve the symptoms you are experiencing; other medications may be used to treat the cause of the symptoms.
- You may not be able to sweat normally while on this drug; use caution in any situation that could lead to overheating.
- Consult your health care provider if you become pregnant or wish to become pregnant, it is not known if this drug affects the fetus.
- If you are breast-feeding, another method of feeding the baby should be used while you are on this drug.
- You may experience these side effects: Dry mouth, GI upset (sucking on sugarless candies and frequent mouth care may help); drowsiness, blurred vision (avoid driving or performing tasks that require alertness while on this drug); constipation (medication may be available to help).
- Report inability to void, fever, blurring of vision, severe constipation.

▽ **darunavir**
See Appendix R, *Less commonly used drugs.*

▽ **dasatinib**
See Appendix R, *Less commonly used drugs.*

▷ DAUNOrubicin citrate

See Appendix R, *Less commonly used drugs.*

▷ decitabine

See Appendix R, *Less commonly used drugs.*

▷ deferasirox

See Appendix R, *Less commonly used drugs.*

▷ deferoxamine mesylate

See Appendix R, *Less commonly used drugs.*

▷ degarelix

See Appendix R, *Less commonly used drugs.*

▷ delavirdine mesylate
(dell ah vur' den)

Rescriptor

PREGNANCY CATEGORY C

Drug classes
Antiviral
Nonnucleoside reverse transcriptase inhibitor

Therapeutic actions
Non-nucleoside inhibitor of HIV reverse transcriptase; binds directly to HIV's reverse transcriptase and blocks RNA-dependent and DNA-dependent DNA polymerase activities.

Indications
• Treatment of HIV-1 infection in combination with other appropriate retroviral drugs when therapy is warranted; not intended as a monotherapy because resistant virus emerges rapidly

Contraindications and cautions
• Contraindicated with life-threatening allergy to any component.
• Use cautiously with compromised or impaired liver function, pregnancy, lactation.

Available forms
Tablets—100, 200 mg

Dosages
Adults and patients older than 16 yr
400 mg PO tid used in combination with appropriate antiretroviral drugs.
Pediatric patients
Not recommended for patients younger than 16 yr.

Pharmacokinetics

Route	Onset	Peak
Oral	Rapid	1 hr

Metabolism: Hepatic; $T_{1/2}$: 2–11 hr
Distribution: May cross placenta; may enter breast milk
Excretion: Urine, feces

Adverse effects
• **CNS:** *Headache,* insomnia, myalgia, *asthenia,* malaise, dizziness, paresthesia, somnolence, fatigue
• **GI:** *Nausea,* GI pain, *diarrhea,* anorexia, vomiting, dyspepsia, increased liver enzymes
• **Skin:** *Rash,* pruritus, maculopapular rash, nodules, urticaria
• **Other:** Anemia, arthralgia, breast enlargement, fat redistribution

Interactions
✳ **Drug-drug** ⊗ *Warning* Potentially serious or life-threatening adverse effects may occur in combination with antiarrhythmics, clarithromycin, dapsone, rifabutin, benzodiazepines, calcium channel blockers, ergot derivatives, indinavir, saquinavir, quinidine or warfarin; avoid these combinations if at all possible; if the combination cannot be avoided, monitor patient very closely and decrease dosage as appropriate.

✳ **Drug-alternative therapy** • Possible loss of antiviral response with St. John's Wort; avoid this combination

■ Nursing considerations
Assessment
• **History:** Life-threatening allergy to any component, impaired liver function, pregnancy, lactation
• **Physical:** Skin rashes, lesions, texture; T; affect, reflexes, peripheral sensation; bowel sounds, LFTs, CBC and differential

Interventions

- Arrange to monitor hematologic indices and liver function periodically during therapy.
- Monitor patient for signs of opportunistic infections that will need to be treated appropriately.
- ⊗ **Black box warning** Administer the drug concurrently with appropriate antiretroviral drugs; not for monotherapy.
- Disperse tablets in water before administration; add four 100-mg tablets to at least 3 oz water; allow to stand for a few minutes, stir until a uniform dispersion occurs; have patient drink immediately. Rinse glass and have patient drink rinse; the 200-mg tablets are not readily soluble in water.
- Offer support and encouragement to deal with the diagnosis; explain that this drug must be taken in combination with other drugs and that the long-term effects of the use of this drug are not known.

Teaching points

- Take drug as prescribed; take with other prescribed drugs; do not change dose or alter routine without consulting your health care provider. If also taking antacids, take at least 1 hour apart.
- Disperse four 100-mg tablets in 3 ounces of water; let stand, then stir and drink immediately, rinse glass with water and drink rinse; the 200-mg tablets are not readily soluble in water.
- These drugs are not a cure for AIDS or AIDS-related complex; opportunistic infections may occur and regular medical care should be sought to deal with the disease.
- Frequent blood tests are needed during the course of treatment; results of blood counts may indicate a need for decreased dosage or discontinuation of the drug for a specific time.
- This drug is not recommended for use in pregnancy; contraceptives are advised.
- Do not breast-feed while taking this drug; adverse effects could occur in the baby.
- This drug may interact with several other drugs; alert any health care provider that you are on this drug. If you are taking antacids, take them at least 1 hour apart from delavirdine.
- Delavirdine does not reduce the risk of transmission of HIV to others by sexual contact or blood contamination; use appropriate precautions.

- You may experience these side effects: Nausea, loss of appetite, change in taste (eat frequent small meals); headache, fever, muscle aches (an analgesic may help; consult your health care provider); rash (skin care will be important).
- Report use of any prescription or over-the-counter drugs or dietary supplements to your physician or pharmacist.
- Report rash, severe headache, severe nausea, vomiting, changes in color of urine or stool, fatigue.

▷ **demeclocycline hydrochloride (demethylchlortetracycline hydrochloride)**

(dem e kloe sye' kleen)

Declomycin

PREGNANCY CATEGORY D

Drug classes

Antibiotic
Tetracycline antibiotic

Therapeutic actions

Bacteriostatic: Inhibits protein synthesis of susceptible bacteria, preventing cell reproduction.

Indications

- Infections caused by susceptible strains of rickettsiae; *Mycoplasma pneumoniae;* agents of psittacosis, ornithosis, lymphogranuloma venereum, and granuloma inguinale; *Borrelia recurrentis; Haemophilus ducreyi; Pasteurella pestis; P. tularensis; Bartonella bacilliformis; Bacteroides; Vibrio cholerae; Vibrio comma; Vibrio fetus; Brucella; Escherichia coli; Enterobacter aerogenes; Shigella; Acinetobacter calcoaceticus; Haemophilus influenzae; Klebsiella; Diplococcus pneumoniae; Staphylococcus aureus; Streptococcus pyogenes; Streptococcus pneumoniae; Mycoplasma* bacteria, *Francisella tularensis, Lersinia pestis*
- When penicillin is contraindicated, infections caused by *Neisseria gonorrhoeae, Treponema pallidum, T. pertenue, Listeria monocytogenes, Clostridium, Bacillus*

anthracis, Fusobacterium fusiforme, Actinomyces, Neisseria meningitidis
- As an adjunct to amebicides in acute intestinal amebiasis
- Treatment of acne or uncomplicated urethral, endocervical, or rectal infections in adults caused by *Chlamydia trachomatis*

Contraindications and cautions
- Contraindicated with allergy to tetracyclines; pregnancy, lactation; in children during tooth-forming years.
- Use cautiously with renal or hepatic impairment.

Available forms
Tablets—150, 300 mg

Dosages
Adults
- *General guidelines:* 150 mg PO qid or 300 mg PO bid.
- *Gonococcal infection:* 600 mg PO then 300 mg every 12 hr for 4 days to a total of 3 g.
- *Streptococcal infections:* Treat for at least 10 days.

Pediatric patients 8 yr and older
3–6 mg/lb/day (6.6–13.2 mg/kg/day) PO in two to four divided doses.

Pediatric patients younger than 8 yr
Not recommended.

Pharmacokinetics

Route	Onset	Peak	Duration
Oral	Varies	3–4 hr	18–20 hr

Metabolism: Hepatic; $T_{1/2}$: 12–16 hr
Distribution: Crosses placenta; enters breast milk
Excretion: Feces, urine

Adverse effects
- **Dental:** *Discoloring and inadequate calcification of primary teeth of fetus if used by pregnant women, discoloring and inadequate calcification of permanent teeth if used during period of dental development*
- **Dermatologic:** *Phototoxic reactions, rash,* exfoliative dermatitis (especially frequent and severe with this tetracycline)

- **GI:** *Fatty liver,* **liver failure,** *anorexia, nausea, vomiting, diarrhea, glossitis,* dysphagia, enterocolitis, esophageal ulcer
- **Hematologic: Hemolytic anemia, thrombocytopenia, neutropenia, eosinophilia, leukocytosis, leukopenia**
- **Other:** Superinfections, nephrogenic diabetes insipidus syndrome (polyuria, polydipsia, weakness) in patients being treated for SIADH

Interactions
* **Drug-drug** • Decreased absorption with antacids, iron, alkali, magnesium • Increased digoxin toxicity • Decreased activity of penicillin • Possibly decreased effectiveness of hormonal contraceptives
* **Drug-food** • Decreased effectiveness of demeclocycline if taken with food, dairy products
* **Drug-lab test** • Interference with culture studies for several days following therapy

■ Nursing considerations
Assessment
- **History:** Allergy to tetracyclines, renal or hepatic impairment, pregnancy, lactation
- **Physical:** Skin status, R and adventitious sounds, GI function and liver evaluation, urinary output and concentration, urinalysis and BUN, LFTs, renal function tests; culture infected area before beginning therapy

Interventions
- Give on an empty stomach; if severe GI upset occurs, give with food. Avoid combination with dairy products, antacids.
- Give with a full 8-oz glass of water.
- Discontinue drug if diabetes insipidus occurs in SIADH patients.
- Recommend the use of barrier contraceptives while on this drug; fetal abnormalities can occur. This drug may decreased the effectiveness of hormonal contraeptives.

Teaching points
- Take drug throughout the day for best results; take on an empty stomach, 1 hour before or 2 hours after meals, unless GI upset occurs; then it can be taken with food. Avoid combining with dairy products or antacids.
- Use of contraceptive measures is advised while on this drug. Hormonal contraceptives may not be effective; fetal harm has been reported.

Adverse effects in *italics* are most common; those in **bold** are life-threatening. ⊞ Do not crush.

- You may experience these side effects: Sensitivity to sunlight (use protective clothing and sunscreen), diarrhea.
- Report rash, itching; difficulty breathing; dark urine or light-colored stools; severe cramps; increased thirst, increased urination, weakness (SIADH patients).

▽denileukin diftitox

See Appendix R, *Less commonly used drugs.*

▽denosumab
(den os you mab)

Prolia, Xgeva

PREGNANCY CATEGORY C

Drug class
Nuclear factor kappa B (RANK) ligand inhibitor

Therapeutic actions
Human monoclonal antibody that prevents the activation of RANK ligand, a protein essential for the formation and function of osteoclasts, which are responsible for bone resorption. This action inhibits osteoclast formation and survival, decreasing bone resorption and increasing bone mass and strength.

Indications
- Treatment of postmenopausal women and men with osteoporosis who are at high risk for fracture (history of osteoporotic fractures, failure on or intolerant to other osteoporosis therapy) (*Prolia* only)
- Prevention of skeletal-related events in patients with bone metastases from solid tumors (*Xgeva* only).
- Treatment of bone loss in breast cancer patients receiving aromatase inhibitors (*Prolia*)
- Treatment of bone loss in prostate cancer patients receiving androgen deprivation therapy (*Prolia*).

Contraindications and cautions
- Contraindicated with known hypersensitivity to components of drug; lactation, hypocalcemia (*Prolia*).
- Use cautiously with current infections, pregnancy.

Available forms
Single-use vial—60 mg/mL; prefilled syringe—60 mg/mL

Dosages
Adults
Osteoporosis (Prolia only): 60 mg by subcutaneous injection in upper arm, thigh, or abdomen every 6 mo.
Bone metastases from solid tumors (Xgeva only): 120 mg by subcutaneous injection every 4 wk.
Pediatric patients younger than 18 yr
Safety and efficacy not established.
Patients with renal impairment
Patients with severe renal impairment or on dialysis are at increased risk for hypocalcemia; carefully weigh benefits vs. risk before using in these patients.

Pharmacokinetics

Route	Onset	Peak
Subcut.	Slow	10 days

Metabolism: Unknown; $T_{1/2}$: 25.4 days
Distribution: May cross placenta; may enter breast milk
Excretion: Tissue

Adverse effects
- **CNS:** *Vertigo*
- **CV:** Angina, atrial fibrillation, peripheral edema
- **Dermatologic:** Dermatitis, eczema, rash
- **GI:** Abdominal pain, flatulence, GERD, **constipation**
- **GU:** *Cystitis*
- **Respiratory:** URI, pneumonia, pharyngitis
- **Other:** *Hypocalcemia,* **serious to life-threatening infection, cancer, osteonecrosis of jaw,** suppression of bone remodeling resulting in fractures and delayed fracture healing, *back pain, extremity pain, musculoskeletal pain, hypercholesterolemia*

Nursing considerations
Assessment
- **History:** Hypersensitivity to components of drug; lactation, pregnancy, hypocalcemia

- **Physical:** Reflexes; skin color, lesions; baseline ECG; R, adventitious sounds; serum calcium levels; cholesterol levels

Interventions

- Obtain baseline serum calcium level before beginning therapy; do not administer if patient has hypocalcemia.
- Assess patient for underlying infections before beginning therapy; encourage patient to have dental follow-up and use good oral hygiene during therapy.
- Ensure that patient is also taking calcium 1,000 mg/day and at least 400 international units of vitamin D.
- Administer by subcutaneous injection into abdomen, upper thigh, or upper arm; rotate injection sites. Injections should be given every 6 mo.
- Ensure that patient has regular cancer screening while on drug.
- Stop drug if signs and symptoms of serious infection, serious dermatologic reaction, or osteonecrosis of the jaw occurs.

Teaching points

- This drug can only be given by subcutaneous injection; it will be given by your health care provider every 6 months for osteoporosis, or every 4 weeks for bone metastases. Mark your calendar for return dates for the injection.
- If you miss an injection, arrange to have your next injection as soon as possible.
- You will need to take calcium and vitamin D while on this drug.
- This drug should not be taken during pregnancy; it can have serious effects on the fetus. Women of childbearing age will need to have a serum pregnancy test before beginning therapy. Use of contraceptive measures is advised.
- If you are breast-feeding, you should use another method of feeding the baby while you are on this drug; this drug could cause serious adverse effects in the baby.
- You will need to have blood tests to monitor the effects of this drug on your calcium level.
- This drug affects your immune system and you may be at increased risk for infections and cancer development. Be alert for signs and symptoms of infection (fever, severe abdominal pain, red or swollen areas, frequency or burning on urination) and report these to your health care provider immediately. Take precautions to avoid exposure to infections. Make sure you have all appropriate cancer screening tests.
- This drug could cause problems with your jaw. Make sure you see your dentist regularly and that you brush and floss your teeth daily.
- You may experience these side effects: Dizziness (use caution when moving about; change position slowly); rash (notify your health care provider if you experience redness, itching, bumps, blisters, or skin peeling); low calcium level (report spasms, twitching, or muscle cramps; make sure you take your calcium and vitamin D daily); constipation (medications may be available if this becomes a problem).
- Report numbness or tingling in extremities or around the mouth, signs and symptoms of infection, jaw pain, severe rash.

▽desipramine hydrochloride

*(dess **ip'** ra meen)*

Alti-Desipramine (CAN), Apo-Desipramine (CAN), Norpramin, Nu-Desipramine (CAN), PMS-Desipramine (CAN), ratio-Desipramine (CAN)

PREGNANCY CATEGORY C

Drug classes

Antidepressant
TCA (secondary amine)

Therapeutic actions

Mechanism of action unknown; inhibits the presynaptic reuptake of the neurotransmitters norepinephrine and serotonin; anticholinergic at CNS and peripheral receptors; sedating.

Indications

- Relief of symptoms of depression (endogenous depression most responsive)
- Unlabeled uses: Treatment of eating disorders, chronic urticaria, diabetic neuropathy, ADHD, enuresis, alcohol dependence, postherpetic neuralgia, traumatic brain injury, Tourette syndrome

Contraindications and cautions

- Contraindicated with hypersensitivity to any tricyclic drug, concomitant therapy with an MAOI, recent MI, myelography within previous 24 hr or scheduled within 48 hr.
- Use cautiously with ECT; preexisting CV disorders (eg, severe coronary heart disease, progressive heart failure, angina pectoris, paroxysmal tachycardia; possibly increased risk of serious CVS toxicity with TCAs); family history of sudden death or rhythm disturbances; angle-closure glaucoma, increased IOP, urinary retention, ureteral or urethral spasm (anticholinergic effects of TCAs may exacerbate these conditions); seizure disorders (TCAs lower the seizure threshold); hyperthyroidism (predisposes to CVS toxicity, including cardiac arrhythmias); impaired hepatic, renal function; psychiatric patients (schizophrenic or paranoid patients may exhibit a worsening of psychosis with TCA therapy); manic-depressive patients (may shift to hypomanic or manic phase); elective surgery (TCAs should be discontinued as long as possible before surgery), pregnancy, lactation.

Available forms

Tablets—10, 25, 50, 75, 100, 150 mg

Dosages
Adults
- *Depression:* 100–200 mg/day PO as single dose or in divided doses initially. May gradually increase to 300 mg/day. Do not exceed 300 mg/day. Patients requiring 300 mg/day should generally have treatment initiated in a hospital. Continue a reduced maintenance dosage after a satisfactory response has been achieved.

Pediatric patients
Not recommended in children younger than 12 yr.

Geriatric patients and adolescents
Initially, 25–100 mg/day PO; dosages more than 100–150 mg are not recommended.

Pharmacokinetics

Route	Onset	Peak	Duration
Oral	Varies	2–4 hr	3–4 days

Metabolism: Hepatic; $T_{1/2}$: 12–24 hr
Distribution: Crosses placenta; enters breast milk
Excretion: Urine

Adverse effects

- **CNS:** *Sedation and anticholinergic effects, confusion* (especially in elderly), *disturbed concentration,* hallucinations, disorientation, decreased memory, feelings of unreality, delusions, anxiety, nervousness, restlessness, agitation, panic, insomnia, nightmares, hypomania, mania, exacerbation of psychosis, drowsiness, weakness, fatigue, headache, numbness, tingling, paresthesias of extremities, incoordination, motor hyperactivity, akathisia, ataxia, tremors, peripheral neuropathy, extrapyramidal symptoms, *seizures,* speech blockage, dysarthria, tinnitus, altered EEG, **stroke,** seizures
- **CV:** *Orthostatic hypotension,* hypertension, syncope, tachycardia, palpitations, **MI,** arrhythmias, heart block, **precipitation of heart failure**
- **Endocrine:** Elevated or depressed blood sugar; elevated prolactin levels; SIADH secretion
- **GI:** *Dry mouth, constipation,* paralytic ileus, *nausea,* vomiting, anorexia, epigastric distress, diarrhea, flatulence, dysphagia, peculiar taste, increased salivation, stomatitis, glossitis, parotid swelling, abdominal cramps, black tongue
- **GU:** Urinary retention, delayed micturition, dilation of the urinary tract, gynecomastia, testicular swelling in men; breast enlargement, menstrual irregularity and galactorrhea in women; increased or decreased libido; impotence
- **Hematologic: Bone marrow depression**
- **Hypersensitivity:** Rash, pruritus, vasculitis, petechiae, photosensitization, edema (generalized or of face and tongue), drug fever
- **Withdrawal:** Symptoms on abrupt discontinuation of prolonged therapy—nausea, headache, vertigo, nightmares, malaise
- **Other:** Nasal congestion, excessive appetite, weight gain or loss; sweating (paradoxical effect in a drug with prominent anticholinergic effects), alopecia, lacrimation, hyperthermia, flushing, chills

Interactions

✱ **Drug-drug** • Increased TCA levels and pharmacologic (especially anticholinergic) effects with cimetidine, fluoxetine • Increased serum levels and risk of bleeding with oral anti-coagulants ● Altered response, including arrhythmias and hypertension with sympatho-mimetics, quinolones ● Risk of severe hypertension with clonidine ● Hyperpyretic crises, severe seizures, hypertensive episodes, and deaths when MAOIs are given with TCAs

■ Nursing considerations
Assessment
- **History:** Hypersensitivity to any tricyclic drug; concomitant therapy with an MAOI; recent MI; myelography within previous 24 hr or scheduled within 48 hr; lactation; ECT; preexisting CV disorders; angle-closure glaucoma, increased IOP, urinary retention, ureteral or urethral spasm; seizure disorders; hyperthyroidism; impaired hepatic, renal function; psychiatric patients; elective surgery; pregnancy, lactation
- **Physical:** Body weight; T; skin color, lesions; orientation, affect, reflexes, vision and hearing; P, BP, orthostatic BP, perfusion; bowel sounds, normal output, liver evaluation; urine flow, normal output; usual sexual function, frequency of menses, breast and scrotal examination; LFTs, urinalysis, CBC, ECG, serum glucose levels in diabetics

Interventions
⊗ **Black box warning** Risk of suicidality in children, adolescents, and young adults; monitor patient, and inform caregivers.
⊗ *Warning* For depressed and potentially suicidal patients, limit access to drug.
- Give major portion of dose at bedtime if drowsiness or severe anticholinergic effects occur.
- Reduce dosage if minor side effects develop; contact health care provider if serious side effects occur.
- Monitor elderly patients for possibly increased adverse effects.
- Arrange for CBC if patient develops fever, sore throat, or other sign of infection.

Teaching points
- Take drug exactly as prescribed; do not stop taking this drug abruptly or without consulting your health care provider.
- Avoid alcohol and other sleep-inducing and over-the-counter drugs while taking this drug.

- Avoid prolonged exposure to sunlight or sun-lamps; use a sunscreen or protective garments with prolonged exposure to sunlight.
- You may experience these side effects: Headache, dizziness, drowsiness, weakness, blurred vision (reversible; if severe, avoid driving or performing tasks that require alertness); nausea, vomiting, loss of appetite, dry mouth (eat frequent small meals, frequent mouth care, and sucking sugarless candies may help); nightmares, inability to concentrate, confusion; changes in sexual function.
- Report dry mouth, difficulty in urination, excessive sedation, suicidal thoughts.

▽desirudin

See Appendix R, *Less commonly used drugs*.

▽desloratadine
(dess lor at' a deen)

Clarinex, Clarinex Reditabs

PREGNANCY CATEGORY C

Drug class
Antihistamine (nonsedating type)

Therapeutic actions
Competitively blocks the effects of histamine at peripheral H_1-receptor sites.

Indications
- Relief of nasal and non-nasal symptoms of seasonal allergic rhinitis in patients 2 yr and older
- Treatment of chronic idiopathic urticaria and perennial allergies caused by indoor and outdoor allergens in patients 6 mo and older

Contraindications and cautions
- Contraindicated with allergy to desloratadine, loratadine, or any components of the product; lactation.
- Use cautiously with hepatic or renal impairment or pregnancy.

Available forms
Tablets—5 mg; rapidly disintegrating tablets—2.5, 5 mg; syrup—2.5 mg/5 mL

Dosages

Adults and children 12 yr and older
5 mg/day PO or 2 tsp (5 mg/10 mL) syrup PO once daily.

Pediatric patients 6–11 yr
1 tsp syrup (2.5 mg/5 mL) PO once daily, or 2.5-mg rapidly disintegrating tablet PO once daily.

Pediatric patients 12 mo–5 yr
1/2 tsp syrup (1.25 mg/2.5 mL) PO once daily.

Pediatric patients 6–11 mo
2 mL syrup (1 mg) PO once daily.

Patients with hepatic or renal impairment
5 mg PO every other day.

Pharmacokinetics

Route	Onset	Peak	Duration
Oral	1 hr	3 hr	24 hr

Metabolism: Hepatic; $T_{1/2}$: 27 hr
Distribution: May cross placenta; enters breast milk
Excretion: Feces, urine

Adverse effects

- **CNS:** Somnolence, nervousness, dizziness, fatigue
- **CV:** Tachycardia
- **GI:** *Dry mouth*, nausea
- **Respiratory: Bronchospasm,** pharyngitis, dry throat
- **Other:** Flulike symptoms, hypersensitivity

■ Nursing considerations

Assessment

- **History:** Allergy to desloratadine, loratadine, other antihistamines; hepatic or renal impairment; pregnancy; lactation
- **Physical:** T, orientation, reflexes, affect, R, adventitious sounds, LFTs, renal function tests

Interventions

- Administer without regard to meals.
- Arrange for use of humidifier if thickening of secretions, throat dryness become bothersome; encourage adequate intake of fluids.
- Provide sugarless candies to suck and regular mouth care if dry mouth is a problem.
- Provide safety measures if CNS effects occur.

Teaching points

- Take this drug exactly as prescribed, with or without food. *Clarinex Reditabs* contain phenylalanine; use caution if you have phenylketonuria.
- Place rapidly disintegrating tablets on tongue immediately after opening blister pack; administer with or without water.
- You may experience these side effects: Dizziness, fatigue (use caution if driving or performing tasks that require alertness); dry throat, thickening of bronchial secretions, dryness of nasal mucosa (use of a humidifier may help if this becomes a problem); dry mouth (sucking on sugarless candies and frequent mouth care may help).
- Report difficulty breathing, tremors, palpitations.

▽**desmopressin acetate (1-deamino-8-D-arginine vasopressin)**
(des moe **press'** *in)*

Apo-Desmopressin (CAN), DDAVP, Octostim (CAN), Stimate, Stimate Nasal Spray

PREGNANCY CATEGORY B

Drug class

Hormone

Therapeutic actions

Synthetic analogue of human ADH; promotes resorption of water in the renal tubule; increases levels of clotting factor VIII.

Indications

- *DDAVP:* Neurogenic diabetes insipidus (not nephrogenic in origin; intranasal and parenteral); hemophilia A (with factor VIII levels exceeding 5%; parenteral); von Willebrand disease (type I; parenteral or intranasal)
- *Stimate:* Treatment of hemophilia A (with factor VIII levels exceeding 5%), von Willebrand disease (type I)
- Unlabeled use (intranasal): Treatment of chronic autonomic failure

Contraindications and cautions

- Contraindicated with allergy to desmopressin acetate; type II von Willebrand disease; severe renal impairment
- Use cautiously with vascular disease or hypertension, lactation, water intoxication, fluid and electrolyte imbalance, pregnancy.

Available forms

Tablets—0.1, 0.2 mg; nasal solution—0.1 mg/mL, 1.5 mg/mL; injection—4 mcg/mL

Dosages

Adults

- *Diabetes insipidus:* 0.1–0.4 mL/day intranasally as a single dose or divided into two to three doses; 0.5–1 mL/day subcutaneously or IV, divided into two doses, adjusted to achieve a diurnal water turnover pattern, or 0.05 mg PO bid—adjust according to water turnover pattern.
- *Hemophilia A or von Willebrand disease:* 0.3 mcg/kg diluted in 50 mL sterile physiologic saline; infuse IV slowly over 15–30 min. If needed preoperatively, infuse 30 min before the procedure. Determine need for repeated administration based on patient response. Intranasal—1 spray per nostril, 2 hr preoperatively for a total dose of 300 mcg.

Pediatric patients

- *Diabetes insipidus:* For patients 3 mo–12 yr, 0.05–0.3 mL/day intranasally as a single dose or divided into two doses; or 0.05 mg PO daily—adjust according to water turnover pattern.
- *Hemophilia A or von Willebrand disease:* For patients 11 mo and older, one spray per nostril (150 mcg), total dose 300 mcg; weighing less than 50 kg, 150 mcg as a single spray.

Pharmacokinetics

Route	Onset	Peak	Duration
Oral	1 hr	4–7 hr	7 hr
IV, Subcut.	30 min	90–120 min	Varies
Nasal	15–60 min	1–5 hr	5–21 hr

Metabolism: $T_{1/2}$: 7.8 min then 75.5 min (IV); 1.5–2.5 hr (oral); 3.3–3.5 hr (nasal)
Distribution: May cross placenta; may enter breast milk
Excretion: Unknown

▼ IV FACTS

Preparation: Use drug as provided; refrigerate vial.
Infusion: Administer by direct IV injection over 1 min; infuse for hemophilia A or von Willebrand disease over 15–30 min. May dilute in normal saline solution.

Adverse effects

- **CNS:** Transient headache
- **CV:** Slight elevation of BP, facial flushing (with high doses)
- **GI:** Nausea, mild abdominal cramps
- **GU:** Vulval pain
- **Local:** *Local erythema, swelling, burning pain* (parenteral injection)
- **Other:** Fluid retention, water intoxication, hyponatremia (rare)

Interactions

✳ **Drug-drug** • Risk of increased antidiuretic effects if combined with carbamazepine, chlorpropamide • Increased risk of hyponatremia related to increased fluid intake if used with TCAs or SSRIs; monitor patient closely and limit fluid intake

■ Nursing considerations

Assessment

- **History:** Allergy to desmopressin acetate; type II von Willebrand disease; vascular disease or hypertension; lactation, pregnancy
- **Physical:** Nasal mucous membranes; skin color; P, BP, edema; R, adventitious sounds; bowel sounds, abdominal examination; urine volume and osmolality, plasma osmolality; factor VIII coagulant activity, skin bleeding times, factor VIII coagulant levels, factor VIII antigen and ristocetin cofactor levels (as appropriate)

Interventions

- Refrigerate nasal solution and injection; *Stimate* will remain stable for up to 3 wk at room temperature.
- Administer intranasally by drawing solution into the rhinal tube or flexible calibrated plastic tube supplied with preparation. Insert one end of tube into nostril; blow on the other end to deposit solution deep into nasal cavity. Administer to infants, young children, or obtunded adults by using an air-filled syringe attached to the plastic tube. Spray form also available.

Adverse effects in *italics* are most common; those in **bold** are life-threatening. ⬛ Do not crush.

- Monitor condition of nasal passages during long-term therapy; inappropriate administration can lead to nasal ulcerations.
⊗ *Warning* Monitor patients with CV diseases carefully for cardiac reactions.
⊗ *Warning* Monitor patient for signs of hyponatremia, which could lead to seizures. Hold drug when patient has fluid or electrolyte disturbances. If using tablets, limit fluid intake 1 hr before and up to 8 hr after dosing.
- Arrange to individualize dosage to establish a diurnal pattern of water turnover; estimate response by adequate duration of sleep and adequate, not excessive, water turnover.
- Monitor P and BP during infusion for hemophilia A or von Willebrand disease. Monitor clinical response and lab reports to determine effectiveness of therapy and need for more desmopressin or use of blood products.

Teaching points
- *Stimate* pump must be primed before first use; prime pump by pressing down on pump four times. Discard after 25 doses. Administer intranasally by drawing solution into the rhinal tube or flexible calibrated plastic tube supplied with preparation. Insert one end of tube into nostril; blow on the other end to deposit solution deep into nasal cavity. Review proper administration technique for nasal use. Do not use intranasal route if you are experiencing nasal congestion or blockage.
- You may experience these side effects: GI cramping, facial flushing, headache, nasal irritation (proper administration may decrease these problems).
- Report drowsiness, listlessness, headache, shortness of breath, heartburn, abdominal cramps, vulval pain, severe nasal congestion or irritation.

---

desvenlafaxine succinate
(des ven la fax' een)

Pristiq ⓄⓇⒸ

PREGNANCY CATEGORY C

Drug classes
Antidepressant
Serotonin-norepinephrine reuptake inhibitor

Therapeutic actions
Potentiates the neurotransmitter activity in the CNS; inhibits serotonin and norepinephrine reuptake at the nerve synapse, leading to prolonged stimulation at the neuroreceptor; this action is thought to decrease the signs and symptoms of depression.

Indications
- Treatment of major depressive disorder in adults

Contraindications and cautions
- Contraindicated with known hypersensitivity to any component of the drug or venlafaxine, with use of an MAOI, or within 14 days of stopping an MAOI.
- Use cautiously with hypertension, glaucoma, abnormal bleeding, use of drugs that alter coagulation, vascular disease, lipid disorders, renal impairment, lung disease, pregnancy, lactation.

Available forms
ER tablets ⓄⓇⒸ—50, 100 mg

Dosages
Adults
50 mg/day PO with or without food; range, 50–400 mg/day.
Pediatric patients
Safety and efficacy not established.
Patients with severe renal impairment
50 mg PO every other day. Do not administer supplemental dose after dialysis.

Pharmacokinetics

Route	Onset	Peak
Oral	Slow	7.5 hr

Metabolism: Hepatic; $T_{1/2}$: 11 hr
Distribution: May cross placenta, enter breast milk
Excretion: Urine

Adverse effects
- **CNS:** *Dizziness, headache,* somnolence, tremor, paresthesia, *insomnia,* anxiety, nervousness, irritability, abnormal dreams, **suicidal ideation,** vision impairment, tinnitus, glaucoma, activation of bipolar symptoms
- **CV:** Palpitations, increased BP, tachycardia

D

- **GI:** *Nausea, dry mouth, diarrhea, constipation, vomiting, decreased appetite*
- **Respiratory: Interstitial lung disease, eosinophilic pneumonia**
- **Other:** *Fatigue, hyperhidrosis,* rash, yawning, increased bleeding, increased cholesterol and triglyceride levels, sexual function disorders (males)

Interactions

✳ **Drug-drug** • Risk of serious adverse reactions if combined with MAOIs; wait 14 days after stopping MAOI before beginning desvenlafaxine, allow 7 days from stopping desvenlafaxine before beginning MAOI • Risk of serotonin syndrome if combined with other drugs that increase serotonin levels; monitor patient closely • Increased risk of bleeding if combined with other drugs that affect coagulation (NSAIDs, aspirin, warfarin); monitor patient closely and adjust dosage as needed • Potential for increased impairment of mental ability if combined with alcohol or other CNS drugs; monitor patient closely • Risk of increased toxicity if combined with venlafaxine; avoid this combination

✳ **Drug-alternative therapy** • Increased risk of serotonin syndrome if combined with St. John's Wort; avoid this combination

■ Nursing considerations

Assessment

- **History:** Hypersensitivity to any component of the drug or venlafaxine, current use of an MAOI or use of an MAOI within 14 days, hypertension, glaucoma, abnormal bleeding or the use of drugs that alter coagulation, vascular disease, lipid disorders, renal impairment, lung disease, pregnancy, lactation
- **Physical:** T; skin—color, lesions; orientation, affect, sensory examination, eye pressure; P, BP; abdominal examination; R, adventitious sounds

Interventions

⊗ **Black box warning** Monitor patient for suicidal ideation, especially when beginning therapy or changing dosage; high risk in children, adolescents, and young adults. Drug is not approved for use in pediatric patients.

- Limit amount of drug available to patient because of increased risk of suicidal ideation.
- Give with food if GI upset occurs.

- Instruct patient to swallow tablet whole; do not cut, crush, or chew.
- Do not administer with an MAOI or within 14 days of stopping an MAOI; allow 7 days after stopping desvenlafaxine before starting an MAOI.
- Monitor patients with glaucoma, hypertension, CV disease, SIADH for potential exacerbation of these problems.
- Inform patient that it may take several weeks to see the effects of this drug.
- Avoid suddenly stopping drug; taper gradually.
- Tell patient that the matrix of the drug may be seen in the stool; assure patient that the active drug has been absorbed.
- Advise women of childbearing age to use contraception.
- Encourage breast-feeding mothers to find a different method of feeding the baby while on this drug.

Teaching points

- Take this drug about the same time each day; swallow the tablet whole; do not cut, crush or chew the tablets.
- If you miss a dose, take it as soon as you remember. If it is almost time for the next dose, just skip the missed dose. Do not make up doses. Do not take more than one dose a day.
- Do not stop taking this drug suddenly; if you are running low on tablets, contact your health care provider about a refill. Your health care provider will reduce the dose over time if the drug is to be stopped.
- It may take several weeks before you see the effects of this drug; keep taking the drug as prescribed.
- You may notice something in your stool that looks like your tablet. This is the empty shell of the tablet; the medicine has already been absorbed into your system.
- Do not use St. John's Wort while on this drug; serious adverse effects could occur.
- Do not drive or operate dangerous machinery until you know how this drug affects you.
- Avoid drinking alcohol while on this drug.
- It is not known whether this drug affects a fetus. Use contraceptive measures while on this drug. If you wish to become pregnant, discuss this with your health care provider. If you become pregnant while taking this drug, consult with your health care provider.

- It is not known how this drug affects a breast-feeding infant. Because of the potential for adverse effects on an infant, another method of feeding the baby should be used while you are on this drug.
- Your health care provider may monitor your eye pressure, blood pressure, and various blood tests while you are on this drug.
- There is a risk of suicidal thoughts, especially when starting the drug or adjusting the dose. Be alert for these thoughts. Call your health care provider if you have any suicidal thoughts or increased depression or anxiety.
- You may experience these side effects: Dry mouth, nausea (eating frequent small meals and sucking sugarless candies may help); dizziness, tremor, changes in ability to concentrate (do not drive a car or operate dangerous machinery until you know how this drug will affect you); constipation (medication may be available to help).
- Report suicidal thoughts, behavioral changes, difficulty breathing, increased bleeding, hallucinations, fever.

▽**dexamethasone**
(dex a meth' a sone)

dexamethasone

Oral, topical dermatologic aerosol and gel, ophthalmic suspension: Aeroseb-Dex, Apo-Dexamethasone (CAN), DexPak TaperPak, Maxidex Ophthalmic, ratio-Dexamethasone (CAN)

dexamethasone sodium phosphate

IV, IM, intra-articular, intralesional injection; respiratory inhalant; intranasal steroid; ophthalmic solution and ointment; topical dermatologic cream: Cortastat, Dalalone, Decadron Phosphate, Decaject, Dexasone, PMS-Dexamethasone (CAN)

PREGNANCY CATEGORY C

Drug classes
Corticosteroid
Glucocorticoid
Hormone

Therapeutic actions
Enters target cells and binds to specific receptors, initiating many complex reactions that are responsible for its anti-inflammatory and immunosuppressive effects.

Indications
- Hypercalcemia associated with cancer
- Cancer chemotherapy–induced nausea and vomiting
- Short-term management of various inflammatory and allergic disorders, such as rheumatoid arthritis, collagen diseases (SLE), dermatologic diseases (pemphigus), status asthmaticus, and autoimmune disorders
- Hematologic disorders: Thrombocytopenic purpura, erythroblastopenia
- Trichinosis with neurologic or myocardial involvement
- Ulcerative colitis, acute exacerbations of MS, and palliation in some leukemias and lymphomas
- Cerebral edema associated with brain tumor, craniotomy, or head injury
- Testing adrenocortical hyperfunction
- Unlabeled uses: Antiemetic for cisplatin-induced vomiting, diagnosis of depression
- Intra-articular or soft-tissue administration: Arthritis, psoriatic plaques
- Respiratory inhalant: Control of bronchial asthma requiring corticosteroids in conjunction with other therapy
- Intranasal: Relief of symptoms of seasonal or perennial rhinitis that responds poorly to other treatments
- Dermatologic preparations: Relief of inflammatory and pruritic manifestations of dermatoses that are steroid responsive
- Ophthalmic preparations: Inflammation of the lid, conjunctiva, cornea, and globe

Contraindications and cautions
- Contraindicated with infections, especially tuberculosis, fungal infections, amebiasis, vaccinia and varicella, and antibiotic-resistant infections, allergy to any component of the preparation used.

- Use cautiously with renal or hepatic disease; hypothyroidism, ulcerative colitis with impending perforation; diverticulitis; active or latent peptic ulcer; inflammatory bowel disease; heart failure, hypertension, thromboembolic disorders; osteoporosis; seizure disorders; diabetes mellitus; lactation.

Available forms
Tablets—0.25, 0.5, 0.75, 1, 1.5, 2, 4, 6 mg; elixir—0.5 mg/5 mL; oral solution concentrate—0.5 mg/0.5 mL; injection—4 mg/mL, 8 mg/mL, 10 mg/mL, 16 mg/mL, 20 mg/mL, 24 mg/mL; aerosol—84 mcg/actuation; ophthalmic solution—0.1%; ophthalmic suspension—0.1%; ophthalmic ointment—0.05%; topical ointment—0.05%; topical cream—0.05%, 0.1%; topical aerosol—0.01%, 0.04%

Dosages
Adults
Systemic administration
Individualize dosage based on severity of condition and response. Give daily dose before 9 AM to minimize adrenal suppression. If long-term therapy is needed, alternate-day therapy with a short-acting steroid should be considered. After long-term therapy, withdraw drug slowly to avoid adrenal insufficiency. For maintenance therapy, reduce initial dose in small increments at intervals until the lowest clinically satisfactory dose is reached.
Oral (dexamethasone)
0.75–9 mg/day.
- *Suppression test for Cushing syndrome:* 1 mg at 11 PM; assay plasma cortisol at 8 AM the next day. For greater accuracy, give 0.5 mg every 6 hr for 48 hr, and collect 24-hr urine to determine 17-hydroxycorticosteroid (17-OHCS) excretion.
- *Suppression test to distinguish Cushing syndrome due to ACTH excess resulting from other causes:* 2 mg every 6 hr for 48 hr. Collect 24-hr urine to determine 17-OHCS excretion.
IV or IM (dexamethasone sodium phosphate)
0.5–9 mg/day.
- *Cerebral edema:* 10 mg IV and then 4 mg IM every 6 hr until cerebral edema symptoms subside; change to oral therapy, 1–3 mg tid, as soon as possible and taper over 5–7 days.

Pediatric patients
Individualize dosage based on severity of condition and response, rather than by strict adherence to formulas that correct adult doses for age or body weight. Carefully observe growth and development in infants and children on long-term therapy.
IV
- *Unresponsive shock:* 1–6 mg/kg as a single IV injection (as much as 20 mg initially followed by repeated injections every 2–6 hr has been reported).
Intra-articular, soft-tissue administration (dexamethasone sodium phosphate)
0.2–6 mg (depending on joint or soft-tissue injection site).
Respiratory inhalant (dexamethasone sodium phosphate)
84 mcg released with each actuation.
Adults
3 inhalations tid–qid, not to exceed 12 inhalations/day.
Pediatric patients
2 inhalations tid–qid, not to exceed 8 inhalations/day.
Intranasal (dexamethasone sodium phosphate)
Each spray delivers 84 mcg dexamethasone.
Adults
2 sprays (168 mcg) into each nostril bid–tid, not to exceed 12 sprays (1,008 mcg)/day.
Pediatric patients
1 or 2 sprays (84–168 mcg) into each nostril bid, depending on age, not to exceed 8 sprays (672 mcg). Arrange to reduce dose and discontinue therapy as soon as possible.
Topical dermatologic preparations
Adults and pediatric patients
Apply sparingly to affected area bid–qid.
Ophthalmic solutions, suspensions
Adults and pediatric patients
Instill 1 or 2 drops into the conjunctival sac every 1 hr during the day and every 2 hr during the night; after a favorable response, reduce dose to 1 drop every 4 hr and then 1 drop tid–qid.
Ophthalmic ointment
Adults and pediatric patients
Apply a thin coating in the lower conjunctival sac tid–qid; reduce dosage to bid and then qid after improvement.

Adverse effects in *italics* are most common; those in **bold** are life-threatening. ⓒⓡⓤ Do not crush.

Pharmacokinetics

Route	Onset	Peak	Duration
Oral	Slow	1–2 hr	2–3 days
IM	Rapid	30–60 min	2–3 days
IV	Rapid	30–60 min	2–3 days

Metabolism: Hepatic; $T_{1/2}$: 110–210 min
Distribution: Crosses placenta; may enter breast milk
Excretion: Urine

▼ IV FACTS

Preparation: No preparation required.
Infusion: Administer by slow, direct IV injection over 1 min.
Incompatibilities: Do not combine with daunorubicin, doxorubicin, metaraminol, vancomycin.

Adverse effects

Adverse effects depend on dose, route, and duration of therapy.

Systemic administration

- **CNS: Seizures,** *vertigo, headaches,* pseudotumor cerebri, *euphoria, insomnia, mood swings, depression,* psychosis, intracerebral hemorrhage, reversible cerebral atrophy in infants, cataracts, IOP, glaucoma
- **CV:** *Hypertension,* heart failure, necrotizing angiitis
- **Endocrine:** Growth retardation, decreased carbohydrate tolerance, diabetes mellitus, cushingoid state, *secondary adrenocortical and pituitary unresponsiveness*
- **GI:** Peptic or esophageal ulcer, pancreatitis, abdominal distention
- **GU:** *Amenorrhea, irregular menses*
- **Hematologic:** *Fluid and electrolyte disturbances,* negative nitrogen balance, increased blood sugar, glycosuria, increased serum cholesterol, decreased serum T_3 and T_4 levels
- **Hypersensitivity:** Anaphylactoid or hypersensitivity reactions
- **Musculoskeletal:** *Muscle weakness,* steroid myopathy, loss of muscle mass, osteoporosis, spontaneous fractures
- **Other:** *Impaired wound healing; petechiae; ecchymoses; increased sweating; thin and fragile skin; acne; immunosuppression and masking of signs of infection;* activation of latent infections, including TB, fungal, and viral eye infections; pneumonia; abscess; septic infection; GI and GU infections

Intra-articular

- **Musculoskeletal:** Osteonecrosis, tendon rupture, infection

Intralesional therapy

- **CNS:** Blindness (when used on face and head—rare)

Respiratory inhalant

- **Endocrine:** Suppression of HPA function due to systemic absorption
- **Respiratory:** Oral, laryngeal, pharyngeal irritation
- **Other:** Fungal infections

Intranasal

- **CNS:** Headache
- **Dermatologic:** Urticaria
- **Endocrine:** Suppression of HPA function due to systemic absorption
- **GI:** Nausea
- **Respiratory:** Nasal irritation, fungal infections, epistaxis, rebound congestion, perforation of the nasal septum, anosmia

Topical dermatologic ointments, creams, sprays

- **Endocrine:** Suppression of HPA function due to systemic absorption, growth retardation in children (children may be at special risk for systemic absorption because of their large skin surface area to body weight ratio)
- **Local:** Local burning, irritation, acneiform lesions, striae, skin atrophy

Ophthalmic preparations

- **Endocrine:** Suppression of HPA function due to systemic absorption; more common with long-term use
- **Local:** Infections, especially fungal; glaucoma, cataracts with long-term use

Interactions

✳ **Drug-drug** • Decreased effects of anticholinesterases with corticotropin; profound muscular depression is possible • Decreased steroid blood levels with phenytoin, phenobarbital, rifampin • Decreased serum levels of salicylates with dexamethasone and increased risk of gastric ulceration

✳ **Drug-lab test** • False-negative nitrobluetetrazolium test for bacterial infection • Suppression of skin test reactions

D

■ Nursing considerations

Assessment

- **History for systemic administration:** Active infections; renal or hepatic disease; hypothyroidism, ulcerative colitis; diverticulitis; active or latent peptic ulcer; inflammatory bowel disease; heart failure, hypertension, thromboembolic disorders; osteoporosis; seizure disorders; diabetes mellitus; lactation
- **History for ophthalmic preparations:** Acute superficial herpes simplex keratitis, fungal infections of ocular structures; vaccinia, varicella, and other viral diseases of the cornea and conjunctiva; ocular TB
- **Physical for systemic administration:** Baseline body weight, T; reflexes, and grip strength, affect, and orientation; P, BP, peripheral perfusion, prominence of superficial veins; R and adventitious sounds; serum electrolytes, blood glucose
- **Physical for topical dermatologic preparations:** Affected area for infections, skin injury

Interventions

- For systemic administration, do not give drug to breast-feeding mothers; drug may be secreted in breast milk.
- ⊗ *Warning* Give daily doses before 9 AM to mimic normal peak corticosteroid blood levels.
- Increase dosage when patient is subject to stress.
- Monitor blood glucose levels; dietary restrictions may be needed.
- Taper doses when discontinuing high-dose or long-term therapy.
- Do not give live virus vaccines with immunosuppressive doses of corticosteroids.
- For respiratory inhalant, intranasal preparation, do not use respiratory inhalant during an acute asthmatic attack or to manage status asthmaticus.
- Do not use intranasal product with untreated local nasal infections, epistaxis, nasal trauma, septal ulcers, or recent nasal surgery.
- ⊗ *Warning* Taper systemic steroids carefully during transfer to inhalational steroids; adrenal insufficiency deaths have occurred.
- For topical dermatologic preparations, use caution when occlusive dressings, tight diapers cover affected area; these can increase systemic absorption.

- Avoid prolonged use near the eyes, in genital and rectal areas, and in skin creases.

Teaching points

Systemic administration

- Do not stop taking the oral drug without consulting your health care provider.
- Avoid exposure to infection.
- Report unusual weight gain, swelling of the extremities, muscle weakness, black or tarry stools, fever, prolonged sore throat, colds or other infections, worsening of this disorder.

Intra-articular administration

- Do not overuse joint after therapy, even if pain is gone.

Respiratory inhalant, intranasal preparation

- Do not use more often than prescribed.
- Do not stop using this drug without consulting your health care provider.
- Use the inhalational bronchodilator drug before using the oral inhalant product when using both.
- Administer decongestant nose drops first if nasal passages are blocked.

Topical

- Apply the drug sparingly.
- Avoid contact with eyes or skin around eyes.
- Report any irritation or infection at the site of application.

Ophthalmic

- Administer as follows: Lie down or tilt head backward and look at ceiling. Warm tube of ointment in hand for several minutes. Apply one-fourth to one-half inch of ointment, or drop suspension inside lower eyelid while looking up. After applying ointment, close eyelids and roll eyeball in all directions. After instilling eye drops, release lower lid, but do not blink for at least 30 seconds; apply gentle pressure to the inside corner of the eye for 1 minute. Do not close eyes tightly, and try not to blink more often than usual; do not touch ointment tube or dropper to eye, fingers, or any surface.
- Wait at least 10 minutes before using any other eye preparations.
- Eyes will become more sensitive to light (use sunglasses).
- Report worsening of the condition, pain, itching, swelling of the eye, failure of the condition to improve after 1 week.

▷dexchlorpheniramine maleate ⓞⓣⓒ

*(dex klor fen **ir**' a meen)*

PREGNANCY CATEGORY B

Drug class
Antihistamine (alkylamine type)

Therapeutic actions
Blocks the effects of histamine at H_1-receptor sites, has atropine-like, antipruritic, and sedative effects.

Indications
• Relief of symptoms associated with perennial and seasonal allergic rhinitis; vasomotor rhinitis; allergic conjunctivitis; mild, uncomplicated urticaria and angioedema; amelioration of allergic reactions to blood or plasma; dermatographism; adjunctive therapy in anaphylactic reactions

Contraindications and cautions
• Contraindicated with allergy to antihistamines, narrow-angle glaucoma, stenosing peptic ulcer, symptomatic prostatic hypertrophy, asthmatic attack, bladder neck obstruction, pyloroduodenal obstruction, MAOI use, third trimester of pregnancy, lactation.
• Use cautiously with pregnancy, COPD.

Available forms
ER tablets ⓞⓣⓒ—4, 6 mg; syrup—2 mg/5 mL

Dosages
Adults and children older than 12 yr
4–6 mg at bedtime PO or every 8–10 hr PO during the day.
Pediatric patients 6–12 yr
4 mg PO once daily at bedtime (syrup only).
Geriatric patients
More likely to cause dizziness, sedation, syncope, toxic confusional states, and hypotension in elderly patients; use with caution.

Pharmacokinetics

Route	Onset	Peak
Oral	15–30 min	3 hr

Metabolism: Hepatic; $T_{1/2}$: 12–15 hr

Distribution: May cross placenta; may enter breast milk
Excretion: Urine

Adverse effects
• **CNS:** *Drowsiness, sedation, dizziness, disturbed coordination,* fatigue, confusion, restlessness, excitation, nervousness, tremor, headache, blurred vision, diplopia, vertigo, tinnitus, acute labyrinthitis, hysteria, tingling, heaviness and weakness of the hands
• **CV:** Hypotension, palpitations, bradycardia, tachycardia, extrasystoles
• **GI:** *Epigastric distress,* anorexia, increased appetite and weight gain, nausea, vomiting, diarrhea or constipation
• **GU:** Urinary frequency, dysuria, urinary retention, early menses, decreased libido
• **Hematologic:** Hemolytic anemia, hypoplastic anemia, **thrombocytopenia, leukopenia, agranulocytosis, pancytopenia**
• **Respiratory:** *Thickening of bronchial secretions,* chest tightness, wheezing, nasal stuffiness, dry mouth, dry nose, dry throat, sore throat
• **Other:** Urticaria, rash, **anaphylactic shock,** photosensitivity, excessive perspiration

Interactions
✳ **Drug-drug** • Increased depressant effects with alcohol, other CNS depressants

■ Nursing considerations
Assessment
• **History:** Allergy to any antihistamines; narrow-angle glaucoma, stenosing peptic ulcer, symptomatic prostatic hypertrophy, asthmatic attack, bladder neck obstruction, pyloroduodenal obstruction, pregnancy, lactation
• **Physical:** Skin color, lesions, texture; orientation, reflexes, affect; vision examination; P, BP; R, adventitious sounds; bowel sounds; prostate palpation; CBC with differential

Interventions
• Administer with food if GI upset occurs.
• Have patient swallow tablets whole—do not cut, crush, or chew.
• Monitor patient response, and adjust dosage to lowest possible effective dose.

D

Teaching points

- Take as prescribed; avoid excessive dosage. Take with food if GI upset occurs; do not crush or chew the tablets; swallow whole.
- Avoid alcohol; serious sedation can occur.
- You may experience these side effects: Dizziness, sedation, drowsiness (use caution driving or performing tasks that require alertness); epigastric distress, diarrhea, or constipation (take with meals); dry mouth (frequent mouth care, sucking sugarless candies may help); thickening of bronchial secretions, dryness of nasal mucosa (use a humidifier).
- Report difficulty breathing; hallucinations, tremors, loss of coordination; unusual bleeding or bruising; visual disturbances; irregular heartbeat.

▷ dexlansoprazole
(**decks**' *lan soh*' *pray zol*)
Dexilant ⬛ⓞⓝⓒ

PREGNANCY CATEGORY B

Drug classes
Antisecretory drug
Proton pump inhibitor

Therapeutic actions
Gastric acid pump inhibitor that suppresses gastric acid secretion by specific inhibition of the hydrogen-potassium ATPase enzyme system at the secretory surface of the gastric parietal cells; blocks the final step in acid production.

Indications
- Healing of all grades of erosive esophagitis
- Maintenance of healing of erosive esophagitis
- Treatment of heartburn associated with nonerosive gastroesophageal reflux disease (GERD)
- Unlabeled use: Prevention of GI bleeding in patients receiving antiplatelet drugs

Contraindications and cautions
- Contraindicated with hypersensitivity to components of drug, lactation.
- Use cautiously with pregnancy.
- Possible increased risk for *C. difficile* infection.

Available forms
DR capsules ⓞⓝⓒ —30, 60 mg

Dosages
Adults
Healing of erosive esophagitis: 60 mg/day PO for up to 8 wk.
Maintenance of healing of erosive esophagitis: 30 mg/day PO.
GERD: 30 mg/day PO for up to 4 wk.
Pediatric patients
Safety and efficacy not established.

Pharmacokinetics

Route	Onset	Peak
Oral	Rapid	1–2 hr, then 4–5 hr

Metabolism: Hepatic; $T_{1/2}$: 1–2 hr
Distribution: May cross placenta; may enter breast milk
Excretion: Urine and feces

Adverse effects
- **CNS:** Headache, dizziness, insomnia, taste changes
- **GI:** Nausea, *diarrhea*, vomiting, abdominal pain, *Clostridium difficile* diarrhea
- **Respiratory:** URI
- **Other:** Fatigue, bone loss, hypomagnesemia

Interactions
✳ **Drug-drug** ● Decreased absorption of atazanavir with resultant loss of effectiveness; avoid this combination ● Potential interference with absorption of drugs that require acidic gastric fluids (ampicillin, digoxin, iron salts, ketoconazole); monitor patient accordingly
● Potential increased effects of warfarin when taken with proton pump inhibitors; if this combination is used, monitor INR regularly and adjust warfarin dosage as needed

■ Nursing considerations
Assessment
- **History:** Hypersensitivity to components of drug; pregnancy, lactation
- **Physical:** Orientation, affect; abdominal examination; respiratory auscultation

Interventions
- Administer without regard to food.
- Capsule should be swallowed whole. Do not cut, crush, or allow patient to chew capsule. If patient cannot swallow capsule, it can be opened and the contents sprinkled over

Adverse effects in *italics* are most common; those in **bold** are life-threatening. ⓞⓝⓒ Do not crush.

1 tablespoon of applesauce and swallowed immediately.

• Monitor patient using drug long term for bone loss, hypomagnesemia.

• Evaluate patients who develop diarrhea for *C. difficile* infection.

• Advise patient to select another method of feeding the baby if breast-feeding.

Teaching points

• Take this drug once a day, with or without food.

• Capsule should be swallowed whole. Do not cut, crush, or chew capsule. If you cannot swallow the capsule, it can be opened and the contents sprinkled over 1 tablespoon of applesauce and swallowed immediately.

• If you miss a dose, take the next dose as soon as you remember.

• It is not known how this drug affects a fetus. If you should become pregnant while taking this drug, consult your health care provider.

• It is not known how this drug affects a breast-feeding infant. Because of the potential for serious adverse effects in an infant, another method of feeding the infant should be used while you are taking this drug.

• You may experience these side effects: Dizziness, headache (do not drive a car or engage in activities that require alertness if these effects occur); diarrhea, nausea, vomiting, abdominal pain (these effects may lessen over time; consult your health care provider if they are too uncomfortable).

• Report persistent or increasing pain, severe diarrhea or vomiting.

▽ dexmedetomidine hydrochloride

See Appendix R, *Less commonly used drugs*.

▽ dexmethylphenidate hydrochloride

*(decks meth ill **fen' i** date)*

Focalin, Focalin XR ⒹⓂⒸ

PREGNANCY CATEGORY C

CONTROLLED SUBSTANCE C-II

Drug class
CNS stimulant

Therapeutic actions
Mild cortical stimulant with CNS actions similar to those of the amphetamines; is thought to block the reuptake of norepinephrine and dopamine, increasing their concentration in the synaptic cleft; mechanism of effectiveness in hyperkinetic syndromes is not understood.

Indications
• Treatment of ADHD in patients 6 yr and older as part of a total treatment program

Contraindications and cautions
• Contraindicated with hypersensitivity to dexmethylphenidate or methylphenidate; marked anxiety, tension, and agitation; glaucoma; motor tics, family history or diagnosis of Tourette syndrome; use of MAOIs within the past 14 days.

• Use cautiously with psychosis, seizure disorders; heart failure, recent MI, hyperthyroidism; drug dependence, alcoholism, severe depression of endogenous or exogenous origin; as treatment of normal fatigue states; pregnancy, lactation.

Available forms
Tablets—2.5, 5, 10 mg; ER capsules ⒹⓂⒸ—5, 10, 15, 20, 30 mg

Dosages
Adults and children 6 yr and older
Individualize dosage. Administer orally twice a day, at least 4 hr apart, without regard to meals. Starting dose, 2.5 mg PO bid; may increase as needed in 2.5- to 5-mg increments to a maximum dose of 10 mg PO bid. ER capsules, initially 5 mg/day for children; increase in 5-mg increments to 30 mg/day; start adults at 10 mg/day; increase in 10-mg increments to 20 mg/day.

• *Patients already on methylphenidate:* Start dose at one-half the methylphenidate dose with a maximum dose of 10 mg PO bid.
Pediatric patients younger than 6 yr
Safety and efficacy not established.

Pharmacokinetics

Route	Onset	Peak
Oral	Varies	1–1.5 hr

Metabolism: Hepatic; $T_{1/2}$: 2.2 hr

Distribution: May cross placenta; may enter breast milk

Excretion: Urine

Adverse effects

- **CNS:** *Nervousness, insomnia,* dizziness, headache, dyskinesia, chorea, drowsiness, Tourette syndrome, toxic psychosis, blurred vision, accommodation difficulties
- **CV:** Increased or decreased pulse and blood pressure; *tachycardia,* angina, arrhythmias, palpitations
- **Dermatologic:** Skin rash, loss of scalp hair
- **GI:** *Anorexia, nausea, abdominal pain;* weight loss, abnormal liver function
- **Hematologic:** Leukopenia, anemia
- **Other:** Fever, tolerance, psychological dependence, abnormal behavior with abuse

Interactions

✳ **Drug-drug** ⊗ *Warning* Risk of severe hypertensive crisis if combined with MAOIs; do not administer dexmethylphenidate with or within 14 days of an MAOI.

• Possible increased serum levels of warfarin, phenobarbital, phenytoin, primidone, TCAs, some SSRIs; if any of these drugs are used with dexmethylphenidate, monitor the patient closely and decrease dose of the other drugs as needed • Risk of adverse effects if combined with pressor drugs (dopamine, epinephrine) or antihypertensives; monitor patients closely

■ Nursing considerations

Assessment

- **History:** Hypersensitivity to dexmethylphenidate or methylphenidate; marked anxiety, tension, and agitation; glaucoma; motor tics, family history or diagnosis of Tourette syndrome; severe depression of endogenous or exogenous origin; seizure disorders; hypertension; drug dependence, alcoholism, emotional instability; pregnancy, lactation
- **Physical:** Body weight, height, T, skin color, lesions, orientation, affect, ophthalmic examination (tonometry), P, BP, auscultation, R, adventitious sounds, bowel sounds, normal output, CBC with differential, platelet count, baseline ECG (as indicated)

Interventions

- Ensure proper diagnosis before administering to children for behavioral syndromes.

Drug should not be used until other causes and concomitants of abnormal behavior (learning disability, EEG abnormalities, neurologic deficits) are ruled out.

- Obtain baseline ECG to rule out cardiac problems before beginning therapy.

⊗ **Black box warning** Use caution with history of substance dependence or alcoholism; dependence, severe depression, psychotic reactions possible with withdrawal.

- Arrange to interrupt drug dosage periodically in children being treated for behavioral disorders to determine if symptoms recur at an intensity that warrants continued drug therapy.
- Monitor growth of children on long-term dexmethylphenidate therapy.

⊗ *Warning* Arrange to dispense the least feasible amount of drug at any one time to minimize risk of overdose.

- Administer drug before 6 PM to prevent insomnia if that is a problem.
- Ensure that ER capsules are swallowed whole or contents are sprinkled over a spoonful of applesauce and taken immediately.
- Arrange to monitor CBC and platelet counts periodically in patients on long-term therapy.
- Monitor BP frequently early in treatment.
- Arrange for consult with school nurse of school-age patients receiving this drug.

Teaching points

- Take this drug exactly as prescribed. Take immediate-release tablets two times a day, at least 4 hours apart. This drug should be part of a total treatment program.
- Take immediate-release tablets before 6 PM to avoid nighttime sleep disturbance.
- Take extended-release capsules once a day, in the morning.
- Swallow extended-release capsules whole; do not cut, crush, or chew. Capsules can be opened and contents sprinkled over applesauce and taken immediately.
- This drug is a controlled substance and should be stored securely and safely out of the reach of children.
- Avoid the use of alcohol and over-the-counter drugs, including nose drops and cold remedies, while taking this drug; some over-the-counter drugs could cause dangerous effects. If you feel that you need one of these preparations, consult your health care provider.

Adverse effects in *italics* are most common; those in **bold** are life-threatening. ⬛ Do not crush.

- You may experience these side effects: Nervousness, restlessness, dizziness, insomnia, impaired thinking (these effects may become less pronounced after a few days, avoid driving a car or engaging in activities that require alertness if these occur, notify your health care provider if these are pronounced or bothersome); headache, loss of appetite, dry mouth.
- Report nervousness, insomnia, palpitations, vomiting, skin rash, depression, chest pain, shortness of breath, fainting, marked changes in behavior or vision.

▷dexpanthenol (dextro-pantothenyl alcohol)

(dex pan' the nole)

Ilopan

PREGNANCY CATEGORY C

Drug classes
Emollient
GI stimulant

Therapeutic actions
Mechanism is unknown; is the alcohol analog of pantothenic acid, a cofactor in the synthesis of the neurotransmitter acetylcholine; acetylcholine is the transmitter released by parasympathetic postganglionic nerves; the parasympathetic nervous system provides stimulation to maintain intestinal function.

Indications
- Prophylactic use immediately after major abdominal surgery to minimize paralytic ileus, intestinal atony causing abdominal distention
- Treatment of intestinal atony causing abdominal distention; postoperative or postpartum retention of flatus; postoperative or postpartum (if not breast-feeding) delay in resumption of intestinal motility; paralytic ileus
- Topical treatment of mild eczema, dermatosis, bee stings, diaper rash, chafing

Contraindications and cautions
- Contraindicated with allergy to dexpanthenol, hemophilia, ileus due to mechanical obstruction.
- Use cautiously in pregnancy, lactation.

Available forms
Injection—250 mg/mL; topical cream—2%

Dosages
Adults
IM
- *Prevention of postoperative adynamic ileus:* 250–500 mg IM; repeat in 2 hr, then every 6 hr until danger of adynamic ileus has passed.
- *Treatment of adynamic ileus:* 500 mg IM; repeat in 2 hr, then every 6 hr as needed.
IV
500 mg diluted in IV solutions.
Topical, adults and children
Apply once or twice daily to affected areas.
Pediatric patients (injection)
Safety and efficacy not established.

Pharmacokinetics

Route	Onset	Peak
IM	Rapid	4 hr

Metabolism: Hepatic; $T_{1/2}$: Unknown
Distribution: May cross placenta; may enter breast milk
Excretion: Feces, urine

▼ IV FACTS
Preparation: Dilute with bulk solutions of glucose or lactated Ringer solution.
Infusion: Infuse slowly over 3–6 hr. Do not administer by direct IV injection.

Adverse effects
- **CV:** *Slight drop in BP*
- **Dermatologic:** Itching, tingling, red patches of skin, generalized dermatitis, urticaria
- **GI:** *Intestinal colic* (30 min after administration), *nausea, vomiting; diarrhea*
- **Respiratory:** Dyspnea

■ Nursing considerations
Assessment
- **History:** Allergy to dexpanthenol, hemophilia, ileus due to mechanical obstruction, lactation
- **Physical:** Skin color, lesions, texture; P, BP; bowel sounds, normal output

Interventions
- Monitor BP carefully during IV administration.

Teaching points

Teaching about this drug should be incorporated into the overall postoperative or postpartum teaching. Intestinal colic may occur within 30 minutes of administration.

• If you are using the topical drug, apply to affected areas once or twice daily.
• You may experience these side effects: Nausea, vomiting, diarrhea, itching, rash.
• Report difficulty breathing, severe itching, or rash.

▽ **dexrazoxane**

See Appendix R, *Less commonly used drugs*.

▽ **dextran, high–molecular-weight**
(dex' tran)

Dextran 70, Gentran 70, Macrodex

PREGNANCY CATEGORY C

Drug class
Plasma volume expander (nonbacteriostatic)

Therapeutic actions
Synthetic polysaccharide used to approximate the colloidal properties of albumin.

Indications
• Adjunctive therapy for treatment of shock or impending shock due to hemorrhage, burns, surgery, or trauma; to be used only in emergency situations when blood or blood products are not available

Contraindications and cautions
• Contraindicated with allergy to dextran (dextran 1 can be used prophylactically in patients known to be allergic to clinical dextran); marked hemostatic defects (risk for increased bleeding effects); severe cardiac congestion; renal failure, anuria, or oliguria.
• Use cautiously in pregnancy and lactation, thrombocytopenia, renal impairment.

Available forms
Injection—6% dextran 70 in 0.9% sodium chloride, 6% dextran 70 in 5% dextrose

Dosages

Adults
500–1,000 mL, given at a rate of 20–40 mL/min IV as an emergency procedure. Do not exceed 20 mL/kg the first 24 hr of treatment.

Pediatric patients
Determine dosage by body weight or surface area of the patient. Do not exceed 20 mL/kg IV total dose.

Patients with renal impairment
Decrease dose for creatinine clearance less than 30 mL/min.

Pharmacokinetics

Route	Onset	Peak	Duration
IV	Minutes	Minutes	12–24 hr

Metabolism: Hepatic; $T_{1/2}$: 24 hr
Distribution: May cross placenta; may enter breast milk
Excretion: Urine

▼ IV FACTS

Preparation: Administer in unit provided. Discard any partially used containers. Do not use unless the solution is clear.
Infusion: Infuse at rate of 20–40 mL/min.

Adverse effects
• **GI:** Nausea, vomiting
• **Hematologic:** *Hypervolemia, coagulation problems*
• **Hypersensitivity:** Urticaria, nasal congestion, wheezing, tightness of chest, mild hypotension (antihistamines may be helpful in relieving these symptoms), anaphylactoid reaction
• **Local:** Infection at injection site, extravasation
• **Other:** Fever, joint pains

Interactions
✳ **Drug-lab test** • Falsely elevated blood glucose assays • Interference with bilirubin assays in which alcohol is used, with total protein assays using biuret reagent • Blood typing and cross-matching procedures using enzyme techniques may give unreliable readings; draw blood samples before giving infusion of dextran

---

Adverse effects in *italics* are most common; those in **bold** are life-threatening. ⬛ Do not crush.

■ Nursing considerations
Assessment
- **History:** Allergy to dextran; marked hemostatic defects; severe cardiac congestion; renal failure or anuria; pregnancy
- **Physical:** T; skin color, lesions; P, BP, peripheral edema; R, adventitious sounds; urinalysis, LFTs, renal function tests, clotting times, PT, PTT, Hgb, Hct, urine output

Interventions
- Administer by IV infusion only; monitor rates based on patient response.
- Do not give more than recommended dose.
- Use only clear solutions. Discard partially used containers; solution contains no bacteriostat.
- ⊗ **Warning** Monitor patients carefully for any sign of hypervolemia or the development of heart failure; supportive measures may be needed.

Teaching points
- Report difficulty breathing, rash, unusual bleeding or bruising, pain at IV site.

▷ dextran, low–molecular-weight
(dex' tran)

Dextran 40, Gentran 40, 10% LMD, Rheomacrodex

PREGNANCY CATEGORY C

Drug class
Plasma volume expander (nonbacteriostatic)

Therapeutic actions
Synthetic polysaccharide used to approximate the colloidal properties of albumin.

Indications
- Adjunctive therapy for treatment of shock or impending shock due to hemorrhage, burns, surgery, or trauma when blood or blood products are not available
- Priming fluid in pump oxygenators during extracorporeal circulation
- Prophylaxis against DVT and PE in patients undergoing procedures known to be associated with a high incidence of thromboembolic complications, such as hip surgery

Contraindications and cautions
- Contraindicated with allergy to dextran (dextran 1 can be used prophylactically in patients known to be allergic to clinical dextran); marked hemostatic defects; severe cardiac congestion; renal failure, anuria, or oliguria.
- Use cautiously with pregnancy, lactation.

Available forms
Injection—10% Dextran 40 in 0.9% sodium chloride, 10% Dextran 40 in 5% dextrose

Dosages
Adults
- *Adjunctive therapy in shock:* Total dosage of 20 mL/kg IV in first 24 hr. The first 10 mL/kg should be infused rapidly, and the remaining dose administered slowly. Beyond 24 hr, total daily dosage should not exceed 10 mL/kg. Do not continue therapy for more than 5 days.
- *Hemodiluent in extracorporeal circulation:* Generally 10–20 mL/kg are added to perfusion circuit. Do not exceed a total dosage of 20 mL/kg.
- *Prophylaxis therapy for DVT, PE:* 500–1,000 mL IV on day of surgery, continue treatment at dose of 500 mL/day for an additional 2–3 days. Thereafter, based on procedure and risk, 500 mL may be administered every second to third day for up to 2 wk.

Pediatric patients
Total dose should not exceed 20 mL/kg.

Pharmacokinetics

Route	Onset	Peak	Duration
IV	Immediate	Minutes	12 hr

Metabolism: Hepatic; $T_{1/2}$: 3 hr
Distribution: Crosses placenta; enters breast milk
Excretion: Urine

▼ IV FACTS
Preparation: Protect from freezing. Use in units provided; no further preparation necessary.
Infusion: Administer first 10 mL/kg rapidly, remainder of solution slowly over 8–24 hr, monitoring patient response.

Adverse effects
- **CV:** Hypotension, anaphylactoid shock, *hypervolemia*

- **GI:** Nausea, vomiting
- **Hypersensitivity:** Ranging from mild cutaneous eruptions to generalized urticaria
- **Local:** Infection at site of injection, extravasation, venous thrombosis or phlebitis
- **Other:** Headache, fever, wheezing

Interactions

✳ **Drug-lab test** • Falsely elevated blood glucose assays • Interference with bilirubin assays in which alcohol is used, with total protein assays using biuret reagent • Blood typing and cross-matching procedures using enzyme techniques may give unreliable readings; draw blood samples before giving infusion of dextran

■ Nursing considerations

Assessment

- **History:** Allergy to dextran; marked hemostatic defects; severe cardiac congestion; renal failure or anuria; lactation, pregnancy
- **Physical:** T; skin color, lesions; P, BP, peripheral edema; R, adventitious sounds; urinalysis, LFTs, renal function tests, clotting times, PT, PTT, Hgb, Hct, urine output

Interventions

- Administer by IV infusion only; monitor rates based on patient response. Do not administer more than recommended dose.
- Monitor urinary output carefully; if no increase in output is noted after 500 mL of dextran, discontinue drug until diuresis can be induced by other means.

⊗ *Warning* Monitor patient for hypervolemia or development of heart failure; slow rate or discontinue drug if rapid CVP increase occurs.

Teaching points

- Report difficulty breathing, rash, unusual bleeding or bruising, pain at IV site.

> ▽ **dextroamphetamine sulfate**
>
> *(dex troe am fet' a meen)*
>
> Dexedrine Spansule█ⓒ,
> DextroStat
>
> **PREGNANCY CATEGORY C**
>
> **CONTROLLED SUBSTANCE C-II**

Drug classes

Amphetamine
CNS stimulant

Therapeutic actions

Acts in the CNS to release norepinephrine from nerve terminals; in higher doses also releases dopamine; suppresses appetite; increases alertness, elevates mood; often improves physical performance, especially when fatigue and sleep deprivation have caused impairment; efficacy in hyperkinetic syndrome, ADHD in children appears paradoxical and is not understood.

Indications

- Narcolepsy
- Adjunct therapy for abnormal behavioral syndrome in children and adults (ADHD, hyperkinetic syndrome) that includes psychological, social, educational measures
- Unlabeled uses: Cocaine-dependence treatment, autism, traumatic brain injury

Contraindications and cautions

- Contraindicated with hypersensitivity to sympathomimetic amines, tartrazine (*DextroStat*); advanced arteriosclerosis, symptomatic CV disease, moderate to severe hypertension, hyperthyroidism, glaucoma, agitated states.
- Use cautiously with history of drug abuse; pregnancy; lactation.

Available forms

Tablets—5, 10 mg; ER capsules█ⓒ—5, 10, 15 mg

Dosages

Adults

- *Narcolepsy:* Start with 10 mg/day PO in divided doses; increase in increments of 10 mg/day at weekly intervals. If insomnia or anorexia occurs, reduce dose. Usual dosage is 5–60 mg/day PO in divided doses. Give first dose on awakening, additional doses (one or two) every 4–6 hr; long-acting forms can be given once a day.
- *ADHD:* 5 mg PO once or twice daily; may be increased at rate of 5 mg weekly to maximum dose of 40 mg/day.

Pediatric patients

- *Narcolepsy:*
  6–12 yr: Condition is rare in children younger than 12 yr; when it does occur,

initial dose is 5 mg/day PO. Increase in increments of 5 mg at weekly intervals until optimal response is obtained.

12 yr and older: Use adult dosage.

• *ADHD:*

Younger than 3 yr: Not recommended.

3–5 yr: 2.5 mg/day PO. Increase in increments of 2.5 mg/day at weekly intervals until optimal response is obtained.

6 yr and older: 5 mg PO daily–bid. Increase in increments of 5 mg/day at weekly intervals until optimal response is obtained. Dosage will rarely exceed 40 mg/day. Give first dose on awakening, additional doses (one or two) every 4–6 hr. Long-acting forms may be used once a day.

Pharmacokinetics

Route	Onset	Peak	Duration
Oral	Rapid	1–5 hr	8–10 hr

Metabolism: Hepatic; $T_{1/2}$: 12 hr
Distribution: May cross placenta; enters breast milk
Excretion: Urine

Adverse effects

• **CNS:** *Overstimulation, restlessness, dizziness, insomnia,* dyskinesia, euphoria, dysphoria, tremor, headache, psychotic episodes
• **CV:** *Palpitations, tachycardia, hypertension*
• **Dermatologic:** Urticaria
• **Endocrine:** Reversible elevations in serum thyroxine with heavy use
• **GI:** *Dry mouth, unpleasant taste, diarrhea,* constipation, anorexia and weight loss
• **GU:** Impotence, changes in libido
• **Other:** Tolerance, psychological dependence, social disability with abuse

Interactions

✳ **Drug-drug** ⊗ *Warning* Hypertensive crisis and increased CNS effects if given within 14 days of MAOIs; do not give dextroamphetamine to patients who are taking or who have recently taken MAOIs.

• Decreased duration of effects if taken with urinary alkalinizers (acetazolamide, sodium bicarbonate), furazolidone • Decreased effects if taken with urinary acidifiers • Decreased efficacy of antihypertensive drugs given with amphetamines

■ Nursing considerations
Assessment

• **History:** Hypersensitivity to sympathomimetic amines, tartrazine; advanced arteriosclerosis, symptomatic CV disease, moderate to severe hypertension, hyperthyroidism, glaucoma, agitated states, history of drug abuse; lactation, pregnancy, use of MAOI in the last 14 days
• **Physical:** Weight; T; skin color, lesions; orientation, affect, ophthalmic examination (tonometry); P, BP, auscultation; R, adventitious sounds; bowel sounds, normal output; thyroid function tests, blood and urine glucose, baseline ECG

Interventions

• Ensure proper diagnosis before administering for behavioral syndromes: Drug should not be used until other causes (learning disability, EEG abnormalities, neurologic deficits) are ruled out.

⊗ *Black box warning* Be aware that drug has a high abuse potential; avoid prolonged use, and prescribe sparingly.

⊗ *Black box warning* Misuse may cause sudden death or serious CV events; increased risk with heart problems or structural heart anomalies.

• Interrupt drug dosage periodically in children being treated for behavioral disorders to determine if symptomatic response still validates drug therapy.
• Monitor growth of children on long-term amphetamine therapy.
• Dispense the lowest feasible dose to minimize risk of overdosage; drug should be stored in a light-resistant container.
• Ensure that patient swallows ER capsules whole; do not cut, crush, or allow patient to chew them.
• Give drug early in the day to prevent insomnia.
• Monitor BP frequently early in therapy.

Teaching points

• Take this drug exactly as prescribed. Do not increase the dosage without consulting your health care provider. If the drug appears ineffective, consult your health care provider.
• Do not crush or chew extended-release or long-acting capsules.
• Take drug (especially sustained-release forms) early in the day to avoid insomnia.

- This drug is a controlled substance; store it in a secure location and safely out of the reach of children.
- Avoid pregnancy while taking this drug. This drug can cause harm to the fetus.
- You may experience these side effects: Nervousness, restlessness, dizziness, insomnia, impaired thinking (may diminish in a few days; avoid driving or engaging in activities that require alertness); headache, loss of appetite, dry mouth.
- Report nervousness, insomnia, dizziness, palpitations, anorexia, GI disturbances.

▽ **dextromethorphan hydrobromide**

(dex troe meth or' fan)

Aerotuss 12, Balminil DM (CAN), Buckley's Cough Mixture, Creomulsion, Creo-Terpin, Delsym, DexAlone, Hold DM, Koffex (CAN), Novahistex DM (CAN), PediaCare Infants Long-Acting Cough, Robitussin Children's (CAN), Robitussin CoughGels, Theraflu Thin Strips Long-Acting Cough, Triaminic Thin Strips Long-Acting Cough, Vicks 44 Cough Relief

PREGNANCY CATEGORY C

Drug class
Nonopioid antitussive

Therapeutic actions
Lacks analgesic and addictive properties; controls cough spasms by depressing the cough center in the medulla; analogue of codeine.

Indications
- Control of nonproductive cough

Contraindications and cautions
- Contraindicated with hypersensitivity to any component (check label of products for flavorings, vehicles); sensitivity to bromides; cough that persists for more than 1 wk, tends to recur, is accompanied by excessive secretions, high fever, rash, nausea, vomiting, or persistent headache (dextromethorphan should not be used; patient should consult a physician).
- Use cautiously with lactation, pregnancy.

Available forms
Gelcaps—15, 30 mg; lozenges—5, 10 mg; liquid—5 mg/5 mL, 10 mg/15 mL, 15 mg/5 mL, 30 mg/5 mL; syrup—5 mg/5 mL, 7.5 mg/5 mL, 10 mg/5 mL, 20 mg/5 mL; sustained-action liquid—30 mg/5 mL; oral disintegrating strips—7.5, 15 mg; freezer pops—7.5 mg/pop

Dosages
Adults and children 12 yr and older
Gelcaps
30 mg every 6–8 hr. Do not exceed 120 mg/day.
Lozenges
5–15 mg every 1–4 hr up to 120 mg/day.
Liquid, syrup, strips
10–20 mg every 4 hr or 30 mg every 6–8 hr up to 120 mg/day.
ER suspension
60 mg every 12 hr up to 120 mg/day.
Pediatric patients (6–11 yr)
Lozenges
5–10 mg every 1–4 hr up to 60 mg/day. Do not give to children younger than 6 yr unless directed by a physician.
Liquid, syrup, strips
15 mg every 6–8 hr up to 60 mg/day.
Freezer pop
2 pops every 6–8 hr.
Pediatric patients (2–6 yr)
Liquid, syrup
7.5 mg every 6–8 hr up to 30 mg/day.
Freezer pop
1 pop every 6–8 hr.

Pharmacokinetics

Route	Onset	Peak	Duration
Oral	15–30 min	2 hr	3–6 hr

Metabolism: Hepatic; T$_{1/2}$: 2–4 hr
Distribution: May cross placenta; enters breast milk
Excretion: Urine

Adverse effects
- **Respiratory: Respiratory depression (with overdose)**

Adverse effects in *italics* are most common; those in **bold** are life-threatening. ⬛▣ Do not crush.

Interactions
❋ **Drug-drug** • Concomitant MAOI use may cause hypotension, fever, nausea, myoclonic jerks, and coma; avoid this combination

■ Nursing considerations
Assessment
- **History:** Hypersensitivity to any component; sensitivity to bromides; cough that persists for more than 1 wk or is accompanied by excessive secretions, high fever, rash, nausea, vomiting, or persistent headache; lactation, pregnancy
- **Physical:** T; R, adventitious sounds

Interventions
- Ensure drug is used only as recommended. Coughs may be symptomatic of a serious underlying disorder that should be diagnosed and properly treated; drug may mask symptoms of serious disease.

Teaching points
- Take this drug exactly as prescribed. Do not take more than recommended or for longer than recommended.
- Be cautious when using over-the-counter products; may contain the same ingredients and overdose can occur.
- Report continued or recurring cough, cough accompanied by fever, rash, persistent headache, nausea, vomiting.

▽ **diazepam**
(dye az' e pam)

Apo-Diazepam (CAN), Diastat AcuDial, Diazemuls (CAN), Diazepam Intensol, Valium

PREGNANCY CATEGORY D

CONTROLLED SUBSTANCE C-IV

Drug classes
Antiepileptic
Anxiolytic
Benzodiazepine
Skeletal muscle relaxant (centrally acting)

Therapeutic actions
Exact mechanisms of action not understood; acts mainly at the limbic system and reticular formation; may act in spinal cord and at supraspinal sites to produce skeletal muscle relaxation; potentiates the effects of GABA, an inhibitory neurotransmitter; anxiolytic effects occur at doses well below those necessary to cause sedation, ataxia; has little effect on cortical function.

Indications
- Management of anxiety disorders or for short-term relief of symptoms of anxiety
- Acute alcohol withdrawal; may be useful in symptomatic relief of acute agitation, tremor, delirium tremens, hallucinosis
- Muscle relaxant: Adjunct for relief of reflex skeletal muscle spasm due to local pathology (inflammation of muscles or joints) or secondary to trauma; spasticity caused by upper motoneuron disorders (cerebral palsy and paraplegia); athetosis, stiff-man syndrome
- Parenteral: Treatment of tetanus
- Antiepileptic: Adjunct in status epilepticus and severe recurrent convulsive seizures (parenteral); adjunct in seizure disorders (oral)
- Preoperative (parenteral): Relief of anxiety and tension and to lessen recall in patients prior to surgical procedures, cardioversion, and endoscopic procedures
- Rectal: Management of selected, refractory patients with epilepsy who require intermittent use to control bouts of increased seizure activity
- Unlabeled use: Treatment of night terrors

Contraindications and cautions
- Contraindicated with hypersensitivity to benzodiazepines; psychoses, acute narrow-angle glaucoma, shock, coma, acute alcoholic intoxication; pregnancy (cleft lip or palate, inguinal hernia, cardiac defects, microcephaly, pyloric stenosis when used in first trimester; neonatal withdrawal syndrome reported in newborns); lactation.
- Use cautiously with elderly or debilitated patients; impaired liver or renal function; and in patients with history of substance abuse.

Available forms
Tablets—2, 5, 10 mg; oral solution—5 mg/mL; oral concentrate solution—5 mg/mL; rectal gel—2.5, 5, 10, 20 mg; injection—5 mg/mL

Dosages

Individualize dosage; increase dosage cautiously to avoid adverse effects.

Adults
Oral
- *Anxiety disorders, skeletal muscle spasm, seizure disorders:* 2–10 mg bid–qid.
- *Alcohol withdrawal:* 10 mg tid–qid first 24 hr; reduce to 5 mg tid–qid, as needed.

Rectal
0.2 mg/kg; treat no more than one episode every 5 days. May give a second dose in 4–12 hr.

Parenteral
Usual dose is 2–20 mg IM or IV. Larger doses may be required for some indications (tetanus). Injection may be repeated in 1 hr.
- *Anxiety:* 2–10 mg IM or IV; repeat in 3–4 hr if necessary.
- *Alcohol withdrawal:* 10 mg IM or IV initially, then 5–10 mg in 3–4 hr if necessary.
- *Endoscopic procedures:* 10 mg or less, up to 20 mg IV just before procedure or 5–10 mg IM 30 min prior to procedure. Reduce or omit dosage of opioids.
- *Muscle spasm:* 5–10 mg IM or IV initially, then 5–10 mg in 3–4 hr if necessary.
- *Status epilepticus:* 5–10 mg, preferably by slow IV. May repeat every 5–10 min up to total dose of 30 mg. If necessary, repeat therapy in 2–4 hr; other drugs are preferable for long-term control.
- *Preoperative:* 10 mg IM.
- *Cardioversion:* 5–15 mg IV 5–10 min before procedure.

Pediatric patients
Oral
Older than 6 mo: 1–2.5 mg PO tid–qid initially. Gradually increase as needed and tolerated. Can be given rectally if needed.

Rectal
Younger than 2 yr: Not recommended.
2–5 yr: 0.5 mg/kg.
6–11 yr: 0.3 mg/kg.
Older than 12 yr: 0.2 mg/kg; may give a second dose in 4–12 hr.

Parenteral
Maximum dose of 0.25 mg/kg IV administered over 3 min; may repeat after 15–30 min. If no relief of symptoms after three doses, adjunctive therapy is recommended.
- *Tetanus (older than 1 mo):* 1–2 mg IM or IV slowly every 3–4 hr as necessary.
- *Tetanus (5 yr and older):* 5–10 mg IV every 3–4 hr.

- *Status epilepticus (older than 1 mo–younger than 5 yr):* 0.2–0.5 mg slowly IV every 2–5 min up to a maximum of 5 mg.
- *Status epilepticus (5 yr and older):* 1 mg IV every 2–5 min up to a maximum of 10 mg; repeat in 2–4 hr if necessary.

Geriatric patients or patients with debilitating disease
2–2.5 mg PO daily–bid or 2–5 mg parenteral initially; reduce rectal dose. Gradually increase as needed and tolerated; use cautiously.

Pharmacokinetics

Route	Onset	Peak	Duration
Oral	30–60 min	1–2 hr	3 hr
IM	15–30 min	30–45 min	3 hr
IV	1–5 min	30 min	15–60 min
Rectal	Rapid	1.5 hr	3 hr

Metabolism: Hepatic; $T_{1/2}$: 20–80 hr
Distribution: Crosses placenta; enters breast milk
Excretion: Urine

▼ IV FACTS

Preparation: Do not mix with other solutions; do not mix in plastic bags or tubing.
Infusion: Inject slowly into large vein, 1 mL/min at most; for children, give over at least 3 min; do not inject intra-arterially; if injected into IV tubing, inject as close to vein insertion site as possible.
Incompatibilities: Do not mix with other solutions; do not mix with any other drugs.
Y-site incompatibilities: Atracurium, heparin, foscarnet, pancuronium, potassium, vecuronium.

Adverse effects
- **CNS:** *Transient, mild drowsiness initially; sedation, depression, lethargy, apathy, fatigue, light-headedness, disorientation, restlessness, confusion,* crying, delirium, headache, slurred speech, dysarthria, stupor, rigidity, tremor, dystonia, vertigo, euphoria, nervousness, difficulty in concentration, vivid dreams, psychomotor retardation, extrapyramidal symptoms; *mild paradoxical excitatory reactions during first 2 wk of treatment,* visual and auditory disturbances, diplopia, nystagmus, depressed hearing, nasal congestion

Adverse effects in *italics* are most common; those in **bold** are life-threatening. ▣ Do not crush.

- **CV:** *Bradycardia, tachycardia,* **CV collapse,** hypertension and hypotension, palpitations, edema
- **Dependence:** *Drug dependence with withdrawal syndrome* when drug is discontinued (common with abrupt discontinuation of higher dosage used for longer than 4 mo); IV diazepam: 1.7% incidence of fatalities; oral benzodiazepines ingested alone; no well-documented fatal overdoses
- **Dermatologic:** Urticaria, pruritus, skin rash, dermatitis
- **GI:** *Constipation; diarrhea,* dry mouth; salivation; nausea; anorexia; vomiting; difficulty in swallowing; gastric disorders; elevations of blood enzymes—LDH, alkaline phosphatase, AST, ALT; hepatic impairment; jaundice
- **GU:** *Incontinence, urinary retention, changes in libido,* menstrual irregularities
- **Hematologic:** Decreased Hct, blood dyscrasias
- **Other:** Phlebitis and thrombosis at IV injection sites, hiccups, fever, diaphoresis, paresthesias, muscular disturbances, gynecomastia; pain, burning, and redness after IM injection

Interactions

✴ **Drug-drug** ● Increased CNS depression with alcohol, omeprazole ● Increased pharmacologic effects of diazepam if combined with cimetidine, disulfiram, hormonal contraceptives ● Decreased effects of diazepam with theophyllines, ranitidine

■ Nursing considerations
Assessment

- **History:** Hypersensitivity to benzodiazepines; psychoses, acute narrow-angle glaucoma, shock, coma, acute alcoholic intoxication; elderly or debilitated patients; impaired liver or renal function; pregnancy, lactation
- **Physical:** Weight; skin color, lesions; orientation, affect, reflexes, sensory nerve function, ophthalmologic examination; P, BP; R, adventitious sounds; bowel sounds, normal output, liver evaluation; normal output; LFTs, renal function tests, CBC

Interventions

⊗ *Warning* Do not administer intra-arterially; may produce arteriospasm, gangrene.

- Change from IV therapy to oral therapy as soon as possible.
- Do not use small veins (dorsum of hand or wrist) for IV injection.
- Reduce dose of opioid analgesics with IV diazepam; dose should be reduced by at least one-third or eliminated.
- Carefully monitor P, BP, respiration during IV administration.

⊗ *Warning* Maintain patients receiving parenteral benzodiazepines in bed for 3 hr; do not permit ambulatory patients to operate a vehicle following an injection.

- Monitor EEG in patients treated for status epilepticus; seizures may recur after initial control, presumably because of short duration of drug effect.
- Monitor liver and renal function, CBC during long-term therapy.
- Taper dosage gradually after long-term therapy, especially in epileptic patients.
- Arrange for epileptic patients to wear medical alert ID indicating that they are epileptics taking this medication.
- Discuss risk of fetal abnormalities with patients desiring to become pregnant.
- Provide safety precautions for older patients who may be at increased risks for falls.

Teaching points

- Take this drug exactly as prescribed. Do not stop taking this drug (long-term therapy, antiepileptic therapy) without consulting your health care provider.
- Caregiver should learn to assess seizures, administer rectal form, and monitor patient.
- Use of barrier contraceptives is advised while on this drug; if you become or wish to become pregnant, consult your health care provider.
- It is advisable to wear a medical alert ID indicating your diagnosis and treatment (as antiepileptic).
- You may experience these side effects: Drowsiness, dizziness (may lessen; avoid driving or engaging in other dangerous activities); GI upset (take drug with food); dreams, difficulty concentrating, fatigue, nervousness, crying (reversible).
- Report severe dizziness, weakness, drowsiness that persists, rash or skin lesions, palpitations, swelling of the ankles, visual or hearing disturbances, difficulty voiding.

▽ diazoxide
(di az ok' side)

Proglycem

PREGNANCY CATEGORY C

Drug class
Glucose-elevating drug

Therapeutic actions
Increases blood glucose by decreasing insulin release and increasing glucose.

Indications
- Management of hypoglycemia due to hyperinsulinism in infants and children and due to inoperable pancreatic islet cell malignancies

Contraindications and cautions
- Contraindicated with allergy to thiazides or other sulfonamide derivatives; pregnancy, lactation, functional hypoglycemia.
- Use extreme caution with decreased cardiac reserve, decreased renal function, gout, or hyperuricemia.

Available forms
Capsules—50 mg; oral suspension—50 mg/mL

Dosages
Adults
3–8 mg/kg/day PO in two to three divided doses every 8–12 hr. Starting dose, 3 mg/kg/day in three equal doses every 8 hr.
Pediatric patients
Infants and newborns: 8–15 mg/kg/day PO in two to three doses every 8–12 hr. Starting dose, 10 mg/kg/day in three equal doses every 8 hr.
Children: 3–8 mg/kg/day PO in two to three doses every 8–12 hr. Starting dose, 3 mg/kg/day in three equal doses every 8 hr.

Pharmacokinetics

Route	Onset	Peak	Duration
Oral	1 hr	8 hr	N/A

Metabolism: Hepatic; $T_{1/2}$: 21–45 hr
Distribution: Crosses placenta; may enter breast milk
Excretion: Urine

Adverse effects
- **CNS:** Anxiety, dizziness, extrapyramidal symptoms, headache, hearing loss, blurred vision, apprehension
- **CV:** *Hypotension* (managed by Trendelenburg position or sympathomimetics), **heart failure** *secondary to fluid and sodium retention*
- **Dermatologic:** Hirsutism, rash
- **GI:** *Nausea, vomiting,* anorexia, constipation, diarrhea, elevated liver enzymes
- **GU:** Renal toxicity, azotemia, reversible nephrotic syndrome
- **Hematologic: Thrombocytopenia,** decreased Hgb, decreased Hct
- **Metabolic:** Hyperglycemia, glycosuria, ketoacidosis, nonketotic hyperosmolar coma, hyperuricemia
- **Respiratory:** Dyspnea, choking sensation
- **Other:** Gout, advanced bone age

Interactions
✳ **Drug-drug** ● Increased therapeutic and toxic effects of diazoxide if taken concurrently with thiazides ● Increased risk of hyperglycemia if taken concurrently with chlorpropamide, glipizide, glyburide, tolazamide, tolbutamide ● Decreased serum levels and effectiveness of hydantoins taken concurrently with diazoxide
✳ **Drug-lab test** ● Hyperglycemic and hyperuricemic effects of diazoxide prevent testing for disorders of glucose and xanthine metabolism ● False-negative insulin response to glucagon

■ Nursing considerations
Assessment
- **History:** Allergy to thiazides or other sulfonamide derivatives; pregnancy; lactation; functional hypoglycemia, decreased cardiac reserve, decreased renal function, gout or hyperuricemia
- **Physical:** Body weight, skin integrity, swelling or limited motion in joints, earlobes; P, BP, edema, peripheral perfusion; R, pattern, adventitious sounds; intake and output; CBC, blood glucose, serum electrolytes and uric acid, urinalysis, urine glucose and ketones, LFTs, renal function tests

Interventions
- Monitor intake and output and weigh patient daily at the same time to check for fluid retention.

Adverse effects in *italics* are most common; those in **bold** are life-threatening. ⊞ Do not crush.

- Check urine or serum glucose and ketones daily.
⊗ **Warning** Have insulin and oral hypoglycemic agents readily available in case hyperglycemic reaction occurs.
- Decrease dose in renal disease.
- Protect oral drug suspensions from light.
- Reassure patient that hirsutism will resolve when drug is discontinued.

Teaching points
- Check blood glucose level daily; report elevated levels.
- Weigh yourself daily at the same time and with the same clothes, and record the results.
- Excessive hair growth may appear on your forehead, back, or limbs; growth will end after drug is stopped.
- Report weight gain of more than 5 pounds in 2–3 days, increased thirst, nausea, vomiting, confusion, fruity odor on breath, abdominal pain, swelling of extremities, difficulty breathing, bruising, bleeding.

▷**diclofenac**
*(dye **kloe'** fen ak)*

diclofenac epolamine
Flector, Pennsaid, Solaraze, Voltaren

diclofenac potassium
Apo-Diclo Rapide (CAN), Cambia, Cataflam, Novo-Difenac-K (CAN), Voltaren Rapide (CAN), Zipsor

diclofenac sodium
Apo-Diclo (CAN), Apo-Diclo SR (CAN)⊞, Novo-Difenac (CAN), Novo-Difenac SR (CAN), Nu-Diclo (CAN), Nu-Diclo SR (CAN)⊞, PMS-Diclofenac (CAN), PMS-Diclofenac SR (CAN)⊞, Solaraze, Voltaren Ophtha (CAN), Voltaren-XR⊞

PREGNANCY CATEGORY C
(FIRST AND SECOND TRIMESTERS)

PREGNANCY CATEGORY D
(THIRD TRIMESTER)

Drug classes
Analgesic (nonopioid)
Anti-inflammatory

Antipyretic
NSAID

Therapeutic actions
Inhibits prostaglandin synthetase to cause antipyretic and anti-inflammatory effects; the exact mechanism is unknown.

Indications
- Acute or long-term treatment of mild to moderate pain, including dysmenorrhea
- Rheumatoid arthritis
- Acute treatment of migraine headache with or without aura (*Cambia*)
- Osteoarthritis
- Ankylosing spondylitis
- Treatment of actinic keratosis in conjunction with sun avoidance (topical only)
- Topical treatment of acute pain due to minor strains, sprains, contusions (*Flector*)
- Ophthalmic: Postoperative inflammation from cataract extraction

Contraindications and cautions
- Contraindicated with allergy to NSAIDs, significant renal impairment, pregnancy, lactation.
- Use cautiously with impaired hearing, allergies, hepatic, CV, GI conditions, and in elderly patients.

Available forms
Tablets—50 mg; DR tablets⊞—25, 50, 75 mg; ER tablets⊞—100 mg; liquid-filled capsules—25 mg; packet for oral solution—50 mg; topical gel—1%, 3%; topical solution—1.5%; ophthalmic solution—0.1%; transdermal patch—180 mg

Dosages
Adults
Oral
- *Pain, including dysmenorrhea:* 50 mg tid PO; initial dose of 100 mg may help some patients (*Cataflam*).
- *Osteoarthritis:* 100–150 mg/day PO in divided doses; 50 mg bid–tid PO (*Cataflam*).
- *Rheumatoid arthritis:* 150–200 mg/day PO in divided doses; 50 mg bid–tid PO (*Cataflam*).
- *Ankylosing spondylitis:* 100–125 mg/day PO. Give as 25 mg qid, with an extra 25-mg dose at bedtime; 25 mg qid PO with an additional 25 mg at bedtime if needed (*Cataflam*).

- *Acute migraine:* 50-mg packet mixed in 30–60 mL water as single dose at onset of headache (*Cambia*).
- *Treatment of mild to moderate pain:* 25 mg liquid-filled capsule PO qid (*Zipsor*). *Not interchangeable with other forms of diclofenac.*

Topical
- *Actinic keratosis:* Cover lesion with gel and smooth into skin; do not cover with dressings or cosmetics (*Solaraze*).
- *Osteoarthritis:* Upper extremities, apply gel (2 g) to affected area qid; lower extremities, apply gel (4 g) to affected area qid (*Voltaren*).

Transdermal patch
1 patch applied to most painful area bid. Use lowest effective dose for shortest time; do not apply to damaged or broken skin (*Flector*).

Ophthalmic
1 drop to affected eye qid starting 24 hr after surgery for 2 wk.

Pediatric patients
Safety and efficacy not established.

Pharmacokinetics

Route	Onset	Peak	Duration
Oral (sodium)	Varies	2–3 hr	12–15 hr
Oral (potassium)	Rapid	20–120 min	12–15 hr

Metabolism: Hepatic; $T_{1/2}$: 1.5–2 hr
Distribution: Crosses placenta; may enter breast milk
Excretion: Feces, urine

Adverse effects
- **CNS:** *Headache, dizziness,* somnolence, insomnia, fatigue, tiredness, tinnitus, ophthalmic effects
- **Dermatologic:** Rash, pruritus, sweating, dry mucous membranes, stomatitis
- **GI:** *Nausea, dyspepsia, GI pain, diarrhea,* vomiting, *constipation,* flatulence, GI bleed
- **GU:** Dysuria, renal impairment
- **Hematologic:** Bleeding, platelet inhibition with higher doses
- **Other:** Peripheral edema, **anaphylactoid reactions to fatal anaphylactic shock**

Interactions
✳ **Drug-drug** • Increased serum levels and increased risk of lithium toxicity • Increased

risk of bleeding with anticoagulants; monitor patient closely

■ Nursing considerations
Assessment
- **History:** Renal impairment; impaired hearing; allergies; hepatic, CV, and GI conditions; lactation, pregnancy
- **Physical:** Skin color and lesions; orientation, reflexes, ophthalmologic and audiometric evaluation, peripheral sensation; P, BP; edema; R, adventitious sounds; liver evaluation; CBC, clotting times, renal function tests, LFTs; serum electrolytes, stool guaiac

Interventions
⊗ **Black box warning** Be aware that patient may be at increased risk for CV events, GI bleed, renal insufficiency; monitor accordingly.
- Administer drug with food or after meals if GI upset occurs. Ensure that patient does not cut, crush, or chew ER or DR tablets. Mix packets for oral suspension in 30–60 mL water.
- Ensure that correct topical gel is being used for indication being treated; gels are not interchangeable.
- Arrange for periodic ophthalmologic examination during long-term therapy.
- Monitor renal function in older patients.
⊗ **Warning** Institute emergency procedures if overdose occurs (gastric lavage, induction of emesis, supportive therapy).
⊗ **Warning** Liquid-filled capsules (*Zipsor*) are not interchangeable with other forms of diclofenac.

Teaching points
- Take drug with food or meals if GI upset occurs. Do not cut, crush, or chew delayed-release or extended-release tablets.
- Apply topical gel as indicated; avoid sun exposure and sun lamps.
- Apply transdermal patch to intact skin. Remove old patch before applying new one.
- Mix packets for oral solution in 30 to 60 mL water. Take at first sign of a migraine.
- Take only the prescribed dosage.
- You may experience these side effects: Dizziness or drowsiness (avoid driving or using dangerous machinery while using this drug).
- Report sore throat, fever, rash, itching, weight gain, swelling in ankles or fingers, changes in vision; black, tarry stools.

▷dicyclomine hydrochloride
(dye sye' kloe meen)

Bentyl, Bentylol (CAN)

PREGNANCY CATEGORY B

Drug classes
Anticholinergic
Antimuscarinic
Antispasmodic
Parasympatholytic

Therapeutic actions
Direct GI smooth muscle relaxant; competitively blocks the effects of acetylcholine at muscarinic cholinergic receptors that mediate the effects of parasympathetic postganglionic impulses, thus relaxing the GI tract.

Indications
- Treatment of functional bowel or IBS (irritable colon, spastic colon, mucous colitis)

Contraindications and cautions
- Contraindicated with glaucoma; adhesions between iris and lens, stenosing peptic ulcer, pyloroduodenal obstruction, paralytic ileus, intestinal atony, severe ulcerative colitis, toxic megacolon, symptomatic prostatic hypertrophy, bladder neck obstruction, bronchial asthma, COPD, cardiac arrhythmias, tachycardia, myocardial ischemia; impaired metabolic, liver, or renal function, myasthenia gravis; lactation, pregnancy.
- Use cautiously with Down syndrome, brain damage, spasticity, hypertension, hyperthyroidism.

Available forms
Capsules—10, 20 mg; tablets—20 mg; syrup—10 mg/5 mL; injection—10 mg/mL.

Dosages
Adults
Oral
The only effective dose is 160 mg/day PO divided into four equal doses; however, begin with 80 mg/day divided into four equal doses; increase to 160 mg/day unless side effects limit dosage.

Parenteral
80 mg/day IM in four divided doses; do not give IV.
Pediatric patients
Not recommended.
Geriatric patients
Use should be avoided; more prone to side effects.

Pharmacokinetics

Route	Onset	Duration
Oral	1–2 hr	4 hr

Metabolism: Hepatic; $T_{1/2}$: 9–10 hr
Distribution: May cross placenta; enters breast milk
Excretion: Urine

Adverse effects
- **CNS:** *Blurred vision,* mydriasis, cycloplegia, photophobia, increased IOP, confusion
- **CV:** Palpitations, tachycardia
- **GI:** *Dry mouth, altered taste perception, nausea, vomiting, dysphagia,* heartburn, constipation, bloated feeling, paralytic ileus, gastroesophageal reflux
- **GU:** *Urinary hesitancy and retention,* impotence
- **Local:** *Irritation at site of IM injection*
- **Other:** Decreased sweating and predisposition to heat prostration, suppression of lactation

Interactions
✳ **Drug-drug** • Decreased effectiveness of all antipsychotic medications when used in combination with dicyclomine • Increased anticholinergic effects when administered with TCAs, amantadine • Possible increased effect of atenolol and digoxin

■ Nursing considerations
Assessment
- **History:** Glaucoma; adhesions between iris and lens, stenosing peptic ulcer, pyloroduodenal obstruction, paralytic ileus, intestinal atony, severe ulcerative colitis, toxic megacolon, symptomatic prostatic hypertrophy, bladder neck obstruction, bronchial asthma, COPD, cardiac arrhythmias, myocardial ischemia; impaired metabolic, liver, or renal function, myasthenia gravis; Down syndrome, brain damage, spasticity, hypertension, hyperthyroidism; lactation, pregnancy

- **Physical:** Bowel sounds, normal output; normal urinary output, prostate palpation; R, adventitious sounds; pulse, BP; IOP, vision; bilateral grip strength, reflexes; liver palpation, LFTs, renal function tests; skin color, lesions, texture

Interventions

- IM use is temporary; switch to oral form as soon as feasible.
- Ensure adequate hydration; control environmental temperature to prevent hyperpyrexia.
- Have patient void before each drug dose if urinary retention is a problem.
- Monitor lighting to minimize discomfort of photophobia.
- Do not give IV.

Teaching points

- Take drug exactly as prescribed.
- Avoid hot environments while taking this drug (heat intolerance may lead to dangerous reactions).
- You may experience these side effects: Constipation (ensure adequate fluid intake, proper diet); dry mouth (sugarless candies, frequent mouth care may help; may lessen with time); blurred vision, sensitivity to light (transient effects; avoid tasks that require acute vision; wear sunglasses); impotence (reversible); difficulty in urination (empty bladder immediately before taking drug).
- Report rash, flushing, eye pain, difficulty breathing, tremors, loss of coordination, irregular heartbeat, palpitations, headache, abdominal distention, hallucinations, severe or persistent dry mouth, difficulty swallowing, difficulty in urination, severe constipation, sensitivity to light.

▽ **didanosine**
(ddI, dideoxyinosine)

(dye dan' oh seen)

Videx, Videx EC ⓞⓝⓒ

PREGNANCY CATEGORY B

Drug class

Antiviral
Nucleoside reverse transcriptase inhibitor

Therapeutic actions

A synthetic nucleoside that inhibits replication of HIV, leading to viral death.

Indications

- Treatment of patients with HIV infection in combination with other antiretroviral drugs

Contraindications and cautions

- Contraindicated with allergy to any component of the formulation, lactation.
- Use cautiously with impaired hepatic or renal function; history of alcohol abuse; history of pancreatitis, lactic acidosis; pregnancy.

Available forms

DR capsules ⓞⓝⓒ—125, 200, 250, 400 mg; powder for oral solution—2, 4 g

Dosages
Adults
DR capsules

- 60 kg or greater: 400 mg/day PO.
- 25–60 kg: 250 mg/day PO.
- 20–25 kg: 200 mg/day PO.

Powder for oral solution

- 60 kg or greater: 200 mg PO bid or 400 mg/day PO.
- Less than 60 kg: 125 mg PO bid or 250 mg/day PO.

Pediatric patients
Older than 8 mo: 120 mg/m^2 bid using buffered formulation or pediatric powder.
2 wk–8 mo: 100 mg/m^2 bid.
DR capsule can be used following adult dosage, based on weight.

Patients with renal impairment

CrCL (mL/min)	60 kg or more		Less than 60 kg	
	DR	Suspension	DR	Suspension
More than 60	400 mg/day	200 mg bid or 400 mg/day	250 mg/day	125 mg bid or 250 mg/day
30–59	200 mg/day	100 mg bid or 200 mg/day	125 mg/day	75 mg bid or 150 mg/day
10–29	125 mg/day	150 mg/day	125 mg/day	100 mg/day
Less than 10	125 mg/day	100 mg/day	—	75 mg/day

Pharmacokinetics

Route	Peak	Onset
Oral	15–90 min	Varies

Metabolism: Hepatic; T$_{1/2}$: 1.6 hr
Distribution: May cross placenta; may enter breast milk
Excretion: Urine

Adverse effects

- **CNS:** Headache, pain, anxiety, confusion, nervousness, twitching, depression, peripheral neuropathy
- **Dermatologic:** Rash, pruritus
- **GI:** *Nausea, vomiting,* **hepatotoxicity,** *abdominal pain,* diarrhea, **pancreatitis,** stomatitis, oral thrush, melena, dry mouth, elevated bilirubin
- **Hematologic:** *Hemopoietic depression*
- **Other:** Chills, fever, infections, dyspnea, myopathy, elevated uric acid, **lactic acidosis**

Interactions

✷ **Drug-drug** • Decreased effectiveness of tetracycline, fluoroquinolone antibiotics • Increased effect of *Videx* when combined with allopurinol • Changed concentrations for either drug when combined with ganciclovir • Decreased effect of *Videx* when combined with methadone • Decreased effect of azole antifungals

✷ **Drug-food** • Decreased absorption and effectiveness of didanosine if taken with food

■ Nursing considerations

Assessment

- **History:** Allergy to any components of formulation, impaired hepatic or renal function, lactation, history of alcohol abuse, pregnancy
- **Physical:** Weight; T; skin color, lesions; orientation, reflexes, muscle strength, affect; abdominal examination; CBC, pancreatic enzymes, LFTs, renal function tests

Interventions

- Arrange for lab tests (CBC, SMA-12) before and frequently during therapy; monitor for bone marrow depression.
- Administer drug on an empty stomach, 1 hr before or 2 hr after meals.
- Ensure patient swallows *Videx EC* whole; do not cut, crush, or chew.

⊗ ***Black box warning*** Monitor patient for signs of pancreatitis—abdominal pain, elevated enzymes, nausea, vomiting. Stop drug, resume only if pancreatitis has been ruled out.

⊗ ***Black box warning*** Monitor patients with hepatic impairment; decreased doses may be needed if toxicity occurs. Fatal liver toxicity with lactic acidosis has been reported. Non-cirrhotic portal hypertension, sometimes fatal, has occurred.

Teaching points

- Take drug on an empty stomach, 1 hour before or 2 hours after meals.
- Pediatric solution should be reconstituted by the pharmacy. Shake admixture thoroughly. Store tightly closed in the refrigerator. If taking a delayed-release capsule, it must be swallowed whole; do not cut, crush, or chew it.
- Have regular blood tests and physical examinations to monitor drug's effects and progress of disease.
- You may experience these side effects: Loss of appetite, nausea, vomiting (frequent mouth care, frequent small meals may help); rash; chills; fever; headache.
- Report abdominal pain, nausea, vomiting, cough, sore throat, change in color of urine or stools.

▷ **diflunisal** ⓄⓉⒸ
(dye floo' ni sal)

Apo-Diflunisal (CAN) ⓄⓉⒸ

PREGNANCY CATEGORY C

Drug classes

Analgesic (nonopioid)
Anti-inflammatory
Antipyretic
NSAID

Therapeutic actions

Exact mechanism of action not known: Inhibition of prostaglandin synthetase, the enzyme that breaks down prostaglandins, may account for its antipyretic and anti-inflammatory effects.

Indications

- Acute or long-term treatment of mild to moderate pain
- Rheumatoid arthritis
- Osteoarthritis

Contraindications and cautions

- Contraindicated with allergy to diflunisal, salicylates or other NSAIDs; with pregnancy, lactation; for treatment of perioperative pain following coronary artery bypass graft (CABG) surgery.
- Use cautiously with CV dysfunction, peptic ulceration, GI bleeding, impaired hepatic or renal function, and in elderly patients.

Available forms

Tablets ⓞⓝⓒ—500 mg

Dosages

Adults

- *Mild to moderate pain:* 1,000 mg PO initially, followed by 500 mg every 8–12 hr PO.
- *Osteoarthritis or rheumatoid arthritis:* 500–1,000 mg/day PO in two divided doses; maintenance dosage should not exceed 1,500 mg/day.

Pediatric patients 12 yr and younger

Safety and efficacy not established.

Pharmacokinetics

Route	Onset	Peak	Duration
Oral	30–60 min	2–3 hr	12 hr

Metabolism: Hepatic; $T_{1/2}$: 8–12 hr
Distribution: Crosses placenta; enters breast milk
Excretion: Urine

Adverse effects

- **CNS:** *Headache, dizziness, somnolence, insomnia,* fatigue, tiredness, dizziness, tinnitus, ophthalmologic effects
- **Dermatologic:** *Rash,* pruritus, sweating, dry mucous membranes, stomatitis
- **GI:** *Nausea, dyspepsia, GI pain, diarrhea,* vomiting, constipation, flatulence
- **GU:** Dysuria, renal impairment
- **Hematologic:** Bleeding, platelet inhibition with higher doses

- **Other:** Peripheral edema, **anaphylactoid reactions to anaphylactic shock**

Interactions

✳ **Drug-drug** • Decreased absorption with antacids (especially aluminum salts) • Decreased serum diflunisal levels with multiple doses of aspirin • Possible increased acetaminophen levels if combined

■ Nursing considerations

Assessment

- **History:** Allergy to diflunisal, salicylates or other NSAIDs, CV dysfunction, peptic ulceration, GI bleeding, impaired hepatic or renal function, lactation, pregnancy
- **Physical:** Skin color, lesions; T; orientation, reflexes, ophthalmologic evaluation; P, BP, edema; R, adventitious sounds; liver evaluation, bowel sounds; CBC, clotting times, urinalysis, LFTs, renal function tests

Interventions

⊗ **Black box warning** Be aware that patient may be at increased risk for CV events, GI bleeding; monitor accordingly.

- Give drug with food or after meals if GI upset occurs.
- Do not crush, and ensure that patient does not chew tablets.

⊗ **Warning** Institute emergency procedures if overdose occurs—gastric lavage, induction of emesis, supportive therapy.

⊗ **Black box warning** Do not use drug to treat perioperative pain following CABG surgery.

- Arrange for ophthalmologic examination if patient offers any eye complaints.

Teaching points

- Take the drug only as recommended to avoid overdose.
- Take the drug with food or after meals if GI upset occurs. Swallow the tablet whole; do not cut, chew, or crush it.
- You may experience these side effects: Nausea, GI upset, dyspepsia (take drug with food); diarrhea or constipation; dizziness, vertigo, insomnia (use caution if driving or operating dangerous machinery).
- Report eye changes, unusual bleeding or bruising, swelling of the feet or hands, difficulty breathing, severe GI pain.

Adverse effects in *italics* are most common; those in **bold** are life-threatening. ⓞⓝⓒ Do not crush.

DANGEROUS DRUG

▽ **digoxin**

(di jox' in)

Lanoxin

PREGNANCY CATEGORY C

Drug classes
Cardiac glycoside
Cardiotonic

Therapeutic actions
Increases intracellular calcium and allows more calcium to enter the myocardial cell during depolarization via a sodium–potassium pump mechanism; this increases force of contraction (positive inotropic effect), increases renal perfusion (seen as diuretic effect in patients with heart failure), decreases heart rate (negative chronotropic effect), and decreases AV node conduction velocity.

Indications
- Heart failure
- Atrial fibrillation

Contraindications and cautions
- Contraindicated with allergy to cardiac glycosides, ventricular tachycardia, ventricular fibrillation, heart block, sick sinus syndrome, IHSS, acute MI, renal insufficiency and electrolyte abnormalities (decreased K+, decreased Mg2+, increased Ca2+).
- Use cautiously with pregnancy and lactation.

Available forms
Tablets—0.125, 0.25 mg; injection—0.25 mg/mL; pediatric injection—0.1 mg/mL

Dosages
Patient response is quite variable. Evaluate patient carefully to determine the appropriate dose.
Adults
Loading dose, 0.25 mg/day IV or PO for patients younger than 70 yr with good renal function; 0.125 mg/day for patients older than 70 yr or with impaired renal function; or 0.0625 mg/day for patients with marked renal impairment. Maintenance dose, 0.125–0.5 mg/day PO.

Pediatric patients
Loading dose:

	Oral (mcg/kg)	IV (mcg/kg)
Premature	20	15–25
Neonate	30	20–30
1–24 mo	40–50	30–50
2–10 yr	30–40	25–35
Older than 10 yr	10–15	8–12

Maintenance dose, 25%–35% of loading dose in divided daily doses. Usually 0.125–0.5 mg/day PO; 20%–30% for premature infants.
Geriatric patients with impaired renal function
For creatinine clearance of 10–50 mL/min, give 25%–75% normal dose every 36 hr. For creatinine clearance of less than 10 mL/min and for patients on hemodialysis, give 10%–25% normal dose, or usual dosage every 48 hr.

Pharmacokinetics

Route	Onset	Peak	Duration
Oral	30–120 min	2–6 hr	6–8 days
IV	5–30 min	1–5 hr	4–5 days

Metabolism: Some hepatic; T$_{1/2}$: 30–40 hr
Distribution: May cross placenta; enters breast milk
Excretion: Urine, unchanged

▼ IV FACTS

Preparation: Give undiluted or diluted in fourfold or greater volume of sterile water for injection, 0.9% sodium chloride injection, 5% dextrose injection. Use diluted product promptly. Do not use if solution contains precipitates.
Infusion: Inject slowly over 5 min or longer.
Incompatibility: Do not mix with dobutamine.

Adverse effects
- **CNS:** *Headache, weakness,* drowsiness, visual disturbances, mental status change
- **CV:** *Arrhythmias*
- **GI:** *GI upset,* anorexia

Interactions
✷ **Drug-drug** • Increased therapeutic and toxic effects of digoxin with thioamines, verapamil, amiodarone, quinidine, erythromycin, cyclosporine (a decrease in digoxin dosage may be

necessary to prevent toxicity; when the interacting drug is discontinued, an increase in the digoxin dosage may be necessary) • Increased incidence of cardiac arrhythmias with potassium-losing (loop and thiazide) diuretics • Increased absorption or increased bioavailability of oral digoxin, leading to increased effects with tetracyclines, erythromycin • Decreased therapeutic effects with thyroid hormones, metoclopramide, penicillamine • Decreased absorption of oral digoxin if taken with cholestyramine, charcoal, colestipol, antineoplastics (bleomycin, cyclophosphamide, methotrexate) • Increased or decreased effects of oral digoxin (adjust the dose of digoxin during concomitant therapy) with oral aminoglycosides

❋ **Drug-alternative therapy** • Increased risk of digoxin toxicity if taken with ginseng, hawthorn, or licorice therapy • Decreased absorption with psyllium • Decreased serum levels with St. John's Wort

■ **Nursing considerations**
Assessment
• **History:** Allergy to cardiac glycosides, ventricular tachycardia, ventricular fibrillation, heart block, sick sinus syndrome, IHSS, acute MI, renal insufficiency, decreased K+, decreased Mg^{2+}, increased Ca^{2+}, pregnancy, lactation
• **Physical:** Weight; orientation, affect, reflexes, vision; P, BP, baseline ECG, cardiac auscultation, peripheral pulses, peripheral perfusion, edema; R, adventitious sounds; abdominal percussion, bowel sounds, liver evaluation; urinary output; electrolyte levels, LFTs, renal function tests

Interventions
⊗ **Warning** Monitor apical pulse for 1 min before administering; hold dose if pulse lower than 60 beats/min in adult or lower than 90 beats/min in infant; retake pulse in 1 hr. If adult pulse remains lower than 60 beats/min or infant pulse remains lower than 90 beats/min, hold drug and notify prescriber. Note any change from baseline rhythm or rate.
• Check dosage and preparation carefully.
• Avoid IM injections, which may be very painful.
• Follow diluting instructions carefully, and use diluted solution promptly.
• Avoid giving with meals; taking this drug with food will delay absorption and alter drug pharmacokinetics.

• Have emergency equipment ready; have K+ salts, lidocaine, phenytoin, atropine, and cardiac monitor readily available in case toxicity develops.
⊗ **Warning** Monitor for therapeutic drug levels: 0.5–2 ng/mL.

Teaching points
• Do not stop taking this drug without notifying your health care provider.
• Take pulse at the same time each day, and record it on a calendar (normal pulse for you is ____; call your health care provider if your pulse rate falls below ____.)
• Weigh yourself every other day with the same clothing and at the same time. Record this on the calendar.
• Do not start taking prescriptions, OTC products, or herbal supplements without talking to your health care provider. Some combinations may increase the risk of digoxin toxicity and may put you at risk of adverse reactions.
• Wear or carry a medical alert tag stating that you are on this drug.
• Have regular medical checkups, which may include blood tests, to evaluate the effects and dosage of this drug.
• Report slow or irregular pulse, rapid weight gain, loss of appetite, nausea, diarrhea, vomiting, blurred or "yellow" vision, unusual tiredness and weakness, swelling of the ankles, legs or fingers, difficulty breathing.

▽ **digoxin immune fab (bovine; digoxin-specific antibody fragments)**
(di jox' in)

DigiFab

PREGNANCY CATEGORY C

Drug class
Antidote

Therapeutic actions
Antigen-binding fragments (fab) derived from specific antidigoxin antibodies; binds molecules of digoxin, making them unavailable at the site of action; fab-fragment complex accumulates in the blood and is excreted by the kidneys.

Indications

- Treatment of potentially life-threatening digoxin toxicity (serum digoxin level exceeding 10 nanograms/mL, serum K+ exceeding 5 mEq/L in setting of digoxin toxicity)

Contraindications and cautions

- Contraindicated with allergy to sheep products.
- Use cautiously with pregnancy or lactation.

Available forms

Powder for injection—40 mg/vial

Dosages

Adults and pediatric patients

Dosage is determined by serum digoxin level or estimate of the amount of digoxin ingested. If no estimate is available and serum digoxin levels cannot be obtained, use 800 mg (20 vials), which should treat most life-threatening ingestions in adults and children.

- Estimated fab fragment dose based on amount of digoxin ingested:

Estimated Number of 0.25-mg Tablets or 0.2-mg Capsules Ingested	Dose (Number of Vials of DigiFab)
25	10
50	20
75	30
100	40
150	60
200	80

- Estimated fab fragments dose based on serum digoxin concentration:

Wt (kg)	Serum Digoxin Concentration (ng/mL)						
	1	2	4	8	12	16	20
Pediatric patients (dose in mg)*							
1	0.4	1	1.5	3	5	6.5	8
3	1	2.5	5	10	14	19	24
5	2	4	8	16	24	32	40
10	4	8	16	32	48	64	80
20	8	16	32	64	96	128	160
Adults (dose in vials)							
40	0.5	1	2	3	5	7	8
60	0.5	1	3	5	7	10	12
70	1	2	3	6	9	11	14
80	1	2	3	7	10	13	16
100	1	2	4	8	12	16	20

* Dilution of reconstituted vial to 1 mg/mL is desirable.

Equations also are available for calculating exact dosage from serum digoxin concentrations.

Pharmacokinetics

Route	Onset	Duration
IV	15–30 min	4–6 hr

Metabolism: $T_{1/2}$: 15–20 hr
Distribution: May cross placenta; may enter breast milk
Excretion: Urine

▼ IV FACTS

Preparation: Dissolve the contents in each vial with 4 mL of sterile water for injection. Mix gently to give an approximate isosmotic solution with a protein concentration of 10 mg/mL. Use reconstituted solution promptly. Store in refrigerator for up to 4 hr. Discard after that time. Reconstituted solution may be further diluted with sterile isotonic saline.
Infusion: Administer IV over 30 min.

Adverse effects

- **CV:** *Low cardiac output states,* **heart failure,** rapid ventricular response in patients with atrial fibrillation
- **Hematologic:** Hypokalemia due to reactivation of Na+, K+, ATPase
- **Hypersensitivity:** Allergic reactions: Drug fever to **anaphylaxis**

■ Nursing considerations

Assessment

- **History:** Allergy to sheep products, digoxin drug history, lactation, pregnancy
- **Physical:** P, BP, auscultation, baseline ECG, serum digoxin levels, serum electrolytes

Interventions

- Arrange for serum digoxin concentration determinations before administration when possible.
- Monitor patient's cardiac response to digoxin overdose and therapy—cardiac rhythm, serum electrolytes, T, BP.
- Keep life-support equipment and emergency drugs (IV inotropes) readily available for severe overdose.

⊗ *Warning* Do not redigitalize patient until digoxin immune-fab has been cleared from the body; several days to a week or longer in cases of renal insufficiency. Serum digoxin levels will be very high and will be unreliable for up to 3 days after administration.

Teaching points
- This drug is given IV to help reduce the level of digoxin in your body.
- Report muscle cramps, dizziness, palpitations.

▽dihydroergotamine mesylate

See Appendix R, *Less commonly used drugs*.

▽diltiazem hydrochloride
(dil tye' a zem)

Apo-Diltiaz (CAN), Apo-Diltiaz CD (CAN) ⊙ⓃⒸ, Apo-Diltiaz SR (CAN) ⊙ⓃⒸ, Cardizem, Cardizem CD ⊙ⓃⒸ, Cardizem LA ⊙ⓃⒸ, Cartia XT ⊙ⓃⒸ, Dilt-CD ⊙ⓃⒸ, Dilt-XR ⊙ⓃⒸ, Diltia XT ⊙ⓃⒸ, Diltzac ⊙ⓃⒸ, Gen-Diltiazem (CAN), Gen-Diltiazem CD (CAN) ⊙ⓃⒸ, Novo-Diltiazem (CAN), Novo-Diltiazem CD (CAN) ⊙ⓃⒸ, Nu-Diltiaz (CAN), Nu-Diltiaz-CD (CAN) ⊙ⓃⒸ, ratio-Diltiazem (CAN), Taztia XT ⊙ⓃⒸ, Tiazac ⊙ⓃⒸ

PREGNANCY CATEGORY C

Drug classes
Antianginal
Antihypertensive
Calcium channel blocker

Therapeutic actions
Inhibits the movement of calcium ions across the membranes of cardiac and arterial muscle cells, resulting in the depression of impulse formation in specialized cardiac pacemaker cells, slowing of the velocity of conduction of the cardiac impulse, depression of myocardial contractility, and dilation of coronary arteries and arterioles and peripheral arterioles; these effects lead to decreased cardiac work, decreased cardiac energy consumption, and in patients with

vasospastic (Prinzmetal) angina, increased delivery of oxygen to myocardial cells.

Indications
- Angina pectoris due to coronary artery spasm (Prinzmetal variant angina)
- Effort-associated angina; chronic stable angina in patients not controlled by beta-adrenergic blockers, nitrates
- ER and SR forms only: Essential hypertension
- Parenteral: Paroxysmal supraventricular tachycardia, atrial fibrillation, atrial flutter

Contraindications and cautions
- Contraindicated with allergy to diltiazem, impaired hepatic or renal function, sick sinus syndrome, heart block (second or third degree), severe hypertension, cardiogenic shock, acute MI with cardiogenic shock (oral), lactation.

Available forms
Tablets—30, 60, 90, 120 mg; ER capsules ⊙ⓃⒸ—60, 90, 120, 180, 240, 300, 360, 420 mg; ER tablets ⊙ⓃⒸ—120, 180, 240, 300, 360, 420 mg; injection—5 mg/mL; powder for injection—25 mg

Dosages
Evaluate patient carefully to determine the appropriate dose of this drug.
Adults
Initially, 30 mg PO qid before meals and at bedtime; gradually increase dose at 1- to 2-day intervals to 180–360 mg PO in three to four divided doses.
ER
Cardizem CD and Cartia XT: 180–240 mg daily PO for hypertension; 120–180 mg daily PO for angina.
Cardizem LA: 120–540 mg daily PO for hypertension; 180–360 mg/day PO for chronic, stable angina. May be given with nitroglycerin or nitrate therapy.
Diltia XT, Dilt-CD, and Dilt-XR: 180–240 mg daily PO as needed; up to 480 mg has been used.
Tiazac, Taztia XT: 120–240 mg daily PO for hypertension—once daily dose; 120–180 mg PO once daily for angina.

IV

Direct IV bolus: 0.25 mg/kg over 2 min (20 mg for the average patient); give second bolus of 0.35 mg/kg over 2 min after 15 min if response is inadequate.

Continuous IV infusion: 5–10 mg/hr with increases up to 15 mg/hr; may be continued for up to 24 hr.

Pediatric patients
Safety and efficacy not established.

Pharmacokinetics

Route	Onset	Peak
Oral	30–60 min	2–3 hr
ER	30–60 min	6–11 hr
IV	Immediate	2–3 min

Metabolism: Hepatic; $T_{1/2}$: 3.5–6 hr; 5–7 hr (ER)
Distribution: May cross placenta; enters breast milk
Excretion: Urine

▼ IV FACTS

Preparation: For continuous infusion, transfer to normal saline, D_5W, $D_5W/0.45\%$ sodium chloride as below. Mix thoroughly. Use within 24 hr. Keep refrigerated.

Diluent Volume (mL)	Quantity of Injection	Final Concentration (mg/mL)	Dose (mg/hr)	Infusion Rate (mL/hr)
100	125 mg	1	10	10
	(25 mL)	—	15	15
250	250 mg	0.83	10	12
	(50 mL)	—	15	18
500	250 mg	0.45	10	22
	(50 mL)	—	15	33

Infusion: Administer bolus dose over 2 min. For continuous infusion, rate of 10 mg/hr is the recommended rate. Do not use continuous infusion longer than 24 hr.
Incompatibility: Do not mix in the same solution with furosemide solution.

Adverse effects

- **CNS:** *Dizziness, light-headedness, headache, asthenia,* fatigue
- **CV:** *Peripheral edema,* hypotension, arrhythmias, *bradycardia, AV block,* **asystole**
- **Dermatologic:** *Flushing,* rash

- **GI:** *Nausea,* hepatic injury, reflux, constipation

Interactions

✳ **Drug-drug** • Increased serum levels and toxicity of cyclosporine if taken with diltiazem • Possible depression of myocardial contractility, AV conduction if combined with beta blockers; use caution and monitor patient closely • Possible increased diltiazem toxicity if combined with amiodarone, cimetidine • Possible decreased diltiazem level with rifampin • Risk of increased statin level and toxicity if statin combined with diltiazem; if this combination is used, monitor patient closely

✳ **Drug-food** • Decreased metabolism and increased risk of toxic effects if taken with grapefruit juice; avoid this combination

■ Nursing considerations
Assessment

- **History:** Allergy to diltiazem, impaired hepatic or renal function, sick sinus syndrome, heart block, lactation, pregnancy
- **Physical:** Skin lesions, color, edema; P, BP, baseline ECG, peripheral perfusion, auscultation; R, adventitious sounds; liver evaluation, normal output; LFTs, renal function tests, urinalysis

Interventions

- Monitor patient carefully (BP, cardiac rhythm, and output) while drug is being titrated to therapeutic dose; dosage may be increased more rapidly in hospitalized patients under close supervision.
- Monitor BP carefully if patient is on concurrent doses of nitrates.
- Monitor cardiac rhythm regularly during stabilization of dosage and periodically during long-term therapy.
- Ensure patient swallows ER or SR preparations whole; do not cut, crush, or chew.

Teaching points

- Swallow extended-release and long-acting preparations whole; do not cut, crush, or chew; do not drink grapefruit juice while using this drug.
- You may experience these side effects: Nausea, vomiting (eat frequent small meals); headache (regulate light, noise, and temperature; medicate if severe).

• Report irregular heart beat, shortness of breath, swelling of the hands or feet, pronounced dizziness, constipation.

▷ **dimenhyDRINATE**
(dye men hye' dri nate)

Oral preparations: Apo-Dimenhydrinate (CAN), Dimetabs, Gravol (CAN), Triptone
Parenteral preparations: Dramanate, Dymenate
PREGNANCY CATEGORY B

Drug classes
Anticholinergic
Antihistamine
Anti–motion-sickness drug

Therapeutic actions
Antihistamine with antiemetic and anticholinergic activity; depresses hyperstimulated labyrinthine function; may block synapses in the vomiting center; peripheral anticholinergic effects may contribute to anti–motion-sickness efficacy.

Indications
• Prevention and treatment of nausea, vomiting, or vertigo of motion sickness
• Unlabeled use: Treatment of nausea and vomiting of pregnancy.

Contraindications and cautions
• Contraindicated with allergy to dimenhydrinate or its components, lactation.
• Use cautiously with narrow-angle glaucoma, stenosing peptic ulcer, symptomatic prostatic hypertrophy, bronchial asthma, bladder neck obstruction, pyloroduodenal obstruction, cardiac arrhythmias, pregnancy.

Available forms
Tablets—50 mg; chewable tablets—50 mg; injection—50 mg/mL; liquid—12.5 mg/4 mL, 12.5 mg/5 mL; 15.62 mg/5 mL

Dosages
Adults
Oral
50–100 mg every 4–6 hr PO; for prophylaxis, first dose should be taken 30 min before exposure to motion. Do not exceed 400 mg in 24 hr.
Parenteral
50 mg IM as needed; 50 mg in 10 mL sodium chloride injection given IV over 2 min.
Pediatric patients 6–12 yr
25–50 mg PO every 6–8 hr, not to exceed 150 mg/day.
Pediatric patients younger than 6 yr
Only on advice of physician; not recommended.
Neonates
Contraindicated.
Geriatric patients
Can cause dizziness, sedation, syncope, confusion, and hypotension in elderly patients; use with caution.

Pharmacokinetics

Route	Onset	Peak	Duration
Oral	15–30 min	2 hr	3–6 hr
IM	20–30 min	1–2 hr	3–6 hr
IV	Immediate	1–2 hr	3–6 hr

Metabolism: Hepatic; $T_{1/2}$: Unknown
Distribution: May cross placenta; enters breast milk
Excretion: Urine

■ IV FACTS
Preparation: Dilute 50 mg in 10 mL sodium chloride injection.
Infusion: Administer by direct IV injection over 2 min.
Incompatibilities: Do not combine with tetracycline, thiopental.
Y-site incompatibilities: Do not mix with aminophylline, heparin, hydrocortisone, hydroxyzine, phenobarbital, phenytoin, prednisolone, promethazine.

Adverse effects
• **CNS:** *Drowsiness, confusion, nervousness, restlessness, headache, dizziness, vertigo, lassitude, tingling, heaviness and weakness of hands; insomnia* and excitement (especially in children), hallucinations, seizures, **death,** blurring of vision, diplopia
• **CV:** Hypotension, palpitations, tachycardia
• **Dermatologic:** Urticaria, drug rash, photosensitivity

Adverse effects in *italics* are most common; those in **bold** are life-threatening. ▣ Do not crush.

- **GI:** Epigastric distress, anorexia, nausea, vomiting, diarrhea or constipation; dryness of mouth, nose, and throat
- **GU:** Urinary hesitancy, urinary retention
- **Respiratory:** Nasal stuffiness, chest tightness, thickening of bronchial secretions
- **Other: Anaphylaxis;** in geriatric patients may cause mental status changes, excessive sedation, constipation; in men, may cause urinary retention

Interactions
❋ **Drug-drug** • Increased depressant effects with alcohol, other CNS depressants

■ Nursing considerations
Assessment
- **History:** Allergy to dimenhydrinate or its components, lactation, narrow-angle glaucoma, stenosing peptic ulcer, symptomatic prostatic hypertrophy, bronchial asthma, bladder neck obstruction, pyloroduodenal obstruction, cardiac arrhythmias
- **Physical:** Skin color, lesions, texture; orientation, reflexes, affect; vision examination; P, BP; R, adventitious sounds; bowel sounds; prostate palpation; CBC

Interventions
⊗ **Warning** Keep epinephrine 1:1,000 readily available when using parenteral preparations; hypersensitivity reactions, including anaphylaxis, have occurred.

Teaching points
- Take drug as prescribed; avoid excessive dosage.
- Drug works best if taken before motion sickness occurs.
- Avoid alcohol; serious sedation could occur.
- You may experience these side effects: Dizziness, sedation, drowsiness (use caution if driving or performing tasks that require alertness); epigastric distress, diarrhea or constipation (take drug with food); dry mouth (use frequent mouth care, suck sugarless candies); thickening of bronchial secretions, dryness of nasal mucosa (try another motion sickness remedy).
- Report difficulty breathing, hallucinations, tremors, loss of coordination, unusual bleeding or bruising, visual disturbances, irregular heartbeat.

▽ **dimercaprol**

See Appendix R, *Less commonly used drugs.*

▽ **dinoprostone (prostaglandin E₂)**
*(dye noe **prost'** ohn)*

Cervidil, Prepidil, Prostin E2

PREGNANCY CATEGORY C

Drug classes
Abortifacient
Prostaglandin

Therapeutic actions
Stimulates the myometrium of the pregnant uterus to contract, similar to the contractions of the uterus during labor, thus evacuating the contents of the uterus.

Indications
- Termination of pregnancy 12–20 wk from the first day of the last menstrual period
- Evacuation of the uterus in the management of missed abortion or intrauterine fetal death up to 28 wk gestational age
- Management of nonmetastatic gestational trophoblastic disease (benign hydatidiform mole)
- Initiation of cervical ripening before induction of labor

Contraindications and cautions
- Contraindicated with allergy to prostaglandin preparations; acute PID; active cardiac, hepatic, pulmonary, renal disease; women in whom prolonged uterine contractions are inappropriate (eg, caesarean delivery, uterine surgery, fetal distress, obstetric emergency).
- Use cautiously with history of asthma; hypotension; hypertension; CV, adrenal, renal, or hepatic disease; anemia; jaundice; diabetes; epilepsy; scarred uterus; cervicitis; infected endocervical lesions, acute vaginitis.

Available forms
Vaginal suppository—20 mg; vaginal gel—0.5 mg; vaginal insert—10 mg

Dosages
Adults
- *Termination of pregnancy:* Insert one suppository (20 mg) high into the vagina; keep supine for 10 min after insertion. Additional suppositories may be given at 3- to 5-hr intervals based on uterine response and tolerance. Do not give longer than 2 days.
- *Cervical ripening:* Give 0.5 mg gel via provided cervical catheter with patient in the dorsal position and cervix visualized using a speculum. Repeat dose may be given if no response in 6 hr. Wait 6–12 hr before beginning oxytocin IV to initiate labor. Insert: Place one insert transversely in the posterior fornix of the vagina. Keep patient supine for 2 hr; one insert delivers 0.3 mg/hr over 12 hr. Remove, using retrieval system, at onset of active labor or 12 hr after insertion.

Pharmacokinetics

Route	Onset	Peak	Duration
Intravaginal	10 min	30–45 min	2–3 hr

Metabolism: Tissue; $T_{1/2}$: 5–10 hr
Distribution: May cross placenta; may enter breast milk
Excretion: Urine

Adverse effects
- **CNS:** *Headache,* paresthesias, anxiety, weakness, syncope, dizziness
- **CV:** *Hypotension,* arrhythmias, chest pain
- **Fetal:** Abnormal heart rates
- **GI:** *Vomiting, diarrhea, nausea*
- **GU:** Endometritis, perforated uterus, uterine rupture, uterine or vaginal pain, incomplete abortion
- **Respiratory:** Coughing, dyspnea
- **Other:** Chills, diaphoresis, backache, breast tenderness, eye pain, skin rash, pyrexia

■ Nursing considerations

★ CLINICAL ALERT!
Name confusion has occurred among *Prostin VR Pediatric* (alprostadil), *Prostin FZ* (dinoprost—available outside the US), *Prostin E₂* (dinoprostone), and *Prostin 15* (carboprost in Europe). Use extreme caution.

Assessment
- **History:** Allergy to prostaglandin preparations; acute PID; active cardiac, hepatic, pulmonary, renal disease; history of asthma; hypotension; hypertension; anemia; jaundice; diabetes; epilepsy; scarred uterus; cervicitis, infected endocervical lesions, acute vaginitis
- **Physical:** T; BP, P, auscultation; R, adventitious sounds; bowel sounds, liver evaluation; vaginal discharge, pelvic examination, uterine tone; LFTs, renal function tests, WBC, urinalysis, CBC

Interventions
- Store suppositories in freezer; bring to room temperature before insertion.
- Store cervical gel in refrigerator. Gel is stable for 24 mo at 2°–8°C.
- Arrange for pre- or concurrent treatment with antiemetic and antidiarrheal drugs to decrease the incidence of GI side effects.
- Ensure that abortion is complete or that other measures are used to complete the abortion if drug effects are not sufficient.
- Monitor temperature, using care to differentiate prostaglandin-induced pyrexia from postabortion endometritis pyrexia.
- Give gel using aseptic technique via cervical catheter to patient in dorsal position. Patient should remain in this position 15–30 min.
- Monitor uterine tone and vaginal discharge throughout procedure and several days after the procedure.
- Ensure adequate hydration throughout procedure.
- Be prepared to support patient through labor (cervical ripening). Give oxytocin infusion 6–12 hr after dinoprostone.

Teaching points
- If you have never had a vaginal suppository, a health care provider will explain the procedure. You will need to lie down for 10 minutes after insertion.
- You will need to stay on your side for 15–30 minutes after injection of gel.
- You may experience these side effects: Nausea, vomiting, diarrhea, uterine or vaginal pain, fever, headache, weakness, dizziness.
- Report severe pain, difficulty breathing, palpitations, eye pain, rash.

▷diphenhydrAMINE hydrochloride

(dye fen hye' dra meen)

Oral: Allerdryl (CAN), AllerMax Caplets, Banophen, Banophen Allergy, Benadryl Allergy, Diphen AF, Diphenhist, Diphenhist Captabs, Genahist, Siladryl

Oral prescription preparations: Benadryl

Parenteral preparations: Benadryl

PREGNANCY CATEGORY B

Drug classes
Antihistamine
Anti–motion-sickness drug
Antiparkinsonian
Cough suppressant
Sedative-hypnotic

Therapeutic actions
Competitively blocks the effects of histamine at H_1-receptor sites, has atropine-like, antipruritic, and sedative effects.

Indications
- Relief of symptoms associated with perennial and seasonal allergic rhinitis; vasomotor rhinitis; allergic conjunctivitis; mild, uncomplicated urticaria and angioedema; amelioration of allergic reactions to blood or plasma; dermatographism; adjunctive therapy in anaphylactic reactions
- Active and prophylactic treatment of motion sickness
- Nighttime sleep aid
- Parkinsonism (including drug-induced parkinsonism and extrapyramidal reactions), in the elderly intolerant of more potent drugs, for milder forms of the disorder in other age groups, and in combination with centrally acting anticholinergic antiparkinsonian drugs
- Syrup formulation: Suppression of cough due to colds or allergy

Contraindications and cautions
- Contraindicated with allergy to antihistamines, third trimester of pregnancy, lactation.

- Use cautiously with narrow-angle glaucoma, stenosing peptic ulcer, symptomatic prostatic hypertrophy, asthmatic attack, bladder neck obstruction, pyloroduodenal obstruction, pregnancy; elderly patients who may be sensitive to anticholinergic effects.

Available forms
Capsule soft gels—25 mg; capsules—25, 50 mg; tablets—25, 50 mg; chewable tablets—12.5 mg; elixir—12.5 mg/5 mL; syrup—12.5 mg/5 mL; liquid—12.5 mg/5 mL; injection—10, 50 mg/mL; solution—12.5 mg/5 mL

Dosages
Adults
Oral
25–50 mg every 4–6 hr PO, not to exceed 300 mg/24 hr.
- *Motion sickness:* Give full dose prophylactically 30 min before exposure to motion, and repeat before meals and at bedtime.
- *Nighttime sleep aid:* 50 mg PO at bedtime.
- *Cough suppression:* 25 mg every 4 hr PO, not to exceed 150 mg in 24 hr (syrup).
Parenteral
10–50 mg IV or deep IM or up to 100 mg if required. Maximum daily dose is 400 mg.
Pediatric patients
Oral
6–12 yr: 12.5–25 mg tid–qid PO or 5 mg/kg/day PO or 150 mg/m² per day PO. Maximum daily dose, 150 mg.
- *Motion sickness:*
  6–12 yr: 12.5–25 mg every 4–6 hr; do not exceed 150 mg/day.
- *Cough suppression:*
  6–12 yr: 12.5 mg every 4 hr PO, not to exceed 75 mg in 24 hr (syrup).
Parenteral
5 mg/kg/day or 150 mg/m² per day IV or by deep IM injection. Maximum daily dose is 300 mg divided into four doses.
Geriatric patients
More likely to cause dizziness, sedation, syncope, toxic confusional states, and hypotension in elderly patients; use with caution.

Pharmacokinetics

Route	Onset	Peak	Duration
Oral	15–30 min	1–4 hr	4–7 hr
IM	20–30 min	1–4 hr	4–8 hr
IV	Rapid	30–60 min	4–8 hr

Metabolism: Hepatic; $T_{1/2}$: 2.5–7 hr
Distribution: May cross placenta; may enter breast milk
Excretion: Urine

▼ IV FACTS

Preparation: No additional preparation required.
Infusion: Administer slowly each 25 mg over 1 min by direct injection or into tubing of running IV.
Incompatibilities: Do not combine with amobarbital, amphotericin B, hydrocortisone, phenobarbital, phenytoin, thiopental.
Y-site incompatibility: Do not mix with foscarnet.

Adverse effects

- **CNS:** *Drowsiness, sedation, dizziness, disturbed coordination,* fatigue, confusion, restlessness, excitation, nervousness, tremor, headache, blurred vision, diplopia
- **CV:** Hypotension, palpitations, bradycardia, tachycardia, extrasystoles
- **GI:** *Epigastric distress,* anorexia, increased appetite and weight gain, nausea, vomiting, diarrhea or constipation
- **GU:** Urinary frequency, dysuria, urinary retention, early menses, decreased libido, impotence
- **Hematologic: Hemolytic anemia, hypoplastic anemia, thrombocytopenia, leukopenia, agranulocytosis, pancytopenia**
- **Respiratory:** *Thickening of bronchial secretions,* chest tightness, wheezing, nasal stuffiness, dry mouth, dry nose, dry throat, sore throat
- **Other:** Urticaria, rash, **anaphylactic shock,** photosensitivity, excessive perspiration

Interactions

* **Drug-drug** • Possible increased and prolonged anticholinergic effects with MAOIs • Risk of increased sedation with alcohol, CNS depressants; avoid this combination

■ Nursing considerations
Assessment

- **History:** Allergy to any antihistamines, narrow-angle glaucoma, stenosing peptic ulcer, symptomatic prostatic hypertrophy, asthmatic attack, bladder neck obstruction, pyloroduodenal obstruction, third trimester of pregnancy, lactation
- **Physical:** Skin color, lesions, texture; orientation, reflexes, affect; vision examination; P, BP; R, adventitious sounds; bowel sounds; prostate palpation; CBC with differential

Interventions

- Administer with food if GI upset occurs.
- Administer syrup form if patient is unable to take tablets.
- Monitor patient response, and arrange for adjustment of dosage to lowest possible effective dose.

Teaching points

- Take as prescribed; avoid excessive dosage.
- Take with food if GI upset occurs.
- Avoid alcohol; serious sedation could occur.
- These side effects may occur: Dizziness, sedation, drowsiness (use caution driving or performing tasks requiring alertness); epigastric distress, diarrhea or constipation (take drug with meals); dry mouth (use frequent mouth care, suck sugarless candies); thickening of bronchial secretions, dryness of nasal mucosa (use a humidifier).
- Report difficulty breathing, hallucinations, tremors, loss of coordination, unusual bleeding or bruising, visual disturbances, irregular heartbeat.

▷ dipyridamole

See Appendix R, *Less commonly used drugs.*

▷ disopyramide phosphate
*(dye soe **peer'** a mide)*

Norpace, Norpace CR, Rythmodan (CAN), Rythmodan-LA (CAN)

PREGNANCY CATEGORY C

Drug class
Antiarrhythmic

Adverse effects in *italics* are most common; those in **bold** are life-threatening. Do not crush.

Therapeutic actions

Type 1a antiarrhythmic: Decreases rate of diastolic depolarization, decreases automaticity, decreases the rate of rise of the action potential, prolongs the refractory period of cardiac muscle cells.

Indications

- Treatment of ventricular arrhythmias considered to be life-threatening
- Unlabeled use: Treatment of paroxysmal supraventricular tachycardia

Contraindications and cautions

- Contraindicated with cardiogenic shock, allergy to disopyramide, cardiac conduction abnormalities (eg, Wolff-Parkinson-White syndrome, sick sinus syndrome, heart block, prolonged QT interval).
- Use cautiously with heart failure, hypotension, cardiac myopathies, urinary retention, glaucoma, myasthenia gravis, renal or hepatic disease, potassium imbalance, pregnancy, lactation.

Available forms

Capsules—100, 150 mg; CR capsules ⒪—100, 150 mg; ER tablets ⒪—150 mg (CAN)

Dosages

Evaluate patient carefully and monitor cardiac response closely to determine the correct dosage for each patient.

Adults
400–800 mg/day PO given in divided doses every 6 hr or every 12 hr if using the CR products.

- *Rapid control of ventricular arrhythmias:* 300 mg PO (immediate release). If no response within 6 hr, give 200 mg PO every 6 hr; may increase to 250–300 mg every 6 hr if no response in 48 hr.
- *Patients with cardiomyopathy:* No loading dose, 100 mg PO every 6–8 hr (immediate release).

Pediatric patients
Give in equal, divided doses every 6 hr PO, adjusting the dose to the patient's need.

Age	Daily Dosage (mg/kg)
Younger than 1 yr	10–30
1–4 yr	10–20
4–12 yr	10–15
12–18 yr	6–15

Patients with renal impairment
Loading dose of 150 mg PO may be given, followed by 100 mg at the intervals shown.

Creatinine Clearance (mL/min)	Interval
30–40	Every 8 hr
15–30	Every 12 hr
Less than 15	Every 24 hr

Pharmacokinetics

Route	Onset	Peak	Duration
Oral	30–60 min	2 hr	1.5–8.5 hr

Metabolism: Hepatic; $T_{1/2}$: 4–10 hr
Distribution: Crosses placenta; enters breast milk
Excretion: Urine

Adverse effects

- **CNS:** Dizziness, fatigue, headache, *blurred vision*
- **CV: HF,** hypotension, cardiac conduction disturbances
- **GI:** *Dry mouth, constipation,* nausea, abdominal pain, gas
- **GU:** *Urinary hesitancy and retention, impotence*
- **Other:** *Dry nose, eyes, and throat; rash; itching; muscle weakness; malaise; aches and pains*

Interactions

✳ **Drug-drug** • Decreased disopyramide plasma levels if used with phenytoins, rifampin
- Risk of increased disopyramide effects with antiarrhythmics, erythromycin, quinidine

■ Nursing considerations
Assessment

- **History:** Allergy to disopyramide, heart failure, hypotension, Wolff-Parkinson-White syndrome, sick sinus syndrome, heart block, cardiac myopathies, urinary retention, glaucoma, myasthenia gravis, renal or hepatic disease, potassium imbalance, labor or delivery, lactation, pregnancy
- **Physical:** Weight; orientation, reflexes; P, BP, auscultation, ECG, edema; R, adventitious sounds; bowel sounds, liver evaluation; urinalysis, LFTs, renal function tests, blood glucose, serum K^+

Interventions

⊗ **Black box warning** Monitor patient for possible refractory arrhythmias that can be life-threatening; reserve use for life-threatening arrhythmias.

- Check that patients with supraventricular tachyarrhythmias have been digitalized before starting disopyramide.
- Reduce dosage in patients weighing less than 110 lb.
- Reduce dosage in patients with hepatic or renal failure.
- Monitor patients with severe refractory tachycardia, who may be given up to 1,600 mg/day continuously.
- Make a pediatric suspension form (1–10 mg/mL) by adding contents of the immediate-release capsule to cherry syrup, if desired. Store in amber glass bottle, and refrigerate. Shake well before using. Stable for 1 mo.
- Take care to differentiate the CR form from the immediate-release preparation. Ensure that patient swallows CR form whole; do not cut, crush, or chew.
- Monitor BP, orthostatic pressure.

⊗ **Warning** Evaluate for safe and effective serum levels (2–8 mcg/mL).

Teaching points

- You will require frequent monitoring of cardiac rhythm and blood pressure.
- Swallow controlled-release capsules whole; do not cut, crush, or chew.
- Take missed dose as soon as possible, unless within 4 hours of next dose. Do not double up on next dose.
- Do not stop taking this drug for any reason without consulting your health care provider.
- Return for regular follow-up visits to check your heart rhythm and blood pressure.
- You may experience these side effects: Dry mouth (try frequent mouth care, suck sugarless candies); constipation (laxatives may be ordered); difficulty voiding (empty the bladder before taking drug); muscle weakness or aches and pains.
- Report swelling of fingers or ankles, difficulty breathing, dizziness, urinary retention, severe headache or visual changes.

▽ **disulfiram**
(dye **sul'** fi ram)

Antabuse

PREGNANCY CATEGORY C

Drug classes
Antialcoholic drug
Enzyme inhibitor

Therapeutic actions
Inhibits the enzyme aldehyde dehydrogenase, blocking oxidation of alcohol and allowing acetaldehyde to accumulate to concentrations in the blood 5–10 times higher than normally achieved during alcohol metabolism; accumulation of acetaldehyde produces the highly unpleasant reaction described below that deters consumption of alcohol.

Indications
- Aids in the management of selected chronic alcoholics who want to remain in a state of enforced sobriety

Contraindications and cautions
- Contraindicated with allergy to disulfiram or other thiuram derivatives used in pesticides and rubber vulcanization, severe myocardial disease or coronary occlusion; psychoses, current or recent treatment with metronidazole, paraldehyde, alcohol, alcohol-containing preparations (eg, cough syrups), pregnancy.
- Use cautiously with diabetes mellitus, hypothyroidism, epilepsy, cerebral damage, chronic and acute nephritis, hepatic cirrhosis or impairment.

Available forms
Tablets—250 mg

Dosages
⊗ **Black box warning** Never administer to an intoxicated patient or without patient's knowledge. Do not administer until patient has abstained from alcohol for at least 12 hr.

Adults
- *Initial dosage:* Administer maximum of 500 mg/day PO in a single dose for 1–2 wk. If a sedative effect occurs, administer at bedtime or decrease dosage.
- *Maintenance regimen:* 125–500 mg/day PO. Do not exceed 500 mg/day. Continue

use until patient fully recovers socially and has basis for permanent self-control.

Pharmacokinetics

Route	Onset	Peak	Duration
Oral	Slow	12 hr	1–2 wk

Metabolism: Hepatic; $T_{1/2}$: Unclear
Distribution: Crosses placenta; enters breast milk
Excretion: Feces, lungs

Adverse effects
Disulfiram with alcohol

- **CNS:** Throbbing headaches, syncope, weakness, vertigo, confusion, seizures, unconsciousness, throbbing in head and neck
- **CV:** Flushing, chest pain, palpitations, tachycardia, hypotension, **arrhythmias, CV collapse, acute HF, MI**
- **Dermatologic:** Sweating
- **EENT:** Blurred vision
- **GI:** Nausea, copious vomiting, thirst
- **Respiratory:** Respiratory difficulty, dyspnea, hyperventilation
- **Other:** Death

Disulfiram alone

- **CNS:** *Drowsiness, fatigability, headache,* restlessness, peripheral neuropathy, optic or retrobulbar neuritis
- **Dermatologic:** *Skin eruptions,* acneiform eruptions, allergic dermatitis
- **GI:** *Metallic or garlic-like aftertaste,* **hepatotoxicity**

Interactions

✳ Drug-drug ● Increased serum levels and risk of toxicity of phenytoin and its congeners, diazepam, chlordiazepoxide ● Increased therapeutic and toxic effects of theophyllines and caffeine ● Increased PT caused by disulfiram may lead to a need to adjust dosage of oral anticoagulants ● Severe alcohol-intolerance reactions with any alcohol-containing liquid medications (eg, elixirs, tinctures) ● Acute toxic psychosis with metronidazole

■ Nursing considerations
Assessment

- **History:** Allergy to disulfiram or other thiuram derivatives; severe myocardial disease or coronary occlusion; psychoses; current or recent treatment with metronidazole, paraldehyde, alcohol, alcohol-containing

preparations (eg, cough syrups, tonics); diabetes mellitus, hypothyroidism, epilepsy, cerebral damage, chronic and acute nephritis, hepatic cirrhosis or impairment; pregnancy
- **Physical:** Skin color, lesions; thyroid palpation; orientation, affect, reflexes; P, auscultation, BP; R, adventitious sounds; liver evaluation; LFTs, renal function tests, CBC, SMA-12

Interventions

- Do not administer until patient has abstained from alcohol for at least 12 hr.
- Administer orally; tablets may be crushed and mixed with liquid beverages.
- Monitor LFTs before, in 10–14 days, and every 6 mo during therapy to evaluate for hepatic impairment.
- Monitor CBC, SMA-12 before and every 6 mo during therapy.
- If patient reports ability to drink alcohol while on this drug, assume noncompliance. Directly observe drug ingestion.
- Inform patient about the seriousness of disulfiram–alcohol reaction and the potential consequences of alcohol use. Disulfiram should not be taken for at least 12 hr after alcohol ingestion, and a reaction may occur up to 2 wk after disulfiram therapy is stopped; all forms of alcohol must be avoided.
- Arrange for treatment with antihistamines if skin reaction occurs.
- ⊗ **Warning** Institute supportive measures if disulfiram-alcohol reaction occurs; oxygen, carbon dioxide combination, massive doses of vitamin C IV, ephedrine have been used.

Teaching points

- Take drug daily; if drug makes you dizzy or tired, take it at bedtime. Tablets may be crushed and mixed with liquid.
- Abstain from forms of alcohol (beer, wine, liquor, vinegars, cough mixtures, sauces, aftershave lotions, liniments, colognes, liquid medications). Using alcohol while taking this drug can cause severe, unpleasant reactions—flushing, copious vomiting, throbbing headache, difficulty breathing, even death.
- Wear or carry a medical ID while you are taking this drug to alert any medical emergency personnel that you are taking it.
- Have periodic blood tests while taking drug to evaluate its effects on the liver.

- You may experience these side effects: Drowsiness, headache, fatigue, restlessness, blurred vision (use caution driving or performing tasks that require alertness); metallic aftertaste (transient).
- Report unusual bleeding or bruising, yellowing of skin or eyes, chest pain, difficulty breathing, ingestion of any alcohol.

DANGEROUS DRUG

▷ **DOBUTamine hydrochloride**
(*doe' byoo ta meen*)

PREGNANCY CATEGORY B

Drug classes
Beta₁-selective adrenergic agonist
Sympathomimetic

Therapeutic actions
Positive inotropic effects are mediated by beta₁-adrenergic receptors in the heart; increases the force of myocardial contraction with relatively minor effects on heart rate, arrhythmogenesis; has minor effects on blood vessels.

Indications
- For inotropic support in the short-term treatment of cardiac decompensation due to depressed contractility, resulting from either organic heart disease or from cardiac surgical procedures
- Unlabeled uses: In children with congenital heart disease undergoing diagnostic cardiac catheterization, to augment CV function

Contraindications and cautions
- Contraindicated with IHSS; hypovolemia (dobutamine is not a substitute for blood, plasma, fluids, electrolytes, which should be restored promptly when loss has occurred and in any case before treatment with dobutamine); acute MI (may increase the size of an infarct by intensifying ischemia); general anesthesia with halogenated hydrocarbons or cyclopropane, which sensitize the myocardium to catecholamines; pregnancy.
- Use cautiously with diabetes mellitus, lactation; allergy to sulfites, more common in asthmatic patients.

Available forms
Injection—12.5 mg/mL; injection in 5% dextrose injection—1 mg/mL, 2 mg/mL, 4 mg/mL

Dosages
Administer only by IV infusion using an infusion pump or other device to control the rate of flow. Titrate on the basis of the patient's hemodynamic and renal responses. Close monitoring is necessary.
Adults
2–20 mcg/kg/min IV is usual rate to increase cardiac output; rarely, rates up to 40 mcg/kg/min are needed.
Pediatric patients
Initially, 0.5–1 mcg/kg/min as continuous IV infusion. Maintenance dose, 2–20 mcg/kg/min; on rare occasions up to 40 mcg/kg/min may be needed.

Pharmacokinetics

Route	Onset	Peak	Duration
IV	1–2 min	Up to 10 min	Length of infusion

Metabolism: Hepatic; T₁/₂: 2 min
Distribution: May cross placenta; may enter breast milk
Excretion: Urine

▼ IV FACTS

Preparation: Dilute vials to at least 50 mL with 5% dextrose injection, 0.9% sodium chloride injection, or sodium lactate injection. Store final diluted solution in glass or Viaflex container at room temperature. Stable for 24 hr. Do not freeze. (Drug solutions may exhibit a pink color that increases with time; this indicates oxidation of the drug, not a loss of potency up to 24 hr.)

Infusion: May be administered through common IV tubing with dopamine, lidocaine, tobramycin, nitroprusside, potassium chloride, or protamine sulfate. Titrate rate based on patient response—P, BP, rhythm; use of an infusion pump is suggested; do not give as an IV bolus.

Incompatibilities: Do not mix drug with alkaline solutions, such as 5% sodium bicarbonate injection; do not mix with hydrocortisone sodium succinate, cefazolin, penicillin, sodium ethacrynate; sodium heparin.

Y-site incompatibilities: Do not mix with acyclovir, alteplase, aminophylline, foscarnet.

Adverse effects in *italics* are most common; those in **bold** are life-threatening. ⬛ Do not crush.

Adverse effects

- **CNS:** *Headache*
- **CV:** *Increase in HR, increase in systolic BP, increase in ventricular ectopic beats (PVCs),* anginal pain, palpitations, shortness of breath
- **GI:** *Nausea*

Interactions

✳ **Drug-drug** • Increased effects with TCAs (eg, imipramine), methyldopa

■ Nursing considerations

CLINICAL ALERT!
Name confusion has occurred between dobutamine and dopamine; use caution.

Assessment

- **History:** IHSS, hypovolemia, acute MI, general anesthesia with halogenated hydrocarbons or cyclopropane, diabetes, lactation, pregnancy
- **Physical:** Weight, skin color, T; P, BP, pulse pressure, auscultation; R, adventitious sounds; urine output; serum electrolytes, Hct, ECG

Interventions

- Arrange to digitalize patients who have atrial fibrillation with a rapid ventricular rate before giving dobutamine—dobutamine facilitates AV conduction.
- ⊗ *Warning* Monitor urine flow, cardiac output, pulmonary wedge pressure, ECG, and BP closely during infusion; adjust dose and rate accordingly.

Teaching points

- Used only in acute emergencies; teaching depends on patient's awareness and emphasizes need for the drug.

DANGEROUS DRUG

▽**docetaxel**
*(dohs eh **tax' ell**)*

Taxotere

PREGNANCY CATEGORY D

Drug class

Antineoplastic (taxoid)

Therapeutic actions

Inhibits the normal dynamic reorganization of the microtubule network that is essential for dividing cells; leads to cell death in rapidly dividing cells.

Indications

- Treatment of patients with locally advanced or metastatic breast cancer after failure of prior chemotherapy
- Treatment of non–small-cell lung cancer after failure with platinum-based chemotherapy, with metastases
- First-line treatment of unresectable, locally advanced, or metastatic non–small-cell lung cancer in patients who have not received prior chemotherapy when used in combination with cisplatin
- Treatment of androgen-independent metastatic prostate cancer with prednisone
- Adjuvant post-surgery treatment of patients with operable node-positive breast cancer in combination with doxorubicin and cyclophosphamide
- Induction treatment of patients with locally advanced squamous cell carcinoma of the head and neck, in combination with cisplatin and 5-FU, before the patient undergoes chemoradiotherapy or radiotherapy
- Treatment of advanced gastric adenocarcinoma in patients who have not received chemotherapy for advanced disease with cisplatin and 5-FU
- Unlabeled uses: Esophageal, ovarian, small-cell lung, urothelial cancers

Contraindications and cautions

- Contraindicated with hypersensitivity to docetaxel or drugs using polysorbate 80; bone marrow depression with neutrophil counts less than 1,500 cells/mm^2, lactation, pregnancy.
- Use cautiously with hepatic impairment, history of treatment with platinum-based chemotherapy.

Available forms

Injection—20 mg/0.5 mL, 80 mg/2 mL

Dosages

Adults

- *Breast cancer:* 60–100 mg/m^2 IV infused over 1 hr every 3 wk.

- *Non–small-cell lung cancer:* 75 mg/m² IV over 1 hr every 3 wk.
- *First-line treatment of non–small-cell lung cancer:* 75 mg/m² of *Taxotere* given over 1 hr followed by 75 mg/m² cisplatin IV given over 30–60 min every 3 wk.
- *Androgen-independent metastatic prostate cancer:* 75 mg/m² IV every 3 wk as a 1-hr infusion with 5 mg prednisone PO bid constantly throughout therapy. Premedicate with dexamethasone 8 mg PO 12 hr, 3 hr, and 1 hr before docetaxel infusion. Reduce dosage to 60 mg/m² if febrile neutropenia, severe or cumulative cutaneous reactions, moderate neurosensory signs or symptoms, or neutrophil count less than 500 mm³ occurs for longer than 1 wk. Stop therapy if reactions continue with reduced dose.
- *Operable node-positive breast cancer:* 75 mg/m² IV given 1 hr after doxorubicin 50 mg/m² and cyclophosphamide 500 mg/m² every 3 wk for 6 courses. Adjust dosage based on neutrophil count.
- *Induction for squamous cell cancer of the head and neck before radiotherapy:* 75 mg/m² as a 1-hr IV infusion followed by cisplatin 75 mg/m² IV over 1 hr on day 1, followed by 5-FU 750 mg/m²/day IV for 5 days. Repeat every 3 wk for four cycles before radiotherapy starts.
- *Induction for squamous cell cancer of the head and neck before chemoradiotherapy:* 75 mg/m² as a 1-hr IV infusion, followed by cisplatin 100 mg/m² as a 30-min–3-hr infusion followed by 5-FU 1,000 mg/m²/day as a continuous infusion on days 1–4. Administer every 3 wk for three cycles before chemoradiotherapy starts. If GI toxicity occurs, consider reducing dosage of 5-FU, docetaxol, or both.
- *Advanced gastric adenocarcinoma:* 75 mg/m² IV as a 1-hr infusion followed by cisplatin 75 mg/m² IV as a 1- to 3-hr infusion (both on day 1), followed by 5-FU 750 mg/m²/day IV as a 24-hr infusion for 5 days. Repeat cycle every 3 wk.

Pediatric patients
Safety and efficacy not established.

Pharmacokinetics

Route	Onset	Duration
IV	Slow	20–24 hr

Metabolism: Hepatic; $T_{1/2}$: 36 min and 11.1 hr
Distribution: Crosses placenta; may enter breast milk
Excretion: Feces, urine

▼ IV FACTS

Preparation: Dilute concentrate with provided diluent; resultant concentration is 10 mg/mL. Stand vials at room temperature for 5 min before diluting; stable at room temperature for 8 hr; refrigerate unopened vials, protect from light; avoid use of PVC infusion bags and tubing. Final dilution: Add to 250 mL normal saline solution or 5% dextrose injection; final concentration is 0.3–0.74 mg/mL. Premedicate patient with oral corticosteroids before beginning infusion.
Infusion: Administer over 1 hr.

Adverse effects

- **CNS:** Neurosensory disturbances, including paresthesias, pain, *asthenia*
- **CV:** Sinus tachycardia, hypotension, arrhythmias, **fluid retention**
- **GI:** *Nausea, vomiting, diarrhea, stomatitis,* constipation
- **Hematologic: Bone marrow depression,** *infection*
- **Other:** *Hypersensitivity reactions, myalgia, arthralgia, alopecia*

Interactions

✳ **Drug-drug** • Possible increase in effectiveness and toxicity with cyclosporine, ketoconazole, erythromycin; avoid these combinations • Avoid giving live vaccines within 3 mo of administration because of immunosuppression

■ Nursing considerations

⚠ CLINICAL ALERT!
Name confusion has occurred between *Taxotere* (docetaxel) and *Taxol* (paclitaxel). Serious adverse effects can occur; use extreme caution.

Assessment

- **History:** Hypersensitivity to docetaxel, polysorbate 80; bone marrow depression; hepatic impairment, pregnancy, lactation

• **Physical:** Neurologic status, T; P, BP, peripheral perfusion; abdominal examination, mucous membranes; LFTs, CBC

Interventions

⊗ **Black box warning** Do not give drug unless blood counts are within acceptable parameters (neutrophils exceed 1,500 cells/m²).

⊗ **Warning** Handle drug with great care; wearing gloves is recommended; if drug comes into contact with skin, wash immediately with soap and water.

⊗ **Warning** Premedicate patient before administration with oral corticosteroids (eg, dexamethasone 16 mg/day PO for 3 days starting 1 day before docetaxel administration) to reduce severity of fluid retention.

• Monitor BP and P during administration.
• Arrange for blood counts before and regularly during therapy.
• Monitor patient's neurologic status frequently during treatment; provide safety measures as needed.

⊗ **Black box warning** Do not give with hepatic impairment; increased risk of toxicity and death. Monitor LFTs carefully.

⊗ **Black box warning** Monitor patient for hypersensitivity reactions, possibly severe; do not give with history of hypersensitivity.

⊗ **Black box warning** Monitor patient carefully for fluid retention and treat accordingly.

Teaching points

• This drug is given IV once every 3 weeks; mark calendar with days to return for treatment.
• You may experience these side effects: Nausea and vomiting (if severe, antiemetics may be helpful; eat frequent small meals); weakness, lethargy (take frequent rest periods); increased susceptibility to infection (avoid crowds, exposure to many people or diseases); numbness and tingling in fingers or toes (avoid injury to these areas; use care if performing tasks that require precision); loss of hair (arrange for a wig or other head covering; keep the head covered at extremes of temperature).
• Report severe nausea and vomiting; fever, chills, sore throat; unusual bleeding or bruising; numbness or tingling in fingers or toes; fluid retention or swelling.

▽dofetilide
(doe fe' ti lyed)

Tikosyn

PREGNANCY CATEGORY C

Drug class
Antiarrhythmic

Therapeutic actions
Selectively blocks potassium channels, widening the QRS complex and prolonging the action potential; has no effect on calcium channels or cardiac contraction; Class III antiarrhythmic.

Indications
• Conversion of atrial fibrillation or flutter to normal sinus rhythm
• Maintenance of normal sinus rhythm in patients with atrial fibrillation or flutter of more than 1-week's duration who have been converted to sinus rhythm

Contraindications and cautions
• Contraindicated with hypersensitivity to dofetilide, ibutilide; second- or third-degree AV heart block; prolonged QT intervals; lactation.
• Use cautiously with ventricular arrhythmias, renal impairment, severe hepatic impairment, pregnancy.

Available forms
Capsules—125, 250, 500 mcg

Dosages
Adults
Dosage is based on ECG response and creatinine clearance. For creatinine clearance greater than 60 mL/min, 500 mcg bid PO; for creatinine clearance 40–60 mL/min, 250 mcg bid PO; for creatinine clearance 20–less than 40 mL/min, 125 mcg bid PO; for creatinine clearance less than 20 mL/min, use is contraindicated.
Pediatric patients
Not recommended.

Pharmacokinetics

Route	Onset	Peak
Oral	Varies	2–3 hr

Metabolism: Hepatic; $T_{1/2}$: 10 hr
Distribution: May cross placenta, may enter breast milk
Excretion: Feces, urine

Adverse effects

- **CNS:** *Headache, fatigue,* light-headedness, dizziness, tingling in arms, numbness
- **CV: Ventricular arrhythmias,** hypotension, hypertension
- **GI:** Nausea, flatulence, diarrhea

Interactions

❋ **Drug-drug** ⊗ *Warning* Increased risk of serious to life-threatening arrhythmias with disopyramide, quinidine, amiodarone, sotalol; do not give together • Increased risk of proarrhythmias if given with phenothiazines, TCAs, antihistamines • Increased risk of serious adverse effects if given with verapamil, cimetidine, trimethoprim, ketoconazole; do not use these combinations

■ Nursing considerations
Assessment

- **History:** Hypersensitivity to dofetilide, ibutilide; second- or third-degree AV heart block, time of onset of atrial arrhythmia; prolonged QT intervals; pregnancy; lactation; ventricular arrhythmias
- **Physical:** Orientation, BP, P, auscultation, ECG, R, adventitious sounds, renal function tests

Interventions

- Dofetilide is only available to those who have completed a *Tikosyn* education program.
- Determine time of onset of arrhythmia and timing of conversion to sinus rhythm before beginning therapy (for maintenance).
- ⊗ **Black box warning** Monitor patient's ECG before and periodically during administration; monitor continually for at least 3 days. Dosage may be adjusted based on the maintenance of sinus rhythm. Risk of induced arrhythmias exist.
- Monitor serum creatinine prior to and every 3 mo during treatment; periodically monitor potassium, magnesium levels.
- Do not attempt electroconversion within 24 hr of starting therapy; if then successful, closely monitor patient for 3 days.
- Provide appointments for continued follow-up including ECG monitoring; tendency to

revert to the atrial arrhythmia after conversion increases with length of time patient was in the abnormal rhythm.

Teaching points

- This drug should be taken twice a day at the same time each day. It will help to keep your heart in a normal rhythm.
- If you miss a dose, skip the dose and resume regular dosing schedule. Do not double up on doses.
- Arrange for follow-up medical evaluation, including ECG, which is important to monitor the effect of this drug on your heart.
- These side effects may occur: Headache, fatigue, dizziness, light-headedness (avoid driving a car or operating dangerous equipment if these effects occur).
- Report chest pain, difficulty breathing, numbness or tingling, palpitations.

▽ **dolasetron mesylate**
(doe laz' e tron)

Anzemet

PREGNANCY CATEGORY B

Drug classes

Antiemetic
Serotonin receptor blocker

Therapeutic actions

Selectively binds to serotonin receptors in the CTZ, blocking the nausea and vomiting caused by the release of serotonin by mucosal cells during chemotherapy, radiotherapy, or surgical invasion (an action that stimulates the CTZ and causes nausea and vomiting).

Indications

- Prevention and treatment of nausea and vomiting associated with emetogenic chemotherapy (oral only)
- Prevention of postoperative nausea and vomiting
- Injection only: Treatment and prevention of postoperative nausea and vomiting
- Unlabeled use: Treatment and prevention of radiation therapy–induced nausea and vomiting

---

Contraindications and cautions

- Contraindicated with allergy to dolasetron or any of its components; markedly prolonged QTc interval, second- or third-degree AV block.
- Use cautiously in any patient at risk of developing prolongation of cardiac conduction intervals, especially QT interval (congenital QT syndrome, hypokalemia, hypomagnesemia), pregnancy, lactation.

Available forms

Tablets—50, 100 mg; injection—12.5 mg/0.625 mL, 20 mg/mL

Dosages

Adults

100 mg PO within 1 hr before chemotherapy or within 2 hr before surgery. For prevention of postoperative nausea and vomiting, 12.5 mg IV about 15 min before stopping anesthesia. For treatment of postoperative nausea and vomiting, 12.5 mg IV as soon as needed.

Pediatric patients 2–16 yr

1.8 mg/kg PO using tablets or injection diluted in apple or apple-grape juice within 1 hr before chemotherapy; for prevention of postoperative nausea and vomiting, 1.2 mg/kg PO using tablets or injection diluted in apple or apple-grape juice within 2 hr before surgery; 0.35 mg/kg IV about 15 min before stopping anesthesia to prevent postoperative nausea and vomiting; 0.35 mg/kg IV as soon as needed to treat postoperative nausea and vomiting; up to a maximum of 12.5 mg per dose.

Pediatric patients younger than 2 yr

Not recommended.

Pharmacokinetics

Route	Onset	Peak
Oral	Rapid	1–2 hr
IV	Immediate	End of infusion

Metabolism: Hepatic; T$_{1/2}$: 3.5–5 hr
Distribution: May cross placenta; may enter breast milk
Excretion: Feces, urine

▼ IV FACTS

Preparation: Dilute in 50 mL 5% dextrose injection, 0.9% sodium chloride injection, 5% dextrose and 0.45% sodium chloride injection, lactated Ringer solution, 10% mannitol; 3% sodium chloride injection; do not mix in any alkaline solution, precipitates may form. Stable at room temperature for 24 hr, or 48 hr if refrigerated, after dilution.

Infusion: Up to 100 mg may be administered IV undiluted over 30 sec or infuse diluted over up to 15 min.

Incompatibilities: Dilute only in recommended solutions. IV infusion line should be flushed before and after administration.

Adverse effects

- **CNS:** *Headache, dizziness,* somnolence, drowsiness, sedation, *fatigue*
- **CV:** *Tachycardia,* ECG changes, **QT-interval prolongation**
- **GI:** *Diarrhea,* constipation, abdominal pain
- **Other:** Fever, pruritus, injection site reaction

Interactions

✳ **Drug-drug** • Possible cardiac arrhythmias with drugs that cause ECG interval prolongation • Potential for severe toxic reaction with high-dose anthracycline therapy • Decreased levels if combined with rifampin

■ Nursing considerations

Assessment

- **History:** Allergy to dolasetron, pregnancy, lactation, QTc prolongation, hypokalemia, hypomagnesemia, pregnancy, lactation
- **Physical:** Orientation, reflexes, affect; BP; P, baseline ECG

Interventions

- Do not use injection (IV) form for chemotherapy-induced nausea and vomiting; risk of serious to fatal arrhythmias. Use oral form only for chemotherapy-induced nausea and vomiting.
- If patient is unable to swallow tablets, dilute injection in apple or apple-grape juice; dosage remains the same; solution is stable for 2 hr at room temperature.
- Provide mouth care, sugarless candies to suck to help alleviate nausea.
- Obtain baseline ECG and periodically monitor ECG in any patient at risk for QTc prolongation.
- Provide appropriate analgesics for headache.

Teaching points

- This drug is given orally when you are receiving your chemotherapy; it will help decrease nausea and vomiting. This drug may be given orally or IV to help control your post operative nausea and vomiting.
- You may experience these side effects: Dizziness, drowsiness (use caution if driving or performing tasks that require alertness), diarrhea; headache (appropriate medication will be arranged to alleviate this problem).
- Report severe headache, fever, numbness or tingling, palpitations, fainting episodes, change in color of stools or urine.

▷ **donepezil hydrochloride**

*(doe **nep'** ah zill)*

Aricept, Aricept ODT

PREGNANCY CATEGORY C

Drug classes

Alzheimer disease drug
Cholinesterase inhibitor

Therapeutic actions

Centrally acting reversible cholinesterase inhibitor leading to elevated acetylcholine levels in the cortex, which slows the neuronal degradation that occurs in Alzheimer disease.

Indications

- Treatment of dementia of the Alzheimer type, including severe dementia
- Unlabeled uses: Possible treatment for vascular dementia; improvement of memory in MS patients

Contraindications and cautions

- Contraindicated with allergy to donepezil.
- Use cautiously with sick sinus syndrome, GI bleeding, seizures, asthma, pregnancy, lactation.

Available forms

Tablets—5, 10, 23 mg; orally disintegrating tablets—5, 10 mg

Dosages

Adults

5 mg PO daily at bedtime for mild to moderate disease. May be increased to 10 mg daily after 4–6 wk. 10 mg PO daily for severe disease. A dose of 23 mg daily may be used after patient has been on 10 mg/day for at least 3 mo.

Pediatric patients

Safety and efficacy not established.

Pharmacokinetics

Route	Onset	Peak
Oral	Varies	3–4 hr

Metabolism: Hepatic; T$_{1/2}$: 70 hr
Distribution: May cross placenta; may enter breast milk
Excretion: Feces, urine

Adverse effects

- **CNS:** *Insomnia, fatigue,* dizziness, confusion, ataxia, somnolence, tremor, agitation, depression, anxiety, abnormal thinking
- **CV:** Bradycardia
- **Dermatologic:** *Rash,* flushing, purpura
- **GI:** *Nausea, vomiting, diarrhea, dyspepsia, anorexia, abdominal pain,* flatulence, constipation, **hepatotoxicity**
- **Other:** *Muscle cramps,* urinary incontinence

Interactions

❋ **Drug-drug** • Increased effects and risk of toxicity with theophylline, cholinesterase inhibitors • Decreased effects of anticholinergics • Increased risk of GI bleeding with NSAIDs • Decreased efficacy with anticholinergics

■ Nursing considerations

 CLINICAL ALERT!
Name confusion has occurred between *Aricept* (donepezil) and *Aciphex* (rabeprazole); use caution.

Assessment

- **History:** Allergy to donepezil, pregnancy, lactation, sick sinus syndrome, GI bleeding, seizures, asthma
- **Physical:** Orientation, affect, reflexes; BP; P; abdominal examination; renal function tests, LFTs

Interventions

- Administer at bedtime each day.
- Provide small, frequent meals if GI upset is severe.
- Place orally disintegrating tablet on tongue; allow to dissolve and follow with water.
- Notify surgeons that patient is on donepezil; exaggerated muscle relaxation may occur if succinylcholine-type drugs are used.

Teaching points

- Take this drug exactly as prescribed, at bedtime.
- Place orally disintegrating tablet on your tongue; allow it to dissolve and then drink water.
- This drug does not cure the disease but is thought to slow down the degeneration associated with the disease.
- Continue taking this drug if no change in symptoms is noted.
- Arrange for regular blood tests and follow-up visits while adjusting to this drug.
- You may experience these side effects: Nausea, vomiting (eat frequent small meals); insomnia, fatigue, confusion (use caution if driving or performing tasks that require alertness).
- Report severe nausea, vomiting, changes in stool or urine color, diarrhea, changes in neurologic functioning, yellowing of eyes or skin.

DANGEROUS DRUG

▷DOPamine hydrochloride

(*doe' pa meen*)

PREGNANCY CATEGORY C

Drug classes

Alpha-adrenergic agonist
Beta₁-selective adrenergic agonist
Dopaminergic drug
Sympathomimetic

Therapeutic actions

Drug acts directly and by the release of norepinephrine from sympathetic nerve terminals; dopaminergic receptors mediate dilation of vessels in the renal and splanchnic beds, which maintains renal perfusion and function; alpha receptors, which are activated by higher doses of dopamine, mediate vasoconstriction, which can override the vasodilating effects; beta₁ receptors mediate a positive inotropic effect on the heart.

Indications

- Correction of hemodynamic imbalances present in the shock syndrome due to MI, trauma, endotoxic septicemia, open heart surgery, renal failure, and chronic cardiac decompensation in heart failure
- Poor perfusion of vital organs
- Low cardiac output
- Hypotension
- Unlabeled uses: COPD, heart failure, RDS in infants

Contraindications and cautions

- Contraindicated with pheochromocytoma, tachyarrhythmias, ventricular fibrillation, hypovolemia (dopamine is not a substitute for blood, plasma, fluids, electrolytes, which should be restored promptly when loss has occurred), general anesthesia with halogenated hydrocarbons or cyclopropane, which sensitize the myocardium to catecholamines.
- Use cautiously with atherosclerosis, arterial embolism, Raynaud disease, cold injury, frostbite, diabetic endarteritis, Buerger disease (monitor color and temperature of extremities), pregnancy, lactation.

Available forms

Injection—40, 80, 160 mg/mL; injection in 5% dextrose—80, 160, 320 mg/100 mL

Dosages

Dilute before using; administer only by IV infusion, using an infusion pump to control the rate of flow. Titrate on the basis of patient's hemodynamic and renal response. Close monitoring is necessary. In titrating to desired systolic BP response, optimum administration rate for renal response may be exceeded, thus necessitating a reduction in rate after hemodynamic stabilization.

Adults

- *Patients likely to respond to modest increments of cardiac contractility and renal perfusion:* Initially, 2–5 mcg/kg/min IV.
- *Patients who are more seriously ill:* Initially, 5 mcg/kg/min IV. Increase in increments of 5–10 mcg/kg/min up to a rate of

20–50 mcg/kg/min. Check urine output frequently if doses exceed 50 mcg/kg/min.

Pediatric patients
Safety and efficacy not established; there is limited experience for use in children.

Pharmacokinetics

Route	Onset	Peak	Duration
IV	1–2 min	10 min	Length of infusion

Metabolism: Hepatic; $T_{1/2}$: 2 min
Distribution: May cross placenta; may enter breast milk
Excretion: Urine

▼ IV FACTS

Preparation: Prepare solution for IV infusion as follows: Add 200–400 mg dopamine to 250–500 mL of one of the following IV solutions: 0.9% sodium chloride solution; 5% dextrose injection; 5% dextrose and 0.45% or 0.9% sodium chloride solution; 5% dextrose in lactated Ringer solution; sodium lactate (1/6 Molar) injection; lactated Ringer injection. Commonly used concentrations are 800 mcg/mL (200 mg in 250 mL) and 1,600 mcg/mL (400 mg in 250 mL). The 160-mg/mL concentrate may be preferred in patients with fluid retention. Protect drug solutions from light; drug solutions should be clear and colorless.
Infusion: Determine infusion rate based on patient response.
Incompatibilities: Do not mix with other drugs; do not add to 5% sodium bicarbonate or other alkaline IV solutions, oxidizing drugs, or iron salts because drug is inactivated in alkaline solution (solutions become pink to violet).
Y-site incompatibilities: Do not give with acyclovir, alteplase, amphotericin B.

Adverse effects

- **CNS:** Headache, anxiety
- **CV:** *Ectopic beats, tachycardia, anginal pain, palpitations, hypotension, vasoconstriction, dyspnea,* bradycardia, hypertension, widened QRS
- **GI:** *Nausea, vomiting*
- **Other:** Piloerection, azotemia, gangrene with prolonged use

Interactions

✳ **Drug-drug** ● Increased effects with MAOIs, TCAs (imipramine) ● Increased risk of hypertension with methyldopa ● Seizures, hypotension, bradycardia when infused with phenytoin

■ Nursing considerations

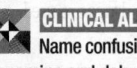 **CLINICAL ALERT!**
Name confusion has occurred between dopamine and dobutamine; use caution.

Assessment

- **History:** Pheochromocytoma, tachyarrhythmias, ventricular fibrillation, hypovolemia, general anesthesia with halogenated hydrocarbons or cyclopropane, occlusive vascular disease, pregnancy, labor, and delivery
- **Physical:** Body weight; skin color, T; P, BP, pulse pressure; R, adventitious sounds; urine output; serum electrolytes, Hct, ECG

Interventions

⊗ **Warning** Exercise extreme caution in calculating and preparing doses; dopamine is a very potent drug; small errors in dosage can cause serious adverse effects. Drug should always be diluted before use if not prediluted.

- Reduce initial dosage to one-tenth of usual dose in patients who have been on MAOIs.
- Administer into large veins of the antecubital fossa in preference to veins in hand or ankle.

⊗ **Black box warning** To prevent sloughing and necrosis after extravasation, infiltrate area with 10–15 mL saline containing 5–10 mg phentolamine. Do so as soon as possible after extravasation occurs.

- Monitor urine flow, cardiac output, and BP closely during infusion.

Teaching points

- Drug is used only in acute emergency; teaching will depend on patient's awareness and will relate mainly to patient's status and monitors, rather than to drug. Instruct patient to report any pain at injection site.

Adverse effects in *italics* are most common; those in **bold** are life-threatening. ⬛ Do not crush.

▽doripenem
*(door ib **pen'** em)*

Doribax

PREGNANCY CATEGORY B

Drug class
Carbapenem antibiotic

Therapeutic actions
Drug inhibits synthesis of bacterial cell wall and causes cell death in susceptible cells. Structure and action are similar to those of beta lactams.

Indications
- Treatment of complicated intra-abdominal infections caused by *Escherichia coli, Klebsiella pneumoniae, Pseudomonas aeruginosa, Bacteroides caccea, Bacteroides fragilis, Bacteroides thetaiotaomicron, Bacteroides uniformis, Bacteroides vulgatus, Streptococcus intermedius, Streptococcus constellatus, Peptostreptococcus micros*
- Treatment of complicated UTI, including pyelonephritis, caused by *E. coli, K. pneumoniae, Proteus mirabilis, P. aeruginosa, Acinetobacter baumannii*
- ◾ NEW INDICATION: Unlabeled uses: Catheter-related bloodstream infections, community-acquired pneumonia, hospital-acquired pneumonia

Contraindications and cautions
- Contraindicated with hypersensitivity to any component of this drug or drugs in this class; history of anaphylactic reaction to beta-lactams.
- Use cautiously with sodium valproate therapy, pregnancy, lactation.

Available forms
Single-use vials—250, 500 mg

Dosages
Adults
500 mg IV over 1 hr every 8 hr for 5–14 days (intra-abdominal infection), for 10 days (UTI or pyelonephritis), or up to 14 days with concurrent bacteremia.
Patients with renal impairment
If creatinine clearance is equal to or greater than 30 and equal to or less than 50 mL/min,

250 mg IV every 8 hr; if creatinine clearance is greater than 10 and less than 30 mL/min, 250 mg IV every 12 hr.

Pharmacokinetics

Route	Onset	Peak	Duration
IV	Rapid	End of infusion	Length of infusion

Metabolism: Hepatic; $T_{1/2}$: 1 hr
Distribution: Does not cross placenta; may enter breast milk
Excretion: Unchanged in urine

▼ IV FACTS
Preparation: Constitute vial with 10 mg sterile water for injection or 0.9% sodium chloride injection; gently shake to form a suspension (concentration is 50 mg/mL). Add suspension to 100 mL normal saline solution or 5% dextrose; gently shake until clear. Infusion concentration is 4.5 mg/mL. If using normal saline solution, drug stays stable for 8 hr at room temperature or 24 hr refrigerated; if using 5% dextrose, stable for 4 hr at room temperature or 24 hr refrigerated. Do not freeze.
Infusion: Infuse over 1 hr.
Incompatibility: Do not mix with or add to solutions containing any other drugs.

Adverse effects
- **CNS:** *Headache*
- **GI:** *Nausea;* diarrhea, including *Clostridium difficile* infection
- **Other:** *Rash, phlebitis,* superinfection, hypersensitivity reaction

Interactions
✳ **Drug-drug** ● Risk for significant reduction in serum valproic acid level and risk of seizures if combined; alternative antibiotic treatment should be considered ● Increased serum doripenem level if combined with probenecid; avoid this combination

■ Nursing considerations
Assessment
- **History:** Hypersensitivity to doripenem, its components, drugs of this class, or beta lactams; pregnancy, lactation
- **Physical:** T, orientation, abdominal examination

Interventions

- Obtain culture and sensitivity tests to ensure appropriate use of the drug.
- Ensure that patient is not controlling seizures with valproic acid therapy; serious drug interaction and seizures could occur.
- Do not administer by inhalation; serious pneumonitis has occurred.
- Administer IV every 8 hr for full length of prescribed dose to prevent emergence of resistant strains of bacteria.
- Monitor injection site for possible phlebitis.
- Encourage women of childbearing age to use barrier contraceptives while on this drug because effects of drug on fetus are not known.
- Advise breast-feeding women to find another method of feeding; potential effects on the baby are not known.
- Monitor patient for possible *C. difficile* diarrhea. Provide fluid and electrolyte management, protein supplements, and antibiotic treatment as needed. Monitor patient for up to 2 mo after therapy.

Teaching points

- This drug is given by IV infusion every 8 hours for 5–14 days, depending on your infection and your response to the drug; it is important to complete the full course of drug therapy.
- If you are being treated as an outpatient and miss a dose, contact your health care provider immediately.
- It is not known how this drug could affect a breast-feeding infant. If you are breast-feeding, another method of feeding the baby should be selected.
- It is not known how this drug could affect a fetus. If you are pregnant or decide to become pregnant while on this drug, consult your health care provider.
- You may experience these side effects: Headache (consult your health care provider, medication may be available to help); nausea (frequent small meals may help); diarrhea (if it becomes severe, contact your health care provider immediately); irritation and inflammation at the injection site.
- Report difficulty breathing; severe or persistent rash, redness, or pain at the injection site; severe diarrhea.

▽dornase alfa

See Appendix R, *Less commonly used drugs*.

▽doxapram hydrochloride
(docks' a pram)

Dopram

PREGNANCY CATEGORY B

Drug classes
Analeptic
Respiratory stimulant

Therapeutic actions
Stimulates the peripheral carotid chemoreceptors to cause an increase in tidal volume and slight increase in respiratory rate; this stimulation also has a pressor effect.

Indications

- To stimulate respiration in patients with drug-induced postanesthesia respiratory depression or apnea; also used to "stir up" patients in combination with oxygen postoperatively
- To stimulate respiration, hasten arousal in patients experiencing drug-induced CNS depression
- As a temporary measure in hospitalized patients with acute respiratory insufficiency superimposed on COPD
- Unlabeled uses: Treatment of apnea of prematurity when methylxanthines have failed, obstructive sleep apnea, laryngospasm secondary to tracheal extubation

Contraindications and cautions

- Contraindicated with newborns (contains benzyl alcohol), epilepsy, incompetence of the ventilatory mechanism, flail chest, hypersensitivity to doxapram, head injury, pneumothorax, acute bronchial asthma, pulmonary fibrosis, severe hypertension, stroke.
- Use cautiously with pregnancy, lactation.

Available forms
Injection—20 mg/mL

Dosages
Adults
IV injection
- *Postanesthetic use:* Single injection of 0.5–1 mg/kg IV; do not exceed 1.5 mg/kg as a total single injection or 2 mg/kg when given as multiple injections at 5-min intervals.

Infusion
250 mg in 250 mL of dextrose or sodium chloride solution; initiate at 5 mg/min until response is seen; maintain at 1–3 mg/min; recommended total dose is 300 mg or 4 mg/kg.

- *COPD associated with acute hypercapnia:* Mix 400 mg in 180 mL of IV infusion; start infusion at 1–2 mg/min (0.5–1 mL/min); check blood gases, and adjust rate accordingly. Do not use for longer than 2 hr. Maximum of 3 mg/min.

- *Management of drug-induced CNS depression:*
Intermittent injection
Priming dose of 1–2 mg/kg IV; repeat in 5 min. Repeat every 1–2 hr until patient awakens; if relapse occurs, repeat at 1–2 hr intervals.

Intermittent IV infusion
Priming dose of 1–2 mg/kg IV; if no response, infuse 250 mg in 250 mL of dextrose or saline solution at a rate of 1–3 mg/min, discontinue at end of 2 hr if patient awakens; repeat in 30 min–2 hr if relapse occurs; do not exceed 3 g/day.

Pediatric patients
Do not give to children younger than 12 yr.

Pharmacokinetics

Route	Onset	Peak	Duration
IV	20–40 sec	1–2 min	5–12 min

Metabolism: Hepatic; $T_{1/2}$: 2.4–4.1 hr
Distribution: May cross placenta; may enter breast milk
Excretion: Urine

▼ IV FACTS

Preparation: Add 250 mg doxapram to 250 mL of 5% or 10% dextrose or 0.9% sodium chloride solution.
Infusion: Initiate infusion at 5 mg/min; once response is seen, 1–3 mg/min is satisfactory.
Incompatibilities: Do not mix in alkaline solutions—precipitate or gas may form; aminophylline, sodium bicarbonate, thiopental.

Adverse effects
- **CNS:** Headache, dizziness, apprehension, disorientation, pupillary dilation, *increased reflexes,* hyperactivity, **seizures,** muscle spasticity, clonus, pyrexia, flushing sweating
- **CV:** Arrhythmias, chest pain, tightness in the chest, *increased BP*
- **GI:** Nausea, vomiting, diarrhea
- **GU:** Urinary retention, spontaneous voiding, proteinuria
- **Hematologic:** Decreased Hgb, Hct
- **Respiratory:** Cough, dyspnea, tachypnea, laryngospasm, **bronchospasm,** hiccups, rebound hypoventilation, hyperventilation

Interactions
✳ **Drug-drug** • Increased pressor effect with sympathomimetics, MAOIs • Increased effects with halothane, enflurane (delay treatment for at least 10 min after discontinuance of anesthesia) • Possible masked residual effects of muscle relaxants if combined with doxapram
• Risk of increased muscle activity, agitation with aminophylline, theophylline; use caution

■ Nursing considerations
Assessment
- **History:** Epilepsy, incompetence of the ventilatory mechanism, flail chest, hypersensitivity to doxapram, head injury, pneumothorax, acute bronchial asthma, pulmonary fibrosis, severe hypertension, stroke, lactation, pregnancy
- **Physical:** T; skin color; weight; R, adventitious sounds; P, BP, ECG; reflexes; urinary output; arterial blood gases, CBC

Interventions
- Administer IV only.
- ⊗ *Warning* Monitor injection site for extravasation. Discontinue, and restart in another vein if extravasation occurs; apply cold compresses.
- Monitor patient carefully until fully awake— P, BP, ECG, reflexes and respiratory status. Patients with COPD should have arterial blood gases monitored during drug use.
- Do not use longer than 2 hr.
- ⊗ *Warning* Discontinue drug and notify physician if deterioration, sudden hypotension, or dyspnea occurs.

Teaching points

• Drug is used in emergency; patient teaching should be general and include procedure and drug.

▽ **doxazosin mesylate**

(dox ay' zoe sin mess' ah late)

Cardura, Cardura XL ⓒ

PREGNANCY CATEGORY C

Drug classes

Alpha-adrenergic blocker
Antihypertensive

Therapeutic actions

Reduces total peripheral resistance through alpha-blockade, causing an antihypertensive effect. The degree of smooth muscle tone in prostate/bladder neck is also mediated by alpha receptors. Its blockade reduces urethral resistance and relieves obstructions.

Indications

• Treatment of mild-to-moderate hypertension, alone or as part of combination therapy
• Treatment of BPH
• Unlabeled use: Pediatric hypertension.

Contraindications and cautions

• Contraindicated with lactation.
• Use cautiously with allergy to doxazosin, heart failure, renal failure, pregnancy, hepatic impairment.

Available forms

Tablets—1, 2, 4, 8 mg; ER tablets ⓒ—4, 8 mg

Dosages

Adults

• *Hypertension:* Initially, 1 mg daily PO, given once daily. For maintenance, 2, 4, 8, or 16 mg daily PO, given once a day; dose may be increased every 2 wk. Do not use ER tablets.
• *BPH:* Initially, 1 mg PO daily; for maintenance, may increase to 2 mg, 4 mg, 8 mg daily, adjusted at 1–2 wk intervals. For ER tablets, 4 mg PO once daily at breakfast; may be increased after 3–4 wk to maximum of 8 mg/day PO.

Pediatric patients
Safety and efficacy not established.

Pharmacokinetics

Route	Onset	Peak
Oral	Varies	2–3 hr

Metabolism: Hepatic; T$_{1/2}$: 22 hr
Distribution: Crosses placenta; enters breast milk
Excretion: Bile, feces, urine

Adverse effects

• **CNS:** *Headache, fatigue, dizziness, postural dizziness, lethargy, vertigo,* asthenia, anxiety, paresthesia, insomnia, eye pain, conjunctivitis
• **CV:** *Tachycardia, palpitations, edema, orthostatic hypotension,* chest pain
• **GI:** *Nausea, dyspepsia, diarrhea,* abdominal pain, flatulence, constipation
• **GU:** *Sexual dysfunction,* increased urinary frequency
• **Other:** Dyspnea, increased sweating, rash, rhinitis, muscle cramps

Interactions

✳ **Drug-drug** • Increased hypotensive effects if taken with alcohol, nitrates, other antihypertensives

■ Nursing considerations

Assessment

• **History:** Allergy to doxazosin, heart failure, renal failure, hepatic impairment, lactation, pregnancy
• **Physical:** Weight; skin color, lesions; orientation, affect, reflexes; ophthalmologic examination; P, BP, orthostatic BP, supine BP, perfusion, edema, auscultation; R, adventitious sounds, status of nasal mucous membranes; bowel sounds, normal output; voiding pattern, normal output; renal function tests, urinalysis

Interventions

• Ensure that patient does not cut, crush, or chew ER tablets.
• Monitor edema, weight in patients with incipient cardiac decompensation, and arrange to add a thiazide diuretic to the drug regimen if sodium and fluid retention, signs of impending heart failure occur.

Adverse effects in *italics* are most common; those in **bold** are life-threatening. ⓒ Do not crush.

⊗ **Warning** Monitor patient carefully with first dose; chance of orthostatic hypotension, dizziness and syncope are great with the first dose. Establish safety precautions.
- Monitor signs and symptoms of BPH to adjust dosage.

Teaching points
- Take this drug exactly as prescribed, once a day. Do not cut, crush, or chew extended-release tablets. Dizziness or syncope may occur at beginning of therapy. Change position slowly to avoid increased dizziness. Taking your first dose at bedtime may decrease excessive dizziness.
- You may experience these side effects: Dizziness, weakness (when changing position, in the early morning, after exercise, in hot weather, and after consuming alcohol; some tolerance may occur after a while; avoid driving or engaging in tasks that require alertness; change position slowly, use caution in climbing stairs, lie down if dizziness persists); GI upset (eat frequent small meals); impotence; stuffy nose; most of these effects gradually disappear with continued therapy.
- Report frequent dizziness or fainting.

▽doxepin hydrochloride
(*dox' e pin*)

Apo-Doxepin (CAN), Sinequan, Zonalon

PREGNANCY CATEGORY C

Drug classes
Antidepressant
TCA (tertiary amine)

Therapeutic actions
Mechanism of action unknown; TCAs inhibit the reuptake of the neurotransmitters norepinephrine and serotonin, leading to an increase in their effects; anticholinergic at CNS and peripheral receptors; sedative.

Indications
- Relief of symptoms of depression (endogenous depression most responsive); sedative effects may help depression associated with anxiety and sleep disturbance

- Treatment of depression in patients with bipolar disorder, psychotic depressive disorders
- Treatment of anxiety
- Treatment of pruritus in adults with atopic dermatitis, lichen chronicus (5% topical cream)
- Unlabeled uses: Neuropathy, neurogenic pain

Contraindications and cautions
- Contraindicated with hypersensitivity to any tricyclic drug; concomitant therapy with an MAOI; recent MI; myelography within previous 24 hr or scheduled within 48 hr; lactation, pregnancy.
- Use cautiously with EST; preexisting CV disorders (severe coronary heart disease, progressive heart failure, angina pectoris, paroxysmal tachycardia); angle-closure glaucoma, increased IOP, urinary retention, ureteral or urethral spasm; seizure disorders; hyperthyroidism; impaired hepatic, renal function; psychiatric patients (schizophrenic or paranoid patients may exhibit a worsening of psychosis); patients with bipolar disorder; patients with suicidal ideation (overdose may be fatal); elective surgery (TCAs should be discontinued as long as possible before surgery); geriatric patients (may be more sensitive to drug and adverse effects).

Available forms
Capsules—10, 25, 50, 75, 100, 150 mg; oral concentrate—10 mg/mL; cream—30-g, 40-g tubes

Dosages
Adults
- *Mild to moderate anxiety or depression:* Initially, 25 mg tid PO; individualize dosage. Usual optimum dosage is 75–150 mg/day; alternatively, total daily dosage, up to 150 mg, may be given at bedtime.
- *More severe anxiety or depression:* Initially, 50 mg tid PO; if needed, may gradually increase to 300 mg/day. Dose may be taken all at once at bedtime.
- *Mild symptomatology or emotional symptoms accompanying organic disease:* 25–50 mg PO is often effective.
- *Pruritus:* Apply cream four times/day at least 3–4 hr apart for 8 days. Do not cover dressing.

Pediatric patients
Not recommended for children younger than 12 yr.

Pharmacokinetics

Route	Onset	Peak
Oral	Varies	4 hr

Metabolism: Hepatic; T$_{1/2}$: 8–25 hr
Distribution: Crosses placenta; enters breast milk
Excretion: Urine

Adverse effects

- **CNS:** *Sedation and anticholinergic (atropine-like) effects; confusion* (especially in elderly), *disturbed concentration,* hallucinations, disorientation, decreased memory, feelings of unreality, delusions, anxiety, nervousness, restlessness, agitation, panic, insomnia, nightmares, hypomania, mania, exacerbation of psychosis, drowsiness, weakness, fatigue, headache, numbness, tingling, paresthesias of extremities, incoordination, motor hyperactivity, akathisia, ataxia, tremors, peripheral neuropathy, extrapyramidal symptoms, seizures, speech blockage, dysarthria, tinnitus, altered EEG
- **CV:** *Orthostatic hypotension,* hypertension, syncope, tachycardia, palpitations, **MI,** arrhythmias, heart block, precipitation of heart failure, **stroke**
- **Endocrine:** Elevated or depressed blood sugar; elevated prolactin levels; inappropriate ADH secretion
- **GI:** *Dry mouth, constipation,* paralytic ileus, *nausea,* vomiting, anorexia, epigastric distress, diarrhea, flatulence, dysphagia, peculiar taste, increased salivation, stomatitis, glossitis, parotid swelling, abdominal cramps, black tongue, hepatitis, jaundice (rare), elevated transaminase, altered alkaline phosphatase
- **GU:** Urinary retention, delayed micturition, dilation of the urinary tract, gynecomastia, testicular swelling; breast enlargement, menstrual irregularity and galactorrhea; changes in libido; impotence
- **Hematologic:** Bone marrow depression, including agranulocytosis; eosinophilia, purpura, thrombocytopenia, leukopenia
- **Hypersensitivity:** Rash, pruritus, vasculitis, petechiae, photosensitization, edema (generalized or of face and tongue), drug fever

- **Withdrawal:** Symptoms on abrupt discontinuation of prolonged therapy: Nausea, headache, vertigo, nightmares, malaise
- **Other:** Nasal congestion, excessive appetite, weight gain or loss; sweating (paradoxical effect in a drug with prominent anticholinergic effects), alopecia, lacrimation, hyperthermia, flushing, chills

Interactions

✳ **Drug-drug** ● Increased TCA levels and pharmacologic (especially anticholinergic) effects with cimetidine, fluoxetine ● Increased TCA levels (due to decreased metabolism) with methylphenidate, phenothiazines, hormonal contraceptives, disulfiram ● Hyperpyretic crises, severe seizures, hypertensive episodes, and deaths with MAOIs ● Increased antidepressant response and cardiac arrhythmias with thyroid medication ● Increased or decreased effects with estrogens ● Delirium with disulfiram ● Sympathetic hyperactivity, sinus tachycardia, hypertension, agitation with levodopa ● Increased biotransformation of TCAs in patients who smoke cigarettes ● Increased sympathomimetic (especially alpha-adrenergic) effects of direct-acting sympathomimetic drugs (norepinephrine, epinephrine), due to inhibition of uptake into adrenergic nerves ● Increased anticholinergic effects of anticholinergic drugs (including anticholinergic antiparkinsonian drugs) ● Increased response (especially CNS depression) to barbiturates ● Increased CNS suppression with alcohol or other CNS depressants; avoid this combination ● Decreased antihypertensive effect of clonidine, other antihypertensives (because the uptake of the antihypertensive drug into adrenergic neurons is inhibited) ● Decreased effects of indirect-acting sympathomimetic drugs (ephedrine) because of inhibition of uptake into adrenergic nerves

■ Nursing considerations

 CLINICAL ALERT!
Name confusion has occurred between *Sinequan* (doxepin) and saquinavir; use caution.

Assessment

- **History:** Hypersensitivity to any tricyclic drug; concomitant therapy with an MAOI; recent MI; myelography within previous 24 hr or scheduled within 48 hr; lactation; EST; preexisting CV disorders; angle-closure glaucoma, increased IOP, urinary retention, ureteral or urethral spasm; seizure disorders; hyperthyroidism; impaired hepatic, renal function; psychiatric treatment; bipolar disorder; elective surgery; pregnancy

- **Physical:** Weight; T; skin color, lesions; orientation, affect, reflexes, vision and hearing; P, BP, orthostatic BP, perfusion; bowel sounds, normal output, liver evaluation; urine flow, normal output; usual sexual function, frequency of menses, breast and scrotal examination; LFTs, urinalysis, CBC, ECG

Interventions

⊗ **Black box warning** Risk of suicidality in children, adolescents, and young adults increases. Monitor patient accordingly.

⊗ **Warning** Limit drug access with depressed and potentially suicidal patients.

- Give most of dose at bedtime if drowsiness or severe anticholinergic effects occur.
- Dilute oral concentrate with approximately 120 mL of water, milk, or fruit juice just prior to administration; do not prepare or store bulk dilutions.
- Expect clinical antianxiety response to be rapidly evident, although antidepressant response may require 2–3 wk.
- Reduce dosage if minor side effects develop; discontinue the drug if serious side effects occur.
- Arrange for CBC if patient develops fever, sore throat, or other sign of infection during therapy.

Teaching points

- Take drug exactly as prescribed; do not stop abruptly or without consulting the health care provider. If using the topical form, do not cover the application area.
- Avoid alcohol, sleep-inducing drugs, over-the-counter drugs.
- Avoid prolonged exposure to sunlight or sunlamps; use a sunscreen or protective garments for exposure to sunlight.
- You may experience these side effects: Headache, dizziness, drowsiness, weakness, blurred vision (reversible; safety measures will be needed if severe; avoid driving or performing tasks that require alertness while these persist); nausea, vomiting, loss of appetite, dry mouth (eat frequent small meals; frequent mouth care and sucking sugarless candies may help); nightmares, inability to

concentrate, confusion; changes in sexual function, suicidal thoughts.
- Report dry mouth, difficulty in urination, excessive sedation, suicidal thoughts.

▷ doxercalciferol

See Appendix R, *Less commonly used drugs.*

DANGEROUS DRUG

▷ DOXOrubicin hydrochloride
(dox oh roo' bi sin)

Adriamycin PFS, Adriamycin RDF, Doxil

PREGNANCY CATEGORY D

Drug classes
Antibiotic
Antineoplastic

Therapeutic actions
Cytotoxic: Binds to DNA and inhibits DNA synthesis in susceptible cells, causing cell death.

Indications

- To produce regression in the following neoplasms: ALL, AML, Wilms tumor, neuroblastoma, soft tissue and bone sarcoma, breast carcinoma, ovarian carcinoma, transitional cell bladder carcinoma, thyroid carcinoma, Hodgkin and non-Hodgkin lymphomas, bronchogenic carcinoma
- Liposomal form: Treatment of AIDS-related Kaposi sarcoma, ovarian cancer that has progressed or recurred after platinum-based chemotherapy

Contraindications and cautions

- Contraindicated with allergy to doxorubicin hydrochloride, malignant melanoma, kidney carcinoma, large bowel carcinoma, brain tumors, CNS metastases, myelosuppression, cardiac disease (may predispose to cardiac toxicity), pregnancy, lactation.
- Use cautiously with impaired hepatic function, previous courses of doxorubicin or daunorubicin therapy (may predispose to cardiac toxicity), prior mediastinal irradiation, concurrent cyclophosphamide therapy (predispose to cardiac toxicity).

Available forms
Powder for injection—10, 20, 50, 100, 150 mg; injection (aqueous)—2 mg/mL; preservative-free injection—2 mg/mL; injection (lipid)—2 mg/mL

Dosages
Adults
60–75 mg/m^2 as a single IV injection administered at 21-day intervals. Alternate schedule: 30 mg/m^2 IV on each of 3 successive days, repeated every 4 wk.
Liposomal form
For AIDS-related Kaposi sarcoma, 20 mg/m^2 IV every 3 wk starting with initial rate of 1 mg/min. If no adverse effects, increase rate to complete dose in 1 hr.
For ovarian cancer, initially 50 mg/m^2 IV at 1 mg/min; if no adverse effects, complete infusion in 1 hr. Repeat every 4 wk.
Patients with elevated bilirubin
For serum bilirubin 1.2–3 mg/100 mL, use 50% of normal dose. For serum bilirubin exceeding 3 mg/100 mL, use 25% of normal dose.

Pharmacokinetics

Route	Onset	Peak	Duration
IV	Rapid	2 hr	24–36 hr

Metabolism: Hepatic; $T_{1/2}$: 12 min, then 3.3 hr, then 29.6 hr
Distribution: May cross placenta; enters breast milk
Excretion: Bile, feces, urine

▼ IV FACTS
Preparation: Reconstitute the 10-mg vial with 5 mL, the 50-mg vial with 25 mL of 0.9% sodium chloride to give a concentration of 2 mg/mL doxorubicin. Reconstituted solution is stable for 7 days at room temperature and normal light or 15 days if refrigerated. Protect from sunlight. Liposomal form: Dilute dose to maximum of 90 mg in 250 mL of 5% dextrose injection; do not use in-line filters; refrigerate and use within 24 hr.
Infusion: Administer slowly into tubing of a freely running IV infusion of sodium chloride injection or 5% dextrose injection; attach the tubing to a butterfly needle inserted into a large vein; avoid veins over joints or in extremities with poor perfusion. Rate of administration will depend on the vein and dosage;

do not give in less than 3–5 min; red streaking over the vein and facial flushing are often signs of too-rapid administration. Liposomal form: Single dose infused over 30 min; rapid infusion increases risk of reaction.
Incompatibilities: Do not mix with heparin, dexamethasone sodium phosphatase (a precipitate forms and the IV solution must not be used), aminophylline, and 5-FU (doxorubicin decomposes) denoted by a color change from red to blue-purple.
Y-site incompatibilities: Do not give with furosemide, heparin.

Adverse effects
• **CV: Cardiac toxicity,** heart failure, phlebosclerosis
• **Dermatologic:** *Complete but reversible alopecia,* hyperpigmentation of nailbeds and dermal creases, facial flushing
• **GI:** *Nausea, vomiting, mucositis,* anorexia, diarrhea
• **GU:** *Red urine*
• **Hematologic:** *Myelosuppression,* hyperuricemia due to cell lysis
• **Hypersensitivity:** Fever, chills, urticaria, **anaphylaxis**
• **Local: Severe local cellulitis,** vesication and tissue necrosis if extravasation occurs
• **Other:** Carcinogenesis (documented in experimental models)

Interactions
✴ Drug-drug • Decreased serum levels and actions of digoxin if taken concurrently with doxorubicin

■ Nursing considerations

◤ CLINICAL ALERT!
Name confusion has been reported between conventional doxorubicin and liposomal doxorubicin; use caution.

Assessment
• **History:** Allergy to doxorubicin hydrochloride, malignant melanoma, kidney carcinoma, large bowel carcinoma, brain tumors, CNS metastases, myelosuppression, cardiac disease, impaired hepatic function, previous courses of doxorubicin or daunorubicin therapy, prior mediastinal irradiation, concurrent cyclophosphamide therapy, lactation, pregnancy

Adverse effects in *italics* are most common; those in **bold** are life-threatening. ▣ Do not crush.

- **Physical:** T; skin color, lesions; weight; hair; nailbeds; local injection site; auscultation, peripheral perfusion, pulses, ECG; R, adventitious sounds; liver evaluation, mucous membranes; CBC, LFTs, uric acid levels

Interventions

⊗ *Black box warning* Accidental substitution of liposomal form for conventional form has resulted in serious adverse reactions. Check drug carefully before administration.

- Do not give IM or subcutaneously because severe local reaction and tissue necrosis occur.

⊗ *Black box warning* Monitor injection site for extravasation and for reports of burning or stinging. If these events occur, discontinue administration and restart in another vein. Local subcutaneous extravasation: Local infiltration with corticosteroid may be ordered; flood area with normal saline; apply cold compress to area. If ulceration begins, arrange consultation with plastic surgeon.

⊗ *Black box warning* Monitor patient's response frequently at beginning of therapy: Serum uric acid level, cardiac output (listen for S_3); CBC changes may require a decrease in the dose; consult with physician; risk of heart failure, myelosuppression, liver damage. Record doses received to monitor total dosage; toxic effects are often dose-related, as total dose approaches 550 mg/m².

- Ensure adequate hydration during the course of therapy to prevent hyperuricemia.

Teaching points

- Prepare a calendar of days to return for drug therapy.
- Avoid pregnancy while using this drug; using barrier contraceptives is advised.
- Arrange for regular medical follow-up, including blood tests.
- You may experience these side effects: Rash, skin lesions, loss of hair, changes in nails (you may want to obtain a wig before hair loss occurs; skin care may help); loss of appetite, nausea, mouth sores (frequent mouth care, eat frequent small meals; try to maintain good nutrition; a dietitian may be able to help; an antiemetic may be ordered); red urine (transient).
- Report difficulty breathing, sudden weight gain, swelling, burning or pain at injection site, unusual bleeding or bruising.

▽ **doxycycline**
(dox i sye' kleen)

Adoxa, Apo-Doxy (CAN), Atridox, Doryx, Doxy 100, Doxy 200, Doxycin (CAN), Monodox, Nu-Doxycycline (CAN), Oracea, Vibramycin

PREGNANCY CATEGORY D

Drug class
Tetracycline antibiotic

Therapeutic actions
Bacteriostatic: Inhibits protein synthesis of susceptible bacteria, causing cell death.

Indications

- Infections caused by rickettsia; *Mycoplasma pneumoniae;* agents of psittacosis, ornithosis, lymphogranuloma venereum, and granuloma inguinale; *Borrelia recurrentis; Haemophilus ducreyi; Pasteurella pestis; Pasteurella tularensis; Bartonella bacilliformis; Bacteroides; Vibrio comma; Vibrio fetus; Brucella; Escherichia coli; Enterobacter aerogenes; Shigella; Acinetobacter calcoaceticus; Haemophilus influenzae, Klebsiella, Streptococcus pneumoniae, Staphylococcus aureus*
- When penicillin is contraindicated, infections caused by *Neisseria gonorrhoeae, Treponema pallidum, Treponema pertenue, Listeria monocytogenes, Clostridium, Bacillus anthracis, Chlamydia psittaci, Chlamydia trachomatis*
- Oral tetracyclines used for acne, uncomplicated adult urethral, endocervical, or rectal infections caused by *C. trachomatis*
- Acute intestinal amebiasis
- Reduction of incidence and progression of disease following exposure to anthrax
- Malaria prophylaxis for malaria due to *Plasmodium falciparum* for short-term use in travelers
- Treatment of inflammatory lesions (papules and pustules) of rosacea in adults; not for generalized erythema of rosacea
- Treatment of periodontal disease as an adjunct to scaling and root planing
- Unlabeled uses: Prevention of traveler's diarrhea commonly caused by enterotoxigenic *E. coli;* Lyme disease; CDC-recommended

treatment of STDs, including granuloma inguinale, syphilis, chlamydial infections in patients older than 8 yr, pelvic inflammatory disease, epididymitis, and sexual assault prophylaxis

Contraindications and cautions

- Contraindicated with allergy to tetracyclines.
- Use cautiously with renal or hepatic impairment, pregnancy, lactation.

Available forms

Tablets—20, 50, 75, 100 mg; DR tablets—75, 100 mg; capsules—50, 100 mg; coated pellets, capsules—75, 100 mg; powder for oral suspension—25 mg; syrup—50 mg/5 mL; powder for injection—100, 200 mg; injection—42.5 mg

Dosages

Adults

- *Rosacea:* 40 mg/day PO in the morning with a full glass of water, on an empty stomach, for up to 9 mo.

Adults and pediatric patients older than 8 yr and weighing more than 45 kg

200 mg IV in one or two infusions (each over 1–4 hr) on the first treatment day, followed by 100–200 mg/day IV, depending on the severity of the infection, or 200 mg PO on day 1, followed by 100 mg/day PO.

- *Primary or secondary syphilis:* 100 mg PO bid for 14 days.
- *Acute gonococcal infection:* 100 mg PO, then 100 mg at bedtime, followed by 100 mg bid for 3 days; or 300 mg PO followed by 300 mg in 1 hr.
- *Traveler's diarrhea:* 100 mg/day PO as prophylaxis.
- *Malaria prophylaxis:* 100 mg PO daily.
- *Anthrax prophylaxis:* 100 mg PO bid for 60 days.
- *CDC recommendations for STDs:* 100 mg bid PO for 7–28 days, depending on disease being treated.
- *Periodontal disease:* 20 mg PO bid, following scaling and root planing.

Pediatric patients older than 8 yr and weighing less than 45 kg

4.4 mg/kg, IV in one or two infusions, followed by 2.2–4.4 mg/kg/day IV in one or two infusions; or 4.4 mg/kg, PO in two divided doses

the first day of treatment, followed by 2.2–4.4 mg/kg/day on subsequent days.

- *Lyme disease:* 100 mg PO bid for 14–21 days.
- *Malaria prophylaxis:* 2 mg/kg/day PO, up to 100 mg/day.
- *Anthrax prophylaxis:* 2.2 mg/kg PO bid for 60 days.

Geriatric patients or patients with renal failure

IV doses of doxycycline may not be as toxic as other tetracyclines in these patients.

Pharmacokinetics

Route	Onset	Peak
Oral	Varies	1.5–4 hr
IV	Rapid	End of infusion

Metabolism: $T_{1/2}$: 15–25 hr
Distribution: Crosses placenta; enters breast milk
Excretion: Feces, urine

▼ IV FACTS

Preparation: Prepare solution of 10 mg/mL, reconstitute with 10 mL (100-mg vial): 20 mL (200-mg vial) of sterile water for injection; dilute further with 100–1,000 mL (100-mg vial) or 200–2,000 mL (200-mg vial) of sodium chloride injection, 5% dextrose injection, Ringer's injection, 10% invert sugar in water, lactated Ringer injection, 5% dextrose in lactated Ringer solution, Normosol-M in D_5W, Normosol-R in D_5W, or Plasma-Lyte 56 or 148 in 5% Dextrose. If mixed in lactated Ringer solution or 5% dextrose in lactated Ringer solution, infusion must be completed within 6 hr after reconstitution; otherwise, may be stored up to 72 hr if refrigerated and protected from light, but infusion should then be completed within 12 hr; discard solution after that time.
Infusion: Infuse slowly over 1–4 hr.

Adverse effects

- **Dental:** *Discoloring and inadequate calcification of primary teeth of fetus if used by pregnant women, discoloring and inadequate calcification of permanent teeth if used during period of dental development*
- **Dermatologic:** *Phototoxic reactions, rash,* **exfoliative dermatitis** (more frequent and more severe with this tetracycline than with any others)

Adverse effects in *italics* are most common; those in **bold** are life-threatening. ⊂⊃ Do not crush.

- **GI:** Fatty liver, **liver failure,** *anorexia, nausea, vomiting, diarrhea, glossitis,* dysphagia, enterocolitis, esophageal ulcer
- **Hematologic: Hemolytic anemia, thrombocytopenia, neutropenia, eosinophilia,** leukocytosis, **leukopenia**
- **Local:** Local irritation at injection site
- **Other:** Superinfections, nephrogenic diabetes insipidus syndrome

Interactions
✳ **Drug-drug** • Decreased absorption with antacids, iron, alkali • Decreased therapeutic effects with barbiturates, carbamazepine, phenytoins • Increased digoxin toxicity with doxycycline • Decreased activity of penicillins
✳ **Drug-food** • Decreased effectiveness of doxycycline if taken with food, dairy products
✳ **Drug-lab test** • Interference with culture studies for several days following therapy

■ Nursing considerations
Assessment
- **History:** Allergy to tetracyclines, renal or hepatic impairment, pregnancy, lactation
- **Physical:** Skin status, R and sounds, GI function and liver evaluation, urinary output and concentration, urinalysis and BUN, LFTs, renal function tests; culture infected area before beginning therapy

Interventions
- Patients on long-term treatment for rosacea should be given drug in the morning, on an empty stomach, with a full glass of water.
- Administer the oral medication without regard to food or meals; if GI upset occurs, give with meals; patients being treated for periodontal disease should receive tablet at least 1 hr before morning and evening meals.
- Protect patient from light and sun exposure.

Teaching points
- Take drug throughout the day for best results; if GI upset occurs, take drug with food. If being treated for periodontal disease, take at least 1 hour before morning and evening meals. If being treated for rosacea, take first thing in the morning, on an empty stomach, with a full glass of water.
- Avoid pregnancy while taking this drug; using barrier contraceptives is advised, because hormonal contraceptives may not be effective.

- You may experience these side effects: Sensitivity to sunlight (wear protective clothing, use sunscreen), diarrhea.
- Report rash, itching, difficulty breathing, dark urine or light-colored stools, pain at injection site.

▷ dronabinol (delta-9-tetrahydrocannabinol, delta-9-THC)
*(droe **nab'** i nol)*

Marinol

PREGNANCY CATEGORY C

CONTROLLED SUBSTANCE C-III

Drug classes
Antiemetic
Appetite stimulant

Therapeutic actions
Principal psychoactive substance in marijuana; has complex CNS effects; mechanism of action as antiemetic is not understood.

Indications
- Treatment of nausea and vomiting associated with cancer chemotherapy in patients who have failed to respond adequately to conventional antiemetic treatment (should be used only under close supervision by a responsible individual because of potential to alter the mental state)
- Treatment of anorexia associated with weight loss in patients with AIDS for appetite stimulation

Contraindications and cautions
- Contraindicated with allergy to dronabinol or sesame oil vehicle in capsules, nausea and vomiting arising from any cause other than cancer chemotherapy, lactation.
- Use cautiously with hypertension; heart disease; manic, depressive, schizophrenic patients (dronabinol may unmask symptoms of these disease states); pregnancy; history of substance abuse; seizures.

Available forms
Capsules—2.5, 5, 10 mg

Dosages

Adults and pediatric patients

- *Antiemetic:* Initially, 5 mg/m^2 PO 1–3 hr prior to the administration of chemotherapy. Repeat dose every 2–4 hr after chemotherapy is given, for a total of four to six doses per day. If the 5 mg/m^2 dose is ineffective and there are no significant side effects, increase dose by 2.5 mg/m^2 increments to a maximum of 15 mg/m^2 per dose.
- *Appetite stimulation:* Initially, give 2.5 mg PO bid before lunch and supper. May reduce dose to 2.5 mg/day as a single evening or bedtime dose; up to 10 mg PO bid (not recommended for pediatric use).

Pharmacokinetics

Route	Onset	Peak	Duration
Oral	30–60 min	2–4 hr	4–6 hr

Metabolism: Hepatic; T$_{1/2}$: 25–36 hr
Distribution: May cross placenta; enters breast milk
Excretion: Bile, feces, urine

Adverse effects

- **CNS:** *Drowsiness; elation, laughing easily, heightened awareness, "high" dizziness; anxiety; muddled thinking; perceptual difficulties; impaired coordination; irritability, depression; weird feeling, weakness, sluggishness, headache; unsteadiness, hallucinations, memory lapse;* paresthesia, visual distortions; ataxia; paranoia, depersonalization; disorientation, confusion; tinnitus, nightmares, speech difficulty
- **CV:** Tachycardia, orthostatic hypotension; syncope
- **Dependence:** Psychological and physical dependence; tolerance to CNS and subjective effects after 30 days of use; withdrawal syndrome (irritability, insomnia, restlessness, hot flashes, sweating, rhinorrhea, loose stools, hiccups, anorexia) beginning 12 hr and ending 96 hr after discontinuation of high doses of the drug
- **Dermatologic:** Facial flushing, perspiring
- **GI:** *Dry mouth,* nausea, vomiting
- **GU:** Decrease in pregnancy rate, spermatogenesis when doses higher than those used clinically were given in preclinical studies

Interactions

❋ **Drug-drug** ● Do not give with ritonavir, alcohol, sedatives, hypnotics, other psychotomimetic substances ● Increased tachycardia, hypertension, drowsiness with anticholinergics, antihistamines, TCAs ● Use caution if combined with dofetilide

■ Nursing considerations

Assessment

- **History:** Allergy to dronabinol or sesame oil vehicle in capsules; nausea and vomiting arising from any cause other than cancer chemotherapy; hypertension; heart disease; manic, depressive, schizophrenic disorders; lactation; pregnancy; seizures; substance abuse
- **Physical:** Skin color, texture; orientation, reflexes, bilateral grip strength, affect; P, BP, orthostatic BP; status of mucous membranes

Interventions

- Store capsules in refrigerator.
- Limit prescriptions to the minimum necessary for a single cycle of chemotherapy because of abuse potential.
- Warn patient about drug's profound effects on mental status and abuse potential before giving drug; patient needs full information regarding the use of this drug.
- Warn patient about drug's potential effects on mood and behavior to prevent panic in case these occur.
- Patient should be supervised by a responsible adult while taking drug; monitor during the first cycle of chemotherapy in which dronabinol is used to determine how long patient will need supervision.

⊗ *Warning* Discontinue drug if psychotic reaction occurs; observe patient closely until evaluated and counseled; patient should participate in decision about further use of drug, perhaps at lower dosage.

Teaching points

- Take drug exactly as prescribed; a responsible adult should be with you at all times while you are taking this drug. This drug is a controlled substance; store in a secure area.
- Avoid alcohol, sedatives, and over-the-counter drugs, including nose drops and cold remedies, while you are taking this drug.
- You may experience these side effects: Mood changes (euphoria, feeling "high" or weird,

---

Adverse effects in *italics* are most common; those in **bold** are life-threatening. ⬛ Do not crush.

laughing, anxiety, depression, hallucinations, memory lapse, impaired thinking); weakness, faintness (change position slowly to avoid injury); dizziness, drowsiness (do not drive or perform tasks that require alertness if you experience these effects).

• Report bizarre thoughts, uncontrollable behavior or thought processes, fainting, dizziness, irregular heartbeat.

▷ **dronedarone**

(droh neb' dah roan)

Multaq

PREGNANCY CATEGORY X

Drug class
Antiarrhythmic

Therapeutic actions
Mechanism of action is not clear. Has properties of all antiarrhythmic classes; affects action potential of cardiac cells to alter conduction.

Indications
• To reduce risk of cardiovascular hospitalization in patients with paroxysmal or persistent atrial fibrillation or atrial flutter with a recent episode of either and associated cardiovascular risk factors (age older than 70 yr, hypertension, diabetes, prior stroke, left atrial diameter 50 mm or more, left ventricular ejection factor less than 40%) who are in sinus rhythm or will be cardioverted

Contraindications and cautions
⊗ *Black box warning* Contraindicated in patients with symptomatic HF or recent decompensation requiring hospitalization; doubled risk of death in these patients.

⊗ *Black box warning* Contraindicated in patients with atrial fibrillation who will not or cannot be cardioverted; doubled risk of death, stroke, and hospitalization for HF in these patients.

• Contraindicated with hypersensitivity to components of drug, class IV HF or recent acute failure requiring hospitalization or referral to a specialized HF clinic, second- or third-degree heart block, sick sinus syndrome, pulse rate less than 50, concomitant use of drugs or herbs that prolong QT interval, prolonged QT interval, severe hepatic impairment, concurrent use of CYP3A inhibitors, pregnancy, lactation, permanent atrial fibrillation.

• Use cautiously with mild to moderate hepatic impairment, hypokalemia, hypomagnesemia, mild to moderate HF.

Available forms
Tablets—400 mg

Dosages
Adults
400 mg PO bid with morning and evening meal.
Pediatric patients
Safety and efficacy not established.

Pharmacokinetics

Route	Onset	Peak
Oral	Slow	3–6 hr

Metabolism: Hepatic; $T_{1/2}$: 13–19 hr
Distribution: Crosses placenta; enters breast milk
Excretion: Feces

Adverse effects
• **CV:** Bradycardia, *prolonged QT interval,* **HF, stroke**
• **GI:** *Nausea, diarrhea,* vomiting, abdominal pain, dyspepsia, **serious liver injury possibly resulting in need for liver transplant**
• **Other:** *Asthenic conditions,* hypokalemia, hypomagnesemia, *rash*

Interactions
✱ **Drug-drug** • Increased risk of serious arrhythmias if combined with other antiarrhythmics; avoid this combination • Risk of digoxin toxicity if combined with dronedarone; cut digoxin dose in half and monitor patient closely • Risk of calcium channel blocker toxicity if combined; start with low dose of calcium channel blocker and monitor patient closely to verify effects and tolerability • Risk of serious bradycardia with beta blockers; start beta blocker with low dose and monitor patient closely • Risk of serious toxicity with CYP3A inhibitors (clarithromycin, itraconazole, ketoconazole, nefazodone, ritonavir; this combination is contraindicated • Decreased effectiveness with CYP3A

inducers (phenobarbital, phenytoin, rifampin); avoid this combination • Increased serum levels of sirolimus, tacrolimus; adjust dosage and monitor patient closely • Risk of increased serum statins levels; adjust dosage accordingly and monitor patient closely

✳ Drug-food • Risk of serious adverse effects if combined with grapefruit juice; avoid this combination

✳ Drug-alternative therapy • Risk of serious arrhythmia if combined with St. John's Wort; avoid this combination

■ Nursing considerations
Assessment
- **History:** Hypersensitivity to components of drug, heart failure or recent acute HF requiring hospitalization or referral to a specialized HF clinic, second- or third-degree heart block, sick sinus syndrome, pulse rate less than 50, concomitant use of drugs or herbs that prolong the QT interval, prolonged QT interval, hepatic impairment, concurrent use of CYP3A inhibitors, hypokalemia, hypomagnesemia, pregnancy, lactation
- **Physical:** Skin color, lesions; P, BP, ECG with QT evaluation, heart sounds, peripheral exam for edema; abdominal exam; LFTs; serum electrolytes

Interventions
- Obtain baseline and periodic ECGs to monitor for QT interval prolongation.
- Ensure that patient does not have serious heart failure; closely monitor patient with mild to moderate heart failure for worsening of condition.
- Monitor liver function prior to and periodically during treatment; risk of serious liver injury possibly resulting in need for liver transplant.
- Administer drug twice a day with morning and evening meal. Do not make up missed doses.
- Encourage patient to avoid grapefruit juice.
- Check patient's complete drug list and ensure that interacting drugs are not being used, and that appropriate dosage adjustments have been considered.
- Advise patient to use contraceptive measures; drug can cause serious fetal abnormalities.
- Advise breast-feeding patient to select another method of feeding.

- Arrange for regular monitoring of heart rhythm, cardiac status.

Teaching points
- Take this drug twice a day with your morning and evening meal.
- If you forget a dose, take the next dose at the regular time. Do not attempt to make up or double doses.
- Do not drink grapefruit juice or use St. John's Wort while taking this drug; serious adverse effects could occur.
- Continue to take this drug as prescribed, even if you are feeling well; you may be feeling well because the drug is working.
- Keep a record of all drugs, herbs, and over-the-counter medications you are taking and review it with your health care provider. This drug interacts with many of these drugs and serious complications could occur. Your health care provider may need to adjust the dosages of these drugs for your safety.
- This drug can cause serious harm to a fetus. The use of contraceptive measures is advised. If you become pregnant or wish to become pregnant, discuss this with your health care provider.
- This drug appears in breast milk and could seriously affect a baby. If you are breast-feeding, use another method of feeding the baby.
- You may experience these side effects: Nausea, vomiting, diarrhea, abdominal pain (small, frequent meals may help; consult your health care provider if abdominal pain becomes too uncomfortable), slow heart rate (you should learn to take your pulse; contact your health care provider if your heart rate becomes markedly slower), rash.
- You will need periodic ECGs to monitor the effects of this drug on your atrial arrhythmias.
- Report shortness of breath, wheezing; difficulty sleeping because of breathing problems; rapid weight gain of 5 pounds or more; swelling in the feet or legs; the need to prop yourself up with many pillows to sleep at night; extreme fatigue; changes in color of urine or stool.

▽ **droperidol**

See Appendix R, *Less commonly used drugs*.

▽ duloxetine hydrochloride
(do locks' ah teen)

Cymbalta ⓞⓡⓒ

PREGNANCY CATEGORY C

Drug classes
Antidepressant
Serotonin and norepinephrine reuptake inhibitor

Therapeutic actions
Inhibits neuronal serotonin and norepinephrine reuptake in the CNS resulting in a potentiation of serotonin and norepinephrine effects with resultant antidepressive effects.

Indications
- Treatment of major depressive disorder
- Management of neuropathic pain associated with diabetic peripheral neuropathy
- Treatment and maintenance therapy of generalized anxiety disorder
- Treatment of fibromyalgia
- Management of chronic musculoskeletal pain; including low back pain and chronic pain due to osteoarthritis
- Unlabeled use: Stress incontinence

Contraindications and cautions
- Contraindicated with allergy to any component of drug, concurrent use of MAOIs, uncontrolled narrow-angle glaucoma, lactation, concurrent substantial alcohol use, end-stage renal disease, hepatic impairment.
- Use cautiously with pregnancy, history of mania, history of seizures, controlled narrow-angle glaucoma.

Available forms
DR capsules ⓞⓡⓒ—20, 30, 60 mg

Dosages
Adults
- *Major depressive disorder:* 20 mg PO bid; up to 60 mg/day given once a day or 30 mg bid has been used; may be increased in 30-mg increments to a maximum of 120 mg/day.
- *Switching from an MAOI:* Allow at least 14 days to elapse between discontinuing the MAOI and beginning duloxetine.

- *Switching to an MAOI:* Allow at least 5 days to elapse between discontinuing duloxetine and starting an MAOI.
- *Diabetic neuropathic pain:* 60 mg/day PO taken as a single dose, without regard to food.
- *Generalized anxiety disorder:* 60 mg/day PO; may be increased in 30-mg increments to maximum of 120 mg/day.
- *Fibromyalgia:* 30 mg/day PO for 1 wk; then increase to 60 mg/day.
- *Chronic musculoskeletal pain:* Initially, 30 mg/day PO for 1 wk, then increase to maintenance dose of 60 mg/day PO.

Pharmacokinetics

Route	Peak	Duration
Oral	2 hr	6 hr

Metabolism: Hepatic; $T_{1/2}$: 8–17 hr
Distribution: May cross placenta; may enter breast milk
Excretion: Feces, urine

Adverse effects
- **CNS:** *Dizziness,* somnolence, tremor, blurred vision, *insomnia,* anxiety, suicidal ideation, agitation, irritability
- **CV:** Increased BP, increased heart rate
- **GI:** *Nausea, dry mouth, constipation, diarrhea,* **hepatoxicity,** vomiting, decreased appetite
- **GU:** Decreased libido, abnormal orgasm, erectile dysfunction, delayed ejaculation, dysuria
- **Other:** Hot flushes, *fatigue, increased sweating,* rash

Interactions
✳ **Drug-drug** • Risk of increased serum levels and toxic effects if combined with fluvoxamine; avoid this combination • Risk of bleeding if taken with NSAIDs, aspirin, warfarin • Risk of serotonin syndrome if combined with other SSRIs, triptans, linezolid, lithium, tramadol; avoid these combinations • Risk of higher serum levels if combined with paroxetine, fluoxetine, quinidine; use caution • Risk of increased levels of TCAs, phenothiazines, propafenone, flecainide if combined with duloxetine; monitor patient closely and adjust dosage as needed • Risk of serious to potentially fatal reactions if combined with MAOIs; avoid this combination and make sure patient has not had an MAOI for at least 14 days before beginning duloxetine • Risk of toxicity if combined with alcohol; avoid this combination

✳ **Drug-alternative therapy** • Risk of serotonin syndrome if combined with St. John's Wort; avoid this combination

■ **Nursing considerations**

Assessment

• **History:** Allergy to any component of the drug, concurrent use of MAOIs, narrow-angle glaucoma, lactation, concurrent substantial alcohol use, end-stage renal disease, hepatic impairment, pregnancy, history of mania, history of seizures

• **Physical:** Skin lesions, orientation, reflexes, affect; BP, P; abdominal examination

Interventions

• Ensure that patient is not taking an MAOI and has not taken one in at least 14 days before starting therapy.

• Monitor patient for signs of hepatotoxicity—darkened urine, right upper quadrant pain, flulike symptoms, elevated liver enzymes—especially if the patient uses alcohol excessively or has a history of liver impairment.

⊗ **Black box warning** Monitor patient for increased depression, including agitation, irritability, and increased suicidal ideation, especially when beginning therapy or changing dosage; especially likely with children, adolescents, and young adults. Provide appropriate interventions and protection. Drug is not approved for pediatric use.

• Ensure that patient swallows capsules whole; they should not be cut, crushed, or chewed, nor should the capsule be opened and the contents sprinkled on food.

• Instruct the patient not to consume considerable amounts of alcohol while on this drug; occurrence of liver damage is much greater when combined with alcohol; if the patient cannot refrain from alcohol intake, a different antidepressant should be used.

• Encourage the use of barrier contraceptives during treatment with this drug: fetal abnormalities are possible.

• Help the breast-feeding patient find another method of feeding the infant.

• Arrange to taper the drug when discontinuing; tapering decreases the risk of adverse events.

Teaching points

• Take this drug two times a day; it may be taken with or without food; if taking for diabetic neuropathy, take once a day.

• If you forget a dose, take it as soon as you remember and return to your usual regimen. Do not make up doses and do not take more than two doses in 24 hours.

• Swallow the capsule whole; do not cut, crush, chew, or sprinkle the contents of the capsule on food.

• Be aware that this drug should not be taken during pregnancy; if you suspect that you are pregnant, or wish to become pregnant, consult your health care provider.

• You should find another method of feeding the baby if you are breast-feeding; it is not known if this drug crosses into breast milk.

• Do not stop this drug abruptly; it should be tapered slowly to decrease adverse effects.

• Avoid alcohol and St. John's Wort while taking this drug; serious adverse effects could occur.

• You may experience impaired judgment, impaired thinking, or impaired motor skills. You should not drive or operate hazardous machinery or sign important documents or make important decisions until you are certain that *Cymbalta* has not affected your ability to engage in these activities safely.

• You may experience these side effects: Dry mouth, diarrhea, abdominal discomfort, nausea (sucking on sugarless candies may help; consult your health care provider if this becomes a problem); depression, thoughts of suicide (you and your family should discuss this possibility and they should be on the alert for signs that this is happening; if this occurs, consult your health care provider); changes in libido or sexual response (discuss this with your health care provider).

• Report depression or thoughts of suicide, changes in color of stool or urine, sexual dysfunction, agitation, fever, hallucinations, rapid heart rate.

▽ **dutasteride**
*(du **tas'** teh ride)*

Avodart ⊙ⁿ

PREGNANCY CATEGORY X

Drug classes

Androgen hormone inhibitor

BPH drug

Adverse effects in *italics* are most common; those in **bold** are life-threatening. ⊙ⁿ Do not crush.

Therapeutic actions

Inhibits the intracellular enzyme (5 alpha-reductase) that converts testosterone into a potent androgen (DHT); does not affect androgen receptors in the body; the prostate gland is dependent on DHT for its development and maintenance.

Indications

- Treatment of symptomatic BPH in men with an enlarged prostate gland
- In combination with tamsulosin for treatment of symptomatic BPH in men with enlarged prostate gland
- Unlabeled use: Prostate cancer prevention.

Contraindications and cautions

- Contraindicated with allergy to any component of the product, other 5-alpha-reductase inhibitors, women, children, pregnancy, lactation.
- Use cautiously with hepatic impairment.

Available forms

Capsule ᴼᵀᶜ—0.5 mg

Dosages

Adults

0.5 mg/day PO. Swallow whole.

- *Combination therapy with tamsulosin:* 0.5 mg/day PO with tamsulosin 0.4. mg/day PO.

Pediatric patients

Contraindicated in pediatric patients.

Pharmacokinetics

Route	Peak	Duration
Oral	2–3 hr	Unknown

Metabolism: Hepatic; $T_{1/2}$: 5 wk
Distribution: Crosses placenta; may enter breast milk (but not indicated for use in women)
Excretion: Feces

Adverse effects

- **GI:** Abdominal upset
- **GU:** Impotence, decreased libido, decreased volume of ejaculation
- **Other:** Breast enlargement, breast tenderness

Interactions

❋ **Drug-drug •** Possible increased serum levels with ketoconazole, ritonavir, verapamil, diltiazem, cimetidine, ciprofloxacin

❋ **Drug-lab test •** Decreased PSA levels; false decrease in PSA does not mean that patient is free of risk of prostate cancer

■ Nursing considerations

Assessment

- **History:** Allergy to any component of the product or other 5 alpha-reductase inhibitors, hepatic impairment, pregnancy, lactation
- **Physical:** Liver evaluation, abdominal examination; LFTs, renal function tests, normal urine output, prostate examination

Interventions

- Assess patient to ensure that problem is BPH and that other disorders (eg, prostate cancer, infection, strictures, hypotonic bladder) have been ruled out.
- Monitor patient periodically; may be at increased risk for an aggressive form of prostate cancer.
- Administer without regard to meals; ensure that the patient swallows capsules whole; do not cut, crush, or chew capsules.
- Arrange for regular follow-up, including prostate examination, PSA levels, and evaluation of urine flow.
- Monitor urine flow and output. Increase in urine flow may not occur in all patients.

⊗ **Warning** Do not allow pregnant women to handle dutasteride capsules because of risk of absorption, which could adversely affect the fetus.

⊗ **Warning** Caution patient that if his sex partner is or may become pregnant, she should be protected from his semen, which contains dutasteride and could adversely affect the fetus. The patient should use a condom or discontinue dutasteride therapy.

- Caution patient that he will not be able to donate blood until at least 6 mo after the last dose of dutasteride.
- Alert patient that libido may be decreased as well as volume of ejaculation; these effects are usually reversible when the drug is stopped.
- Provide counseling to help patient deal with effects on sexuality.

Teaching points

- Take this drug without regard to meals. Swallow the capsule whole; do not cut, crush, or chew capsules. If you miss a dose, take the capsule as soon as you remember and take the next dose the following day. Do not take more than one capsule each day.

- Arrange to have regular medical follow-up while you are on this drug to evaluate your response.
- This drug has serious adverse effects on unborn babies; do not allow a pregnant woman to handle the drug; if your sex partner is or may become pregnant, protect her from exposure to your semen by using a condom; you may need to discontinue the drug if this is not acceptable.
- You will not be able to donate blood until at least 6 months after your last dose of dutasteride to prevent inadvertently giving dutasteride to a pregnant woman in a blood transfusion.
- You may experience these side effects: Loss of libido, impotence, decreased amount of ejaculate (these effects are usually reversible when the drug is stopped).
- Report inability to void, groin pain, sore throat, fever, weakness.

▷ dyphylline
(dihydroxypropyl
theophyllin)
(dye' fi lin)

Dylix, Lufyllin, Lufyllin-400

PREGNANCY CATEGORY C

Drug classes
Bronchodilator
Xanthine

Therapeutic actions
A theophylline derivative that is not metabolized to theophylline; relaxes bronchial smooth muscle, causing bronchodilation and increasing vital capacity, which has been impaired by bronchospasm and air trapping; at high doses it also inhibits the release of slow-reacting substance of anaphylaxis and histamine.

Indications
- Symptomatic relief or prevention of bronchial asthma and reversible bronchospasm associated with chronic bronchitis and emphysema

Contraindications and cautions
- Contraindicated with hypersensitivity to any xanthine or to ethylenediamine, peptic ulcer, active gastritis.
- Use cautiously with cardiac arrhythmias, acute myocardial injury, heart failure, cor pulmonale, severe hypertension, severe hypoxemia, renal or hepatic disease, hyperthyroidism, alcoholism, pregnancy, lactation.

Available forms
Tablets—200, 400 mg; elixir—100 mg/15 mL

Dosages
Individualize dosage based on clinical responses with monitoring of serum dyphylline levels; serum theophylline levels do not measure dyphylline; equivalence of dyphylline to theophylline is not known.
Adults
Up to 15 mg/kg, PO every 6 hr.
Pediatric patients
Safety and efficacy not established.
Geriatric patients or impaired adults
Use cautiously in elderly men and with cor pulmonale, heart failure, or renal disease.

Pharmacokinetics

Route	Peak	Duration
Oral	1 hr	6 hr

Metabolism: Hepatic; $T_{1/2}$: 2 hr
Distribution: Crosses placenta; enters breast milk
Excretion: Urine

Adverse effects
- **CNS:** *Headache, insomnia,* irritability; restlessness, dizziness, muscle twitching, seizures, severe depression, stammering speech; abnormal behavior: Withdrawal, mutism, and unresponsiveness alternating with hyperactivity; brain damage, **death**
- **CV:** Palpitations, sinus tachycardia, ventricular tachycardia, life-threatening ventricular arrhythmias, circulatory failure, hypotension
- **GI:** *Nausea, vomiting, diarrhea,* loss of appetite, hematemesis, epigastric pain, gastroesophageal reflux during sleep, increased AST

Adverse effects in *italics* are most common; those in **bold** are life-threatening. ⊂⊃ Do not crush.

- **GU:** Proteinuria, increased excretion of renal tubular cells and RBCs; diuresis (dehydration), urinary retention in men with prostate enlargement
- **Respiratory:** Tachypnea, respiratory arrest
- **Other:** Fever, flushing, hyperglycemia, SIADH, rash

Interactions

✳ **Drug-drug** • Increased effects with probenecid, mexiletine • Increased cardiac toxicity with halothane • Decreased effects of benzodiazepines, nondepolarizing neuromuscular blockers • Mutually antagonistic effects of beta blockers and dyphylline

■ Nursing considerations
Assessment

- **History:** Hypersensitivity to any xanthine or to ethylenediamine, peptic ulcer, active gastritis, cardiac arrhythmias, acute myocardial injury, heart failure, cor pulmonale, severe hypertension, severe hypoxemia, renal or hepatic disease, hyperthyroidism, alcoholism, labor, lactation
- **Physical:** Bowel sounds, normal output; P, auscultation, BP, perfusion, ECG; R, adventitious sounds; frequency, voiding, normal output pattern, urinalysis, renal function tests; liver palpation, LFTs; thyroid function tests; skin color, texture, lesions; reflexes, bilateral grip strength, affect, EEG

Interventions

- Give with food if GI effects occur.
- Monitor patient carefully for clinical signs of adverse effects.
- Keep diazepam readily available to treat seizures.

Teaching points

- Take this drug exactly as prescribed (around the clock for adequate control of asthma attacks).
- Avoid excessive intake of coffee, tea, cocoa, cola beverages, and chocolate.
- Keep all appointments for monitoring of response to this drug.
- You may experience these side effects: Nausea, loss of appetite (take with food); difficulty sleeping, depression, emotional lability.

- Report nausea, vomiting, severe GI pain, restlessness, seizures, irregular heartbeat.

▷ ecallantide
See Appendix R, *Less commonly used drugs*.

▷ eculizumab
See Appendix R, *Less commonly used drugs*.

▷ edetate calcium disodium (calcium EDTA)
(**ed' e tate**)

Calcium Disodium Versenate

PREGNANCY CATEGORY B

Drug class
Antidote

Therapeutic actions
Calcium in this compound is easily displaced by heavy metals, such as lead, to form stable complexes that are excreted in the urine; edetate disodium has strong affinity to calcium, lowering calcium levels and pulling calcium out of extracirculatory stores during slow infusion.

Indications
- Acute and chronic lead poisoning and lead encephalopathy

Contraindications and cautions
- Contraindicated with sensitivity to EDTA preparations, anuria, active renal disease, hepatitis, increased intracranial pressure (rapid IV infusion).
- Use cautiously with cardiac disease, heart failure, lactation, renal impairment, pregnancy.

Available forms
Injection—200 mg/mL

Dosages
Effective by IV, IM routes; IM route is safest in children and patients with lead encephalopathy.
Adults and pediatric patients
- *Lead poisoning:* For blood levels 20–70 mcg/dL, 1,000 mg/m²/day IV or IM for

5 days. Interrupt therapy for 2–4 days; follow with another 5 days of treatment if indicated. For blood levels higher than 70 mcg/dL, combine with dimercaprol therapy.

Pharmacokinetics

Route	Onset	Peak
IM, IV	1 hr	24–48 hr

Metabolism: $T_{1/2}$: 20–60 min (IV), 90 min (IM)
Distribution: May cross placenta; may enter breast milk
Excretion: Urine

▼ IV FACTS

Preparation: *Lead poisoning:* Dilute the 5 mL ampule with 250–500 mL of 0.9% sodium chloride or 5% dextrose solution. *Pediatric:* Dissolve dose in a sufficient volume of 5% dextrose injection or 0.9% sodium chloride injection to bring the final concentration to not more than 3%.
Infusion: *Lead poisoning:* Infuse the total daily dose over 4–24 hr. *Pediatric:* Infuse over 3 hr or more. Do not exceed the patient's cardiac reserve.

Adverse effects

- **CNS:** Headache, transient circumoral paresthesia, numbness
- **CV:** Heart failure, blood pressure changes, thrombophlebitis
- **GI:** *Nausea, vomiting, diarrhea* (edetate disodium)
- **GU:** Renal tubular necrosis
- **Hematologic:** *Electrolyte imbalance* (hypocalcemia, hypokalemia, hypomagnesemia, altered blood sugar)

Interactions

✳ Drug-drug • Decreased effectiveness of zinc insulin with edetate calcium disodium; suggest use of other insulin preparation

■ Nursing considerations

Assessment

- **History:** Sensitivity to EDTA preparations; anuria; increased intracranial pressure; cardiac disease, HF, active renal disease, hepatitis, lactation, pregnancy
- **Physical:** Pupillary reflexes, orientation; P, BP; urinalysis, BUN, serum electrolytes

Interventions

⊗ **Black box warning** Reserve use for serious conditions that require aggressive therapy; serious toxicity can occur.
- Administer IM or IV.
- Avoid excess fluids in patients with lead encephalopathy and increased intracranial pressure; for these patients, mix edetate calcium disodium 20% solution with procaine to give a final concentration of 0.5% procaine, and administer IM.
- Establish urine flow by IV infusion prior to first dose to those dehydrated from vomiting. Once urine flow is established, restrict further IV fluid. Stop EDTA when urine flow ceases.
- Arrange for periodic BUN and serum electrolyte determinations before and during each course of therapy. Stop drug if signs of increasing renal damage occur.
- Do not administer in larger than recommended doses.

⊗ **Warning** Keep patient supine for a short period because of the possibility of orthostatic hypotension.

Teaching points

- Prepare a schedule of rest and drug days.
- Arrange for periodic blood tests during the course of therapy.
- Constant monitoring of heart rhythm may be needed during drug administration.
- Report pain at injection site, difficulty voiding, markedly decreased urine production.

▷ edrophonium chloride

(ed roe foe' nee um)

Enlon, Reversol

PREGNANCY CATEGORY C

Drug classes

Antidote
Cholinesterase inhibitor (anticholinesterase)
Diagnostic agent
Muscle stimulant

Therapeutic actions

Increases the concentration of acetylcholine at the sites of cholinergic transmission;

prolongs and exaggerates the effects of acetylcholine by reversibly inhibiting the enzyme acetylcholinesterase, facilitating transmission at the skeletal neuromuscular junction.

Indications
- Differential diagnosis and adjunct in evaluating treatment of myasthenia gravis
- Antidote for nondepolarizing neuromuscular junction blockers (curare, tubocurarine) after surgery

Contraindications and cautions
- Contraindicated with hypersensitivity to anticholinesterases, intestinal or urogenital tract obstruction, peritonitis, sulfite sensitivity, lactation.
- Use cautiously with asthma, peptic ulcer, bradycardia, cardiac arrhythmias, recent coronary occlusion, vagotonia, hyperthyroidism, epilepsy, pregnancy near term.

Available forms
Injection—10 mg/mL

Dosages
Adults
IM
- *Differential diagnosis of myasthenia gravis:* If veins are inaccessible, inject 10 mg IM. Patients who demonstrate cholinergic reaction (see table) should be retested with 2 mg IM after 30 min to rule out false-negative results.

IV
- *Differential diagnosis of myasthenia gravis:* Prepare tuberculin syringe containing 10 mg edrophonium with IV needle. Inject 2 mg IV in 15–30 sec; leave needle in vein. If no reaction occurs after 45 sec, inject the remaining 8 mg. If a cholinergic reaction (parasympathomimetic effects, muscle fasciculations, or increased muscle weakness) occurs after 2 mg, discontinue the test, and administer atropine sulfate 0.4–0.5 mg IV. May repeat test after 30 min.
- *Evaluation of treatment requirements in myasthenia gravis:* 1–2 mg IV 1 hr after oral intake of the treatment drug. Responses are summarized below:

Response to Edrophonium Test	Myasthenia (Under-treated)	Cholinergic (Over-treated)
Muscle strength: ptosis, diplopia, respiration, limb strength	Increased	Decreased
Fasciculations: orbicularis oculi facial and limb muscles	Absent	Present or absent
Side reactions: lacrimation, sweating, salivating, nausea, vomiting, diarrhea, abdominal cramps	Absent	Severe

- *Edrophonium test in crisis:* Secure controlled respiration immediately if patient is apneic, then administer test. If patient is in cholinergic crisis, administration of edrophonium will increase oropharyngeal secretions and further weaken respiratory muscles. If crisis is myasthenic, administration of edrophonium will improve respiration, and patient can be treated with longer-acting IV anticholinesterase medication. To administer the test, draw up no more than 2 mg edrophonium into the syringe. Give 1 mg IV initially. Carefully observe cardiac response. If after 1 min this dose does not further impair the patient, inject the remaining 1 mg. If after a 2-mg dose no clear improvement in respiration occurs, discontinue all anticholinesterase drug therapy, and control ventilation by tracheostomy and assisted respiration.
- *Antidote for nondepolarizing neuromuscular junction blockers:* 10 mg given slowly IV over 30–45 sec so that onset of cholinergic reaction can be detected; repeat when necessary. Maximal dose for any patient is 40 mg.

Pediatric patients
IV
- *Differential diagnosis of myasthenia gravis:*
  Infants: 0.5 mg.
  Child weighing 34 kg or less: 1 mg.
  Child weighing more than 34 kg: 2 mg.
If child does not respond in 45 sec, dose may be titrated up to 5 mg in child less than 34 kg, up to 10 mg in child more than 34 kg, given in increments of 1 mg every 30–45 sec.

IM

- *Differential diagnosis of myasthenia gravis:*
  Child weighing 34 kg or less: 2 mg.
  Child weighing more than 34 kg: 5 mg.
  A delay of 2–10 min occurs until reaction.
  Maximum dose: total of 10 mg.

Pharmacokinetics

Route	Onset	Duration
IM	2–10 min	5–30 min
IV	30–60 sec	5–20 min

Metabolism: $T_{1/2}$: 5–10 min
Distribution: May cross placenta; may enter breast milk
Excretion: Unknown

▼ IV FACTS

Preparation: No preparation is required.
Infusion: Rate of infusion varies with reason for administration; see Dosages.

Adverse effects
Parasympathomimetic effects

- **CV:** *Bradycardia, cardiac arrhythmias,*
  AV block and nodal rhythm, **cardiac arrest;** decreased cardiac output, leading to
  hypotension, syncope
- **Dermatologic:** Diaphoresis, flushing
- **EENT:** *Lacrimation, miosis,* spasm of accommodation, diplopia, conjunctival hyperemia
- **GI:** *Salivation, dysphagia, nausea, vomiting, increased peristalsis, abdominal cramps,* flatulence, diarrhea
- **GU:** *Urinary frequency and incontinence,*
  urinary urgency
- **Respiratory:** *Increased pharyngeal and tracheobronchial secretions,* laryngospasm, bronchospasm, bronchiolar constriction, dyspnea

General effects

- **CNS:** Seizures, dysarthria, dysphonia, drowsiness, dizziness, headache, loss of consciousness
- **Dermatologic:** Rash, urticaria, **anaphylaxis**
- **Local:** Thrombophlebitis after IV use
- **Peripheral:** Skeletal muscle weakness, fasciculations, muscle cramps, arthralgia
- **Respiratory:** Respiratory muscle paralysis, central respiratory paralysis

Interactions

✳ **Drug-drug** • Risk of profound muscular
depression refractory to anticholinesterases if given concurrently with corticosteroids, succinylcholine

■ Nursing considerations
Assessment

Administering edrophonium for diagnostic purposes is generally supervised by a neurologist or other physician skilled and experienced in dealing with myasthenic patients; administering edrophonium to reverse neuromuscular blocking drugs is generally supervised by an anesthesiologist. Any nurse participating in the care of a patient receiving anticholinesterases should keep these points in mind.

- **History:** Hypersensitivity to anticholinesterases; intestinal or urogenital tract obstruction, peritonitis, lactation, asthma, peptic ulcer, cardiac arrhythmias, recent coronary occlusion, vagotonia, hyperthyroidism, epilepsy, pregnancy near term
- **Physical:** Bowel sounds, normal output; frequency, voiding pattern, normal output; R, adventitious sounds; P, auscultation, BP; reflexes, bilateral grip strength, EEG; thyroid function tests; skin color, texture, lesions

Interventions

- Administer IV slowly with constant monitoring of patient's response.
- Overdosage with anticholinesterase drugs can cause muscle weakness (cholinergic crisis) that is difficult to differentiate from myasthenic weakness; edrophonium is used to help make this diagnostic distinction. The administration of atropine may mask the parasympathetic effects of anticholinesterases and confound the diagnosis.

⊗ **Warning** Keep atropine sulfate readily available as an antidote and antagonist to edrophonium.

Teaching points

- The patient should know what to expect during diagnostic test with edrophonium (patients receiving drug to reverse neuromuscular blockers will not be aware of drug effects and do not require specific teaching about the drug).

efavirenz
(eff ah vye' renz)

Sustiva ⓒⓐⓝ

PREGNANCY CATEGORY D

Drug classes
Antiviral
Non-nucleoside reverse transcriptase inhibitor

Therapeutic actions
A non-nucleoside reverse transcriptase inhibitor shown to be effective in suppressing the HIV virus in adults and children.

Indications
• Treatment of HIV and AIDS in adults and children when used in combination with other antiretroviral drugs

Contraindications and cautions
• Contraindicated with life-threatening allergy to any component, lactation.
• Use cautiously with hepatic impairment, hypercholesterolemia, psychiatric disorders, pregnancy.

Available forms
Capsules ⓒⓐⓝ—50, 200 mg; tablets ⓒⓐⓝ—600 mg

Dosages
Adults
600 mg PO daily in conjunction with a protease inhibitor or other nucleoside reverse transcriptase inhibitor. In combination with voriconazole 400 mg PO every 12 hr: 300 mg/day efavirenz PO. In combination with rifampin, patients weighing 50 kg or more, increase efavirenz to 800 mg/day PO.
Pediatric patients 3 yr and older
Dosage, given at bedtime, is based on weight of child as follows:

Weight (kg)	Daily Dosage (mg)
10–less than 15	200 PO
15–less than 20	250 PO
20–less than 25	300 PO
25–less than 32.5	350 PO
32.5–less than 40	400 PO
40 or more	600 PO

Pediatric patients younger than 3 yr
Not recommended.

Pharmacokinetics

Route	Onset	Peak
Oral	Varies	3–5 hr

Metabolism: Hepatic; $T_{1/2}$: 52–76 hr
Distribution: Crosses placenta; may enter breast milk
Excretion: Urine

Adverse effects
• **CNS:** *Headache,* insomnia, *drowsiness, asthenia,* malaise, *dizziness,* paresthesia, somnolence, impaired concentration, depression, suicidal ideation
• **GI:** *Nausea, diarrhea,* anorexia, vomiting, dyspepsia, liver impairment
• **Other:** Increased cholesterol, *rash*

Interactions
✳ **Drug-drug** ⊗ *Warning* Possible severe adverse effects if taken with bepridil, cisapride, pimozide, midazolam, rifabutin, triazolam, ergot derivatives; avoid these combinations, which are contraindications • Possible increased hepatic impairment if combined with alcohol or hepatotoxic drugs; avoid this combination • Decreased levels of voriconazole if combined; adjust dosages of both drugs • Decreased effectiveness of indinavir, saquinavir; consider dosage adjustments • Decreased serum levels of efavirenz if combined with rifampin • Risk of increased levels of ritonavir when combined • Risk of decreased methadone levels and withdrawal symptoms of methadone if taken with efavirenz
✳ **Drug-food** • Decreased absorption and therapeutic effects if taken with a high-fat meal; avoid taking with food
✳ **Drug-lab test** • False-positive urine cannabinoid test
✳ **Drug-alternative therapy** • Decreased effectiveness of efavirenz with St. John's Wort; avoid this combination

■ Nursing considerations
Assessment
• **History:** Life-threatening allergy to any component, impaired hepatic function, pregnancy, lactation, hypercholesterolemia
• **Physical:** Rashes, lesions, texture; body T; affect, reflexes, peripheral sensation; bowel sounds, liver evaluation; LFTs, CBC and differential, serum cholesterol

Interventions

- Arrange to monitor hematologic indices every 2 wk during therapy.
- Ensure that patient is taking this drug as part of a combination therapy program.
- ⊗ **Warning** Administer the drug at bedtime for the first 2–4 wk of therapy to minimize the CNS effects of the drug.
- Monitor patient for signs of opportunistic infections that will need to be treated appropriately.
- Administer the drug once a day, with meals if GI effects occur. Avoid high-fat meals.
- Provide comfort measures to help patient to cope with drug's effects—environmental control (temperature, lighting), back rubs, mouth care.
- Recommend patient use barrier contraceptives while taking this drug; serious fetal deformities have occurred.
- Establish safety precautions if CNS effects occur, especially likely during the first few days of treatment.
- Offer support and encouragement to the patient to deal with the diagnosis as well as the effects of drug therapy.

Teaching points

- Take drug once a day. Take the drug at bedtime to cut down some of the unpleasant effects of the drug. You may take the drug with meals if GI upset is a problem. Avoid taking this drug with high-fat meals. Be sure to take your other drugs regularly along with the efavirenz. Do not break tablets; swallow them whole.
- Efavirenz is not a cure for AIDS or HIV; opportunistic infections may occur and regular medical care should be sought to deal with the disease.
- Efavirenz does not reduce the risk of transmission of HIV to others by sexual contact or blood contamination; use appropriate precautions.
- Use barrier contraceptives while you are taking this drug; serious fetal deformities can occur. If you wish to become pregnant, consult your health care provider.
- Report any medications or herbs you are taking to your health care provider; avoid St. John's Wort while taking this drug.
- You may experience these side effects: Nausea, loss of appetite, GI upset (eat frequent small meals; consult your health care provider if this becomes severe); dizziness,

drowsiness (this is more likely at the beginning of drug therapy; avoid driving and operating machinery if these occur).
- Report extreme fatigue, lethargy, severe headache, severe nausea, vomiting, difficulty breathing, rash, depression, changes in color of stools, thoughts of suicide.

▷ eletriptan hydrobromide
*(ell ah **trip'** tan)*

Relpax

PREGNANCY CATEGORY C

Drug classes

Antimigraine drug
5-HT receptor selective agonist
Triptan

Therapeutic actions

Binds to serotonin receptors to cause vascular constrictive effects on cranial blood vessels, causing the relief of migraine in selective patients.

Indications

- Treatment of acute migraines with or without aura in adults

Contraindications and cautions

- Contraindicated with hypersensitivity to any component of eletriptan, allergy to other triptans, ischemic heart disease, cerebrovascular syndrome, peripheral vascular disease, uncontrolled hypertension, hemiplegic or basilar migraine, severe hepatic impairment, within 24 hr of using any other triptan- or ergotamine-containing medication.
- Use cautiously with pregnancy, lactation, hepatic impairment.

Available forms

Tablets—20, 40 mg

Dosages
Adults

Individualize dosage; 20–40 mg PO. If the headache improves but then returns, a second dose may be given after waiting at least 2 hr. Maximum daily dose, 80 mg.
Pediatric patients

Safety and efficacy not established.

Adverse effects in *italics* are most common; those in **bold** are life-threatening. ⊞ Do not crush.

Pharmacokinetics

Route	Onset	Peak
Oral	Rapid	1.5–2 hr

Metabolism: Hepatic; $T_{1/2}$: 4 hr
Distribution: May cross placenta; enters breast milk
Excretion: Urine, nonrenal processes

Adverse effects

- **CNS:** *Hypertonia, hypesthesia, vertigo,* abnormal dreams, anxiety
- **CV: Palpitations,** hypertension, tachycardia, angina, **MI**
- **GI:** Nausea, anorexia, constipation, esophagitis, flatulence
- **Respiratory:** *Pharyngitis,* dyspnea, asthma, URI, rhinitis
- **Other:** Fever, chills, *sweating,* bone pain

Interactions

✳ **Drug-drug** ● Risk of prolonged vasospastic reactions if combined with ergot-containing drugs; do not use within 24 hr of each other ● Risk of greatly elevated serum levels of CYP3A4 inhibitors—ketoconazole, itraconazole, nefazodone, clarithromycin, ritonavir, nelfinavir—and of eletriptan if combined; do not use within 72 hr of each other ● Risk of combined effects if used within 24 hr of other triptans; do not use within 24 hr of each other ● Risk of serotonin syndrome if combined with other serotonergic drugs, such as SSRIs

■ Nursing considerations
Assessment

- **History:** Hypersensitivity to any component of eletriptan, allergy to other triptans, presence of ischemic heart disease, cerebrovascular syndrome, peripheral vascular disease, uncontrolled hypertension, hemiplegic or basilar migraine, severe hepatic impairment, use within 24 hr of any other triptan- or ergotamine-containing medication, pregnancy, lactation, hepatic impairment
- **Physical:** T, orientation, reflexes, peripheral sensation; P, BP; R, adventitious sounds; abdominal examination; LFTs

Interventions

- Administer to relieve acute migraine, not as a prophylactic measure; supervise first dose of drug.

- Ensure that the patient has not taken an ergot-containing compound or other triptan within 24 hr.
- Do not administer more than two doses in a 24-hr period.
- Establish safety measures if CNS or visual disturbances occur.
- Control environment (eg, lighting, temperature) as appropriate to help relieve migraine.

⊗ **Warning** Monitor BP of patients with possible coronary artery disease; discontinue at any sign of angina, prolonged high BP, tachycardia, chest discomfort.

Teaching points

- Take this drug exactly as prescribed, at the onset of headache or aura. Do not take this drug to prevent a migraine; it is used only to treat migraines that are occurring. If the headache persists after you take this drug, you may repeat the dose 2 hours later.
- Do not take more than two doses in 24-hour period. Do not take any other migraine medication while you are taking this drug. If your headache is not relieved, consult your health care provider.
- Maintain your usual procedures during a migraine—eg, control lighting, noise.
- Contact your health care provider immediately if you experience chest pain or pressure that is severe or does not go away.
- This drug interacts with many other drugs; consult with your health care provider if you are taking any other medications or if you add any drugs to your drug regimen.
- This drug should not be taken during pregnancy; if you suspect that you are pregnant, contact your health care provider and refrain from using drug.
- You may experience these side effects: Dizziness, drowsiness (avoid driving and using dangerous machinery while taking this drug); numbness, tingling, feelings of tightness or pressure.
- Report chest pain, numbness, chills.

▽ **eltrombopag**

See Appendix R, *Less commonly used drugs.*

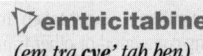

▷ emtricitabine

(em tra cye' tah ben)

Emtriva

PREGNANCY CATEGORY B

Drug classes
Anti-HIV drug
Antiviral
Nucleoside reverse transcriptase inhibitor

Therapeutic actions
HIV-1 reverse transcriptase inhibitor; competes with a natural substrate and is incorporated into the viral DNA, leading to chain termination.

Indications
- In combination with other antiretroviral drugs for the treatment of HIV-1 infection in adults and children

Contraindications and cautions
- Contraindicated with allergy to any components of the product; lactation (HIV-infected mothers are discouraged from breast-feeding); concurrent use of lamivudine, *Atripla*, *Truvada*.
- Use cautiously with pregnancy; hepatic impairment; signs of lactic acidosis, risk factors for lactic acidosis including female gender and obesity; infection with hepatitis B virus; impaired renal function.

Available forms
Capsules—200 mg; oral solution—10 mg/mL

Dosages
Adults
200 mg daily PO, with or without food or 240 mg (24 mL) oral solution/day PO.
Pediatric patients 3 mo–17 yr
6 mg/kg/day PO to a maximum 240 mg (24 mL) oral solution; children weighing more than 33 kg and able to swallow a capsule may take one 200-mg capsule/day PO.
Pediatric patients up to 3 mo
3 mg/kg oral solution PO once daily
Patients with renal impairment
For dialysis patients, 200 mg PO every 96 hr. For renally impaired patients, use these dosages:

CrCl (mL/min)	Capsule Dosage (mg)	Oral Solution Dosage (mg)
50 or more	200 daily	240 daily
30–49	200 every 48 hr	120 daily
15–29	200 every 72 hr	80 daily
Less than 15	200 every 96 hr	60 daily

Pharmacokinetics

Route	Onset	Peak
Oral	Rapid	1–2 hr

Metabolism: Hepatic; $T_{1/2}$: 10 hr
Distribution: May cross placenta; may enter breast milk
Excretion: Feces, urine

Adverse effects
- **CNS:** *Headache, asthenia,* depression, *insomnia, dizziness,* peripheral neurologic symptoms, neuritis, fatigue, paresthesia, *abnormal dreams*
- **GI:** *Nausea, diarrhea, abdominal pain,* vomiting, dyspepsia, **severe hepatomegaly with steatosis, sometimes fatal;** *elevated liver enzymes and bilirubin*
- **Metabolic: Lactic acidosis, sometimes severe;** hyperglycemia
- **Respiratory:** *Cough, rhinitis*
- **Other:** *Rash,* arthralgia, myalgia, fat redistribution

■ Nursing considerations
Assessment
- **History:** Allergy to any components of the product, lactation, pregnancy, hepatic impairment, signs of lactic acidosis, obesity, renal impairment, hepatitis B infection
- **Physical:** T; orientation, reflexes; R, adventitious sounds; abdominal examination, LFTs, renal function tests

Interventions
- Ensure that HIV antibody testing has been done before initiating therapy to reduce risk of emergence of HIV resistance.
- Ensure that patient is taking this drug in combination with other antiretroviral drugs.
- Ensure that patient is not taking combination drugs *Atripla, Complera, Truvada;* concurrent use is contraindicated.
- Monitor patients regularly to evaluate liver and renal function.

⊗ Black box warning Use caution if patient has or is suspected of having hepatitis B; serious resurgence of the disease can occur.

• Administer this drug without regard to food.

⊗ Black box warning Withdraw drug and monitor patient if patient develops signs of lactic acidosis or hepatotoxicity, including hepatomegaly and steatosis.

• Encourage women of childbearing age to use barrier contraceptives while taking this drug because the effects of the drug on the fetus are not known.

• Advise women who are breast-feeding to find another method of feeding the infant; HIV-infected woman are advised not to breast-feed.

• Advise patient that this drug does not cure the disease and there is still a risk of transmitting the disease to others.

Teaching points

• Take this drug once a day with or without food and in combination with your other antiviral drugs.

• Take the drug every day; if you miss a dose, take it as soon as you remember and then take the next dose at the usual time the next day. Do not double any doses.

• This drug does not cure your HIV infection and you will still be able to pass it to others; using condoms is advised. Women of childbearing age are encouraged not to become pregnant while taking this drug; barrier contraceptives are recommended.

• This drug may enter breast milk; if you are breast-feeding, you should find another method of feeding.

• With some antiviral drugs, there is a redistribution of body fat—a "buffalo hump" appears and fat is distributed around the trunk and lost in the limbs; the long-term effects of this redistribution are not known.

• You may experience these side effects: Nausea, diarrhea, abdominal pain, headache (try to maintain your intake of nutrition and fluid as much as possible; eat frequent small meals and take the drug with food).

• Report severe weakness, muscle pain, trouble breathing, dizziness, cold feelings in your arms or legs, palpitations, yellowing of the eyes or skin, darkened urine or light-colored stools.

▷**enalapril maleate**
(e nal' a pril)

Vasotec

enalaprilat
Vasotec I.V.

PREGNANCY CATEGORY D

E

Drug classes
ACE inhibitor
Antihypertensive

Therapeutic actions
Renin, synthesized by the kidneys, is released into the circulation where it acts on a plasma precursor to produce angiotensin I, which is converted by ACE to angiotensin II, a potent vasoconstrictor that also causes release of aldosterone from the adrenals; both of these actions increase BP. Enalapril blocks the conversion of angiotensin I to angiotensin II, decreasing BP, decreasing aldosterone secretion, slightly increasing serum K+ levels, and causing Na+ and fluid loss; increased prostaglandin synthesis also may be involved in the antihypertensive action. In patients with heart failure, peripheral resistance, afterload, preload, and heart size are decreased.

Indications
Oral

• Treatment of hypertension alone or in combination with other antihypertensives, especially thiazide-type diuretics

• Treatment of acute and chronic heart failure

• Treatment of asymptomatic left ventricular dysfunction (LVD)

■ **NEW INDICATION:** Unlabeled use: Raynaud phenomenon in adults

Parenteral

• Treatment of hypertension when oral therapy is not possible

Contraindications and cautions

• Contraindicated with pregnancy, allergy to enalapril, history of hereditary or idiopathic angioedema.

• Use cautiously with impaired renal function; salt or volume depletion (hypotension may occur); lactation.

Available forms

Tablets—2.5, 5, 10, 20 mg; injection—1.25 mg/mL

Dosages

Adults

Oral

- *Hypertension:*
  Patients not taking diuretics: Initial dose is 5 mg/day PO. Adjust dosage based on patient response. Usual range is 10–40 mg/day as a single dose or in two divided doses.
  Patients taking diuretics: Discontinue diuretic for 2–3 days if possible. If it is not possible to discontinue diuretic, give initial dose of 2.5 mg, and monitor for excessive hypotension for at least 2 hr.
  Converting to oral therapy from IV therapy: 5 mg daily with subsequent doses based on patient response.
- *Heart failure:* 2.5 mg PO daily or bid in conjunction with diuretics and digitalis. Maintenance dose is 2.5–20 mg/day given in two divided doses. Maximum daily dose is 40 mg.
- *Asymptomatic LVD:* 2.5 mg PO bid; target maintenance dose 20 mg/day in two divided doses.

Parenteral

Give IV only. 1.25 mg every 6 hr given IV over 5 min. A response is usually seen within 15 min, but peak effects may not occur for 4 hr.

- *Hypertension:*
  Converting to IV therapy from oral therapy: 1.25 mg every 6 hr; monitor patient response.
  Patients taking diuretics: 0.625 mg IV over 5 min. If adequate response is not seen after 1 hr, repeat the 0.625-mg dose. Give additional doses of 1.25 mg every 6 hr.

Pediatric patients 2 mo–16 yr

Oral

- *Hypertension:* Initial dose is 0.08 mg/kg PO once daily; maximum dose is 5 mg.

Geriatric patients and patients with renal impairment and heart failure

Oral

Excretion is reduced in renal failure; use smaller initial dose, and adjust upward to a maximum of 40 mg/day PO. For patients on dialysis, use 2.5 mg on dialysis days.

CrCl (mL/min)	Serum Creatinine	Initial Dose
More than 80	Not applicable	5 mg/day
80 or less– more than 30	Less than 3 mg/dL	5 mg/day
Less than 30	More than 3 mg/dL	2.5 mg/day

IV

If creatinine clearance is less than 30 mL/min, the initial dose is 0.625 mg, which may be repeated after 1 hr. Additional doses of 1.25 mg every 6 hr may be given with careful patient monitoring.

Pharmacokinetics

Route	Onset	Peak	Duration
Oral	60 min	4–6 hr	24 hr
IV	15 min	1–4 hr	6 hr

Metabolism: $T_{1/2}$: 11 hr
Distribution: Crosses placenta; enters breast milk
Excretion: Urine

▼ IV FACTS

Preparation: Enalaprilat can be given as supplied or mixed with up to 50 mL of 5% dextrose injection, 0.9% sodium chloride injection, 0.9% sodium chloride injection in 5% dextrose, 5% dextrose in lactated Ringer solution, *Isolyte E.* Stable at room temperature for 24 hr.
Infusion: Give by slow IV infusion over at least 5 min.

Adverse effects

- **CNS:** *Headache, dizziness, fatigue,* insomnia, paresthesia, vertigo
- **CV:** Syncope, chest pain, palpitations, hypotension in salt- or volume-depleted patients
- **GI:** Gastric irritation, *nausea,* vomiting, *diarrhea,* abdominal pain, dyspepsia, elevated liver enzymes
- **GU:** Proteinuria, renal insufficiency, renal failure, polyuria, oliguria, urinary frequency, impotence
- **Hematologic:** *Decreased Hct and Hgb*
- **Other:** *Cough,* muscle cramps, hyperhidrosis, increased BUN and serum creatinine, hyperkalemia

Interactions

✸ **Drug-drug** ● Decreased hypotensive effect if taken concurrently with indomethacin, rifampin, NSAIDs

Adverse effects in *italics* are most common; those in **bold** are life-threatening. ⬛ Do not crush.

■ Nursing considerations
Assessment
- **History:** Allergy to enalapril, impaired renal function, salt or volume depletion, lactation, pregnancy
- **Physical:** Skin color, lesions, turgor; T; orientation, reflexes, affect, peripheral sensation; P, BP, peripheral perfusion; mucous membranes, bowel sounds, liver evaluation; urinalysis, LFTs, renal function tests, CBC, and differential

Interventions
⊗ *Warning* Alert surgeon, and mark the patient's chart with notice that enalapril is being taken; the angiotensin II formation subsequent to compensatory renin release during surgery will be blocked; hypotension may be reversed with volume expansion.

⊗ **Black box warning** Be aware that use of this drug in the second and third trimesters can cause serious injury or death to the fetus; advise contraceptive use.
- Monitor patients on diuretic therapy for excessive hypotension after the first few doses of enalapril.
- Monitor patient closely in any situation that may lead to a drop in BP secondary to reduced fluid volume (excessive perspiration and dehydration, vomiting, diarrhea) because excessive hypotension may occur.
- Arrange for reduced dosage in patients with impaired renal function.

⊗ *Warning* Monitor patient carefully because peak effect may not be seen for 4 hr. Do not administer second dose until BP has been checked.

Teaching points
- Do not stop taking the medication without consulting your health care provider.
- Be careful in any situation that may lead to a drop in blood pressure (diarrhea, sweating, vomiting, dehydration).
- Avoid over-the-counter medications, especially cough, cold, and allergy medications that may interact with this drug.
- You may experience these side effects: GI upset, loss of appetite, change in taste perception (will pass with time); mouth sores (frequent mouth care may help); rash; fast heart rate; dizziness, light-headedness (usually passes in a few days;

change position slowly, limit activities to those not requiring alertness and precision).
- Use of contraception is advised while taking this drug; fetal abnormalities or death may occur.
- Report mouth sores; sore throat, fever, chills; swelling of the hands, feet; irregular heartbeat, chest pains; swelling of the face, eyes, lips, tongue; difficulty breathing.

▽ enfuvirtide
*(en foo **veer'** tide)*

Fuzeon

PREGNANCY CATEGORY B

Drug classes
Anti-HIV drug
Fusion inhibitor

Therapeutic actions
Prevents the entry of the HIV-1 virus into cells by inhibiting the fusion of the virus membrane with the viral and cellular membrane.

Indications
- In combination with other antiretrovirals for the treatment of HIV-1 infection in treatment-experienced patients with evidence of HIV-1 replication despite ongoing antiretroviral therapy

Contraindications and cautions
- Contraindicated with hypersensitivity to any component of enfuvirtide, lactation.
- Use cautiously with history of lung disease, pregnancy.

Available forms
Powder for injection—90 mg/mL

Dosages
Adults
90 mg bid by subcutaneous injection into the upper arm, anterior thigh, or abdomen.
Pediatric patients 6–16 yr
2 mg/kg bid by subcutaneous injection, up to a maximum of 90 mg/dose into the upper arm, anterior thigh, or abdomen.

Pharmacokinetics

Route	Onset	Peak
Subcut.	Slow	4–8 hr

Metabolism: Hepatic; $T_{1/2}$: 3.2–4.4 hr
Distribution: May cross placenta; may enter breast milk
Excretion: Tissue recycling of amino acids, not excreted

Adverse effects

- **CNS:** Dizziness, insomnia, depression, anxiety, peripheral neuropathy
- **GI:** Nausea, diarrhea, constipation, pancreatitis, abdominal pain, taste perversion, increased appetite
- **Respiratory: Pneumonia,** cough
- **Other:** Injection site reactions—pain, discomfort, redness, nodules; hypersensitivity reactions, fatigue, rash

■ Nursing considerations
Assessment

- **History:** Allergy to any components of the product, lactation, pregnancy, lung disease
- **Physical:** T; orientation, reflexes; R, adventitious sounds; skin evaluation

Interventions

- Make sure that the patient is taking this drug in combination with other antiretrovirals.
- Monitor patients regularly to evaluate lung function and viral load.
- Administer this drug by subcutaneous injection only; rotate sites regularly.
- Encourage women of childbearing age to use barrier contraceptives while taking this drug because the effects of the drug on the fetus are not known.
- Advise women who are breast-feeding to find another method of feeding the baby; HIV-infected women are advised not to breast-feed.
- Advise patient that this drug does not cure the disease and there is still a risk of transmitting the disease to others.

Teaching points

- Administer this drug by subcutaneous injection; you and a significant other should learn the proper method for preparing and administering the drug and for properly disposing of the syringes and needles.

- Administer the drug every day; if you miss a dose, contact your health care provider immediately.
- Rotate injection sites among the upper arm, abdomen, and anterior thigh; keep a record of the sites.
- Keep any reconstituted drug in the refrigerator; use within 24 hours.
- Bring refrigerated solution to room temperature before injecting; discard any unused portions.
- Continue taking your other antiviral drugs; the drugs are designed to be taken in combination.
- This drug does not cure the HIV infection and you will still be able to pass it to others; using condoms is advised. Women of childbearing age are discouraged from becoming pregnant while taking this drug; using barrier contraceptives is recommended.
- Select another method of feeding the baby if you are breast-feeding.
- Local reactions at the site of the injection occur commonly. Review the proper administration technique regularly, and rotate injection sites. If you experience severe pain, redness, or hardness at the site, consult your health care provider.
- You may experience these side effects: Nausea, diarrhea, abdominal pain, headache (try to maintain your intake of nutrition and fluid as much as possible; eat frequent small meals); dizziness, lack of sleep (avoid driving and operating dangerous machinery if this occurs).
- Report chills, fever, any sign of infection, difficulty breathing or signs of respiratory infection, cough with fever, rapid breathing, shortness of breath.

DANGEROUS DRUG

▽ **enoxaparin**
(en ocks' a par in)

Lovenox

PREGNANCY CATEGORY B

Drug classes
Antithrombotic
Low–molecular-weight heparin

Therapeutic actions
Low–molecular-weight heparin that inhibits thrombus and clot formation by blocking

factor Xa, factor IIa, preventing the formation of clots.

Indications

- Prevention of DVT, which may lead to pulmonary embolism following hip replacement, knee replacement surgery, abdominal surgery
- Prevention of ischemic complications of unstable angina and non–Q-wave MI
- Treatment of DVT, pulmonary embolus with warfarin
- Prevention of DVT in medical patients who are at risk for thromboembolic complications due to severely restricted mobility during acute illnesses
- Treatment of acute ST-segment elevation MI, managed medically or with subsequent percutaneous coronary intervention
- Unlabeled uses: Venous thromboembolism prevention in cancer patients with central venous catheters; DVT prevention in general surgery or gynecologic surgery; prevention of exercise-induced bronchoconstriction

Contraindications and cautions

- Contraindicated with hypersensitivity to enoxaparin, heparin, pork products; severe thrombocytopenia; uncontrolled bleeding.
- Use cautiously with pregnancy or lactation, history of GI bleed, spinal tap, spinal/epidural anesthesia.

Available forms

Injection—30 mg/0.3 mL; 40 mg/0.4 mL; 60 mg/0.6 mL; 80 mg/0.8 mL; 100 mg/mL; 120 mg/0.8 mL; 150 mg/mL; 300 mg/3 mL

Dosages
Adults

- *DVT prophylaxis after hip or knee replacement surgery:* 30 mg subcutaneously bid with initial dose 12–24 hr after surgery. Continue throughout the postoperative period for 7–10 days; then 40 mg daily subcutaneously for up to 3 wk may be used.
- *Patients undergoing abdominal surgery:* 40 mg/day subcutaneously begun within 2 hr preoperatively and continued for 7–10 days.
- *Outpatient DVT treatment:* 1 mg/kg subcutaneously every 12 hr.
- *Inpatient DVT treatment:* 1.5 mg/kg subcutaneously once daily or 1 mg/kg every 12 hr.

- *Unstable angina and non–Q-wave MI:* 1 mg/kg subcutaneously every 12 hr for 2–8 days.
- *Prevention of DVT in high-risk medical patients:* 40 mg/day subcutaneously for 6–11 days; has been used up to 14 days.
- *Treatment of MI:*
  Younger than 75 yr: 30-mg IV bolus plus 1 mg/kg subcutaneous dose followed by 1 mg/kg subcutaneously every 12 hr with aspirin. (Maximum 100 mg for first two doses only.)
  75 yr and older: 0.75 mg/kg subcutaneously every 12 hr. (Maximum 75 mg for first two doses only.)

Pediatric patients
Safety and efficacy not established.

Patients with renal impairment (creatinine clearance less than 30 mL/min)

- *DVT prophylaxis:* 30 mg/day subcutaneously.
- *DVT treatment:* 1 mg/kg subcutaneously once daily.
- *MI treatment:* For patient younger than 75 yr, 30-mg IV bolus; then 1 mg/kg subcutaneously followed by 1 mg/kg/day subcutaneously. For patient 75 yr and older, 1 mg/kg/day subcutaneously.

Pharmacokinetics

Route	Onset	Peak	Duration
Subcut.	20–60 min	3–5 hr	12 hr

Metabolism: $T_{1/2}$: 4.5 hr
Distribution: May cross placenta; may enter breast milk
Excretion: Urine

Adverse effects

- **Hematologic: Hemorrhage;** *bruising;* thrombocytopenia; elevated AST, ALT levels; hyperkalemia
- **Hypersensitivity:** Chills, fever, urticaria, asthma
- **Other:** Fever; pain; local irritation, hematoma, erythema at site of injection, epidural or spinal hematoma with spinal tap, spinal/epidural anesthesia

Interactions

❋ **Drug-drug** • Increased bleeding tendencies with oral anticoagulants, salicylates, SSRIs,

NSAIDs, penicillins, cephalosporins ● Risk of severe bleeding if combined with heparin

✳ **Drug-lab test** ● Increased AST, ALT levels

✳ **Drug-alternative therapy** ● Increased risk of bleeding if combined with chamomile, garlic, ginger, ginkgo, and ginseng therapy, high-dose vitamin E

■ **Nursing considerations**
Assessment
● **History:** Recent surgery or injury; sensitivity to heparin, pork products, enoxaparin; lactation; history of GI bleed; pregnancy
● **Physical:** Peripheral perfusion, R, stool guaiac test, PTT or other tests of blood coagulation, platelet count, renal function tests

Interventions
● Give drug as soon as possible after hip surgery, within 12 hr of knee surgery, and within 2 hr preoperatively for abdominal surgery.
⊗ *Black box warning* Be aware of increased risk of spinal hematoma and neurologic damage if used with spinal/epidural anesthesia; if must be used, monitor patient closely.
● Give deep subcutaneous injections; do not give enoxaparin by IM injection.
● Administer by deep subcutaneous injection; patient should be lying down. Alternate between the left and right anterolateral and posterolateral abdominal wall. Introduce the whole length of the needle into a skinfold held between the thumb and forefinger; hold the skinfold throughout the injection.
● Apply pressure to all injection sites after needle is withdrawn; inspect injection sites for signs of hematoma; do not massage injection sites.
● Do not mix with other injections or infusions.
● Store at room temperature; fluid should be clear, colorless to pale yellow.
● Provide for safety measures (electric razor, soft toothbrush) to prevent injury to patient who is at risk for bleeding.
● Check patient for signs of bleeding; monitor blood tests.
● Alert all health care providers that patient is taking enoxaparin.
● Discontinue and initiate appropriate therapy if thromboembolic episode occurs despite enoxaparin therapy.
⊗ *Warning* Have protamine sulfate (enoxaparin antidote) readily available in case of overdose.

● Treat overdose as follows: Protamine sulfate (1% solution). Each mg of protamine neutralizes 1 mg enoxaparin. Give very slowly IV over 10 min.

Teaching points
● Have periodic blood tests to monitor your response to this drug.
● You and a significant other may need to learn to give the drug by subcutaneous injection and how to properly dispose of needles and syringes. Rotate injection sites.
● Avoid injury while you are taking this drug: Use an electric razor; avoid activities that might lead to injury.
● Report nosebleed, bleeding of the gums, unusual bruising, black or tarry stools, cloudy or dark urine, abdominal or lower back pain, severe headache.

▽**entacapone**
*(en tab **kap'** own)*

Comtan

PREGNANCY CATEGORY C

Drug class
Antiparkinsonian

Therapeutic actions
Selectively and reversibly inhibits COMT, an enzyme that eliminates biologically active catecholamines, including dopa, dopamine, norepinephrine, epinephrine; when given with levodopa, entacapone's inhibition of COMT is believed to increase the plasma concentrations and duration of action of levodopa.

Indications
● Adjunct with levodopa and carbidopa in the treatment of the signs and symptoms of idiopathic Parkinson disease in patients who are experiencing "wearing off" of drug effects

Contraindications and cautions
● Contraindicated with hypersensitivity to drug or its component.
● Use cautiously with hypertension, hypotension, hepatic or renal impairment, pregnancy, lactation.

Available forms
Tablets—200 mg

Dosages
Adults
200 mg PO taken concomitantly with the dose of levodopa-carbidopa, a maximum of eight times/day (1,400 mg).
Pediatric patients
Safety and efficacy not established.

Pharmacokinetics

Route	Onset	Peak
Oral	Varies	1 hr

Metabolism: Hepatic; $T_{1/2}$: 0.4–0.7 hr, then 2.4 hr
Distribution: May cross placenta; may enter breast milk
Excretion: Feces, urine

Adverse effects
- **CNS:** *Disorientation, confusion,* memory loss, **hallucinations,** psychoses, agitation, nervousness, delusions, delirium, paranoia, euphoria, excitement, *light-headedness, dizziness,* depression, drowsiness, weakness, giddiness, paresthesias, hypokinesia, heaviness of the limbs, numbness of fingers, *dyskinesias, hyperkinesia*
- **CV:** *Hypotension, orthostatic hypotension*
- **Dermatologic:** Rash, urticaria, other dermatoses
- **GI:** *Nausea, vomiting,* epigastric distress, flatulence, diarrhea, abdominal pain, constipation
- **Respiratory:** URIs, dyspnea, sinus congestion, **rhabdomyolysis**
- **Other:** *Fever,* urine discoloration

Interactions
✴ Drug-drug ● Increased toxicity and serum levels if combined with MAOIs; avoid this combination ● Possible decreased excretion if combined with probenecid, cholestyramine, erythromycin, rifampin, ampicillin, or chloramphenicol; if one of these combinations is used, monitor patient closely ● Risk of increased heart rate, arrhythmias, excessive BP changes if combined with norepinephrine, dopamine, dobutamine, isoetharine, isoproterenol, methyldopa, apomorphine, or epinephrine; administer with extreme caution and monitor patient closely

■ Nursing considerations
Assessment
- **History:** Hypersensitivity to drug or its components, hypertension, hypotension, hepatic or renal impairment, pregnancy, lactation
- **Physical:** Body weight; body T; skin color, lesions; orientation, affect, reflexes, bilateral grip strength, visual examination; P, BP, orthostatic BP, auscultation; bowel sounds, normal output, liver evaluation; urinary output, voiding pattern, LFTs, renal function tests

Interventions
⊗ **Warning** Administer only in conjunction with levodopa and carbidopa. Monitor patient response, customary levodopa dosage may need to be decreased.
- Provide sugarless candies or ice chips to suck if dry mouth is a problem.
- Give with meals if GI upset occurs; give before meals to patients bothered by dry mouth; give after meals if drooling is a problem or if drug causes nausea.
- Advise patient to use barrier contraceptives, serious birth defects can occur while using this drug; advise breast-feeding mothers to use another means of feeding the infant because drug can enter breast milk and adversely affect the infant.
- Establish safety precautions if CNS, vision changes, hallucinations, or hypotension occurs (use side rails, accompany patient when ambulating).
- Provide additional comfort measures appropriate to patient with parkinsonism.

Teaching points
- Take this drug exactly as prescribed. Always take with your levodopa and carbidopa.
- Use barrier contraceptives while taking this drug; serious birth defects can occur. Do not breast-feed while on this drug; the drug enters breast milk and can adversely affect the infant.
- You may experience these side effects: Drowsiness, dizziness, confusion, blurred vision (avoid driving a car or engaging in activities that require alertness and visual acuity; if these occur, rise slowly when changing positions to help decrease dizziness); nausea (eat frequent small meals); dry mouth (suck sugarless candies or ice chips); hallucinations (this is a side effect of the drug; use care and have someone stay with you if this occurs); constipation (maintain adequate

fluid intake and exercise regularly; if this does not help, consult your health care provider); reddish brown discoloration of urine (a drug effect).

- Report constipation, rapid or pounding heartbeat, confusion, eye pain, hallucinations, rash.

▽entecavir
(en tek' ah veer)

Baraclude

PREGNANCY CATEGORY C

Drug classes
Antiviral
Nucleoside analogue

Therapeutic actions
Blocks activities of hepatitis B virus reverse transcriptases by competing with a natural substrate and leading to decreased viral load associated with hepatitis B.

Indications
- Treatment of chronic hepatitis B infection in adults with evidence of active viral replication and either evidence of persistent elevations in serum aminotransferases or histologically active disease

Contraindications and cautions
- Contraindicated with known hypersensitivity to entecavir or any of its components, lactation, co-infection with HIV in patients not receiving highly active antiretroviral therapy.
- Use cautiously with pregnancy, renal impairment, liver transplant, concurrent use of drugs that alter renal function.

Available forms
Tablets—0.5, 1 mg; oral solution—0.05 mg/mL

Dosages
Adults and children 16 yr and older with no previous nucleoside treatment
0.5 mg/day PO on an empty stomach at least 2 hr after a meal or 2 hr before the next meal.

Adults and children 16 yr and older with a history of viremia also receiving lamivudine or with known resistance mutations
1 mg/day PO on an empty stomach at least 2 hr after a meal or 2 hr before the next meal.
Pediatric patients younger than 16 yr
Safety and efficacy not established.
Patients with renal impairment
Creatinine clearance of 50 mL/min or more, 0.5 mg/day PO (1 mg/day PO with lamivudine resistance); creatinine clearance of 30–less than 50 mL/min, 0.25 mg/day PO or 0.5 mg PO every 48 hr (0.5 mg/day PO or 1 mg every 48 hr with lamivudine resistance); creatinine clearance of 10–less than 30 mL/min, 0.15 mg/day PO or 0.5 mg PO every 72 hr (0.3 mg/day PO or 1 mg every 72 hr with lamivudine resistance); creatinine clearance less than 10 mL/min, 0.05 mg/day PO or 0.5 mg PO every 7 days (0.1 mg/day PO or 1 mg every 7 days with lamivudine resistance); in hemodialysis, 0.05 mg/day PO or 0.5 mg PO every 7 days (0.1 mg/day PO or 1 mg every 7 days with lamivudine resistance, given after hemodialysis).

Pharmacokinetics

Route	Onset	Peak
Oral	Rapid	0.5–1.5 hr

Metabolism: $T_{1/2}$: 128–149 hr
Distribution: May cross placenta; may pass into breast milk
Excretion: Urine, unchanged

Adverse effects
- **CNS:** *Dizziness, headache, fatigue,* somnolence, insomnia
- **GI:** *Nausea,* vomiting, diarrhea, dyspepsia, lactic acidosis, and severe hepatomegaly with steatosis
- **Other:** Acute exacerbations of hepatitis B (with discontinuation of therapy)

Interactions
✳ **Drug-drug** • Risk of decreased excretion and toxic effects if combined with drugs that alter renal function; monitor patient carefully and adjust dosages as needed

Adverse effects in *italics* are most common; those in **bold** are life-threatening. ⊂⊃ Do not crush.

■ **Nursing considerations**
Assessment
- **History:** Allergy to any components of the product, lactation, pregnancy; renal impairment; signs of lactic acidosis
- **Physical:** T; orientation, reflexes; abdominal examination, LFTs, renal function tests

Interventions
- Assess renal function before beginning therapy; adjust dosage as appropriate.
- Maintain other measures used to help patient deal with chronic hepatitis B.
- Monitor patient regularly to evaluate effects of drug on the body.
- Administer this drug on an empty stomach, at least 2 hr after a meal or 2 hr before the next meal.

⊗ **Black box warning** Withdraw drug and monitor patient if patient develops signs of lactic acidosis or hepatotoxicity, including hepatomegaly and steatosis.

⊗ **Black box warning** Do not use in patients co-infected with HIV unless patient is receiving highly active antiretroviral therapy because of high risk of HIV resistance. HIV testing should be offered to all patients before starting entecavir therapy.

⊗ **Black box warning** Severe, acute exacerbations of hepatitis B have occurred in patients who discontinue antihepatitis therapy. Monitor patients for several mo following cessation of drug; restarting antihepatitis therapy may be warranted.

- Effects of the drug on a fetus are not known. Advise women of childbearing age to use barrier contraceptives while on this drug.
- Advise women who are breast-feeding to find another method of feeding the baby; potential effects on the baby are not known.
- Advise patient that this drug does not cure the disease and there is still a risk of transmitting the disease to others.
- Monitor for worsening of hepatitis if drug is withdrawn.

Teaching points
- This drug is no cure for hepatitis B. It may decrease the number of viruses in your body and may improve the condition of your liver.

⊗ **Warning** You should still take precautions to prevent the spread of hepatitis B; do not share any personal items that may have blood or body fluids on them; use condoms if having intercourse.

- Always take *Baraclude* on an empty stomach at least 2 hours after a meal and at least 2 hours before the next meal.
- If you are using the oral solution, use the measuring spoon provided to measure out your dose. Swallow the medicine directly from the measuring spoon. Rinse the spoon with water and allow to air dry after each use. Store the solution at room temperature.
- If you forget a dose of the drug, take that dose as soon as you remember, then take your next dose at the usual time. Do not take two doses at the same time.
- Do not run out of *Baraclude*. If you are running low, contact your health care provider; if you stop taking this drug, your hepatitis symptoms could get worse and become very serious.
- You will need to have regular health care, including blood tests, to monitor the effects of this drug on your body.
- It is not known how this drug could affect a breast-feeding infant. If you are breast-feeding, another method of feeding should be selected.
- It is not known how this drug could affect a fetus. If you are pregnant or decide to become pregnant while on this drug, consult your health care provider.
- You may experience the following side effects: Headache (consult your health care provider, medication may be available to help); dizziness (avoid driving a car or operating hazardous equipment if this occurs); nausea (frequent small meals may help).
- Report unusual muscle pain, trouble breathing, stomach pain with nausea and vomiting, feeling cold, light-headedness, fast or irregular heartbeat, dark urine, yellowing of the eyes or skin, light-colored stools.

DANGEROUS DRUG

▽**ephedrine sulfate**
(*e fed' rin*)

PREGNANCY CATEGORY C

Drug classes
Bronchodilator
Sympathomimetic
Vasopressor

Therapeutic actions

Peripheral effects are mediated by receptors in target organs and are due in part to the release of norepinephrine from nerve terminals. Effects mediated by these receptors include vasoconstriction (increased BP, decreased nasal congestion alpha receptors), cardiac stimulation (beta$_1$), and bronchodilation (beta$_2$). Longer acting but less potent than epinephrine; also has CNS stimulant properties.

Indications
Parenteral

- Treatment of hypotensive states, especially those associated with spinal anesthesia; Stokes-Adams syndrome with complete heart block; CNS stimulant in narcolepsy and depressive states; acute bronchospasm; myasthenia gravis
- Pressor drug in hypotensive states following sympathectomy, overdosage with ganglionic-blocking drugs, antiadrenergic drugs, or other drugs used for lowering BP
- Relief of acute bronchospasm (epinephrine is the preferred drug)

Oral

- Treatment of allergic disorders, such as bronchial asthma, and temporary relief of wheezing, shortness of breath, and tightness of the chest

Contraindications and cautions

- Contraindicated with allergy to ephedrine, angle-closure glaucoma, anesthesia with cyclopropane or halothane, thyrotoxicosis, diabetes, hypertension, CV disorders, women in labor whose BP is lower than 130/80 mm Hg.
- Use cautiously with angina, arrhythmias, prostatic hypertrophy, unstable vasomotor syndrome, lactation.

Available forms

Capsules—25 mg; injection—50 mg/mL

Dosages

May be given PO, IM, slow IV, or subcutaneously.
Adults
Parenteral

- *Hypotensive episodes, allergic disorders:* 25–50 mg IM (fast absorption), subcutaneously (slower absorption), or 5–25 mg IV given slowly; may be repeated in 5–10 min.

Oral

- *Acute asthma:* Administer the smallest effective dose (12.5–25 mg PO every 4 hr).

Pediatric patients
Parenteral

0.5 mg/kg or 16.7 mg/m^2 IM or subcutaneously every 4–6 hr.

Oral

Not recommended for children younger than 12 yr.

Geriatric patients

More likely to experience adverse reactions; use with caution.

Pharmacokinetics

Route	Onset	Duration
Oral	30–40 min	3–5 hr
IM	10–20 min	1 hr
IV	Instant	1 hr

Metabolism: Hepatic; T$_{1/2}$: 3–6 hr
Distribution: May cross placenta; enters breast milk
Excretion: Urine

▼ IV FACTS

Preparation: Administer as provided; no preparation required.
Infusion: Administer directly into vein or tubing of running IV; administer slowly, each 10 mg over at least 1 min.

Adverse effects

- **CNS:** *Fear, anxiety, tenseness, restlessness, headache, light-headedness, dizziness,* drowsiness, tremor, insomnia, hallucinations, psychological disturbances, **seizures,** CNS depression, weakness, blurred vision, ocular irritation, tearing, photophobia, symptoms of paranoid schizophrenia
- **CV:** Arrhythmias, **hypertension resulting in intracranial hemorrhage, CV collapse with hypotension, palpitations, tachycardia, precordial pain in patients with ischemic heart disease**
- **GI:** *Nausea,* vomiting, anorexia
- **GU:** Constriction of renal blood vessels and *decreased urine formation* (initial parenteral administration), *dysuria, vesical sphincter spasm* resulting in difficult and

painful urination, urinary retention in males with prostatism
- **Other:** *Pallor,* respiratory difficulty, orofacial dystonia, sweating

Interactions

⁕ **Drug-drug** • Severe hypertension with MAOIs, TCAs • Additive effects and increased risk of toxicity with urinary alkalinizers • Decreased vasopressor response with reserpine, methyldopa, urinary acidifiers

⁕ **Drug-alternative therapy** • Administration with ephedra, ma huang, guarana, and caffeine leads to additive effects and may lead to overstimulation, increased BP, stroke, and death

■ Nursing considerations
Assessment
- **History:** Allergy to ephedrine; angle-closure glaucoma; anesthesia with cyclopropane or halothane; thyrotoxicosis, diabetes, hypertension, CV disorders; prostatic hypertrophy, unstable vasomotor syndrome; lactation
- **Physical:** Skin color, T; orientation, reflexes, peripheral sensation, vision; P, BP, auscultation, peripheral perfusion; R, adventitious sounds; urinary output pattern, bladder percussion, prostate palpation

Interventions
- Protect solution from light; give only if clear; discard any unused portion.
- Monitor urine output with parenteral administration; initially renal blood vessels may be constricted and urine formation decreased.
- Avoid prolonged use of systemic ephedrine (a syndrome resembling an anxiety effect may occur); temporary cessation of the drug usually reverses this syndrome.
- Monitor CV effects carefully; patients with hypertension may experience changes in BP because of the additional vasoconstriction. If a nasal decongestant is needed, give pseudoephedrine.

Teaching points
- Do not exceed recommended dose.
- Avoid OTC medications. Many of them contain the same or similar drugs and serious overdosage can occur.

- You may experience these side effects: Dizziness, weakness, restlessness, tremor, light-headedness (avoid driving or operating dangerous equipment); urinary retention (empty your bladder before taking drug).
- Report nervousness, palpitations, sleeplessness, sweating.

E

DANGEROUS DRUG

▽**epinephrine (adrenaline)**
(ep i nef´ rin)

epinephrine bitartrate
Aerosol: Primatene Mist

epinephrine hydrochloride

Insect-sting emergencies:
EpiPen Auto-Injector (delivers 0.3 mg IM adult dose), EpiPen Jr. Auto-Injector (delivers 0.15 mg IM for children)
OTC solutions for nebulization:
AsthmaNefrin, S_2

PREGNANCY CATEGORY C

Drug classes
Alpha-adrenergic agonist
Antiasthmatic
$Beta_1$- and $beta_2$-adrenergic agonists
Bronchodilator
Cardiac stimulant
Sympathomimetic
Vasopressor

Therapeutic actions
Naturally occurring neurotransmitter, the effects of which are mediated by alpha or beta receptors in target organs. Effects on alpha receptors include vasoconstriction, contraction of dilator muscles of iris. Effects on beta receptors include positive chronotropic and inotropic effects on the heart ($beta_1$ receptors); bronchodilation, vasodilation, and uterine relaxation ($beta_2$ receptors); decreased production of aqueous humor.

Indications
- IV: In ventricular standstill after all other measures have failed to restore circulation,

given by trained personnel by intracardiac puncture and intramyocardial injection; treatment and prophylaxis of cardiac arrest and attacks of transitory AV heart block with syncopal seizures (Stokes-Adams syndrome); syncope due to carotid sinus syndrome; acute hypersensitivity (anaphylactoid) reactions, serum sickness, urticaria, angioneurotic edema; in acute asthmatic attacks to relieve bronchospasm not controlled by inhalation or subcutaneous injection; relaxation of uterine musculature; additive to local anesthetic solutions for injection to prolong their duration of action and limit systemic absorption

- Injection: Relief from respiratory distress of bronchial asthma.
- Aerosols and solutions for nebulization: Temporary relief from acute attacks of bronchial asthma, COPD

Contraindications and cautions

- Contraindicated with allergy or hypersensitivity to epinephrine or components of preparation (many of the inhalant and ophthalmic products contain sulfites: Sodium bisulfite, sodium or potassium metabisulfite; check label before using any of these products in a sulfite-sensitive patient); narrow-angle glaucoma; shock other than anaphylactic shock; hypovolemia; general anesthesia with halogenated hydrocarbons or cyclopropane; organic brain damage, cerebral arteriosclerosis; cardiac dilation and coronary insufficiency; tachyarrhythmias; ischemic heart disease; hypertension; renal impairment (drug may initially decrease renal blood flow); COPD patients who have developed degenerative heart disease; diabetes mellitus; hyperthyroidism; lactation.
- Use cautiously with prostatic hypertrophy (may cause bladder sphincter spasm, difficult and painful urination), history of seizure disorders, psychoneurotic individuals, labor and delivery (may delay second stage of labor; can accelerate fetal heart beat; may cause fetal and maternal hypoglycemia), children (syncope has occurred when epinephrine has been given to asthmatic children). Use EpiPen Auto-Injector cautiously with hyperthyroidism, CAD, hypertension, diabetes, elderly patients, pregnancy, and patients weighing less than 30 kg.

Available forms

Solution for inhalation—1:100, 1:1,000, 1.125%, 2.25 %, 1%; aerosol—0.35 mg, 0.5%, 0.22 mg; injection—1, 5 mg/mL; solution for injection—1:1,000, 1:2,000, 1:10,000, 1:100,000; suspension for injection—1:200; injection device—0.15 mg/0.15 mL, 0.15 mg/0.3 mL, 0.3 mg/0.3 mL

Dosages
Adults
Epinephrine injection

- *Hypersensitivity or bronchospasm:* 0.1–0.25 mg (1–2.5 mL of 1:10,000 solution) IV injected slowly.
- *Cardiac arrest:* 0.1–1 mg (5–10 mL of 1:10,000 solution) IV during resuscitation. 0.5 mg every 5 min. Intracardiac injection into left ventricular chamber, 0.3–0.5 mg (3–5 mL of 1:10,000 solution).

Intraspinal

0.2–0.4 mL added to anesthetic spinal fluid mixture. Concentrations of 1:100,000–1:20,000 are usually used.

1:1,000 solution

- *Respiratory distress:* 0.2–1 mL of 1:1,000 solution subcutaneously or IM every 5–15 min as needed; or 1–2.5 mL IV, repeated every 3–5 min or injected via endotracheal tube.

1:200 suspension (for subcutaneous administration only)

- *Respiratory distress:* 0.1–0.3 mL (0.5–1.5 mg) subcutaneously.

Auto-injector

15–29 kg, 0.15 mg IM. 30 kg or more, 0.3 mg IM; may repeat as necessary.

Inhalation (aerosol)

Begin treatment at first symptoms of bronchospasm. Individualize dosage. Wait 1–5 min between inhalations to avoid overdose.

Inhalation (nebulization)

Place not more than 10 drops into the nebulizer reservoir. Place nebulizer nozzle into partially opened mouth. Patient inhales deeply while bulb is squeezed one to three times (not more than every 3 hr).

Pediatric patients
Epinephrine injection

- *1:1,000 solution, children:* 0.01 mg/kg or 0.3 mL/m^2 (0.01 mg/kg or 0.3 mg/m^2) subcutaneously; repeat every 4 hr if needed. Do not exceed 0.5 mL (0.5 mg) in a single dose. For infants, use 0.05 mg subcutaneously as initial dose, repeat every 20–30 min as needed. For neonates, use 0.01 mg/kg subcutaneously.

- *1:200 suspension, infants and children (1 mo–1 yr):* 0.005 mL/kg (0.025 mg/kg) subcutaneously.
- *Children 30 kg or less:* 0.15 mg or 0.01 mg/kg by autoinjector.
- *Hypersensitivity or bronchospasm:* For neonates, use 0.01 mg/kg IV. For infants, use 0.05 mg IV as initial dose and repeat every 20–30 min as needed with 1:10,000 solution.

Geriatric patients or patients with renal failure
Use with caution.

Pharmacokinetics

Route	Onset	Peak	Duration
Subcut.	5–10 min	20 min	20–30 min
IM	5–10 min	20 min	20–30 min
IV	Instant	20 min	20–30 min
Inhalation	3–5 min	20 min	1–3 hr

Metabolism: Neural
Distribution: Crosses placenta; enters breast milk
Excretion: Urine

▼ IV FACTS

Preparation: 0.5 mL dose may be diluted to 10 mL with sodium chloride injection for direct injection; prepare infusion by mixing 1 mg in 250 mL D₅W (4 mcg/mL).
Infusion: Administer by direct IV injection or into the tubing of a running IV, each 1 mg over 1 min, or run infusion at 1–4 mcg/min (15–60 mL/hr).

Adverse effects
Systemic administration

- **CNS:** *Fear, anxiety, tenseness, restlessness, headache, light-headedness, dizziness,* drowsiness, tremor, insomnia, hallucinations, psychological disturbances, seizures, CNS depression, weakness, blurred vision, ocular irritation, tearing, photophobia, symptoms of paranoid schizophrenia
- **CV:** Arrhythmias, **hypertension resulting in intracranial hemorrhage, CV collapse with hypotension,** palpita-

tions, tachycardia, precordial pain in patients with ischemic heart disease
- **GI:** *Nausea,* vomiting, anorexia
- **GU:** Constriction of renal blood vessels and *decreased urine formation* (initial parenteral administration), *dysuria, vesical sphincter spasm* resulting in difficult and painful urination, urinary retention in males with prostatism
- **Other:** *Pallor,* respiratory difficulty, orofacial dystonia, sweating

Local injection
- **Local:** Necrosis at sites of repeat injections (due to intense vasoconstriction)

Interactions

✳ **Drug-drug** • Increased sympathomimetic effects with TCAs (eg, imipramine) • Excessive hypertension with propranolol, beta-blockers • Decreased cardiostimulating and bronchodilating effects with beta-adrenergic blockers (eg, propranolol) • Decreased vasopressor effects with chlorpromazine, phenothiazines • Decreased antihypertensive effect of methyldopa

■ Nursing considerations
Assessment

- **History:** Allergy or hypersensitivity to epinephrine or components of drug preparation; narrow-angle glaucoma; shock other than anaphylactic shock; hypovolemia; general anesthesia with halogenated hydrocarbons or cyclopropane; organic brain damage, cerebral arteriosclerosis; cardiac dilation and coronary insufficiency; tachyarrhythmias; ischemic heart disease; hypertension; renal impairment; COPD; diabetes mellitus; hyperthyroidism; prostatic hypertrophy; history of seizure disorders; psychoneuroses; labor and delivery; lactation
- **Physical:** Weight; skin color, T, turgor; orientation, reflexes, IOP; P, BP; R, adventitious sounds; prostate palpation, normal urine output; urinalysis, renal function tests, blood and urine glucose, serum electrolytes, thyroid function tests, ECG

Interventions

⊗ *Warning* Use extreme caution when calculating and preparing doses; epinephrine is a very potent drug; small errors in dosage can cause serious adverse effects. Double-check pediatric dosage.

- Use minimal doses for minimal periods of time; "epinephrine-fastness" (a form of drug tolerance) can occur with prolonged use.
- Protect drug solutions from light, extreme heat, and freezing; do not use pink or brown solutions. Drug solutions should be clear and colorless (does not apply to suspension for injection).
- Shake the suspension for injection well before withdrawing the dose.
- Rotate subcutaneous injection sites to prevent necrosis; monitor injection sites frequently.
- ⊗ **Warning** Keep a rapidly acting alpha-adrenergic blocker (phentolamine) or a vasodilator (a nitrate) readily available in case of excessive hypertensive reaction.
- ⊗ **Warning** Have an alpha-adrenergic blocker or facilities for intermittent positive pressure breathing readily available in case pulmonary edema occurs.
- ⊗ **Warning** Keep a beta-adrenergic blocker (propranolol; a cardioselective beta-adrenergic blocker, such as atenolol, should be used in patients with respiratory distress) readily available in case cardiac arrhythmias occur.
- Do not exceed recommended dosage of inhalation products; administer pressurized inhalation drug forms during second half of inspiration, because the airways are open wider and the aerosol distribution is more extensive. If a second inhalation is needed, administer at peak effect of previous dose, 3–5 min.

Teaching points

- Do not exceed recommended dosage; adverse effects or loss of effectiveness may result. Read the instructions that come with respiratory inhalant products, and consult your health care provider or pharmacist if you have any questions.
- You may experience these side effects: Dizziness, drowsiness, fatigue, apprehension (use caution if driving or performing tasks that require alertness); anxiety, emotional changes; nausea, vomiting, change in taste (eat frequent small meals); fast heart rate.
- Report chest pain, dizziness, insomnia, weakness, tremor or irregular heart beat (respiratory inhalant), difficulty breathing, productive cough, failure to respond to usual dosage (respiratory inhalant).

▽ **epirubicin hydrochloride**

See Appendix R, *Less commonly used drugs*.

▽ **eplerenone**
(ep ler' eh nown)

Inspra

PREGNANCY CATEGORY B

Drug classes
Aldosterone receptor blocker
Antihypertensive

Therapeutic actions
Binds to aldosterone receptors, blocking the binding of aldosterone, leading to increased loss of sodium and water and lowering of BP.

Indications

- Treatment of hypertension, alone or in combination with other antihypertensive drugs
- HF, post-MI, improvement in the survival of patients with left ventricular dysfunction after a heart attack
- Unlabeled uses: Alone or with ACE inhibitors to reduce left ventricular hypertrophy; adjunct in diabetic hypertensives with microalbuminuria

Contraindications and cautions

- Contraindicated with allergy to eplerenone, hyperkalemia (exceeding 5.5 mEq/L), type 2 diabetes with microalbuminuria, severe renal impairment (creatinine clearance less than 50 mL/min or serum creatinine level higher than 2 mg/dL in males or 1.8 mg/dL in females), lactation.
- Use cautiously with hepatic impairment, pregnancy, concurrent treatment with potassium supplements, potassium-sparing diuretics, CYP450 and CYP3A4 inhibitors (eg, ketoconazole).

Available forms
Tablets—25, 50 mg

Dosages
Adults
- *Hypertension:* Initially, 50 mg/day PO as a single daily dose; if necessary, may be

increased to 50 mg PO bid after a minimum of a 4-wk trial period. Maximum, 100 mg/day.

• *Heart failure post-MI:* Start with 25 mg/day PO titrate to 50 mg/day over 4 wk.

• *Heart failure:* If serum K+ is lower than 5, increase dose; if 5–5.4, no adjustment necessary; if 5.5–5.9, decrease dose; if 6 or higher, withhold dose.

Pediatric patients
Safety and efficacy not established.

Pharmacokinetics

Route	Onset	Peak
Oral	Slow	1.5 hr

Metabolism: Hepatic; $T_{1/2}$: 4-6 hr
Distribution: May cross placenta; may enter breast milk
Excretion: Feces, urine

Adverse effects

CNS: Headache, dizziness, fatigue
CV: Angina, **MI**
GI: Diarrhea, abdominal pain
GU: Abnormal vaginal bleeding, albuminuria, changes in sexual function
Metabolic: Hypercholesterolemia, **hyperkalemia**
Respiratory: Cough
Other: Gynecomastia and breast pain in men, flulike symptoms

Interactions

✳ **Drug–drug** ⊗ *Warning* Risk of serious toxic effects if combined with strong inhibitors of the CYP450 3A4 system (ketoconazole, itraconazole, erythromycin, verapamil, saquinavir, fluconazole); if any of these drugs are being used, initiate treatment with 25 mg eplerenone and monitor patient closely.

• Increased risk of hyperkalemia if combined with ACE inhibitors and ARBs; monitor patient closely • Possible risk of lithium toxicity if combined with lithium; monitor serum lithium levels closely if this combination is necessary • Possible risk of decreased antihypertensive effect if combined with NSAIDs; monitor BP carefully • Risk of hyperkalemia also with potassium supplements, potassium-sparing diuretics such as spironolactone, amiloride, triamterene; avoid concomitant use

✳ **Drug-alternative therapy** • Decreased serum levels and lessened therapeutic effect if taken with St. John's Wort

■ Nursing considerations
Assessment

• **History:** Allergy to eplerenone, hyperkalemia, type 2 diabetes mellitus, severe renal impairment, lactation, hepatic impairment, pregnancy, concurrent treatment with potassium supplements, CYP450 or CYP3A4 inhibitors

• **Physical:** Orientation, reflexes; BP; R; urinary output; LFTs, renal function tests, serum potassium levels, serum cholesterol

Interventions

• Arrange for pretreatment and periodic evaluation of serum potassium and renal function.

• Establish baseline patient weight to monitor drug effect.

• Administer once a day, in the morning, so increased urination will not interrupt sleep.

• Avoid giving patient any foods rich in potassium (see Appendix D, *Important Dietary Guidelines for Patient Teaching,* for a complete list).

• Establish appropriate safety precautions if patient experiences adverse CNS effects.

• Suggest another method of feeding the baby if the drug is needed in a lactating woman.

Teaching points

• Take this drug early in the morning so any increase in urination will not affect sleep.

• Weigh yourself on a regular basis, at the same time of day and in the same clothes, and record this weight on your calendar.

• This drug may interact with many other medications. Alert any health care provider caring for you that you are taking this drug.

• This drug should not be taken during pregnancy or when breast-feeding; using barrier contraceptives is suggested.

• You will need periodic blood tests to evaluate the effect of this drug on your serum potassium level and cholesterol level.

• Avoid foods that are high in potassium (fruits, *Sanka* coffee).

• You may experience these side effects: Dizziness (use caution and avoid driving a car or performing other tasks that require alertness if you experience dizziness); enlargement or pain of the breasts (it may help to know that this is a drug effect and will pass when drug therapy is ended).

• Report weight change of more than 3 pounds in 1 day, severe dizziness, trembling, numbness, muscle weakness or cramps, palpitations.

▷epoetin alfa
(EPO, erythropoietin)
(e poe e' tin)

Epogen, Eprex (CAN), Procrit

PREGNANCY CATEGORY C

Drug class
Recombinant human erythropoietin

Therapeutic actions
A natural glycoprotein produced in the kidneys, which stimulates red blood cell production in the bone marrow.

Indications
- Treatment of anemia associated with chronic renal failure, including patients older than 1 mo on dialysis
- Treatment of anemia related to therapy with zidovudine (AZT) in HIV-infected patients
- Treatment of anemia related to chemotherapy in cancer patients
- Reduction of allogenic blood transfusions in surgical patients
- Unlabeled uses: Pruritus associated with renal failure; myelodysplastic syndromes; chronic inflammation associated with rheumatoid arthritis

Contraindications and cautions
- Contraindicated with uncontrolled hypertension; hypersensitivity to mammalian cell-derived products or to albumin human; contains benzyl alcohol, which can be fatal in premature infants.
- Use cautiously with pregnancy, lactation, sickle cell anemia, myelodysplastic syndromes, porphyria, hypercoagulable disorders.

Available forms
Injection—2,000, 3,000, 4,000, 10,000, 20,000, 40,000 units/mL

Dosages
Monitor patient closely; target Hgb 10–12 g/dL.
Adults
- *Anemia of chronic renal failure:* Starting dose, 50–100 units/kg three times weekly IV for dialysis patients and IV or subcutaneously for nondialysis patients. Reduce dose if Hgb increases more than 1 g/dL in any 2-wk period. Reduce dose by 25% if Hgb is

12 g/dL. Increase dose if Hgb does not increase by 1 g/dL after 4 wk of therapy or if Hgb is less than 10 g/dL. For maintenance dose, individualized based on Hgb—generally, 75–100 units/kg three times weekly. If on dialysis, median dose is 75 units/kg three times weekly. Target Hgb range is 10–12 g/dL.
- *Treatment of anemia in HIV-infected patients on AZT therapy:* For patients receiving AZT dose of 4,200 mg/wk or less with serum erythropoietin levels of 500 milliunits/mL or less, use 100 units/kg IV or subcutaneously three times/wk for 8 wk; when desired response is achieved, titrate dose to maintain Hgb with lowest possible dose.
- *Treatment of anemia in cancer patients on chemotherapy (Procrit only):* 150 units/kg subcutaneously three times/wk or 40,000 units subcutaneously weekly; after 8 wk, can be increased to 300 units/kg or 60,000 units subcutaneously weekly if Hgb increases by less than 1 g/dL and remains below 10 g/dL.
- *Reduction of allogenic blood transfusions in surgery:* 300 units/kg/day subcutaneously for 10 days before surgery, on day of surgery, and 4 days after surgery. Or, 600 units/kg/day subcutaneously 21, 14, and 7 days before surgery and on day of surgery. Make sure that Hgb is higher than 10 g/dL and lower than 13 g/dL.

Pediatric patients 1 mo–16 yr
- *Anemia of chronic renal failure:* 50 units/kg IV or subcutaneously 3 times/wk (for patients on dialysis only).
- *Anemia of prematurity:* 25–100 units/kg/dose subcutaneously 3 times/wk.
- *Anemia with cancer:* 600 units/kg/wk IV. Maximum dose, 60,000 units in children 5 yr and older.

Pharmacokinetics

Route	Onset	Peak	Duration
Subcut.	7–14 days	5–24 hr	24 hr

Metabolism: Serum; $T_{1/2}$: 4–13 hr
Distribution: Crosses placenta; enters breast milk
Excretion: Urine

▼ IV FACTS
Preparation: As provided; no additional preparation. Enter vial only once; do not shake

Adverse effects in *italics* are most common; those in **bold** are life-threatening. ⬛ Do not crush.

vial. Discard any unused solution. Refrigerate.

Infusion: Administer by direct IV injection or into tubing of running IV.

Incompatibilities: Do not mix with any other drug solution.

Adverse effects

- **CNS:** *Headache, arthralgias, fatigue, asthenia, dizziness,* **seizure, stroke,** TIA
- **CV:** *Hypertension, edema, chest pain,* **DVT**
- **GI:** *Nausea, vomiting, diarrhea*
- **Other:** Clotting of access line, **development of anti-erythropoietin antibodies with subsequent pure red cell aplasia and extreme anemia, tumor progression and shortened survival (with cancers)**

■ Nursing considerations

Assessment

- **History:** Uncontrolled hypertension, hypersensitivity to mammalian cell-derived products or to albumin human, lactation
- **Physical:** Reflexes, affect; BP, P; urinary output, renal function tests; CBC, Hct, iron levels, electrolytes

Interventions

⊗ *Black box warning* Risk of death and serious CV events is increased if Hgb target is higher than 11 g/dL. Use lowest levels of drug needed to increase Hgb to lowest level needed to avoid transfusion.

⊗ *Black box warning* Incidence of DVT is higher in patients who are receiving erythropoietin-stimulating agents preoperatively to reduce need for transfusion; consider antithrombotic prophylaxis if used for this purpose.

⊗ *Black box warning* Patients with cancer are at risk for more rapid tumor progression, shortened survival, and death when Hgb level target is more than 12 g/dL. Risk of death is increased in cancer patients not receiving radiation or chemotherapy.

- Confirm chronic, renal nature of anemia; not intended as a treatment of severe anemia or substitute for emergency transfusion.
- Patients with chronic renal failure on hemodialysis should receive the drug IV, not by subcutaneous injection, to decrease the risk of developing anti-erythropoietin antibodies.

- Gently mix; do not shake, shaking may denature the glycoprotein. Use only one dose per vial; do not re-enter the vial. Discard unused portions.
- Do not give with any other drug solution.
- Administer dose three times per week. If administered independent of dialysis, administer into venous access line. If patient is not on dialysis, administer IV or subcutaneously.
- Monitor access lines for signs of clotting.
- Arrange for Hgb reading before administration of each dose to determine dosage. If patient fails to respond within 8 wk of therapy, evaluate patient for other etiologies of the problem.
- Monitor patient for sudden loss of response and severe anemia with low reticulocyte count; withhold drug and check patient for anti-erythropoietin antibodies. If antibodies are present, discontinue drug permanently and do not switch to any other erythropoietic agent; cross-sensitivity can occur.
- Monitor Hgb levels; target range is 10–12 g/dL; do not exceed 12 g/dL.
- Evaluate iron stores before and periodically during therapy. Supplemental iron may need to be ordered.
- Institute seizure precautions.

Teaching points

- Drug must be given three times per week and can only be given IV, subcutaneously, or into a dialysis access line. Prepare a schedule of administration dates.
- If you will be giving yourself injections, you and a significant other should learn proper administration technique; dispose of syringes and needles appropriately.
- Keep appointments for blood tests needed to determine the effects of the drug on your blood count and to determine dosage.
- Maintain all of the usual activities and restrictions that apply to your chronic renal failure. If this becomes difficult, consult your health care provider.
- You may experience these side effects: Dizziness, headache, seizures (avoid driving or performing hazardous tasks); fatigue, joint pain (may be medicated); nausea, vomiting, diarrhea (proper nutrition is important).
- Report difficulty breathing, numbness or tingling, chest pain, seizures, severe headache.

▽ epoprostenol sodium (prostacyclin, PGX, PGI₂)

See Appendix R, *Less commonly used drugs*.

▽ eprosartan mesylate
(ep row sar' tan)

Teveten

PREGNANCY CATEGORY C
(FIRST TRIMESTER)

PREGNANCY CATEGORY D
(SECOND AND THIRD TRIMESTERS)

Drug classes
Antihypertensive
ARB

Therapeutic actions
Selectively blocks the binding of angiotensin II to specific tissue receptors found in the vascular smooth muscle and adrenal gland; this action blocks the vasoconstriction effect of the renin–angiotensin system as well as the release of aldosterone leading to decreased BP.

Indications
- Treatment of hypertension, alone or in combination with other antihypertensive drugs, particularly diuretics and calcium channel blockers
- Unlabeled uses: Heart failure, left ventricular hypertrophy, diabetic nephropathy

Contraindications and cautions
- Contraindicated with hypersensitivity to any ARB, pregnancy (use during the second or third trimester can cause injury or even death to the fetus), lactation.
- Use cautiously with renal impairment, hypovolemia, hyperkalemia.

Available forms
Tablets—400, 600 mg

Dosages
Adults
Usual starting dose is 600 mg PO daily. Can be administered in divided doses bid with a total daily dose of 400–800 mg/day being effective. Patients with moderate and severe renal impairment, maximum dose is 600 mg/day. If used as part of combination therapy, eprosartan should be added to established dose of other antihypertensive, starting at the lowest dose and increasing dosage based on patient response.

Pediatric patients
Safety and efficacy not established.

Pharmacokinetics

Route	Onset	Peak
Oral	Rapid	1–2 hr

Metabolism: Hepatic; $T_{1/2}$: 5–9 hr
Distribution: Crosses placenta; may enter breast milk
Excretion: Feces, urine

Adverse effects
- **CNS:** Headache, dizziness, syncope, muscle weakness, *fatigue, depression*
- **CV:** Hypotension
- **Dermatologic:** Rash, inflammation, urticaria, pruritus, alopecia, dry skin
- **GI:** Diarrhea, *abdominal pain,* nausea, constipation
- **Renal:** Hyperkalemia, increased BUN
- **Respiratory:** *URI symptoms,* cough, sinus disorders
- **Other:** Cancer (in preclinical studies), UTIs, **angioedema**

Interactions
✳ **Drug-drug** • Use caution when combining with other drugs that may elevate serum potassium concentrations—potassium-sparing diuretics, potassium supplements, or potassium-containing salt substitutes • Do not use in combination with aliskiren in diabetic patients

■ Nursing considerations
Assessment
- **History:** Hypersensitivity to any ARB, pregnancy, lactation, renal impairment, hypovolemia, hyperkalemia
- **Physical:** Skin lesions, turgor; T; reflexes, affect; BP; R, respiratory auscultation; renal function tests

Interventions
- Administer without regard to meals.
- ⊗ **Black box warning** Ensure that patient is not pregnant before beginning therapy, suggest the use of barrier birth control while

using eprosartan; fetal injury and deaths have been reported.

- For breast-feeding patients, find an alternate method of feeding the infant. Depression of the renin–angiotensin system in infants is potentially very dangerous.

⊗ *Warning* Alert surgeon and mark the patient's chart with notice that eprosartan is being taken. The blockage of the renin–angiotensin system following surgery can produce problems. Hypotension may be reversed with volume expansion.

- If BP control does reach desired levels, diuretics or other antihypertensives may be added to the drug regimen. Monitor patient's BP carefully.
- Monitor patient closely in any situation that may lead to a decrease in BP secondary to reduction in fluid volume—excessive perspiration, dehydration, vomiting, diarrhea—excessive hypotension can occur.

Teaching points

- Take drug without regard to meals. Do not stop taking this drug without consulting your health care provider.
- Use a barrier method of birth control while taking this drug; if you become pregnant or desire to become pregnant, consult your health care provider.
- You may experience these side effects: Dizziness (avoid driving a car or performing hazardous tasks); nausea, abdominal pain (proper nutrition is important, consult with your dietitian to maintain nutrition); symptoms of upper respiratory tract or urinary tract infection, cough (do not self-medicate, consult your health care provider if this becomes uncomfortable).
- Report fever, chills, dizziness, pregnancy, prolonged episodes of severe nausea, vomiting, and diarrhea.

DANGEROUS DRUG

▽eptifibatide
*(ep tiff **ib**' ah tide)*

Integrilin

PREGNANCY CATEGORY B

Drug classes
Antiplatelet drug
Glycoprotein IIb/IIIa receptor agonist

Therapeutic actions
Inhibits platelet aggregation by binding to the glycoprotein IIb/IIIa receptor on the platelet, which prevents the binding of fibrinogen and other adhesive ligands to the platelet.

Indications
- Treatment of acute coronary syndrome
- Prevention of cardiac ischemic complications in patients undergoing elective, emergency, or urgent percutaneous coronary intervention

Contraindications and cautions
- Contraindicated with allergy to eptifibatide, bleeding diathesis, hemorrhagic stroke, active, abnormal bleeding or stroke within 30 days, uncontrolled or severe hypertension, major surgery within 6 wk, dialysis, severe renal impairment, low platelet count.
- Use cautiously in the elderly; with pregnancy, lactation, renal insufficiency.

Available forms
Injection—0.75, 2 mg/mL

Dosages
Adults
- *Acute coronary syndrome:* 180 mcg/kg IV (maximum of 22.6 mg) over 1–2 min as soon as possible after diagnosis, then 2 mcg/kg/min (maximum 15 mg/hr) by continuous IV infusion for up to 72 hr. If patient is to undergo percutaneous coronary intervention, continue for 18–24 hr after the procedure, up to 96 hr of therapy. Reduce infusion dose to 1 mcg/kg/min if serum creatinine is greater than 2 mg/dL.
- *Percutaneous coronary intervention:* 180 mcg/kg IV as a bolus immediately before the procedure, then 2 mcg/kg/min by continuous IV infusion for 18–24 hr. May give a second bolus of 180 mcg/kg 10 min after the first bolus is given.

Pediatric patients
Not recommended.

Pharmacokinetics

Route	Onset	Peak	Duration
IV	15 min	45 min	2–4 hr

Metabolism: Tissue; $T_{1/2}$: 1.5–2.5 hr
Distribution: May cross placenta; may enter breast milk
Excretion: Urine

▼ IV FACTS

Preparation: Withdraw bolus from 10-mL vial. No preparation needed for continuous infusion. Spike the 100-mL vial with a vented infusion set. Protect from light.

Infusion: Infuse bolus quickly; infuse as continuous infusion using guidelines under Dosages section.

Compatibilities: May be given with alteplase, atropine, dobutamine, heparin, lidocaine, meperidine, metoprolol, morphine, nitroglycerin, verapamil.

Incompatibility: Do not mix with furosemide.

Adverse effects

- **CNS:** *Headache, dizziness,* weakness, syncope, flushing
- **Dermatologic:** *Rash,* pruritus
- **GI:** Nausea, GI distress, constipation, diarrhea
- **Hematologic:** Thrombocytopenia
- **Other:** *Bleeding, hypotension*

Interactions

✳ Drug-drug • Use caution when combining with other drugs that affect blood clotting—thrombolytics, anticoagulants, ticlopidine, dipyridamole, clopidogrel, NSAIDs; increased risk of bleeding or hemorrhage

■ Nursing considerations
Assessment

- **History:** Allergy to eptifibatide; bleeding diathesis; hemorrhagic stroke; active, abnormal bleeding or stroke within 30 days; uncontrolled or severe hypertension; major surgery within 6 wk; dialysis; severe renal impairment; low platelet count; pregnancy, lactation
- **Physical:** Skin color, temperature, lesions; orientation, reflexes, affect; P, BP, orthostatic BP, baseline ECG, peripheral perfusion; respiratory rate, adventitious sounds, aPTT, PT, active clotting time

Interventions

- Use eptifibatide in conjunction with heparin and aspirin.
- ⊗ **Warning** As much as possible, avoid arterial and venous puncture, IM injection, catheterization, and intubation in patient using this drug to minimize blood loss.

- Avoid the use of noncompressible IV access sites to prevent excessive, uncontrollable bleeding.
- Arrange for baseline and periodic tests of CBC, PT, aPTT, and active clotting time. Maintain aPTT of 50–70 sec and active bleeding time of 300–350 sec.
- Properly care for femoral access site to minimize bleeding. Document aPTT lower than 45 sec or activated clotting time lower than 150 sec, and stop heparin for 3–4 hr before pulling sheath.
- Provide comfort measures and arrange for analgesics if headache occurs.

Teaching points

- This drug is given to minimize blood clotting and cardiac damage. It must be given IV.
- You will be monitored closely and periodic blood tests will be done to monitor the effects of this drug on your body.
- You may experience these side effects: Dizziness, light-headedness, bleeding.
- Report light-headedness, palpitations, pain at IV site, bleeding.

▽ ergotamine tartrate

See Appendix R, *Less commonly used drugs.*

▽ erlotinib

See Appendix R, *Less commonly used drugs.*

▽ ertapenem
*(er tah **pen'** em)*

Invanz

PREGNANCY CATEGORY B

Drug classes
Antibiotic
Methyl-carbapenem

Therapeutic actions
Bactericidal: Inhibits synthesis of susceptible bacterial cell wall causing cell death.

Indications

- Community-acquired pneumonia caused by *Streptococcus pneumoniae* (penicillin-susceptible strains only), *Haemophilus*

influenzae (beta-lactamase–negative strains only), *Moraxella catarrhalis*
- Complicated skin and skin-structure infections including diabetic foot infections without osteomyelitis caused by *Staphylococcus aureus* (methicillin-susceptible strains only), *Streptococcus pyogenes, Escherichia coli, Streptococcus agalactiae, Klebsiella pneumoniae, Proteus mirabilis, Bacteroides fragilis, Porphyromonas asaccharolytica, Prevotella bivia, Peptostreptococcus* species
- Complicated GU infections, including pyelonephritis caused by *E. coli* or *K. pneumoniae.*
- Complicated intra-abdominal infections due to *E. coli, Clostridium clostridiiforme, Eubacterium lentum, Peptostreptococcus* species, *B. fragilis, Bacteroides distasonis, Bacteroides ovatus, Bacteroides thetaiotaomicron, Bacteroides uniformis*
- Acute pelvic infections, including postpartum endomyometritis, septic abortion, postsurgical gynecologic infections due to *S. agalactiae, E. coli, B. fragilis, P. asaccharolytica, Peptostreptococcus* species, *P. bivia*
- Prophylaxis of surgical-site infection after elective colorectal surgery in adults
- Unlabeled use: Hospital-acquired pneumonia, catheter-related bloodstream infections

Contraindications and cautions
- Contraindicated with allergies to any component of the drug and to beta-lactam antibiotics; allergy to amide-type local anesthetics (IM use); allergy to penicillins, cephalosporins, other allergens.
- Use cautiously with pregnancy; lactation, seizure disorder.

Available forms
Vials for reconstitution—1 g/vial

Dosages
Adults and children 13 yr and older
1 g IM or IV each day; length of treatment varies with infection—intra-abdominal, 5–14 days; urinary tract, 10–14 days; skin and skin structure, 7–14 days; community-acquired pneumonia, 10–14 days; acute pelvic infections, 3–10 days.
Prophylaxis: 1 g IV 1 hr before surgical incision.

Pediatric patients 3 mo to 12 yr
15 mg/kg IV or IM bid for 3–14 days; do not exceed 1 g/day. Length of treatment varies by infection (see dosage above).
Patients with renal impairment
For creatinine clearance of 30 mL/min or less, use 500 mg IV or IM daily.

Pharmacokinetics

Route	Onset	Peak
IV	Rapid	30 min
IM	10 min	2 hr

Metabolism: $T_{1/2}$: 4 hr
Distribution: Crosses the placenta; enters breast milk
Excretion: Urine, unchanged

▼ IV FACTS
Preparation: Reconstitute 1-g vial with 10 mL of water for injection, 0.9% sodium chloride injection or bacteriostatic water for injection; do not dilute with diluents containing dextrose. Shake well to dissolve and transfer to 50 mL of 0.9% sodium chloride injection; use within 6 hr of reconstitution, or store refrigerated for up to 24 hr, but use within 4 hr of removal from refrigeration; inspect solution for particulate matter.
Infusion: Infuse over 30 min.
Incompatibilities: Do not mix in solution or in the same line as any other medications or any solution containing dextrose.

Adverse effects
- **CNS:** *Headache,* dizziness, asthenia, fatigue, insomnia, altered mental status, anxiety, **seizures**
- **CV:** Heart failure, arrhythmias, edema, swelling, hypotension, hypertension, chest pain
- **GI:** *Nausea,* vomiting, *diarrhea,* abdominal pain, constipation, dyspepsia, **pseudomembranous colitis,** liver toxicity, GERD, *Clostridium difficile* diarrhea
- **GU:** Vaginitis
- **Hypersensitivity:** *Ranging from rash* to *fever* to **anaphylaxis;** serum sickness reaction
- **Local:** *Pain, phlebitis,* thrombophlebitis, inflammation at IV site
- **Respiratory:** Pharyngitis, rales, respiratory distress, cough, dyspnea, rhonchi
- **Other:** Fever, rash, vaginitis

■ Nursing considerations

 CLINICAL ALERT!
Name confusion has occurred between *Avinza* (extended-release morphine) and *Invanz* (ertapenem); use extreme caution.

Assessment

- **History:** Allergies to any component of the drug and to beta-lactam antibiotics; allergy to amide-type local anesthetics (IM use), penicillins, cephalosporins, other allergens; pregnancy, lactation, seizures
- **Physical:** T, skin status, swelling, orientation, reflexes, R, adventitious sounds, P, BP, peripheral perfusion, culture of affected area, sensitivity tests

Interventions

- Culture infected area and arrange for sensitivity tests before beginning drug therapy and during therapy if expected response is not seen.
- Prepare IM solution as follows: Reconstitute 1-g vials with 3.2 mL of 1% lidocaine injection without epinephrine; shake to form solution; immediately withdraw contents for injection.
- Administer IM injections deeply into large muscle mass within 1 hr of reconstitution.
- ⊗ *Warning* Have emergency and life-support equipment readily available in case of severe hypersensitivity reaction.
- Discontinue drug if hypersensitivity reaction occurs.
- Monitor injection site for adverse reactions.
- Ensure ready access to bathroom facilities and provide frequent small meals if GI complications occur.
- Evaluate patient for *C. difficile* infection if diarrhea occurs.
- Arrange for treatment of superinfections if they occur.

Teaching points

- This drug is given IV or IM to treat your specific infection.
- You may experience these side effects: Nausea, diarrhea, dizziness, headache (consult your health care provider if any of these are severe).
- Report severe diarrhea, difficulty breathing, unusual tiredness or fatigue, pain at injection site.

▷**erythromycin**
(er ith roe mye' sin)

erythromycin base
Oral, ophthalmic ointment, topical dermatologic solution for acne, topical dermatologic ointment: Akne-mycin, A/T/S, Apo-Erythro (CAN), Apo-Erythro E-C (CAN), Erybid (CAN), EryDerm, Erygel, EryPads, Ery-Tab, Erythromycin Film-tabs, PCE Dispertab

erythromycin estolate (CAN)
Novo-Rythro Estolate (CAN)

erythromycin ethylsuccinate
Oral: Apo-Erythro ES (CAN), E.E.S. 400, E.E.S. Granules, EryPed, EryPed 200, EryPed 400, EryPed Drops, Novo-Rhythro Ethylsuccinate (CAN)

erythromycin gluceptate

erythromycin lactobionate
Erythrocin I.V. (CAN), Erythrocin Lactobionate

erythromycin stearate
Apo-Erythro-S (CAN)

PREGNANCY CATEGORY B

Drug class
Macrolide antibiotic

Therapeutic actions
Bacteriostatic or bactericidal in susceptible bacteria; binds to cell membrane, causing change in protein function, leading to cell death.

Indications
Systemic administration

- Acute infections caused by sensitive strains of *Streptococcus pneumoniae, Mycoplasma pneumoniae, Listeria monocytogenes, Legionella pneumophila*

Adverse effects in *italics* are most common; those in **bold** are life-threatening. ⊕ Do not crush.

- URIs, lower respiratory tract infections, skin and soft-tissue infections caused by group A beta-hemolytic streptococci when oral treatment is preferred to injectable benzathine penicillin
- PID caused by *Neisseria gonorrhoeae* in patients allergic to penicillin
- In conjunction with sulfonamides in URIs caused by *Haemophilus influenzae*
- As an adjunct to antitoxin in infections caused by *Corynebacterium diphtheriae* and *Corynebacterium minutissimum*
- Prophylaxis against alpha-hemolytic streptococcal endocarditis before dental or other procedures in patients allergic to penicillin who have valvular heart disease
- Oral erythromycin: Treatment of intestinal amebiasis caused by *Entamoeba histolytica;* infections in the newborn and in pregnancy that are caused by *Chlamydia trachomatis* and in adult chlamydial infections when tetracycline cannot be used; primary syphilis (*Treponema pallidum*) in penicillin-allergic patients; eliminating *Bordetella pertussis* organisms from the nasopharynx of infected individuals and as prophylaxis in exposed and susceptible individuals
- Unlabeled uses: Erythromycin base is used with neomycin before colorectal surgery to reduce wound infection; treatment of severe diarrhea associated with *Campylobacter* enteritis or enterocolitis; treatment of genital, inguinal, or anorectal lymphogranuloma venereum infection; treatment of *Haemophilus ducreyi* (chancroid)

Ophthalmic ointment
- Treatment of superficial ocular infections caused by susceptible strains of microorganisms; prophylaxis of ophthalmia neonatorum caused by *N. gonorrhoeae* or *C. trachomatis*

Topical dermatologic solutions for acne
- Treatment of acne vulgaris

Topical dermatologic
- Granules used with flexible hydroactive dressings for dermal ulcers, pressure ulcers, leg ulcers, superficial wounds, and postoperative wounds
- Treatment of skin infections caused by sensitive microorganisms

Contraindications and cautions
Systemic administration
- Contraindicated with allergy to erythromycin.
- Use cautiously with hepatic impairment, lactation (secreted and may be concentrated in breast milk; may modify bowel flora of nursing infant and interfere with fever workups).

Ophthalmic ointment
- Contraindicated with allergy to erythromycin; viral, fungal, mycobacterial infections of the eye.

Available forms
Base: Tablets—250, 500 mg; DR tablets—250, 333, 500 mg; DR capsules—250 mg; ophthalmic ointment—5 mg/g. Stearate tablets—250 mg ethylsuccinate: Ethylsuccinate tablets—400 mg; suspension—200, 400 mg/5 mL; powder for suspension—200 mg/5 mL, 400 mg/5mL; granules for suspension—200 mg/5 mL; topical solution—2%; topical gel, ointment—2%; topical pad—2%. Lactobionate injection—500, 1,000 mg.

Dosages
Systemic administration
Oral preparations of the different erythromycin salts differ in pharmacokinetics: 400 mg erythromycin ethylsuccinate produces the same free erythromycin serum levels as 250 mg of erythromycin base, stearate, or estolate.

Adults
15–20 mg/kg/day in continuous IV infusion or up to 4 g/day in divided doses every 6 hr; 250 mg (400 mg of ethylsuccinate) every 6 hr PO or 500 mg every 12 hr PO or 333 mg every 8 hr PO, up to 4 g/day, depending on the severity of the infection.

- *Streptococcal infections:* 250 mg every 6 hr or 500 mg every 12 hr (for group A beta-hemolytic streptococcal infections, continue therapy for at least 10 days).
- *Legionnaires disease:* 1–4 g/day PO or IV in divided doses for 10–21 days (ethylsuccinate 1.6 g/day; optimal doses not established).
- *Dysenteric amebiasis:* 250 mg (400 mg of ethylsuccinate) PO every 6 hr or 333 mg every 8 hr or 500 mg every 12 hr for 10–14 days.
- *Acute PID* (N. gonorrhoeae): 500 mg of lactobionate or glucepate IV every 6 hr for

3 days and then 250 mg stearate or base PO every 6 hr or 333 mg every 8 hr or 500 mg every 12 hr for 7 days.

- *Chlamydial infections:* Urogenital infections during pregnancy: 500 mg PO qid or 666 mg every 8 hr for at least 7 days, one-half this dose every 8 hr or 250 mg bid for at least 14 days if intolerant to first regimen. Urethritis in males: 800 mg of ethylsuccinate PO tid for 7 days.
- *Primary syphilis:* 30–40 g (48–64 g of ethylsuccinate) in divided doses over 10–15 days.
- *CDC recommendations for STDs:* 500 mg PO qid for 7–30 days, depending on the infection.

Pediatric patients
30–50 mg/kg/day PO in divided doses. Specific dosage determined by severity of infection, age, and weight. Maximum dose should not exceed 4 g/day.

- *Dysenteric amebiasis:* 30–50 mg/kg/day in divided doses for 10–14 days.
- *Pertussis:* 40–50 mg/kg/day PO daily in divided doses for 5–14 days.
- *Chlamydial infections:* 50 mg/kg/day PO in divided doses, for at least 2 (conjunctivitis of newborn) or 3 (pneumonia of infancy) wk.

Ophthalmic ointment
Adults and pediatric patients
One-half–inch ribbon instilled into conjunctival sac of affected eye two to six times per day, depending on severity of infection.

Topical
Adults and pediatric patients
- *Dermatologic ointment for acne:* Apply a thin layer sparingly to affected areas morning and evening.
- *Topical dermatologic:* Flexible hydroactive dressings and granules applied and kept in place for 1–7 days.
- *Pledgets:* Rub over affected area bid; use each pledget once, then discard.

Pharmacokinetics

Route	Onset	Peak
Oral	1–2 hr	1–4 hr
IV	Rapid	1 hr

Metabolism: Hepatic; $T_{1/2}$: 1.5–2 hr
Distribution: Crosses placenta; enters breast milk
Excretion: Bile, urine

▼ IV FACTS

Preparation: Reconstitute powder for IV infusion only with sterile water for injection without preservatives—10 mL for 250- and 500-mg vials, 20 mL for 1-g vials. Prepare intermittent infusion as follows: Dilute 250–500 mg in 100–250 mL of 0.9% sodium chloride injection or 5% dextrose in water. Prepare for continuous infusion by adding reconstituted drug to 0.9% sodium chloride injection, lactated Ringer injection, or D_5W that will make a solution of 1 g/L.

Infusion: *Intermittent infusion:* Administer over 20–60 min qid; infuse slowly to avoid vein irritation. Administer continuous infusion within 4 hr, or buffer the solution to neutrality if administration is prolonged.

Incompatibilities: *Gluceptate*—do not add to aminophylline, pentobarbital, secobarbital, tetracycline. *Lactobionate*—do not mix with heparin, metoclopramide, tetracycline.

Y-site incompatibilities: Avoid chloramphenicol, heparin, phenobarbital, phenytoin.

Adverse effects
Systemic administration
- **CNS:** Reversible hearing loss, confusion, uncontrollable emotions, abnormal thinking, **seizures**
- **CV: Ventricular arrhythmias** (with IV)
- **GI:** *Abdominal cramping, anorexia, nausea, diarrhea, vomiting,* **pseudomembranous colitis,** hepatotoxicity, pancreatitis
- **Hypersensitivity:** Allergic reactions ranging from rash to **anaphylaxis**
- **Other:** *Superinfections*

Ophthalmic ointment
- **Dermatologic:** Edema, urticaria, dermatitis, angioneurotic edema
- **Local:** *Irritation, burning, itching* at site of application

Topical dermatologic preparations
- **Local:** *Superinfections,* particularly with long-term use

Interactions
Systemic administration
✱ **Drug-drug** • Increased serum levels of digoxin • Increased effects of oral anticoagulants, theophylline, carbamazepine, ergot derivatives, disopyramide, calcium blockers, HMG-CoA reductase inhibitors, midazolam, proton

---

Adverse effects in *italics* are most common; those in **bold** are life-threatening. ⊞ Do not crush.

pump inhibitors, quinidine • Increased therapeutic and toxic effects of corticosteroids • Increased levels of cyclosporine and risk of renal toxicity

＊ Drug-food • Decreased metabolism and increased risk of toxic effects if taken with grapefruit juice; avoid this combination

＊ Drug-lab test • Interferes with fluorometric determination of urinary catecholamines • Decreased urinary estriol levels due to inhibition of hydrolysis of steroids in the gut

Topical dermatologic solution for acne

＊ Drug-drug • Increased irritant effects with peeling, desquamating, or abrasive agents

■ **Nursing considerations**
Assessment

• **History:** Allergy to erythromycin, hepatic impairment, lactation; viral, fungal, mycobacterial infections of the eye (ophthalmologic), pregnancy
• **Physical:** Site of infection; skin color, lesions; orientation, affect, hearing tests; R, adventitious sounds; GI output, bowel sounds, liver evaluation; culture and sensitivity tests of infection, urinalysis, LFTs

Interventions
Systemic administration

• Culture site of infection before therapy.
• Administer oral erythromycin base or stearate on an empty stomach, 1 hr before or 2–3 hr after meals, with a full glass of water (oral erythromycin estolate, ethylsuccinate, and certain enteric-coated tablets [review the manufacturer's instructions] may be given without regard to meals).
• Administer around the clock to maximize effect; adjust schedule to minimize sleep disruption.
• Monitor liver function in patients on prolonged therapy.
• Give some preparations with meals, as directed, or substitute one of these preparations, if GI upset occurs with oral therapy.

Topical dermatologic solution for acne

• Wash affected area, rinse well, and dry before application.

Ophthalmic and topical dermatologic preparation

• Use topical products only when needed. Sensitization produced by the topical use of an an-

tibiotic may preclude its later systemic use in serious infections. Topical antibiotic preparations not normally used systemically are best.
• Culture site before beginning therapy.
• Cover the affected area with a sterile bandage if needed (topical).

Teaching points
Systemic administration

• Take oral drug on an empty stomach, 1 hour before or 2–3 hours after meals, with a full glass of water; some forms may be taken without regard to meals. Do not drink grapefruit juice while on this drug. The drug should be taken around the clock; schedule to minimize sleep disruption. Finish the full course of the drug therapy.
• You may experience these side effects: Stomach cramping, discomfort (take the drug with meals, if appropriate); uncontrollable emotions, crying, laughing, abnormal thinking (reversible).
• Report severe or watery diarrhea, severe nausea or vomiting, dark urine, yellowing of the skin or eyes, loss of hearing, rash or itching.

Ophthalmic ointment

• Pull the lower eyelid down gently and squeeze a one-half–inch ribbon of the ointment into the sac, avoid touching the eye or lid. A mirror may be helpful. Gently close the eye, and roll the eyeball in all directions.
• Drug may cause temporary blurring of vision, stinging, or itching.
• Report stinging or itching that becomes pronounced.

Topical dermatologic agents for acne

• Wash and rinse area, and pat it dry before applying solution.
• Use fingertips or an applicator to apply; wash hands thoroughly after application.
• Use pledgets once and discard.

▽**escitalopram oxalate**
*(ess si **tal'** oh pram)*

Lexapro

PREGNANCY CATEGORY C

Drug classes
Antidepressant
SSRI

E

Therapeutic actions
Potentiates serotonergic activity in the CNS by inhibiting reuptake of serotonin resulting in antidepressant effect with little effect on norepinephrine or dopamine; an isomer of citalopram.

Indications
- Acute and maintenance treatment for patients with major depressive disorder
- Treatment of generalized anxiety disorder
- Unlabeled uses: Panic disorder, PTSD insomnia in adults, IBS

Contraindications and cautions
- Contraindicated with MAOI, pimozide use; with allergy to drug or to citalopram or any component of the drug.
- Use cautiously in the elderly and with renal or hepatic impairment, illnesses of metabolism or hemodynamic response, pregnancy, lactation, suicidal patients, patients with mania or seizure disorders.

Available forms
Tablets—5, 10, 20 mg; oral solution—1 mg/5 mL

Dosages
Adults
- *Major depressive disorder:* Initially, 10 mg/day PO as a single daily dose; if needed, may be increased to 20 mg/day after a minimum of 1-wk trial period. For maintenance, 10–20 mg/day PO; reassess periodically.
- *Generalized anxiety disorder:* 10 mg/day PO; may be increased to 20 mg/day after 1 wk if needed. Treatment beyond 8 wk not tested.

Pediatric patients 12–17 yr
- *Major depressive disorder:* 10 mg/day PO as a single dose. Increase dose slowly over a minimum of 3 wk. Maximum dose, 20 mg/day.

Geriatric patients or adults with hepatic impairment
10 mg/day PO as a single dose; do not increase dose.

Pharmacokinetics

Route	Onset	Peak
Oral	Slow	3.5–6.5 hr

Metabolism: Hepatic; $T_{1/2}$: 27–32 hr
Distribution: Crosses placenta; enters breast milk
Excretion: Urine

Adverse effects
- **CNS:** *Somnolence, dizziness,* insomnia, fatigue, headache, lethargy, complex sleep disorders, serotonin syndrome (with abrupt discontinuation)
- **Dermatologic:** Sweating
- **GI:** *Nausea,* dry mouth, constipation, diarrhea, indigestion, abdominal pain, decreased appetite
- **GU:** *Ejaculatory disorders,* impotence, anorgasmia in females, decreased libido
- **Respiratory:** Rhinitis, sinusitis, flulike symptoms
- **Other: Anaphylaxis, angioedema,** serotonin syndrome

Interactions
✴ **Drug-drug** ● Risk of serious toxic effects if combined with citalopram; do not use these drugs concomitantly ● Increased escitalopram levels and toxicity if taken with MAOIs; ensure that patient has been off the MAOI for at least 14 days before administering escitalopram ● Risk of serotonin syndrome—a syndrome characterized by increased BP, T, severe anxiety, agitation, rigidity, and can occur when multiple serotonin elevating drugs are used. Monitor patient carefully ● Possible severe adverse effects if combined with other centrally acting CNS drugs including alcohol; use caution ● Possible decreased effects of escitalopram if combined with carbamazepine, lithium; monitor patient closely
✴ **Drug-alternative therapy** ● Increased risk of severe reaction if combined with St. John's Wort; avoid this combination

■ Nursing considerations

CLINICAL ALERT!
There is potential for name confusion between escitalopram and citalopram and between *Lexapro* (escitalopram) and *Loxitane* (loxapine); use caution.

Assessment
- **History:** MAOI use; allergy to drug, citalopram, or any component of the drug; renal or hepatic impairment; older age; pregnancy; lactation; suicidal tendencies; metabolic illnesses or problems with hemodynamic response; alcoholism
- **Physical:** Orientation, reflexes; P, BP, perfusion; R, bowel sounds, normal output;

urinary output; liver evaluation; LFTs, renal function tests

Interventions

⊗ **Black box warning** Monitor patient for risk of suicidality, especially when starting or altering dosage; children, adolescents, and young adults are at increased risk.

- Give once a day, in the morning or in the evening; may be taken with food if desired.
- Encourage patient to continue use for 4–6 wk, as directed, to ensure adequate levels to affect depression.

⊗ **Warning** Limit amount of drug given in prescription to potentially suicidal patients.

⊗ **Warning** If discontinuing drug after long-term use, taper dosage gradually to avoid withdrawal syndrome.

⊗ **Warning** Use during third trimester of pregnancy has led to prolonged hospitalization, need for respiratory support, and tube feedings for the baby.

- Advise any depressed patients to avoid the use of alcohol while being treated with antidepressive drugs.
- Establish appropriate safety precautions if patient experiences adverse CNS effects.
- Institute appropriate therapy for patient suffering from depression.

Teaching points

- Take this drug exactly as directed, and as long as directed; it may take several weeks to realize the benefits of the drug. The drug may be taken with food if desired.
- Do not stop taking this medication without consulting your health care provider.
- Avoid the use of alcohol while you are taking this drug.
- This drug should not be taken during pregnancy or when breast-feeding; using barrier contraceptives is suggested.
- You may experience these side effects: Drowsiness, dizziness, tremor (use caution and avoid driving a car or performing other tasks that require alertness if you experience daytime drowsiness); GI upset (frequent small meals, frequent mouth care may help); alterations in sexual function (this is a drug effect and will pass when drug therapy is ended); allergic reaction; swelling; complex sleep disorders.
- Report severe nausea, vomiting; blurred vision; excessive sweating, suicidal ideation, sexual dysfunction, insomnia.

DANGEROUS DRUG

▽ **esmolol hydrochloride**
(*ess' moe lol*)

Brevibloc

PREGNANCY CATEGORY C

E

Drug classes
Antiarrhythmic
Beta₁-selective adrenergic blocker

Therapeutic actions
Blocks beta-adrenergic receptors in the heart and juxtaglomerular apparatus, reducing the influence of the sympathetic nervous system on these tissues; decreasing the excitability of the heart, cardiac output, and release of renin; and lowering BP and heart rate. At low doses, acts relatively selectively at the beta₁-adrenergic receptors of the heart; has very rapid onset and short duration.

Indications
- Supraventricular tachycardia, when rapid but short-term control of ventricular rate is desirable (atrial fibrillation, flutter, perioperative or postoperative situations)
- Noncompensatory tachycardia when heart rate requires specific intervention
- Intraoperative and postoperative tachycardia and hypertension when intervention is needed
- Unlabeled use: Unstable angina

Contraindications and cautions
- Contraindicated with decompensated heart failure, cardiogenic shock, second- or third-degree heart block (in the absence of a pacemaker), bradycardia.
- Use cautiously with bronchospastic disease, pregnancy, lactation.

Available forms
Injection—10 mg/mL, 20 mg/mL

Dosages
Adults
Individualize dosage by titration (loading dose followed by a maintenance dose). Initial loading dose of 500 mcg/kg/min IV for 1 min followed by a maintenance dose of 50 mcg/kg/min for 4 min. If adequate response is not observed

in 5 min, repeat loading dose and follow with maintenance infusion of 100 mcg/kg/min. Repeat titration as necessary, increasing rate of maintenance dose in increments of 50 mcg/kg/min. As desired heart rate or safe end point is approached, omit loading infusion and decrease incremental dose in maintenance infusion to 25 mcg/kg/min (or less), or increase interval between titration steps from 5 to 10 min. Usual range is 50–200 mcg/kg/min. Infusions for up to 24 hr have been used; up to 48 hr may be well tolerated. Dosage should be individualized based on patient response; do not exceed 300 mcg/kg/min.

Pediatric patients
Safety and efficacy not established.

Pharmacokinetics

Route	Onset	Peak	Duration
IV	< 5 min	10–20 min	10–30 min

Metabolism: RBC esterases; $T_{1/2}$: 9 min
Distribution: Crosses placenta; may enter breast milk
Excretion: Urine

▼ IV FACTS

Preparation: Dilute drug before infusing as follows: Add the contents of 2 ampules of esmolol (2.5 g) to a compatible diluent: 5% dextrose injection, 5% dextrose in Ringer injection; 5% dextrose and 0.9% or 0.45% sodium chloride injection; lactated Ringer injection; 0.9% or 0.45% sodium chloride injection after removing 20 mL from a 500 mL bottle, to make a drug solution with a concentration of 10 mg/mL. Diluted solution is stable for 24 hr at room temperature.
Infusion: Rate of infusion is determined by patient response; see Dosages section above.
Incompatibilities: Do not mix in solution with diazepam, furosemide, thiopental, or sodium bicarbonate.

Adverse effects
- **CNS:** *Light-headedness,* speech disorder, *midscapular pain, weakness, rigors,* somnolence, confusion
- **CV:** *Hypotension,* pallor, bradycardia
- **GI:** Taste perversion
- **GU:** Urine retention

- **Local:** *Inflammation,* induration, edema, erythema, burning at the site of infusion
- **Other:** Fever, rhonchi, flushing

Interactions
✳ **Drug-drug** • Increased therapeutic and toxic effects with verapamil • Impaired antihypertensive effects with ibuprofen, indomethacin, piroxicam

■ **Nursing considerations**
Assessment
- **History:** Cardiac, cerebrovascular disease; bronchospastic disease; pregnancy, lactation
- **Physical:** P, BP, ECG; orientation, reflexes; R, adventitious sounds; urinary output

Interventions
- Ensure that drug is not used in chronic settings when transfer to another drug is anticipated.
- Do not give undiluted drug.
- ⊗ **Warning** Do not mix with sodium bicarbonate, diazepam, furosemide, or thiopental.
- Monitor BP, HR, and ECG closely.

Teaching points
- This drug is reserved for emergency use; incorporate information about this drug into an overall teaching plan.

▽ **esomeprazole magnesium (perprazole, S-omeprazole)**
*(ess oh **me'** pray zol)*

Nexium⊕, Nexium IV

PREGNANCY CATEGORY B

Drug classes
Antisecretory drug
Proton pump inhibitor

Therapeutic actions
Gastric acid-pump inhibitor: Suppresses gastric acid secretion by specific inhibition of the hydrogen–potassium ATPase enzyme system at the secretory surface of the gastric parietal cells; blocks the final step of acid production; is broken down less in the first pass through

the liver than the parent compound omeprazole, allowing for increased serum levels.

Indications

- GERD—treatment of heartburn and other related symptoms
- Erosive esophagitis—short-term (4–8 wk) treatment for healing and symptom relief; also used for maintenance therapy following healing of erosive esophagitis
- Short-term treatment of GERD with a history of erosive esophagitis by IV route for up to 10 days, when oral therapy is not possible for patients 1 mo and older
- As part of combination therapy for the treatment of duodenal ulcer associated with *Helicobacter pylori*
- Reduction in occurrence of gastric ulcers associated with continuous NSAID use in patients at risk (60 yr and older, history of gastric ulcers) for developing gastric ulcers
- Treatment of pathologic hypersecretory conditions, including Zollinger-Ellison syndrome
- Unlabeled uses: Non-GERD dyspepsia, Barrett esophagus, stress ulcer prophylaxis, prevention of GI bleeding in patients receiving antiplatelet drugs

Contraindications and cautions

- Contraindicated with hypersensitivity to omeprazole, esomeprazole, or other proton pump inhibitor.
- Use cautiously with hepatic impairment, pregnancy, lactation.
- Possible increased risk of *Clostridium difficile* infection.

Available forms

DR capsules ⊙ⓡⓔ—20, 40 mg; DR powder for suspension—2.5, 5, 10, 20, 40 mg; injection—20, 40 mg/vial

Dosages
Adults

- *Healing of erosive esophagitis:* 20–40 mg PO daily for 4–8 wk. An additional 4–8 wk course of therapy can be considered for patients who have not healed.
- *Maintenance of healing of erosive esophagitis:* 20 mg PO daily.
- *Symptomatic GERD:* 20 mg daily for 4 wk. An additional 4-wk course of therapy can be considered if symptoms have not resolved.

- *Short-term treatment of GERD when oral therapy is not possible:* 20–40 mg IV by injection over at least 3 min or IV infusion over 10–30 min.
- *Duodenal ulcer:* 40 mg/day PO for 10 days with 1,000 mg PO bid amoxicillin and 500 mg PO bid clarithromycin.
- *Reduction of risk of gastric ulcers with NSAID use:* 20–40 mg PO daily for 6 mo.

Pediatric patients (12–17 yr)

- *Short-term treatment of GERD:* 20–40 mg/day PO for up to 8 wk.

Pediatric patients (1–11 yr)

- *Treatment of GERD:* 10 mg/day PO for up to 8 wk.
- *Healing of erosive esophagitis:*
Weight less than 20 kg: 10 mg/day PO for up to 8 wk.
Weight of 20 kg or more: 10–20 mg/day PO for up to 8 wk.

Pediatric patients (1 mo–17 yr)

- *Treatment of GERD when oral therapy is not possible:* 20–40 mg IV daily for up to 8 wk.

Patients with hepatic impairment

Do not exceed 20 mg/day in patients with severe hepatic impairment.

Pharmacokinetics

Route	Onset	Peak	Duration
Oral	1–2 hr	1.5 hr	17 hr

Metabolism: Hepatic; $T_{1/2}$: 1–1.5 hr
Distribution: May cross placenta; may enter breast milk
Excretion: Bile, urine

▼ IV FACTS

Preparation: Reconstitute with 5 mL of 0.9% sodium chloride injection; withdraw 5 mL of reconstituted solution. May be further diluted with 0.9% sodium chloride, lactated Ringer, or 5% dextrose to a volume of 50 mL for infusion. Do not use if particulate matter is seen in solution, or solution is discolored. May be stored at room temperature for up to 12 hr; protect from light.
Injection: Inject 5 mL directly or into line of running IV over no less than 3 min.
Infusion: Infuse dilute solution (50 mL) over 10–30 min.
Incompatibilities: Do not mix with other medications; flush tubing before and after each

dose with 0.9% sodium chloride, lactated Ringer, 5% dextrose.

Adverse effects

- **CNS:** *Headache, dizziness,* asthenia, vertigo, insomnia, apathy, anxiety, paresthesias, dream abnormalities
- **Dermatologic:** Rash, inflammation, urticaria, pruritus, alopecia, dry skin
- **GI:** *Diarrhea, abdominal pain, nausea, vomiting,* constipation, dry mouth, tongue atrophy, flatulence, *C. difficile* diarrhea
- **Respiratory:** *URI symptoms, sinusitis,* cough, epistaxis
- **Other:** Bone loss, increased risk of fractures with long-term use, hypomagnesemia

Interactions

✳ **Drug-drug** • Increased serum levels and potential increase in toxicity of benzodiazepines when taken concurrently • May interfere with absorption of drugs dependent upon presence of acidic environment (eg, ketoconazole, iron salts, digoxin) • Decreased levels of atazanavir if combined.

■ Nursing considerations

⭐ **CLINICAL ALERT!**
Potential for name confusion exists between esomeprazole and omeprazole; use caution. Name confusion has been reported between *Nexium* (esomeprazole) and *Nexavar* (sorafenib); use caution.

Assessment

- **History:** Hypersensitivity to any proton pump inhibitor; hepatic impairment; pregnancy, lactation
- **Physical:** Skin lesions; T; reflexes; affect; urinary output, abdominal examination; respiratory auscultation, LFTs

Interventions

⊗ **Warning** Arrange for further evaluation of patient after 4 wk of therapy for gastroesophageal reflux disorders. Symptomatic improvement does not rule out gastric cancer.

- If administering antacids, they may be administered concomitantly with esomeprazole.
- Administer IV for maximum of 10 days; switch to oral form as soon as possible.

- Prepare suspension by emptying packet into 15 mL water. Stir, let thicken 2–3 min, stir, and administer within 30 min. Rinse container with water and have patient drink.
- Ensure that the patient swallows capsule whole; do not crush, or chew; patients having difficulty swallowing may open capsule and sprinkle in applesauce or disperse in tap water, orange or apple juice, or yogurt; do not crush or chew pellets.
- To administer through a nasogastric (NG) tube, capsules can be opened and granules emptied into a syringe and delivered through the tube. For suspension form, add 15 mL of water to syringe, add packet, shake syringe, let thicken for 2–3 min, shake syringe, and inject through NG tube. Use within 30 min of preparation.
- Obtain baseline liver function tests and monitor periodically during therapy.
- Maintain supportive treatment as appropriate for underlying problem.
- Evaluate patient for *C. difficile* infection if diarrhea occurs.
- Provide additional comfort measures to alleviate discomfort from GI effects and headache.
- Establish safety precautions if dizziness or other CNS effects occur (use side rails, accompany patient).

Teaching points

- Take the drug at least 1 hour before meals. Swallow the capsules whole; do not chew or crush. If you cannot swallow the capsule, it can be opened and sprinkled in applesauce or mixed in tap water, orange or apple juice, or yogurt; do not crush or chew the pellets. If using suspension, add 1 tablespoon water to packet, stir, let stand for 2–3 minutes to set, stir again, and drink within 30 minutes of preparing. Then rinse container with water and immediately drink remaining granules. This drug will need to be taken for 4–8 weeks, at which time your condition will be re-evaluated.
- Arrange to have regular medical follow-up visits while you are using this drug.
- Maintain all of the usual activities and restrictions that apply to your condition. If this becomes difficult, consult your health care provider.
- You may experience these side effects: Dizziness (avoid driving a car or performing hazardous tasks); headaches (consult your

health care provider if these become bothersome; medications may be available to help); nausea, vomiting, diarrhea (proper nutrition is important; consult with your dietitian to maintain nutrition; ensure ready access to bathroom); symptoms of upper respiratory tract infection, cough (it may help to know that this is a drug effect; do not self-medicate; consult your health care provider if this becomes uncomfortable).

• Report severe headache, worsening of symptoms, fever, chills, darkening of the skin, changes in color of urine or stool, diarrhea.

▽estazolam
(es taz' e lam)

PREGNANCY CATEGORY X

CONTROLLED SUBSTANCE C-IV

Drug classes
Benzodiazepine
Sedative-hypnotic

Therapeutic actions
Exact mechanisms of action not understood; acts mainly at subcortical levels of the CNS, leaving the cortex relatively unaffected; potentiates the effects of GABA, an inhibitory neurotransmitter.

Indications
• Insomnia characterized by difficulty in falling asleep, frequent nocturnal awakenings, or early morning awakening
• Recurring insomnia or poor sleeping habits
• Acute or chronic medical situations requiring restful sleep

Contraindications and cautions
• Contraindicated with hypersensitivity to benzodiazepines, psychoses, acute narrow-angle glaucoma, shock, coma, acute alcoholic intoxication with depression of vital signs, pregnancy (increased risk of congenital malformations, neonatal withdrawal syndrome), labor and delivery ("floppy infant" syndrome reported), lactation (secreted in breast milk; long-term administration of diazepam, another benzodiazepine, to breast-feeding mothers has caused infants to become lethargic and lose weight).

• Use cautiously with impaired liver or renal function, debilitation, depression, suicidal tendencies, history of substance abuse.

Available forms
Tablets—1, 2 mg

Dosages
Individualize dosage.
Adults
1 mg PO before bedtime; up to 2 mg may be needed.
Pediatric patients
Not for use in patients younger than 18 yr.
Geriatric patients or patients with debilitating disease
1 mg PO if healthy; start with 0.5 mg in debilitated patients.

Pharmacokinetics

Route	Onset	Peak
Oral	45–60 min	2 hr

Metabolism: Hepatic; $T_{1/2}$: 10–24 hr
Distribution: Crosses placenta; may enter breast milk
Excretion: Feces, urine

Adverse effects
• **CNS:** *Transient, mild drowsiness initially; sedation, depression, lethargy, apathy, fatigue, light-headedness, disorientation, restlessness, asthenia,* crying, delirium, headache, slurred speech, dysarthria, stupor, rigidity, tremor, dystonia, vertigo, euphoria, nervousness, difficulty in concentration, vivid dreams, psychomotor retardation, extrapyramidal symptoms, *mild paradoxical excitatory reactions during first 2 wk of treatment* (especially in psychiatric patients, aggressive children, and with high dosage), visual and auditory disturbances, diplopia, nystagmus, depressed hearing, nasal congestion, complex sleep disorders
• **CV:** *Bradycardia, tachycardia,* **CV collapse,** hypertension and hypotension, palpitations, edema
• **Dependence:** *Drug dependence with withdrawal syndrome* when drug is discontinued (more common with abrupt discontinuation of higher dosage used for longer than 4 mo)
• **Dermatologic:** Urticaria, pruritus, skin rash, dermatitis

- **GI:** *Constipation, diarrhea, dyspepsia,* dry mouth, salivation, nausea, anorexia, vomiting, difficulty in swallowing, gastric disorders, elevations of blood enzymes: LDH, alkaline phosphatase, AST, ALT; hepatic impairment, jaundice
- **GU:** *Incontinence, urinary retention, changes in libido,* menstrual irregularities
- **Hematologic:** Decreased Hct, blood dyscrasias
- **Other:** Hiccups, fever, diaphoresis, paresthesia, muscular disturbances, gynecomastia, **anaphylaxis, angioedema**

Interactions
✳ **Drug-drug** • Increased CNS depression when taken with alcohol, phenothiazines, opioids, barbiturates • Decreased sedative effects of estazolam if taken concurrently with theophylline, aminophylline, rifampin, and TCAs

■ Nursing considerations
Assessment
- **History:** Hypersensitivity to benzodiazepines; psychoses; acute narrow-angle glaucoma; shock; coma; acute alcoholic intoxication; pregnancy; labor; lactation; impaired liver or renal function, debilitation, depression, suicidal tendencies
- **Physical:** Skin color, lesions; T, orientation, reflexes, affect, ophthalmologic examination; P, BP; R, adventitious sounds; liver evaluation, abdominal examination, bowel sounds, normal output; CBC, LFTs, renal function tests

Interventions
- Arrange to monitor liver and renal function and CBC during long-term therapy.
⊗ *Warning* Taper dosage gradually after long-term therapy, especially in epileptic patients.

Teaching points
- Take drug exactly as prescribed; do not stop taking this drug without consulting your health care provider.
- Avoid alcohol, sleep-inducing, or over-the-counter drugs while taking this drug.
- Be aware that this drug provides symptomatic relief and is not a cure for insomnia. It may be habit-forming; it works best if used on an "as needed" basis and not every night.

- You may experience these side effects: Transient drowsiness, dizziness (avoid driving or engaging in dangerous activities); complex sleep disorders; allergic reaction; swelling; GI upset (take the drug with water); depression, dreams, emotional upset, crying; sleep may be disturbed for several nights after discontinuing the drug.
- Report severe dizziness, weakness, drowsiness that persists, rash or skin lesions, palpitations, swelling of the extremities, visual changes, difficulty voiding.

▷ estradiol
*(ess tra **dye'** ole)*

estradiol
Oral: Estrace, Gynodiol
Transdermal system: Alora, Climara, Estraderm, Menostar, Vivelle, Vivelle Dot
Topical vaginal cream: Estrace
Vaginal ring: Estring
Topical emulsion: Estrasorb
Gel: Divigel, Elestrin, Estrogel
Topical spray: Evamist

estradiol acetate
Tablets: Femtrace
Vaginal ring: Femring

estradiol cypionate
Injection in oil: Depo-Estradiol

estradiol hemihydrate
Vaginal tablet: Vagifem

estradiol valerate
Injection in oil: Delestrogen

PREGNANCY CATEGORY X

Drug classes
Estrogen
Hormone

Therapeutic actions
Estradiol is the most potent endogenous female sex hormone. Estrogens are important in the development of the female reproductive system and secondary sex characteristics; affect the

---

Adverse effects in *italics* are most common; those in **bold** are life-threatening. ⊞ Do not crush.

release of pituitary gonadotropins; cause capillary dilatation, fluid retention, protein anabolism and thin cervical mucus; conserve calcium and phosphorus and encourage bone formation; inhibit ovulation and prevent postpartum breast discomfort. They are responsible for proliferation of the endometrium; absence or decline of estrogen produces signs and symptoms of menopause on the uterus, vagina, breasts, cervix; relief in androgen-dependent prostatic carcinoma is attributable to competition with androgens for receptor sites, decreasing influence of the androgens.

Indications

• *Femtrace, Estrasorb,* estradiol cypionate, estradiol valerate: Vasomotor symptoms
• Estradiol acetate tablets (*Femtrace*), estradiol gel 0.1% (*Divigel*), estradiol spray (*Evamist*): Treatment of moderate to severe vasomotor symptoms associated with menopause
• *Vagifem, Estrace, Estring:* Vaginal atrophy
• *Femring,* tablets, transdermal (except *Menostar*), *Estrogel:* Vasomotor symptoms and vaginal atrophy
• Estradiol oral, transdermal, estradiol valerate: Prevention of postmenopausal osteoporosis
• Estradiol oral, transdermal, estradiol cypionate, valerate: Treatment of female hypogonadism, female castration, primary ovarian failure
• Estradiol oral, estradiol valerate: Palliation of inoperable prostatic cancer
• Estradiol oral: Palliation of inoperable, progressing breast cancer

Contraindications and cautions

• Contraindicated with allergy to estrogens, allergy to tartrazine (in 2-mg oral tablets), breast cancer (with exceptions), estrogen-dependent neoplasm, undiagnosed abnormal genital bleeding, active or past history of thrombophlebitis or thromboembolic disorders, pregnancy (potential serious fetal defects; women of childbearing age should be advised of risks and birth control measures suggested), history of breast cancer.
• Use cautiously with metabolic bone disease, renal or hepatic insufficiency, heart failure, lactation.

Available forms

Transdermal—release rates of 0.014, 0.025, 0.0375, 0.05, 0.06, 0.075, 0.1 mg/24 hr;

tablets—0.5, 1, 2 mg; *Femtrace*—0.45, 0.9, 1.8 mg; injection—5, 10, 20, 40 mg/mL; vaginal cream—0.1 mg/g; vaginal ring—2 mg; *Femring*—0.05 mg/day, 0.1 mg/day; vaginal tablet—10, 25 mcg; topical emulsion—2.5 mg/g; gel—0.06%, 0.1%; topical spray—1.53 mg

Dosages
Adults

• *Moderate to severe vasomotor symptoms, atrophic vaginitis, kraurosis vulvae associated with menopause:* 1–2 mg/day PO. Adjust dose to control symptoms. For gel, 0.25 g of 0.1% gel applied to right or left upper thigh on alternating days; may be increased to 0.5 or 1 g/day to control symptoms. For topical spray (*Evamist*), 1 spray once daily to forearm; may be increased to 2–3 sprays daily. Cyclic therapy (3 wk on/1 wk off) is recommended, especially in women who have not had a hysterectomy. 1–5 mg estradiol cypionate in oil IM every 3–4 wk. 10–20 mg estradiol valerate in oil IM, every 4 wk. The 0.014- to 0.05-mg system is applied to the skin weekly or twice weekly. If oral estrogens have been used, start transdermal system 1 wk after withdrawal of oral form. Given on a cyclic schedule (3 wk on/1 wk off). Attempt to taper or discontinue medication every 3–6 mo.

• *Female hypogonadism, female castration, primary ovarian failure:* 1–2 mg/day PO. Adjust dose to control symptoms. Cyclic therapy (3 wk on/1 wk off) is recommended. 1.5–2 mg estradiol cypionate in oil IM at monthly intervals. 10–20 mg estradiol valerate in oil IM every 4 wk. The 0.05-mg system is applied to skin twice weekly as above.

Vaginal

• *Vaginal cream:* 2–4 g intravaginally daily for 1–2 wk, then reduce to one-half dosage for similar period followed by maintenance doses of 1 g one to three times/wk thereafter. Discontinue or taper at 3- to 6-mo intervals.

• *Vaginal ring:* Insert one ring high into vagina. Replace every 90 days.

• *Vaginal tablet:* 1 tablet inserted vaginally daily for 2 wk; then twice weekly.

Oral

• *Prostatic cancer (inoperable):* 1–2 mg PO tid. Administer long-term. 30 mg or more estradiol valerate in oil IM every 1–2 wk.

- *Breast cancer (inoperable, progressing):* 10 mg tid PO for at least 3 mo.
- *Prevention of postpartum breast engorgement:* 10–25 mg estradiol valerate in oil IM as a single injection at the end of the first stage of labor.
- *Osteoporosis prevention:* 0.5 mg/day PO given cyclically—23 days on, 5 days rest—starting as soon after menopause as possible.

Topical emulsion

Relief of menopausal symptoms: Apply lotion to legs, thighs, or calves once daily. Apply gel to one arm once daily.

Pediatric patients

Not recommended due to effect on growth of the long bones.

Pharmacokinetics

Route	Onset	Peak
Oral	Slow	Days

Metabolism: Hepatic; $T_{1/2}$: Not known
Distribution: Crosses placenta; enters breast milk
Excretion: Urine

Adverse effects

- **CNS:** Steepening of the corneal curvature with a resultant change in visual acuity and intolerance to contact lenses, *headache,* migraine, dizziness, mental depression, chorea, **seizures**
- **CV:** Increased BP, thromboembolic and thrombotic disease
- **Dermatologic:** *Photosensitivity, peripheral edema, chloasma,* erythema nodosum or multiforme, hemorrhagic eruption, loss of scalp hair, hirsutism, urticaria, dermatitis
- **GI:** Gallbladder disease (in postmenopausal women), **hepatic adenoma,** *nausea, vomiting, abdominal cramps, bloating,* **cholestatic jaundice, colitis, acute pancreatitis**
- **GU:** Increased risk of postmenopausal endometrial cancer, *breakthrough bleeding, change in menstrual flow, dysmenorrhea, premenstrual-like syndrome,* amenorrhea, vaginal candidiasis, cystitis-like syndrome, endometrial cystic hyperplasia
- **Hematologic:** Hypercalcemia, decreased glucose tolerance
- **Local:** *Pain at injection site,* sterile abscess, postinjection flare

- **Other:** Weight changes, reduced carbohydrate tolerance, aggravation of porphyria, edema, changes in libido, breast tenderness

Topical vaginal cream

Systemic absorption may cause uterine bleeding in menopausal women and may cause serious bleeding of remaining endometrial foci in sterilized women with endometriosis

Interactions

✳ Drug-drug ● Increased therapeutic and toxic effects of corticosteroids ● Decreased serum levels of estradiol with drugs that enhance hepatic metabolism of the drug—barbiturates, phenytoin, rifampin, carbamazepine

✳ Drug-lab test ● Increased prothrombin and factors VII, VIII, IX, and X; thyroid-binding globulin with increased PBI, T_4, increased uptake of free T_3 resin (free T_4 is unaltered), serum triglycerides and phospholipid concentration ● Decreased antithrombin III, pregnanediol excretion, response to metyrapone test, serum folate concentration ● Impaired glucose tolerance

■ Nursing considerations

Assessment

- **History:** Allergy to estrogens, tartrazine; breast cancer, estrogen-dependent neoplasm; undiagnosed abnormal genital bleeding; active or previous thrombophlebitis or thromboembolic disorders; pregnancy; lactation; metabolic bone disease; renal insufficiency; heart failure
- **Physical:** Skin color, lesions, edema; breast examination; injection site; orientation, affect, reflexes; P, auscultation, BP, peripheral perfusion; R, adventitious sounds; bowel sounds, liver evaluation, abdominal examination; pelvic examination; serum calcium, phosphorus; LFTs, renal function tests; Papanicolaou (Pap) test, glucose tolerance test

Interventions

⊗ *Black box warning* Arrange for pretreatment and periodic (at least annual) history and physical, which should include BP, breasts, abdomen, pelvic organs, and a Pap test; may increase risk of endometrial cancer.

⊗ *Black box warning* Do not use to prevent CV events or dementia; may increase risk, including thrombophlebitis, pulmonary embolism, stroke, MI.

Adverse effects in *italics* are most common; those in **bold** are life-threatening. ▭ Do not crush.

⊗ **Black box warning** Caution patient of the risks of estrogen use, the need to prevent pregnancy during treatment, for frequent medical follow-up, and for periodic rests from drug treatment.

- Administer cyclically for short-term only when treating postmenopausal conditions because of the risk of endometrial neoplasm; taper to the lowest effective dose, and provide a drug-free week each month.
- Apply transdermal system to a clean, dry area of skin on the trunk of the body, preferably the abdomen; do not apply to breasts; rotate the site at least 1 wk between applications; avoid the waistline because clothing may rub the system off; apply immediately after opening and compress for about 10 sec to attach.
- Apply topical gel to upper thighs, alternating right and left daily. Do not apply to irritated skin, and do not wash site for at least 1 hr.
- Apply topical spray to forearm. Let dry for at least 30 min.
- Insert vaginal ring as deeply as possible into upper one-third of vagina. Ring will remain in place for 3 months. Then, remove and evaluate need for continued therapy. If a ring falls out during 3 mo, rinse with warm water and reinsert.
- Insert vaginal tablet as high into vagina as is comfortable for patient; use supplied applicator.

⊗ **Warning** Arrange for the concomitant use of progestin therapy during long-term estrogen therapy in women with a uterus; this will mimic normal physiologic cycling and allow for a cyclic uterine bleeding that may decrease the risk of endometrial cancer. Women without a uterus do not need progestin.

- Administer parenteral preparations by deep IM injection only. Monitor injection sites and rotate with each injection to decrease development of abscesses.

Teaching points

- Use this drug in cycles or short term; prepare a calendar of drug days, rest days, and drug-free periods.
- Apply transdermal system and vaginal cream properly; insert vaginal tablet as high into the vagina as is comfortable.
- Apply gel to upper thighs, alternating right and left daily. Do not apply to irritated skin, and do not wash site for at least 1 hour.

- Apply one spray to forearm each day. Let dry for at least 30 minutes.
- Insert vaginal ring high in vagina; it should remain in place for 3 months. If it falls out before that time, rinse with warm water and reinsert.
- Potentially serious side effects include cancers, blood clots, and liver problems; it is very important to have periodic medical examinations throughout therapy.
- This drug cannot be given to pregnant women because of serious toxic effects to the baby; use of contraceptives is advised.
- You may experience these side effects: Nausea, vomiting, bloating; headache, dizziness, mental depression (use caution if driving or performing tasks that require alertness); sensitivity to sunlight (use a sunscreen and wear protective clothing); rash, loss of scalp hair, darkening of the skin on the face; changes in menstrual patterns.
- Report pain in the groin or calves of the legs, chest pain or sudden shortness of breath, abnormal vaginal bleeding, lumps in the breast, sudden severe headache, dizziness or fainting, changes in vision or speech, weakness or numbness in the arm or leg, severe abdominal pain, yellowing of the skin or eyes, severe mental depression, pain at injection site.

▷ **estrogens, conjugated**
(*ess' troe jenz*)

Oral, topical vaginal cream:
C.E.S. (CAN), Premarin
Parenteral: Premarin Intravenous
Synthetic: Cenestin, Enjuvia

PREGNANCY CATEGORY X

Drug classes
Estrogen
Hormone

Therapeutic actions
Estrogens are endogenous female sex hormones important in the development of the female reproductive system and secondary sex characteristics. They affect the release of pituitary gonadotropins; cause capillary dilation, fluid retention, protein anabolism, and thin cervical mucus; conserve calcium and

phosphorus; encourage bone formation; inhibit ovulation and prevent postpartum breast discomfort. They are responsible for the proliferation of the endometrium; absence or decline of estrogen produces signs and symptoms of menopause on the uterus, vagina, breasts, cervix. Their efficacy as palliation in male patients with androgen-dependent prostatic carcinoma is attributable to their competition with androgens for receptor sites, thus decreasing the influence of androgens.

Indications
Oral
- Palliation of moderate to severe vasomotor symptoms, atrophic vaginitis, or kraurosis vulvae associated with menopause
- Treatment of female hypogonadism; female castration; primary ovarian failure
- Osteoporosis: To retard progression
- Palliation of inoperable prostatic cancer
- Palliation of metastatic breast cancer
- *Cenestin, Enjuvia:* Treatment of moderate to severe vasomotor symptoms associated with menopause

Parenteral
- Treatment of uterine bleeding due to hormonal imbalance in the absence of organic pathology

Vaginal cream
- Treatment of atrophic vaginitis and kraurosis vulvae associated with menopause

Contraindications and cautions
- Contraindicated with allergy to estrogens, breast cancer (with exceptions), estrogen-dependent neoplasm, undiagnosed abnormal genital bleeding, active or past thrombophlebitis or thromboembolic disorders from previous estrogen use, pregnancy (serious fetal defects; women of childbearing age should be advised of risks and birth control measures suggested).
- Use cautiously with metabolic bone disease, renal or hepatic insufficiency, heart failure, lactation.

Available forms
Tablets—0.3, 0.45, 0.625, 0.9, 1.25 mg; injection—25 mg; vaginal cream—0.625 mg/g

Dosages
Oral drug should be given cyclically (3 wk on/1 wk off) except in selected cases of carci-

noma and prevention of postpartum breast engorgement.

Adults
- *Moderate to severe vasomotor symptoms associated with menopause:* 0.3–0.625 mg/day PO.
- *Atrophic vaginitis, kraurosis vulvae associated with menopause:* 0.5–2 g vaginal cream daily intravaginally or topically, depending on severity of condition. Taper or discontinue at 3- to 6-mo intervals. Or, 0.3 mg/day PO continually.
- *Female hypogonadism:* 0.3–0.625 mg/day PO for 3 wk followed by 1 wk of rest. Adjust dose depending on severity of symptoms and responsiveness of endometrium.
- *Female castration, primary ovarian failure:* 1.25 mg/day PO. Adjust dosage by patient response to lowest effective dose.
- *Prostatic cancer (inoperable):* 1.25–2.5 mg tid PO. Judge effectiveness by phosphatase determinations and by symptomatic improvement.
- *Osteoporosis:* Start with lowest dose, 0.3 mg/day PO given continuously or cyclically (25 days on/5 days off). Adjust dosage based on individual response.
- *Breast cancer (inoperable, progressing):* 10 mg tid PO for at least 3 mo.
- *Abnormal uterine bleeding due to hormonal imbalance:* 25 mg IV or IM. Repeat in 6–12 hr as needed. IV route provides a more rapid response.

Pediatric patients
Not recommended due to effect on growth of the long bones.

Pharmacokinetics

Route	Onset	Peak
Oral	Slow	Days
IV	Gradual	Hours

Metabolism: Hepatic; $T_{1/2}$: Unknown
Distribution: Crosses placenta; enters breast milk
Excretion: Urine

▼ IV FACTS
Preparation: Reconstitute with provided diluent; add to normal saline, dextrose, and invert sugar solutions. Refrigerate unreconstituted parenteral solution; use reconstituted solution within a few hours. Refrigerated

reconstituted solution is stable for 60 days; do not use solution if darkened or precipitates have formed.

Infusion: Inject slowly over 2–5 min.

Incompatibilities: Do not mix with protein hydrolysate, ascorbic acid, or any solution with an acid pH.

Adverse effects

- **CNS:** Steepening of the corneal curvature with a resultant change in visual acuity and intolerance to contact lenses, *headache,* migraine, dizziness, mental depression, chorea, **seizures**
- **CV:** Increased BP, thromboembolic and thrombotic disease
- **Dermatologic:** *Photosensitivity, peripheral edema, chloasma,* erythema nodosum or multiforme, hemorrhagic eruption, loss of scalp hair, hirsutism, urticaria, dermatitis
- **GI:** Gallbladder disease (in postmenopausal women), **hepatic adenoma,** *nausea, vomiting, abdominal cramps, bloating,* **cholestatic jaundice,** *colitis,* **acute pancreatitis**
- **GU:** Increased risk of endometrial cancer in postmenopausal women, *breakthrough bleeding, change in menstrual flow, dysmenorrhea, premenstrual-like syndrome,* amenorrhea, vaginal candidiasis, cystitis-like syndrome, endometrial cystic hyperplasia
- **Hematologic:** Hypercalcemia, decreased glucose tolerance
- **Local:** *Pain at injection site,* sterile abscess, postinjection flare
- **Other:** Weight changes, reduced carbohydrate tolerance, aggravation of porphyria, edema, changes in libido, breast tenderness

Topical vaginal cream

Systemic absorption may cause uterine bleeding in menopausal women and serious bleeding of remaining endometrial foci in sterilized women with endometriosis

Interactions

✻ **Drug-drug** • Increased therapeutic and toxic effects of corticosteroids • Decreased serum levels of estrogen with drugs that enhance hepatic metabolism of the drug: Barbiturates, phenytoin, rifampin, carbamazepine

✻ **Drug-lab test** • Increased prothrombin and factors VII, VIII, IX, and X; thyroid-binding globulin with increased PBI, T_4, increased uptake of free T_3 resin (free T_4 is unaltered), serum triglycerides and phospholipid concentration • Decreased antithrombin III, pregnanediol excretion, response to metyrapone test, serum folate concentration • Impaired glucose tolerance

■ Nursing considerations
Assessment

- **History:** Allergy to estrogens; breast cancer, estrogen-dependent neoplasm; undiagnosed abnormal genital bleeding; active or previous thrombophlebitis or thromboembolic disorders; pregnancy; lactation; metabolic bone disease; renal insufficiency; heart failure
- **Physical:** Skin color, lesions, edema; breast examination; injection site; orientation, affect, reflexes; P, auscultation, BP, peripheral perfusion; R, adventitious sounds; bowel sounds, liver evaluation, abdominal examination; pelvic examination; serum calcium, phosphorus; LFTs, renal function tests; Papanicolaou (Pap) test; glucose tolerance test

Interventions

⊗ *Black box warning* Arrange for pretreatment and periodic (at least annual) history and physical, which should include BP, breasts, abdomen, pelvic organs, and a Pap test; increased risk of endometrial cancer.

⊗ *Black box warning* Do not use to prevent CV events or dementia; may increase risk, including thrombophlebitis, pulmonary embolism, stroke, MI.

⊗ *Black box warning* Caution patient of the risks involved with estrogen use, the need to prevent pregnancy during treatment, for frequent medical follow-up, and periodic rests from drug treatment.

⊗ *Warning* Give cyclically for short term only when treating postmenopausal conditions because of the risk of endometrial neoplasm; taper to the lowest effective dose, and provide a drug-free week each month.

- Refrigerate unreconstituted parenteral solution; use reconstituted solution within a few hours.
- Refrigerated reconstituted solution is stable for 60 days; do not use solution if darkened or precipitates have formed.

⊗ *Warning* Arrange for the concomitant use of progestin therapy during long-term estrogen therapy in women with a uterus; this will mimic normal physiologic cycling and allow for cyclic uterine bleeding, which may decrease the risk of endometrial cancer. Women without a uterus do not need progestin.

Teaching points

- Use this drug cyclically or short term; prepare a calendar of drug days, rest days, and drug-free periods.
- Use vaginal cream properly.
- Potentially serious side effects can occur: Cancers, blood clots, liver problems; it is very important that you have periodic medical examinations throughout therapy.
- This drug cannot be given to pregnant women because of serious toxic effects to the baby; use of contraceptives is advised.
- You may experience these side effects: Nausea, vomiting, bloating; headache, dizziness, mental depression (use caution if driving or performing tasks that require alertness); sensitivity to sunlight (use a sunscreen and wear protective clothing); rash, loss of scalp hair, darkening of the skin on the face; changes in menstrual patterns.
- Report pain in the groin or calves of the legs, chest pain or sudden shortness of breath, abnormal vaginal bleeding, lumps in the breast, sudden severe headache, dizziness or fainting, changes in vision or speech, weakness or numbness in the arm or leg, severe abdominal pain, yellowing of the skin or eyes, severe mental depression, pain at injection site.

▷ estrogens, esterified
(ess' troe jenz)

Menest

PREGNANCY CATEGORY X

Drug classes
Estrogen
Hormone

Therapeutic actions
Estrogens are endogenous hormones important in the development of the female reproductive system and secondary sex characteristics. They cause capillary dilatation, fluid retention, protein anabolism, and thin cervical mucus; conserve calcium and phosphorus

and encourage bone formation; inhibit ovulation and prevent postpartum breast discomfort. They are responsible for the proliferation of the endometrium; absence or decline of estrogen produces signs and symptoms of menopause on the uterus, vagina, breasts, cervix. Palliation with androgen-dependent prostatic carcinoma is attributable to competition for androgen receptor sites, decreasing the influence of androgens.

Indications

- Palliation of moderate to severe vasomotor symptoms, atrophic vaginitis, or kraurosis vulvae associated with menopause
- Treatment of female hypogonadism; female castration; primary ovarian failure
- Palliation of inoperable prostatic cancer
- Palliation of inoperable, metastatic breast cancer in men, postmenopausal women

Contraindications and cautions

- Contraindicated with allergy to estrogens, breast cancer (with exceptions), estrogen-dependent neoplasm, undiagnosed abnormal genital bleeding, active or past thrombophlebitis or thromboembolic disorders from previous estrogen use, pregnancy (serious fetal defects; women of childbearing age should be advised of the risks and birth control measures suggested).
- Use cautiously with metabolic bone disease, renal or hepatic insufficiency, heart failure, lactation.

Available forms
Tablets—0.3, 0.625, 1.25, 2.5 mg

Dosages
Administer PO only.
Adults
- *Moderate to severe vasomotor symptoms, atrophic vaginitis, kraurosis vulvae associated with menopause:* 0.3–1.25 mg/day PO for atrophic vaginitis and kraurosis vulvae. 1.25 mg/day PO for vasomotor symptoms. Adjust to lowest effective dose. Cyclic therapy (3 wk of daily estrogen followed by 1 wk of rest from drug therapy) is recommended. If patient has not menstruated in 2 mo, start at any time. If patient is still menstruating, start therapy on day 5 of bleeding.
- *Female hypogonadism:* 2.5–7.5 mg/day PO in divided doses for 20 days on/10 days

off. If bleeding does not occur by the end of that period, repeat the same dosage schedule. If bleeding does occur before the end of the 10-day rest, begin a 20-day estrogen-progestin cyclic regimen with progestin given orally during the last 5 days of estrogen therapy. If bleeding occurs before this cycle is finished, restart course on day 5 of bleeding.

• *Female castration, primary ovarian failure:* 1.25 mg/day PO cyclically. Adjust dosage by patient response to lowest effective dose.
• *Prostatic cancer (inoperable):* 1.25–2.5 mg tid PO. In long-term therapy, judge effectiveness by symptomatic response and serum phosphatase determinations.
• *Breast cancer (inoperable, progressing):* 10 mg tid PO for at least 3 mo in select men and postmenopausal women.

Pediatric patients
Not recommended due to effect on growth of the long bones.

Pharmacokinetics

Route	Onset	Peak
Oral	Slow	Days

Metabolism: Hepatic; $T_{1/2}$: Unknown
Distribution: Crosses placenta; enters breast milk
Excretion: Urine

Adverse effects

• **CNS:** Steepening of the corneal curvature with a resultant change in visual acuity and intolerance to contact lenses, *headache,* migraine, dizziness, mental depression, chorea, **seizures**
• **CV:** Increased BP, thromboembolic and thrombotic disease (with high doses in certain groups of susceptible women and in men receiving estrogens for prostatic cancer)
• **Dermatologic:** *Photosensitivity, peripheral edema, chloasma,* erythema nodosum or multiforme, hemorrhagic eruption, loss of scalp hair, hirsutism, urticaria, dermatitis
• **GI:** Gallbladder disease (in postmenopausal women), **hepatic adenoma** (rarely occurs, but may rupture and cause death), *nausea, vomiting, abdominal cramps, bloating,* cholestatic jaundice, colitis, acute pancreatitis
• **GU:** Increased risk of endometrial cancer in postmenopausal women, *breakthrough bleeding, change in menstrual flow, dysmenorrhea, premenstrual-like syndrome,* amenorrhea, vaginal candidiasis, cystitis-like syndrome, endometrial cystic hyperplasia
• **Hematologic:** Hypercalcemia (in breast cancer patients with bone metastases), decreased glucose tolerance
• **Other:** Weight changes, reduced carbohydrate tolerance, aggravation of porphyria, edema, changes in libido, breast tenderness

Interactions

✴ **Drug-drug** • Increased therapeutic and toxic effects of corticosteroids • Decreased serum levels of estrogen if taken with drugs that enhance hepatic metabolism of the drug: Barbiturates, phenytoin, rifampin, carbamazepine
✴ **Drug-lab test** • Increased prothrombin and factors VII, VIII, IX, and X; thyroid-binding globulin with increased PBI, T_4 increased uptake of free T_3 resin (free T_4 is unaltered), serum triglycerides and phospholipid concentration • Decreased antithrombin III, pregnanediol excretion, response to metyrapone test, serum folate concentration • Impaired glucose tolerance

■ Nursing considerations
Assessment

• **History:** Allergy to estrogens; breast cancer, estrogen-dependent neoplasm; undiagnosed abnormal genital bleeding; thrombophlebitis or thromboembolic disorders; pregnancy; lactation; metabolic bone disease; renal insufficiency; heart failure
• **Physical:** Skin color, lesions, edema; breast examination; injection site; orientation, affect, reflexes; P, auscultation, BP, peripheral perfusion; R, adventitious sounds; bowel sounds, liver evaluation, abdominal examination; pelvic examination; serum calcium, phosphorus; LFTs, renal function tests; Papanicolaou (Pap) test; glucose tolerance test

Interventions
⊗ **Black box warning** Arrange for pretreatment and periodic (at least annual) history and physical examination, which should include BP, breasts, abdomen, pelvic organs, and a Pap test; increased risk of endometrial cancer.
⊗ **Black box warning** Do not use to prevent CV events or dementia; may increase risk, including thrombophlebitis, pulmonary embolism, stroke, MI.

⊗ **Black box warning** Caution patient of the risks involved with estrogen use; the need to prevent pregnancy during treatment, for frequent medical follow-up, and for periodic rests from drug treatment.

⊗ **Black box warning** Give cyclically for short term only when treating postmenopausal conditions because of the risk of endometrial neoplasm; taper to the lowest effective dose, and provide a drug-free week each month.

⊗ **Warning** Arrange for progestin therapy during long-term estrogen therapy in postmenopausal women with a uterus; this will mimic normal physiologic cycling and allow for cyclic uterine bleeding, which may decrease the risk of endometrial cancer. Women without a uterus do not need progestin.

Teaching points

- Use this drug in cycles or short term; prepare a calendar of drug days, rest days, and drug-free periods (as appropriate).
- Potentially serious side effects can occur, including cancers, blood clots, liver problems; it is very important that you have periodic medical examinations throughout therapy.
- This drug cannot be given to pregnant women because of serious toxic effects to the baby; use of contraceptives is advised.
- You may experience these side effects: Nausea, vomiting, bloating; headache, dizziness, mental depression (use caution if driving or performing tasks that require alertness); sensitivity to sunlight (use a sunscreen and wear protective clothing); rash, loss of scalp hair, darkening of the skin on the face; changes in menstrual patterns.
- Report pain in the groin or calves of the legs, chest pain or sudden shortness of breath, abnormal vaginal bleeding, lumps in the breast, sudden severe headache, dizziness or fainting, changes in vision or speech, weakness or numbness in the arm or leg, severe abdominal pain, yellowing of the skin or eyes, severe mental depression.

▷ **estropipate
(piperazine estrone
sulfate)**
(*ess' troe pi' pate*)

PREGNANCY CATEGORY X

Drug classes
Estrogen
Hormone

Therapeutic actions
Estrogens are endogenous female sex hormones important in the development of the female reproductive system and secondary sex characteristics. They cause capillary dilatation, fluid retention, protein anabolism, and thin cervical mucus; conserve calcium and phosphorus and encourage bone formation; inhibit ovulation and prevent postpartum breast discomfort. They are responsible for the proliferation of the endometrium; absence or decline of estrogen produces signs and symptoms of menopause on the uterus, vagina, breasts, cervix. Palliation with androgen-dependent prostatic carcinoma is attributable to competition with androgens for receptor sites, decreasing the influence of androgens.

Indications
- Palliation of moderate to severe vasomotor symptoms, atrophic vaginitis, or kraurosis vulvae associated with menopause
- Treatment of female hypogonadism, female castration, primary ovarian failure
- Prevention of osteoporosis

Contraindications and cautions
- Contraindicated with allergy to estrogens, breast cancer (with exceptions), estrogen-dependent neoplasm, undiagnosed abnormal genital bleeding, active or past thrombophlebitis or thromboembolic disorders from previous estrogen use, pregnancy (serious fetal defects; advise women of childbearing age of the potential risks and suggest birth control measures).
- Use cautiously with metabolic bone disease, renal or hepatic insufficiency, heart failure, lactation.

Available forms
Tablets—0.625, 1.25, 2.5, 5 mg

Dosages
Adults
- *Moderate to severe vasomotor symptoms, atrophic vaginitis, kraurosis vulvae associated with menopause:* 0.75–6 mg/day PO given cyclically (3 wk on and 1 wk off). Use lowest possible dose.

Adverse effects in *italics* are most common; those in **bold** are life-threatening. ⊡ Do not crush.

- *Female hypogonadism, female castration, primary ovarian failure:* 1.5–9 mg/day PO for the first 3 wk, followed by a rest period of 8–10 days. Repeat if bleeding does not occur at end of rest period.
- *Prevention of osteoporosis:* 0.75 mg daily PO for 25 days of a 31-day cycle per month.

Pediatric patients
Not recommended due to effect on growth of the long bones.

Pharmacokinetics

Route	Onset	Peak
Oral	Slow	Days

Metabolism: Hepatic; $T_{1/2}$: Unknown
Distribution: Crosses placenta; enters breast milk
Excretion: Urine

Adverse effects

- **CNS:** Steepening of the corneal curvature with a resultant change in visual acuity and intolerance to contact lenses, *headache,* migraine, dizziness, mental depression, chorea, **seizures**
- **CV:** Increased BP, thromboembolic and thrombotic disease
- **Dermatologic:** *Photosensitivity, peripheral edema, chloasma,* erythema nodosum or multiforme, hemorrhagic eruption, loss of scalp hair, hirsutism, urticaria, dermatitis
- **GI:** Gallbladder disease (in postmenopausal women), **hepatic adenoma,** *nausea, vomiting, abdominal cramps, bloating,* **cholestatic jaundice,** *colitis,* acute pancreatitis
- **GU:** Increased risk of endometrial cancer in postmenopausal women, *breakthrough bleeding, change in menstrual flow, dysmenorrhea, premenstrual-like syndrome,* amenorrhea, vaginal candidiasis, cystitis-like syndrome, endometrial cystic hyperplasia
- **Hematologic:** Hypercalcemia, decreased glucose tolerance
- **Other:** Weight changes, reduced carbohydrate tolerance, aggravation of porphyria, edema, changes in libido, breast tenderness

Interactions

✴ **Drug-drug** • Increased therapeutic and toxic effects of corticosteroids • Decreased serum levels of estrogens if taken with drugs that enhance hepatic metabolism of the drug: barbiturates, phenytoin, rifampin, carbamazepine

✴ **Drug-lab test** • Increased prothrombin and factors VII, VIII, IX, and X; thyroid-binding globulin with increased PBI, T_4, increased uptake of free T_3 resin (free T_4 is unaltered), serum triglycerides and phospholipid concentration • Decreased antithrombin III, pregnanediol excretion, response to metyrapone test, serum folate concentration • Impaired glucose tolerance

■ Nursing considerations

Assessment

- **History:** Allergy to estrogens; breast cancer, estrogen-dependent neoplasm; undiagnosed abnormal genital bleeding; thrombophlebitis or thromboembolic disorders; pregnancy; lactation; metabolic bone disease; renal insufficiency; heart failure
- **Physical:** Skin color, lesions, edema; breast examination; injection site; orientation, affect, reflexes; P, auscultation, BP, peripheral perfusion; R, adventitious sounds; bowel sounds, liver evaluation, abdominal examination; pelvic examination; serum calcium, phosphorus; LFTs, renal function tests; Papanicolaou (Pap) test; glucose tolerance test

Interventions

⊗ *Black box warning* Arrange for pretreatment and periodic (at least annual) history and physical examination, which should include BP, breasts, abdomen, pelvic organs, and a Pap test; increased risk of endometrial cancer.

⊗ *Black box warning* Do not use to prevent CV events or dementia; may increase risk, including thrombophlebitis, pulmonary embolism, stroke, MI.

⊗ *Black box warning* Caution patient of the risks involved with estrogen use, the need to prevent pregnancy during treatment, for frequent medical follow-up, and for periodic rests from drug treatment.

⊗ *Black box warning* Give cyclically for short term only when treating postmenopausal conditions because of the risk of endometrial neoplasm. Taper to the lowest effective dose and provide a drug-free week each month.

⊗ *Warning* Arrange for the concomitant use of progestin therapy during long-term estrogen therapy in postmenopausal women with a uterus; this will mimic normal physiologic cycling and allow for a cyclic uterine bleeding, which may decrease the risk of endometrial cancer. Women without a uterus do not need progestin.

Teaching points

• Prepare a calendar of drug days, rest days, and drug-free periods.
• This drug cannot be given to pregnant women because of serious toxic effects to the baby; use of contraceptives is advised.
• Potentially serious side effects can occur, including cancers, blood clots, and liver problems; it is very important that you have periodic medical examinations throughout therapy.
• You may experience these side effects: Nausea, vomiting, bloating; headache, dizziness, mental depression (use caution driving or performing tasks that require alertness); sensitivity to sunlight (use a sunscreen and wear protective clothing); rash, loss of scalp hair, darkening of the skin on the face; changes in menstrual patterns.
• Report pain in the groin or calves of the legs, chest pain or sudden shortness of breath, abnormal vaginal bleeding, lumps in the breast, sudden severe headache, dizziness or fainting, changes in vision or speech, weakness or numbness in the arm or leg, severe abdominal pain, yellowing of the skin or eyes, severe mental depression.

▽ eszopiclone

(ess zop' ah klone)

Lunesta ⓒ

PREGNANCY CATEGORY C

CONTROLLED SUBSTANCE
SCHEDULE IV

Drug classes
Nonbenzodiazepine hypnotic
Sedative-hypnotic

Therapeutic actions
Exact mechanism of action is not known. It is thought to interact with GABA receptors at binding domains near benzodiazepine receptor sites, leading to sedation.

Indications
• Treatment of insomnia

Contraindications and cautions
• No known contraindications.
• Use cautiously with geriatric or debilitated patients, diseases or conditions that could affect metabolism or hemodynamics, signs or symptoms of depression, pregnancy, or lactation; history of substance abuse (may be habit-forming).

Available forms
Tablets ⓒ—1, 2, 3 mg

Dosage
Adult
Initial dose—2 mg PO taken immediately before bedtime. Dosage may be increased to 3 mg PO immediately before bedtime if clinically needed. The tablet should be swallowed whole, not cut or crushed. Avoid taking with meals.
Pediatric patients
Safety and efficacy not established.
Geriatric patients
Initial dose—1 mg PO taken immediately before bedtime if the primary complaint is falling asleep. If the primary complaint is difficulty staying asleep, 2 mg PO immediately before bedtime may be used.
Patients with severe hepatic impairment
1 mg PO immediately before bedtime. Use caution and monitor the patient closely.
Patients concurrently using CYP3A4 inhibitors
1 mg PO immediately before bedtime. May be increased to 2 mg with caution.

Pharmacokinetics

Route	Onset	Peak
Oral	Rapid	1 hr

Metabolism: Hepatic; $T_{1/2}$: 6 hr
Distribution: May cross placenta; may pass into breast milk
Excretion: Urine

Adverse effects
• **CNS:** *Dizziness, somnolence, nervousness,* anxiety, depression, hallucinations, *headache,* complex sleep disorders, abnormal thinking, suicidal thoughts

---

Adverse effects in *italics* are most common; those in **bold** are life-threatening. ⓒ Do not crush.

- **GI:** Unpleasant taste, dry mouth, dyspepsia, nausea, vomiting
- **GU:** Dysmenorrhea, gynecomastia
- **Respiratory:** Respiratory infection
- **Other:** Viral infection, rash, **anaphylaxis, angioedema**

Interactions

✳ **Drug-drug** • Risk of additional effects on psychomotor performance if combined with ethanol • Increased serum levels and risk of adverse effects if combined with potent CYP3A4 inhibitors (ketoconazole, itraconazole, clarithromycin, nefazodone, ritonavir, nelfinavir) • Risk of decreased serum levels and effectiveness if combined with rifampin

■ Nursing considerations
Assessment

- **History:** Lactation, pregnancy, depression, underlying medical conditions that could affect metabolism or hemodynamics
- **Physical:** Orientation, reflexes, affect; R, adventitious sounds; abdominal examination

Interventions

- Ensure that the patient swallows the tablet whole; do not cut, crush or allow patient to chew tablet.
- Administer drug only if patient is in bed and able to stay in bed for up to 8 hr; changes in cognition and motor function can be a safety issue.
- Monitor patients using drug for suicidal thoughts.
- Do not administer this drug after a fatty or large meal, absorption can be affected.
- Effects of the drug on a fetus are not known. Advise women of childbearing age to use barrier contraceptives while on this drug.
- It is not known if this drug would affect a breast-feeding infant. Advise breast-feeding women to use another method of feeding the infant.

Teaching points

- Take this drug exactly as prescribed. Do not use it longer than advised by your health care provider.
- Swallow the tablet whole, do not break or crush the tablet.
- Do not share this drug with anyone else. Store the drug in its original container and keep it out of the reach of children.

- Do not take this drug unless you are about to get into bed and are able to get 8 or more hours of sleep before you need to be alert again.
- Do not take this drug with or immediately after a high-fat or heavy meal, which could interfere with the absorption and effectiveness of the drug.
- Do not combine this drug with other sleep-inducing drugs, including over-the-counter products.
- It is not known how this drug would affect a pregnancy. If you think you are pregnant or would like to become pregnant, consult your health care provider.
- This drug should not be taken while breast-feeding. If you are breast-feeding, another method of feeding should be used while you are using this drug.
- Do not drink alcohol while you are using this drug.
- You may experience sleeping problems the first night or two after stopping any sleep medicine, including *Lunesta*.
- You may experience these side effects: Changes in thinking, alertness (do not drive a car, operate potentially dangerous equipment, or make important legal decisions the day after you take this drug); complex sleep disorders; allergic reaction; swelling; headache (consult your health care provider for potential pain medications if this occurs); unpleasant taste, nausea (frequent mouth care, frequent small meals may help).
- Report depression, thoughts of suicide or disturbing thoughts, rash, severe headache, changes in behavior.

▽ etanercept
(ee tan er' sept)

Enbrel

PREGNANCY CATEGORY B

Drug classes
Antiarthritic
Disease-modifying antirheumatic drug
Immunomodulator

Therapeutic actions
Genetically engineered tumor necrosis factor receptors from Chinese hamster ovary cells;

keep inflammatory response to autoimmune disease in check by reacting with and deactivating free-floating tumor necrosis factor released by active leukocytes.

Indications

- Reduction of the signs and symptoms, inducing major clinical response, inhibiting the progression of structural damage, and improving physical function in patients with moderately to severely active rheumatoid arthritis; to delay the structural damage associated with rheumatoid arthritis; or may be used in combination with methotrexate when patients do not respond to methotrexate alone
- Reduction of signs and symptoms of moderately to severely active polyarticular juvenile idiopathic arthritis in patients 2 yr and older
- Reduction of signs and symptoms and to improve function in patients with psoriatic arthritis; may be used alone or in combination with methotrexate
- Treatment of ankylosing spondylitis
- Treatment of adult patients with chronic moderate to severe plaque psoriasis who are candidates for systemic therapy or phototherapy
- Unlabeled uses: Heart failure, Crohn disease, graft-versus-host disease, hidradenitis suppurativa, nephrotic syndrome, pyoderma gangrenosum

Contraindications and cautions

- Contraindicated with allergy to etanercept or Chinese hamster ovary products, lactation, pregnancy, cancer, severe infection including sepsis, CNS demyelinating disorders, myelosuppression, sepsis.
- Use cautiously with renal or hepatic disorders, any infection, heart failure, latex allergy.

Available forms

Powder for injection—25 mg; prefilled single-use syringe—25, 50 mg/mL.

Dosages
Adults

- *Plaque psoriasis:* 50 mg/dose subcutaneously twice weekly 3 or 4 days apart for 3 mo; then maintenance dose of 50 mg/wk subcutaneously.

- *Ankylosing spondylitis, rheumatoid arthritis, psoriatic arthritis:* 50 mg/wk subcutaneously.

Pediatric patients 2–17 yr
0.8 mg/kg subcutaneously once weekly. Maximum dose, 50 mg/wk.

Pediatric patients younger than 2 yr
Safety and efficacy not established.

Pharmacokinetics

Route	Onset	Peak
Subcut.	Slow	72 hr

Metabolism: Tissue; $T_{1/2}$: 115 hr
Distribution: Crosses placenta; may enter breast milk
Excretion: Tissues

Adverse effects

- **CNS: CNS demyelinating disorders (MS, myelitis, optic neuritis),** dizziness, headache
- **CV:** Hypotension, DVT, MI, heart failure
- **GI:** Abdominal pain, dyspepsia
- **Hematologic: Pancytopenia**
- **Respiratory:** *URIs,* congestion, rhinitis, cough, pharyngitis
- **Other:** *Irritation at injection site;* **increased risk of serious infections, cancers;** ANA development; autoimmune diseases, rash

Interactions

✱ **Drug-drug** • Increased risk of serious infection with other immunosuppressants; monitor patient closely

■ Nursing considerations
Assessment

- **History:** Allergy to etanercept or Chinese hamster ovary products; pregnancy, lactation; serious infections; cancer; CNS demyelinating disorders, myelosuppression
- **Physical:** Skin lesions, color; R, adventitious sounds; injection site evaluation; range-of-motion to monitor drug effectiveness; CNS—neurologic evaluation, reflexes; CBC

Interventions

⊗ *Warning* Obtain a baseline and periodic CBC; discontinue drug at signs of severe bone marrow suppression.

⊗ *Warning* Obtain baseline values of neurologic function; discontinue drug at any sign of CNS demyelinating disorders.

- Advise patient that this drug does not cure the disease and appropriate therapies for rheumatoid arthritis should be used.
- Reconstitute for injection by slowly injecting 1 mL sterile bacteriostatic water provided with powder into the vial; swirl gently, do not shake; avoid foaming; liquid should be clear and free of particulate matter; use within 6 hr of reconstitution. Do not mix with any other medications.
- Rotate injection sites between abdomen, thigh, and upper arm. Maintain a chart to ensure that sites are rotated regularly.
- Teach patient and a significant other how to reconstitute and administer subcutaneous injections; observe the process periodically.

⊗ **Black box warning** Monitor patient for any sign of infection; discontinue drug if infection occurs; risk of serious infections, including TB, or death exists.

⊗ **Black box warning** There is an increased risk of lymphoma and other cancers in children taking this drug for juvenile rheumatoid arthritis, Crohn disease, or other inflammatory conditions; monitor patient accordingly.

- Evaluate drug effectiveness periodically; 1–2 wk may be required before any change is noted; if no response has occurred within 3 mo, discontinue drug.
- Do not administer drug with any vaccinations; allow at least 2–3 wk between starting this drug and a vaccination.
- Stop drug if patient develops lupus-like symptoms.
- Protect patient from exposure to infections and ensure routine physical examinations and monitoring for potential cancers and autoimmune diseases.

Teaching points

- Take this drug exactly as prescribed. Note that this drug does not cure rheumatoid arthritis and appropriate therapies to deal with the disease should be followed. You and a significant other should learn how to prepare the drug and to administer subcutaneous injections. Prepare a chart of injection sites to ensure that sites are rotated on a regular basis. Consult your health care provider about proper disposal of needles and syringes.

- Arrange for frequent, regular medical follow-up visits, including blood tests to follow the effects of the drug on your body.
- You may experience these side effects: Signs and symptoms of upper respiratory infections, cough, sore throat (consult your health care provider for potential treatment if this becomes severe); headache (analgesics may be available to help); increased susceptibility to infections (avoid crowded areas and people who might have infections; use strict handwashing and good hygiene).
- Report fever, chills, lethargy; rash, difficulty breathing; swelling; worsening of arthritis; severe diarrhea; numbness, tingling; bruising, bleeding.

▷ ethacrynic acid

See Appendix R, *Less commonly used drugs.*

▷ ethambutol hydrochloride

(*e tham' byoo tole*)

Etibi (CAN), Myambutol

PREGNANCY CATEGORY C

Drug class

Antituberculotic (second line)

Therapeutic actions

Inhibits the synthesis of metabolites in growing mycobacterium cells, impairing cell metabolism, arresting cell multiplication, and causing cell death.

Indications

- Treatment of pulmonary TB in conjunction with at least one other antituberculotic

Contraindications and cautions

- Contraindicated with allergy to ethambutol; optic neuritis.
- Use cautiously with impaired renal function, lactation, pregnancy (use other antituberculotics), visual problems (cataracts, diabetic retinopathy).

Available forms

Tablets—100, 400 mg

Dosages

Ethambutol is not administered alone; use in conjunction with other antituberculotics.

Adults

- *Initial treatment:* 15 mg/kg/day PO as a single daily oral dose. Continue therapy until bacteriologic conversion has become permanent and maximal clinical improvement has occurred.
- *Retreatment:* 25 mg/kg/day as a single daily oral dose. After 60 days, reduce dose to 15 mg/kg/day as a single daily dose.

Pediatric patients

Not recommended for patients younger than 13 yr.

Pharmacokinetics

Route	Onset	Peak	Duration
Oral	Rapid	2–4 hr	20–24 hr

Metabolism: Hepatic; T$_{1/2}$: 3.3 hr
Distribution: Crosses placenta; enters breast milk
Excretion: Feces, urine

Adverse effects

- **CNS:** *Optic neuritis* (loss of visual acuity, changes in color perception), *fever, malaise, headache,* dizziness, mental confusion, disorientation, hallucinations, peripheral neuritis
- **GI:** *Anorexia, nausea, vomiting,* GI upset, abdominal pain, transient liver impairment
- **Hypersensitivity:** Allergic reactions—dermatitis, pruritus, anaphylactoid reaction
- **Other: Toxic epidermal necrolysis, thrombocytopenia,** joint pain, acute gout

Interactions

✳ **Drug-drug** • Decreased absorption with aluminum salts

■ Nursing considerations

Assessment

- **History:** Allergy to ethambutol, optic neuritis, impaired renal function, pregnancy, lactation
- **Physical:** Skin color, lesions; T, orientation, reflexes, ophthalmologic examination; liver evaluation, bowel sounds; CBC, LFTs, renal function tests

Interventions

- Administer with food if GI upset occurs.
- Administer in a single daily dose; must be used in combination with other antituberculotics.
- Arrange for follow-up of LFTs, renal function tests, CBC, ophthalmologic examinations.

Teaching points

- Take drug in a single daily dose; it may be taken with meals if GI upset occurs.
- Take this drug regularly; avoid missing doses. Do not discontinue this drug without first consulting your health care provider. This drug must be taken in combination with other drugs used to treat tuberculosis.
- Avoid using aluminum-containing antacids within at least 4 hours of taking drug.
- Arrange to have periodic medical checkups, which will include an eye examination and blood tests.
- You may experience these side effects: Nausea, vomiting, epigastric distress; skin rashes or lesions; visual changes, disorientation, confusion, drowsiness, dizziness (use caution if driving or operating dangerous machinery; use precautions to avoid injury).
- Report changes in vision (blurring, altered color perception), rash.

▷ethionamide

(e thye on am' ide)

Trecator

PREGNANCY CATEGORY C

Drug class

Antituberculotic (third line)

Therapeutic actions

Bacteriostatic against *Mycobacterium tuberculosis;* mechanism of action is not known.

Indications

- TB—any form that is not responsive to first-line antituberculotics—in conjunction with other antituberculotics

Contraindications and cautions

- Contraindicated with allergy to ethionamide, pregnancy.

• Use cautiously with hepatic impairment, diabetes mellitus, lactation.

Available forms
Tablets—250 mg

Dosages
Adults
Always use with at least one other antituberculotic. 15–20 mg/kg/day PO up to a maximum 1 g/day; dosage may be divided if GI upset is intolerable. Concomitant use of pyridoxine is recommended to prevent or minimize the symptoms of peripheral neuritis. Alternative dosing: 250 mg/day PO; gradually titrate to optimal dose.
Pediatric patients
10–20 mg/kg/day PO in two or three divided doses after meals (not to exceed 1 g/day) or 15 mg/kg/24 hr as a single daily dose.

Pharmacokinetics

Route	Peak	Duration
Oral	3 hr	9 hr

Metabolism: Hepatic; $T_{1/2}$: 2 hr
Distribution: Crosses placenta; may enter breast milk
Excretion: Urine

Adverse effects
• **CNS:** *Depression, drowsiness, asthenia,* seizures, peripheral neuritis, neuropathy, olfactory disturbances, blurred vision, diplopia, optic neuritis, dizziness, headache, restlessness, tremors, psychosis
• **CV:** Orthostatic hypotension
• **Dermatologic:** Rash, acne, alopecia, thrombocytopenia, pellagra-like syndrome
• **GI:** *Anorexia, nausea, vomiting, diarrhea, metallic taste,* stomatitis, hepatitis
• **Other:** Gynecomastia, impotence, menorrhagia, difficulty managing diabetes mellitus

■ Nursing considerations
Assessment
• **History:** Allergy to ethionamide; hepatic impairment, diabetes mellitus; pregnancy, lactation
• **Physical:** Skin color, lesions; orientation, reflexes, ophthalmologic examination, affect; BP, orthostatic BP; liver evaluation; LFTs, blood and urine glucose

Interventions
• Arrange for culture and sensitivity tests before use.
• Give only with other antituberculotics.
⊗ **Warning** Arrange for follow-up of LFTs before and every 2–4 wk during therapy.
• Monitor diabetic patients carefully.
• Caution patient to avoid pregnancy.

Teaching points
• Take drug once a day; take with food if GI upset occurs. Dose may be divided if GI upset is severe.
• Take this drug regularly; avoid missing doses. Do not discontinue this drug without first consulting your health care provider. This drug must be taken in combination with other drugs used to treat tuberculosis.
• Do not use this drug during pregnancy; serious fetal abnormalities have been reported. Use of barrier contraceptives is advised.
• Arrange to have regular, periodic medical checkups, including blood tests.
• You may experience these side effects: Loss of appetite, nausea, vomiting, metallic taste in mouth, increased salivation (take the drug with food, frequent mouth care, frequent small meals may help), diarrhea; drowsiness, depression, dizziness, blurred vision (use caution operating a car or dangerous machinery; change position slowly; avoid injury); impotence, menstrual difficulties.
• Report unusual bleeding or bruising, severe GI upset, severe changes in vision.

▽ ethosuximide
*(eth oh **sux**' i mide)*

Zarontin

PREGNANCY CATEGORY C

Drug classes
Antiepileptic
Succinimide

Therapeutic actions
Suppresses the EEG pattern associated with lapses of consciousness in absence (petit mal) seizures; reduces frequency of attacks; mechanism of action not understood, but may act in inhibitory neuronal systems.

E

Indications

- Control of absence (petit mal) seizures; may be given in combination with other antiepileptics especially when other forms of epilepsy coexist with absence seizures

Contraindications and cautions

- Contraindicated with hypersensitivity to succinimides, lactation.
- Use cautiously with hepatic, renal abnormalities; pregnancy, blood dyscrasias, intermittent porphyria.

Available forms

Capsules—250 mg; syrup—250 mg/5 mL

Dosages

Adults and pediatric patients 6 yr and older

Initial dose is 500 mg/day PO. Increase by small increments to maintenance level. One method is to increase the daily dose by 250 mg every 4–7 days until control is achieved with minimal side effects. Give dosage of more than 1.5 g/day in divided doses only under strict supervision (compatible with other antiepileptics when other forms of epilepsy coexist with absence seizures).

Pediatric patients 3–6 yr

Initial dose is 250 mg/day PO. Increase as described for adults above. The optimal dose for most children is 20 mg/kg/day in one dose or two divided doses.

Pharmacokinetics

Route	Peak
Oral	3–7 hr

Metabolism: Hepatic; $T_{1/2}$: 30 hr in children, 60 hr in adults
Distribution: Crosses placenta; enters breast milk
Excretion: Bile, urine

Adverse effects

- **CNS:** *Drowsiness, ataxia, dizziness, irritability, nervousness, headache, blurred vision,* myopia, photophobia, hiccups, euphoria, dreamlike state, lethargy, hyperactivity, fatigue, insomnia, increased frequency of **grand mal seizures** may occur when used alone in some patients with mixed types of epilepsy, confusion, instability, mental slowness, depression,

hypochondriacal behavior, sleep disturbances, night terrors, aggressiveness, inability to concentrate
- **Dermatologic: Stevens-Johnson syndrome,** *pruritus, urticaria,* pruritic erythematous rashes, skin eruptions, erythema multiforme, systemic lupus erythematosus, alopecia, hirsutism
- **GI:** *Nausea, vomiting, vague gastric upset, epigastric and abdominal pain, cramps, anorexia, diarrhea, constipation, weight loss,* swelling of tongue, gum hypertrophy
- **Hematologic: Eosinophilia, granulocytopenia, leukopenia, agranulocytosis, aplastic anemia, monocytosis, pancytopenia**
- **Other:** Vaginal bleeding, periorbital edema, hyperemia, muscle weakness, abnormal LFTs, renal function tests

Interactions

✳ **Drug-drug** • Decreased serum levels of primidone • Risk of increased effects if combined with other CNS depressants including alcohol

■ Nursing considerations

Assessment

- **History:** Hypersensitivity to succinimides; hepatic, renal abnormalities; lactation, pregnancy
- **Physical:** Skin color, lesions; orientation, affect, reflexes, bilateral grip strength, vision examination; bowel sounds, normal output, liver evaluation; LFTs, renal function tests, urinalysis, CBC with differential, EEG

Interventions

⊗ *Warning* Reduce dosage, discontinue, or substitute other antiepileptic gradually; abrupt discontinuation may precipitate absence (petit mal) status.
- Monitor CBC and differential before and frequently during therapy.
⊗ *Warning* Discontinue drug if rash, depression of blood count, or unusual depression, aggressiveness, or behavioral alterations occur.
- Arrange counseling for women of childbearing age who need long-term maintenance therapy with antiepileptics and who wish to become pregnant.
⊗ *Warning* Evaluate for therapeutic serum levels (40–100 mcg/mL).

Adverse effects in *italics* are most common; those in **bold** are life-threatening. ⏸ Do not crush.

Teaching points

- Take this drug exactly as prescribed. Do not discontinue this drug abruptly or change dosage.
- Avoid alcohol, sleep-inducing, or over-the-counter drugs while you are using this drug.
- Arrange for frequent checkups to monitor this drug; keep all appointments for checkups.
- Wear a medical ID at all times so that any emergency medical personnel will know that you have epilepsy and are taking antiepileptic medication.
- You may experience these side effects: Drowsiness, dizziness, confusion, blurred vision (avoid driving or performing tasks requiring alertness or visual acuity); GI upset (take the drug with food or milk and eat frequent small meals).
- Report rash, joint pain, unexplained fever, sore throat, unusual bleeding or bruising, drowsiness, dizziness, blurred vision, pregnancy.

▽**ethotoin**
(*eth' i toe in*)

Peganone

PREGNANCY CATEGORY D

Drug classes

Antiepileptic
Hydantoin

Therapeutic actions

Has antiepileptic activity without causing general CNS depression; stabilizes neuronal membranes and prevents hyperexcitability caused by excessive stimulation; limits the spread of seizure activity from an active focus.

Indications

- Control of tonic-clonic and complex partial (psychomotor) seizures; may be combined with other antiepileptics

Contraindications and cautions

- Contraindicated with hypersensitivity to hydantoins, pregnancy, lactation, hepatic abnormalities, hematologic disorders.
- Use cautiously with acute intermittent porphyria; hypotension, severe myocardial insufficiency; diabetes mellitus, hyperglycemia.

Available forms

Tablets—250 mg

Dosages

Administer in four to six divided doses daily. Take after eating; space as evenly as possible.
Adults
Initial dose should be 1 g/day PO in four to six divided doses. Increase gradually over several days; usual maintenance dose is 2–3 g/day PO in four to six divided doses; less than 2 g/day is ineffective in most adults. If replacing another drug, reduce the dose of the other drug gradually as ethotoin dose is increased.
Pediatric patients 1 yr and older
Initial dose should not exceed 750 mg/day PO in four to six divided doses; maintenance doses range from 500 mg/day to 1 g/day PO in four to six divided doses.

Pharmacokinetics

Route	Onset	Peak
Oral	Rapid	1–3 hr

Metabolism: Hepatic; $T_{1/2}$: 3–9 hr
Distribution: Crosses placenta; enters breast milk
Excretion: Urine

Adverse effects

- **CNS:** *Nystagmus, ataxia, dysarthria, slurred speech, mental confusion, dizziness, drowsiness, insomnia, transient nervousness, motor twitchings, fatigue, irritability, depression, numbness, tremor, headache,* photophobia, diplopia, conjunctivitis
- **Dermatologic:** Scarlatiniform, morbilliform, maculopapular, urticarial and nonspecific rashes; also serious and sometimes fatal dermatologic reactions: Bullous, exfoliative, or purpuric dermatitis, lupus erythematosus, and **Stevens-Johnson syndrome; toxic epidermal necrolysis,** hirsutism, alopecia, coarsening of the facial features, enlargement of the lips, Peyronie disease
- **GI:** *Nausea,* vomiting, diarrhea, constipation, *gingival hyperplasia,* toxic hepatitis, **liver damage,** hypersensitivity reactions with hepatic involvement, including hepatocellular degeneration and **hepatocellular necrosis**

- **GU:** Nephrosis
- **Hematologic: Thrombocytopenia, leukopenia, granulocytopenia, agranulocytosis, pancytopenia; macrocytosis and megaloblastic anemia that usually respond to folic acid therapy;** eosinophilia, monocytosis, leukocytosis, simple anemia, hemolytic anemia, aplastic anemia, hyperglycemia
- **Respiratory: Pulmonary fibrosis,** acute pneumonitis
- **Other:** Lymph node hyperplasia, sometimes progressing to **frank malignant lymphoma,** monoclonal gammopathy and **multiple myeloma** (prolonged therapy), polyarthropathy, osteomalacia, weight gain, chest pain, periarteritis nodosa

Interactions

✳ Drug-drug • Increased pharmacologic effects with chloramphenicol, cimetidine, disulfiram, isoniazid, phenacemide, phenylbutazone, sulfonamides, trimethoprim **•** Complex interactions and effects when hydantoins and valproic acid are given together: Toxicity with apparently normal serum ethotoin levels; decreased plasma levels of valproic acid given with hydantoins; breakthrough seizures when the two drugs are given together **•** Decreased pharmacologic effects with antineoplastics, diazoxide, folic acid, rifampin, theophyllines **•** Increased pharmacologic effects and toxicity with primidone, fluconazole, amiodarone **•** Increased hepatotoxicity with acetaminophen **•** Decreased pharmacologic effects of these drugs: Corticosteroids, cyclosporine, disopyramide, doxycycline, estrogens, levodopa, methadone, metyrapone, mexiletine, hormonal contraceptives, carbamazepine
✳ Drug-lab test • Interference with the metyrapone and the 1-mg dexamethasone tests; avoid the use of hydantoins for at least 7 days prior to metyrapone testing

■ Nursing considerations

Assessment

- **History:** Hypersensitivity to hydantoins; hepatic abnormalities; hematologic disorders; acute intermittent porphyria; hypotension, severe myocardial insufficiency; diabetes mellitus, hyperglycemia; pregnancy; lactation
- **Physical:** T; skin color, lesions; lymph node palpation; orientation, affect, reflexes, vision examination; P, BP; R, adventitious sounds; bowel sounds, normal output, liver evaluation; periodontal examination;

LFTs, urinalysis, CBC and differential, blood proteins, blood and urine glucose, EEG, ECG

Interventions

- Give after food to enhance absorption and reduce GI upset; give in four to six divided doses as evenly spaced as possible.
- Administer with other antiepileptics to regulate seizures as needed.
- ⊗ **Warning** Reduce dosage, discontinue, or substitute other antiepileptic gradually; abrupt discontinuation may precipitate status epilepticus.
- ⊗ **Warning** Discontinue drug if rash, depression of blood count, enlarged lymph nodes, hypersensitivity reaction, signs of liver damage, or Peyronie disease (induration of the corpora cavernosa of the penis) occurs. Institute another antiepileptic promptly.
- Monitor hepatic function periodically during long-term therapy; monitor blood counts, urinalysis monthly.
- Monitor urine sugar of patients with diabetes mellitus regularly. Adjustment of dosage of hypoglycemic drug may be needed because antiepileptic may inhibit insulin release and induce hyperglycemia.
- ⊗ **Warning** Arrange to have lymph node enlargement occurring during therapy evaluated carefully. Lymphadenopathy, which simulates Hodgkin disease, has occurred. Lymph node hyperplasia may progress to lymphoma.
- Monitor blood proteins to detect early malfunction of the immune system (multiple myeloma).
- Arrange dental consultation for patients on long-term therapy; proper oral hygiene can prevent development of gum hyperplasia.
- Arrange counseling for women of childbearing age who need long-term maintenance therapy with antiepileptics and who wish to become pregnant.
- ⊗ **Warning** Evaluate for therapeutic serum levels (15–50 mcg/mL).

Teaching points

- Take this drug exactly as prescribed, after food to enhance absorption and reduce GI upset. Space doses as evenly apart as possible throughout the day.
- Do not discontinue this drug abruptly or change dosage.
- Maintain good oral hygiene—regular brushing and flossing—to prevent gum disease while you are taking this drug.

Adverse effects in *italics* are most common; those in **bold** are life-threatening. ⬛ Do not crush.

- Arrange frequent dental checkups to prevent serious gum disease.
- Arrange for frequent checkups to monitor your response to this drug; keep all appointments for checkups.

⊗ **Warning** Monitor your blood sugar regularly, and report any abnormality if you are a diabetic.

⊗ **Warning** Use some form of contraception, other than birth control pills, while you are on this drug. This drug is not recommended for use during pregnancy. If you wish to become pregnant, discuss with your health care provider.

- Wear or carry a medical alert tag at all times so that any emergency medical personnel will know that you have epilepsy and are taking antiepileptic medication.
- You may experience these side effects: Drowsiness, dizziness, confusion, blurred vision (avoid driving or performing tasks requiring alertness or visual acuity); GI upset (take the drug with food and eat frequent small meals).
- Report rash, severe nausea or vomiting, drowsiness, slurred speech, impaired coordination, swollen glands, bleeding, swollen or tender gums, yellowish discoloration of the skin or eyes, joint pain, unexplained fever, sore throat, unusual bleeding or bruising, persistent headache, malaise, any indication of an infection or bleeding tendency, abnormal erection, pregnancy.

▽ **etidronate disodium**
(e tid′ ro nate)

CO Etidronate (CAN), Didronel, Gen-Etidronate (CAN)

PREGNANCY CATEGORY C

Drug classes
Bisphosphonate
Calcium regulator

Therapeutic actions
Slows normal and abnormal bone resorption; reduces bone formation and bone turnover.

Indications
- Treatment of Paget disease of bone
- Treatment of heterotopic ossification

- Unlabeled uses: Prevention and treatment of corticosteroid-induced osteoporosis, prevention of osteoporosis with spinal cord injury

Contraindications and cautions
- Contraindicated with allergy to bisphosphonates, hypocalcemia, pregnancy, lactation, severe renal impairment, clinically overt osteomalacia.
- Use cautiously with renal impairment, upper GI disease, enterocolitis.

Available forms
Tablets—200, 400 mg

Dosages
Adults
- *Paget disease:* 5–10 mg/kg/day PO for up to 6 mo; or 11–20 mg/kg/day PO for up to 3 mo. Doses above 10 mg/kg/day should be reserved for when lower doses are ineffective or when there is an urgent need to suppress rapid bone turnover or reduce elevated cardiac output. If retreatment is needed, wait at least 90 days between treatment regimens.
- *Heterotopic ossification:* 20 mg/kg/day PO for 2 wk followed by 10 mg/kg/day PO for 10 wk (following spinal cord injury); 20 mg/kg/day PO for 1 mo preoperatively if due to total hip replacement, then 20 mg/kg/day PO for 3 mo postoperatively.

Pediatric patients
Safety and efficacy not established.

Patients with renal impairment
Use caution and monitor patient frequently.

Pharmacokinetics

Route	Onset	Duration
Oral	Slow	90 days

Metabolism: Not metabolized; $T_{1/2}$: 1–6 hr
Distribution: Crosses placenta; may enter breast milk
Excretion: Urine

Adverse effects
- **CNS:** *Headache*
- **GI:** *Nausea, diarrhea,* altered taste, metallic taste
- **Hematologic:** Elevated BUN, serum creatinine
- **Skeletal:** *Increased or recurrent bone pain,* focal osteomalacia

Interactions

✳ **Drug-drug** • Increased risk of GI distress with aspirin • Decreased absorption with antacids, calcium, iron, multivalent cations; separate dosing by at least 2 hr

✳ **Drug-food** • Significantly decreased absorption and serum levels if taken with any food; administer on an empty stomach 2 hr before meals

■ Nursing considerations

Assessment

- **History:** Allergy to bisphosphonates, renal failure, upper GI disease, lactation, pregnancy
- **Physical:** Muscle tone, bone pain; bowel sounds; urinalysis, serum calcium, serum alkaline phosphatase, serum phosphate, renal function tests

Interventions

- Administer with a full glass of water, 2 hr before meals.
- Monitor serum calcium levels before, during, and after therapy.
- ⊗ **Warning** Ensure 3-mo rest period after treatment for Paget disease if retreatment is required, 7 days between treatments for hypercalcemia of malignancy.
- Ensure adequate vitamin and calcium intake.
- Provide comfort measures if bone pain returns.

Teaching points

- Take this drug with a full glass of water 2 hours before meals. Avoid eating food before and 2 hours after taking this drug.
- Periodic blood tests may be required to monitor your calcium levels.
- You may experience these side effects: Nausea, diarrhea, bone pain, headache (analgesics may be available to help).
- Report twitching, muscle spasms, dark-colored urine, severe diarrhea.

▽ **etodolac**
(ee toe doe' lak)

PREGNANCY CATEGORY C

Drug classes

Analgesic (nonopioid)
NSAID

Therapeutic actions

Inhibits prostaglandin synthesis by inhibiting the enzyme, cyclo-oxygenase.

Indications

- Acute or long-term use in the management of signs and symptoms of osteoarthritis, rheumatoid arthritis, and juvenile rheumatoid arthritis
- Management of pain

Contraindications and cautions

- Contraindicated with significant renal impairment, pregnancy, lactation, hypersensitivity to aspirin, etodolac, or other NSAIDs.
- Use cautiously with impaired hearing; allergies; hepatic, hypertension, and GI conditions.

Available forms

Capsules—200, 300 mg; tablets—400, 500 mg; ER tablets—400, 500, 600 mg

Dosages

Adults

- *Osteoarthritis, rheumatoid arthritis:* Initially, 600–1,000 mg/day PO in divided doses; maintenance ranges, 600–1,200 mg/day in divided doses. Do not exceed 1,200 mg/day. Patients less than 60 kg: Do not exceed 20 mg/kg. ER: 400–1,000 mg/day PO; adjust based on patient response. Do not exceed 1,200 mg/day.
- *Analgesia, acute pain:* 200–400 mg every 6–8 hr PO. Do not exceed 1,200 mg/day.

Patients 6–16 yr

- *Juvenile rheumatoid arthritis:* The daily dose (given as single dose, extended-release tablets) should be based upon body weight as follows:
  20–30 kg: 400 mg/day PO.
  31–45 kg: 600 mg/day PO.
  46–60 kg: 800 mg/day PO given as 400 mg PO bid.
  More than 60 kg: 1,000 mg/day PO given as 500 mg PO bid.

Pharmacokinetics

Route	Onset	Peak
Oral	Varies	1–2 hr
Oral (ER)	Slow	6–7 hr

Metabolism: Hepatic; $T_{1/2}$: 7.3 hr, 8.3 hr (ER)
Distribution: Crosses placenta; enters breast milk
Excretion: Feces, urine

Adverse effects in *italics* are most common; those in **bold** are life-threatening. ⊞ Do not crush.

Adverse effects

- **CNS:** *Dizziness,* somnolence, insomnia, fatigue, tiredness, tinnitus, blurred vision
- **Dermatologic:** Rash, pruritus, sweating, dry mucous membranes, stomatitis
- **GI:** *Nausea, dyspepsia, GI pain, diarrhea,* vomiting, *constipation,* flatulence, **bleeding ulcers,** elevated liver enzymes, **hepatic failure**
- **GU:** Dysuria, **renal impairment or insufficiency**
- **Hematologic:** Bleeding, platelet inhibition with higher doses
- **Other:** Peripheral edema, **anaphylactoid reactions** to fatal anaphylactic shock

Interactions

✳ Drug-drug ● Increased risk of bleeding if combined with anticoagulants, antiplatelet drugs ● Possible decreased effectiveness of antihypertensives if taken with etodolac

■ Nursing considerations
Assessment

- **History:** Renal impairment, impaired hearing, allergy to aspirin or NSAIDs, hepatic, CV, and GI conditions, lactation, pregnancy
- **Physical:** Skin color and lesions; orientation, reflexes, ophthalmologic and audiometric evaluations, peripheral sensation; P, edema; R, adventitious sounds; liver evaluation; CBC, clotting times, LFTs, renal function tests; serum electrolytes, stool guaiac

Interventions

⊗ **Black box warning** Be aware that patient may be at increased risk for CV events and GI bleeding; monitor accordingly.
- Give with food or after meals if GI upset occurs.
- Arrange for periodic ophthalmologic examination during long-term therapy.

⊗ *Warning* Institute emergency procedures if overdose occurs (gastric lavage, induction of emesis, supportive therapy).

Teaching points

- Take with food or meals if GI upset occurs.
- Take only the prescribed dosage.
- You may experience dizziness or drowsiness (avoid driving or the use of dangerous machinery while on this drug).

- Report sore throat, fever, rash, itching, weight gain, swelling in ankles or fingers; changes in vision; black, tarry stools; bleeding.

DANGEROUS DRUG

▽etoposide (VP-16)
*(e toe **poe**' side)*

Etopophos, Toposar

PREGNANCY CATEGORY D

Drug classes
Antineoplastic
Mitotic inhibitor

Therapeutic actions
G2-specific cell toxic: Lyses cells entering mitosis; inhibits cells from entering prophase; inhibits DNA synthesis, leading to cell death.

Indications
- Refractory testicular tumors as part of combination therapy (IV)
- First-line treatment of small-cell lung carcinoma as part of combination therapy (oral, IV)
- Unlabeled uses: Bladder cancer, lymphomas, leukemias, Ewing sarcoma, Kaposi sarcoma, brain tumors, gestational trophoblastic tumors, ovarian germ-cell tumors, rhabdomyosarcomas, Wilms tumors, bone marrow transplants

Contraindications and cautions
- Contraindicated with allergy to etoposide, teniposide, *Cremophor EL;* pregnancy, lactation.
- Use cautiously with bone marrow suppression.

Available forms
Capsules—50 mg; injection—20 mg/mL; powder for injection—100 mg

Dosages
Modify dosage based on myelosuppression.
Adults
Parenteral
- *Testicular cancer:* 50–100 mg/m^2 per day IV on days 1 to 5 or 100 mg/ m^2 per day IV on days 1, 3, and 5, every 3–4 wk in combination with other chemotherapeutics.

- *Small-cell lung cancer:* 35 mg/m^2 per day IV for 4 days to 50 mg/ m^2 per day for 5 days; repeat every 3–4 wk after recovery from toxicity.

Oral
Small-cell lung cancer: Two times the IV dose rounded to the nearest 50 mg.

Pediatric patients
Safety and efficacy not established.

Patients with renal impairment
For creatinine clearance of 15–50 mL/min, give 75% of dose. For creatinine clearance of less than 15 mL/min, consider further dosage reduction.

Pharmacokinetics

Route	Onset	Peak	Duration
Oral	30–60 min	60–90 min	20–30 hr
IV	30 min	60 min	20–30 hr

Metabolism: Hepatic; T$_{1/2}$: 4–11 hr
Distribution: Crosses placenta; enters breast milk
Excretion: Bile, urine

▼ IV FACTS
Preparation: Dilute with 5% dextrose injection or 0.9% sodium chloride injection to give a concentration of 0.2 or 0.4 mg/mL. Unopened vials are stable at room temperature for 2 yr; diluted solutions are stable at room temperature for 2 (0.4 mg/mL) or 4 (0.2 mg/mL) days.
Infusion: Administer slowly over 30–60 min. Etoposide phosphate solutions may be administered over 5–20 min. Do not give by rapid IV push.

Adverse effects
- **CNS:** *Somnolence, fatigue,* peripheral neuropathy
- **CV:** Hypotension (after rapid IV administration)
- **Dermatologic:** *Alopecia*
- **GI:** *Nausea, vomiting, anorexia, diarrhea,* stomatitis, aftertaste, liver toxicity
- **Hematologic:** *Myelotoxicity*
- **Hypersensitivity:** Chills, fever, tachycardia, **anaphylactic-like reaction, bronchospasm,** dyspnea
- **Other:** Carcinogenesis

■ Nursing considerations
Assessment
- **History:** Allergy to etoposide, teniposide, *Cremophor EL;* bone marrow suppression; pregnancy; lactation
- **Physical:** T; weight; hair; orientation, reflexes; BP, P; mucous membranes, abdominal examination; CBC

Interventions
- Do not administer IM or subcutaneously; severe local reaction and tissue necrosis occur.
- ⊗ *Warning* Avoid skin contact with this drug; use rubber gloves; if contact occurs, immediately wash with soap and water.
- Monitor BP during administration; if hypotension occurs, discontinue dose and consult with physician. Fluids and other supportive therapy may be needed.
- ⊗ **Black box warning** Obtain platelet count, Hgb, Hct, WBC count, differential before starting therapy and prior to each dose. If severe response occurs, discontinue therapy and consult with physician; severe myelosuppression is possible.
- ⊗ **Black box warning** Monitor patient for severe hypersensitivity reaction with any dose; arrange supportive care.
- Arrange for an antiemetic for severe nausea and vomiting.
- Arrange for wig or other suitable head covering before alopecia occurs. Teach patient the importance of covering the head at extremes of temperature.

Teaching points
- Keep a calendar for specific treatment days and additional courses of therapy.
- Avoid pregnancy while using this drug; you should use barrier contraceptives.
- Have regular blood tests to monitor the drug's effects.
- Avoid exposures to other people with infections, especially during periods of low blood counts.
- You may experience these side effects: Loss of appetite, nausea, vomiting, mouth sores (frequent mouth care, frequent small meals may help; try to maintain good nutrition; a dietitian may be able to help, and an antiemetic may be ordered); loss of hair (arrange for a wig or other suitable head covering before

the hair loss occurs; it is important to keep the head covered at extremes of temperature).
- Report severe GI upset, diarrhea, vomiting, unusual bleeding or bruising, fever, chills, sore throat, difficulty breathing.

▽etravirine
(eh tra vye' rin)

Intelence ⬤

PREGNANCY CATEGORY B

Drug classes
Antiviral
Non-nucleoside reverse transcriptase inhibitor

Therapeutic actions
Binds directly to reverse transcriptase and blocks both RNA and DNA dependent polymerase activity leading to inability for viral replication, a decrease in viral load and subsequent increase, increases number of healthy $CD4^+$ cells; does not inhibit human DNA polymerase.

Indications
- In combination with other antiretroviral drugs, for treatment of HIV-1 infection in treatment-experienced patients 6 yr and older who have evidence of viral replication and HIV-1 strains resistant to nonnucleotide reverse transcriptase inhibitors and other antiretroviral drugs

Contraindications and cautions
- No known contraindications.
- Women are advised not to nurse a baby while taking drug. Use cautiously with pregnancy.

Available forms
Tablets ⬤ —25, 100, 200 mg

Dosages
Adults
200 mg PO bid following a meal.
Pediatric patients 6 to younger than 18 yr
- 16 to less than 20 kg: 100 mg PO bid.
- 20 to less than 25 kg: 125 mg PO bid.
- 25 to less than 30 kg: 150 mg PO bid.
- 30 kg or more: 200 mg PO bid.

Pharmacokinetics

Route	Onset	Peak
Oral	Slow	2.5–4 hr

Metabolism: Hepatic; $T_{1/2}$: 21–61 hr
Distribution: May cross placenta, may enter breast milk
Excretion: Feces and urine

Adverse effects
- **CNS:** Headache, peripheral neuropathy, vertigo, blurred vision, insomnia, anxiety, paresthesias
- **CV:** Hypertension
- **Dermatologic: Stevens-Johnson syndrome, epidermal necrolysis,** *rash*
- **GI:** *Diarrhea,* nausea, abdominal pain, vomiting, dry mouth, flatulence
- **Other:** Fatigue; altered fat distribution, immune reconstitution syndrome; **severe hypersensitivity reactions**

Interactions
✻ **Drug-drug** ● Risk of decreased serum levels and loss of effectiveness if used with efavirenz, nevirapine rifampin, rifapentine, rifabutin; avoid these combinations ● Risk of increased serum levels and risk of toxic effects if used with delavirdine; avoid this combination ● Risk of significant alteration in serum level of protease inhibitors (atazanavir, fosamprenavir, nelfinavir, indinavir) if combined; also use low dose ritonavir if this combination is used ● Possible loss of therapeutic effect if combined with 600 mg bid ritonavir; avoid this combination ● Risk of decreased effectiveness of maraviroc; increase maraviroc dosage to 600 mg bid if this combination is used ● Risk of significant changes in therapeutic effect if combined with tipranavir and ritonavir; fosamprenavir and ritonavir; atazanavir and ritonavir; avoid these combinations ● Risk of decreased effectiveness of antiarrhythmics; monitor patient closely if this combination is needed ● Risk of increased bleeding tendencies with warfarin: if this combination is used; monitor patient closely and adjust dosage of warfarin as needed ● Risk of decreased effectiveness of clopidogrel; suggest use of a different drug of etravirine is needed ● Risk of significant decrease in effectiveness if combined with carbamazepine, phenobarbital, phenytoin; avoid these combinations ● Risk of serum level concentration of azole antifungals if combined; monitor

patient carefully and adjust antifungal dosage as appropriate • Risk of decreased effectiveness of clarithromycin if combined; suggest use of an alternate antibiotic

✴ **Drug-alternative therapy** • Risk of decreased serum levels and loss of effectiveness if combined with St. John's Wort; avoid this combination

■ Nursing considerations
Assessment
- **History:** Hypersensitivity to any component of the drug, pregnancy, lactation, previous or current anti-HIV regimen
- **Physical:** T; skin color, lesions; orientation, affect; BP; abdominal examination

Interventions
- Give this drug with other antiretrovirals.
⊗ *Warning* Discontinue drug at first sign of severe skin or hypersensitivity reaction; fatalities have been reported.
- Review antiviral therapy and adjust dosage as needed to take into account effects on liver enzymes and numerous drug-drug interactions.
- Have patient swallow tablets whole with liquid, following a meal. Do not administer on an empty stomach. If patient is unable to swallow tablets, put them in a glass of water and stir; when water appears milky have the patient drink the whole glass and rinse several times and drink the rinse each time to get the full dose.
- Encourage breast-feeding mothers to find a different method of feeding the infant while on this drug.

Teaching points
- Take this drug twice a day following a meal; never take on an empty stomach. Swallow the tablets whole; do not cut, crush, or chew the tablets.
- If you or your child cannot swallow the tablets, you can place them in a glass of water, stir well, and when the water looks milky, drink immediately. Fill the glass with water several times and completely swallow each time to get any residue to make sure that you receive the entire dose.
- Always take this drug with other anti-HIV drugs that have been prescribed for you.
- Do not use St. John's Wort while taking this drug; antiviral activity could be lost.

- If you miss a dose within 6 hours of the time you usually take it, take the dose following a meal, as soon as possible. Then take your next dose at the regular time. If you miss a dose by more than 6 hours, wait and take the next regularly scheduled dose. Do not double up doses and do not take more than the prescribed amount each day.
- Do not stop taking this drug; if you are running low, talk to your health care provider about a refill; the drug could stop working if stopped for even a short period.
- This drug does not cure HIV or AIDS; opportunistic infections may occur and regular medical care should be sought to deal with the disease.
- This drug does not reduce the risk of transmission of HIV to others by sexual contact or blood contamination; use appropriate precautions.
- It is not known if this drug could affect a fetus. If you wish to become pregnant, discuss this with your health care provider. If you become pregnant while taking this drug, consult your health care provider about enrolling in the *Antiretroviral Pregnancy Registry*.
- It is not known how this drug could affect a breast-feeding infant. Because of the potential for passing the virus on to an infant, women with HIV infection are advised not to breast-feed; another method of feeding should be used while you are taking this drug.
- Your health care provider will monitor $CD4^+$ levels regularly while you are taking this drug.
- You may experience these side effects: Headache, fever, rash (medication may be available to relieve these symptoms); dizziness (do not drive a car or operate dangerous machinery until you know how this drug will affect you); changes in fat distribution (decreased fat in the face, legs and arms; increased fat on the back, neck, chest).
- Report rash of any kind, any signs of infection (fever, swelling, redness), inability to eat, any changes in your prescribed medications, severe diarrhea.

▽ everolimus
See Appendix R, *Less commonly used drugs*.

▷ exemestane

See Appendix R, *Less commonly used drugs*.

▷ exenatide
(ex enn' ah tyde)

Bydureon, Byetta

PREGNANCY CATEGORY C

Drug classes
Antidiabetic
Incretin mimetic drug

Therapeutic actions
An incretin that mimics the enhancement of glucose-dependent insulin secretion by pancreatic beta cells, depresses inappropriately elevated glucagon secretion, and slows gastric emptying, leading to lower blood glucose levels. Also associated with appetite suppression and weight loss.

Indications
- Adjunct to diet and exercise, to improve glycemic control in adults with type 2 diabetes
- ▪ NEW INDICATION: Add-on therapy with insulin glargine, with or without metformin, with diet and exercise to help improve glycemic control in adults with type 2 diabetes

Contraindications and cautions
- Contraindicated with hypersensitivity to exenatide or any of its components, end stage renal disease, severe GI disease, type 1 diabetes, diabetic ketoacidosis, lactation, history of pancreatitis.
- Use cautiously with pregnancy.

Available forms
Solution for injection, solution in a pre-filled pen—250 mcg/mL as 5 mcg/dose or 10 mcg/dose; extended-release injectable suspension—2 mg

Dosage
Adult
5 mcg by subcutaneous injection bid at any time within 60 min before the morning and evening meals or the two main meals of the day, approximately 6 hr apart. May be increased to 10 mcg bid after 1 month of therapy, if needed. May be given in combina-

tion with oral antidiabetic drugs. ER form: 2 mg by subcutaneous injection once every 7 days.
Patients with renal impairment
For creatinine clearance of 30–50 mL/min, use caution when increasing dosage from 5 to 10 mcg. For creatine clearance of less than 30 mL/min, use not recommended.

Pharmacokinetics

Route	Onset	Peak	Duration
Subcut.	Rapid	2 hr	8–10 hr

Metabolism: $T_{1/2}$: 2.4 hr
Distribution: Crosses placenta; may pass into breast milk
Excretion: Urine, unchanged

Adverse effects
- **CNS:** Headache, feeling jittery, dizziness
- **GI:** *Nausea,* vomiting, dyspepsia, diarrhea, **pancreatitis**
- **Other:** **Hypoglycemia,** injection site reaction, **hemorrhagic** or **necrotizing pancreatitis**

Interactions
✳ **Drug-drug** • Slowed gastric emptying and reduced absorption of some oral drugs; use with caution with oral drugs that require rapid absorption; space oral contraceptives and antibiotics at least 1 hr before administering exenatide
- Risk of increased bleeding and increased INR with warfarin; if this combination is used, monitor INR carefully

■ Nursing considerations
Assessment
- **History:** Hypersensitivity to exenatide or any of its components; end-stage renal disease, severe GI disease; type 1 diabetes, diabetic ketoacidosis; pancreatitis; lactation, pregnancy
- **Physical:** Orientation, reflexes, affect; abdominal examination; injection site; blood glucose levels, serum calcitonin levels

Interventions
⊗ *Black box warning* ER form (*Bydureon*) increases risk of thyroid C-cell tumors, including medullary thyroid carcinoma, in animals. Contraindicated with history or family history of medullary thyroid cancer or multiple endocrine neoplasia syndrome.

- Inject subcutaneously within 60 min before the morning and evening meals or the two main meals of the day. If using ER form, inject once every 7 days without regard to food.
- Maintain other antidiabetic drugs, diet, and exercise regimen for control of diabetes.
- Monitor serum glucose levels and glycosylated Hgb levels to evaluate effectiveness of drug on controlling glucose levels.
- Monitor for pancreatitis. Stop drug and do not restart if signs of pancreatitis develop.
- Monitor serum calcitonin levels if using ER form; changes in calcitonin levels or development of thyroid nodules should lead to a referral to an endocrinologist.
- Arrange for thorough diabetic teaching program to include disease, dietary control, exercise, signs and symptoms of hypoglycemia and hyperglycemia, avoidance of infection, and hygiene.

Teaching points

- If you are using the prefilled pen, review your manual before each use. Be advised that the needles for the pen need to be purchased separately. Dispose of needles appropriately.
- Do not use solution that appears cloudy.
- Inject it into a site on your thigh, abdomen, or upper arm; rotate injection sites periodically.
- Discard the pen after 30 days, even if solution remains in the pen.
- Inject this drug within 1 hour of your morning and evening meals or your two main meals of the day; do not use if you are not going to be eating. If you forget a dose, do not inject after you have eaten.
- If you are using the extended-release form (*Bydureon*), inject it subcutaneously immediately after the powder is suspended in the diluent and transferred to the syringe. Change injection sites each week. Dispose of needles and syringes appropriately. You may take this drug without regard to meals.
- Alcohol consumption can change your blood glucose levels and may alter your response to this drug.
- Do not take the daily drug if you are not able to eat, if you plan to skip a meal, or if your blood sugar is too low.
- Do not change the dosage of this drug without consulting with your health care provider.

- It is not known how this drug would affect a pregnancy. If you think you are pregnant or would like to become pregnant, consult your health care provider.
- It is not known how this drug could affect a breast-feeding infant. If you are breast-feeding, consult your health care provider.
- You will need to regularly monitor your blood glucose levels. Your health care provider may change the dose of exenatide or your other antidiabetic drugs, based on your blood glucose response.
- It is important that you follow the diet and exercise guidelines related to your disease.
- Review the signs and symptoms of hypoglycemia. Be prepared to treat hypoglycemia with fast-acting sugar or glucagon.
- Do not drive a car or operate potentially dangerous machinery until you are aware of how exenatide will affect your blood sugar. Low blood sugar can cause dizziness and changes in thinking.
- Using the ER form may increase the risk of medullary thyroid cancer; blood tests will be done periodically to screen for this.
- You may experience these side effects: Injection site reactions (proper injection and rotation of injection sites should help; if bothersome, consult your health care provider); hypoglycemia (use fast acting sugars or glucagons if this occurs; proper use and eating of meals should prevent this effect); nausea (this usually passes after a few days).
- Report continued nausea; hypoglycemic reactions; redness, pain or swelling at injection sites; stomach pain; vomiting.

▽ ezetimibe
(ee zet' ah mibe)

Zetia

PREGNANCY CATEGORY C

Drug classes
Cholesterol absorption inhibitor
Cholesterol-lowering drug

Therapeutic actions
Localizes in the brush border of the small intestine and inhibits the absorption of cholesterol from the small intestine; this leads to a

decrease delivery of dietary cholesterol to the liver, which will then increase the clearance of cholesterol from the blood and lead to a decrease in serum cholesterol.

Indications

- As an adjunct to diet and exercise to lower the cholesterol, LDL, and Apo-B levels in patients with primary hypercholesterolemia as monotherapy or in combination with HMG-CoA reductase inhibitors (statins)
- In combination with fenofibrate as adjunct to diet to reduce elevated total cholesterol, LDL cholesterol, apolipoprotein B, and non-HDL cholesterol levels in patients with mixed hyperlipidemia
- In combination with atorvastatin or simvastatin for the treatment of homozygous familial hypercholesterolemia as adjuncts to other lipid-lowering treatments
- As adjunctive therapy to diet for the treatment of homozygous sitosterolemia to reduce elevated sitosterol and campesterol levels
- As an adjunct to diet for the reduction of elevated total cholesterol, LDL, and apolipoprotein B as monotherapy in patients with primary hypercholesterolemia

Contraindications and cautions

- Contraindicated with allergy to any component of the drug. If given in combination with an HMG-CoA reductase inhibitor, contraindicated with pregnancy, lactation, active liver disease, or unexplained persistent increases in serum transaminase, alkaline phosphorus levels.
- In monotherapy, use cautiously in the elderly and with hepatic impairment, pregnancy, lactation.

Available forms

Tablets—10 mg

Dosages

Adults and children 10 yr and older
10 mg/day PO taken without regard to food; may be taken at the same time as an HMG-CoA reductase inhibitor or fenofibrate; if combined with a bile acid sequestrant, should be taken at least 2 hr before or 4 hr after the bile acid sequestrant.

Pediatric patients younger than 10 yr
Safety and efficacy not established.

Pharmacokinetics

Route	Onset	Peak
Oral	Moderate	4–12 hr

Metabolism: Small intestine and hepatic; $T_{1/2}$: 22 hr
Distribution: May cross placenta; may enter breast milk
Excretion: Feces, urine

Adverse effects

- **CNS:** Headache, dizziness, fatigue
- **GI:** Abdominal pain, diarrhea
- **Respiratory:** Pharyngitis, sinusitis, *URI, cough*
- **Other:** Back pain, myalgia, arthralgia, viral infection

Interactions

✳ **Drug-drug** • Decreased serum levels and decreased effectiveness of ezetimibe if combined with cholestyramine; monitor patient closely and space ezetimibe dosing at least 2 hr before or 4 hr or more after the other drug • Increased serum levels of ezetimibe if combined with fenofibrate or gemfibrozil • Risk of cholelithiasis if combined with fibrates • Risk of increased levels and toxicity of ezetimibe and cyclosporine if combined with cyclosporine; if this combination is used monitor patient very carefully.

■ Nursing considerations
Assessment

- **History:** Allergy to any component of the drug; pregnancy, hepatic impairment, lactation, evidence of diet and exercise program
- **Physical:** Skin lesions, color, T; orientation, affect; liver evaluation, bowel sounds; lipid studies, LFTs

Interventions

- Monitor serum cholesterol, LDLs, triglycerides before starting treatment and periodically during treatment.
- Determine that the patient has been on a low-cholesterol diet and exercise program for at least 2 wk before starting ezetimibe.
- If used as part of combination therapy; give drug at the same time as HMG-CoA reductase inhibitors or fenofibrate and at least 2 hr before or 4 hr or more after bile acid sequestrants.

- Encourage the use of barrier contraceptives if used with an HMG-CoA reductase inhibitor.
- Help mother to find another method of feeding her baby if this drug is needed for a breast-feeding woman; it is not known if the drug enters breast milk.
- Consult with dietitian regarding low-cholesterol diets and provide information about exercise programs.
- Arrange for regular follow-up during long-term therapy.

Teaching points
- Take drug once each day at a time that is easy for you to remember. Do not take more than one tablet per day.
- Continue to take any other lipid-lowering drugs that have been prescribed for you. If you are also taking a bile acid sequestrant, take this drug at least 2 hours before or at least 4 hours after the bile acid sequestrant.
- Continue to follow your low-fat diet and participate in an exercise program.
- If you are breast-feeding, you should find another method of feeding the infant.
- Plan to return for periodic blood tests, including tests of liver function and cholesterol levels, to evaluate the effectiveness of this drug.
- You may experience these side effects: Abdominal pain, diarrhea (these usually pass with time, notify your health care provider if this becomes a problem); dizziness, (avoid driving and operating dangerous machinery until you know how this drug affects you); headache (analgesics may help).
- Report unusual muscle pain, weakness, or tenderness; severe diarrhea; respiratory infections.

▽**ezogabine**
(ee zog' a been)

Potiga

PREGNANCY CATEGORY C

Drug classes
Antiepileptic
Potassium channel opener

Therapeutic actions
Enhances transmembrane potassium currents, leading to stabilization of the resting membrane potential and reducing brain excitability; may also augment GABA effects.

Indications
- Adjunct treatment of partial-onset seizures in adults

Contraindications and cautions
- Contraindicated with history of serious hypersensitivity reactions to ezogabine.
- Use cautiously with urine retention, prolonged QT interval, pregnancy, lactation.

Available forms
Tablets—50, 200, 300, 400 mg

Dosages
Adults
100 mg PO tid for 1 wk; titrate to maintenance dose of 200–400 mg PO tid at weekly intervals by no greater than 50 mg tid each wk.
Geriatric patients, patients with renal impairment
Initially, 50 mg PO tid; increase by no more than 50 mg tid at weekly intervals. Target dose, 250 mg PO tid for elderly patients, 200 mg PO tid for patients with renal impairment (CrCl less than 50 mL/min).

Pharmacokinetics

Route	Onset	Peak
Oral	Rapid	1–2 hr

Metabolism: Cellular; $T_{1/2}$: 7–11 hr
Distribution: May cross placenta; may enter breast milk
Excretion: Urine

Adverse effects
- **CNS:** *Sedation, somnolence, dizziness, insomnia, fatigue, confusion, abnormal coordination, blurred vision, memory impairment, aphasia, balance disorder,* **suicidality**
- **CV: Prolonged QT interval**
- **Renal:** Urine retention, dysuria, hematuria
- **Other:** *Dysarthria, withdrawal (with rapid dose reduction),* physical dependence, *fever*

Adverse effects in *italics* are most common; those in **bold** are life-threatening. ⬛ Do not crush.

Interactions

✳ **Drug-drug** • Increased toxicity if combined with alcohol • Decreased effectiveness if combined with carbamazepine, phenytoin; if these combinations are used, consider increase in ezogabine dosage • Increased digoxin serum level and toxicity; monitor digoxin level closely

■ Nursing considerations

Assessment

• **History:** Hypersensitivity to any component of the drug, pregnancy, lactation
• **Physical:** Orientation, affect; vision; ECG

Interventions

• Arrange to taper gradually over at least 3 wk after long-term use; risk of withdrawal reaction with rapid dose reduction.
• Have patient swallow tablets whole; do not cut, crush, or allow patient to chew tablets.
• Be aware of suicidality risk; monitor patient accordingly.
• Provide safety measures for CNS effects.
• Encourage patient to empty bladder before each dose; urine retention can occur.

Teaching points

• Take this drug three times a day. Swallow the tablets whole; do not cut, crush, or chew them.
• Do not stop taking this drug suddenly. Make sure you have a supply on hand; suddenly stopping the drug can cause serious effects.
• Empty your bladder before each dose; this drug may cause urine retention.
• It is not known if this drug could harm a fetus. If you are pregnant or thinking about becoming pregnant, discuss this with your health care provider.
• This drug appears in breast milk; if you are breast-feeding, you will need to find another method of feeding the baby.
• Do not drink alcohol while taking this drug; increased sedation and dizziness may occur.
• This drug can lead to increased thoughts of suicide; report thoughts of suicide or worsening depression.
• You may experience these side effects: Dizziness, sleepiness, slowed thinking (do not drive or operate hazardous machinery if these effects occur); changes in memory, thought processes (do not make important decisions until you know how this drug is affecting you).
• Report abnormal heartbeat, thoughts of suicide, severe urine retention.

▷ factor IX concentrates

AlphaNine SD, Bebulin VH, BeneFIX, Mononine, Profilnine SD

PREGNANCY CATEGORY C

Drug class

Antihemophilic

Therapeutic actions

Human factor IX complex consists of plasma fractions involved in the intrinsic pathway of blood coagulation; causes an increase in blood levels of clotting factors II, VII, VIII, IX, and X.

Indications

• Factor IX deficiency (hemophilia B, Christmas disease) to prevent or control bleeding

Contraindications and cautions

• Contraindicated with factor VII deficiencies; liver disease with signs of intravascular coagulation or fibrinolysis; do not use if hypersensitive to mouse or hamster protein (*Mononine* or *BeneFIX*).
• Use cautiously with pregnancy, lactation.

Available forms

Injection—varies with brand; see label

Dosages

For factor IX deficiency, dosage depends on severity of deficiency and severity of bleeding; follow treatment carefully with factor IX level assays. Dosage should be calculated based on body weight and plasma factor IX levels and will vary for each preparation and intended use. See manufacturers' details.
Adults
• *BeneFIX, Bebulin VH:* Administer IV daily–bid: minor hemorrhage—for 1–2 days; moderate hemorrhage—for 2–7 days; major hemorrhage—for 7–10 days.

- *Others:* 1 international unit/kg × body weight (kg) × desired increase (% of normal).
- *BeneFIX:* 1.3 units/kg × body weight (kg) × desired increase (% of normal).
- *Bebulin VH:* body weight (kg) × desired increase (% of normal) × 1.2 units/kg.

Adults and pediatric patients
- *Prophylaxis of factor IX deficiency:* 20–30 units/kg IV once or twice a week may prevent spontaneous bleeding in hemophilia B patients. Individualize dose. Increase dose if patient is exposed to trauma or surgery.

Pharmacokinetics

Route	Onset	Duration
IV	Immediate	1–2 days

Metabolism: Plasma; $T_{1/2}$: 24–32 hr
Distribution: Crosses placenta; enters breast milk
Excretion: Unknown

▼ IV FACTS

Preparation: Prepare using diluents and needles supplied with product. Refrigerate.
Infusion: ⊗ *Warning* Infuse slowly. 100 units/min and 2–3 mL/min have been suggested. Do not exceed 3 mL/min, and stop or slow the infusion at any sign of headache; pulse, or BP changes.

Adverse effects

- **CNS:** *Headache,* flushing, chills, tingling, somnolence, lethargy
- **GI:** *Nausea,* vomiting, **hepatitis** (risk associated with use of blood products)
- **Hematologic:** *Thrombosis,* DIC, **AIDS** (risk associated with use of blood products; risk is lower with preparations treated with solvent detergents)
- **Other:** Chills, fever; BP changes, urticaria, *Creutzfeldt-Jakob disease*

■ Nursing considerations
Assessment

- **History:** Factor VII, factor IX deficiencies; liver disease with signs of intravascular coagulation or fibrinolysis; pregnancy; lactation
- **Physical:** Skin color, lesions; T; orientation, reflexes, affect; P, BP, peripheral perfusion; clotting factor levels, LFTs

Interventions

- Administer by IV route only.
- ⊗ *Warning* Decrease rate of infusion if headache, flushing, fever, chills, tingling, or urticaria occur; in some patients, the drug will need to be discontinued.
- Monitor patient's clinical response and factors II, VII, IX, and X levels regularly, and regulate dosage based on response.
- Monitor patient for any sign of thrombosis; use comfort and preventive measures when possible (eg, exercise, support stockings, ambulation, positioning).

Teaching points

- Dosage varies widely.
- Safety precautions are taken to ensure that this blood product is pure and the risk of AIDS and hepatitis is minimal.
- Wear or carry a medical ID to alert emergency medical personnel that you require this treatment.
- Report headache, rash, chills, calf pain, swelling, unusual bleeding, or bruising.

▽ factor XIII concentrate (human)

See Appendix R, *Less commonly used drugs.*

▽ famciclovir sodium
(fam sye' kloe vir)

Famvir

PREGNANCY CATEGORY B

Drug class
Antiviral

Therapeutic actions
Antiviral activity; inhibits viral DNA replication in acute herpes zoster.

Indications

- Management of acute herpes zoster (shingles)
- Treatment or suppression of recurrent episodes of genital herpes
- Treatment of recurrent herpes labialis (cold sores) in immunocompetent patients
- Treatment of recurrent mucocutaneous orolabial or genital herpes simplex infections in HIV-infected patients

Adverse effects in *italics* are most common; those in **bold** are life-threatening. ⬛⬛ Do not crush.

- Unlabeled use: Initial management of herpes genitalis
- ◼ **NEW INDICATION:** Unlabeled use: Infection prophylaxis in neutropenia.

Contraindications and cautions

- Contraindicated with hypersensitivity to famciclovir or penciclovir, lactation.
- Use cautiously with pregnancy, impaired renal function.

Available forms

Tablets—125, 250, 500 mg

Dosages

Adults

- *Herpes zoster:* 500 mg every 8 hr PO for 7 days.
- *Genital herpes, first episode in immunecompetent patients:* 230 mg tid for 7–10 days.
- *Treatment of recurrent genital herpes:* 125 mg PO bid for 5 days or 1,000 mg PO bid for 1 day.
- *Chronic suppression of recurrent genital herpes:* 250 mg PO bid for up to 1 yr.
- *Recurrent orolabial or genital herpes simplex infection in HIV-infected patients:* 500 mg every 12 hr PO for 7 days.
- *Recurrent herpes labialis:* 1,500 mg PO as a single dose.

Pediatric patients

Safety and efficacy not established.

Patients with renal impairment

- *Herpes zoster:* Treat for 7 days as indicated below.

CrCl (mL/min)	Dose
60 or more	500 mg every 8 hr
40–59	500 mg every 12 hr
20–39	500 mg every 24 hr
Less than 20	250 mg every 24 hr
Dialysis	250 mg as a single dose after dialysis

- *Recurrent herpes labialis:* Give a single dose as indicated below.

CrCl (mL/min)	Dose
60 or more	1,500 mg
40–59	750 mg
20–39	500 mg
Less than 20	250 mg
Dialysis	250 mg after dialysis

- *Treatment of recurrent genital herpes as single-day dosing:* Give drug as indicated below.

CrCl (mL/min)	Dose
60 and over	1,000 mg every 12 hr for 1 day
40–59	500 mg every 12 hr for 1 day
20–39	500 mg single dose
Less than 20	250 mg single dose
Dialysis	250 mg single dose after dialysis

- *Treatment of recurrent genital herpes:* Treat for 5 days as indicated below.

CrCl (mL/min)	Dose
40 or more	125 mg every 12 hr
20–39	125 mg every 24 hr
Less than 20	125 mg every 24 hr
Dialysis	125 mg after dialysis

- *Suppression of recurrent genital herpes:*

CrCl (mL/min)	Dose
40 or more	250 mg every 12 hr
20–39	125 mg every 12 hr
Less than 20	125 mg every 24 hr
Dialysis	125 mg after dialysis

- *Recurrent orolabial or genital herpes simplex infection in HIV-infected patients:*

CrCl (mL/min)	Dose
40 or more	500 mg every 12 hr
20–39	500 mg every 24 hr
Less than 20	250 mg every 24 hr
Dialysis	250 mg after dialysis

Pharmacokinetics

Route	Onset	Peak
Oral	Varies	30–60 min

Metabolism: $T_{1/2}$: 2 hr
Distribution: Crosses placenta; may enter breast milk
Excretion: Feces, urine

Adverse effects

- **CNS:** Dreams, ataxia, coma, confusion, dizziness, *headache*
- **CV:** Arrhythmia, hypertension, hypotension
- **Dermatologic:** *Rash,* alopecia, pruritus, urticaria
- **GI:** Abnormal liver function tests, nausea, vomiting, anorexia, *diarrhea,* abdominal pain
- **Hematologic: Granulocytopenia, thrombocytopenia,** anemia
- **Other:** *Fever,* chills, **cancer,** sterility

Interactions

✳ **Drug-drug** • Increased serum concentration of famciclovir if taken with cimetidine • Increased digoxin levels if taken together

■ Nursing considerations
Assessment

- **History:** Hypersensitivity to famciclovir or penciclovir, cytopenia; impaired renal function; lactation, pregnancy
- **Physical:** Skin color, lesions; orientation; BP, P, auscultation, perfusion, edema; R, adventitious sounds; urinary output; CBC, Hct, BUN, creatinine clearance, LFTs

Interventions

- Decrease dosage in patients with impaired renal function.
- ⊗ **Warning** Arrange for CBC before and every 2 days during therapy and at least weekly thereafter. Consult with physician to reduce dosage if WBC or platelet counts fall.

Teaching points

- Take drug for 1, 5, or 7 full days as prescribed.
- Famciclovir does not cure genital herpes; use precautions to prevent transmission.
- If using drug for treatment of cold sores (herpes labialis), begin treatment at first sign of cold sore (tingling, itching, burning, pain, or lesion).
- You may experience these side effects: Decreased blood count leading to susceptibility to infection (blood tests may be needed; avoid crowds and exposure to disease), headache (analgesics may be ordered), diarrhea.
- Report bruising, bleeding, worsening of condition, fever, infection.

▽famotidine

*(fa **moe'** ti deen)*

Apo-Famotidine (CAN), Apo-Famotidine Injectable (CAN), Gen-Famotidine (CAN), Nu-Famotidine (CAN), Pepcid, Pepcid AC, Pepcid AC Maximum Strength, Pepcid RPD

PREGNANCY CATEGORY B

Drug class

Histamine-2 (H_2) receptor antagonist

Therapeutic actions

Competitively blocks the action of histamine at the H_2 receptors of the parietal cells of the stomach; inhibits basal gastric acid secretion and chemically induced gastric acid secretion.

Indications

- Short-term treatment and maintenance of duodenal ulcer
- Short-term treatment of benign gastric ulcer
- Treatment of pathologic hypersecretory conditions (eg, Zollinger-Ellison syndrome)
- Short-term treatment of GERD, esophagitis due to GERD
- OTC: Relief of symptoms of heartburn, acid indigestion, sour stomach
- Unlabeled uses: Part of combination therapy for *Helicobacter pylori,* perioperative suppression of gastric acid secretion, prevention of stress ulcers, prevention of aspiration pneumonitis, treatment of certain types of urticaria

Contraindications and cautions

- Contraindicated with allergy to famotidine; other known allergies (cross-sensitivities have been observed); renal failure; lactation.
- Use cautiously with pregnancy, renal or hepatic impairment.

Available forms

Tablets—10, 20, 40 mg; chewable tablets—10 mg; orally disintegrating tablets—20, 40 mg; gelcaps—10 mg; powder for oral suspension—40 mg/5 mL; injection—10 mg/mL; injection, premixed—20 mg/50 mL in 0.9% sodium chloride

Dosages
Adults

- *Acute treatment of active duodenal ulcer:* 40 mg PO or IV at bedtime *or* 20 mg bid PO or IV. Therapy at full dosage should generally be discontinued after 6–8 wk. May be used with antacids for pain relief.
- *Maintenance therapy for duodenal ulcer:* 20 mg PO at bedtime.
- *Benign gastric ulcer:* 40 mg PO daily at bedtime.
- *Hypersecretory syndrome:* 20 mg every 6 hr PO initially. Doses up to 160 mg every 6 hr have been administered. 20 mg IV every 12 hr in patients unable to take oral drugs.

- *GERD:* 20 mg bid PO for up to 6 wk. For patients with esophagitis, the dose is 20–40 mg bid PO for up to 12 wk.
- *Heartburn, acid indigestion:* 10–20 mg PO for relief; 10–20 mg PO, 15–60 min before eating for prevention. Do not exceed 20 mg/24 hr.

Pediatric patients 1–12 yr
- *Peptic ulcer:* 0.5 mg/kg/day PO at bedtime or divided in two doses up to 40 mg/day; 0.25 mg/kg every 12 hr IV up to 40 mg/day if unable to take orally or for pathologic hypersecretory conditions.
- *GERD with or without esophagitis:* 1 mg/kg/day PO divided in two doses up to 40 mg bid.

Infants
- *Younger than 3 mo:* 0.5 mg/kg/dose oral suspension once daily for up to 8 wk.
- *3 mo–1 yr:* 0.5 mg /kg PO bid for up to 8 wk.

Patients with renal impairment
Reduce dosage to 20 mg PO at bedtime or 40 mg PO every 36–48 hr.

Pharmacokinetics

Route	Onset	Peak	Duration
Oral	Slow	1–3 hr	6–12 hr
IV	Less than 1 hr	0.5–3 hr	8–15 hr

Metabolism: Hepatic; $T_{1/2}$: 2.5–3.5 hr
Distribution: Crosses placenta; enters breast milk
Excretion: Urine

▼ IV FACTS

Preparation: For direct injection, dilute 2 mL (solution contains 10 mg/mL) with 0.9% sodium chloride injection, water for injection, 5% or 10% dextrose injection, lactated Ringer injection, or 5% sodium bicarbonate injection to a total volume of 5–10 mL. For infusion, 2 mL diluted with 100 mL 5% dextrose solution or other IVs. Stable for 48 hr at room temperature, 14 days if refrigerated.
Infusion: Inject directly slowly, over not less than 2 min. Infuse over 15–30 min; continuous infusion: 40 mg/24 hr.

Adverse effects
- **CNS:** *Headache,* malaise, *dizziness,* somnolence, insomnia
- **Dermatologic:** Rash

- **GI:** *Diarrhea, constipation,* anorexia, abdominal pain
- **Other:** Muscle cramp, increase in total bilirubin, sexual impotence

■ Nursing considerations
Assessment
- **History:** Allergy to famotidine; renal failure; lactation, pregnancy, hepatic impairment
- **Physical:** Skin lesions; liver evaluation, abdominal examination, normal output; renal function tests, serum bilirubin

Interventions
- If using one dose a day, administer drug at bedtime.
- Decrease doses with renal failure.
- Arrange for administration of concurrent antacid therapy to relieve pain.
- Reserve IV use for hospitalized patients not able to take oral medications; switch to oral medication as soon as possible.

Teaching points
- Take this drug at bedtime (or in the morning and at bedtime). Therapy may continue for 4–6 weeks or longer. Place rapidly disintegrating tablet on tongue and swallow with or without water.
- If needed, take antacid exactly as prescribed, being careful of the times of administration.
- Have regular medical follow-up while on this drug to evaluate your response.
- Take over-the-counter drug 1 hour before eating to prevent indigestion. Do not take more than two per day.
- You may experience these side effects: Constipation or diarrhea; loss of libido or impotence (reversible); headache (adjust lights, temperature, noise levels).
- Report sore throat, fever, unusual bruising or bleeding, severe headache, muscle or joint pain.

▽fat emulsion, intravenous

Intralipid 20%, 30%; Liposyn II 10%, 20%; Liposyn III 10%, 20%, 30%

PREGNANCY CATEGORY C

Drug classes
Caloric drug
Nutritional drug

Therapeutic actions
A preparation from soybean or safflower oil that provides neutral triglycerides, mostly unsaturated fatty acids; these are used as a source of energy, causing an increase in heat production, decrease in respiratory quotient, and increase in oxygen consumption.

Indications
- Source of calories and essential fatty acids for patients requiring parenteral nutrition for extended periods
- Essential fatty acid deficiency

Contraindications and cautions
- Contraindicated with disturbance of normal fat metabolism (hyperlipemia, lipoid nephrosis, acute pancreatitis), allergy to eggs.
- Use cautiously with severe liver damage, pulmonary disease, anemia, blood coagulation disorders, pregnancy, jaundiced or premature infants.

Available forms
Injection—10% (100, 200, 500 mL), 20% (50, 100, 250, 500 mL); 30% (500 mL)

Dosages
Adults
- *Parenteral nutrition:* Should not constitute more than 60% of total calorie intake. *10%:* Infuse IV at 1 mL/min for the first 15–30 min; may be increased to 2 mL/min. Infuse only 500 mL the first day, and increase the following day. Do not exceed 2.5 g/kg/day. *20%:* Infuse at 0.5 mL/min for the first 15–30 min; infuse only 250 mL *Liposyn II* or 500 mL *Intralipid* the first day, and increase the following day. Do not exceed 3 g/kg/day. *30%:* Infuse at 1 mL/min (0.1 g fat/min) for first 15–30 min; do not exceed 2.5 g/kg/day.
- *Fatty acid deficiency:* Supply 8%–10% of the caloric intake by IV fat emulsion.

Pediatric patients
- *Parenteral nutrition:* Should not constitute more than 60% of total calorie intake. *10%:* Initial IV infusion rate is 0.1 mL/min for the first 10–15 min. *20%:* Initial infusion rate is 0.05 mL/min for the first 10–15 min. If no untoward reactions occur,

increase rate to 1 g/kg in 4 hr. Do not exceed 3 g/kg/day. *30%:* Initial infusion, 0.1 mL/min (0.01 g fat/min) for first 10–15 min; do not exceed 3 g/kg/day.

Pharmacokinetics

Route	Onset
IV	Rapid

Metabolism: Hepatic and tissue; $T_{1/2}$: Varies
Distribution: Crosses placenta; may enter breast milk
Excretion: Unknown

▼ IV FACTS
Preparation: ⊗ *Warning* Supplied in single-dose containers; do not store partially used bottles; do not resterilize for later use; do not use with filters; do not use any bottle in which there appears to be separation from the emulsion. Do not add anything to bottle, with the exception of heparin.
Infusion: Infusion rate is 1 mL/min for 10% solution, monitor for 15–30 min; if no adverse reaction occurs, may be increased to 2 mL/min; 0.5 mL/min for 20% solution; 1 mL/min for 30%; may be increased if no adverse reactions. May be infused simultaneously with amino acid-dextrose mixtures by means of Y-connector located near the infusion site using separate flow rate; keep the lipid solution higher than the amino acid-dextrose line.
Incompatibilities: Do not mix or inject at Y site with amikacin, tetracycline. Monitor electrolyte and acid content; fat emulsion separates in acid solution.

Adverse effects
- **CNS:** *Headache,* flushing, fever, sweating, sleepiness, pressure over the eyes, dizziness
- **GI:** *Nausea,* vomiting
- **Hematologic:** *Thrombophlebitis,* **sepsis,** hyperlipidemia, hypercoagulability, **thrombocytopenia, leukopenia,** elevated liver enzymes
- **Other:** Irritation at infusion site, brown pigmentation in RES (IV fat pigment), cyanosis, infection

■ Nursing considerations
Assessment
- **History:** Disturbance of normal fat metabolism, allergy to eggs, severe liver damage,

pulmonary disease, anemia, blood coagulation disorders, pregnancy, jaundiced or premature infants

- **Physical:** Skin color, lesions; T; orientation; P, BP, peripheral perfusion; CBC, plasma lipid profile (especially triglycerides), clotting factor levels, LFTs

Interventions

⊗ Black box warning Administer to preterm infants only if benefit clearly outweighs risk; deaths have occurred.

- Administer by IV route only.

⊗ Warning Inspect admixture for "breaking or oiling out" of the emulsion—seen as yellow streaking or accumulation of yellow droplets—or for the formation of any particulates; discard any admixture if these occur.

⊗ Warning Monitor patient carefully for fluid or fat overloading during infusion: Diluted serum electrolytes, overhydration, pulmonary edema, elevated jugular venous pressure, metabolic acidosis, impaired pulmonary diffusion capacity. Discontinue the infusion; re-evaluate patient before restarting infusion at a lower rate.

- Monitor patient's clinical response, serum lipid profile (obtain triglycerides every week), weight gain, improved nitrogen balance.
- Monitor patient for thrombosis or sepsis; use comfort and preventive measures (such as exercise, support stockings, ambulation, positioning).

Teaching points

- Report pain at infusion site, difficulty breathing, chest pain, calf pain, excessive sweating.

▽febuxostat

*(feb **bux'** ob stat)*

Uloric

PREGNANCY CATEGORY C

Drug classes

Antigout drug
Xanthine oxidase inhibitor

Therapeutic actions

Blocks xanthine oxidase, an important enzyme in the process of uric acid formation; not thought to affect other enzymes involved in purine or pyrimidine synthesis.

Indications

- Long-term management of hyperuricemia in patients with gout

Contraindications and cautions

- Contraindicated with hypersensitivity to components of drug, concurrent treatment with azathioprine, mercaptopurine, or theophyllines.
- Use cautiously with severe renal or hepatic impairment, history of heart attack or stroke, pregnancy, lactation.

Available forms

Tablets—40, 80 mg

Dosages

Adults
Initially, 40 mg/day PO; if serum uric acid level is not less than 6 mg/dL in 2 weeks, dosage may be increased to 80 mg/day PO.

Pediatric patients
Safety and efficacy not established.

Patients with renal or hepatic impairment
No dosage change required with mild to moderate impairment; use caution with severe impairment (Child-Pugh Class C).

Pharmacokinetics

Route	Onset	Peak
Oral	Rapid	1–1.5 hr

Metabolism: Hepatic; T$_{1/2}$: 5–8 hr
Distribution: May cross placenta; may enter breast milk
Excretion: Urine, feces

Adverse effects

- **CNS:** Dizziness
- **CV:** Thromboembolic events, **MI, stroke**
- **GI:** Nausea, liver function abnormalities
- **Other:** Arthralgia, rash, gout flares

Interactions

✳ Drug-drug • Risk of decreased metabolism and increased serum levels of azathioprine, mercaptopurine, theophyllines when given with these drugs, causing toxicity; avoid these combinations; concurrent use is contraindicated

■ Nursing considerations

Assessment

- **History:** Hypersensitivity to components of drug, liver or renal dysfunction, heart attack or stroke, pregnancy, lactation
- **Physical:** Orientation, affect; skin—color, lesions; abdominal exam; serum uric acid level, liver and renal function tests, baseline ECG

Interventions

- Administer without regard to food. May be taken with antacids.
- Obtain baseline and periodic serum uric acid levels.
- Arrange for other medication if gout flare occurs.
- Monitor for signs and symptoms of heart attack or stroke; patient may be at increased risk.

Teaching points

- Take this drug once a day, with or without food. You may take this drug with antacids.
- Store this drug at room temperature, protected from light.
- If you miss a dose, take the next dose as soon as you remember.
- You may experience a flare-up of your gout symptoms when you start taking this drug. Do not stop taking the drug; contact your health care provider, who may give you other medications to handle the flare-up.
- You will be asked to have periodic blood tests to evaluate the effects of this drug on your body.
- It is not known how this drug affects a fetus. If you become pregnant while taking this drug, consult your health care provider.
- It is not known how this drug affects a breast-feeding infant. Discuss the risks and benefits with your health care provider if you are breast-feeding.
- You may experience these side effects: Dizziness (do not drive a car or engage in activities that require alertness if these effects occur); nausea, joint pain, rash (these may lessen over time; consult your health care provider if they become too uncomfortable).
- Report chest pain, difficulty breathing, numbness or tingling, changes in the color of urine or stool, yellowing of the eyes or skin.

▷ felodipine ⓪Ⓝ

(fell ob' di peen)

Plendil ⓞⓃⒸ, Renedil (CAN) ⓞⓃⒸ

PREGNANCY CATEGORY C

Drug classes

Antihypertensive
Calcium channel blocker

Therapeutic actions

Inhibits the movement of calcium ions across the membranes of cardiac and vascular smooth muscle cells; greater selectivity for vascular smooth muscle as compared to cardiac muscle; leads to arterial and coronary artery vasodilation and decreased peripheral vascular resistance.

Indications

- Essential hypertension, alone or in combination with other antihypertensives

Contraindications and cautions

- Contraindicated with allergy to felodipine or other calcium channel blockers, sick sinus syndrome, heart block (second or third degree), lactation.
- Use cautiously with pregnancy, impaired hepatic function.

Available forms

ER tablets ⓞⓃⒸ—2.5, 5, 10 mg

Dosages

Adults

Initially, 5 mg PO daily; dosage may be gradually increased over at least 14 days. Usual dose is 2.5–10 mg PO daily. Doses greater than 10 mg PO daily are associated with an increased risk of peripheral edema.

Pediatric patients

Safety and efficacy not established.

Geriatric patients or patients with hepatic impairment

Monitor carefully; begin with 2.5 mg daily, and do not exceed 10 mg daily PO.

Pharmacokinetics

Route	Onset	Peak
Oral	2–5 hr	2.5–5 hr

Metabolism: Hepatic; $T_{1/2}$: 11–16 hr

Adverse effects in *italics* are most common; those in **bold** are life-threatening. ⓞⓃⒸ Do not crush.

Distribution: Crosses placenta; may enter breast milk
Excretion: Urine

Adverse effects

- **CNS:** *Dizziness, light-headedness, head-ache,* asthenia, *fatigue, lethargy*
- **CV:** *Peripheral edema,* arrhythmias
- **Dermatologic:** *Flushing,* rash
- **GI:** *Nausea,* abdominal discomfort, reflux, constipation

Interactions

✴ **Drug-drug** • Decreased serum levels with barbiturates, hydantoins, carbamazepine • Increased serum levels and toxicity with erythromycin, cimetidine, ranitidine, antifungals

✴ **Drug-food** • Decreased metabolism and increased risk of toxic effects if taken with grapefruit juice; avoid this combination

■ Nursing considerations

Assessment

- **History:** Allergy to felodipine, impaired hepatic function, sick sinus syndrome, heart block, lactation, pregnancy
- **Physical:** Skin lesions, color, edema; P, BP, baseline ECG, peripheral perfusion, auscultation, R, adventitious sounds; liver evaluation, GI normal output; LFTs, urinalysis

Interventions

- Have patient swallow tablet whole; do not chew or crush.
- Monitor patient carefully (BP, cardiac rhythm and output) while drug is being adjusted to therapeutic dose.
- Monitor cardiac rhythm regularly during stabilization of dosage and periodically during long-term therapy.
- Administer drug without regard to meals.

Teaching points

- Take this drug with light meals if upset stomach occurs; swallow tablet whole, do not cut, crush, or chew. Do not drink grapefruit juice while using this drug.
- You may experience these side effects: Nausea, vomiting (eat frequent small meals); headache (adjust lighting, noise, and temperature; medication may be ordered if severe).
- Report irregular heart beat, shortness of breath, swelling of the hands or feet, pronounced dizziness, constipation.

▷**fenofibrate**
(fee no fye' brate)

Antara, Apo-Fenofibrate (CAN), Fenoglide, Gen-Fenofibrate (CAN), Lipofen, Lofibra, PMS-Fenofibrate (CAN), ratio-Fenofibrate MC (CAN), TriCor, Triglide, Trilipix ⒪ⓡⒸ

PREGNANCY CATEGORY C

Drug class
Antihyperlipidemic

Therapeutic actions
Inhibits triglyceride synthesis in the liver resulting in a reduction in VLDL released into circulation; may also stimulate the breakdown of triglyceride-rich lipoproteins.

Indications

- Adjunct to diet in treating adults with primary hypercholesterolemia or mixed dyslipidemia
- Adjunct to diet for treatment of adults with hypertriglyceridemia
- As adjunct to diet with a statin to reduce triglycerides and increase HDLs in patients with mixed dyslipidemia and coronary heart disease or at high risk for coronary heart disease
- Unlabeled use: Hyperuricemia

Contraindications and cautions

- Contraindicated with allergy to fenofibrate, hepatic or severe renal impairment, primary biliary cirrhosis, gall bladder disease, pregnancy.
- Use cautiously with lactation and in the elderly.

Available forms
Tablets—35, 40, 48, 50, 54, 105, 107, 120, 145, 160 mg; capsules—43, 50, 67, 100, 130, 134, 150, 200 mg; DR capsules—45, 135 mg ⒪ⓡⒸ

Dosages
Adults

- *Hypertriglyceridemia:* Initially, 48–145 mg (*TriCor*) or 67–200 mg (*Lofibra*) with a meal or 50–160 mg/day (*Triglide*) daily PO or 43–130 mg/day PO (*Antara*), or 50–150 mg/day PO (*Lipofen*), or 40–120 mg/day PO (*Fenoglide*), or 45–135 mg/day PO (*Trilipix*)

- *Primary hypercholesterolemia or mixed dys-lipidemia:* 145 mg/day PO (*TriCor*) or 200 mg/day (*Lofibra*) with a meal or 160 mg/day (*Triglide*) or 130 mg/day PO (*Antara*), or 150 mg/day PO (*Lipofen*), or 120 mg /day PO (*Fenoglide*), or 135 mg/day PO (*Trilipix*)
- *Combination with a statin:* 135 mg/day PO (*Trilipix*)

Pediatric patients
Safety and efficacy not established.

Geriatric patients
Initial dose, 48 mg/day PO (*TriCor*), 67 mg/day (*Lofibra*) with a meal or 50 mg/day (*Triglide*) or 43 mg/day PO (*Antara*), or 50 mg/day PO (*Lipofen*); adjust slowly with close monitoring.

Patients with renal impairment
Initiate therapy with 48 mg/day PO (*TriCor*), 67 mg/day (*Lofibra*) with a meal or 50 mg/day (*Triglide*) or 43 mg/day PO (*Antara*), or 50 mg/day PO (*Lipofen*), or 40 mg/day PO (*Fenoglide*), or 45 mg/day PO (*Trilipix*); monitor renal function tests for 4–8 wk before increasing.

Pharmacokinetics

Route	Onset	Peak	Duration
Oral	Varies	6–8 hr	Wks

Metabolism: Hepatic; $T_{1/2}$: 20 hr
Distribution: Crosses placenta; enters breast milk
Excretion: Urine

Adverse effects

- **CV:** Angina, arrhythmias, swelling, phlebitis, thrombophlebitis
- **Dermatologic:** *Rash,* alopecia, dry skin, dry and brittle hair, pruritus, urticaria
- **GI:** *Nausea,* vomiting, diarrhea, dyspepsia, flatulence, bloating, stomatitis, gastritis, cholelithiasis, abnormal LFTs, **pancreatitis,** peptic ulcer, GI hemorrhage
- **GU:** *Impotence, decreased libido,* dysuria, hematuria, proteinuria, decreased urine output
- **Hematologic:** Leukopenia, anemia, eosinophilia, increased AST and ALT, increased CPK
- **Other:** *Myalgia, flulike symptoms,* arthralgia, weight gain, polyphagia, increased perspiration, systemic lupus erythematosus, blurred vision, gynecomastia

Interactions

❋ **Drug-drug** • Increased bleeding tendencies if oral anticoagulants are given with fenofibrate; reduce dosage of anticoagulant • Possible rhabdomyolysis, acute renal failure if given with any statins; avoid this combination • Decreased absorption and effectiveness if given with bile acid sequestrants; administer at least 1 hr before or 4–6 hr after these drugs • Increased risk of renal toxicity if combined with immunosuppressants or other nephrotoxic drugs; use caution and monitor patient carefully

■ Nursing considerations
Assessment

- **History:** Allergy to fenofibrate, hepatic impairment, primary biliary cirrhosis, gallbladder disease, pregnancy, renal impairment, lactation
- **Physical:** Skin lesions, color, T; P, BP, auscultation, baseline ECG, peripheral perfusion, edema; bowel sounds, normal urine output, liver evaluation; lipid studies, CBC, LFTs, renal function tests, urinalysis

Interventions

- Differentiate between brand names used; dosage varies.
- Administer drug with meals (*Lofibra, Lipofen, Fenoglide*).
- Do not allow patient to cut, crush, or chew DR capsules; capsules must be swallowed whole.
- Monitor patient carefully.
- Ensure that patient continues strict dietary restrictions and exercise program.
- Arrange for regular follow-up, including blood tests for lipids, liver function, and CBC during long-term therapy.
- Give frequent skin care to deal with rashes and dryness.
- Suggest alternative method of feeding the infant if patient is breast-feeding.
- Monitor patient for muscle weakness, aches, especially if patient takes *TriCor* in combination with other cholesterol-lowering drugs.

Teaching points

- Take the drug with meals (*Lofibra, Lipofen, Fenoglide*).
- If you miss a dose, take it as soon as you remember. If you remember at about the same time as your next scheduled dose, just take

the next dose. Do not double up doses. Do not take more than one dose each day (*Trilipix*).
- Continue to follow strict dietary regimen and exercise program.
- Arrange to have regular follow-up visits to your health care provider, which will include blood tests.
- It is not known how this drug affects a fetus. If you are pregnant or thinking of becoming pregnant, consult your health care provider.
- It is not known how this drug affects a breast-feeding infant. Because of the potential for adverse effects, you should use a different method of feeding the infant while taking this drug.
- You may experience these side effects: Diarrhea, loss of appetite (ensure ready access to the bathroom if this occurs; frequent small meals may help).
- Report chest pain, shortness of breath, palpitations, myalgia, malaise, excessive fatigue, fever.

▽**fenoprofen calcium**
*(fen oh **proe'** fen)*

Nalfon

PREGNANCY CATEGORY B
(FIRST AND SECOND TRIMESTERS)

PREGNANCY CATEGORY D
(THIRD TRIMESTER)

Drug classes
Analgesic (nonopioid)
NSAID
Propionic acid derivative

Therapeutic actions
Analgesic, anti-inflammatory, and antipyretic activities largely related to inhibition of prostaglandin synthesis by inhibiting cyclooxygenase; exact mechanisms of action are not known.

Indications
- Acute and long-term treatment of rheumatoid arthritis and osteoarthritis
- Relief of mild to moderate pain
- Unlabeled uses: Treatment of juvenile rheumatoid arthritis; symptomatic treatment of sunburn, migraine headache

Contraindications and cautions
- Contraindicated with significant renal impairment, pregnancy, lactation, hypersensitivity to aspirin, fenoprofen, or other NSAIDs.
- Use cautiously with impaired hearing; hepatic, hypertension, and GI conditions.

Available forms
Capsules—200, 300, 400 mg; tablets—600 mg

Dosages
Do not exceed 3,200 mg/day.
Adults
- *Rheumatoid arthritis or osteoarthritis:* 400–600 mg PO tid or qid. Treatment for 2–3 wk may be required to see improvement.
- *Mild to moderate pain:* 200 mg every 4–6 hr PO, as needed.
Pediatric patients
Safety and efficacy not established.

Pharmacokinetics

Route	Onset	Peak
Oral	15–30 min	1–2 hr

Metabolism: Hepatic; $T_{1/2}$: 2–3 hr
Distribution: Crosses placenta; enters breast milk
Excretion: Urine

Adverse effects
NSAIDs
- **CNS:** *Headache, dizziness, somnolence, insomnia,* fatigue, tiredness, tinnitus, ophthalmologic effects
- **Dermatologic:** *Rash,* pruritus, sweating, dry mucous membranes, stomatitis
- **GI:** *Nausea, dyspepsia, GI pain,* diarrhea, vomiting, constipation, flatulence, **ulcer, GI bleed**
- **GU:** Dysuria, **renal impairment** (fenoprofen is one of the most nephrotoxic NSAIDs)
- **Hematologic:** Bleeding, platelet inhibition with higher doses, **neutropenia, eosinophilia, leukopenia, pancytopenia, thrombocytopenia, agranulocytosis, granulocytopenia, aplastic anemia,** decreased Hgb or Hct, menorrhagia
- **Respiratory:** Dyspnea, hemoptysis, pharyngitis, **bronchospasm,** rhinitis

- **Other:** Peripheral edema, **anaphylactoid reactions to fatal anaphylactic shock**

Interactions

✳ **Drug-drug** • Increased risk of bleeding with anticoagulants, antiplatelet drugs • Decreased effect when used with phenobarbital • Risk of decreased antihypertensive effects if combined with ACE inhibitors • Increased risk of serious GI events if combined with aspirin; combination is not recommended

■ Nursing considerations

Assessment

- **History:** Renal impairment; impaired hearing; allergy to aspirin or NSAIDs; hepatic, CV, and GI conditions; lactation; pregnancy
- **Physical:** Skin color and lesions; orientation, reflexes, ophthalmologic and audiometric evaluations, peripheral sensation; P, edema; R, adventitious sounds; liver evaluation; CBC, clotting times, LFTs, renal function tests; serum electrolytes, stool guaiac

Interventions

⊗ **Black box warning** Be aware that patient may be at increased risk for CV events, GI bleeding; monitor patient accordingly.
- Administer drug with food or after meals if GI upset occurs.
- Arrange for periodic ophthalmologic examination during long-term therapy.

⊗ **Warning** If overdose occurs, institute emergency procedures—gastric lavage, induction of emesis, supportive therapy.

Teaching points

- Take drug with food or meals if GI upset occurs.
- Take only the prescribed dosage.
- Do not take this drug during pregnancy; using contraceptives is advised.
- Dizziness or drowsiness can occur (avoid driving or using dangerous machinery).
- Report sore throat, fever, rash, itching, weight gain, swelling in ankles or fingers; changes in vision; black, tarry stools; bleeding.

DANGEROUS DRUG

▽**fentanyl**
(fen' ta nil)

Abstral, Actiq; Duragesic 12, 25, 50, 75, 100; Duragesic Patch 12; Fentora, Lazanda, Onsolis, SUBSYS

PREGNANCY CATEGORY C

CONTROLLED SUBSTANCE C-II

Drug class
Opioid agonist analgesic

Therapeutic actions
Acts at specific opioid receptors, causing analgesia, respiratory depression, physical depression, euphoria.

Indications
- Analgesic action of short duration during anesthesia and immediate postoperative period
- Analgesic supplement in general or regional anesthesia
- Administration with a neuroleptic as an anesthetic premedication, for induction of anesthesia, and as an adjunct in maintenance of general and regional anesthesia
- For use as an anesthetic drug with oxygen in select high-risk patients
- Transdermal system: Management of chronic pain in patients requiring continuous opioid analgesia over an extended period of time who cannot be managed by other means and who are already receiving opioid therapy
- *Abstral, Actiq, Fentora, Lazanda, Onsolis, SUBSYS:* Treatment of breakthrough pain in cancer patients being treated with and tolerant to opioids for underlying cancer pain

Contraindications and cautions
- Contraindicated with hypersensitivity to opioids, diarrhea caused by poisoning, acute bronchial asthma, upper airway obstruction, pregnancy. Transdermal and nasal forms contraindicated in patients not opioid-tolerant and not meeting indication criteria.
- Use cautiously with bradycardia, history of seizures, lactation, renal impairment; history of drug addiction.

Adverse effects in *italics* are most common; those in **bold** are life-threatening. ⬛ Do not crush.

Available forms

Lozenge on a stick (*Actiq*)—200, 400, 600, 800, 1,200, 1,600 mcg; transdermal—12.5, 25, 50, 75, 100 mcg/hr; injection—50 mcg/mL; buccal tablets—100, 200, 400, 600, 800 mcg; buccal soluble film—200, 400, 600, 800, 1,200 mcg; sublingual tablets—100, 200, 300, 400, 600, 800 mcg; nasal spray—100, 400 mcg; sublingual spray—100, 200, 400, 600, 800 mcg/spray

Dosages

Individualize dosage; monitor vital signs.

Adults
Parenteral

- *Premedication:* 50–100 mcg IM 30–60 min before surgery.
- *Adjunct to general anesthesia:* Initial dosage is 2–20 mcg/kg. Maintenance dose, 2–50 mcg IV or IM; 25–100 mcg IV or IM when changes in vital signs indicate surgical stress or lightening of analgesia.
- *With oxygen for anesthesia:* Total high dose is 50–100 mcg/kg IV.
- *Adjunct to regional anesthesia:* 50–100 mcg IM or slowly IV over 1–2 min.
- *Postoperatively:* 50–100 mcg IM for the control of pain, tachypnea, or emergence delirium; repeat in 1–2 hr if needed.

Transdermal

Initiate therapy with 25 mcg/hr system; adjust dose as needed and tolerated. Apply to nonirritated and nonirradiated skin on a flat surface of the upper torso; may require replacement in 72 hr if pain has not subsided; do not use torn or damaged systems, serious overdose can occur.

Lozenges

- *Actiq:* Place unit in mouth between cheek and lower gum. Start with initial dose of 200 mcg. Until appropriate dose is reached, an additional dose can be used to treat an episode of breakthrough pain. Redosing may start 15 min after the previous lozenge has been completed. No more than two lozenges should be used for each breakthrough pain episode. Can consider increasing dose if requiring more than one lozenge for treatment of several consecutive breakthrough pain episodes. If more than four lozenges are needed daily, increase the dosage of long-acting opioid. *Actiq* should be sucked slowly over 15 min.

Buccal forms

- *Buccal tablets:* Initially, 100-mcg tablet between cheek and gum for 14–25 min; may be repeated in 30 min if needed. Adjust slowly to control pain.
- *Buccal soluble film:* Remove film and place inside cheek; will dissolve within 5–30 min. Available only through FOCUS program.
- *Sublingual tablets:* Initially, 100 mcg sublingually; increase dose to achieve control of pain. Once at maintenance dose, wait at least 2 hr between doses when treating breakthrough pain.
- *Sublingual spray:* 100 mcg by sublingual spray; if pain is not relieved within 30 min, repeat dose. Wait at least 4 hr before treating another episode of pain. Individualize dose based on patient report; up to 800 mcg/spray has been used.

Nasal spray

Initially, 100 mcg as a single spray in one nostril. Titrate to a maximum dose of 800 mcg, as a single spray in one nostril or single spray in each nostril per episode. Wait at least 2 hr before treating new episode. Give no more than four doses in 24 hr.

Pediatric patients 2–12 yr
Transdermal system

Children 2 yr and older initiating therapy on 25 mcg/hr system should be opioid tolerant and receiving at least 60 mg oral morphine equivalents/day.

Parenteral

2–3 mcg/kg IV as vital signs indicate.

Pharmacokinetics

Route	Onset	Duration
IV	1–2 min	0.5–1 hr
IM	7–8 min	1–2 hr
Transdermal	Gradual	72 hr
Transmucosal	15 min	1 hr
Nasal	15–20 min	6 hr

Metabolism: Liver; $T_{1/2}$: 1.5–6 hr
Distribution: Crosses placenta; may enter breast milk
Excretion: Unknown

▼ IV FACTS

Preparation: May be used undiluted or diluted with 250 mL of D_5W. Protect vials from light.

Infusion: Administer slowly by direct injection, each milliliter over at least 1 min, or into running IV tubing.

Incompatibilities: Do not mix with methohexital, pentobarbital, thiopental.

Adverse effects

- **CNS:** *Sedation, clamminess, sweating, headache, vertigo, floating feeling, dizziness, lethargy, confusion, light-headedness,* nervousness, unusual dreams, agitation, euphoria, hallucinations, delirium, insomnia, anxiety, fear, disorientation, impaired mental and physical performance, mood changes, coma, weakness, headache, tremor, seizures
- **CV:** Palpitation, increase or decrease in BP, circulatory depression, **cardiac arrest, shock,** tachycardia, bradycardia, arrhythmia, palpitations
- **Dermatologic:** Rash, hives, pruritus, flushing, warmth, sensitivity to cold
- **EENT:** Diplopia, blurred vision
- **GI:** *Nausea, vomiting,* dry mouth, anorexia, *constipation,* biliary tract spasm
- **GU:** Ureteral spasm, spasm of vesical sphincters, urinary retention or hesitancy, oliguria, antidiuretic effect, reduced libido or potency
- **Local:** Phlebitis following IV injection, pain at injection site; tissue irritation and induration (subcutaneous injection)
- **Respiratory:** Slow, shallow respiration, **apnea,** suppression of cough reflex, laryngospasm, bronchospasm
- **Other:** Physical tolerance and dependence; psychological dependence; local skin irritation with transdermal system

Interactions

✳ **Drug-drug** • Potentiation of effects when given with other CNS acting drugs or barbiturate anesthetics; decrease dose of fentanyl when co-administering • Do not administer an MAOI within 14 days of fentanyl (increased CNS effects) • Increased risk of adverse effects and toxicity if combined with alcohol

⊗ **Black box warning** Potentiation of effects may occur when given with CYP4503A4 inhibitors such as macrolide antibiotics, ketoconazole, itraconazole, and protease inhibitors. Potentially fatal respiratory depression may occur. Monitor patient for an extended period and adjust dosage if combination is needed.

✳ **Drug-food** • Decreased metabolism and risk of toxic effects if taken with grapefruit juice; avoid this combination

✳ **Drug-lab test** • Elevated biliary tract pressure may cause increases in plasma amylase, lipase; determinations of these levels may be unreliable for 24 hr after administration of opioids

■ Nursing considerations

★ **CLINICAL ALERT!**
Name confusion has occurred between fentanyl and sufentanil; use extreme caution.

Assessment

- **History:** Hypersensitivity to fentanyl or opioids, physical dependence on an opioid analgesic, pregnancy, labor, lactation, COPD, respiratory depression, anoxia, increased intracranial pressure, acute MI, ventricular failure, coronary insufficiency, hypertension, biliary tract surgery, renal or hepatic impairment
- **Physical:** Orientation, reflexes, bilateral grip strength, affect; pupil size, vision; P, auscultation, BP; R, adventitious sounds; bowel sounds, normal output; LFTs, renal function tests

Interventions

- Administer to breast-feeding women 4–6 hr before the next scheduled feeding to minimize the amount in milk.

⊗ **Black box warning** Keep opioid antagonist and facilities for assisted or controlled respiration readily available during parenteral administration; ensure appropriate use of drug because it is potentially dangerous. Respiratory depression and death can occur.

⊗ **Black box warning** Use caution when switching between forms of delivery; dosages vary.

⊗ **Black box warning** Transdermal and nasal forms not for use in opioid–nontolerant patients; not for acute or postoperative pain; do not substitute for any other fentanyl product. Keep out of reach of children; can be fatal to children.

- Prepare site for transdermal form by clipping (not shaving) hair at site; do not use soap, oils, lotions, alcohol; let skin dry completely before application. Apply immediately after removal from the sealed package;

Adverse effects in *italics* are most common; those in **bold** are life-threatening. ⊙ Do not crush.

firmly press the transdermal system in place with the palm of the hand for 10–20 sec, making sure the contact is complete. Must be worn continually for 72 hr. Do not use any system that has been torn or damaged. Remove old patch before applying a new one.

- Note that the patch doesn't work quickly. It may take up to 12 hr to get the full therapeutic effect. Breakthrough medications may need to be used.
- Do not use *Actiq* in patients who never received opioids before; should be used only in opioid-tolerant patients.
- Use caution with *Actiq* form to keep this drug out of the reach of children (it looks like a lollipop) and follow the distribution restrictions in place with this drug very carefully.
- Buccal soluble film is only available through FOCUS limited-access program. Dispose of unused films by removing from foil pack and flushing down toilet.
- Nasal form is only available through a restricted access program.
- Sublingual spray is only available through a restricted-access program. Open blister pack with scissors immediately before use. Spray contents of unit under the tongue. Dispose of unit systems in provided disposal bottle.

Teaching points

- Do not drink grapefruit juice while using this drug. If using the patch, do not use any patch that has been torn or damaged. Remove old patch before applying a new one. If using buccal soluble film, remove from the foil pack and place inside your cheek; it will dissolve within 5 to 30 minutes. Dispose of unused films by removing them from the foil pack, depositing them in the toilet and then flushing the toilet.
- When using nasal form, if relief is not achieved within 30 minutes, you may use a rescue medication as prescribed by your health care provider.
- When using the sublingual spray, open the blister pack with scissors and immediately spray contents of unit under your tongue. Dispose of the unit in the disposal bottle provided. Keep out of reach of children.
- You may experience these side effects: Dizziness, sedation, drowsiness, impaired visual acuity (ask for assistance if you need to

move); nausea, loss of appetite (lie quietly, eat frequent small meals); constipation (a laxative may help).

- Report severe nausea, vomiting, palpitations, shortness of breath, or difficulty breathing.

▷**ferrous salts**
(fair' us)

ferrous asparate
FE Asparate

ferrous fumarate
Femiron, Ferretts, Ferro-Sequels, Hemocyte, Palafer (CAN)

ferrous gluconate
Apo-Ferrous Gluconate (CAN), Fergon

ferrous sulfate
Apo-Ferrous Sulfate (CAN), Enfamil Fer-in-Sol, Feosol, Fer-Gen-Sol, Ferosul

ferrous sulfate exsiccated
Feosol, Ferodan (CAN), Slow Fe, Slow Release Iron

PREGNANCY CATEGORY A

Drug class
Iron preparation

Therapeutic actions
Elevates the serum iron concentration, and is then converted to Hgb or trapped in the reticuloendothelial cells for storage and eventual conversion to a usable form of iron.

Indications
- Prevention and treatment of iron deficiency anemias
- Dietary supplement for iron
- Unlabeled use: Supplemental use during epoetin therapy to ensure proper hematologic response to epoetin

Contraindications and cautions
- Contraindicated with allergy to any ingredient; sulfite allergy; hemochromatosis, hemosiderosis, hemolytic anemias.

- Use cautiously with normal iron balance; peptic ulcer, regional enteritis, ulcerative colitis.

Available forms

Tablets—asparate—112 mg; sulfate, 324, 325 mg; sulfate exsiccated, 200, 300 mg; gluconate, 240, 325 mg; fumarate, 63, 200, 324, 325, 350 mg; timed-release capsules—sulfate exsiccated, 160 mg; timed-release tablets—sulfate exsiccated, 160 mg; syrup—fumarate (*Ferro-Sequels*), 150 mg; sulfate, 90 mg/5 mL; elixir—sulfate, 220 mg/5 mL; drops—sulfate, 75 mg/0.6 mL, 125 mg/mL; fumarate, 45 mg/0.6 mL; tablet, chewable—fumarate, 100 mg; suspension—fumarate, 100 mg/5 mL

Dosages

Adults

- *Daily requirements:* Men, 8–11 mg/day PO; women, 8–18 mg/day PO; pregnant and lactating women, 9–27 mg/day PO.
- *Replacement in deficiency states:* 150–300 mg/day (6 mg/kg/day) PO for approximately 6–10 mo may be required.

Pediatric patients

- *Daily requirement:* 7–11 mg/day PO.
- *Replacement:* 3–6 mg/kg/day PO.

Pharmacokinetics

Route	Onset	Peak	Duration
Oral	4 days	7–10 days	2–4 mo

Metabolism: Recycled for use; $T_{1/2}$: Not known

Distribution: Crosses placenta; enters breast milk

Excretion: Unknown

Adverse effects

- **CNS:** CNS toxicity, acidosis, **coma and death with overdose**
- **GI:** *GI upset, anorexia, nausea, vomiting, constipation,* diarrhea, dark stools, temporary staining of the teeth (liquid preparations)

Interactions

✳ **Drug-drug** • Decreased anti-infective response to ciprofloxacin, norfloxacin, ofloxacin; separate doses by at least 2 hr • Decreased absorption with antacids, cimetidine • Decreased effects of levodopa if taken with iron • Increased serum iron levels with chloramphenicol • Decreased absorption of levothyroxine; separate doses by at least 2 hr

✳ **Drug-food** • Decreased absorption with antacids, eggs or milk, coffee and tea; avoid concurrent administration of any of these

■ **Nursing considerations**

Assessment

- **History:** Allergy to any ingredient, sulfite; hemochromatosis, hemosiderosis, hemolytic anemias; normal iron balance; peptic ulcer, regional enteritis, ulcerative colitis
- **Physical:** Skin lesions, color; gums, teeth (color); bowel sounds; CBC, Hgb, Hct, serum ferritin and iron levels

Interventions

- Confirm that patient does have iron deficiency anemia before treatment.
- Give drug with meals (avoiding milk, eggs, coffee, and tea) if GI discomfort is severe; slowly increase to build up tolerance.
- Administer liquid preparations in water or juice to mask the taste and prevent staining of teeth; have the patient drink solution with a straw.
- Warn patient that stool may be dark or green.
- Arrange for periodic monitoring of Hct and Hgb levels.

⊗ **Black box warning** Warn patient to keep drug out of children's reach; leading cause of fatal poisoning in children younger than 6 yr.

Teaching points

- Take drug on an empty stomach with water. Take after meals if GI upset is severe (avoid milk, eggs, coffee, and tea).
- Take liquid preparations diluted in water or juice, and sip them through a straw to prevent staining of the teeth.
- Treatment may not be necessary if cause of anemia can be corrected. It may be needed for several months to reverse anemia.
- Have periodic blood tests during therapy to determine the appropriate dosage.
- Do not take this preparation with antacids or tetracyclines. If these drugs are needed, they will be prescribed.
- You may experience these side effects: GI upset, nausea, vomiting (take drug with meals); diarrhea or constipation; dark or green stools.
- Keep this drug out of the reach of children.
- Report severe GI upset, lethargy, rapid respirations, constipation.

▽ferumoxytol

See Appendix R, *Less commonly used drugs.*

▽fesoterodine fumarate
*(fess oh **tear'** oh deen)*

Toviaz ⓒⓐⓝ

PREGNANCY CATEGORY C

Drug class
Antimuscarinic

Therapeutic actions
Competitively blocks muscarinic receptor sites: Bladder contraction is mediated by muscarinic receptors; blocking these receptors decreases bladder contraction and signs and symptoms of bladder overactivity.

Indications
- Treatment of overactive bladder with symptoms of urinary incontinence, urgency, and frequency in adults

Contraindications and cautions
- Contraindicated with known hypersensitivity to any component of the drug; urinary retention; gastric retention; uncontrolled narrow-angle glaucoma.
- Use cautiously with bladder outlet obstruction, decreased GI motility, controlled narrow-angle glaucoma, reduced hepatic function, myasthenia gravis, impaired renal function, pregnancy, lactation.

Available forms
ER tablets ⓒⓐⓝ—4, 8 mg

Dosages
Adults
4 mg/day PO; may be increased to a maximum of 8 mg/day if needed and tolerated.
Pediatric patients
Safety and efficacy not established.
Patients with renal impairment
No dosage adjustment needed in mild to moderate renal impairment. Limit dose to 4 mg/day PO in severe renal impairment.
Patients with hepatic impairment
Not recommended for patients with severe hepatic impairment.

Pharmacokinetics

Route	Onset	Peak
Oral	Rapid	5 hr

Metabolism: Hepatic; $T_{1/2}$: 7 hr
Distribution: May cross placenta; may enter breast milk
Excretion: Urine

Adverse effects
- **CNS:** Dry eyes, insomnia, drowsiness, blurred vision
- **CV:** Tachycardia
- **GI:** *Dry mouth, constipation,* dyspepsia, nausea, abdominal pain
- **GU:** Dysuria, urinary retention, UTI
- **Respiratory:** URI, cough, dry throat
- **Other:** Back pain, rash, decreased sweating

Interactions
✳ **Drug-drug** • Risk of increased serum levels and toxicity if given with any potent CYP3A4 inhibitor (ketoconazole, itraconazole, clarithromycin); dosage of fesoterodine should not exceed 4 mg/day and patient should be monitored closely • Increased risk of drowsiness if combined with alcohol; advise patient to avoid this combination

■ Nursing considerations
Assessment
History: Hypersensitivity to any component of the drug, urinary retention, gastric retention, narrow-angle glaucoma, bladder outlet obstruction, decreased GI motility, reduced hepatic function, myasthenia gravis, impaired renal function, pregnancy, lactation
Physical: IOP reading; orientation; skin color and lesions; R, adventitious sounds; P; bowel sounds; urinary output, prostate palpation, LFT, renal function tests

Interventions
- Monitor IOP before and periodically during treatment if patient has glaucoma.
- Administer tablet with water. Ensure that tablet is swallowed whole, not cut, crushed, or chewed.
- Provide frequent mouth hygiene and sugarless candies if dry mouth is a problem.
- Provide frequent small meals if GI upset is a problem.

F

- Arrange for safety precautions if visual changes are a problem.
- Monitor bowel function and institute a bowel program if constipation becomes an issue.
- Monitor patient in hot environments; decreased ability to sweat can lead to heat prostration.

Teaching points
- Take this drug with water once a day as prescribed. Swallow the tablet whole; do not cut, crush, or chew it.
- You may experience these side effects: Dry mouth (sucking sugarless candies, frequent mouth care may help), constipation (ensure adequate fluid intake and fiber in the diet, consult your health care provider if this becomes a serious problem), dry eyes (this effect may pass with time; consult with your health care provider for possible treatment if this becomes severe), blurred vision (avoid driving or operating dangerous machinery until you know how this drug will affect you), difficulty emptying the bladder (it may help to empty your bladder before taking each dose of the drug), decreased ability to sweat (use caution in hot environments, make sure you have plenty of fluids and take precautions to avoid overheating).
- Be aware that alcohol may increase the sedation effects of this drug. Avoid drinking alcohol while on this drug.
- Report tremors, restlessness, thoughts of suicide, increased depression, inability to stay alert, sudden behavioral changes.

▽ **fexofenadine hydrochloride**

(fecks oh fen' a deen)

Allegra, Allegra ODT, Children's Allegra Allergy, Children's Allegra Hives

PREGNANCY CATEGORY C

Drug class
Antihistamine (nonsedating type)

Therapeutic actions
Competitively blocks the effects of histamine at peripheral H_1-receptor sites; has no anticholinergic (atropine-like) or sedating effects.

Indications
- Symptomatic relief of symptoms associated with seasonal allergic rhinitis in adults and children 2 yr and older
- Chronic idiopathic urticaria in adults and children 6 mo and older

Contraindications and cautions
- Contraindicated with allergy to any antihistamines, pregnancy, lactation.
- Use cautiously with hepatic or renal impairment, in geriatric patients.

Available forms
Tablets—30, 60, 180 mg; suspension—6 mg/mL; orally disintegrating tablets—30 mg

Dosages
Adults and patients 12 yr and older
- *Allergic rhinitis:* 60 mg PO bid or 180 mg PO once daily; or 10 mL suspension PO bid.
- *Chronic idiopathic urticaria:* 60 mg PO bid or 180 mg PO once daily.

Pediatric patients 6–12 yr
- *Allergic rhinitis and chronic idiopathic urticaria:* 30 mg orally disintegrating tablet PO bid, or 5 mL suspension PO bid.

Pediatric patients 2–12 yr
- *Allergic rhinitis and chronic idiopathic urticaria:* 5 mL suspension PO bid.

Geriatric patients or patients with renal impairment
For geriatric patients or adults with renal impairment, use 60 mg PO daily. For children 2–12 yr with renal impairment, use 30 mg PO daily. For children 6 mo–2 yr with renal impairment, use 15 mg/day PO.

Pharmacokinetics

Route	Onset	Peak
Oral	Rapid	2.6 hr

Metabolism: Hepatic; $T_{1/2}$: 14.4 hr
Distribution: Crosses placenta; may enter breast milk
Excretion: Feces, urine

Adverse effects
- **CNS:** Fatigue, drowsiness
- **GI:** Nausea, dyspepsia
- **Other:** Dysmenorrhea, flulike symptoms

Adverse effects in *italics* are most common; those in **bold** are life-threatening. ⬛ Do not crush.

Interactions

❋ **Drug-drug** • Increased levels and possible toxicity with ketoconazole, itraconazole, erythromycin; fexofenadine dose may need to be decreased • Decreased effects when taken with antacids

■ Nursing considerations

Assessment

- **History:** Allergy to any antihistamines, renal impairment, pregnancy, lactation
- **Physical:** Mucous membranes, oropharynx, R, adventitious sounds; skin color, lesions; orientation, affect; renal function tests

Interventions

- Arrange for use of humidifier if thickening of secretions, nasal dryness become bothersome; encourage adequate intake of fluids.
- Provide supportive care for flulike symptoms.

Teaching points

- Avoid excessive dosage; take as prescribed.
- Do not take at the same time as antacids.
- Place orally disintegrating tablet on tongue; let disintegrate and then swallow with or without water.
- To maximize effects, take this medication in the morning before exposure to allergens.
- You may experience these side effects: Dizziness, sedation, drowsiness (use caution if driving or performing tasks that require alertness); thickening of bronchial secretions, dryness of nasal mucosa (use of a humidifier may help); menstrual irregularities; flulike symptoms (medication may be helpful).
- Report difficulty breathing, severe nausea, fever.

▽**fibrinogen concentrate, human**

See Appendix R, *Less commonly used drugs.*

▽**fidaxomicin**

(fah dax oh my' sin)

Dificid

PREGNANCY CATEGORY B

Drug class

Macrolide antibiotic

Therapeutic actions

Bactericidal; inhibits RNA synthesis by RNA polymerases, causing cell death. Works primarily against *Clostridium difficile* locally in the GI tract.

Indications

- Treatment of *C. difficile* diarrhea in patients 18 yr and older

Contraindications and cautions

- Contraindicated with history of serious hypersensitivity reactions to fidaxomicin.
- Use cautiously with pregnancy, lactation.

Available forms

Tablets—200 mg

Dosages

Adults

200 mg PO bid for 10 days without regard for food.

Pediatric patients

Safety and efficacy not established.

Pharmacokinetics

Drug undergoes minimal systemic absorption; exerts its effects locally in the GI tract.

Adverse effects

- **GI:** *Nausea, vomiting, abdominal pain,* **gastric hemorrhage,** flatulence, dyspepsia
- **Hematologic:** Anemia, neutropenia
- **Other:** Rash, pruritus, hyperglycemia

Interactions

None known.

■ Nursing considerations

Assessment

History: Hypersensitivity to components of drug; pregnancy, lactation
Physical: GI exam, skin status, stool culture, sensitivity tests

Interventions

- Obtain stool culture and arrange for sensitivity tests before beginning therapy. Ensure that appropriate infection is proven before fidaxomicin use to decrease the development of resistant strains.
- Do not use for systemic infections; drug is intended only for *C. difficile* diarrhea.

- Administer without regard to food.
- Encourage small, frequent meals and comfort measures if GI upset is severe.

Teaching points
- This drug has been prescribed specifically to treat the infection causing your diarrhea. It is not meant to treat any other infection, including viral infection.
- Take this drug twice a day, without regard for food. If you miss a dose, take the next dose as soon as you remember. Do not take more than two doses in one day.
- Take the full, prescribed dose of this drug. You may begin to feel better after you start treatment, but it is very important to continue the full course of drug therapy. Not completing the full prescription can lead to ineffective treatment and the development of resistant strains that might not be treatable.
- You may experience these side effects: GI upset, vomiting, nausea (small frequent meals may help). Notify your health care provider if these become severe.
- Report severe vomiting, bloody diarrhea, rash.

▷ filgrastim (granulocyte colony-stimulating factor, G-CSF)
*(fill **grass' stim**)*

Neupogen

PREGNANCY CATEGORY C

Drug class
Colony-stimulating factor

Therapeutic actions
Human granulocyte colony-stimulating factor produced by recombinant DNA technology; increases the production of neutrophils within the bone marrow with little effect on the production of other hematopoietic cells.

Indications
- To decrease the incidence of infection in patients with nonmyeloid malignancies receiving myelosuppressive anticancer drugs associated with a significant incidence of severe neutropenia with fever
- To reduce the time to neutrophil recovery and duration of fever, following induction or consolidation chemotherapy treatment of acute myeloid leukemia
- To reduce the duration of neutropenia following bone marrow transplant
- Treatment of severe chronic neutropenia
- Mobilization of hematopoietic progenitor cells into the blood for leukapheresis collection
- Orphan drug uses: Treatment of myelodysplastic syndrome, aplastic anemia, graft failure after bone marrow transplant, hairy cell leukemia, AIDS–drug-induced neutropenias, neutropenic fever

Contraindications and cautions
- Contraindicated with hypersensitivity to *Escherichia coli* products.
- Use cautiously with lactation, pregnancy.

Available forms
Injection—300 mcg/mL, 480 mcg/1.6 mL; prefilled syringes—300 mcg/0.5 mL, 480 mcg/0.8 mL.

Dosages
Adults
Starting dose is 5 mcg/kg/day subcutaneously or IV as a single daily injection. May be increased in increments of 5 mcg/kg for each chemotherapy cycle; 4–8 mcg/kg/day is usually effective.
- *Bone marrow transplant:* 10 mcg/kg/day IV or continuous subcutaneous infusion.
- *Severe chronic neutropenia:* 6 mcg/kg subcutaneously bid (congenital neutropenia); 5 mcg/kg/day subcutaneously as single injection (idiopathic or cyclic neutropenia).
- *Mobilization for harvesting:* 10 mcg/kg/day subcutaneously at least 4 days before first leukapheresis; continue to last leukapheresis.

Pediatric patients
Safety and efficacy not established.

Pharmacokinetics

Route	Peak	Duration
Subcut.	8 hr	4 days
IV	2 hr	4 days

Metabolism: Unknown; $T_{1/2}$: 210–231 min
Distribution: Crosses placenta; may enter breast milk
Excretion: Unknown

▼ IV FACTS

Preparation: No special preparation required. Refrigerate; avoid shaking. Before injection, allow to warm to room temperature. Discard vial after one use, and do not reenter vial; discard any vial that has been at room temperature longer than 24 hr.
Infusion: Inject directly IV slowly over 15–30 min, or inject slowly into tubing of running IV over 4–24 hr.
Incompatibilities: Do not mix in solutions other than D_5W. Incompatible with numerous drugs in solution; check manufacturer's details before any combination.

Adverse effects
- **CNS:** Headache, fever, generalized weakness, fatigue
- **Dermatologic:** *Alopecia,* rash, mucositis
- **GI:** *Nausea, vomiting,* stomatitis, anorexia, *diarrhea,* constipation
- **Other:** *Bone pain,* generalized pain, sore throat, cough

■ Nursing considerations
Assessment
- **History:** Hypersensitivity to *E. coli* products, pregnancy, lactation
- **Physical:** Skin color, lesions, hair; T; abdominal examination, status of mucous membranes; CBC with differential, platelets

Interventions
- Obtain CBC and platelet count before and twice weekly during therapy; doses may be increased after chemotherapy cycles according to the duration and severity of bone marrow suppression.
- ⊗ *Warning* Do not give within 24 hr before and after chemotherapy.
- Give daily for up to 2 wk until the neutrophil count is 10,000/mm³; discontinue therapy if this number is exceeded.
- Store in refrigerator; allow to warm to room temperature before use; if vial is at room temperature for longer than 24 hr, discard. Use each vial for one dose; do not reenter the vial. Discard any unused drug.

- Do not shake vial before use. If subcutaneous dose exceeds 1 mL, consider using two sites.

Teaching points
- Store drug in refrigerator; do not shake vial. Each vial can be used only once; do not reuse syringes or needles (proper container for disposal will be provided). Another person should be instructed in the proper administration technique. Use sterile technique.
- Avoid exposure to infection while you are receiving this drug (avoid crowds and people known to have infections).
- Keep appointments for frequent blood tests to evaluate effects of drug on your blood count.
- You may experience these side effects: Bone pain (analgesia may be ordered), nausea and vomiting (eat frequent small meals), loss of hair (it is very important to cover head in extreme temperatures).
- Report fever, chills, severe bone pain, sore throat, weakness, pain or swelling at injection site.

▽ finasteride
(fin as' teh ride)

Propecia, Proscar

PREGNANCY CATEGORY X

Drug class
Androgen hormone inhibitor

Therapeutic actions
Inhibits the intracellular enzyme that converts testosterone into a potent androgen (DHT); does not affect androgen receptors in the body; the prostate gland depends on DHT for its development and maintenance.

Indications
- *Proscar:* Treatment of symptomatic BPH; most effective with long-term use; reduces the need for prostate surgery and reduces the risk of urinary retention; with doxazosin, to reduce the risk of progression of BPH symptoms
- *Propecia:* Prevention of male pattern baldness (androgenetic alopecia) in patients with family history or early signs of loss

F

- Unlabeled uses: Adjuvant monotherapy following radical prostatectomy; prevention of the progression of first-stage prostate cancer; hirsutism; male chronic pelvic pain syndrome

Contraindications and cautions
- Contraindicated with allergy to finasteride or any component of the product, pregnancy, lactation.
- Use cautiously with hepatic impairment.

Available forms
Tablets—1 mg (*Propecia*), 5 mg (*Proscar*)

Dosages
Adults
- *BPH:* 5 mg daily PO with or without meals; may take 6–12 mo for response (*Proscar*).
- *Male pattern baldness:* 1 mg/day PO for 3 mo or more before benefit is observed (*Propecia*).

Pediatric patients
Safety and efficacy not established.

Geriatric patients or patients with hepatic insufficiency
No dosage adjustment is needed.

Pharmacokinetics

Route	Onset	Peak	Duration
Oral	Rapid	8 hr	24 hr

Metabolism: Hepatic; $T_{1/2}$: 6 hr
Distribution: Crosses placenta; may enter breast milk (not used in women)
Excretion: Feces, urine

Adverse effects
- **GI:** Abdominal upset
- **GU:** *Impotence, decreased libido,* decreased volume of ejaculation
- **Other:** Gynecomastia

Interactions
❋ **Drug-lab test** • Decreased PSA levels when measured; false decrease does not mean patient is free of risk of prostate cancer

■ Nursing considerations
Assessment
- **History:** Allergy to finasteride or any component, hepatic impairment, pregnancy, lactation

- **Physical:** Liver evaluation, abdominal examination; renal function tests, normal urine output, prostate examination

Interventions
- Confirm that problem is BPH, and other disorders (prostate cancer, infection, strictures, hypotonic bladder) have been ruled out.
- Administer without regard to meals; protect container from light.
- Arrange for regular follow-up, including prostate examination, PSA levels, and evaluation of urine flow. Be aware that patient could be at increased risk for aggressive prostate cancer; monitor closely.
- Monitor urine flow and output; increase in urine flow may not occur in all situations.
- ⊗ *Warning* Do not allow pregnant women to handle crushed or broken tablets because of risk of inadvertent absorption, adversely affecting the fetus.
- Alert patient that libido may be decreased as well as the volume of ejaculate; usually reversible when the drug is stopped.

Teaching points
- Take this drug once a day without regard to meals; protect from light.
- Have regular medical follow-up to evaluate your response. Your health care provider will monitor your liver and kidney function as well as prostate-specific antigen levels.
- This drug has serious adverse effects on unborn babies. Do not allow a pregnant woman to handle the tablet if it is crushed or broken.
- You may experience these side effects: Loss of libido, impotence, decreased amount of ejaculate (usually reversible when the drug is stopped); breast enlargement, tenderness.
- Report inability to void, groin pain, sore throat, fever, weakness, changes in breast tissue.

▽ fingolimod
(fin gol ih mod)

Gilenya

PREGNANCY CATEGORY C

Drug classes
MS drug
Sphingosine 1-phosphate receptor modulator

Adverse effects in *italics* are most common; those in **bold** are life-threatening. ⬛ Do not crush.

Therapeutic actions

By blocking sphingosine 1-phosphate receptors, drug blocks the capacity of lymphocytes to egress from lymph nodes, reducing the number of lymphocytes in peripheral blood. Mechanism of action in MS is not known; thought to be related to the reduction of lymphocyte migration into the CNS.

Indications

- Treatment of relapsing forms of MS to reduce the frequency of clinical exacerbations and to delay the accumulation of physical disability

Contraindications and cautions

- Contraindicated with known hypersensitivity to components of drug; lactation.
- Use cautiously with hepatic impairment, slow heart rate, active infection, diabetes with macular edema or uveitis, hypertension, preexisting or recent heart conditions, concurrent use of antiarrhythmics, pregnancy.

Available forms

Capsules—0.5 mg

Dosages
Adults

0.5 mg/day PO; monitor patient for bradycardia for at least 6 hr after first dose.

Pediatric patients younger than 18 yr

Safety and efficacy not established.

Pharmacokinetics

Route	Onset	Peak
Oral	Slow	12–16 hr

Metabolism: Hepatic; $T_{1/2}$: 6–9 days
Distribution: May cross placenta; may enter breast milk
Excretion: Urine

Adverse effects

- **CNS:** *Headache,* dizziness, paresthesia, migraine, asthenia, macular edema, *depression*
- **CV:** Bradycardia, *hypertension*
- **GI:** *Diarrhea, liver enzyme elevation*
- **Respiratory:** Bronchitis, sinusitis, decreased lung capacity, *cough, dyspnea*
- **Other:** Infections, *influenza, back pain*

Interactions

✳ **Drug-drug** • Possible increased risk of bradycardia if taken with Class 1A or III antiarrhythmics (amiodarone, quinidine, sotalol), beta blockers, calcium channel blockers; closely monitor patients receiving this combination • Increased risk of toxic effects if combined with ketoconazole; monitor patient closely if this combination must be used • Decreased effectiveness of vaccines during and for 2 months after discontinuing therapy; avoid use of live vaccines • Increased risk of infection if combined with antineoplastic, immunosuppressive, or immunomodulating therapy; monitor patient closely and protect from infection

■ Nursing considerations
Assessment

History: Known hypersensitivity to components of drug, lactation, hepatic impairment, slow heart rate, active infection, diabetes with macular edema or uveitis, hypertension, pregnancy

Physical: T; orientation, affect, eye exam; P, BP; R, adventitious sounds, spirometry; GI exam; liver function tests

Interventions

- Administer at about the same time each day without regard to meals.
- Monitor patient for bradycardia for at least 6 hr after first dose; bradycardia may last up to 20 hr in some cases. If drug is discontinued and restarted, observe patient again at the first dose.
- Arrange for pretreatment and periodic ophthalmic evaluation because of the risk of macular edema.
- Arrange for spirometry studies if patient experiences shortness of breath or dyspnea during therapy.
- Help breast-feeding patient find an alternative method of feeding the baby during therapy.
- Encourage women of childbearing age to use effective contraception during and for 2 mo after completion of therapy.
- Protect patient from exposure to infections and encourage complying with all cancer screening tests as appropriate; patient is at increased risk for infections and cancer development.

- Warn patient not to have vaccines while taking this drug and for 2 months after therapy ends.

Teaching points

- Take this drug without regard to meals. Take it daily at about the same time each day. You will need to be observed for at least 6 hours after taking the first dose because the drug may cause your heart rate to become very slow.
- Do not take this drug if you are pregnant; it can seriously affect the fetus or even cause fetal death. You should use a barrier contraceptive while taking this drug. If you become pregnant, consult your health care provider immediately.
- If you are breast-feeding, you should use another method of feeding the baby during therapy because this drug could cause serious adverse effects in the baby.
- You may experience these side effects: Infection (avoid exposure to infections, crowded areas, and people you know to be ill; wear protective gloves when digging in the dirt); cancer (because of the suppression of your immune system, you may be at increased risk for cancer development; make sure you follow through with all cancer screening); dizziness (avoid driving a car or using dangerous machinery if this occurs); diarrhea (small, frequent meals may help; medication may be available to relieve these symptoms); eye changes (macular edema may occur; report any changes in vision); difficulty breathing (take frequent rest periods; report any difficulty breathing).
- Report severe diarrhea, pregnancy, vision changes, shortness of breath, very slow heart rate, signs of infection (fever, muscle aches and pains), abdominal pain accompanied by fatigue, anorexia, dark urine, yellowing of the eyes or skin.

▽flavoxate hydrochloride

(fla vox' ate)

PREGNANCY CATEGORY B

Drug classes

Parasympathetic blocker
Urinary antispasmodic

Therapeutic actions

Counteracts smooth muscle spasm of the urinary tract by relaxing the detrusor and other muscles through action at the parasympathetic receptors; has local anesthetic and analgesic properties.

Indications

- Symptomatic relief of dysuria, urgency, nocturia, suprapubic pain, frequency and incontinence due to cystitis, prostatitis, urethritis, urethrocystitis, urethrotrigonitis

Contraindications and cautions

- Contraindicated with allergy to flavoxate, pyloric or duodenal obstruction, obstructive intestinal lesions or ileus, achalasia, GI hemorrhage, obstructive uropathies of the lower urinary tract.
- Use cautiously with glaucoma, pregnancy, lactation.

Available forms

Tablets—100 mg

Dosages

Adults and patients 12 yr and older
100–200 mg PO tid or qid. Reduce dose when symptoms improve. Use up to 1,200 mg/day in severe urinary urgency following pelvic radiotherapy.
Pediatric patients younger than 12 yr
Safety and efficacy not established.

Pharmacokinetics

Route	Onset	Duration
Oral	Slow	6 hr

Metabolism: $T_{1/2}$: 2–3 hr
Distribution: May cross placenta
Excretion: Feces, urine

Adverse effects

- **CNS:** *Nervousness, vertigo, headache, drowsiness,* mental confusion, hyperpyrexia, *blurred vision,* increased ocular tension, disturbance in accommodation
- **CV:** Tachycardia, palpitations
- **Dermatologic:** Urticaria, dermatoses
- **GI:** *Nausea, vomiting, dry mouth*
- **GU:** Dysuria
- **Hematologic: Eosinophilia, leukopenia**

Adverse effects in *italics* are most common; those in **bold** are life-threatening. ▣ Do not crush.

Interactions

✳ **Drug-drug** • Risk of toxic effects if combined with anticholinergic drugs • Loss of effectiveness of cholinergic drugs such as Alzheimer disease drugs if combined

■ Nursing considerations
Assessment

• **History:** Allergy to flavoxate, pyloric or duodenal obstruction, obstructive intestinal lesions or ileus, achalasia, GI hemorrhage, obstructive uropathies of the lower urinary tract, glaucoma, pregnancy, lactation
• **Physical:** Skin color, lesions; T; orientation, affect, reflexes, ophthalmic examination, ocular pressure measurement; P; bowel sounds, oral mucous membranes; CBC, stool guaiac

Interventions

• Arrange for definitive treatment of UTIs causing the symptoms being managed by flavoxate.
• Arrange for ophthalmic examination before and during therapy.

Teaching points

• Take drug three or four times a day.
• This drug is meant to relieve the symptoms you are experiencing; other medications will be used to treat the cause.
• You may experience these side effects: Dry mouth, GI upset (suck on sugarless candies and use frequent mouth care); drowsiness, blurred vision (avoid driving or performing tasks requiring alertness).
• Report blurred vision, fever, rash, nausea, vomiting.

▽ flecainide acetate
(fle ka' nide)

Tambocor

PREGNANCY CATEGORY C

Drug class
Antiarrhythmic

Therapeutic actions
Type 1c antiarrhythmic: Acts selectively to depress fast sodium channels, decreasing the height and rate of rise of cardiac action potentials and slowing conduction in all parts of the heart.

Indications

• Prevention and treatment of life-threatening ventricular arrhythmias, such as sustained ventricular tachycardia (not recommended for less severe ventricular arrhythmias)
• Prevention of paroxysmal atrial fibrillation or flutter (PAF) associated with symptoms and paroxysmal supraventricular tachycardias (PSVT), including atrioventricular nodal and atrioventricular re-entrant tachycardia; other supraventricular tachycardias of unspecified mechanism with disabling symptoms in patients without structural heart disease

Contraindications and cautions

• Contraindicated with allergy to flecainide; heart failure; cardiogenic shock; cardiac conduction abnormalities (heart blocks of any kind, unless an artificial pacemaker is present to maintain heartbeat); MI; sick sinus syndrome; lactation; pregnancy.
• Use cautiously with endocardial pacemaker (permanent or temporary—stimulus parameters may need to be increased); heart failure; hepatic or renal disease; potassium imbalance.

Available forms
Tablets—50, 100, 150 mg

Dosages
Evaluation with close monitoring of cardiac response necessary for determining the correct dosage.
Adults

• *PSVT and PAF:* Starting dose of 50 mg every 12 hr PO; may be increased in increments of 50 mg bid every 4 days until efficacy is achieved; maximum dose is 300 mg/day.
• *Sustained ventricular tachycardia:* 100 mg every 12 hr PO. Increase in 50-mg increments twice a day every fourth day until efficacy is achieved. Maximum dose is 400 mg/day.
• *Transfer to flecainide:* Allow at least 2–4 plasma half-lives to elapse after other antiarrhythmic drugs discontinued before starting flecainide. Consider hospitalization because withdrawal of a previous

F

antiarrhythmic is likely to produce life-threatening arrhythmias.

Pediatric patients
Safety and efficacy in patients younger than 18 yr have not been established.

Patients with renal impairment
Initial dose, 100 mg daily PO or 50 mg every 12 hr. Wait about 4 days to reach a steady state, then increase dose cautiously.

Geriatric patients
Elimination may be slower. Usual dose should be used in patients up to 80 yr.

Pharmacokinetics

Route	Onset	Peak	Duration
Oral	30–60 min	3 hr	24 hr

Metabolism: Hepatic; $T_{1/2}$: 20 hr
Distribution: Crosses placenta; may enter breast milk
Excretion: Feces, urine

Adverse effects

- **CNS:** *Dizziness, fatigue, drowsiness, visual changes, headache,* tinnitus, paresthesias
- **CV:** *Cardiac arrhythmias,* heart failure, slowed cardiac conduction, *palpitations, chest pain*
- **GI:** *Nausea, vomiting, abdominal pain, constipation,* diarrhea
- **GU:** Polyuria, urinary retention, decreased libido
- **Other:** *Dyspnea,* sweating, hot flashes, night sweats, **leukopenia**

Interactions

✳ **Drug-drug** ⊗ *Warning* Risk of marked drop in cardiac output if combined with disopyramide or verapamil; avoid these combinations if possible.
- Risk of increased flecainide levels if combined with amiodarone, cimetidine, propranolol

■ Nursing considerations
Assessment

- **History:** Allergy to flecainide, heart failure, MI, cardiogenic shock, cardiac conduction abnormalities, sick sinus syndrome, endocardial pacemaker, hepatic or renal disease, potassium imbalance, lactation, pregnancy

- **Physical:** Weight; orientation, reflexes, vision; P, BP, auscultation, ECG, edema, R, adventitious sounds; bowel sounds, liver evaluation; urinalysis, CBC, serum electrolytes, LFTs, renal function tests

Interventions

⊗ **Black box warning** In patients with recent MI or chronic atrial fibrillation, treatment increases risk of nonfatal cardiac arrest and death.
- Monitor patient response carefully, especially when beginning therapy.
- Reduce dosage in patients with renal disease or hepatic failure.
- Check serum K⁺ levels before giving.

⊗ **Black box warning** Monitor cardiac rhythm carefully; risk of potentially fatal proarrhythmias.

⊗ *Warning* Evaluate for therapeutic serum levels of 0.2–1 mcg/mL.

⊗ *Warning* Keep life support equipment, including pacemaker, readily available in case serious CVS, CNS effects occur—also keep dopamine, dobutamine, isoproterenol, or other positive inotropics nearby.

Teaching points

- You will need frequent monitoring of cardiac rhythm.
- Do not stop taking this drug for any reason without checking with your health care provider. Drug is taken at 12-hour intervals; work out a schedule so you take the drug as prescribed without waking up at night.
- Return for regular follow-up visits to check your heart rhythm and have a blood test to check your blood levels of this drug.
- You may experience these side effects: Drowsiness, dizziness, numbness, visual disturbances (avoid driving or using dangerous machinery); nausea, vomiting (frequent small meals may help); diarrhea, polyuria; sweating, night sweats, hot flashes, loss of libido (reversible after stopping the drug); palpitations.
- Report swelling of ankles or fingers, palpitations, fainting, chest pain.

▽ **floxuridine**

See Appendix R, *Less commonly used drugs.*

Adverse effects in italics *are most common; those in* **bold** *are life-threatening.* ⊙ *Do not crush.*

▷fluconazole

*(floo **kon'** a zole)*

Apo-Fluconazole (CAN), Diflucan,
Gen-Fluconazole (CAN), PMS-
Fluconazole (CAN)

PREGNANCY CATEGORY D

Drug class
Antifungal

Therapeutic actions
Binds to sterols in the fungal cell membrane,
changing membrane permeability; fungicidal or fungistatic depending on concentration
and organism.

Indications
- Treatment of oropharyngeal, esophageal,
  vaginal, and systemic candidiasis, UTI and
  peritonitis caused by *Candida*
- Treatment of cryptococcal meningitis
- Prophylaxis of candidiasis in bone marrow
  transplants

Contraindications and cautions
- Contraindicated with hypersensitivity to fluconazole, lactation.
- Use cautiously with renal or hepatic impairment.

Available forms
Tablets—50, 100, 150, 200 mg; powder for
oral suspension—10, 40 mg/mL; injection—
2 mg/mL

Dosages
Individualize dosage; same for oral or IV routes
because of rapid and almost complete absorption.

Adults
- *Oropharyngeal candidiasis:* 200 mg PO or
  IV on the first day, followed by 100 mg daily. Continue treatment for at least 2 wk to
  decrease likelihood of relapse.
- *Esophageal candidiasis:* 200 mg PO or IV
  on the first day, followed by 100 mg daily.
  Dosage up to 400 mg/day may be used in
  severe cases. Treat for a minimum of 3 wk;
  at least 2 wk after resolution.
- *Vaginal candidiasis:* 150 mg PO as a single dose.

- *Systemic candidiasis:* 400 mg PO or IV
  daily.
- Candida *UTI and peritonitis:* 50–200
  mg/day PO.
- *Cryptococcal meningitis:* 400 mg PO or IV
  on the first day, followed by 200 mg daily.
  400 mg daily may be needed. Continue treatment for 10–12 wk after cultures of CSF become negative.
- *Suppression of cryptococcal meningitis in
  AIDS patients:* 200 mg daily PO or IV.
- *Prevention of candidiasis in bone marrow transplants:* 400 mg PO daily for several days before onset of neutropenia and for
  7 days after neutrophil count rises above 1,000
  cells/mm^3.

Pediatric patients
Maximum daily dosage for children is 600
mg/day.
- *Oropharyngeal candidiasis:* 6 mg/kg PO
  or IV on the first day, followed by 3 mg/kg
  once daily for at least 2 wk.
- *Esophageal candidiasis:* 6 mg/kg PO or IV
  on the first day, followed by 3 mg/kg once
  daily. Treat for a minimum of 3 wk; at least
  2 wk after resolution.
- *Systemic* Candida *infections:* Daily doses of
  6–12 mg/kg/day PO or IV.
- *Cryptococcal meningitis:* 12 mg/kg PO or
  IV on the first day, followed by 6 mg/kg once
  daily. Continue treatment for 10–12 wk after cultures of CSF become negative.
- *Suppression of cryptococcal meningitis
  in children with AIDS:* 6 mg/kg daily PO
  or IV.

Patients with renal impairment
Initial dose of 50–400 mg PO or IV. If creatinine clearance is greater than 50 mL/min, use
100% of recommended dose; for creatinine
clearance less than or equal to 50 mL/min,
use 50% of recommended dose; for patients on
hemodialysis, use one full dose after each dialysis.

Pharmacokinetics

Route	Onset	Peak	Duration
Oral	Slow	1–2 hr	2–4 days
IV	Rapid	1 hr	2–4 days

Metabolism: Hepatic; $T_{1/2}$: 30 hr
Distribution: Crosses placenta; may enter
breast milk
Excretion: Urine

▼ IV FACTS

Preparation: Do not remove overwrap until ready for use. Inner bag maintains sterility of product. Do not use plastic containers in series connections. Tear overwrap down side at slit, and remove solution container. Some opacity of plastic may occur; check for minute leaks, squeezing bag firmly. Discard solution if any leaks are found.

Infusion: Infuse at a maximum rate of 200 mg/hr given as a continuous infusion.

Incompatibilities: Do not add any supplementary medications.

Adverse effects

- **CNS:** *Headache*
- **GI:** *Nausea, vomiting, diarrhea, abdominal pain,* AST/ALT elevations
- **Other:** Rash

Interactions

✳ **Drug-drug** • Increased serum levels and therefore therapeutic and toxic effects of cyclosporine, phenytoin, benzodiazepines, oral hypoglycemics, warfarin anticoagulants, zidovudine • Decreased serum levels with rifampin, cimetidine

■ Nursing considerations

Assessment

- **History:** Hypersensitivity to fluconazole and other azoles, renal impairment, lactation, pregnancy
- **Physical:** Skin color, lesions; T; injection site; orientation, reflexes, affect; bowel sounds; LFTs, renal function tests; CBC and differential; culture of area involved

Interventions

- Culture infection before therapy; begin treatment before lab results are returned.
- Decrease dosage in cases of renal failure.
- Infuse IV only; not intended for IM or subcutaneous use.
- Do not add supplement medication to fluconazole.
- Administer through sterile equipment at a maximum rate of 200 mg/hr given as a continuous infusion.

⊗ *Warning* Monitor renal function tests weekly, discontinue or decrease dosage of drug at any sign of increased renal toxicity. Monitor liver function tests monthly during therapy.

Teaching points

- Drug may be given orally or IV as needed. The drug will need to be taken for the full course and may need to be taken long term.
- Use hygiene measures to prevent reinfection or spread of infection.
- Arrange for frequent follow-up while you are taking this drug. Be sure to keep all appointments, including those for blood tests.
- You may experience these side effects: Nausea, vomiting, diarrhea (frequent small meals may help); headache (analgesics may be ordered).
- Report rash, changes in stool or urine color, difficulty breathing, increased tears or salivation.

▷ flucytosine
(5-FC, 5-fluorocytosine)
(floo sye' toe seen)

Ancobon

PREGNANCY CATEGORY C

Drug class

Antifungal

Therapeutic actions

Affects cell membranes of susceptible fungi to cause fungus death; exact mechanism of action is not understood.

Indications

- Treatment of serious infections caused by susceptible strains of *Candida, Cryptococcus*

Contraindications and cautions

- Contraindicated with allergy to flucytosine, pregnancy, lactation.
- Use cautiously with renal impairment (drug accumulation and toxicity may occur), hepatic impairment, bone marrow depression.

Available forms

Capsules—250, 500 mg

Dosages

Adults
50–150 mg/kg/day PO at 6-hr intervals.
Pediatric patients
Safety and efficacy not established.

Adverse effects in *italics* are most common; those in **bold** are life-threatening. ⊞ Do not crush.

Patients with renal impairment
Adjust dosing interval based on creatinine clearance: maintain blood levels below 100 mcg/mL.

CrCl (mg/mL)	Dosing interval
20–40	Every 12 hr
10–20	Every 24 hr
Less than 10	Every 24–48 hr

Pharmacokinetics

Route	Onset	Peak	Duration
Oral	Varies	2 hr	10–12 hr

Metabolism: Not significantly metabolized; $T_{1/2}$: 2–5 hr
Distribution: Crosses placenta; may enter breast milk
Excretion: Urine

Adverse effects

- **CNS:** Confusion, hallucinations, headache, sedation, vertigo
- **CV: Cardiac arrest,** chest pain
- **Dermatologic:** *Rash*
- **GI:** *Nausea, vomiting, diarrhea*
- **Hematologic:** *Anemia,* **leukopenia, thrombocytopenia,** elevation of liver enzymes, BUN, creatinine
- **Respiratory: Respiratory arrest,** shortness of breath

■ **Nursing considerations**
Assessment
- **History:** Allergy to flucytosine, renal impairment, bone marrow depression, lactation, pregnancy
- **Physical:** Skin color, lesions; orientation, reflexes, affect; bowel sounds, liver evaluation; LFTs, renal function tests; CBC and differential; serum flucytosine levels (in patients with renal impairment)

Interventions
- Administer capsules a few at a time over a 15-min period to decrease the GI upset and diarrhea.
- Monitor LFTs, renal function tests and hematologic function periodically throughout treatment.

⊗ **Black box warning** Monitor serum flucytosine levels in patients with renal impairment (levels higher than 100 mcg/mL associated with toxicity).

Teaching points
- Take the capsules a few at a time over a 15-minute period to decrease GI upset.
- You may experience these side effects: Nausea, vomiting, diarrhea (take capsules a few at a time over 15 minutes); sedation, dizziness, confusion (avoid driving or performing tasks that require alertness).
- Report rash, severe nausea, vomiting, diarrhea, fever, sore throat, unusual bleeding or bruising.

DANGEROUS DRUG

▷**fludarabine phosphate**
*(floo **dar'** a been)*

Fludara, Oforta⬛

PREGNANCY CATEGORY D

Drug classes
Antimetabolite
Antineoplastic

Therapeutic actions
Inhibits DNA polymerase alpha, ribonucleotide reductase and DNA primase, which inhibits DNA synthesis and prevents cell replication.

Indications
- Chronic lymphocytic leukemia (CLL); unresponsive B-cell CLL or no progress during treatment with at least one standard regimen that contains an alkylating drug

Contraindications and cautions
- Contraindicated with allergy to fludarabine or any component, lactation, pregnancy, severe bone marrow depression.
- Use cautiously with renal impairment.

Available forms
Tablets⬛—10 mg; powder for reconstitution—50 mg; injection—25 mg/mL

Dosages
Adults
40 mg/m² PO or 25 mg/m² IV over 30 min for 5 consecutive days. Begin each 5-day course every 28 days. Recommendation is to use three additional cycles after a maximal response is achieved, then to discontinue drug.

Patients with renal impairment
Creatinine clearance of 30–70 mL/min, reduce dosage by 20%; creatinine clearance of less than 30 mL/min, do not administer IV form, and reduce dose by 50% for oral doses.

Pharmacokinetics

Route	Onset	Peak
IV	Rapid	1–2 hr

Metabolism: Hepatic; $T_{1/2}$: 10 hr
Distribution: Crosses placenta; enters breast milk
Excretion: Urine

▼ IV FACTS

Preparation: Reconstitute with 2 mL of sterile water for injection; the solid cake should dissolve in less than 15 sec; each mL of resulting solution will contain 25 mg fludarabine; may be further diluted in 100 or 125 mL of 5% dextrose injection or 0.9% sodium chloride; use within 8 hr of reconstitution; discard after that time. Store unreconstituted drug in refrigerator.
Infusion: Infuse slowly over no less than 30 min.

Adverse effects

- **CNS:** *Weakness, paresthesia, headache, visual disturbance,* hearing loss, sleep disorder, depression, **CNS toxicity including blindness, coma, death**
- **CV:** *Edema,* angina
- **Dermatologic:** *Rash, pruritus,* seborrhea
- **GI:** *Diarrhea, anorexia, nausea, vomiting, stomatitis,* esophagopharyngitis, GI bleeding, mucositis
- **GU:** Dysuria, urinary infection, hematuria, **renal failure**
- **Hematologic:** *Bone marrow toxicity,* **autoimmune hemolytic anemia**
- **Respiratory:** *Cough, pneumonia, dyspnea, sinusitis,* URI, epistaxis, bronchitis, hypoxia, **pulmonary toxicity**
- **Other:** *Fever, chills, fatigue, infection, pain, malaise,* diaphoresis, hemorrhage, myalgia, arthralgia, osteoporosis, **tumor lysis syndrome**

Interactions

✴ **Drug-drug** • Risk of fatal pulmonary toxicity with pentostatin; avoid this combination

■ Nursing considerations

Assessment

- **History:** Allergy to fludarabine or any component, lactation, pregnancy, severe bone marrow depression, renal impairment
- **Physical:** Weight; T; skin lesions, color, edema; hair; vision, speech, orientation, reflexes, sensation; R, adventitious sounds; mucous membranes, liver evaluation, abdominal examination; CBC, differential; Hgb, Hct, uric acid, LFTs, renal function tests; urinalysis, chest X-ray

Interventions

- Evaluate hematologic status before therapy and before each dose.
- ⊗ **Black box warning** Discontinue therapy if any sign of toxicity occurs (CNS complaints, stomatitis, esophagopharyngitis, rapidly falling WBC count, intractable vomiting, diarrhea, GI ulceration and bleeding, thrombocytopenia, hemorrhage, hemolytic anemia); serious to life-threatening infections have occurred. Consult physician.
- Do not crush tablets. Avoid direct contact with skin or mucous membranes.
- Caution patient to avoid pregnancy while taking this drug.

Teaching points

- Prepare a calendar of treatment days.
- If using oral form, do not cut or crush tablets. Avoid direct contact of skin or mucous membranes with tablets. Wear gloves when handling tablets. If contact occurs, wash with soap and water; if eyes are involved, wash with flowing water for at least 15 minutes. Consult health care provider for proper disposal of unused drug.
- Use birth control while taking this drug; may cause birth defects or miscarriages.
- Have frequent, regular medical follow-up visits, including blood tests.
- You may experience these side effects: Nausea, vomiting, loss of appetite (medication; eat frequent small meals; maintain your nutrition while you are taking this drug); headache, fatigue, malaise, weakness, lethargy (avoid driving or operating dangerous machinery); mouth sores (practice frequent mouth care); diarrhea; increased susceptibility to infection (avoid crowds, exposure to infection; report any sign of infection—fever, fatigue).

Adverse effects in *italics* are most common; those in **bold** are life-threatening. ⊕⊞ Do not crush.

- Report black, tarry stools; fever; chills; sore throat; unusual bleeding or bruising; chest pain; mouth sores; changes in vision; dizziness.

▷fludrocortisone acetate

See Appendix R, *Less commonly used drugs.*

▷flumazenil
*(floo **maz**' eh nill)*

Anexate (CAN), Romazicon

PREGNANCY CATEGORY C

Drug classes
Antidote
Benzodiazepine receptor antagonist

Therapeutic actions
Antagonizes the actions of benzodiazepines on the CNS and inhibits activity at GABA-benzodiazepine receptor sites.

Indications
- Complete or partial reversal of the sedative effects of benzodiazepines when general anesthesia has been induced or maintained with them, and when sedation has been produced for diagnostic and therapeutic procedures
- Management of benzodiazepine overdose

Contraindications and cautions
- Contraindicated with hypersensitivity to flumazenil or benzodiazepines; patients who have been given benzodiazepines to control potentially life-threatening conditions; patients showing signs of serious cyclic antidepressant overdose.
- Use cautiously with history of seizures, hepatic impairment, panic disorders, head injury, history of drug or alcohol dependence, pregnancy, lactation.

Available forms
Injection—0.1 mg/mL

Dosages
Use smallest effective dose possible.

Adults
- *Reversal of conscious sedation or in general anesthesia:* Give initial dose of 0.2 mg (2 mL) IV over 15 sec then wait 45 sec; if ineffectual, repeat dose at 60-sec intervals. Maximum cumulative dose of 1 mg (10 mL).
- *Management of suspected benzodiazepine overdose:* Give initial dose of 0.2 mg IV over 30 sec; repeat with 0.3 mg IV every 30 sec; can give further doses of 0.5 mg over 30 sec at 1-min intervals, up to a maximum cumulative dose of 3 mg.

Pediatric patients younger than 1 yr
Safety and efficacy not established.

Pediatric patients older than 1 yr
- *Reversal of conscious sedation with benzodiazepines:* 0.01 mg/kg (up to 0.2 mg) IV over 15 sec; if ineffectual after 45 sec, repeat dose at 60-sec intervals. Maximum cumulative dose, 0.05 mg/kg or 1 mg, whichever is lowest.

Pharmacokinetics

Route	Onset	Peak	Duration
IV	1–2 min	6–10 min	72 hr

Metabolism: Hepatic; $T_{1/2}$: 54 min
Distribution: Crosses placenta; may enter breast milk
Excretion: Unknown

▼ IV FACTS
Preparation: Can be drawn into syringe with D_5W, lactated Ringer and normal saline solutions. Discard within 24 hr if mixed in solution. Do not remove from vial until ready for use.

Infusion: Infuse slowly over 15 sec for general anesthesia, over 30 sec for overdose. To reduce pain of injection, administer through a freely running IV infusion in a large vein.

Compatibilities: Stable with aminophylline, dobutamine, cimetidine, famotidine, ranitidine, heparin, lidocaine, procainamide.

Adverse effects
- **CNS:** *Dizziness, vertigo,* agitation, nervousness, dry mouth, tremor, palpitations, emotional lability, confusion, crying, vision changes, seizures

- **CV:** Vasodilation, flushing, arrhythmias, chest pain
- **GI:** *Nausea, vomiting,* hiccups
- **Other:** *Pain at injection site, increased sweating*

Interactions

❋ **Drug-food** • Ingestion of food during IV infusion decreases serum levels and effectiveness

■ Nursing considerations
Assessment

- **History:** Hypersensitivity to flumazenil or benzodiazepines; use of benzodiazepines for control of potentially life-threatening conditions; signs of serious cyclic antidepressant overdose, history of seizures, hepatic impairment, panic disorders, head injury, history of drug or alcohol dependence, pregnancy, lactation
- **Physical:** Skin color, lesions; T; orientation, reflexes, affect; P, BP, peripheral perfusion; serum drug levels

Interventions

- Administer by IV route only.

⊗ **Warning** Have emergency equipment ready, secure airway during administration.

⊗ **Black box warning** Drug may increase the risk of seizures, especially in patients on long-term benzodiazepine therapy and patients with serious cyclic antidepressant overdose; take appropriate precautions.

- Monitor clinical response carefully to determine effects of drug and need for repeated doses.
- Inject into running IV in a large vein to decrease pain of injection.
- Provide patient with written information after use; amnesia may be long-term, and teaching may not be remembered, including safety measures.

Teaching points

- Do not use any alcohol or over-the-counter drugs for 18–24 hours after use of this drug.
- Drug may cause changes in vision, dizziness, changes in alertness (avoid driving or operating hazardous machinery for at least 18–24 hours after drug use).
- Report difficulty breathing, pain at IV site, changes in vision, severe headache.

▽ **flunisolide**

*(floo **niss'** oh lide)*

AeroBid, AeroSpan HFA,
Apo-Flunisolide (CAN),
ratio-Flunisolide (CAN)

PREGNANCY CATEGORY C

Drug classes
Corticosteroid
Glucocorticoid
Hormone

Therapeutic actions
Anti-inflammatory effect; local administration into lower respiratory tract or nasal passages maximizes beneficial effects while decreasing possible adverse effects from systemic absorption.

Indications

- Intranasal: Relief and management of nasal symptoms of seasonal or perennial allergic rhinitis
- Inhalation: Maintenance treatment of asthma

Contraindications and cautions

- Contraindicated with systemic fungal infections, untreated local nasal infections, epistaxis, nasal trauma, septal ulcers, recent nasal surgery.
- Use cautiously with pregnancy, lactation, status asthmaticus.

Available forms
Intranasal solution, spray—25 mcg/actuation; inhalation—80 mcg/actuation

Dosages
Intranasal
Each actuation of the inhaler delivers 25 mcg.
Adults
Initial dosage, two sprays (50 mcg) in each nostril bid (total dose 200 mcg/day); may be increased to two sprays in each nostril tid (total dose 300 mcg/day). Maximum daily dose, eight sprays in each nostril (400 mcg/day).
Pediatric patients 6–14 yr
Initial dosage, one spray in each nostril tid or two sprays in each nostril bid (total dose 150–200 mcg/day). Maximum daily dose,

four sprays in each nostril (200 mcg/day). For maintenance dosage, reduce to smallest effective dose. Discontinue therapy after 3 wk if no significant symptomatic improvement.

Pediatric patients younger than 6 yr

Not recommended.

Inhalation

Each actuation of the inhaler delivers 80 mcg.

Adults

Two inhalations by mouth bid. Maximum *AeroBid* dosage 2 mg/day; maximum *AeroSpan* dosage 640 mcg.

Pediatric patients

- *AeroBid:* For 6–15 yr, dosage same as for adults. Maximum dosage 1 mg/day.
- *AeroSpan:* For 12 yr and older, dosage same as for adults. For 6–11 yr, one inhalation bid. Maximum, 160 mcg bid. For younger than 6 yr, not recommended.

Pharmacokinetics

Route	Onset	Peak	Duration
Intranasal	Slow	10–30 min	4–6 hr
Inhalation	Fast	Unknown	Unknown

Metabolism: Hepatic; $T_{1/2}$: 1–2 hr
Distribution: Crosses placenta; enters breast milk
Excretion: Feces, urine

Adverse effects

- **CNS:** *Headache*
- **Dermatologic:** Urticaria
- **Endocrine:** HPA suppression, Cushing syndrome with overdosage
- **GI:** Nausea
- **Local:** *Nasal irritation, fungal infection*
- **Respiratory:** *Epistaxis, rebound congestion,* perforation of the nasal septum, anosmia

■ Nursing considerations
Assessment

- **History:** Systemic fungal infections, untreated local nasal infections, epistaxis, nasal trauma, septal ulcers, recent nasal surgery, lactation
- **Physical:** Weight; T; BP, P, auscultation, R, adventitious sounds, examination of nares

Interventions

- Do not use during an acute asthmatic attack or to manage status asthmaticus.
- ⊗ **Black box warning** Taper systemic steroids carefully during transfer to inhalational steroids; deaths from adrenal insufficiency have occurred.
- Use decongestant nose drops to facilitate penetration if edema or excessive secretions are present.

Teaching points

- Do not use this drug more often than prescribed. Do not use this drug during an acute asthmatic attack.
- Do not stop using this drug without consulting your health care provider.
- Use decongestant nose drops first if nasal passages are blocked when using intranasal form.
- After using the inhaler, rinse your mouth with water or mouthwash to prevent oral candidiasis.
- You may experience these side effects: Local irritation (make sure you are using your device correctly), headache.
- Report sore mouth, sore throat.

DANGEROUS DRUG

▷fluorouracil (5-fluorouracil, 5-FU)

*(flure oh **yoor**' a sill)*

Adrucil, Carac, Efudex, Fluoroplex

PREGNANCY CATEGORY D

Drug classes
Antimetabolite
Antineoplastic

Therapeutic actions
Inhibits thymidylate synthetase, leading to inhibition of DNA synthesis and cell death.

Indications

- Parenteral: Palliative management of carcinomas of the colon, rectum, breast, stomach, pancreas in select patients considered incurable by surgery or other means
- Topical treatment of multiple actinic or solar keratoses

- Topical treatment of superficial basal cell carcinoma
- Orphan drug uses: In combination with interferon alfa 2-a recombinant for esophageal and advanced colorectal carcinoma; with leucovorin for colon or rectum metastatic adenocarcinoma
- Unlabeled use: Topical treatment of condylomata acuminata

Contraindications and cautions

- Contraindicated with allergy to 5-FU; poor nutritional status; serious infections; lactation.
- Use cautiously with hematopoietic depression secondary to radiation or chemotherapy; impaired liver function; pregnancy.

Available forms

Injection—50 mg/mL; cream—0.5%, 1%, 5%; topical solution—2%, 5%

Dosages

IV
Adults
Initial dosage, 12 mg/kg IV daily for 4 successive days; do not exceed 800 mg/day. If no toxicity occurs, give 6 mg/kg on the days 6, 8, 10, and 12, with no drug therapy on days 5, 7, 9, and 11. Discontinue therapy at end of day 12, even if no toxicity.

- *For patients without toxicity:* Repeat dosage every 30 days after the last day of the previous treatment.
- *For patients with toxicity:* Give 10–15 mg/kg/wk as a single dose after signs of toxicity subside. Do not exceed 1 g/wk. Adjust dosage based on patient response; therapy may be prolonged (12–60 mo).

Poor-risk or undernourished patients
6 mg/kg/day IV for 3 days. If no toxicity develops, give 3 mg/kg on the days 5, 7, and 9. No drug is given on days 4, 6, and 8. Do not exceed 400 mg/day.

Topical

Adults

- *Actinic or solar keratoses:* Apply bid to cover lesions. Usually, 0.5% and 1% preparations are used on head, neck, and chest while 2% and 5% preparations are used on hands. Continue until inflammatory response reaches erosion, necrosis, and ulceration stage, then discontinue. Usual course of therapy is

2–4 wk. Complete healing may not be evident for 1–2 mo after cessation of therapy.

- *Superficial basal cell carcinoma:* Apply 5% strength bid in an amount sufficient to cover the lesions. Continue treatment for at least 3–6 wk. Treatment may be required for 10–12 wk.

Pharmacokinetics

Route	Onset	Peak	Duration
IV	Immediate	1–2 hr	6 hr

Metabolism: Hepatic; $T_{1/2}$: 18–20 min
Distribution: Crosses placenta; enters breast milk
Excretion: Lungs, urine

▼ IV FACTS

Preparation: Store vials at room temperature; solution may discolor during storage with no adverse effects. Protect ampule from light. Precipitate may form during storage, heat to 60° C, and shake vigorously to dissolve. Cool to body temperature before administration. No dilution is required.
Infusion: Infuse slowly over 24 hr; inject into tubing of running IV to avoid pain on injection; direct injection over 1–3 min.
Incompatibilities: Do not mix with IV additives or other chemotherapeutic drugs.
Y-site incompatibility: Do not inject with droperidol.

Adverse effects

Parenteral

- **CNS:** *Lethargy, malaise, weakness,* euphoria, acute cerebellar syndrome, photophobia, lacrimation, decreased vision, nystagmus, diplopia
- **CV:** Myocardial ischemia, angina
- **Dermatologic:** *Alopecia, dermatitis, maculopapular rash, photosensitivity,* nail changes including nail loss, dry skin, fissures
- **GI:** *Diarrhea, anorexia, nausea, vomiting, cramps, enteritis, duodenal ulcer, duodenitis, gastritis, glossitis, stomatitis,* pharyngitis, esophagopharyngitis
- **Hematologic: Leukopenia, thrombocytopenia,** elevations in alkaline phosphatase, serum transaminase, serum bilirubin, lactate dehydrogenase
- **Other:** Fever, epistaxis

Adverse effects in *italics* are most common; those in **bold** are life-threatening. ⊞ Do not crush.

Topical
- **Hematologic:** Leukocytosis, **thrombocytopenia, toxic granulation,** eosinophilia
- **Local:** *Local pain, pruritus, hyperpigmentation, irritation, inflammation and burning at the site of application,* allergic contact dermatitis, scarring, soreness, tenderness, suppuration, scaling and swelling

Interactions
✳ **Drug-lab test** • 5-HIAA urinary excretion may increase • Plasma albumin may decrease due to protein malabsorption

■ Nursing considerations
Assessment
- **History:** Allergy to 5-FU, poor nutritional status, serious infections, hematopoietic depression, impaired liver function, pregnancy, lactation
- **Physical:** Weight; T; skin lesions, color; hair; vision, speech, orientation, reflexes, sensation; R, adventitious sounds; mucous membranes, liver evaluation, abdominal examination; CBC, differential; LFTs, renal function tests; urinalysis, chest X-ray

Interventions
- Evaluate hematologic status before beginning therapy and before each dose.

⊗ **Black box warning** Discontinue drug therapy at any sign of toxicity (stomatitis, esophagopharyngitis, rapidly falling WBC count, intractable vomiting, diarrhea, GI ulceration and bleeding, thrombocytopenia, hemorrhage); serious to life-threatening reactions have occurred. Consult physician.

- Arrange for biopsies of skin lesions to rule out frank neoplasm before beginning topical therapy and in all patients who do not respond to topical therapy.

⊗ **Warning** Thoroughly wash hands immediately after application of topical preparations. Use caution in applying near the nose, eyes, and mouth.

- Avoid occlusive dressings with topical application; the incidence of inflammatory reactions in adjacent skin areas is increased with these dressings. Use porous gauze dressings for cosmetic reasons.

Teaching points
- Prepare a calendar of treatment days. If using the topical application, wash hands

thoroughly after application. Do not use occlusive dressings; a porous gauze dressing may be used for cosmetic reasons.
- Have frequent, regular medical follow-up visits, including frequent blood tests to evaluate drug effects.
- You may experience these side effects: Nausea, vomiting, loss of appetite (request medication; frequent small meals may help; maintain nutrition); decreased vision, tearing, double vision, malaise, weakness, lethargy (reversible; avoid driving or operating dangerous machinery); mouth sores (practice frequent mouth care); diarrhea; loss of hair (obtain a wig or other head covering; keep the head covered in extremes of temperature); rash, sensitivity of skin and eyes to sun and ultraviolet light (avoid exposure to the sun; use a sunscreen and protective clothing. With topical application, ultraviolet light will increase the severity of the local reaction); birth defects or miscarriages (use birth control); unsightly local reaction to topical application (transient; use a porous gauze dressing to cover areas); pain, burning, stinging, swelling at local application.
- Report black, tarry stools; fever; chills; sore throat; unusual bleeding or bruising; chest pain; mouth sores; severe pain; tenderness; scaling at site of local application.

▽ **fluoxetine hydrochloride**
(floo ox' e teen)

Apo-Fluoxetine (CAN), Co-Fluoxetine (CAN), Gen-Fluoxetine (CAN), Novo-Fluoxetine (CAN), PMS-Fluoxetine (CAN), Prozac, Prozac Pulvules, Prozac Weekly, ratio-Fluoxetine (CAN), Sarafem, Sarafem Pulvules

PREGNANCY CATEGORY C

Drug classes
Antidepressant
SSRI

Therapeutic actions
Acts as an antidepressant by inhibiting CNS neuronal uptake of serotonin; blocks uptake of serotonin with little effect on norepinephrine;

little affinity for muscarinic, histaminergic, and alpha$_1$-adrenergic receptors.

Indications

- Treatment of depression; most effective in patients with major depressive disorder
- Treatment of depressive episodes associated with bipolar I disorder in combination with olanzapine
- Short-term treatment of treatment-resistant depression with olanzapine
- Treatment of OCD
- Treatment of bulimia
- Treatment of PMDD (*Sarafem*)
- Treatment of panic disorder with or without agoraphobia
- Unlabeled uses: Raynaud phenomenon, alcoholism, borderline personality disorder, fibromyalgia, hot flashes, diabetic neuropathy, nocturnal enuresis, post-herpetic neuralgia, PTSD, migraine prevention

Contraindications and cautions

- Contraindicated with hypersensitivity to fluoxetine, pregnancy.
- Use cautiously with impaired hepatic or renal function, diabetes mellitus, lactation, seizures; history of suicide attempts.

Available forms

Tablets—10, 15, 20 mg; capsules—10, 20, 40 mg; liquid—20 mg/5 mL; DR capsules—90 mg

Dosages
Adults

- *Antidepressant:* The full antidepressant effect may not be seen for up to 4–6 wk. Initially, 20 mg/day PO in the morning. If no clinical improvement is seen, increase dose after several weeks. Administer doses larger than 20 mg/day on a bid schedule or once a day in the morning. Do not exceed 80 mg/day. Once stabilized, may switch to 90-mg DR capsules once a week.
- *OCD:* Initially, 20 mg/day PO. If no clinical improvement is seen, increase the dose after several weeks. Usual dosage range is 20–60 mg/day PO; may require up to 5 wk for effectiveness. Do not exceed 80 mg/day.
- *Bulimia:* 60 mg/day PO in the morning.
- *PMDD (Sarafem):* 20 mg/day PO or 20 mg/day PO starting 14 days before the anticipated beginning of menses and

continuing through the first full day of menses, then no drug until 14 days before next menses; do not exceed 80 mg/day.
- *Panic disorder:* 10 mg/day PO for the first week; increase to 20 mg/day if needed. Maximum dose, 60 mg/day.
- *Depressive episodes of bipolar I disorder:* 20 mg/day PO with 5 mg olanzapine.
- *Treatment of treatment-resistant depression:* 20–50 mg/day PO with 5–20 mg olanzapine.

Pediatric patients 8–18 yr

- *Major depressive disorder:* 10 mg/day PO; may be increased to 20 mg/day after 1 wk or after several weeks for lower-weight children.

Adolescents and higher-weight children

- *OCD:* Initially, 10 mg/day PO. After 2 wk increase to 20 mg/day. Suggested range, 20–60 mg/day PO.

Adolescents and lower-weight children

- *OCD:* Initially, 10 mg/day PO. Range, 20–30 mg/day.

Pediatric patients younger than 7 yr
Safety and efficacy not established.

Geriatric patients or patients with hepatic impairment
Give a lower or less frequent dose. Monitor response to guide dosage.

Pharmacokinetics

Route	Onset	Peak
Oral	Slow	6–8 hr

Metabolism: Hepatic; T$_{1/2}$: 9 days
Distribution: Crosses placenta; enters breast milk
Excretion: Feces, urine

Adverse effects

- **CNS:** *Headache, nervousness, insomnia, drowsiness, anxiety, tremor, dizziness, light-headedness,* agitation, sedation, abnormal gait, **seizures**
- **CV:** Hot flashes, palpitations
- **Dermatologic:** *Sweating, rash, pruritus,* acne, alopecia, contact dermatitis
- **GI:** *Nausea, vomiting, diarrhea, dry mouth, anorexia, dyspepsia, constipation, taste changes,* flatulence, gastroenteritis, dysphagia, gingivitis
- **GU:** *Painful menstruation, sexual dysfunction, frequency,* cystitis, impotence, urgency, vaginitis

Adverse effects in *italics* are most common; those in **bold** are life-threatening. ▭ Do not crush.

- **Respiratory:** *URIs, pharyngitis,* cough, dyspnea, bronchitis, rhinitis
- **Other:** *weight changes, asthenia, fever*

Interactions
✳ **Drug-drug** ⊗ *Warning* Possible fatal reactions with MAOIs; do not administer together; 2-wk washout period needed ● Toxic effects of fluoxetine may be increased if combined with opioids ● Possible severe effects with linezolid; allow at least 2 wk after stopping linezolid before starting fluoxetine.

● Increased therapeutic and toxic effects of TCAs ● Do not use with thioridazine (increased levels of thioridazine) ● Decreased effectiveness if taken while smoking ● Increased toxicity of lithium; avoid this combination ● Additive CNS effects if combined with benzodiazepines, alcohol; avoid these combinations ● Avoid administration with other serotonergic drugs; may lead to serotonin syndrome ● Reduce dosage of PDE5 inhibitors if combining with fluoxetine.

✳ **Drug-alternative therapy** ● Increased risk of severe reaction if combined with St. John's Wort therapy

■ Nursing considerations

 CLINICAL ALERT!
Name confusion has occurred between *Sarafem* (fluoxetine) and *Serophene* (clomiphene); use caution.

Assessment
- **History:** Hypersensitivity to fluoxetine, impaired hepatic or renal function, diabetes mellitus, lactation, pregnancy, seizures
- **Physical:** Weight, T; skin rash, lesions; reflexes, affect; bowel sounds, liver evaluation; P, peripheral perfusion; urinary output, LFTs, renal function tests

Interventions
● Arrange for lower or less frequent doses in elderly patients and patients with hepatic impairment.

⊗ *Black box warning* Establish suicide precautions for severely depressed patients. Limit quantity of capsules dispensed; high risk of suicidality in children, adolescents, and young adults.

● Administer drug in the morning.
● Monitor patient for response to therapy for up to 4 wk before increasing dose.

● Switch to once a week therapy by starting weekly dose 7 days after last 20 mg/day dose. If response is not satisfactory, reconsider daily dosing.

⊗ *Warning* If discontinuing drug, dosage should be tapered gradually to avoid withdrawal syndrome.

Teaching points
● It may take up to 4 weeks before the full effect occurs. Take in the morning. If you feel sleepy or tired, you may take it at night. If you are taking the once-weekly capsule, mark calendar with reminders of drug day.
● Do not stop taking this drug without consulting your health care provider.
● Do not take this drug during pregnancy. If you think that you are pregnant or wish to become pregnant, consult your health care provider.
● Keep this drug, and all medications, out of the reach of children.
● Do not use St. John's Wort while taking this drug.
● You may experience these side effects: Dizziness, drowsiness, nervousness, insomnia (avoid driving or performing hazardous tasks); nausea, vomiting, weight loss (eat small frequent meals; monitor your weight loss); sexual dysfunction; flulike symptoms.
● Report rash, mania, seizures, severe weight loss, thoughts of suicide.

▽**fluphenazine**
(floo fen' a zeen)

fluphenazine decanoate
Injection: Modecate Concentrate (CAN)

fluphenazine hydrochloride
Oral tablets, concentrate, elixir, injection: Apo-Fluphenazine (CAN)

PREGNANCY CATEGORY C

Drug classes
Antipsychotic
Dopaminergic blocker
Phenothiazine

Therapeutic actions

Mechanism not fully understood: Antipsychotic drugs block postsynaptic dopamine receptors in the brain, depress the RAS, including the parts of the brain involved with wakefulness and emesis; anticholinergic, antihistaminic (H_1), and alpha-adrenergic blocking activity also may contribute to some of its therapeutic (and adverse) actions.

Indications

- Management of manifestations of psychotic disorders; the longer acting parenteral dosage forms, fluphenazine enanthate and fluphenazine decanoate, indicated for management of patients (chronic schizophrenics) who require prolonged parenteral therapy
- Fluphenazine decanoate: Long-term or parenteral neuroleptic therapy
- Unlabeled use: Post-herpetic neuralgia

Contraindications and cautions

- Contraindicated with hypersensitivity to fluphenazine, other phenothiazines, tartrazine, or aspirin; coma or severe CNS depression; bone marrow depression; blood dyscrasia; circulatory collapse; subcortical brain damage; Parkinson disease; liver damage; cerebral arteriosclerosis; coronary disease; severe hypotension or hypertension; pregnancy.
- Use cautiously with respiratory disorders ("silent pneumonia"); glaucoma, prostatic hypertrophy (anticholinergic effects may exacerbate glaucoma and urinary retention); epilepsy or history of epilepsy (drug lowers seizure threshold); breast cancer (elevations in prolactin may stimulate a prolactin-dependent tumor); thyrotoxicosis; peptic ulcer, decreased renal function; myelography within previous 24 hr or myelography scheduled within 48 hr; exposure to heat or phosphorous insecticides; pregnancy; lactation; children younger than 12 yr, especially those with chickenpox, CNS infections (children are especially susceptible to dystonias that may confound the diagnosis of Reye syndrome).

Available forms

Tablets—1, 2.5, 5, 10 mg; injection—25 mg/mL (decanoate); 2.5 mg/mL (hydrochloride); oral elixir—2.5 mg/5 mL; solution (concentrate)—5 mg/mL

Dosages

Full clinical effects may require 6 wk–6 mo of therapy. Patients who have never taken phenothiazines, poor-risk patients (those with disorders that predispose to undue reactions) should be treated initially with this shorter acting dosage form and then switched to the longer-acting parenteral forms, fluphenazine enanthate, or decanoate.

The duration of action of the esterified forms of fluphenazine is markedly longer than those of fluphenazine hydrochloride; the duration of action of fluphenazine enanthate is estimated to be 1–3 wk; the duration of action of fluphenazine decanoate is estimated to be 4 wk. No precise formula is available for the conversion of fluphenazine hydrochloride dosage to fluphenazine decanoate dosage, but one study suggests that 20 mg of fluphenazine hydrochloride daily was equivalent to 25 mg decanoate every 3 wk.

Adults

fluphenazine hydrochloride

Individualize dosage; begin with low dosage, and gradually increase.

Oral

2.5–10 mg/day PO in divided doses every 6–8 hr; usual maintenance dose is 1–5 mg/day, often as a single dose. Oral concentrate solution should be diluted in 60 mL of a suitable diluent that does not contain caffeine, tannic acid (eg, tea), or pectinates (eg, apple juice). Give daily doses greater than 20 mg with caution. When symptoms are controlled, gradually reduce dosage.

IM

Average starting dose is 1.25 mg IM (range 2.5–10 mg), divided and given every 6–8 hr; parenteral dose is one-third to one-half the oral dose. Give daily doses greater than 10 mg with caution.

fluphenazine decanoate

IM or subcutaneous: Initial dose, 12.5–25 mg IM or subcutaneously; determine subsequent doses and dosage interval based on patient response. If doses above 50 mg are needed, increase cautiously in 12.5-mg increments. Dose should not exceed 100 mg.

Pediatric patients

Generally not recommended for children younger than 12 yr.

Adverse effects in *italics* are most common; those in **bold** are life-threatening. ⬛ Do not crush.

Geriatric patients
Oral
Initial dose is 1–2.5 mg/day PO.

Pharmacokinetics

Route	Onset	Peak	Duration
Oral	1 hr	2 hr	6–8 hr
IM (HCl)	1 hr	1–2 hr	6–8 hr
IM (decanoate)	24–72 hr	Unknown	1–6 wk

Metabolism: Hepatic; $T_{1/2}$: 4.5–15.3 hr (fluphenazine hydrochloride), 6.8–9.6 days (fluphenazine decanoate)
Distribution: Crosses placenta; enters breast milk
Excretion: Urine, unchanged

Adverse effects

- **Autonomic:** Dry mouth, salivation, nasal congestion, nausea, vomiting, anorexia, fever, pallor, flushed facies, sweating, constipation, paralytic ileus, urinary retention, incontinence, polyuria, enuresis, priapism, ejaculation inhibition, male impotence
- **CNS:** *Drowsiness,* insomnia, vertigo, headache, weakness, tremor, ataxia, slurring, cerebral edema, **seizures,** exacerbation of psychotic symptoms, extrapyramidal syndromes *(pseudoparkinsonism); dystonias; akathisia,* tardive dyskinesias, potentially irreversible, **neuroleptic malignant syndrome,** hyperthermias, **autonomic disturbances** (rare, but 20% fatal)
- **CV:** Hypotension, orthostatic hypotension, hypertension, tachycardia, bradycardia, **cardiac arrest,** heart failure, cardiomegaly, **refractory arrhythmias,** pulmonary edema
- **Endocrine:** Lactation, breast engorgement in females, galactorrhea; SIADH; amenorrhea, menstrual irregularities; gynecomastia in males; changes in libido; hyperglycemia or **hypoglycemia;** glycosuria; hyponatremia; pituitary tumor with hyperprolactinemia; inhibition of ovulation, infertility, pseudopregnancy; reduced urinary levels of gonadotropins, estrogens, progestins
- **Hematologic:** Eosinophilia, leukopenia, leukocytosis, anemia; **aplastic anemia; hemolytic anemia; thrombocytopenic or nonthrombocytopenic purpura; pancytopenia**

- **Hypersensitivity:** Urticaria, angioneurotic edema, **laryngeal edema,** photosensitivity, eczema, asthma, **anaphylactoid reactions,** exfoliative dermatitis
- **Respiratory: Bronchospasm, laryngospasm,** dyspnea; suppression of cough reflex and potential for aspiration **(sudden death related to asphyxia or cardiac arrest has been reported)**
- **Other:** Risk of structural defects, growth retardation, functional or behavioral dysfunction, extrapyramidal effects in newborn if used during last trimester of pregnancy, photosensitivity

Interactions

✳ **Drug-drug** • Additive CNS depression with alcohol, barbiturates, or other sedatives • Additive anticholinergic effects and possibly decreased antipsychotic efficacy with anticholinergic drugs • Increased likelihood of seizures with metrizamide (contrast agent used in myelography)

✳ **Drug-lab test** • False-positive pregnancy tests (less likely if serum test is used)

■ Nursing considerations
Assessment

- **History:** Coma or severe CNS depression; bone marrow depression; blood dyscrasia; circulatory collapse; subcortical brain damage; Parkinson disease; liver damage; cerebral arteriosclerosis; coronary disease; severe hypotension or hypertension; respiratory disorders; glaucoma; prostatic hypertrophy; epilepsy; breast cancer; thyrotoxicosis; peptic ulcer, decreased renal function; myelography within previous 24 hr or myelography scheduled within 48 hr; exposure to heat or phosphorous insecticides; age younger than 12 yr; chickenpox; CNS infections; pregnancy
- **Physical:** Weight; T; reflexes, orientation, IOP; P, BP, orthostatic BP; R, adventitious sounds; bowel sounds and normal output, liver evaluation; urinary output, prostate size; CBC, urinalysis, thyroid, LFTs, renal function tests

Interventions

- Oral concentrate solution should be diluted in 60 mL of a suitable diluent that does not contain caffeine, tannic acid (eg, tea), or pectinates (eg, apple juice).

- Arrange for discontinuation of drug if serum creatinine or BUN become abnormal or if WBC count is depressed.
- Monitor elderly patients for dehydration; institute remedial measures promptly. Sedation and decreased sensation of thirst related to CNS effects can lead to severe dehydration.
- Consult physician regarding appropriate warning of patient or patient's guardian about tardive dyskinesias.
- Consult physician about dosage reduction, use of anticholinergic antiparkinsonian drugs (controversial) if extrapyramidal effects occur.

Teaching points
- Take drug exactly as prescribed.
- Avoid driving or engaging in other dangerous activities if drowsiness, weakness, tremor, extrapyramidal symptoms, or vision changes occur.
- Avoid prolonged exposure to sun; use a sunscreen or cover skin if exposure is unavoidable.
- Maintain fluid intake, and use precautions against heatstroke in hot weather.
- Report sore throat, fever, unusual bleeding or bruising, rash, weakness, tremors, impaired vision, dark urine (pink or reddish brown urine is expected), pale stools, yellowing of skin or eyes.

▷ flurazepam hydrochloride
(flur az' e pam)

Apo-Flurazepam (CAN)

PREGNANCY CATEGORY X

CONTROLLED SUBSTANCE C-IV

Drug classes
Benzodiazepine
Sedative-hypnotic

Therapeutic actions
Exact mechanisms not understood; acts mainly at subcortical levels of the CNS, leaving the cortex relatively unaffected; potentiates the effects of GABA, an inhibitory neurotransmitter.

Indications
- Insomnia characterized by difficulty in falling asleep, frequent nocturnal awakenings, or early morning awakening
- Recurring insomnia or poor sleeping habits
- Acute or chronic medical situations requiring restful sleep

Contraindications and cautions
- Contraindicated with hypersensitivity to benzodiazepines, psychoses, acute narrow-angle glaucoma, shock, coma, acute alcoholic intoxication with depression of vital signs, pregnancy (risk of congenital malformations, neonatal withdrawal syndrome), labor and delivery ("floppy infant" syndrome), lactation (infants become lethargic and lose weight).
- Use cautiously in the elderly or with impaired liver or renal function, debilitation, depression, suicidal tendencies.

Available forms
Capsules—15, 30 mg

Dosages
Individualize dosage.
Adults
30 mg PO at bedtime; 15 mg may suffice.
Pediatric patients
Not for use in patients younger than 15 yr.
Geriatric patients or patients with debilitating disease
Initially, 15 mg PO; adjust as needed.

Pharmacokinetics

Route	Onset	Peak
Oral	Fast	30–60 min

Metabolism: Hepatic; $T_{1/2}$: 47–100 hr
Distribution: Crosses placenta; enters breast milk
Excretion: Urine

Adverse effects
- **CNS:** *Transient, mild drowsiness initially; sedation, depression, lethargy, apathy, fatigue, light-headedness, disorientation, restlessness, asthenia,* crying, delirium, headache, slurred speech, dysarthria, stupor, rigidity, tremor, dystonia, vertigo, euphoria, nervousness, difficulty in concentration, vivid dreams, psychomotor retardation, extrapyramidal

symptoms; *mild paradoxical excitatory reactions during first 2 wk of treatment* (psychiatric patients, aggressive children, with high dosage), visual and auditory disturbances, diplopia, nystagmus, depressed hearing, nasal congestion, complex sleep disorders

- **CV:** *Bradycardia, tachycardia,* **CV collapse,** hypertension and hypotension, palpitations, edema
- **Dependence:** *Drug dependence with withdrawal syndrome* when drug is discontinued (common with abrupt cessation of high dosage used more than 4 mo)
- **Dermatologic:** Urticaria, pruritus, rash, dermatitis
- **GI:** *Constipation, diarrhea, dyspepsia,* dry mouth, salivation, nausea, anorexia, vomiting, difficulty in swallowing, gastric disorders, elevations of blood enzymes: LDH, alkaline phosphatase, AST, ALT, hepatic impairment, jaundice
- **GU:** *Incontinence, urine retention, changes in libido,* menstrual irregularities
- **Hematologic:** Decreased Hct, blood dyscrasias
- **Other: Anaphylaxis, angioedema,** hiccups, fever, diaphoresis, paresthesias, muscular disturbances, gynecomastia

Interactions
✴ **Drug-drug** • Increased CNS depression with alcohol, phenothiazines, opioids, barbiturates, TCAs • Increased pharmacologic effects of flurazepam with cimetidine, disulfiram, hormonal contraceptives, SSRIs • Decreased sedative effects of flurazepam with theophylline, aminophylline, rifampin

■ Nursing considerations
Assessment
- **History:** Hypersensitivity to benzodiazepines; psychoses; acute narrow-angle glaucoma; shock; coma; acute alcoholic intoxication; pregnancy; labor; lactation; impaired liver or renal function, debilitation, depression, suicidal tendencies
- **Physical:** Skin color, lesions; T; orientation, reflexes, affect, ophthalmologic examination; P, BP; R, adventitious sounds; liver evaluation, abdominal examination, bowel sounds, normal output; CBC, LFTs, renal function tests

Interventions
- Monitor liver and renal function and CBC during long-term therapy.
⊗ **Warning** Taper dosage gradually after long-term therapy, especially in epileptic patients.
- Do not administer to pregnant women.

Teaching points
- Take drug exactly as prescribed.
- In long-term therapy, do not stop taking without consulting your health care provider.
- Avoid pregnancy while taking this drug; using barrier contraceptives is advised.
- You may experience these side effects: Drowsiness, dizziness (may lessen; avoid driving or engaging in other dangerous activities); GI upset (take with water); depression, dreams, emotional upset, crying; nocturnal sleep disturbance (may be prolonged after drug cessation).
- Report severe dizziness, weakness, drowsiness that persists, rash or skin lesions, palpitations, swelling of the extremities, visual changes, difficulty voiding.

▷ flurbiprofen
*(flure **bi'** proe fen)*

Ophthalmic solution: Ocufen
Oral: Ansaid, Apo-Flurbiprofen (CAN)

PREGNANCY CATEGORY B (ORAL), C (OPHTHALMIC)

Drug classes
Analgesic (nonopioid)
Anti-inflammatory
NSAID

Therapeutic actions
Analgesic, anti-inflammatory, and antipyretic activities largely related to inhibition of cyclo-oxygenase and prostaglandin synthesis; exact mechanisms of action are not known.

Indications
- Oral: Acute or long-term treatment of the signs and symptoms of rheumatoid arthritis and osteoarthritis
- Oral: Relief of moderate to mild pain
- Ophthalmic solution: Inhibition of intraoperative miosis

- Unlabeled uses of ophthalmic solution: Topical treatment of cystoid macular edema, inflammation after cataract surgery and uveitis syndromes; oral—juvenile rheumatoid arthritis, sunburn, migraine headache

Contraindications and cautions

- Contraindicated with allergy to aspirin, flurbiprofen, or other NSAIDs, significant renal impairment, pregnancy, lactation.
- Use cautiously with impaired hearing, allergies, hepatic, CV, and GI conditions.

Available forms

Tablets—50, 100 mg; ophthalmic solution—0.03%

Dosages
Adults
Oral
Initial recommended daily dose of 200–300 mg PO, give in divided doses bid, tid, or qid. Largest recommended single dose is 100 mg. Doses above 300 mg/day PO are not recommended. Taper to lowest possible dose.
Ophthalmic solution
Instill 1 drop approximately every 30 min, beginning 2 hr before surgery (total of 4 drops).
Pediatric patients
Safety and efficacy not established.

Pharmacokinetics

Route	Onset	Peak
Oral	30–60 min	90 min

Metabolism: Hepatic; $T_{1/2}$: 5.7 hr
Distribution: Crosses placenta; enters breast milk
Excretion: Urine

Adverse effects
Oral
- **CNS:** *Headache, dizziness, somnolence, insomnia,* fatigue, tiredness, dizziness, tinnitus, ophthalmologic effects
- **CV:** Hypertension, heart failure
- **Dermatologic:** Rash, pruritus, sweating, dry mucous membranes, stomatitis
- **GI:** *Nausea, dyspepsia, GI pain,* diarrhea, vomiting, *constipation,* flatulence, **ulcer**
- **GU:** Dysuria, **renal impairment**
- **Hematologic: Bleeding,** platelet inhibition with higher doses, **neutropenia,**

eosinophilia, leukopenia, pancytopenia, thrombocytopenia, agranulocytosis, granulocytopenia, aplastic anemia, decreased Hgb or Hct, **bone marrow depression,** menorrhagia
- **Respiratory:** Dyspnea, hemoptysis, pharyngitis, **bronchospasm,** rhinitis
- **Other:** Peripheral edema, **fatal anaphylactic shock**
Ophthalmic solution
- **Local:** *Transient stinging and burning on instillation, ocular irritation*

■ Nursing considerations
Assessment
- **History:** Renal impairment; impaired hearing; allergies; hepatic, CV, and GI conditions; lactation, pregnancy
- **Physical:** Skin color and lesions; orientation, reflexes, ophthalmologic and audiometric evaluation, peripheral sensation; P, edema; R, adventitious sounds; liver evaluation; CBC, clotting times, LFTs, renal function tests; serum electrolytes, stool guaiac

Interventions
⊗ **Black box warning** Be aware that patient may be at increased risk for CV event, GI bleeding; monitor accordingly.
⊗ **Black box warning** Contraindicated for treatment of perioperative pain in setting of coronary artery bypass graft.
- Administer drug with food or after meals if GI upset occurs.
- Assess patient receiving ophthalmic solutions for systemic effects because absorption does occur.
- Arrange for periodic ophthalmologic examinations during long-term therapy.
⊗ **Warning** If overdose occurs, institute emergency procedures—gastric lavage, induction of emesis, supportive therapy.

Teaching points
- Take drug with food or meals if GI upset occurs; take only the prescribed dosage.
- If using eyedrops, review proper administration.
- Avoid use during pregnancy, serious adverse effects could occur. Using barrier contraceptives is advised.
- Dizziness or drowsiness can occur (avoid driving or using dangerous machinery).

Adverse effects in *italics* are most common; those in **bold** are life-threatening. ⬛ Do not crush.

- Report sore throat, fever, rash, itching, weight gain, swelling in ankles or fingers, changes in vision, black or tarry stools, bleeding.

DANGEROUS DRUG

▽ **flutamide**

(floo' ta mide)

Euflex (CAN), Novo-Flutamide (CAN)

PREGNANCY CATEGORY D

Drug classes
Antiandrogen
Antineoplastic

Therapeutic actions
Exerts potent antiandrogenic activity by inhibiting androgen uptake or by inhibiting nuclear binding of androgen in target tissues.

Indications
- Treatment of locally advanced and metastatic prostatic carcinoma in combination with LH-RH agonistic analogues (leuprolide acetate, goserelin)
- Unlabeled use: Treatment of hirsutism in women (250 mg/day)

Contraindications and cautions
- Contraindicated with hypersensitivity to flutamide or any component of the preparation, severe hepatic impairment, pregnancy, lactation.
- Use cautiously with smoking, G6PD deficiencies.

Available forms
Capsules—125 mg; tablets—250 mg (CAN)

Dosages
Adults
- *Locally advanced or metastatic prostatic cancer:* 250 mg PO tid. Treatment should begin at same as initiation of therapy with LH-RH analogue.
Pediatric patients
Safety and efficacy not established.

Pharmacokinetics

Route	Onset	Peak	Duration
Oral	Varies	2 hr	72 hr

Metabolism: Hepatic; $T_{1/2}$: 6 hr
Distribution: Crosses placenta; enters breast milk
Excretion: Urine

Adverse effects
- **CNS:** Drowsiness, confusion, depression, anxiety, nervousness
- **Dermatologic:** *Rash,* photosensitivity
- **Endocrine:** *Gynecomastia, hot flashes*
- **GI:** *Nausea, vomiting, diarrhea, GI disturbances,* jaundice, **hepatitis, hepatic necrosis,** elevated AST, ALT
- **GU:** *Impotence, loss of libido*
- **Hematologic:** *Anemia, leukopenia,* thrombocytopenia
- **Other:** Carcinogenesis, mutagenesis

■ Nursing considerations
Assessment
- **History:** Hypersensitivity to flutamide or any component of the preparation, hepatic impairment, smoking, G6PD deficiencies, pregnancy, lactation
- **Physical:** Skin color, lesions; reflexes, affect; urinary output; bowel sounds, liver evaluation; CBC, Hct, electrolytes, LFTs, PSA

Interventions
- Give flutamide with other drugs used for medical castration (LH-RH analogue).
- ⊗ **Black box warning** Arrange for periodic monitoring of liver function tests during long-term therapy; severe hepatic toxicity can occur.

Teaching points
- Take this drug with other drugs to treat your problem. Do not interrupt dosing or stop taking these medications without consulting your health care provider.
- Periodic blood tests will be needed to monitor the drug effects. Keep appointments for these tests.
- You may experience these side effects: Dizziness, drowsiness (avoid driving or performing hazardous tasks); nausea, vomiting, diarrhea (maintain nutrition, consult dietitian); impotence, loss of libido (reversible); sensitivity to light (use sunscreen or protective clothing).
- Report change in stool or urine color, yellow skin, difficulty breathing, malaise.

F

▽fluvastatin sodium
*(flue va **sta' tin**)*

Lescol, Lescol XL⊙

PREGNANCY CATEGORY X

Drug classes
Antihyperlipidemic
Statin

Therapeutic actions
Inhibits the enzyme HMG-CoA that catalyzes the first step in the cholesterol synthesis pathway, resulting in a decrease in serum cholesterol, serum LDL (associated with increased risk of CAD), and either an increase or no change in serum HDL (associated with decreased risk of CAD).

Indications
• Adjunct to diet in the treatment of elevated total cholesterol and LDL cholesterol with primary hypercholesterolemia and mixed dyslipidemia (types IIa and IIb) where response to dietary restriction of saturated fat and cholesterol and other nonpharmacologic measures has not been adequate
• To slow progression of coronary atheroscleroses in patients with CAD, along with diet and exercise
• Reduction of the risk of undergoing coronary revascularization procedures in patients with CAD
• Treatment of heterozygous familial hypercholesterolemia in children 9–16 yr

Contraindications and cautions
• Contraindicated with allergy to fluvastatin, allergy to fungal byproducts, pregnancy, lactation.
• Use cautiously with impaired hepatic function, cataracts, myopathy.

Available forms
Capsules—20, 40 mg; extended-release tablets⊙—80 mg

Dosages
Adults
Initial dosage, 40 mg/day PO administered in the evening. Maintenance doses, 20–80 mg/day PO; give 80 mg/day as two 40-mg doses, or use 80-mg ER form.

Pediatric patients 9–16 yr
Initial dose, 20 mg/day PO. Adjust every 6 wk to a maximum dose of 40 mg bid or 80 mg of ER form PO once a day.

Pharmacokinetics

Route	Onset	Peak
Oral	Fast	4–8 hr

Metabolism: Hepatic; $T_{1/2}$: 3–7 hr
Distribution: Crosses placenta; enters breast milk
Excretion: Bile, feces

Adverse effects
• **CNS:** *Headache, blurred vision,* dizziness, insomnia, fatigue, muscle cramps, cataracts
• **GI:** *Flatulence, abdominal pain, cramps, constipation, nausea,* dyspepsia, heartburn
• **Hematologic:** Elevations of CPK, alkaline phosphatase, and transaminases
• **Other: Rhabdomyolysis**

Interactions
✷ **Drug-drug** ⊗ *Warning* Possible severe myopathy or rhabdomyolysis if taken with azole antifungals, cyclosporine, erythromycin, gemfibrozil, niacin, other statins.
• Increased levels of phenytoin, warfarin
✷ **Drug-food** • Decreased metabolism and increased risk of toxic effects if taken with grapefruit juice; avoid this combination

■ Nursing considerations
Assessment
• **History:** Allergy to fluvastatin, fungal byproducts; impaired hepatic function; cataracts (use caution); pregnancy; lactation
• **Physical:** Orientation, affect, ophthalmologic examination; liver evaluation; lipid studies, LFTs, muscle pain, CPK

Interventions
• Give in the evening; highest rates of cholesterol synthesis are between midnight and 5 AM. Doses of 80 mg/day of immediate-release product should be taken as two 40-mg doses.
• Before administering, ensure that patient is not pregnant and understands need to avoid pregnancy.
• Do not cut or crush ER tablets; ensure that patient swallows tablets whole.
• Arrange for regular follow-up during long-term therapy, including liver function tests.

Adverse effects in *italics* are most common; those in **bold** are life-threatening. ⊙ Do not crush.

- Arrange for periodic ophthalmologic examination to check for cataract development.

Teaching points
- Take drug in the evening. Do not drink grapefruit juice while taking this drug. Do not cut, crush, or chew tablets.
- Institute dietary changes, and maintain a low-cholesterol diet while taking this drug.
- This drug cannot be taken during pregnancy; using barrier contraceptives is advised.
- Arrange to have periodic ophthalmic examinations while you are taking this drug.
- You may experience these side effects: Nausea (eat frequent small meals); headache, muscle and joint aches and pains (may lessen).
- Report severe GI upset, changes in vision, unusual bleeding or bruising, dark urine or light-colored stools, muscle pain, fever.

▽fluvoxamine maleate
(floo vox' a meen)

Apo-Fluvoxamine (CAN),
CO Fluvoxamine (CAN),
Luvox, Luvox CR⊙ⓝ⊙,
PMS-Fluvoxamine (CAN),
ratio-Fluvoxamine (CAN)

PREGNANCY CATEGORY C

Drug classes
Antidepressant
SSRI

Therapeutic actions
Selectively inhibits CNS neuronal uptake of serotonin; blocks uptake of serotonin with weak effect on norepinephrine; little affinity for muscarinic, histaminergic, and alpha$_1$-adrenergic receptors.

Indications
- Treatment of OCD
- Treatment of social anxiety disorder (CR capsules)
- Unlabeled uses: Treatment of depression, bulimia nervosa, panic disorder, PTSD, migraine prevention

Contraindications and cautions
- Contraindicated with hypersensitivity to fluvoxamine, lactation.

- Use cautiously with impaired hepatic or renal function, suicidal tendencies, seizures, mania, ECT therapy, CV disease, labor and delivery, pregnancy.

Available forms
Tablets—25, 50, 100 mg; CR capsules⊙ⓝ⊙—100, 150 mg

Dosages
Adults
Initially, 50 mg PO at bedtime. Increase in 50-mg increments at 4–7 day intervals. Usual range, 100–300 mg/day. Divide doses over 100 mg/day; give larger dose at bedtime. If symptoms do not improve within 10–12 wk, form of treatment should be reconsidered. CR capsules: 100–300 mg/day PO.
Pediatric patients 8–17 yr
Initially, 25 mg PO at bedtime. Increase dose by 25 mg/day every 4–7 days to achieve desired effect. Divide doses over 50 mg/day and give larger dose at bedtime. Maximum dose for children up to age 11 yr is 200 mg/day.
Geriatric patients or patients with hepatic impairment
Give a reduced dose (25 mg PO at bedtime), adjust more slowly.

Pharmacokinetics

Route	Onset	Peak
Oral	3–10 wk	2–8 hr

Metabolism: Hepatic; $T_{1/2}$: 15–20 hr
Distribution: Crosses placenta; enters breast milk
Excretion: Urine

Adverse effects
- **CNS:** *Headache, nervousness, insomnia, drowsiness, anxiety, tremor, dizziness, light-headedness,* agitation, *sedation,* abnormal gait, **seizures**
- **Dermatologic:** *Sweating, rash, pruritus,* acne, alopecia, contact dermatitis
- **GI:** *Nausea, vomiting, diarrhea, dry mouth, anorexia, dyspepsia, constipation, taste changes,* flatulence, gastroenteritis, dysphagia, gingivitis
- **GU:** *Sexual dysfunction, frequency,* cystitis, impotence, urgency, vaginitis
- **Respiratory:** *URIs, pharyngitis,* cough, dyspnea, bronchitis, rhinitis

F

Interactions

✴ **Drug-drug** • Do not administer with MAOIs (during or within 14 days) • Increased effects of triazolam, alprazolam, warfarin, carbamazepine, methadone, beta blockers, statins, diltiazem, TCAs, theophylline, clozapine; reduced dosages of these drugs will be needed • Decreased effects due to increased metabolism in cigarette smokers • Increased risk of serotonin syndrome if combined with other serotonergic drugs such as linezolid • Increased risk of neuroleptic malignant syndrome if combined with quetiapine

✴ **Drug-alternative therapy** • Increased risk of severe reaction if combined with St. John's Wort therapy

■ Nursing considerations
Assessment

• **History:** Hypersensitivity to fluvoxamine; lactation; impaired hepatic function; suicidal tendencies; seizures; mania; CV disease; labor and delivery; pregnancy
• **Physical:** Weight; T; skin rash, lesions; reflexes; affect; bowel sounds; liver evaluation; P, peripheral perfusion; LFTs, renal function tests

Interventions

• Give lower or less frequent doses in elderly patients and with hepatic or renal impairment.

⊗ **Black box warning** Establish suicide precautions for severely depressed patients, children, adolescents, and young adults. Limit quantity of tablets dispensed. Risk of suicidal ideation and behavior is related.

• Administer drug at bedtime. If dose exceeds 100 mg, divide dose and administer the largest dose at bedtime.
• Ensure that patient does not cut, crush, or chew CR capsules.
• Monitor patient for therapeutic response for up to 4–7 days before increasing dose.
• Monitor patient for serotonin hypertension syndrome, elevated fever, severe anxiety, rigidity.

⊗ **Warning** When discontinuing the drug, taper dose by 50 mg/day every 5–7 days.

Teaching points

• Take this drug at bedtime; if a large dose is needed, the dose may be divided but take the largest dose at bedtime. Do not cut, crush, or chew controlled-release capsules.

• Do not stop taking this drug abruptly; it should be discontinued slowly.
• Do not use St. John's Wort while taking this drug.
• You may experience these side effects: Dizziness, drowsiness, nervousness, insomnia (avoid driving or performing hazardous tasks), nausea, vomiting, weight loss (eat frequent small meals), sexual dysfunction (reversible).
• Report rash, mania, seizures, severe weight loss, suicidal thoughts.

▽folic acid (folate)
(foe' lik)

PREGNANCY CATEGORY A

Drug classes

Folic acid
Vitamin supplement

Therapeutic actions

Required for nucleoprotein synthesis and maintenance of normal erythropoiesis.

Indications

• Treatment of megaloblastic anemias due to sprue, nutritional deficiency, pregnancy, infancy, and childhood

Contraindications and cautions

• Contraindicated with allergy to folic acid preparations; pernicious, aplastic, normocytic anemias.
• Use cautiously during lactation.

Available forms

Tablets—0.4, 0.8, 1 mg; injection—5 mg/mL

Dosages

Administer orally unless patient has severe intestinal malabsorption.
Adults
• *Therapeutic dose:* Up to 1 mg/day PO, IM, IV, or subcutaneously. Larger doses may be needed in severe cases.
• *Maintenance dose:* 0.4 mg/day.
• *Pregnancy and lactation:* 0.8 mg/day.
Pediatric patients
• *Maintenance dose:*
 Infants: 0.1 mg/day.
 Younger than 4 yr: Up to 0.3 mg/day.
 Older than 4 yr: 0.4 mg/day.

Pharmacokinetics

Route	Onset	Peak
Oral, IM, Subcut., IV	Varies	30–60 min

Metabolism: Hepatic; $T_{1/2}$: Unknown
Distribution: Crosses placenta; enters breast milk
Excretion: Urine

▼ IV FACTS

Preparation: Solution is yellow to yellow-orange; may be added to hyperalimentation solution or dextrose solutions.
Infusion: Infuse at rate of 5 mg/min by direct IV injection; may be diluted in hyperalimentation for continuous infusion.

Adverse effects

• **Hypersensitivity:** Allergic reactions
• **Local:** *Pain and discomfort at injection site*

Interactions

✳ **Drug-drug** • Decrease in serum phenytoin and increase in seizure activity with folic acid preparations • Decreased absorption with sulfasalazine, aminosalicylic acid

■ Nursing considerations

✦ CLINICAL ALERT!

Name confusion has occurred between folinic acid (leucovorin) and folic acid; use extreme caution.

Assessment

• **History:** Allergy to folic acid preparations; pernicious, aplastic, normocytic anemias; lactation
• **Physical:** Skin lesions, color; R, adventitious sounds; CBC, Hgb, Hct, serum folate levels, serum vitamin B_{12} levels, Schilling test

Interventions

• Administer orally if at all possible. With severe GI malabsorption or very severe disease, give IM, IV, or subcutaneously.
• Test using Schilling test and serum vitamin B_{12} levels to rule out pernicious anemia. Therapy may mask signs of pernicious anemia while the neurologic deterioration continues.
⊗ **Warning** Use caution when giving the parenteral preparations to premature infants.

These preparations contain benzyl alcohol and may produce a fatal gasping syndrome in premature infants.
⊗ **Warning** Monitor patient for hypersensitivity reactions, especially if drug previously taken. Keep supportive equipment and emergency drugs readily available in case of serious allergic response.

Teaching points

• When the cause of megaloblastic anemia is treated or passes (infancy, pregnancy), there may be no need for folic acid because it normally exists in sufficient quantities in the diet.
• Report rash, difficulty breathing, pain or discomfort at injection site.

▽follitropin alfa

See Appendix R, *Less commonly used drugs.*

▽follitropin beta

See Appendix R, *Less commonly used drugs.*

▽fomepizole

See Appendix R, *Less commonly used drugs.*

DANGEROUS DRUG

▽fondaparinux

*(fon dah **pear'** ah nucks)*

Arixtra

PREGNANCY CATEGORY B

Drug classes

Antithrombotic
Factor Xa inhibitor

Therapeutic actions

Blocks naturally occurring factor Xa, leading to an alteration in the clot formation process; decreasing the risk of clot and thrombus formation.

Indications

• Prevention of venous thromboembolic events (including DVT and pulmonary emboli) in patient undergoing surgery for hip fracture, hip replacement, knee replacement or undergoing abdominal surgery

• Extended prophylaxis of DVT, which may lead to pulmonary embolism in patients undergoing hip fracture surgery
• Treatment of acute DVT in conjunction with warfarin
• Treatment of acute pulmonary embolism when administered in conjunction with warfarin when initial therapy is administered in the hospital

Contraindications and cautions

• Contraindicated with hypersensitivity to fondaparinux, severe renal impairment, adults weighing less than 50 kg, active major bleeding, bacterial endocarditis, thrombocytopenia.
• Use cautiously with pregnancy or lactation, mild to moderate renal impairment, adults older than 65 yr, bleeding disorders, history of heparin-induced thrombocytopenia, uncontrolled arterial hypertension, GI ulcers, diabetic retinopathy, spinal puncture, neuroaxial anesthesia.

Available forms

Prefilled syringes—2.5 mg/0.5 mL, 5 mg/0.4 mL, 7.5 mg/0.6 mL, 10 mg/0.8 mL

Dosages

Adults
• *Prevention of DVT:* 2.5 mg/day subcutaneously starting 6–8 hr following surgical closure and continuing for 5–9 days. An additional 24 days may be added after the initial course for patients undergoing hip fracture surgery.
• *Treatment of DVT, acute pulmonary embolism in conjunction with warfarin:*
Weight less than 50 kg: 5 mg/day subcutaneously for 5–9 days.
Weight 50–100 kg: 7.5 mg/day subcutaneously for 5–9 days.
Weight more than 100 kg: 10 mg/day subcutaneously for 5–9 days.
Warfarin therapy should begin within 72 hr. Treatment should continue for at least 5 days until INR of 2 to 3 is achieved with heparin therapy.
Pediatric patients
Safety and efficacy not established.
Geriatric patients or patients with renal impairment
Contraindicated with severe renal impairment. Use caution with moderate renal impairment and with elderly patients. Monitor patient

closely and discontinue drug if renal impairment increases or severe bleeding occurs.

Pharmacokinetics

Route	Onset	Peak
Subcut.	Rapid	3 hr

Metabolism: $T_{1/2}$: 17–21 hr
Distribution: May cross placenta; may enter breast milk
Excretion: Urine, unchanged

Adverse effects

• **CNS:** Insomnia, dizziness, confusion, headache
• **CV:** Edema, hypotension
• **GI:** *Nausea,* constipation, diarrhea, vomiting, dyspepsia
• **GU:** UTI, urinary retention
• **Hematologic: Hemorrhage;** *bruising;* thrombocytopenia; *anemia*
• **Hypersensitivity:** Chills, fever, urticaria, asthma
• **Metabolic:** Elevated AST, ALT levels; hypokalemia
• **Renal:** Impaired renal functions
• **Other:** *Fever;* pain; local irritation, hematoma, erythema at site of injection, rash

Interactions

✳ **Drug-drug** • Increased bleeding tendencies with oral anticoagulants, salicylates, penicillins, cephalosporins, NSAIDs
✳ **Drug-alternative therapy** • Increased bleeding with high dose of vitamin E, garlic, ginkgo

■ Nursing considerations
Assessment

• **History:** Recent surgery or injury; sensitivity to fondaparinux; renal impairment; pregnancy, lactation; recent bleeding, thrombocytopenia, bacterial endocarditis, spinal puncture
• **Physical:** Weight, peripheral perfusion, R, stool guaiac test, PTT or other tests of blood coagulation, platelet count, CBC, renal function tests

Interventions

• Arrange to give drug 6–8 hr following surgical closure; continue for 5–9 days. An additional 24-day course may be added for patients undergoing hip fracture surgery.

Adverse effects in *italics* are most common; those in **bold** are life-threatening. ⚫ Do not crush.

⊗ *Black box warning* Carefully monitor patients receiving spinal/epidural anesthesia; risk of spinal hematoma and neurologic damage.

- Give deep subcutaneous injections; do not give by IM injection.
- To administer by deep subcutaneous injection, patient should be lying down, and alternate administration between the left and right anterolateral and left and right posterolateral abdominal wall. Introduce the whole length of the needle into a skinfold held between the thumb and forefinger; hold the skinfold throughout the injection.
- Apply pressure to all injection sites after needle is withdrawn; inspect injection sites for signs of hematoma.
- Do not massage injection sites.
- Do not mix with other injections or infusions.
- Store at room temperature; fluid should be clear, colorless to pale yellow.
- Provide for safety measures (electric razor, soft toothbrush) to prevent injury to patient who is at risk for bleeding.
- Check patient for signs of bleeding; monitor blood tests.

Teaching points

- This drug must be given by subcutaneous injection; it is not taken orally. You and a significant other will be instructed in how to administer the drug if you are being discharged with it. Arrange for proper disposal of syringes and needles.
- Arrange for periodic blood tests that will be needed to monitor your response to this drug.
- Be careful to avoid injury while taking this drug: Use an electric razor; avoid activities that might lead to injury.
- Report nose bleed, bleeding of the gums, unusual bruising, black or tarry stools, cloudy or dark urine, abdominal or lower back pain, severe headache.

▽formoterol fumarate
*(for **mob**' te rol)*

Foradil Aerolizer, Perforomist

PREGNANCY CATEGORY C

Drug classes
Antiasthmatic
Beta$_2$ agonist

Therapeutic actions
Long-acting agonist that binds to beta$_2$ receptors in the lungs, causing bronchodilation; may also inhibit the release of inflammatory mediators in the lung, blocking swelling and inflammation.

Indications
- Long-term maintenance treatment of asthma in adults and children 5 yr and older when used in combination with other drugs such as inhaled corticosteroids
- Prevention of exercise-induced bronchospasm in adults and children 5 yr and older when used on an occasional, as-needed basis
- Long-term maintenance treatment of bronchoconstriction in patients with COPD

Contraindications and cautions
- Contraindicated with hypersensitivity to adrenergics, amines, or formoterol; acute asthma attack; acute airway obstruction; asthma, without concomitant use of other drugs such as inhaled corticosteroids
- Use cautiously in the elderly and with pregnancy, lactation.

Available forms
Inhalation powder in capsules—12 mcg; inhalation solution—20 mcg/2 mL

Dosages
Adults
- *Maintenance treatment of COPD:* Oral inhalation of contents of 1 capsule (12 mcg) using *Aerolizer Inhaler* every 12 hr; do not exceed a total daily dose of 24 mcg. Or, one 20-mcg/2 mL vial by oral inhalation using a jet nebulizer connected to an air compressor twice daily, morning and evening; do not exceed 40 mcg/day.

Adults and pediatric patients 12 yr and older
- *Prevention of exercise-induced bronchospasm:* Oral inhalation of contents of one capsule (12 mcg) using the *Aerolizer Inhaler* 15 min before exercise. Additional doses should not be used for 72 hr. Use on an occasional, as-needed basis.

Adults and pediatric patients 5 yr and older
- *Maintenance treatment of asthma:* Oral inhalation of contents of 1 capsule (12 mcg) using the *Aerolizer Inhaler* every 12 hr. Do not exceed 1 capsule every 12 hr.

Pharmacokinetics

Route	Onset	Peak	Duration
Inhalation	1–3 min	1–3 hr	8–20 hr

Metabolism: Hepatic; $T_{1/2}$: 10–14 hr
Distribution: Crosses placenta; may enter breast milk
Excretion: Feces, urine

Adverse effects

- **CNS:** Tremor, dizziness, insomnia, dysphonia, *headache, nervousness*
- **CV:** Hypertension, tachycardia, chest pain
- **GI:** Nausea, dyspepsia, abdominal pain, *irritation of the throat and mouth*
- **Respiratory:** Bronchitis, respiratory infection, dyspnea, tonsillitis
- **Other:** *Viral infection* (most likely in children)

Interactions

✳ **Drug-drug** ● Beta blockers and formoterol may inhibit each other's effects; avoid use together ● Risk of prolonged QTc interval if combined with other drugs that prolong QTc interval; use with extreme caution

■ Nursing considerations

 CLINICAL ALERT!
Name confusion has occurred between *Foradil* (formoterol) and *Toradol* (ketorolac); use extreme caution.

Assessment

- **History:** Hypersensitivity to adrenergics, amines, or formoterol; acute asthma attack, acute airway obstruction, pregnancy, lactation
- **Physical:** R, adventitious sounds, P, BP, ECG, orientation, reflexes

Interventions

⊗ **Black box warning** Long-acting beta-agonists may increase risk of asthma-related deaths; use only if clearly warranted. Use without a concomitant inhaled corticosteroid is contraindicated. Risk increases in children and adolescents; suggest use of a fixed combination drug with an inhaled corticosteroid to ensure combination compliance.

- Instruct patient in the proper use of *Aerolizer Inhaler*. Ensure that patient does not swallow the capsule.

- Monitor use of inhaler. Patient should not wash the inhaler but should keep it dry; it should not be used for delivering any other medication. If a bronchodilator is needed between doses, consult with health care provider. Do not use more often than every 12 hr.
- Use a jet nebulizer connected to an air compressor for oral inhalation.
- Encourage patient who experiences exercise-induced asthma to use drug 15 min before activity, and to reserve this drug for occasional, as-needed use.
- Ensure that patient continues with appropriate use of corticosteroids or other drugs used to block bronchospasm, as appropriate.
- Arrange for periodic evaluation of respiratory condition during therapy.
- Arrange for analgesics as appropriate for headache.
- Establish safety precautions if tremor becomes a problem.

Teaching points

- This medication should not be used to relieve acute symptoms. For that purpose, use a short-acting beta$_2$-agonist.
- Always use this medication with an inhaled corticosteroid as part of the treatment program.
- Use the *Aerolizer Inhaler* as instructed. This is the only inhaler that can be used with this drug.
- Use only twice a day. Do not wash the inhaler; keep it dry at all times. Do not use this inhaler to deliver any other drugs. Check the "use by" date on your drug and discard any capsules that have expired.
- For oral inhalation formulation, use a jet nebulizer connected to an air compressor.
- If drug is to be used periodically for exercise-induced asthma, use 15 minutes before activity.
- Arrange for periodic evaluation of your respiratory problem while using this drug; continue to use any other therapies that have been prescribed to control your asthma.
- You may experience these side effects: Headache (appropriate analgesics may be ordered); tremors (use care in performing dangerous tasks if this occurs); fast heartbeat, palpitations (monitor activity if this occurs, rest frequently).
- Report severe headache, irregular heartbeat, worsening of asthma, difficulty breathing.

Adverse effects in *italics* are most common; those in **bold** are life-threatening. ▣ Do not crush.

▷fosamprenavir calcium

*(foss am **pren'** ah ver)*

Lexiva

PREGNANCY CATEGORY C

Drug classes
Antiviral
Protease inhibitor

Therapeutic actions
Antiviral activity; inhibits HIV protease activity, leading to the formation of immature, noninfectious virus particles.

Indications
- Treatment of HIV infection in adults in combination with other antiretrovirals (the use of fosamprenavir with ritonavir is not recommended for protease inhibitor–experienced patients)

Contraindications and cautions
- Contraindicated with allergy to any component of the drug or to amprenavir; concurrent use of drugs dependent on the CYP3A4 system for clearance, lactation; if used with ritonavir, use of flecainide and propafenone is contraindicated.
- Use cautiously with pregnancy, hepatic impairment, diabetes mellitus, lipid abnormalities, hemophilia, sulfonamide allergy.

Available forms
Tablets—700 mg; suspension—50 mg/mL

Dosages
Adults
1,400 mg PO bid.
- **With ritonavir:** 1,400 mg/day PO plus ritonavir 100 mg/day PO, 1,400 mg/day PO plus ritonavir 200 mg/day PO, or 700 mg PO bid with ritonavir 100 mg PO bid.
- *Protease-experienced patients:* 700 mg PO bid with ritonavir 100 mg PO bid.
Pediatric patients
- *Therapy-naïve children 2–5 yr:* 30 mg/kg oral suspension PO bid; do not exceed 1,400 mg bid.
- *Therapy-naïve children 6 yr and older:* 30 mg/kg oral suspension PO bid; do not exceed 1,400 mg bid. Or, 18 mg/kg oral sus-

pension PO with ritonavir 3 mg/kg PO bid; do not exceed 700 mg fosamprenavir plus 100 mg ritonavir bid.
- *Therapy-experienced children 2–5 yr:* Safety and efficacy not established.
- *Therapy-experienced children 6 yr and older:* 18 mg/kg oral suspension with 3 mg/kg ritonavir PO bid; do not exceed 700 mg fosamprenavir with 100 mg ritonavir bid.
Patients with hepatic impairment
- *Child-Pugh score 5–6:* 700 mg PO bid without ritonavir (therapy-naïve patients) or 700 mg PO bid plus 100 mg/day ritonavir (therapy-naïve or protease-inhibitor–experienced patients).
- *Child-Pugh score 7–9:* 700 mg PO bid without ritonavir (therapy naïve) or 450 mg PO bid with 100 mg/day ritonavir PO.
- *Child-Pugh score 10–15:* 350 mg PO bid without ritonavir (therapy naïve) or 300 mg PO bid with ritonavir 100 mg/day PO.

Pharmacokinetics

Route	Onset	Peak
Oral	Varies	1.5–4 hr

Metabolism: Hepatic; $T_{1/2}$: 7.7 hr
Distribution: Crosses placenta; may enter breast milk
Excretion: Feces, urine

Adverse effects
- **CNS:** Headache, oral paresthesias, depression, mood disorders
- **CV:** MI, dyslipidemia
- **Dermatologic:** Rash, **Stevens-Johnson syndrome,** pruritus
- **GI:** Nausea, vomiting, diarrhea, anorexia, abdominal pain, elevated liver enzymes
- **Hematologic:** Hyperglycemia, hypercholesterolemia, hypertriglyceridemia, neutropenia
- **Other:** Fatigue, redistribution of body fat (buffalo hump, thinning of arms and legs)

Interactions
❋ **Drug-drug** ⊗ *Warning* Potentially large increases in the serum concentration of flecainide, piroxicam, propafenone, rifabutin, simvastatin, lovastatin, midazolam, triazolam, dihydroergotamine, ergotamine, methylergonovine, pimozide, when taken with fosamprenavir. Potential for serious arrhythmias, seizure, rhabdomyolysis, and fatal reactions. Do

not administer fosamprenavir with any of these drugs.

• Potentially large increases in the serum concentration of the following: Antiarrhythmics—amiodarone, lidocaine, quinidine—monitor patient closely and adjust antiarrhythmic dosage as needed; antifungals—ketoconazole, itraconazole—reduced dosage of antifungals may be needed; rifabutin—reduce dosage to half recommended dose and monitor for neutropenia weekly; calcium channel blockers—diltiazem, felodipine, nifedipine, nicardipine, nimodipine, verapamil, amlodipine, nisoldipine, isradipine—increases calcium channel blocker concentrations; monitor patient very closely and use caution; atorvastatin—suggest use of a different HMG-CoA inhibitor; immunosuppressants—cyclosporine, tacrolimus—monitor serum concentration carefully and consider need for dosage reduction; sildenafil, vardenafil—reduce dosage and monitor patient carefully for adverse effects; TCAs—amitriptyline, imipramine—monitor serum concentrations closely and consider need for dosage reduction • Risk of decreased antiviral effectiveness when used with saquinavir, carbamazepine, phenobarbital, phenytoin, rifampin, delavirdine, efavirenz, nevirapine, lopinavir and ritonavir—check that appropriate dosage changes have been made; if any of these drugs are used together; monitor patient for progression of disease, adverse effects • Risk of decreased effectiveness of hormonal contraceptives; advise patient to use barrier contraceptives

✳ **Drug-alternative therapy** • Loss of virologic response if combined with St. John's Wort; avoid this combination

■ **Nursing considerations**
Assessment
• **History:** Allergy to any component of the drug or to amprenavir; concurrent use of drugs dependent on the CYP3A4 system for clearance, lactation, pregnancy, hepatic impairment, diabetes mellitus, lipid abnormalities, hemophilia, sulfonamide allergy
• **Physical:** Orientation, affect, reflexes; bowel sounds; skin color, perfusion; LFTs, CBC, serum triglycerides and cholesterol

Interventions
⊗ **Warning** Do not administer with any of the drugs listed as contraindications. Check all

other drugs in drug regimen for potential interaction and arrange for appropriate monitoring or dosage adjustment as needed.
• Use cautiously with any history of sulfonamide allergy; cross-reactivity may occur.
• Administer this drug with other antiretrovirals.
• Administer tablets without regard to food. Adults should take suspension without food; children should take suspension with food.
• Redose oral suspension if vomiting occurs within 30 min of dose.
• Be aware of increased risk of dyslipidemia, MI; monitor patient accordingly.
• Monitor liver function and blood glucose levels before and periodically during therapy.
• Monitor patient for rash; arrange to discontinue drug if severe skin reaction occurs.

Teaching points
• Take this drug without regard to meals. Adults should take suspension without food; children should take suspension with food.
• Take the full course of therapy as prescribed; do not take double doses if one is missed; if you forget to take a dose for more than 4 hours, wait and take the next dose at the regular time; if you miss a dose by less than 4 hours, take your missed dose right away and your next dose at the regular time.
• Shake suspension vigorously before each use. Drug may be stored in refrigerator or at room temperature.
• Do not change dosage without consulting your health care provider. Take this drug with other antivirals as prescribed.
• This drug does not cure HIV infection; long-term effects are not yet known. Continue to take precautions as the risk of transmission is not reduced by this drug.
• Do not take other prescription or over-the-counter drugs without consulting your health care provider. This drug interacts with many other drugs; serious problems can occur.
• Consider using barrier contraceptives while taking this drug; hormonal contraceptives may not be effective.
• Use caution if taking sildenafil (*Viagra*), tadalafil (*Cialis*), or vardenafil (*Levitra*). There is an increased risk of adverse effects; consult your health care provider if adverse effects occur.
• Some diabetic patients may have changes in blood glucose while taking this drug;

check your blood sugar often and consult your health care provider if control becomes a problem.

- Do not use St. John's Wort while you are using this drug; consult your health care provider before using any herbal therapies.
- You may experience these side effects: Nausea, vomiting, diarrhea, abdominal pain (eat frequent small meals); headache, numbness and tingling (use caution if driving or operating dangerous machinery); redistribution of body fat with thinning of arms and legs, development of a buffalo hump (it may help to know that this is a drug effect).
- Report severe diarrhea, severe nausea, rash, changes in the color of urine or stool; increased thirst or urination.

▽fosfomycin
tromethamine
*(foss foe my' sin
troh meth' ah meen)*

Monurol

PREGNANCY CATEGORY B

Drug classes
Antibacterial
Urinary tract anti-infective

Therapeutic actions
Bactericidal; interferes with bacterial cell wall synthesis, blocks adherence of bacteria to uroepithelial cells.

Indications
- Uncomplicated UTIs in women caused by susceptible strains of *Escherichia coli* and *Enterococcus faecalis;* not indicated for the treatment of pyelonephritis or perinephric abscess

Contraindications and cautions
- Contraindicated with allergy to fosfomycin.
- Use cautiously with pregnancy, lactation.

Available forms
Granule packet—3 g

Dosages
Adults
1 packet dissolved in water PO as a single dose.

Pediatric patients younger than 12 yr
Not recommended.

Pharmacokinetics

Route	Onset	Peak
Oral	Rapid	2–4 hr

Metabolism: Hepatic; $T_{1/2}$: 5.7 hr
Distribution: Crosses placenta; may enter breast milk
Excretion: Feces, urine

Adverse effects
- **CNS:** *Headache, dizziness,* back pain, asthenia
- **GI:** *Nausea,* abdominal cramps, dyspepsia, diarrhea
- **GU:** Vaginitis, dysmenorrhea
- **Other:** Rhinitis, rash

Interactions
✳ **Drug-drug** • Lowered serum concentration and urinary tract excretion with metoclopramide

■ Nursing considerations
Assessment
- **History:** Allergy to fosfomycin, pregnancy, lactation
- **Physical:** Skin color, lesions; orientation, reflexes; urine for analysis

Interventions
- Arrange for culture and sensitivity tests.
- Administer drug with food if GI upset occurs.
- ⊗ *Warning* Do not administer dry; mix a single dose packet in 90–120 mL of water and stir to dissolve; do not use hot water. Administer immediately.
- Monitor clinical response; if no improvement is seen or a relapse occurs, send urine for repeat culture and sensitivity tests.
- Encourage patient to observe other measures (avoid bubble baths, alkaline ash foods, sexual intercourse; drink lots of fluids) to decrease risk of UTI.

Teaching points
- This drug is meant to be a one-dose treatment for urinary tract infection; improvement should be seen in 2–3 days. If no improvement occurs, consult your health care provider.

F

- Take drug with food if GI upset occurs. Do not take in the dry form; mix a single dose packet in 90–120 milliliters of water and stir to dissolve; do not use hot water. Drink immediately after mixing.
- You may experience these side effects: Nausea, abdominal pain (eat frequent small meals; take the drug with meals); dizziness (observe caution if driving or using dangerous equipment).
- Report rash, visual changes, severe GI problems, weakness, tremors, worsening of urinary tract symptoms.

▷ fosinopril sodium
(foh sin' oh pril)

Monopril

PREGNANCY CATEGORY C
(FIRST TRIMESTER)

PREGNANCY CATEGORY D
(SECOND AND THIRD TRIMESTERS)

Drug classes
ACE inhibitor
Antihypertensive

Therapeutic actions
Renin, synthesized by the kidneys, is released into the circulation where it acts on a plasma precursor to produce angiotensin I, which is converted by ACE to angiotensin II, a potent vasoconstrictor that also causes release of aldosterone from the adrenals; fosinopril blocks the conversion of angiotensin I to angiotensin II, leading to decreased BP, decreased aldosterone secretion, an increase in serum potassium levels, and sodium and fluid loss; increased prostaglandin synthesis may be involved in the antihypertensive action.

Indications
- Treatment of hypertension, alone or in combination with thiazide-type diuretics
- Management of heart failure as adjunctive therapy

Contraindications and cautions
- Contraindicated with allergy to fosinopril or other ACE inhibitors; pregnancy.

- Use cautiously with impaired renal or hepatic function, hyperkalemia, salt or volume depletion, lactation.

Available forms
Tablets—10, 20, 40 mg

Dosages
Adults
- *Hypertension:* Initial dose, 10 mg PO daily. Maintenance dose, 20–40 mg/day PO as a single dose or two divided doses. In patients receiving diuretic therapy, begin fosinopril therapy with 10 mg. Do not exceed maximum dose of 80 mg.
- *Heart failure:* Initially, 10 mg/day PO; observe for 2 hr for hypotension. If patient has moderate to severe renal failure, 5 mg/day PO. Do not exceed maximum dose of 40 mg/day.

Pediatric patients
Safety and efficacy not established.

Pharmacokinetics

Route	Onset	Peak	Duration
Oral	1 hr	3 hr	24 hr

Metabolism: Hepatic; $T_{1/2}$: 12 hr
Distribution: Crosses placenta; enters breast milk
Excretion: Feces, urine

Adverse effects
- **CV:** Angina pectoris, orthostatic hypotension in salt- or volume-depleted patients, palpitations
- **Dermatologic:** Rash, pruritus, diaphoresis, flushing
- **GI:** *Nausea,* abdominal pain, vomiting, diarrhea
- **Respiratory:** *Cough,* asthma, bronchitis, dyspnea, sinusitis
- **Other: Angioedema,** asthenia, myalgia, arthralgia, hyperkalemia

Interactions
✳ **Drug-drug** ● Decreased effectiveness if combined with indomethacin or other NSAIDs ● Risk of lithium toxicity if combined with ACE inhibitors ● Risk of increased potassium levels if taken with potassium-sparing diuretics ● Decreased absorption when given with antacids; separate by at least 2 hr

Adverse effects in *italics* are most common; those in **bold** are life-threatening. ⬛ Do not crush.

■ Nursing considerations

CLINICAL ALERT!

Name confusion has occurred between fosinopril and lisinopril; use caution.

Assessment

- **History:** Allergy to fosinopril and other ACE inhibitors, impaired renal or hepatic function, hyperkalemia, salt or volume depletion, lactation, pregnancy
- **Physical:** Skin color, lesions, turgor; T; P; BP, peripheral perfusion; mucous membranes, bowel sounds, liver evaluation; urinalysis, LFTs, renal function tests, CBC, and differential

Interventions

⊗ *Warning* Alert surgeon and mark the patient's chart with notice that fosinopril is being taken; the angiotensin II formation subsequent to compensatory renin release during surgery will be blocked; hypotension may be reversed with volume expansion.

⊗ **Black box warning** Suggest use of a contraceptive. Pregnancy should be avoided; fetal damage can occur if drug is used in the second or third trimester. Arrange to switch to a different drug if pregnancy occurs.

- Monitor patient closely for a drop in BP secondary to reduction in fluid volume (excessive perspiration and dehydration, vomiting, diarrhea); excessive hypotension may occur.

Teaching points

- Do not stop taking the medication without consulting your health care provider.
- Avoid pregnancy while taking this drug; using barrier contraceptives is advised.
- Be careful with any conditions that may lead to a drop in blood pressure (such as diarrhea, sweating, vomiting, dehydration); if light-headedness or dizziness occurs, consult your health care provider.
- You may experience these side effects: GI upset, loss of appetite (these may be transient); light-headedness (transient; change position slowly and limit activities to those that do not require alertness and precision); dry cough (not harmful).
- Report mouth sores; sore throat, fever, chills; swelling of the hands, feet; irregular heartbeat, chest pains; swelling of the face, eyes, lips, tongue; difficulty breathing; persistent cough.

▷fosphenytoin sodium
(faws fen' i toe in)

Cerebyx

PREGNANCY CATEGORY D

Drug classes
Antiepileptic
Hydantoin

Therapeutic actions
A prodrug that is converted to phenytoin; has antiepileptic activity without causing general CNS depression; stabilizes neuronal membranes and prevents hyperexcitability caused by excessive stimulation; limits the spread of seizure activity from an active focus.

Indications
- Short-term control of general convulsive status epilepticus
- Prevention and treatment of seizures occurring during or following neurosurgery
- Short-term substitute for oral phenytoin

Contraindications and cautions
- Contraindicated with hypersensitivity to hydantoins, sinus bradycardia, sinoatrial block, second- or third-degree AV heart block, Stokes-Adams syndrome, pregnancy (data suggest an association between use of antiepileptic drugs by women with epilepsy and an elevated incidence of birth defects in children born to these women; however, do not discontinue antiepileptic therapy in pregnant women who are receiving therapy to prevent major seizures—this is likely to precipitate status epilepticus, with attendant hypoxia and risk to both mother and unborn child), lactation.
- Use cautiously with hypotension, severe myocardial insufficiency, porphyria, hepatic dysfunction.

Available forms
Injection—75 mg/mL (50 mg/mL phenytoin equivalents [PE])

Dosages
Dosage is given as PEs to facilitate transfer from phenytoin.

Adults
- *Status epilepticus:* Loading dose of 15–20 mg PE/kg administered at 100–150 mg PE/min IV.
- *Neurosurgery (prophylaxis):* Loading dose of 10–20 mg PE/kg IM or IV; maintenance dose of 4–6 mg PE/kg/day.
- *Substitution for oral phenytoin therapy:* Substitute IM or IV at the same total daily dose as phenytoin, for short-term use only.

Pediatric patients
Not recommended; off-label use only.

Patients with renal or hepatic impairment
Use caution and monitor for early signs of toxicity—changes in the metabolism of the drug may result in increased risk of adverse effects.

Pharmacokinetics

Route	Onset	Peak
IV	Rapid	End of infusion

Metabolism: Hepatic; $T_{1/2}$: 15 min
Distribution: Crosses placenta; enters breast milk
Excretion: Urine

▼ IV FACTS

Preparation: Dilute in 5% dextrose or 0.9% saline solution to a concentration of 1.5–25 mg PE/mL. Refrigerate; stable at room temperature for less than 48 hr.
Infusion: Infuse for status epilepticus at rate of 100–150 mg PE/min; never administer at a rate that exceeds 150 mg PE/min. Usually takes 5–20 min, depending on dose.

Adverse effects

- **CNS:** *Nystagmus, ataxia, dizziness, somnolence,* drowsiness, insomnia, transient nervousness, motor twitchings, fatigue, irritability, depression, numbness, tremor, headache, photophobia, diplopia, asthenia, back pain, suicidal ideation
- **CV:** *Hypotension,* vasodilation, tachycardia
- **Dermatologic:** *Pruritus*
- **GI:** *Nausea,* vomiting, dry mouth, taste perversion
- **Other:** Lymph node hyperplasia, sometimes progressing to frank malignant lymphoma, monoclonal gammopathy and multiple myeloma (prolonged therapy), polyarthropathy, osteomalacia, weight gain, chest pain, periarteritis nodosa

Interactions

No specific drug interactions have been reported, but because fosphenytoin is a metabolite of phenytoin, documented interactions with that drug should be considered.

✳ **Drug-drug** • Increased pharmacologic effects of hydantoins with chloramphenicol, cimetidine, disulfiram, phenacemide, sulfonamides, trimethoprim; reduced fosphenytoin dose may be needed • Complex interactions and effects when phenytoin and valproic acid are given together; phenytoin toxicity with apparently normal serum phenytoin levels; decreased plasma levels of valproic acid given with phenytoin; breakthrough seizures when the two drugs are given together • Increased pharmacologic effects and toxicity when primidone, amiodarone, chloramphenicol, fluconazole, isoniazid are given with hydantoins • Decreased pharmacologic effects of the following with hydantoins: Corticosteroids, cyclosporine, dicumarol, disopyramide, doxycycline, estrogens, furosemide, levodopa, methadone, metyrapone, mexiletine, hormonal contraceptives, quinidine, atracurium, pancuronium, tubocurarine, vecuronium, carbamazepine, diazoxide

✳ **Drug-lab test** • Interference with metyrapone and 1-mg dexamethasone tests for at least 7 days

■ Nursing considerations

CLINICAL ALERT!
Name confusion has occurred between *Cerebyx* (fosphenytoin), *Celebrex* (celecoxib), *Celexa* (citalopram), and *Xanax* (alprazolam); use caution.

Assessment

- **History:** Hypersensitivity to hydantoins; sinus bradycardia, sinoatrial block, second- or third-degree AV heart block, Stokes-Adams syndrome, pregnancy, lactation, hepatic failure, severe myocardial insufficiency, porphyria
- **Physical:** T; skin color, lesions; orientation, affect, reflexes, vision examination; P, BP; bowel sounds, normal output, liver evaluation; LFTs, CBC and differential, EEG and ECG

Adverse effects in *italics* are most common; those in **bold** are life-threatening. ⓒⓃⓒ Do not crush.

Interventions

• Continue supportive measures, including use of an IV benzodiazepine, until drug becomes effective against seizures.

• Possible increased risk of suicidal ideation; monitor patient accordingly.

⊗ **Warning** Administer IV slowly to prevent severe hypotension; margin of safety between full therapeutic and toxic doses is small. Continually monitor cardiac rhythm and check BP frequently and regularly during IV infusion and for 10–20 min after infusion.

• Monitor infusion site carefully—drug solutions are very alkaline and irritating.

• This drug is recommended for short-term use only (up to 5 days); switch to oral phenytoin as soon as possible.

⊗ **Black box warning** Suggest use of a contraceptive. Pregnancy should be avoided; fetal damage can occur.

Teaching points

• This drug can only be given IV and will be stopped as soon as you are able to take an oral drug.

• Use of a contraceptive is advised; drug should not be used during pregnancy. This drug may cause hormonal contraceptives to be ineffective, use of barrier contraceptives is advised.

• You may experience these side effects: Drowsiness, dizziness, GI upset.

• Report rash, severe nausea or vomiting, drowsiness, slurred speech, impaired coordination (ataxia), sore throat, unusual bleeding or bruising, persistent headache, malaise, pain at injection site, thoughts of suicide.

▽ **fospropofol disodium**
*(foss **prob'** poh fall)*

Lusedra

PREGNANCY CATEGORY B

Drug class
Sedative-hypnotic

Therapeutic actions
Thought to increase sensitivity to GABA, leading to inhibition of neurotransmission and CNS depression.

Indications

• Monitored anesthesia care sedation in adults undergoing diagnostic and therapeutic procedures

Contraindications and cautions

• Contraindicated in hypersensitivity to components of drug.

• Use cautiously in elderly patients; severe systemic diseases, dehydration, decreased myocardial function or reduced vascular tone; pregnancy, lactation.

Available forms
Single-use vial—35 mg/mL

Dosages
Adults
6.5 mg/kg IV bolus followed by 1.6 mg/kg IV to maintain desired sedation. Bolus should not exceed 16.5 mL and IV infusion should not exceed 4 mL.
Pediatric patients
Safety and efficacy not established.
Geriatric patients and patients with severe systemic disease
75% of the standard dose is recommended.

▼ IV FACTS

Preparation: Drug is ready to use and does not require further reconstitution. May be given with 5% dextrose, 5% dextrose with 0.2% or 0.45% sodium chloride injection; 0.9% sodium chloride injection; lactated Ringer solution; lactated Ringer with 5% dextrose; 0.45% sodium chloride injection; 5% dextrose, 0.45% sodium chloride, and 20 mEq potassium chloride, USP. Does not need to be protected from light or infused through a filter. Solution should be clear, with no particulate matter. Discard vial after withdrawing drug.

Infusion: Administer through a freely flowing IV using a compatible solution. Flush line with normal saline before and after administering drug.

Incompatibilities: Do not mix with other drugs or solutions; physically incompatible with midazolam, meperidine.

Pharmacokinetics

Route	Onset	Peak
IV	Rapid	4–13 min

Metabolism: Hepatic; T$_{1/2}$: 0.8–0.9 hr
Distribution: May cross placenta; enters breast milk
Excretion: Urine

Adverse effects

- **CNS:** Headache, *paresthesia* (burning, tingling) *in perianal region,* **loss of responsiveness**
- **CV:** Hypotension
- **GI:** Nausea, vomiting
- **Respiratory: Hypoxemia, respiratory depression**
- **Other:** *Perianal pruritus*

Interactions

✶ **Drug-drug** • Risk of increased cardiac or respiratory depression if combined with other sedative-hypnotics (benzodiazepines, opioid analgesics)

■ Nursing considerations
Assessment

- **History:** Systemic diseases, pregnancy, lactation
- **Physical:** Orientation, affect; R, adventitious sounds; BP, ECG, state of hydration, skin lesions

Interventions

- Drug should only be administered by persons trained in administration of anesthesia who can continually monitor patient and are not involved in the diagnostic procedure or treatment being performed.
- Patient will require oxygen administration and continuous monitoring of pulse oximetry, ECG, and frequent blood pressure checks.
- Patients weighing more than 90 kg should be dosed as if they weigh 90 kg; patients less than 60 kg should be dosed as if they weigh 60 kg.
- Emergency equipment should be readily available.
- Patient should be escorted after the procedure; driving is not advised.
- Alert patient that perianal burning, stinging, and tingling are common after injection of the drug and that these symptoms will pass and no treatment is required.

Teaching points

- You will be very relaxed and unaware during the procedure; you will require an escort at discharge because no driving is permitted immediately after the use of this drug.
- You may experience perianal burning, stinging, tingling, and rash, which are common effects when the drug is given. These symptoms are usually mild, last only a short time, and do not require treatment.

▷ **frovatriptan succinate**
*(frow vah **trip'** tan)*

Frova

PREGNANCY CATEGORY C

Drug classes
Antimigraine drug
Serotonin selective agonist
Triptan

Therapeutic actions
Binds to serotonin receptors to cause vascular constrictive effects on cranial blood vessels, causing the relief of migraine in selective patients.

Indications
- Treatment of acute migraines with or without aura in adults

Contraindications and cautions
- Contraindicated with allergy to frovatriptan, active CAD, ischemic heart disease, Prinzmetal angina, peripheral or cerebral vascular syndromes, uncontrolled hypertension, hemiplegic or basilar migraine, use of an ergot compound or other triptan within 24 hr.
- Use cautiously with hepatic or renal impairment, risk factors for CAD, lactation, pregnancy.

Available forms
Tablets—2.5 mg

Dosages
Adults
2.5 mg PO as a single dose at first sign of migraine; if headache returns, may be repeated after 2 hr. Do not use more than 3 doses/24 hr. Safety of treating more than four headaches/30 days has not been established.

Pediatric patients
Safety and efficacy not established for patients younger than 18 yr.

Pharmacokinetics

Route	Onset	Peak
Oral	Varies	2–4 hr

Metabolism: Hepatic; $T_{1/2}$: 26 hr
Distribution: Crosses placenta; may enter breast milk
Excretion: Feces, urine

Adverse effects
- **CNS:** Dizziness, headache, anxiety, malaise, fatigue, weakness, myalgia, somnolence, paresthesia (tingling, burning, prickling, itching sensation), loss of sensation, abnormal vision, tinnitus
- **CV:** Palpitations, tightness or pressure in chest, flushing, **MI, cerebrovascular events, ventricular arrhythmias**
- **GI:** Vomiting, diarrhea, abdominal pain, dry mouth, dyspepsia, nausea
- **Musculoskeletal:** Skeletal pain
- **Other:** Warm or hot sensations, cold sensation, pain, increased sweating, rhinitis

Interactions
✳ Drug-drug ⊗ **Warning** Increased risk of weakness, hyperreflexia, CNS effects if combined with an SSRI (fluoxetine, fluvoxamine, paroxetine, sertraline); if combined with these drugs, appropriate safety precautions should be observed and patient monitored closely.

• Prolonged vasoactive reactions when taken concurrently with ergot-containing drugs or other triptans; space these drugs at least 24 hr apart

■ Nursing considerations
Assessment
- **History:** Allergy to frovatriptan, active coronary artery disease, Prinzmetal angina, pregnancy, lactation, peripheral or cerebral vascular syndromes, uncontrolled hypertension, hemiplegic or basilar migraine, use of an ergot compound or other triptan within 24 hr, risk factors for CAD
- **Physical:** Skin color and lesions, orientation, reflexes, peripheral sensation, P, BP, LFTs, ECG

Interventions
- Ensure that the patient has been diagnosed with migraine headaches.
- Administer to relieve acute migraine, not as a prophylactic measure.
- Ensure that the patient has not taken an ergot-containing compound or other triptan within 24 hr.
- Do not administer more than three doses in a 24-hr period; space them at least 2 hr apart.
- Establish safety measures if CNS or visual disturbances occur.
- Provide environmental (lighting, temperature) control as appropriate to help relieve migraine.

⊗ **Warning** Monitor BP of patients with possible CAD; discontinue at any sign of angina, prolonged high BP, tachycardia, chest pain.

Teaching points
- Take drug exactly as prescribed, at the onset of headache or aura. Do not take this drug to prevent a migraine; it is only used to treat migraines that are occurring. If the headache persists after you take this drug, you may repeat the dose after 2 hours have passed.
- Do not take more than three doses in a 24-hour period. Do not take any other migraine medication while you are taking this drug. If the headache is not relieved, call your health care provider.
- This drug should not be taken during pregnancy; if you suspect that you are pregnant, contact your health care provider and refrain from using the drug.
- Maintain any procedures you usually use during a migraine (such as controlling lighting and noise).
- Contact your health care provider immediately if you experience chest pain or pressure that is severe or does not go away.
- You may experience these side effects: Dizziness, drowsiness (avoid driving or the use of dangerous machinery while taking this drug); numbness, tingling, feelings of tightness or pressure.
- Report feelings of heat, flushing, tiredness, feelings of sickness, swelling of lips or eyelids.

DANGEROUS DRUG

▷fulvestrant
(full ves' trant)

Faslodex

PREGNANCY CATEGORY D

Drug classes
Antineoplastic
Estrogen receptor antagonist

Therapeutic actions
Binds to estrogen receptors, has anti-estrogen effects; and inhibits growth of estrogen receptor–positive breast cancer cell lines.

Indications
- Treatment of hormone receptor–positive breast cancer in postmenopausal women with disease progression following anti-estrogen therapy

Contraindications and cautions
- Contraindicated with allergy to any component of the drug, pregnancy.
- Use cautiously with bleeding disorders, thrombocytopenia, hepatic impairment, lactation.

Available forms
Injection—50 mg/mL

Dosages
Adults
500 mg IM on days 1, 15, 29 and then monthly as two concomitant 5-mL injections, one in each buttock.
Patients with hepatic impairment (Child-Pugh Class B)
250 mg IM on days 1, 15, 29 and then monthly.

Pharmacokinetics

Route	Onset	Peak
IM	Slow	7 days

Metabolism: Hepatic; $T_{1/2}$: 40 days
Distribution: Crosses placenta; may enter breast milk
Excretion: Feces

Adverse effects
- **CNS:** Depression, light-headedness, dizziness, *headache*, hallucinations, vertigo, insomnia, paresthesia, anxiety, *asthenia*

- **CV:** Chest pain, *vasodilation*
- **Dermatologic:** *Hot flashes,* rash
- **GI:** *Nausea, vomiting,* food distaste, constipation, *diarrhea,* anorexia, *abdominal pain*
- **GU:** UTI, *pelvic pain*
- **Respiratory:** *Dyspnea, increased cough*
- **Other:** Peripheral edema, fever, pharyngitis, injection site reactions, pain, flulike symptoms, *increased sweat, anemia, back pain, bone pain, arthritis*

Interactions
✳ Drug-drug • Increased risk of bleeding if taken with oral anticoagulants

■ Nursing considerations
Assessment
- **History:** Allergy to any component of the drug; pregnancy, lactation; hepatic impairment, bleeding disorders, thrombocytopenia
- **Physical:** Skin color, lesions, turgor; pelvic examination; orientation, affect, reflex; BP, peripheral pulses, edema; LFTs

Interventions
- Ensure that the patient is not pregnant before administering drug.
- Counsel patient about the need to use contraceptives to avoid pregnancy while taking this drug. Inform patient that serious fetal harm could occur.
- Suggest an alternative method of feeding the baby if this drug is prescribed for a breast-feeding patient.
- Use caution when handling drug; it is a potential teratogen.
- Warm solution before injecting by storing at room temperature for an hour or gently rolling before use.
- Administer by slow IM injection (1–2 min) into buttocks; use two injections per dose, with one in each buttock.
- Mark a calendar for dates for monthly injections; periodically monitor injection sites if patient is self-administering drug.
- Provide comfort measures to help patient deal with drug effects: Hot flashes (environmental temperature control); headache, depression (monitoring light and noise); vaginal bleeding (hygiene measures); nausea, food distaste (eat frequent small meals).

Adverse effects in *italics* are most common; those in **bold** are life-threatening. ▭▭▭ Do not crush.

Teaching points

• You and a significant other should learn the proper technique for administering an intramuscular injection. You will administer by slow injection over 1 to 2 minutes. You will need two injections for each dose; administer one in each buttock. Proper disposal of needles and syringes is important and should be reviewed.

• Mark your calendar with the date of your injection. If you are not able to self-administer the injection, mark your calendar with the dates to return to your health care provider for injections.

• This drug can cause serious fetal harm and must not be taken during pregnancy. Use contraceptives while you are taking this drug. If you become pregnant or decide that you would like to become pregnant, consult your health care provider immediately.

• You may experience these side effects: Hot flashes (staying in cool environment may help); nausea, vomiting (eat frequent small meals); weight gain; dizziness, headache, light-headedness (use caution if driving or performing tasks that require alertness if these occur).

• Report marked weakness, sleepiness, mental confusion, changes in color of urine or stool, pregnancy.

▷furosemide
(fur oh' se mide)

Apo-Furosemide (CAN), Furosemide Special (CAN), Lasix

PREGNANCY CATEGORY C

Drug class
Loop diuretic

Therapeutic actions
Inhibits reabsorption of sodium and chloride from the proximal and distal tubules and ascending limb of the loop of Henle, leading to a sodium-rich diuresis.

Indications
• Oral, IV: Edema associated with heart failure, cirrhosis, renal disease
• IV: Acute pulmonary edema
• Oral: Hypertension

Contraindications and cautions

• Contraindicated with allergy to furosemide, sulfonamides; allergy to tartrazine (in oral solution); anuria, severe renal failure; hepatic coma; pregnancy; lactation.
• Use cautiously with SLE, gout, diabetes mellitus.

Available forms
Tablets—20, 40, 80 mg; oral solution—10 mg/mL, 40 mg/5 mL; injection—10 mg/mL

Dosages
Adults
• *Edema:* Initially, 20–80 mg/day PO as a single dose. If needed, a second dose may be given in 6–8 hr. If response is unsatisfactory, dose may be increased in 20- to 40-mg increments at 6- to 8-hr intervals. Up to 600 mg/day may be given. Intermittent dosage schedule (2–4 consecutive days/wk) is preferred for maintenance, *or* 20–40 mg IM or IV (slow IV injection over 1–2 min). May increase dose in increments of 20 mg in 2 hr. High-dose therapy should be given as infusion at rate not exceeding 4 mg/min.
• *Acute pulmonary edema:* 40 mg IV over 1–2 min. May be increased to 80 mg IV given over 1–2 min if response is unsatisfactory after 1 hr.
• *Hypertension:* 40 mg bid PO. If needed, additional antihypertensives may be added.
Pediatric patients
Premature infants, **do not exceed 1 mg/kg/day.** Stimulates prostaglandin E_2 synthesis and may increase incidence of patent ductus arteriosus and complicate RDS.
• *Edema:* Initially, 2 mg/kg/day PO. If needed, increase by 1–2 mg/kg in 6–8 hr. **Do not exceed 6 mg/kg.** Adjust maintenance dose to lowest effective level.
• *Pulmonary edema:* 1 mg/kg IV or IM. May increase by 1 mg/kg in 2 hr until the desired effect is seen. **Do not exceed 6 mg/kg.**
Patients with renal impairment
Up to 4 g/day has been tolerated. IV bolus injection should not exceed 1 g/day given over 30 min.

Pharmacokinetics

Route	Onset	Peak	Duration
Oral	60 min	60–120 min	6–8 hr
IV, IM	5 min	30 min	2 hr

Metabolism: Hepatic; $T_{1/2}$: 30–60 min
Distribution: Crosses placenta; enters breast milk
Excretion: Feces, urine

▼ IV FACTS

Preparation: Store at room temperature; exposure to light may slightly discolor solution.
Infusion: Inject directly or into tubing of actively running IV; inject slowly over 1–2 min.
Incompatibilities: Do not mix with acidic solutions. Isotonic saline, lactated Ringer injection, and 5% dextrose injection may be used after pH has been adjusted (if necessary); precipitates form with gentamicin, milrinone in 5% dextrose, 0.9% sodium chloride.

Adverse effects

- **CNS:** *Dizziness, vertigo, paresthesias, xanthopsia, weakness,* headache, drowsiness, fatigue, blurred vision, tinnitus, irreversible hearing loss
- **CV:** *Orthostatic hypotension,* volume depletion, cardiac arrhythmias, *thrombophlebitis*
- **Dermatologic:** *Photosensitivity, rash, pruritus, urticaria,* purpura, exfoliative dermatitis, erythema multiforme
- **GI:** *Nausea, anorexia, vomiting, oral and gastric irritation, constipation,* diarrhea, acute pancreatitis, jaundice
- **GU:** Polyuria, nocturia, glycosuria, *urinary bladder spasm*
- **Hematologic:** *Leukopenia, anemia, thrombocytopenia,* fluid and electrolyte imbalances, hyperglycemia, hyperuricemia
- **Other:** *Muscle cramps and muscle spasms*

Interactions

✳ Drug-drug • Increased risk of cardiac arrhythmias with cardiac glycosides (due to electrolyte imbalance) • Increased risk of ototoxicity with aminoglycoside antibiotics, cisplatin • Decreased absorption of furosemide with phenytoin • Decreased natriuretic and antihypertensive effects with indomethacin, ibuprofen, other NSAIDs • Decreased GI absorption with charcoal • May reduce effect of insulin or oral antidiabetics because blood glucose levels can become elevated

■ Nursing considerations

> ⚡ **CLINICAL ALERT!**
> Name confusion has occurred between furosemide and torsemide; use extreme caution.

Assessment

- **History:** Allergy to furosemide, sulfonamides, tartrazine; electrolyte depletion anuria, severe renal failure; hepatic coma; SLE; gout; diabetes mellitus; lactation, pregnancy
- **Physical:** Skin color, lesions, edema; orientation, reflexes, hearing; pulses, baseline ECG, BP, orthostatic BP, perfusion; R, pattern, adventitious sounds; liver evaluation, bowel sounds; urinary output patterns; CBC, serum electrolytes (including calcium), blood sugar, LFTs, renal function tests, uric acid, urinalysis, weight

Interventions

⊗ **Black box warning** Profound diuresis with water and electrolyte depletion can occur; careful medical supervision is required.
- Administer with food or milk to prevent GI upset.
- Reduce dosage if given with other antihypertensives; readjust dosage gradually as BP responds.
- Give early in the day so that increased urination will not disturb sleep.
- Avoid IV use if oral use is at all possible.

⊗ **Warning** Do not mix parenteral solution with highly acidic solutions with pH below 3.5.
- Do not expose to light, which may discolor tablets or solution; do not use discolored drug or solutions.
- Discard diluted solution after 24 hr.
- Keep oral solution at room temperature; discard any solution left 60 days after opening bottle.
- Measure and record weight to monitor fluid changes.
- Arrange to monitor serum electrolytes, hydration, liver and renal function.
- Arrange for potassium-rich diet or supplemental potassium as needed.

Teaching points

- Record intermittent therapy on a calendar or dated envelopes. When possible, take the drug early so increased urination will not disturb sleep. Take with food or meals to prevent GI upset.

- Weigh yourself on a regular basis, at the same time and in the same clothing, and record the weight on your calendar.
- Blood glucose levels may become temporarily elevated in patients with diabetes after starting this drug.
- You may experience these side effects: Increased volume and frequency of urination; dizziness, feeling faint on arising, drowsiness (avoid rapid position changes; hazardous activities, like driving; and consumption of alcohol); sensitivity to sunlight (use sunglasses, wear protective clothing, or use a sunscreen); increased thirst (suck on sugarless candies; use frequent mouth care); loss of body potassium (a potassium-rich diet or potassium supplement will be needed).
- Report loss or gain of more than 1.5 kg in 1 day, swelling in your ankles or fingers, unusual bleeding or bruising, dizziness, trembling, numbness, fatigue, muscle weakness or cramps.

▷ gabapentin
(gab ah pen' tin)

Apo-Gabapentin (CAN), CO Gabapentin (CAN), Gen-Gabapentin (CAN), Gralise⬛Ⓖ, Neurontin, Novo-Gabapentin (CAN), PMS Gabapentin (CAN), ratio-Gabapentin (CAN)

gabapentin enacarbil
Horizant⬛Ⓖ

PREGNANCY CATEGORY C

Drug class
Antiepileptic

Therapeutic actions
Mechanism of action not understood; antiepileptic activity may be related to its ability to inhibit polysynaptic responses and block posttetanic potentiation.

Indications
- Adjunctive therapy in the treatment of partial seizures with and without secondary generalization in adults and children older than 12 yr with epilepsy

- ◾ NEW INDICATION: Adjunctive therapy for treatment of partial seizures in children 3–12 yr
- Orphan drug use: Treatment of amyotrophic lateral sclerosis
- Management of post-herpetic neuralgia or pain in the area affected by herpes zoster after the disease has been treated
- Treatment of moderate to severe primary restless legs syndrome in adults (*Horizant*)
- Unlabeled uses: Hot flashes, neuropathic pain, diabetic neuropathy, pruritus

Contraindications and cautions
- Contraindicated with hypersensitivity to gabapentin.
- Use cautiously with pregnancy, lactation.

Available forms
Capsules—100, 300, 400 mg; tablets—100, 300, 400, 600, 800 mg; oral solution—250 mg/5 mL; ER tablets—600 mgⒼ; tabletsⒼ—300, 600 mg (*Gralise*)

Dosages
Adults
- *Epilepsy:* Starting dose is 300 mg PO tid, then titrated up as needed. *Maintenance:* 900–1,800 mg/day PO in divided doses tid PO; maximum interval between doses should not exceed 12 hr. Up to 2,400–3,600 mg/day has been used
- *Post-herpetic neuralgia:* Initial dose of 300 mg/day PO; 300 mg bid PO on day 2; 300 mg tid PO on day 3. Or, 1,800 mg/day PO with the evening meal (*Gralise*).
- *Moderate to severe restless legs syndrome:* 600–800 mg/day PO with food, around 5 PM; maximum dose, 2,400 mg/day (*Horizant*).

Pediatric patients 3–12 yr
Initially, 10–15 mg/kg/day PO in three divided doses; adjust upward over about 3 days to 25–35 mg/kg daily in three divided doses in children 5 yr and older, and up to 40 mg/kg/day in three divided doses in children 3–4 yr.

Geriatric patients or patients with renal impairment

CrCl (mL/min)	Dosage (mg/day)
More than 60	900–3,600 in three divided doses
More than 30–59	400–1,400 in two divided doses
More than 15–29	200–700 in one dose
Less than 15	100–300 in one dose

Postdialysis supplemental dosing, 125–350 mg PO following each 4 hr of dialysis.

Pharmacokinetics

Route	Onset	Duration
Oral	Varies	6–8 hr

Metabolism: Hepatic; $T_{1/2}$: 5–7 hr
Distribution: Crosses placenta; enters breast milk
Excretion: Urine, unchanged

Adverse effects

- **CNS:** *Dizziness, insomnia,* nervousness, fatigue, *somnolence, ataxia,* diplopia, tremor
- **Dermatologic:** Pruritus, abrasion
- **GI:** Dyspepsia, vomiting, nausea, constipation, dry mouth, diarrhea
- **Respiratory:** Rhinitis, pharyngitis
- **Other:** Weight gain, facial edema, cancer, impotence, suicidal ideation

Interactions

* **Drug-drug** • Decreased serum levels with antacids
* **Drug-lab test** • False-positives may occur with *Ames N-Multistix SG* dipstick test for protein in the urine

■ Nursing considerations
Assessment

- **History:** Hypersensitivity to gabapentin; lactation, pregnancy
- **Physical:** Weight; T; skin color, lesions; orientation, affect, reflexes; P; R, adventitious sounds; bowel sounds, normal output

Interventions

- Be aware that *Gralise* is not interchangeable with any other form of gabapentin.
- Ensure that patient does not cut, crush, or chew *Gralise* or ER tablets; tablets must be swallowed whole.
- Give drug with food to prevent GI upset.
- Be aware that patient may be at increased risk for suicidality; monitor accordingly.
- Arrange for consultation with support groups for people with epilepsy.
- Taper *Gralise* over 1 wk or longer if discontinuing or substituting a new drug.
- ⊗ *Warning* If overdose occurs, hemodialysis may be an option.

Teaching points

- Take this drug exactly as prescribed; do not discontinue abruptly or change dosage, except on the advice of your health care provider.
- If taking *Gralise* or ER tablet, swallow tablet whole; do not cut, crush, or chew tablets.
- Wear a medical alert ID at all times so that any emergency medical personnel will know that you have epilepsy and are taking antiepileptic medication.
- You may experience these side effects: Dizziness, blurred vision (avoid driving or performing other tasks requiring alertness or visual acuity); GI upset (take drug with food or milk, eat frequent small meals); headache, nervousness, insomnia; fatigue (periodic rest periods may help).
- Report severe headache, sleepwalking, rash, severe vomiting, chills, fever, difficulty breathing, thoughts of suicide.

▽ gadobutrol

See Appendix R, *Less commonly used drugs.*

▽ galantamine hydrobromide
(gah lan' tah meen)

Razadyne, Razadyne ER ⃟

PREGNANCY CATEGORY B

Drug classes
Alzheimer disease drug
Cholinesterase inhibitor

Therapeutic actions
Centrally acting, selective, long-acting, reversible cholinesterase inhibitor; causes elevated acetylcholine levels in the cortex, which is thought to slow the neuronal degradation that occurs in Alzheimer disease.

Indications
- Treatment of mild to moderate dementia of the Alzheimer type
- Unlabeled use: Vascular dementia

Contraindications and cautions
- Contraindicated with allergy to galantamine, severe hepatic impairment, severe renal impairment.

- Use cautiously with moderate renal or hepatic impairment, GI bleeding, seizures, asthma, COPD, pregnancy, lactation, and CV conditions.

Available forms

Tablets—4, 8, 12 mg; oral solution with dosing syringe—4 mg/mL; ER capsules ⊙ᴺ⊙—8, 16, 24 mg

Dosages
Adults
Initially, 4 mg PO bid. If well tolerated after 4 wk, increase to 8 mg PO bid. If well tolerated after 4 more wk, increase to 12 mg PO bid. Range: 16–32 mg/day in two divided doses; ER capsules—initial dose, 8 mg/day PO; titrate to 16–24 mg/day PO.
Pediatric patients
Safety and efficacy not established.
Patients with hepatic or renal impairment
Do not exceed 16 mg/day. Contraindicated if creatinine clearance less than 9 mL/min or if Child-Pugh score is 10–15.

Pharmacokinetics

Route	Onset	Peak	Duration
Oral	Varies	1 hr	8 hr

Metabolism: Hepatic; $T_{1/2}$: 7 hr
Distribution: Crosses placenta; may enter breast milk
Excretion: Urine

Adverse effects

- **CNS:** *Insomnia,* tremor, *dizziness,* fatigue, sedation, somnolence, tremor, headache
- **CV:** Bradycardia, syncope
- **GI:** *Nausea, vomiting, diarrhea, dyspepsia, anorexia, abdominal pain,* weight loss
- **GU:** UTI, hematuria

Interactions

✳ **Drug-drug** • Increased galantamine concentration with drugs that are potent inhibitors of CYP2D6 or CYP3A4 • Increased effects and risk of galantamine toxicity if combined with cimetidine, ketoconazole, paroxetine, erythromycin, succinylcholine, or bethanechol; if any of these combinations are used, monitor patient closely and adjust dosage as needed

■ Nursing considerations

⚡ CLINICAL ALERT!
Because of name confusion, the manufacturer has changed the drug name *Reminyl* to *Razadyne.*

Assessment
- **History:** Allergy to galantamine, pregnancy, lactation, impaired renal or hepatic function, GI bleeding, seizures, asthma, COPD, CV conditions
- **Physical:** Orientation, affect, reflexes, BP, P, abdominal examination, LFTs, renal function tests

Interventions
- Establish baseline functional profile to allow evaluation of drug effectiveness.
- Ensure at least 4 wk at each dosage level to establish effectiveness and tolerance of adverse effects.
- Administer with food in the morning and evening to decrease GI discomfort.
- Mix solution with water, fruit juice, or soda to improve compliance.
- Ensure that patient swallows ER capsules whole; do not cut, crush, or allow patient to chew capsule. Capsule can be opened and contents sprinkled over soft food.
- Monitor patient for weight loss, diarrhea, and arrhythmias before use and periodically with prolonged use.
- Provide frequent small meals if GI upset is severe; antiemetics may be used if necessary.
- Provide patient safety measures if CNS effects occur.
⊗ **Warning** Notify surgeon that patient takes galantamine; exaggerated muscle relaxation may occur if succinylcholine-type drugs are used.

Teaching points
- Take drug exactly as prescribed, with food, in the morning and evening to decrease GI upset.
- Switch to oral solution if swallowing becomes difficult; mix with water, fruit juice, or soda to improve taste.
- Swallow capsules whole; do not cut, crush, or chew. Contents can be sprinkled over soft food if swallowing is difficult.
- This drug does not cure the disease but is thought to slow the degeneration associated with the disease.

- Dosage changes may be needed to achieve the best effects. If the drug is stopped for more than a few days, consult your health care provider; it should be restarted at the original, lower dose.
- You may experience these side effects: Nausea, vomiting (eat frequent small meals); insomnia, fatigue, confusion (use caution if driving or performing tasks that require alertness).
- Report severe nausea, vomiting, changes in stool or urine color, diarrhea, changes in neurologic functioning, palpitations.

▽ **galsulfase**

See Appendix R, *Less commonly used drugs.*

▽ **ganciclovir sodium (DHPG)**

(gan sye' kloe vir)

Cytovene, Vitrasert, Zirgan

PREGNANCY CATEGORY C

Drug class
Antiviral

Therapeutic actions
Antiviral activity; inhibits viral DNA replication in cytomegalovirus (CMV).

Indications
- IV and implant: Treatment of CMV retinitis in immunocompromised patients, including patients with AIDS
- IV: Prevention of CMV disease in transplant recipients at risk for CMV disease
- Oral: Alternative to IV for maintenance treatment of CMV retinitis
- Oral: Prevention of CMV disease in individuals with advanced HIV infection at risk of developing CMV disease
- Ophthalmic: Treatment of acute herpetic keratitis
- Unlabeled use: Treatment of other CMV infections in immunocompromised patients

Contraindications and cautions
- Contraindicated with hypersensitivity to ganciclovir or acyclovir, lactation.
- Use cautiously with cytopenia, history of cytopenic reactions, impaired renal function, pregnancy.

Available forms
Capsules ⊙⊙⊙—250, 500 mg; powder for injection—500 mg/vial; ocular implant—4.5 mg; ophthalmic gel—0.15%

Dosages
Adults
- *CMV retinitis:* Initial dose, 5 mg/kg given IV at a constant rate over 1 hr, every 12 hr for 14–21 days. For maintenance, 5 mg/kg given by IV infusion over 1 hr once daily, 7 days/wk *or* 6 mg/kg once daily, 5 days/wk; or 1,000 mg PO tid with food or 500 mg PO 6 times per day every 3 hr with food while awake. Implant surgically placed in affected eye every 5–8 mo.
- *Prevention of CMV disease in transplant recipients:* 5 mg/kg IV over 1 hr every 12 hr for 7–14 days; then 5 mg/kg/day once daily for 7 days/wk, *or* 6 mg/kg/day once daily for 5 days/wk. Prophylactic oral dose is 1,000 mg tid with food. Duration depends on duration and degree of immunosuppression.
- *Prevention of CMV disease with advanced AIDS:* 1,000 mg PO tid with food.

Patients 2 yr and older
Ophthalmic gel: 1 drop in affected eye(s) five times daily (approximately every 3 hr while awake) until ulcer heals. Maintenance dose, 1 drop three times daily for 7 days.

Pediatric patients
Safety and efficacy not established. Use only if benefit outweighs potential carcinogenesis and reproductive toxicity.

Patients with renal impairment
Initial IV dose

CrCl (mL/min)	Dose IV (mg/kg)	Dosing Intervals
70 or more	5	12 hr
50–69	2.5	12 hr
25–49	2.5	24 hr
10–24	1.25	24 hr
<10	1.25	Three times/wk following hemodialysis

Maintenance

CrCl (mL/min)	Dose IV (mg/kg)	Dosing Intervals
70 or more	5	24 hr
50–69	2.5	24 hr
25–49	1.25	24 hr
10–24	0.625	24 hr
<10	0.625	Three times/wk following hemodialysis

Adverse effects in *italics* are most common; those in **bold** are life-threatening. ⊙⊙⊙ Do not crush.

Oral dose CrCl (mL/min)	Dose PO (mg)
70 or more	1,000 tid or 500 every 3 hr six times/day
50–69	1,500 daily or 500 tid
25–49	1,000 daily or 500 bid
10–24	500 daily
<10	500 three times/wk following dialysis

Pharmacokinetics

Route	Onset	Peak
IV	Slow	1 hr
Oral	Slow	2–4 hr

Metabolism: Hepatic; $T_{1/2}$: 2–4 hr (IV), 4.8 hr (PO)
Distribution: Crosses placenta; may enter breast milk
Excretion: Feces, urine

▼ IV FACTS

Preparation: Reconstitute vial by injecting 10 mL of sterile water for injection into vial; do not use bacteriostatic water for injection; shake vial to dissolve the drug. Discard vial if any particulate matter or discoloration is seen. Reconstituted solution in the vial is stable at room temperature for 12 hr. Do not refrigerate reconstituted solution. Drug is stable for 14 days after mixing with 0.9% normal saline.
Infusion: Infuse slowly over 1 hr.
Compatibilities: Compatible with 0.9% sodium chloride, 5% dextrose, Ringer injection, and lactated Ringer injection.
Y-site incompatibilities: Do not combine with foscarnet, ondansetron.

Adverse effects

- **CNS:** Dreams, ataxia, coma, confusion, dizziness, headache
- **CV:** Arrhythmia, hypertension, hypotension
- **Dermatologic:** *Rash,* alopecia, pruritus, urticaria
- **GI:** *Abnormal liver function tests,* nausea, vomiting, anorexia, diarrhea, abdominal pain
- **Hematologic:** *Granulocytopenia, thrombocytopenia, anemia,* neutropenia
- **Local:** *Pain, inflammation at injection site,* phlebitis
- **Other:** *Fever,* chills, **cancer,** sterility

Interactions

✳ **Drug-drug** ⊗ *Warning* Use with extreme caution with cytotoxic drugs because the accumulation effect could cause severe bone marrow depression and other GI and dermatologic problems.
- Increased effects if taken with probenecid • Increased risk of seizures with imipenem-cilastatin • Extreme drowsiness and risk of bone marrow depression with zidovudine

■ Nursing considerations

Assessment

- **History:** Hypersensitivity to ganciclovir or acyclovir; cytopenia; impaired renal function; lactation, pregnancy
- **Physical:** Skin color, lesions; orientation; BP, P, auscultation, perfusion, edema; R, adventitious sounds; urinary output; CBC, Hct, BUN, creatinine clearance, LFTs

Interventions

- Give by IV infusion only. Do not give IM or subcutaneously; drug is very irritating to tissues.
- Do not exceed the recommended dosage, frequency, or infusion rates.
- Monitor infusion carefully; infuse at concentrations no greater than 10 mg/mL.
- Decrease dosage in patients with impaired renal function.
- Give oral doses with food.

⊗ **Black box warning** Obtain CBC before therapy, every 2 days during daily dosing, and at least weekly thereafter. Consult with physician and arrange for reduced dosage if WBC or platelet counts fall.

⊗ **Black box warning** IV therapy is *only* for treatment of CMV retinitis in immunocompromised patients and for the prevention of CMV disease in transplant patients at risk for CMV.

⊗ *Warning* Consult with pharmacy for proper disposal of unused solution. Precautions are required for disposal of nucleoside analogues.

⊗ *Warning* Avoid direct contact with skin or mucous membranes.

⊗ *Warning* Do not open or crush capsules.

- Provide patient with a calendar of drug days, and arrange convenient times for the IV infusion in outpatients.
- Advise patients having surgical implant of ganciclovir that procedure will need to be repeated every 5–8 mo.

- Arrange for periodic ophthalmic examinations. Drug is not a cure for the disease, and deterioration may occur.
- Advise patients that ganciclovir can decrease sperm production and cause birth defects in fetuses. Advise the patient to use contraception during ganciclovir therapy. Men receiving ganciclovir therapy should use barrier contraception during and for at least 90 days after ganciclovir therapy.
- Advise patient that ganciclovir has caused cancer in animals and that risk is possible in humans.

Teaching points

- Appointments will be made for you if you are an outpatient on IV therapy. Long-term therapy is frequently needed. Take the oral drug with food; do not open, crush, cut, or chew capsules. Surgical implant of drug will need to be repeated every 5–8 months. Store eyedrops at room temperature.
- Frequent blood tests will be necessary to determine drug effects on your blood count and to adjust drug dosage. Keep appointments for these tests.
- Arrange for periodic ophthalmic examinations during therapy to evaluate progress of the disease. This drug is not a cure for your retinitis.
- Do not wear contact lenses while using eyedrops or if you have signs and symptoms of herpetic keratitis.
- If you also are receiving zidovudine, the two drugs cannot be given at the same time; severe adverse effects may occur.
- You may experience these side effects: Rash, fever, pain at injection site; decreased blood count leading to susceptibility to infection (frequent blood tests will be needed; avoid crowds and exposure to disease); birth defects and decreased sperm production (drug must not be taken during pregnancy; if pregnant or intending to become pregnant, consult your health care provider; use some form of contraception during therapy; male patients should use barrier contraception during therapy and for at least 90 days after therapy).
- Report bruising, bleeding, pain at injection site, fever, infection.

▽ **ganirelix acetate**

See Appendix R, *Less commonly used drugs.*

▽ **gefitinib**

See Appendix R, *Less commonly used drugs.*

> **DANGEROUS DRUG**

▽ **gemcitabine hydrochloride**

(jem site' ah ben)

Gemzar

PREGNANCY CATEGORY D

Drug classes
Antimetabolite
Antineoplastic
Pyrimidine analogue

Therapeutic actions
Cytotoxic: A nucleoside analogue that is cell cycle S–specific; causes cell death by disrupting and inhibiting DNA synthesis.

Indications

- First-line treatment of locally advanced or metastatic adenocarcinoma of pancreas; indicated for patients who have previously received 5-FU
- In combination with cisplatin as the first-line treatment of inoperable, locally advanced or metastatic non–small-cell lung cancer
- First-line therapy for metastatic breast cancer after failure of other adjuvant chemotherapy with an anthracycline, with paclitaxel
- In combination with carboplatin for the treatment of advanced ovarian cancer that has relapsed at least 6 mo after completion of a platinum-based therapy
- Unlabeled uses: Treatment of biliary cancer, bladder cancer, relapsed or refractory testicular cancer, squamous cell carcinoma of the head and neck

Contraindications and cautions

- Contraindicated with hypersensitivity to gemcitabine.
- Use cautiously with bone marrow suppression, renal or hepatic impairment, pregnancy, lactation.

Available forms
Powder for injection—200 mg, 1 g, 2 g

Dosages
Adults
- *Pancreatic cancer:* 1,000 mg/m² IV over 30 min given once weekly for up to 7 wk or until bone marrow suppression requires withholding treatment; subsequent cycles of once weekly for 3 out of 4 consecutive weeks can be given after 1-wk rest from treatment. For a patient who has completed the 7-wk course of initial therapy, the dose may be increased by 25% provided there is no significant hematologic toxicity.
- *Non–small-cell lung cancer:* 1,000 mg/m² IV over 30 min, days 1, 8, and 15 of each 28-day cycle with 100 mg/m² cisplatin on day 1 after gemcitabine infusion, *or* 1,250 mg/m² IV over 30 min, days 1 and 8 of each 21-day cycle with 100 mg/m² cisplatin on day 1 after gemcitabine infusion.
- *Metastatic breast cancer:* 1,250 mg/m² IV given over 30 min on days 1 and 8 of each 21-day cycle; with 175 mg/m² paclitaxel IV as a 3-hr infusion given before gemcitabine on day 1 of the cycle. Adjust dosage based on total granulocyte and platelet counts taken on day 8 of the cycle for that dose.
- *Advanced ovarian cancer:* 1,000 mg/m² IV given over 30 min on days 1 and 8 of each 21-day cycle. Carboplatin is given on day 1 after gemcitabine.

Pediatric patients
Safety and efficacy not established.

Pharmacokinetics

Route	Onset	Peak
IV	Rapid	30 min

Metabolism: Hepatic; $T_{1/2}$: 42–70 min; half-life is linearly dependent on infusion time
Distribution: Crosses placenta; may enter breast milk
Excretion: Bile, urine

▼ IV FACTS
Preparation: Use 0.9% sodium chloride injection as diluent for reconstitution of powder, 5 mL of 0.9% sodium chloride injection added to the 200-mg vial or 25 mL added to the 1-g vial. This will yield a concentration of 38 mg/mL; higher concentrations may lead to inadequate dissolution of powder. Resultant drug can be injected as reconstituted or further diluted in 0.9% sodium chloride injection. Stable for 24 hr at room temperature after reconstitution.
Infusion: Infuse slowly over 30 min; do not allow prolonged infusion; toxicity increases with length of infusion.

Adverse effects
- **CNS:** Somnolence, paresthesias
- **GI:** *Nausea, vomiting,* diarrhea, constipation, mucositis, GI bleeding, stomatitis, hepatic impairment
- **Hematologic: Bone marrow depression,** *infections*
- **Hepatic:** Elevated ALT
- **Pulmonary:** Dyspnea, **interstitial pneumonitis**
- **Renal:** Hematuria, proteinuria, elevated BUN and creatinine
- **Other:** *Fever, alopecia, pain, rash, edema, flulike symptoms*

■ Nursing considerations
Assessment
- **History:** Hypersensitivity to gemcitabine; bone marrow depression; renal or hepatic impairment; pregnancy, lactation
- **Physical:** T; skin color, lesions; R, adventitious sounds; abdominal examination, mucous membranes; LFTs, renal function tests, CBC with differential, urinalysis

Interventions
⊗ *Warning* Infuse over 30 min; longer infusions (more than 60 min) cause increased half-life and severe toxicity.
⊗ *Warning* Follow CBC, LFTs, and renal function tests carefully before and frequently during therapy; dosage adjustment may be needed if myelosuppression becomes severe or hepatic or renal impairment occurs.
- Protect patient from exposure to infection; monitor occurrence of infection at any site and arrange for appropriate treatment.
- Provide medication, frequent small meals for severe nausea and vomiting; monitor nutritional status.

Teaching points
- This drug must be given IV over 30 minutes once a week or as protocol dosing. Mark calendar with days to return for treatment. Regular blood tests will be needed to evaluate the effects of treatment.

- You may experience these side effects: Nausea and vomiting (may be severe; antiemetics may be helpful; eat frequent small meals); increased susceptibility to infection (avoid crowds and situations that may expose you to diseases); loss of hair (arrange for a wig or other head covering; keep the head covered at extremes of temperature).
- Report severe nausea and vomiting, fever, chills, sore throat, unusual bleeding or bruising, changes in color of urine or stool.

▽gemfibrozil

(jem fi' broe zil)

Apo-Gemfibrozil (CAN),
Gen-Gemfibrozil (CAN), Lopid,
PMS-Gemfibrozil (CAN)

PREGNANCY CATEGORY C

Drug class
Antihyperlipidemic

Therapeutic actions
Inhibits peripheral lipolysis and decreases the hepatic excretion of free fatty acids; this reduces hepatic triglyceride production; inhibits synthesis of VLDL carrier apolipoprotein; decreases VLDL production; increases HDL concentration.

Indications
- As adjunct to diet and exercise for hypertriglyceridemia in adult patients with very high elevations of triglyceride levels (types IV and V hyperlipidemia) at risk of pancreatitis unresponsive to diet therapy
- As adjunct to diet and exercise in reduction of coronary heart disease risk in patients who have not responded to diet, exercise, and other drugs and have low HDL levels in addition to high LDL and triglyceride levels

Contraindications and cautions
- Contraindicated with allergy to gemfibrozil, hepatic or renal impairment, primary biliary cirrhosis, gallbladder disease.
- Use cautiously with pregnancy, lactation, cholelithiasis, and renal impairment.

Available forms
Tablets—600 mg

Dosages
Adults
⊗ *Warning* 1,200 mg/day PO in two divided doses, 30 min before morning and evening meals. Caution: Use only if strongly indicated and lipid studies show a definite response; hepatic tumorigenicity occurs in laboratory animals.
Pediatric patients
Safety and efficacy not established.
Patients with renal or hepatic impairment
Contraindicated with hepatic impairment or severe renal impairment. Use caution with mild to moderate renal impairment.

Pharmacokinetics

Route	Onset	Peak
Oral	Varies	1–2 hr

Metabolism: Hepatic; $T_{1/2}$: 90 min
Distribution: Crosses placenta; enters breast milk
Excretion: Feces, urine

Adverse effects
- **CNS:** *Headache, dizziness, blurred vision,* vertigo, insomnia, paresthesia, tinnitus, *fatigue,* malaise, syncope
- **Dermatologic:** *Eczema, rash,* dermatitis, pruritus, urticaria
- **GI:** *Abdominal pain, epigastric pain, diarrhea, nausea, vomiting,* flatulence, dry mouth, constipation, anorexia, *dyspepsia,* cholelithiasis, elevated ALT and AST
- **GU:** Impairment of fertility
- **Hematologic:** Anemia, **eosinophilia, leukopenia,** hypokalemia, liver function changes, hyperglycemia
- **Other:** Painful extremities, back pain, arthralgia, muscle cramps, myalgia, swollen joints, myopathy

Interactions
✱ **Drug-drug** • Risk of rhabdomyolysis from 3 wk to several mo after therapy when combined with HMG-CoA reductase inhibitors (eg, lovastatin, simvastatin) • Risk of increased bleeding when combined with anticoagulants; monitor patient closely • Risk of hypoglycemia if combined with sulfonylureas and repaglinide; monitor closely

■ Nursing considerations

Assessment

- **History:** Allergy to gemfibrozil, hepatic or renal impairment, primary biliary cirrhosis, gallbladder disease, pregnancy, lactation
- **Physical:** Skin lesions, color, T; gait, range of motion; orientation, affect, reflexes; bowel sounds, normal output, liver evaluation; lipid studies, CBC, LFTs, renal function tests, blood glucose

Interventions

- Administer drug with meals or milk if GI upset occurs.
- Ensure that patient continues diet and exercise programs.
- Arrange for regular follow-up visits, including blood tests for lipids, liver function, CBC, and blood glucose during long-term therapy.

Teaching points

- Take the drug with meals or with milk if GI upset occurs; changes in diet will be needed.
- Continue to follow diet and exercise recommendations for your high lipid levels.
- Have regular follow-up visits to your health care provider for blood tests to evaluate drug effectiveness.
- You may experience these side effects: Diarrhea, loss of appetite, flatulence (eat frequent small meals); muscular aches and pains, bone and joint discomfort; dizziness, faintness, blurred vision (use caution if driving or operating dangerous equipment).
- Report severe stomach pain with nausea and vomiting, fever and chills or sore throat, severe headache, vision changes.

▽ **gemifloxacin mesylate**

(jem ab flox' a sin)

Factive ⓞⓝⓒ

PREGNANCY CATEGORY C

Drug classes

Antibiotic
Fluoroquinolone

Therapeutic actions

Bactericidal; interferes with DNA replication, repair, transcription, and recombination in susceptible gram-negative and gram-positive bacteria, preventing cell reproduction and leading to cell death.

Indications

- Treatment of acute bacterial exacerbation of chronic bronchitis caused by *Streptococcus pneumoniae, Haemophilus influenzae, H. parainfluenzae, Moraxella catarrhalis*
- Treatment of community-acquired pneumonia caused by *S. pneumoniae* (including multi-drug–resistant strains), *H. influenzae, Moraxella catarrhalis, Mycoplasma pneumonia, Chlamydia pneumoniae, Klebsiella pneumoniae*

Contraindications and cautions

- Contraindicated with history of sensitivity to gemifloxacin or any fluoroquinolone antibiotic; history of tendinitis, tendon rupture; history of prolonged QTc interval; uncorrected hypokalemia or hypomagnesemia; use of quinidine, procainamide, amiodarone, or sotalol antiarrhythmics.
- Use cautiously with epilepsy or predisposition to seizures; pregnancy; lactation.

Available forms

Tablets ⓞⓝⓒ—320 mg

Dosages

Adults

- *Acute bacterial exacerbation of chronic bronchitis:* 320 mg/day PO for 5 days.
- *Community-acquired pneumonia:* 320 mg/day PO for 5 days for known or suspected *S. pneumoniae, H. influenzae, M. pneumoniae,* or *C. pneumoniae* and 7 days for known or suspected multi-drug–resistant *S. pneumoniae, K. pneumoniae,* or *M. catarrhalis.*

Pediatric patients

Safety and efficacy not established.

Patients with renal impairment

For creatinine clearance greater than 40 mL/min, use usual dose; for creatinine clearance of 40 mL/min or less, use 160 mg/day PO.

Pharmacokinetics

Route	Onset	Peak
Oral	Rapid	0.5–2 hr

Metabolism: Hepatic; $T_{1/2}$: 4–12 hr

Distribution: May cross the placenta; may enter breast milk

Excretion: Feces, urine

Adverse effects

- **CNS:** Headache, dizziness, anorexia, tremor, vertigo, nervousness, insomnia
- **CV:** Increased QT interval
- **GI:** Diarrhea, **ulcerative colitis,** nausea, abdominal pain, vomiting, taste perversion, gastroenteritis, dry mouth, dyspepsia, flatulence, elevated ALT
- **GU:** Fungal infection, genital moniliasis, vaginitis
- **Respiratory:** Pharyngitis, pneumonia
- **Other:** Rash, fatigue, back pain, eczema, urticaria, myalgia, photosensitivity, ruptured tendons, tendinitis

Interactions

✱ **Drug-drug** • Decreased absorption and serum levels if taken with calcium, sucalfrate, iron, didanosine, aluminum- or potassium-containing antacids; take these drugs 3 hr before or 2 hr after taking gemifloxacin • Increased risk of prolonged QT interval if combined with disopropamide, butilide, quinidine, amiodarone or sotalol, erythromycin, antipsychotics, antidepressants; avoid these combinations

■ Nursing considerations

Assessment

- **History:** Allergy to fluoroquinolones; prolonged QT interval, uncorrected hypokalemia or hypomagnesemia; use of quinidine, procainamide, amiodarone, or sotalol antiarrhythmics; epilepsy or predisposition to seizures, pregnancy, lactation, myasthenia gravis
- **Physical:** Skin color, lesions; T; orientation, reflexes, affect; R, adventitious sounds; mucous membranes, bowel sounds; LFTs, renal function tests, ECG, serum electrolytes

Interventions

⊗ **Black box warning** There is a risk of tendinitis and tendon rupture with drug administration. Risk increases in patients older than 60 yr, with concurrent corticosteroid use, and with kidney, heart, or lung transplant. Monitor these patients accordingly.

⊗ **Black box warning** Risk of exacerbation of muscle weakness and potential crisis in patients with myasthenia gravis; contraindicated for use in any patient with a history of myasthenia gravis.

- Arrange for culture and sensitivity tests before beginning therapy.
- Continue therapy as indicated for condition being treated.
- Ensure that the tablet is swallowed whole, not cut, crushed, or chewed.

⊗ **Warning** Administer drug 3 hr before or at least 2 hr after antacids, iron, multivitamins, didanosine, or sucralfate.

⊗ **Warning** Discontinue drug at any sign of hypersensitivity (rash, photophobia) or with severe diarrhea.

- Discontinue drug and monitor ECG if palpitations or dizziness occurs.
- Monitor clinical response; if no improvement or a relapse occurs, repeat culture and sensitivity tests.

Teaching points

- Take drug once a day, at the same time each day, for the period prescribed, even if you are feeling much better. Swallow the tablet whole; do not cut, crush, or chew the tablet.
- If antacids, iron, multivitamins, sucralfate, or didanosine are being taken, you should take gemifloxacin 3 hours before or at least 2 hours after these drugs.
- Do not save tablets to self-treat other infections because this drug is very specific for the infection you have now.
- Drink plenty of fluids while you are taking this drug.
- Find another method of feeding your baby if you are breast-feeding; the effects of this drug on the baby are not known.
- Stop the drug and notify your health care provider immediately if you experience acute pain or tenderness in a muscle or tendon; if you develop severe or bloody diarrhea or a severe rash.
- You may experience these side effects: Nausea, vomiting, abdominal pain (eat frequent small meals); diarrhea or constipation (consult your health care provider if this occurs); drowsiness, blurring of vision, dizziness (use caution if driving or using dangerous equipment); sensitivity to the sun (avoid exposure or use a sunscreen).
- Report palpitations, severe diarrhea, rash, fainting spells, sudden tendon pain or weakness.

Adverse effects in *italics* are most common; those in **bold** are life-threatening. ⬚ Do not crush.

▽gentamicin sulfate
(jen ta mye' sin)

Parenteral, intrathecal: Alcomicin
(CAN), Pediatric Gentamicin Sulfate
Ophthalmic: Gentak

PREGNANCY CATEGORY D

PREGNANCY CATEGORY C
(OPHTHALMIC)

Drug class
Aminoglycoside

Therapeutic actions
Bactericidal: Inhibits protein synthesis in susceptible strains of gram-negative bacteria; appears to disrupt functional integrity of bacterial cell membrane, causing cell death.

Indications
Parenteral
- Serious infections caused by susceptible strains of *Pseudomonas aeruginosa, Proteus* species, *Escherichia coli, Klebsiella-Enterobacter-Serratia* species, *Citrobacter, Staphylococcus* species
- Serious infections when causative organisms are not known (often in conjunction with a penicillin or cephalosporin)
- Unlabeled use: With clindamycin as alternative regimen in PID

Intrathecal
- Gram-negative infections
- Serious CNS infections, such as meningitis, ventriculitis, infections caused by susceptible *Pseudomonas* species

Ophthalmic preparations
- Treatment of superficial ocular infections due to strains of microorganisms susceptible to gentamicin

Topical dermatologic preparation
- Infection prophylaxis in minor skin abrasions and treatment of superficial infections of the skin due to susceptible organisms amenable to local treatment

Contraindications and cautions
- Contraindicated with allergy to any aminoglycosides.
- Use cautiously with renal or hepatic disease; sulfite sensitivity; pre-existing hearing loss;

active infection with herpes, vaccinia, varicella, fungal infections, mycobacterial infections (ophthalmic preparations); myasthenia gravis; parkinsonism; infant botulism; burn patients; lactation, pregnancy.

Available forms
Injection—10, 40 mg/mL; injection in 0.9% sodium chloride—0.6, 0.8, 0.9, 1, 1.2, 1.4, 1.6 mg/mL; ophthalmic solution—3 mg/mL; ophthalmic ointment—3 mg/g; topical ointment—0.1%; topical cream—0.1%; ointment—1 mg; cream—1 mg

G

Dosages
Dosage should be based on estimated lean body mass.
Parenteral
Adults
3 mg/kg/day in three equal doses every 8 hr IM or IV. Up to 5 mg/kg/day in three to four equal doses in severe infections, usually for 7–10 days. For IV use, a loading dose of 1–2 mg/kg may be infused over 30–60 min.
- *PID:* 2 mg/kg IV followed by 1.5 mg/kg tid plus clindamycin 600 mg IV qid. Continue for at least 4 days and at least 48 hr after patient improves, then continue clindamycin 450 mg orally qid for 10–14 days total therapy.
- *Surgical prophylaxis regimens:* Several complex, multidrug prophylaxis regimens are available for preoperative use; consult manufacturer's instructions.
Pediatric patients
2–2.5 mg/kg every 8 hr IM or IV.
Infants and neonates: 2.5 mg/kg every 8 hr.
Preterm or full-term neonates 1 wk or younger: 2.5 mg/kg every 12 hr.
Preterm neonates younger than 32 wk gestatinal age: 2.5 mg/kg every 18 hr or 3 mg/kg every 24 hr.
Geriatric patients or patients with renal failure
Reduce dosage or extend dosage intervals, and carefully monitor serum drug levels and renal function tests.
Ophthalmic solution
Adults and pediatric patients
1–2 drops into affected eye or eyes every 4 hr; use up to 2 drops hourly in severe infections.
Ophthalmic ointment
Adults and pediatric patients
Apply about ½″ to affected eye bid–tid.

Dermatologic preparations
Adults and pediatric patients
Apply tid–qid. Cover with sterile bandage if needed.

Pharmacokinetics

Route	Onset	Peak
IM, IV	Rapid	30–90 min

Metabolism: Hepatic; $T_{1/2}$: 2–3 hr
Distribution: Crosses placenta; enters breast milk
Excretion: Urine

▼ IV FACTS
Preparation: Dilute single dose in 50–200 mL of sterile isotonic saline or D₅W. Do not mix in solution with any other drugs.
Infusion: Infuse over 30–120 min.
Incompatibilities: Do not mix in solution with any other drugs.

Adverse effects
- **CNS:** Ototoxicity—*tinnitus, dizziness,* vertigo, deafness (partially reversible to irreversible), vestibular paralysis, confusion, disorientation, depression, lethargy, nystagmus, visual disturbances, headache, *numbness, tingling,* tremor, paresthesias, muscle twitching, **seizures,** muscular weakness, **neuromuscular blockade**
- **CV:** Palpitations, hypotension, hypertension
- **GI:** Hepatic toxicity, *nausea, vomiting, anorexia,* weight loss, stomatitis, increased salivation
- **GU:** Nephrotoxicity
- **Hematologic:** *Leukemoid reaction,* **agranulocytosis, granulocytosis, leukopenia,** leukocytosis, **thrombocytopenia, eosinophilia, pancytopenia,** anemia, hemolytic anemia, increased or decreased reticulocyte count, electrolyte disturbances
- **Hypersensitivity:** *Purpura, rash,* urticaria, exfoliative dermatitis, itching
- **Local:** *Pain, irritation, arachnoiditis at IM injection sites*
- **Other:** Fever, **apnea,** splenomegaly, joint pain, *superinfections*

Ophthalmic preparations
- **Local:** *Transient irritation, burning, stinging, itching,* angioneurotic edema, urticaria, vesicular and maculopapular dermatitis, bacterial and fungal corneal ulcers

Topical dermatologic preparations
- **Local:** *Photosensitization,* superinfections

Interactions
✷ **Drug-drug** • Increased ototoxic, nephrotoxic, neurotoxic effects with other aminoglycosides, potent diuretics, cephalosporins, vancomycin, methoxyflurane, enflurane • Increased neuromuscular blockade and muscular paralysis with anesthetics, nondepolarizing neuromuscular blocking drugs, succinylcholine, citrate-anticoagulated blood • Potential inactivation of both drugs if mixed with beta-lactam–type antibiotics (space doses with concomitant therapy) • Increased bactericidal effect with penicillins, cephalosporins (to treat some gram-negative organisms and enterococci), carbenicillin, ticarcillin (to treat *Pseudomonas* infections)

■ Nursing considerations
Assessment
- **History:** Allergy to any aminoglycosides; renal or hepatic disease; pre-existing hearing loss; active infection with herpes, vaccinia, varicella, fungal infections, mycobacterial infections (ophthalmic preparations); myasthenia gravis; parkinsonism; infant botulism; lactation, pregnancy
- **Physical:** Site of infection; skin color, lesions; orientation, reflexes, eighth cranial nerve function; P, BP; R, adventitious sounds; bowel sounds, liver evaluation; urinalysis, BUN, serum creatinine, serum electrolytes, LFTs, CBC

Interventions
- Monitor serum concentrations when feasible to avoid potentially toxic levels. Peak levels should not exceed 12 mcg/mL (6–8 mcg/mL is usually adequate for most infections). Trough levels should not exceed 2 mcg/mL.
- Give by IM route if at all possible; give by deep IM injection.
- Culture infected area before therapy.
- Use 2 mg/mL intrathecal preparation without preservatives, for intrathecal use.
- Avoid long-term therapies because of increased risk of toxicities. Reduction in dose may be clinically indicated.
- Patients with edema or ascites may have lower peak concentrations due to expanded extracellular fluid volume.
- Cleanse area before application of dermatologic preparations.

Adverse effects in *italics* are most common; those in **bold** are life-threatening. ▭ Do not crush.

- Ensure adequate hydration of patient before and during therapy.

⊗ **Black box warning** Monitor hearing with long-term therapy; ototoxicity can occur.

⊗ **Black box warning** Monitor renal function tests, CBC, and serum drug levels during long-term therapy. Consult with prescriber to adjust dosage as needed.

⊗ **Black box warning** Carefully monitor patient if combined with any other neurotoxic or nephrotoxic drug.

Teaching points

- Apply ophthalmic preparations by tilting head back; place medications into conjunctival sac and close eye; apply light pressure on lacrimal sac for 1 minute.
- Cleanse area before applying dermatologic preparations; area may be covered if necessary.
- You may experience these side effects: Ringing in the ears, headache, dizziness (reversible; use safety measures if severe); nausea, vomiting, loss of appetite (eat frequent small meals, perform frequent mouth care); burning, blurring of vision with ophthalmic preparations (avoid driving or performing dangerous activities if visual effects occur); photosensitization with dermatologic preparations (wear sunscreen and protective clothing).
- Report pain at injection site, severe headache, dizziness, loss of hearing, changes in urine pattern, difficulty breathing, rash or skin lesions; itching or irritation (ophthalmic preparations); worsening of the condition, rash, irritation (dermatologic preparations).

▽**glatiramer acetate**

See Appendix R, *Less commonly used drugs.*

DANGEROUS DRUG

▽**glimepiride**

(*glye **meh'** per ide*)

Amaryl, CO-Glimepiride (CAN), ratio-Glimepiride (CAN)

PREGNANCY CATEGORY C

Drug classes

Antidiabetic
Sulfonylurea (second generation)

Therapeutic actions

Stimulates insulin release from functioning beta cells in the pancreas; may improve binding between insulin and insulin receptors or increase the number of insulin receptors; thought to be more potent in effect than first-generation sulfonylureas.

Indications

- As an adjunct to diet to lower blood glucose in patients with type 2 diabetes mellitus whose hyperglycemia cannot be controlled by diet and exercise alone
- In combination with metformin or insulin to better control glucose as an adjunct to diet and exercise in patients with type 2 diabetes mellitus

Contraindications and cautions

- Contraindicated with allergy to sulfonylureas; diabetes complicated by fever, severe infections, severe trauma, major surgery, ketosis, acidosis, coma (insulin is indicated in these conditions); type 1 or juvenile diabetes, serious hepatic or renal impairment, uremia, thyroid or endocrine impairment, glycosuria, hyperglycemia associated with primary renal disease; labor and delivery—if glimepiride is used during pregnancy, discontinue drug at least 1 mo before delivery; lactation, safety not established.
- Use cautiously with pregnancy.

Available forms

Tablets—1, 2, 4 mg

Dosages

Dose conservatively in elderly patients, debilitated or malnourished patients, and patients with renal or hepatic impairment.

Adults

Usual starting dose is 1–2 mg PO once daily with breakfast or first meal of the day; usual maintenance dose is 1–4 mg PO once daily, depending on patient response and glucose levels. Do not exceed an increase of 2 mg/dose at 1- to 2-wk intervals based on glucose levels; do not exceed total daily dose of 8 mg.

- *Combination with insulin therapy:* 8 mg PO daily with first meal of the day with low-dose insulin.
- *Transfer from other hypoglycemics:* No transition period is necessary.

Pediatric patients

Safety and efficacy not established.

Patients with renal or hepatic impairment; elderly, debilitated, malnourished patients; patients with adrenal or pituitary insufficiency

Usual starting dose is 1 mg PO once daily; adjust dose carefully, lower maintenance doses may be sufficient to control blood sugar.

Pharmacokinetics

Route	Onset	Peak
Oral	1 hr	2–3 hr

Metabolism: Hepatic; $T_{1/2}$: 5.5–7 hr
Distribution: Crosses placenta; enters breast milk
Excretion: Bile, urine

Adverse effects

- **CNS:** Drowsiness, asthenia, nervousness, tremor, insomnia, blurred vision
- **CV: Increased risk of CV mortality** (possible)
- **Endocrine:** *Hypoglycemia,* SIADH
- **GI:** *Anorexia, nausea,* vomiting, *epigastric discomfort, heartburn, diarrhea*
- **Hematologic: Leukopenia, thrombocytopenia,** anemia
- **Hypersensitivity:** *Allergic skin reactions,* eczema, pruritus, erythema, urticaria, photosensitivity, fever, **eosinophilia,** jaundice
- **Other:** Diuresis, tinnitus, fatigue, weight gain, hyponatremia

Interactions

✳ **Drug-drug** • Increased risk of hypoglycemia with androgens, anticoagulants, azole antifungals, beta blockers, chloramphenicol, clofibrate, fluconazole, gemfibrozil, histamine-2 blockers, magnesium salts, MAOIs, methyldopa, probenecid, salicylates, sulfinpyrazone, sulfonamides, TCAs, urinary acidifiers • Decreased effectiveness of both glimepiride and diazoxide if taken concurrently • Increased risk of hyperglycemia with rifampin, thiazides • Risk of hypoglycemia and hyperglycemia with alcohol; "disulfiram reaction" has also been reported • Possible decreased hypoglycemic effect with calcium channel blockers, cholestyramine, corticosteroids, diazoxide, estrogens, hydantoins, hormonal contraceptives, isoniazid, nicotinic acid, phenothiazines, rifampin, sympathomimetics, thiazide diuretics, thyroid drugs, urinary alkalinizers

✳ **Drug-alternative therapy** • Increased risk of hypoglycemia if taken with juniper berries, ginseng, garlic, fenugreek, coriander, dandelion root, celery

■ Nursing considerations
Assessment

- **History:** Allergy to sulfonylureas; diabetes complicated by fever, severe infections, severe trauma, major surgery, ketosis, acidosis, coma (insulin is indicated in these conditions); type 1 or juvenile diabetes, serious hepatic or renal impairment, uremia, thyroid or endocrine impairment, glycosuria, hyperglycemia associated with primary renal disease; pregnancy
- **Physical:** Skin color, lesions; T; orientation, reflexes, peripheral sensation; R, adventitious sounds; liver evaluation, bowel sounds; urinalysis, BUN, serum creatinine, LFTs, blood glucose, CBC

Interventions

- Monitor serum glucose levels frequently to determine effectiveness of drug and dosage being used.
- ⊗ *Warning* Transfer to insulin therapy during periods of high stress (eg, infections, surgery, trauma).
- Use IV glucose if severe hypoglycemia occurs as a result of overdose.
- Arrange for consultation with dietitian to establish weight-loss program and dietary control.
- Arrange for thorough diabetic teaching program, including disease, dietary control, exercise, signs and symptoms of hypoglycemia and hyperglycemia, avoidance of infection, hygiene.
- Consider adding metformin to drug regimen if response is not adequate; monitor patient closely.

Teaching points

- Take this drug once a day with breakfast or the first main meal of the day.
- Do not discontinue this drug without consulting your health care provider.
- Continue with diet and exercise program for diabetes control.
- Monitor blood for glucose as prescribed.
- Do not use this drug if you are pregnant.
- Avoid alcohol while taking this drug.

- Report fever, sore throat, unusual bleeding or bruising, rash, dark urine, light-colored stools, hypoglycemic or hyperglycemic reactions.

DANGEROUS DRUG

▽ **glipiZIDE**

(glip' i zide)

Glucotrol, Glucotrol XL ⓞⓡ

PREGNANCY CATEGORY C

Drug classes
Antidiabetic
Sulfonylurea (second generation)

Therapeutic actions
Stimulates insulin release from functioning beta cells in the pancreas; may improve binding between insulin and insulin receptors or increase the number of insulin receptors; more potent in effect than first-generation sulfonylureas.

Indications
- Adjunct to diet and exercise to lower blood glucose with type 2 diabetes mellitus

Contraindications and cautions
- Contraindicated with allergy to sulfonylureas, diabetes with ketoacidosis, sole therapy of type 1 diabetes or diabetes complicated by pregnancy; diabetes complicated by fever, severe infections, severe trauma, major surgery, ketosis, acidosis, coma (insulin is indicated); type 1 diabetes, serious hepatic impairment, serious renal impairment.
- Use cautiously with uremia, thyroid or endocrine impairment, glycosuria, hyperglycemia associated with primary renal disease; labor and delivery (if glipizide is used during pregnancy, discontinue drug at least 1 mo before delivery); lactation; pregnancy.

Available forms
Tablets—5, 10 mg; ER tablets ⓞⓡ—2.5, 5, 10 mg

Dosages
Dose conservatively in elderly patients, debilitated or malnourished patients, and patients with renal or hepatic impairment.

Give approximately 30 min before breakfast to achieve greatest reduction in postprandial hyperglycemia; if using extended-release form, give with breakfast.

Adults
- *Initial therapy:* 5 mg PO before breakfast. Adjust dosage in increments of 2.5–5 mg as determined by blood glucose response. At least several days should elapse between adjustments. Maximum once-daily dose should not exceed 15 mg; above 15 mg, divide dose, and administer before meals. Do not exceed 40 mg/day. ER tablets: 5 mg/day. Adjust dosage in 5-mg increments every 3 mo; maximum dose—20 mg/day.
- *Maintenance therapy:* Total daily doses above 15 mg PO should be divided; total daily doses above 30 mg are given in divided doses bid.
- *ER form:* 5 mg/day with breakfast, may be increased to 10 mg/day after 3 mo if indicated.

Pediatric patients
Safety and efficacy not established.

Geriatric patients
Geriatric patients tend to be more sensitive to the drug. Start with initial dose of 2.5 mg/day PO. Monitor for 24 hr and gradually increase dose after several days as needed.

Pharmacokinetics

Route	Onset	Peak	Duration
Oral	1–1.5 hr	1–3 hr	10–24 hr
Oral (ER)	2–3 hr	6–12 hr	24 hr

Metabolism: Hepatic; $T_{1/2}$: 2–4 hr
Distribution: Crosses placenta; enters breast milk
Excretion: Bile, urine

Adverse effects
- **CNS:** Drowsiness, asthenia, nervousness, tremor, insomnia, tinnitus, fatigue, headache
- **CV: Increased risk of CV mortality,** syncope, blurred vision
- **Endocrine:** *Hypoglycemia,* SIADH
- **GI:** *Anorexia, nausea,* vomiting, *epigastric discomfort, heartburn, diarrhea,* flatulence
- **Hematologic: Leukopenia, thrombocytopenia,** anemia
- **Hypersensitivity:** *Allergic skin reactions,* eczema, pruritus, erythema, urticaria, photosensitivity, fever, eosinophilia, jaundice
- **Other:** Weight gain, arthralgia, leg cramps, hyponatremia

Interactions

❋ **Drug-drug** • Increased risk of hypoglycemia with sulfonamides, chloramphenicol, salicylates, clofibrate, beta blockers • Decreased effectiveness of glipizide and diazoxide if taken concurrently • Increased risk of hyperglycemia with rifampin, thiazides • Risk of hypoglycemia and hyperglycemia with alcohol; "disulfiram reaction" also has been reported

❋ **Drug-alternative therapy** • Increased risk of hypoglycemia if taken with juniper berries, ginseng, garlic, fenugreek, coriander, dandelion root, celery, karela

■ Nursing considerations
Assessment

- **History:** Allergy to sulfonylureas; diabetes mellitus with complications; type 1 diabetes mellitus, serious hepatic or renal impairment, uremia, thyroid or endocrine impairment, glycosuria, hyperglycemia associated with primary renal disease; pregnancy
- **Physical:** Skin color, lesions; T; orientation, reflexes, peripheral sensation; R, adventitious sounds; liver evaluation, bowel sounds; urinalysis, BUN, serum creatinine, LFTs, blood glucose, CBC

Interventions

- Give drug 30 min before breakfast; if severe GI upset occurs or more than 15 mg/day is required, dose may be divided and given before meals.
- Ensure that patient swallows ER tablets whole; do not allow patient to cut, crush, or chew them.
- Monitor serum glucose levels frequently to determine drug effectiveness and dosage.

⊗ **Warning** Transfer to insulin therapy during periods of high stress (eg, infections, surgery, trauma).

⊗ **Warning** Use IV glucose if severe hypoglycemia occurs as a result of overdose.

Teaching points

- Take this drug 30 minutes before breakfast for best results.
- Do not discontinue this drug without consulting your health care provider.
- Monitor blood for glucose as prescribed.
- If taking ER tablets, swallow them whole; do not crush, chew, or divide tablets. The empty tablet may appear in your stool.

- Continue the prescribed diet and exercise regimen.
- Do not use this drug during pregnancy; consult your health care provider.
- Avoid alcohol while using this drug.
- Report fever, sore throat, unusual bleeding or bruising, rash, dark urine, light-colored stools, hypoglycemic or hyperglycemic reactions.

▽ **glucagon (rDNA origin)**

(*gloo' ka gon*)

GlucaGen Diagnostic Kit,
GlucaGen HypoKit,
Glucagon Emergency Kit

PREGNANCY CATEGORY B

Drug classes

Diagnostic agent
Glucose-elevating drug
Hormone

Therapeutic actions

Accelerates the breakdown of glycogen to glucose (glycogenolysis) in the liver, causing an increase in blood glucose level; relaxes smooth muscle of the GI tract and increases the force of contraction of the heart.

Indications

- Hypoglycemia: Counteracts severe hypoglycemic reactions in diabetic patients treated with insulin
- Diagnostic aid in the radiologic examination of the stomach, duodenum, small bowel, or colon when a hypotonic state is advantageous
- Unlabeled uses: Treatment of beta blocker and calcium channel blocker overdose and in anaphylactic reactions

Contraindications and cautions

- Contraindicated with hypersensitivity, pheochromocytoma, insulinoma.
- Use cautiously with pregnancy, lactation, insulinoma.

Available forms

Powder for injection—1 mg

Adverse effects in *italics* are most common; those in **bold** are life-threatening. ▣▣ Do not crush.

Dosages
Adults and pediatric patients weighing more than 20 kg
- *Hypoglycemia:* 0.5–1 mg IV, IM, or subcutaneously; severe hypoglycemia: 1 mL IV, IM, or subcutaneously. Response is usually seen in 5–20 min. If response is delayed, dose may be repeated one to two times. Use IV if possible.
- *Diagnostic aid:* Suggested dose, route, and timing of dose vary with the segment of GI tract to be examined and duration of effect needed. Carefully check manufacturer's literature before use. Usual dose is 0.25–2 mg IV or 1–2 mg IM.

Pediatric patients weighing less than 20 kg
0.5 mg IM, IV, or subcutaneously, or a dose equivalent to 20–30 mcg/kg.

Pharmacokinetics

Route	Onset	Peak	Duration
IV	1 min	15 min	9–20 min
IM	8–10 min	20–30 min	19–32 min

Metabolism: Hepatic; T$_{1/2}$: 3–10 min
Distribution: Crosses placenta; enters breast milk
Excretion: Bile, urine

▼ IV FACTS

Preparation: Reconstitute with vial provided. Use immediately; refrigerated solution stable for 48 hr. If doses higher than 2 mg, reconstitute with sterile water for injection and use immediately.
Infusion: Inject directly into the IV tubing of an IV drip infusion, each 1 mg over 1 min.
Incompatibilities: Compatible with dextrose solutions, but precipitates may form in solutions of sodium chloride, potassium chloride, or calcium chloride.

Adverse effects
- **CV:** Hypotension, hypertension, tachycardia
- **GI:** *Nausea, vomiting*
- **Hematologic:** Hypokalemia in overdose
- **Hypersensitivity:** Urticaria, **respiratory distress**, hypotension

Interactions
❋ **Drug-drug** • Increased anticoagulant effect and risk of bleeding with oral anticoagulants

■ Nursing considerations
Assessment
- **History:** Insulinoma, pheochromocytoma, lactation, pregnancy
- **Physical:** Skin color, lesions, T; orientation, reflexes; P, BP, peripheral perfusion; R; liver evaluation, bowel sounds; blood and urine glucose, serum potassium

Interventions
⊗ *Warning* Arouse hypoglycemic patient as soon as possible after drug injection, and provide supplemental carbohydrates to restore liver glycogen and prevent secondary hypoglycemia.
- Arrange for evaluation of insulin dosage in cases of hypoglycemia as a result of insulin overdosage; insulin dosage may need to be adjusted.

Teaching points
- You and significant others should learn to administer the drug subcutaneously in case of hypoglycemia, and know when to notify your health care provider.

▽ glucarpidase
See Appendix R, *Less commonly used drugs.*

DANGEROUS DRUG
▽ glyBURIDE
(glye' byoor ide)

Apo-Glyburide (CAN), DiaBeta, Gen-Glybe (CAN), Glibenclamide (CAN), Glynase PresTab, Novo-Glyburide (CAN), PMS-Glyburide (CAN), ratio-Glyburide (CAN)

PREGNANCY CATEGORY B (GLYNASE)

PREGNANCY CATEGORY C (DIABETA)

Drug classes
Antidiabetic
Sulfonylurea

Therapeutic actions
Stimulates insulin release from functioning beta cells in the pancreas; may improve binding between insulin and insulin receptors or

increase the number of insulin receptors; more potent in effect than first-generation sulfonylureas.

Indications

• Adjunct to diet and exercise to lower blood glucose with type 2 diabetes mellitus

Contraindications and cautions

• Contraindicated with allergy to sulfonylureas; diabetes mellitus with ketoacidosis, sole therapy of type 1 diabetes mellitus or diabetes mellitus complicated by pregnancy, serious hepatic or renal impairment, uremia; diabetes mellitus complicated by fever, severe infections, severe trauma, major surgery, ketosis, acidosis, coma (insulin is contraindicated).

• Use cautiously with pregnancy, lactation, thyroid or endocrine impairment, glycosuria, hyperglycemia associated with primary renal disease; labor and delivery (if glyburide is used during pregnancy, discontinue drug at least 1 mo before delivery).

Available forms

Tablets—1.25, 2.5, 5 mg; micronized tablets—1.5, 3, 4.5, 6 mg

Dosages

Adults

• *Initial therapy:* 2.5–5 mg PO with breakfast (*DiaBeta*); 1.5–3 mg/day PO (*Glynase*).

• *Maintenance therapy:* 1.25–20 mg/day PO given as a single dose or in divided doses. Increase in increments of no more than 2.5 mg (1.5 mg micronized) at weekly intervals based on patient's blood glucose response (*DiaBeta*); 0.75–12 mg/day PO (*Glynase*).

Debilitated or malnourished patients

Start with 1.25 mg daily (nonmicronized) or 0.75 mg daily (micronized).

Pediatric patients

Safety and efficacy not established.

Geriatric patients

Geriatric patients tend to be more sensitive to the drug; start with initial dose of 1.25 mg/day PO (*DiaBeta*); 0.75 mg/day PO (*Glynase*). Monitor for 24 hr, and gradually increase dose after at least 1 wk as needed.

Pharmacokinetics

Route	Onset	Peak	Duration
Oral			
Micronized	1 hr	2–3 hr	12–24 hr
Nonmicronized	2–4 hr	4 hr	12–24 hr

Metabolism: Hepatic; $T_{1/2}$: 4 hr
Distribution: Crosses placenta; enters breast milk
Excretion: Bile, urine

Adverse effects

• **CNS:** Drowsiness, tinnitus, fatigue, asthenia, nervousness, tremor, insomnia
• **CV: Increased risk of CV mortality**
• **Endocrine: Hypoglycemia**
• **GI:** *Anorexia, nausea,* vomiting, *epigastric discomfort, heartburn,* diarrhea, weight gain
• **Hematologic: Leukopenia, thrombocytopenia,** anemia
• **Hypersensitivity:** *Allergic skin reactions,* eczema, pruritus, erythema, urticaria, photosensitivity, fever, eosinophilia, jaundice
• **Other:** Blurred vision

Interactions

✳ **Drug-drug** • Increased risk of hypoglycemia with sulfonamides, chloramphenicol, salicylates, clofibrate • Decreased effectiveness of glyburide and diazoxide if taken concurrently • Increased risk of hyperglycemia with rifampin, thiazides • Risk of hypoglycemia and hyperglycemia with alcohol; "disulfiram reaction" has been reported

✳ **Drug-alternative therapy** • Increased risk of hypoglycemia if taken with juniper berries, ginseng, garlic, fenugreek, coriander, dandelion root, celery, karela

■ Nursing considerations

CLINICAL ALERT!
Name confusion has occurred between *DiaBeta* (glyburide) and *Zebeta* (bisoprolol); use caution.

Assessment

• **History:** Allergy to sulfonylureas; diabetes with complications; type 1 diabetes, serious hepatic or renal impairment, uremia, thyroid or endocrine impairment, glycosuria, hyperglycemia associated with primary renal disease, pregnancy

- **Physical:** Skin color, lesions; T; orientation, reflexes, peripheral sensation; R, adventitious sounds; liver evaluation, bowel sounds; urinalysis, BUN, serum creatinine, LFTs, blood glucose, CBC

Interventions

- Give drug before breakfast. If severe GI upset occurs, dose may be divided and given before meals.
- Monitor serum glucose levels frequently to determine drug effectiveness and dosage.
- Monitor dosage carefully if switching to or from *Glynase*.
- ⊗ **Warning** Transfer to insulin therapy during periods of high stress (eg, infections, surgery, trauma).
- ⊗ **Warning** Use IV glucose if severe hypoglycemia occurs as a result of overdose.

Teaching points

- Do not discontinue this medication without consulting your health care provider.
- Monitor blood for glucose as prescribed; continue diet and exercise regimen for your diabetes.
- Do not use this drug during pregnancy; consult your health care provider.
- Avoid alcohol while using this drug.
- Report fever, sore throat, unusual bleeding or bruising, rash, dark urine, light-colored stools, hypoglycemic or hyperglycemic reactions.

▽ **glycopyrrolate**
*(glye koe **pye'** roe late)*

Cuvposa, Robinul, Robinul Forte

PREGNANCY CATEGORY B

Drug classes
Anticholinergic (quaternary)
Antimuscarinic
Antispasmodic
Parasympatholytic

Therapeutic actions
Competitively blocks the effects of acetylcholine at receptors that mediate the effects of parasympathetic postganglionic impulses; depresses salivary and bronchial secretions; dilates the bronchi; inhibits vagal influences on the heart;

relaxes the GI and GU tracts; inhibits gastric acid secretion.

Indications

- Oral: Adjunctive therapy in the treatment of peptic ulcer
- Oral solution: Treatment of chronic, severe drooling caused by neurologic disorders in children 3–16 yr
- Parenteral: Reduction of salivary, tracheobronchial, and pharyngeal secretions preoperatively; reduction of the volume and free acidity of gastric secretions; and blocking of cardiac vagal inhibitory reflexes during induction of anesthesia and intubation; may be used intraoperatively to counteract drug-induced or vagal traction reflexes with the associated arrhythmias
- Parenteral: Protection against the peripheral muscarinic effects (eg, bradycardia, excessive secretions) of cholinergics (neostigmine, pyridostigmine) that are used to reverse the neuromuscular blockade produced by nondepolarizing neuromuscular junction blockers

Contraindications and cautions

- Contraindicated with glaucoma; adhesions between iris and lens; stenosing peptic ulcer; pyloroduodenal obstruction; paralytic ileus; intestinal atony; severe ulcerative colitis; toxic megacolon; symptomatic prostatic hypertrophy; bladder neck obstruction; bronchial asthma; COPD; cardiac arrhythmias; tachycardia; myocardial ischemia; lactation; impaired metabolic, liver, or kidney function; myasthenia gravis.
- Use cautiously in the elderly and with Down syndrome, brain damage, spasticity, hypertension, hyperthyroidism, pregnancy.

Available forms
Tablets—1, 2, mg; injection—0.2 mg/mL; oral solution—1 mg/5 mL

Dosages
Adults
Oral
1 mg tid or 2 mg bid–tid. For maintenance, 1 mg bid. Maximum daily dose is 8 mg PO.
Parenteral
- *Peptic ulcer:* 0.1–0.2 mg IM or IV tid–qid.
- *Preanesthetic medication:* 0.004 mg/kg IM 30–60 min before anesthesia.

- *Intraoperative:* 0.1 mg IV; repeat as needed at 2- to 3-min intervals.
- *Reversal of neuromuscular blockade:* With neostigmine, pyridostigmine: 0.2 mg for each 1 mg neostigmine or 5 mg pyridostigmine; administer IV simultaneously.

Pediatric patients
Not recommended for children younger than 12 yr for peptic ulcer.

Oral
Pediatric patients 3–16 yr
- *Chronic, severe drooling:* Initially, 0.02 mg/kg PO tid; titrate in 0.02-mg increments every 5–7 days. Maximum dose, 0.1 mg/kg PO tid; do not exceed 1.5–3 mg/dose.

Parenteral
- *Preanesthetic medication:*
  1 mo–2 yr: Up to 0.009 mg/kg IM may be needed.
  2 yr and older: 0.004 mg/kg IM 30 min to 1 hr before anesthesia.
  Younger than 12 yr: 0.002–0.004 mg/kg IM.

Pediatric patients older than 1 mo
- *Intraoperative:* 0.004 mg/kg IV, not to exceed 0.1 mg in a single dose. May be repeated at 2- to 3-min intervals.
- *Reversal of neuromuscular blockade:* 0.2 mg for each 1 mg neostigmine or 5 mg pyridostigmine. Give IV simultaneously.

Pharmacokinetics

Route	Onset	Peak	Duration
Oral	60 min	60 min	8–12 hr
IM, Subcut.	15–30 min	30–45 min	2–7 hr
IV	1 min	End of infusion	Unknown

Metabolism: Hepatic; $T_{1/2}$: 2.5 hr
Distribution: Crosses placenta; enters breast milk
Excretion: Urine

▼ IV FACTS

Preparation: No additional preparation required.
Infusion: Administer slowly into tubing of a running IV, each 0.2 mg over 1–2 min.
Incompatibilities: Do not combine with methylprednisolone; sodium succinate. May be incompatible with drugs that have more alkaline pH (greater than 6)—eg, barbiturates, diazepam, lactated Ringer solution.

Adverse effects
- **CNS:** Headache, flushing, nervousness, drowsiness, fever, mental confusion
- **CV:** Palpitations, tachycardia
- **GI:** *Dry mouth, altered taste perception, nausea, vomiting, dysphagia,* heartburn, constipation, bloated feeling, paralytic ileus, gastroesophageal reflux
- **GU:** *Urinary hesitancy and retention,* impotence
- **Local:** *Irritation at site of IM injection*
- **Ophthalmic:** *Blurred vision,* mydriasis, cycloplegia, photophobia, increased IOP
- **Other:** Decreased sweating and predisposition to heat prostration, suppression of lactation, nasal congestion

Interactions
✳ **Drug-drug** ● Decreased antipsychotic effectiveness of haloperidol with anticholinergic drugs ● Increased anticholinergic side effects (dry mouth, constipation, urinary retention) with amantadine and TCAs ● Decreased antipsychotic effects and increased anticholinergic effects with phenothiazines ● Risk of increased digoxin level with oral glycopyrrolate; monitor patient closely ● Increased toxic effects with amantadine; dosage may need to be decreased

■ Nursing considerations
Assessment
- **History:** Glaucoma; adhesions between iris and lens, stenosing peptic ulcer, pyloroduodenal obstruction, paralytic ileus, intestinal atony, severe ulcerative colitis, toxic megacolon, symptomatic prostatic hypertrophy, bladder neck obstruction, COPD, cardiac arrhythmias, myocardial ischemia, impaired metabolic, liver or kidney function, myasthenia gravis; lactation; Down syndrome, brain damage, spasticity, hypertension, hyperthyroidism, pregnancy
- **Physical:** Bowel sounds, normal output; normal urinary output, prostate palpation; R, adventitious sounds; P, BP; IOP, vision; bilateral grip strength, reflexes; hepatic palpation, LFTs, renal function tests; skin color, lesions, texture

Interventions
- Ensure adequate hydration; provide environmental control (temperature) to prevent hyperpyrexia.

Adverse effects in *italics* are most common; those in **bold** are life-threatening. ⬛ Do not crush.

- Check pediatric dosage carefully; may be in mg/lb or mg/kg.
- Have patient void before each dose if urinary retention is a problem.

Teaching points
- Take this drug exactly as prescribed.
- Avoid hot environments (you will be heat-intolerant; dangerous reactions may occur).
- You may experience these side effects: Constipation (ensure adequate fluid intake, proper diet); dry mouth (suck sugarless candies, use frequent mouth care; this effect may lessen); blurred vision, sensitivity to light (reversible; avoid tasks that require acute vision; wear sunglasses in bright light); impotence (reversible); difficulty in urination (empty bladder immediately before taking each dose).
- Report rash, flushing, eye pain, difficulty breathing, tremors, loss of coordination, irregular heartbeat, palpitations, headache, abdominal distention, hallucinations, severe or persistent dry mouth, difficulty swallowing, difficulty urinating, severe constipation, sensitivity to light.

▽gold sodium thiomalate

See Appendix R, *Less commonly used drugs.*

▽golimumab
(*goh lim' yoo mab*)

Simponi

PREGNANCY CATEGORY B

Drug classes
Antiarthritic
Monoclonal antibody
Tumor necrosis factor inhibitor

Therapeutic actions
Tumor necrosis factor antibody that binds to tumor necrosis factor, blocking an important mediator in the inflammatory response seen in chronic inflammatory diseases, such as rheumatoid arthritis, psoriatic arthritis, and ankylosing spondylitis.

Indications
- Treatment of moderately to severely active rheumatoid arthritis in adults in combination with methotrexate

- Treatment of active psoriatic arthritis in adults, as monotherapy or in combination with methotrexate
- Treatment of ankylosing spondylitis in adults

Contraindications and cautions
- Contraindicated with hypersensitivity to components of drug, active infection, active tuberculosis, lactation.
- Use cautiously with heart failure, history of exposure to fungal infections, hepatitis B, TB, bacterial infections, malignancies, demyelinating disorders such as multiple sclerosis, pregnancy.

Available forms
Single-use prefilled syringe—50 mg/0.5 mL; single-use autoinjector—50 mg/0.5 mL

Dosages
Adults
50 mg by subcutaneous injection once a month.
Pediatric patients
Safety and efficacy not established.

Pharmacokinetics

Route	Onset	Peak
Subcut.	Slow	2–6 days

Metabolism: Hepatic; $T_{1/2}$: 2 wk
Distribution: May cross placenta; may enter breast milk
Excretion: Tissues

Adverse effects
- **CNS:** Dizziness, **increased risk of demyelinating disorders**
- **CV:** Hypertension, heart failure
- **Respiratory:** *URI, nasopharyngitis,* bronchitis, sinusitis, rhinitis
- **Other:** Fever, injection-site reaction, **risk of infection,** psoriasis

Interactions
✳ **Drug-drug** • Increased risk of potentially serious infection if combined with anakinra, abatacept, rituximab, other TNF blockers (infliximab, adalimumab, etanercept, certolizumab); avoid this combination • Risk of infection if live vaccines are given while patient is taking this drug; avoid this combination

■ **Nursing considerations**
Assessment
• **History:** Tuberculosis, malignancy, heart failure, multiple sclerosis, travel exposure to invasive fungal infections, hepatitis B, pregnancy, lactation
• **Physical:** T, orientation; R, adventitious sounds; BP

Interventions

⊗ **Black box warning** Potentially serious infections are possible with drug administration, including TB, sepsis, invasive fungal infections *legionella* and *listeria* infections, recurrent infections. Discontinue drug if patient develops infection or sepsis. Perform TB test before beginning therapy. If TB is present, start TB treatment and monitor patient carefully throughout therapy.

⊗ **Black box warning** There is increased risk of lymphoma and other cancers in children and adolescents being treated with golimumab; monitor accordingly.

• Store syringes in refrigerator. Allow prefilled syringe or autoinjector to sit at room temperature for 30 min before giving subcutaneous injection. Solution should be clear and free of particles. Discard unused solution.
• Rotate injection sites; do no inject into areas that are bruised, red, or hard. Monitor sites for infection.
• Monitor patient with history of hepatitis B for possible reactivation; if reactivation occurs, stop golimumab and begin antiviral therapy.
• Monitor patient for possible demyelinating disorders.
• Do not administer live vaccines to patient taking this drug.
• Monitor patient for signs and symptoms of infection and discontinue drug if infection occurs.
• Protect patient from exposure to infections and ensure regular physical examinations and monitoring for infections or cancer development.

Teaching points
• You will need to have a TB test before beginning therapy with this drug.
• Take this drug exactly as prescribed, once a month by subcutaneous injection. Mark your calendar with the injection dates. This drug does not cure your rheumatic disease, and you may be taking other drugs to help with the signs and symptoms.

• You and a significant other should learn how to administer subcutaneous injections. Store the syringes in the refrigerator. Let the syringe sit at room temperature for 30 minutes before injecting drug. Make sure the solution is clear and free of particles. Discard any leftover solution. Consult your health care provider about the proper disposal of needles and syringes.
• Arrange for periodic medical follow-up to evaluate the effects of the drug on your body.
• This drug may appear in breast milk and cause adverse effects in a breast-feeding infant; if you are breast-feeding, you should use another method of feeding the infant.
• You should not receive live vaccines while you are taking this drug.
• You may experience these side effects: dizziness (avoid driving or operating hazardous machinery if this occurs); upper respiratory infection, runny nose (consult your health care provider for potential treatments if this becomes uncomfortable); increased susceptibility to infections (avoid people who might have infections and crowded areas; use strict hand-washing technique and good hygiene).
• Report fever, rash, chills, lethargy, swelling, numbness, tingling, worsening of arthritis symptoms, difficulty breathing.

DANGEROUS DRUG

▽ **goserelin acetate**
(*goe' se rel in*)

Zoladex, Zoladex LA (CAN)

PREGNANCY CATEGORY X

PREGNANCY CATEGORY D
(IN BREAST CANCER)

Drug classes
Antineoplastic
Hormone

Therapeutic actions
An analogue of LH-RH or gonadotropin-releasing hormone; potent inhibitor of pituitary gonadotropin secretion; initial administration causes an increase in FSH and LH and resultant increase in testosterone levels; with long-term administration, these hormone levels fall to levels normally seen

with surgical castration within 2–4 wk, as pituitary is inhibited. In women this leads to a decrease in serum estradiol levels and therefore a reduction in ovarian size and function, uterus and mammary gland size, and a repression of sex hormone–responsive tumors.

Indications

- Palliative treatment of advanced prostatic cancer when orchiectomy or estrogen administration is not indicated or is unacceptable
- Stage B_2–C prostatic cancer with flutamide for locally confined T2b–T4 carcinoma
- Management of endometriosis, including pain relief and reduction of endometriotic lesions
- Palliative treatment of advanced breast cancer in premenopausal and perimenopausal women
- Endometrial thinning drug before endometrial ablation

Contraindications and cautions

- Contraindicated with pregnancy, lactation, hypersensitivity to LH-RH or any component, undiagnosed vaginal bleeding.
- Use cautiously with hypercalcemia, high lipid levels.

Available forms

Implant—3.6, 10.8 mg

Dosages

Adults

3.6 mg subcutaneously every 28 days or 10.8 mg every 3 mo into the upper abdominal wall.

- *Prostatic or breast carcinoma:* Long-term use of 3.6 mg.
- *Endometriosis:* Continue therapy with 3.6 mg for 6 mo.
- *Endometrial thinning:* One to two 3.6-mg subcutaneous depots 4 wk apart; surgery should be done 4 wk after first dose— within 2–4 wk after second depot if two are used.
- *Stage B_2–C prostatic cancer:* Start therapy 8 wk before initiating radiation therapy and continue during radiation therapy. Treatment regimen is one 3.6-mg depot 8 wk before radiation followed by one 10.8-mg depot 28 days later. Or, four injections of 3.6-mg depot at 28-day intervals, two depots preceding and two during radiotherapy.

Pediatric patients

Safety and efficacy not established.

Pharmacokinetics

Route	Onset	Peak
Subcut.	Slow (men)	12–15 days (men)
	8–22 days (women)	8–22 days (women)

Metabolism: Hepatic; $T_{1/2}$: 4.2 hr (men), 2.3 hr (women)
Distribution: Crosses placenta; may enter breast milk
Excretion: Urine

Adverse effects

- **CNS:** Insomnia, dizziness, lethargy, anxiety, depression, headache, emotional lability
- **CV:** Heart failure, edema, hypertension, arrhythmia, chest pain, vasodilation, hypotension
- **GI:** Nausea, anorexia
- **GU:** *Hot flashes, sexual dysfunction, dysmenorrhea, decreased erections, lower urinary tract symptoms, vaginitis,* gynecomastia
- **Other:** Rash, sweating, **cancer,** pain, breast atrophy, peripheral edema

■ Nursing considerations

Assessment

- **History:** Pregnancy, lactation
- **Physical:** Skin T, lesions; reflexes, affect; BP, P; urinary output; pregnancy test if appropriate, calcium levels, lipid levels

Interventions

⊗ **Warning** Ensure that patient is not pregnant before use; advise patient to use barrier contraceptives.

- Use syringe provided. Discard if package is damaged. Remove sterile syringe immediately before use. Use a local anesthetic before injection to decrease pain and discomfort.
- Administer using aseptic technique under the supervision of a physician familiar with the implant technique.
- Bandage area after injection of implant.
- Repeat injection in 28 days; keep as close to this schedule as possible.

Teaching points

- This drug will be implanted into your upper abdomen every 28 days or 3 months as

appropriate. It is important to keep to this schedule. Mark a calendar of injection dates.
- Do not take this drug if you are pregnant; if you think you are pregnant or wish to become pregnant, consult your health care provider.
- You may experience these side effects: Hot flashes (keep environment cool); sexual dysfunction—regression of sex organs, impaired fertility, decreased erections; pain at injection site (a local anesthetic will be used; if discomfort is severe, analgesics may be ordered).
- Report chest pain, increased signs and symptoms of your cancer, difficulty breathing, dizziness, severe pain at injection site.

▽granisetron hydrochloride
(gran iz' e tron)

Kytril, Sancuso

PREGNANCY CATEGORY B

Drug classes
Antiemetic
5-HT$_3$ receptor antagonist

Therapeutic actions
Selectively binds to serotonin (5-HT$_3$) receptors in the CTZ, blocking the nausea and vomiting caused by the release of serotonin by mucosal cells during chemotherapy, which stimulates the CTZ and causes nausea and vomiting.

Indications
- Prevention and treatment of nausea and vomiting associated with emetogenic chemotherapy and radiation
- Prevention and treatment of postoperative nausea and vomiting (injection)
- Unlabeled uses: Postanesthetic shivering, cancer-related pruritus

Contraindications and cautions
- Contraindicated with history of hypersensitivity, concurrent use of apomorphine.
- Use cautiously with colitis, hepatic or renal impairment, pregnancy, lactation.

Available forms
Tablets—1 mg; injection—0.1, 1 mg/mL; oral solution—1 mg/5 mL; transdermal system—3.1 mg/24 hr

Dosages
Adults and patients 2 yr and older
IV
- *Chemotherapy-induced nausea and vomiting:* 10 mcg/kg IV over 5 min starting within 30 min of chemotherapy; only on days of chemotherapy.
- *Postoperative nausea and vomiting:* 1 mg IV over 30 seconds before induction or reversal of anesthesia.

Oral
1 mg PO bid or 2 mg/day as 1 dose, beginning up to 1 hr before chemotherapy and second dose 12 hr after chemotherapy; only on days of chemotherapy.
- *Radiation therapy:* 2 mg once daily taken 1 hr before radiation.

Transdermal
Apply 1 patch to clean, dry skin on the upper, outer arm 24–48 hr before chemotherapy. Keep patch in place a minimum of 24 hr after completion of chemotherapy and then remove it. Patch may be left in place for up to 7 days.

Pediatric patients younger than 18 yr
Safety and efficacy of transdermal use not established.

Pediatric patients younger than 2 yr
Oral and IV use not recommended.

Pharmacokinetics

Route	Onset	Peak
IV	Rapid	30–45 min
Oral	Moderate	60–90 min

Metabolism: Hepatic; T$_{1/2}$: 5 hr (IV), 6.2 hr (oral)
Distribution: Crosses placenta; enters breast milk, protein-bound
Excretion: Urine

▼ IV FACTS
Preparation: Dilute in 0.9% sodium chloride or 5% dextrose to a total volume of 20–50 mL; stable up to 24 hr refrigerated; protect from light.
Infusion: Inject slowly over 5 min.
Incompatibilities: Do not mix in solution with other drugs.

Adverse effects
- **CNS:** *Headache,* asthenia, somnolence, dizziness, insomnia
- **CV:** Hypertension, angina

Adverse effects in *italics* are most common; those in **bold** are life-threatening. ▭ Do not crush.

- **GI:** Diarrhea or constipation, nausea, abdominal pain, vomiting, decreased appetite, dyspepsia
- **Other:** Fever, chills, shivering, increased AST and ALT, alopecia

■ Nursing considerations
Assessment
- **History:** Allergy to granisetron, pregnancy, lactation, liver or renal impairment, colitis
- **Physical:** Orientation, reflexes, affect; BP; bowel sounds; T

Interventions
- Provide mouth care and sugarless candies to suck to help alleviate nausea.
- Give drug only on days of chemotherapy, or before radiation therapy, or before surgery or reversal of anesthesia.

Teaching points
- This drug may be given IV, orally, or as a transdermal patch when you are receiving your chemotherapy; it will help decrease nausea and vomiting.
- If using the transdermal patch, apply one patch to clean, dry skin on the upper, outer arm 24–48 hr before chemotherapy. Keep patch in place a minimum of 24 hr after completion of chemotherapy and then remove it. Patch may be left in place for up to 7 days.
- You may experience these side effects: Lack of sleep, drowsiness (use caution if driving or performing tasks that require alertness); diarrhea or constipation; headache (ask for medication).
- Report severe headache, fever, numbness or tingling, severe diarrhea or constipation.

▽ guaifenesin
(glyceryl guaiacolale)
(gwye fen' e sin)

Allfen; Altarussin; Diabetic Tussin; Ganidin NR; Guiatuss; Liquibid; Mucinex; Naldecon Senior Ex; Organidin NR; Robitussin; Scot-Tussin Expectorant; Siltussin DAS, Siltussin SA

PREGNANCY CATEGORY C

Drug class
Expectorant

Therapeutic actions
Enhances the output of respiratory tract fluid by reducing adhesiveness and surface tension, facilitating the removal of viscous mucus.

Indications
- Symptomatic relief of respiratory conditions characterized by dry, nonproductive cough and when there is mucus in the respiratory tract

Contraindications and cautions
- Contraindicated with allergy to guaifenesin.
- Use cautiously with pregnancy, lactation, and persistent coughs.

Available forms
Syrup—100 mg/5 mL; liquid—100, 200 mg/5 mL; capsules—200 mg; tablets—100, 200, 400 mg; ER tablets—600, 1,200 mg; granules—50, 100 mg per packet

Dosages
Adults and patients older than 12 yr
200–400 mg PO every 4 hr; do not exceed 2.4 g/day. For 600-mg ER tablets, 1–2 tablets every 12 hr; do not exceed 2.4 g/day.
Pediatric patients 6–12 yr
100–200 mg PO every 4 hr. Do not exceed 1.2 g/day or 600 mg (ER) PO every 12 hr.
Pediatric patients 2–6 yr
50–100 mg PO every 4 hr. Do not exceed 600 mg/day.

Pharmacokinetics

Route	Onset	Duration
Oral	30 min	4–6 hr

Metabolism: Not known; $T_{1/2}$: 1 hr
Distribution: Not known
Excretion: Urine

Adverse effects
- **CNS:** Headache, dizziness
- **Dermatologic:** Rash, urticaria
- **GI:** *Nausea, vomiting,* GI discomfort

Interactions
* **Drug-lab test** • Color interference and false results of 5-HIAA and VMA urinary determinations

■ Nursing considerations

CLINICAL ALERT!
Name confusion has been reported between *Mucinex* (guaifenesin) and *Mucomyst* (acetylcysteine); use caution.

Assessment
- **History:** Allergy to guaifenesin; persistent cough due to smoking, asthma, or emphysema; very productive cough; pregnancy
- **Physical:** Skin lesions, color; T; orientation, affect; R, adventitious sounds

Interventions
⊗ *Warning* Monitor reaction to drug; persistent cough for longer than 1 wk, fever, rash, or persistent headache may indicate a more serious condition.

Teaching points
- Some extended-release formulations may be cut in half but cannot be crushed or chewed. *Mucinex* cannot be crushed, chewed, or cut.
- Do not take for longer than 1 week; if fever, rash, or headache occur, consult your health care provider.
- You may experience these side effects: Nausea, vomiting (eat frequent small meals); dizziness, headache (avoid driving or operating dangerous machinery).
- Report fever, rash, severe vomiting, persistent cough.

▽ **guanfacine
hydrochloride**
(gwahn' fa seen)

Intuniv ᴏᴍᴄ, Tenex

PREGNANCY CATEGORY B

Drug classes
Antihypertensive
Sympatholytic (centrally acting)

Therapeutic actions
Stimulates central (CNS) alpha₂-adrenergic receptors, reduces sympathetic nerve impulses from the vasomotor center to the heart and blood vessels, decreases peripheral vascular resistance, and lowers systemic BP.

Indications
- Management of hypertension, alone or with a thiazide diuretic
- Treatment of ADHD as monotherapy or as adjunctive therapy with stimulants (ER tablets)
- Unlabeled uses: Amelioration of symptoms in heroin withdrawal; reduced frequency of migraine headaches and reduced nausea and vomiting; Tourette syndrome

Contraindications and cautions
- Contraindicated with hypersensitivity to guanfacine, labor and delivery, lactation.
- Use cautiously with severe coronary insufficiency, recent MI, CV disease, chronic renal or hepatic failure, pregnancy.

Available forms
Tablets—1, 2 mg; ER tablets ᴏᴍᴄ—1, 2, 3, 4 mg

Dosages
Adults and children 12 yr and older
- *Hypertension:* Recommended dose is 1 mg/day PO given at bedtime to minimize somnolence. If 1 mg/day does not give a satisfactory result after 3–4 wk of therapy, doses of 2 mg and then 3 mg may be given, although most of the drug's effect is seen at 1 mg. If BP rises toward the end of the dosing interval, divided dosage should be used. Higher daily doses (rarely up to 4 mg/day in divided doses) have been used, but adverse reactions increase with doses larger than 3 mg/day, and there is no evidence of increased efficacy. Taper ER form when discontinuing; decrease by no more than 1 mg every 3–7 days.

Adults and children 6 yr and older
- *ADHD:* 1 mg/day PO; titrate at increments of 1 mg/wk to a range of 1–4 mg/day. Taper at dose reduction of no more than 1 mg every 3–7 days if discontinuing.

Geriatric patients
Use with caution, starting at lower end of dosage range. Safety and efficacy of extended-release forms not established.

Patients with renal or hepatic impairment
Extended-release forms: Dosage may need adjustment; monitor patient closely.

Adverse effects in *italics* are most common; those in **bold** are life-threatening. ᴏᴍᴄ Do not crush.

Pharmacokinetics

Route	Onset	Peak	Duration
Oral	2 hr	1–4 hr	24 hr

Metabolism: Hepatic; $T_{1/2}$: 10–30 hr
Distribution: Crosses placenta; enters breast milk
Excretion: Urine

Adverse effects

- **CNS:** *Sedation, weakness, dizziness,* headache, insomnia, amnesia, confusion, depression, conjunctivitis, iritis, vision disturbance, malaise, paresthesia, paresis, taste perversion, tinnitus, hypokinesia, somnolence
- **CV:** Bradycardia, palpitations, substernal pain, hypotension
- **Dermatologic:** Dermatitis, pruritus, purpura, sweating
- **GI:** *Dry mouth, constipation,* abdominal pain, diarrhea, dyspepsia, dysphagia, nausea
- **GU:** *Impotence,* libido decrease, testicular disorder, urinary incontinence
- **Other:** Rhinitis, leg cramps, taste alterations, fatigue

■ Nursing considerations
Assessment

- **History:** Hypersensitivity to guanfacine; severe coronary insufficiency, cerebrovascular disease; chronic renal or hepatic failure; pregnancy; lactation
- **Physical:** Skin color, lesions; orientation, affect, reflexes; ophthalmologic examination; P, BP, orthostatic BP, perfusion, auscultation; R, adventitious sounds; bowel sounds, normal output; normal urinary output, voiding pattern; LFTs, renal function tests, ECG

Interventions

⊗ *Warning* Do not discontinue drug abruptly; discontinue therapy by reducing the dosage gradually over 2–4 days to avoid rebound hypertension (much less likely than with clonidine; BP usually returns to pretreatment levels in 2–4 days without ill effects).

- If switching from immediate-release to ER form, discontinue immediate-release form and titrate to desired dose of ER form.
- Assess compliance with drug regimen in a nonthreatening, supportive manner.
- Ensure that patient does not cut, crush, or chew ER tablets. Administer ER tablets first

thing in the morning. Do not administer with a high-fat meal.
- Administer immediate-release tablets at bedtime to minimize daytime somnolence.

Teaching points

- Take this drug exactly as prescribed; it is important that you do not miss doses. Swallow ER tablets whole with water, milk, or other liquid. Do not cut, crush, or chew tablets; take extended-release forms first thing in the morning. Do not take with a high-fat meal. Do not discontinue the drug unless instructed to do so by your health care provider. Do not discontinue drug abruptly. This drug must be tapered to prevent serious adverse effects.
- If taking this drug for ADHD, continue all other therapies being used for this disorder.
- You may experience these side effects: Drowsiness, dizziness, light-headedness, headache, weakness (transient; observe caution while driving or performing other tasks that require alertness or physical dexterity); dry mouth (suck sugarless candies or ice chips); GI upset (eat frequent small meals); dizziness, light-headedness when you change position (get up slowly; use caution when climbing stairs); impotence, other sexual dysfunction, decreased libido; palpitations.
- Report urinary incontinence, changes in vision, rash.

▽ haloperidol
*(ha loe **per**' i dole)*

haloperidol
Apo-Haloperidol (CAN),
Haldol, Haloperidol LA (CAN),
Novo-Peridol (CAN)

haloperidol decanoate
Haldol Decanoate,
Haldol Decanoate 50,
Haldol Decanoate 100

haloperidol lactate
PREGNANCY CATEGORY C

Drug classes
Antipsychotic
Dopaminergic blocker

Therapeutic actions

Mechanism not fully understood; antipsychotics block postsynaptic dopamine receptors in the brain, depress the RAS, including those parts of the brain involved with wakefulness and emesis; chemically resembles the phenothiazines.

Indications

- Management of manifestations of psychotic disorders
- Control of tics and vocalizations in Tourette syndrome in adults and children
- Behavioral problems in children with combative, explosive hyperexcitability that cannot be attributed to immediate provocation
- Short-term treatment of hyperactive children with excessive motor activity, mood lability
- Haloperidol decanoate and lactate: Prolonged parenteral therapy of chronic schizophrenia
- Unlabeled uses: Control of nausea and vomiting, treatment of intractable hiccoughs

Contraindications and cautions

- Contraindicated with hypersensitivity to typical antipsychotics, coma or severe CNS depression, bone marrow depression, blood dyscrasia, circulatory collapse, subcortical brain damage, Parkinson disease, liver damage, cerebral arteriosclerosis, coronary disease, severe hypotension or hypertension, dementia-related psychosis.
- Use cautiously with pregnancy; lactation; respiratory disorders ("silent pneumonia"); glaucoma, prostatic hypertrophy (anticholinergic effects may exacerbate glaucoma and urinary retention); epilepsy or history of epilepsy (drug lowers seizure threshold); tardive dyskinesia; NMS; breast cancer (elevations in prolactin may stimulate a prolactin-dependent tumor); thyrotoxicosis; peptic ulcer; decreased renal function; myelography within previous 24 hr or scheduled within 48 hr; exposure to heat or phosphorous insecticides; children younger than 12 yr, especially those with chickenpox, CNS infections (children are especially susceptible to dystonias that may confound the diagnosis of Reye syndrome); allergy to aspirin if giving the 1-, 2-, 5-, and 10-mg tablets (these tablets contain tartrazine).

Available forms

Tablets—0.5, 1, 2, 5, 10, 20 mg; oral concentrate—2 mg/mL; injection—50, 100 mg/mL as decanoate, 5 mg/mL as lactate

Dosages

Full clinical effects may require 6 wk–6 mo of therapy. Children, debilitated and geriatric patients, and patients with a history of adverse reactions to neuroleptic drugs may require lower dosage.

Adults

Oral

- *Psychiatric disorders, Tourette syndrome:* Initial dosage range, 0.5–2 mg bid–tid PO with moderate symptoms; 3–5 mg bid–tid PO for more resistant patients. Daily dosages up to 100 mg/day (or more) have been used, but safety of prolonged use has not been demonstrated. For maintenance, reduce dosage to lowest effective level.

IM, haloperidol lactate injection

2–5 mg (up to 10–30 mg) every 60 min or every 4–8 hr IM as necessary for prompt control of acutely agitated patients with severe symptoms. Switch to oral dosage as soon as feasible, using total IM dosage in previous 24 hr as a guide to total daily oral dosage.

IM, haloperidol decanoate injection

Maintenance, 10–15 times the daily oral dose in elderly patients stabilized on 10 mg/day or less; 20 times the daily oral dose in patients stabilized on high doses and tolerant to oral haloperidol. Do not exceed 3 mL per injection site; repeat at 4-wk intervals. Initial dose should not exceed 100 mg. If more than 100 mg is needed, divide into two doses of 100 mg on day 1 and give rest of dose 3–7 days later.

Pediatric patients 3–12 yr or 15–40 kg

Initial dose, 0.5 mg/day (25–50 mcg/kg/day) PO; may increase in increments of 0.5 mg every 5–7 days as needed. Total daily dose may be divided and given bid–tid.

- *Psychiatric disorders:* 0.05–0.15 kg/day PO given bid–tid. Severely disturbed psychotic children may require higher dosage.
- *Nonpsychotic and Tourette syndromes, behavioral disorders, hyperactivity:* 0.05–0.075 mg/kg/day PO given bid–tid.

In severely disturbed nonpsychotic children, short-term administration may suffice. There is little evidence of improved effects at doses greater than 6 mg/day.

Geriatric patients

Use lower doses (0.5–2.0 mg bid–tid), and increase dosage more gradually than in younger patients.

Pharmacokinetics

Route	Onset	Peak
Oral	Varies	3–5 hr
IM	Rapid	20 min
IM, decanoate	Slow	6 days

Metabolism: Hepatic; $T_{1/2}$: 21–24 hr, 3 wk for decanoate

Distribution: Crosses placenta; enters breast milk

Excretion: Bile, urine

Adverse effects

Not all effects have been reported with haloperidol; however, because haloperidol has certain pharmacologic similarities to the phenothiazine class of antipsychotic drugs, all adverse effects associated with phenothiazine therapy should be kept in mind when haloperidol is used.

- **Autonomic:** Dry mouth, salivation, nasal congestion, nausea, vomiting, anorexia, fever, pallor, facial flushing, sweating, constipation, paralytic ileus, urinary retention, incontinence, polyuria, enuresis, priapism, ejaculation inhibition
- **CNS:** *Drowsiness,* insomnia, vertigo, headache, weakness, tremor, ataxia, slurring, cerebral edema, seizures, exacerbation of psychotic symptoms, extrapyramidal syndromes—*pseudoparkinsonism; dystonias; akathisia,* tardive dyskinesias, potentially irreversible (no known treatment), **NMS**—extrapyramidal symptoms, hyperthermia, autonomic disturbances
- **CV:** Hypotension, orthostatic hypotension, hypertension, tachycardia, bradycardia, **cardiac arrest,** cardiomegaly, **refractory arrhythmias,** pulmonary edema
- **Endocrine:** Lactation, breast engorgement in females, galactorrhea; SIADH; amenorrhea, menstrual irregularities; gynecomastia in males; changes in libido; hyperglycemia or hypoglycemia; glyco-

suria; hyponatremia; pituitary tumor with hyperprolactinemia; inhibition of ovulation, infertility, pseudopregnancy

- **Hematologic:** Eosinophilia, leukopenia, leukocytosis, anemia; aplastic anemia; hemolytic anemia; thrombocytopenic or nonthrombocytopenic purpura; pancytopenia
- **Hypersensitivity:** Jaundice, urticaria, angioneurotic edema, laryngeal edema, photosensitivity, eczema, asthma, **anaphylactoid reactions,** exfoliative dermatitis
- **Respiratory:** Bronchospasm, laryngospasm, dyspnea; **suppression of cough reflex and potential for aspiration**

Interactions

✳ Drug-drug • Additive anticholinergic effects and possibly decreased antipsychotic efficacy with anticholinergic drugs • Increased risk of toxic side effects with lithium • Decreased effectiveness with carbamazepine

✳ Drug-lab test • False-positive pregnancy tests (less likely if serum test is used) • Increase in PBI, not attributable to an increase in thyroxine

✳ Drug-alternative therapy • With ginkgo biloba, increased drug effectiveness and decreased extrapyramidal effects of haloperidol

■ Nursing considerations
Assessment

- **History:** Severe CNS depression; bone marrow depression; blood dyscrasia; circulatory collapse; subcortical brain damage; Parkinson disease; liver damage; cerebral arteriosclerosis; coronary disease; severe hypotension or hypertension; respiratory disorders; glaucoma, prostatic hypertrophy; epilepsy or history of epilepsy; breast cancer; thyrotoxicosis; peptic ulcer, decreased renal function; myelography within previous 24 hr or scheduled within 48 hr; exposure to heat or phosphorus insecticides; children younger than 12 yr, especially those with chickenpox, CNS infections; allergy to aspirin, pregnancy, lactation
- **Physical:** Weight, T; reflexes, orientation, IOP; P, BP, orthostatic BP; R, adventitious sounds; bowel sounds and normal output, liver evaluation; urinary output,

prostate size, CBC, urinalysis, thyroid, LFTs, renal function tests

Interventions

⊗ **Black box warning** There is an increased risk of death in elderly patients with dementia-related psychosis; drug is not approved for this use.
• Do not give children IM injections.
• Do not use haloperidol for IV injections.
• Note that dosing of haloperidol decanoate injection and haloperidol lactate injection is very different; use caution.
⊗ **Warning** Gradually withdraw drug when patient has been on maintenance therapy to avoid withdrawal-emergent dyskinesias.
⊗ **Warning** Discontinue drug if serum creatinine or BUN become abnormal or if WBC count is depressed.
⊗ **Warning** Monitor elderly patients for dehydration; institute remedial measures promptly; sedation and decreased thirst related to CNS effects can lead to severe dehydration.
• Consult physician regarding appropriate warning of patient or patient's guardian about tardive dyskinesias.
• Consult physician about reducing dosage and using anticholinergic antiparkinsonians (controversial) if extrapyramidal effects occur.

Teaching points

• Take this drug exactly as prescribed.
• Avoid driving or engaging in other dangerous activities if dizziness or drowsiness or vision changes occur.
• Avoid prolonged exposure to sun, or use a sunscreen or covering garments.
• Maintain fluid intake, and use precautions against heatstroke in hot weather.
• You may experience these side effects: dry mouth (sucking sugarless candies may help); urinary retention (empty your bladder before taking the drug), constipation (medication may be available to help).
• Report sore throat, fever, unusual bleeding or bruising, rash, weakness, tremors, impaired vision, dark-colored urine (pink or reddish brown urine is to be expected), pale stools, yellowing of the skin or eyes.

DANGEROUS DRUG

▷ **heparin sodium**
(*hep' ah rin*)

heparin sodium and 0.9% sodium chloride

heparin sodium and 0.45% sodium chloride

heparin sodium injection
Hepalean (CAN), Heparin LEO (CAN)

heparin sodium lock flush solution
Hepalean-Lok (CAN), Heparin Lock Flush, Hepflush-10, Hep-Lock, Hep-Lock U/P

PREGNANCY CATEGORY C

Drug class
Anticoagulant

Therapeutic actions
Heparin inactivates factor Xa, therefore inhibiting thrombus and clot formation by blocking the conversion of prothrombin to thrombin and fibrinogen to fibrin, the final steps in the clotting process. Heparin also inhibits the activation of factor XIII and thrombin-induced activation of factors V and VIII

Indications
• Prevention and treatment of venous thrombosis, pulmonary embolism, and peripheral arterial embolism
• Treatment of atrial fibrillation with embolization
• Diagnosis and treatment of DIC
• Prevention of clotting in blood samples and heparin lock sets and during dialysis procedures
• Unlabeled uses: Adjunct in therapy of coronary occlusion with acute MI, prevention of left ventricular thrombi and stroke post-MI, prevention of cerebral thrombosis in the evolving stroke

Contraindications and cautions
• Contraindicated with hypersensitivity to heparin; severe thrombocytopenia; uncontrolled

bleeding; any patient who cannot be monitored regularly with blood coagulation tests; in pediatric patients if using injection preserved with benzyl alcohol, which can lead to death in pediatric patients; labor and immediate postpartum period.

- Use cautiously with pregnancy; women older than 60 yr who are at high risk for hemorrhaging, dysbetalipoproteinemia; recent surgery or injury.

Available forms

Injection—1,000, 2,500, 5,000, 10,000, 20,000 units/mL; also single-dose and unit-dose forms; lock flush solution—1, 10, 100 units/mL

Dosages

Adjust dosage according to coagulation tests. Dosage is adequate when WBCT = 2.5–3 times control—or aPTT = 1.5–2 times control value. The following are guidelines to dosage:

Adults

Subcutaneous (deep subcutaneous injection)

- *For general anticoagulation:* IV loading dose of 5,000 units and then 10,000–20,000 units subcutaneously followed by 8,000–10,000 units every 8 hr or 15,000–20,000 units every 12 hr.
- *Prophylaxis of postoperative thromboembolism:* 5,000 units by deep subcutaneous injection 2 hr before surgery and every 8–12 hr thereafter for 7 days or until patient is fully ambulatory.

IV

- *Intermittent IV:* Initial dose of 10,000 units and then 5,000–10,000 units every 4–6 hr.
- *Continuous IV infusion:* Loading dose of 5,000 units and then 20,000–40,000 units/day.
- *Surgery of heart and blood vessels for patients undergoing total body perfusion:* Not less than 150 units/kg; guideline often used is 300 units/kg for procedures less than 60 min, 400 units/kg for longer procedures. Add 400–600 units to 100 mL whole blood.
- *Clot prevention in blood samples:* 70–150 units/10–20 mL of whole blood.
- *Heparin lock and extracorporal dialysis:* See manufacturers' instructions.

Pediatric patients

Initial IV bolus of 50 units/kg and then 100 units/kg IV every 4 hr, or 20,000 units/m^2 per 24 hr by continuous IV infusion.

Pharmacokinetics

Route	Onset	Peak	Duration
IV	Immediate	Minutes	2–6 hr
Subcut.	20–60 min	2–4 hr	8–12 hr

Metabolism: $T_{1/2}$: 30–180 min
Distribution: Does not cross placenta, does not enter breast milk; broken down in liver
Excretion: Urine

▼ IV FACTS

Continuous infusion: Can be mixed in normal saline, D_5W, Ringer; mix well; invert bottle numerous times to ensure adequate mixing. Monitor patient closely; infusion pump is recommended.

Single dose: Direct, undiluted IV injection of up to 5,000 units (adult) or 50 units/kg (pediatric), given over 60 seconds.

Monitoring: Blood should be drawn for coagulation testing 30 min before each intermittent IV dose or every 4–6 hr if patient is on continuous infusion pump.

Incompatibilities: Heparin should not be mixed in solution with any other drug unless specifically ordered; direct incompatibilities in solution and at Y-site seen with amikacin, codeine, chlorpromazine, cytarabine, diazepam, dobutamine, doxorubicin, droperidol, ergotamine, erythromycin, gentamicin, haloperidol, hydrocortisone, kanamycin, levorphanol, meperidine, methadone, methicillin, methotrimeprazine, morphine, netilmicin, pentazocine, phenytoin, polymyxin B, promethazine, streptomycin, tetracycline, tobramycin, vancomycin.

Adverse effects

- **Dermatologic:** Loss of hair
- **Hematologic: Hemorrhage;** *bruising;* thrombocytopenia; elevated AST, ALT levels, hyperkalemia
- **Hypersensitivity:** Chills, fever, urticaria, asthma
- **Other:** Osteoporosis, suppression of renal function (long-term, high-dose therapy), **white clot syndrome**

Interactions

✳ **Drug-drug** • Increased bleeding tendencies with oral anticoagulants, salicylates, penicillins, cephalosporins, low–molecular-weight heparins, platelet inhibitors • Decreased anticoagulation effects if taken concurrently with nitroglycerin, nicotine, digoxin, tetracycline

✳ **Drug-lab test** • Increased AST, ALT levels • Increased thyroid function tests • Altered blood gas analyses, especially levels of carbon dioxide, bicarbonate concentration, and base excess

✳ **Drug-alternative therapy** • Increased risk of bleeding if combined with chamomile, garlic, ginger, ginkgo, and ginseng therapy; high-dose vitamin E

■ Nursing considerations
Assessment

• **History:** Recent surgery or injury; sensitivity to heparin; hyperlipidemia; pregnancy
• **Physical:** Peripheral perfusion, R, stool guaiac test, PTT or other tests of blood coagulation, platelet count, renal function tests

Interventions

• Adjust dose according to coagulation test results performed just before injection (30 min before each intermittent dose or every 4–6 hr if continuous IV dose). Therapeutic range aPTT: 1.5–2.5 times control.
• Always check compatibilities with other IV solutions.
• Evaluate patient's use of herbal products; many interact with heparin and a dosage change may be needed.
• Do not confuse injection with catheter lock flush; dosage varies.
• Use heparin lock needle to avoid repeated injections.
• Give deep subcutaneous injections; do not give heparin by IM injection.
• Do not give IM injections to patients on heparin therapy (heparin predisposes to hematoma formation).

⊗ **Warning** Apply pressure to all injection sites after needle is withdrawn; inspect injection sites for signs of hematoma; do not massage injection sites.
• Mix well when adding heparin to IV infusion.
• Do not add heparin to infusion lines of other drugs, and do not piggyback other drugs into heparin line. If this must be done, ensure drug compatibility.

• Provide for safety measures (electric razor, soft toothbrush) to prevent injury from bleeding.
• Check for signs of bleeding; monitor blood tests.
• Alert all health care providers of heparin use.

⊗ **Warning** Have protamine sulfate (heparin antidote) readily available in case of overdose. Each mg of protamine neutralizes 100 USP heparin units. Give very slowly IV over 10 min, not to exceed 50 mg. Establish dose based on blood coagulation studies.

Teaching points

• This drug must be given by a parenteral route (cannot be taken orally).
• Frequent blood tests are needed to determine whether blood clotting time is within the correct range.
• Report any use of herbal products; many interact with heparin and a dosage adjustment may be needed.
• Be careful to avoid injury: Use an electric razor, avoid contact sports, and avoid other activities that might lead to injury.
• You may experience loss of hair.
• Report nose bleed, bleeding of the gums, unusual bruising, black or tarry stools, cloudy or dark urine, abdominal or lower back pain, severe headache.

⊳ hetastarch
(hydroxyethyl starch, HES)
(het' a starch)

Hespan, Voluven

PREGNANCY CATEGORY C

Drug class
Plasma expander

Therapeutic actions

Complex mixture of various-sized molecules with colloidal properties that approximate those of human albumin and raise human plasma volume when administered IV; increases the erythrocyte sedimentation rate and improves the efficiency of granulocyte collection by centrifugal means.

Indications
- Adjunctive therapy for plasma volume expansion in shock due to hemorrhage, burns, surgery, sepsis, trauma
- Adjunctive therapy in leukapheresis to improve harvesting and increase the yield of granulocytes

Contraindications and cautions
- Contraindicated with allergy to hetastarch, severe bleeding disorders, severe cardiac failure, renal failure with anuria or oliguria.
- Use cautiously with hepatic impairment, pregnancy, lactation.

Available forms
Injection—6 g/100 mL in 500 mL IV infusion bottle

Dosages
Adults
- *Plasma volume expansion:* 500–1,000 mL IV. Do not usually exceed 1,500 mL/day. In acute hemorrhagic shock, rates approaching 20 mL/kg/hr are often needed (*Hespan*); up to 50 mL/kg/day *Voluven* injection.
- *Leukapheresis (Hespan):* 250–700 mL hetastarch infused at a constant fixed ratio of 1:8 to 1:13 to venous whole blood. Safety of up to two procedures per week and a total of seven to ten procedures using hetastarch have been established.

Pediatric patients
Safety and efficacy not established.

Pharmacokinetics

Route	Onset	Peak	Duration
IV	Immediate	24 hr	24–36 hr

Metabolism: Renal; $T_{1/2}$: 17 days, then 48 days
Distribution: Crosses placenta; enters breast milk
Excretion: Urine

▼ IV FACTS
Preparation: Use as prepared by manufacturer; store at room temperature; do not use if turbid deep brown or if crystalline precipitate forms.
Infusion: Rate of infusion should be determined by patient response; start at approximately 20 mL/kg, reduce rate to lowest possible needed to maintain hemodynamics.

Incompatibilities: Do not mix in solution with any other drug and do not add at Y-site with any other drugs.

Adverse effects
- **CNS:** *Headache,* muscle pain
- **GI:** *Vomiting, submaxillary and parotid glandular enlargement*
- **Hematologic:** Prolongation of PT, PTT; **bleeding and increased clotting times**
- **Hypersensitivity:** Periorbital edema, urticaria, wheezing
- **Other:** *Mild temperature elevations, chills, itching, mild influenza-like symptoms,* peripheral edema of the lower extremities

■ Nursing considerations
Assessment
- **History:** Allergy to hetastarch, severe bleeding disorders, severe cardiac congestion, renal failure or anuria; hepatic impairment; pregnancy, lactation
- **Physical:** T; submaxillary and parotid gland evaluation; P, BP, adventitious sounds, peripheral and periorbital edema; R, adventitious sounds; liver evaluation; urinalysis, LFTs, renal function tests, clotting times, PT, PTT, Hgb, Hct, CBC with differential

Interventions
- Administer by IV infusion only; monitor rates based on patient response.
- ⊗ **Warning** Keep life-support equipment readily available in cases of shock.
- ⊗ **Warning** Ensure that no other drugs are mixed with or added to hetastarch.

Teaching points
- This drug can only be given IV.
- Report difficulty breathing, headache, muscle pain, rash, unusual bleeding or bruising.

▽ histrelin implant
See Appendix R, *Less commonly used drugs.*

▽ hyaluronic acid derivatives
See Appendix R, *Less commonly used drugs.*

▽ hyaluronidase
See Appendix R, *Less commonly used drugs.*

▷ hydrALAZINE hydrochloride
(bye dral' a zeen)

Apo-Hydralazine (CAN), Apresoline

PREGNANCY CATEGORY C

Drug classes
Antihypertensive
Vasodilator (peripheral)

Therapeutic actions
Acts directly on vascular smooth muscle to cause vasodilation, primarily arteriolar, decreasing peripheral resistance; maintains or increases renal and cerebral blood flow.

Indications
- Oral: Essential hypertension alone or in combination with other drugs
- Parenteral: Severe essential hypertension when drug cannot be given orally or when need to lower BP is urgent
- Unlabeled uses: Reducing afterload in the treatment of heart failure, severe aortic insufficiency, and after valve replacement (doses up to 800 mg tid)

Contraindications and cautions
- Contraindicated with hypersensitivity to hydralazine, tartrazine (in 100-mg tablets marketed as *Apresoline*); CAD, mitral valvular rheumatic heart disease (implicated in MI).
- Use cautiously with stroke; increased intracranial pressure (drug-induced BP decrease increases risk of cerebral ischemia); severe hypertension with uremia; advanced renal damage; slow acetylators (higher plasma levels may be achieved; lower dosage may be adequate); lactation, pregnancy, pulmonary hypertension.

Available forms
Tablets—10, 25, 50, 100 mg; injection—20 mg/mL

Dosages
Adults
Oral
Initiate therapy with gradually increasing dosages. Start with 10 mg qid PO for the first 2–4 days; increase to 25 mg qid PO for the first

week. Second and subsequent weeks: 50 mg qid. For maintenance, adjust to lowest effective dosage; twice-daily dosage may be adequate. Some patients may require up to 300 mg/day. Incidence of toxic reactions, particularly the lupus-like syndrome, is high in patients receiving large doses.
Parenteral
- *Hypertension:* Patient should be hospitalized. Give IV or IM. Use parenteral therapy only when drug cannot be given orally. Usual dose is 20–40 mg, repeated as necessary. Monitor BP frequently; average maximal decrease occurs in 10–80 min. Transfer to oral form as soon as possible.
- *Eclampsia:* 5–10 mg every 20 min via IV bolus; if no response after 20 mg, try another drug.
Pediatric patients
Although safety and efficacy have not been established by controlled clinical trials, hydralazine has been used in children.
Oral
0.75 mg/kg/day PO, given in divided doses every 6 hr. Dosage may be gradually increased over the next 3–4 wk to a maximum of 7.5 mg/kg/day PO in four divided doses or 200 mg/day PO.
Parenteral
1.7–3.5 mg/kg divided into 4–6 doses.

Pharmacokinetics

Route	Onset	Peak	Duration
Oral	Rapid	1–2 hr	6–12 hr
IM, IV	Rapid	10–20 min	2–4 hr

Metabolism: Hepatic; $T_{1/2}$: 3–7 hr
Distribution: Crosses placenta; may enter breast milk
Excretion: Urine

▼ IV FACTS
Preparation: No further preparation required, use as provided.
Infusion: Inject slowly over 1 min, directly into vein or into tubing of running IV; monitor BP response continually.
Incompatibilities: Do not mix with aminophylline, ampicillin, chlorothiazide, edetate, hydrocortisone, nitroglycerin, phenobarbital, verapamil.
Y-site incompatibilities: Do not mix with aminophylline, ampicillin, diazoxide, furosemide.

Adverse effects in *italics* are most common; those in **bold** are life-threatening. ⦿ Do not crush.

Adverse effects

- **CNS:** *Headache,* peripheral neuritis, dizziness, tremors; psychotic reactions characterized by depression, disorientation, or anxiety
- **CV:** *Palpitations, tachycardia, angina pectoris,* hypotension, paradoxical pressor response, orthostatic hypotension
- **GI:** *Anorexia, nausea, vomiting, diarrhea,* constipation, paralytic ileus
- **GU:** Difficult micturition, impotence
- **Hematologic:** Blood dyscrasias
- **Hypersensitivity:** Rash, urticaria, pruritus; fever, chills, arthralgia, eosinophilia; rarely, hepatitis, obstructive jaundice
- **Other:** Nasal congestion, flushing, edema, muscle cramps, lymphadenopathy, splenomegaly, dyspnea, lupus-like syndrome, possible carcinogenesis, lacrimation, conjunctivitis

Interactions

✳ **Drug-drug** • Increased pharmacologic effects of beta-adrenergic blockers and hydralazine when given concomitantly; dosage of beta blocker may need adjustment

✳ **Drug-food** • Increased bioavailability of oral hydralazine given with food

■ Nursing considerations

Assessment

- **History:** Hypersensitivity to hydralazine, tartrazine; heart disease; stroke; increased intracranial pressure; severe hypertension; advanced renal damage; slow acetylators; lactation, pregnancy
- **Physical:** Weight; T; skin color, lesions; lymph node palpation; orientation, affect, reflexes; examination of conjunctiva; P, BP, orthostatic BP, supine BP, perfusion, edema, auscultation; R, adventitious sounds, status of nasal mucous membranes; bowel sounds, normal output; voiding pattern, normal output; CBC with differential, lupus-like cell preparations, ANA determinations, renal function tests, urinalysis

Interventions

- Give oral drug with food to increase bioavailability (drug should be given in a consistent relationship to ingestion of food for consistent response to therapy).

⊗ **Warning** Use parenteral drug immediately after opening ampule. Use as quickly as possible after drawing through a needle into a syringe.

Hydralazine changes color after contact with metal, and discolored solutions should be discarded.

⊗ **Warning** Withdraw drug gradually, especially from patients who have experienced marked BP reduction. Rapid withdrawal may cause a sudden increase in BP.

- Drug may cause a syndrome resembling SLE. Arrange for CBC, lupus erythematosus (LE) cell preparations, and ANA titers before and periodically during prolonged therapy, even in the asymptomatic patient. Discontinue if blood dyscrasias occur. Re-evaluate therapy if ANA or LE tests are positive.

⊗ **Warning** Discontinue or re-evaluate therapy if patient develops arthralgia, fever, chest pain, or continued malaise.

- Arrange for pyridoxine therapy if patient develops symptoms of peripheral neuritis.
- Monitor patient for orthostatic hypotension, which is most marked in the morning and in hot weather, and with consumption of alcohol or during exercise.

Teaching points

- Take this drug exactly as prescribed. Take with food. Do not discontinue or reduce dosage without consulting your health care provider.
- You may experience these side effects: Dizziness, weakness (these are most likely when changing position, in the early morning, after exercise, in hot weather, and when you have consumed alcohol; some tolerance may occur; avoid driving or engaging in tasks that require alertness; change position slowly; use caution in climbing stairs; lie down for a while if dizziness persists); GI upset (eat frequent small meals); constipation; impotence; numbness, tingling (vitamin supplements may ameliorate symptoms); stuffy nose.
- Report persistent or severe constipation; unexplained fever or malaise, muscle or joint aching; chest pain; rash; numbness, tingling.

▽ **hydrochlorothiazide**
*(hye droe klor oh **thye'** a zide)*

Apo-Hydro (CAN), Ezide, HydroDIURIL, Hydro-Par, Microzide Capsules

PREGNANCY CATEGORY B

Drug class

Thiazide diuretic

Therapeutic actions

Inhibits reabsorption of sodium and chloride in distal renal tubule, increasing the excretion of sodium, chloride, and water by the kidney.

Indications

- Adjunctive therapy in edema associated with heart failure, cirrhosis, corticosteroid, and estrogen therapy; renal impairment
- Hypertension as sole therapy or in combination with other antihypertensives
- Unlabeled uses: Calcium nephrolithiasis alone or with amiloride or allopurinol to prevent recurrences in hypercalciuric or normal calciuric patients; diabetes insipidus, especially nephrogenic diabetes insipidus; osteoporosis

Contraindications and cautions

- Contraindicated with allergy to thiazides, sulfonamides; fluid or electrolyte imbalance; renal disease (can lead to azotemia); liver disease (risk of hepatic coma); anuria.
- Use cautiously with gout (risk of attack); SLE; glucose tolerance abnormalities, diabetes mellitus; hyperparathyroidism; manic-depressive disorder (aggravated by hypercalcemia); pregnancy; lactation, elevated triglyceride levels.

Available forms

Tablets—12.5, 25, 50, 100 mg; capsules—12.5 mg

Dosages
Adults

- *Edema:* 25–100 mg daily PO until dry weight is attained. Then, 25–100 mg daily PO or intermittently, up to 200 mg/day.
- *Hypertension:* 12.5–50 mg PO; maximum dose, 50 mg/day.
- *Calcium nephrolithiasis:* 50 mg daily or bid PO.

Pediatric patients
General guidelines: 1–2 mg/kg/day PO in 1 or 2 doses.
Maximum dose:
2–12 yr: 100 mg/day in 2 doses.
6 mo–2 yr: 37.5 mg/day in 2 doses.
Younger than 6 mo: Up to 3 mg/kg/day in 2 doses.

Geriatric patients
Initiate with 12.5 mg/day; increase in 12.5-mg increments, monitoring patient closely.

Pharmacokinetics

Route	Onset	Peak	Duration
Oral	2 hr	4–6 hr	6–12 hr

Metabolism: Hepatic; $T_{1/2}$: 5.6–14.8 hr
Distribution: Crosses placenta; enters breast milk
Excretion: Urine

Adverse effects

- **CNS:** *Dizziness, vertigo,* paresthesias, weakness, headache, drowsiness, fatigue
- **CV:** Orthostatic hypotension, venous thrombosis, volume depletion, cardiac arrhythmias, chest pain
- **Dermatologic:** Photosensitivity, rash, purpura, exfoliative dermatitis, hives, alopecia
- **GI:** *Nausea, anorexia, vomiting, dry mouth,* diarrhea, constipation, jaundice, hepatitis, pancreatitis
- **GU:** *Polyuria, nocturia,* impotence, loss of libido, hyperuricemia
- **Hematologic:** Leukopenia, thrombocytopenia, agranulocytosis, aplastic anemia, neutropenia
- **Other:** Muscle cramps and muscle spasms, fever, gouty attacks, flushing, weight loss, rhinorrhea, electrolyte imbalances, hyperglycemia

Interactions

✳ **Drug-drug** • Altered electrolytes with loop diuretics, amphotericin B, corticosteroids • Increased neuromuscular blocking effects and respiratory depression with nondepolarizing muscle relaxants • Decreased absorption with cholestyramine, colestipol • Increased risk of cardiac glycoside toxicity if hypokalemia occurs • Increased risk of lithium toxicity • Decreased effectiveness of antidiabetic drugs

✳ **Drug-lab test** • Decreased PBI levels without clinical signs of thyroid disturbance

■ Nursing considerations
Assessment

- **History:** Allergy to thiazides, sulfonamides; fluid or electrolyte imbalance; renal or liver disease; gout; SLE; glucose tolerance abnormalities, diabetes mellitus; hyperparathyroidism; manic-depressive disorders; lactation, pregnancy

- **Physical:** Skin color, lesions, edema; orientation, reflexes, muscle strength; pulses, baseline ECG, BP, orthostatic BP, perfusion; R, pattern, adventitious sounds; liver evaluation, bowel sounds, urinary output patterns; CBC, serum electrolytes, blood glucose, LFTs, renal function tests, serum uric acid, urinalysis

Interventions

- Give with food or milk if GI upset occurs.
- Mark calendars or provide other reminders of drug for alternate day or 3–5 days/wk therapy.
- Reduce dosage of other antihypertensives by at least 50% if given with thiazides; readjust dosages gradually as BP responds.
- Administer early in the day so increased urination will not disturb sleep.
- Measure and record weights to monitor fluid changes.

Teaching points

- Record intermittent therapy on a calendar, or use prepared, dated envelopes. Take drug early so increased urination will not disturb sleep. Drug may be taken with food or meals if GI upset occurs.
- Weigh yourself on a regular basis, at the same time and in the same clothing: Record weight on your calendar.
- You may experience these side effects: Increased volume and frequency of urination; dizziness, feeling faint on arising, drowsiness (avoid rapid position changes; hazardous activities, like driving; alcohol); sensitivity to sunlight (use sunglasses, wear protective clothing, or use a sunscreen); decrease in sexual function; increased thirst (sucking on sugarless candies and frequent mouth care may help); gout attack (report any sudden joint pain).
- Report weight change of more than 3 pounds in 1 day, swelling in your ankles or fingers, unusual bleeding or bruising, dizziness, trembling, numbness, fatigue, muscle weakness or cramps.

▽ **hydrocortisone**
*(bye droe **kor'** ti zone)*

hydrocortisone acetate

Dermatologic cream, ointment:
Cortaid with Aloe, Cortef Cream
(CAN), Cortef Feminine Itch,
Cortoderm (CAN), Gynecort Female
Creme, Lanacort-5, Lanacort-10,
Maximum Strength Caldecort,
Maximum Strength Cortaid, Tucks,
U-Cort

hydrocortisone butyrate

Dermatologic ointment and cream: Locoid

hydrocortisone probutate

Pandel

hydrocortisone sodium succinate

IV, IM injection: A-Hydrocort,
Solu-Cortef

hydrocortisone valerate

Dermatologic cream, ointment, lotion: Westcort

PREGNANCY CATEGORY C

Drug classes

Adrenocortical steroid
Corticosteroid (short-acting)
Glucocorticoid
Hormone

Therapeutic actions

Enters target cells and binds to cytoplasmic receptors; initiates many complex reactions that are responsible for its anti-inflammatory, immunosuppressive (glucocorticoid), and salt-retaining (mineralocorticoid) actions. Some actions may be undesirable, depending on drug use.

Indications

- Replacement therapy in adrenal cortical insufficiency

- Allergic states—severe or incapacitating allergic conditions
- Hypercalcemia associated with cancer
- Short-term inflammatory and allergic disorders, such as rheumatoid arthritis, collagen diseases (SLE), dermatologic diseases (pemphigus), status asthmaticus, and autoimmune disorders
- Hematologic disorders—thrombocytopenic purpura, erythroblastopenia
- Trichinosis with neurologic or myocardial involvement
- Ulcerative colitis, acute exacerbations of MS, and palliation in some leukemias and lymphomas
- Intra-articular or soft-tissue administration: Arthritis, psoriatic plaques
- Retention enema: For ulcerative colitis, proctitis
- Topical preparations: Minor skin irritation and rashes due to seborrheic dermatitis and psoriasis
- Dermatologic preparations: To relieve inflammatory and pruritic manifestations of dermatoses that are steroid responsive
- Anorectal cream, suppositories: To relieve discomfort of hemorrhoids and perianal itching or irritation

Ophthalmic
- Ophthalmic diseases: Acute and chronic severe allergic or inflammatory conditions including herpes zoster ophthalmicus, iritis, iridocyclitis, chorioretinitis, uveitis and choroiditis, optic neuritis, sympathetic ophthalmia, allergic conjunctivitis, keratitis, allergic corneal marginal ulcers, anterior segment inflammation

Contraindications and cautions
Systemic administration
- Contraindicated with allergy to any component of the drug, fungal infections, amebiasis, hepatitis B, vaccinia, or varicella, and antibiotic-resistant infections, immunosuppression.
- Use cautiously with kidney disease (risk for edema); liver disease, cirrhosis, hypothyroidism; ulcerative colitis with impending perforation; diverticulitis; recent GI surgery; active or latent peptic ulcer; inflammatory bowel disease (risks exacerbations or bowel perforation); hypertension, heart failure; thromboembolic tendencies, thrombophle-

bitis, osteoporosis, convulsive disorders, metastatic carcinoma, diabetes mellitus; TB; lactation.

Retention enemas, intrarectal foam
- Contraindicated with systemic fungal infections, recent intestinal surgery, extensive fistulas.
- Use cautiously with pregnancy.

Topical dermatologic administration
- Contraindicated with fungal, tubercular, herpes simplex skin infections; vaccinia, varicella; ear application when eardrum is perforated.
- Use cautiously with pregnancy, lactation.

Available forms
Tablets—5, 10, 20 mg; injection—25, 50 mg/mL, 100, 250, 500, 1,000 mg/vial; topical lotion—0.25%, 0.5%, 1%, 2%, 2.5%; topical liquid—1%; topical oil—1%; topical solution—1%; topical spray—1%; cream—0.2%, 0.5%, 1%, 2.5%; ointment—0.5%, 1%, 2.5%; topical gel—1%, 2%; stick, roll-on—1%; pump spray—1%

Dosages
Adults
Individualize dosage, based on severity and response. Give daily dose before 9 AM to minimize adrenal suppression. If long-term therapy is needed, alternate-day therapy should be considered. After long-term therapy, withdraw drug slowly to avoid adrenal insufficiency. For maintenance therapy, reduce initial dose in small increments at intervals until lowest clinically satisfactory dose is reached.

IM, IV (hydrocortisone sodium succinate)
100–500 mg initially and every 2, 4, or 6 hr, based on condition and response.

Pediatric patients
Individualize dosage based on severity and response rather than on formulas that correct adult doses for age or weight. Carefully observe growth and development in infants and children on prolonged therapy.

Adults and pediatric patients
IM, IV (hydrocortisone sodium succinate)
Reduce dose, based on condition and response, but give no less than 25 mg/day.

*Retention enema
(hydrocortisone)*
100 mg nightly for 21 days.
*Intrarectal foam
(hydrocortisone acetate)*
1 applicator daily or bid for 2 or 3 wk and every
second day thereafter.
*Topical dermatologic
preparations*
Apply sparingly to affected area bid–qid.

Pharmacokinetics

Route	Onset	Peak	Duration
Oral	1–2 hr	1–2 hr	1–1.5 days
IM	Rapid	4–8 hr	1–1.5 days
IV	Immediate	Unknown	1–1.5 days
Rectal	Slow	3–5 days	4–6 days

Metabolism: Hepatic; $T_{1/2}$: 80–120 min
Distribution: Crosses placenta; enters breast
milk
Excretion: Urine

▼ IV FACTS

Preparation: Give directly or dilute in normal saline or D_5W. Administer within 24 hr of
diluting.
Infusion: Inject slowly, directly or dilute, and
infuse hydrocortisone phosphate at a rate of
25 mg/min; hydrocortisone sodium succinate
at rate of each 500 mg over 30 sec–10 min.
Incompatibilities: Do not mix or inject at
Y-site with amobarbital, ampicillin, bleomycin,
dimenhydrinate, doxapram, doxorubicin,
ephedrine, ergotamine, heparin, hydralazine,
metaraminol, nafcillin, pentobarbital, phenobarbital, phenytoin, prochlorperazine,
promethazine, secobarbital.

Adverse effects
Systemic

• **CNS:** *Vertigo, headache,* paresthesias, insomnia, seizures, psychosis
• **CV:** *Hypotension, shock,* hypertension and
heart failure secondary to fluid retention,
thromboembolism, thrombophlebitis, fat
embolism, cardiac arrhythmias secondary
to electrolyte disturbances
• **Dermatologic:** *Thin, fragile skin; petechiae; ecchymoses;* purpura; striae; subcutaneous fat atrophy
• **EENT:** Cataracts, glaucoma (long-term
therapy), increased IOP

• **Endocrine:** *Amenorrhea, irregular menses,* growth retardation, decreased carbohydrate tolerance and diabetes mellitus,
cushingoid state (long-term therapy), HPA
suppression systemic with therapy longer than
5 days, Cushing syndrome, hyperglycemia
• **GI:** *Peptic or esophageal ulcer, pancreatitis,* abdominal distention, nausea, vomiting, increased appetite and weight gain
(long-term therapy)
• **Hematologic:** *Na+ and fluid retention,
hypokalemia,* hypocalcemia, increased
blood sugar, increased serum cholesterol,
decreased serum T_3 and T_4 levels
• **Hypersensitivity:** Anaphylactoid or hypersensitivity reactions
• **Musculoskeletal:** *Muscle weakness,*
steroid myopathy and loss of muscle mass,
osteoporosis, spontaneous fractures (long-
term therapy)
• **Other:** *Immunosuppression, aggravation or masking of infections, impaired
wound healing*

*Adverse effects related to
specific routes of
administration*

• **IM repository injections:** Atrophy at
injection site
• **Intra-articular:** Osteonecrosis, tendon
rupture, infection
• **Intralesional therapy, head and
neck:** Blindness (rare)
• **Intraspinal:** Meningitis, adhesive arachnoiditis, conus medullaris syndrome
• **Intrathecal administration:** Arachnoiditis
• **Retention enema:** Local pain, burning;
rectal bleeding; systemic absorption and adverse effects (see Systemic Adverse Effects)
• **Topical dermatologic ointments,
creams, sprays:** Local burning, irritation, acneiform lesions, striae, skin atrophy

Interactions

✳ **Drug-drug** • Increased steroid blood levels with hormonal contraceptives, ketoconazole, estrogen • Decreased steroid blood levels
with phenytoin, phenobarbital, rifampin,
cholestyramine • Decreased serum level of salicylates • Decreased effectiveness of anticholinesterases (ambenonium, edrophonium,
neostigmine, pyridostigmine); ketoconazole,
estrogen • Use cautiously with anticoagulants;
monitor PT/INR

H

✳ **Drug-lab test** • False-negative nitroblue tetrazolium test for bacterial infection (with systemic absorption) • Suppression of skin test reactions • May decrease serum potassium levels, T_3, and T_4 levels

■ Nursing considerations
Assessment
• **History:** Infections; kidney disease; liver disease, hypothyroidism; ulcerative colitis with impending perforation; diverticulitis; recent GI surgery; active or latent peptic ulcer; inflammatory bowel disease; hypertension, heart failure; thromboembolic tendencies, thrombophlebitis, osteoporosis, seizure disorders, metastatic carcinoma, diabetes mellitus; lactation. *Retention enemas, intrarectal foam:* Systemic fungal infections; recent intestinal surgery, extensive fistulas. *Topical dermatologic administration:* Fungal, tubercular, herpes simplex skin infections; vaccinia, varicella; ear application when eardrum is perforated
• **Physical:** *Systemic administration:* Weight, T; reflexes, affect, bilateral grip strength, ophthalmologic examination; BP, P, auscultation, peripheral perfusion, discoloration, pain or prominence of superficial vessels; R, adventitious sounds, chest X-ray; upper GI X-ray (history or symptoms of peptic ulcer), liver palpation; CBC, serum electrolytes, 2-hr postprandial blood glucose, urinalysis, thyroid function tests, serum cholesterol. *Topical, dermatologic preparations:* Affected area, integrity of skin

Interventions
Systemic administration
⊗ *Warning* Give daily before 9 AM to mimic normal peak diurnal corticosteroid levels and minimize HPA suppression.
• Space multiple doses evenly throughout the day.
• Do not give IM injections if patient has thrombocytopenic purpura.
• Rotate sites of IM repository injections to avoid local atrophy.
• Use minimal doses for minimal duration to minimize adverse effects.
• Taper doses when discontinuing high-dose or long-term therapy.
• Arrange for increased dosage when patient is subject to unusual stress.

• Ensure that adequate amount of Ca^{2+} is taken if prolonged administration of steroids.
• Use alternate-day maintenance therapy with short-acting corticosteroids whenever possible.
⊗ *Warning* Do not give live virus vaccines with immunosuppressive doses of hydrocortisone.
• Provide antacids between meals to help avoid peptic ulcer.

Topical dermatologic administration
• Use caution with occlusive dressings; tight or plastic diapers over affected area can increase systemic absorption.
• Avoid prolonged use, especially near eyes, in genital and rectal areas, on face, and in skin creases.

Teaching points
Systemic administration
• Take this drug exactly as prescribed. Do not stop taking this drug without notifying your health care provider; slowly taper dosage to avoid problems.
• Dosage reductions may create adrenal insufficiency. Report any fatigue, muscle and joint pains, anorexia, nausea, vomiting, diarrhea, weight loss, weakness, dizziness, or low blood sugar (if you monitor blood sugar).
• Take with meals or snacks if GI upset occurs.
• Take single daily or alternate-day doses before 9 AM; mark calendar or use other measures as reminder of treatment days.
• Do not overuse joint after intra-articular injections, even if pain is gone.
• Frequent follow-up visits to your health care provider are needed to monitor drug response and adjust dosage.
• Wear a medical alert ID (if you are using long-term therapy) so that any emergency medical personnel will know that you are taking this drug.
• You may experience these side effects: Increase in appetite, weight gain (some of gain may be fluid retention; monitor intake); heartburn, indigestion (eat frequent small meals, use of antacids may help); increased susceptibility to infection (avoid crowds during peak cold or flu seasons, and

avoid anyone with a known infection); poor wound healing (if injured or wounded, consult health care provider); muscle weakness, fatigue (frequent rest periods may help).

• Report unusual weight gain, swelling of lower extremities, muscle weakness, black or tarry stools, vomiting of blood, epigastric burning, puffing of face, menstrual irregularities, fever, prolonged sore throat, cold or other infection, worsening of symptoms.

Intra-articular, intralesional administration

• Do not overuse the injected joint even if the pain is gone. Adhere to rules of proper rest and exercise.

Topical dermatologic administration

• Apply sparingly, and rub in lightly.
• Avoid contacting your eye with the medication.
• Report burning, irritation, or infection of the site, worsening of the condition.
• Avoid prolonged use.

Anorectal preparations

• Maintain normal bowel function with proper diet, adequate fluid intake, and regular exercise.
• Use stool softeners or bulk laxatives if needed.
• Notify your health care provider if symptoms do not improve in 7 days or if bleeding, protrusion, or seepage occurs.

DANGEROUS DRUG

▷ **hydromorphone hydrochloride**

*(hye droe **mor' **fone)*

Dilaudid, Dilaudid-HP, Exalgo ⓔⓡ
Hydromorph Contin (CAN),
Hydromorph HP 10, 20, 50 (CAN),
Hydromorph HP Forte (CAN),
PMS-Hydromorphone (CAN)

PREGNANCY CATEGORY C

PREGNANCY CATEGORY D
(LABOR AND DELIVERY)

CONTROLLED SUBSTANCE C-II

Drug class
Opioid agonist analgesic (phenanthrene)

Therapeutic actions
Acts as agonist at specific mu-opioid receptors in the CNS to produce analgesia, euphoria, sedation; the receptors mediating these effects are thought to be the same as those mediating the effects of endogenous opioids (enkephalins, endorphins).

Indications
• Relief of moderate to severe pain, acute and chronic pain
• Treatment of moderate to severe pain when round-the-clock analgesia is needed for an extended period (ER tablets)

Contraindications and cautions
• Contraindicated with hypersensitivity to opioids, tartrazine (2- and 4-mg tablets, *Dilaudid*); physical dependence on an opioid analgesic (drug may precipitate withdrawal); severe or acute bronchial asthma, upper airway obstruction. Liquid and tablets contraindicated in labor and delivery and status asthmaticus. Extended-release tablets contraindicated with paralytic ileus, impaired pulmonary function, narrowed or obstructed GI tract, opioid nontolerant patients, mild pain or pain not expected to persist.
• Use cautiously with pregnancy (readily crosses placenta; neonatal withdrawal if mother used drug during pregnancy); bronchial asthma, COPD, respiratory depression, anoxia, increased intracranial pressure, acute MI, ventricular failure, coronary insufficiency, hypertension, biliary tract disease, renal or hepatic impairment, lactation.

Available forms
Injection—1, 2, 4, 10 mg/mL; tablets—2, 4, 8 mg; ER tablets ⓔⓡ—8, 12, 16 mg; suppositories—3 mg; powder for injection—250 mg/vial; oral solution—1 mg/mL; injection—1, 2, 4 mg/mL; injection concentrate—10 mg/mL

Dosages
Individualize to each patient.
Adults
Oral
Tablet, 2–4 mg every 4–6 hr; more than 4 mg may be needed for severe pain. Liquid, 2.5–10 mg every 3–6 hr. ER tablets, 8–64 mg PO

once a day, titrated to patient needs; for opioid-tolerant patients only. (*Exalgo*)

Parenteral

1–2 mg IM, subcutaneously every 4–6 hr as needed. May be given by slow IV injection over 2–3 min if no other route is tolerated.

Rectal

3 mg every 6–8 hr.

Pediatric patients

Safety and efficacy not established. Contraindicated in premature infants.

Geriatric patients or patients with renal or hepatic impairment

Use caution; respiratory depression may occur in elderly, the very ill, those with respiratory problems. Reduced dosage may be necessary.

Pharmacokinetics

Route	Onset	Peak	Duration
Oral	Varies	30–60 min	4–5 hr
IM	15–30 min	30–60 min	4–5 hr

Metabolism: Hepatic; $T_{1/2}$: 2–3 hr; ER capsules, 18 hr

Distribution: Crosses placenta; enters breast milk

Excretion: Urine

▼ IV FACTS

Preparations: Administer undiluted or diluted in normal saline or D_5W.

Infusion: Inject slowly, each 2 mg over 2–5 min, directly into vein or into tubing of running IV.

Adverse effects

- **CNS:** *Light-headedness, dizziness, sedation,* euphoria, dysphoria, delirium, insomnia, agitation, anxiety, fear, hallucinations, disorientation, drowsiness, lethargy, impaired mental and physical performance, coma, mood changes, weakness, headache, tremor, seizures, miosis, visual disturbances, suppression of cough reflex
- **CV:** Facial flushing, peripheral circulatory collapse, tachycardia, bradycardia, arrhythmia, palpitations, chest wall rigidity, hypertension, hypotension, orthostatic hypotension, syncope
- **Dermatologic:** Pruritus, urticaria, laryngospasm, bronchospasm, edema, diaphoresis

- **GI:** *Nausea, vomiting,* dry mouth, anorexia, *constipation,* biliary tract spasm; increased colonic motility in patients with chronic ulcerative colitis
- **GU:** Ureteral spasm, spasm of vesical sphincters, urinary retention or hesitancy, oliguria, antidiuretic effect, reduced libido or potency
- **Hypersensitivity:** Anaphylactoid reactions (IV administration)
- **Local:** Phlebitis following IV injection pain at injection site; tissue irritation and induration (subcutaneous injection)
- **Major hazards: Respiratory depression, apnea, circulatory depression, respiratory arrest, shock, cardiac arrest**
- **Other:** *Sweating,* physical tolerance and dependence, psychological dependence

Interactions

✳ **Drug-drug** ● Potentiation of effects of hydromorphone with barbiturate anesthetics, alcohol; decrease dose of hydromorphone when coadministering ● Opioid agonist/antagonists may reduce effects of hydromorphone; use caution ● Extended-release tablets are not for use with MAOIs or within 14 days of their use ● Increased urine retention or severe constipation if extended-release tablets are combined with anticholinergics; monitor patient closely

✳ **Drug-lab test** ● Elevated biliary tract pressure (an effect of opioids) may cause increases in plasma amylase, lipase; determinations of these levels may be unreliable for 24 hr after administration of opioids

■ Nursing considerations
Assessment

- **History:** Hypersensitivity to opioids, tartrazine; physical dependence on an opioid analgesic; pregnancy; lactation; COPD, respiratory depression, anoxia, increased intracranial pressure, acute MI, ventricular failure, coronary insufficiency, hypertension, biliary tract surgery, GI obstruction or narrowing, renal or hepatic impairment
- **Physical:** Orientation, reflexes, bilateral grip strength, affect; pupil size, vision; P, auscultation, BP; R, adventitious sounds; bowel sounds, normal output; thyroid, LFTs, renal function tests

Adverse effects in *italics* are most common; those in **bold** are life-threatening. ⬛ Do not crush.

Interventions

⊗ **Black box warning** Monitor dosage and intended use; it varies with form. Serious effects can occur. Drug can be abused or misused.

⊗ **Black box warning** Extended-release form is for opioid-tolerant patients only; fatal respiratory depression can occur. Extended-release form is not for use with acute or postoperative pain or as an as-needed drug. Extended-release tablets must be swallowed whole; broken, chewed, or crushed tablets allow rapid release of drug and could cause fatal overdose.

• Avoid use in breast-feeding women; another method of feeding the baby should be used.

⊗ **Warning** Ensure opioid antagonist and facilities for assisted or controlled respiration are readily available during parenteral administration.

⊗ **Warning** Use caution when injecting subcutaneously into chilled body areas or in patients with hypotension or in shock; impaired perfusion may delay absorption. With repeated doses, an excessive amount may be absorbed when circulation is restored.

• Refrigerate rectal suppositories.
• Ensure that patient swallows extended-release tablets whole; do not cut, crush, or dissolve tablets.

Teaching points

• Learn how to administer rectal suppositories; refrigerate suppositories.
• Take drug exactly as prescribed. Extended-release tablets are taken once a day and must be swallowed whole. Do not cut, crush, chew, or dissolve tablets.
• Avoid alcohol, antihistamines, sedatives, tranquilizers, and over-the-counter drugs.
• Do not take leftover medication; do not let anyone else take the prescription. Store in a secure area.
• Do not use this drug if you are breast-feeding; you should use another method of feeding the baby.
• You may experience these side effects: Nausea, loss of appetite (take drug with food, lie quietly, eat frequent small meals); constipation (laxative may help); dizziness, sedation, drowsiness, impaired vision (avoid tasks that require alertness, visual acuity); difficulty voiding (empty your bladder before taking drug; notify your health care provider if this becomes a problem).

• Report severe nausea, vomiting, constipation, shortness of breath or difficulty breathing.

▽hydroxocobalamin

See Appendix R, *Less commonly used drugs*.

▽hydroxyethyl starch in sodium choride

See Appendix R, *Less commonly used drugs*.

▽hydroxyprogesterone caproate

(hye drox' ee proe jess' ter own)

Makena

PREGNANCY CATEGORY B

Drug class
Progestin

Therapeutic actions
Endogenous female hormone substance that inhibits spontaneous uterine contractions

Indications
• Reduction of the risk of preterm birth in women with a singleton pregnancy and a history of singleton spontaneous preterm birth; not indicated for use in multiple gestations

Contraindications and cautions
• Contraindicated with known hypersensitivity to components of drug (hydroxyprogesterone, castor oil, benzyl benzoate, benzyl alcohol); history of thrombosis or thromboembolic disorders; known or suspected breast cancer or other hormone-sensitive cancer; undiagnosed abnormal vaginal bleeding; cholestatic jaundice of pregnancy; liver tumors, active liver disease; uncontrolled hypertension.
• Use cautiously with prediabetic or diabetic states, pre-eclampsia, cardiac or renal dysfunction, clinical depression, lactation, seizure disorder.

Available forms
Solution for injection—250 mg/mL

Dosages

Adults

250 mg IM once weekly, beginning between 16 wk, 0 days' and 20 wk, 6 days' gestation. Continue weekly injections until week 37 of gestation, or until delivery, whichever comes first.

Pediatric patients

Safety and efficacy not established.

Pharmacokinetics

Route	Onset	Peak
IM	Rapid	4.6 days

Metabolism: Hepatic; $T_{1/2}$: 7.5-8.1 days
Distribution: May cross placenta; may enter breast milk
Excretion: Urine, feces

Adverse effects

- **CNS:** Depression
- **CV:** Fluid retention, **thromboembolic events,** hypertension
- **GI:** *Nausea,* diarrhea, jaundice
- **Other:** *Urticaria, pruritus,* hyperglycemia, *injection-site reactions,* hypersensitivity reactions

Interactions

None known.

■ Nursing considerations

Assessment

History: Hypersensitivity to components of drug; thrombosis or thromboembolic disorders; known or suspected breast cancer or other hormone-sensitive cancer; undiagnosed abnormal vaginal bleeding; cholestatic jaundice of pregnancy; liver tumors, active liver disease; uncontrolled hypertension; prediabetic or diabetic states; pre-eclampsia; cardiac or renal dysfunction; clinical depression; lactation; seizure disorder

Physical: Affect; T, P; GI exam; skin status; liver function tests; pregnancy evaluation

Interventions

- Administer as an IM injection into the upper outer area of the buttocks once each wk; vial is stable for 5 wk at room temperature, protected from light.
- Monitor injection site for possible reactions.
- Monitor patient for signs and symptoms of hypersensitivity reaction, thromboembolic events.

- Monitor blood glucose level before and periodically during treatment; glucose intolerance is possible.
- Encourage small, frequent meals and comfort measures if GI upset is severe.

Teaching points

- This drug is given by injection into your hip to help prevent early labor in women with a singleton pregnancy and a history of preterm labor.
- Continue all therapies, cautions, and dietary changes that have been part of your pregnancy regimen.
- Mark your calendar for weekly injections; the injection must be given to you. If you are keeping the vial at home, it must be kept at room temperature and protected from light. It must be discarded after 5 weeks.
- The injections must be given each week until the 37th week of your pregnancy or until you deliver the baby, whichever comes first. If you miss a week, consult your health care provider as soon as possible to discuss how to get back on schedule.
- You may experience these side effects: GI upset, diarrhea, nausea (small, frequent meals may help; notify your health care provider if these become severe); depression (be aware that this could occur and consult your health care provider if you experience depression); allergic reaction (immediately report hives, itching, swelling of the face); blood clots (be aware of leg pain that worsens when you bend your foot, leg swelling, leg redness); injection-site reactions (hot packs may help; consult your health care provider if you notice a problem at the site).
- Report swelling, pain, or bleeding at injection site; hives, itching, face swelling; yellowing of skin or eyes; increasing depression; leg pain with swelling, redness; severe nausea.

DANGEROUS DRUG

▽ hydroxyurea

(hye drox ee yoor ee' a)

Droxia ⓄⓇⒸ, Gen-Hydroxyurea (CAN) ⓄⓇⒸ, Hydrea ⓄⓇⒸ

PREGNANCY CATEGORY D

Drug class

Antineoplastic

Adverse effects in *italics* are most common; those in **bold** are life-threatening. ⒹⓃⒸ Do not crush.

Therapeutic actions

Cytotoxic: Inhibits an enzyme that is crucial for DNA synthesis, but exact mechanism of action is not fully understood.

Indications

- Melanoma
- Resistant chronic myelocytic leukemia (*Hydrea*)
- Recurrent, metastatic, or inoperable ovarian cancer (*Hydrea*)
- Concomitant therapy with irradiation for primary squamous cell carcinoma of the head and neck, excluding the lip
- To reduce the frequency of painful crises and to reduce the need for blood transfusions in adult patients with sickle cell anemia (*Droxia*)
- Unlabeled uses: Essential thrombocythemia, psoriasis, HIV treatment with didanosine

Contraindications and cautions

- Contraindicated in severe bone marrow suppression, allergy to hydroxyurea.
- Use cautiously in patients with impaired hepatic and renal functions, mild to moderate bone marrow suppression, pregnancy, lactation.

Available forms

Capsules ⊕—500 mg; *Droxia* capsules ⊕—200, 300, 400 mg

Dosages

Adults

⊗ **Warning** Base dosage on ideal or actual body weight, whichever is less. Interrupt therapy if WBC count falls below 2,500/mm³ or platelet count below 100,000/mm³. Recheck in 3 days and resume therapy when counts approach normal (*Hydrea*).

- *Solid tumors:* Intermittent therapy: 80 mg/kg PO as a single dose every third day. Continuous therapy: 20–30 mg/kg PO as a single daily dose.
- *Concomitant therapy with irradiation:* 80 mg/kg as a single daily dose every third day. Begin hydroxyurea 7 days before irradiation, and continue during and for a prolonged period after radiation therapy (*Hydrea*).
- *Resistant chronic myelocytic leukemia:* 20–30 mg/kg as a single daily dose (*Hydrea*).

- *Reduction of sickle cell anemia crises (Droxia):* 15 mg/kg/day PO as a single dose; may be increased by 5 mg/kg/day PO as a single dose; may be increased by 5 mg/kg/day every 12 wk until maximum tolerated dose or 35 mg/kg/day is reached. If blood levels become toxic, stop drug and resume at 2.5 mg/kg/day less than the dose that resulted in toxicity when blood levels return to normal. May increase every 12 wk in 2.5-mg/kg/day intervals if blood levels stay acceptable. (Acceptable levels are neutrophils, at least 2,500 cells/mm³; platelets, at least 95,000/mm³; hemoglobin, at least 5.3 g/dL, reticulocytes, at least 95,000/mm³ if hemoglobin concentration is less than 9 g/dL.)

Pediatric patients

Dosage regimen not established.

Patients with renal impairment

Consider need to decrease dosage, and monitor patient closely.

Pharmacokinetics

Route	Onset	Peak	Duration
Oral	Varies	1–4 hr	18–20 hr

Metabolism: Hepatic; $T_{1/2}$: 3–4 hr
Distribution: Crosses placenta; enters breast milk
Excretion: Urine

Adverse effects

- **CNS:** *Headache, dizziness,* disorientation, hallucinations
- **Dermatologic:** Maculopapular rash, facial erythema
- **GI:** *Stomatitis, anorexia, nausea, vomiting,* diarrhea, constipation, elevated hepatic enzymes
- **GU:** Impaired renal tubular function
- **Hematologic:** *Bone marrow depression*
- **Local:** Mucositis at the site, especially in combination with irradiation
- **Other:** Fever, chills, malaise, **cancer,** pulmonary reactions

Interactions

✳ **Drug-drug** • Uricosuric agents may increase uric acid levels; adjust dose of uricosuric agent

✳ **Drug-lab test** • Serum uric acid, BUN, and creatinine levels may increase with hydroxyurea therapy • Drug causes self-limited abnormalities in erythrocytes that resemble those of pernicious anemia but are not related to vitamin B_{12} or folate deficiency

■ **Nursing considerations**
Assessment
- **History:** Allergy to hydroxyurea, irradiation, leukopenia, impaired hepatic and renal function, lactation, pregnancy
- **Physical:** Weight; T; skin color, lesions; reflexes, orientation, affect; mucous membranes, abdominal examination; CBC, LFTs, renal function tests

Interventions
⊗ *Warning* Handle with extreme care; may cause cancer. Secondary leukemia has been reported with long-term treatment of myeloproliferative disorder.
- Give in oral form only. Do not cut, crush, or allow patient to chew capsules. If patient is unable to swallow capsules, empty capsules into a glass of water, and give immediately (inert products may not dissolve).
- Encourage patient to drink 10–12 glasses of fluid each day.
- Check CBC before administration before therapy and every 2 wk.
- Caution patient to avoid pregnancy while using this drug; using barrier contraceptives is advised.

Teaching points
- Prepare a calendar for dates to return for diagnostic testing and treatment days. If you are unable to swallow the capsule, empty the capsule into a glass of water and take immediately (some of the material may not dissolve).
- This medication can cause serious adverse effects. Avoid handling it, store it safely away from children and pets, and dispose of it in a closed container.
- You should wear gloves when touching this medication or bottle; wash hands immediately after dosing.
- Avoid pregnancy while using this drug, fetal abnormalities have been reported; using barrier contraceptives is advised.
- Arrange for regular blood tests at least every 2 weeks to monitor the drug's effects.
- Drink at least 10–12 glasses of fluid each day while using this drug.

- You may experience these side effects: Loss of appetite, nausea, vomiting, mouth sores (frequent mouth care, frequent small meals may help; maintain good nutrition; an antiemetic may be ordered); constipation or diarrhea (a bowel program may be established); disorientation, dizziness, headache (take precautions to avoid injury); red face, rash (reversible).
- Report fever, chills, sore throat, unusual bleeding or bruising, severe nausea, vomiting, loss of appetite, sores in the mouth or on the lips, pregnancy (it is advisable to use birth control while on this drug).

▷ **hydrOXYzine**
(bye drox' i zeen)

hydrOXYzine hydrochloride
Oral preparations: Apo-Hydroxyzine (CAN), Vistaril
Parenteral preparations: Vistaril

hydrOXYzine pamoate
Oral preparation: Vistaril

PREGNANCY CATEGORY C

Drug classes
Antiemetic
Antihistamine
Anxiolytic

Therapeutic actions
Mechanisms of action not understood; actions may be due to suppression of subcortical areas of the CNS; has clinically demonstrated antihistaminic, analgesic, antispasmodic, antiemetic, mild antisecretory, and bronchodilator activity.

Indications
- Symptomatic relief of anxiety and tension associated with psychoneurosis; adjunct in organic disease states in which anxiety is manifested; alcoholism and asthma; before dental procedures
- Management of pruritus due to allergic conditions, such as chronic urticaria, atopic and contact dermatosis, and in histamine-mediated pruritus

- Sedation when used as premedication and following general anesthesia
- Control of nausea and vomiting and as adjunct to analgesia preoperatively and postoperatively to allow decreased opioid dosage
- Management of the acutely disturbed or hysterical patient; the acute or chronic alcoholic with anxiety withdrawal symptoms or delirium tremens; as preoperative and postoperative adjunct to permit reduction in opioid dosage, allay anxiety, and control emesis

Contraindications and cautions

- Contraindicated with allergy to hydroxyzine or cetirizine; pregnancy, lactation.
- Use cautiously with uncomplicated vomiting in children (may contribute to Reye syndrome or unfavorably influence its outcome; extrapyramidal effects may obscure diagnosis of Reye syndrome).

Available forms

Tablets—10, 25, 50 mg; syrup—10 mg/5 mL; capsules—25, 50, 100 mg; injection—25, 50 mg/mL

Dosages

Start patients on IM therapy when indicated; use oral therapy for maintenance. Adjust dosage to patient's response.

Adults

Oral

- *Symptomatic relief of anxiety:* 50–100 mg qid.
- *Management of pruritus:* 25 mg tid–qid.
- *Sedative (preoperative and postoperative):* 50–100 mg.

IM

- *Psychiatric and emotional emergencies:* 50–100 mg immediately and every 4–6 hr as needed.
- *Preoperative and postoperative sedation:* 50–100 mg.
- *Pruritus:* 25 mg tid–qid.

Pediatric patients

Oral

- *Anxiety, pruritus:*

Younger than 6 yr: 50 mg/day in divided doses.

Older than 6 yr: 50–100 mg/day in divided doses.

- *Sedative:* 0.6 mg/kg.

IM

- *Preoperative and postoperative sedation:* 0.6 mg/kg.

Pharmacokinetics

Route	Onset	Peak	Duration
Oral, IM	15–30 min	3 hr	4–6 hr

Metabolism: Hepatic; $T_{1/2}$: 3 hr
Distribution: Crosses placenta; may enter breast milk
Excretion: Urine

Adverse effects

- **CNS:** *Drowsiness,* involuntary motor activity, including tremor and seizures
- **GI:** *Dry mouth,* reflux, constipation
- **GU:** Urinary retention
- **Hypersensitivity:** Wheezing, dyspnea, chest tightness

Interactions

✳ **Drug-drug** ● Potentiating action when used concomitantly with CNS depressants (opioids, barbiturates)

■ Nursing considerations

Assessment

- **History:** Allergy to hydroxyzine or cetirizine, uncomplicated vomiting in children, lactation, pregnancy
- **Physical:** Skin color, lesions, texture; orientation, reflexes, affect; R, adventitious sounds

Interventions

⊗ *Warning* Determine and treat underlying cause of vomiting. Drug may mask signs and symptoms of serious conditions, such as brain tumor, intestinal obstruction, or appendicitis.

⊗ *Warning* Do not administer parenteral solution subcutaneously, IV, or intra-arterially; tissue necrosis has occurred with subcutaneous and intra-arterial injection, and hemolysis with IV injection.

- Give IM injections deep into a large muscle: In adults, use upper outer quadrant of buttocks or midlateral thigh; in children, use midlateral thigh muscles; use deltoid area only if well developed.

Teaching points

- Take as prescribed. Avoid excessive dosage.

H

- You may experience these side effects: Dizziness, sedation, drowsiness (use caution if performing tasks that require alertness); avoid alcohol, sedatives, sleep aids (serious overdosage could result); dry mouth (mouth care, sucking sugarless candies may help).
- Report difficulty breathing, tremors, loss of coordination, sore muscles, or muscle spasm.

▷hyoscyamine sulfate (L-hyoscyamine)
(high ah' ska meen)

IB-Stat, Levbid ⬭, Levsin/SL, Mar-Spas, Neosol, NuLev, Symax Duotab, Symax Fastab, Symax-SL ⬭, Symax-SR ⬭

PREGNANCY CATEGORY C

Drug classes
Anticholinergic
Antimuscarinic
Antispasmodic
Belladonna alkaloid
Parasympatholytic

Therapeutic actions
Direct GI smooth muscle relaxant; competitively blocks the effects of acetylcholine at muscarinic cholinergic receptors that mediate the effects of parasympathetic postganglionic impulses, thus relaxing the GI tract. Also has antisecretory effects along the GI.

Indications
- Adjunctive therapy in IBS, peptic ulcer, spastic or functional GI disorders, cystitis, neurogenic bladder or bowel disorders, parkinsonism, biliary or renal colic
- Rhinitis and anticholinesterase poisoning
- Reduction of rigidity and tremors and control of sialorrhea and hyperhidrosis associated with parkinsonism
- Partial heart block associated with vagal activity
- Preoperatively to decrease secretions
- Parenterally to improve radiologic imaging tests

Contraindications and cautions
- Contraindicated with hypersensitivity to anticholinergic drugs, glaucoma, adhesions between iris and lens, stenosing peptic ulcer, pyloroduodenal obstruction, paralytic ileus, intestinal atony, severe ulcerative colitis, toxic megacolon, symptomatic prostatic hypertrophy, bladder neck obstruction, bronchial asthma, COPD, myocardial ischemia, myasthenia gravis, tachycardia, renal disease.
- Use cautiously with high environmental temperatures, fever, diarrhea, hyperthyroidism, CV disease, hypertension, heart failure, arrhythmias, renal disease, hiatal hernia, pregnancy, lactation.

Available forms
Tablets—0.125 mg, 0.15 mg; sublingual tablets—0.125 mg; ER tablets ⬭—0.375 mg; ER capsules ⬭—0.375 mg; orally disintegrating tablets—0.125 mg; oral spray—0.125 mg/mL; elixir—0.125 mg/5 mL; solution—0.125 mg/mL; injection—0.5 mg/mL

Dosages
Adults
Oral or sublingual
0.125–0.25 mg every 4 hr or as needed.
Oral solution: 1–2 mL every 4 hr as needed; do not exceed 12 mL per day.
Oral spray: 1–2 sprays every 4 hr as needed; do not exceed 12 sprays per day.
Orally disintegrating tablets: ½–1 tablet 3–4 times per day 30 min–1 hr before meals and at bedtime.
Elixir: 1–2 teaspoons every 4 hr as needed; do not exceed 12 teaspoons per day.
ER
0.375–0.75 mg PO every 12 hr. May give 1 capsule every 8 hr if needed; do not exceed 4 capsules per day.
Parenteral
- *GI disorders:* 0.25–0.5 mg subcutaneously, IM, or IV 2–4 times per day at 4-hr intervals as needed.
- *Preanesthetic:* 0.005 mg/kg IV or IM 30–60 min before induction.
- *Treatment of bradycardia:* 0.125 mg (0.25 mL) IV. Repeat as needed.
- *Reversal of neuromuscular blockade:* 0.2 mg IV, IM, or subcutaneously for every 1 mg neostigmine.

Adverse effects in *italics* are most common; those in **bold** are life-threatening. ⬭ Do not crush.

Pediatric patients
Regular and sublingual tablets, orally disintegrating tablets (except Mar-Spas)
12 yr and older: 1–2 tablets PO every 4 hr as needed; do not exceed 12 tablets in 24 hr.
2 yr to younger than 12 yr: ½–1 tablet PO every 4 hr as needed; do not exceed 6 tablets in 24 hr.
Mar-Spas *orally disintegrating tablets*
12 yr and older: ½–1 tablet PO tid–qid 30 min–1 hr before meals and at bedtime.
Younger than 12 yr: Not recommended.
Extended release and timed-release capsules
12 yr and older: 1–2 capsules PO every 12 hr; adjust to 1 capsule every 8 hr if needed. Do not exceed 4 capsules in 24 hr.
Oral solution
12 yr and older: 1–2 mL PO every 4 hr or as needed; do not exceed 12 mL in 24 hr.
2 yr to younger than 12 yr: 0.25–1 mL PO every 4 hr or as needed; do not exceed 6 mL in 24 hr.
Younger than 2 yr:

Weight (kg)	Dose (drops)	Maximum drops/day
3.4	4	24
5	5	30
7	6	36
10	8	48

Elixir
12 yr and older: 1–2 tsp PO every 4 hr or as needed; do not exceed 12 tsp in 24 hr.
2 yr to younger than 12 yr: Give dose based on weight every 4 hr as needed; do not exceed 6 tsp PO in 24 hr.

Weight (kg)	Dose (tsp) (mL)
10	0.25 (1.25 mL)
20	0.5 (2.5 mL)
40	0.75 (3.75 mL)
50	1 (5 mL)

Oral spray
12 yr and older: 1–2 sprays every 4 hr as needed.
Injectable
Older than 2 yr:
Preanesthetic: 5 mcg/kg IV 30–60 min before anesthesia.

Treatment of drug-induced bradycardia: 0.25 mL IV during surgery; repeat as needed.
Reversal of neuromuscular blockade: 0.2 mg IV for every 1 mg neostigmine.

Pharmacokinetics

Route	Onset	Peak	Duration
Oral tablets	20–30 min	30–60 min	4 hr
Sublingual	5–20 min	30–60 min	4hr
ER	20–30 min	40–90 min	12 hr
Parenteral	2–3 min	15–30 min	4 hr

Metabolism: Hepatic; $T_{1/2}$: 9–10 hr (injection, 3.5 hr)
Distribution: Crosses placenta; enters breast milk
Excretion: Urine

Adverse effects
- **CNS:** *Dizziness,* blurred vision, dilated pupils, confusion, *drowsiness,* psychosis, headache
- **CV:** *Palpitations,* hypertension, chest pain, tachycardia
- **GI:** *Nausea, dry mouth,* taste loss, *constipation,* vomiting
- **GU:** *Urinary hesitancy,* impotence
- **Other:** *Decreased sweating, fever, anaphylaxis, urticaria,* heat prostration

Interactions
✷ Drug-drug • Additive effects with other anticholinergics, amantadine, haloperidol, phenothiazines, MAOIs, TCAs, or antihistamines; monitor patient closely and adjust dosages as needed • Decreased absorption if combined with antacids; space 2–4 hr apart

■ Nursing considerations
Assessment
- **History:** Glaucoma, adhesions between iris and lens, stenosing peptic ulcer, pyloroduodenal obstruction, paralytic ileus, intestinal atony, severe ulcerative colitis, toxic megacolon, symptomatic prostatic hypertrophy, bladder neck obstruction, bronchial asthma, COPD, myocardial ischemia, myasthenia gravis, fever, diarrhea, hyperthyroidism, CV disease, hypertension, heart failure, arrhythmias, renal disease, hiatal hernia, pregnancy, lactation

- **Physical:** Bowel sounds, normal output; normal urinary output, prostate palpation; R, adventitious sounds; P, BP; IOP, vision; bilateral grip strength, reflexes; liver palpation, LFTs, renal function tests; skin color, lesions, texture

Interventions

- Ensure adequate hydration; control environment (temperature) to prevent hyperpyrexia.
- Use caution in geriatric patients who may be more sensitive to anticholinergic effects.
- Encourage patient to void before each dose if urinary retention becomes a problem.
- Ensure ER forms are not cut, crushed, or chewed.
- Monitor lighting to minimize discomfort of photophobia.
- Establish safety precautions (side rails, assistance with ambulation, proper lighting) if visual effects occur.
- Provide sugarless candies, ice chips to suck (if permitted) if dry mouth occurs.
- Provide frequent small meals if GI upset is severe.

Teaching points

- Take drug exactly as prescribed; do not cut, crush, or chew ER tablets.
- Take 30–60 minutes before meals.
- Avoid hot environments while taking this drug (you will be heat intolerant and dangerous reactions may occur).
- You may experience these side effects: Dry mouth (sugarless candies, frequent mouth care may help; this effect sometimes lessens over time); blurred vision, sensitivity to light (these effects will go away when you discontinue the drug; avoid tasks that require acute vision and wear sunglasses when in bright light); impotence (this effect will go away when you discontinue the drug; you may wish to discuss it with your health care provider); difficulty in urination (it may help to empty the bladder immediately before taking each dose).
- Report skin rash, flushing, eye pain, difficulty breathing, tremors, loss of coordination, irregular heartbeat, palpitations, headache, abdominal distention, hallucinations, difficulty swallowing, difficulty urinating.

▷ ibandronate sodium

(eh ban' drow nate)

Boniva ⓞⓝⓒ

PREGNANCY CATEGORY C

Drug classes

Bisphosphonate
Calcium regulator

Therapeutic actions

Inhibits osteoclast activity and reduces bone resorption and turnover, without inhibiting bone formation or mineralization.

Indications

- Treatment and prevention of osteoporosis in postmenopausal women
- Unlabeled use: Treatment of metastatic bone disease in breast cancer

Contraindications and cautions

- Contraindicated with known allergy to any component of the tablet, uncorrected hypocalcemia, inability to stand or sit upright for at least 60 minutes (oral form).
- Use caution with known upper GI abnormalities, pregnancy, lactation.

Available forms

Prefilled syringe—1 mg/mL; tablets ⓞⓝⓒ— 150 mg

Dosages

Adults

One 2.5-mg tablet/day PO or one 150-mg tablet PO once per month on the same date each month or 3 mg IV, given over 15–30 sec, every 3 mo.

Pediatric patients

Safety and efficacy not established.

For patients with renal impairment

Not recommended with severe renal impairment (creatinine clearance less than 30 mL/min).

Pharmacokinetics

Route	Onset	Peak
Oral	Rapid	0.5–2 hr
IV	Rapid	Unknown

Metabolism: $T_{1/2}$: 37–157 hr

Distribution: May cross placenta; may pass into breast milk

Excretion: Urine, unchanged

Adverse effects

- **CNS:** *Headache,* dizziness, vertigo, nerve root lesion, asthenia, insomnia
- **CV:** Angina, *hypertension*
- **GI:** *Diarrhea, dyspepsia, abdominal pain,* constipation, vomiting, gastritis, tooth disorder, dysphagia, esophagitis, esophageal ulcers, gastric ulcers
- **Respiratory:** *URI, bronchitis, pneumonia,* pharyngitis
- **Other: Jaw osteonecrosis** (increased risk with cancer, chemotherapy, radiation therapy, pre-existing dental disease), *back pain,* infection, *myalgia,* joint pain, hypercholesterolemia, long-bone fractures

Interactions

✳ **Drug-drug** ● Decreased absorption of ibandronate if taken at the same time as multivalent cations (aluminum, iron, magnesium), antacids

✳ **Drug-food** ● Milk or food; ibandronate should be taken on an empty stomach, first thing in the morning, 60 min before any food or other medications (patient may have water)

■ Nursing considerations

Assessment

- **History:** Allergy to any component of the tablet, uncorrected hypocalcemia, inability to stand or sit upright for at least 60 min, upper GI abnormalities, pregnancy, lactation
- **Physical:** Orientation, reflexes; BP; respiratory evaluation; abdominal examination, serum calcium levels, renal function tests

Interventions

⊗ *Warning* Administer in the morning with a full glass of water at least 60 min before the first beverage, food, or medication of the day. Patient must stay upright for 60 min after taking the tablet to avoid potentially serious esophageal erosion.

- Monitor serum calcium levels before, during, and after therapy. Consider limiting drug use to no more than 3–5 yr.
- Ensure adequate intake of vitamin D and calcium.

- Make calendar for patient using once-a-month or once every 3 mo dosing as a reminder to take drug.
- Provide comfort measures and possible analgesics for headache and pain.
- Encourage frequent small meals if GI effects are uncomfortable.

Teaching points

- Take this drug in the morning with a full glass of water, at least 60 minutes before any food, beverage, or other medications. You must stay upright for at least 60 minutes after taking the tablet to prevent potentially serious problems with your esophagus. If you are taking the once a month dose, be sure to mark your calendar as a reminder of when to take the drug. Swallow the tablet whole; do not suck on it or chew it. If taking once every 3 months IV and you miss a dose, reschedule the missed dose as soon as possible. Subsequent injections should be rescheduled for once every 3 months from that month.
- If you miss a dose of the daily medication, do not take the dose later in the day. Return to your usual routine the next morning. Do not take more than 1 tablet each day. If you miss a dose of the monthly medication or if the next scheduled dose is more than 7 days away, take the 150-mg tablet the morning following the day that you remembered. Then return to taking the tablet every month on your original date. If your next scheduled dose is 1–7 days away, wait and take the tablet on the scheduled day, then every month on that same date as scheduled. Never take two 150-mg tablets in the same week.
- Take vitamin D and calcium to increase the effectiveness of this drug.
- If you experience pain or burning in your esophagus, stop drug and contact your health care provider.
- You may need to have periodic bone density tests to evaluate the effects of this drug on your body. Use of this drug may be limited to 3–5 years.
- It is not known how this drug could affect a breast-feeding infant. If you are breast-feeding, you should choose another method of feeding the infant.
- It is not known how this drug could affect a fetus. If you are pregnant or would like to

become pregnant while on this drug, consult your health care provider.

• You may experience these side effects: Headache (consult with your health care provider; medication may be available to help); nausea, diarrhea (frequent small meals may help).

• Report pain or trouble swallowing, chest pain, very bad heartburn, or heartburn that does not get better.

▷ibritumomab

See Appendix R, *Less commonly used drugs*.

▷ibuprofen
(eye byoo' proe fen)

Advil, Advil Liqui-Gels, Advil Migraine, Advil Pediatric Drops, Apo-Ibuprofen (CAN), Apo-Ibuprofen Prescription (CAN), Caldolor, Children's Advil, Children's Motrin, Ibutab, Infants' Motrin, Junior Strength Motrin, Midol Maximum Strength Cramp Formula, Motrin, Motrin IB, Motrin Migraine Pain, PediaCare Fever, Pediatric Advil Drops

PREGNANCY CATEGORY B

PREGNANCY CATEGORY D
(THIRD TRIMESTER)

Drug classes
Analgesic (nonopioid)
NSAID
Propionic acid derivative

Therapeutic actions
Anti-inflammatory, analgesic, and antipyretic activities largely related to inhibition of prostaglandin synthesis; exact mechanisms of action are not known. Inhibits both cyclooxygenase (COX) 1 and 2. Ibuprofen is slightly more selective for COX-1.

Indications
• Relief of signs and symptoms of rheumatoid arthritis and osteoarthritis
• Relief of mild to moderate pain
• Treatment of primary dysmenorrhea

• Prevention and treatment of migraine headache
• Fever reduction
• Unlabeled use: Prevention of adverse reactions with DTP vaccine in patients at risk for seizures

Contraindications and cautions
• Contraindicated with allergy to ibuprofen, salicylates, or other NSAIDs (more common in patients with rhinitis, asthma, chronic urticaria, nasal polyps).

⊗ **Black box warning** Contraindicated for treatment of perioperative pain after coronary artery bypass graft.

• Use cautiously with CV dysfunction, hypertension, peptic ulceration, GI bleeding, pregnancy, lactation, impaired hepatic or renal function.

Available forms
Tablets—100, 200, 400, 600, 800 mg; chewable tablets—50, 100 mg; capsules—200 mg; suspension—100 mg/2.5 mL, 100 mg/5 mL; oral drops—40 mg/mL; injection—10 mg/mL, 100 mg/mL

Dosages
Adults
Do not exceed 3,200 mg/day.
• *Mild to moderate pain:* 400 mg every 4–6 hr PO.
• *Migraine:* 400 mg PO at onset of headache.
• *Osteoarthritis or rheumatoid arthritis:* 1,200–3,200 mg/day PO (300 mg qid or 400, 600, 800 mg tid or qid; individualize dosage. Therapeutic response may occur in a few days, but often takes 2 wk).
• *Primary dysmenorrhea:* 400 mg every 4 hr PO.
• *IV use:* 400–800 mg IV over 30 min every 6 hr for pain; 400 mg IV over 30 min for fever, can be followed by 400 mg every 4–6 hr or 100–200 mg every 4 hr to control fever.
• *OTC use:* 200–400 mg every 4–6 hr PO while symptoms persist; do not exceed 1,200 mg/day. Do not take for more than 10 days for pain or 3 days for fever, unless so directed by health care provider.
Pediatric patients 6 mo–11 yr
Give dose every 6–8 hr according to weight (shown below) but no more than four times/day.

Adverse effects in *italics* are most common; those in **bold** are life-threatening. ⬛ Do not crush.

Weight (kg)	Dose (mg)
5–7	50
8–10	75
11–15	100
16–21	150
22–26	200
27–31	250
32–43	300

- *Juvenile arthritis:* 30–50 mg/kg/day PO in three to four divided doses; 20 mg/kg/day for milder disease.

Oral drops
5–8 kg (12–17 lb) or age 6–11 months: 1.25 mL (50 mg)
9–11 kg (18–23 lb) or age 12–23 months: 1.875 mL (75 mg)

Pharmacokinetics

Route	Onset	Peak	Duration
Oral	30 min	1–2 hr	4–6 hr

Metabolism: Hepatic; $T_{1/2}$: 1.8–2.5 hr
Distribution: Crosses placenta; may enter breast milk
Excretion: Urine

▼ IV FACTS

Preparation: Dilute to a concentration of 4 mg/mL or less using 0.9% sodium chloride, 5% dextrose, or lactated Ringer. Solution should be particulate matter–free and not discolored. Diluted solution is stable for up to 24 hr at room temperature.
Infusion: Infuse over no less than 30 min.

Adverse effects

- **CNS:** *Headache, dizziness, somnolence, insomnia,* fatigue, tiredness, dizziness, tinnitus, ophthalmologic effects
- **CV:** Hypertension, palpitations, arrhythmia, **heart failure**
- **Dermatologic:** *Rash,* pruritus, sweating, dry mucous membranes, stomatitis
- **GI:** *Nausea, dyspepsia, GI pain,* diarrhea, vomiting, *constipation,* flatulence, **GI bleeding**
- **GU:** Dysuria, renal impairment, menorrhagia
- **Hematologic:** Bleeding, platelet inhibition with higher doses, neutropenia, eosinophilia, leukopenia, **pancytopenia,** thrombocytopenia, **agranulocytosis,** granulocytopenia, **aplastic anemia,** decreased Hgb or Hct, bone marrow depression
- **Respiratory:** Dyspnea, hemoptysis, pharyngitis, **bronchospasm,** rhinitis
- **Other:** Peripheral edema, **anaphylactoid reactions to anaphylactic shock**

Interactions

✳ **Drug-drug** • Increased toxic effects of lithium with ibuprofen • Decreased diuretic effect with loop diuretics—bumetanide, furosemide, ethacrynic acid • Potential decrease in antihypertensive effect of beta-adrenergic blocking drugs and ACE inhibitors • Increased risk of gastric ulceration with bisphosphonates • Increased risk of bleeding with anticoagulants
✳ **Drug-alternative therapy** • Increased risk of bleeding with concurrent use of ginkgo biloba

■ Nursing considerations
Assessment

- **History:** Allergy to ibuprofen, salicylates or other NSAIDs; CV dysfunction, hypertension; peptic ulceration, GI bleeding; impaired hepatic or renal function; pregnancy; lactation
- **Physical:** Skin color, lesions; T; orientation, reflexes, ophthalmologic evaluation, audiometric evaluation, peripheral sensation; P, BP, edema; R, adventitious sounds; liver evaluation, bowel sounds; CBC, clotting times, urinalysis, LFTs, renal function tests, serum electrolytes, stool guaiac

Interventions

⊗ *Black box warning* Be aware that patient may be at increased risk of CV event, GI bleeding; monitor accordingly.
- Ensure that patient is well hydrated if using IV form.
- Administer drug with food or after meals if GI upset occurs.
- Arrange for periodic ophthalmologic examination during long-term therapy.
- Discontinue drug if eye changes, symptoms of hepatic impairment, or renal impairment occur.
⊗ *Warning* Institute emergency procedures if overdose occurs: Gastric lavage, induction of emesis, and supportive therapy.

Teaching points

- Use drug only as suggested; avoid overdose. Take the drug with food or after meals if GI upset occurs. Do not exceed the prescribed dosage.

- Avoid over-the-counter drugs. Many of these drugs contain similar medication, and serious overdosage can occur.
- You may experience these side effects: Nausea, GI upset, dyspepsia (take drug with food); diarrhea or constipation; drowsiness, dizziness, vertigo, insomnia (use caution when driving or operating dangerous machinery).
- Report sore throat, fever, rash, itching, weight gain, swelling in ankles or fingers, changes in vision, black or tarry stools.

DANGEROUS DRUG

▽**ibutilide fumarate**
(*eye byu' ti lyed foo' mah rate*)

Corvert

PREGNANCY CATEGORY C

Drug class
Antiarrhythmic (predominantly class III)

Therapeutic actions
Prolongs cardiac action potential, increases atrial and ventricular refractoriness; produces mild slowing of sinus rate and AV conduction; delays repolarization by activating inward current rather than blocking outward current.

Indications
- Rapid conversion of atrial fibrillation or flutter of recent onset to sinus rhythm; most effective in arrhythmias of less than 90 days' duration

Contraindications and cautions
- Contraindicated with hypersensitivity to ibutilide; second- or third-degree AV heart block, prolonged QTc intervals.
- Use cautiously with ventricular arrhythmias, pregnancy, lactation, renal and hepatic impairment.

Available forms
Solution—0.1 mg/mL

Dosages
Adults weighing 60 kg or more
1 vial (1 mg) infused IV over 10 min; may be repeated after 10 min if arrhythmia is not terminated.

Adults weighing less than 60 kg
0.1 mL/kg (0.01 mg/kg) infused IV over 10 min; may be repeated after 10 min if arrhythmia is not terminated.
Pediatric patients
Not recommended.

Pharmacokinetics

Route	Onset	Peak
IV	Immediate	10 min

Metabolism: Hepatic; $T_{1/2}$: 6 hr
Distribution: Crosses placenta, may enter breast milk
Excretion: Feces, urine

▼ IV FACTS

Preparation: May be diluted in 50 mL of diluent, 0.9% sodium chloride, or 5% dextrose injection; one 10-mL vial added to 50 mL of diluent yields a concentration of 0.017 mg/mL; may also be infused undiluted; diluted solution is stable for 24 hr at room temperature or for 48 hr refrigerated.
Infusion: Infuse slowly over 10 min.
Compatibilities: Compatible with 5% dextrose injection, 0.9% sodium chloride injection.
Incompatibilities: Do not mix in solution with any other drugs.

Adverse effects
- **CNS:** Headache, light-headedness, dizziness, tingling in arms, numbness
- **CV: Ventricular arrhythmias,** hypotension, hypertension, tachycardia
- **GI:** *Nausea*

Interactions
✳ **Drug drug** • Increased risk of serious to life-threatening arrhythmias with disopyramide, quinidine, procainamide, amiodarone, sotalol; do not give together • Increased risk of proarrhythmias with phenothiazines, TCAs, antihistamines • Use cautiously with digoxin because ibutilide may mask digoxin cardiotoxicity

■ Nursing considerations
Assessment
- **History:** Hypersensitivity to ibutilide; second- or third-degree AV heart block, time of onset of atrial arrhythmia; prolonged QTc

---

intervals; pregnancy, lactation; ventricular arrhythmias

- **Physical:** Orientation; BP, P, auscultation, ECG; R, adventitious sounds

Interventions

- Determine time of onset of arrhythmia and potential benefit before beginning therapy. Conversion is more likely in patients with arrhythmias of short (fewer than 90 days') duration.

⊗ *Warning* Ensure that patient is adequately anticoagulated, generally for at least 2 wk, if atrial fibrillation lasts more than 2–3 days.

- Monitor ECG continually during and for at least 4 hr after administration. Be alert for possible arrhythmias, including PVCs, sinus tachycardia, sinus bradycardia, and varying degrees of block at time of conversion.

⊗ **Black box warning** Keep emergency equipment readily available during and for at least 4 hr after administration; can cause potentially life-threatening arrhythmias. Use caution when selecting patients for this drug treatment.

- Provide appointments for continued follow-up care, including ECG monitoring; tendency to revert to atrial arrhythmia after conversion increases with length of time patient was in abnormal rhythm.

Teaching points

- This drug can only be given by intravenous infusion. You will need electrocardiographic monitoring during and for 4 hours after administration.
- Arrange for follow-up medical evaluation, including electrocardiography, which is important to monitor the effect of the drug on your heart.
- You may experience these side effects: Rapid or irregular heartbeat (usually passes shortly), headache.
- Report chest pain, difficulty breathing, numbness, or tingling.

▷**icatibant**

See Appendix R, *Less commonly used drugs*.

▷**icosapent**

See Appendix R, *Less commonly used drugs*.

DANGEROUS DRUG

▷**idarubicin hydrochloride**
(eye da roo' bi sin)

Idamycin PFS

PREGNANCY CATEGORY D

Drug classes

Antibiotic (anthracycline)
Antineoplastic

Therapeutic actions

Cytotoxic: Binds to DNA and inhibits DNA synthesis in susceptible cells.

Indications

- In combination with other approved antileukemic drugs for the treatment of AML in adults
- Orphan drug uses: Acute nonlymphocytic leukemia and ALL in pediatric patients
- Unlabeled uses: Breast cancer, autologous hematopoietic stem-cell transplantation, chronic myelogenous leukemia

Contraindications and cautions

- Contraindicated with allergy to idarubicin, other anthracycline antibiotics; myelosuppression; cardiac disease; pregnancy; lactation.
- Use cautiously with impaired hepatic or renal function.

Available forms

Injection—1 mg/mL

Dosages

Adults

- *Induction therapy in adults with AML:* 12 mg/m² daily for 3 days by slow IV injection (10–15 min) in combination with cytarabine. Cytarabine may be administered as 100 mg/m² daily given by continuous infusion for 7 days or as a 25-mg/m² IV bolus followed by 200 mg/m² daily for 5 days by continuous infusion. A second course may be administered when toxicity has subsided, if needed, at a 25% dose reduction.

Pediatric patients

Safety and efficacy not established.

Patients with renal or hepatic impairment

Reduce dosage by 25%. Do not administer if bilirubin level exceeds 5 mg/dL.

Pharmacokinetics

Route	Onset	Peak
IV	Rapid	Minutes

Metabolism: Hepatic; $T_{1/2}$: 22 hr
Distribution: Crosses placenta; enters breast milk
Excretion: Bile, urine

▼ IV FACTS

Preparing drug: Use extreme caution when preparing drug. Using goggles and gloves is recommended as drug can cause severe skin reactions. If skin is accidentally exposed to idarubicin, wash with soap and water; use standard irrigation techniques if eyes are contaminated. Store solution in the refrigerator and protect from light.

Infusion: Administer slowly (over 10–15 min) into tubing of a freely running IV infusion of sodium chloride injection or 5% dextrose injection. Attach the tubing to a butterfly needle inserted into a large vein; avoid veins over joints or in extremities with poor perfusion.

Incompatibilities: ⊗ *Warning* Do not mix idarubicin with other drugs, especially heparin (a precipitate form, and the IV solution must not be used) and any alkaline solution.

Adverse effects

- **CV: Cardiac toxicity, heart failure,** phlebosclerosis
- **Dermatologic:** *Complete but reversible alopecia,* hyperpigmentation of nailbeds and dermal creases, facial flushing
- **GI:** *Nausea, vomiting, mucositis,* anorexia, diarrhea, abdominal cramping
- **Hematologic: Myelosuppression,** hyperuricemia due to cell lysis
- **Hypersensitivity:** Fever, chills, urticaria, **anaphylaxis**
- **Local:** Severe local cellulitis, vesication, and tissue necrosis if extravasation occurs
- **Other:** Carcinogenesis, infertility, infection, headache

■ Nursing considerations

Assessment

- **History:** Allergy to idarubicin, other anthracycline antibiotics; myelosuppression; cardiac disease; impaired hepatic or renal function; pregnancy; lactation
- **Physical:** T; skin color, lesions; weight; hair; nailbeds; local injection site; cardiac auscultation, peripheral perfusion, pulses, ECG; R, adventitious sounds; liver evaluation, mucous membranes; CBC, LFTs, renal function tests, uric acid levels

Interventions

⊗ **Black box warning** Do not give IM or subcutaneously because severe local reaction and tissue necrosis occur. Give IV only.

⊗ **Black box warning** Be aware that patient is at risk for myocardial toxicity; monitor accordingly.

⊗ *Warning* Monitor injection site for extravasation; ask about burning or stinging. If extravasation occurs, discontinue infusion immediately, and restart in another vein. For local subcutaneous extravasation, local infiltration with corticosteroid may be ordered; flood area with normal saline, and apply cold compress to area. If ulceration begins, arrange consultation with plastic surgeon.

⊗ **Black box warning** Monitor the patient's response to therapy frequently at beginning of therapy: Serum uric acid level, CBC, cardiac output (listen for S_3), liver function tests, changes in uric acid levels may require a decrease in the dose; consult physician.

- Ensure adequate hydration to prevent hyperuricemia.
- Ensure that patient is not pregnant; explain the importance of avoiding pregnancy.

Teaching points

- Prepare a calendar for days to return for drug therapy. Drug can only be given IV.
- This drug should not be used during pregnancy; using barrier contraceptives is advised.
- Have regular medical follow-up care, including blood tests to monitor the drug's effects.
- You may experience these side effects: Rash, skin lesions, loss of hair, changes in nails (obtain a wig before hair loss occurs; skin care may help); loss of appetite, nausea, mouth sores (perform frequent mouth care,

frequent small meals may help; maintain good nutrition; consult a dietitian; an antiemetic may be ordered); red urine (transient).
• Report difficulty breathing, sudden weight gain, swelling, burning or pain at injection site, unusual bleeding or bruising; chest pain.

▽ **idursulfase**

See Appendix R, *Less commonly used drugs*.

DANGEROUS DRUG

▽ **ifosfamide**

(eye foss' fa mide)

Ifex

PREGNANCY CATEGORY D

Drug classes

Alkylating drug
Antineoplastic
Nitrogen mustard

Therapeutic actions

Cytotoxic: Exact mechanism of action is not known, although metabolite of ifosfamide alkylates DNA and interferes with the replication of susceptible cells; immunosuppressive: Lymphocytes are especially sensitive to drug effects.

Indications

• In combination with other approved neoplastic drugs for third-line chemotherapy of germ cell testicular cancer; prophylactically with mesna to prevent hemorrhagic cystitis
• Orphan drug uses: Third-line chemotherapy in the treatment of bone sarcomas, soft-tissue sarcomas
• Unlabeled uses: Possible effectiveness in the treatment of lung, breast, ovarian, pancreatic, and gastric cancers; sarcomas; acute leukemias; malignant lymphomas; bladder and cervical cancer

Contraindications and cautions

• Contraindicated with allergy to ifosfamide, hematopoietic depression, pregnancy, lactation.
• Use cautiously with impaired hepatic or renal function.

Available forms

Powder for injection—1, 3 g

Dosages

Adults

Administer IV at a dose of 1.2 g/m²/day over at least 30 min for 5 consecutive days. Treatment is repeated every 3 wk or after recovery from hematologic toxicity. For prevention of bladder toxicity, give more than 2 L of fluid per day IV or PO. Also use mesna IV to prevent hemorrhagic cystitis.

Pediatric patients

Safety and efficacy not established.

Patients with renal impairment

Data not available on appropriate dosage. Reduced dosage is advisable; use caution.

Pharmacokinetics

Route	Onset
IV	Rapid

Metabolism: Hepatic; $T_{1/2}$: 15 hr
Distribution: Crosses placenta; enters breast milk
Excretion: Urine

▼ IV FACTS

Preparation: Add sterile water for injection or bacteriostatic water for injection to the vial, and shake gently. Use 20 mL diluent with 1-g vial, giving a final concentration of 50 mg/mL, or use 60-mL diluent with 3-g vial, giving a final concentration of 50 mg/mL. Solutions may be further diluted to achieve concentrations of 0.6–20 mg/mL in 5% dextrose injection, 0.9% sodium chloride injection, lactated Ringer injection, and sterile water for injection. Solution is stable for at least 1 wk at room temperature or 6 wk if refrigerated. Dilutions not prepared with bacteriostatic water for injection should be refrigerated and used within 6 hr.
Infusion: Administer as a slow IV infusion lasting a minimum of 30 min.

Adverse effects

• **CNS:** *Somnolence, confusion, hallucinations,* coma, depressive psychosis, dizziness, seizures
• **Dermatologic:** *Alopecia,* darkening of skin and fingernails
• **GI:** *Anorexia, nausea, vomiting,* diarrhea, stomatitis

- **GU:** *Hemorrhagic cystitis,* bladder fibrosis, *hematuria* to **potentially fatal hemorrhagic cystitis,** increased urine uric acid levels, gonadal suppression
- **Hematologic:** *Leukopenia,* thrombocytopenia, anemia (rare), increased serum uric acid levels
- **Other:** Immunosuppression, secondary neoplasia, hepatic impairment, infection

Interactions
✳ **Drug-food** • Decreased metabolism and risk of toxic effects if taken with grapefruit juice; avoid this combination

■ Nursing considerations
Assessment
- **History:** Allergy to ifosfamide, hematopoietic depression, impaired hepatic or renal function, pregnancy, lactation
- **Physical:** Reflexes, affect; skin lesions, hair; urinary output, renal function; LFTs, renal function tests, CBC, Hct

Interventions
⊗ **Black box warning** Arrange for blood tests to evaluate hematopoietic function before beginning therapy and weekly during therapy; serious hemorrhagic toxicities have occurred.

⊗ **Black box warning** Arrange for extensive hydration consisting of at least 2 L of oral or IV fluid per day to prevent bladder toxicity.

⊗ **Black box warning** Arrange to administer a protector, such as mesna, to prevent hemorrhagic cystitis.

- Counsel male patients not to father a child during or immediately after therapy; infant cardiac and limb abnormalities have occurred. Counsel female patients not to become pregnant while using this drug; severe birth defects have occurred.

Teaching points
- This drug can only be given IV.
- Have frequent blood tests to monitor your response to this drug. All appointments for follow-up care should be kept.
- Avoid grapefruit juice while using this drug.
- Men or women should use birth control while using drug and for a time afterward; this drug can cause severe birth defects.
- You may experience these side effects: Nausea, vomiting, loss of appetite (take drug with food, eat frequent small meals); maintain your fluid intake and nutrition (drink at least 10–12 glasses of fluid each day); darkening of the skin and fingernails, loss of hair (obtain a wig or arrange for some other head covering before hair loss occurs; keep head covered in extreme temperatures).
- Report unusual bleeding or bruising, fever, chills, sore throat, cough, shortness of breath, blood in the urine, painful urination, unusual lumps or masses, flank, stomach or joint pain, sores in mouth or on lips, yellow discoloration of skin or eyes.

▽ **iloperidone**
*(il oh **pair'** ih dohn)*

Fanapt

PREGNANCY CATEGORY C

Drug classes
Atypical antipsychotic
Benzisoxazole derivative

Therapeutic actions
Mechanism of action not fully understood; blocks dopamine and serotonin receptors in the brain, depresses the reticular activating system; suppresses many of the negative aspects of schizophrenia, including blunted affect, social withdrawal, lack of motivation, anger.

Indications
- Acute treatment of schizophrenia in adults. Consider first using drugs that do not prolong QT interval. Consider need to slowly titrate drug, prolonging time until therapeutic effect is seen; faster-acting drugs may be more appropriate.

Contraindications and cautions
- Contraindicated with hypersensitivity to components of drug, pregnancy, lactation.
- Use cautiously with prolonged QT interval, history of seizures, diabetes, suicidal ideation.

Available forms
Tablets—1, 2, 4, 6, 8 10, 12 mg

Adverse effects in *italics* are most common; those in **bold** are life-threatening. ⬛ Do not crush.

Dosages

Adults

Target dose: 12–24 mg/day PO. Titrate based on orthostatic hypotension tolerance—initially, 1 mg PO bid; then 2, 4, 6, 8, 10, and 12 mg PO bid on days 2, 3, 4, 5, 6, and 7, respectively.

Pediatric patients

Safety and efficacy not established.

Patients with hepatic impairment

Not recommended.

Pharmacokinetics

Route	Onset	Peak
Oral	Rapid	2–4 hr

Metabolism: Hepatic; $T_{1/2}$: 18–23 hr
Distribution: May cross placenta; may enter breast milk
Excretion: Urine, feces

Adverse effects

- **CNS:** *Dizziness, somnolence,* extrapyramidal disorders, tremor, lethargy, blurred vision, altered thinking
- **CV:** Orthostatic hypotension, hypotension, tachycardia, **prolonged QT interval**
- **GI:** *Nausea,* diarrhea, dry mouth, abdominal discomfort
- **GU:** Priapism, ejaculation failure
- **Respiratory:** URI, nasal pharyngitis
- **Other:** Fatigue, lethargy, bone marrow suppression, **neuroleptic malignant syndrome,** hyperglycemia, weight gain, gynecomastia, galactorrhea

Interactions

✳ **Drug-drug** ● Increased risk of serious cardiac arrhythmias if taken with other drugs that prolong QT interval; avoid this combination. If combination must be used, monitor patient carefully ● Possible increased serum levels and toxicity if combined with ketoconazole, fluoxetine, itraconazole, paroxetine; iloperidone dosage should be halved if these drug combinations are used ● Risk of increased effectiveness of antihypertensives if used with iloperidone; monitor patient closely and adjust antihypertensive dosage as needed ● Risk of increased CNS effects if combined with centrally acting drugs or alcohol; use caution if this combination is used

✳ **Drug-alternative therapy** ● Possible increased toxicity if combined with St. John's Wort

■ Nursing considerations

Assessment

- **History:** Hypersensitivity to components of drug; prolonged QT interval, history of seizures, diabetes, suicidal ideation, pregnancy, lactation
- **Physical:** Orientation, affect, reflexes; BP, P; abdominal exam; liver evaluation; ECG, LFTs, CBC

Interventions

⊗ **Black box warning** There is an increased risk of death if used in elderly patients with dementia-related psychosis. Do not use for these patients; not approved for this use.

- Obtain baseline ECG to rule out prolonged QT interval; monitor patient periodically throughout therapy.
- Titrate drug over first week to decrease effect of orthostatic hypotension.
- Monitor patient regularly for signs and symptoms of increased blood glucose level.
- Use drug in pregnancy only if benefits outweigh risks; if used in third trimester, alert patient that baby may exhibit abnormal movements.
- Advise patient who is breast-feeding to select another method of feeding the baby.
- Monitor patient for signs and symptoms of neuroleptic malignant syndrome (high temperature, muscle rigidity, altered mental status, high or low blood pressure, diaphoresis, tachycardia); discontinue drug and support patient if these occur. Carefully consider reintroduction of drug because recurrence is likely.
- Provide safety measures as needed if patient develops extrapyramidal effects or orthostatic hypotension.
- Because of the risk of suicidal ideation with treatment, limit amount of drug dispensed to the smallest effective amount to decrease chances of overdose.
- Continue other measures used to deal with schizophrenia.

Teaching points

- Take this drug once a day, exactly as prescribed. Carefully follow directions for increasing the dosage over the first week.
- If you miss a dose, take the next dose as soon as you remember. Do not take more than the prescribed amount each day.

- Avoid alcohol while taking this drug. Tell your health care provider about other drugs, over-the-counter drugs, or herbal therapies that you are using because serious drug interactions are possible.
- If you are diabetic, monitor your blood glucose level very carefully and adjust treatment as ordered.
- It is not known how this drug affects a fetus. If you become pregnant while taking this drug, consult your health care provider.
- It is not known how this drug affects a breast-feeding baby. Because of the potential for serious adverse effects in an infant, you should use another method of feeding the baby while you are taking this drug.
- This drug may cause your blood pressure to fall when you stand up; this is called *orthostatic hypotension*. Use care when standing or changing positions. Orthostatic hypotension is most likely to occur when starting the drug and when changing dosage.
- You may experience these side effects: Dizziness, changes in motor performance and impaired thinking (do not drive a car or engage in activities that require alertness if these effects occur); nausea, dry mouth (small, frequent meals may help; sucking sugarless candies may also be helpful).
- Report fever accompanied by sweating, changes in mental status, muscle rigidity; heart palpitations, feeling faint, loss of consciousness, thoughts of suicide.

▷**iloprost**

See Appendix R, *Less commonly used drugs*.

DANGEROUS DRUG

▷**imatinib mesylate**
(eh mat' eh nib mess' ah late)

Gleevec ⊙⊞⊙

PREGNANCY CATEGORY D

Drug classes
Antineoplastic
Protein tyrosine kinase inhibitor

Therapeutic actions
A protein tyrosine kinase inhibitor that selectively inhibits the Bcr-Abl tyrosine kinase cre-

ated by the Philadelphia chromosome abnormality in CML; this inhibits proliferation and induces apoptosis in the Bcr-Abl positive cell lines as well as fresh leukemic cells, leading to an inhibition of tumor growth in CML patients in blast crisis.

Indications
- Treatment of patients with Philadelphia-chromosome–positive CML in blast crisis, accelerated phase or in chronic phase after failure with interferon-alfa therapy
- Treatment of patients with Kit (CD117) positive unresectable or metastatic malignant GI stromal tumors (GISTs)
- Treatment of adults with newly diagnosed or relapsed or refractory Philadelphia-chromosome–positive ALL
- Treatment of aggressive systemic mastocytosis (ASM)
- Treatment of adults with unresectable, recurrent, or metastatic dermatofibrosarcoma protuberans (DFSP)
- Treatment of adults with myelodysplastic/myeloproliferative diseases (MDS/MPD)
- Treatment of hypereosinophilic syndrome and chronic eosinophilic leukemia (HES/CEL) in adults
- Treatment of pediatric patients with Philadelphia chromosome positive CML in chronic phase, whose disease recurred after stem cell transplant or who are resistant to interferon alfa therapy
- Unlabeled use: Rectal administration of twice-daily doses

Contraindications and cautions
- Contraindicated with allergy to imatinib or any of its components, pregnancy, lactation.
- Use cautiously with hepatic or renal impairment; bone marrow suppression; cardiac disease, risk factors for heart failure.

Available forms
Tablets ⊙⊞⊙ —100, 400 mg

Dosages
Dosage should be adjusted based on bone marrow function and liver toxicity.

When used with CYP3A4 inducers, increase imatinib dosage by 50% and carefully monitor patient. For dosages of 800 mg or more, use 400 mg tablets to avoid increase in iron.

Adults

- *Chronic phase CML:* 400 mg/day PO as a once-a-day dose; increase to 600 mg/day may be considered if response is not satisfactory and patient can tolerate the drug.
- *Accelerated phase or blast crisis CML:* 600 mg/day PO as a single dose; increase to 400 mg PO bid may be considered if response is not satisfactory and patient can tolerate the drug.
- *ALL:* 600 mg/day PO.
- *ASM:* 400 mg/day PO.
- *ASM with eosinophilia:* 100 mg/day PO.
- *DFSP:* 800 mg/day PO.
- *HES/CEL:* 400 mg/day PO.
- *MDS/MPD:* 400 mg/day PO.
- *GIST:* 400 mg/day PO or 400 mg PO bid.

Pediatric patients older than 2 yr

Newly diagnosed CML: 340 mg/m^2 PO; maximum dose 600 mg/day.

Chronic phase CML: 260 mg/m^2/day PO given as one dose, or divided and given morning and evening.

Patients with hepatic impairment

Severe impairment, decrease dosage by 25%.

Patients with renal impairment

For creatinine clearance of 20–39 mL/min, reduce starting dose by 50%; increase as tolerated. Doses of 400 mg not recommended. For creatinine clearance of 40–59 mL/min, doses of 600 mg not recommended.

Pharmacokinetics

Route	Onset	Peak
Oral	Slow	2–4 hr

Metabolism: Hepatic; T$_{1/2}$: 14–17 hr
Distribution: Crosses placenta; may enter breast milk; 95% protein-bound
Excretion: Feces, urine

Adverse effects

- **CNS:** Malaise, insomnia, *headache,* dizziness
- **CV: Severe heart failure, left ventricular dysfunction**
- **GI:** Abdominal pain, *vomiting, nausea, diarrhea,* dyspepsia, anorexia, constipation, hepatotoxicity, GI irritation
- **Hematologic:** *Neutropenia, thrombocytopenia*
- **Respiratory:** Pulmonary edema, pneumonia, URI, cough

- **Other:** Myalgia, fever, *rash, sudden weight gain, fluid retention,* night sweats, joint pain, muscle cramps, fatigue, hemorrhage, pruritus, rigors, hemorrhage

Interactions

✳ **Drug-drug** ⊗ *Warning* Increased serum levels of simvastatin, cyclosporine, or pimozide when combined with imatinib; avoid these combinations if possible.
- Risk of increased imatinib effects with ketoconazole, itraconazole, azithromycin, or clarithromycin; use caution if this combination is used • Risk of decreased imatinib effects if combined with dexamethasone, phenytoin, carbamazepine, rifampin, or phenobarbital; use caution if this combination is required
- Increased risk of bleeding with warfarin; if anticoagulation is needed, use of a heparin is recommended • Increased clearance of levothyroxine; monitor thyroid function if this combination is used

✳ **Drug-food** • Increased risk of toxic effects with grapefruit juice; avoid this combination

✳ **Drug-alternative therapy** • Decreased effectiveness of imatinib if taken with St. John's Wort; avoid this combination

■ Nursing considerations

Assessment

- **History:** Allergy to imatinib or any of its components, pregnancy, lactation, hepatic or renal impairment
- **Physical:** T, body weight, P, BP, R, adventitious sounds, CBC with differential, LFTs, Hgb, Hct, cardiac function

Interventions

- Administer once a day with a meal and a large glass of water. Pediatric patients may have the dose divided and given half in the morning and half in the evening.
- If patient cannot swallow tablets, they may be dispersed in a glass of water or apple juice and given immediately. Use 50 mL for 10-mg tablet and 200 mL for 400-mg tablet. Do not cut or crush tablet.
- Provide frequent small meals if GI upset occurs.
- Arrange for nutritional consult if nausea and vomiting are persistent.
- Provide analgesics if headache or muscle pain is a problem.

- Advise women of child-bearing age to use a barrier form of contraception while taking this drug.
- Closely monitor children using the drug; growth retardation has been reported.
- Increase imatinib dose by at least 50% when administering with a potent CYP3A4 inducer such as rifampin or phenytoin.

⊗ **Warning** Monitor CBC before and periodically during therapy; arrange for dosage adjustment as indicated if bone marrow suppression occurs.

⊗ **Warning** Monitor patient for tumor lysis syndrome and manage appropriately.

⊗ **Warning** Monitor patient for fluid retention and edema; severe cases may require dosage reduction or discontinuation of drug.

- Arrange for appropriate consultation to help patient cope with the high cost of drug.

Teaching points

- This drug should be taken once a day as a single dose, with a meal and a large glass of water. Do not crush tablet. If tablet is crushed, avoid contact with skin and mucous membranes. If contact occurs, flush area immediately with water. Children may split the dose in two, taking half in the morning and half in the evening.
- This drug has been linked to serious fetal abnormalities; women of childbearing age who are taking this drug should use a barrier contraceptive.
- Avoid infection while taking this drug; avoid crowded areas or people with known infections.
- Do not use any alternative therapy, including St. John's Wort, while you are in this treatment program; it may decrease the effectiveness of the drug.
- Do not drink grapefruit juice while taking this drug.
- Children taking this drug should have growth monitored closely.
- You will need regular blood tests to monitor the effects of this drug on your blood.
- You may experience these side effects: Nausea, vomiting (eat frequent small meals, suck on sugarless candies, or chew gum); headache, muscle cramps, pain (use of an analgesic may help; consult your health care provider); fluid retention and sudden weight gain (monitor daily weights and report sudden increases or difficulty breathing).

- Report fever, chills, unusual bleeding or bruising, difficulty breathing, yellowing of your skin or eyes, any signs of infection, sudden weight gain, severe swelling.

▽**imipramine**
(im **ip'** ra meen)

imipramine hydrochloride
Tofranil

imipramine pamoate
Tofranil-PM

PREGNANCY CATEGORY C

Drug class
TCA (tertiary amine)

Therapeutic actions
Mechanism of action unknown; the TCAs are structurally related to the phenothiazine antipsychotic drugs (eg, chlorpromazine), but unlike the phenothiazines, TCAs inhibit the presynaptic reuptake of the neurotransmitters norepinephrine and serotonin; anticholinergic at CNS and peripheral receptors; sedative; the relation of these effects to clinical efficacy is unknown.

Indications
- Relief of symptoms of depression (endogenous depression most responsive); sedative effects of tertiary amine TCAs may be helpful in patients whose depression is associated with anxiety and sleep disturbance
- Enuresis in children 6 yr and older
- Unlabeled uses: Control of chronic pain (eg, intractable pain of cancer, peripheral neuropathies, post-herpetic neuralgia, tic douloureux, central pain syndromes), migraine prophylaxis, ADHD, bulimia, cocaine dependence

Contraindications and cautions
- Contraindicated with hypersensitivity to any tricyclic drug or to tartrazine (in preparations marketed as *Tofranil, Tofranil-PM*; patients with aspirin allergy are commonly allergic to tartrazine); concomitant therapy with an MAOI; EST with coadministration of TCAs; recent MI; myelography within

previous 24 hr or scheduled within 48 hr; pregnancy.
- Use cautiously with pre-existing CV disorders; seizure disorders (TCAs lower the seizure threshold); hyperthyroidism; angle-closure glaucoma, increased IOP, urinary retention, ureteral or urethral spasm; impaired hepatic, renal function; psychiatric patients (schizophrenic or paranoid patients may exhibit a worsening of psychosis with TCA therapy; manic-depressive patients may shift to hypomanic or manic phase); elective surgery; lactation; history of suicide attempts; use with alcohol.

Available forms
Tablets (imipramine hydrochloride, imipramine pamoate)—10, 25, 50 mg; capsules (imipramine pamoate)—75, 100, 125, 150 mg

Dosages
Adults
- *Depression:* Hospitalized patients—Initially, 100–150 mg/day PO in divided doses. Gradually increase to 200 mg/day as required. If no response after 2 wk, increase to 250–300 mg/day. Total daily dosage may be given at bedtime. Outpatients—Initially, 75 mg/day PO, increasing to 150 mg/day. Dosages more than 200 mg/day not recommended. Total daily dosage may be given at bedtime. Maintenance dose is 50–150 mg/day.

Adolescent and geriatric patients
- *Depression:* 30–40 mg/day PO; doses greater than 100 mg/day generally are not needed.

Pediatric patients 6 yr and older
Imipramine pamoate capsules should not be used in children because of potential for overdose. Capsules can be used in adults if daily dosage is 75 mg or higher.
- *Childhood enuresis:* Initially, 25 mg/day 1 hr before bedtime. If response is not satisfactory after 1 wk, increase to 50 mg nightly in children younger than 12 yr, 75 mg nightly in children older than 12 yr. Doses or more than 75 mg/day do not have greater efficacy but are more likely to increase side effects. Do not exceed 2.5 mg/kg per day. Early-night bedwetters may be more effectively treated with earlier and divided dosage (25 mg midafternoon, repeated at bedtime). Institute drug-free period after successful therapy, gradually tapering dosage.

Pharmacokinetics

Route	Onset	Peak
Oral	Varies	2–4 hr

Metabolism: Hepatic; $T_{1/2}$: 8–16 hr
Distribution: Crosses placenta; enters breast milk
Excretion: Urine

Adverse effects
Adult use
- **CNS:** *Sedation and anticholinergic effects,* dry mouth, blurred vision, disturbance of accommodation for near vision, mydriasis, increased IOP; *confusion, disturbed concentration,* hallucinations, disorientation, decreased memory, feelings of unreality, delusions, anxiety, nervousness, restlessness, agitation, panic, insomnia, nightmares, hypomania, mania, exacerbation of psychosis, drowsiness, weakness, fatigue, headache, numbness, tingling, paresthesias of extremities, incoordination, motor hyperactivity, akathisia, ataxia, tremors, peripheral neuropathy, extrapyramidal symptoms, *seizures,* dysarthria, tinnitus, altered EEG, suicidal ideation
- **CV:** *Orthostatic hypotension,* hypertension, syncope, tachycardia, palpitations, **MI,** arrhythmias, heart block, precipitation of heart failure, **stroke**
- **Endocrine:** Elevated or depressed blood sugar, elevated prolactin levels, inappropriate ADH secretion
- **GI:** *Dry mouth, constipation,* paralytic ileus, *nausea,* vomiting, anorexia, epigastric distress, diarrhea, flatulence, dysphagia, peculiar taste, increased salivation, stomatitis, glossitis, parotid swelling, abdominal cramps, black tongue, hepatitis
- **GU:** Urinary retention, delayed micturition, dilation of the urinary tract, gynecomastia, testicular swelling in men; breast enlargement, menstrual irregularity and galactorrhea in women; increased or decreased libido; impotence
- **Hematologic: Bone marrow depression,** including agranulocytosis; eosinophilia, purpura, thrombocytopenia, leukopenia
- **Hypersensitivity:** Rash, pruritus, vasculitis, petechiae, photosensitization, edema (generalized, facial, tongue), drug fever

- **Withdrawal:** Abrupt discontinuation of prolonged therapy—nausea, headache, vertigo, nightmares, malaise
- **Other:** Nasal congestion, excessive appetite, weight gain or loss; sweating (paradoxic effect in a drug with prominent anticholinergic effects), alopecia, lacrimation, hyperthermia, flushing, chills

Pediatric use for enuresis

- **CNS:** *Nervousness, sleep disorders, tiredness,* seizures, anxiety, emotional instability, syncope, collapse
- **CV:** ECG changes of unknown significance when given in doses of 5 mg/kg/day
- **GI:** Constipation, *mild GI disturbances*
- **Other:** Adverse reactions reported with adult use

Interactions

✳ **Drug-drug** • Increased TCA levels and pharmacologic (especially anticholinergic) effects with cimetidine, fluoxetine, or ranitidine • Increased serum levels and risk of bleeding with oral anticoagulants • Altered response, including arrhythmias and hypertension, with sympathomimetics • Risk of severe hypertension with clonidine • Hyperpyretic crises, severe seizures, hypertensive episodes, and deaths when MAOIs are given with TCAs • Decreased hypotensive activity of guanethidine with imipramine

Note: MAOIs and TCAs have been used successfully in some patients resistant to therapy with single drugs; however, the combination can cause serious and potentially fatal adverse effects.

✳ **Drug-alternative therapy** • Plasma imipramine levels may be reduced with St. John's Wort

■ Nursing considerations
Assessment

- **History:** Hypersensitivity to any tricyclic drug or to tartrazine; concomitant therapy with an MAOI; EST with coadministration of TCAs; recent MI; myelography within previous 24 hr or scheduled within 48 hr; preexisting CV disorders; seizure disorders; hyperthyroidism; angle-closure glaucoma, increased IOP, urinary retention, ureteral or urethral spasm; impaired hepatic, renal function; psychiatric patients; elective surgery; pregnancy; lactation

- **Physical:** Weight; T; skin color, lesions; orientation, affect, reflexes, vision and hearing; P, BP, auscultation, orthostatic BP, perfusion; bowel sounds, normal output, liver evaluation; urine flow, normal output; usual sexual function, frequency of menses, breast and scrotal examination; LFTs, urinalysis, CBC, ECG

Interventions

- Obtain baseline ECG to monitor cardiac arrhythmias.

⊗ **Black box warning** Limit drug access for depressed and potentially suicidal patients; increased risk of suicidality especially in children, adolescents, and young adults; monitor patients accordingly.

- Give IM only when oral therapy is impossible. Do not give IV.
- Give major portion of dose at bedtime if drowsiness, severe anticholinergic effects occur (note that elderly may not tolerate single-daily-dose therapy).

⊗ **Warning** Reduce dosage if minor side effects develop; discontinue if serious side effects occur.

- Arrange for CBC if fever, sore throat, or other sign of infection develops during therapy.

Teaching points

- Take drug exactly as prescribed. Do not stop taking drug abruptly or without consulting your health care provider; clinical effects may take 4–6 weeks to be seen.
- Do not use St. John's Wort while taking this drug.
- Avoid prolonged exposure to sunlight or sunlamps; use a sunscreen or wear protective garments.
- Use of barrier contraceptives is recommended. If breast-feeding, choose another method to feed the baby.
- You may experience these side effects: Headache, dizziness, drowsiness, weakness, blurred vision (reversible; safety measures may need to be taken if severe; avoid driving or performing tasks that require alertness); nausea, vomiting, constipation, loss of appetite (eat frequent small meals; frequent mouth care may help); dry mouth (sucking sugarless candies may help); disorientation, difficulty concentrating, emotional changes; changes in sexual function, impotence, changes in libido.

- Report dry mouth, difficulty in urination, excessive sedation, fever, chills, sore throat, palpitations, suicidal thoughts.

▽**indacaterol**

*(in da **ka'** ter ol)*

Arcapta Neohaler

PREGNANCY CATEGORY C

Drug classes

Beta₂ agonist, long-acting
Bronchodilator

Therapeutic actions

Long-acting agonist that binds to beta₂ receptors in the lungs, causing bronchodilation; may also inhibit the release of inflammatory mediators in the lungs, blocking swelling and inflammation.

Indications

- Long-term maintenance for treatment of airflow obstruction in patients with COPD, including chronic bronchitis and emphysema

Contraindications and cautions

- Contraindicated with history of serious hypersensitivity reactions to indacaterol, asthma, deteriorating COPD.
- Use cautiously with convulsive disorders, thyrotoxicosis, CV disorders, known sensitivity to sympathomimetics, pregnancy, lactation.

Available forms

Inhalation powder—75 mcg

Dosages

Adults

75 mcg/day by oral inhalation using the *Neohaler* only.

Pediatric patients

Not recommended.

Pharmacokinetics

Route	Onset	Peak
Inhalation	Rapid	15 min

Metabolism: Hepatic; T₁/₂: 45–56 hr
Distribution: May cross placenta; may enter breast milk
Excretion: Feces

Adverse effects

- **CNS: Seizures,** headache, nervousness, tremor
- **CV: Arrhythmias, hypertension,** edema
- **GI:** Nausea
- **Respiratory: Asthma-related deaths, paradoxical bronchospasm,** cough, oropharyngeal pain, nasopharyngitis, URI
- **Other:** Hyperglycemia, hypokalemia, musculoskeletal pain

Interactions

✳ **Drug-drug** • Increased risk of hypokalemia with xanthines, corticosteroids, diuretics; monitor patient carefully • Increased risk of serious arrhythmias with MAOIs, TCAs, drugs that prolong QT interval; use extreme caution and monitor patient accordingly • Lack of effectiveness if used with beta blocker • Increased risk of toxicity if combined with other beta agonists

■ Nursing considerations

Assessment

- **History:** Hypersensitivity to components of drug, convulsive disorders, thyrotoxicosis, CV disorders, known sensitivity to sympathomimetics, asthma; pregnancy; lactation
- **Physical:** BP, P; R and adventitious sounds; ECG; serum potassium, glucose levels

Interventions

⊗ *Black box warning* Long-acting beta agonists increase the risk of asthma-related deaths. Not for use in asthma; not approved for use in children.

- Do not initiate use with deteriorating COPD.
- Do not use for acute symptoms; do not exceed recommended dose.
- Teach patient appropriate care and use of *Neohaler;* capsule should not be swallowed.
- Continue other treatments for COPD as needed.
- Taper drug if discontinuing; condition can worsen if drug is stopped suddenly.

Teaching points

- This drug is only for long-term use in COPD to help dilate your bronchi. It is not for use in asthma or for acute breathing issues.
- Store capsules in the blister packs; remove only one capsule at a time and use immediately. Discard capsules exposed to air and not used.

I

- Do not swallow the capsule. Learn the proper care and use of the *Neohaler*. Do not use more than the recommended dose.
- Do not stop this drug suddenly. Consult your health care provider; sudden stopping can worsen your condition.
- It is not known if this drug could harm a fetus if taken during pregnancy. If you are pregnant or thinking about becoming pregnant, discuss this with your health care provider.
- This drug appears in breast milk; if you are breast-feeding, discuss the risk with your health care provider.
- Tell your health care provider about all drugs you are taking; dosage adjustments may be needed. Do not use with other long-acting beta agonists.
- You may experience these side effects: Nervousness, rapid heartbeat, tremor (these are effects of the drug and should pass; if these effects become uncomfortable, contact your health care provider).
- Report difficulty breathing, increased use of a rescue inhaler, worsening of condition.

▽indapamide
(in dap' a mide)

Apo-Indapamide (CAN),
Gen-Indapamide (CAN),
PMS-Indapamide (CAN)

PREGNANCY CATEGORY B

Drug class
Thiazide-like diuretic (indoline)

Therapeutic actions
Inhibits reabsorption of sodium and chloride in distal renal tubule, increasing excretion of sodium, chloride, and water by the kidneys; may decrease peripheral resistance.

Indications
- Edema associated with heart failure
- Hypertension, as sole therapy or in combination with other antihypertensives
- Unlabeled use: Diabetes insipidus, especially nephrogenic diabetes insipidus

Contraindications and cautions
- Contraindicated with allergy to thiazides, sulfonamides; hepatic coma or precoma, anuria.

- Use cautiously with fluid or electrolyte imbalance; renal disease (risk of azotemia); liver disease (may precipitate hepatic coma); gout (risk of precipitation of attack); SLE; glucose tolerance abnormalities, diabetes mellitus; hyperparathyroidism; bipolar disorder (aggravated by hypercalcemia); pregnancy; lactation.

Available forms
Tablets—1.25, 2.5 mg

Dosages
Adults
- *Edema:* 2.5 mg/day PO as single dose in the morning. May be increased to 5 mg/day if response is not satisfactory after 1 wk.
- *Hypertension:* 1.25 mg/day PO. May be increased up to 2.5 mg/day if response is not satisfactory after 4 wk. May increase to a maximum of 5 mg/day or consider adding another antihypertensive. If combination antihypertensive therapy is needed, reduce the dosage of other drugs by 50%, then adjust according to patient's response.

Pediatric patients
Safety and efficacy not established.

Pharmacokinetics

Route	Onset	Peak	Duration
Oral	1–2 hr	2 hr	36 hr

Metabolism: Hepatic; $T_{1/2}$: 14 hr
Distribution: Crosses placenta; enters breast milk
Excretion: Urine

Adverse effects
- **CNS:** *Dizziness, vertigo,* paresthesias, weakness, headache, drowsiness, fatigue, anxiety, nervousness
- **CV:** Orthostatic hypotension, venous thrombosis, volume depletion, cardiac arrhythmias, chest pain
- **Dermatologic:** Photosensitivity, rash, purpura, exfoliative dermatitis, hives
- **GI:** *Nausea, anorexia, vomiting, dry mouth,* diarrhea, constipation, jaundice, hepatitis, pancreatitis, dyspepsia
- **GU:** *Polyuria, nocturia,* impotence, decreased libido
- **Hematologic:** Leukopenia, thrombocytopenia, **agranulocytosis, aplastic anemia,** neutropenia

Adverse effects in *italics* are most common; those in **bold** are life-threatening. ⬛ Do not crush.

- **Other:** Hypokalemia, muscle cramps and muscle spasms, fever, gouty attacks, flushing, weight loss, rhinorrhea, infection, pain, back pain

Interactions

✳ **Drug-drug** • Consider risk of interactions seen with all thiazides • Increased thiazide effects if taken with diazoxide • Decreased absorption with cholestyramine, colestipol • Increased risk of cardiac glycoside toxicity if hypokalemia occurs • Increased risk of lithium toxicity • Decreased effectiveness of antidiabetics

✳ **Drug-lab test** • Decreased protein-bound iodine levels without clinical signs of thyroid disturbance

■ Nursing considerations
Assessment

- **History:** Allergy to thiazides, sulfonamides; fluid or electrolyte imbalance; renal or liver disease; gout; SLE; glucose tolerance abnormalities, diabetes mellitus; hyperparathyroidism; manic-depressive disorders; lactation, pregnancy
- **Physical:** Skin color, lesions, edema; orientation, reflexes, muscle strength; pulses, baseline ECG, BP, orthostatic BP, perfusion; R, pattern, adventitious sounds; liver evaluation, bowel sounds, urinary output patterns; CBC, serum electrolytes, blood glucose, LFTs, renal function tests, serum uric acid, urinalysis

Interventions

- Give with food or milk if GI upset occurs.
- Mark calendars or provide other reminders for outpatients on alternate-day or 3–5 days/wk therapy.
- Give early in the day so increased urination will not disturb sleep.
- Measure and record regular weight to monitor fluid changes.

Teaching points

- Record intermittent therapy on a calendar, or use prepared, dated envelopes. Take the drug early in the day so increased urination will not disturb sleep. The drug may be taken with food or meals if GI upset occurs.
- Weigh yourself on a regular basis, at the same time of the day and in the same clothing; record the weight on your calendar.
- You may experience these side effects: Increased volume and frequency of urination;

dizziness, feeling faint on arising, drowsiness (avoid rapid position changes; hazardous activities, like driving a car; and alcohol, which can intensify these problems); sensitivity to sunlight (use sunglasses, wear protective clothing, or use a sunscreen); decrease in sexual function; increased thirst (sucking on sugarless candies, frequent mouth care may help).

- Report weight change of more than 3 pounds in 1 day, swelling in ankles or fingers, unusual bleeding or bruising, dizziness, trembling, numbness, fatigue, muscle weakness or cramps.

▷ indinavir sulfate
(in din' ah ver)

Crixivan

PREGNANCY CATEGORY C

Drug classes
Antiretroviral
Antiviral
Protease inhibitor

Therapeutic actions
Antiviral activity; inhibits HIV protease activity, leading to production of immature, noninfective HIV particles.

Indications
- Treatment of HIV infection in adults; used in combination with other drugs

Contraindications and cautions
- Contraindicated with allergy to component of indinavir.
- Use cautiously with pregnancy, hepatic or renal impairment, lactation.

Available forms
Capsules—100, 200, 400 mg

Dosages
Adults
800 mg PO every 8 hr. With delavirdine, 600 mg PO every 8 hr with delavirdine 400 mg tid; with didanosine, administer more than 1 hr apart on an empty stomach; with itraconazole, 600 mg PO every 8 hr with itraconazole 200 mg bid; with ketoconazole, 600 mg PO every 8 hr; with rifabutin, 1,000 mg PO every 8 hr, reduce rifabutin by 50%.

Pediatric patients
Safety and efficacy not established in children younger than 12 yr.

Patients with hepatic impairment
600 mg PO every 8 hr with mild to moderate hepatic impairment.

Pharmacokinetics

Route	Onset	Peak
Oral	Rapid	0.8 hr

Metabolism: Hepatic; $T_{1/2}$: 3–4 hr
Distribution: Crosses placenta; enters breast milk; 60% bound to human plasma proteins
Excretion: Feces, urine

Adverse effects

- **CNS:** *Headache,* dizziness, insomnia, somnolence
- **CV:** Palpitations
- **Dermatologic:** Acne, dry skin, contact dermatitis, rash, body odor
- **GI:** *Nausea, vomiting, diarrhea,* anorexia, dry mouth, acid regurgitation, *hyperbilirubinemia,* abdominal pain, increased appetite
- **GU:** Dysuria, hematuria, nocturia, pyelonephritis, nephrolithiasis, urolithiasis
- **Respiratory:** Cough, dyspnea, sinusitis
- **Other:** Hypothermia, chills, back pain, flank pain, flulike symptoms, appetite increase, fever, back pain, fatigue, taste perversion

Interactions

✳ **Drug-drug** ⊗ *Warning* Potentially large increase in serum concentration of triazolam, midazolam, pimozide and ergot derivatives with indinavir; potential for serious arrhythmias, seizure, and fatal reactions; do not administer indinavir with any of these drugs.
• Azole antifungals, delavirdine, nelfinavir, ritonavir, interleukins may increase indinavir concentrations and cause toxicity • Decreased effectiveness with didanosine; give these two drugs 1 hr apart on empty stomach to decrease effects of interaction • Significant decrease in serum levels with nevirapine—avoid this combination; if combination is necessary, increase indinavir to 1,000 mg every 8 hr with nevirapine 200 mg bid; carefully monitor effectiveness of indinavir if starting or stopping nevirapine • Decreased indinavir concentrations with atazanavir, efavirenz, carbamazepine,

phenobarbital, phenytoin, rifabutin, rifampin, venlafaxine • Indinavir may cause increased concentrations of fentanyl, rifamycin, benzodiazepines, ritonavir, and sildenafil

✳ **Drug-food** • Absorption is decreased by presence of food and grapefruit juice; give on empty stomach with full glass of water

✳ **Drug-alternative therapy** • Decreased effectiveness if combined with St. John's Wort

■ Nursing considerations

Assessment

- **History:** Allergy to indinavir, hepatic or renal impairment, pregnancy, lactation
- **Physical:** T; orientation, reflexes; BP, P, peripheral perfusion; R, adventitious sounds; bowel sounds; urinary output; skin color, perfusion; LFTs, renal function tests

Interventions

- Capsules should be protected from moisture; store in container provided and keep desiccant in bottle. Give drug every 8 hr around the clock.
- Give on an empty stomach, 1 hr before or 2 hr after meal with a full glass of water. If GI upset is severe, give with a light meal; avoid grapefruit juice and foods high in calories, fat, or protein.
- ⊗ **Warning** Carefully screen drug history to avoid potentially dangerous drug interactions.
- Monitor patient to maintain hydration; if nephrolithiasis occurs, therapy will need to be interrupted or stopped.

Teaching points

- Take this drug on an empty stomach, 1 hour before or 2 hours after a meal, with a full glass of water. If GI upset is severe, take with a light meal; avoid grapefruit juice and foods high in calories, fat, or protein.
- Avoid St. John's Wort while taking this drug.
- Store the capsules in the original container and leave the desiccant in the bottle. These capsules are very sensitive to moisture.
- Take the full course of therapy as prescribed; do not take double doses if one is missed; do not change dosage without consulting your health care provider. Take drug every 8 hours around the clock.
- Drink 1.5 liters or more of water per day to ensure adequate hydration.
- This drug does not cure HIV infection; long-term effects are not yet known; continue to

take precautions as the risk of transmission is not reduced by this drug.
- Do not take any other prescription or over-the-counter drugs without consulting your health care provider; this drug interacts with many other drugs and serious problems can occur.
- You may experience these side effects: Nausea, vomiting, loss of appetite, diarrhea, abdominal pain, headache, dizziness, insomnia.
- Report severe diarrhea, severe nausea, personality changes, changes in color of urine or stool, flank pain, fever or chills.

▷indomethacin
*(in **mdoe eth**' a sin)*

indomethacin
Indocid P.D.A. (CAN), Indocin

indomethacin sodium trihydrate
Apo-Indomethacin (CAN), Indocin I.V.

PREGNANCY CATEGORY B

PREGNANCY CATEGORY D
(THIRD TRIMESTER)

Drug class
NSAID

Therapeutic actions
Anti-inflammatory, analgesic, and antipyretic activities largely related to inhibition of prostaglandin synthesis; exact mechanisms of action are not known. Inhibits both cyclooxygenase (COX) 1 and 2. Indomethacin is mainly COX-1 selective.

Indications
- Oral, topical, suppositories: Relief of signs and symptoms of moderate to severe rheumatoid arthritis and moderate to severe osteoarthritis, moderate to severe ankylosing spondylitis, acute painful shoulder (bursitis, tendinitis), acute gouty arthritis (*not* SR form)
- Parenteral use: Closure of hemodynamically significant patent ductus arteriosus in premature infants weighing 500–1,750 g, if 48 hr of usual medical management is not effective

- Unlabeled uses for oral form: Pharmacologic closure of persistent patent ductus arteriosus in premature infants; juvenile rheumatoid arthritis; prevention of premature labor
- Unlabeled use of topical eyedrops: Cystoid macular edema
- Unlabeled uses: To reduce incidence of patent ductus arteriosus in patients at risk for the condition.

Contraindications and cautions
Oral and rectal
- Contraindicated with allergy to indomethacin, salicylates, or other NSAIDs; history of proctitis or rectal bleeding (suppositories); pregnancy in the third trimester, lactation, labor; pain associated with coronary artery bypass graft surgery.
- Use cautiously with CV dysfunction, hypertension, peptic ulceration, GI bleeding, impaired renal or hepatic function, pregnancy.
IV
- Contraindicated with proven or suspected infection; bleeding, thrombocytopenia, coagulation defects; necrotizing enterocolitis; neonates with significant renal impairment, congenital heart disease when patency of ductus arteriosus is needed for blood flow.
- Use cautiously with renal impairment.

Available forms
Capsules—25, 50 mg; SR capsules—75 mg; oral suspension—25 mg/5 mL; suppositories—50 mg; powder for injection—1 mg

Dosages
Adults
- *Osteoarthritis or rheumatoid arthritis, ankylosing spondylitis:* 25 mg PO bid or tid. If tolerated, increase dose by 25- or 50-mg increments if needed up to total daily dose of 150–200 mg/day PO. SR dose may be used.
- *Acute painful shoulder:* 75–150 mg/day PO, in three or four divided doses. Discontinue drug after inflammation is controlled, usually 7–14 days. SR dose may be used.
- *Acute gouty arthritis:* 50 mg PO, tid until pain is tolerable, then rapidly decrease dose until no longer needed, usually within 3–5 days. Do not use SR dose. In those who have persistent night pain or morning stiffness, a total daily dose of 100 mg may be given at bedtime. Do not exceed 200 mg.

Pediatric patients
Safety and efficacy not established. When special circumstances warrant use in children older than 2 yr, initial dose is 2 mg/kg/day in divided doses PO. Do not exceed 4 mg/kg/day or 150–200 mg/day, whichever is less.

IV
Three IV doses given at 12- to 24-hr intervals.

Age	1st Dose	2nd Dose	3rd Dose
Younger than 48 hr	0.2 mg/kg	0.1 mg/kg	0.1 mg/kg
2–7 days	0.2 mg/kg	0.2 mg/kg	0.2 mg/kg
Older than 7 days	0.2 mg/kg	0.25 mg/kg	0.25 mg/kg

If marked anuria or oliguria occurs, do not give additional doses. If ductus reopens, repeat course of therapy at 12- to 24-hr intervals.

Pharmacokinetics

Route	Onset	Peak	Duration
Oral	30 min	1–2 hr	4–6 hr
IV	Immediate	Unknown	15–30 min

Metabolism: Hepatic; $T_{1/2}$: 4.5–6 hr
Distribution: Crosses placenta; enters breast milk
Excretion: Urine

▼ IV FACTS

Preparation: Reconstitute solution with 1–2 mL of 0.9% sodium chloride injection or water for injection; diluents should be preservative free. If 1 mL of diluent is used, concentration is 0.1 mg/0.1 mL. If 2 mL of diluent is used, concentration is 0.05 mg/0.1 mL. Discard any unused portion of the solution; prepare fresh solution before each dose.
Infusion: Inject reconstituted solution IV over 20–30 min; further dilution is not recommended.

Adverse effects
Oral, suppositories
- **CNS:** *Headache, dizziness, somnolence, insomnia,* fatigue, tiredness, dizziness, tinnitus, ophthalmologic effects
- **CV: Thrombotic events, MI, stroke**
- **Dermatologic:** *Rash,* pruritus, sweating, dry mucous membranes, stomatitis
- **GI:** *Nausea, dyspepsia, GI pain,* diarrhea, vomiting, *constipation,* flatulence, **GI bleed**

- **GU:** Dysuria, renal impairment
- **Hematologic: Bleeding ulcer,** platelet inhibition with higher doses, neutropenia, eosinophilia, leukopenia, **pancytopenia,** thrombocytopenia, **agranulocytosis,** granulocytopenia, **aplastic anemia,** decreased Hgb or Hct, bone marrow depression, menorrhagia
- **Respiratory:** Dyspnea, hemoptysis, pharyngitis, **bronchospasm,** rhinitis
- **Other:** Peripheral edema, **anaphylactoid reactions to anaphylactic shock**

IV preparation
- **GI: GI bleeding,** *vomiting,* abdominal distention, transient ileus
- **GU:** Renal impairment
- **Hematologic:** *Increased bleeding problems,* including intracranial bleed, **DIC,** hyponatremia, hyperkalemia, hypoglycemia, fluid retention
- **Respiratory:** *Apnea, exacerbation of pulmonary infection,* **pulmonary hemorrhage**
- **Other:** Retrolental fibroplasia, local irritation with extravasation

Interactions
✳ **Drug-drug** • Increased toxic effects of lithium • Decreased diuretic effect with loop diuretics: Bumetanide, furosemide, ethacrynic acid • Potential decrease in antihypertensive effect of beta-adrenergic blocking drugs, ACE inhibitors, and ARBs • Increased risk of gastric ulceration with bisphosphonates • Increased risk of bleeding with anticoagulants • Indomethacin may potentiate potassium-sparing properties of potassium-sparing diuretics
✳ **Drug-lab test** • False-negative results in dexamethasone suppression test

■ Nursing considerations
Assessment
- **History:** Oral and rectal preparations: Allergy to indomethacin, salicylates, or other NSAIDs; CV dysfunction, hypertension, recent history of coronary artery bypass surgery; peptic ulceration, GI bleeding; history of proctitis or rectal bleeding; impaired hepatic or renal function; pregnancy; labor and delivery. IV preparations: Proven or suspected infection; bleeding, thrombocytopenia, coagulation defects; necrotizing enterocolitis; renal impairment; local irritation if extravasation occurs

Adverse effects in *italics* are most common; those in **bold** are life-threatening. ▣ Do not crush.

- **Physical:** Skin color, lesions; T; orientation, reflexes, ophthalmologic evaluation, audiometric evaluation, peripheral sensation; P, BP, edema; R, adventitious sounds; liver evaluation, bowel sounds; CBC, clotting times, urinalysis, LFTs, renal function tests, serum electrolytes, stool guaiac

Interventions
Oral and rectal preparations
⊗ **Black box warning** Be aware that patient may be at increased risk for CV events, GI bleeding; monitor accordingly. Adverse reactions are dose-related; use lowest effective dose.

- Do not give SR tablets for gouty arthritis.
- Give drug with food or after meals if GI upset occurs.
- Arrange for periodic ophthalmologic examination during long-term therapy.

⊗ **Warning** Discontinue drug if eye changes or symptoms of hepatic or renal impairment occur.

⊗ **Warning** For overdose, use emergency procedures—gastric lavage, induction of emesis, support.

⊗ **Warning** Test renal function between doses. If severe renal impairment is noted, do not give the next dose.

Teaching points
- Parents of infants receiving IV therapy for patent ductus arteriosus will need support and encouragement and an explanation of the drug's action; this is best incorporated into the teaching about the disease.
- Use the drug only as suggested; avoid overdose. Take with food or after meals if GI upset occurs. Do not exceed the prescribed dosage. Do not use with over-the-counter analgesics; serious toxicity can occur.
- You may experience these side effects: Nausea, GI upset, dyspepsia (take drug with food); diarrhea or constipation; drowsiness, dizziness, vertigo, insomnia (use caution if driving or operating dangerous machinery).
- Report sore throat, fever, rash, itching, weight gain, swelling in ankles or fingers, changes in vision, black tarry stools.

▽infliximab
See Appendix R, *Less commonly used drugs.*

▽insoluble Prussian blue
See Appendix R, *Less commonly used drugs.*

DANGEROUS DRUG

▽insulin
(in´ su lin)
Insulin injection: Humulin R, Novolin Toronto (CAN), Novolin R
Insulin injection concentrate: Humulin R Regular U-500
Insulin lispro: Humalog
Isophane insulin suspension (NPH): Humulin N, Novolinge (CAN), Novolin NPH (CAN), Novolin N
Insulin aspart: NovoLog
Insulin detemir: Levemir
Insulin glargine: Lantus
Insulin glulisine: Apidra, Apidra SoloSTAR
Combination insulins: Humalog 50/50, Humalog 75/25, Humulin 70/30, Novolin 70/30, Novolinge 10/90, 20/80, 30/70, 40/60, 50/50 (CAN), NovoLog 70/30

PREGNANCY CATEGORY B

PREGNANCY CATEGORY C (INSULIN GLARGINE, INSULIN ASPART, INSULIN GLULISINE)

Drug classes
Antidiabetic
Hormone

Therapeutic actions
Insulin is a hormone secreted by beta cells of the pancreas that, by receptor-mediated effects, promotes the storage of the body's fuels, facilitating the transport of metabolites and ions (potassium) through cell membranes and stimulating the synthesis of glycogen from glucose, of fats from lipids, and proteins from amino acids.

Indications
- Treatment of type 1 diabetes mellitus

- Treatment of type 2 diabetes mellitus that cannot be controlled by diet or oral drugs
- Regular insulin injection: Treatment of severe ketoacidosis or diabetic coma
- Treatment of hyperkalemia with infusion of glucose to produce a shift of potassium into the cells
- Highly purified and human insulins promoted for short courses of therapy (surgery, intercurrent disease), newly diagnosed patients, patients with poor metabolic control, and patients with gestational diabetes
- Insulin injection concentrated: Treatment of diabetic patients with marked insulin resistance (requiring more than 200 units/day)
- Glargine (*Lantus*): Treatment of adult patients with type 2 diabetes mellitus who require basal insulin control of hyperglycemia
- Treatment of adults and children 6 yr and older who require basal insulin control
- Detemir (*Levemir*): Treatment of adults with diabetes who require basal insulin for the control of hyperglycemia
- Aspart (*NovoLog*): To maintain glycemic control in children 4–18 yr using a continuous subcutaneous infusion pump

Contraindications and cautions

- Contraindicated with allergy to pork products (varies with preparations; human insulin not contraindicated with pork allergy); during episodes of hypoglycemia.
- Use cautiously with pregnancy (keep patients under close supervision; rigid control is desired; following delivery, requirements may drop for 24–72 hr, rising to normal levels during next 6 wk); lactation (monitor mother carefully; insulin requirements may decrease during lactation).

Available forms

Injection—100 units/mL, 500 units/mL (concentrated); prefilled cartridges and pens—100 units/mL

Dosages
Adults and pediatric patients
General guidelines, 0.5–1 unit/kg/day. The number and size of daily doses, times of administration, and type of insulin preparation are determined after close medical scrutiny of the patient's blood and urine glucose, diet, exercise, and intercurrent infections and other

stresses. Usually given subcutaneously. Regular insulin and insulin glulisine may be given IV in diabetic coma or ketoacidosis. Insulin injection concentrated may be given subcutaneously or IM but do not administer IV.

Adults with type 2 diabetes mellitus requiring basal insulin control
10 units/day subcutaneously, given at the same time each day. Range, 2–100 units/day (*Lantus*) or 0.1–0.2 units/kg subcutaneously in the evening or 10 units once or twice a day (*Levemir*).

Pharmacokinetics

Type	Onset	Peak	Duration
Regular	30–60 min	2–3 hr	6–12 hr
NPH	1–1.5 hr	4–12 hr	24 hr
Lente	1–2.5 hr	7–15 hr	24 hr
Ultralente	4–8 hr	10–30 hr	> 36 hr
Lispro	< 15 min	30–90 min	2–5 hr
Aspart	10–20 min	1–3 hr	3–5 hr
Detemir	Slow	3–6 hr	6–23 hr
Glargine	60 min	None	24 hr
Glulisine	2–5 min	30–90 min	1–2 hr
Combination insulins	30–60 min, then 1–2 hr	2–4 hr, then 6–12 hr	6–8 hr, then 18–24 hr

Metabolism: Cellular; $T_{1/2}$: Varies with preparation
Distribution: Crosses placenta; does not enter breast milk
Excretion: Unknown

▼ IV FACTS
Preparation: May be mixed with standard IV solutions; use of plastic tubing or bag will change the amount of insulin delivered.
Infusion: Use of a monitored delivery system is suggested. Rate should be determined by patient response and glucose levels.
Incompatibilities: Do not add to aminophylline, amobarbital, chlorothiazide, cytarabine, dobutamine, methylprednisolone, pentobarbital, phenobarbital, phenytoin, secobarbital, sodium bicarbonate, thiopental.

Adverse effects
- **Hypersensitivity:** Rash, **anaphylaxis or angioedema**
- **Local:** Allergy—local reactions at injection site—redness, swelling, itching; usually resolves in a few days to a few weeks; a

change in type or species source of insulin may be tried; lipodystrophy; pruritus

- **Metabolic:** Hypoglycemia; ketoacidosis
- **Respiratory:** Decline in pulmonary function (inhaled insulin)

Interactions

✳ **Drug-drug** • Increased hypoglycemic effects of insulin with MAOIs, beta blockers, salicylates, or alcohol • Delayed recovery from hypoglycemic episodes and masked signs and symptoms of hypoglycemia if taken with beta-adrenergic blocking drugs • Decreased effectiveness of insulin with corticosteroids, diuretics, atypical antipsychotics

✳ **Drug-alternative therapy** • Increased risk of hypoglycemia if taken with juniper berries, ginseng, garlic, fenugreek, coriander, dandelion root, celery

■ Nursing considerations

Assessment

- **History:** Allergy to pork products; pregnancy; lactation
- **Physical:** Skin color, lesions; eyeball turgor; orientation, reflexes, peripheral sensation; P, BP; R, adventitious sounds; urinalysis, blood glucose

Interventions

- Ensure uniform dispersion of insulin suspensions by rolling the vial gently between hands; avoid vigorous shaking.
- Give maintenance doses subcutaneously, rotating injection sites regularly to decrease incidence of lipodystrophy; give regular insulin IV or IM in severe ketoacidosis or diabetic coma.
- Monitor patients receiving insulin IV carefully; plastic IV infusion sets have been reported to remove 20%–80% of the insulin; dosage delivered to the patient will vary.
- Do not give insulin injection concentrated IV; severe anaphylactic reactions can occur.
- Use caution when mixing two types of insulin; always draw the regular insulin into the syringe first; if mixing with insulin lispro, draw the lispro first; use mixtures of regular and NPH or regular and Lente insulins within 5–15 min of combining them; *Lantus* (insulin glargine) and *Levemir* (insulin detemir) cannot be mixed in solution with any other drug, including other insulins.

⊗ *Warning* Double-check, or have a colleague check, the dosage drawn up for pediatric patients, for patients receiving concentrated insulin injection, or patients receiving very small doses; even small errors in dosage can cause serious problems.

- Carefully monitor patients being switched from one type of insulin to another; dosage adjustments are often needed. Human insulins often require smaller doses than beef or pork insulin; monitor cautiously if patients are switched; lispro insulin is given 15 min before a meal. *Levemir* is given in the evening.
- Store insulin in a cool place away from direct sunlight. Refrigeration is preferred. Do not freeze insulin. Insulin prefilled in glass or plastic syringes is stable for 1 wk refrigerated; this is a safe way of ensuring proper dosage for patients with limited vision or who have problems with drawing up insulin.
- Monitor serum glucose levels frequently to determine effectiveness of drug and dosage. Patients can learn to adjust insulin dosage on a sliding scale based on test results.
- Monitor insulin needs during times of trauma or severe stress; dosage adjustments may be needed.

⊗ *Warning* Keep life-support equipment and glucose readily available to deal with ketoacidosis or hypoglycemic reactions.

Teaching points

- Use the same type and brand of syringe; use the same type and brand of insulin to avoid dosage errors. Arrange for proper disposal of syringes.
- Do not change the order of mixing insulins. Rotate injection sites regularly (keep a chart of sites used) to prevent breakdown at injection sites.
- Dosage may vary with activities, stress, or diet. Monitor blood glucose levels, and consult your health care provider if problems arise.
- Store drug in the refrigerator or in a cool place out of direct sunlight; do not freeze insulin.
- If refrigeration is not possible, drug is stable at controlled room temperature and out of direct sunlight for up to 1 month.
- Wear a medical alert tag stating that you have diabetes and are taking insulin so that

emergency medical personnel will take proper care of you.
- Avoid alcohol; serious reactions can occur.
- Report fever, sore throat, vomiting, hypoglycemic or hyperglycemic reactions, rash.

DANGEROUS DRUG

▷**interferon alfa-2b (IFN-a2, rIFN-a2, a-2-interferon)**
(in ter feer' on)

Intron-A

PREGNANCY CATEGORY C

Drug classes
Antineoplastic
Immunomodulator
Interferon

Therapeutic actions
Inhibits growth of tumor cells; mechanism of action is not clearly understood; prevents the replication of tumor cells and enhances host immune response. Interferons are produced by human leukocytes in response to viral infections and other stimuli. Interferon alfa-2b is produced by recombinant DNA technology using *Escherichia coli.*

Indications
- Hairy cell leukemia in patients 18 yr and older
- Intralesional treatment of condylomata acuminata in patients 18 yr and older
- AIDS-related Kaposi sarcoma in patients 18 yr and older
- Adjunct to surgical treatment of malignant melanoma in patients older than 18 yr who are free of disease, but at high risk of recurrence with 56 days of surgery
- Treatment of chronic hepatitis C in patients 18 yr and older
- Treatment of chronic hepatitis B in patients 1 yr and older
- Follicular lymphoma, as initial treatment of clinically aggressive follicular non-Hodgkin lymphoma with other chemotherapy in patient 18 yr and older
- Orphan drug uses: CML, metastatic renal cell carcinoma, ovarian carcinoma, invasive carcinoma of cervix, primary malig-

nant brain tumors, laryngeal papillomatosis, carcinoma in situ of urinary bladder, chronic delta hepatitis, acute hepatitis B

Contraindications and cautions
- Contraindicated with allergy to interferon-alfa or any components of the product, severe hepatic impairment.
- Use cautiously with cardiac disease, pulmonary disease, diabetes mellitus prone to ketoacidosis, coagulation disorders, bone marrow depression, pregnancy, neuropsychiatric disorders, autoimmune diseases, lactation.

Available forms
Powder for injection—10, 18, 50 million international units/vial; solution for injection— 18, 25 million international units/vial; injection—3, 5, 10 million international units/dose (in multidose pens)

Dosages
Adults
- *Hairy cell leukemia:* 2 million international units/m^2 subcutaneously or IM three times/wk for up to 6 mo. Continue for several months, depending on clinical and hematologic response. Patient with platelet count less than 50,000/mm^3 should not receive IM injection.
- *Condylomata acuminata:* 1 million international units/lesion three times/wk for 3 wk intralesionally. Maximum response occurs 4–8 wk after initiation of therapy. Up to five lesions can be treated at one time. May repeat course at 12–16 wk.
- *Chronic hepatitis C:* 3 million international units subcutaneously or IM, three times/wk for 18–24 mo.
- *AIDS-related Kaposi sarcoma:* 30 million international units/m^2 three times/wk subcutaneously or IM. Maintain dosage until disease progresses rapidly or severe intolerance occurs. Do not use the multidose pens or multidose vials due to inappropriate concentration.
- *Chronic hepatitis B:* 30–35 million international units/wk subcutaneously or IM either as 5 million international units daily or 10 million international units three times/wk for 16 wk.
- *Follicular lymphoma:* 5 million international units subcutaneously, three times/wk

for 18 mo with other chemotherapy. Adjust dosage based on blood counts.
- *Malignant melanoma:* 20 million international units/m^2 IV over 20 min on 5 consecutive days/wk for 4 wk; maintenance, 10 million international units/m^2 IV three times/wk for 48 wk.

Pediatric patients
- *Chronic hepatitis B:* 3 million international units/m^2 subcutaneously three times/wk for the first wk, then increase to 6 million international units/m^2 subcutaneously three times/wk for a total of 16–24 wk (maximum dose, 10 million international units, three times/wk). Adjust dosage based on blood counts.

Pharmacokinetics

Route	Onset	Peak
IM, Subcut.	Rapid	3–12 hr
IV	Rapid	End of infusion

Metabolism: Renal; T$_{1/2}$: 2–3 hr
Distribution: Crosses placenta; may enter breast milk
Excretion: Unknown

▼ IV FACTS

Powder for injection is not indicated for pediatric patients because diluent contains benzyl alcohol.
Preparation: Inject diluent (bacteriostatic water for injection) into vial using chart provided by manufacturer; agitate gently, withdraw with sterile syringe, inject into 100 mL of normal saline.
Infusion: Administer each dose slowly over 20 min.

Adverse effects

- **CNS:** *Dizziness, confusion,* paresthesias, numbness, lethargy, decreased mental status, depression, visual disturbances, sleep disturbances, nervousness
- **CV:** Hypotension, edema, hypertension, chest pain, arrhythmias, palpitations
- **Dermatologic:** *Rash,* dryness or inflammation of the oropharynx, *dry skin, pruritus,* partial alopecia
- **GI:** *Anorexia, nausea,* diarrhea, vomiting, change in taste
- **GU:** Impaired fertility in women, transient impotence

- **Hematologic:** Leukopenia, neutropenia, thrombocytopenia, anemia, decreased Hgb; increased levels of AST, LDH, alkaline phosphatase, bilirubin, uric acid, serum creatinine, BUN, blood sugar, serum phosphorus, neutralizing antibodies; hypocalcemia
- **Other:** *Flulike symptoms,* weight loss, diaphoresis, arthralgia

■ Nursing considerations
Assessment
- **History:** Allergy to interferon-alfa or product components, cardiac or pulmonary disease, diabetes mellitus prone to ketoacidosis, coagulation disorders, bone marrow depression, pregnancy, lactation
- **Physical:** Weight; T; skin color, lesions; orientation, reflexes; P, BP, edema, ECG; liver evaluation; CBC, blood glucose, LFTs, renal function tests, urinalysis

Interventions
- Obtain laboratory tests (CBC, differential, granulocytes and hairy cells, bone marrow and hairy cells, LFTs) before therapy and monthly during therapy.
- Prepare solution as follows (see manufacturer's guidelines for specific indications and dilutions):

Vial Strength (Million International Units)	Final Amount of Diluent (mL)	Concentration (Million International Units/mL)
3	1	3
5	1	5
10	2	5
25	5	5
10	1	10
50	1	50

- Use bacteriostatic water for injection as diluent. Agitate gently. After reconstitution, stable for 1 mo if refrigerated.
- Administer IM or subcutaneously.
- ⊗ **Black box warning** Monitor for severe reactions, including hypersensitivity reactions and neuropsychiatric, autoimmune, ischemic, and infectious disorders; notify physician immediately; dosage reduction or discontinuation may be necessary; risk of serious to life-threatening reactions.
- Ensure that patient is well hydrated, especially during initiation of treatment.

Teaching points

- Prepare a calendar to check off as drug is given. You and a significant other should learn proper subcutaneous or IM injection technique for outpatient use. Do not change brands of interferon without consulting your health care provider. Arrange for proper disposal of syringes and needles.
- Arrange for regular blood tests to monitor the drug's effects.
- You may experience these side effects: Loss of appetite, nausea, vomiting (frequent mouth care, frequent small meals may help; maintain good nutrition; a dietitian may be able to help; an antiemetic also may be ordered); fatigue, confusion, dizziness, numbness, visual disturbances, depression (use special precautions to avoid injury; avoid driving or using dangerous machinery); flu-like symptoms (take drug at bedtime; ensure rest periods for yourself; a medication may be ordered for fever).
- Report fever, chills, sore throat, unusual bleeding or bruising, chest pain, palpitations, dizziness, changes in mental status.

▽**interferon alfacon-1**

See Appendix R, *Less commonly used drugs.*

▽**interferon beta-1a**
(in ter feer' on)

Avonex, Rebif

PREGNANCY CATEGORY C

Drug classes

Immunomodulator
Interferon
MS drug

Therapeutic actions

Interferons are produced by human leukocytes in response to viral infections and other stimuli; interferon beta-1a blocks replication of viruses and stimulates the host immunoregulatory activities. It is produced by Chinese hamster ovary cells.

Indications

- MS—treatment of relapsing forms of MS to slow accumulation of physical disability and decrease frequency of clinical exacerbations

Contraindications and cautions

- Contraindicated with allergy to beta interferon, human albumin, or any components of product, lactation.
- Use cautiously with chronic progressive MS, suicidal tendencies or mental disorders, cardiac disease, seizures, pregnancy.

Available forms

Powder for injection—33 mcg (*Avonex*), prefilled syringe—30 mcg/0.5 mL (*Avonex*); injection—8.8 mcg/0.2 mL, 22 mcg/0.5 mL, 44 mcg/0.5 mL (*Rebif*)

Dosages
Adults

30 mcg IM once per week (*Avonex*)—22 or 44 mcg subcutaneously 3 times per week (*Rebif*)—start with 8.8 mcg 3 times per week and titrate up over 5 wk to full dose of 22–44 mcg.
Pediatric patients

Safety and efficacy not established in patients younger than 18 yr.

Pharmacokinetics

Route	Onset	Peak	Duration
IM	12 hr	48 hr	4 days

Metabolism: Hepatic and renal; $T_{1/2}$: 10 hr
Distribution: Crosses placenta; may enter breast milk
Excretion: Urine

Adverse effects

- **CNS:** *Dizziness, confusion,* paresthesias, numbness, lethargy, decreased mental status, depression, visual disturbances, sleep disturbances, nervousness, asthenia
- **CV:** Hypotension, edema, hypertension, chest pain, arrhythmias, palpitations
- **Dermatologic:** *Photosensitivity,* rash, alopecia, sweating
- **GI:** *Anorexia, nausea,* diarrhea, vomiting, change in taste
- **GU:** Impairment of fertility in women, transient impotence
- **Hematologic:** Leukopenia, neutropenia, thrombocytopenia, anemia, decreased Hgb; increased levels of AST, LDH, alkaline phosphatase, bilirubin, uric acid, serum creatinine,

---

Adverse effects in *italics* are most common; those in **bold** are life-threatening. ▨ Do not crush.

BUN, blood sugar, serum phosphorus, neutralizing antibodies; hypocalcemia
- **Other:** *Flulike symptoms,* weight loss, diaphoresis, arthralgia, injection site reaction

■ **Nursing considerations**
Assessment
- **History:** Allergy to beta interferon or any component of product, mental disorders, suicidal tendencies, cardiac disease, seizures, depression, pregnancy, lactation
- **Physical:** Weight; T; skin color, lesions; orientation, reflexes; P, BP, edema, ECG; liver evaluation; CBC, blood glucose, LFTs, renal function tests, urinalysis

Interventions
- Arrange for laboratory tests—CBC, differential, granulocytes and hairy cells and bone marrow hairy cells, and liver function tests—before and monthly during therapy.
- Reconstitute with 1.1 mL of diluent and swirl gently to dissolve; use within 6 hr (*Avonex*).
- Ensure that patient is well hydrated, especially during initiation of treatment.
- Ensure regular follow-up and treatment of MS; this drug is not a cure.
- If flulike symptoms occur, arrange for supportive treatment—rest, acetaminophen for fever and headache, environmental control.
- Carefully monitor patients with any history of mental disorders or suicidal tendencies.
- Counsel female patients to use birth control while using this drug. Drug should not be used in pregnancy.

Teaching points
- *Avonex* needs to be taken weekly. If you or a significant other can give an IM injection: Store vial in refrigerator, reconstitute with 1.1 milliliters of diluent and swirl gently, use within 6 hours. Do not give in the same site each week.
- *Rebif* needs to be given three times per week subcutaneously, preferably at the same time of day and on the same days of the week. Store in refrigerator, reconstitute with solution provided, and discard any solution remaining in the syringe. Rotate injection sites.
- Keep a chart of injection sites to prevent overuse of one area. Arrange for proper disposal of needles and syringes.
- Have regular treatment and follow-up of MS; this drug is not a cure.

- You may experience these side effects: Loss of appetite, nausea, vomiting (use frequent mouth care; eat frequent small meals; maintain good nutrition if possible—dietitian may be able to help; antiemetics may be ordered); fatigue, confusion, dizziness, numbness, visual disturbances, depression (use caution to avoid injury; avoid driving or using dangerous machinery); impotence (usually transient); sensitivity to sunlight (use a sunscreen, wear protective clothing if exposure to sun cannot be prevented).
- Report fever, chills, sore throat, unusual bleeding or bruising, chest pain, palpitations, dizziness, changes in mental status.

▽**interferon beta-1b (rIFN-B)**
(in ter feer' on)

Betaseron, Extavia

PREGNANCY CATEGORY C

Drug classes
Immunomodulator
Interferon
MS drug

Therapeutic actions
Interferons are produced by human leukocytes in response to viral infections and other stimuli; interferon beta-1b block replication of viruses and stimulate the host immunoregulatory activities. Interferon beta-1b is produced by recombinant DNA technology using *Escherichia coli.*

Indications
- Reduce the frequency of clinical exacerbations in relapsing, remitting MS

Contraindications and cautions
- Contraindicated with allergy to beta interferon, human albumin, or product components; lactation.
- Use cautiously with chronic progressive MS, suicidal tendencies, mental disorders, pregnancy.

Available forms
Powder for injection—0.3 mg

Dosages

Adults

0.25 mg subcutaneously every other day; discontinue use if disease is unremitting for more than 6 mo. Initially, 0.0625 mg subcutaneously every other day, weeks 1–2; then 0.125 mg subcutaneously every other day, weeks 3–4; 0.1875 mg subcutaneously every other day, weeks 5–6; target 0.25 mg subcutaneously every other day by week 7.

Pediatric patients

Safety and efficacy not established in patients younger than 18 yr.

Pharmacokinetics

Route	Onset	Peak
Subcut.	Slow	1–8 hr

Metabolism: Hepatic and renal; $T_{1/2}$: 8 min–4.3 hr
Distribution: Crosses placenta; may enter breast milk
Excretion: Urine

Adverse effects

- **CNS:** *Dizziness, confusion,* paresthesias, numbness, lethargy, decreased mental status, depression, visual disturbances, sleep disturbances, nervousness
- **CV:** Hypotension, edema, hypertension, chest pain, arrhythmias, palpitations
- **Dermatologic:** *Photosensitivity,* rash, alopecia, sweating
- **GI:** *Anorexia, nausea,* diarrhea, vomiting, change in taste, abdominal pain
- **GU:** Impairment of fertility in women, transient impotence, metrorrhagia
- **Hematologic:** Leukopenia, neutropenia, thrombocytopenia, anemia, decreased Hgb; increased levels of AST, LDH, alkaline phosphatase, bilirubin, uric acid, serum creatinine, BUN, blood sugar, serum phosphorus, neutralizing antibodies; hypocalcemia
- **Other:** *Flulike symptoms,* weight loss, diaphoresis, arthralgia, injection site reaction

■ Nursing considerations

Assessment

- **History:** Allergy to interferon beta or any components of the product, mental disorders, suicidal tendencies, pregnancy, lactation
- **Physical:** Weight; T; skin color, lesions; orientation, reflexes; P, BP, edema, ECG; liver evaluation; CBC, blood glucose, LFTs, renal function tests, urinalysis

Interventions

- Obtain laboratory tests (CBC, differential, granulocytes and hairy cells, bone marrow hairy cells, and liver function tests) before therapy and monthly during therapy.
- ⊗ *Warning* Monitor for severe reactions; notify physician immediately; you may need to reduce dosage or discontinue drug.
- Reconstitute by using a sterile syringe and needle to inject 1.2 mL supplied diluent into vial; gently swirl vial to dissolve drug completely; do not shake. Discard if any particulate matter or discoloration has occurred. After reconstitution, vial contains 0.25 mg/mL solution. Withdraw 1 mL of reconstituted solution with a sterile syringe fitted with a 27-gauge needle. Inject subcutaneously into arms, abdomen, hips, or thighs. Vial is for single use only. Discard any unused portions. Drug is stable at room temperature before reconstitution. Refrigerate reconstituted solution and use within 3 hr.
- Ensure that patient is well hydrated, especially during initiation of treatment.
- Ensure regular follow-up and treatment of MS; this drug is not a cure.
- ⊗ *Warning* Carefully monitor patients with any mental disorders or suicidal tendencies.
- Counsel female patients to use birth control. Drug should not be used in pregnancy.

Teaching points

- Reconstitute by using a sterile syringe and needle to inject 1.2 mL supplied diluent into vial; gently swirl the vial to dissolve the drug completely; do not shake. Discard if any particulate matter or discoloration has occurred. After reconstitution, vial contains 0.25 mg/mL solution. Withdraw 1 mL of reconstituted solution with a sterile syringe fitted with a 27-gauge needle. Inject subcutaneously into arms, abdomen, hips, or thighs. Vial is for single use only. Discard any unused portions. Drug is stable at room temperature before reconstitution. Refrigerate reconstituted solution and use within 3 hours.
- Keep a chart of injection sites to prevent overuse of one area. Arrange for proper disposal of needles and syringes.

Adverse effects in *italics* are most common; those in **bold** are life-threatening. ⬛ Do not crush.

- Have regular treatment and follow-up of MS; this drug is not a cure.
- Using barrier contraceptives is advised; the drug should not be used during pregnancy.
- You may experience these side effects: Loss of appetite, nausea, vomiting (frequent mouth care, frequent small meals may help; maintain good nutrition; a dietitian may be able to help; an antiemetic also may be ordered); fatigue, confusion, dizziness, numbness, visual disturbances, depression (use special precautions to avoid injury; avoid driving or using dangerous machinery); impotence (transient and reversible); sensitivity to the sun (use sunscreen and wear protective clothing if exposed to sun).
- Report fever, chills, sore throat, unusual bleeding or bruising, chest pain, palpitations, dizziness, changes in mental status, thoughts of suicide.

▽ interferon gamma-1b
(in ter feer' on)

Actimmune

PREGNANCY CATEGORY C

Drug classes
Immunomodulator
Interferon

Therapeutic actions
Interferons are produced by human leukocytes in response to viral infections and other stimuli; interferon gamma-1b block has potent phagocyte-activating effects; acts as an interleukin; produced by *Escherichia coli* bacteria.

Indications
- For reducing the frequency and severity of serious infections associated with chronic granulomatous disease
- For delaying time to disease progression in patients with severe, malignant osteopetrosis
- Orphan drug use: Renal cell carcinoma

Contraindications and cautions
- Contraindicated with allergy to interferon gamma, *E. coli,* or product components; lactation.

- Use cautiously with seizure disorders, compromised CNS function, cardiac disease, myelosuppression, pregnancy.

Available forms
Injection—100 mcg/0.5 mL (2 million international units)

Dosages
Adults
50 mcg/m^2 (1 million international units/m^2) subcutaneously three times/wk in patients who have a body surface area greater than 0.5 m^2; 1.5 mcg/kg per dose in patients who have a body surface area less than or equal to 0.5 m^2 subcutaneously three times/wk. Reduce dose by 50% or hold therapy for severe reactions.
Pediatric patients
Safety and efficacy not established in patients younger than 18 yr.

Pharmacokinetics

Route	Onset	Peak
Subcut.	Slow	7 hr

Metabolism: Hepatic and renal; T$_{1/2}$: 2.9–5.9 hr
Distribution: Crosses placenta; may enter breast milk
Excretion: Urine

Adverse effects
- **CNS:** *Dizziness, confusion,* paresthesias, headache, numbness, lethargy, decreased mental status, depression, visual disturbances, sleep disturbances, nervousness
- **CV:** Hypotension, edema, hypertension, chest pain, arrhythmias, palpitations
- **GI:** *Anorexia, nausea,* diarrhea, vomiting, change in taste, pancreatitis
- **Other:** *Flulike symptoms,* weight loss, diaphoresis, arthralgia, injection site reaction, fever, rash, chills, fatigue, myalgia

■ Nursing considerations
Assessment
- **History:** Allergy to interferon gamma, *E. coli,* or product components; pregnancy, lactation, seizure disorders, compromised CNS function, cardiac disease, myelosuppression

- **Physical:** Weight; T; skin color, lesions; orientation, reflexes; P, BP, edema, ECG; liver evaluation; CBC, blood glucose, LFTs, renal function tests, urinalysis

Interventions

- Obtain laboratory tests (CBC, differential, granulocytes and hairy cells, bone marrow and hairy cells, and liver function tests) before therapy and monthly during therapy.
- ⊗ **Warning** Monitor for severe reactions and notify physician immediately; dosage may need to be reduced or drug discontinued.
- Store in refrigerator; each vial is for one use only, discard after that time. Discard any vial that has been unrefrigerated for 12 hr.
- Give drug at bedtime if flulike symptoms become a problem.
- Advise women of childbearing age to use barrier contraceptives; drug should not be used during pregnancy.

Teaching points

- Store in refrigerator; each vial is for one use only; discard after that time. Discard vial that has been unrefrigerated for 12 hours. You and a significant other should learn the proper technique for subcutaneous injections. Product does not contain a preservative.
- Keep a chart of injection sites to prevent overuse of one area. Arrange for proper disposal of needles and syringes.
- Using barrier contraceptives is advised; this drug should not be used in pregnancy.
- You may experience these side effects: Loss of appetite, nausea, vomiting (frequent mouth care, frequent small meals may help; maintain good nutrition; a dietitian may be able to help; an antiemetic also may be ordered); fatigue, confusion, dizziness, numbness, visual disturbances, depression (use special precautions to avoid injury; avoid driving or using dangerous machinery); flulike symptoms (fever, chills, aches, pains; rest, take acetaminophen for fever and headache; take drug at bedtime).
- Report fever, chills, sore throat, unusual bleeding or bruising, chest pain, palpitations, dizziness, changes in mental status.

▽ iodine thyroid products

(eye' oh dine)

Iosat, Lugol's Solution, Pima, SSKI, Strong Iodine Solution, ThyroSafe, ThyroShield

PREGNANCY CATEGORY D

Drug class
Thyroid suppressant

Therapeutic actions
Inhibits synthesis of the active thyroid hormones T_3 and T_4 and inhibits the release of these hormones into circulation.

Indications

- Hyperthyroidism: Adjunctive therapy with antithyroid drugs in preparation for thyroidectomy, treatment of thyrotoxic crisis, or neonatal thyrotoxicosis
- Thyroid blocking in a radiation emergency (*Iosat, ThyroSafe, ThyroShield*)
- Unlabeled uses: Potassium iodide has been effective with Sweet syndrome, treatment of lymphocutaneous sporotrichosis in combination with a potent topical steroid

Contraindications and cautions

- Contraindicated with allergy to iodides.
- Use cautiously with pulmonary edema, pulmonary TB (sodium iodide); pregnancy; lactation.

Available forms
Solution—5% iodine, 10% potassium iodide; tablets—65, 130 mg potassium iodide; solution—65 mg/mL. 1 g/mL; syrup—325 mg/5 mL. *Note:* Potassium iodide tablets and drops are available only to state and federal agencies.

Dosages
Adults and pediatric patients older than 1 yr

- *RDA:* 150 mcg PO.
- *Hyperthyroidism:* 0.3 mL PO tid (*Strong Iodine Solution, Lugol Solution*); range may be 0.1–0.9 mL/day.

Adults and pediatric patients (birth–18 yr)
- *Thyroid blocking in a radiation emergency used as directed by state or local health authorities* (Iosat, ThyroSafe, ThyroShield): 130 mg PO every 24 hr.

Pediatric patients 12–18 yr weighing 150 lb or more: 130 mg/day PO.

Pediatric patients 1–18 yr weighing less than 150 lb: 65 mg/day PO.

Pediatric patients older than 3 yr to 12 yr: 65 mg/day PO.

Pediatric patients older than 1 mo to 3 yr: 32.5 mg/day PO.

Pediatric patients from birth to 1 mo: 16.25 mg/day PO.

Pharmacokinetics

Route	Onset	Peak	Duration
Oral	24 hr	10–15 days	6 wk

Metabolism: Hepatic; $T_{1/2}$: Unknown
Distribution: Crosses placenta; may enter breast milk
Excretion: Urine

Adverse effects
- **Dermatologic:** *Rash*
- **Endocrine:** Hypothyroidism, hyperthyroidism, goiter
- **GI:** *Swelling of the salivary glands, iodism* (metallic taste, burning mouth and throat, sore teeth and gums, head cold symptoms, stomach upset, diarrhea)
- **Hypersensitivity:** Allergic reactions— fever, joint pains, swelling of the face or body, shortness of breath

Interactions
✳ **Drug-drug** • Increased risk of hypothyroidism if taken concurrently with lithium

■ Nursing considerations
Assessment
- **History:** Allergy to iodides, pulmonary edema, pulmonary TB, lactation
- **Physical:** Skin color, lesions, edema; R, adventitious sounds; gums, mucous membranes; T_3 and T_4

Interventions
- Test skin for idiosyncrasy to iodine before giving parenteral doses.

- Dilute strong iodine solution with fruit juice or water to improve taste.
- Crush tablets for small children.

⊗ **Warning** Discontinue drug if symptoms of acute iodine toxicity occur: Vomiting, abdominal pain, diarrhea, or circulatory collapse.

Teaching points
- Drops may be diluted in fruit juice or water. Tablets may be crushed.
- Discontinue use and report fever, rash, swelling of the throat, metallic taste, sore teeth and gums, head cold symptoms, severe GI distress, enlargement of the thyroid gland.

▽ **iodoquinol**
(diiodohydroxyquinoline)
*(eye oh doe **kwin'** ole)*

Yodoxin

PREGNANCY CATEGORY C

Drug class
Amebicide

Therapeutic actions
Directly amebicidal by an unknown mechanism; is poorly absorbed in the GI tract and is able to exert its amebicidal action directly in the large intestine.

Indications
- Acute or chronic intestinal amebiasis

Contraindications and cautions
- Contraindicated with hepatic failure, allergy to iodine preparations or 8-hydroxyquinolines.
- Use cautiously with thyroid disease, pregnancy, lactation.

Available forms
Tablets—210, 650 mg; powder—25 g

Dosages
Adults
650 mg tid PO after meals for 20 days.

Pediatric patients
10–13.3 mg/kg/day PO, in 3 divided doses for 20 days. Maximum dose, 650 mg/dose. Do not exceed 1.95 g in 24 hr for 20 days.

Pharmacokinetics

Route	Onset
Oral	Slow

Very poorly absorbed; exerts effects locally in the intestine.
Excretion: Feces

Adverse effects

- **CNS:** Blurring of vision, weakness, fatigue, optic atrophy, peripheral neuropathy, vertigo, numbness, headache
- **Dermatologic:** *Rash, pruritus,* urticaria
- **GI:** *Nausea, vomiting, diarrhea,* anorexia, abdominal cramps, pruritus ani
- **Other:** Thyroid enlargement, fever, chills

Interactions

✳ **Drug-lab test** ● Interferes with many tests of thyroid function; interference may last up to 6 mo after drug is discontinued

■ Nursing considerations
Assessment

- **History:** Hepatic failure, allergy to iodine preparations or 8-hydroxyquinolines, thyroid disease, lactation, pregnancy
- **Physical:** Rashes, lesions; check reflexes, ophthalmologic examination; BP, P, R; LFTs, thyroid function tests (PBI, T_3, and T_4)

Interventions

- Administer drug after meals.
- Administer for full course of therapy.
- Maintain patient's nutrition.

Teaching points

- Take drug after meals.
- You may experience these side effects: GI upset, nausea, vomiting, diarrhea (eat frequent small meals; frequent mouth care often helps).
- Report severe GI upset, rash, blurring of vision, unusual fatigue, fever.

▽ipilimumab

See Appendix R, *Less commonly used drugs.*

▽ipratropium bromide
*(i pra **troe'** pee um)*

Apo-Ipravent (CAN), Atrovent, Atrovent HFA, Gen-Ipratropium (CAN), ratio-Ipratropium (CAN), ratio-Ipratropium UDV (CAN)

PREGNANCY CATEGORY B

Drug classes
Anticholinergic
Antimuscarinic
Bronchodilator
Parasympatholytic

Therapeutic actions
Anticholinergic, chemically related to atropine, which blocks vagally mediated reflexes by antagonizing the action of acetylcholine. Causes bronchodilation and inhibits secretion from serous and seromucous glands lining the nasal mucosa.

Indications

- Bronchodilator for maintenance treatment of bronchospasm associated with COPD (solution, aerosol), chronic bronchitis, and emphysema
- Nasal spray: Symptomatic relief of rhinorrhea associated with perennial rhinitis, common cold, seasonal allergic rhinitis

Contraindications and cautions

- Contraindicated with hypersensitivity to atropine or its derivatives, soybean or peanut allergies (aerosol).
- Use cautiously with narrow-angle glaucoma, prostatic hypertrophy, bladder neck obstruction, pregnancy, lactation.

Available forms
Aerosol—17 mcg/actuation; solution for inhalation—0.02%; (500 mcg/vial); nasal spray—0.03% (21 mcg/spray), 0.06% (42 mcg/spray)

Dosages
Aerosol
Adults
The usual dosage is 2 inhalations qid. Patients may take additional inhalations as required. Do not exceed 12 inhalations/24 hr.

Solution for inhalation
Adults and pediatric patients 12 yr and older
500 mcg tid–qid via nebulizer, with doses 6–8 hr apart.

Nasal spray
Adults and pediatric patients 12 yr and older
2 sprays 0.06% per nostril tid–qid for relief with common cold.
Adults and pediatric patients 6 yr and older
2 sprays 0.03% per nostril bid–tid for rhinitis.
Adults and pediatric patients older than 5 yr
• *Rhinorrhea in seasonal allergic rhinitis:* 2 sprays 0.06% qid for 3 wk.
Pediatric patients 5–11 yr
2 sprays 0.06% per nostril tid for relief with common cold.

Pharmacokinetics

Route	Onset	Peak	Duration
Inhalation	15 min	1–2 hr	3–4 hr

Metabolism: Hepatic, $T_{1/2}$: 2 hr
Distribution: May cross placenta; may enter breast milk
Excretion: Unknown

Adverse effects
• **CNS:** *Nervousness, dizziness, headache,* fatigue, insomnia, *blurred vision*
• **GI:** *Nausea,* GI distress, *dry mouth*
• **Respiratory:** Dyspnea, bronchitis, bronchospasms, URI, *cough,* exacerbation of symptoms, hoarseness, pharyngitis
• **Other:** Back pain, chest pain, allergic-type reactions, palpitations, rash

■ Nursing considerations
Assessment
• **History:** Hypersensitivity to atropine, soybeans, peanuts (aerosol preparation); acute bronchospasm, narrow-angle glaucoma, prostatic hypertrophy, bladder neck obstruction, pregnancy, lactation
• **Physical:** Skin color, lesions, texture, T; orientation, reflexes, bilateral grip strength; affect; ophthalmic examination; P, BP; R, adventitious sounds; bowel sounds, normal output; normal urinary output, prostate palpation

Interventions
• Protect solution for inhalation from light. Store unused vials in foil pouch.
• Use nebulizer mouthpiece instead of face mask to avoid blurred vision or aggravation of narrow-angle glaucoma.
• Can mix with albuterol in nebulizer for up to 1 hr.
• Ensure adequate hydration; control environment (temperature) to prevent hyperpyrexia.
• Have patient void before taking medication to avoid urinary retention.
• Teach patient proper use of inhaler.

Teaching points
• Use this drug as an inhalation product. Review the proper use of inhaler; for nasal spray, initiation of pump requires 7 actuations; if not used for 24 hours, 2 actuations will be needed before use. If not used for more than 7 days, reprime pump with 7 sprays. Protect from light; do not freeze.
• For *Atrovent HFA,* use only the supplied HFA aerosol inhalation mouthpiece.
• You may experience these side effects: Dizziness, headache, blurred vision (avoid driving or performing hazardous tasks); nausea, vomiting, GI upset (proper nutrition is important; consult with a dietitian to maintain nutrition); cough.
• Report rash, eye pain, difficulty voiding, palpitations, vision changes.

▷ irbesartan
(er bah sar' tan)

Avapro

PREGNANCY CATEGORY C
(FIRST TRIMESTER)

PREGNANCY CATEGORY D
(SECOND AND THIRD TRIMESTERS)

Drug classes
Antihypertensive
ARB

Therapeutic actions
Selectively blocks the binding of angiotensin II to specific tissue receptors found in the

vascular smooth muscle and adrenal gland; this action blocks the vasoconstriction effect of the renin-angiotensin system as well as the release of aldosterone, leading to decreased BP.

Indications

- Treatment of hypertension as monotherapy or in combination with other antihypertensives
- Slowing of the progression of nephropathy in patients with hypertension and type 2 diabetes

Contraindications and cautions

- Contraindicated with hypersensitivity to irbesartan, pregnancy (use during the second or third trimester can cause injury or even death to the fetus).
- Use cautiously with hepatic or renal impairment, hypovolemia, volume or sodium depletion, lactation.

Available forms

Tablets—75, 150, 300 mg

Dosages
Adults
- *Diabetic nephropathy:* 300 mg/day PO as a single dose.
- *Hypertension:* 150 mg PO daily as one dose; adjust slowly to determine effective dose; maximum daily dose, 300 mg.

Pediatric patients 13–16 yr
150 mg/day PO; maximum dose, 300 mg.

Pediatric patients 6–12 yr
75 mg/day PO, titrate to a maximum of 150 mg/day.

Pediatric patients younger than 6 yr
Not recommended.

Volume- or salt-depleted patients
75 mg/day PO.

Pharmacokinetics

Route	Onset	Peak
Oral	Varies	1–3 hr

Metabolism: Hepatic; $T_{1/2}$: 11–15 hr
Distribution: Crosses placenta; enters breast milk
Excretion: Feces, urine

Adverse effects

- **CNS:** *Headache, dizziness,* syncope, muscle weakness, sleep disturbance
- **CV:** Hypotension, orthostatic hypotension, flushing
- **Dermatologic:** Rash, inflammation, urticaria, pruritus, alopecia, dry skin
- **GI:** *Diarrhea, abdominal pain, nausea,* constipation, dry mouth, dental pain, dyspepsia
- **Respiratory:** *URI symptoms, cough,* sinus disorders
- **Other:** Cancer in preclinical studies, back pain, fever, gout, *fatigue,* neutropenia, **angioedema**

Interactions

＊ **Drug-drug** ● Use caution with drugs metabolized by CYP2C9; anticipated effects may be altered

■ Nursing considerations
Assessment
- **History:** Hypersensitivity to irbesartan, pregnancy, lactation, hepatic or renal impairment, hypovolemia
- **Physical:** Skin lesions, turgor; T; reflexes, affect; BP; R, respiratory auscultation; LFTs, renal function tests

Interventions
- Administer without regard to meals.

⊗ **Black box warning** Ensure that patient is not pregnant before beginning therapy; suggest using barrier birth control while using irbesartan; fetal injury and deaths have been reported.

- Find an alternative method of feeding the baby if giving drug to a nursing mother. Depression of the renin-angiotensin system in infants is potentially very dangerous.

⊗ **Warning** Alert surgeon and mark the patient's chart with notice that irbesartan is being taken. The blockage of the renin-angiotensin system following surgery can produce problems. Hypotension may be reversed with volume expansion.

- Monitor patient closely in any situation that may lead to a decrease in BP secondary to reduction in fluid volume (excessive perspiration, dehydration, vomiting, diarrhea); excessive hypotension can occur.

Teaching points

- Take this drug without regard to meals. Do not stop taking this drug without consulting your health care provider.
- Use a barrier method of birth control while using this drug; if you become pregnant or desire to become pregnant, consult your health care provider. If you are breast-feeding, you should find another method of feeding the infant.
- You may experience these side effects: Dizziness (more likely to occur in any situation where you may be fluid depleted [extreme heat, exertion]; avoid driving or performing hazardous tasks); headache (medications may be available to help); nausea, vomiting, diarrhea (proper nutrition is important; consult a dietitian); symptoms of upper respiratory tract infection, cough (do not self-medicate; consult your health care provider if this becomes uncomfortable).
- Report fever, chills, dizziness, pregnancy.

DANGEROUS DRUG

▽irinotecan hydrochloride

(eh rin oh' te kan)

Camptosar

PREGNANCY CATEGORY D

Drug classes

Antineoplastic
DNA topoisomerase inhibitor

Therapeutic actions

Cytotoxic: Causes death of cells during cell division by causing damage to the DNA strand during DNA synthesis; specific to cells using topoisomerase I, DNA, and irinotecan complexes.

Indications

- First-line therapy in combination with 5-FU and leucovorin for patients with metastatic colon or rectal carcinomas
- Treatment of patients with metastatic colon or rectal cancer whose disease has recurred or progressed following 5-FU therapy
- Unlabeled uses: Cervical cancer, lung cancer, gastric cancer, CNS tumor

Contraindications and cautions

- Contraindicated with allergy to irinotecan, lactation, pregnancy.
- Use cautiously with bone marrow depression, severe diarrhea.

Available forms

Injection—20 mg/mL

Dosages

Adults

Monitor patient for toxicity at each visit, and modify dose based on patient tolerance.

- *Single-drug use:* 125 mg/m² IV over 90 min once weekly for 4 wk, then a 2-wk rest; repeat 6-wk regimen or 350 mg/m² IV over 90 min once every 3 wk.
- *Combination drugs:* 125 mg/m² IV over 90 min, days 1, 8, 15, and 22 with leucovorin 20 mg/m² IV bolus days 1, 8, 15, and 22 and 5-FU, 500 mg/m² IV days 1, 8, 15, and 22. Restart cycle on day 43. *Or* 180 mg/m² IV over 90 min days 1, 15, and 29 with leucovorin—200 mg/m² IV over 2 hr days 1, 2, 15, 16, 29, and 30 and 5-FU—400 mg/m² as IV bolus days 1, 2, 15, 16, 29, and 30 followed by 5-FU 600 mg/m² IV infusion over 22 hr on days 1, 2, 15, 16, 29, and 30. Restart cycle on day 43.

Pediatric patients

Not recommended.

Pharmacokinetics

Route	Onset	Peak
IV	Immediate	1–2 hr

Metabolism: Hepatic; $T_{1/2}$: 6–12 hr
Distribution: Crosses placenta; may enter breast milk, binds to albumin
Excretion: Bile, urine

▼ IV FACTS

Preparation: Dilute in 5% dextrose injection or 0.9% sodium chloride injection to final concentration of 0.12–2.8 mg/mL. Store diluted drug protected from light; use within 48 hr if refrigerated or within 24 hr if at room temperature (5% dextrose only). Store vials at room temperature, protected from light.
Infusion: Infuse total dose over 90 min.
Incompatibilities: Do not add any other drugs to solution.

Adverse effects

- **CNS:** Insomnia, dizziness, asthenia, confusion
- **Dermatologic:** *Alopecia,* sweating, flushing, rashes
- **GI:** *Nausea, vomiting, diarrhea,* constipation, stomatitis, flatulence, dyspepsia, abdominal pain, anorexia, mucositis
- **Hematologic: Neutropenia, leukopenia, anemia, thrombocytopenia**
- **Respiratory:** *Dyspnea,* cough, rhinitis
- **Other:** Fatigue, malaise, pain, infections, fever, cramping, weight loss, pain, infection

Interactions

✳ **Drug-drug** • Irinotecan used with other antineoplastics may cause excessive diarrhea, myelosuppression, and other associated adverse reactions • Increased risk of dehydration if patient is also on diuretics; withhold diuretics if patient has nausea and vomiting • Risk of severe toxicity with ketoconazole; combination is contraindicated

✳ **Drug-alternative therapy** • May decrease irinotecan plasma levels and efficacy if taken with St. John's Wort; combination is contraindicated

■ Nursing considerations

Assessment

- **History:** Allergy to irinotecan, diarrhea, pregnancy, lactation, bone marrow depression
- **Physical:** T; skin lesions, color, turgor; orientation, affect, reflexes; R; abdominal examination, bowel sounds; CBC with differential

Interventions

⊗ **Black box warning** Obtain CBC before each infusion; do not give to patients with a baseline neutrophil count of less than 1,500 cells/mm^2; consult with physician for reduction in dose or withholding of drug if bone marrow depression becomes evident; severe bone marrow depression can occur.

⊗ *Warning* Ensure that patient is not pregnant before beginning therapy; advise the use of barrier contraceptives.

- Monitor infusion site; if extravasation occurs, flush with sterile water and apply ice.

⊗ **Black box warning** Monitor for diarrhea; assess hydration and arrange to decrease dose if 4–6 stools/day; omit a dose if 7–9 stools/day; if 10 or more stools/day, consult a physician. Early diarrhea may be prevented or ameliorated by atropine 0.25–1 mg IV or subcutaneously; treat late diarrhea lasting more than 24 hr with loperamide; late diarrhea can be severe to life-threatening.

- Protect patient from any exposure to infection.
- Arrange for wig or other appropriate head covering when alopecia occurs.

Teaching points

- This drug can only be given by IV infusion, which should run over 90 minutes. Mark calendar with days to return for infusion. A blood test will be required before each dose.
- Do not use St. John's Wort while taking this drug.
- This drug cannot be used during pregnancy; using barrier contraceptives is suggested.
- You may experience these side effects: Increased susceptibility to infection (avoid crowded areas or people with known infections; report any injury); nausea, vomiting (eat frequent small meals; medication may be ordered); headache; loss of hair (arrange for a wig or other head covering; it is important to protect the head from extreme temperatures); diarrhea.
- Report pain at injection site, any injury or illness, fatigue, severe nausea or vomiting, increased, severe, or bloody diarrhea.

▽ iron dextran

DexFerrum, INFeD, Infufer (CAN)

PREGNANCY CATEGORY C

Drug class

Iron preparation

Therapeutic actions

Elevates the serum iron concentration and is then converted to Hgb or trapped in the reticuloendothelial cells for storage and eventual conversion to usable form of iron.

Indications

- Treatment of iron deficiency anemia only when oral administration of iron is unsatisfactory or impossible

---

- Unlabeled use: May be required for patients receiving epoetin therapy

Contraindications and cautions

- Contraindicated with allergy to iron dextran, anemias other than iron deficiency anemia, acute phase of infectious renal disease.
- Use cautiously with impaired hepatic function, rheumatoid arthritis, allergies, asthma, lactation, pregnancy.

Available forms

Injection—50 mg/mL

Dosages
Adults and pediatric patients

- *Iron deficiency anemia:* Administer a 0.5 mL IM or IV test dose before therapy. Base dosage on hematologic response with frequent Hgb determinations.

For patients weighing more than 15 kg:
Use the following formula:
Dose (mL) = [0.0442 (desired Hgb − observed Hgb) × LBW] + (0.26 × LBW), where Hgb = Hgb in g/dL and LBW = lean body weight.
Determine LBW as follows:
For males: LBW = 50 kg + 2.3 kg for each inch of patient's height over 5 ft.
For females: LBW = 45.5 kg + 2.3 kg for each inch of patient's height over 5 ft.
For children 5–15 kg and older than 4 mo:
Use the following formula:
Dose (mL) = 0.0442 (desired Hgb − observed Hgb) × W + (0.26 × W), where W = actual weight in kg.

- *Iron replacement for blood loss:* Determine dosage by the following formula: Replacement iron (in mg) = blood loss (in mL) × Hct

IM

Inject only into the upper outer quadrant of the buttocks. Give test dose of 0.5 mL IM. If tolerated, do not exceed 0.5 mL (25 mg) for infants weighing less than 5 kg; 1 mL for those more than 5 to less than 10 kg; 2 mL for all others.

IV injection

Give a test dose of 0.5 mL over at least 5 min before beginning therapy. May give up to 2 mL per daily dose (100 mg). Give slowly at 50 mg/min or less, undiluted.

Pharmacokinetics

Route	Onset	Peak
IM	Slow	1–2 wk

Metabolism: $T_{1/2}$: 6 hr
Distribution: Crosses placenta; enters breast milk
Excretion: Blood loss

▼ IV FACTS

Preparation: *Intermittent IV:* Calculate dose from formula. Give individual doses of 2 mL or less per day. Use single-dose ampules without preservatives. *IV infusion:* Dilute needed dose in 200–250 mL of normal saline.
Infusion: *Intermittent IV:* Give undiluted and slowly—1 mL or less/min. *IV infusion (not approved by the FDA):* Infuse over 1–2 hr after a test dose of 25 mL. Do not mix with other drugs or add to parenteral nutrition.

Adverse effects

- **CNS:** Headache, backache, dizziness, malaise, transitory paresthesias, seizures, numbness, syncope, unconsciousness
- **CV:** Hypotension, chest pain, shock, tachycardia, **cardiac arrest,** hypertension, arrhythmias
- **GI:** *Nausea, vomiting,* diarrhea, abdominal pain, altered taste
- **Hypersensitivity:** Hypersensitivity reactions, including **anaphylaxis;** dyspnea, urticaria, rash and itching, arthralgia and myalgia, fever, sweating, purpura
- **Local:** *Pain, inflammation and sterile abscesses at injection site, brown skin discoloration* (IM use); *lymphadenopathy, local phlebitis, peripheral vascular flushing* (IV administration)
- **Other:** *Arthritic reactivation,* fever, shivering, sweating, rash, pruritus, arthritis, iron overload, cyanosis

Interactions

✳ **Drug-drug** • Delayed response to iron dextran therapy in patients taking chloramphenicol
✳ **Drug-lab test** • Use caution when interpreting serum iron levels when done within 4 hr of iron dextran injection • Serum may be discolored to a brownish color following IV injection • Bone scans using Tc-99m diphosphonate may have abnormal areas following IM injection

■ Nursing considerations

Assessment

- **History:** Allergy to iron dextran, anemias other than iron deficiency anemia, impaired liver function, rheumatoid arthritis, allergies or asthma, lactation, pregnancy
- **Physical:** Skin lesions, color; T; injection site examination; range of motion, joints; R, adventitious sounds; liver evaluation; CBC, Hgb, Hct, serum ferritin assays, LFTs

Interventions

- Verify that patient has iron deficiency anemia before treatment.
- Arrange treatment of underlying cause of iron deficiency anemia.
- Give IM injections using the Z-track technique (displace skin laterally before injection) to avoid injection into the tissue and tissue staining. Use a large-gauge needle; if patient is standing, have patient support leg not receiving the injection. If patient is lying down, have the injection site uppermost.
- ⊗ **Black box warning** Monitor patient for hypersensitivity reactions; test dose is highly recommended. Keep epinephrine readily available in case severe hypersensitivity reaction occurs.
- Monitor serum ferritin levels periodically; these correlate well with iron stores. Do not give with oral iron preparations.
- Caution patients with rheumatoid arthritis that acute exacerbation of joint pain and swelling may occur; provide appropriate comfort measures.

Teaching points

- This drug must be given by injection (IV or intramuscularly).
- Treatment will end if anemia is corrected.
- Have periodic blood tests during therapy to assess drug response and determine appropriate dosage.
- Do not take oral iron products or vitamins with iron added while using this drug.
- You may experience these side effects: Pain at injection site, headache, joint and muscle aches, GI upset.
- Report difficulty breathing, pain at injection site, rash, itching.

▽ iron sucrose

See Appendix R, *Less commonly used drugs*.

▽ isocarboxazid

See Appendix R, *Less commonly used drugs*.

▽ isoniazid (isonicotinic acid hydrazide, INH)

*(eye soe **nye'** a zid)*

Isotamine (CAN), Nydrazid

PREGNANCY CATEGORY C

Drug class

Antituberculotic

Therapeutic actions

Bactericidal: Interferes with lipid and nucleic acid biosynthesis in actively growing tubercle bacilli.

Indications

- TB, all forms in which organisms are susceptible
- Prophylaxis in specific patients who are tuberculin reactors or household members of recently diagnosed tuberculars or who are considered to be high risk (patients with HIV, IV drug users, recent converters [5 mm or more increase on skin test within 2 yr in patients younger than 35 yr or 15 mm or more increase in patients older than 35 yr] and children younger than 4 yr with 10 mm or more induration on purified protein derivative tuberculin skin test)
- Unlabeled use: 300–400 mg/day, increased over 2 wk to 20 mg/kg/day, for improvement of severe tremor in patients with MS

Contraindications and cautions

- Contraindicated with allergy to isoniazid, isoniazid-associated hepatic injury or other severe adverse reactions to isoniazid, acute hepatic disease.
- Use cautiously with renal impairment, lactation, pregnancy.

Available forms

Tablets—100, 300 mg; syrup—50 mg/5 mL; injection—100 mg/mL

Adverse effects in *italics* are most common; those in **bold** are life-threatening.   ⊞ Do not crush.

Dosages
Adults
- *Treatment of active TB:* 5 mg/kg/day (up to 300 mg) PO in a single dose, with other effective drugs or 15 mg/kg (up to 900 mg) PO two or three times per week. "First-line treatment" is considered to be 300 mg INH plus 600 mg rifampin, each given in a single daily oral dose. Consult manufacturer's guidelines for other possible combinations.
- *Prophylaxis for TB:* 300 mg/day PO in a single dose.
- Concomitant administration of 10–50 mg/day of pyridoxine is recommended for those who are malnourished or predisposed to neuropathy (alcoholics, diabetics).

Pediatric patients
- *Treatment of active TB:* 10–15 mg/kg/day (up to 300 mg) PO in a single dose, with other effective drugs or 20–40 mg/kg (up to 900 mg/day) two or three times per week.
- *Prophylaxis for TB:* 10 mg/kg/day (up to 300 mg) PO in a single dose.

Pharmacokinetics

Route	Onset	Peak	Duration
Oral	Varies	1–2 hr	24 hr

Metabolism: Hepatic; $T_{1/2}$: 1–4 hr
Distribution: Crosses placenta; enters breast milk
Excretion: Urine

Adverse effects
- **CNS:** *Peripheral neuropathy,* seizures, toxic encephalopathy, optic neuritis and atrophy, memory impairment, toxic psychosis
- **GI:** *Nausea, vomiting, epigastric distress,* bilirubinemia, bilirubinuria, *elevated AST,* ALT levels, jaundice, **hepatitis**
- **Hematologic:** Agranulocytosis, hemolytic or aplastic anemia, **thrombocytopenia,** eosinophilia, pyridoxine deficiency, pellagra, hyperglycemia, metabolic acidosis, hypocalcemia, hypophosphatemia due to altered vitamin D metabolism
- **Hypersensitivity:** Fever, skin eruptions, lymphadenopathy, vasculitis
- **Local:** *Local irritation at IM injection site*
- **Other:** Gynecomastia, rheumatic syndrome, SLE syndrome

Interactions
* **Drug-drug** • Increased incidence of isoniazid-related hepatitis with alcohol and possibly if taken in high doses with rifampin • Increased serum levels of phenytoin • Increased effectiveness and risk of toxicity of carbamazepine • Risk of high output renal failure in fast INH acetylators with enflurane • Increased risk of hepatotoxicity with acetaminophen, rifampin
* **Drug-food** • Risk of sympathetic-type reactions with tyramine-containing foods and exaggerated response (headache, palpitations, sweating, hypotension, flushing, diarrhea, itching) to histamine-containing food (fish [skipjack, tuna] sauerkraut juice, yeast extracts)

■ Nursing considerations
Assessment
- **History:** Allergy to isoniazid, isoniazid-associated adverse reactions; acute hepatic disease; renal impairment; lactation, pregnancy
- **Physical:** Skin color, lesions; T; orientation, reflexes, peripheral sensitivity, bilateral grip strength; ophthalmologic examination; R, adventitious sounds; liver evaluation; CBC, LFTs, renal function tests, blood glucose

Interventions
- Give on an empty stomach, 1 hr before or 2 hr after meals; may be given with food if GI upset occurs.
- Give in a single daily dose. Reserve parenteral dose for patients unable to take oral medications.
- Decrease foods containing tyramine or histamine in patient's diet.
- Consult with physician and arrange for daily pyridoxine in diabetic, alcoholic, or malnourished patients; also for patients who develop peripheral neuritis, and those with HIV.
- ⊗ *Warning* Discontinue drug, and consult with physician if signs of hypersensitivity occur.
- ⊗ **Black box warning** Monitor liver enzymes monthly; risk of serious to fatal hepatitis.

Teaching points
- Take this drug in a single daily dose. Take drug on an empty stomach, 1 hour before

or 2 hours after meals. If GI distress occurs, may be taken with food.

- Take this drug regularly; avoid missing doses; do not discontinue without first consulting your health care provider.
- Do not drink alcohol, or drink as little as possible. There is an increased risk of hepatitis if these two drugs are combined.
- Avoid foods containing tyramine; consult a dietitian to obtain a list of foods containing tyramine or histamine.
- Have periodic medical check-ups, including an eye examination and blood tests, to evaluate the drug effects.
- You may experience these side effects: Nausea, vomiting, epigastric distress (take drug with meals); skin rashes or lesions; numbness, tingling, loss of sensation (use caution to prevent injury or burns).
- Report weakness, fatigue, loss of appetite, nausea, vomiting, yellowing of skin or eyes, darkening of the urine, numbness or tingling in hands or feet.

DANGEROUS DRUG

▷**isoproterenol**
*(eye soe proe **ter'** e nole)*

**isoproterenol
hydrochloride**
Isuprel

PREGNANCY CATEGORY C

Drug classes
Antiasthmatic
Beta$_1$- and beta$_2$-adrenergic agonist
Bronchodilator
Sympathomimetic
Vasopressor in shock

Therapeutic actions
Effects are mediated by beta$_1$- and beta$_2$-adrenergic receptors; acts on beta$_1$-receptors in the heart to produce positive chronotropic and positive inotropic effects and to increase automaticity; acts on beta$_2$-receptors in the bronchi to cause bronchodilation; acts on beta$_2$-receptors in smooth muscle in the walls of blood vessels in skeletal muscle and splanchnic beds to cause dilation (cardiac stimulation, va-

sodilation may be adverse effects when drug is used as bronchodilator).

Indications
- Management of bronchospasm during anesthesia; a vasopressor in shock
- Adjunct in the management of shock (hypoperfusion syndrome) and in the treatment of cardiac standstill or arrest; carotid sinus hypersensitivity; heart block; Stokes-Adams syndrome; heart failure; ventricular tachycardia and ventricular arrhythmias that require increased inotropic activity for therapy

Contraindications and cautions
- Contraindicated with hypersensitivity to isoproterenol; tachyarrhythmias, tachycardia caused by digoxin toxicity; acute angina; general anesthesia with halogenated hydrocarbons or cyclopropane (sensitize the myocardium to catecholamines); labor and delivery (may delay second stage of labor; can accelerate fetal heart beat; may cause hypoglycemia, hypokalemia, pulmonary edema in the mother, and hypoglycemia in the neonate).
- Use cautiously with unstable vasomotor system disorders, hypertension, coronary insufficiency, history of stroke, COPD patients with degenerative heart disease, diabetes mellitus, hyperthyroidism, history of seizure disorders, psychoneuroses, lactation, pregnancy.

Available forms
Injection—0.02 mg/mL (1:50,000), 0.2 mg/mL (1:5,000)

Dosages
Adults
Injection
- *Bronchospasm during anesthesia:* 0.01–0.02 mg (0.5–1 mL of diluted solution) bolus IV; repeat when necessary.
- *Shock:* 0.5–5 mcg/min; infuse IV at a rate adjusted on the basis of HR, CVP, systemic BP, and urine flow.
- *Cardiac standstill and arrhythmias:* IV injection, 0.02–0.06 mg using diluted solution. IV infusion, 5 mcg/min using diluted solution.

Pediatric patients
There are no well-controlled studies in children. The American Heart Association recommends an infusion of 0.1 mcg/kg/min as an initial dose; range, 0.1–1 mcg/kg/min.

• *Bronchospasm during anesthesia (patients 7–19 yr):* 0.05–0.17 mcg/kg/min. Maximum dose, 1.3–2.7 mcg/kg/min. Postoperative cardiac patients will need a lower dose than patients with asthma.

Geriatric patients
Patients older than 60 yr are more likely to experience side effects; use with extreme caution.

Pharmacokinetics

Route	Onset	Duration
IV	Immediate	1–2 min

Metabolism: Tissue; $T_{1/2}$: Unknown
Distribution: Crosses placenta; enters breast milk
Excretion: Urine

▼ IV FACTS

Preparation: Dilute the 1:5,000 solutions for IV injection or infusion with 5% dextrose or sodium chloride injection; a convenient dilution is 1 mg isoproterenol (5 mL) in 500 mL diluent (final concentration 1:500,000 or 2 mcg/mL).
Infusion: Dosage of 5 mcg/min is provided by infusing 2.5 mL/min; adjust dosage to keep heart rate less than 110 beats per min.
Incompatibilities: Do not combine with aminophylline, barbiturates, lidocaine, sodium bicarbonate.

Adverse effects

• **CNS:** *Restlessness, apprehension, anxiety, fear,* CNS stimulation, hyperkinesia, insomnia, tremor, drowsiness, irritability, weakness, vertigo, headache
• **CV:** *Cardiac arrhythmias, tachycardia, palpitations,* anginal pain, changes in BP, paradoxic precipitation of Stokes-Adams seizures during normal sinus rhythm or transient heart block
• **GI:** *Nausea, vomiting, heartburn,* unusual or bad taste, swelling of the parotid glands
• **Respiratory:** *Respiratory difficulties,* dyspnea, **pulmonary edema,** *coughing, bronchospasm, paradoxic airway resistance with repeated, excessive use*
• **Other:** *Sweating, pallor,* flushing, muscle cramps, blurred vision

Interactions

❋ **Drug-drug** • Increased peripheral vasoconstriction if given with ergot alkaloids; if this combination is used, monitor BP and perfusion carefully • Increased BP response may occur if combined with TCAs, halogenated hydrocarbon anesthetics, oxytocic drugs; monitor patient closely and adjust dosage as needed
• Possible arrhythmias with epinephrine; do not administer together

■ Nursing considerations
Assessment

• **History:** Hypersensitivity to isoproterenol; tachyarrhythmias; general anesthesia with halogenated hydrocarbons or cyclopropane; unstable vasomotor system disorders; hypertension; CAD; history of stroke; COPD patients with degenerative heart disease; diabetes mellitus; hyperthyroidism; seizure disorders; psychoneurotic disorders; labor and delivery; lactation
• **Physical:** Weight; skin color, T, turgor; orientation, reflexes; P, BP; R, adventitious sounds; blood and urine glucose, serum electrolytes, thyroid function tests, ECG

Interventions

• Protect drug from light, and keep in original carton until use.
• Use minimal doses for minimum periods; drug tolerance can occur with prolonged use.
⊗ *Warning* Keep a beta-adrenergic blocker (a cardioselective beta-adrenergic blocker, such as atenolol, should be used in patients with respiratory distress) readily available in case cardiac arrhythmias occur.

Teaching points

• This drug is given IV.
• You may experience these side effects: Drowsiness, dizziness, inability to sleep (use caution); nausea, vomiting (eat frequent small meals); anxiety; rapid heart rate.
• Report chest pain, dizziness, insomnia, weakness, tremor or irregular heartbeat.

▷ isosorbide nitrates
(eye soe sor' bide)

isosorbide dinitrate
Apo-ISDN (CAN), Dilatrate SR ⊞, Isochron ⊞, Isordil Titradose

isosorbide mononitrate
Imdur ⊞, ISMO, Monoket

PREGNANCY CATEGORY C

PREGNANCY CATEGORY B
(IMDUR, MONOKET)

Drug classes
Antianginal
Nitrate
Vasodilator

Therapeutic actions
Relaxes vascular smooth muscle with a resultant decrease in venous return and decrease in arterial BP, which reduces left ventricular workload and decreases myocardial oxygen consumption.

Indications
• Dinitrate: Treatment and prevention of angina pectoris
• Mononitrate: Prevention of angina pectoris; treatment of angina pectoris (*Monoket*)
• Unlabeled uses (dinitrate): Used with hydralazine in black patients with advanced heart failure; acute angle-closure glaucoma in emergent situations; achalasia
• Unlabeled use (mononitrate): Used with nadolol to prevent recurrent variceal bleeding

Contraindications and cautions
• Contraindicated with allergy to nitrates, severe anemia, head trauma, cerebral hemorrhage, hypertrophic cardiomyopathy, narrow-angle glaucoma, orthostatic hypotension.
• Use cautiously with pregnancy, lactation, acute MI, heart failure.

Available forms
Dinitrate: Tablets—5, 10, 20, 30, 40 mg; ER tablets ⊞—40 mg; SR capsules ⊞—40 mg; SL tablets—2.5, 5 mg
Mononitrate: Tablets —10, 20 mg; ER tablets ⊞—30, 60, 120 mg

Dosages
Adults
To avoid tolerance to drug, take short-acting products bid or tid with last dose no later than 7 PM and ER or SR products once daily or bid at 8 AM and 2 PM. This creates a nitrate-free period.
Isosorbide dinitrate
• *Angina pectoris:* Starting dose, 2.5–5 mg sublingual or 5- to 20-mg oral tablets. For maintenance, 10–40 mg every 6 hr or tid oral tablets or capsules; SR or ER, initially 40 mg, then 40–80 mg PO every 8–12 hr.
• *Acute prophylaxis:* Initial dosage, 2.5–5 mg sublingually every 2–3 hr. Give 15 min before activity that may cause angina.
Isosorbide mononitrate
• *Prevention of angina:* 20 mg PO bid given 7 hr apart. In smaller patients, start with 5 mg (one-half of 10-mg tablet) but then increase to at least 10 mg by day 2 or 3 of therapy. Give first dose when waking and second dose 7 hr later. This creates a nitrate-free period and minimizes tolerance to drug. ER tablets—30–60 mg/day PO may be increased to 120 mg/day if needed.
Pediatric patients
Safety and efficacy not established.

Pharmacokinetics

Route	Onset	Duration
Oral	15–45 min	4–6 hr
Oral SR, ER	Up to 4 hr	6–8 hr
SL	2–5 min	1–2 hr

Metabolism: Hepatic; $T_{1/2}$: 5 min, then 2–5 hr
Distribution: May cross placenta; may enter breast milk
Excretion: Urine

Adverse effects
• **CNS:** *Headache, apprehension, restlessness, weakness,* vertigo, dizziness, faintness
• **CV:** *Tachycardia, retrosternal discomfort, palpitations, hypotension,* **syncope,** *collapse, orthostatic hypotension, angina, rebound hypertension,* atrial fibrillation
• **Dermatologic:** Rash, exfoliative dermatitis, cutaneous vasodilation with flushing
• **GI:** *Nausea,* vomiting, incontinence of feces, abdominal pain, diarrhea, ulcer

Adverse effects in *italics* are most common; those in **bold** are life-threatening. ⊞ Do not crush.

- **GU:** Dysuria, impotence, urinary frequency
- **Other:** Muscle twitching, pallor, perspiration, cold sweat, arthralgia, bronchitis, thrombocytopenia

Interactions
✲ Drug-drug • Increased systolic BP and decreased antianginal effect if taken concurrently with ergot alkaloids
✲ Drug-lab test • False report of decreased serum cholesterol if done by the Zlatkis-Zak color reaction

■ Nursing considerations

CLINICAL ALERT!
Name confusion has occurred between *Isordil* (isosorbide) and *Plendil* (felodipine); use caution.

Assessment
- **History:** Allergy to nitrates, severe anemia, GI hypermobility, head trauma, cerebral hemorrhage, hypertrophic cardiomyopathy, pregnancy, lactation
- **Physical:** Skin color, T, lesions; orientation, reflexes, affect; P, BP, orthostatic BP, baseline ECG, peripheral perfusion; R, adventitious sounds; liver evaluation, normal output; CBC, Hgb

Interventions
- Give sublingual preparations under the tongue or in the buccal pouch; discourage the patient from swallowing.
- Create a nitrate-free period to minimize tolerance.
⊗ **Warning** Give chewable tablets slowly, only 5 mg initially, because severe hypotension can occur; ensure that patient does not chew or crush SR or ER preparations.
- Give oral preparations on an empty stomach, 1 hr before or 2 hr after meals; take with meals if severe, uncontrolled headache occurs.
⊗ **Warning** Keep life-support equipment readily available if overdose occurs or cardiac condition worsens.
⊗ **Warning** Gradually reduce dose if anginal treatment is being terminated; rapid discontinuation can lead to problems of withdrawal.

Teaching points
- Place sublingual tablets under your tongue or in your cheek; do not chew, swallow, or

crush the tablet. Take the isosorbide before chest pain begins, when activities or situation may precipitate an attack. Take oral isosorbide dinitrate on an empty stomach, 1 hour before or 2 hours after meals; do not chew or crush extended- or sustained-release preparations; do not take isosorbide mononitrate to relieve acute anginal episodes.
- You may experience these side effects: Dizziness, light-headedness (may be transient; use care to change positions slowly); headache (lie down in a cool environment, rest; over-the-counter preparations may not help; take drug with meals); flushing of the neck or face (reversible).
- Report blurred vision, persistent or severe headache, rash, more frequent or more severe angina attacks, fainting.

▷ **isotretinoin** (13-*cis*-retinoic acid, vitamin A metabolite)
(*eye so* **tret'** *i noyn*)

Amnesteem ⓒⓐⓝ, Claravis ⓒⓐⓝ, Sotret ⓒⓐⓝ

PREGNANCY CATEGORY X

Drug classes
Acne product
Retinoid (first generation)
Vitamin metabolite

Therapeutic actions
Decreases sebaceous gland size and inhibits sebaceous gland differentiation, resulting in a reduction in sebum secretion; inhibits follicular keratinization; exact mechanism of action is not known.

Indications
- Treatment of severe recalcitrant nodular acne unresponsive to conventional treatments
- Unlabeled uses: Treatment of cutaneous disorders of keratinization, cutaneous T-cell lymphoma and leukoplakia, psoriasis, rosacea, pityriasis rubra pilaris, keratoacanthomas

Contraindications and cautions
- Contraindicated with allergy to isotretinoin, parabens, or product component; pregnancy

(has caused severe fetal malformations and spontaneous abortions); lactation.
• Use cautiously with history of severe depression, suicidal ideation, diabetes mellitus, pediatric patients with genetic predisposition to age-related osteoporosis, a history of childhood osteoporosis, osteomalacia, other diseases of bone metabolism.

Available forms

Capsules ⊕ᴅᴺᴳ—10, 20, 30, 40 mg; soft gel capsules ⊕ᴅᴺᴳ—10, 20, 30, 40 mg

Dosages

Adults and pediatric patients 12 yr and older

Individualize dosage based on side effects and disease response. Initial dose, 0.5–1 mg/kg/day PO; usual dosage range is 0.5–2 mg/kg/day divided into two doses for 15–20 wk. Maximum daily dose, 2 mg/kg. If a second course of therapy is needed, allow a rest period of at least 8 wk between courses. Must take with food or absorption of drug will decrease.

Pharmacokinetics

Route	Onset	Peak	Duration
Oral	Varies	2.9–3.2 hr	6–20 hr

Metabolism: Hepatic; $T_{1/2}$: 10–20 hr
Distribution: Crosses placenta; may enter breast milk
Excretion: Urine

Adverse effects

• **CNS:** *Lethargy, insomnia, fatigue, headache,* pseudotumor cerebri (papilledema, headache, nausea, vomiting, visual disturbances); depression, psychoses, **suicide,** aggressive or violent behavior
• **CV:** Palpitations, tachycardia, vascular thrombotic disease
• **Dermatologic:** *Skin fragility, dry skin, pruritus, rash,* thinning of hair, peeling of palms and soles, skin infections, photosensitivity, nail brittleness, petechiae
• **EENT:** *Cheilitis, eye irritation, conjunctivitis,* corneal opacities, epistaxis
• **GI:** *Nausea, vomiting, abdominal pain,* anorexia, inflammatory bowel disease, dry mouth, gum irritation
• **GU:** *White cells in the urine, proteinuria, hematuria*

• **Hematologic:** Elevated sedimentation rate, hypertriglyceridemia, abnormal liver function tests, increased fasting serum glucose
• **Musculoskeletal:** Skeletal hyperostosis, arthralgia, bone and joint pain and stiffness
• **Respiratory:** *Epistaxis, dry nose, bronchospasms*

Interactions

❋ **Drug-drug** • Increased toxicity when taken with vitamin A; avoid this combination • Risk of increased adverse effects if combined with systemic corticosteroids, phenytoin; use caution if these combinations are used • Risk of pseudotumor cerebri with concomitant tetracycline use

■ Nursing considerations

Assessment

• **History:** Allergy to isotretinoin, parabens, or product component; diabetes mellitus; pregnancy; lactation; history of depression
• **Physical:** Skin color, lesions, turgor, texture; joint range of motion; orientation, reflexes, affect, ophthalmologic examination; mucous membranes, bowel sounds; serum triglycerides, HDL, sedimentation rate, CBC and differential, urinalysis, pregnancy test

Interventions

⊗ *Black box warning* Ensure that patient reads and signs the consent form that comes with this drug. Place this form in the patient's permanent record.
⊗ *Black box warning* Ensure that patient is not pregnant before therapy; test for pregnancy within 2 wk of beginning therapy. Advise patient to use two forms of contraception starting 1 mo before therapy, during treatment, and for 1 mo after treatment is discontinued. Patient must sign consent form acknowledging this information; form should be kept in patient's medical record. Pharmacists must register patients in iPLEDGE program before dispensing drug. Patient may obtain no more than a 30-day supply.
• Do not give a second course of therapy within 8 wk of first course.
• Give drug with meals; do not crush capsules.
• Do not give vitamin supplements that contain vitamin A.

Adverse effects in *italics* are most common; those in **bold** are life-threatening. ⊕ᴅᴺᴳ Do not crush.

⊗ **Warning** Discontinue drug if signs of papilledema occur; consult with a neurologist for further care.

⊗ **Warning** Discontinue drug at any indication of severe depression or psychoses. Patient must sign informed consent concerning risk of suicide; form should be kept in patient's medical record.

• Discontinue drug if visual disturbances occur; arrange for an ophthalmologic examination.

⊗ **Warning** Discontinue drug if abdominal pain, rectal bleeding, or severe diarrhea occurs; consult with physician.

• Monitor triglycerides during therapy; if elevation occurs, institute measures to lower serum triglycerides: Reduce weight, reduce dietary fat, exercise, increase intake of insoluble fiber, decrease alcohol consumption.
• Monitor diabetic patients with frequent blood glucose determinations.
• Do not allow blood donation from patients taking isotretinoin due to the teratogenic effects of the drug.

Teaching points

• Only 1 month's prescription can be given at a time. You will need to complete a consent form before this drug is prescribed.
• Take drug with meals; do not crush capsules.
• Transient flare-ups of acne may occur at beginning of therapy.
• There is a risk of injury in pediatric patients who participate in sports that involve repetitive impact; parents should monitor activity and alert coaches.
• Use two forms of contraception 1 month before treatment, during treatment, and for 1 month after treatment is discontinued. This drug has been associated with severe birth defects and miscarriages; it is contraindicated in pregnant women. If you think that you are pregnant, consult your health care provider immediately. You must sign a consent form stating your understanding of the need for contraception.
• Do not donate blood while using this drug because of its potential effects on the fetus of a blood recipient.
• Avoid vitamin supplements containing vitamin A; serious toxic effects may occur. Limit your consumption of alcohol. You also may need to limit your intake of fats and

increase exercise to limit drug effects on blood triglyceride levels.
• Avoid wax expilation and skin resurfacing during and for 6 months after therapy; scarring could occur.
• You may experience these side effects: Dizziness, lethargy, headache, visual changes (avoid driving or performing tasks that require alertness); sensitivity to the sun (avoid sunlamps, exposure to the sun; use sunscreens, protective clothing); diarrhea, abdominal pain, loss of appetite (take drug with meals); dry mouth (suck sugarless candies); eye irritation and redness, inability to wear contact lenses; dry skin, itching, redness, nose bleeds.
• Report headache with nausea and vomiting, severe diarrhea or rectal bleeding, visual difficulties, depression, suicidal ideation, violent or aggressive behavior.

▽ **isradipine**
(eyes rad' i peen)

DynaCirc CR ⓞⓡⓒ

PREGNANCY CATEGORY C

Drug classes
Antihypertensive
Calcium channel blocker

Therapeutic actions
Inhibits the movement of calcium ions across the membranes of cardiac and arterial muscle cells; calcium is involved in the generation of the action potential in specialized automatic and conducting cells in the heart and in arterial smooth muscle and excitation-contraction coupling in cardiac muscle cells; inhibition of transmembrane calcium flow results in the depression of impulse formation in specialized cardiac pacemaker cells, slowing of the velocity of conduction of the cardiac impulse, the depression of myocardial contractility, and the dilation of coronary arteries and arterioles and peripheral arterioles. These effects lead to decreased cardiac work, cardiac energy consumption, and BP.

Indications
• Management of hypertension alone or in combination with thiazide-type diuretics

Contraindications and cautions

- Contraindicated with allergy to isradipine; sick sinus syndrome, except with ventricular pacemaker; heart block (second or third degree); IHSS; cardiogenic shock.
- Use cautiously in the elderly and with hypotension, impaired hepatic or renal function (repeated doses may accumulate), pregnancy, lactation, heart failure.

Available forms

Capsules—2.5, 5 mg; CR tablets ⓄⓃⒸ—5, 10 mg

Dosages

Adults
Initial dose of 2.5 mg PO bid. An antihypertensive effect is usually seen within 2–3 hr; maximal response may require 2–4 wk. Dosage may be increased in increments of 5 mg/day at 2- to 4-wk intervals. Maximum dose, 20 mg/day. CR: 5–10 mg PO daily as monotherapy or combined with thiazide diuretic.

Pediatric patients
Safety and efficacy are not established.

Geriatric patients and patients with hepatic or renal impairment
Starting dose is 5 mg/day PO for CR tablets; 2.5 mg PO bid for capsules.

Pharmacokinetics

Route	Onset	Peak
Oral	40 min	90 min
CR	NA	7–8 hr

Metabolism: Hepatic; $T_{1/2}$: 8 hr
Distribution: Crosses placenta; enters breast milk; 95% protein-bound
Excretion: Feces, urine

Adverse effects

- **CNS:** *Dizziness,* vertigo, emotional depression, sleepiness, *headache*
- **CV:** *Peripheral edema, hypotension,* arrhythmias, bradycardia, **AV heart block, angina, MI, stroke** (increased risk with isradipine than with other calcium channel blockers)
- **GI:** *Nausea,* constipation, abdominal discomfort, diarrhea
- **Other:** Muscle fatigue, diaphoresis, fatigue, rash

Interactions

✴ **Drug-drug** ● Increased cardiac depression with beta-adrenergic blocking drugs ● Increased serum levels of digoxin, carbamazepine, prazosin, and quinidine ● Increased respiratory depression with atracurium, pancuronium, tubocurarine, and vecuronium ● Decreased effects with calcium and rifampin ● Increased isradipine levels with azole antifungals and H_2 antagonists ● Risk of severe hypotension with fentanyl anesthesia; use caution

■ Nursing considerations

Assessment

- **History:** Allergy to isradipine; sick sinus syndrome, heart block; IHSS; cardiogenic shock, severe heart failure; hypotension; impaired hepatic or renal function; pregnancy; lactation
- **Physical:** Skin color, edema; orientation, reflexes; P, BP, baseline ECG, peripheral perfusion, auscultation; R, adventitious sounds; liver evaluation, normal output; LFTs, renal function tests, urinalysis

Interventions

- Consider increased risk of angina, MI, and stroke with use of this drug; select patients carefully.
- ⊗ **Warning** Monitor patient carefully (BP, cardiac rhythm, and output) while drug is being adjusted to therapeutic dose.
- Monitor BP very carefully with concurrent doses of other antihypertensive drugs.
- Monitor cardiac rhythm regularly during stabilization of dosage and periodically during long-term therapy.
- ⊗ **Warning** Monitor patients with renal or hepatic impairment carefully for drug accumulation and adverse reactions.

Teaching points

- Swallow controlled-release tablets whole. Do not crush, chew, or divide them. The empty shell is eliminated in the stool.
- You may experience these side effects: Nausea, vomiting (eat frequent small meals); headache (monitor lighting, noise, and temperature; medication may be ordered if severe); dizziness, sleepiness (avoid driving or operating dangerous equipment); emotional depression (should pass when the drug is stopped); constipation (measures may be taken to alleviate this problem).

- Report irregular heartbeat, shortness of breath, swelling of the hands or feet, pronounced dizziness, constipation.

▽itraconazole
*(eye tra **kon'** a zole)*

Sporanox

PREGNANCY CATEGORY C

Drug class
Antifungal—triazole

Therapeutic actions
Binds to sterols in the fungal cell membrane, changing membrane permeability; fungicidal or fungistatic depending on concentration and organism.

Indications
- Parenteral and oral: Treatment of blastomycosis, histoplasmosis in immunocompromised and nonimmunocompromised patients
- Parenteral and oral: Treatment of aspergillosis in patients intolerant or refractory to amphotericin B
- Treatment of onychomycosis due to dermatophytes (capsules only)
- Parenteral and oral: Treatment of febrile neutropenic patients with suspected fungal infections
- Oral solution: Treatment of fungal, candidiasis infections of the esophagus or mouth
- Unlabeled uses: Treatment of superficial and systemic mycoses, fungal keratitis, cutaneous leishmaniasis; used as an alternative to fluconazole for HIV patients to prevent candiasis, cryptococcosis, and coccidiodomycosis

Contraindications and cautions
- Contraindicated with hypersensitivity to itraconazole or other azoles, lactation, heart failure, history of prolonged QTc interval.
- Use cautiously with hepatic or renal impairment, arrhythmias, pregnancy.

Available forms
Capsules—100 mg; oral solution—10 mg/mL

Dosages
Adults
- *Empiric febrile neutropenia:* 200 mg PO bid until clinically significant neutropenia resolves.
- *Candidiasis:* 200 mg/day PO (oral solution only) for 1–2 wk (oropharyngeal); 100 mg/day for a minimum of 3 wk (esophageal); 200 mg/day in AIDS patients and neutropenic patients.
- *Blastomycosis or chronic histoplasmosis:* 200 mg/day PO for a minimum of 3 mo, may increase to a maximum of 400 mg/day.
- *Other systemic mycoses:* 100–200 mg/day PO for 3–6 mo.
- *Dermatophytoses:* 100–200 mg/day to bid for 7–28 days, determined by specific infection.
- *Fingernail onychomycosis:* 200 mg bid PO for 1 wk, followed by 3-wk rest period; repeat.
- *Toenail onychomycosis:* 200 mg/day PO for 12 wk.
- *Aspergillosis:* 200–400 mg/day PO.

Oral solution
100–200 mg (10–20 mL), rinse and hold, swallow solution daily for 1–3 wk.

Pediatric patients
Safety and efficacy not established.

Patients with renal impairment
Do not give to patients if creatinine clearance less than 30 mL/min.

Pharmacokinetics

Route	Onset	Peak	Duration
Oral	Slow	4.6 hr	4–6 days

Metabolism: Hepatic; $T_{1/2}$: 21 hr, then 64 hr
Distribution: Crosses placenta; may enter breast milk, highly protein-bound
Excretion: Feces, urine

Adverse effects
- **CNS:** *Headache,* dizziness
- **CV:** **Heart failure**
- **GI:** *Nausea, vomiting, diarrhea, abdominal pain,* anorexia, hepatic function abnormality
- **Other:** *Rash, edema,* fever, malaise

Interactions
✳ **Drug-drug** ⊗ ***Black box warning***
Potential for serious CV events, including ventricular tachycardia and death, if taken with lovastatin, simvastatin, triazolam, midazolam,

nisoldipine, felodipine, methadone, ergots, cisapride, levomethadyl, pimozide, dofetilide, and quinidine due to significant CYP450 inhibition; avoid these combinations • Increased serum levels and therefore therapeutic and toxic effects of cyclosporine, digoxin, oral hypoglycemics, warfarin anticoagulants, phenytoin, and buspirone • Decreased serum levels with histamine-2 antagonists, antacids, proton pump inhibitors, isoniazid, phenytoin, rifampin, carbamazepine, phenobarbital, and nevirapine • Increased plasma level of itraconazole with macrolide antibiotics and protease inhibitors • Potential for prolonged sedation if combined with benzodiazepines • Increased risk of rhabdomyolysis with lovastatin

✳ **Drug-food** • Risk of decreased effectiveness if combined with grapefruit juice, orange juice • Risk of increased effects if combined with cola beverages; avoid this combination

■ Nursing considerations
Assessment
- **History:** Hypersensitivity to itraconazole, hepatic impairment, lactation, heart failure, prolonged QTc interval, pregnancy
- **Physical:** Skin color, lesions; T; orientation, reflexes, affect; bowel sounds, BP, P, auscultation; LFTs; culture of area involved, ECG

Interventions
- Culture of infection before beginning therapy; begin treatment before laboratory results are returned.
- Screen medications to prevent serious drug interactions.
- Decrease dosage in cases of hepatic failure.
- ⊗ *Black box warning* Do not administer to patients with evidence of cardiac dysfunction or heart failure; risk of severe heart failure.
- Give oral capsules with meals to facilitate absorption.
- ⊗ *Warning* Monitor LFTs regularly in patients with a history of hepatic impairment; discontinue or decrease dosage at signs of increased liver toxicity.
- Discontinue drug at any sign of active liver disease—elevated enzymes, hepatitis; or signs of heart failure.

Teaching points
- Take the full course of drug therapy that has been prescribed. Therapy may need to be long term.
- Take capsules with food; take oral solution without food.
- Do not use grapefruit juice, orange juice, or cola beverages while taking this drug.
- Adopt hygiene measures to prevent reinfection or spread of infection.
- Have frequent follow-up visits while you are using this drug. Keep all appointments, which may include those for blood tests.
- Women of childbearing age should use contraceptives during therapy and for 1 month after therapy is stopped.
- You may experience these side effects: Nausea, vomiting, diarrhea (eat frequent small meals); headache (analgesics may be ordered); rash, itching (appropriate medication may help).
- Report unusual fatigue, anorexia, vomiting, jaundice, dark urine, pale stool, edema, difficulty breathing.

▽ **ivacaftor**

See Appendix R, *Less commonly used drugs.*

▽ **ivermectin**

See Appendix R, *Less commonly used drugs.*

▽ **ixabepilone**

See Appendix R, *Less commonly used drugs.*

▽ **ketoconazole**
*(kee toe **koe'** na zole)*

Apo-Ketoconazole (CAN), Extina, Nizoral A-D, Xolegel, Xolegel Care Pack, Xolegel Duo Convenience Pack

PREGNANCY CATEGORY C

Drug class
Antifungal (imidazole)

Therapeutic actions

Impairs the synthesis of ergosterol, the main sterol of fungal cell membranes, allowing increased permeability and leakage of cellular components and causing cell death.

Indications

- Treatment of systemic fungal infections: Candidiasis, chronic mucocutaneous candidiasis, oral thrush, candiduria, blastomycosis, coccidioidomycosis, histoplasmosis, chromomycosis, paracoccidioidomycosis
- Treatment of dermatophytosis (recalcitrant infections not responding to topical or griseofulvin therapy)
- Topical treatment of seborrheic dermatitis in patients older than 12 yr
- Cream, gel: Tinea corporis (ringworm), tinea cruris (jock itch), and tinea pedis (athlete's foot)
- Shampoo: Reduction of scaling due to dandruff
- Orphan drug use: With cyclosporine to diminish cyclosporine-induced nephrotoxicity in organ transplant
- Unlabeled uses: Treatment of onychomycosis, pityriasis versicolor, vaginal candidiasis, tinea pedis, tinea corporis, tinea cruris, tinea capitis; CNS fungal infections at high doses (800–1,200 mg/day); advanced prostate cancer at doses of 400 mg every 8 hr; Cushing syndrome (800–1,200 mg/day); refractory depression

Contraindications and cautions

- Contraindicated with allergy to ketoconazole; fungal meningitis; administration with terfenadine, astemizole, oral triazolam; pregnancy; lactation.
- Use cautiously with hepatic failure (increased risk of hepatocellular necrosis).

Available forms

Tablets—200 mg; shampoo—1% (OTC), 2%; topical gel—2%; cream—2%; topical foam—2%

Dosages

Adults

200 mg PO daily. Up to 400 mg/day in severe infections. Treatment period must be long enough to prevent recurrence, 1 wk–6 mo, depending on infecting organism and site.

Pediatric patients older than 2 yr

3.3–6.6 mg/kg/day PO as a single dose.

Pediatric patients younger than 2 yr

Safety and efficacy not established.

Shampoo

Moisten hair and scalp thoroughly with water; apply sufficient shampoo to produce a lather; leave on hair for 5 min. Shampoo twice a week for 4 wk with at least 3 days between shampooing. Up to 8 wk may be needed.

Topical

Patients older than 12 yr

- *Tinea pedis, tinea corporis, tinea cruris, cutaneous candidiasis:* Apply thin film of gel, foam, or cream once daily to affected areas for 2 wk; do not wash this area for 3 hr after applying. Wait 20 min before applying makeup or sunscreen. May require 6 wk of treatment.

Foam

- *Seborrheic dermatitis:* Apply foam bid for 4 wk.

Pharmacokinetics

Route	Onset	Peak
Oral	Varies	1–2 hr
Topical	Slow	Unknown

Metabolism: Hepatic; $T_{1/2}$: 8 hr
Distribution: Crosses placenta; enters breast milk
Excretion: Bile, urine

Adverse effects

- **CNS:** Headache, dizziness, somnolence, photophobia
- **GI:** Hepatotoxicity, *nausea, vomiting,* abdominal pain
- **GU:** Impotence, oligospermia (with very high doses)
- **Hematologic:** Thrombocytopenia, leukopenia, hemolytic anemia
- **Hypersensitivity:** Urticaria to **anaphylaxis**
- **Local:** Severe irritation, *pruritus, stinging* with topical application
- **Other:** *Pruritus,* fever, chills, gynecomastia

Interactions

✳ **Drug-drug** • Decreased blood levels of ketoconazole with rifampin due to significant CYP 450 inhibition • Increased blood levels of cyclosporine and risk of toxicity • Increased duration of adrenal suppression with corticosteroids ● Decreased absorption if taken with antacids, histamine-2 blockers, proton pump inhibitors; space these at least 2 hr apart ● Potent inhibitor of CYP3A4 enzyme system. Use with drugs metabolized via this system (eg, tacrolimus, warfarin) may lead to increased plasma levels and toxicity; use is contraindicated.

■ Nursing considerations

Assessment

- **History:** Allergy to ketoconazole, fungal meningitis, hepatic failure, pregnancy, lactation
- **Physical:** Skin color, lesions; orientation, reflexes, affect; bowel sounds; LFTs; CBC and differential; culture of area involved

Interventions

- Culture fungus before therapy; begin treatment before return of laboratory results.

⊗ *Warning* Keep epinephrine readily available in case of severe anaphylaxis after first dose.

⊗ **Black box warning** Risk of serious to fatal hepatic toxicity; monitor patient closely.

- Administer oral drug with food to decrease GI upset.
- Do not administer with antacids, H₂-blockers, proton pump inhibitors; ketoconazole requires an acidic environment for absorption; if antacids are required, administer at least 2 hr apart.
- Continue administration for long-term therapy until infection is eradicated: Candidiasis, 1–2 wk; other systemic mycoses, 6 mo; chronic mucocutaneous candidiasis, often requires maintenance therapy; tinea versicolor, 2 wk of topical application.
- Stop treatment, and consult physician about diagnosis if no improvement is seen within 2 wk of topical application.
- Administer shampoo as follows: Moisten hair and scalp thoroughly with water; apply sufficient shampoo to produce a lather; gently massage for 1 min; rinse hair with warm water; repeat, leaving on hair for 3 min.
- Arrange to monitor hepatic function tests before therapy and monthly or more frequently throughout treatment.

Teaching points

- Take the full course of drug therapy. Long-term use of the drug will be needed; beneficial effects may not be seen for several weeks.

- Take oral drug with meals to decrease GI upset.
- If using shampoo, moisten hair and scalp thoroughly with water; apply sufficient shampoo to produce a lather; leave on hair for 5 minutes. Shampoo twice a week for 4 weeks with at least 3 days between shampooing.
- Apply thin layer of gel, foam, or cream to affected area for 2 weeks. Wait 20 minutes before applying makeup or sunscreen to area, and do not wash area for 3 hours.
- Use appropriate hygiene measures to prevent reinfection or spread of infection.
- Do not take antacids, histamine-2 blockers, proton pump inhibitors with this drug; if they are needed, take this drug at least 2 hours after their administration.
- You may experience these side effects: Nausea, vomiting, diarrhea (take drug with food); sedation, dizziness, confusion (avoid driving or performing tasks that require alertness); stinging, irritation (local application).
- Report rash, severe nausea, vomiting, diarrhea, fever, sore throat, unusual bleeding or bruising, yellow skin or eyes, dark urine or pale stools, severe irritation (local application).

▷ketoprofen
*(kee toe **proe'** fen)*

PREGNANCY CATEGORY B
(FIRST AND SECOND TRIMESTERS)

PREGNANCY CATEGORY D
(THIRD TRIMESTER)

Drug classes
Nonopioid analgesic
NSAID

Therapeutic actions
Anti-inflammatory and analgesic activity; inhibits prostaglandin and leukotriene synthesis and has antibradykinin and lysosomal membrane-stabilizing actions.

Indications
- Acute and long-term treatment of rheumatoid arthritis and osteoarthritis
- Relief of mild to moderate pain

Adverse effects in *italics* are most common; those in **bold** are life-threatening. ⬛ Do not crush.

- Treatment of dysmenorrhea
- Reduction of fever (OTC indication)
- Unlabeled use: Juvenile idiopathic arthritis

Contraindications and cautions

- Contraindicated with significant renal impairment, pregnancy, lactation; allergy to ketoprofen, aspirin; immediate coronary artery bypass procedure.
- Use cautiously with impaired hearing; allergies; hepatic, CV, and GI conditions.

Available forms

Capsules—50, 75 mg; ER capsules—100, 150, 200 mg

Dosages
Adults
Do not exceed 300 mg/day, or 200 mg/day ER.
- *Rheumatoid arthritis, osteoarthritis:* Starting dose, 75 mg tid or 50 mg qid PO. Maintenance dose, 150–300 mg PO in three or four divided doses. ER, 200 mg PO daily.
- *Mild to moderate pain, primary dysmenorrhea:* 25–50 mg PO every 6–8 hr as needed.
Pediatric patients
Safety and efficacy not established.
Geriatric patients or patients with hepatic or renal impairment
Reduce starting dose by one-half or one-third; maximum dose, 100 mg/day.

Pharmacokinetics

Route	Onset	Peak
Oral	30–60 min	0.5–2 hr
ER oral	30–60 min	6–7 hr

Metabolism: Hepatic; $T_{1/2}$: 2–4 hr, 5–6 hr for ER
Distribution: Crosses placenta; enters breast milk
Excretion: Urine

Adverse effects

- **CNS:** *Headache, dizziness,* somnolence, *insomnia,* fatigue, tiredness, tinnitus, ophthalmologic effects
- **Dermatologic:** *Rash,* pruritus, sweating, dry mucous membranes
- **GI:** *Nausea, dyspepsia, GI pain,* diarrhea, vomiting, *constipation,* flatulence, **gastric or duodenal ulcer**

- **GU:** Dysuria, **renal impairment**
- **Hematologic:** Bleeding, platelet inhibition with higher doses, neutropenia, eosinophilia, leukopenia, thrombocytopenia, agranulocytosis, aplastic anemia, menorrhagia
- **Respiratory:** Dyspnea, hemoptysis, pharyngitis, bronchospasm, rhinitis
- **Other:** Peripheral edema, **anaphylactoid reactions to anaphylactic shock**

Interactions

✳ **Drug-drug** ● Increased risk of nephrotoxicity with other nephrotoxins (aminoglycosides, cyclosporine, diuretics) ● Increased risk of bleeding with anticoagulants (warfarin) and aspirin

■ Nursing considerations
Assessment

- **History:** Renal impairment, impaired hearing, allergies, hepatic, CV, and GI conditions, lactation, pregnancy
- **Physical:** Skin color and lesions; orientation, reflexes, ophthalmologic and audiometric evaluation, peripheral sensation; P, BP, edema; R, adventitious sounds; liver evaluation; CBC, clotting times, LFTs, renal function tests; serum electrolytes, stool guaiac

Interventions

⊗ **Black box warning** Be aware that patient may be at increased risk for CV events, GI bleeding; monitor accordingly.

⊗ **Black box warning** Contraindicated for the treatment of perioperative pain following coronary artery bypass graft; serious adverse effects have been reported.

- Administer drug with food or after meals if GI upset occurs.
- Arrange for periodic ophthalmologic examination during long-term therapy.

⊗ **Warning** If overdose occurs, institute emergency procedures: Gastric lavage, induction of emesis, supportive therapy.

Teaching points

- Take drug with food or meals if GI upset occurs; take only the prescribed dosage.
- Use during pregnancy is not advised; if an analgesic is needed, consult your health care provider.
- Dizziness, drowsiness can occur (avoid driving or using dangerous machinery).

- For over-the-counter use: Do not take for more than 3 days for fever or for more than 10 days for pain. If symptoms persist, contact your health care provider.
- Report sore throat, fever, rash, itching, weight gain, swelling in ankles or fingers; changes in vision; black, tarry stools; easy bruising.

▷ketorolac tromethamine

(kee' toe role ak)

Acular LS, Acuvail, Sprix

PREGNANCY CATEGORY C
(FIRST AND SECOND TRIMESTERS)

PREGNANCY CATEGORY D
(THIRD TRIMESTER)

Drug classes
Antipyretic
Nonopioid analgesic
NSAID

Therapeutic actions
Anti-inflammatory and analgesic activity; inhibits prostaglandins and leukotriene synthesis.

Indications
- Short-term management of pain (up to 5 days)
- Ophthalmic: Relief of ocular itching due to seasonal conjunctivitis and relief of postoperative inflammation and pain after cataract surgery

Contraindications and cautions
- Contraindicated with significant renal impairment, during labor and delivery, lactation; patients wearing soft contact lenses (ophthalmic); aspirin allergy; concurrent use of NSAIDs; active peptic ulcer disease, recent GI bleed or perforation, history of peptic ulcer disease or GI bleeding; hypersensitivity to ketorolac; as prophylactic analgesic before major surgery; treatment of perioperative pain in CABG; suspected or confirmed cerebrovascular bleeding; hemorrhagic diathesis, incomplete hemostasis, high risk of bleeding; use with probenecid, pentoxyphylline.

- Use cautiously with impaired hearing; allergies; hepatic, CV and GI conditions.

Available forms
Ophthalmic solution—0.4%, 0.45%, 0.5%; tablets—10 mg; injection—15, 30 mg/mL; nasal spray—15.75 mg/spray

Dosages
For short-term use only (up to 5 days). Potent NSAID with many adverse effects.
Adults
Parenteral
- *Single-dose treatment:* 60 mg IM or 30 mg IV.
- *Multiple-dose treatment:* 30 mg IM or IV every 6 hr to a maximum 120 mg/day.
Oral
- *Transfer to oral:* 20 mg PO as a first dose for patients who received 60 mg IM or 30 mg IV as a single dose or 30-mg multiple dose, followed by 10 mg every 4–6 hr; do not exceed 40 mg/24 hr.
Nasal spray
- *Patients younger than 65 yr:* 1 spray (15.75 mg) in each nostril every 6–8 hr; maximum daily dose, 126 mg.
- *Patients 65 yr and older, patients with renal impairment, and patients weighing less than 50 kg:* 1 spray in one nostril every 6–8 hr; maximum daily dose, 63 mg.
Ophthalmic
- *Itching from allergic conjunctivitis:* 1 drop qid.
- *Acular:* For cataract surgery, begin 1 drop qid 24 hr after and continue for 2 wk.
- *Acular LS:* 1 drop qid prn for burning and stinging for up to 4 days after surgery. For pain and photophobia, use for 3 days.
- *Acuvail:* 1 drop twice a day beginning 1 day before cataract surgery; continue the day of surgery and for the next 2 weeks.
Pediatric patients 2–16 yr
Use one single-dose injection—1 mg/kg IM up to a maximum of 30 mg, or 0.5 mg/kg IV up to a maximum of 15 mg.
Geriatric patients 65 yr and older, patients with renal impairment, and patients weighing less than 50 kg
Parenteral
- *Single-dose treatment:* 30 mg IM or 15 mg IV.
- *Multiple-dose treatment:* 15 mg IM or IV every 6 hr to a maximum of 60 mg/day.

Oral
- *Transfer to oral:* 10 mg PO as first dose for patients who received 30 mg IM or 15 mg IV single dose or 15 mg IM or IV multiple dose, then 10 mg PO every 4–6 hr; do not exceed 40 mg/24 hr.

Pharmacokinetics

Route	Onset	Peak	Duration
Oral	Varies	30–60 min	6 hr
IM, IV	30 min	1–2 hr	6 hr

Metabolism: Hepatic; $T_{1/2}$: 2.4–8.6 hr
Distribution: Crosses placenta; enters breast milk
Excretion: Urine

▼ IV FACTS
Preparation: No further preparation is required.
Infusion: Infuse slowly as a bolus over no less than 15 sec.
Incompatibilities: Do not mix with morphine, sulfate, meperidine, promethazine, or hydroxyzine; a precipitate will form. Protect injection from light.

Adverse effects
- **CNS:** *Headache, dizziness, somnolence, insomnia,* fatigue, tinnitus, ophthalmologic effects
- **Dermatologic:** *Rash,* pruritus, sweating, dry mucous membranes
- **GI:** *Nausea, dyspepsia, GI pain,* diarrhea, vomiting, *constipation,* flatulence, **gastric or duodenal ulcers**
- **GU:** Dysuria, **renal impairment**
- **Hematologic:** Bleeding, platelet inhibition with higher doses, neutropenia, eosinophilia, leukopenia, pancytopenia, thrombocytopenia, agranulocytosis, granulocytopenia, aplastic anemia, decreased Hgb or Hct, bone marrow depression, menorrhagia
- **Respiratory:** Dyspnea, hemoptysis, pharyngitis, bronchospasm, rhinitis
- **Other:** Peripheral edema; anaphylactoid reactions to anaphylactic shock; local burning, stinging (ophthalmic)

Interactions
✴ **Drug-drug** • Increased risk of nephrotoxicity with other nephrotoxins (aminoglycosides, cyclosporine) • Increased risk of bleeding with anticoagulants (warfarin), aspirin

■ Nursing considerations
Assessment
- **History:** Renal impairment; impaired hearing; allergies; hepatic, CV, and GI conditions; lactation, pregnancy
- **Physical:** Skin color and lesions; orientation, reflexes, ophthalmologic and audiometric evaluation, peripheral sensation; P, edema, BP; R, adventitious sounds; liver evaluation; CBC, clotting times, LFTs, renal function tests; serum electrolytes, stool guaiac

Interventions
⊗ **Black box warning** Be aware that patient may be at increased risk for CV events, GI bleeding, renal toxicity; monitor accordingly.
⊗ **Black box warning** Do not use during labor or delivery or in breast-feeding patients; serious adverse effects to the fetus or baby are possible.
⊗ **Black box warning** May increase risk of bleeding. Do not use with high risk of bleeding or prophylactically before surgery.
⊗ **Black box warning** There is increased risk of severe hypersensitivity with known hypersensitivity to aspirin, NSAIDs. Contraindicated for use with aspirin or NSAIDs because of risk of serious cumulative NSAID effects.
⊗ **Warning** Keep emergency equipment readily available at time of initial dose, in case of severe hypersensitivity reaction.
- Protect drug vials from light.
- Discard bottle from nasal spray within 24 hr of opening.
- Administer every 6 hr to maintain serum levels and control pain.

Teaching points
- Every effort will be made to administer the drug on time to control pain; dizziness, drowsiness can occur (avoid driving or using dangerous machinery); burning and stinging on application (ophthalmic).
- Do not use ophthalmic drops with contact lenses.
- Discard bottle from nasal spray within 24 hours of opening, even if medication remains in the bottle.
- Report sore throat, fever, rash, itching, weight gain, swelling in ankles or fingers; changes in vision; black, tarry stools; easy bruising.

K

DANGEROUS DRUG

▽ **labetalol hydrochloride**
(la **bet**' a lol)

Trandate

PREGNANCY CATEGORY C

Drug classes
Alpha- and beta-adrenergic blocker
Antihypertensive

Therapeutic actions
Competitively blocks alpha$_1$- and beta$_1$- and beta$_2$-adrenergic receptors, and has some sympathomimetic activity at beta$_2$-receptors. Alpha- and beta-blocking actions contribute to the BP-lowering effect; beta blockade prevents the reflex tachycardia seen with most alpha-blocking drugs and decreases plasma renin activity.

Indications
• Hypertension, alone or with other oral drugs, especially diuretics
• Parenteral preparations: Severe hypertension
• Unlabeled uses: Control of BP in pheochromocytoma; clonidine withdrawal hypertension

Contraindications and cautions
• Contraindicated with sinus bradycardia, second- or third-degree heart block, cardiogenic shock, heart failure, asthma.
• Use cautiously with diabetes or hypoglycemia (can mask cardiac signs of hypoglycemia), nonallergic bronchospasm (oral drug—IV is absolutely contraindicated), pheochromocytoma (paradoxic increases in BP have occurred), hepatic impairment, pregnancy, lactation.

Available forms
Tablets—100, 200, 300 mg; injection—5 mg/mL

Dosages
Adults
Oral
Initial dose, 100 mg bid. After 2–3 days, using standing BP as indicator, adjust dosage in increments of 100 mg bid every 2–3 days. For maintenance, 200–400 mg bid. May need up to 2,400 mg/day; to improve tolerance, divide total daily dose and give tid.

Parenteral
• Severe hypertension: For repeated IV injection, 20 mg (0.25 mg/kg) slowly over 2 min. Individualize dosage using supine BP; additional doses of 40 or 80 mg can be given at 10-min intervals until desired BP is achieved or until a 300-mg dose has been injected. For continuous IV infusion, dilute ampule (see IV facts), infuse at a rate of up to 2 mg/min, adjust according to BP response up to 300 mg total dose. Transfer to oral therapy as soon as possible.
Pediatric patients
Safety and efficacy not established.
Geriatric patients
Generally require lower maintenance doses between 100 and 200 mg bid.

Pharmacokinetics

Route	Onset	Peak	Duration
Oral	Varies	1–2 hr	8–12 hr
IV	Immediate	5 min	5.5 hr

Metabolism: Hepatic; T$_{1/2}$: 6–8 hr
Distribution: Crosses placenta; enters breast milk
Excretion: Urine

▼ **IV FACTS**

Preparation: Add 200 mg to 160 mL of a compatible IV fluid to make a 1 mg/mL solution; infuse at 2 mL/min, or add 200 mg (2 ampules) to 250 mg of IV fluid to make a 2 mg/3 mL solution, infuse at 3 mL/min. Compatible IV fluids include Ringer, lactated Ringer, 0.9% sodium chloride, 2.5% dextrose and 0.45% sodium chloride, 5% dextrose, 5% dextrose and Ringer, 5% dextrose and 5% lactated Ringer, and 5% dextrose and 0.2%, 0.33%, or 0.9% sodium chloride. Stable for 24 hr in these solutions at concentrations between 1.25 and 3.75 mg/mL.
Infusion: Administer infusion at 2–3 mL/min; inject slowly over 2 min.
Incompatibilities: Do not dilute drug in 5% sodium bicarbonate injection or other alkaline solutions, including furosemide.
Y-site incompatibilities: Do not give with nafcillin.

Adverse effects
• **CNS:** Dizziness, vertigo, fatigue, depression, paresthesias, sleep disturbances,

Adverse effects in *italics* are most common; those in **bold** are life-threatening. ⬛ Do not crush.

hallucinations, disorientation, memory loss, slurred speech
- **CV:** Heart failure, cardiac arrhythmias, peripheral vascular insufficiency, claudication, **stroke,** pulmonary edema, hypotension
- **Dermatologic:** Rash, pruritus, sweating, dry skin
- **EENT:** Eye irritation, dry eyes, conjunctivitis, blurred vision
- **GI:** *Gastric pain, flatulence, constipation, diarrhea, nausea, vomiting,* anorexia, ischemic colitis, renal and mesenteric arterial thrombosis, retroperitoneal fibrosis, hepatomegaly, acute pancreatitis, taste alteration
- **GU:** *Impotence, decreased libido,* Peyronie disease, dysuria, nocturia, polyuria, priapism, urinary retention
- **Respiratory: Bronchospasm,** *dyspnea, cough,* bronchial obstruction, nasal stuffiness, rhinitis, pharyngitis
- **Other:** *Decreased exercise tolerance,* development of antinuclear antibodies, hyperglycemia or hypoglycemia, elevated liver enzymes

Interactions

✳ **Drug-drug** • Risk of excessive hypotension with enflurane or isoflurane • Potential for added antihypertensive effects with nitroglycerin • Additive AV block with calcium channel blockers

✳ **Drug-lab test** • Possible falsely elevated urinary catecholamines in lab tests using a trihydroxyindole reaction

■ Nursing considerations

Assessment

- **History:** Sinus bradycardia, second- or third-degree heart block, cardiogenic shock, heart failure, asthma, pregnancy, lactation, diabetes or hypoglycemia, nonallergic bronchospasm, pheochromocytoma
- **Physical:** Weight, skin condition, neurologic status, P, BP, ECG, respiratory status, renal and thyroid function, blood and urine glucose

Interventions

⊗ **Warning** Do not discontinue drug abruptly after long-term therapy. (Hypersensitivity to catecholamines may have developed, causing exacerbation of angina, MI and ventricular arrhythmias; taper drug gradually over 2 wk with monitoring.)

- Consult physician about withdrawing the drug if the patient is to undergo surgery (withdrawal is controversial).
- Keep patient supine during parenteral therapy, and assist initial ambulation.
- Position to decrease effects of edema.
- Provide support and encouragement to deal with drug effects and disease.

Teaching points

- Take drug with meals.
- Do not stop taking drug unless instructed to do so by your health care provider.
- If you have diabetes, monitor your blood glucose carefully. This drug may mask usual symptoms of hypoglycemia.
- You may experience these side effects: Dizziness, light-headedness, loss of appetite, nightmares, depression, sexual impotence.
- Report difficulty breathing, night cough, swelling of extremities, slow pulse, confusion, depression, rash, fever, sore throat.

▽ **lacosamide**
(lah koss' ah mide)

Vimpat

PREGNANCY CATEGORY C

Drug class

Antiepileptic

Therapeutic actions

Mechanism of action not fully understood; inhibits voltage-sensitive sodium channels, resulting in stabilization of neuronal membranes and inhibition of repetitive neuronal firing.

Indications

- Adjunctive therapy for the treatment of partial-onset seizures in patients 17 yr and older; IV use is indicated for short-term treatment when oral administration is not feasible

Contraindications and cautions

- Contraindicated with hypersensitivity to components of drug, pregnancy, lactation.
- Use cautiously with cardiac conduction problems, MI, heart failure, drugs that prolong

the PR interval, suicidal ideation, hepatic dysfunction, renal impairment.

Available forms

Tablets—50, 100, 150, 200 mg; single-use vial—10 mg/mL; solution—10 mg/mL

Dosages
Adults

Initially, 50 mg PO bid; may be increased, if needed and tolerated, at weekly intervals by 100 mg/day given in two divided doses. Usual effective dosage is 200–400 mg/day PO. IV dosage is the same as oral dosage and may be used short-term if oral dosing is not feasible; transfer patient to oral form as soon as feasible.

Pediatric patients younger than 17 yr

Safety and efficacy not established.

Patients with renal impairment

Patients with severe renal impairment (CrCl ≤30 mL/min) should receive a maximum of 300 mg/day.

Patients with hepatic impairment

Increase dosage with caution. Maximum dosage is 300 mg/day with mild to moderate hepatic impairment; not recommended for use with severe hepatic impairment.

Pharmacokinetics

Route	Onset	Peak
Oral	Rapid	1–4 hr
IV	Rapid	End of infusion

Metabolism: Hepatic; $T_{1/2}$: 13 hr
Distribution: May cross placenta; may enter breast milk
Excretion: Urine

▼ IV FACTS

Preparation: Solution may be given as provided or diluted in 0.9% sodium chloride injection, 5% dextrose injection, or lactated Ringer injection. Solution should be clear; discard solution that is discolored or contains particulate matter. Discard unused portion. Stable for 24 hr at room temperature when diluted in appropriate solutions.
Infusion: Infuse slowly over 30–60 min.
Incompatibilities: Do not administer in the same line as other medications.

Adverse effects

- **CNS:** *Dizziness, ataxia, diplopia,* somnolence, tremor, *headache,* nystagmus, gait disorder, balance disorder, blurred vision, vertigo
- **CV:** Prolonged PR interval
- **GI:** *Nausea, vomiting,* diarrhea
- **Other:** Fatigue, pruritus

Interactions

✳ **Drug-drug** • Increased risk of prolonged PR interval if combined with other drugs known to prolong PR interval; monitor patient closely if such a combination is needed

■ Nursing considerations
Assessment

- **History:** Hypersensitivity to components of drug, cardiac conduction problems, MI, heart failure, use of drugs that prolong PR interval, suicidal ideation, hepatic dysfunction, renal impairment, pregnancy, lactation
- **Physical:** Orientation, affect, reflexes; BP, P, bowel sounds, LFTs, renal function tests, baseline ECG

Interventions

⊗ **Black box warning** There is an increased risk of suicidal ideation when used in children, adolescents, or young adults; monitor patient accordingly.

⊗ **Warning** Taper drug slowly when discontinuing; risk of seizures increases if drug is stopped abruptly.

- Be aware that dosage is the same for PO and IV routes. IV route should be reserved for short-term use when oral dosing is not feasible. Switch to oral route as soon as possible.
- Provide safety measures if CNS effects occur.

Teaching points

- Take this drug exactly as prescribed; be aware that the dosage may be slowly increased.
- Do not discontinue this drug abruptly. If the drug is discontinued, it will need to be slowly tapered to prevent seizures.
- You will need to have regular medical follow-up to monitor your response to this drug.
- It is not known how this drug affects a fetus; use of contraceptives is advised when you are taking this drug.

Adverse effects in *italics* are most common; those in **bold** are life-threatening. ⬛ Do not crush.

- If you are breast-feeding, you should use another method of feeding the infant while you are taking this drug because the drug could cause serious adverse effects in the infant.
- You may experience these side effects: Headache (medications may be available to help); nausea and vomiting (small, frequent meals may help; medication may be available to relieve these symptoms); dizziness, sleepiness, problems with vision and balance (avoid driving or performing tasks that require alertness or visual acuity until you know how this drug will affect you; take special precautions to avoid falls); thoughts of suicide, depression (be aware of changes in thoughts or thoughts of suicide; report changes to your health care provider immediately).
- Report thoughts of suicide, sudden changes in personality, excessive activity or thoughts of aggression, severe nausea or vomiting.

▽lactulose
(lak' tyoo lose)

Ammonia-reducing drug:
Apo-Lactulose (CAN), Cephulac, Enulose
Laxative: Chronulac, Constilac, Constulose, Duphalac, Kristalose, PMS-Lactulose (CAN), ratio-Lactulose (CAN)

PREGNANCY CATEGORY B

Drug classes
Ammonia reduction drug
Laxative

Therapeutic actions
The drug passes unchanged into the colon where bacteria break it down to organic acids that increase the osmotic pressure in the colon and slightly acidify the colonic contents, resulting in an increase in stool water content, stool softening, laxative action. This also results in migration of blood ammonia into the colon contents with subsequent trapping and expulsion in the feces.

Indications
- Treatment of constipation
- Prevention and treatment of portal-systemic encephalopathy

Contraindications and cautions
- Contraindicated with allergy to lactulose, low-galactose diet.
- Use cautiously with diabetes, pregnancy, and lactation.

Available forms
Syrup, solution—10 g/15 mL

Dosages
Adults
Laxative
15–30 mL/day (10–20 g) PO; may be increased to 60 mL/day as needed.
Oral
- *Portal-systemic encephalopathy:* 30–45 mL (20–30 g) PO tid or qid. Adjust dosage every 1–2 days to produce two or three soft stools/day. 30–45 mL/hr may be used if needed. Return to standard dose as soon as possible.
Rectal
- *Portal-systemic encephalopathy:* 300 mL (20 g) lactulose mixed with 700 mL water or physiologic saline as a retention enema, retained for 30–60 min. May be repeated every 4–6 hr. Start oral drug as soon as feasible and before stopping enemas.
Pediatric patients
Laxative
Safety and efficacy not established.
Oral
- *Portal-systemic encephalopathy:* Standards not clearly established. Initial dose of 2.5–10 mL/day PO in divided dose for small children or 40–90 mL/day for older children is suggested. Attempt to produce two or three soft stools daily.

Pharmacokinetics

Route	Onset	Peak	Duration
Oral	Varies	20 hr	24–48 hr

Very minimal systemic absorption

Adverse effects
- **GI:** *Transient flatulence, distention, intestinal cramps, belching,* diarrhea, nausea

- **Other:** Acid-base imbalances, electrolyte imbalance

■ **Nursing considerations**
Assessment
- **History:** Allergy to lactulose, low-galactose diet, diabetes, lactation, pregnancy
- **Physical:** Abdominal examination, bowel sounds, serum electrolytes, serum ammonia levels

Interventions
⊗ *Warning* Do not freeze laxative form. Extremely dark or cloudy syrup may be unsafe; do not use.
- Give laxative syrup orally with fruit juice, water, or milk to increase palatability.
- Administer retention enema using a rectal balloon catheter. Do not use cleansing enemas containing soapsuds or other alkaline drugs that counteract the effects of lactulose.
- Do not administer other laxatives while using lactulose.
- Monitor serum ammonia levels.
- Monitor with long-term therapy for potential electrolyte and acid–base imbalances.
- Carefully monitor blood glucose levels in diabetic patients.

Teaching points
- Do not use other laxatives. The drug may be mixed in water, juice, or milk to make it more tolerable.
- For laxative use, do not use continuously for longer than 1 week unless directed by your health care provider.
- Make sure you have ready access to bathroom; bowel movements will be increased to two or three per day.
- You may experience these side effects: Abdominal fullness, flatulence, belching.
- Report diarrhea, severe belching, abdominal fullness.

▽**lamivudine (3TC)**
(lam ah vew' den)

Epivir, Epivir-HBV

PREGNANCY CATEGORY C

Drug classes
Antiviral
Reverse transcriptase inhibitor

Therapeutic actions
Nucleoside analogue inhibitor of HIV reverse transcriptase via DNA viral chain termination and HBV polymerase.

Indications
- Treatment of HIV infection in combination with other antiretroviral drugs
- Treatment of chronic hepatitis B (*Epivir-HBV*) with active liver inflammation

Contraindications and cautions
- Contraindicated with life-threatening allergy to any component.
- Use cautiously with compromised bone marrow function, impaired renal function, hepatic impairment, obesity, pregnancy, lactation.

Available forms
Tablets—100 (*Epivir–HBV*); 150, 300 mg (*Epivir*); oral solution—5 mg/mL (*Epivir–HBV*), 10 mg/mL (*Epivir*)

Dosages
Adults
- *Hepatitis B:* 100 mg PO daily.
Adults and patients 16 yr and older
- *HIV infection:* 150 mg PO bid or 300 mg/day PO as a single dose in combination with other antiretroviral drugs.
Pediatric patients
- *HIV infection:*
3 mo–16 yr: 4 mg/kg PO bid; up to a maximum of 150 mg bid.
or:
Patients weighing 14–21 kg: 75 mg (one-half tablet) PO bid.
Patients weighing more than 21 kg but less than 30 kg: 75 mg (one-half tablet) PO in the morning and then 150 mg (1 tablet) PO in the evening.
Patients weighing 30 kg or more: 150 mg (1 tablet) PO bid.
- *Hepatitis B:*
2–17 yr: 3 mg/kg PO daily up to a maximum of 100 mg daily.
Patients with impaired renal function
- *HIV infection:*

CrCl (mL/min)	Dosage (PO)
50 or more	150 mg bid or 300 mg daily
30–49	150 mg daily
15–29	150 mg first dose, then 100 mg daily
5–14	150 mg first dose, then 50 mg daily
Less than 5	50 mg first dose, then 25 mg daily

- *Hepatitis B:*

CrCl (mL/min)	Dosage (PO)
50 or more	100 mg daily
30–49	100 mg first dose, then 50 mg daily
15–29	100 mg first dose, then 25 mg daily
5–14	35 mg first dose, then 15 mg daily
Less than 5	35 mg first dose, then 10 mg daily

Pharmacokinetics

Route	Onset	Peak
Oral	Slow	2–4 hr

Metabolism: Unknown; $T_{1/2}$: 5–7 hr
Distribution: Crosses placenta; enters breast milk
Excretion: Urine

Adverse effects

- **CNS:** *Headache,* insomnia, myalgia, *asthenia,* malaise, dizziness, paresthesias, somnolence
- **GI:** *Nausea, GI pain, diarrhea,* anorexia, vomiting, dyspepsia, **pancreatitis** (children), **hepatomegaly with lactic acidosis, steatosis**
- **Hematologic:** *Agranulocytosis*
- **Respiratory:** *Nasal signs and symptoms, cough*
- **Other:** Fever, rash, taste perversion

Interactions

✳ **Drug-drug** • Increased levels of lamivudine taken concurrently with trimethoprim-sulfamethoxazole • Lamivudine and zalcitabine inhibit the effects of each other; avoid concurrent use

■ Nursing considerations
Assessment

- **History:** Life-threatening allergy to any component, compromised bone marrow function, impaired renal function, pregnancy, lactation, hepatic impairment, obesity

- **Physical:** Skin rashes, lesions, texture; T; affect, reflexes, peripheral sensation; bowel sounds, liver evaluation; renal function tests, CBC and differential

Interventions

⊗ **Black box warning** Arrange to monitor hematologic indices and liver function every 2 wk during therapy; severe hepatomegaly with steatosis, lactic acidosis has occurred.

⊗ **Black box warning** Counsel and periodically test patients receiving *Epivir-HBV.* Severe, acute exacerbations of HBV have been reported in patients with both HIV and HBV infection who stop taking lamivudine.

- Monitor children for any sign of pancreatitis and discontinue immediately if it occurs.
- Monitor patient for signs of opportunistic infections that will need to be treated appropriately.
- Administer the drug concurrently with other antiretrovirals for HIV infection.
- Offer support and encouragement to the patient to deal with the diagnosis as well as the effects of drug therapy and the high expense of treatment.

Teaching points

- Take drug as prescribed; take concurrently with other drugs prescribed for HIV treatment.
- These drugs are not a cure for AIDS, AIDS-related complex, or hepatitis B; opportunistic infections may occur and regular medical care should be sought to deal with the disease.
- Arrange for frequent blood tests during the course of treatment; results of blood counts may indicate a need to decrease dosage or discontinue the drug for a time.
- Lamivudine does not reduce the risk of transmission of HIV or hepatitis B to others by sexual contact or blood contamination—use appropriate precautions.
- Avoid pregnancy while using this drug; using barrier contraceptives is urged.
- You may experience these side effects: Nausea, loss of appetite, change in taste (eat frequent small meals); dizziness, loss of feeling (take appropriate precautions); headache, fever, muscle aches (an analgesic may help, consult your health care provider).
- Report extreme fatigue, lethargy, severe headache, severe nausea, vomiting, difficulty breathing, rash.

▽ lamotrigine
(la mo' tri geen)

Apo-Lamotrigine (CAN), Gen-
Lamotrigine (CAN), Lamictal,
Lamictal CD, Lamictal ODT,
Lamictal XR ⊕, PMS-Lamotrigine
(CAN), ratio-Lamotrigine (CAN)

PREGNANCY CATEGORY C

Drug class
Antiepileptic

Therapeutic actions
Mechanism not well understood; may inhibit voltage-sensitive sodium channels, stabilizing the neuronal membrane and modulating calcium-dependent presynaptic release
of excitatory amino acids.

Indications
• ER form—once-daily adjunctive therapy
  for patients 13 yr and older with partial onset seizures and primary generalized tonic-
  clonic seizures
• Adjunctive therapy for the treatment of
  Lennox-Gastaut syndrome in infants, children, and adults; primary generalized tonic-
  clonic seizures and partial seizures in adults
  and children 2 yr and older
• Monotherapy in adults with partial seizures
  that have not been controlled by other therapies
• Conversion to monotherapy in patients 13
  yr and older (ER form, immediate-release)
  with partial seizures receiving treatment
  with a single enzyme-inducing antiepileptic drug
• Long-term maintenance of bipolar I disorder in adults, to delay the occurrence of acute
  mood episodes in patients on standard therapy (immediate-release only)
• Unlabeled uses: Absence seizures (children), temporal lobe seizures, migraine
  headache, post-poliomyelitis syndrome
  obesity, depression

Contraindications and cautions
• Contraindicated with allergy to drug, lactation.
• Use cautiously with impaired hepatic, renal,
  or cardiac function; patients younger than
  16 yr, pregnancy.

Available forms
Tablets—25, 100, 150, 200 mg; chewable
tablets—2, 5, 25, 100 mg; orally disintegrating tablets—25, 50, 100, 200 mg; ER
tablets ⊕—25, 50, 100, 200 mg

Dosages
Adults
• *Epilepsy*
  Patients taking enzyme-inducing anti-
  epileptics (ie, carbamazepine, phenytoin,
  phenobarbital) and not valproic acid:
  50 mg PO daily for 2 wk; then 100 mg PO
  daily in two divided doses for 2 wk; may increase by 100 mg/day every wk up to a maintenance dose of 300–500 mg/day in two divided doses. Patients older than 13 yr (ER
  tablets): wk 1–2, 50 mg/day PO; wk 3–4,
  100 mg/day PO; wk 5, 200 mg/day PO; wk
  6, 300 mg/day PO; wk 7, 400 mg/day PO.
  Range, 400–600 mg/day.
  Patients taking enzyme-inducing anti-
  epileptics (ie, carbamazepine, phenytoin,
  phenobarbital) and also valproic acid:
  25 mg PO every other day for 2 wk; then
  25 mg PO daily for 2 wk, then may increase
  by 25–50 mg every 1–2 wk up to a maintenance dose of 100–400 mg/day PO in two
  divided doses.
  Conversion of patients to lamotrigine
  monotherapy: Titrate as above to a target
  dose of 500 mg/day in two divided doses,
  then attempt to decrease other antiepileptic
  by 20% weekly.
• *Bipolar I disorder*
  Patients taking valproic acid: 25 mg every
  other day for 2 wk; then 25 mg once daily for 2 wk. After 4 wk, dose may be doubled at weekly intervals to target of 100
  mg/day.
  Patients taking enzyme-inducing anti-
  epileptics but not valproic acid: 50 mg/day
  for 2 wk; then 100 mg daily in two divided
  doses for 2 wk. After 4 wk, dose may be increased in 100-mg increments at weekly
  intervals to target maintenance dosage of
  400 mg/day in two divided doses.
  Patients taking neither enzyme-induc-
  ing antiepileptics nor valproic acid: 25
  mg/day for 2 wk; then 50 mg daily for 2 wk.
  After 4 wk, dose may be doubled at weekly
  intervals to maintenance dosage of 200
  mg/day.

Adverse effects in *italics* are most common; those in **bold** are life-threatening. ⊕ Do not crush.

Pediatric patients 2–12 yr

- *Patients taking non–enzyme-inducing antiepileptics with valproic acid*—0.15 mg/kg/day in one to two divided doses for 2 wk. Then 0.3 mg/kg/day in one to two divided doses, rounded down to nearest 5 mg for 2 wk. For maintenance, 1–5 mg/kg/day in one to two divided doses, to a maximum of 200 mg/day.
- *Single enzyme-inducing antiepileptic without valproic acid:* 0.6 mg/kg/day in two divided doses for 2 wk, then 1.2 mg/kg/day in two divided doses for 2 wk. For maintenance, 5–15 mg/kg/day in two divided doses, to a maximum of 400 mg/day.

Pediatric patients older than 12 yr

- *Patients taking valproic acid*—25 mg PO every other day for 2 wk, then 25 mg PO daily for 2 wk. For maintenance, 100–400 mg/day in one to two divided doses. *Without valproic acid:* 50 mg/day PO for 2 wk, then 100 mg/day in two divided doses for 2 wk. For maintenance, 300–500 mg/day in one to two divided doses, to a maximum of 500 mg/day.

Pharmacokinetics

Route	Onset	Peak
Oral	Rapid	2–5 hr

Metabolism: Hepatic; $T_{1/2}$: 25–33 hr
Distribution: Crosses placenta; may enter breast milk
Excretion: Urine

Adverse effects

- **CNS:** *Dizziness,* insomnia, headache, somnolence, *ataxia,* diplopia, blurred vision, aseptic meningitis
- **Dermatologic: Stevens-Johnson syndrome, rash, toxic epidermal necrosis with multiorgan failure**
- **GI:** *Nausea,* vomiting, abdominal pain, constipation, diarrhea

Interactions

✳ Drug-drug • Decrease in lamotrigine levels of 40%–50% with enzyme-inducing antiepileptics—carbamazepine, phenytoin, phenobarbital, primidone • Decreased clearance of lamotrigine, requiring a lower dose, if taken with valproic acid

■ Nursing considerations

⚡ CLINICAL ALERT!
Name confusion has occurred between *Lamictal* (lamotrigine) and *Lamisil* (terbinafine); use extreme caution.

Assessment

- **History:** Lactation; impaired hepatic, renal or cardiac function; pregnancy
- **Physical:** Weight; T; skin color, lesions; orientation, affect, reflexes; P, BP, perfusion; bowel sounds, normal output; LFTs, renal function tests

Interventions

- Be aware that patient may have increased risk of suicidality; monitor accordingly.
- Be aware that patient may be at risk for aseptic meningitis (headache, fever, chills, nausea, stiff neck, sensitivity to light); monitor patient accordingly.
- Monitor renal and hepatic function before and periodically during therapy; if abnormal, re-evaluate therapy.
- ⊗ *Warning* Monitor drug doses carefully when starting therapy and with each increase in dose; special care will be needed when changing the dose or frequency of any other antiepileptic.
- Ensure that extended-release tablets are not cut, crushed, or chewed.
- ⊗ **Black box warning** Monitor patient for any sign of rash; discontinue lamotrigine immediately if rash appears and be prepared with appropriate life support if needed; potential for serious or life-threatening rash.
- Administer only whole dispersible tablets.
- Administer chewable, dispersible tablets with a small amount of water or fruit juice if chewed; to disperse, add tablet to 1 tsp water, wait 1 min, swirl and administer immediately.
- Taper drug slowly over a 2-wk period when discontinuing.

Teaching points

- Take this drug exactly as prescribed. Swallow extended-release tablets whole; do not cut, crush, or chew tablets.
- Do not discontinue this drug abruptly or change dosage, except on the advice of your health care provider.

- Wear or carry a medical ID tag to alert emergency medical personnel that you are an epileptic taking antiepileptic medication.
- If rash occurs, notify your health care provider immediately.
- You may experience these side effects: Dizziness, drowsiness (avoid driving or performing tasks requiring alertness or visual acuity); GI upset (take drug with food or milk, eat frequent small meals); headache (medication can be ordered).
- Report yellowing of skin, abdominal pain, changes in color of urine or stools, fever, sore throat, mouth sores, unusual bleeding or bruising, rash; headache, fever, chills, nausea, stiff neck, sensitivity to light.

▽lanreotide acetate

See Appendix R, *Less commonly used drugs.*

▽lansoprazole
(lanz ah' pray zol)

Prevacid ⬤,
Prevacid 24 Hr

PREGNANCY CATEGORY B

Drug classes
Antisecretory drug
Proton pump inhibitor

Therapeutic actions
Gastric acid-pump inhibitor: Suppresses gastric acid secretion by specific inhibition of the hydrogen–potassium ATPase enzyme system at the secretory surface of the gastric parietal cells; blocks the final step of acid production.

Indications
- Short-term treatment (up to 4 wk) of active duodenal ulcer
- Short-term treatment (up to 8 wk) of gastric ulcers
- Healing of NSAID-related gastric ulcer
- Risk reduction for NSAID-related gastric ulcer
- Short-term treatment (up to 8 wk) of GERD: Severe erosive esophagitis; poorly responsive symptomatic GERD
- Long-term treatment of pathologic hypersecretory conditions (eg, Zollinger-Ellison

syndrome, multiple adenomas, systemic mastocytosis)
- Maintenance therapy for healing of erosive esophagitis, duodenal ulcers
- Eradication of *Helicobacter pylori* infection in patients with active or recurrent duodenal ulcers in combination with clarithromycin and amoxicillin
- Treatment of frequent heartburn (*Prevacid 24 Hr*)
- Unlabeled uses: Alternate-day dosing for management of reflux esophagitis, laryngitis

Contraindications and cautions
- Contraindicated with hypersensitivity to lansoprazole or its components.
- Use cautiously with pregnancy, lactation.
- Use cautiously because of possible increased risk of *Clostridium difficile* infection.

Available forms
DR capsules ⬤—15, 30 mg; orally disintegrating DR tablets—15, 30 mg

Dosages
Adults
- *Active duodenal ulcer:* 15 mg PO daily before eating for 4 wk. For maintenance, 15 mg PO daily.
- *Gastric ulcer:* 30 mg/day PO for up to 8 wk.
- *Risk reduction of gastric ulcer with NSAIDs:* 15 mg/day PO for up to 12 wk.
- *Duodenal ulcers associated with* H. pylori: 30 mg lansoprazole, 500 mg clarithromycin, 1 g amoxicillin, all given PO bid for 10–14 days; or 30 mg lansoprazole and 1 g amoxicillin PO tid for 14 days.
- *GERD:* 15 mg/day PO for up to 8 wk.
- *Erosive esophagitis or poorly responsive GERD:* 30 mg PO daily before eating for up to 8 wk. An additional 8-wk course may be helpful for patients who do not heal with 8-wk therapy.
- *Maintenance of healing of erosive esophagitis:* 15 mg/day PO.
- *Pathologic hypersecretory conditions:* Individualize dosage. Initial dose is 60 mg PO daily. Doses up to 90 mg bid have been used. Administer daily doses of more than 120 mg in divided doses.
- *Heartburn:* 1 capsule *Prevacid 24 Hr* taken with a full glass of water in the morning before eating for 14 days; 14-day course can be repeated every 4 mo.

Adverse effects in *italics* are most common; those in **bold** are life-threatening. ⬤ Do not crush.

Pediatric patients 12–17 yr
Nonerosive GERD: 15 mg/day PO for up to 8 wk.
Erosive esophagitis: 30 mg/day PO for up to 8 wk.
Pediatric patients 1–11 yr
Capsules may be opened and the granules sprinkled on soft food. Do not cut, crush, or allow patient to chew granules.
Patients weighing 30 kg or less: 15 mg/day PO for up to 12 wk.
Patients weighing more than 30 kg: 30 mg/day PO for up to 12 wk.
Patients with hepatic impairment
Consider reducing dose and monitoring patient response.

Pharmacokinetics

Route	Onset	Peak
Oral	Varies	1.7 hr
IV	Rapid	End of transfusion

Metabolism: Hepatic; T$_{1/2}$: 2 hr, 1.3 hr (IV)
Distribution: Crosses placenta; may enter breast milk
Excretion: Bile

Adverse effects
- **CNS:** *Headache,* dizziness, asthenia, vertigo, insomnia, anxiety, paresthesias, dream abnormalities
- **Dermatologic:** Rash, inflammation, urticaria, pruritus, alopecia, dry skin, acne
- **GI:** *Diarrhea, abdominal pain, nausea, vomiting,* constipation, dry mouth
- **Respiratory:** *URI symptoms,* cough, epistaxis
- **Other:** Gastric cancer in preclinical studies, back pain, fever, bone loss

Interactions
✴ **Drug-drug** • Decreased serum levels if taken concurrently with sucralfate • Decreased serum levels of ketoconazole, theophylline when taken with lansoprazole

■ Nursing considerations
Assessment
- **History:** Hypersensitivity to lansoprazole or any of its components; pregnancy; lactation
- **Physical:** Skin lesions; body T; reflexes, affect; urinary output; abdominal examination; respiratory auscultation

Interventions
- Administer before meals. Caution patient to swallow capsules whole, not to chew or crush. If patient has difficulty swallowing, open capsule and sprinkle granules on applesauce, *Ensure,* yogurt, cottage cheese, or strained pears. For nasogastric tube, place 15- or 30-mg tablet in a syringe and draw 4 or 10 mL of water; shake gently for quick dispersal. After dispersal, inject through nasogastric tube into the stomach within 15 min. If using capsules with nasogastric tube, mix granules from capsule with 40 mL apple juice and inject through tube, flush tube with more apple juice. Place orally disintegrating tablet on tongue; follow with water after it dissolves.
- ⊗ *Warning* Arrange for further evaluation of patient after 4 wk of therapy for acute gastroesophageal reflux disorders if symptomatic improvement does not rule out gastric cancer, which did occur in preclinical studies.

Teaching points
- Take the drug before meals. Swallow the capsules whole—do not chew, open, or crush. If you are unable to swallow capsule, open and sprinkle granules on applesauce, or use granules, which can be added to 30 mL water, stirred, and drunk immediately. If using orally disintegrating tablet, place on your tongue and allow to dissolve. Follow with a drink of water.
- Arrange to have regular medical follow-up care while you are taking this drug.
- You may experience these side effects: Dizziness (avoid driving a car or performing hazardous tasks); headache (medications may be available to help); nausea, vomiting, diarrhea (proper nutrition is important; consult with a dietitian to maintain nutrition); symptoms of upper respiratory tract infection, cough (reversible; do not self-medicate, consult your health care provider if this becomes uncomfortable).
- Report severe headache, worsening of symptoms, fever, chills.

▷ lanthanum carbonate
See Appendix R, *Less commonly used drugs.*

▷ lapatinib
See Appendix R, *Less commonly used drugs.*

▷laronidase

See Appendix R, *Less commonly used drugs*.

▷leflunomide
(leh flew' no mide)

Arava

PREGNANCY CATEGORY X

Drug classes
Antiarthritic
Pyrimidine synthesis inhibitor

Therapeutic actions
Reversibly inhibits the enzyme dihydroorotate dehydrogenase, which is active in the autoimmune process that leads to rheumatoid arthritis; blocking this enzyme relieves the signs and symptoms of inflammation and blocks the structural damage caused by the inflammatory response to the autoimmune process.

Indications
- Treatment of active rheumatoid arthritis; to relieve symptoms and slow progression
- Improvement in physical functioning in adults with active rheumatoid arthritis

Contraindications and cautions
- Contraindicated with allergy to leflunomide, lactation, pregnancy, childbearing age when not using a reliable method of contraception, significant hepatic impairment, hepatitis B or C, severe immune deficiency.
- Use cautiously with renal or hepatic disorders.

Available forms
Tablets—10, 20, 100 mg

Dosages
Adults
Loading dose, 100 mg PO daily for 3 days; maintenance dose, 20 mg PO daily. If not well tolerated or if ALT elevates to more than two times upper level of normal, may reduce to 10 mg PO daily. If elevation of ALT is between two and three times upper limit of normal, monitor closely if continued therapy is desired; if it is three times or greater than up-

per limit of normal, use of cholestyramine may decrease absorption; consider discontinuation.
Pediatric patients
Safety and efficacy not established.
Patients with hepatic impairment
Do not use with serious hepatic impairment. Decrease dosage and monitor patient closely with mild to moderate hepatic impairment.

Pharmacokinetics

Route	Onset	Peak
Oral	Varies	6–12 hr

Metabolism: Hepatic; $T_{1/2}$: 14–18 days
Distribution: Crosses placenta; enters breast milk
Excretion: Urine

Adverse effects
- **CNS:** *Headache,* drowsiness, blurred vision, fatigue, dizziness, paresthesias
- **Dermatologic:** *Erythematous rashes,* pruritus, urticaria, *transient alopecia*
- **GI:** Nausea, vomiting, *diarrhea,* **hepatic toxicity**
- **Other:** Serious birth defects, pancytopenia, agranulocytosis, thrombocytopenia

Interactions
✳ **Drug-drug** • Possible severe hepatic impairment if combined with other hepatotoxic drugs; use with caution • Decreased absorption and effectiveness if combined with charcoal, cholestyramine • Increased risk of toxicity if combined with rifampin; monitor patient closely if this combination is used

■ Nursing considerations
Assessment
- **History:** Allergy to leflunomide, childbearing age, pregnancy, lactation, hepatitis B or C, severe hepatic impairment
- **Physical:** Weight; skin lesions, color; hair; orientation, liver evaluation, abdominal examination; LFTs

Interventions
- Advise patient that this drug does not cure the disease and appropriate therapies for rheumatoid arthritis should be used.
- Arrange for patient to obtain a wig or some other suitable head covering if alopecia occurs; ensure that head is covered at extreme

temperatures; loss of hair is usually reversible.
- Provide appropriate skin care; arrange for treatment of skin lesions as needed.

⊗ **Black box warning** Advise women of childbearing age of the risks associated with becoming pregnant while using this drug. Arrange for counseling for appropriate contraceptive measures while this drug is being used. If patient decides to become pregnant, a withdrawal program to rid the body of leflunomide is recommended. Cholestyramine may be used to rapidly decrease serum levels if unplanned pregnancy occurs.

⊗ **Black box warning** There is a risk of severe liver injury; check LFTs before and periodically during treatment. Drug is not recommended for patients with pre-existing liver disease or with liver enzyme levels greater than two times the upper limit of normal. Use caution with other drugs that cause liver injury; start cholestyramine washout if ALT increases to three times the upper limit of normal.

Teaching points
- Take this drug exactly as prescribed. Note that this drug does not cure rheumatoid arthritis, and appropriate therapies to deal with the disease should be followed.
- This drug may cause birth defects or miscarriages. It is advisable to use birth control while using this drug and for 8 weeks thereafter. Consult your health care provider if you decide to become pregnant; a withdrawal program is available.
- Arrange for frequent, regular medical follow-up care, including frequent blood tests to follow the effects of the drug on your body.
- You may experience these side effects: Nausea, vomiting, diarrhea (medication may be ordered to help; eat frequent small meals); dizziness, drowsiness (these are all effects of the drug; consult with your nurse or physician if these occur; dosage adjustment may be needed; avoid driving or operating dangerous machinery if these occur); loss of hair (you may wish to obtain a wig or other suitable head covering; it is important to keep the head covered at extremes of temperature); rash (avoid exposure to the sun, use a sunscreen and protective clothing if exposed to sun).
- Report black, tarry stools; fever, chills, sore throat; unusual bleeding or bruising; cough or shortness of breath; darkened or bloody urine; abdominal, flank, or joint pain; yellow color to the skin or eyes; mouth sores.

▽lenalidomide
See Appendix R, *Less commonly used drugs.*

▽lepirudin
See Appendix R, *Less commonly used drugs.*

▽letrozole
(le' tro zol)

Femara

PREGNANCY CATEGORY D

Drug classes
Antiestrogen
Antineoplastic
Aromatase inhibitor

Therapeutic actions
Inhibits the conversion of androgens to estrogens by the aromatase enzyme system (in postmenopausal women, the aromatase system is the main source of estrogens); reduces estrogen levels in all tissues, including tumors.

Indications
- Treatment of advanced breast cancer in postmenopausal women as a first-line treatment and with disease progression following traditional antiestrogen therapy
- Adjuvant treatment of early, receptor-positive breast cancer in postmenopausal women
- Extended adjuvant treatment of breast cancer in postmenopausal women who have received 5 yr of tamoxifen therapy

Contraindications and cautions
- Contraindicated with allergy to letrozole, pregnancy.
- Use cautiously with hepatic impairment, lactation.

Available forms
Tablets—2.5 mg

Dosages
Adults
2.5 mg PO daily; continue until tumor progression is evident.

Patients with hepatic impairment
Reduce dose by 50% in patients with cirrhosis
or severe hepatic impairment; give 2.5 mg
every other day. No adjustment needed for mild
to moderate impairment.

Pharmacokinetics

Route	Onset	Peak
Oral	Varies	2–6 wk

Metabolism: Hepatic; $T_{1/2}$: 2 days
Distribution: Crosses placenta; may enter
breast milk
Excretion: Urine

Adverse effects

- **CNS:** Depression, *headache,* fatigue, somnolence, anxiety, vertigo, dizziness, insomnia
- **CV:** Thromboembolic events, CV events, cerebrovascular events
- **Dermatologic:** Alopecia, *hot flashes,*
  rash
- **GI:** *Nausea, GI upset,* elevated liver enzymes, diarrhea, vomiting, constipation, abdominal pain, dyspepsia
- **Respiratory:** Cough, dyspnea, chest wall
  pain
- **Other:** Peripheral edema; arthralgia, bone
  pain, back pain, decreased bone density; increased cholesterol levels

■ Nursing considerations

Assessment

- **History:** Allergy to letrozole, hepatic impairment, pregnancy, lactation
- **Physical:** Skin lesions, color, turgor; orientation, affect, reflexes; peripheral pulses,
  edema; LFTs, estrogen receptor evaluation
  of tumor cells

Interventions

⊗ **Warning** Counsel patient about the need
to use contraceptive measures to avoid pregnancy while taking this drug; inform patient
that serious fetal harm could occur.

- Provide comfort measures to help patient
  deal with drug effects: Hot flashes (control
  environmental temperature); headache, depression (monitor light and noise); vaginal
  bleeding (hygiene measures).
- Discontinue drug at signs that tumor is progressing.

Teaching points

- This drug can cause serious fetal harm and
  must not be taken during pregnancy. Contraceptive measures should be used while
  you are taking this drug. If you become
  pregnant or decide that you would like to
  become pregnant, consult your health care
  provider immediately.
- You may experience these side effects: Hot
  flashes (stay in cool temperatures); nausea,
  GI upset (eat frequent small meals); headache, light-headedness (use caution if driving or performing tasks that require alertness).
- Report changes in color of urine or stool,
  increased fatigue, rash, fever, chills, severe
  depression.

▽ **leucovorin calcium
(citrovorum factor,
folinic acid)**
(loo koe vor' in)

PREGNANCY CATEGORY C

Drug class

Folic acid derivative

Therapeutic actions

Active reduced form of folic acid; required for
nucleoprotein synthesis and maintenance of
normal hematopoiesis.

Indications

- "Leucovorin rescue"—after high-dose
  methotrexate therapy for various cancers
- Parenteral form: Treatment of megaloblastic
  anemias due to sprue, nutritional deficiency,
  pregnancy, and infancy when oral folic acid
  therapy is not feasible
- IV: With 5-FU for palliative treatment of
  metastatic colorectal cancer
- To decrease toxicity of methotrexate caused
  by decreased elimination or for inadvertent
  overdose of folic acid antagonists such as
  trimethoprim

Contraindications and cautions

- Contraindicated with allergy to leucovorin
  on previous exposure, pernicious anemia or
  other megaloblastic anemias in which vitamin B_{12} is deficient.
- Use cautiously with pregnancy, lactation.

Available forms

Tablets—5, 10, 15, 25 mg; injection—10 mg/mL; powder for injection—50, 100, 200, 350, 500 mg/vial

Dosages
Adults

- *Rescue after methotrexate therapy:* Begin therapy within 24 hr of methotrexate dose. 10 mg/m^2 PO every 6 hr for 10 doses or until methotrexate level is less than 0.05 micromolar. If at 24 hr following methotrexate administration, serum creatinine is 100% greater than the pretreatment level, or based on methotrexate levels, increase the leucovorin dose to 150 mg IV every 3 hr until the serum methotrexate level is less than 1.0 micromolar; then 15 mg IV every 3 hr until methotrexate level is less than 0.05 micromolar.
- *Megaloblastic anemia:* Up to 1 mg/day IM may be used. Do not exceed 1 mg/day.
- *Metastatic colon cancer:* Give 200 mg/m^2 by slow IV injection over up to 3 min, followed by 5-FU 370 mg/m^2 IV *or* 20 mg/m^2 IV, followed by 5-FU 425 mg/m^2 IV. Repeat daily for 5 days; may be repeated at 4-wk intervals.

Pharmacokinetics

Route	Onset	Peak	Duration
Oral	30 min	2.4 hr	3–6 hr
IM	Rapid	52 min	3–6 hr
IV	Immediate	10 min	3–6 hr

Metabolism: Hepatic; $T_{1/2}$: 5.7 hr (oral), 6.2 hr (IV, IM)
Distribution: Crosses placenta; enters breast milk
Excretion: Urine

▼ IV FACTS

Preparation: Prepare solution by diluting a 50-mg vial of powder with 5 mL bacteriostatic water for injection that contains benzyl alcohol and use within 7 days, or reconstitute with water for injection and use immediately. Protect from light.
Infusion: Infuse slowly over 3–5 min; not more than 160 mg/min.
Incompatibility: Do not mix with floxuridine or 5-FU.
Y-site incompatibility: Do not inject with droperidol.

Adverse effects

- **Hypersensitivity:** Allergic reactions
- **Local:** *Pain, discomfort at injection site*

Interactions

✻ **Drug-drug** • Leucovorin increases the efficacy and potential side effects of 5-FU; adjust dosage of 5-FU and monitor.

■ Nursing considerations

 CLINICAL ALERT!
Name confusion has occurred between leucovorin and *Leukeran* (chlorambucil) and between folinic acid (leucovorin) and folic acid; use extreme caution.

Assessment

- **History:** Allergy to leucovorin on previous exposure, pernicious anemia or other megaloblastic anemias, lactation, pregnancy
- **Physical:** Skin lesions, color; R, adventitious sounds; CBC, Hgb, Hct, serum folate levels, serum methotrexate levels

Interventions

⊗ *Warning* Do not use benzyl alcohol solutions when giving leucovorin to premature infants; a fatal gasping syndrome has occurred.
- Begin leucovorin rescue within 24 hr of methotrexate administration. Arrange for fluid loading and urine alkalinization during this procedure to decrease methotrexate toxicity.
- Give drug orally unless intolerance to oral route develops due to nausea and vomiting from chemotherapy or clinical condition. Switch to oral drug when feasible. Doses more than 25 mg should be divided or given IV.
⊗ *Warning* Monitor patient for hypersensitivity reactions, especially if drug has been used previously. Keep supportive equipment and emergency drugs readily available in case of serious allergic response.
⊗ *Warning* Do not administer intrathecally; doing so can be fatal.

Teaching points

- Leucovorin "rescues" normal cells from the effects of methotrexate and allows them to survive.

- Leucovorin used to treat anemias or colorectal cancer must be given IV. Mark calendars with treatment days.
- Report rash, difficulty breathing, pain, or discomfort at injection site.

▷leuprolide acetate
*(loo **proe'** lide)*

Eligard, Lupron Depot,
Lupron Depot-PED,
Lupron Depot—3 Month,
Lupron Depot—4 Month,
Lupron Depot—6 Month,
Lupron for Pediatric Use

PREGNANCY CATEGORY X

Drug class
Gonadotropin-releasing hormone (GnRH) analogue

Therapeutic actions
An LH-RH agonist that occupies pituitary gonadotropin-releasing hormone receptors and desensitizes them; inhibits gonadotropin secretion when given continuously, leading to an initial increase, then profound decrease in LH and FSH levels.

Indications
- Advanced prostatic cancer—palliation, alternative to orchiectomy or estrogen therapy
- Depot only: Endometriosis
- Central precocious puberty
- Depot only: Uterine leiomyomata
- Unlabeled uses: Treatment of breast, ovarian, and endometrial cancers; infertility; prostatic hypertrophy

Contraindications and cautions
- Contraindicated with allergy to leuprolide, pregnancy, undiagnosed vaginal bleeding, lactation.

Available forms
Injection—5 mg/mL; *Depot*—3.75, 7.5 mg; *Depot-Ped*—7.5, 11.25, 15 mg; 3-mo *Depot*—11.25, 22.5, 45 mg; 4-mo *Depot*—30 mg, 72 mg; 6-mo *Depot*—45 mg; powder for injection—7.5 mg

Dosages
Adults
- *Advanced prostate cancer:* 1 mg/day subcutaneously; use only the syringes that come with the drug.
  Depot: 7.5 mg IM monthly (every 28–33 days). Do not use needles smaller than 22 gauge.
  3-mo Depot: 22.5 mg IM or subcutaneously every 3 mo (84 days).
  4-mo Depot: 30 mg IM or subcutaneously every 4 mo.
  6-mo Depot: 45 mg subcutaneously every 6 mo.
- *Endometriosis:* 3.75 mg as a single monthly IM injection or 11.25 mg IM every 3 mo. Continue for 6 mo.
- *Uterine leiomyomata:* 3.75 mg as a single monthly injection for 3 mo *or* 11.25 mg IM once; give with concomitant iron treatment.

Pediatric patients
- *Central precocious puberty:* 50 mcg/kg/day subcutaneously; may be titrated up by 10 mcg/kg/day increments.
  Depot: 0.3 mg/kg IM monthly every 4 wk. Round to nearest depot size; minimum, 7.5 mg.

Pharmacokinetics

Route	Onset	Peak	Duration
IM depot	4 hr	Variable	1, 3, or 4 mo

Metabolism: Unknown; $T_{1/2}$: 3 hr (subcutaneous injection)
Distribution: Crosses placenta; may enter breast milk
Excretion: Unknown

Adverse effects
- **CNS:** *Dizziness, headache, pain,* paresthesia, blurred vision, lethargy, fatigue, insomnia, memory disorder
- **CV:** *Peripheral edema,* cardiac arrhythmias, thrombophlebitis, heart failure, **MI**
- **Dermatologic:** Rash, alopecia, itching, erythema
- **GI:** GI bleeding, *nausea, vomiting, anorexia,* sour taste, *constipation*
- **GU:** *Frequency, hematuria,* decreases in sizes of testes, increased BUN and creatinine, impotence, decreased libido, gynecomastia
- **Local:** Ecchymosis at injection site

Adverse effects in *italics* are most common; those in **bold** are life-threatening. ▧ Do not crush.

- **Respiratory:** Difficulty breathing, pleural rub, worsening of pulmonary fibrosis
- **Other:** *Hot flashes, sweats,* bone pain, diabetes

■ **Nursing considerations**
Assessment
- **History:** Allergy to leuprolide; pregnancy, lactation
- **Physical:** Skin lesions, color, turgor; testes; injection sites; orientation, affect, reflexes, peripheral sensation; peripheral pulses, edema, P; R, adventitious sounds; serum testosterone and serum PSA levels

Interventions
- Administer only with the syringes provided with the drug.
- Administer subcutaneously; monitor injection sites for bruising and rash; rotate injection sites to decrease local reaction.
- Give depot injection deep into muscle. Prepare a calendar of monthly (28–33 days every 3, 4, or 6 mo) return visits for new injection.
- Store below room temperature (25° C or 77° F); avoid freezing. Depot suspension is stable for 24 hr following reconstitution; product does not contain preservatives, so discard if not used properly.
- Arrange for periodic serum testosterone and PSA determinations in males.

⊗ *Warning* Consider stopping therapy for central precocious puberty before 11 yr in females, 12 yr in males. Monitor patient with GnRH stimulation test, sex steroids, and Tanner staging.

⊗ *Warning* There is a possible increased risk of diabetes and CV disease in men treated for prostate cancer; monitor patient closely.

- Advise patient to use barrier contraceptives; serious fetal harm can occur.
- Teach patient and significant other the technique for subcutaneous injection, and observe administration before home administration of daily doses.

Teaching points
- Administer subcutaneously only, using the syringes that come with the drug; arrange to dispose of needles and syringes appropriately. If Depot is used, drug may be given IM or subcutaneously; prepare calendar for return dates, stressing the importance of receiving each injection.

- Do not stop taking this drug without first consulting your health care provider.
- This drug cannot be taken during pregnancy; using barrier contraceptives is advised.
- You may experience these side effects: Bone pain, difficulty urinating (usually transient); hot flashes (stay in cool places); nausea, vomiting (eat frequent small meals); dizziness, headache, light-headedness (use caution when driving or performing tasks that require alertness); decreased libido, impotence.
- Report injection site pain, burning, itching, swelling, numbness, tingling, severe GI upset, pronounced hot flashes, chest pain.

▽**levalbuterol**
*(lev al **byoo'** ter ole)*

levalbuterol hydrochloride
Xopenex

levalbuterol tartrate
Xopenex HFA

PREGNANCY CATEGORY C

Drug classes
Antiasthmatic
Beta$_2$-selective adrenergic agonist
Bronchodilator
Sympathomimetic

Therapeutic actions
In low doses, acts relatively selectively at beta$_2$-adrenergic receptors to cause bronchodilation and vasodilation; at higher doses, beta$_2$-selectivity is lost and the drug also acts at beta$_1$ receptors to cause typical sympathomimetic cardiac effects.

Indications
- Treatment and prevention of bronchospasm in adults and children 4 yr and older, (tartrate) and 6 yr and older (hydrochloride) with reversible obstructive pulmonary disease
- Unlabeled uses: Treatment of acute asthma, asthma exacerbations

Contraindications and cautions
- Contraindicated with hypersensitivity to albuterol or levalbuterol; tachyarrhythmias,

tachycardia caused by digoxin toxicity; general anesthesia with halogenated hydrocarbons or cyclopropane (these sensitize the myocardium to catecholamines); unstable vasomotor system disorders; hypertension; coronary insufficiency, coronary artery disease; history of stroke; COPD in patients who have developed degenerative heart disease.

• Use cautiously in psychoneurotic individuals and with hyperthyroidism; history of seizure disorders; pregnancy; lactation.

Available forms

Solution for inhalation—0.31 mg/3 mL, 0.63 mg/3 mL, 1.25 mg/3 mL; solution for inhalation concentrate—1.25 mg/0.5 mL; aerosol inhalation—45 mcg/actuation

Dosages
Levalbuterol hydrochloride (Xopenex)
Adults and patients 12 yr and older
0.63 mg tid, every 6–8 hr by nebulization; if patient does not respond, the dose may be increased to up to 1.25 mg tid by nebulization.
Pediatric patients 6–11 yr
0.31 mg tid by nebulization; do not exceed 0.63 mg tid.
Pediatric patients younger than 6 yr
Safety and efficacy not established.
Levalbuterol tartrate (Xopenex HFA)
Adults and children 4 yr and older
Two inhalations (90 mcg) repeated every 4–6 hr; some patients may respond to 1 inhalation (45 mcg) every 4 hr.

Pharmacokinetics

Route	Onset	Peak	Duration
Inhalation	5 min	1 hr	6–8 hr

Metabolism: Hepatic; $T_{1/2}$: 4–6 hr
Distribution: Crosses placenta; enters breast milk
Excretion: Urine

Adverse effects

• **CNS:** *Apprehension, anxiety, fear, CNS stimulation,* hyperkinesia, insomnia, tremor, dizziness, irritability, weakness, vertigo, headache

• **CV:** Cardiac arrhythmias, tachycardia, palpitations, PVCs (rare), anginal pain (less likely with bronchodilator doses of this drug than with bronchodilator doses of a nonselective beta-agonist, eg, isoproterenol), increases or decreases in BP
• **Dermatologic:** Sweating, pallor, flushing
• **GI:** *Nausea,* vomiting, heartburn, unusual or bad taste
• **Respiratory:** Respiratory difficulties, pulmonary edema, coughing, URI, **bronchospasm**

Interactions

✳ **Drug-drug** • Risk of increased sympathomimetic effects when given with other sympathomimetics • Risk of increased toxicity, especially cardiac, when used in combination with theophylline, aminophylline • Possible decreased bronchodilating effects when given with beta-adrenergic blockers (eg, propranolol) • Risk of severe toxicity if combined with MAO inhibitors; use extreme caution

■ Nursing considerations
Assessment

• **History:** Hypersensitivity to levalbuterol or albuterol; tachyarrhythmias, tachycardia caused by digoxin toxicity; general anesthesia with halogenated hydrocarbons or cyclopropane; unstable vasomotor system disorders; hypertension; coronary artery disease; history of stroke; COPD in patients who have developed degenerative heart disease; diabetes mellitus; hyperthyroidism; history of seizure disorders; history of psychiatric illness; pregnancy, lactation
• **Physical:** Weight, skin color, T, turgor; orientation, reflexes, affect; P, BP; R, adventitious sounds; blood and urine glucose, serum electrolytes, thyroid function tests, ECG

Interventions

⊗ **Warning** Keep unopened drug in foil pouch until ready to use; protect from heat and light. Once foil pouch is open, use the vial within 2 wk, protected from light and heat. Once a vial is removed from foil pouch, use immediately. If not used, protect from light and use within 1 wk. Discard vial if solution is not colorless.
• Teach patient correct use of inhaler and maintenance of actuator (*Xopenex HFA*).

Adverse effects in *italics* are most common; those in **bold** are life-threatening. ⏞ Do not crush.

- Continue use to control recurrent bouts of bronchospasm; most effective with regular use.
- Do not exceed recommended dosage; administer inhalation drug forms during second half of inspiration, because the airways are open wider and the aerosol distribution is more extensive.

⊗ **Warning** Monitor patient response; if usual effective dosage regimen does not provide relief, this usually indicates a serious worsening of the asthma and indicates need for reassessment of drug regimen.

- Establish safety precautions if CNS changes occur.
- Reassure patients with acute respiratory distress; provide appropriate supportive measures.
- Monitor environmental temperature if patient has flushing or sweating.

Teaching points

- Do not exceed recommended dosage—adverse effects or loss of effectiveness may result; read the instructions for use that come with the product for proper administration of nebulized drug.
- Keep unopened drug in foil pouch until ready to use; protect from heat and light. Once foil pouch is open, use the vial within 2 weeks, protected from light and heat. Once a vial is removed from its foil pouch, use immediately. If not used, protect from light and use within 1 week. Discard the vial if the solution is not colorless.
- If using a metered inhaler (*Xopenex HFA*), prime the inhaler before use; blow out all the air you can expel, place the actuator in your mouth and slowly breathe in while pressing down on the top of the metal canister. Hold your breath for 10 seconds. If you are prescribed two inhalations, wait 10 seconds and then repeat the process. Wash and air dry the actuator at least once a week. Discard the metal canister after 200 sprays, even if you think the canister is not empty.
- You may experience these side effects: Dizziness, fatigue, headache (use caution if driving or performing tasks that require alertness if these effects occur); nausea, vomiting, change in taste (eat frequent small meals; consult your health care provider if this is prolonged); rapid heart rate, anxiety, sweating, flushing.

- Report chest pain, dizziness, insomnia, weakness, tremors or irregular heartbeat, difficulty breathing, productive cough, failure to respond to usual dosage.

▽ levetiracetam
*(lev ah ty **ray' ca** tam)*

Keppra, Keppra XR ⒞

PREGNANCY CATEGORY C

Drug class
Antiepileptic

Therapeutic actions
Mechanism of action not well understood; antiepileptic activity may be related to its ability to inhibit polysynaptic responses and block post-tetanic potentiation.

Indications

- Adjunctive therapy in the treatment of partial-onset seizures in adults and children 4 yr and older with epilepsy, when used with other epilepsy medication
- Adjunctive therapy in the treatment of myoclonic seizures in patients 12 yr and older
- Adjunctive therapy in treatment of primary generalized tonic-clonic seizures in adults and children 6 yr and older with idiopathic generalized epilepsy
- Unlabeled uses: Migraine, adjunctive therapy for bipolar disease, monotherapy for new-onset pediatric epilepsy.

Contraindications and cautions

- Contraindicated with hypersensitivity to levetiracetam.
- Use cautiously with lactation, pregnancy, renal impairment.

Available forms
Tablets—250, 500, 750, 1,000 mg; oral solution—100 mg/mL; injection—500 mg/5 mL; ER tablets ⒞ —500 mg

Dosages
Adults and children older than 16 yr

- *Partial-onset seizures:* 1,000 mg/day given as 500 mg PO or IV bid; may be increased in 1,000-mg/day increments every 2 wk;

maximum dose, 3,000 mg/day. ER tablets: 1,000 mg/day PO; increase every 2 wk in 1,000 mg/day intervals to maximum dosage 3,000 mg/day.

- *Generalized tonic-clonic seizures:* Initially, 1,000 mg/day PO given as 500 mg bid; increase by 1,000 mg/day every 2 wk to recommended 3,000 mg/day.

Adults and children 12 yr and older

- *Myoclonic seizures:* 1,000 mg/day given as 500 mg PO bid; slowly increase to recommended maximum dose, 3,000 mg/day.

Pediatric patients 6–15 yr

- *Generalized tonic-clonic seizures:* Initially, 20 mg/kg/day PO in two divided doses of 10 mg/kg. Increase every 2 wk by 20-mg/kg increments to recommended dosage of 60 mg/kg/day given as 30 mg/kg bid.

Pediatric patients 4–16 yr

- *Partial-onset seizures:* 10 mg/kg PO bid (500–1,000 mg/day), may be increased every 2 wk in 20 mg/kg increments to 30 mg/kg bid (1,500–3,000 mg/day). To determine daily dose of oral solution: total dose (mL/day) = daily dose (mg/kg/day) × patient weight (kg) divided by 100 mg/mL.

Patients with renal impairment

CrCl (mL/min)	Dosage (mg)
More than 80	500–1,500 every 12 hr
50–80	500–1,000 every 12 hr
30–50	250–750 every 12 hr
Less than 30	250–500 every 12 hr

For patients on dialysis, use 500–1,000 mg every 24 hr.

Pharmacokinetics

Route	Onset	Peak
Oral	Rapid	1 hr

Metabolism: $T_{1/2}$: 6–8 hr
Distribution: Crosses placenta; may enter breast milk
Excretion: Urine, unchanged

▼ IV FACTS

Preparation: Dilute desired dose in 100 mL of 0.9% sodium chloride, lactated Ringer solution, or 5% dextrose solution.
Infusion: Infuse over 15 min.
Compatibilities: Compatible with lorazepam, diazepam, valproate sodium.

Adverse effects

- **CNS:** *Dizziness, headache,* vertigo, nervousness, fatigue, *somnolence, ataxia,* diplopia, suicidal ideation
- **Dermatologic:** Pruritus
- **GI:** Dyspepsia, vomiting, nausea, constipation, anorexia
- **Respiratory:** Rhinitis, pharyngitis
- **Other:** Weight gain, facial edema, impotence

■ Nursing considerations

◤ CLINICAL ALERT!
Name confusion has occurred between *Keppra* (levetiracetam) and *Kaletra* (lopinavir and ritonavir); use extreme caution.

Assessment

- **History:** Hypersensitivity to levetiracetam; lactation, renal impairment, pregnancy
- **Physical:** Body weight; body T; skin color, lesions; orientation, affect, reflexes; P, R, adventitious sounds; bowel sounds, normal output, renal function tests

Interventions

- Reserve IV use for short-term, when oral administration is not feasible; revert to oral use as soon as patient is able.
- Give drug with food to prevent GI upset; use oral solution for children or adults with difficulty swallowing. Ensure that patient does not cut, crush, or chew ER tablets.
- If CNS, vision, or coordination changes occur, establish safety precautions (use side rails, accompany patient when ambulating).
- Advise using barrier contraceptives while this drug is being used.
- ⊗ *Warning* Do not stop drug abruptly. Risk of seizure precipitation; withdraw gradually.
- Offer support and encouragement for dealing with epilepsy and adverse drug effects; arrange for consultation with support groups for people with epilepsy as needed.

Teaching points

- Take this drug exactly as prescribed. Do not cut, crush, or chew ER tablets; swallow them whole.
- Do not discontinue this drug abruptly or change dosage, except on the advice of your health care provider.

Adverse effects in *italics* are most common; those in **bold** are life-threatening. ⊞ Do not crush.

- Do not take this drug if you are pregnant or plan to become pregnant, serious fetal effects can occur, using barrier contraceptives is recommended.
- Wear or carry a medical alert tag at all times so that any emergency medical personnel taking care of you will know that you have epilepsy and are taking an antiepileptic.
- You may experience these side effects: Dizziness, blurred vision (avoid driving a car or performing other tasks requiring alertness or visual acuity if this occurs); GI upset (taking the drug with food or milk and eating frequent small meals may help); headache, nervousness (if these become severe, consult your health care provider); fatigue (periodic rest periods may be helpful).
- Report severe headache, sleepwalking, rash, severe vomiting, chills, fever, difficulty breathing.

▽levocetirizine dihydrochloride

*(lev oh seh **teer'** ih zeen)*

Xyzal

PREGNANCY CATEGORY B

Drug class
Antihistamine

Therapeutic actions
Potent histamine (H_1) receptor antagonist; inhibits histamine release and eosinophil chemotaxis during inflammation, reducing swelling and inflammatory response.

Indications
- Relief from symptoms of seasonal and perennial allergic rhinitis in adults and children 6 mo and older
- Treatment of uncomplicated skin effects in chronic idiopathic urticaria in patients 2 yr and older

Contraindications and cautions
- Contraindicated with hypersensitivity to levocetirizine, any of its components, or cetirizine; end-stage renal disease; renal impairment in children 6–11 yr; lactation.
- Use cautiously with pregnancy and with use of CNS depressants.

Available forms
Tablets—5 mg; oral solution—2.5 mg/5 mL

Dosages
Adults and children 12 yr and older
5 mg/day PO, taken in the evening.
Children 6–11 yr
2.5 mg/day PO taken in the evening.
Children 6 mo–5 yr
1.25 mg (½ tsp oral solution) PO once daily in the evening.
Patients with renal impairment
12 yr and older: If creatinine clearance is 50–80 mL/min, give 2.5 mg/day PO; if creatinine clearance is 30–50 mL/min, give 2.5 mg PO every other day; if creatinine clearance is 10–30 mL/min, give 2.5 mg PO twice weekly (once every 3–4 days); if creatinine clearance is less than 10 mL/min, drug is not recommended.

Pharmacokinetics

Route	Onset	Peak
Oral	Rapid	1 hr

Metabolism: $T_{1/2}$: 8 hr
Distribution: May cross placenta; enters breast milk
Excretion: Urine, unchanged

Adverse effects
- **CNS:** *Somnolence,* asthenia
- **GI:** Dry mouth
- **Respiratory:** *Nasopharyngitis,* cough, pharyngitis, epistaxis
- **Other:** *Fatigue,* fever

Interactions
✳ **Drug-drug** • Risk of increased CNS depression and altered mental alertness if combined with alcohol or other CNS depressing drugs; avoid this combination

■ Nursing considerations
Assessment
- **History:** Hypersensitivity to any component of the drug or to cetirizine, renal impairment, pregnancy, lactation, use of CNS depressants
- **Physical:** T; orientation, affect, reflexes; R, adventitious sounds; renal function tests

Interventions
- Administer once each day, in the evening.
- Alert patient to possible alterations in mental alertness while taking this drug.

- Encourage use of humidifiers and adequate intake of fluids to help prevent severe dryness of mucous membranes.
- Provide skin care for urticaria.

Teaching points

- Take this drug once each day, in the evening. Do not take more than the prescribed dose in any one day.
- It is not known how this drug could affect a breast-feeding infant. If you are breast-feeding, another method of feeding the infant should be selected.
- It is not known how this drug could affect a fetus; if you are pregnant, consult your health care provider.
- Avoid the use of alcohol or any CNS depressants while you are using this drug; these could increase the effects on mental alertness.
- You may experience these side effects: Sleepiness, decreased mental alertness (avoid driving a car, operating dangerous machinery, or engaging in tasks that require mental alertness while you are on this drug); cough, nosebleed, sore throat (use a humidifier, and make sure you drink plenty of fluids to help prevent severe drying of your mucous membranes).
- Report difficulty breathing, nosebleeds, and marked changes in mental functioning.

▽ levodopa
*(lee voe **doe' **pa)*

PREGNANCY CATEGORY C

Drug class
Antiparkinsonian

Therapeutic actions
Biochemical precursor of the neurotransmitter dopamine, which is deficient in the basal ganglia of parkinsonism patients; unlike dopamine, levodopa penetrates the blood–brain barrier. It is transformed in the brain to dopamine; thus, levodopa is a form of replacement therapy. It is efficacious for 2–5 yr in relieving the symptoms of parkinsonism but not drug-induced extrapyramidal disorders.

Indications

- Treatment of parkinsonism (postencephalitic, arteriosclerotic, and idiopathic types) and symptomatic parkinsonism following injury to the nervous system by carbon monoxide or manganese intoxication
- Given with carbidopa (*Lodosyn;* fixed combinations, *Sinemet*), an enzyme inhibitor that decreases the activity of dopa decarboxylase in the periphery, thus reducing blood levels of levodopa and decreasing the intensity and incidence of many of the adverse effects of levodopa
- Unlabeled uses: Relief of herpes zoster (shingles) pain; restless legs syndrome

Contraindications and cautions

- Contraindicated with hypersensitivity to levodopa; glaucoma, especially angle-closure glaucoma; lactation.
- Use cautiously in psychiatric patients, especially the depressed or psychotic; and with severe CV or pulmonary disease; occlusive cerebrovascular disease; history of MI with residual arrhythmias; bronchial asthma; renal, hepatic, endocrine disease; history of peptic ulcer; pregnancy.

Available forms
Available only in combination products

Dosages
Adults
Individualize dosage. Increase dosage gradually to minimize side effects; titrate dosage carefully to optimize benefits and minimize side effects. Initially, 0.5–1 g PO daily divided into two or more doses given with food. Increase gradually in increments not exceeding 0.75 g/day every 3–7 days as tolerated. Do not exceed 8 g/day, except for exceptional patients. A significant therapeutic response may not be obtained for 6 mo. Only available in combination forms.
Pediatric patients
Safety for use in children younger than 12 yr not established.

Pharmacokinetics

Route	Onset	Peak
Oral	Varies	0.5–2 hr

Metabolism: Hepatic; $T_{1/2}$: 1–3 hr

Adverse effects in *italics* are most common; those in **bold** are life-threatening. ⊞ Do not crush.

Distribution: Crosses placenta; enters breast milk
Excretion: Urine

Adverse effects

- **CNS:** *Adventitious movement (eg, dystonic movements), ataxia, increased hand tremor, headache, dizziness, numbness, weakness and faintness,* bruxism, confusion, insomnia, nightmares, hallucinations and delusions, agitation and anxiety, malaise, fatigue, euphoria, mental changes (including paranoid ideation), psychotic episodes, depression with or without suicidal tendencies, dementia, bradykinesia ("on-off" phenomenon), muscle twitching and blepharospasm, diplopia, blurred vision, dilated pupils
- **CV:** Cardiac irregularities, palpitations, orthostatic hypotension
- **Dermatologic:** Flushing, hot flashes, increased sweating, rash
- **GI:** *Anorexia, nausea, vomiting, abdominal pain or distress, dry mouth, dysphagia, dysgeusia,* bitter taste, sialorrhea, trismus, burning sensation of the tongue, diarrhea, constipation, flatulence, weight change, upper GI hemorrhage in patients with history of peptic ulcer
- **GU:** Urinary retention, urinary incontinence
- **Hematologic:** Leukopenia, anemia, elevated BUN, AST, ALT, LDH, bilirubin, alkaline phosphatase, protein-bound iodine
- **Respiratory:** Bizarre breathing patterns

Interactions

✳ **Drug-drug** ⊗ *Warning* Increased therapeutic effects and possible hypertensive crisis with MAOIs; withdraw MAOIs at least 14 days before starting levodopa therapy
• Decreased efficacy with pyridoxine (vitamin B_6), phenytoin, papaverine, TCAs, benzodiazepines
✳ **Drug-lab test** • May interfere with urine tests for sugar or ketones • False Coombs test results • False elevations of uric acid when using colorimetric method

■ Nursing considerations
Assessment

- **History:** Hypersensitivity to levodopa, tartrazine; glaucoma; history of melanoma; suspicious or undiagnosed skin lesions; severe CV or pulmonary disease; occlusive cerebrovascular disease; history of MI with residual arrhythmias; bronchial asthma; renal, hepatic, endocrine disease; history of peptic ulcer; psychiatric disorders; lactation, pregnancy
- **Physical:** Weight; T; skin color, lesions; orientation, affect, reflexes, bilateral grip strength, vision examination; P, BP, orthostatic BP, auscultation; R, depth, adventitious sounds; bowel sounds, normal output, liver evaluation; voiding pattern, normal output, prostate palpation; LFTs, renal function tests; CBC with differential

Interventions

⊗ *Warning* Arrange to decrease dosage if therapy is interrupted; observe for the development of suicidal tendencies.
- Give with meals if GI upset occurs.
- Ensure that patient voids before receiving dose if urinary retention is a problem.
- Monitor hepatic, renal, hematopoietic, and CV function.
- For patients who take multivitamins, provide a preparation without pyridoxine.

Teaching points

- Take this drug exactly as prescribed.
- Do not take multivitamin preparations with pyridoxine. These may prevent any therapeutic effect of levodopa. Notify your health care provider if you need vitamins.
- You may experience these side effects: Drowsiness, dizziness, confusion, blurred vision (avoid driving or engaging in activities that require alertness and visual acuity); nausea (take with meals, eat frequent small meals); dry mouth (suck sugarless candies or ice chips); painful or difficult urination (empty bladder before each dose); constipation (maintain adequate fluid intake and exercise regularly, request correctives); dark sweat or urine (not harmful); dizziness or faintness when you get up (change position slowly and use caution when climbing stairs).
- Report fainting, light-headedness, dizziness; uncontrollable movements of the face, eyelids, mouth, tongue, neck, arms, hands, or legs; mental changes; irregular heartbeat or palpitations; difficult urination; severe or persistent nausea or vomiting.

▷ levofloxacin
(lee voe flox' a sin)

Levaquin

PREGNANCY CATEGORY C

Drug classes
Antibiotic
Fluoroquinolone

Therapeutic actions
Bactericidal: Interferes with DNA by inhibiting DNA gyrase replication in susceptible gram-negative and gram-positive bacteria, preventing cell reproduction.

Indications
• Treatment of adults with community-acquired pneumonia, bacterial sinusitis caused by susceptible bacteria including multidrug resistant strains
• Treatment of acute exacerbation of chronic bronchitis caused by susceptible bacteria
• Treatment of complicated and uncomplicated skin and skin structure infections caused by susceptible bacteria
• Treatment of complicated and uncomplicated UTIs and acute pyelonephritis caused by susceptible bacteria
• Treatment of complicated UTIs caused by *Escherichia coli, Klebsiella pneumoniae,* or *Proteus mirabilis* and acute pyelonephritis caused by *E. coli*
• Treatment of chronic bacterial prostatitis caused by *E. coli, Enterococcus faecalis, Staphylococcus*
• Treatment of nosocomial pneumonia due to methicillin-sensitive *Staphylococcus aureus, Pseudomonas* strains, *Serratia, E. coli, Klebsiella, Haemophilus influenzae, Streptococcus pneumoniae*
• Treatment of postexposure inhalational anthrax
•■ NEW INDICATION: Prophylaxis and treatment of plague due to *Yersinia pestis* in patients 6 mo and older
• Unlabeled uses: Epididymitis, gonococcal infection, infective endocarditis, TB, traveler's diarrhea

Contraindications and cautions
• Contraindicated with allergy to fluoroquinolones, lactation, myasthenia gravis, tendinitis, tendon rupture.
• Use cautiously with renal impairment, seizures, pregnancy.

Available forms
Tablets—250, 500, 750 mg; oral solution—25 mg/mL; injection—5 mg/mL; injection concentrate—25 mg/mL

Dosages
Adults
• *Community-acquired pneumonia:* 500 mg daily PO or IV for 7–14 days.
• *Sinusitis:* 500 mg daily PO or IV for 10–14 days or 750 mg/day PO or IV for 5 days.
• *Chronic bronchitis:* 500 mg daily PO or IV for 7 days.
• *Skin infection:* 500–750 mg daily PO or IV for 7–14 days.
• *UTIs:* 250 mg daily PO or IV for 3–10 days; complicated, 750 mg/day PO or IV for 5 days.
• *Pyelonephritis:* 250 mg daily PO or IV for 10 days or 750 mg PO or IV for 5 days.
• *Nosocomial pneumonia:* 750 mg daily PO or IV for 7–14 days.
• *Chronic prostatitis:* 500 mg/day PO for 28 days or 500 mg/day by slow IV infusion over 60 min for 28 days.
• *Postexposure anthrax:* 500 mg/day PO or IV for 60 days.
• *Plague:* 500 mg/day PO for 10–14 days.
Pediatric patients
• *Inhalational anthrax:* 6 mo or older weighing more than 50 kg: 500 mg/day PO for 60 days; 6 mo or older weighing less than 50 kg: 8 mg/kg every 12 hr PO for 60 days. Do not exceed 250 mg/dose.
• *Plague:* More than 50 kg: 500 mg/day PO for 10–14 days; 6 mo and older weighing less than 50 kg: 8 mg/kg PO every 12 hr for 10–14 days. Maximum dose, 250 mg.
Patients with renal impairment

CrCl (mL/min)	Dose
50–80	No adjustment
20–49	500 mg initially, then 250 mg daily; or 750 mg then 750 mg every 48 hr
10–19	500 mg initially, then 250 mg every 48 hr; or 750 mg, then 500 mg every 48 hr

For patients on dialysis, 750 mg initially, then 500 mg every 48 hr; or 500 mg initially, then 250 mg every 48 hr.

Pharmacokinetics

Route	Onset	Peak	Duration
Oral	Varies	1–2 hr	3–5 hr
IV	Rapid	End of infusion	3–5 hr

Metabolism: Hepatic; $T_{1/2}$: 6–8 hr
Distribution: Crosses placenta; enters breast milk
Excretion: Urine

▼ IV FACTS

Preparation: No further preparation is needed if using the premixed solution; dilute single-use vials in 50–100 mL D_5W.
Infusion: Administer slowly over at least 60–90 min. Do not administer IM or subcutaneously.
Compatibilities: Can be further diluted in 0.9% sodium chloride injection, 5% dextrose injection, 5% dextrose/0.9% sodium chloride, 5% dextrose in lactated Ringer, *Plasma-Lyte 56* and *5% Dextrose* injection, 5% dextrose/ 0.45% sodium chloride, 0.15% potassium chloride, sodium lactate injection.

Adverse effects

- **CNS:** *Headache,* dizziness, *insomnia,* fatigue, somnolence, blurred vision
- **CV:** Prolonged QT interval
- **GI:** *Nausea,* vomiting, dry mouth, *diarrhea,* abdominal pain (occur less with this drug than with ofloxacin), constipation, flatulence, abnormal liver function
- **GU:** Abnormal renal function, acute renal failure, UTI, urine retention
- **Hematologic:** Elevated BUN, serum creatinine, and alkaline phosphatase; neutropenia, anemia
- **Other:** Fever, rash, photosensitivity, *muscle and joint tenderness,* increased serum glucose, tendinitis, tendon rupture, blood glucose alterations

Interactions

✳ **Drug-drug** • Decreased therapeutic effect with iron salts, sucralfate, antacids, zinc, magnesium (separate by at least 2 hr) • Increased risk of seizures with NSAIDs; avoid this combination • Risk of prolonged QT interval if combined with other drugs known to prolong QT interval; use caution

✳ **Drug-alternative therapy** • Increased risk of severe photosensitivity reactions if combined with St. John's Wort therapy

■ Nursing considerations
Assessment

- **History:** Allergy to fluoroquinolones, renal impairment, seizures, lactation, pregnancy, myasthenia gravis, tendinitis
- **Physical:** Skin color, lesions; T; orientation, reflexes, affect; mucous membranes, bowel sounds; LFTs, renal function tests; blood glucose (patients with diabetes)

Interventions

⊗ **Black box warning** There is a risk of tendinitis and tendon rupture with drug administration. Risk increase in patients older than 60 yr, with concurrent corticosteroids use, and with kidney, heart, or lung transplant.

⊗ **Black box warning** Risk of exacerbation of myasthenia gravis with serious muscle weakness; do not administer to patients with a history of myasthenia gravis.

- Arrange for culture and sensitivity tests before beginning therapy.
- Continue therapy as indicated for condition being treated.
- Administer oral drug without regard to meals with a glass of water; separate oral drug from other cation administration, including antacids, by at least 2 hr.
- Ensure that patient is well hydrated during course of therapy.

⊗ **Warning** Discontinue drug at any sign of hypersensitivity (rash, photophobia) or at complaint of tendon pain, inflammation, or rupture.

- Monitor clinical response; if no improvement is seen or a relapse occurs, repeat culture and sensitivity test.

Teaching points

- Take oral drug without regard to meals. If an antacid is needed, do not take it within 2 hours of levofloxacin dose.
- Drink plenty of fluids while you are taking this drug. Do not use St. John's Wort while taking this drug.
- You may experience these side effects: Nausea, vomiting, abdominal pain (eat frequent

small meals); diarrhea or constipation (consult your health care provider); drowsiness, blurred vision, dizziness (use caution if driving or operating dangerous equipment); sensitivity to sunlight (avoid exposure, use a sunscreen if needed).
- Report rash, visual changes, severe GI problems, weakness, tremors, muscle pain.

▽levoleucovorin

See Appendix R, *Less commonly used drugs.*

DANGEROUS DRUG
▽levorphanol tartrate
(lee vor' fa nole)

PREGNANCY CATEGORY C

CONTROLLED SUBSTANCE C-II

Drug class
Opioid agonist analgesic

Therapeutic actions
Acts as agonist at specific opioid receptors in the CNS to produce analgesia, euphoria, sedation; the receptors are thought to be the same as those mediating the effects of endogenous opioids (enkephalins, endorphins).

Indications
- Relief of moderate to severe acute and chronic pain

Contraindications and cautions
- Contraindicated with hypersensitivity to opioids, diarrhea caused by poisoning (before toxins are eliminated), pregnancy (neonatal withdrawal), labor or delivery (respiratory depression of neonate—premature infants are especially at risk; may prolong labor), bronchial asthma, acute alcoholism, increased intracranial pressure, respiratory depression, anoxia.
- Use cautiously with COPD, cor pulmonale, acute abdominal conditions, CV disease, supraventricular tachycardias, myxedema, seizure disorders, delirium tremens, cerebral arteriosclerosis, ulcerative colitis, kyphoscoliosis, Addison disease, prostatic hypertrophy, urethral stricture, recent GI or GU surgery, toxic psychosis, and renal or hepatic impairment.

Available forms
Tablets—2 mg

Dosages
Adults
Starting dose is 2 mg PO repeated every 3–6 hr. Higher doses may be needed in opioid-tolerant patients or patients with severe pain. Usual dose, 8–16 mg/day.
Geriatric patients or impaired adults
Use caution—respiratory depression may occur in the elderly, the very ill, and those with respiratory problems. Reduced dosage (by up to 50%) may be necessary.

Pharmacokinetics

Route	Onset	Peak	Duration
Oral	30–90 min	0.5–1 hr	6–8 hr

Metabolism: Hepatic; $T_{1/2}$: 12–16 hr
Distribution: Crosses placenta; enters breast milk
Excretion: Urine

Adverse effects
- **CNS:** *Light-headedness, dizziness, sedation,* euphoria, dysphoria, delirium, insomnia, agitation, anxiety, fear, hallucinations, disorientation, drowsiness, lethargy, impaired mental and physical performance, coma, mood changes, weakness, headache, tremor, seizures, miosis, visual disturbances, suppression of cough reflex
- **CV:** Facial flushing, peripheral circulatory collapse, tachycardia, bradycardia, arrhythmia, palpitations, chest wall rigidity, hypertension, hypotension, orthostatic hypotension, syncope
- **Dermatologic:** Pruritus, urticaria, edema, hemorrhagic urticaria (rare)
- **GI:** *Nausea, vomiting,* dry mouth, anorexia, *constipation,* biliary tract spasm; increased colonic motility in patients with chronic ulcerative colitis
- **GU:** Ureteral spasm, spasm of vesicle sphincters, urinary retention or hesitancy, oliguria, antidiuretic effect, reduced libido or potency
- **Respiratory:** Bronchospasm, laryngospasm
- **Major hazards:** Respiratory depression, apnea, circulatory depression, **respiratory arrest, shock, cardiac arrest**

Adverse effects in *italics* are most common; those in **bold** are life-threatening. ⬛ Do not crush.

- **Other:** *Sweating* (more common in ambulatory patients and those without severe pain), physical tolerance and dependence, psychological dependence

Interactions

✳ **Drug-drug** • Potentiation of effects of levorphanol when given with barbiturate anesthetics; decrease dose of levorphanol when coadministering • Increased risk of CNS effects with ethanol, barbiturates, antihistamines, and other sedating drugs

✳ **Drug-lab test** • Elevated biliary tract pressure may cause increases in plasma amylase and lipase; determinations of these levels may be unreliable for 24 hr after administration of opioids

■ Nursing considerations
Assessment

- **History:** Hypersensitivity to opioids, diarrhea caused by poisoning, labor or delivery, bronchial asthma, acute alcoholism, increased intracranial pressure, respiratory depression, cor pulmonale, acute abdominal conditions, CV disease, myxedema, seizure disorders, delirium tremens, cerebral arteriosclerosis, ulcerative colitis, fever, kyphoscoliosis, Addison disease, prostatic hypertrophy, urethral stricture, recent GI or GU surgery, toxic psychosis, renal or hepatic impairment
- **Physical:** T; skin color, texture, lesions; orientation, reflexes, pupil size, bilateral grip strength, affect; P, auscultation, BP, orthostatic BP, perfusion; R, adventitious sounds; bowel sounds, normal output; frequency and pattern of voiding, normal output; ECG; EEG; thyroid, LFTs, renal function tests

Interventions

- Give to lactating women 4–6 hr before the next feeding to minimize the amount in milk.
- Reassure patient that most people who receive opiates for medical reasons do not develop psychological dependency.

Teaching points

- Take drug exactly as prescribed.
- Do not take leftover medication for other disorders, and do not let anyone else take your prescription. Dispose of leftover medication appropriately.
- Do not breast-feed while taking this drug.
- You may experience these side effects: Nausea, loss of appetite (take with food, lie quietly, eat frequent small meals); constipation (laxative may help); dizziness, sedation, drowsiness, impaired visual acuity (avoid driving, performing other tasks that require alertness or visual acuity).
- Report severe nausea, vomiting, constipation, shortness of breath, or difficulty breathing.

▷ levothyroxine sodium (L-thyroxine, T_4)
(lee voe thye rox' een)

Levothroid, Levoxine, Levoxyl, Synthroid, Thyro-Tabs

PREGNANCY CATEGORY A

Drug class
Thyroid hormone

Therapeutic actions
Increases the metabolic rate of body tissues, thereby increasing oxygen consumption; respiration and HR; rate of fat, protein, and carbohydrate metabolism; and growth and maturation.

Indications

- Replacement therapy in hypothyroidism
- Pituitary TSH suppression in the treatment and prevention of euthyroid goiters and in the management of thyroid cancer
- Treatment of thyrotoxicosis in conjunction with antithyroid drugs and to prevent goitrogenesis, hypothyroidism, and thyrotoxicosis during pregnancy
- Treatment of myxedema coma

Contraindications and cautions

- Contraindicated with allergy to active or extraneous constituents of drug, untreated thyrotoxicosis, and acute MI uncomplicated by hypothyroidism.
- Use cautiously with Addison disease (treat hypoadrenalism with corticosteroids before thyroid therapy), lactation, patients with coronary artery disease or angina.

Available forms

Tablets—25, 50, 75, 88, 100, 112, 125, 137, 150, 175, 200, 300 mcg; powder for injection—200, 500 mcg/vial; capsules—13, 25, 50, 75, 100, 125, 150 mcg

Dosages

50–100 mcg equals approximately 60 mg (1 grain) desiccated thyroid.

Adults

• *Hypothyroidism:* Initial dose, 12.5–25 mcg PO, with increasing increments of 25 mcg PO every 2–4 wk; maintenance up to 200 mcg/day. IV or IM injection can be substituted for the oral dosage form when oral ingestion is not possible. Usual IV dose is 50% of oral dose. Start at 25 mcg/day or less in patients with long-standing hypothyroidism or known cardiac disease. Usual replacement 1.7 mcg/kg per day.

• *Myxedema coma without severe heart disease:* 200–500 mcg IV as initial dose. An additional 100–300 mcg or more may be given the second day if necessary. Switch to PO once patient is able. Full effect not seen for 24 hr; dose based on improvement.

• *TSH suppression in thyroid cancer, nodules, and euthyroid goiters:* Doses should be individualized based on specific disease and patient. Larger amounts than used for normal suppression.

• *Thyroid suppression therapy:* 2.6 mcg/kg/day PO for 7–10 days.

• Older patients may require less than 1 mcg/kg/day. For most patients older than 50 yr or under age 50 with cardiac disease, an initial dose of 12.5 to 25 mcg/day with increases of 25 mcg/day every 6–8 wk.

Pediatric patients

• *Congenital hypothyroidism:* Infants require replacement therapy from birth.

0–3 mo: 10–15 mcg/kg/day.
3–6 mo: 8–10 mcg/kg/day.
6–12 mo: 6–8 mcg/kg/day.
1–5 yr: 5–6 mcg/kg/day.
6–12 yr: 4–5 mcg/kg/day.
Older than 12 yr: 2–3 mcg/kg/day.

Pharmacokinetics

Route	Onset	Peak
Oral	Slow	1–3 wk
IV	6–8 hr	24–48 hr

Metabolism: Hepatic; $T_{1/2}$: 6–7 days

Distribution: Crosses placenta; enters breast milk
Excretion: Urine

▼ IV FACTS

Preparation: Add 5 mL 0.9% sodium chloride injection. Shake the vial to ensure complete mixing. Use immediately after reconstitution. Discard any unused portion.
Infusion: Inject directly, each 100 mcg over 1 min.
Incompatibilities: Do not mix with any other IV fluids.

Adverse effects

• **CNS:** Tremors, headache, nervousness, insomnia
• **CV:** Palpitations, tachycardia, angina, **cardiac arrest**
• **Dermatologic:** Allergic skin reactions, partial loss of hair in first few months of therapy in children
• **GI:** Diarrhea, nausea, vomiting, gagging, tablet stuck in throat, choking, esophageal atresia

Interactions

✳ **Drug-drug** • Decreased absorption of oral thyroid preparation with cholestyramine, clolestipol, aluminum- and magnesium-containing antacids, iron, sucralfate • Increased risk of bleeding with warfarin—reduce dosage of anticoagulant when T_4 is begun • Decreased effectiveness of cardiac glycosides if taken with thyroid replacement • Decreased theophylline clearance when patient is in hypothyroid state; monitor levels and patient response as euthyroid state is achieved

■ Nursing considerations

Assessment

• **History:** Allergy to active or extraneous constituents of drug, thyrotoxicosis, acute MI uncomplicated by hypothyroidism, Addison disease, lactation
• **Physical:** Skin lesions, color, T, texture; muscle tone, orientation, reflexes; P, auscultation, baseline ECG; BP; R, adventitious sounds; thyroid function tests

Interventions

⊗ *Black box warning* Do not use for weight loss; large doses may cause serious adverse effects.

Adverse effects in *italics* are most common; those in **bold** are life-threatening. ⬚ Do not crush.

- Monitor response carefully at start of therapy, and adjust dosage. Full therapeutic effect may not be seen for several days.
- Do not change brands of T_4 products, due to possible bioequivalence problems.
- Do not add IV doses to other IV fluids.
- Use caution in patients with CV disease.
- Administer oral drug as a single daily dose before breakfast.
- Arrange for regular, periodic blood tests of thyroid function.
- For children and other patients who cannot swallow tablets, crush and suspend in a small amount of water or formula, or sprinkle over soft food. Administer immediately.

⊗ **Warning** Most CV and CNS adverse effects indicate that the dose is too high. Check thyroid function tests and arrange to adjust dosage as necessary.

Teaching points

- Take as a single dose before breakfast. Store drug in a dry place. Do not use drug past expiration date because potency may be lost.
- This drug replaces an important hormone and will need to be taken for life. Do not discontinue drug without consulting your health care provider; serious problems can occur.
- Carry a medical ID tag to alert emergency medical personnel that you use this drug.
- Arrange to have periodic blood tests and medical evaluations. Keep your scheduled appointments.
- Report headache, chest pain, palpitations, fever, weight loss, sleeplessness, nervousness, irritability, unusual sweating, intolerance to heat, diarrhea.

DANGEROUS DRUG

▽**lidocaine hydrochloride**
(lye' doe kane)

lidocaine HCl in 5% dextrose

lidocaine HCl without preservatives

Antiarrhythmic preparations:

Xylocaine HCl IV for Cardiac Arrhythmias

Local anesthetic preparations:
Octocaine, Xylocaine HCl (injectable)

Topical for mucous membranes: Anestacon, Burn-O-Jel, Xylocaine, Zilactin-L

Topical Dermatologic: L-M-X4, Lidamantle, Numby Stuff, Regenecare, Solarcaine, Xylocaine

Transdermal: Lidoderm

PREGNANCY CATEGORY B

Drug classes
Antiarrhythmic
Local anesthetic

Therapeutic actions
Type 1b antiarrhythmic: Decreases diastolic depolarization, decreasing automaticity of ventricular cells; increases ventricular fibrillation threshold.
Local anesthetic: Blocks the generation and conduction of action potentials in sensory nerves by reducing sodium permeability, reducing height and rate of rise of the action potential, increasing excitation threshold, and slowing conduction velocity.

Indications
- As antiarrhythmic: Management of acute ventricular arrhythmias during cardiac surgery and MI (IV use). Use IM when IV administration is not possible or when ECG monitoring is not available and the danger of ventricular arrhythmias is great (single-dose IM use, for example, by paramedics in a mobile coronary care unit)
- As alternative to amiodarone to treat ventricular fibrillation or tachycardia with cardiac arrest
- As anesthetic: Infiltration anesthesia, peripheral and sympathetic nerve blocks, central nerve blocks, spinal and caudal anesthesia, retrobulbar and transtracheal injection; topical anesthetic for skin disorders and accessible mucous membranes
- As local analgesia for pain associated with post-herpetic neuralgia

Contraindications and cautions
- Contraindicated with allergy to lidocaine or amide-type local anesthetics, heart failure,

cardiogenic shock, second- or third-degree heart block (if no artificial pacemaker), Stokes-Adams syndrome, Wolff-Parkinson-White syndrome.
- Use cautiously with hepatic or renal disease, inflammation or sepsis in the region of injection (local anesthetic), labor and delivery (epidural anesthesia may prolong the second stage of labor; monitor for fetal and neonatal CV and CNS toxicity), and lactation.

Available forms

Direct injection—10, 20 mg/mL; IV injection (admixture)—5, 10, 15, 20, 40, 100 mg/mL; IV infusion—2, 4, 8 mg/mL; topical liquid—2.5%; topical ointment—5%; topical cream—0.5%, 3%, 4%; topical gel—0.5%, 2%, 2.5%, 4%, 5%; topical spray—0.5%, 10%; topical solution—2%, 4%; transdermal system—5%; topical lotion—3%

Dosages
Adults
IM
- *Arrhythmia:* Use only the 10% solution for IM injection. 300 mg in deltoid or thigh muscle. Switch to IV lidocaine or oral antiarrhythmic as soon as possible. Repeat dose in 60–90 min if necessary.

IV bolus
- *Arrhythmia:* Use only lidocaine injection labeled for IV use and without preservatives or catecholamines. Monitor ECG constantly. Give 50–100 mg at rate of 25–50 mg/min. Give second bolus dose after 5 min if needed. Do not exceed 200–300 mg in 1 hr.

IV, continuous infusion
- *Arrhythmia:* Give 1–4 mg/min (or 20–50 mcg/kg/min). Titrate the dose down as soon as the cardiac rhythm stabilizes. Use lower doses in patients with heart failure, liver disease, and in patients older than 70 yr.

Topical, intratissue, epidural
- *Local anesthesia:* Preparations containing preservatives should not be used for spinal or epidural anesthesia. Drug concentration and diluent should be appropriate to particular local anesthetic use: 5% solution with glucose is used for spinal anesthesia, 1.5% solution with dextrose for low spinal or "saddle block" anesthesia. Dosage varies with the area to be anesthetized and the reason for the anesthesia; use the lowest dose possible to achieve results.

Topical analgesia
- *Transdermal:* Apply up to 3 patches to area of pain for up to 12 hr within 24 hr.
- *Cream, ointment, gel, solution, oral patch, spray:* Apply as directed 1–3 times per day.

Pediatric patients
IV
- *Arrhythmia:* Safety and efficacy have not been established. American Heart Association recommends bolus of 0.5–1 mg/kg IV, followed by 30 mcg/kg/min with caution.

Topical, intratissue, epidural
- *Local anesthesia:* See adult dosage discussion. Use lower concentrations.

Geriatric or debilitated patients, patients with liver disease or heart failure
Use lower concentrations in these patients.

Pharmacokinetics

Route	Onset	Peak	Duration
IM	5–10 min	5–15 min	2 hr
IV	Immediate	Immediate	10–20 min

Metabolism: Hepatic; $T_{1/2}$: 10 min, then 1.5–3 hr
Distribution: Crosses placenta; may enter breast milk
Excretion: Urine

▼ IV FACTS

Preparation: Prepare solution for IV infusion as follows: 1–2 g lidocaine to 1 L D_5W = 0.1%–0.2% solution; 1–2 mg lidocaine/mL. Stable for 24 hr after dilution.
Infusion: IV bolus: Give 50–100 mg at rate of 25–50 mg/min. Continuous infusion: Given at a rate of 1–4 mL/min of a 1 mg/mL solution will provide 1–4 mg lidocaine/min. Use only preparations of lidocaine specifically labeled for IV infusion.

Adverse effects
Antiarrhythmic with systemic administration
- **CNS:** *Dizziness or light-headedness, fatigue, drowsiness,* unconsciousness, tremors, twitching, vision changes; may progress to **seizures**
- **CV:** **Cardiac arrhythmias, cardiac arrest,** vasodilation, *hypotension*
- **GI:** *Nausea,* vomiting

- **Hypersensitivity:** Rash, **anaphylactoid reactions**
- **Respiratory:** Respiratory depression, **Respiratory arrest**
- **Other:** Malignant hyperthermia, fever, local injection site reaction

Injectable local anesthetic for epidural or caudal anesthesia

- **CNS:** *Headache; backache;* septic meningitis; persistent sensory, motor, or autonomic deficit of lower spinal segments, sometimes with incomplete recovery
- **CV:** *Hypotension* due to sympathetic block
- **Dermatologic:** Urticaria, pruritus, erythema, edema
- **GU:** *Urinary retention, urinary or fecal incontinence*

Topical local anesthetic

- **Dermatologic:** Contact dermatitis, urticaria, cutaneous lesions
- **Hypersensitivity: Anaphylactoid reactions**
- **Local:** *Burning, stinging, tenderness, swelling, tissue irritation,* tissue sloughing and necrosis
- **Other:** Methemoglobinemia, **seizures** (children)

Interactions

✳ **Drug-drug** • Increased lidocaine levels with beta blockers (propranolol, metoprolol, nadolol, pindolol, atenolol), cimetidine • Prolonged neuromuscular blockade with succinylcholine

✳ **Drug-lab test** • Increased CPK if given IM

■ **Nursing considerations**
Assessment

- **History:** Allergy to lidocaine or amide-type local anesthetics, heart failure, cardiogenic shock, second- or third-degree heart block, Wolff-Parkinson-White syndrome, Stokes-Adams syndrome, hepatic or renal disease, inflammation or sepsis in region of injection, lactation, pregnancy
- **Physical:** T; skin color, rashes, lesions; orientation, speech, reflexes, sensation and movement (local anesthetic); P, BP, auscultation, continuous ECG monitoring during use as antiarrhythmic; edema; R, adventitious sounds; bowel sounds, liver evaluation; urine output; serum electrolytes, LFTs, renal function tests

Interventions

⊗ *Warning* Check drug concentration carefully; many concentrations are available.
- Reduce dosage with hepatic or renal failure.
- Continuously monitor response when used as antiarrhythmic or injected as local anesthetic.

⊗ *Warning* Keep life-support equipment and vasopressors readily available in case severe adverse reaction (CNS, CV, or respiratory) occurs when lidocaine is injected.

⊗ *Warning* Establish safety precautions if CNS changes occur; have IV diazepam or short-acting barbiturate (thiopental) readily available in case of seizures.

⊗ *Warning* Monitor for malignant hyperthermia (jaw muscle spasm, rigidity); have life-support equipment and IV dantrolene readily available.

- Titrate dose to minimum needed for cardiac stability, when using lidocaine as antiarrhythmic.
- Reduce dosage when treating arrhythmias in heart failure, digoxin toxicity with AV block, and geriatric patients.
- Monitor fluid load carefully; more concentrated solutions can be used to treat arrhythmias in patients on fluid restrictions.
- Have patients who have received lidocaine as a spinal anesthetic remain lying flat for 6–12 hr afterward, and ensure that they are adequately hydrated to minimize risk of headache.

⊗ *Warning* Large amounts of anesthetics used during cosmetic procedures may result in severe, life-threatening adverse effects. Amount used should be as small as possible and monitored by an experienced physician.

⊗ *Warning* Check lidocaine preparation carefully; epinephrine is added to solutions of lidocaine to retard the absorption of the local anesthetic from the injection site. Make sure that such solutions are used only to produce local anesthesia. These solutions should be injected cautiously in body areas supplied by end arteries and used cautiously in patients with peripheral vascular disease, hypertension, thyrotoxicosis, or diabetes.

- Use caution to prevent choking. Patient may have difficulty swallowing after using oral topical anesthetic. Do not give food or drink for 1 hr after use of oral anesthetic.
- Apply lidocaine ointments or creams to a gauze or bandage before applying to the skin.

⊗ **Warning** Monitor for safe and effective serum drug concentrations (antiarrhythmic use: 1–5 mcg/mL). Concentrations of 6 or more mcg/mL are usually toxic.

Teaching points
- Dosage is changed frequently in response to cardiac rhythm on monitor.
- Oral lidocaine can cause numbness of the tongue, cheeks, and throat. Do not eat or drink for 1 hour after using oral lidocaine to prevent biting the inside of your mouth or tongue and choking.
- You may experience these side effects: Drowsiness, dizziness, numbness, double vision; nausea, vomiting; stinging, burning, local irritation (local anesthetic).
- Report difficulty speaking, thick tongue, numbness, tingling, difficulty breathing, pain or numbness at IV site, swelling, or pain at site of local anesthetic use.

▽ **linaclotide**

See Appendix R, *Less commonly used drugs.*

▽ **linagliptin**
(lin ah glip' tin)

Tradjenta

PREGNANCY CATEGORY B

Drug classes
Antidiabetic
Dipeptidyl peptidase-4 (DPP-4) inhibitor

Therapeutic actions
Slows the inactivation of the incretin hormones by DPP-4, increasing these hormone levels and prolonging their activity. The incretin hormones stimulate insulin release in response to a meal and help regulate glucose homeostasis throughout the day. This action increases and prolongs insulin release and reduces hepatic glucose production to help achieve glycemic control.

Indications
- As an adjunct to diet and exercise to improve glycemic control in adults with type 2 diabetes

Contraindications and cautions
- Contraindicated with history of serious hypersensitivity reactions to linagliptin.
- Use cautiously with concurrent use of strong CYP3A inducers; pregnancy, lactation.

Available forms
Tablets—5 mg

Dosages
Adults
5 mg PO once a day without regard to food.
Pediatric patients
Safety and efficacy not established.

Pharmacokinetics

Route	Onset	Peak
Oral	Rapid	1.5 hr

Metabolism: Minimal; $T_{1/2}$: 12 hr
Distribution: May cross placenta; may enter breast milk
Excretion: Urine

Adverse effects
- **GI:** Pancreatitis
- **Respiratory:** *Nasopharyngitis*
- **Other:** Hypoglycemia, hypertriglyceridemia, rash

Interactions
✳ **Drug-drug** ● Possible loss of effectiveness if combined with potent CYP3A inhibitors (such as rifampin); this combination is not advised and another drug should be used
✳ **Drug-herb** ● Increased risk of hypoglycemia if taken with celery, coriander, dandelion root, fenugreek, garlic, ginger, juniper berries

■ Nursing considerations
Assessment
- **History:** Hypersensitivity to components of drug, pregnancy, lactation.
- **Physical:** R, adventitious sounds; blood glucose, HbA1c levels

Interventions
- Monitor blood glucose and HbA1c levels before and periodically during therapy.
- Ensure that patient continues diet and exercise program for the management of type 2 diabetes.

- If appropriate, ensure that patient continues use of other prescribed drugs to manage type 2 diabetes; safety of use with insulin has not been established.
- Arrange for thorough diabetic teaching program, including diet and exercise, signs and symptoms of hypoglycemia and hyperglycemia, and safety measures to avoid infections and injuries.

Teaching points

- Take this drug once a day with or without food.
- Report the use of any herbal products; many interact and dosage may need to be adjusted.
- If you forget a dose, take it as soon as you remember; then begin your usual dosage the next day. Do not make up skipped doses and do not take more than one dose each day.
- Monitor and maintain your blood glucose level as directed by your health care provider.
- Arrange for periodic monitoring of your fasting blood glucose and HbA1c levels.
- Continue the diet and exercise program designed for the treatment of your type 2 diabetes. Continue other drugs you may be using to treat your diabetes if instructed to do so by your health care provider.
- It is not known how this drug affects a fetus. If you are pregnant or thinking about becoming pregnant, discuss this with your health care provider.
- It is not known if this drug enters breast milk; if you are breast-feeding, discuss this with your health care provider.
- During times of stress (such as surgery, severe infection) the needs of your body change. Consult your health care provider immediately if you experience severe stress. The dosages of your antidiabetic medication and other medication that may be needed could change.
- Tell your health care provider about herbal supplements, over-the-counter products, or other prescription drugs you may be using. Many of these products may change your glucose level and dosages may need to be changed.
- Report signs of infection, uncontrolled glucose levels, trauma, severe stress.

▷**lincomycin hydrochloride**

See Appendix R, *Less commonly used drugs.*

▷**linezolid**
*(lah **nez**' oh lid)*

Zyvox

PREGNANCY CATEGORY C

Drug class
Oxazolidinone antibiotic

Therapeutic actions
Bacteriostatic and bacteriocidal: Interferes with protein synthesis on the bacterial ribosome; effective in VRE, *Staphylococcus,* and methicillin-resistant *S. aureus* (MRSA) and penicillin-resistant *pneumococci* and *S. aureus;* is a reversible, nonselective MAOI.

Indications
- Treatment of infections due to vancomycin-resistant *Enterococcus faecium* (VREF)
- Treatment of nosocomial and community-acquired pneumonia due to *S. aureus* and penicillin-susceptible *Streptococcus pneumoniae*
- Treatment of complicated and uncomplicated skin and skin-structure infections including those caused by MRSA
- Treatment of diabetic foot infections without osteomyelitis caused by gram-positive organisms including MRSA, *Streptococcus pyogenes,* or *Streptococcus agalactiae*

Contraindications and cautions
- Contraindicated with allergy to linezolid; lactation; phenylketonuria (oral suspension).
- Use cautiously with bone marrow suppression, hepatic impairment, hypertension, hyperthyroidism, pheochromocytoma, carcinoid syndrome, pregnancy.

Available forms
Tablets—600 mg; powder for oral suspension—100 mg/5 mL; injection—2 mg/mL

Dosages
No dosage adjustment is needed if switching between oral and IV forms.
Adults and children 12 yr and older
- *VREF, MRSA, pneumonia, complicated skin and skin structure infections, including diabetic foot ulcers without*

osteomyelitis: 600 mg IV or PO every 12 hr for 10–28 days, depending on infection.

• *Uncomplicated skin and skin structure infections:* 400 mg PO every 12 hr for 10–14 days.

Pediatric patients

• *VREF, CAP, nosocomial pneumonia, complicated skin, and skin structure infections:*
11 yr or younger: 10 mg/kg IV or PO every 8 hr for 10–14 days.

• *Uncomplicated skin and skin structure infections:*
5–11 yr: 10 mg/kg PO every 12 hr for 10–14 days.
Younger than 5 yr: 10 mg/kg PO every 8 hr.

Pharmacokinetics

Route	Onset	Peak
Oral	Rapid	1–2 hr
IV	Rapid	30 min

Metabolism: Hepatic; $T_{1/2}$: 5 hr
Distribution: Crosses placenta; enters breast milk
Excretion: Urine

▼ IV FACTS

Preparation: Use premixed solution—available in 100, 200, and 300 mL forms; store at room temperature, protect from light, leave overwrap in place until ready to use; appears yellow.
Infusion: Infuse over 30–120 min, switch to oral form as soon as appropriate. May be infused into line using 5% dextrose injection, 0.9% sodium chloride, or lactated Ringer.
Incompatibilities: ⊗ *Warning* Do not introduce additives into this solution; do not mix in solution or at Y-connection with any other drugs. If other drugs are being given through the same line, the line should be flushed before and after linezolid administration.

Adverse effects

• **CNS:** *Headache,* dizziness, *insomnia,* fatigue, somnolence, depression, nervousness
• **GI:** *Nausea,* vomiting, dry mouth, *diarrhea,* anorexia, gastritis, **pseudomembranous colitis**
• **Hematologic: Thrombocytopenia**
• **Other:** Fever, rash, sweating, photosensitivity, tendinitis

Interactions

✳ **Drug-drug** • Risk of hypertension and related adverse effects if combined with drugs containing pseudoephedrine, SSRIs, MAOIs; use caution and monitor patient carefully if any of these combinations are used • Increased risk of bleeding and thrombocytopenia if combined with antiplatelet drugs (aspirin, dipyridamole, NSAIDs); monitor platelet counts carefully • Risk of potentially serious serotonin syndrome if combined with serotonergic drugs; do not use with serotonergic drugs except in emergency cases of VRE infection, complicated skin infections and nosocomial pneumonia caused by MRSA; use other drugs if possible. If combination is needed, stop serotonergic drug 2 wk before therapy (with fluoxetine allow 5 wk); may resume therapy 24 hr after last linezolid dose. Teach patient to be alert for signs and symptoms of serotonin syndrome (confusion, memory problems, muscle twitching, excessive sweating, shivering, shaking, diarrhea, fever).

✳ **Drug-food** ⊗ *Warning* Risk of severe hypertension if combined with large amounts of food containing tyramine (see Appendix B, *Important dietary guidelines for patient teaching,* for tyramine food lists); patient should be cautioned to avoid eating large amounts of these foods.

■ Nursing considerations

✖ CLINICAL ALERT!
Name confusion has occurred between *Zyvox* (linezolid) and *Zovirax* (acyclovir); use caution.

Assessment

• **History:** Allergy to linezolid; hepatic impairment, bone marrow depression, hypertension, phenylketonuria, hyperthyroidism, carcinoid syndrome, pheochromocytoma, pregnancy, lactation
• **Physical:** Culture site; skin color, lesions; T; orientation, reflexes, affect; P, BP; mucous membranes, bowel sounds; LFTs, CBC, and differential

Interventions

• Arrange for culture and sensitivity tests before beginning therapy.
• Reserve use of this drug for cases of well-documented bacteria-sensitive infections.

Adverse effects in *italics* are most common; those in **bold** are life-threatening. ▭ Do not crush.

- Continue therapy as indicated for condition being treated.
- Monitor platelet counts regularly if drug is used for 2 wk or longer.
- Monitor BP before and periodically during therapy if patient is on antidepressants or drugs containing sympathomimetics.
- Advise patient to avoid foods high in tyramine to avoid risk of severe hypertension.
- Advise patient of high cost of drug and refer for financial support as needed.
- Monitor clinical response—if no improvement is seen or a relapse occurs, repeat culture and sensitivity tests.

Teaching points

- Take drug every 12 hours or every 8 hours as prescribed; take the full course of the drug; drug may be taken with or without food.
- Avoid foods high in tyramine (a list will be provided) while you are using this drug.
- You may experience these side effects: Nausea, vomiting, abdominal pain (eat frequent small meals; take the drug with food); diarrhea (consult your health care provider if this occurs).
- Report rash, severe GI problems, weakness, tremors, anxiety, increased bleeding.

▷**liothyronine sodium**
(T$_3$, triiodithyronine)
(lye' oh thye' roe neen)

Cytomel, Triostat

PREGNANCY CATEGORY A

Drug class
Thyroid hormone

Therapeutic actions
Increases the metabolic rate of body tissues, thereby increasing oxygen consumption; respiratory and HR; rate of fat, protein, and carbohydrate metabolism; and growth and maturation.

Indications
- Replacement therapy in hypothyroidism
- Pituitary TSH suppression in the treatment and prevention of euthyroid goiters and in the management of thyroid cancer

- Thyrotoxicosis in conjunction with antithyroid drugs and to prevent goitrogenesis, hypothyroidism, and thyrotoxicosis during pregnancy
- Synthetic hormone used with patients allergic to desiccated thyroid or thyroid extract derived from pork or beef
- Diagnostic use: T$_3$ suppression test to differentiate suspected hyperthyroidism from euthyroidism
- IV: Treatment of myxedema coma and precoma

Contraindications and cautions
- Contraindicated with allergy to active or extraneous constituents of drug, untreated thyrotoxicosis, and acute MI uncomplicated by hypothyroidism.
- Use cautiously with Addison disease (treat hypoadrenalism with corticosteroids before thyroid therapy), lactation, patients with coronary artery disease or angina, pregnancy.

Available forms
Tablets—5, 25, 50 mcg; injection—10 mcg/mL

Dosages
15–37.5 mcg equals approximately 60 mg (1 grain) desiccated thyroid.
Adults
- *Hypothyroidism:* Initial dosage, 25 mcg/day PO. May be increased every 1–2 wk in increments of 12.5–25-mcg. For maintenance, 25–75 mcg/day.
- *Myxedema:* Initial dosage, 5 mcg/day PO. Increase in increments of 5–10 mcg every 1–2 wk. For maintenance, 50–100 mcg/day.
- *Myxedema coma and precoma:* 25–50 mcg IV every 4–12 hr; do not give IM or subcutaneously. In patients with cardiac disease, start at 10–20 mcg IV. Do not exceed 100 mcg/24 hr.
- *Simple goiter:* Initial dosage, 5 mcg/day PO. May be increased by increments of 5–10 mcg every 1–2 wk. For maintenance, 75 mcg/day.
- *T$_3$ suppression test:* 75–100 mcg/day PO for 7 days, then repeat iodine 131 (^{131}I) uptake test. ^{131}I uptake will be unaffected in the hyperthyroid patient but will be decreased by 50% or more in the euthyroid patient.

L

Pediatric patients
- *Congenital hypothyroidism:* Infants require replacement therapy from birth. Starting dose is 5 mcg/day PO with 5-mcg increments every 3–4 days until the desired dosage is reached. Usual maintenance dosage, 20 mcg/day PO up to age 1 yr; 50 mcg/day for age 1–3 yr. Use adult dosage after age 3 yr.

Geriatric patients
Start therapy with 5 mcg/day PO. Increase by only 5-mcg increments at 2-wk intervals, and monitor patient response.

Pharmacokinetics

Route	Onset	Peak	Duration
Oral	Varies	2–3 days	3–4 days
IV	Rapid	End of infusion	Unkown

Metabolism: Hepatic; $T_{1/2}$: 1–2 days
Distribution: Does not cross placenta; enters breast milk
Excretion: Urine

▼ IV FACTS

Preparation: No further preparation is needed; refrigerate vials before use; discard unused portions.
Infusion: Infuse slowly, each 10 mcg over 1 min. Switch to oral form as soon as possible.

Adverse effects
- **Dermatologic:** Allergic skin reactions, partial loss of hair in first few months of therapy in children
- **Endocrine:** Mainly symptoms of hyperthyroidism: *Palpitations, elevated pulse pressure, tachycardia, arrhythmias,* angina pectoris, **cardiac arrest;** tremors, *headache, nervousness, insomnia; nausea,* diarrhea, changes in appetite; weight loss, menstrual irregularities, sweating, heat intolerance, fever
- **Other:** Esophageal atresia

Interactions
✳ **Drug-drug** ● Decreased absorption of oral thyroid preparation with cholestyramine ● Increased risk of bleeding with warfarin; reduce dosage of anticoagulant when thyroid hormone is begun ● Decreased effectiveness of cardiac glycosides with thyroid replacement ● Decreased

clearance of theophyllines if patient is in hypothyroid state; monitor response and adjust dosage as patient approaches euthyroid state

■ Nursing considerations
Assessment
- **History:** Allergy to active or extraneous constituents of drug, thyrotoxicosis, acute MI uncomplicated by hypothyroidism, Addison disease, lactation, pregnancy
- **Physical:** Skin lesions, color, T, texture; T; muscle tone, orientation, reflexes; P, auscultation, baseline ECG, BP; R, adventitious sounds; thyroid function tests

Interventions
⊗ ***Black box warning*** Do not use for weight loss; large doses may cause serious adverse effects.
- Monitor patient response carefully at start of therapy; adjust dosage.
- Monitor exchange from one form of thyroid replacement to T_3. Discontinue the other medication, then begin this drug at a low dose with gradual increases based on the patient's response.
⊗ *Warning* Most CV and CNS adverse effects indicate a too-high dose. Stop medication for several days and reinstitute at a lower dose.
- Administer as a single daily dose before breakfast with a full glass of water.
- Arrange for regular, periodic blood tests of thyroid function.
- Monitor cardiac response.

Teaching points
- Take as a single dose before breakfast with a full glass of water. Store in dry place. Do not use drug past the expiration date because potency may be lost.
- This drug replaces an important hormone and will need to be taken for life. Do not discontinue drug for any reason without consulting your health care provider; serious problems can occur.
- Wear or carry a medical ID tag to alert emergency medical personnel that you are using this drug.
- Have periodic blood tests and medical evaluations.
- Nausea and diarrhea may occur (dividing the dose may help).
- Report headache, chest pain, palpitations, fever, weight loss, sleeplessness, nervousness,

Adverse effects in *italics* are most common; those in **bold** are life-threatening. ⬛ Do not crush.

irritability, unusual sweating, intolerance to heat, diarrhea.

▷liotrix
(lye' oh trix)

Thyrolar

PREGNANCY CATEGORY A

Drug class
Thyroid hormone (contains synthetic T_3 and T_4 in a ratio of 1 to 4 by weight)

Therapeutic actions
Increases the metabolic rate of body tissues, thereby increasing oxygen consumption; respiratory and HR; rate of fat, protein, and carbohydrate metabolism; and growth and maturation.

Indications
- Replacement therapy in hypothyroidism
- Congenital hypothyroidism
- Pituitary TSH suppression in the treatment and prevention of euthyroid goiters and in the management of thyroid cancer
- Treatment of thyrotoxicosis in conjunction with antithyroid drugs and to prevent goitrogenesis, hypothyroidism, and thyrotoxicosis during pregnancy
- Diagnostic test for thyroid disease

Contraindications and cautions
- Contraindicated with allergy to active or extraneous constituents of drug, untreated thyrotoxicosis, and acute MI uncomplicated by hypothyroidism.
- Use cautiously with Addison disease (hypoadrenalism; treat with corticosteroids before thyroid therapy), lactation, coronary artery disease, or angina, pregnancy.

Available forms
Tablets—¼, ½, 1, 2, 3 grains equivalent to 15, 30, 60, 120, 180 mg thyroid, respectively

Dosages
60 mg equals 65 mg (1 grain) desiccated thyroid; administered only PO.
Adults
- *Hypothyroidism:* Initial dosage, 30 mg/day PO. Increase gradually every 2–3 wk in 15-mg (thyroid equivalent) increments (2 wk in children). In patients with cardiac disease, start with 15 mg/day (thyroid equivalent).
- *Maintenance dose:* 60–120 mg/day PO (thyroid equivalent).
- *Thyroid cancer:* Use larger doses than required for replacement surgery.
- *Diagnostic test:* 1.56 mcg/kg/day PO for 7–10 days.

Pediatric patients older than 12 yr
More than 90 mg/day (thyroid equivalent PO).
Pediatric patients 6–12 yr
60–90 mg/day (thyroid equivalent PO).
Pediatric patients 1–5 yr
45–60 mg/day (thyroid equivalent PO).
Pediatric patients 6–12 mo
30–45 mg/day (thyroid equivalent PO).
Pediatric patients 0–6 mo
15–30 mg/day (thyroid equivalent PO).

Pharmacokinetics

Route	Onset	Peak	Duration
Oral	Varies	2–3 days	3 days

Metabolism: Hepatic; $T_{1/2}$: 1–6 days
Distribution: Does not cross placenta; enters breast milk
Excretion: Urine

Adverse effects
- **Dermatologic:** Allergic skin reactions, partial hair loss in first few months of therapy in children
- **Endocrine:** Mainly symptoms of hyperthyroidism: *Palpitations, elevated pulse pressure, tachycardia, arrhythmias,* angina pectoris, **cardiac arrest;** tremors, *headache, nervousness, insomnia; nausea,* diarrhea, changes in appetite; weight loss, menstrual irregularities, sweating, heat intolerance, fever
- **Other:** Esophageal atresia

Interactions
✳ **Drug-drug** • Decreased absorption of oral thyroid preparation with cholestyramine • Increased risk of bleeding with warfarin; reduce dosage of anticoagulant when T_4 is begun • Decreased effectiveness of cardiac glycosides if taken with thyroid replacement • Decreased clearance of theophyllines in hypothyroid state; monitor response and adjust dosage as patient approaches euthyroid state

＊ **Drug-lab test •** Androgens, corticosteroids, estrogens, oral contraceptives, iodine-containing preparations may alter thyroid tests

■ Nursing considerations
Assessment
- **History:** Allergy to active or extraneous constituents of drug, thyrotoxicosis, acute MI uncomplicated by hypothyroidism, Addison disease, lactation, pregnancy
- **Physical:** Skin lesions, color, T, texture; T; muscle tone, orientation, reflexes; P, auscultation, baseline ECG, BP; R, adventitious sounds; thyroid function tests

Interventions
⊗ **Black box warning** Do not use for weight loss; large doses may cause serious adverse effects.
- Monitor response carefully at start of therapy, and adjust dosage.
⊗ **Warning** Most CV and CNS adverse effects indicate a dose that is too high. Stop drug for several days and reinstitute at a lower dose.
- Administer as a single daily dose before breakfast with a full glass of water.
- Carefully check dosage; dosing can be confusing when converting from grains to thyroid-equivalent dosages.
- Arrange for regular, periodic blood tests of thyroid function.
- Monitor cardiac response.

Teaching points
- Take as a single dose before breakfast with a full glass of water. Store drug in dry place. Do not use after expiration date because potency may be lost.
- This drug replaces an important hormone and will need to be taken for life. Do not discontinue without consulting your health care provider; serious problems can occur.
- If you are also diabetic, dosages of your diabetic medications may need to be changed.
- Wear a medical ID tag to alert emergency medical personnel that you take this drug.
- Have periodic blood tests and medical evaluations.
- Nausea and diarrhea may occur (divide the dose).
- Report headache, chest pain, palpitations, fever, weight loss, sleeplessness, nervousness, irritability, unusual sweating, intolerance to heat, diarrhea.

DANGEROUS DRUG
▷liraglutide
*(lir ah **gloo'** tide)*

Victoza

PREGNANCY CATEGORY C

Drug classes
Antidiabetic
Glucagon-like peptide receptor agonist

Therapeutic actions
Increases intracellular cyclic AMP in pancreatic beta cells, leading to insulin release in the presence of elevated glucose concentrations; this insulin secretion subsides as blood glucose levels approach normal; it also decreases glucagon secretion in a glucose-dependent manner; this mechanism of glucose lowering also causes a delay in gastric emptying, helping to achieve glucose control.

Indications
- As adjunct to diet and exercise to improve glycemic control in adults with type 2 diabetes

Contraindications and cautions
- Contraindicated with history of serious hypersensitivity reactions to liraglutide, personal or family history of medullary thyroid cancer, multiple endocrine neoplasia syndrome (MENS) type 2, type 1 diabetes, diabetic ketoacidosis.
- Use cautiously with pancreatitis, pregnancy, lactation.

Available forms
Solution for injection in prefilled pens—6 mg/mL (delivers 0.6, 1.2, or 1.8 mg)

Dosages
Adults
Initially, 0.6 mg by subcutaneous injection once a day, without regard to meals, for 1 wk; then increase to 1.2 mg/day by subcutaneous injection. May be increased to 1.8 mg/day if needed.
Pediatric patients
Safety and efficacy not established.

Pharmacokinetics

Route	Onset	Peak
Oral	Moderate	8–12 hr

Metabolism: Endogenous; $T_{1/2}$: 13 hr
Distribution: May cross placenta; may enter breast milk
Excretion: Urine, feces

Adverse effects

- **CNS:** Headache, dizziness
- **GI:** *Nausea, diarrhea, vomiting,* constipation, **pancreatitis**
- **GU:** UTI
- **Respiratory:** URI, sinusitis, nasopharyngitis
- **Other:** Urticaria, hypoglycemia, injection-site reactions, **papillary thyroid carcinoma**

Interactions

✳ **Drug-drug** • Possible altered absorption of oral drugs related to delay in gastric emptying; use caution when using oral drugs with liraglutide • Increased risk of hypoglycemia when combined with antidiabetic secretagogues (such as sulfonylureas); consider lowering secretagogue dosage

✳ **Drug-alternative therapies** • Increased risk of hypoglycemia if taken with juniper berries, ginseng, garlic, fenugreek, coriander, dandelion root, celery

Nursing considerations

Assessment

- **History:** Hypersensitivity to components of drug, personal or family history of medullary thyroid cancer, MENS type 2, pancreatitis, pregnancy, lactation
- **Physical:** R, adventitious sounds; GI exam; blood glucose, HbA1c levels

Interventions

⊗ **Black box warning** Drug causes thyroid medullary cancer in rodents; not for use with personal or family history of thyroid medullary cancer or MENS type 2; monitor patient closely.

- Monitor blood glucose and HbA1c levels before and periodically during therapy.
- Ensure patient continues diet and exercise program for management of type 2 diabetes.
- Alert patient to risk of medullary thyroid cancer and pancreatitis.

- If appropriate, ensure patient continues use of other drugs prescribed to manage type 2 diabetes.
- Arrange for thorough diabetic teaching program, including diet, exercise, signs and symptoms of hypoglycemia and hyperglycemia, and safety measures to avoid infections and injuries.

Teaching points

- Liraglutide should be taken once a day, with or without food. It must be injected by subcutaneous injection. You and a significant other should learn to give these injections. Drug is supplied in a prefilled pen. You must dispose of needles appropriately.
- Before use, store pen in refrigerator. After first use, store at room temperature or in refrigerator. Mark date of first use on pen; pen can only be used for a total of 30 days after first use and should then be discarded. Protect pen from exposure to heat and light. Remove needle after each use and dispose of it properly; store pen with cap in place. Do not share pen with other patients.
- If you forget a dose, take it as soon as you remember, then begin your usual dosage the next day. Do not make up skipped doses and do not take more than one dose each day.
- Maintain your blood glucose level as directed by your health care provider.
- Continue the diet and exercise program designed for treatment of your type 2 diabetes; continue taking other drugs used to treat your diabetes if instructed to do so by your health care provider.
- Arrange for periodic monitoring of your fasting blood glucose and glycosylated hemoglobin levels.
- It is not known how drug affects a fetus. If you are pregnant or thinking about becoming pregnant, discuss this with your health care provider.
- Drug enters breast milk, but it is not known how this could affect a breast-feeding infant. If you are breast-feeding, discuss this with your health care provider.
- During times of stress (surgery, infection, injury), the needs of your body change. Consult your health care provider immediately if you experience times of stress. The dosage of your antidiabetic drugs and

L

the actual drugs that are needed may change.
- Tell your health care provider if you are taking herbal or over-the-counter products or other prescription drugs; many of these products may change your glucose level and dosage adjustments will be needed.
- Report uncontrolled glucose levels; severe abdominal pain that radiates to the back and may be accompanied by vomiting; severe headache; lump in the neck; hoarseness; difficulty swallowing; increased stress; trauma.

▷ **lisdexamfetamine dimesylate**

(liss dex am fet' a meen)

Vyvanse

PREGNANCY CATEGORY C
CONTROLLED SUBSTANCE C-II

Drug classes
Amphetamine
CNS stimulant

Therapeutic actions
Thought to block reuptake of norepinephrine and dopamine in the presynaptic neuron and increase release of these monamines into the extraneuronal space, stimulating CNS activity and leading to suppressed appetite, increased alertness, elevated mood, improved physical performance when fatigue and sleep deprivation have caused impairment; mode of action in attention deficit hyperactivity disorder (ADHD) is not understood.

Indications
- Treatment of ADHD in patients 6 yr and older as part of an integrated treatment plan

Contraindications and cautions
- Contraindicated with hypersensitivity to any component of the drug, advanced arteriosclerosis, symptomatic CV disease, moderate to severe hypertension, hyperthyroidism, hypersensitivity or idiosyncratic reaction to sympathetic amines, glaucoma, agitated states, history of drug abuse, during or within 14 days following treatment with an MAOI, lactation.

- Use cautiously with history of seizures, pre-existing psychosis or bipolar disorder, pregnancy.

Available forms
Capsules—20, 30, 40, 50, 60, 70 mg

Dosages
Adults and children 6 yr and older
30 mg/day PO in the morning; may increase at weekly intervals in increments of 10–20 mg/day to a maximum of 70 mg/day.

Pharmacokinetics

Route	Onset	Peak
Oral	Rapid	3.5 hr

Metabolism: Hepatic; $T_{1/2}$: 1 hr
Distribution: May cross placenta; enters breast milk
Excretion: Urine

Adverse effects
- **CNS:** *Headache,* dizziness, somnolence, *insomnia,* tics, *irritability,* aggression, mania, affect lability, seizures, visual disturbances
- **CV: Serious cardiac events, sudden death,** hypertension, tachycardia
- **GI:** *Abdominal pain, diarrhea,* nausea, *vomiting,* dry mouth, *decreased appetite*
- **Other:** Fever, *weight loss,* rash, drug dependence, slowed growth

Interactions
✳ **Drug-drug** • Risk of decreased effectiveness if combined with urine acidifying agents, methenamine • Risk of increased activity of TCAs and sympathomimetic agents and increased risk of CV events • Risk of toxic neurologic effects and potentially fatal malignant hyperpyrexia if combined with MAOIs; do not use for 14 days after stopping MAOI • Blocked effects if combined with chlorpromazine; do not use this combination (chlorpromazine may be used to treat amphetamine poisoning) • Decreased CNS stimulation if combined with haloperidol • Enhanced effects of meperidine, norepinephrine if combined with lisdexamfetamine • Risk of excessive CNS stimulation and fatal seizures if combined with propoxyphene overdose

✳ **Drug-lab test** • Significant elevation in plasma corticosteroid level, particularly in the evening

Adverse effects in *italics* are most common; those in **bold** are life-threatening. ⬛ Do not crush.

■ Nursing considerations

⊗ *Black box warning* High risk of abuse could lead to drug dependence; misuse of amphetamines has caused serious CV events and sudden death.

Assessment

- **History:** Hypersensitivity to any component of the drug, advanced arteriosclerosis, symptomatic CV disease, moderate to severe hypertension, hyperthyroidism, known hypersensitivity or idiosyncrasy to sympathetic amines, glaucoma, agitated states, history of drug abuse, during or within 14 days following treatment with an MAOI, lactation; history of seizures, pre-existing psychosis or bipolar disorder, pregnancy
- **Physical:** Skin color, lesions; orientation, affect, reflexes; BP, P; height and weight; baseline ECG suggested.

Interventions

- Ensure proper diagnosis before administering to children for behavioral syndromes; drug should not be used until other causes (learning disabilities, EEG abnormalities, neurologic deficits) are ruled out.
- Drug therapy should be part of a comprehensive program to help with the problem.
- Interrupt drug therapy periodically to determine if symptomatic response still validates drug therapy.
- Monitor growth of children on long-term therapy; failure to grow may indicate need to stop drug.
- Dispense the lowest feasible dose to minimize risk of overdosage; drug should be stored securely out of the reach of anyone who might abuse drug (drug is a controlled substance).
- If child cannot swallow capsules, empty the capsule contents into a glass of water and have the child drink it right away. Do not try to divide doses or save contents.
- Administer drug early in the day to help prevent insomnia.
- Provide small, frequent meals if GI upset is a problem.
- Monitor BP periodically.

Teaching points

- Store this drug at room temperature in a dry place (not in the bathroom or near the kitchen sink). It is a controlled substance with abuse potential; store it out of the reach of children.
- Give this drug once a day in the morning. If you or your child cannot swallow the capsule, open it, dissolve the entire contents in a glass of water, and drink or have the child drink it right away.
- You or your child will need to have periodic blood tests, blood pressure checks, and height and weight checks to monitor the effects of this drug.
- This drug should be used as part of a comprehensive ADHD treatment program that includes behavior modification.
- The effectiveness of this drug may be changed by combining with certain other drugs, especially antidepressants such as MAOIs, antipsychotic drugs, blood pressure drugs, seizure drugs, and opioid pain relievers. Tell all of you or your child's health care providers that your child is taking this drug so that appropriate dosage adjustments and precautions can be taken.
- You or your child may experience the following side effects: Irritability, insomnia (monitor the child, especially at the start of drug therapy); dry mouth, loss of appetite, abdominal pain (sucking sugarless candies may help, but make sure to safeguard the child's nutrition); slowing of growth, weight loss (report any marked changes to your health care provider).
- Report aggression, vision changes, manic symptoms, marked weight loss, seizures.

▽ lisinopril
*(lyse **in**' oh pril)*

Prinivil, Zestril

PREGNANCY CATEGORY C (FIRST TRIMESTER)

PREGNANCY CATEGORY D (SECOND AND THIRD TRIMESTERS)

Drug classes
ACE inhibitor
Antihypertensive

Therapeutic actions
Renin, synthesized by the kidneys, is released into the circulation where it acts on a plasma precursor to produce angiotensin I, which is converted by ACE to angiotensin II, a potent vasoconstrictor that also causes release of

aldosterone from the adrenals. Lisinopril blocks the conversion of angiotensin I to angiotensin II, leading to decreased BP, decreased aldosterone secretion, a small increase in serum potassium levels, and sodium and fluid loss.

Indications

- Treatment of hypertension alone or in combination with other antihypertensives
- Adjunctive therapy in heart failure for patients unresponsive to diuretics and digoxin alone
- Treatment of stable patients within 24 hr of acute MI to improve survival with standard treatments

Contraindications and cautions

- Contraindicated with allergy to lisinopril, other ACE inhibitors, history of angioedema.
- Use cautiously with impaired renal function, heart failure, salt or volume depletion, IHSS, pregnancy, lactation.

Available forms

Tablets—2.5, 5, 10, 20, 30, 40 mg

Dosages

Adults not taking diuretics

Initial dose, 10 mg/day PO. Adjust dosage based on response. Usual range is 20–40 mg/day as a single dose.

Adults taking diuretics

Discontinue diuretic for 2–3 days. If it is not possible to discontinue, give initial dose of 5 mg, and monitor for excessive hypotension.

- *Heart failure:* 5 mg PO daily with diuretics and digitalis. Effective range, 5–20 mg/day (*Prinivil*) and 5–40 mg/day (*Zestril*).
- *Acute MI:* Start within 24 hr of MI with 5 mg PO followed in 24 hr by 5 mg PO; 10 mg PO after 48 hr, then 10 mg PO daily for 6 wk. Give with other recommended treatments.

Pediatric patients 6 yr and older

Usual starting dose is 0.07 mg/kg once daily up to 5 mg total.

Pediatric patients younger than 6 yr

Safety and efficacy not established; drug usually not recommended.

Geriatric patients and patients with renal impairment

Excretion is reduced in renal failure. Use smaller initial dose, and adjust upward to a maximum of 40 mg/day PO.

CrCl (mL/min)	Initial Dose
More than 30	10 mg/day
10–30	5 mg/day (2.5 mg for HF)
Less than 10	2.5 mg/day

For patients on dialysis, give 2.5 mg on day of dialysis.

Pharmacokinetics

Route	Onset	Peak	Duration
Oral	1 hr	7 hr	24 hr

Metabolism: Hepatic; $T_{1/2}$: 12 hr
Distribution: Crosses placenta; may enter breast milk
Excretion: Urine

Adverse effects

- **CNS:** *Headache, dizziness, insomnia, fatigue,* paresthesias
- **CV:** *Orthostatic hypotension,* tachycardia, angina pectoris, **MI,** Raynaud syndrome, heart failure, severe hypotension in salt- or volume-depleted patients
- **GI:** *Gastric irritation, nausea, diarrhea,* peptic ulcers, dysgeusia, cholestatic jaundice, hepatocellular injury, anorexia, constipation
- **GU:** Proteinuria, renal insufficiency, renal failure, polyuria, oliguria, frequency
- **Hematologic:** Neutropenia, agranulocytosis, thrombocytopenia, hemolytic anemia, **pancytopenia,** hyperkalemia
- **Other:** *Angioedema* (particularly of the face, extremities, lips, tongue, larynx); death has been reported with **airway obstruction;** cough, muscle cramps, impotence, rash, pruritus

Interactions

✳ **Drug-drug** • Decreased antihypertensive effects and increased risk of renal damage if taken with NSAIDs • Exacerbation of cough if combined with capsaicin

■ Nursing considerations

CLINICAL ALERT!
Name confusion has occurred between lisinopril and fosinopril; use caution.

Assessment

- **History:** Allergy to lisinopril or other ACE inhibitors, impaired renal function, heart

Adverse effects in *italics* are most common; those in **bold** are life-threatening. ⬛ Do not crush.

failure, salt or volume depletion, lactation, pregnancy
- **Physical:** Skin color, lesions, turgor; T; P, BP, peripheral perfusion; mucous membranes, bowel sounds, liver evaluation; urinalysis, LFTs, renal function tests, CBC and differential, potassium

Interventions
- Begin drug within 24 hr of acute MI; ensure that patient is also receiving standard treatment (eg, aspirin, beta-adrenergic blockers, thrombolytics).

⊗ *Warning* Keep epinephrine readily available in case of angioedema of the face or neck region; if breathing difficulty occurs, consult physician, and administer epinephrine.

⊗ *Warning* Alert surgeon, and mark the patient's chart with notice that lisinopril is being taken. The angiotensin II formation subsequent to compensatory renin release during surgery will be blocked. Hypotension may be reversed with volume expansion.

- Monitor patients on diuretic therapy for excessive hypotension following the first few doses of lisinopril.
- Monitor patients closely in any situation that may lead to a decrease in BP secondary to reduction in fluid volume (excessive perspiration and dehydration, vomiting, diarrhea) because excessive hypotension may occur.
- Arrange for reduced dosage in patients with impaired renal function.

⊗ **Black box warning** Suggest the use of contraceptives; if pregnancy should occur, discontinue drug as soon as possible; fetal injury or death may occur.

Teaching points
- Take this drug once a day. It may be taken with meals. Do not stop taking drug without consulting your health care provider.
- Be careful with any conditions that may lead to a drop in blood pressure (such as diarrhea, sweating, vomiting, dehydration). If light-headedness or dizziness occurs, consult your health care provider.
- Do not take this during pregnancy; use of contraceptive measures is advised.
- You may experience these side effects: GI upset, loss of appetite, change in taste perception (may be transient; take with meals); rash; fast heart rate; dizziness, light-headedness (transient; change position slowly,

and limit activities to those that do not require alertness and precision); headache, fatigue, sleeplessness.
- Report mouth sores; sore throat; fever; chills; swelling of the hands or feet; irregular heartbeat; chest pains; swelling of the face, eyes, lips, or tongue; and difficulty breathing.

▷**lithium**
(lith' ee um)

lithium carbonate
Apo-Lithium Carbonate (CAN), Carbolith (CAN), Duralith (CAN), Lithane (CAN), Lithobid ⓒⓡ, Lithonate, Lithotabs, PMS-Lithium Carbonate (CAN)

lithium citrate
PREGNANCY CATEGORY D

Drug class
Antimanic drug

Therapeutic actions
Mechanism is not known; alters sodium transport in nerve and muscle cells; inhibits release of norepinephrine and dopamine, but not serotonin, from stimulated neurons; slightly increases intraneuronal stores of catecholamines; decreases intraneuronal content of second messengers and may thereby selectively modulate the responsiveness of hyperactive neurons that might contribute to the manic state.

Indications
- Treatment of manic episodes of bipolar disorder; maintenance therapy to prevent or diminish frequency and intensity of subsequent manic episodes
- Unlabeled uses: Prophylaxis of cluster headache and cyclic migraine headache, treatment of SIADH, hypothyroidism (doses of 600–900 mg/day), borderline personality disorder, major depression

Contraindications and cautions
- Contraindicated with hypersensitivity to tartrazine; significant renal or CV disease; severe debilitation, dehydration; sodium

depletion, patients on diuretics (lithium decreases sodium reabsorption, and hyponatremia increases lithium retention); use of ACE inhibitors; pregnancy; lactation.

• Use cautiously with protracted sweating and diarrhea; suicidal or impulsive patients; infection with fever.

Available forms
Capsules—150, 300, 600 mg; tablets—300 mg; SR tablets ⊞—300 mg; syrup—300 mg/5 mL

Dosages
Individualize dosage according to serum levels and clinical response.

Adults
• *Acute mania:* 600 mg PO tid or 900 mg slow-release form PO bid to produce effective serum levels between 1 and 1.5 mEq/L. Serum levels should be determined twice per week in samples drawn immediately before a dose (at least 8–12 hr after previous dose).

• *Long-term use:* 300 mg PO tid–qid to produce a serum level of 0.6–1.2 mEq/L. Serum levels should be determined at least every 2 mo in samples drawn immediately before a dose (at least 8–12 hr after previous dose).

• *Conversion from conventional to slow-release dosage forms:* Give the same total daily dose divided into two or three doses.

Pediatric patients
Safety and efficacy for children younger than 12 yr not established.

Geriatric patients and patients with renal impairment
Reduced dosage may be needed. Elderly patients often respond to reduced dosage and may exhibit signs of toxicity at serum levels tolerated by other patients. Plasma half-life is prolonged in renal impairment.

Pharmacokinetics

Route	Onset	Peak
Oral (tablets, capsules)	Unknown	0.5–3 hr
Oral (SR, CR tablets, capsules)	Unknown	4–12 hr

Metabolism: $T_{1/2}$: 24 hr
Distribution: Crosses placenta; enters breast milk
Excretion: Urine

Adverse effects
Reactions are related to serum lithium levels. (Toxic lithium levels are close to therapeutic levels: Therapeutic levels in acute mania range between 1 and 1.5 mEq/L; therapeutic levels for maintenance are 0.6–1.2 mEq/L.)

Less than 1.5 mEq/L
• **CNS:** *Lethargy, slurred speech, muscle weakness, fine hand tremor*
• **GI:** Nausea, vomiting, diarrhea, thirst
• **GU:** Polyuria

1.5–2 mEq/L (mild to moderate toxic reactions)
• **CNS:** Coarse hand tremor, mental confusion, hyperirritability of muscles, drowsiness, incoordination
• **CV:** ECG changes
• **GI:** Persistent GI upset, gastritis, salivary gland swelling, abdominal pain, excessive salivation, flatulence, indigestion

2–2.5 mEq/L (moderate to severe toxic reactions)
• **CNS:** Ataxia, giddiness, fasciculations, tinnitus, blurred vision, clonic movements, seizures, stupor, coma
• **CV:** Serious ECG changes, severe hypotension with **cardiac arrhythmias**
• **GU:** Large output of dilute urine
• **Respiratory:** Fatalities secondary to **pulmonary complications**

Greater than 2.5 mEq/L (life-threatening toxicity)
• **General:** Complex involvement of multiple organ systems, including seizures, arrhythmias, **CV collapse,** stupor, coma

Reactions unrelated to serum levels
• **CNS:** Headache, worsening of organic brain syndromes, fever, reversible short-term memory impairment, dyspraxia
• **CV:** ECG changes; hyperkalemia associated with ECG changes; syncope; tachycardia-bradycardia syndrome; rarely, arrhythmias, heart failure, diffuse myocarditis, **death**
• **Dermatologic:** Pruritus with or without rash; maculopapular, acneiform, and follicular eruptions; cutaneous ulcers; edema of ankles or wrists

Adverse effects in *italics* are most common; those in **bold** are life-threatening. ⊞ Do not crush.

- **Endocrine:** Diffuse nontoxic goiter; hypothyroidism; hypercalcemia associated with hyperparathyroidism; transient hyperglycemia; irreversible nephrogenic diabetes insipidus, which improves with diuretic therapy; impotence or sexual dysfunction
- **GI:** Dysgeusia (taste distortion), salty taste; swollen lips; dental caries
- **Other:** Weight gain (5–10 kg); chest tightness; swollen or painful joints, eye irritation, worsening of cataracts, disturbance of visual accommodation, leukocytosis

Interactions

✳ **Drug-drug** • Increased risk of toxicity with diuretics due to decreased renal clearance of lithium—reduced lithium dosage may be needed • Increased plasma lithium levels with indomethacin and some other NSAIDs (phenylbutazone, piroxicam, ibuprofen) and fluoxetine, methyldopa, and metronidazole • Increased CNS toxicity with carbamazepine • Encephalopathic syndrome (weakness, lethargy, fever, tremulousness, confusion, extrapyramidal symptoms, leukocytosis, elevated serum enzymes) with irreversible brain damage when taken with haloperidol • Greater risk of hypothyroidism with iodide salts • Decreased effectiveness due to increased excretion of lithium with urinary alkalinizers, including antacids, tromethamine • Risk of increased adverse effects with SSRIs

✳ **Drug-alternative therapy** • Increased effects and toxicity with juniper, dandelion

■ Nursing considerations
Assessment

- **History:** Hypersensitivity to tartrazine; significant renal or CV disease; severe debilitation, dehydration; sodium depletion, patients on diuretics; protracted sweating, diarrhea; suicidal or impulsive patients; infection with fever; pregnancy; lactation
- **Physical:** Weight and T; skin color, lesions; orientation, affect, reflexes; ophthalmic examination; P, BP, R, adventitious sounds; bowel sounds, normal output; normal fluid intake, normal output, voiding pattern; thyroid, renal glomerular and tubular function tests, urinalysis, CBC and differential, baseline ECG

Interventions

- Give with caution and frequent monitoring of serum lithium levels to patients with renal or CV disease, debilitation, or dehydration or life-threatening psychiatric disorders.
- Give drug with food or milk or after meals.

⊗ *Black box warning* Monitor clinical status closely, especially during initial stages of therapy; monitor for therapeutic serum levels of 0.6–1.2 mEq/L; toxicity is closely related to serum levels.

- Individuals vary in their response to this drug; some patients may exhibit toxic signs at serum lithium levels considered within the therapeutic range.
- Advise patient that this drug may cause serious fetal harm and cannot be used during pregnancy; urge use of barrier contraceptives.
- Decrease dosage after the acute manic episode is controlled; lithium tolerance is greater during the acute manic phase and decreases when manic symptoms subside.

⊗ *Warning* Ensure that patient maintains adequate intake of salt and adequate intake of fluid (2,500–3,000 mL/day).

Teaching points

- Take this drug exactly as prescribed, after meals or with food or milk. Swallow sustained-release tablets whole; do not chew or crush.
- Eat a normal diet with normal salt intake; maintain adequate fluid intake (at least 2.5 quarts/day).
- Arrange for frequent checkups, including blood tests. Keep all appointments for checkups to get the most benefits with the least toxicity.
- Use contraception to avoid pregnancy. If you wish to become pregnant or believe that you have become pregnant, consult your health care provider.
- Discontinue drug and notify your health care provider if toxicity occurs—diarrhea, vomiting, ataxia, tremor, drowsiness, lack of coordination or muscular weakness.
- You may experience these side effects: Drowsiness, dizziness (avoid driving or performing tasks that require alertness); GI upset (eat frequent small meals); mild

thirst, greater than usual urine volume, fine hand tremor (may persist throughout therapy; notify your health care provider if severe).
• Report diarrhea, fever, tremor, unsteady walking.

DANGEROUS DRUG

▷**lomustine (CCNU)**
(loe mus' teen)

CeeNU

PREGNANCY CATEGORY D

Drug classes
Alkylating drug, nitrosourea
Antineoplastic

Therapeutic actions
Cytotoxic: Exact mechanism of action not known, but it involves alkylation of DNA, thus inhibiting DNA, RNA, and protein synthesis; cell-cycle nonspecific.

Indications
• Treatment with other drugs for primary and metastatic brain tumors and secondary treatment of Hodgkin disease in patients who relapse following primary therapy

Contraindications and cautions
• Contraindicated with allergy to lomustine, myelosuppression, pregnancy (teratogenic and embryotoxic in preclinical studies), and lactation.
• Use cautiously with impaired renal or hepatic function.

Available forms
Capsules—10, 40, 100 mg

Dosages
Adults and pediatric patients
130 mg/m^2 PO as a single dose every 6 wk. Adjustments must be made with bone marrow suppression; initially reduce the dose to 100 mg/m^2 PO every 6 wk; do not give a repeat dose until platelets exceed 100,000/mm^2 and leukocytes exceed 4,000/mm^2; adjust dosage after initial dose based on hematologic response as follows:
Minimum (nadir) count after prior dose:

Leukocytes/ mm^3	Platelets/ mm^3	Percentage of Prior Dose to Give
More than 4,000	More than 100,000	100
3,000–3,999	75,000–99,999	100
2,000–2,999	25,000–74,999	70
Less than 2,000	Less than 25,000	50

Pharmacokinetics

Route	Onset	Peak	Duration
Oral	10 min	1.6 hr	48 hr

Metabolism: Hepatic; T$_{1/2}$: 16–72 hr
Distribution: Crosses placenta; enters breast milk
Excretion: Urine

Adverse effects
• **CNS:** Ataxia, lethargy
• **Dermatologic:** Alopecia
• **GI:** *Nausea, vomiting,* stomatitis, hepatotoxicity
• **GU:** Renal toxicity
• **Hematologic:** *Leukopenia; thrombocytopenia; anemia,* delayed for 4–6 wk; immunosuppression
• **Respiratory:** Pulmonary fibrosis
• **Other:** Secondary malignancies

■ Nursing considerations
Assessment
• **History:** Allergy to lomustine, radiation therapy, chemotherapy, hematopoietic depression, impaired renal or hepatic function, pregnancy, lactation
• **Physical:** T; weight; mucous membranes, liver evaluation; CBC, differential; urinalysis, LFTs, renal function tests

Interventions
⊗ **Black box warning** Arrange for blood tests to evaluate hematopoietic function before therapy and weekly for at least 6 wk thereafter; severe bone marrow suppression is possible. Delayed suppression at or beyond 6 wk is also possible.
⊗ **Warning** Do not give full dosage within 2–3 wk after a full course of radiation therapy or chemotherapy due to risk of severe bone marrow depression; reduced dosage may be needed.

Adverse effects in *italics* are most common; those in **bold** are life-threatening. ⊂⊃ Do not crush.

- Advise patient that drug cannot be taken during pregnancy; suggest using barrier contraceptives.
- Reduce dosage in patients with depressed bone marrow function.
- Administer tablets on an empty stomach to decrease GI upset; antiemetics may be needed for nausea and vomiting.
- Monitor pulmonary function because of risk of pulmonary fibrosis.

Teaching points

- Take this drug on an empty stomach.
- Maintain your fluid intake and nutrition.
- Use contraceptives; this drug can cause severe birth defects.
- You may experience these side effects: Nausea, vomiting, loss of appetite (take on an empty stomach, an antiemetic may be ordered; frequent small meals may help), hair loss.
- Report unusual bleeding or bruising, fever, chills, sore throat, stomach or flank pain, sores on your mouth or lips, unusual tiredness, confusion, difficulty breathing.

▽**loperamide hydrochloride**

(loe per' a mide)

Prescription: Apo-Loperamide (CAN), Imodium
OTC: Diar-Aid Caplets, Imodium A-D, K-Pek II, Neo-Diaral, Pepto Diarrhea Control

PREGNANCY CATEGORY B

Drug class
Antidiarrheal

Therapeutic actions
Slows intestinal motility and affects water and electrolyte movement through the bowel by inhibiting peristalsis through direct effects on the circular and longitudinal muscles of the intestinal wall.

Indications
- Control and symptomatic relief of acute nonspecific diarrhea and chronic diarrhea associated with inflammatory bowel disease

- Reduction of volume of discharge from ileostomies
- OTC use: Control of diarrhea, including traveler's diarrhea

Contraindications and cautions
- Contraindicated with allergy to loperamide, patients who must avoid constipation, diarrhea associated with organisms that penetrate the intestinal mucosa (*Escherichia coli, Salmonella, Shigella, Clostridium difficile*).
- Use cautiously with hepatic impairment, acute ulcerative colitis, pregnancy, and lactation.

Available forms
Tablets—2 mg; capsules—2 mg; liquid—1 mg/5 mL; 1 mg/7.5 mL

Dosages
Adults
- *Acute diarrhea:* Initial dose of 4 mg PO followed by 2 mg after each unformed stool. Do not exceed 16 mg/day unless directed by a physician. Clinical improvement is usually seen within 48 hr.
- *Chronic diarrhea:* Initial dose of 4 mg PO followed by 2 mg after each unformed stool until diarrhea is controlled. Individualize dose based on patient response. Average daily maintenance dose is 4–8 mg. If no clinical improvement is seen with dosage of 16 mg/day for 10 days, further treatment will probably not be effective.
- *Traveler's diarrhea (OTC):* 4 mg PO after first loose stool, followed by 2 mg after each subsequent stool; do not exceed 16 mg/day.

Pediatric patients
Avoid use in children younger than 2 yr, and use extreme caution in younger children.

- *Acute diarrhea:* First-day dosage schedule:

Age	Weight	Dose Form	Dosage
2–5 yr	13–20 kg	Liquid	1 mg tid
6–8 yr	20–30 kg	Liquid or capsule	2 mg bid
8–12 yr	More than 30 kg	Liquid or capsule	2 mg tid

Subsequent doses: Administer 1 mg/10 kg PO only after a loose stool. Daily dosage should not exceed recommended first-day dosage.

- *Chronic diarrhea:* Dosage schedule has not been established.
- *Traveler's diarrhea (OTC):*
  Younger than 6 yr (21 kg and less): Consult with physician; not recommended.
  6–8 yr (22–26 kg): 2 mg PO after first loose stool, followed by 1 mg after each subsequent loose stool; do not exceed 4 mg/day for more than 2 days.
  9–11 yr (27–43 kg): 2 mg PO after first loose stool followed by 1 mg after each subsequent stool; do not exceed 6 mg/day for more than 2 days.

Pharmacokinetics

Route	Onset	Peak
Oral	Varies	1–6 hr

Metabolism: Hepatic; $T_{1/2}$: first phase, 6 hr; second phase, 1–2 days
Distribution: May cross placenta and enter breast milk
Excretion: Feces, urine

Adverse effects

- **CNS:** Tiredness, drowsiness, dizziness
- **GI: Toxic megacolon** (in patients with ulcerative colitis), *abdominal pain, distention or discomfort, constipation, dry mouth, nausea,* vomiting
- **Hematologic:** Myelosuppression
- **Hypersensitivity:** Rash
- **Respiratory:** Pulmonary infiltrates, pulmonary fibrosis

■ Nursing considerations
Assessment

- **History:** Allergy to loperamide, patients who must avoid constipation, diarrhea associated with organisms that penetrate the intestinal mucosa (*E. coli, Salmonella, Shigella*); hepatic impairment, acute ulcerative colitis, lactation
- **Physical:** Skin color, lesions; orientation, reflexes; abdominal examination, bowel sounds, liver evaluation; serum electrolytes (with extended use)

Interventions

- Monitor for response. If improvement is not seen within 48 hr, discontinue treatment and notify health care provider.

- Give drug after each unformed stool. Keep track of amount given to avoid exceeding the recommended daily dosage unless directed by a physician.

⊗ **Warning** Have the opioid antagonist naloxone readily available in case of overdose and CNS depression.

Teaching points

- Take drug as prescribed. Do not exceed prescribed dosage or recommended daily dosage.
- Drink clear fluids to prevent dehydration.
- You may experience these side effects: Abdominal fullness, nausea, vomiting; dry mouth (suck on sugarless candies); dizziness.
- Report abdominal pain or distention, fever, and diarrhea that does not stop after a few days.

▽ lopinavir
(lopinavir and ritonavir)
*(low **pin**' ah ver)*

Kaletra ⓒ

PREGNANCY CATEGORY C

Drug classes
Antiviral
Protease inhibitor combination

Therapeutic actions
Lopinavir in this combination exhibits antiviral activity; inhibits HIV protease activity, leading to the decrease in production of HIV particles; ritonavir in this preparation inhibits metabolism of lopinavir, allowing for increased plasma levels of lopinavir.

Indications
- Treatment of HIV infection in combination with other antiretrovirals

Contraindications and cautions
- Contraindicated with allergy to lopinavir, ritonavir; in preterm infants.
- Use cautiously with pregnancy, hepatic impairment, pancreatitis, lactation.

Available forms

Tablets ⊕—100 mg lopinavir/25 mg ritonavir, 200 mg lopinavir/50 mg ritonavir; capsules—133.3 mg lopinavir/133.3 mg ritonavir; oral solution—80 mg lopinavir/20 mg ritonavir/5 mL

Dosages

Dose is based on lopinavir component of lopinavir/ritonavir solution (400 mg/100 mg/5 mL).

Once-daily lopinavir/ritonavir can be used in patients with less than three lopinavir-resistance-associated substitutions.

Adults and pediatric patients older than 12 yr and weighing more than 40 kg

• *HIV infection, with other antiretrovirals in treatment-naïve patients:* 800 mg lopinavir and 200 mg ritonavir (four tablets or 10 mL) PO once daily or 400 mg lopinavir and 100 mg ritonavir PO bid with food (two tablets, or three capsules, or 5 mL)

• *HIV infection, with other antiretrovirals in treatment-experienced patients:* 400 mg lopinavir and 100 mg ritonavir (two tablets, or three capsules, or 5 mL) PO bid.

• *Taken with efavirenz, nevirapine, fosamprenavir without ritonavir, or nelfinavir:* 533 mg lopinavir and 133 mg ritonavir (four capsules or 6.5 mL) PO bid for treatment-experienced patients. No dosage adjustment needed for treatment-naïve patients.

Pediatric patients 6 mo to 12 yr
Dosage is usually based on weight.

Weight (kg)	Dosage	Volume of oral solution bid
7–less than 15	12 mg/kg bid	
7–10		1.25 mL
More than 10–less than 15		1.75 mL
15–40	10 mg/kg bid	
15–20		2.25 mL
More than 20–25		2.75 mL
More than 25–30		3.5 mL
More than 30–35		4 mL
More than 35–40		4.75 mL
More than 40	Adult dose	5 mL

• *Concomitant therapy with efavirenz, nevirapine, amprenavir*

Weight (kg)	Dosage	Volume of oral solution bid
7–less than 15	13 mg/kg bid	
7–10		1.5 mL
More than 10–less than 15		2 mL
15–40	11 mg/kg bid	
15–20		2.5 mL
More than 20–25		3.25 mL
More than 25–30		4 mL
More than 30–35		4.5 mL
More than 35–40		5 mL
More than 40–45		5.75 mL
More than 45	Adult dose	6.5 mL

Pharmacokinetics

Route	Onset	Peak
Oral	Varies	3–4 hr

Metabolism: Hepatic; $T_{1/2}$: 5–6 hr
Distribution: Crosses placenta; may enter breast milk
Excretion: Feces and urine

Adverse effects

• **CNS:** *Asthenia, peripheral and circumoral paresthesias,* anxiety, dreams, *headache,* dizziness, hallucinations, personality changes
• **CV:** DVTs, hypotension, syncope, tachycardia, chest pain, prolonged P-R interval, prolonged QTc interval
• **Dermatologic:** Rash, acne, alopecia, dry skin, exfoliative dermatitis
• **Endocrine:** *Increased triglycerides and cholesterol,* hyperglycemia, hyperuricemia, gynecomastia, hypothyroidism, hypogonadism
• **GI:** *Nausea, vomiting, diarrhea, anorexia, abdominal pain,* pancreatitis, *taste perversion,* dry mouth, hepatitis, hepatic impairment, dehydration
• **Hematologic:** Leukopenia, anemia
• **Other:** Hypothermia, chills, back pain, edema, cachexia, redistribution of body fat

Interactions

✳ **Drug-drug** ⊗ *Warning* Potentially large increase in serum concentration of drugs metabolized by CYP450 3A4 (caused by ritonavir). Do not administer lopinavir with any of these drugs, including amiodarone, bepridil, bupropion, clozapine, encainide, flecainide, meperidine, piroxicam, propafenone, propoxyphene, quinidine, and rifabutin. Potential for serious arrhythmias, seizures, and fatal reactions.

⊗ **Warning** Potentially large increases in serum concentration of these sedatives and hypnotics: Alprazolam, clonazepam, diazepam, estazolam, flurazepam, midazolam, triazolam, zolpidem. Extreme sedation and respiratory depression could occur. Do not administer lopinavir with any of these drugs.

• May increase level and adverse effects of phosphodiesterase-5 inhibitors (eg, sildenafil, vardenafil, tadalafil) including hypotension and prolonged erection • May decrease effectiveness of hormonal contraceptives; using barrier contraceptives is advised

✳ **Drug-food** • Absorption of lopinavir oral solution is increased by the presence of food; taking the oral solution with food is strongly recommended

✳ **Drug-alternative therapy** • Potential for reduced effectiveness if combined with St. John's Wort; avoid this combination

■ Nursing considerations

CLINICAL ALERT!
Name confusion has occurred between *Kaletra* (lopinavir/ritonavir) and *Keppra* (levetiracetam); use extreme caution.

Assessment

• **History:** Allergy to lopinavir, ritonavir, hepatic impairment, pancreatitis, pregnancy, lactation

• **Physical:** T; orientation, reflexes; BP, P, peripheral perfusion; R, adventitious sounds; bowel sounds; skin color, perfusion; LFTs, serum amylase levels, triglycerides, cholesterol, electrolytes

Interventions

⊗ **Warning** No safe or effective dose has been established for preterm infants. Do not use in preterm infants until 14 days after their actual due date or in full-term infants until they are 14 days of age; serious toxicity has been reported. Monitor all infants for an increase in serum osmolality or serum creatinine or for signs and symptoms of toxicity.

• Solution should be stored in the refrigerator; may be left at room temperature but should be used within 60 days; protect from

light and extreme heat. Oral solution contains 42% alcohol.

• Obtain baseline triglycerides, cholesterol levels, electrolytes, and glucose levels. Monitor periodically during therapy.

⊗ **Warning** Screen medication history before administration to avoid potentially serious drug interactions.

• Administer oral solution with meals or food to increase absorption. Tablets may be taken without regard to food; ensure that tablets are swallowed whole and are not cut, crushed, or chewed.

• Didanosine and lopinavir/ritonavir tablets may be administered simultaneously without food.

• Administer didanosine 1 hr before or 2 hr after lopinavir solution.

Teaching points

• Take the oral solution with meals or food; store the solution in the refrigerator. The taste of the solution may be improved if mixed with chocolate milk, *Ensure,* or *Advera* 1 hour before taking.

• Tablets must be swallowed whole and may be taken with or without food. Do not crush, chew, or divide tablets.

• Take the full course of therapy as prescribed; do not take a double dose if one is missed; do not change dosage without consulting your health care provider. Take this drug with your other HIV medications.

• This drug does not cure HIV infection; long-term effects are not yet known; continue to take precautions because the risk of transmission is not reduced by this drug.

• This drug may cause hormonal contraceptives to be ineffective; using barrier contraceptives is advised.

• Do not take any other drug, prescription or over-the-counter, or use any herbal therapies without consulting with your health care provider; this drug interacts with many other drugs and serious problems can occur. Do not use St. John's Wort while taking this drug.

• You may experience these side effects: Nausea, vomiting, loss of appetite, diarrhea, abdominal pain; headache, dizziness, numbness, and tingling.

• Report severe diarrhea, severe nausea, personality changes, changes in the color of urine or stool, fever or chills, severe abdominal pain.

▽loratadine
(lor at' a deen)

Alavert, Alavert Childrens,
Apo-Loratadine (CAN), Claritin,
Claritin Hives Relief,
Claritin Reditabs, Claritin Syrup,
Claritin 24-Hour Allergy,
Dimetapp Children's ND
Non-Drowsy Allergy,
Triaminic Allerchews

PREGNANCY CATEGORY B

Drug class
Antihistamine (nonsedating type)

Therapeutic actions
Competitively blocks the effects of histamine at peripheral histamine-1 receptor sites; has anticholinergic (atropine-like) and antipruritic effects.

Indications
- Symptomatic relief of perennial and seasonal allergic rhinitis, vasomotor rhinitis, allergic conjunctivitis, and mild, uncomplicated urticaria and angioedema
- Treatment of rhinitis and chronic urticaria in children 2 yr and older

Contraindications and cautions
- Contraindicated with allergy to any antihistamines.
- Use cautiously with lactation, pregnancy.

Available forms
Tablets—10 mg; syrup—5 mg/5 mL; chewable tablets—5 mg; orally disintegrating tablets—5, 10 mg

Dosages
Place rapid dissolving tablets on tongue. Administer with or without water.
Adults and pediatric patients 6 yr and older
10 mg daily PO on an empty stomach.
Pediatric patients 2–5 yr
5 mg PO daily (syrup, chewable tablets).
Geriatric patients or patients with renal or hepatic impairment
10 mg PO every other day.

Pharmacokinetics

Route	Onset	Peak	Duration
Oral	1–3 hr	8–12 hr	24 hr

Metabolism: Hepatic; $T_{1/2}$: 8.4 hr
Distribution: Crosses placenta; enters breast milk
Excretion: Feces, urine

Adverse effects
- **CNS:** *Headache, nervousness, dizziness,* depression, drowsiness
- **CV:** Palpitations, edema
- **GI:** *Appetite increase,* nausea, diarrhea, abdominal pain
- **Respiratory: Bronchospasm,** pharyngitis
- **Other:** Fever, photosensitivity, rash, myalgia, arthralgia, angioedema, *weight gain,* dry mouth

Interactions
✴ **Drug-drug** • Additive CNS depressant effects with alcohol or other CNS depressants
✴ **Drug-lab test** • False skin testing procedures if done while patient is taking antihistamines

■ Nursing considerations
Assessment
- **History:** Allergy to any antihistamines; lactation, pregnancy
- **Physical:** Skin color, lesions, texture; orientation, reflexes, affect; vision examinations; R, adventitious sounds; prostate palpation; serum transaminase levels

Interventions
- Administer without regard to meals.

Teaching points
- If using rapid or orally disintegrating tablets, place on tongue; tablet will dissolve within seconds. Swallow with or without water.
- Avoid the use of alcohol; serious sedation could occur.
- You may experience these side effects: Dizziness, sedation, drowsiness (use caution if driving or performing tasks that require alertness); headache; thickening of bronchial secretions, dryness of nasal mucosa (use a humidifier).

- Report difficulty breathing, hallucinations, tremors, loss of coordination, irregular heartbeat.

▷ lorazepam
(lor a' ze pam)

Apo-Lorazepam (CAN), Ativan,
Lorazepam Intensol,
PMS-Lorazepam (CAN)

PREGNANCY CATEGORY D

CONTROLLED SUBSTANCE C-IV

Drug classes
Anxiolytic
Benzodiazepine
Sedative-hypnotic

Therapeutic actions
Exact mechanisms are not understood; acts mainly at subcortical levels of the CNS, binding to benzodiazepine receptors on postsynaptic GABA neurons in the CNS, leaving the cortex relatively unaffected. Main sites of action may be the limbic system and reticular formation; benzodiazepines potentiate the effects of GABA, an inhibitory neurotransmitter; anxiolytic effects occur at doses well below those needed to cause sedation and ataxia.

Indications
- Oral: Management of anxiety disorders or for short-term relief of symptoms of anxiety or anxiety associated with depression; insomnia due to anxiety or transient situational stress
- Parenteral: Preanesthetic medication in adults to produce sedation, relieve anxiety, and decrease recall of events related to surgery; treatment of status epilepticus

Contraindications and cautions
- Contraindicated with hypersensitivity to benzodiazepines, propylene glycol, polyethylene glycol or benzyl alcohol (parenteral lorazepam); psychoses; acute narrow-angle glaucoma; shock; coma; acute alcoholic intoxication with depression of vital signs; pregnancy (crosses placenta; risk of congenital malformations and neonatal withdrawal syndrome); labor

and delivery ("floppy infant" syndrome); lactation.
- Use cautiously with impaired hepatic or renal function.

Available forms
Injection—2, 4 mg/mL; oral solution—2 mg/mL; tablets—0.5, 1, 2 mg

Dosages
Adults
Oral
Usual dose is 2–6 mg/day; range, 1–10 mg/day in divided doses with largest dose at bedtime.
- *Insomnia due to transient stress:* 2–4 mg given at bedtime.

IM
0.05 mg/kg up to a maximum of 4 mg administered at least 2 hr before operative procedure.

IV
Initial dose is 2 mg total or 0.044 mg/kg, whichever is smaller. Do not exceed this dose in patients older than 50 yr. Doses as high as 0.05 mg/kg up to a total of 4 mg may be given 15–20 min before the procedure to those benefited by a greater lack of recall.
- *Status epilepticus:* For patients older than 18 yr, 4 mg slowly at 2 mg/min. May give another 4 mg after 10–15 min if needed.

Pediatric patients
Drug should not be used in children younger than 12 yr.

Patients with renal or hepatic impairment
Initially, 1–2 mg/day in divided doses. Adjust as needed and tolerated.

Pharmacokinetics

Route	Onset	Peak	Duration
Oral	Intermediate	1 hr	12–24 hr
IM	15–30 min	60–90 min	12–24 hr
IV	1–5 min	10–15 min	12–24 hr

Metabolism: Hepatic; $T_{1/2}$: 10–20 hr
Distribution: Crosses placenta; enters breast milk
Excretion: Urine

▼ IV FACTS
Preparation: Dilute lorazepam immediately before IV use. For direct IV injection or injection

into IV line, dilute with an equal volume of compatible solution (sterile water for injection, sodium chloride injection, or 5% dextrose injection); do not use if solution is discolored or contains a precipitate. Protect from light.

Infusion: Direct inject slowly, or infuse at maximum rate of 2 mg/min.

Y-site incompatibilities: Do not mix with foscarnet, ondansetron, aztreonam, imipenem/cilastatin, omeprazole.

Adverse effects

- **CNS:** *Transient, mild drowsiness initially; sedation, depression, lethargy, apathy, fatigue, light-headedness, disorientation, anger, hostility,* episodes of mania and hypomania, *restlessness, confusion,* crying, delirium, *headache,* slurred speech, dysarthria, stupor, rigidity, tremor, dystonia, vertigo, euphoria, nervousness, difficulty concentrating, vivid dreams, psychomotor retardation, extrapyramidal symptoms; *mild paradoxic excitatory reactions during first 2 wk of treatment,* anterograde amnesia
- **CV:** Bradycardia, tachycardia, **CV collapse,** hypertension and hypotension, palpitations, edema
- **Dermatologic:** Urticaria, pruritus, rash, dermatitis
- **EENT:** Visual and auditory disturbances, diplopia, nystagmus, depressed hearing, nasal congestion
- **GI:** Constipation, diarrhea, *dry mouth,* salivation, *nausea,* anorexia, vomiting, difficulty in swallowing, gastric disorders, hepatic impairment
- **GU:** Incontinence, urinary retention, libido changes, menstrual irregularities
- **Other:** Hiccups, fever, diaphoresis, paresthesias, muscular disturbances, gynecomastia; *drug dependence with withdrawal syndrome when drug is discontinued; more common with abrupt discontinuation of higher dosage used for longer than 4 mo*

Interactions

✳ **Drug-drug** • Increased CNS depression with alcohol and other sedating medications, such as barbiturates and opioids • Decreased effectiveness with theophyllines • Risk of toxicity if combined with probenecid, valproate; reduce lorazepam dose by 50%

✳ **Drug-alternative therapy** • Kava kava increases the sedative effects of benzodiazepines; coma has been reported with concurrent use

■ Nursing considerations

 CLINICAL ALERT!
Name confusion has occurred between lorazepam and alprazolam; use caution.

Assessment

- **History:** Hypersensitivity to benzodiazepines, propylene glycol, polyethylene glycol or benzyl alcohol; psychoses; acute narrow-angle glaucoma; shock; coma; acute alcoholic intoxication with depression of vital signs; pregnancy; lactation; impaired liver or renal function, debilitation
- **Physical:** Skin color, lesions; T; orientation, reflexes, affect, ophthalmologic examination; P, BP; R, adventitious sounds; liver evaluation, abdominal examination, bowel sounds, normal output; CBC, LFTs, renal function tests

Interventions

- Sublingual administration has more rapid absorption than PO, and bioavailability compares to IM use.
- Do not administer intra-arterially; arteriospasm or gangrene may result.
- Give IM injections of undiluted drug deep into muscle mass, monitor injection sites.
- Do not use solutions that are discolored or contain a precipitate. Protect drug from light, and refrigerate oral solution.
- Oral solution may be mixed with water, juice, soda, applesauce, or pudding.
- ⊗ *Warning* Keep equipment to maintain a patent airway readily available when drug is given IV.
- Refrigerate injection and oral solution (36° F to 46° F). Can be stored at room temperature for 60 days.
- Reduce dose of opioid analgesics by at least half in patients who have received parenteral lorazepam.
- Keep patients who have received parenteral doses under close observation, preferably in bed, up to 3 hr. Do not permit ambulatory patients to drive following an injection.

⊗ **Warning** Taper dosage gradually after long-term therapy, especially in patients with epilepsy.

Teaching points
- Take drug exactly as prescribed; do not stop taking drug (in long-term therapy) without consulting your health care provider.
- You may experience these side effects: Drowsiness, dizziness (may be transient; avoid driving or engaging in dangerous activities); GI upset (take drug with food); nocturnal sleep disturbances for several nights after discontinuing the drug if used as a sedative and hypnotic; depression, dreams, emotional upset, crying.
- Report severe dizziness, weakness, drowsiness that persists, rash or skin lesions, palpitations, edema of the extremities; visual changes; difficulty voiding.

▽lorcaserin hydrochloride
*(lore **cass'** ah rin)*

Belviq

PREGNANCY CATEGORY X

Drug classes
Serotonin receptor agonist
Weight loss drug

Therapeutic actions
Thought to decrease food consumption and promote satiety by selectively activating the serotonin-2C receptors in the anorexigenic neurons in the hypothalamus.

Indications
- Adjunct to diet and exercise for long-term weight management in adults with initial body mass index (BMI) of 30 kg/m² or greater or 27 kg/m² or greater with at least one weight-related condition, such as hypertension or dyslipidemia

Contraindications and cautions
- Contraindicated with history of serious hypersensitivity to components of drug, severe renal impairment, pregnancy, lactation.
- Use cautiously with concurrent use of other serotonergic or antidopaminergic agents,

history of depression, history of priapism, moderate renal impairment, severe hepatic impairment, heart failure.

Available forms
Tablets—10 mg

Dosages
Adults
10 mg PO bid without regard to food; if patient has not lost 5% of baseline weight within 12 wk, drug should be discontinued.

Pharmacokinetics

Route	Onset	Peak
Oral	Rapid	1.5–2 hr

Metabolism: Hepatic: $T_{1/2}$: 11 hr
Distribution: May cross placenta; may enter breast milk
Excretion: Urine

Adverse effects
- **CNS:** Headache, *dizziness, fatigue,* cognitive impairment, euphoria, dissociation, **suicidality**
- **CV:** Bradycardia, **valvular heart disease**
- **GI:** *Nausea, dry mouth, constipation*
- **Respiratory:** Cough, *URI,* nasopharyngitis, **pulmonary hypertension**
- **Other:** *Hypoglycemia, back pain,* **neuroleptic malignant syndrome,** elevated prolactin level, low WBC count, priapism

Interactions
✳ **Drug-drug** • Increased risk of neuroleptic malignant syndrome if combined with SSRIs, selective serotonin norepinephrine reuptake inhibitors, TCAs, MAOIs, linezolid, dextromethorphan, lithium, tramadol, tryptophan, bupropion; combination is not recommended; use extreme caution and monitor patient closely
✳ **Drug-alternative therapy** • Increased risk of toxicity with St. John's Wort; avoid this combination

■ Nursing considerations
Assessment
- **History:** Hypersensitivity to components of drug, renal or hepatic impairment, priapism, heart failure, depression, pregnancy, lactation

- **Physical:** Weight, BMI; T; orientation, affect; P, cardiac auscultation; R, adventitious sounds; renal function tests, LFTs, CBC

Interventions

- Establish baseline weight and BMI; ensure that patient meets the criteria for use of this drug.
- Ensure that patient is following a reduced-calorie diet and exercise program before beginning therapy.
- Advise women of childbearing age to avoid pregnancy; fetal harm has been reported.
- Instruct breast-feeding women that they must use another method of feeding the baby during therapy.
- Monitor weight and discontinue the drug if patient has not lost 5% of baseline body weight in 12 wk.
- Have diabetic patients monitor blood glucose level carefully; weight loss may result in hypoglycemia.
- Do not administer with other weight loss drugs; safety has not been established.
- Be aware of risk of cognitive and emotional changes and suicidality; monitor patient accordingly.
- Monitor patient for signs and symptoms of valvular heart disease; discontinue drug and provide appropriate support if this occurs.
- Be aware that the effect of this drug on CV morbidity and mortality has not been established.
- Monitor patient for signs and symptoms of neuroleptic malignant syndrome; discontinue drug and provide supportive treatment if this occurs.

Teaching points

- Take this drug twice a day with or without food. Do not increase your dose for any reason. If you have not lost 5% of your baseline weight within 12 weeks, this drug will be stopped.
- If you forget a dose, take the drug at the next scheduled time; do not take more than two tablets/day.
- This drug is used in combination with a low-calorie diet and exercise program; be sure to follow these guidelines.
- This drug could cause harm to a fetus if taken during pregnancy. Use of contraceptives is advised. If you are thinking about becoming pregnant, discuss this with your health care provider.

- This drug may appear in breast milk. If you are breast-feeding, you will need to find another method of feeding the baby.
- If you have diabetes, you may experience episodes of low blood sugar while taking this drug; monitor your blood sugar very closely.
- This drug may interact with many other drugs; tell your health care provider about all other prescription drugs, over-the-counter drugs, and herbal products you may be using.
- Do not use St. John's Wort while taking this drug.
- Serious adverse effects may occur while you are taking this drug, such as neuroleptic malignant syndrome (report mental changes, coordination problems, restlessness, sweating, stiff muscles, changes in heart rate) and valvular heart problems (report trouble breathing, swelling, dizziness, irregular heartbeat, weakness).
- You may experience these side effects: Dizziness, sleepiness, slowed thinking (do not drive or operate hazardous machinery if these effects occur); changes in attention or memory, thoughts of suicide (if these occur, consult your health care provider); headache (medications may be available to help); dry mouth (sucking on sugarless candies may help).
- Report changes in mental status, trouble breathing, severe dizziness, fever, changes in heart rate or rhythm, thoughts of suicide, erection that lasts more than 6 hours, enlarged breasts, discharge from the breasts.

▽losartan potassium
(low sar' tan)

Cozaar

PREGNANCY CATEGORY C (FIRST TRIMESTER)

PREGNANCY CATEGORY D (SECOND AND THIRD TRIMESTERS)

Drug classes
Antihypertensive
ARB

Therapeutic actions

Selectively blocks the binding of angiotensin II to specific tissue receptors found in the vascular smooth muscle and adrenal gland; this action blocks the vasoconstriction effect of the renin-angiotensin system as well as the release of aldosterone leading to decreased BP.

Indications

- Treatment of hypertension, alone or in combination with other antihypertensives
- Treatment of diabetic nephropathy with an elevated serum creatinine and proteinuria in patients with type 2 (non–insulin-dependent) diabetes and a history of hypertension
- Reduction of the risk of stroke in patients with hypertension and left ventricular hypertrophy

Contraindications and cautions

- Contraindicated with hypersensitivity to losartan, pregnancy (use during the second or third trimester can cause injury or even death to the fetus), lactation.
- Use cautiously with hepatic or renal impairment, hypovolemia, history of angioedema.

Available forms

Tablets—25, 50, 100 mg

Dosages

Adults

- *Hypertension:* Starting dose of 50 mg PO daily. Patients on diuretics or hypovolemic patients may only require 25 mg daily. Dosage ranges from 25–100 mg daily PO given once or twice a day have been used.
- *Diabetic nephropathy:* 50 mg/day PO once daily; may be increased to 100 mg/day once daily based on BP response.
- *Hypertension with left ventricular hypertrophy:* 50 mg/day PO with 12.5 mg/day hydrochlorothiazide. May be increased to 100 mg/day PO with 25 mg/day hydrochlorothiazide if needed.

Pediatric patients 6 yr and older

- *Hypertension:* 0.7 mg/kg once daily up to 50 mg/day total.

Pharmacokinetics

Route	Onset	Peak
Oral	Varies	1–3 hr

Metabolism: Hepatic; $T_{1/2}$: 2 hr, then 6–9 hr
Distribution: Crosses placenta; enters breast milk
Excretion: Feces, urine

Adverse effects

- **CNS:** Headache, *dizziness,* syncope, insomnia
- **CV:** Hypotension
- **Dermatologic:** Rash, urticaria, pruritus, alopecia, dry skin
- **GI:** *Diarrhea, abdominal pain, nausea,* constipation, dry mouth
- **Respiratory:** *URI symptoms, cough,* sinus disorders
- **Other:** Back pain, fever, gout, muscle weakness

Interactions

✳ **Drug-drug** ● Decreased serum levels and effectiveness if taken concurrently with phenobarbital, indomethacin, and rifamycin ● Losartan is converted to an active metabolite by CYP450 3A4, and 2C9 (fluconazole); drugs that inhibit 3A4 (ketoconazole, fluconazole) may increase antihypertensive effects of losartan

■ Nursing considerations

Assessment

- **History:** Hypersensitivity to losartan, pregnancy, lactation, hepatic or renal impairment, hypovolemia
- **Physical:** Skin lesions, turgor; T; reflexes, affect; BP; R, respiratory auscultation; LFTs, renal function tests

Interventions

- Administer without regard to meals.

⊗ **Black box warning** Ensure that patient is not pregnant before beginning therapy, suggest the use of barrier birth control while using losartan; fetal injury and deaths have been reported.

- Find an alternative method of feeding the infant if given to a breast-feeding patient. Depression of the renin-angiotensin system in infants is potentially very dangerous.

⊗ *Warning* Alert surgeon and mark the patient's chart with notice that losartan is being taken. The blockage of the renin-angiotensin system following surgery can produce problems.

Hypotension may be reversed with volume expansion.

- Monitor patient closely in any situation that may lead to a decrease in BP secondary to reduction in fluid volume—excessive perspiration, dehydration, vomiting, diarrhea—excessive hypotension can occur.

Teaching points

- Take drug without regard to meals. Do not stop taking this drug without consulting your health care provider.
- Use a barrier method of birth control while using this drug; if you become pregnant or desire to become pregnant, consult with your health care provider. If you are breast-feeding, you should find another method of feeding the infant.
- You may experience these side effects: Dizziness (avoid driving a car or performing hazardous tasks); headache (request medications); nausea, vomiting, diarrhea (proper nutrition is important, consult a dietitian to maintain nutrition); symptoms of upper respiratory tract infection, cough (do not self-medicate; consult your health care provider if uncomfortable).
- Report fever, chills, dizziness, pregnancy.

▷lovastatin (mevinolin)
(loe va sta' tin)

Altoprev⦿, Apo-Lovastatin (CAN), Co-Lovastatin (CAN), Gen-Lovastatin (CAN), Mevacor, Nu-Lovastatin (CAN), PMS-Lovastatin (CAN), ratio-Lovastatin (CAN)

PREGNANCY CATEGORY X

Drug classes
Antihyperlipidemic
HMG-CoA reductase inhibitor

Therapeutic actions
Inhibits the enzyme that catalyzes the rate-limiting step in the cholesterol synthesis pathway, resulting in a decrease in serum cholesterol, serum LDLs (the lipids associated with the development of coronary artery disease), and either an increase or no change in serum HDLs (the lipids associated with decreased risk of CAD).

Indications
- Treatment of familial hypercholesterolemia
- Adjunctive treatment of type II hyperlipidemia (ER only)
- To slow the progression of atherosclerosis in patients with CAD
- Primary prevention of coronary heart disease in patients without symptomatic disease; average to moderately elevated total cholesterol and LDL cholesterol, and low HDLs
- Treatment of primary hypercholesterolemia with diet and exercise to decrease total and LDL cholesterol
- As adjunct to diet to reduce total cholesterol, LDLs, apolipoprotein B levels in adolescent boys and girls who are at least 1 yr postmenarche who have heterozygous familial hypercholesterolemia

Contraindications and cautions
- Contraindicated with allergy to lovastatin, active liver disease, unexplained persistent serum transaminase, pregnancy.
- Use cautiously with impaired hepatic function, cataracts, lactation.

Available forms
Tablets—10, 20, 40 mg; ER tablets⦿—10, 20, 40, 60 mg

Dosages
Adults
Initially, 20 mg/day PO given in the evening with meals. Maintenance range, 10–80 mg/day PO single or divided doses. Do not exceed 80 mg/day. For ER tablets, 10–60 mg/day as single dose PO, taken in the evening. Adjust at intervals of 4 wk or more. Maximum daily dose, 40 mg/day if taking amiodarone or verapamil. Patients receiving cyclosporine should start at 10 mg daily and not exceed 20 mg daily. May be combined with bile acid sequestrants. If combined with fibrates or niacin, do not exceed 20 mg daily.
Pediatric patients
- *Adolescent boys and postmenarchal girls, 10–17 yr:* 10–40 mg/day PO; may increase to a maximum of 40 mg/day.
Patients with renal impairment
For creatinine clearance less than 30 mL/min, use doses more than 20 mg/day with caution.

Pharmacokinetics

Route	Onset	Peak
Oral	2 wk	4–6 wk

Metabolism: Hepatic; $T_{1/2}$: 2–4 hr
Distribution: Crosses placenta; enters breast milk
Excretion: Bile, feces

Adverse effects

- **CNS:** *Headache,* blurred vision, dizziness, insomnia, fatigue, muscle cramps, cataracts
- **GI:** *Flatulence, abdominal pain, cramps, constipation, nausea,* dyspepsia, heartburn, elevations of alkaline phosphatase, transaminases
- **Other:** Myalgia, rhabdomyolysis, rash, glucose intolerance

Interactions

٭ Drug-drug ⊗ *Warning* Possibility of severe myopathy or rhabdomyolysis with cyclosporine, amiodarone, verapamil, or gemfibrozil or other HMG-CoA inhibitors, or niacin and azole antifungals; avoid these combinations.

- Increased serum levels and risk of myopathy if combined with drugs that inhibit CYP450 3A4 (eg, itraconazole, ketoconazole); reduce lovastatin dose or interrupt treatment if these drugs are needed

٭ Drug-food • Decreased metabolism and increased risk of toxic effects if taken with grapefruit juice; avoid this combination

■ Nursing considerations

Assessment

- **History:** Allergy to lovastatin, impaired hepatic function, cataracts, pregnancy, lactation
- **Physical:** Orientation, affect, ophthalmologic examination; liver evaluation; lipid studies, LFTs

Interventions

- Give in the evening; highest rates of cholesterol synthesis are between midnight and 5 AM. Ensure that extended-release tablets are not cut, crushed, or chewed.
- Arrange for regular checkups.
- Advise patient that this drug cannot be taken during pregnancy; urge the use of barrier contraceptives.
- Arrange for periodic ophthalmologic examinations to check for cataract develop-

ment, and liver function studies every 4–6 wk during first 15 mo and then periodically.

- Monitor patient closely in any situation
- Administer only when diet restricted in cholesterol and saturated fats fails to lower cholesterol and lipids adequately.
- Discontinue lovastatin if LFTs increase to three times the upper limit of normal.

Teaching points

- Take drug in the evening. Continue following a cholesterol-lowering diet while taking this medication. Avoid drinking grapefruit juice while taking this drug.
- Do not cut, crush, or chew extended-release tablets.
- Use a barrier contraceptive while you are taking this drug; if you think you are pregnant or wish to become pregnant, consult your health care provider.
- Have periodic ophthalmologic examinations.
- You may experience these side effects: Nausea (eat frequent small meals), headache, muscle and joint aches and pains (may lessen).
- Report severe GI upset, changes in vision, unusual bleeding or bruising, dark urine, or light-colored stools, severe muscle pain, soreness.

▽**loxapine**
(lox' a peen)

loxapine hydrochloride

loxapine succinate

Apo-Loxapine (CAN),
Loxapac (CAN), Loxitane,
PMS-Loxapine (CAN)

PREGNANCY CATEGORY C

Drug classes

Antipsychotic
Dopaminergic blocker

Therapeutic actions

Mechanism of action is not fully understood: Antipsychotic drugs block postsynaptic dopamine receptors in the brain, but this may not be necessary and sufficient for antipsychotic activity.

Adverse effects in *italics* are most common; those in **bold** are life-threatening. ⬛ Do not crush.

Indications
• Treatment of schizophrenia

Contraindications and cautions
• Contraindicated with coma or severe CNS depression; bone marrow depression; blood dyscrasia; circulatory collapse; subcortical brain damage; Parkinson disease; liver disease; cerebral arteriosclerosis; coronary disease; severe hypotension or hypertension; known hypersensitivity to dibenzoxazepines.
• Use cautiously with respiratory disorders ("silent pneumonia"); glaucoma, prostatic hypertrophy; epilepsy or history of epilepsy; breast cancer (elevations in prolactin may stimulate a prolactin-dependent tumor); thyrotoxicosis; peptic ulcer, decreased renal function; exposure to heat or phosphorus insecticides; pregnancy; and lactation.

Available forms
Capsules—5, 10, 25, 50 mg

Dosages
Adults
Oral
Individualize dosage, and administer in divided doses bid–qid, initially 10 mg bid. Severely disturbed patients may need up to 50 mg/day. Increase dosage fairly rapidly over the first 7–10 days until symptoms are controlled. Usual dosage range is 60–100 mg/day; dosage greater than 250 mg/day is not recommended. For maintenance, reduce to minimum effective dose. Usual range is 20–60 mg/day.
Pediatric patients
Not recommended for patients younger than 16 yr.
Geriatric patients
Use lower doses, and increase dosage more gradually than in younger patients.

Pharmacokinetics

Route	Onset	Peak	Duration
Oral	30 min	1.5–3 hr	12 hr

Metabolism: Hepatic; $T_{1/2}$: 1–14 hr
Distribution: Unknown
Excretion: Urine

Adverse effects
Adverse effects listed are those of antipsychotic drugs.

• **Autonomic:** Dry mouth, salivation, nasal congestion, nausea, vomiting, anorexia, fever, pallor, facial flushing, sweating, constipation, paralytic ileus, urinary retention, incontinence, polyuria, enuresis, priapism, ejaculation inhibition, male impotence
• **CNS:** *Drowsiness,* insomnia, vertigo, headache, weakness, tremor, ataxia, slurring, cerebral edema, seizures, exacerbation of psychotic symptoms, extrapyramidal syndromes—*pseudoparkinsonism; dystonias; akathisia,* tardive dyskinesias, potentially irreversible, **neuroleptic malignant syndrome**
• **CV:** Hypotension, orthostatic hypotension, hypertension, tachycardia, bradycardia, cardiac arrest, heart failure, cardiomegaly, **refractory arrhythmias,** pulmonary edema
• **Endocrine:** Lactation, breast engorgement, galactorrhea; SIADH; amenorrhea, menstrual irregularities; gynecomastia; changes in libido; hyperglycemia or hypoglycemia; glycosuria; hyponatremia; pituitary tumor with hyperprolactinemia; inhibition of ovulation, infertility, pseudopregnancy; reduced urinary levels of gonadotropins, estrogens, progestins
• **Hematologic:** Eosinophilia, leukopenia, leukocytosis, anemia; aplastic anemia; hemolytic anemia; thrombocytopenic or nonthrombocytopenic purpura; pancytopenia
• **Hypersensitivity:** Jaundice, urticaria, angioneurotic edema, laryngeal edema, photosensitivity, eczema, asthma, anaphylactoid reactions, exfoliative dermatitis
• **Respiratory: Bronchospasm, laryngospasm,** dyspnea; suppression of cough reflex and potential for aspiration

Interactions
✳ **Drug-drug** • Increased risk of CNS effects if combined with other CNS medications

■ Nursing considerations

⚡ CLINICAL ALERT!
Name confusion has been reported between *Loxitane* (loxapine), *Lexapro* (escitalopram), and Soriatane (acitretin); use caution.

Assessment
• **History:** Coma or severe CNS depression; blood dyscrasia; circulatory collapse; subcortical brain damage; Parkinson disease; liver damage; cerebral arteriosclerosis; coronary

disease; severe hypotension or hypertension; respiratory disorders; glaucoma, prostatic hypertrophy; epilepsy; breast cancer; thyrotoxicosis; peptic ulcer, decreased renal function; myelography within previous 24 hr or myelography scheduled within 48 hr; exposure to heat or phosphorus insecticides; pregnancy, lactation

• **Physical:** Weight, T; reflexes, orientation, IOP; P, BP, orthostatic BP; R, adventitious sounds; bowel sounds and normal output, liver evaluation; urinary output, prostate size; CBC, urinalysis, thyroid, LFTs, renal function tests

Interventions

⊗ **Black box warning** There is increased risk of mortality when antipsychotics are used in elderly patients with dementia-related psychosis. Avoid this use; not approved for this use.

⊗ **Warning** Arrange for discontinuation if WBC count is depressed.

⊗ **Warning** Monitor elderly patients for dehydration; institute remedial measures promptly; sedation and decreased thirst sensation due to CNS effects can lead to severe dehydration (drug may impair heat regulation).

• Alert patient that there is a risk of extrapyramidal effects in newborns if drug is taken during the last trimester of pregnancy.

• Consult physician about appropriate warning of patient or patient's guardian about tardive dyskinesias.

• Consult physician about dosage reduction and use of anticholinergic antiparkinsonian drugs (controversial) if extrapyramidal effects occur.

Teaching points

• Take drug exactly as prescribed.

• Avoid driving or engaging in dangerous activities if dizziness or vision changes occur.

• Avoid prolonged exposure to sun or use a sunscreen or covering garments.

• Maintain fluid intake, and use precautions against heatstroke in hot weather.

• Be aware that infants born to mothers taking this drug in the last trimester may exhibit abnormal movements and shaking.

• Report sore throat, fever, unusual bleeding or bruising, rash, weakness, tremors, impaired vision, dark urine, pale stools, and yellowing of the skin or eyes.

▽**lucinactant**
*(loo sin **ak'** tant)*

Surfaxin

PREGNANCY CATEGORY UNKNOWN

Drug class
Lung surfactant

Therapeutic actions
Nonpyrogenic pulmonary surfactant containing lipids and peptides that reduce surface tension and all expansion of the alveoli; replaces the surfactant missing from the lungs of preterm infants

Indications
• Prevention of RDS in preterm infants at high risk for RDS

Contraindications and cautions
None known.

Available forms
Suspension—8.5 mL/vial

Dosages
Pediatric patients
5.8 mL/kg birth weight by intratracheal administration; up to four doses may be given in the first 48 hours of life, spaced at not less than every 6 hours.

Pharmacokinetics
Effects occur at the terminal bronchi. Pharmacokinetic studies have not been done.

Adverse effects
• **CV:** Bradycardia
• **Respiratory: Endotracheal (ET) tube reflux, ET tube obstruction, acute change in lung compliance, oxygen desaturation**
• **Other:** Pallor

■ Nursing considerations
Assessment
• **History:** Time of birth, accurate birth weight
• **Physical:** BP, P; R and adventitious sounds, oximeter reading, ET tube position and patency, ECG, responsiveness

Interventions

- Ensure proper placement and patency of ET tube.
- Warm vial in dry block heater to 111° F (44° C) for 15 min; once warmed, shake vial vigorously. May store for up to 2 hr at room temperature, protected from light. Discard after 2 hr; discard any leftover solution. Vial is for single use only.
- Inspect solution; it should be opaque to off-white and free flowing. Draw into syringe using strict aseptic technique. Patient may be suctioned before beginning procedure.
- Place infant in right lateral decubitus position with head and thorax inclined upward at 30 degrees. Attach syringe to #5 French end-hole catheter. Thread catheter through a valve device to maintain end pressure and thread into ET tube, extending just beyond end of tube. Dose is delivered in 4 aliquots while maintaining positive pressure with mechanical ventilation; stabilize infant to oxygen saturation of 90% and P over 120 beats/min after each dose. Repeat with second dose in left position; switch to right lateral positions for doses three and four. After last dose, remove catheter and keep head elevated at least 10 degrees for next 1–2 hr, maintaining mechanical ventilation. Do not suction during first hour after dosing unless significant airway obstruction occurs.
- Continually monitor color, breath sounds, oximetry, ECG, and blood gas readings. Provide all support needed for a preterm infant.

Teaching points

- Details of drug's effects and administration are best incorporated into parents' and/or caregivers' comprehensive teaching program for the preterm infant.

▽**lurasidone hydrochloride**
(loo *ras' ih dohn*)

Latuda

PREGNANCY CATEGORY B

Drug class
Atypical antipsychotic

Therapeutic actions
Acts as an antagonist at central dopamine and serotonin receptor sites, which is thought to account for its antischizophrenic effects, although the actual mechanism of action is not understood.

Indications
- Treatment of adults with schizophrenia

Contraindications and cautions
- Contraindicated with history of serious hypersensitivity reactions to lurasidone; concurrent use of CYP3A4 inhibitors (such as ketoconazole) or inducers (such as rifampin); lactation.
- Use cautiously with cardiovascular or cerebrovascular disorders, history of seizures, diabetes, liver or renal dysfunction, pregnancy.

Available forms
Tablets—40, 80 mg

Dosages
Adults
Initially, 40 mg/day PO with food; may titrate to a maximum 80 mg/day PO with food. If administering with moderate CYP3A4 inhibitors (such as diltiazem and others), dosage should not exceed 40 mg/day.
Pediatric patients
Safety and efficacy not established.
Patients with renal or hepatic impairment
Do not exceed 40 mg/day PO.

Pharmacokinetics

Route	Onset	Peak
Oral	Rapid	1–3 hr

Metabolism: Hepatic; $T_{1/2}$: 18 hr
Distribution: May cross placenta; may enter breast milk
Excretion: Urine

Adverse effects
- **CNS:** *Somnolence, akathisia, parkinsonism,* agitation, *dystonia,* dizziness, *insomnia,* seizures, suicidality
- **CV:** Tachycardia, blood pressure changes
- **GI:** *Nausea,* diarrhea, *vomiting, dyspepsia,* constipation, anorexia
- **Hematologic:** Leukopenia, neutropenia

- **Respiratory:** URI, sinusitis, nasopharyngitis
- **Other:** Hyperglycemia, weight gain, dyslipidemia, hyperprolactinemia, **neuroleptic malignant syndrome,** heat intolerance, back pain

Interactions

✳ Drug-drug • Possible serious adverse effects if combined with strong CYP3A4 inhibitors (diltiazem, ketoconazole); this combination is contraindicated • Risk of ineffective therapeutic levels if combined with CYP3A4 inducers (rifampin) or lithium; these combinations are contraindicated • Risk of increased CNS effects if combined with alcohol; avoid this combination

✳ Drug-food • Decreased metabolism and increased toxic effects if taken with grapefruit juice; do not exceed 40 mg/day if using this combination

■ Nursing considerations

Assessment

- **History:** History of serious hypersensitivity reactions to lurasidone; concurrent use of CYP3A4 inhibitors (ketoconazole) or inducers (rifampin); cardiovascular or cerebrovascular disorders; history of seizures; diabetes; renal or liver dysfunction; pregnancy; lactation
- **Physical:** Orientation, reflexes, BP, P, weight; abdominal exam; blood glucose; renal and liver function tests

Interventions

⊗ **Black box warning** Increased risk of death in elderly patients with dementia-related psychosis who are treated with this drug; lurasidone is not indicated for use in these patients

- Dispense the least amount possible to potentially suicidal patients.
- Establish baseline orientation and neurologic functioning, weight, and blood glucose levels.
- Provide safety measures if neurologic changes or orthostatic hypotension occurs.
- Monitor patient for signs and symptoms of hyperglycemia and for weight gain.
- Monitor patient with pre-existing low WBC count before and periodically during therapy.
- Protect patient from overheating and ensure adequate hydration.

Teaching points

- Take this drug once a day at approximately the same time each day.
- If you forget a dose, take it as soon as you remember; then begin your usual dosage the next day. Do not make up skipped doses and do not take more than one dose each day.
- Avoid consuming alcohol while taking this drug; serious effects could occur.
- You will need periodic blood tests to check your blood glucose level and blood counts.
- It is not known how this drug affects a fetus. If you are pregnant or thinking about becoming pregnant, discuss this with your health care provider.
- This drug may enter breast milk, but it is not known how this could affect a breast-feeding baby. If you are breast-feeding, you should use another method of feeding the baby during therapy.
- You may experience these side effects: Weight gain, high blood glucose level (monitor your weight and be alert for increased thirst, increased urination, increased appetite, fatigue; dietary measures may be needed); dizziness (change position slowly and take care to avoid falls); changes in mental functioning (avoid driving or operating hazardous machinery if this occurs); intolerance to heat (make sure you avoid overheating and maintain an adequate intake of fluids).
- Report weight gain; increased urination; thirst, appetite, fatigue; dizziness; thoughts of suicide.

▷**lutropin**

See Appendix R, *Less commonly used drugs.*

▷**magnesium salts**
(mag nee' zee um)

magnesia

magnesium citrate
Citro-Mag (CAN), Citroma

magnesium hydroxide
Milk of Magnesia, Phillips' Chewable, Pedia-Lax

magnesium oxide
Mag-Ox 400, Maox 420, Uro-Mag

PREGNANCY CATEGORY C

PREGNANCY CATEGORY A
(ANTACID)

PREGNANCY CATEGORY B
(LAXATIVE)

Drug classes
Antacid
Laxative

Therapeutic actions
Antacid (magnesium hydroxide, magnesium oxide): Neutralizes or reduces gastric acidity, resulting in an increase in the pH of the stomach and duodenal bulb and inhibition of the proteolytic activity of pepsin. Laxative (magnesium citrate, magnesium hydroxide): Attracts and retains water in intestinal lumen and distends bowel; causes the duodenal secretion of cholecystokinin, which stimulates fluid secretion and intestinal motility.

Indications
- Symptomatic relief of upset stomach associated with hyperacidity
- Hyperacidity associated with peptic ulcer, gastritis, peptic esophagitis, gastric hyperacidity, and hiatal hernia
- Prophylaxis of GI bleeding, stress ulcers, aspiration pneumonia
- Short-term relief of constipation; evacuation of the colon for rectal and bowel examination

Contraindications and cautions
- Contraindicated with allergy to magnesium products.
- Use cautiously with renal insufficiency, pregnancy, lactation.

Available forms
Tablets—311 (chewable), 400, 420, 500 mg; capsules—140 mg; liquid—various

Dosages
Adults
Magnesium citrate
- *Laxative:* 300 mL or in divided doses with a full glass of water.

Magnesium hydroxide
- *Antacid:* 5–15 mL liquid or 622–1,244 mg tablets PO qid (adult and patients older than 12 yr).
- *Laxative:* 15–60 mL PO taken with liquid.
  6–11 yr: 15–30 mL (400 mg/5 mL) PO once daily at bedtime or 7.5–15 mL/day (800 mg/5 mL) PO once daily at bedtime.
  2–5 yr: 5–15 mL (400 mg/5 mL) PO once daily at bedtime.

Magnesium oxide
- *Capsules:* 140 mg PO tid–qid.
- *Tablets:* 400–800 mg/day PO.

Pediatric patients
Magnesium citrate
- *Laxative:* 90–210 mL for ages 6–12 yr with full glass of water; 60 mL for ages 2–6 yr with full glass of water.

Magnesium hydroxide
- *Laxative:*
  12 yr and older: 30–60 mL (400 mg/5 mL) PO with water or 15–30 mL/day (800 mg/5 mL) PO once daily at bedtime, or eight 311-mg tablets PO once daily at bedtime or in divided doses.
  6–11 yr: four 311-mg tablets PO once daily at bedtime.
  3–5 yr: two 311-mg tablets PO once daily at bedtime.
  Younger than 2 yr: Do not administer unless directed by a physician.

Pharmacokinetics

Route	Onset
Oral	20–60 min

Minimal systemic absorption
Excretion: Renal

Adverse effects
- **CNS:** Dizziness, fainting, sweating
- **GI:** *Diarrhea, nausea, perianal irritation*
- **Metabolic:** Hypermagnesemia and toxicity in patients with renal failure

Interactions
✳ **Drug-drug** ⊗ **Warning** Do not give other oral drugs within 1–2 hr of antacid administration; change in gastric pH may interfere with absorption.
- Decreased pharmacologic effect of tetracyclines, penicillamine, nitrofurantoin, fluoroquinolones, ketoconazole

M

■ **Nursing considerations**
Assessment
• **History:** Allergy to magnesium products; renal insufficiency
• **Physical:** Abdominal examination, bowel sounds; renal function tests, serum magnesium

Interventions
• Do not administer other oral drugs within 1–2 hr of antacid administration.
• Have patient chew antacid tablets thoroughly before swallowing; follow with a glass of water.
• Give antacid between meals and at bedtime.

Teaching points
• Take antacid between meals and at bedtime. If tablets are being used, chew thoroughly before swallowing, and then drink a glass of water.
• Do not use laxatives if you have abdominal pain, nausea, or vomiting.
• Refrigerate magnesium citrate solutions to keep them effective and improve their taste.
• Do not take with any other oral medications; absorption of those medications can be inhibited. Take other oral medications at least 1–2 hours after aluminum salt.
• Diarrhea may occur with antacid therapy.
• Do not use laxatives long-term. Prolonged or excessive use can lead to serious problems. You should increase your intake of water (to 6–8 glasses/day) and fiber, and exercise regularly.
• You may experience these side effects: Excessive bowel activity, cramping, diarrhea, nausea, dizziness (be careful not to fall).
• With antacid use, report diarrhea; coffee-ground vomitus; black, tarry stools; no relief from symptoms being treated. With laxative use, report rectal bleeding, muscle cramps or pain, weakness, dizziness (not related to abdominal cramps and bowel movement), unrelieved constipation.

DANGEROUS DRUG (IV)

▷ **magnesium sulfate (epsom salt)**
(*mag nee' zee um*)

PREGNANCY CATEGORY A

PREGNANCY CATEGORY B
(LAXATIVE)

Drug classes
Antiepileptic
Electrolyte
Laxative

Therapeutic actions
Cofactor of many enzyme systems involved in neurochemical transmission and muscular excitability; prevents or controls seizures by blocking neuromuscular transmission; attracts and retains water in the intestinal lumen and distends the bowel to promote mass movement and relieve constipation.

Indications
• Acute nephritis (children), to control hypertension
• IV: Hypomagnesemia, replacement therapy
• IV or IM: Pre-eclampsia or eclampsia
• PO: Short-term treatment of constipation
• PO: Evacuation of the colon for rectal and bowel examinations
• To correct or prevent hypomagnesemia in patients on parenteral nutrition
• Unlabeled uses: Inhibition of premature labor (parenteral), adjunct treatment of exacerbations of acute asthma; treatment torsades de pointes, atypical ventricular arrhythmias

Contraindications and cautions
• Contraindicated with allergy to magnesium products; heart block, myocardial damage; abdominal pain, nausea, vomiting, or other symptoms of appendicitis; acute surgical abdomen, fecal impaction, intestinal and biliary tract obstruction, hepatitis. Do not give during 2 hr preceding delivery because of risk of magnesium toxicity in the neonate.
• Use cautiously with renal insufficiency.

Available forms
Granules—40 mEq/5 g; injection—0.081, 0.162, 0.325, 0.65, 1, 4 mEq/mL

Dosages
Adults

- *Parenteral nutrition:* 8–24 mEq/day IV.
- *Mild magnesium deficiency:* 1 g IM or IV every 6 hr for 4 doses (32.5 mEq/24 hr).
- *Severe hypomagnesemia:* Up to 246 mg/kg IM within 4 hr or 5 g (40 mEq)/1,000 mL D₅W or 0.9% normal saline IV infused over 3 hr.
- *Eclampsia, severe pre-eclampsia:* Total initial dose of 10–14 g. May infuse 4–5 g in 250 mL 5% dextrose injection or 0.9% sodium chloride while giving IM doses up to 10 g (5 g or 10 mL of undiluted 50% solution in each buttock). Or, may give initial IV dose of 4 g by diluting 50% solution to 10% or 20%; may inject diluted fluid (40 mL of 10% or 20 mL of 20% solution) IV over 3–4 min. Then inject 4–5 g (8 to 10 mL of 50% solution) IM into alternate buttocks every 4 hr as needed depending on patellar reflex and respiratory function. Or, after initial IV dose, may give 1–2 g/hr by constant IV infusion. Continue until paroxysms stop. To control seizures, optimal serum magnesium level is 6 mg/100 mL. Do not exceed 30–40 g in 24 hr.

IM

- *Toxemia:* 4–5 g of a 50% solution every 4 hr as needed.

IV

1–4 g of a 10%–20% solution. Do not exceed 1.5 mL/min of a 10% solution. Or, 4–5 g in 250 mL of 5% dextrose. Do not exceed 3 mL/min.
- *Arrhythmias:* 3–4 g IV over several min; then 3–20 mg/min continuous infusion for 5–48 hr.
- *Acute MI:* 2 g IV over 5–15 min followed by 18 g IV over 24 hr.

PO

- *Laxative:* 10–30 g daily given as single dose or divided doses.

Pediatric patients
- *Laxative:*
  - *6–11 yr:* 5–10 g daily in single dose or divided doses; 15–30 mL/day.
  - *2–5 yr:* 2.5–5 g daily in single dose or divided doses; 5–15 mL/day.

IM

100 mg/kg (0.8 mEq/kg or 0.2 mL/kg of a 50% solution) IM every 4–6 hr as needed. Or, 20–40 mg/kg (0.16–0.32 mEq/kg or 0.1–0.2 mL/kg of a 20% solution).

IV

For severe symptoms, 100–200 mg/kg of a 1%–3% solution IV over 1 hr with half of dose given in first 15–20 min (seizure control).

Patients with renal impairment
- *Severe pre-eclampsia, eclampsia:* In severe impairment, maximum dosage is 20 g in 48 hr. Check serum magnesium level often.

Pharmacokinetics

Route	Onset	Duration
IV	Immediate	30 min
IM	60 min	3–4 hr
Oral	1–2 hr	3–4 hr

Metabolism: $T_{1/2}$: Unknown
Distribution: Crosses placenta, enters breast milk
Excretion: Urine

▼ IV FACTS

Preparation: Dilute IV infusion to a concentration of 20% or less before IV administration; dilute 4–5 g in 250 mL D₅W or sodium chloride solution.
Infusion: Do not exceed 1.5 mL of a 10% solution per minute IV or 3 mL/min IV infusion.
Incompatibilities: Do not mix with other IV drugs.

Adverse effects
- **CNS:** *Weakness, dizziness,* fainting, sweating (PO)
- **CV:** Palpitations
- **GI:** *Excessive bowel activity, perianal irritation* (PO)
- **Metabolic:** *Magnesium intoxication* (flushing, sweating, hypotension, depressed reflexes, flaccid paralysis, hypothermia, circulatory collapse, cardiac and CNS depression—parenteral); hypocalcemia with tetany (secondary to treatment of eclampsia—parenteral)

Interactions
❋ **Drug-drug** ● Potentiation of neuromuscular blockade produced by nondepolarizing neuromuscular relaxants (atracurium, pancuronium, vecuronium). Potential for hypomagnesia if combined with alcohol, aminoglycosides, amphotericin B, cisplatin, cyclosporine, digoxin, diuretics; monitor patient closely.

■ Nursing considerations
Assessment

- **History:** Allergy to magnesium products; renal insufficiency; heart block, myocardial damage; symptoms of appendicitis; acute surgical abdomen, fecal impaction, intestinal and biliary tract obstruction, hepatitis
- **Physical:** Skin color, texture; muscle tone; T; orientation, affect, reflexes, peripheral sensation; P, auscultation, BP, rhythm strip; abdominal examination, bowel sounds; renal function tests, serum magnesium and calcium, LFTs (oral use)

Interventions

- Reserve IV use in eclampsia for immediate life-threatening situations.
- Give IM route by deep IM injection of the undiluted (50%) solution for adults; dilute to a 20% solution for children.
- ⊗ **Warning** Monitor serum magnesium levels during parenteral therapy. Arrange to discontinue administration as soon as levels are within normal limits (1.5–3 mEq/L) and desired clinical response is obtained.
- ⊗ **Warning** Monitor knee-jerk reflex before repeated parenteral administration. If knee-jerk reflexes are suppressed, do not administer magnesium because respiratory center failure may occur.
- Give oral magnesium sulfate as a laxative only as a temporary measure. Arrange for dietary measures (fiber, fluids), exercise, and environmental control to return to normal bowel activity.
- Do not give oral magnesium sulfate with abdominal pain, nausea, or vomiting.
- Monitor bowel function; if diarrhea and cramping occur, discontinue oral drug.
- Maintain urine output at a level of 100 mL every 4 hr during parenteral administration.

Teaching points

- Use only as a temporary measure to relieve constipation. Do not take if abdominal pain, nausea, or vomiting occurs.
- You may experience diarrhea with oral use. If this occurs, discontinue drug and consult your health care provider.
- Report sweating, flushing, muscle tremors or twitching, inability to move extremities.

▽ mannitol
(man' i tole)

Osmitrol

PREGNANCY CATEGORY B

Drug classes

Diagnostic agent
Osmotic diuretic
Urinary irrigant

Therapeutic actions

Elevates the osmolarity of the glomerular filtrate, thereby hindering the reabsorption of water and leading to a loss of water, sodium, chloride (used for diagnosis of glomerular filtration rate); creates an osmotic gradient in the eye between plasma and ocular fluids, thereby reducing IOP; creates an osmotic effect, leading to decreased swelling in posttransurethral prostatic resection.

Indications

- Prevention and treatment of the oliguric phase of renal failure
- Reduction of intracranial pressure and treatment of cerebral edema; of elevated IOP when the pressure cannot be lowered by other means
- Promotion of the urinary excretion of toxic substances
- Diagnostic use: Measurement of GFR

Contraindications and cautions

- Contraindicated with anuria due to severe renal disease.
- Use cautiously with pulmonary congestion, active intracranial bleeding (except during craniotomy), dehydration, renal disease, heart failure, pregnancy, lactation.

Available forms

Injection—5%, 10%, 15%, 20%, 25%

Dosages
Adults

IV infusion only; individualize concentration and rate of administration. Dosage is 50–200 g/day. Adjust dosage to maintain urine flow of 30–50 mL/hr.

- *Prevention of oliguria:* 50–100 g IV as a 5%–25% solution.

Adverse effects in *italics* are most common; those in **bold** are life-threatening. ⊂⊃ Do not crush.

- *Treatment of oliguria:* 50–100 g IV of a 15%–25% solution.

- *Reduction of intracranial pressure and cerebral edema:* 1.5–2 g/kg IV as a 15%–25% solution over 30–60 min. Evidence of reduced pressure should be seen in 15 min.

- *Reduction of IOP:* Infuse 1.5–2 g/kg IV as a 25% solution, 20% solution, or 15% solution over 30 min. If used preoperatively, use 60–90 min before surgery for maximal effect.

- *Adjunctive therapy to promote diuresis in intoxications:* Maximum of 200 g IV of mannitol with other fluids and electrolytes.

- *Measurement of glomerular filtration rate:* Dilute 100 mL of a 20% solution with 180 mL of sodium chloride injection. Infuse this 280 mL of 7.2% solution IV at a rate of 20 mL/min. Collect urine with a catheter for the specified time for measurement of mannitol excreted in mg/min. Draw blood at the start and at the end of the time for measurement of mannitol in mg/mL plasma.

- *Test dose of mannitol for patients with inadequate renal function:* 0.2 g/kg IV (about 50 mL of a 25% solution, 75 mL of a 20% solution) in 3–5 min to produce a urine flow of 30–50 mL/hr. If urine flow does not increase, repeat dose. If no response to second dose, re-evaluate patient situation.

Pediatric patients
Dosage for children younger than 12 yr not established.

Pharmacokinetics

Route	Onset	Peak	Duration
IV	30–60 min	1 hr	6–8 hr
Irrigant	Rapid	Rapid	Short

Metabolism: $T_{1/2}$: 15–100 min
Distribution: Crosses placenta; may enter breast milk
Excretion: Urine

▼ IV FACTS

Preparation: Mannitol may crystallize at low temperatures, especially solutions of more than 15%. If crystals are observed, warm solution to dissolve.
Infusion: Infuse at rates listed (above). Use an infusion set with a filter if concentrated mannitol is used.
Incompatibilities: Do not add to blood products.

Adverse effects

- **CNS:** *Dizziness,* headache, blurred vision, **seizures**
- **CV:** Hypotension, hypertension, edema, HF, thrombophlebitis, tachycardia, chest pain
- **Dermatologic:** Urticaria, skin necrosis with infiltration
- **GI:** *Nausea, anorexia, dry mouth, thirst*
- **GU:** *Diuresis,* urine retention
- **Hematologic:** Fluid and electrolyte imbalances, hyponatremia
- **Respiratory:** Pulmonary congestion, rhinitis

■ Nursing considerations
Assessment

- **History:** Pulmonary congestion, active intracranial bleeding, dehydration, renal disease, heart failure, pregnancy, lactation
- **Physical:** Skin color, lesions, edema, hydration; orientation, muscle strength, reflexes, pupils; pulses, BP, perfusion; R, pattern, adventitious sounds; urinary output patterns; serum electrolytes, urinalysis, renal function tests

Interventions
⊗ **Warning** Do not give electrolyte-free mannitol with blood. If blood must be given, add at least 20 mEq of sodium chloride to each liter of mannitol solution.

- Do not expose solutions to low temperatures; crystallization may occur. If crystals are seen, warm the bottle in a hot water bath, then cool to body temperature before administering.

- Make sure the infusion set contains a filter if giving concentrated mannitol.

- Monitor serum electrolytes periodically with prolonged therapy.

Teaching points
- This drug must be given by IV infusion.
- You may experience these side effects: Increased urination; GI upset (eat frequent small meals); dry mouth (suck on sugarless candies); headache, blurred vision (use caution when moving, ask for assistance).
- Report difficulty breathing, pain at the IV site, chest pain.

M

▽ **maprotiline hydrochloride**
(ma **proe'** ti leen)

Novo-Maprotiline (CAN)

PREGNANCY CATEGORY B

Drug class
Antidepressant (tetracyclic)

Therapeutic actions
Mechanism of action unknown; appears to act similarly to TCAs; the TCAs act to inhibit the presynaptic reuptake of the neurotransmitters norepinephrine (primarily) and serotonin; anticholinergic at CNS and peripheral receptors; sedating; the relation of these effects to clinical efficacy is unknown.

Indications
• Treatment of depressive illness in patients with depressive neurosis (dysthymic disorder)
• Treatment of depression in patients with bipolar disorder (depressed type)
• Treatment of anxiety associated with depression
• Unlabeled use: Treatment of post-herpetic neuralgia

Contraindications and cautions
• Contraindicated with hypersensitivity to tricyclic drugs, concomitant therapy with an MAOI, recent MI, myelography within previous 24 hr or scheduled within 48 hr, known or suspected seizure disorder, pregnancy (limb reduction abnormalities reported), lactation.
• Use cautiously with EST; pre-existing CV disorders (increased risk of serious CV toxicity); angle-closure glaucoma, increased IOP, urine retention, ureteral or urethral spasm; seizure disorders (lowers seizure threshold); hyperthyroidism (predisposes to CV toxicity, including cardiac arrhythmias); impaired hepatic, renal function; psychiatric disorders (schizophrenic or paranoid patients may worsen); manic-depression (may shift to hypomanic or manic phase); elective surgery (stop use as soon as possible before surgery).

Available forms
Tablets—25, 50, 75 mg

Dosages
Adults
• *Mild to moderate depression:* Initially, 75 mg/day PO in outpatients. Maintain initial dosage for 2 wk due to long drug half-life. Dosage may then be increased gradually in 25-mg increments. Most patients respond to 150 mg/day.
• *More severe depression:* Initially, 100–150 mg/day PO in hospitalized patients. If needed, gradually increase to 225 mg/day.
• *Maintenance:* Reduce dosage to lowest effective level, usually 75–150 mg/day PO.
Pediatric patients
Not recommended in patients younger than 18 yr.
Geriatric patients
Give lower doses to patients older than 60 yr; begin at 25 mg PO daily and gradually increase to 50–75 mg/day PO for maintenance.

Pharmacokinetics

Route	Onset	Peak	Duration
Oral	Slow	12 hr	2–4 wk

Metabolism: Hepatic; $T_{1/2}$: 51 hr
Distribution: Crosses placenta; enters breast milk
Excretion: Feces, urine

Adverse effects
• **CNS:** *Sedation and anticholinergic (atropine-like) effects; confusion* (especially in elderly), *disturbed concentration,* hallucinations, disorientation, decreased memory, feelings of unreality, delusions, anxiety, nervousness, restlessness, agitation, panic, insomnia, nightmares, hypomania, mania, exacerbation of psychosis, drowsiness, weakness, fatigue, headache, numbness, tingling, paresthesias of extremities, incoordination, motor hyperactivity, akathisia, ataxia, tremors, peripheral neuropathy, extrapyramidal symptoms, **seizures,** speech blockage, dysarthria, tinnitus, altered EEG, **suicidal ideation**
• **CV:** *Orthostatic hypotension,* hypertension, syncope, tachycardia, palpitations, **MI,** arrhythmias, heart block, precipitation of HF, **stroke**
• **Endocrine:** Elevated or depressed blood sugar, elevated prolactin levels, inappropriate ADH secretion

Adverse effects in *italics* are most common; those in **bold** are life-threatening. ▭ Do not crush.

- **GI:** *Dry mouth, constipation,* paralytic ileus, *nausea,* vomiting, anorexia, epigastric distress, diarrhea, flatulence, dysphagia, peculiar taste, increased salivation, stomatitis, glossitis, parotid swelling, abdominal cramps, black tongue, hepatitis, jaundice (rare), elevated transaminases, altered alkaline phosphatase
- **GU:** Urine retention, delayed micturition, dilation of the urinary tract, gynecomastia, testicular swelling; breast enlargement, menstrual irregularity and galactorrhea; increased or decreased libido; impotence
- **Hematologic:** Bone marrow depression, eosinophilia, thrombocytopenia, leukopenia
- **Hypersensitivity:** Rash, pruritus, vasculitis, petechiae, photosensitization, edema
- **Withdrawal:** Symptoms with abrupt discontinuation of prolonged therapy: Nausea, headache, vertigo, nightmares, malaise
- **Other:** Nasal congestion, excessive appetite, weight gain or loss; sweating (paradoxic effect in a drug with prominent anticholinergic effects), alopecia, lacrimation, hyperthermia, flushing, chills

Interactions

✴ **Drug-drug** ● Risk of seizures if taken with benzodiazepines (or if benzodiazepines are rapidly tapered during maprotiline therapy), phenothiazines ● Additive atropine-like effects if combined with anticholinergics, sympathomimetics; monitor patient closely and adjust dosages as needed ● Increased risk of cardiotoxicity if taken with thyroid medications; monitor patient closely

■ Nursing considerations
Assessment

- **History:** Hypersensitivity to any tricyclic drug; concomitant therapy with an MAOI; recent MI; myelography within previous 24 hr or scheduled within 48 hr; lactation; EST; preexisting CV disorders; angle-closure glaucoma, increased IOP, urine retention, ureteral or urethral spasm; seizure disorders; hyperthyroidism; impaired hepatic, renal function; psychiatric problems; bipolar disorder; elective surgery, pregnancy, lactation
- **Physical:** Weight; T; skin color, lesions; orientation, affect, reflexes, vision and hearing; P, BP, orthostatic BP, perfusion; bowel sounds, normal output, liver evaluation; urine flow, normal output; usual sexual function,

frequency of menses, breast and scrotal examination; LFTs, urinalysis, CBC, ECG

Interventions

⊗ **Warning** Limit drug access to depressed and potentially suicidal patients.

⊗ **Black box warning** Monitor children, adolescents, and young adults for increased risk of suicidal thinking and behavior.
- Expect clinical response in 3 wk, although some have improved in 3–7 days.
- Give major portion of dose at bedtime if drowsiness or severe anticholinergic effects occur.
- Reduce dosage with minor side effects; discontinue drug if serious side effects occur.
- Arrange for CBC if patient develops fever, sore throat, or signs of infection.

Teaching points

- Take drug exactly as prescribed, and do not stop taking this drug without consulting your health care provider.
- Avoid pregnancy while taking this drug, fetal abnormalities have been reported; using barrier contraceptive is advised.
- Avoid alcohol, sleep-inducing drugs, and over-the-counter drugs.
- Avoid prolonged exposure to sunlight or sunlamps, use sunscreen or protective garments if exposure is unavoidable.
- You may experience these side effects: Headache, dizziness, drowsiness, weakness, blurred vision (reversible; use caution if severe, avoid driving or performing tasks that require alertness); nausea, vomiting, loss of appetite, dry mouth (frequent small meals, frequent mouth care, sucking sugarless candies may help); nightmares, inability to concentrate, confusion; changes in sexual function.
- Report dry mouth, difficulty in urination, excessive sedation, chest pain, thoughts of suicide.

▽ **maraviroc**
(mar ah vye' rock)

Selzentry Ⓒᴺᴰ

Pregnancy Category B

Drug classes
Antiviral
CCR5 coreceptor antagonist

Therapeutic actions

Selectively binds to the human chemokine receptor CCR5 on the cell membrane, preventing interaction of HIV-1 and CCR5 needed for HIV to enter the cell and multiply.

Indications

- Combination antiretroviral treatment of adults infected only with detectable CCR5-tropic HIV-1

Contraindications and cautions

- Contraindicated with hypersensitivity to any component of the drug, lactation.
- Use cautiously with co-infection with hepatitis B, liver disease, increased risk of CV events, hypotension, pregnancy.

Available forms

Tablets ⊚ⓝⓒ—150, 300 mg

Dosages

Adults

When given with strong CYP3A inhibitors, protease inhibitors (except tipranavir/ritonavir), delavirdine, 150 mg PO bid. When given with tipranavir/ritonavir, nevirapine, enfuvirtide, nucleoside reverse transcriptase inhibitors, other drugs that are not strong CYP3A inhibitors, 300 mg PO bid. When given with efavirenz, rifampin, carbamazepine, phenobarbital, phenytoin, 600 mg PO bid.

Pediatric patients younger than 16 yr

Safety and efficacy not established.

Patients with renal impairment

With potent CYP3A inhibitors: If creatinine clearance ranges from 30–80 mL/min or more, give 150 mg PO bid. With other concomitant medications, give 300 mg PO bid. With CYP3A inducers, give 600 mg PO bid. Drug is not recommended if creatinine clearance is less than 30 mL/min or if patient is on dialysis.

Pharmacokinetics

Route	Onset	Peak
Oral	Slow	0.5–4 hr

Metabolism: Hepatic; $T_{1/2}$: 14–18 hr
Distribution: May cross placenta; enters breast milk
Excretion: Feces, urine

Adverse effects

- **CNS:** *Dizziness,* paresthesias, dysesthesias, peripheral neuropathies, sensory abnormalities, depression, sleep disturbances
- **GI:** *Abdominal pain,* constipation, dyspepsia, stomatitis, appetite disorder, **hepatotoxicity**
- **Respiratory:** *Cough,* URI, sinusitis, bronchitis, pneumonia
- **Other:** *Fever, musculoskeletal symptoms,* pruritus, dermatitis, infections

Interactions

✴ **Drug-drug** • Increased serum levels and toxicity when combined with CYP3A inhibitors (ketoconazole, lopinavir/ritonavir, ritonavir, saquinavir, atazanavir, delavirdine); adjust maraviroc dosage accordingly • Decreased serum levels and loss of effectiveness if combined with CYP3A inducers (nevirapine, rifampin, efavirenz); adjust maraviroc dose accordingly

✴ **Drug-alternative therapy** • Loss of effectiveness if taken with St. John's Wort; avoid this combination

■ Nursing considerations

⊗ **Black box warning** Risk of severe hepatotoxicity, possibly preceded by evidence of systemic allergic reaction (rash, eosinophilia, elevated IgE level); immediately evaluate and support patient with any sign of hepatitis or allergic reaction.

Assessment

- **History:** Hypersensitivity to any component of the drug, history of liver impairment, hepatitis B infection, risk factors for cardiovascular events, pregnancy, lactation
- **Physical:** T; orientation, affect; BP; R, lung sounds; abdominal exam; LFTs

Interventions

- Give this drug with other antiretroviral drugs.
- Review antiviral therapy and adjust dosage according to effects on liver enzyme systems.
- Ensure that patient swallows tablet whole; do not cut, crush, or allow patient to chew tablet.
- Monitor patient for any sign of allergic reaction or hepatitis; severe hepatoxicity could occur. Check CBC and IgE markers.
- Encourage breast-feeding mothers to find a different method of feeding the baby while on this drug.

- Protect patient from exposure to infection, and encourage patient to avoid situations that increase risk of infection.

Teaching points

- Take this drug twice a day without regard to food. Swallow the tablets whole; do not cut, crush, or chew them.
- Always take this drug with other anti-HIV drugs that have been prescribed for you.
- Do not take St. John's Wort while on this drug; antiviral activity could be lost.
- If you miss a dose, take it as soon as you remember and then take the regularly scheduled dose at the regular time. If it is less than 6 hours until the next scheduled dose, skip the missed dose and just take the next scheduled dose. Do not double doses. Do not take more than two doses on any one day.
- Do not stop taking this drug; it could lose effectiveness if stopped for even a short period of time. If you are running low, talk to your health care provider about a refill.
- This drug does not cure HIV or AIDS; you may still develop opportunistic infections, and you should seek regular medical care to manage the disease.
- Maraviroc does not reduce the risk of transmitting HIV to others by sexual contact or blood contamination; use appropriate precautions.
- It is not known if this drug could affect a fetus. If you wish to become pregnant, discuss this with your health care provider. If you become pregnant while taking this drug, consult your health care provider about enrolling in the Antiretroviral Pregnancy Registry.
- It is not known how this drug could affect a breast-feeding infant. Because of the risk of serious adverse effects on an infant, you should choose another method of feeding the infant while you are on this drug.
- Your health care provider will monitor your CD4 levels and your liver function regularly while you are on this drug.
- You may experience these side effects: Headache, fever, rash (medication may be available to relieve these symptoms); dizziness (do not drive a car or operate dangerous machinery until you know how this drug will affect you); increased risk of infection, cancer (have regular screenings, and consult your health care provider at the first sign of infection).

- Report rash, difficulty breathing, changes in the color of your stool or urine, fainting, yellowing of the eyes or skin, infections.

DANGEROUS DRUG

▷**mechlorethamine hydrochloride (HN₂, nitrogen mustard)**
(me klor eth' a meen)

Mustargen

PREGNANCY CATEGORY D

Drug classes
Alkylating drug
Antineoplastic
Nitrogen mustard

Therapeutic actions
Cytotoxic: Reacts chemically with DNA, RNA, other proteins to prevent replication and function of susceptible cells, causing cell death; cell-cycle nonspecific.

Indications

- IV use: Palliative treatment of bronchogenic carcinoma, Hodgkin disease, lymphosarcoma, chronic myelogenous leukemia, chronic lymphocytic leukemia, mycosis fungoides, polycythemia vera
- Intrapleural, intraperitoneal, intrapericardial use: Palliative treatment of effusion secondary to metastatic carcinoma
- Unlabeled use: Topical treatment of cutaneous mycosis fungoides

Contraindications and cautions

- Contraindicated with allergy to mechlorethamine, active infection, pregnancy, lactation.
- Use cautiously with amyloidosis, hematopoietic depression, concomitant steroid therapy.

Available forms
Powder for injection—10 mg

Dosages
Individualize dosage based on hematologic profile and response.
Adults
IV
Usual dose, total of 0.4 mg/kg IV for each course of therapy as a single dose or in two to

four divided doses of 0.1–0.2 mg/kg/day. Give at night in case sedation is required for side effects. Interval between courses of therapy is usually 3–6 wk.

Intracavitary

Dose and preparation vary greatly with cavity and disease treated. Consult manufacturer's label; usual dose 0.2–0.4 mg/kg.

Pharmacokinetics

Route	Onset	Peak	Duration
IV	Immediate	Seconds	Minutes

Metabolism: $T_{1/2}$: A few minutes
Distribution: Crosses placenta; may enter breast milk
Excretion: Urine

▼ IV FACTS

Preparation: Reconstitute vial with 10 mL of sterile water for injection or sodium chloride injection; resultant solution contains 1 mg/mL of mechlorethamine hydrochloride. Prepare solution immediately before use; decomposes on standing.
Infusion: Inject into tubing of a flowing IV infusion slowly over 3–5 min.

Adverse effects

- **CNS:** *Weakness,* vertigo, tinnitus, diminished hearing
- **Dermatologic:** Maculopapular rash, alopecia, herpes zoster
- **GI:** *Nausea, vomiting, anorexia,* diarrhea, jaundice
- **GU:** *Impaired fertility*
- **Hematologic:** *Bone marrow depression,* immunosuppression, hyperuricemia
- **Local:** *Vesicant thrombosis, thrombophlebitis,* tissue necrosis if extravasation occurs

Interactions

✷ **Drug-drug** • Risk of serious to fatal infections if combined with adalimumab, denosumab, infliximab; monitor patient closely • Risk of multifocal leukoencephalopathy with natalizumab; avoid this combination • Increased risk of toxic effects with leflunomide; do not use a leflunomide loading dose • Increased immunosuppresive effects with pimecrolimus, roflumilast, topical tacrolimus; avoid these combinations

■ Nursing considerations
Assessment

- **History:** Allergy to mechlorethamine, active infection, amyloidosis, hematopoietic depression, concomitant steroid therapy, pregnancy, lactation
- **Physical:** T; weight; skin color, lesions; injection site; orientation, reflexes, hearing evaluation; CBC, differential, uric acid

Interventions

- Arrange for blood tests to evaluate hematopoietic function before and during therapy.

⊗ **Black box warning** Use caution when preparing drug for administration; use chemosafe nonpermeable gloves for handling drug; drug is highly toxic and a vesicant. Avoid inhalation of dust or vapors and contact with skin or mucous membranes (especially the eyes). If eye contact occurs, immediately irrigate with copious amount of ophthalmic irrigating solution, and obtain an ophthalmologic consultation. If skin contact occurs, irrigate with copious amount of water for 15 min, followed by application of 2% sodium thiosulfate.

⊗ **Warning** Use caution when determining correct amount of drug for injection. The margin of safety is very small; double check dosage before administration.

⊗ **Black box warning** Monitor injection site for any sign of extravasation. Painful inflammation and induration or sloughing of skin may occur. If leakage is noted, promptly infiltrate with sterile isotonic sodium thiosulfate (1/6M), and apply an ice compress for 6–12 hr. Notify physician.

- Consult physician for premedication with antiemetics or sedatives to prevent severe nausea and vomiting. Giving at night may help alleviate the problem.
- Ensure that patient is well hydrated before treatment.
- Caution patient to avoid pregnancy while taking this drug; advise using barrier contraceptives.
- Monitor uric acid levels; ensure adequate fluid intake, and prepare for appropriate treatment if hyperuricemia occurs.

Teaching points

- This drug must be given IV or directly into a body cavity.
- Use birth control. This drug cannot be taken during pregnancy; serious fetal effects

---

Adverse effects in *italics* are most common; those in **bold** are life-threatening. ⏚ Do not crush.

can occur. If you think you are pregnant or wish to become pregnant, consult your health care provider.

- You may experience these side effects: Nausea, vomiting, loss of appetite (use antiemetic or sedative at night; maintain fluid intake and nutrition); weakness, dizziness, ringing in the ears or loss of hearing (use special precautions to avoid injury); infertility, from irregular menses to complete amenorrhea; men may stop producing sperm (may be irreversible).
- Report pain, burning at IV site, severe GI distress, sore throat, rash, joint pain, fever.

▷meclizine hydrochloride
(mek' li zeen)

Bonamine (CAN), Bonine
Oral prescription tablets:
Antivert, Antirizine, Dramamine Less Drowsy Formula, Vertin-32

PREGNANCY CATEGORY B

Drug classes
Anticholinergic
Antiemetic
Antihistamine
Anti–motion-sickness drug

Therapeutic actions
Reduces sensitivity of the labyrinthine apparatus; probably acts at least partly by blocking cholinergic synapses in the vomiting center, which receives input from the CTZ and from peripheral nerve pathways; peripheral anticholinergic effects may contribute to efficacy.

Indications
- Prevention and treatment of nausea, vomiting, motion sickness
- Possibly effective for the management of vertigo associated with diseases affecting the vestibular system

Contraindications and cautions
- Contraindicated with allergy to meclizine or cyclizine; tartrazine sensitivity (more common in patients with aspirin hypersensitivity).

- Use cautiously with lactation, narrow-angle glaucoma, stenosing peptic ulcer, symptomatic prostatic hypertrophy, bronchial asthma, bladder neck obstruction, pyloroduodenal obstruction, cardiac arrhythmias, postoperative state (hypotensive effects may be confusing and dangerous), pregnancy.

Available forms
Tablets—12.5, 25, 32, 50 mg; chewable tablets—25 mg; capsules—25 mg

Dosages
Adults and children older than 12 yr
- *Motion sickness:* 25–50 mg PO 1 hr before travel. May repeat dose every 24 hr for the duration of the journey.
- *Vertigo:* 25–100 mg PO daily in divided doses.

Pediatric patients
Not recommended for children younger than 12 yr.

Geriatric patients
More likely to cause dizziness, sedation, syncope, toxic confusional states, and hypotension in elderly patients; use with caution.

Pharmacokinetics

Route	Onset	Peak	Duration
Oral	1 hr	1–2 hr	4–24 hr

Metabolism: $T_{1/2}$: 6 hr
Distribution: Crosses placenta; may enter breast milk
Excretion: Feces

Adverse effects
- **CNS:** *Drowsiness, confusion,* euphoria, nervousness, restlessness, insomnia and excitement, seizures, vertigo, tinnitus, blurred vision, diplopia, auditory and visual hallucinations
- **CV:** Hypotension, palpitations, tachycardia
- **Dermatologic:** Urticaria, rash
- **GI:** *Dry mouth, anorexia, nausea,* vomiting, diarrhea or constipation
- **GU:** *Urinary frequency, difficult urination,* urine retention

- **Respiratory: Respiratory depression, death** (due to overdose, especially in young children), dry nose and throat

Interactions
* **Drug-drug** • Increased sedation with alcohol or other CNS depressants

■ Nursing considerations
Assessment
- **History:** Allergy to meclizine or cyclizine, pregnancy, narrow-angle glaucoma, stenosing peptic ulcer, symptomatic prostatic hypertrophy, bronchial asthma, bladder neck obstruction, pyloroduodenal obstruction, cardiac arrhythmias, postoperative patients, lactation, pregnancy
- **Physical:** Skin color, lesions, texture; orientation, reflexes, affect; ophthalmic examination; P, BP; R, adventitious sounds; bowel sounds, normal output, status of mucous membranes; prostate palpation, urinary output

Interventions
- Monitor I & O, and take appropriate measures with urine retention.

Teaching points
- Take as prescribed. Avoid excessive dosage. If you are using chewable tablets, chew them carefully before swallowing.
- Anti–motion-sickness drugs work best if used ahead of time for prevention.
- Avoid alcohol; serious sedation could occur.
- You may experience these side effects: Dizziness, sedation, drowsiness (use caution driving or performing tasks that require alertness); epigastric distress, diarrhea, or constipation (take with food); dry mouth (practice frequent mouth care, suck sugarless candies); dryness of nasal mucosa (try another motion-sickness or anti-vertigo remedy).
- Report difficulty breathing, hallucinations, tremors, loss of coordination, visual disturbances, irregular heartbeat.

DANGEROUS DRUG

▷ **medroxyPROGESTERone acetate**

(me drox' ee proe jess' te rone)

Oral: Apo-Medroxyprogesterone (CAN), Gen-Medroxy (CAN), Provera

Parenteral: Depo-Provera, depo-subQ provera 104

PREGNANCY CATEGORY X

Drug classes
Antineoplastic
Contraceptive
Hormone
Progestin

Therapeutic actions
Progesterone derivative; endogenous progesterone transforms proliferative endometrium into secretory endometrium; inhibits the secretion of pituitary gonadotropins, which prevents follicular maturation and ovulation; inhibits spontaneous uterine contraction.

Indications
- Reduction of endometrial hyperplasia in postmenopausal women
- Oral: Treatment of secondary amenorrhea
- Oral: Abnormal uterine bleeding due to hormonal imbalance in the absence of organic pathology
- Parenteral: Adjunctive therapy and palliation of inoperable, recurrent, and metastatic endometrial carcinoma or renal carcinoma; long acting contraceptive (*Depo-Provera*)
- Subcutaneous depot: Long-acting contraceptive; management of endometriosis-associated pain (*depo-subQ provera 104*)
- Unlabeled use for depot form: Treatment of breast cancer

Contraindications and cautions
- Contraindicated with allergy to progestins; thrombophlebitis, thromboembolic disorders, cerebral hemorrhage or history of these conditions; hepatic disease, carcinoma of the breast, ovaries, or endometrium, undiagnosed vaginal bleeding, missed abortion; pregnancy (fetal abnormalities, including masculinization of the female fetus have been reported); lactation.

Adverse effects in *italics* are most common; those in **bold** are life-threatening. ⬟ Do not crush.

- Use cautiously with epilepsy; migraine; asthma; cardiac or renal impairment.

Available forms
Tablets—2.5, 5, 10 mg; injection—150, 400 mg/mL; 104 mg/0.65 mL (depo-subQ)

Dosages
Adults
- *Contraception monotherapy:* 150 mg IM every 3 mo. For *depo-subQ Provera:* 104 mg subcutaneously into thigh or abdomen every 12–14 wk.
- *Secondary amenorrhea:* 5–10 mg/day PO for 5–10 days. A dose for inducing an optimum secretory transformation of an endometrium that has been primed with exogenous or endogenous estrogen is 10 mg/day for 10 days. Start therapy at any time; withdrawal bleeding usually occurs 3–7 days after therapy ends.
- *Abnormal uterine bleeding:* 5–10 mg/day PO for 5–10 days, beginning on the 16th or 21st day of the menstrual cycle. To produce an optimum secretory transformation of an endometrium that has been primed with estrogen, give 10 mg/day PO for 10 days, beginning on the 16th day of the cycle. Withdrawal bleeding usually occurs 3–7 days after discontinuing therapy. If bleeding is controlled, administer two subsequent cycles.
- *Endometrial or renal carcinoma:* 400–1,000 mg/wk IM. If improvement does not occur within a few weeks or months and the disease appears stabilized, it may be possible to maintain improvement with as little as 400 mg/mo IM.
- *Reduction of endometrial hyperplasia:* 5–10 mg/day PO for 12–14 consecutive days/mo. Start on 1st or 16th day of cycle.
- *Management of endometriosis-associated pain:* 104 mg subcutaneously (depo-subQ Provera) into anterior thigh or abdomen every 12–14 wk; do not use for longer than 2 yr.

Pharmacokinetics

Route	Onset	Peak
Oral	Slow	Unknown
IM	Weeks	Months

Metabolism: Hepatic; $T_{1/2}$: 50 days (IM)
Distribution: Crosses placenta; enters breast milk
Excretion: Unknown

Adverse effects
- **CNS:** Sudden, partial, or complete loss of vision; proptosis, diplopia, migraine, precipitation of acute intermittent porphyria, mental depression, pyrexia, insomnia, somnolence, nervousness, fatigue
- **CV:** Thrombophlebitis, cerebrovascular disorders, retinal thrombosis, pulmonary embolism, thromboembolic and thrombotic disease, increased BP
- **Dermatologic:** *Rash with or without pruritus, acne,* melasma or chloasma, alopecia, hirsutism, photosensitivity, pruritus, urticaria
- **GI:** Cholestatic jaundice, nausea
- **GU:** *Breakthrough bleeding, spotting, change in menstrual flow, amenorrhea,* changes in cervical erosion and cervical secretions, breast tenderness and secretion
- **Other:** *Fluid retention, edema, increase or decrease in weight,* decreased glucose tolerance; bone loss

Interactions
✳ **Drug-lab test** • Inaccurate tests of hepatic and endocrine function

■ Nursing considerations
Assessment
- **History:** Allergy to progestins; thrombophlebitis; thromboembolic disorders; cerebral hemorrhage; hepatic disease; carcinoma of the breasts, ovaries, or endometrium; undiagnosed vaginal bleeding; missed abortion; epilepsy; migraine; asthma; cardiac dysfunction; renal impairment; pregnancy; lactation
- **Physical:** Skin color, lesions, turgor; hair; breasts; pelvic examination; orientation, affect; ophthalmologic examination; P, auscultation, peripheral perfusion, edema; R, adventitious sounds; liver evaluation; LFTs, renal function tests, glucose tolerance, Papanicolaou (Pap) test

Interventions
- Arrange for pretreatment and periodic (at least annual) history and physical, which should include BP, breasts, abdomen, pelvic organs, and a Pap test.
- ⊗ **Black box warning** Before therapy begins, ensure that patient is not pregnant and caution patient to prevent pregnancy and to have frequent medical follow-up visits.

M

⊗ Black box warning Alert patients using contraceptive injections that drug does not protect them from HIV or other STDs; precautions should be used.

⊗ Warning Discontinue medication and consult physician if sudden, partial, or complete loss of vision occurs; if papilledema or retinal vascular lesions are present, discontinue drug.

⊗ Warning Discontinue medication and consult physician at the first sign of thromboembolic disease (leg pain, swelling, peripheral perfusion changes, shortness of breath).

Teaching points

- If you are taking the oral form of this drug, mark days you should take the medication on a calendar.
- If using the subcutaneous depot form of this drug, mark your calendar for days you should receive new injections. This drug does not protect you from HIV or other STDs; use precautions.
- This drug should not be taken during pregnancy due to risk of serious fetal abnormalities. If drug is used for indications other than contraception, using barrier contraceptives is suggested. If using the drug as a contraceptive, be aware of other medications that may decrease effectiveness and use other methods of contraception.
- You may experience these side effects: Sensitivity to light (avoid exposure to the sun; use sunscreen and protective clothing); dizziness, sleeplessness, depression (use caution driving or performing tasks that require alertness); rash, color changes, loss of hair; fever; nausea.
- Report pain or swelling and warmth in the calves, acute chest pain or shortness of breath, sudden severe headache or vomiting, dizziness or fainting, visual disturbances, numbness or tingling in the arm or leg.

> ▽ **mefenamic acid**
> *(me fe **nam'** ik)*
>
> Apo-Mefenamic (CAN), Ponstel
>
> PREGNANCY CATEGORY C

Drug class
NSAID

Therapeutic actions
Anti-inflammatory, analgesic, and antipyretic activities related to inhibition of prostaglandin synthesis; exact mechanisms of action are not known.

Indications
- Relief of moderate pain when therapy will not exceed 1 wk
- Treatment of primary dysmenorrhea
- ▪▀ **NEW INDICATION:** Unlabeled uses: Migraine, PMS

Contraindications and cautions
- Contraindicated with hypersensitivity to mefenamic acid, aspirin or NSAID allergy, and as treatment of perioperative pain with coronary artery bypass grafting.
- Use cautiously with asthma, renal or hepatic impairment, peptic ulcer disease, GI bleeding, hypertension, heart failure, pregnancy, lactation.

Available forms
Capsules—250 mg

Dosages
Adults and patients older than 14 yr
- *Acute pain:* Initially, 500 mg PO followed by 250 mg every 6 hr as needed. Do not exceed 1 wk of therapy.
- *Primary dysmenorrhea:* Initially, 500 mg PO then 250 mg every 6 hr starting with the onset of bleeding. Can be initiated at start of menses and should not be necessary for longer than 2–3 days.

Pediatric patients
Safety and efficacy for patients younger than 14 yr not established.

Geriatric patients
Use caution in treating patients 65 yr and older. Elderly patients are at greater risk for serious GI events.

Pharmacokinetics

Route	Onset	Peak	Duration
Oral	Varies	2–4 hr	6 hr

Metabolism: Hepatic; $T_{1/2}$: 2–4 hr
Distribution: Crosses placenta; enters breast milk
Excretion: Feces, urine

Adverse effects in *italics* are most common; those in **bold** are life-threatening. ⊗ Do not crush.

Adverse effects

- **CNS:** *Headache, dizziness,* somnolence, *insomnia,* fatigue, tiredness, dizziness, tinnitus, ophthalmic effects
- **CV: HF**, hypertension, tachycardia
- **Dermatologic:** *Rash,* pruritus, sweating, dry mucous membranes, stomatitis
- **GI:** *Nausea, dyspepsia, GI pain, diarrhea,* vomiting, *constipation,* flatulence, ulcers, GI bleed
- **GU:** Dysuria, **renal impairment**
- **Hematologic:** Bleeding, platelet inhibition with higher doses, neutropenia, eosinophilia, leukopenia, pancytopenia, thrombocytopenia, agranulocytosis, granulocytopenia, aplastic anemia, decreased Hgb or Hct, bone marrow depression, menorrhagia
- **Respiratory:** Dyspnea, hemoptysis, pharyngitis, bronchospasm, rhinitis
- **Other:** Peripheral edema, **anaphylactoid reactions** to **anaphylactic shock**

Interactions

＊ **Drug-drug** • Increased risk of GI bleeds with ASA, anticoagulants, other NSAIDs • Increased risk of methotrexate toxicity if combined with methotrexate; use caution

＊ **Drug-lab test** • False-positive reaction for urinary bile using the Diazo tablet test

■ Nursing considerations

Assessment

- **History:** Allergies; renal, hepatic, CV, GI conditions; pregnancy; lactation
- **Physical:** Skin color and lesions; orientation, reflexes, ophthalmologic and audiometric evaluation, peripheral sensation; P, edema; R, adventitious sounds; liver evaluation; CBC, clotting times, LFTs, renal function tests; serum electrolytes, stool guaiac

Interventions

⊗ **Black box warning** Be aware that patient may be at increased risk for CV events, GI bleeding; monitor accordingly.

⊗ **Black box warning** Do not use for the treatment of perioperative pain in the setting of coronary artery bypass graft surgery.

- Give with milk or food to decrease GI upset.
- Arrange for periodic ophthalmologic examinations during long-term therapy.

⊗ **Warning** If overdose occurs, institute emergency procedures—supportive therapy and induced emesis, activated charcoal, and/or an osmotic cathartic.

Teaching points

- Take drug with food; take only the prescribed dosage; do not take the drug longer than 1 week.
- Discontinue drug and consult your health care provider if rash, diarrhea, or digestive problems occur.
- Dizziness or drowsiness can occur (avoid driving and using dangerous machinery).
- Report sore throat, fever, rash, itching, weight gain, swelling in ankles or fingers; changes in vision; black, tarry stools; severe diarrhea, right upper abdominal pain, flulike symptoms, chest pain.

DANGEROUS DRUG

(as antineoplastic)

▽ **megestrol acetate**
(me jess' trole)

Apo-Megestrol (CAN), Megace, Megace ES, Megace OS (CAN)

PREGNANCY CATEGORY X
(ORAL SUSPENSION)

PREGNANCY CATEGORY D
(TABLETS)

Drug classes

Antineoplastic
Hormone
Progestin

Therapeutic actions

Inhibits secretion of pituitary gonadotropins with resulting decrease in estrogen secretion; exerts cytotoxic effects on tumor cells.

Indications

- Tablets: Palliation of advanced carcinoma of the breast or endometrium and as an adjunct to surgery or radiation
- Suspension: Appetite stimulant in HIV-related cachexia, anorexia or unexplained weight loss
- Unlabeled uses: Appetite stimulant for cachexia in advanced cancer; treatment for hot flashes

Contraindications and cautions

- Contraindicated with allergy to progestins; thrombophlebitis, thromboembolic disorders, cerebral hemorrhage or history of these conditions; hepatic disease, undiagnosed vaginal bleeding, missed abortion; pregnancy (masculinization of female fetus); lactation.
- Use cautiously with epilepsy, migraine, asthma, cardiac dysfunction, renal impairment.

Available forms

Tablets—20, 40 mg; suspension—40 mg/mL; extra strength suspension—125 mg/mL

Dosages

Adults

- *Breast cancer:* 160 mg/day PO (40 mg qid).
- *Endometrial cancer:* 40–320 mg/day PO in divided doses.
- *Cachexia with HIV:* Initially, 800 mg/day; normal range, 400–800 mg/day (suspension only) or 625 mg/day ES suspension.

Pharmacokinetics

Route	Onset	Peak
Oral	Slow	Weeks

Metabolism: Hepatic; $T_{1/2}$: 13–105 hr (tablets)
Distribution: Crosses placenta; enters breast milk
Excretion: Urine, feces

Adverse effects

- **CNS:** Paresthesia, confusion, seizures, depression, neuropathy, hypesthesia, abnormal thinking
- **CV:** Thrombophlebitis, cerebrovascular disorders, retinal thrombosis, **pulmonary embolism,** thromboembolic and thrombotic disease, increased BP
- **Dermatologic:** *Rash with or without pruritus, acne,* melasma or chloasma, alopecia, hirsutism, photosensitivity, pruritus, urticaria
- **GI:** Cholestatic jaundice, nausea
- **GU:** *Breakthrough bleeding, spotting, change in menstrual flow, amenorrhea,* changes in cervical erosion and cervical secretions, breast tenderness and secretion
- **Other:** *Fluid retention, edema, increase in weight,* decreased glucose tolerance

Interactions

✴ Drug-lab test • Inaccurate tests of hepatic and endocrine function

■ Nursing considerations

Assessment

- **History:** Allergy to progestins; thrombophlebitis, thromboembolic disorders, cerebral hemorrhage; hepatic disease; carcinoma of the breast or genital organs, undiagnosed vaginal bleeding, missed abortion; epilepsy, migraine, asthma, cardiac dysfunction, renal impairment; pregnancy; lactation
- **Physical:** Skin color, lesions, turgor; hair; breasts; pelvic examination; orientation, affect; ophthalmologic examination; P, auscultation, peripheral perfusion, edema; R, adventitious sounds; liver evaluation; LFTs, renal function tests, glucose tolerance, Papanicolaou (Pap) test

Interventions

⊗ **Warning** Discontinue drug and consult physician at signs of thromboembolic disease—leg pain, swelling, peripheral perfusion changes, shortness of breath.

⊗ **Black box warning** Caution patient to avoid using drug during pregnancy because of risks to the fetus; advise using barrier contraceptives.

- Shake suspension well before use; store in a tightly closed bottle in a cool place.

Teaching points

- If the suspension form is ordered, store in a cool place in a tightly closed bottle; shake well before each use. Take care to differentiate long-acting from regular suspension.
- This drug causes serious fetal abnormalities or fetal death; avoid pregnancy. Use of barrier contraceptives is advised.
- You may experience these side effects: Sensitivity to light (avoid exposure to the sun; use sunscreen and protective clothing); dizziness, sleeplessness, depression (use caution if driving or performing tasks that require alertness); skin rash, color changes, loss of hair; fever; nausea.
- Report pain or swelling and warmth in the calves, acute chest pain or shortness of breath, sudden severe headache or vomiting, dizziness or fainting, numbness or tingling in the arm or leg.

Adverse effects in *italics* are most common; those in **bold** are life-threatening. ⬤ Do not crush.

▽ meloxicam
(mel ox' i kam)

Apo-Meloxicam (CAN),
CO Meloxicam (CAN), Gen-
Meloxicam (CAN), Mobic,
Mobicox (CAN), Novo-Meloxicam (CAN),
PMS-Meloxicam (CAN),
ratio-Meloxicam (CAN)

PREGNANCY CATEGORY C
(FIRST AND SECOND TRIMESTERS)

PREGNANCY CATEGORY D
(THIRD TRIMESTER)

Drug class
NSAID (oxicam derivative)

Therapeutic actions
Anti-inflammatory, analgesic, and antipyretic activities related to inhibition of the enzyme cyclooxygenase (COX), which is required for the synthesis of prostaglandins and thromboxanes. Somewhat more selective for COX-2 sites (found in the brain, kidneys, ovaries, uterus, cartilage, bone, and at sites of inflammation) than for COX-1 sites, which are found throughout the tissues and are related to protection of the GI mucosa.

Indications
- Relief from the signs and symptoms of osteoarthritis and rheumatoid arthritis
- Relief from the signs and symptoms of pauciarticular or polyarticular course juvenile rheumatoid arthritis in patients 2 yr or older
- Unlabeled uses: Treatment of ankylosing spondylitis, acute shoulder pain

Contraindications and cautions
- Contraindicated with allergy to aspirin or meloxicam; for perioperative pain after coronary artery bypass surgery.
- Use cautiously with allergies; renal, hepatic, CV, GI conditions; bleeding disorders; pregnancy; lactation.

Available forms
Tablets—7.5, 15 mg; oral suspension—7.5 mg/5 mL

Dosages
Adults
Starting dose, 7.5 mg PO daily. Maximum dosage, 15 mg PO daily.
Pediatric patients
0.125 mg/kg PO once daily up to a maximum dose of 7.5 mg, using oral suspension.

Pharmacokinetics

Route	Onset	Peak
Oral	1 hr	5–6 hr

Metabolism: Hepatic; $T_{1/2}$: 15–20 hr
Distribution: Crosses placenta; enters breast milk
Excretion: Feces, urine

Adverse effects
- **CNS:** *Headache, dizziness,* somnolence, *insomnia,* fatigue, tiredness, tinnitus, ophthalmologic effects
- **Dermatologic:** *Rash,* pruritus, sweating, dry mucous membranes, stomatitis
- **GI:** *Nausea, dyspepsia, GI pain, diarrhea,* vomiting, constipation, flatulence
- **GU:** Dysuria, renal impairment
- **Hematologic:** Bleeding, platelet inhibition (with higher doses), neutropenia, eosinophilia, leukopenia, pancytopenia, thrombocytopenia, agranulocytosis, granulocytopenia, aplastic anemia, decreased Hgb or Hct, bone marrow depression, menorrhagia
- **Respiratory:** Dyspnea, hemoptysis, pharyngitis, bronchospasm, rhinitis
- **Other:** Peripheral edema, anaphylactoid reactions to **anaphylactic shock**

Interactions
✳ **Drug-drug** • Increased serum lithium levels and risk of toxicity if taken concurrently; monitor patient carefully • Possible increased risk of renal failure if combined with ACE inhibitors, diuretics • Increased risk of GI bleeding if combined with aspirin, anticoagulants, oral corticosteroids • Possible increased risk of methotrexate toxicity if combined with methotrexate

■ Nursing considerations
Assessment
- **History:** Allergies; renal, hepatic, CV, and GI bleeding; history of ulcers; pregnancy; lactation; bleeding disorders

- **Physical:** Skin color and lesions; orientation, reflexes, peripheral sensation; P, edema; R, adventitious sounds; liver evaluation; CBC, clotting times, LFTs, renal function tests; serum electrolytes, stool guaiac

Interventions

⊗ **Black box warning** Be aware that patient may be at increased risk for CV events, GI bleeding; monitor accordingly.

⊗ **Black box warning** Do not use for the treatment of perioperative pain in the setting of coronary artery bypass graft.

- Administer drug with food or milk if GI upset occurs.
- Establish safety measures if CNS disturbances occur.
- Monitor patient on prolonged therapy for signs of GI bleeding or hepatic toxicity.

⊗ **Warning** If overdose occurs, institute emergency procedures—gastric lavage followed by activated charcoal, supportive therapy.

- Provide further comfort measures to reduce pain (positioning, environmental control), and to reduce inflammation (warmth, positioning, rest).

Teaching points

- Take drug with food if GI upset occurs.
- Take only the prescribed dosage.
- You may experience these side effects: Dizziness, drowsiness (avoid driving or using dangerous machinery while taking this drug).
- Report sore throat, fever, rash, itching, weight gain, swelling in ankles or fingers, changes in vision; black, tarry stools.

DANGEROUS DRUG

▽ **melphalan (L-Pam, L-Phenylalanine Mustard, L-Sarcolysin)**

(mel' fa lan)

Alkeran

PREGNANCY CATEGORY D

Drug classes

Alkylating drug
Antineoplastic
Nitrogen mustard

Therapeutic actions

Cytotoxic: Alkylates cellular DNA, thus interfering with the replication of susceptible cells, causing cell death; cell-cycle nonspecific.

Indications

- Treatment of multiple myeloma, nonresectable epithelial ovarian carcinoma; use IV only when oral therapy is not possible
- Unlabeled uses: Breast cancer, testicular cancer, bone marrow transplantation

Contraindications and cautions

- Contraindicated with allergy to melphalan, lactation.
- Use cautiously with radiation therapy, chemotherapy, pregnancy (potentially mutagenic and teratogenic; avoid use in the first trimester).

Available forms

Tablets—2 mg; powder for injection—50 mg

Dosages

Individualize dosage based on hematologic profile and response.

Adults

Oral

- *Multiple myeloma:* 6 mg/day PO. After 2–3 wk, stop drug for up to 4 wk, and monitor blood counts. When blood counts are rising, institute maintenance dose of 2 mg/day PO. Response may occur gradually over many months (many alternative regimens, some including prednisone, are used).
- *Epithelial ovarian carcinoma:* 0.2 mg/kg/day PO for 5 days as a single course. Repeat courses every 4–5 wk, depending on hematologic response.

IV

- *Multiple myeloma:* 16 mg/m^2 administered as a single infusion over 15–20 min; administered at 2-wk intervals for 4 doses, then at 4-wk intervals.

Pediatric patients

Safety and efficacy not established.

Patients with renal impairment

Consider reducing initial oral dosage in patients with moderate to severe impairment; reduce IV dosage by 50% in patients with BUN of 30 mg/dL or more.

Pharmacokinetics

Route	Onset	Peak
Oral	Varies	2 hr
IV	Rapid	1 hr

Metabolism: $T_{1/2}$: 90 min (oral)
Distribution: Crosses placenta; enters breast milk
Excretion: Urine

▼ IV FACTS

Preparation: Reconstitute with 10 mL of supplied diluent, and shake vigorously until a clear solution is obtained; this provides 5 mg/mL solution. Immediately dilute in 0.9% sodium chloride injection to a dilution of less than 0.45 mg/mL. Complete infusion within 60 min of reconstitution. Protect from light. Dispense in glass containers. Do not refrigerate reconstituted solution.

Infusion: Administer dilute product over a minimum of 15 min; complete within 60 min of reconstitution.

Adverse effects

- **Dermatologic:** Maculopapular rash, urticaria, *alopecia*
- **GI:** *Nausea, vomiting,* oral ulceration, diarrhea
- **Hematologic: Bone marrow depression,** hyperuricemia
- **Respiratory:** Bronchopulmonary dysplasia, **pulmonary fibrosis**
- **Other:** *Amenorrhea,* cancer, acute leukemia, **anaphylaxis**

Interactions

✳ **Drug-lab test** ● Increased urinary 5-HIAA levels due to tumor cell destruction

■ Nursing considerations

Assessment

- **History:** Allergy to melphalan or chlorambucil, radiation therapy, chemotherapy, pregnancy, lactation
- **Physical:** T; weight; skin color, lesions; R, adventitious sounds; liver evaluation; CBC, differential, Hgb, renal function tests

Interventions

⊗ **Black box warning** Arrange for blood tests to evaluate hematopoietic function before therapy and weekly during therapy;

severe bone marrow suppression may occur.

⊗ **Warning** Do not give full dosage until 4 wk after a full course of radiation therapy or chemotherapy due to risk of severe bone marrow depression.

- Consider dosage reductions in patients with impaired renal function.
- Ensure that patient is well hydrated before treatment.

⊗ **Black box warning** Caution patient to avoid pregnancy while taking this drug; drug is considered to be mutagenic.

- Divide single daily dose if nausea and vomiting occur.

Teaching points

- Take drug once a day. If nausea and vomiting occur, consult with your health care provider about dividing the dose.
- Refrigerate tablets in glass bottle.
- This drug causes severe birth defects; use of barrier contraceptives is advised.
- You may experience these side effects: Nausea, vomiting, loss of appetite (divided dose, frequent small meals may help; maintain fluid intake and nutrition; drink at least 10–12 glasses of fluid each day); skin rash, loss of hair (obtain a wig if hair loss occurs; head should be covered at extremes of temperature).
- Report unusual bleeding or bruising, fever, chills, sore throat, cough, shortness of breath, black tarry stools, flank or stomach pain, joint pain.

▽ memantine hydrochloride

(meh *man' teen*)

Ebixa (CAN), Namenda, Namenda XR ⓞⓡⓒ

PREGNANCY CATEGORY B

Drug classes

Alzheimer disease drug
N-methyl-D-aspartate (NMDA) receptor antagonist

Therapeutic actions

Exerts a low to moderate affinity for NMDA receptor sites with no effects on GABA, dopamine, histamine, glycine, or adrenergic receptor sites; persistent activation of the CNS NMDA receptors by the excitatory amino acid glutamate has been suggested to contribute to the symptomatology of Alzheimer disease.

Indications
- Treatment of moderate to severe dementia of the Alzheimer type
- Unlabeled uses: Treatment of vascular dementia, treatment of ADHD, prevention of migraines, treatment of post-herpetic neuralgia

Contraindications and cautions
- Contraindicated with allergy to memantine or any component of the drug.
- Use cautiously with pregnancy, lactation, renal impairment.

Available forms
Tablets—5, 10 mg; ER capsules ⊞—7, 14, 21, 28 mg; oral solution—2 mg/mL

Dosages
Adults
Initially, 5 mg/day PO, increase at weekly intervals to 5 mg bid (10 mg/day), 15 mg/day (5 mg and 10 mg doses) with at least 1 week between increases; target dose is 20 mg/day (10 mg bid). Use solution-dosing device if solution is used. If using ER form: Initially 7 mg PO once a day; may be increased by 7 mg/day after at least 1 week. Maintenance dose is 28 mg PO once daily.
Pediatric patients
Safety and efficacy not established.
Patients with renal impairment
Consider dosage reduction and closely monitor the patient; avoid use with severe renal impairment. If using ER form, maximum dose of 14 mg once a day is recommended.

Pharmacokinetics

Route	Onset	Peak
Oral	Varies	3–7 hr

Metabolism: Hepatic metabolism; T$_{1/2}$: 60–80 hr
Distribution: May cross placenta; may enter breast milk
Excretion: Urine

Adverse effects
- **CNS:** Fatigue, *headache, dizziness, confusion,* somnolence, hallucinations, agitation, insomnia, anxiety
- **CV:** Hypertension, peripheral edema
- **GI:** Vomiting, diarrhea, *constipation*
- **GU:** UTI, urinary incontinence
- **Respiratory:** Cough, dyspnea, URI, bronchitis
- **Other:** Pain, back pain, arthralgia

Interactions
✳ **Drug-drug** • Increased effects and risk of toxicity of memantine if taken with drugs that alkalinize the urine, including carbonic anhydrase inhibitors, sodium bicarbonate; monitor patient closely and make dosage adjustments as needed • Potential for increased effects and toxicity if combined with amantadine, ketamine, or dextromethorphan; use caution if this combination is used

■ Nursing considerations
Assessment
- **History:** Allergy to memantine or component of the drug, pregnancy, lactation, renal impairment
- **Physical:** Orientation, affect, reflexes; BP; R, adventitious sounds, assessment of normal function

Interventions
- Establish baseline functional profile to follow evaluation of drug effectiveness.
- Administer without regard to food; may take with food if GI upset is a problem; switch to oral solution if swallowing is difficult. If using ER form, make sure patient swallows capsule whole; do not cut, crush, or allow patient to chew capsule. Capsule may be opened and contents sprinkled on applesauce and then swallowed.
- Provide patient safety measures if CNS effects occur.
- Establish bowel program if constipation becomes an issue.

Teaching points
- Take drug exactly as prescribed; take with food to decrease GI upset; learn to use the solution-dosing device rather than spoon to determine exact dose of solution. If using ER capsule, swallow capsule whole;

do not cut, crush, or chew capsule. If swallowing is difficult, you can open capsule and sprinkle contents on applesauce, then swallow.
- This drug does not cure the disease; it is not thought to prevent or slow the degeneration associated with the disease.
- Dosage changes will be needed and will be made on a weekly basis until the target dosage is reached.
- You may experience these side effects: Headache (an analgesic may be available); dizziness, fatigue, confusion (use caution if driving or performing tasks that require alertness); constipation (consult your health care provider for an appropriate bowel program).
- Report severe nausea, vomiting, severe headache, swelling of the legs, respiratory problems, lack of improvement in day-to-day functioning.

▷ menotropins
*(men oh **troe'** pins)*

Menopur, Repronex

PREGNANCY CATEGORY X

Drug classes
Fertility drug
Hormone

Therapeutic actions
A purified preparation of human gonadotropins; in women, produces ovarian follicular growth; when followed by administration HCG, produces ovulation; used with HCG for at least 3 mo to induce spermatogenesis in men with primary or secondary pituitary hypofunction who have previously achieved adequate masculinization with HCG administration.

Indications
- Women: Given with HCG sequentially to induce ovulation and pregnancy in anovulatory infertile patients without primary ovarian failure; used with HCG to stimulate multiple follicles for in vitro fertilization programs
- Unlabeled use: Treatment of male infertility caused by hypogonotropic hypogonadism

Contraindications and cautions
- Contraindicated with known sensitivity to menotropins; high gonadotropin levels, indicating primary ovarian failure; overt thyroid or adrenal dysfunction; abnormal bleeding of undetermined origin; ovarian cysts or enlargement not due to polycystic ovary syndrome; intracranial lesion, such as pituitary tumor; pregnancy (women); normal gonadotropin levels, indicating pituitary function; elevated gonadotropin levels, indicating primary testicular failure; infertility disorders other than hypogonadotropin hypogonadism (men).
- Use cautiously with lactation.

Available forms
Powder or pellet for injection—75 international units FSH/75 international units LH

Dosages
Women
To achieve ovulation, HCG must be given following menotropins when clinical assessment indicates sufficient follicular maturation as indicated by urinary excretion of estrogens.
Menopur, Repronex
225 units IM; then 75–150 units/day by subcutaneous injection up to a maximum of 450 units/day for no longer than 12 days (*Repronex*) or 20 days (*Menopur*). Base actual dose on follicular development.
Repronex
Patients who have received gonadotropin-releasing hormone agonists or pituitary suppression: Initially, 150 international units subcutaneously or IM daily for first 5 days; adjust dosage as needed after 2 or more days. Do not adjust by more than 150 international units per adjustment and do not exceed maximum daily dose of 450 international units. Do not use for longer than 12 days. If patient response is adequate, give HCG 5,000–10,000 units 1 day following last dose of menotropins.

Pharmacokinetics

Route	Onset	Peak	Duration
IM	Slow	Weeks	Months

Metabolism: $T_{1/2}$: 11–13 hr (*Menopur*), 53–59 hr (*Repronex*)
Distribution: Crosses placenta
Excretion: Urine

Adverse effects
Women
- **CNS:** Dizziness
- **CV:** Arterial thromboembolism, tachycardia
- **GI:** Nausea, vomiting, abdominal pain, bloating
- **GU:** *Ovarian enlargement,* hyperstimulation syndrome, hemoperitoneum
- **Hypersensitivity:** Hypersensitivity reactions
- **Other:** *Febrile reactions;* birth defects in resulting pregnancies, *multiple pregnancies*

■ Nursing considerations
Assessment
- **History:** Sensitivity to menotropins; high gonadotropin levels; overt thyroid or adrenal dysfunction, abnormal bleeding of undetermined origin, ovarian cysts or enlargement not due to polycystic ovary syndrome, intracranial lesion, pregnancy, lactation (women); normal gonadotropin levels; elevated gonadotropin levels; infertility disorders other than hypogonadotropin hypogonadism (men)
- **Physical:** Abdominal examination, pelvic examination; testicular examination; serum gonadotropin levels; 24-hr urinary estrogens and estriol excretion (women); T; masculinization, serum testosterone levels (men)

Interventions
- Dissolve contents of 1–6 vials in 1–2 mL of sterile saline. Administer subcutaneously immediately. *Repronex* may also be given IM. Discard any unused portion.
- Store ampules at room temperature or in refrigerator; do not freeze.
- Monitor women for any sign of ovarian enlargement at least every other day during treatment and for 2 wk after treatment.
- ⊗ **Warning** Discontinue drug at any sign of ovarian overstimulation, and arrange to have patient admitted to the hospital for observation and supportive measures. Do not attempt to remove ascitic fluid because of the risk of injury to the ovaries. Have the patient refrain from intercourse if ovarian enlargement occurs.
- Provide calendar of treatment days and explanations about what signs of estrogen and progesterone activity to watch for. Caution patient that 24-hr urine collections will be needed periodically, that HCG also must be given

to induce ovulation, and that daily intercourse should begin 1 day prior to HCG administration and until ovulation occurs.
- Alert patient to risks and hazards of multiple births.

Teaching points
- Prepare a calendar showing the treatment schedule; drug can only be given intramuscularly and must be used with human chorionic gonadotropin (HCG) to achieve the desired effects. If you are administering the drug yourself, dispose of needles and syringes properly.
- Know that there is a risk of multiple pregnancy when using this drug.
- Have intercourse daily beginning on the day prior to HCG therapy until ovulation occurs.
- Report pain at injection site, severe abdominal or lower back pain, fever, fluid in the abdomen.

DANGEROUS DRUG

▷meperidine hydrochloride (pethidine)
(me per' i deen)

Demerol

PREGNANCY CATEGORY B

PREGNANCY CATEGORY D (PROLONGED USE)

CONTROLLED SUBSTANCE C-II

Drug class
Opioid agonist analgesic

Therapeutic actions
Acts as agonist at specific opioid receptors in the CNS to produce analgesia, euphoria, sedation; the receptors mediating these effects are thought to be the same as those mediating the effects of endogenous opioids (enkephalins, endorphins).

Indications
- Oral, parenteral: Relief of moderate to severe acute pain
- Parenteral: Preoperative medication, support of anesthesia, and obstetric analgesia

Contraindications and cautions

- Contraindicated with hypersensitivity to opioids, diarrhea caused by poisoning (before toxins are eliminated), bronchial asthma, COPD, cor pulmonale, respiratory depression, anoxia, kyphoscoliosis, acute alcoholism, increased intracranial pressure, pregnancy, seizure disorder, renal impairment. Contraindicated in premature infants.
- Use cautiously with acute abdominal conditions, CV disease, supraventricular tachycardias, myxedema, delirium tremens, cerebral arteriosclerosis, ulcerative colitis, fever, Addison disease, prostatic hypertrophy, urethral stricture, recent GI or GU surgery, toxic psychosis, labor or delivery (opioids given to the mother can cause respiratory depression of neonate; premature infants are especially at risk), renal or hepatic impairment, lactation.

Available forms

Tablets—50, 100 mg; syrup—50 mg/5 mL; injection—10, 25, 50, 75, 100 mg/mL; oral solution—50 mg/5 mL

Dosages

Adults

- Relief of pain: Individualize dosage; 50–150 mg IM, subcutaneously, or PO every 3–4 hr as needed. Diluted solution may be given by slow IV injection. IM route is preferred for repeated injections.
- Preoperative medication: 50–100 mg IM or subcutaneously, 30–90 min before beginning anesthesia.
- Support of anesthesia: Dilute to 10 mg/mL, and give repeated doses by slow IV injection, or dilute to 1 mg/mL and infuse continuously. Individualize dosage.
- Obstetric analgesia: When contractions become regular, 50–100 mg IM or subcutaneously; repeat every 1–3 hr.

Pediatric patients

Contraindicated in premature infants.

- Relief of pain: 1.1–1.75 mg/kg IM, subcutaneously, or PO up to adult dose every 3–4 hr as needed.
- Preoperative medication: 1.1–2.2 mg/kg IM or subcutaneously, up to adult dose, 30–90 min before beginning anesthesia.

Geriatric or debilitated patients

Use caution; respiratory depression may occur in elderly, the very ill, and those with respiratory problems. Reduced dosage may be needed.

Patients with renal impairment

Reduce dose with severe renal impairment: for creatinine clearance of 10–50 mL/min, give 75% of normal dose; for creatinine clearance of less than 10 mL/min, give 25%–50% of normal dose. Not recommended for patients on dialysis.

Patients with hepatic impairment

Give with caution; reduce initial dose for patients with severe impairment.

Pharmacokinetics

Route	Onset	Peak	Duration
Oral	15 min	60–90 min	2–4 hr
IM, Subcut.	10–15 min	3–50 min	2–4 hr
IV	Immediate	5–7 min	2–4 hr

Metabolism: Hepatic; $T_{1/2}$: 3–4 hr
Distribution: Crosses placenta; enters breast milk
Excretion: Urine

▼ IV FACTS

Preparation: Dilute parenteral solution prior to IV injection using 5% dextrose and lactated Ringer dextrose-saline combinations; 2.5%, 5%, or 10% dextrose in water, Ringer or lactated Ringer 0.45% or 0.9% sodium chloride; 1/6M sodium lactate.

Infusion: Administer by slow IV injection over 4–5 min or by continuous infusion when diluted to 1 mg/mL.

Incompatibilities: ⊗ Warning Do not mix meperidine solutions with solutions of barbiturates, aminophylline, heparin, morphine sulfate, methicillin, phenytoin, sodium bicarbonate, iodide, sulfadiazine, sulfisoxazole.

Y-site incompatibilities: Do not give with other drugs.

Adverse effects

- **CNS:** Light-headedness, dizziness, sedation, euphoria, dysphoria, delirium, insomnia, agitation, anxiety, fear, hallucinations, disorientation, drowsiness, lethargy, impaired mental and physical performance, coma, mood changes, weakness, headache, tremor, seizures, miosis, visual disturbances, suppression of cough reflex
- **CV:** Facial flushing, peripheral circulatory collapse, tachycardia, bradycardia,

arrhythmia, palpitations, chest wall rigidity, hypertension, hypotension, orthostatic hypotension, syncope
- **Dermatologic:** Pruritus, urticaria, laryngospasm, bronchospasm, edema
- **GI:** *Nausea, vomiting,* dry mouth, anorexia, *constipation,* biliary tract spasm, increased colonic motility in patients with chronic ulcerative colitis
- **GU:** Ureteral spasm, spasm of vesical sphincters, urine retention or hesitancy, oliguria, antidiuretic effect, reduced libido or potency
- **Local:** Tissue irritation and induration (subcutaneous injection)
- **Major hazards: Respiratory depression, apnea, circulatory depression, respiratory arrest, shock, cardiac arrest**
- **Other:** *Sweating,* physical tolerance and dependence, psychological dependence

Interactions

✳ Drug-drug ⊗ *Warning* Severe and sometimes fatal reactions (resembling opioid overdose; characterized by seizures, hypertension, hyperpyrexia) when given to patients receiving or who have recently received MAOIs; do not give meperidine to patients on MAOIs • Potentiation of effects with barbiturate anesthetics; decrease dose of meperidine when coadministering • Increased likelihood of respiratory depression, hypotension, profound sedation, or coma with phenothiazines

✳ Drug-lab test • Elevated biliary tract pressure may cause increases in plasma amylase, lipase; determinations of these levels may be unreliable for 24 hr after administration of opioids

■ Nursing considerations
Assessment

- **History:** Hypersensitivity to opioids, diarrhea caused by poisoning, bronchial asthma, COPD, cor pulmonale, respiratory depression, anoxia, kyphoscoliosis, acute alcoholism, increased intracranial pressure, acute abdominal conditions, CV disease, supraventricular tachycardias, myxedema, seizure disorders, delirium tremens, cerebral arteriosclerosis, ulcerative colitis, fever, Addison disease, prostatic hypertrophy, urethral stricture, recent GI or GU surgery, toxic psychosis, renal or hepatic impairment, pregnancy, lactation

- **Physical:** T; skin color, texture, lesions; orientation, reflexes, bilateral grip strength, affect, pupil size; P, auscultation, BP, orthostatic BP, perfusion; R, adventitious sounds; bowel sounds, normal output; frequency and pattern of voiding, normal output; ECG; EEG; LFTs, renal and thyroid function tests

Interventions

- Administer to lactating women 4–6 hr before the next feeding to minimize the amount in milk.
- ⊗ *Warning* Keep opioid antagonist and facilities for assisted or controlled respiration readily available during parenteral administration.
- ⊗ *Warning* Use caution when injecting subcutaneously into chilled areas of the body or in patients with hypotension or in shock; impaired perfusion may delay absorption; with repeated doses, an excessive amount may be absorbed when circulation is restored.
- Reduce dosage of meperidine by 25%–50% in patients receiving phenothiazines or other tranquilizers.
- Give each dose of the oral syrup in half a glass of water. If taken undiluted, it may exert a slight local anesthetic effect on mucous membranes.
- Reassure patient that addiction is unlikely; most patients who receive opiates for medical reasons do not develop dependence syndromes.
- ⊗ *Warning* Use meperidine with extreme caution in patients with renal impairment or those requiring repeated dosing due to accumulation of normeperidine, a toxic metabolite that may cause seizures.

Teaching points

- Take drug exactly as prescribed.
- Avoid alcohol, antihistamines, sedatives, tranquilizers, and over-the-counter drugs.
- Do not take leftover medication for other disorders, and do not let anyone else take this prescription.
- You may experience these side effects: Nausea, loss of appetite (take with food and lie quietly, eat frequent small meals); constipation (request a laxative); dizziness, sedation, drowsiness, impaired visual acuity (avoid driving, performing other tasks that require alertness or visual acuity).
- Report severe nausea, vomiting, constipation, shortness of breath, or difficulty breathing.

▽ meprobamate
(me proe ba' mate)

Novo-Mepro (CAN)

PREGNANCY CATEGORY D

CONTROLLED SUBSTANCE C-IV

Drug class
Anxiolytic

Therapeutic actions
Has effects at many sites in the CNS, including the thalamus and limbic system; inhibits multineuronal spinal reflexes; is mildly tranquilizing; has some antiepileptic and central skeletal muscle relaxing properties.

Indications
• Management of anxiety disorders for the short-term relief of the symptoms of anxiety (anxiety or tension associated with the stress of everyday life usually does not require treatment with anxiolytic drugs); effectiveness for longer than 4 mo not established.

Contraindications and cautions
• Contraindicated with hypersensitivity to meprobamate or to related drugs, such as carisoprodol; acute intermittent porphyria; hepatic or renal impairment; pregnancy; lactation.
• Use cautiously with epilepsy (drug may precipitate seizures).

Available forms
Tablets—200, 400 mg

Dosages
Adults
1,200–1,600 mg/day PO in three or four divided doses. Do not exceed 2,400 mg/day.
Pediatric patients 6–12 yr
100–200 mg PO bid–tid.
Pediatric patients younger than 6 yr
Safety and efficacy not established.
Geriatric patients
Use lowest effective dose to avoid oversedation.

Pharmacokinetics

Route	Onset	Peak
Oral	Varies	1–3 hr

Metabolism: Hepatic; $T_{1/2}$: 6–14 hr
Distribution: Crosses placenta; enters breast milk
Excretion: Urine

Adverse effects
• **CNS:** *Drowsiness, ataxia, dizziness, headache, slurred speech, vertigo, weakness, impairment of visual accommodation,* euphoria, overstimulation, paradoxic excitement, paresthesias
• **CV:** *Palpitations, tachycardia,* various arrhythmias, syncope, **hypotensive crisis**
• **GI:** *Nausea, vomiting, diarrhea*
• **Hematologic:** Agranulocytosis, aplastic anemia; thrombocytopenic purpura; exacerbation of porphyric symptoms
• **Hypersensitivity:** Allergic or idiosyncratic reactions (usually seen between first and fourth doses in patients without previous drug exposure): *Itchy, urticarial or erythematous maculopapular rash;* leukopenia, acute nonthrombocytopenic purpura, petechiae, ecchymoses, eosinophilia, peripheral edema, adenopathy, fever, fixed drug eruption; hyperpyrexia, chills, angioneurotic edema, bronchospasm, oliguria, anuria, anaphylaxis, erythema multiforme, exfoliative dermatitis, stomatitis, proctitis; **Stevens-Johnson syndrome,** bullous dermatitis
• **Other:** Physical, psychological dependence; withdrawal reaction

Interactions
✳ **Drug-drug** • Additive CNS depression with alcohol, opioids, barbiturates, and other CNS depressants

■ Nursing considerations
Assessment
• **History:** Hypersensitivity to meprobamate or to related drugs; acute intermittent porphyria; hepatic or renal impairment; epilepsy; pregnancy; lactation
• **Physical:** T; skin color, lesions; orientation, affect, reflexes, vision examination; P, BP; R, adventitious sounds; bowel sounds, normal output, liver evaluation; LFTs, renal function tests, CBC and differential, EEG and ECG

Interventions

- Supervise dose and amount for patients who are addiction-prone or alcoholic.
- ⊗ **Warning** Dispense least amount of drug feasible to patients who are depressed or suicidal.
- Withdraw gradually over 2 wk if patient has been maintained on high doses for weeks or months.
- Withdraw drug if allergic or idiosyncratic reactions occur.
- Caution patient about the need to avoid pregnancy while taking this drug.
- ⊗ **Warning** Keep epinephrine, antihistamines, corticosteroids, and life-support equipment readily available in case allergic or idiosyncratic reaction occurs.

Teaching points

- Take this drug exactly as prescribed. This drug may not be effective after several months of therapy; continue to see your health care provider.
- Avoid alcohol, sleep-inducing, or over-the-counter drugs; these could cause dangerous effects.
- Use barrier method of birth control while taking this drug; do not take this drug during pregnancy. Consult your health care provider immediately if you decide to become pregnant or find that you are pregnant.
- You may experience these side effects: Drowsiness, dizziness, light-headedness, blurred vision (avoid driving or performing other tasks requiring alertness or visual acuity); GI upset (eat frequent small meals).
- Report rash, sore throat, fever, easy bruising, bleeding, thoughts of suicide.

DANGEROUS DRUG

▷**mercaptopurine (6-mercaptopurine, 6-MP)**

(mer kap toe pyoor' een)

Purinethol

PREGNANCY CATEGORY D

Drug classes

Antimetabolite
Antineoplastic

Therapeutic actions

Tumor-inhibiting properties, probably due to interference with purine nucleotide synthesis and hence with RNA and DNA synthesis, leading to cell death; cell-cycle specific.

Indications

- Maintenance therapy of acute lymphatic leukemia (lymphocytic, lymphoblastic) as part of combination therapy
- ◢ **NEW INDICATION:** Unlabeled uses: Non-Hodgkin lymphoma, Crohn disease, ulcerative colitis

Contraindications and cautions

- Contraindicated with allergy to mercaptopurine, prior resistance to mercaptopurine (cross-resistance with thioguanine is frequent), hematopoietic depression, pregnancy, lactation.
- Use cautiously with impaired renal function (slower elimination and greater accumulation; reduce dosage).

Available forms

Tablets—50 mg

Dosages
Adults

- *Induction therapy:* Usual initial dose is 2.5 mg/kg/day PO (about 100–200 mg in adults, 50 mg in the average 5-yr-old child). Continue daily for several wk. After 4 wk, if no clinical improvement or toxicity, increase to 5 mg/kg/day.
- *Maintenance therapy after complete hematologic remission:* 1.5–2.5 mg/kg/day PO as a single daily dose.

Pediatric patients

- *Induction therapy:* 2.5 mg/kg/day PO or 70–100 mg/m^2/day PO; titrate up to 5 mg/kg/day PO or 75 mg m^2/day PO.
- *Maintenance therapy after complete hematologic remission:* 1.5–2.5 mg/kg/day PO as a single daily dose.

Patients with renal impairment

Reduce dosage and monitor patient closely. For creatinine clearance less than 50 mL/min, administer every 48 hr.

Pharmacokinetics

Route	Onset	Peak
Oral	Varies	2 hr

Adverse effects in *italics* are most common; those in **bold** are life-threatening. ⬛ Do not crush.

Metabolism: Hepatic; $T_{1/2}$: 47 min (adults)
Distribution: Crosses placenta; may enter breast milk
Excretion: Urine

Adverse effects

- **GI:** Hepatotoxicity; oral lesions (resembling thrush); nausea; vomiting; anorexia, pancreatitis
- **Hematologic: *Bone marrow depression, immunosuppression, hyperuricemia*** as consequence of antineoplastic effect and cell lysis
- **Other:** Drug fever, **cancer,** chromosomal aberrations, rash, hyperpigmentation **hepatosplenic T-cell lymphoma**

Interactions

✳ Drug-drug ⊗ *Warning* Increased risk of severe toxicity with allopurinol, tumor necrosis factor blockers; reduce mercaptopurine to one-third to one-fourth the usual dose

■ Nursing considerations

CLINICAL ALERT!
Name confusion has occurred between *Purinethol* (mercaptopurine) and propylthiouracil; use extreme caution.

Assessment

- **History:** Allergy to mercaptopurine; prior resistance to mercaptopurine; hematopoietic depression; impaired renal function; pregnancy; lactation
- **Physical:** T; mucous membranes, liver evaluation; abdominal examination; CBC, differential, Hgb, platelet counts; LFTs, renal function tests; urinalysis; serum uric acid

Interventions

⊗ **Black box warning** Reserve use for patients with established diagnosis of acute lymphatic leukemia; serious adverse effects can occur.

- Evaluate hematopoietic status before and frequently during therapy.
- Round dose to nearest 25 mg (tablets are scored).
- Ensure that patient is well hydrated before and during therapy to minimize adverse effects of hyperuricemia.
- Caution patient about the risk of serious fetal harm while taking this drug; advise patient to use barrier contraceptives.

- Discuss increased risk of hepatosplenic T-cell lymphoma with patient. Caution patient to report signs or symptoms of this cancer (night sweats, persistent fever, abdominal pain, hepatomegaly, splenomegaly).
- Administer as a single daily dose.

Teaching points

- Drink adequate fluids; drink at least 8–10 glasses of fluid each day.
- Have frequent, regular medical follow-up visits, including blood tests to follow the drug effects.
- This drug is not for use during pregnancy; use of contraceptives is advised.
- If you are breast-feeding, you should use another method of feeding the infant; serious reactions can occur in the infant.
- You may experience these side effects: Mouth sores (practice frequent mouth care); miscarriages (use barrier contraceptives); nausea, vomiting.
- Report fever, chills, sore throat, unusual bleeding or bruising, yellow discoloration of the skin or eyes, abdominal pain, flank pain, joint pain, fever, weakness, diarrhea, night sweats, weight loss.

▽ **meropenem**
*(mare oh **pen**' ehm)*

Merrem IV

PREGNANCY CATEGORY B

Drug class

Antibiotic (carbapenem)

Therapeutic actions

Bactericidal: Inhibits synthesis of bacterial cell wall and causes cell death in susceptible cells.

Indications

- Susceptible intra-abdominal infections caused by viridans group streptococci, *Escherichia coli, Klebsiella pneumoniae, Pseudomonas aeruginosa, Bacteroides fragilis, Bacteroides thetaiotaomicron,* and *Peptostreptococcus*
- Bacterial meningitis caused by *Streptococcus pneumoniae, Haemophilus influenzae, Neisseria meningitidis* in pediatric patients 3 mo and older

M

- Treatment of complicated skin and skin structure infections due to *Staphylococcus aureus* (beta-lactamase and non–beta-lactamase–producing methicillin-susceptible isolates only), *Streptococcus pyogenes, Streptococcus agalactiae,* viridans group streptococci, *Enterococcus faecalis* (excluding vancomycin-resistant isolates), *Pseudomonas aeruginosa, E. coli, Proteus mirabilis, Bacteroides fragilis, Peptostreptococcus* species
- Unlabeled uses: Community-acquired pneumonia, therapy for patients with febrile neutropenia, nosocomial pneumonia, catheter-related bloodstream infections

Contraindications and cautions
- Contraindicated with allergy to cephalosporins, penicillins, beta-lactams; lactation.
- Use cautiously with CNS disorders, seizures, renal or hepatic impairment, pregnancy.

Available forms
Powder for injection—500 mg, 1 g

Dosages
Adults
- *Meningitis, intra-abdominal infections:* 1 g IV every 8 hr.
- *Skin and skin structure infections:* 500 mg IV every 8 hr.
Pediatric patients 3 mo and older
- *Intra-abdominal infections:* If less than 50 kg, 20 mg/kg IV every 8 hr. If more than 50 kg, 1 g IV every 8 hr.
- *Meningitis:* If less than 50 kg, 40 mg/kg IV every 8 hr; if more than 50 kg, 2 g IV every 8 hr.
- *Skin and skin structure infections:* If less than 50 kg, 10 mg/kg IV every 8 hr; if more than 50 kg, 500 mg IV every 8 hr.
Pediatric patients younger than 3 mo
Not recommended.
Patients with impaired renal function

CrCl (mL/min)	Dose (meningitis, intra-abdominal infections)	Dose (skin, skin structure infections)
26–50	1 g IV every 12 hr	500 mg IV every 12 hr
10–25	500 mg IV every 12 hr	250 mg IV every 12 hr
Less than 10	500 mg IV every 24 hr	250 mg IV every 24 hr

Pharmacokinetics

Route	Onset	Peak	Duration
IV	Immediate	5 min	10–12 min

Metabolism: T$_{1/2}$: 1 hr
Distribution: Unknown whether crosses placenta; may enter breast milk
Excretion: Urine, unchanged

▼ IV FACTS

Preparation: Dilute in 0.9% sodium chloride injection; 5% or 10% dextrose injection; dextrose in sodium chloride, potassium chloride, sodium bicarbonate, Normosol-M, Ringer lactate; 2.5% mannitol injection; Ringer injection; Ringer lactate injection; sodium lactate injection 1/6N; sodium bicarbonate. Store at room temperature or 39° F (4° C); stability in each solution varies—consult manufacturer's instructions if not used immediately.
Infusion: Infuse over 15–30 min or give by direct IV injection over 3–5 min.
Incompatibilities: Do not mix in solution with other drugs.

Adverse effects
- **CNS:** *Headache,* dizziness, lethargy, paresthesias, **seizures,** insomnia
- **GI:** *Nausea, vomiting, diarrhea, anorexia, abdominal pain, flatulence,* **pseudomembranous colitis,** liver toxicity
- **Other:** *Superinfections,* abscess (redness, tenderness, heat, tissue sloughing), inflammation at injection site, *phlebitis, rash,* urticaria, pruritus

Interactions
✳ **Drug-drug** • Possible toxic levels if combined with probenecid; avoid this combination. Increased risk of seizures if taken with valproic acid; if this combination is used, monitor patient very closely (valproic acid levels may decrease 45%–95%)

■ Nursing considerations
Assessment
- **History:** Allergy to cephalosporins, penicillins, beta lactams; renal failure; CNS disorders, seizures, renal or hepatic impairment; pregnancy, lactation
- **Physical:** Orientation, affect; skin color, lesions; culture site of infection; R, adventitious sounds; bowel sounds, abdominal examination; LFTs, renal function tests

Interventions

- Culture infected area and arrange for sensitivity tests before beginning therapy.
- Monitor for superinfections and arrange treatment as appropriate.

⊗ **Warning** Discontinue drug at any sign of colitis and arrange for appropriate supportive treatment.

Teaching points

- This drug can only be given IV.
- You may experience these side effects: Stomach upset, loss of appetite, nausea (take drug with food); diarrhea (stay near bathroom); headache, dizziness.
- Report severe diarrhea, difficulty breathing, unusual tiredness, pain at injection site.

▽**mesalamine**
(5-aminosalicylic acid,
5-ASA)

(me sal' a meen)

Apriso, Asacol ⓒ, Asacol HD,
CANASA, Lialda ⓒ, Mesasal (CAN),
Pentasa ⓒ, Rowasa, Salofalk (CAN)

PREGNANCY CATEGORY B

Drug class
Anti-inflammatory

Therapeutic actions
Mechanism of action is unknown; thought to be a direct, local anti-inflammatory effect in the colon where mesalamine blocks cyclooxygenase and inhibits prostaglandin production in the colon.

Indications

- Oral: Remission, treatment and maintenance treatment, and induction of remission with one daily dose, of active mild to moderate ulcerative colitis
- Suppository: Treatment of active, distal, mild to moderate ulcerative colitis, ulcerative proctitis, or proctosigmoiditis

Contraindications and cautions

- Contraindicated with hypersensitivity to mesalamine, salicylates, any component of the formulation.
- Use cautiously with renal impairment, pregnancy, lactation.

Available forms
DR tablets ⓒ—400, 800 (*Asacol HD*) mg, 1.2 g; CR capsules ⓒ—250, 500 mg; ER capsules ⓒ—375 mg; suppositories—1 g; rectal suspension—4 g/60 mL

Dosages
Adults
Rectal

- *Suspension enema:* 60 mL units in one rectal instillation (4 g) once a day, preferably at bedtime, and retained for approximately 8 hr. Usual course of therapy is 3–6 wk. Effects may be seen within 3–21 days.
- *Rectal suppository:* 1 g (1 suppository) bid. Retain suppository for 1–3 hr or longer. Usual course is 3–6 wk.

Oral

- *DR tablets:* 2–4 1.2 g tablets PO once daily with food for total dose of 2.4–4.8 g. Treatment beyond 8 wk has not been studied (*Lialda*).
- *ER capsules:* 1.5 g/day PO (4 capsules) in the morning (*Apriso*). Treatment for up to 6 mo.
- *CR capsules:* 1 g PO qid for a total daily dose of 4 g for up to 8 wk (*Pentasa*).
- *DR tablets:* 1.6 g/day PO in divided doses (*Asacol*) or 800 mg PO tid for 6 wk (*Asacol HD*).

Pediatric patients
Safety and efficacy not established.

Pharmacokinetics

Route	Onset	Peak
Oral	Varies	3–6 hr
Rectal	Slow	3–6 hr

Metabolism: $T_{1/2}$: 5–10 hr
Distribution: Crosses placenta; may enter breast milk
Excretion: Feces

Adverse effects

- **CNS:** *Headache, fatigue, malaise,* dizziness, asthenia, insomnia
- **GI:** *Abdominal pain, cramps, discomfort; gas; flatulence; nausea;* diarrhea, bloating, hemorrhoids, rectal pain, constipation
- **GU:** Urinary urgency, dysmenorrhea
- **Other:** *Flulike symptoms, fever, cold,* rash, back pain, hair loss, peripheral edema, pruritus

M

■ Nursing considerations

⭐ CLINICAL ALERT!

Name confusion has occurred between mesalamine and methenamine and memantine; use caution.

Assessment

- **History:** Hypersensitivity to mesalamine, salicylates, any component of the formulation; renal impairment; lactation, pregnancy
- **Physical:** T, hair status; reflexes; affect; abdominal examination, rectal examination; urinary output; renal function tests

Interventions

- Administer enemas as follows: Shake bottle well to ensure suspension is homogeneous. Remove protective applicator sheath; hold bottle at the neck to ensure that none of the dose is lost. Have patient lie on the left side (to facilitate migration of drug into the sigmoid colon) with the lower leg extended and the upper leg flexed forward. Knee-chest position can be used if more acceptable to the patient. Gently insert the application tip into the rectum pointing toward the umbilicus; steadily squeeze the bottle to discharge the medication. Patient must retain medication for approximately 8 hr.
- ⊗ **Warning** Be aware the *Asacol HD* 800-mg tablets are not bioequivalent to two *Asacol* 400-mg tablets. Check drug name carefully before administering.
- Administer rectal suppository as follows: Remove the foil wrapper; avoid excessive handling (suppository will melt at body temperature); insert completely into the rectum with pointed end first; have patient retain for 1–3 hr or longer.
- Caution patient not to chew tablet or capsule; swallow whole. Notify physician if intact tablets are found in the stool.
- Monitor patients with renal impairment for possible side effects.

Teaching points

- This drug may be given as a suspension enema, so the medication must be retained for approximately 8 hours; it is best given at bedtime to facilitate the retention; the effects of the drug are usually seen within 3–21 days, but a full course of therapy is about 6 weeks. (Review administration with patient and significant other.)
- Administer rectal suppository as follows: Remove the foil wrapper; avoid excessive handling (suppository will melt at body temperature); insert completely into the rectum with pointed end first; retain for 3 hours or longer; staining of clothing may occur, using a protective pad is suggested.
- Do not chew oral tablets or capsules; swallow whole. If intact tablets are seen in the stool, notify your health care provider.
- You may experience these side effects: Abdominal cramping, discomfort, pain, gas (relax; maintain the position used for insertion to relieve pressure on the abdomen); headache, fatigue, fever, flulike symptoms (request medication); hair loss (usually mild and transient).
- Report difficulty breathing, rash, severe abdominal pain, fever, headache.

▽ mesna

See Appendix R, *Less commonly used drugs*.

▽ metaproterenol sulfate

(met a proe ter' e nole)

PREGNANCY CATEGORY C

Drug classes

Antiasthmatic
Beta$_2$-selective adrenergic agonist
Bronchodilator
Sympathomimetic

Therapeutic actions

In low doses, acts relatively selectively at beta$_2$-adrenergic receptors to cause bronchodilation; at higher doses, beta$_2$ selectivity is lost and the drug also acts at beta$_1$ receptors to cause typical sympathomimetic cardiac effects.

Indications

- Prophylaxis and treatment of bronchial asthma and reversible bronchospasm that may occur with bronchitis and emphysema

Contraindications and cautions

- Contraindicated with hypersensitivity to metaproterenol; tachyarrhythmias; tachycardia caused by digitalis intoxication.
- Use cautiously with unstable vasomotor system disorders; hypertension; CAD; **history of stroke;** COPD in patients who have developed degenerative heart disease; hyperthyroidism; history of seizure disorders; psychoneurotic individuals; pregnancy; labor and delivery (may inhibit labor; parenteral use of beta$_2$-adrenergic agonists can accelerate fetal heartbeat, cause hypoglycemia, hypokalemia, and pulmonary edema in the mother and hypoglycemia in the neonate); lactation.

Available forms

Tablets—10, 20 mg; syrup—10 mg/5 mL

Dosages

Adults and children 12 yr and older
Oral
20 mg PO three to four times a day.
Pediatric patients
Oral
Younger than 6 yr: Not recommended.
6–9 yr or weight less than 27 kg: 10 mg PO three to four times a day.
Older than 9 yr or weight more than 27 kg: 20 mg PO three to four times a day.
Geriatric patients
Patients older than 60 yr are more likely to develop side effects; use extreme caution.

Pharmacokinetics

Route	Onset	Peak	Duration
Oral	1 hr	2–3 hr	3–6 hr

Metabolism: Liver and tissue; T$_{1/2}$: Unknown
Excretion: Feces

Adverse effects

- **CNS:** *Restlessness, apprehension, anxiety, fear, CNS stimulation,* hyperkinesia, insomnia, tremor, drowsiness, irritability, weakness, vertigo, headache
- **CV:** Cardiac arrhythmias, *tachycardia,* palpitations, PVCs (rare), anginal pain—less likely with bronchodilator doses of this drug than with bronchodilator doses of a nonselective beta-agonist (isoproterenol), changes in BP

- **GI:** *Nausea, vomiting, heartburn,* unusual or bad taste in mouth
- **Respiratory:** Respiratory difficulties, pulmonary edema, coughing, **bronchospasm,** paradoxic airway resistance with repeated, excessive use of inhalation preparations
- **Other:** *Sweating, pallor, flushing*

■ Nursing considerations

Assessment

- **History:** Hypersensitivity to metaproterenol; tachyarrhythmias; unstable vasomotor system disorders; hypertension; CAD; stroke; COPD patients who have developed degenerative heart disease; hyperthyroidism; seizure disorders; psychoneuroses; pregnancy; labor; lactation
- **Physical:** Weight; skin color, T, turgor; orientation, reflexes; P, BP; R, adventitious sounds; blood and urine glucose, serum electrolytes, thyroid function tests, ECG

Interventions

- Use minimal doses for minimal periods—drug tolerance can occur with prolonged use.
- Switch to syrup if swallowing is difficult.
- ⊗ **Warning** Keep a beta-adrenergic blocker (a cardioselective beta blocker such as atenolol should be used in patients with respiratory distress) readily available in case cardiac arrhythmias occur.
- Do not exceed recommended dosage.

Teaching points

- If taking tablets, protect from moisture.
- Do not exceed recommended dosage; adverse effects or loss of effectiveness may result. Read product instructions and ask your health care provider or pharmacist if you have any questions.
- You may experience these side effects: Nausea, vomiting, change in taste (eat small frequent meals); dizziness, drowsiness, fatigue, weakness (use caution if driving or performing tasks that require alertness); irritability, apprehension, sweating, flushing.
- Report chest pain, dizziness, insomnia, weakness, tremor or irregular heartbeat, difficulty breathing, productive cough, failure to respond to usual dosage.

M

▷ **metaxalone**
(me tax' ah lone)

Skelaxin

PREGNANCY CATEGORY C

Drug class
Skeletal muscle relaxant (centrally acting)

Therapeutic actions
Precise mechanism of action not known, but may be due to general CNS depression; does not directly relax tense skeletal muscles or directly affect the motor endplate or motor nerves.

Indications
• Adjunct to rest, physical therapy, and other measures for the relief of discomfort associated with acute, painful musculoskeletal disorders

Contraindications and cautions
• Contraindicated with hypersensitivity to metaxalone; tendency for hemolytic or other anemias; severe renal or hepatic impairment, lactation.
• Use cautiously with mild hepatic impairment, pregnancy.

Available forms
Tablets—800 mg

Dosages
Adults and patients 12 yr and older
800 mg PO three to four times a day.
Pediatric patients younger than 12 yr
Not recommended.

Pharmacokinetics

Route	Onset	Peak	Duration
Oral	60 min	3 hr	4–6 hr

Metabolism: Hepatic; $T_{1/2}$: 2–4 hr
Distribution: Crosses placenta; may enter breast milk
Excretion: Urine

Adverse effects
• **CNS:** *Light-headedness, dizziness, drowsiness,* headache, fever, blurred vision
• **Dermatologic:** Urticaria, pruritus, rash

• **GI:** *Nausea,* vomiting, GI upset, hepatic impairment
• **Other: Hemolytic anemia, leukopenia**

Interactions
✳ **Drug-drug** • Increased risk of sedation with other CNS depressants and alcohol
✳ **Drug-lab test** • False-positive Benedict test; use of a more specific glucose test is advised

■ Nursing considerations
Assessment
• **History:** Hypersensitivity to metaxalone; tendency for hemolytic or other anemias; severe renal or hepatic impairment; lactation, pregnancy
• **Physical:** T; skin color, lesions; orientation, affect, vision examination, reflexes; bowel sounds, normal output; CBC, LFTs, renal function tests

Interventions
• Establish safety precautions if dizziness, drowsiness, or blurred vision occurs (use side rails, accompany patient when ambulating).
• Arrange for analgesics if headache occurs (and possibly as adjunct for relief of discomfort of muscle spasm).
• Provide positioning, massage, and warm soaks as appropriate for relief of pain of muscle spasm.
• Provide support and encouragement to deal with discomfort of underlying condition and drug effects.

Teaching points
• Take this drug exactly as prescribed. Do not take a higher dosage than that prescribed.
• Continue the use of rest, physical therapy, and other measures to relieve the discomfort.
• Avoid the use of alcohol, sleep-inducing, or over-the-counter drugs while you are taking this drug. These could cause dangerous effects. If you feel that you need one of these preparations, consult your health care provider.
• You may experience these side effects: Drowsiness, dizziness (avoid driving a car or engaging in activities that require alertness if these occur); nausea (take drug with food and eat frequent small meals).
• Report rash, itching, yellow discoloration of the skin or eyes.

DANGEROUS DRUG

▷**metformin hydrochloride**

(met **fore'** min)

Apo-Metformin (CAN), CO Metformin Coated (CAN), Fortamet, Gen-Metformin (CAN), Glucophage, Glucophage XR ⓞⓝⓒ, Glumetza ⓞⓝⓒ, Metformin HCl ER ⓞⓝⓒ, Nu-Metformin (CAN), PMS-Metformin (CAN), ratio-Metformin (CAN), Riomet

PREGNANCY CATEGORY B

Drug class

Antidiabetic
Biguanide

Therapeutic actions

Exact mechanism is not understood; possibly increases peripheral utilization of glucose, decreases hepatic glucose production, and alters intestinal absorption of glucose.

Indications

- Adjunct to diet to lower blood glucose with type 2 diabetes mellitus in patients 10 yr and older; ER in patients 17 yr and older; 18 yr and older for *Glumetza*
- As part of combination therapy with a sulfonylurea or insulin when either drug alone cannot control glucose levels in patients with type 2 diabetes mellitus
- Unlabeled uses: Treatment of anovulation in women with polycystic ovary syndrome; treatment of antipsychotic drug-induced weight gain

Contraindications and cautions

- Contraindicated with allergy to metformin; heart failure; diabetes complicated by fever, severe infections, severe trauma, major surgery, ketosis, acidosis, coma (use insulin); type 1 diabetes, serious hepatic impairment, serious renal impairment, uremia, thyroid or endocrine impairment, glycosuria, hyperglycemia associated with primary renal disease; labor and delivery (if metformin is used during pregnancy, discontinue drug at least 1 mo before delivery); lactation (safety not established).
- Use cautiously with the elderly.

Available forms

Tablets—500, 850, 1,000 mg; ER tablets ⓞⓝⓒ—500, 750, 1,000 mg; oral solution—500 mg/5 mL

Dosages

Adults

500 mg bid or 850 mg once daily PO. May increase 500 mg/wk or 850 mg/2 wk to maximum of 2,550 mg/day in divided doses. Dosage should be adjusted based on response and blood glucose level. ER tablet: Initially, 1,000 mg/day PO with evening meal; may be increased by 500 mg/wk to a maximum of 2,000 mg once daily (2,500 mg *Fortamet*). If higher doses are required, use immediate-release tablets.

Pediatric patients 10–16 yr

500 mg bid with meals. May increase 500 mg/wk to maximum of 2,000 mg/day in divided doses. ER tablet is not recommended.

Geriatric patients and patients with renal impairment

Smaller doses may be necessary; monitor closely and adjust slowly.

Pharmacokinetics

Route	Peak	Duration
Oral	2–2.5 hr	10–16 hr

Metabolism: $T_{1/2}$: 6.2 and 17.6 hr
Distribution: Crosses placenta; enters breast milk
Excretion: Urine

Adverse effects

- **Endocrine:** Hypoglycemia, **lactic acidosis**
- **GI:** *Anorexia, nausea,* vomiting, *epigastric discomfort, heartburn, diarrhea,* flatulence
- **Hypersensitivity:** *Allergic skin reactions,* eczema, pruritus, erythema, urticaria

Interactions

✳ **Drug-drug** • Increased risk of hypoglycemia with sulfonylureas, cimetidine, furosemide, cationic drugs such as digoxin, amiloride, vancomycin • Increased risk of lactic acidosis with ethanol • Increased risk of acute renal failure and lactic acidosis with iodinated contrast material used in radiologic studies; stop metformin at or before time of procedure and hold for 48 hr afterward

M

✳ **Drug-alternative therapy** • Increased risk of hypoglycemia if taken with juniper berries, ginseng, garlic, fenugreek, coriander, dandelion root, celery

■ **Nursing considerations**

Assessment

• **History:** Allergy to metformin; diabetes complicated by fever, severe infections, severe trauma, major surgery, ketosis, acidosis, coma; type 1 diabetes, serious hepatic or renal impairment, uremia, thyroid or endocrine impairment, glycosuria, hyperglycemia associated with primary renal disease; HF; pregnancy, lactation

• **Physical:** Skin color, lesions; T, orientation, reflexes, peripheral sensation; R, adventitious sounds; liver evaluation, bowel sounds; urinalysis, BUN, serum creatinine, LFTs, blood glucose, CBC

Interventions

⊗ **Black box warning** Risk of severe lactic acidosis; monitor patient, and treat any suspicion of lactic acidosis.

• Monitor serum glucose levels frequently to determine effectiveness of drug and dosage.

⊗ **Warning** Arrange for transfer to insulin therapy during periods of high stress (infections, surgery, trauma).

⊗ **Warning** Use IV glucose if severe hypoglycemia occurs as a result of overdose.

• Ensure that patient swallows ER forms whole; do not cut, crush, or allow patient to chew tablets.

• Give drug at night or split dose (morning and evening) if diarrhea is a problem.

Teaching points

• Do not discontinue this medication without consulting your health care provider.

• Monitor blood for glucose as prescribed.

• Swallow extended-release tablets whole; do not cut, crush, or chew.

• Do not use this drug during pregnancy; if you become pregnant, consult your health care provider for appropriate therapy.

• Avoid using alcohol while taking this drug.

• Report fever, sore throat, unusual bleeding or bruising, rash, dark urine, light-colored stools, hypoglycemic or hyperglycemic reactions.

DANGEROUS DRUG

▷ **methadone hydrochloride**
(meth' a done)

Diskets, Dolophine, Methadone HCl Intensol, Methadose

PREGNANCY CATEGORY C

CONTROLLED SUBSTANCE C-II

Drug class
Opioid agonist analgesic

Therapeutic actions
Acts as agonist at specific opioid receptors in the CNS to produce analgesia, euphoria, sedation; the receptors mediating these effects are thought to be the same as those mediating the effects of endogenous opioids (enkephalins, endorphins); when used in approved methadone maintenance programs, can substitute for heroin, other illicit opioids in patients who want to terminate a drug use.

Indications

• Relief of severe pain not responsive to non-opioid analgesics

• Detoxification and temporary maintenance treatment of opioid addiction (ineffective for relief of general anxiety)

Contraindications and cautions

• Contraindicated with hypersensitivity to opioids, diarrhea caused by poisoning (before toxins are eliminated), bronchial asthma, COPD, cor pulmonale, respiratory depression, anoxia, kyphoscoliosis, acute alcoholism, increased intracranial pressure.

• Use cautiously with acute abdominal conditions, CV disease, supraventricular tachycardias, myxedema, seizure disorders, delirium tremens, cerebral arteriosclerosis, ulcerative colitis, fever, Addison disease, prostatic hypertrophy, urethral stricture, recent GI or GU surgery, toxic psychosis, pregnancy before labor (crosses placenta; neonatal withdrawal observed in infants born to drug-using mothers; safety in pregnancy before labor not established), labor or delivery (administration of opioids to mother can cause respiratory

2014 LIPPINCOTT'S
Nursing Drug Guide

Photoguide to tablets and capsules

This photoguide includes nearly 450 tablets and capsules, representing the most commonly prescribed generic and trade name drugs. These drugs, organized alphabetically by generic name, are shown in actual size and color with cross-references to drug information. Each product is labeled with its trade name and its strength.

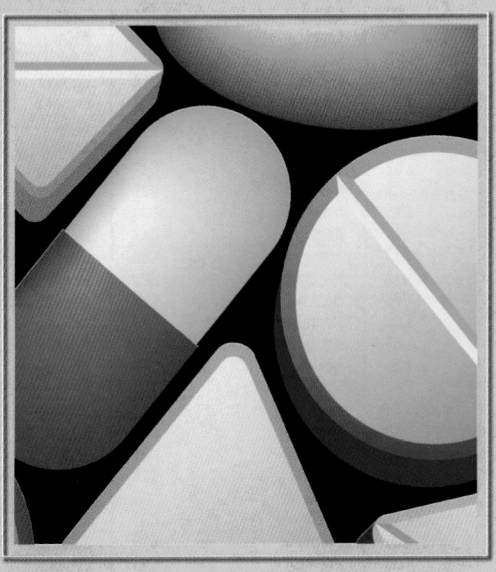

INDEX OF TRADE NAMES IN PHOTOGUIDE TO TABLETS AND CAPSULES

ACAMPROSATE CALCIUM

Campral
(Page 69)

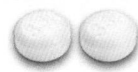

333 mg

ALENDRONATE SODIUM

Fosamax
(Page 88)

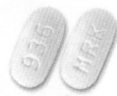 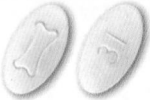

10 mg   40 mg   70 mg

ALFUZOSIN HYDROCHLORIDE

Uroxatral
(Page 90)

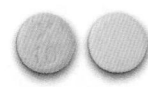

10 mg

ALPRAZOLAM

Xanax
(Page 98)

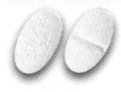   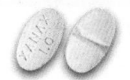

0.25 mg   0.5 mg   1 mg

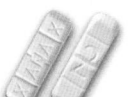

2 mg

AMLODIPINE BESYLATE

Norvasc
(Page 122)

          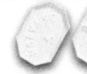

2.5 mg   5 mg

ANASTROZOLE

Arimidex
(Page 135)

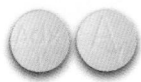

1 mg

ARIPIPRAZOLE

Abilify
(Page 142)

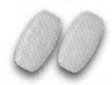
10 mg

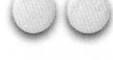
15 mg

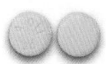
30 mg

ATAZANAVIR SULFATE

Reyataz
(Page 151)

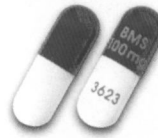
100 mg

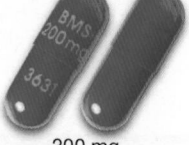
200 mg

ATENOLOL

Tenormin
(Page 153)

25 mg

50 mg

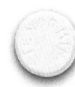
100 mg

ATOMOXETINE HYDROCHLORIDE

Strattera
(Page 154)

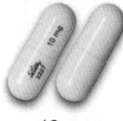
10 mg

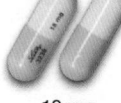
18 mg

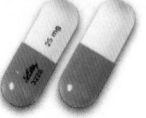
25 mg

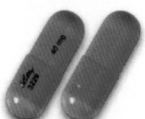
40 mg

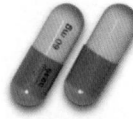
60 mg

ATORVASTATIN CALCIUM

Lipitor
(Page 156)

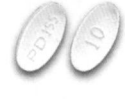
10 mg

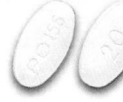
20 mg

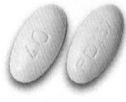
40 mg

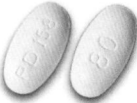
80 mg

AZITHROMYCIN

Zithromax
(Page 166)

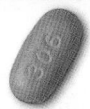 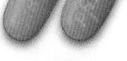 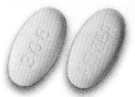

250 mg   500 mg   600 mg

BENAZEPRIL HYDROCHLORIDE

Lotensin
(Page 177)

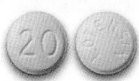 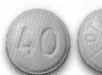

20 mg   40 mg

BUPROPION HYDROCHLORIDE

Wellbutrin
(Page 208)

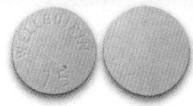 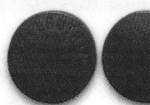

75 mg   100 mg

Wellbutrin SR
(Page 208)

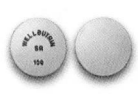 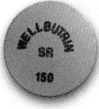  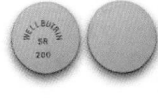

100 mg   150 mg   200 mg

Zyban
(Page 208)

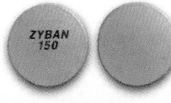

150 mg

CARISOPRODOL

Soma
(Page 233)

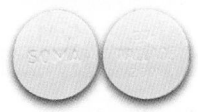

350 mg

CELECOXIB

Celebrex
(Page 259)

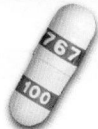 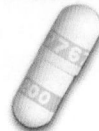

100 mg   200 mg

CIPROFLOXACIN

Cipro
(Page 285)

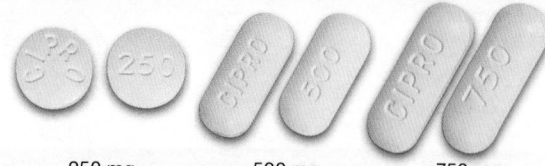

250 mg   500 mg   750 mg

CITALOPRAM HYDROBROMIDE

Celexa
(Page 289)

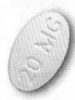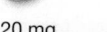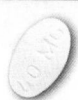

20 mg   40 mg

CLARITHROMYCIN

Biaxin
(Page 292)

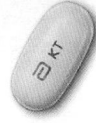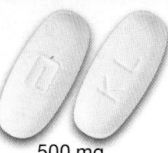

250 mg   500 mg

Biaxin XL
(Page 292)

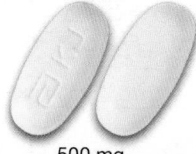

500 mg

CLONAZEPAM

Klonopin
(Page 303)

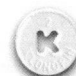

0.5 mg   1 mg   2 mg

CLOPIDOGREL BISULFATE

Plavix
(Page 308)

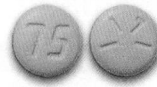

75 mg

CLOZAPINE

Clozaril
(Page 312)

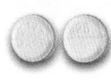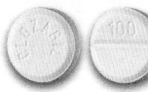

25 mg   100 mg

CODEINE PHOSPHATE—ACETAMINOPHEN

Tylenol with Codeine #3
(Page 1272)

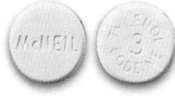

30 mg/300 mg

DARIFENACIN HYDROBROMIDE

Enablex
(Page 346)

7.5 mg   15 mg

DESLORATADINE

Clarinex
(Page 354)

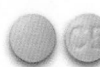

5 mg

DESVENLAFAXINE SUCCINATE

Pristiq
(Page 357)

50 mg   100 mg

DEXLANSOPRAZOLE

Dexilant
(Page 364)

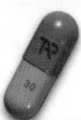   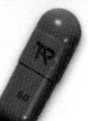

30 mg   60 mg

DEXMETHYLPHENIDATE HYDROCHLORIDE

Focalin XR
(Page 365)

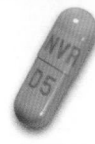   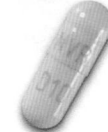   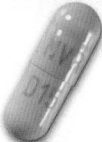

5mg   10 mg   15 mg

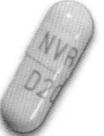   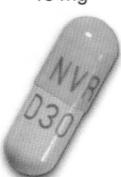   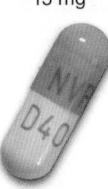

20 mg   30 mg   40 mg

DIAZEPAM

Valium
(Page 373)

2 mg   5 mg   10 mg

DILTIAZEM HYDROCHLORIDE

Cardizem
(Page 386)

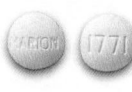

30 mg   90 mg

Cardizem CD
(Page 386)

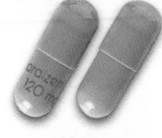 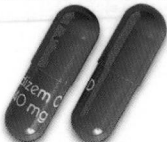

120 mg   180 mg   240 mg

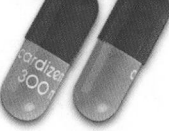 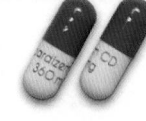

300 mg   360 mg

Cardizem LA
(Page 386)

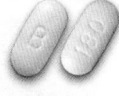 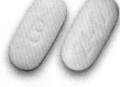 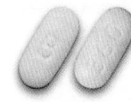

180 mg   240 mg   360 mg

DIVALPROEX SODIUM

Depakote
(Page 1183)

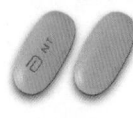 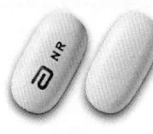 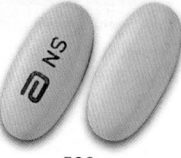

125 mg   250 mg   500 mg

Depakote Sprinkle
(Page 1183)

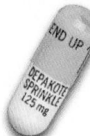

125 mg

DONEPEZIL HYDROCHLORIDE

Aricept
(Page 402)

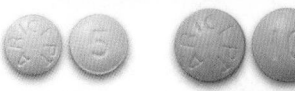

5 mg   10 mg

DOXAZOSIN MESYLATE

Cardura
(Page 408)

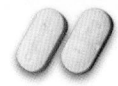   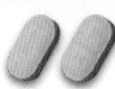   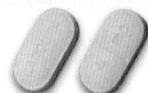

1 mg   2 mg   4 mg

8 mg

DULOXETINE HYDROCHLORIDE

Cymbalta
(Page 419)

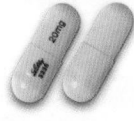   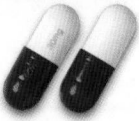   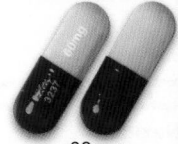

20 mg   30 mg   60 mg

DUTASTERIDE

Avodart
(Page 420)

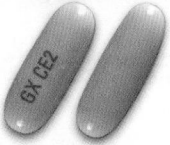

0.5 mg

ELETRIPTAN HYDROBROMIDE

Relpax
(Page 428)

20 mg   40 mg

ENALAPRIL MALEATE

Vasotec
(Page 431)

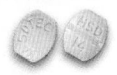   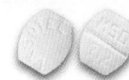   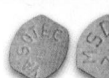

2.5 mg   5 mg   10 mg

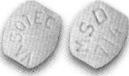

20 mg

ERYTHROMYCIN BASE

Eryc
(Page 452)

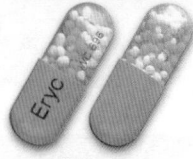

250 mg

Ery-Tab
(Page 452)

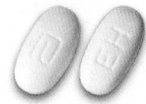

333 mg

ESCITALOPRAM OXALATE

Lexapro
(Page 455)

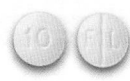 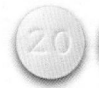

10 mg   20 mg

ESOMEPRAZOLE MAGNESIUM

Nexium
(Page 458)

 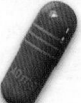

20 mg   40 mg

ESTRADIOL

Estrace
(Page 462)

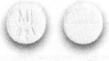

0.5 mg   1 mg   2 mg

ESTROGENS (CONJUGATED)

Premarin
(Page 465)

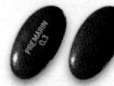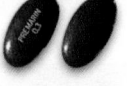 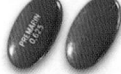

0.3 mg   0.45 mg   0.625 mg

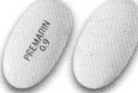 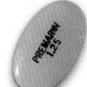

0.9 mg   1.25 mg

ESZOPICLONE

Lunesta
(Page 472)

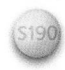

1 mg   2 mg   3 mg

EZETIMIBE

Zetia
(Page 488)

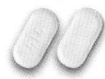

10 mg

EZETIMIBE—SIMVASTATIN

Vytorin
(Page 1312)

10 mg/10 mg   10 mg/20 mg   10 mg/40 mg

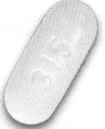

10 mg/80 mg

FAMCICLOVIR

Famvir
(Page 492)

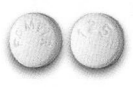 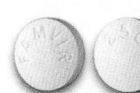 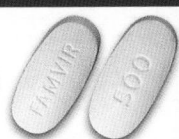

125 mg   250 mg   500 mg

FAMOTIDINE

Pepcid
(Page 494)

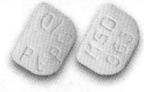 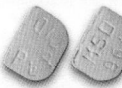

20 mg   40 mg

FENOFIBRATE

TriCor
(Page 499)

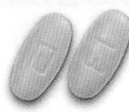 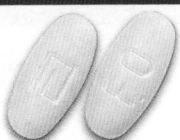

48 mg   145 mg

FINASTERIDE

Proscar
(Page 511)

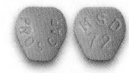

5 mg

FLUCONAZOLE

Diflucan
(Page 517)

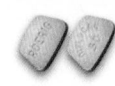

50 mg

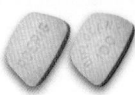

100 mg

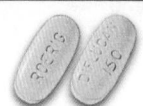

150 mg

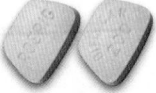

200 mg

FLUOXETINE HYDROCHLORIDE

Prozac
(Page 525)

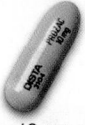

10 mg

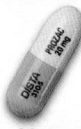

20 mg

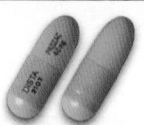

40 mg

Prozac Weekly
(Page 525)

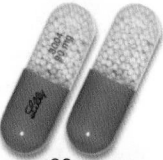

90 mg

Sarafem
(Page 525)

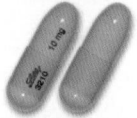

10 mg

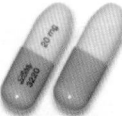

20 mg

FLUVASTATIN SODIUM

Lescol
(Page 534)

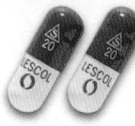

20 mg

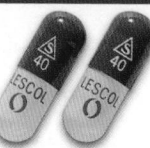

40 mg

FROVATRIPTAN SUCCINATE

Frova
(Page 548)

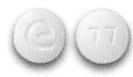

2.5 mg

FUROSEMIDE

Lasix
(Page 551)

 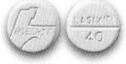 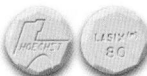

20 mg   40 mg   80 mg

GABAPENTIN

Neurontin
(Page 553)

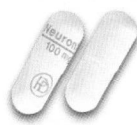 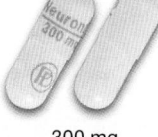 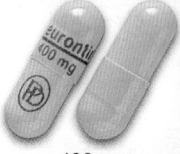

100 mg   300 mg   400 mg

GEMFIBROZIL

Lopid
(Page 560)

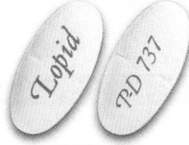

600 mg

GLIMEPIRIDE

Amaryl
(Page 565)

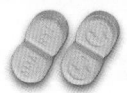 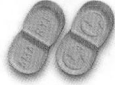 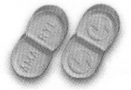

1 mg   2 mg   4 mg

GLIPIZIDE

Glucotrol
(Page 567)

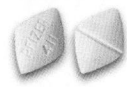 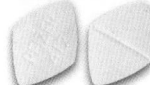

5 mg   10 mg

Glucotrol XL
(Page 567)

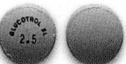

2.5 mg   5 mg   10 mg

GLYBURIDE

DiaBeta
(Page 569)

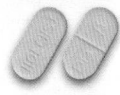

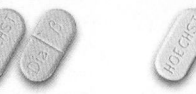

| 1.25 mg | 2.5 mg | 5 mg |

HYDROCODONE BITARTRATE—ACETAMINOPHEN

Lortab
(Page 1273)

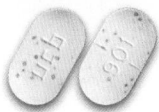

5 mg/500 mg

Vicodin
(Page 1273)

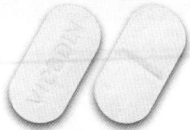

5 mg/500 mg

Vicodin ES
(Page 1273)

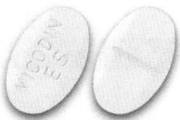

7.5 mg/750 mg

IBANDRONATE SODIUM

Boniva
(Page 602)

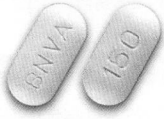

150 mg

INDINAVIR SULFATE

Crixivan
(Page 619)

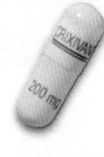

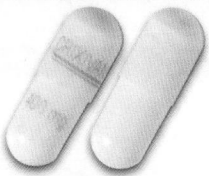

| 200 mg | 400 mg |

IRBESARTAN

Avapro
(Page 635)

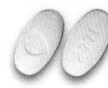

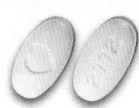

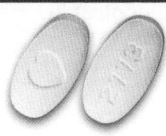

| 75 mg | 150 mg | 300 mg |

LAMIVUDINE—ZIDOVUDINE

Combivir
(Page 1295)

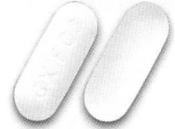

150 mg/300 mg

LANSOPRAZOLE

Prevacid
(Page 664)

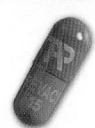 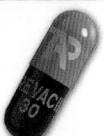

15 mg   30 mg

LEVODOPA— CARBIDOPA

Sinemet
(Page 1292)

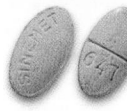 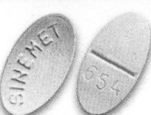

100 mg/10 mg   250 mg/25 mg

Sinemet CR
(Page 1292)

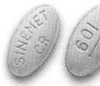

100 mg/25 mg

LEVODOPA—CARBIDOPA—ENTACAPONE

Stalevo
(Page 1293)

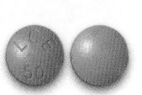 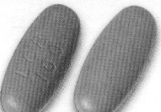 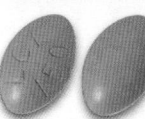

50 mg/12.5 mg/   100 mg/25 mg/   150 mg/37.5 mg/
200 mg   200 mg   200 mg

LEVOFLOXACIN

Levaquin
(Page 678)

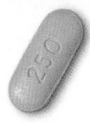 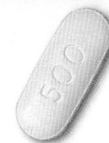

250 mg   500 mg

LEVOTHYROXINE SODIUM

Levoxyl
(Page 681)

25 mcg

50 mcg

75 mcg

88 mcg

100 mcg

112 mcg

125 mcg

137 mcg

150 mcg

175 mcg

200 mcg

300 mcg

Synthroid
(Page 681)

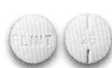
25 mcg

50 mcg

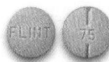
75 mcg

88 mcg

100 mcg

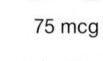
112 mcg

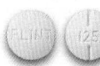
125 mcg

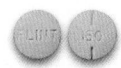
150 mcg

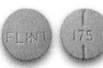
175 mcg

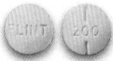
200 mcg

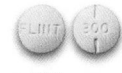
300 mcg

LISDEXAMFETAMINE DIMESYLATE

Vyvanse
(Page 694)

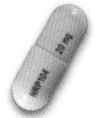 20 mg

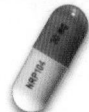 30 mg

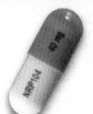 40 mg

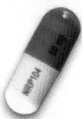 50 mg

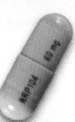 60 mg

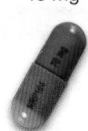 70 mg

LISINOPRIL

Prinivil
(Page 695)

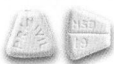 5 mg

 10 mg

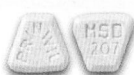 20 mg

 40 mg

Zestril
(Page 695)

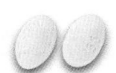 2.5 mg

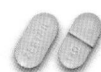 5 mg

 10 mg

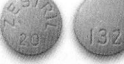 20 mg

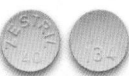 40 mg

LOPINAVIR—RITONAVIR

Kaletra
(Page 702)

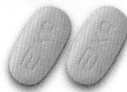 200 mg/50 mg

LORAZEPAM

Ativan
(Page 706)

 0.5 mg

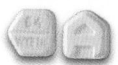 1 mg

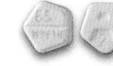 2 mg

LOSARTAN POTASSIUM

Cozaar
(Page 709)

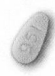

25 mg   50 mg

LOVASTATIN

Mevacor
(Page 711)

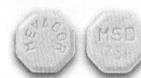

20 mg   40 mg

LUBIPROSTONE

Amitiza
(Page 1268)

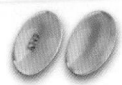

24 mcg

MEDROXYPROGESTERONE ACETATE

Provera
(Page 728)

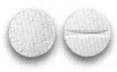 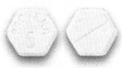 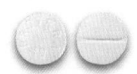

2.5 mg   5 mg   10 mg

MEMANTINE HYDROCHLORIDE

Namenda
(Page 735)

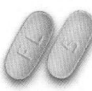 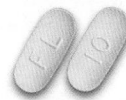

5 mg   10 mg

MEPERIDINE HYDROCHLORIDE

Demerol
(Page 738)

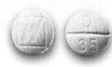 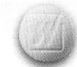

50 mg   100 mg

METFORMIN HYDROCHLORIDE

Glucophage
(Page 749)

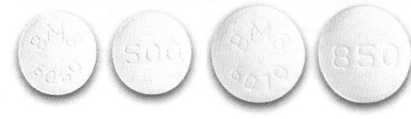

500 mg   850 mg

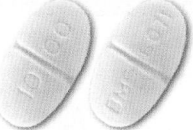

1,000 mg

Glucophage XR
(Page 749)

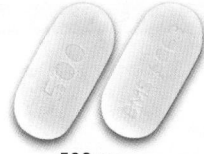

500 mg

METHYLPHENIDATE HYDROCHLORIDE

Concerta
(Page 765)

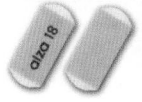   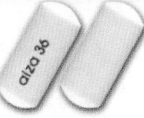   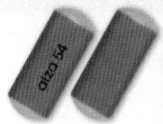

18 mg   36 mg   54 mg

Ritalin
(Page 765)

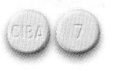   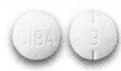   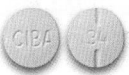

5 mg   10 mg   20 mg

Ritalin-SR
(Page 765)

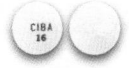

20 mg

METHYLPREDNISOLONE

Medrol
(Page 768)

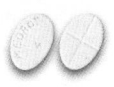   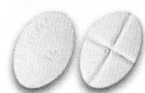

4 mg   16 mg

METOPROLOL SUCCINATE

Toprol-XL
(Page 773)

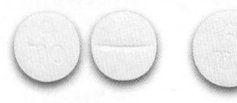 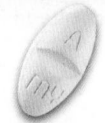

50 mg   100 mg   200 mg

METOPROLOL TARTRATE

Lopressor
(Page 773)

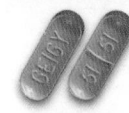   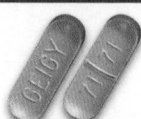

50 mg   100 mg

MONTELUKAST SODIUM

Singulair
(Page 802)

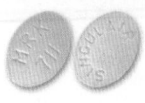

4 mg   5 mg   10 mg

MOXIFLOXACIN HYDROCHLORIDE

Avelox
(Page 807)

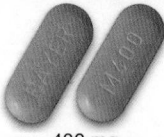

400 mg

NAPROXEN

Naprosyn
(Page 822)

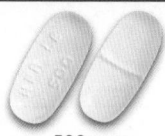

500 mg

NEBIVOLOL HYDROCHLORIDE

Bystolic
(Page 827)

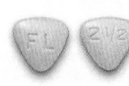

2.5 mg   5 mg   10 mg

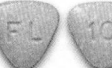

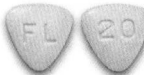

20 mg

NIFEDIPINE

Procardia XL
(Page 841)

30 mg   60 mg   90 mg

NITROFURANTOIN MACROCRYSTALS

Macrobid
(Page 844)

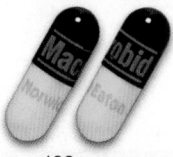

100 mg

NITROGLYCERIN

Nitrostat
(Page 845)

0.4 mg

NORTRIPTYLINE HYDROCHLORIDE

Pamelor
(Page 857)

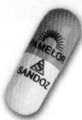 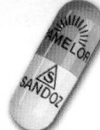 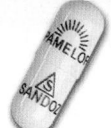

10 mg   25 mg   50 mg

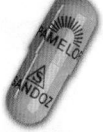

75 mg

OLANZAPINE

Zyprexa
(Page 864)

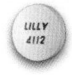 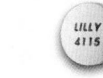 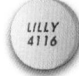

2.5 mg   5 mg   7.5 mg

10 mg   15 mg   20 mg

OLMESARTAN MEDOXOMIL

Benicar
(Page 866)

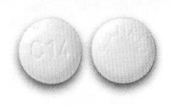

20 mg　　　　　40 mg

OLMESARTAN MEDOXOMIL—HYDROCHLOROTHIAZIDE

Benicar HCT
(Page 1290)

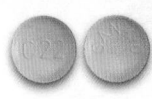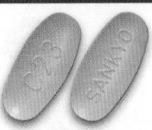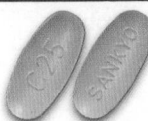

20 mg/12.5 mg　　　40 mg/12.5 mg　　　40 mg/25 mg

OMEGA-3-ACID ETHYL ESTERS

Lovaza
(Page 867)

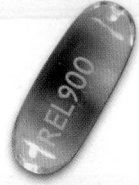

1 g

OMEPRAZOLE

Prilosec
(Page 868)

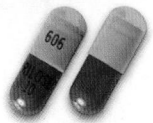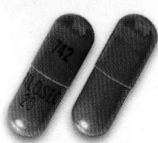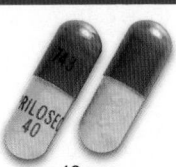

10 mg　　　　　20 mg　　　　　40 mg

OXYCODONE HYDROCHLORIDE

OxyContin
(Page 887)

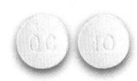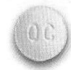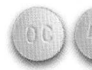

10 mg　　　　　20 mg　　　　　40 mg

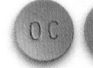

80 mg

PANTOPRAZOLE SODIUM

Protonix
(Page 904)

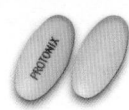

20 mg　　　　　40 mg

PENTOXIFYLLINE

Trental
(Page 923)

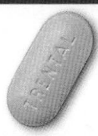

400 mg

PIOGLITAZONE HYDROCHLORIDE

Actos
(Page 943)

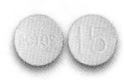 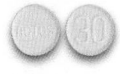 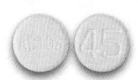

| 15 mg | 30 mg | 45 mg |

PRASUGREL

Effient
(Page 959)

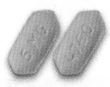 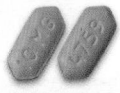

5 mg 10 mg

PRAVASTATIN SODIUM

Pravachol
(Page 961)

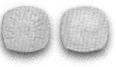 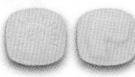 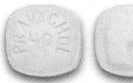

10 mg 20 mg 40 mg

PREGABALIN

Lyrica
(Page 968)

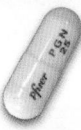 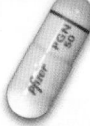 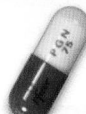

25 mg 50 mg 75 mg

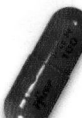 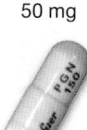 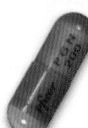

100 mg 150 mg 200 mg

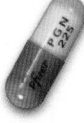 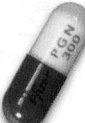

225 mg 300 mg

PROPRANOLOL HYDROCHLORIDE

Inderal
(Page 981)

    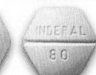

40 mg   60 mg   80 mg

Inderal LA
(Page 981)

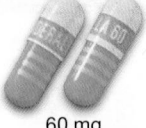 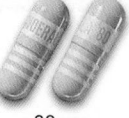 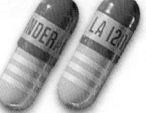

60 mg   80 mg   120 mg

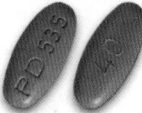

160 mg

QUETIAPINE FUMARATE

Seroquel
(Page 994)

25 mg   50 mg   100 mg

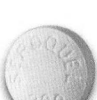 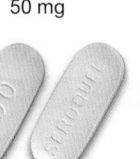 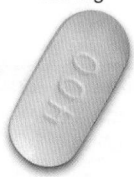

200 mg   300 mg   400 mg

QUINAPRIL HYDROCHLORIDE

Accupril
(Page 996)

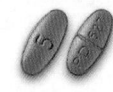

5 mg   10 mg   20 mg

40 mg

RABEPRAZOLE SODIUM

Aciphex
(Page 1000)

20 mg

RALOXIFENE HYDROCHLORIDE

Evista
(Page 1001)

60 mg

RANITIDINE HYDROCHLORIDE

Zantac
(Page 1007)

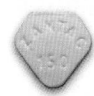 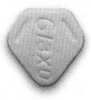 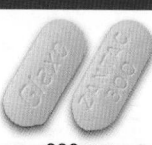

150 mg   300 mg

RANOLAZINE

Ranexa
(Page 1008)

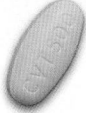

500 mg

RASAGILINE MESYLATE

Azilect
(Page 1010)

0.5 mg   1 mg

RISEDRONATE SODIUM

Actonel
(Page 1021)

 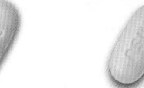

5 mg   35 mg

RISPERIDONE

Risperdal
(Page 1023)

  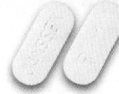

0.25 mg 0.5 mg 1 mg

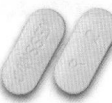 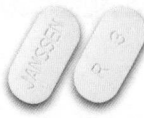 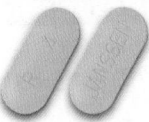

2 mg 3 mg 4 mg

ROSIGLITAZONE MALEATE

Avandia
(Page 1388)

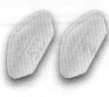 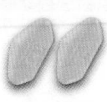 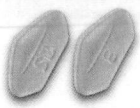

2 mg 4 mg 8 mg

ROSUVASTATIN CALCIUM

Crestor
(Page 1034)

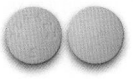 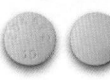 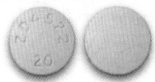

5 mg 10 mg 20 mg

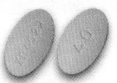

40 mg

SERTRALINE HYDROCHLORIDE

Zoloft
(Page 1051)

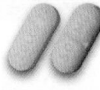 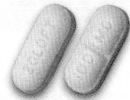

50 mg 100 mg

SILDENAFIL CITRATE

Viagra
(Page 1053)

25 mg 50 mg 100 mg

SIMVASTATIN

Zocor
(Page 1057)

5 mg   10 mg   20 mg

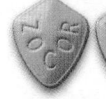

40 mg

SITAGLIPTIN PHOSPHATE

Januvia
(Page 1059)

100 mg

SOLIFENACIN SUCCINATE

VESIcare
(Page 1067)

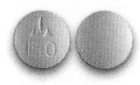   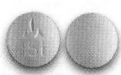

5 mg   10 mg

SPIRONOLACTONE

Aldactone
(Page 1073)

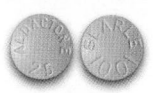   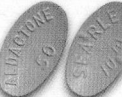   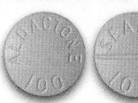

25 mg   50 mg   100 mg

SUCRALFATE

Carafate
(Page 1077)

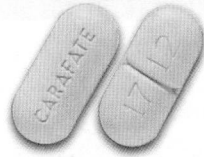

1 g

SULFAMETHOXAZOLE—TRIMETHOPRIM

Bactrim DS
(Page 1277)

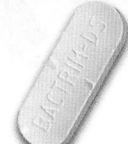

800 mg/160 mg

SUMATRIPTAN SUCCINATE

Imitrex
(Page 1084)

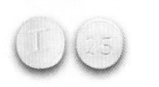

25 mg

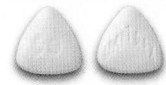

50 mg

SUNITINIB MALATE

Sutent
(Page 1391)

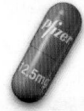

12.5 mg

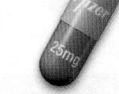

25 mg

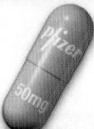

50 mg

TADALAFIL

Cialis
(Page 1088)

2.5 mg

5 mg

10 mg

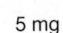

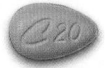

20 mg

TAMSULOSIN HYDROCHLORIDE

Flomax
(Page 1091)

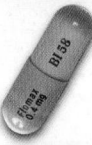

0.4 mg

TELMISARTAN

Micardis
(Page 1099)

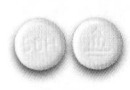

20 mg

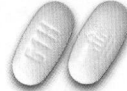

40 mg

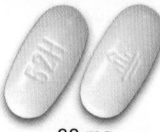

80 mg

TEMAZEPAM

Restoril
(Page 1100)

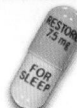

7.5 mg

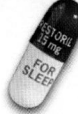

15 mg

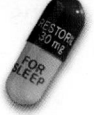

30 mg

TENOFOVIR DISOPROXIL FUMARATE

Viread
(Page 1103)

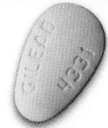

300 mg

TERAZOSIN HYDROCHLORIDE

Hytrin
(Page 1105)

1 mg

2 mg

5 mg

10 mg

TOLTERODINE TARTRATE

Detrol
(Page 1147)

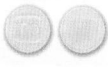

1 mg

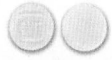

2 mg

TOPIRAMATE

Topamax
(Page 1148)

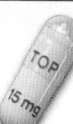

15 mg

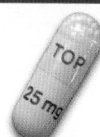

25 mg

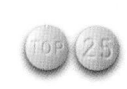

25 mg

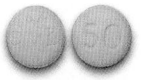

50 mg

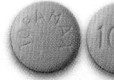

100 mg

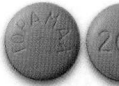

200 mg

TORSEMIDE

Demadex
(Page 1151)

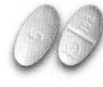

5 mg

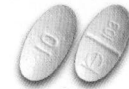

10 mg

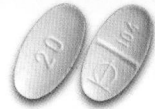

20 mg

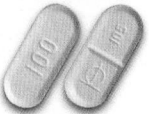

100 mg

TRAMADOL HYDROCHLORIDE—ACETAMINOPHEN

Ultracet
(Page 1276)

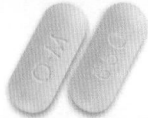

37.5 mg/325 mg

TRANDOLAPRIL

Mavik
(Page 1154)

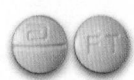 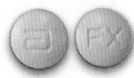 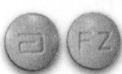

1 mg   2 mg   4 mg

VALACYCLOVIR HYDROCHLORIDE

Valtrex
(Page 1179)

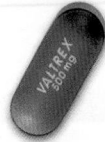 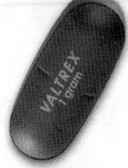

500 mg   1,000 mg

VALSARTAN

Diovan
(Page 1185)

 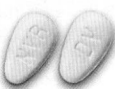 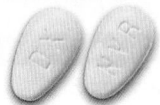

40 mg   80 mg   160 mg

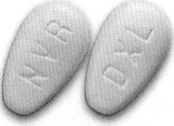

320 mg

VALSARTAN—HYDROCHLOROTHIAZIDE

Diovan HCT
(Page 1291)

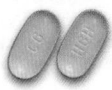 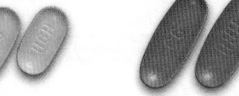 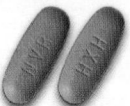

80 mg/12.5 mg   160 mg/12.5 mg   160 mg/25 mg

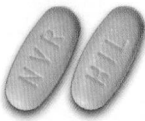 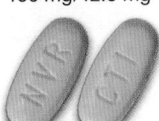

320 mg/12.5 mg   320 mg/25 mg

VARDENAFIL HYDROCHLORIDE

Levitra
(Page 1188)

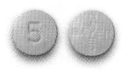
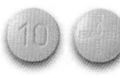
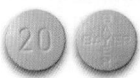

| 5 mg | 10 mg | 20 mg |

VARENICLINE TARTRATE

Chantix
(Page 1190)

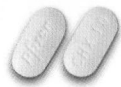

| 0.5 mg | 1 mg |

VENLAFAXINE HYDROCHLORIDE

Effexor XR
(Page 1191)

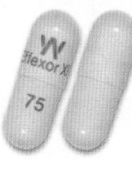
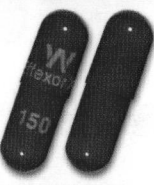

| 75 mg | 150 mg |

VERAPAMIL HYDROCHLORIDE

Calan
(Page 1193)

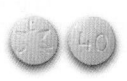
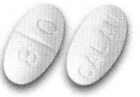
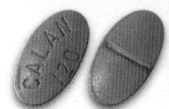

| 40 mg | 80 mg | 120 mg |

Verelan
(Page 1193)

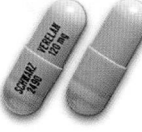
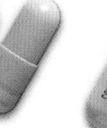
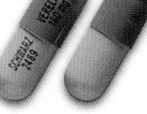
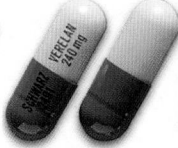

| 120 mg | 180 mg | 240 mg |

WARFARIN SODIUM

Coumadin
(Page 1204)

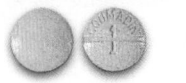

1 mg

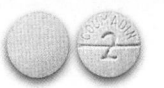

2 mg

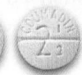

2.5 mg

3 mg

4 mg

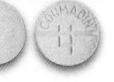

5 mg

6 mg

7.5 mg

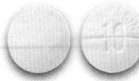

10 mg

ZIDOVUDINE

Retrovir
(Page 1209)

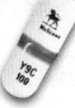

100 mg

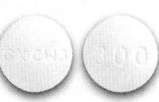

300 mg

ZIPRASIDONE HYDROCHLORIDE

Geodon
(Page 1212)

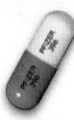

20 mg

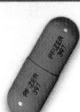

40 mg

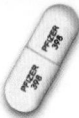

60 mg

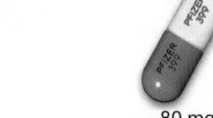

80 mg

ZOLPIDEM TARTRATE

Ambien
(Page 1216)

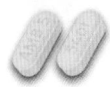

5 mg

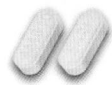

10 mg

depression of neonate—risk greatest for premature neonates), renal or hepatic impairment, lactation.

Available forms

Tablets—5, 10 mg; oral solution—5 mg/5 mL, 10 mg/5 mL; oral concentrate—10 mg/mL; injection—10 mg/mL; dispersible tablets—40 mg

Dosages

Oral methadone is approximately one-half as potent as parenteral methadone.

Adults

• *Relief of pain:* 2.5–10 mg IM, subcutaneously, or PO every 8–12 hr as necessary. IM route is preferred to subcutaneous for repeated doses (subcutaneous use may cause local irritation). Individualize dosage; patients with excessively severe pain and those who have become tolerant to the analgesic effect of opioids may need higher dosage.

• *Detoxification:* Initially 20–30 mg PO or parenteral; PO preferred. Increase dose to suppress withdrawal signs. 40 mg/day in single or divided doses is usually an adequate stabilizing dose for those physically dependent on high doses. Continue stabilizing doses for 2–3 days, then gradually decrease dosage every day or every 2 days. A daily reduction of 20% of the total dose may be tolerated. Provide sufficient dosage to keep withdrawal symptoms at tolerable level. Treatment should not exceed 21 days and may not be repeated earlier than 4 wk after completion of previous course. Detoxification treatment continued longer than 21 days becomes maintenance treatment, which may be undertaken only by approved programs (addicts hospitalized for other medical conditions may receive methadone maintenance treatment).

• *Maintenance treatment:* For patients who had been heavy heroin users up until hospital admission, initial dose of 20 mg 4–8 hr after heroin is stopped or 40 mg in a single dose PO. For patients with little or no opioid tolerance, half this dose may suffice. Dosage should suppress withdrawal symptoms but not produce acute opioid effects of sedation, respiratory depression. Give additional 10-mg doses if needed to suppress withdrawal syndrome. Adjust dosage, up to 120 mg/day.

Pediatric patients

Not recommended for relief of pain in children due to insufficient documentation.

Geriatric patients or impaired adults

Use caution. Respiratory depression may occur in the elderly, the very ill, and those with respiratory problems. Reduced dosage may be necessary.

Pharmacokinetics

Route	Onset	Peak	Duration
Oral	30–60 min	1.5–2 hr	4–12 hr
IM	10–20 min	1–2 hr	4–8 hr
Subcut.	10–20 min	1–2 hr	4–8 hr

Metabolism: Hepatic; $T_{1/2}$: 25 hr
Distribution: Crosses placenta; enters breast milk
Excretion: Bile, feces, urine

Adverse effects

• **CNS:** *Light-headedness, dizziness, sedation,* euphoria, dysphoria, delirium, insomnia, agitation, anxiety, fear, hallucinations, disorientation, drowsiness, lethargy, impaired mental and physical performance, coma, mood changes, weakness, headache, tremor, seizures, miosis, visual disturbances, suppression of cough reflex

• **CV:** Facial flushing, peripheral circulatory collapse, arrhythmia, palpitations, chest wall rigidity, hypertension, hypotension, orthostatic hypotension, syncope, prolonged QT interval

• **Dermatologic:** Pruritus, urticaria, laryngospasm, bronchospasm, edema, hemorrhagic urticaria (rare)

• **GI:** *Nausea, vomiting,* dry mouth, anorexia, constipation, biliary tract spasm; increased colonic motility in patients with chronic ulcerative colitis

• **GU:** Ureteral spasm, spasm of vesical sphincters, urine retention or hesitancy, oliguria, antidiuretic effect, reduced libido or potency

• **Local:** Tissue irritation and induration (subcutaneous injection)

• **Major hazards: Respiratory depression, apnea, circulatory depression, respiratory arrest, shock, cardiac arrest**

• **Other:** Sweating (more common in ambulatory patients and those without severe

M

pain), physical tolerance and dependence, psychological dependence

Interactions

✳ **Drug-drug** • Potentiation of effects of methadone with barbiturate anesthetics—decrease dose of methadone when coadministering • Decreased effectiveness of methadone with hydantoins, rifampin, urinary acidifiers (ammonium chloride, potassium acid phosphate, sodium acid phosphate) • Numerous interactions with HIV antiretrovirals, especially protease inhibitors • Increased risk of prolonged QT interval if combined with other drugs that prolong QT interval

✳ **Drug-lab test** • Elevated biliary tract pressure (opioid effect) may cause increases in plasma amylase, lipase; determinations of these levels may be unreliable for 24 hr after administration of opioids

■ Nursing considerations

Assessment

• **History:** Hypersensitivity to opioids, diarrhea caused by poisoning, bronchial asthma, COPD, cor pulmonale, respiratory depression, kyphoscoliosis, acute alcoholism, increased intracranial pressure; acute abdominal conditions, CV disease, supraventricular tachycardias, myxedema, seizure disorders, delirium tremens, cerebral arteriosclerosis, ulcerative colitis, fever, Addison disease, prostatic hypertrophy, urethral stricture, recent GI or GU surgery, toxic psychosis; pregnancy; labor; lactation

• **Physical:** T; skin color, texture, lesions; orientation, reflexes, bilateral grip strength, affect, pupil size; pulse, auscultation, BP, orthostatic BP, perfusion; R, adventitious sounds; bowel sounds, normal output; frequency and pattern of voiding; ECG; EEG; LFTs, renal and thyroid function tests

Interventions

⊗ **Black box warning** Use for opioid addiction should be part of an approved program. Deaths have been reported during initiation of treatment for opioid dependence. Use care to determine all drugs patient is using, and keep emergency services on standby.

⊗ **Black box warning** Monitor patient for QT interval prolongation, especially at higher doses.

• Give to breast-feeding women 4–6 hr before the next feeding to minimize the amount in milk.

⊗ **Warning** Keep opioid antagonist and equipment for assisted or controlled respiration readily available during parenteral administration. Monitor respirations carefully.

⊗ **Warning** Use caution when injecting subcutaneously into chilled body areas or in patients with hypotension or in shock—impaired perfusion may delay absorption; with repeated doses, an excessive amount may be absorbed when circulation is restored.

Teaching points

• Take drug exactly as prescribed.

• Avoid alcohol—serious adverse effects may occur.

• Do not take leftover medication for other disorders; do not let anyone else take the prescription.

• Avoid pregnancy while taking this drug; using barrier contraceptives is advised.

• You may experience these side effects: Nausea, loss of appetite (take with food, lie quietly, eat frequent small meals); constipation (laxative may help); dizziness, sedation, drowsiness, impaired visual acuity (avoid driving, performing other tasks that require alertness or visual acuity).

• Report severe nausea, vomiting, constipation, shortness of breath, or difficulty breathing.

▽ **methazolamide**

See Appendix R, *Less commonly used drugs.*

▽ **methenamine**
(meth en' a meen)

methenamine
Dehydral (CAN)

methenamine hippurate
Hiprex, Urex

PREGNANCY CATEGORY C

Drug classes

Antibacterial
Urinary tract anti-infective

Therapeutic actions

Hydrolyzed in acid urine to ammonia and formaldehyde, which is bactericidal; the hippurate and mandelate salts help to maintain an acid urine.

Indications

- Suppression or elimination of bacteriuria associated with pyelonephritis, cystitis, chronic UTIs, residual urine (accompanying some neurologic disorders), and in anatomic abnormalities of the urinary tract

Contraindications and cautions

- Contraindicated with allergy to methenamine, tartrazine (in methenamine hippurate marketed as *Hiprex*), aspirin (associated with tartrazine allergy), lactation.
- Use cautiously with hepatic or renal impairment, gout (causes urate crystals to precipitate in urine), pregnancy, severe dehydration.

Available forms

Tablets—0.5, 1 g

Dosages

Adults
Methenamine
1 g four times a day PO after meals and at bedtime.
Methenamine hippurate
1 g bid PO.
Pediatric patients
Methenamine
Younger than 6 yr: 50 mg/kg/day PO divided into three doses.
6–12 yr: 500 mg four times a day PO.
Methenamine hippurate
6–12 yr: 0.5–1 g bid PO.
Older than 12 yr: 1 g bid PO.

Pharmacokinetics

Route	Onset	Peak
Oral	Rapid	30–90 min
Oral (hippurate)	Rapid	2 hr

Metabolism: Hepatic; $T_{1/2}$: 3–6 hr
Distribution: Crosses placenta; enters breast milk
Excretion: Urine

Adverse effects

- **Dermatologic:** Pruritus, urticaria, erythematous eruptions, rash

- **GI:** Nausea, abdominal cramps, vomiting, diarrhea, anorexia, stomatitis
- **GU:** *Bladder irritation, dysuria,* proteinuria, hematuria, frequency, urgency, crystalluria
- **Other:** Headache, dyspnea, generalized edema, elevated serum transaminase (with hippurate salt)

Interactions

✳ Drug-lab test ● False increase in 17-hydroxycorticosteroids, catecholamines ● False decrease in 5-HIAA ● Inaccurate measurement of urine estriol levels by acid hydrolysis procedures during pregnancy

■ Nursing considerations

 CLINICAL ALERT!
Name confusion has occurred between methimazole and mesalamine; use caution.

Assessment

- **History:** Allergy to methenamine, tartrazine, aspirin; renal or hepatic impairment; dehydration; gout; pregnancy, lactation
- **Physical:** Skin color, lesions; hydration; ear lobes—tophi; joints; liver evaluation; urinalysis, LFTs; serum uric acid

Interventions

- Arrange for culture and sensitivity tests before and during therapy.
- Administer drug with food to prevent GI upset; give drug around-the-clock for best effects.
- Ensure patient avoids foods and medications that alkalinize the urine.
- Ensure adequate hydration for patient.
- Monitor clinical response; if no improvement is seen or a relapse occurs, repeat urine culture and sensitivity tests.
- Monitor LFTs with methenamine hippurate.

Teaching points

- Take drug with food. Complete the full course of therapy to resolve the infection.
- Take this drug at regular intervals around-the-clock; develop a schedule with the help of your health care provider.
- Avoid alkalinizing foods: Citrus fruits, milk products; or alkalinizing medications (sodium bicarbonate).
- Review other medications with your health care provider.
- Drink plenty of fluids.

M

- You may experience these side effects: Nausea, vomiting, abdominal pain (eat frequent small meals); diarrhea; painful urination, frequency, blood in urine (drink plenty of fluids).
- Report rash, painful urination, severe GI upset.

▽ **methimazole**
*(meth **im'** a zole)*

Tapazole

PREGNANCY CATEGORY D

Drug class
Antithyroid drug

Therapeutic actions
Inhibits the synthesis of thyroid hormones.

Indications
- Treatment of hyperthyroidism
- Palliation of certain thyroid cancers

Contraindications and cautions
- Contraindicated with allergy to antithyroid products, pregnancy (use only if absolutely necessary and when mother has been informed about potential harm to the fetus; if an antithyroid drug is required, propylthiouracil is the drug of choice), lactation.
- Use cautiously with bone marrow depression.

Available forms
Tablets—5, 10, 15, 20 mg

Dosages
Adults
Initial dose, 15–60 mg/day PO in three equal doses every 8 hr. Maintenance dose, 5–15 mg/day PO.
Pediatric patients
Initially, give 0.4 mg/kg/day PO, followed by maintenance dose of approximately one-half the initial dose; actual dose is determined by the patient's response. Alternatively, give initial dose of 0.5–0.7 mg/kg/day or 15–20 mg/m²/day PO in three divided doses, followed by maintenance dose of one-third to two-thirds of initial dose, starting when patient becomes euthyroid. Maximum dose is 30 mg/24 hr.

Pharmacokinetics

Route	Onset	Peak	Duration
Oral	30–40 min	60 min	2–4 hr

Metabolism: $T_{1/2}$: 6–13 hr
Distribution: Crosses placenta; enters breast milk
Excretion: Urine

Adverse effects
- **CNS:** *Paresthesias, neuritis,* vertigo, drowsiness, neuropathies, depression, headache
- **Dermatologic:** *Rash,* urticaria, pruritus, skin pigmentation, exfoliative dermatitis, lupus-like syndrome, loss of hair
- **GI:** Nausea, vomiting, epigastric distress, loss of taste, sialadenopathy, jaundice, hepatitis
- **GU:** Nephritis
- **Hematologic:** *Agranulocytosis, granulocytopenia, thrombocytopenia, hypoprothrombinemia, bleeding,* vasculitis, periarteritis
- **Other:** Arthralgia, myalgia, edema, lymphadenopathy, drug fever

Interactions
✳ **Drug-drug** ● Increased theophylline clearance and decreased effectiveness if given to hyperthyroid patients; clearance will change as patient approaches euthyroid state ● Altered effects of oral anticoagulants with methimazole ● Increased therapeutic effects and toxicity of cardiac glycosides, metoprolol, propranolol when hyperthyroid patients become euthyroid

■ Nursing considerations
Assessment
- **History:** Allergy to antithyroid products; pregnancy, lactation
- **Physical:** Skin color, lesions, pigmentation; orientation, reflexes, affect; liver evaluation; CBC, differential, PT, LFTs, renal function tests

Interventions
- Give drug in three equally divided doses at 8-hr intervals; try to schedule to allow patient to sleep at his or her regular time.
- Obtain regular, periodic blood tests to monitor bone marrow depression and bleeding tendencies.
- Advise medical and surgical personnel that patient is taking this drug, which increases the risk of bleeding problems.

Adverse effects in *italics* are most common; those in **bold** are life-threatening. ⬛ Do not crush.

- Ensure patient is not pregnant before giving this drug; advise patient to use barrier contraceptives.

Teaching points

- Take this drug around-the-clock at 8-hour intervals. Establish a schedule, with the aid of your health care provider, which fits your routine.
- This drug will need to be taken for a prolonged period to achieve the desired effects.
- Using barrier contraceptives is advised while taking this drug; serious fetal abnormalities may occur.
- If you are breast-feeding, another method of feeding the infant should be used.
- You may experience these side effects: Dizziness, weakness, vertigo, drowsiness (use caution driving or operating dangerous machinery); nausea, vomiting, loss of appetite (eat frequent small meals); rash, itching.
- Report fever, sore throat, unusual bleeding or bruising, headache, general malaise.

▷ methocarbamol
*(meth oh **kar**' ba mole)*

Robaxin, Robaxin-750

PREGNANCY CATEGORY C

Drug class
Skeletal muscle relaxant (centrally acting)

Therapeutic actions
Precise mechanism of action not known but may be due to general CNS depression; does not directly relax tense skeletal muscles or directly affect the motor end plate or motor nerves.

Indications
- Relief of discomfort associated with acute, painful musculoskeletal conditions, as an adjunct to rest, physical therapy, and other measures
- Control of neuromuscular manifestations of tetanus

Contraindications and cautions
- Contraindicated with hypersensitivity to methocarbamol; known or suspected renal pathology (parenteral methocarbamol is contraindicated because of polyethylene glycol 300 in vehicle).
- Use cautiously in patients with epilepsy, pregnancy, lactation.

Available forms
Tablets—500, 750 mg; injection—100 mg/mL

Dosages
Adults
Oral
Initially, 1.5 g four times a day PO. For the first 48–72 hr, 6 g/day or up to 8 g/day is recommended. For maintenance, 1 g four times a day or 750 mg every 4 hr PO or 1.5 g tid for total dosage of 4–4.5 g/day.
- *Tetanus:* Up to 24 g/day may be needed.
Parenteral
1 g IM or IV; 2–3 g may be needed in severe cases. Do not exceed 3 g for longer than 3 days except when treating tetanus.
Pediatric patients
Oral
Not recommended.
Parenteral
- *Tetanus:* 15 mg/kg IV, repeated every 6 hr as needed.

Pharmacokinetics

Route	Onset	Peak
Oral	30 min	2 hr
IM, IV	Unknown	Unknown

Metabolism: Hepatic; $T_{1/2}$: 1–2 hr
Distribution: Crosses placenta; may enter breast milk
Excretion: Feces, urine

▼ IV FACTS
Preparation: Administer undiluted, as provided.
Infusion: Administer at maximum rate of 300 mg/min (3 mL/min). May dilute 1 vial in no more than 250 mL sodium chloride injection or 5% dextrose solution. For tetanus, inject 1–2 g directly into IV tubing; add 1–2 g to infusion bottle for total dose of 3 g or less. May repeat every 6 hr.

Adverse effects
- **CNS:** *Light-headedness, dizziness, drowsiness,* headache, fever, blurred vision

M

- **CV:** Bradycardia, flushing, hypotension, syncope
- **Dermatologic:** *Urticaria,* pruritus, rash
- **GI:** *Nausea,* vomiting, dyspepsia
- **Other:** Conjunctivitis with nasal congestion

Interactions

✱ **Drug-lab test** • May cause interference with color reactions in tests for 5-HIAA and vanillylmandelic acid

■ Nursing considerations

CLINICAL ALERT!
Name confusion has occurred between methocarbamol and mephobarbital; use caution.

Assessment
- **History:** Hypersensitivity to methocarbamol; known or suspected renal pathology, epilepsy (use caution with parenteral administration), pregnancy, lactation
- **Physical:** T; skin color, lesions; nasal mucous membranes, conjunctival examination; orientation, affect, vision examination, reflexes; P, BP; bowel sounds, normal output; urinalysis, renal function tests

Interventions
- Do not exceed 3 g total dosage for longer than 3 days except when treating tetanus.
- Have patient remain recumbent during and for at least 15 min after IV injection.
- For IM use, do not inject more than 5 mL into each gluteal region; repeat at 8-hr intervals.
- Switch from parenteral to oral route as soon as possible.
- Ensure patient is not pregnant before use; use in pregnancy only if benefits clearly outweigh risk to the fetus.
- Patient's urine may darken on standing.

Teaching points
- Take this drug exactly as prescribed. Do not take a higher dosage than prescribed, and do not take it longer than prescribed.
- Avoid alcohol, sleep-inducing, or over-the-counter drugs; these could cause dangerous effects.
- Your urine may darken to a brown, black, or green color on standing.

- You may experience these side effects: Drowsiness, dizziness, blurred vision (avoid driving or engaging in activities that require alertness); nausea (take with food, eat frequent small meals).
- Report rash, itching, fever, or nasal congestion.

DANGEROUS DRUG

▷methotrexate (amethopterin, MTX)
(meth oh **trex'** *ate)*

ratio-Methotrexate (CAN), Rheumatrex, Rheumatrex Dose Pack, Trexall

PREGNANCY CATEGORY X

Drug classes
Antimetabolite
Antineoplastic
Antipsoriatic
Antirheumatic

Therapeutic actions
Inhibits dihydrofolic acid reductase, leading to inhibition of DNA synthesis and inhibition of cellular replication; selectively affects the most rapidly dividing cells (neoplastic and psoriatic cells).

Indications
- Treatment of gestational choriocarcinoma, chorioadenoma destruens, hydatidiform mole
- Treatment and prophylaxis of meningeal leukemia, mycosis fungoides
- Symptomatic control of severe, recalcitrant, disabling psoriasis
- Management of severe, active, classic, or definite rheumatoid arthritis
- Management of polyarticular course juvenile rheumatoid arthritis
- High-dose regimen followed by leucovorin rescue for adjuvant therapy of nonmetastatic osteosarcoma (orphan drug designation)
- Unlabeled uses: To reduce corticosteroid requirements in patients with severe corticosteroid-dependent asthma; as a maintenance regimen for Wegener agranulomatosis, dermatomyositis, relapsing-remitting MS, myositis, ulcerative colitis, refractory Crohn disease, uveitis, SLE, psoriatic arthritis

Adverse effects in *italics* are most common; those in **bold** are life-threatening. ▭ Do not crush.

Contraindications and cautions

- Contraindicated with pregnancy, lactation, alcoholism, chronic liver disease, immune deficiencies, blood dyscrasias, hypersensitivity to methotrexate.
- Use cautiously with renal disease, infection, peptic ulcer, ulcerative colitis, debility.

Available forms

Tablets—2.5, 5, 7.5, 10, 15 mg; powder for injection—20 mg, 1 g per vial; injection—25 mg/mL

Dosages
Adults

- *Choriocarcinoma and other trophoblastic diseases:* 15–30 mg PO or IM daily for a 5-day course. Repeat courses three to five times with rest periods of 1 wk or longer between courses until toxic symptoms subside. Continue one to two courses of methotrexate after chorionic gonadotropin hormone levels are normal.
- *Leukemia:* Induction: 3.3 mg/m^2 of methotrexate PO or IM with 60 mg/m^2 of prednisone daily for 4–6 wk. Maintenance: 30 mg/m^2 methotrexate PO or IM twice weekly or 2.5 mg/kg IV every 14 days. If relapse occurs, return to induction doses.
- *Meningeal leukemia:* Give methotrexate intrathecally in cases of lymphocytic leukemia as prophylaxis. 12 mg/m^2 (maximum 15 mg) intrathecally at intervals of 2–5 days; repeat until cell count of CSF is normal, then give one additional dose.
- *Lymphomas:* Burkitt tumor, stages I and II: 10–25 mg/day PO for 4–8 days. In stage III, combine with other neoplastic drugs. All usually require several courses of therapy with 7- to 10-day rest periods between doses.
- *Mycosis fungoides:* 2.5–10 mg/day PO for weeks or months or 50 mg IM once weekly or 25 mg IM twice weekly. Alternatively, in early stage, 5–50 mg PO or IM once weekly, or 15–37.5 mg PO or IM twice weekly; can also give IV with combination chemotherapy regimens in advanced disease.
- *Osteosarcoma:* Starting dose is 12 g/m^2 or up to 15 g/m^2 IV to give a peak serum concentration of 1,000 micromol. Must be used as part of a cytotoxic regimen with leucovorin rescue.
- *Severe psoriasis:* 10–25 mg/wk PO, IM, or IV as a single weekly dose. Do not exceed 30 mg/wk. Or 2.5 mg PO at 12-hr intervals for three doses each wk. Do not exceed 30 mg/wk. After optimal clinical response is achieved, reduce dosage to lowest possible with longest rest periods and consider return to conventional, topical therapy.
- *Severe rheumatoid arthritis:* Starting dose: Single doses of 7.5 mg/wk PO or divided dosage of 2.5 mg PO at 12-hr intervals for three doses given as a course once weekly. Dosage may be gradually increased, based on response. Do not exceed 20 mg/wk. Therapeutic response usually begins within 3–6 wk, and improvement may continue for another 12 wk. Improvement may be maintained for up to 2 yr with continued therapy.

Pediatric patients

- *Meningeal leukemia:*
  Younger than 1 yr: 6 mg intrathecally every 2–5 days.
  1–2 yr: 8 mg intrathecally every 2–5 days.
  2–3 yr: 10 mg intrathecally every 2–5 days.
  3 yr or older: 12 mg intrathecally every 2–5 days.
- *Polyarticular course juvenile rheumatoid arthritis (2–16 yr):* Initially, 10 mg/m^2 PO weekly. Dosage may be increased based on patient response. Maximum 20 mg/m^2/wk. Therapeutic response usually begins in 3–6 wk.

Pharmacokinetics

Route	Onset	Peak
Oral	Varies	1–2 hr
IM, IV	Rapid	0.5–1 hr

Metabolism: $T_{1/2}$: 3–15 hr
Distribution: Crosses placenta; enters breast milk
Excretion: Urine

▼ IV FACTS

Preparation: Reconstitute 20-mg vials with an appropriate sterile preservative-free medium, 5% dextrose solution, or sodium chloride injection to a concentration no greater than 25 mg/mL; reconstitute 1-g vial with 19.4 mL to a concentration of 50 mg/mL.

Infusion: Administer diluted drug by direct IV injection at a rate of not more than 10 mg/min. ⊗ *Warning* Do not give formulations with benzyl alcohol or preservatives intrathecally or for high-dose therapy.

Incompatibilities: Do not combine with bleomycin, prednisolone.
Y-site incompatibility: Do not give with droperidol.

Adverse effects

- **CNS:** Headache, drowsiness, blurred vision, aphasia, hemiparesis, paresis, seizures, *fatigue, malaise, dizziness*
- **Dermatologic:** *Erythematous rashes,* pruritus, urticaria, photosensitivity, depigmentation, *alopecia,* ecchymosis, telangiectasia, acne, furunculosis
- **GI:** *Ulcerative stomatitis,* gingivitis, pharyngitis, anorexia, *nausea,* vomiting, diarrhea, hematemesis, melena, GI ulceration and bleeding, enteritis, **hepatic toxicity**
- **GU:** Renal failure, *effects on fertility* (defective oogenesis, defective spermatogenesis, transient oligospermia, menstrual dysfunction, infertility, abortion, fetal defects)
- **Hematologic: Severe bone marrow depression,** *increased susceptibility to infection*
- **Hypersensitivity: Anaphylaxis, sudden death**
- **Respiratory: Interstitial pneumonitis,** chronic interstitial obstructive pulmonary disease
- **Other:** *Chills and fever,* metabolic changes (diabetes, osteoporosis), cancer

Interactions

✳ **Drug-drug** ⊗ *Warning* Potentially serious to fatal reactions when given with NSAIDs; use extreme caution if this combination is used.
⊗ *Warning* Risk of toxicity if combined with alcohol; avoid this combination.
- Increased risk of toxicity with salicylates, phenytoin, probenecid, sulfonamides ● Decreased serum levels and therapeutic effects of digoxin ● May decrease theophylline clearance

■ Nursing considerations

Assessment

- **History:** Allergy to methotrexate, hematopoietic depression, severe hepatic or renal disease, infection, peptic ulcer, ulcerative colitis, debility, psoriasis, pregnancy, lactation
- **Physical:** Weight; T; skin lesions, color; hair; vision, speech, orientation, reflexes, sensation; R, adventitious sounds; mucous membranes, liver evaluation, abdominal examination; CBC, differential; LFTS, renal function tests; urinalysis, blood and urine glucose, glucose tolerance test, chest X-ray

Interventions

⊗ *Black box warning* Arrange for tests to evaluate CBC, urinalysis, renal and liver function tests, and chest X-ray before therapy, during therapy, and for several weeks after therapy; severe toxicity could occur.

⊗ *Black box warning* Ensure that patient is not pregnant before administering this drug; counsel patient about the severe risks of fetal abnormalities associated with this drug.

⊗ *Black box warning* Reserve use for life-threatening neoplastic diseases or severe psoriasis or rheumatoid arthritis unresponsive to other therapies.

⊗ *Black box warning* Monitor liver function carefully with long-term use; serious liver toxicity can occur.

⊗ *Black box warning* Drug is associated with high risk of serious opportunistic infections. Monitor patient closely during therapy.

⊗ *Black box warning* Use with caution in patients who have malignant lymphomas or rapidly growing tumors as worsening of malignancy may result.

⊗ *Warning* Reduce dosage or discontinue if renal failure occurs.

- Reconstitute powder for intrathecal use with preservative-free sterile sodium chloride injection; intended for one dose only; discard remainder. The solution for injection contains benzyl alcohol and should not be given intrathecally.

⊗ *Warning* Arrange to have leucovorin or levoleucovorin readily available as antidote for methotrexate overdose or when large doses are used. In general, doses of leucovorin (calcium leucovorin or levoleucovorin) should be equal or higher than doses of methotrexate and should be given within the first hour. Up to 75 mg IV within 12 hr, followed by 12 mg IM every 6 hr for four doses. For average doses of methotrexate that cause adverse effects, give 6–12 mg leucovorin IM, every 6 hr for four doses or 10 mg/m^2 PO followed by 10 mg/m^2 every 6 hr for 72 hr.
- Arrange for an antiemetic if nausea and vomiting are severe.
- Arrange for adequate hydration during therapy to reduce the risk of hyperuricemia.
- Do not administer any other medications containing alcohol.

Teaching points

- Prepare a calendar of treatment days.
- This drug may cause birth defects or miscarriages. Use birth control while taking this drug and for 3 months thereafter. Men using this drug should also use barrier contraceptives.
- Avoid alcohol and NSAIDs; serious side effects may occur.
- Arrange for frequent, regular medical follow-up visits, including blood tests to follow the drug's effects.
- You may experience these side effects: Nausea, vomiting (request medication; eat frequent small meals); numbness, tingling, dizziness, drowsiness, blurred vision, difficulty speaking (drug effects; seek dosage adjustment; avoid driving or operating dangerous machinery); mouth sores (frequent mouth care is needed); infertility; loss of hair (obtain a wig or other suitable head covering; keep the head covered at extremes of temperature); rash, sensitivity to sun and ultraviolet light (avoid sun; use a sunscreen and protective clothing).
- Report black, tarry stools; fever; chills; sore throat; unusual bleeding or bruising; cough or shortness of breath; darkened or bloody urine; abdominal, flank, or joint pain; yellow color to the skin or eyes; mouth sores.

▽ **methoxsalen**

See Appendix R, *Less commonly used drugs.*

▽ **methscopolamine bromide**

*(meth skoe **pol'** a meen)*

Pamine, Pamine Forte

PREGNANCY CATEGORY C

Drug classes

Anticholinergic
Antimuscarinic
Antispasmodic
Parasympatholytic

Therapeutic actions

Competitively blocks the effects of acetylcholine at muscarinic cholinergic receptors that mediate the effects of parasympathetic postganglionic impulses, relaxing the GI tract and inhibiting gastric acid secretion.

Indications

- Adjunctive therapy in the treatment of peptic ulcer
- Unlabeled use: Treatment of cholinergic-induced bronchospasm

Contraindications and cautions

- Contraindicated with known hypersensitivity to the drug; glaucoma; adhesions between iris and lens; stenosing peptic ulcer, pyloroduodenal obstruction, paralytic ileus, intestinal atony, severe ulcerative colitis, toxic megacolon, symptomatic prostatic hypertrophy, bladder neck obstruction; bronchial asthma, COPD; cardiac arrhythmias, myocardial ischemia; sensitivity to anticholinergic drugs, bromides, tartrazine (tartrazine sensitivity is more common with allergy to aspirin); impaired metabolic, liver, or renal function; myasthenia gravis.
- Use cautiously with hypertension, hyperthyroidism, pregnancy, lactation.

Available forms

Tablets—2.5, 5 mg

Dosages

Adults
2.5 mg PO 30 min before meals and 2.5–5 mg PO at bedtime.
Pediatric patients
Safety and efficacy not established.

Pharmacokinetics

Route	Onset	Duration
Oral	1 hr	4–6 hr

Metabolism: Hepatic; $T_{1/2}$: 2–3 hr
Distribution: Crosses placenta; may enter breast milk
Excretion: Bile, urine

Adverse effects

- **CNS:** *Blurred vision,* mydriasis, cycloplegia, photophobia, increased IOP
- **CV:** Palpitations, tachycardia
- **GI:** *Dry mouth, altered taste perception, nausea, vomiting, dysphagia,* heartburn, constipation, bloated feeling, paralytic ileus, gastroesophageal reflux

M

- **GU:** *Urinary hesitancy and retention;* impotence
- **Other:** Decreased sweating and predisposition to heat prostration, suppression of lactation, nasal congestion, xerostomia

Interactions

❋ **Drug-drug** • Decreased antipsychotic effectiveness of haloperidol with anticholinergic drugs • Additive anticholinergic effects with concomitant use of antipsychotics, TCAs, other drugs with anticholinergic effects

■ Nursing considerations
Assessment

- **History:** Hypersensitivity to methscopolamine; glaucoma, adhesions between iris and lens; stenosing peptic ulcer, pyloroduodenal obstruction, paralytic ileus, intestinal atony, severe ulcerative colitis, toxic megacolon, symptomatic prostatic hypertrophy, bladder neck obstruction; bronchial asthma, COPD; cardiac arrhythmias, myocardial ischemia; sensitivity to anticholinergic drugs, bromides, tartrazine, impaired metabolic, liver, or renal function; myasthenia gravis; hypertension; hyperthyroidism; pregnancy; lactation
- **Physical:** Bowel sounds, normal output; urinary output, prostate palpation; R; adventitious sounds; P, BP; IOP, vision; bilateral grip strength, reflexes; liver palpation, LFTs, renal function tests; skin color, lesions, texture

Interventions

- Ensure adequate hydration; control environment (temperature) to prevent hyperpyrexia.
- Encourage patient to void before each dose of medication if urine retention becomes a problem.

Teaching points

- Take drug exactly as prescribed.
- Avoid hot environments (you will be heat intolerant, and dangerous reactions may occur).
- You may experience these side effects: Constipation (ensure adequate fluid intake, proper diet); dry mouth (suck on sugarless candies, use frequent mouth care); blurred vision, sensitivity to light (avoid tasks that require acute vision; wear sunglasses when in bright light); impotence (reversible); difficulty with urination (empty bladder immediately before taking dose).

- Report rash, flushing, eye pain, difficulty breathing, tremors, loss of coordination, irregular heartbeat, palpitations, headache, abdominal distention, hallucinations, severe or persistent dry mouth, difficulty swallowing, difficulty in urination, severe constipation, sensitivity to light.

▽ methsuximide

See Appendix R, *Less commonly used drugs.*

▽ methyclothiazide
*(meth i kloe **thye'** a zide)*

Enduron

PREGNANCY CATEGORY B

Drug class
Thiazide diuretic

Therapeutic actions
Inhibits reabsorption of sodium and chloride in distal renal tubule, thereby increasing excretion of sodium, chloride, and water by the kidneys.

Indications

- Adjunctive therapy in edema associated with heart failure, cirrhosis, corticosteroid and estrogen therapy, renal impairment
- Hypertension, as sole therapy or in combination with other antihypertensives

Contraindications and cautions

- Contraindicated with hypersensitivity to thiazides.
- Use cautiously with fluid or electrolyte imbalances, renal or liver disease, gout, SLE, glucose tolerance abnormalities, hyperparathyroidism.

Available forms
Tablets—2.5, 5 mg

Dosages
Adults

- *Edema:* 2.5–10 mg daily PO. Maximum single dose is 10 mg.
- *Hypertension:* 2.5–5 mg daily PO. If BP is not controlled by 5 mg daily within 8–12 wk, another antihypertensive may be needed.

Adverse effects in *italics* are most common; those in **bold** are life-threatening. ⬛ Do not crush.

Pharmacokinetics

Route	Onset	Peak	Duration
Oral	2 hr	6 hr	24 hr

Metabolism: T$_{1/2}$: Unknown
Distribution: Crosses placenta; enters breast milk
Excretion: Urine

Adverse effects

- **CNS:** *Dizziness, vertigo,* paresthesias, weakness, headache, drowsiness, fatigue
- **CV:** Orthostatic hypotension, volume depletion
- **Dermatologic:** Photosensitivity, rash, purpura, hives
- **GI:** *Nausea, anorexia, vomiting, dry mouth,* diarrhea, constipation, jaundice
- **GU:** *Polyuria, nocturia*
- **Hematologic:** Leukopenia, thrombocytopenia, agranulocytosis, aplastic anemia, neutropenia
- **Other:** Muscle cramp, hyperglycemia, hyperuricemia, electrolyte imbalance

Interactions

✳ **Drug-drug** • Risk of hyperglycemia with diazoxide • Decreased absorption with cholestyramine, colestipol • Increased risk of digoxin toxicity if hypokalemia occurs • Increased risk of lithium toxicity when taken with thiazides • Increased fasting blood glucose leading to need to adjust dosage of antidiabetics
✳ **Drug-lab test** • Decreased PBI levels without clinical signs of thyroid disturbances

■ Nursing considerations

Assessment
- **History:** Fluid or electrolyte imbalances, renal or liver disease, gout, SLE, glucose tolerance abnormalities, hyperparathyroidism, bipolar disorders, pregnancy, lactation
- **Physical:** Skin color and lesions; orientation, reflexes, muscle strength; pulses, BP, orthostatic BP, perfusion, edema, baseline ECG; R, adventitious sounds; liver evaluation, bowel sounds; CBC, serum electrolytes, blood glucose, LFTs, renal function tests, serum uric acid, urinalysis

Interventions
- Give with food or milk if GI upset occurs.
- Administer early in the day so increased urination will not disturb sleep.

- Measure and record regular body weights to monitor fluid changes.

Teaching points
- Take drug early in the day so sleep will not be disturbed by increased urination.
- Weigh yourself daily, and record weight on a calendar.
- Protect skin from exposure to sun or bright lights (sensitivity may occur).
- Increased urination will occur.
- Use caution if you feel dizzy, drowsy, or faint.
- Report rapid weight change, swelling in ankles or fingers, unusual bleeding or bruising, muscle cramps.

▽ **methyldopa**
(meth ill doe' pa)

methyldopa
Apo-Methyldopa (CAN)

methyldopate hydrochloride

PREGNANCY CATEGORY B (ORAL)

PREGNANCY CATEGORY C (IV)

M

Drug classes
Antihypertensive
Sympatholytic (centrally acting)

Therapeutic actions
Mechanism of action not conclusively demonstrated; probably due to drug's metabolism, which lowers arterial BP by stimulating CNS alpha$_2$-adrenergic receptors, which in turn decreases sympathetic outflow from the CNS.

Indications
- Hypertension
- IV methyldopate: Acute hypertensive crisis; not drug of choice because of slow onset of action
- Unlabeled use: Hypertension of pregnancy

Contraindications and cautions
- Contraindicated with hypersensitivity to methyldopa, active hepatic disease, previous methyldopa therapy associated with liver disorders.
- Use cautiously with previous liver disease, renal failure, dialysis, bilateral cerebrovascular disease, pregnancy, lactation.

Available forms

Tablets—250, 500 mg; injection—50 mg/mL

Dosages

Adults

Oral therapy (methyldopa)

- *Initial therapy:* 250 mg bid–tid in the first 48 hr. Adjust dosage at minimum intervals of at least 2 days until response is adequate. Increase dosage in the evening to minimize sedation. For maintenance, 500 mg–2 g/day in two to four doses. Usually given in two to four doses; some patients may be controlled with a single dose at bedtime.
- *Concomitant therapy:* With antihypertensives other than thiazides, limit initial dosage to 500 mg/day in divided doses. When added to a thiazide, dosage of thiazide need not be changed.

IV therapy (methyldopate)

250–500 mg every 6 hr as required (maximum 1 g every 6 hr). Switch to oral therapy as soon as control is attained; use the dosage schedule used for parenteral therapy.

Pediatric patients

Oral therapy (methyldopa)

Individualize dosage; initial dosage is based on 10 mg/kg/day in two to four doses. Maximum dosage is 65 mg/kg/day or 3 g/day, whichever is less.

IV therapy (methyldopate)

20–40 mg/kg/day in divided doses every 6 hr. Maximum dosage is 65 mg/kg or 3 g/day, whichever is less.

Geriatric patients and patients with impaired renal function

Reduce dosage. Drug is largely excreted by the kidneys.

Pharmacokinetics

Route	Onset	Peak	Duration
Oral	Varies	2–4 hr	12–24 hr
IV	4–6 hr	4–6 hr	10–16 hr

Metabolism: Hepatic; $T_{1/2}$: 1.8 hr
Distribution: Crosses placenta; enters breast milk
Excretion: Urine

▼ IV FACTS

Preparation: Add the dose to 100 mL of 5% dextrose, or give in D_5W in a concentration of 10 mg/mL.
Infusion: Administer over 30–60 min.

Incompatibilities: Do not combine with barbiturates or sulfonamides.

Adverse effects

- **CNS:** *Sedation, headache, asthenia, weakness* (usually early and transient), dizziness, light-headedness, symptoms of cerebrovascular insufficiency, paresthesias, parkinsonism, Bell palsy, decreased mental acuity, involuntary choreoathetotic movements, psychic disturbances
- **CV:** *Bradycardia,* prolonged carotid sinus hypersensitivity, aggravation of angina pectoris, paradoxical pressor response, pericarditis, **myocarditis,** orthostatic hypotension, edema
- **Dermatologic:** Rash seen as eczema or lichenoid eruption, toxic epidermal necrolysis fever, lupus-like syndrome
- **Endocrine:** Breast enlargement, gynecomastia, lactation, hyperprolactinemia, amenorrhea, galactorrhea, impotence, failure to ejaculate, decreased libido
- **GI:** *Nausea, vomiting, distention, constipation,* flatus, diarrhea, colitis, dry mouth, sore or black tongue, pancreatitis, sialadenitis, abnormal liver function tests, jaundice, hepatitis, **hepatic necrosis**
- **Hematologic:** Positive Coombs test, hemolytic anemia, bone marrow depression, leukopenia, granulocytopenia, thrombocytopenia, positive tests for antinuclear antibody, lupus-like syndrome, and rheumatoid factor
- **Other:** Nasal stuffiness, mild arthralgia, myalgia, septic shock–like syndrome

Interactions

✳ **Drug-drug** • Potentiation of the pressor effects of sympathomimetic amines • Increased hypotension with levodopa • Risk of hypotension during surgery with central anesthetics; monitor patient carefully • Risk of increased lithium toxicity if taken concurrently; monitor patient closely

✳ **Drug-lab test** • Methyldopa may interfere with tests for urinary uric acid, serum creatinine, AST, urinary catecholamines

■ Nursing considerations

Assessment

- **History:** Hypersensitivity to methyldopa; hepatic disease; previous methyldopa therapy associated with liver disorders; renal failure; dialysis; bilateral cerebrovascular disease; lactation, pregnancy

- **Physical:** Weight; T; skin color, lesions; mucous membrane color, lesions; orientation, affect, reflexes; P, BP, orthostatic BP, perfusion, edema, auscultation; bowel sounds, normal output, liver evaluation; breast examination; LFTs, renal function tests, urinalysis, CBC and differential, direct Coombs test

Interventions

- Administer IV slowly over 30–60 min; monitor injection site.

⊗ *Warning* Monitor hepatic function, especially in the first 6–12 wk of therapy or if unexplained fever appears. Discontinue drug if fever, abnormalities in liver function tests, or jaundice occurs. Ensure that methyldopa is not reinstituted in such patients.

⊗ *Warning* Monitor blood counts periodically to detect hemolytic anemia; a direct Coombs test before therapy and 6 and 12 mo later may be helpful. Discontinue drug if Coombs-positive hemolytic anemia occurs. If hemolytic anemia is related to methyldopa, ensure that drug is not reinstituted.

⊗ *Warning* Discontinue therapy if involuntary choreoathetotic movements occur.

⊗ *Warning* Discontinue if edema progresses or signs of HF occur.

- Add a thiazide to drug regimen or increase dosage if methyldopa tolerance occurs (second and third month of therapy).

⊗ *Warning* Monitor BP carefully when discontinuing methyldopa; drug has short duration of action, and hypertension usually returns within 48 hr.

Teaching points

- Take this drug exactly as prescribed; it is important that you not miss doses.
- You may experience these side effects: Drowsiness, dizziness, light-headedness, headache, weakness (often transient; avoid driving or engaging in tasks that require alertness); GI upset (eat frequent small meals); dreams, nightmares, memory impairment (reversible); dizziness, light-headedness when you get up (get up slowly; use caution when climbing stairs); urine that darkens on standing (expected effect); impotence, failure of ejaculation, decreased libido; breast enlargement, sore breasts.
- Report unexplained, prolonged general tiredness; yellowing of the skin or eyes; fever; bruising; rash.

▽methylene blue
(meth' i leen)
Methblue 65

PREGNANCY CATEGORY C

Drug classes
Antidote
Diagnostic agent
Urinary tract anti-infective

Therapeutic actions
Oxidation-reduction agent that converts the ferrous iron of reduced Hgb to the ferric form, producing methemoglobin; weak germicide in lower doses; tissue staining.

Indications
- Treatment of cyanide poisoning and drug-induced methemoglobinemia
- May be useful in the management of patients with oxalate urinary tract calculi
- GU antiseptic for cystitis and urethritis
- Unlabeled uses: Delineation of body structures and fistulas through dye effect; neonatal glutaric aciduria II unresponsive to riboflavin

Contraindications and cautions
- Contraindicated with allergy to methylene blue, renal insufficiency, intraspinal injections.
- Use cautiously with G6PD deficiency; anemias; CV deficiencies; pregnancy, lactation.

Available forms
Tablets—65 mg; injection—10 mg/mL

Dosages
Adults and children
Oral
65–130 mg tid with a full glass of water.
IV
1–2 mg/kg or 25–50 mg/m² injected over several minutes. May repeat after 1 hour as needed.

Pharmacokinetics

Route	Onset	Peak
Oral	Varies	Unknown
IV	Immediate	End of infusion

Metabolism: Tissue; $T_{1/2}$: Unknown
Excretion: Bile, feces, urine

▼ IV FACTS

Preparation: No preparation required.
Infusion: Inject directly IV or into tubing of actively running IV; inject slowly over several minutes.

Adverse effects

- **CNS:** Dizziness, headache, mental confusion, sweating
- **CV:** Precordial pain
- **GI:** *Nausea,* vomiting, diarrhea, abdominal pain, *blue-green stool*
- **GU:** *Discolored urine* (blue-green); bladder irritation
- **Other:** Necrotic abscess (subcutaneous injection); fetal anemia and distress (amniotic injection); neural damage, paralysis (intrathecal injection); *skin stained blue*

Interactions

✳ **Drug-drug** • Risk of serotonin syndrome if combined with serotogenic drugs (SSRIs, norepinephrine reuptake inhibitors); avoid this combination except in emergency situations

■ Nursing considerations
Assessment

- **History:** Allergy to methylene blue, renal insufficiency, presence of G6PD deficiency; anemias; CV deficiencies; pregnancy, lactation
- **Physical:** Skin color, lesions; urinary output, bladder palpation; abdominal examination, normal output; CBC with differential

Interventions

- Give oral drug after meals with a full glass of water.
- Give IV slowly over several minutes; avoid exceeding recommended dosage.
- ⊗ *Warning* Use care to avoid subcutaneous injection; monitor intrathecal sites used for diagnostic injection for necrosis and damage.
- Contact with skin will dye the skin blue; stain may be removed by hypochlorite solution.
- Monitor CBC for signs of marked anemia.

Teaching points

- Take drug after meals with a full glass of water.
- Avoid bubble baths, excessive ingestion of citrus juice, and sexual contacts if bladder infection or urethritis is being treated.

- You may experience these side effects: Urine or stool discolored blue-green; abdominal pain, nausea, vomiting (eat frequent small meals).
- Report difficulty breathing, severe nausea or vomiting, fatigue.

▽ methylergonovine maleate

*(meth ill er goe **noe' veen**)*

Methergine

PREGNANCY CATEGORY C

Drug class

Oxytocic

Therapeutic actions

A partial agonist or antagonist at alpha receptors; as a result, it increases the strength, duration, and frequency of uterine contractions, which shortens the third stage of labor and reduces blood loss.

Indications

- Routine management after delivery of the placenta
- Treatment of postpartum atony and hemorrhage; subinvolution of the uterus
- Uterine stimulation during the second stage of labor following the delivery of the anterior shoulder, under strict medical supervision

Contraindications and cautions

- Contraindicated with allergy to methylergonovine, hypertension, toxemia, lactation, pregnancy.
- Use cautiously with sepsis, obliterative vascular disease, hepatic or renal impairment.

Available forms

Tablets—0.2 mg; injection—0.2 mg/mL

Dosages
Adults
IM
0.2 mg after delivery of the placenta, after delivery of the anterior shoulder, or during puerperium. May be repeated every 2–4 hr.
IV
Same dosage as IM; infuse slowly over at least 60 sec. Monitor BP very carefully as severe

hypertensive reaction can occur; reserve this route for emergency situations.

Oral

0.2 mg PO three or four times daily in the puerperium for up to 1 wk.

Pharmacokinetics

Route	Onset	Peak	Duration
Oral	5–10 min	30–60 min	3 hr
IM	2–5 min	30 min	3 hr
IV	Immediate	2–3 min	1–3 hr

Metabolism: Hepatic; $T_{1/2}$: 1.5–12.7 hr
Distribution: Crosses placenta; enters breast milk
Excretion: Feces

▼ IV FACTS

Preparation: No additional preparation required.
Infusion: Inject directly IV or into tubing of running IV; inject very slowly, over no less than 60 sec; rapid infusion can result in sudden hypertension or cerebral events.

Adverse effects

- **CNS:** *Dizziness, headache,* tinnitus, diaphoresis
- **CV:** *Hypertension,* palpitations, chest pain, dyspnea
- **GI:** *Nausea,* vomiting

Interactions

✳ **Drug-drug** • Risk of severe hypertension, vasoconstriction, MI if combined with vasoconstrictors, ergot alkaloids; use extreme caution • Avoid use with potent CYP3A4 inhibitors (such as clarithromycin, erythromycin, itraconazole, ritonavir) • Use caution with mild CYP3A4 inhibitors (such as fluoxetine, fluvoxamine, nefazodone)

■ Nursing considerations

Assessment

- **History:** Allergy to methylergonovine, hypertension, toxemia, sepsis, obliterative vascular disease, hepatic or renal impairment, lactation, pregnancy
- **Physical:** Uterine tone, vaginal bleeding; orientation, reflexes, affect; P, BP, edema; CBC, LFTs, renal function tests; fetal monitoring when used during labor

Interventions

- Administer by IM injection or orally unless emergency requires IV use. Complications are more frequent with IV use.
- Monitor postpartum women for BP changes and amount and character of vaginal bleeding.
- Discontinue if signs of toxicity occur.
- Avoid prolonged use of the drug.

Teaching points

- This drug should not be needed for longer than 1 week.
- The patient receiving a parenteral oxytocic is usually receiving it as part of an immediate medical situation, and the drug teaching should be incorporated into the teaching about delivery. The patient needs to know the name of the drug and what she can expect after it is administered.
- You may experience these side effects: Nausea, vomiting, dizziness, headache, ringing in the ears (short-term use may make it tolerable).
- Report difficulty breathing, headache, numb or cold extremities, severe abdominal cramping.

▽ **methylnaltrexone bromide**

See Appendix R, *Less commonly used drugs.*

▽ **methylphenidate hydrochloride**
(meth ill fen' i date)

Apo-Methylphenidate (CAN),
Apo-Methylphenidate SR (CAN),
Biphentin (CAN), Concerta ⓒⓝⓒ,
Daytrana, Metadate CD ⓒⓝⓒ, Metadate
ER ⓒⓝⓒ, Methylin, Methylin ER ⓒⓝⓒ,
PMS-Methylphenidate (CAN),
Ritalin, Ritalin LA ⓒⓝⓒ, Ritalin-SR ⓒⓝⓒ

PREGNANCY CATEGORY C

CONTROLLED SUBSTANCE C-II

Drug class

CNS stimulant

M

Therapeutic actions
Mild cortical stimulant with CNS actions similar to those of the amphetamines; efficacy in hyperkinetic syndrome, attention-deficit disorders in children appear paradoxic and are not understood.

Indications
- Narcolepsy (*Ritalin, Ritalin SR, Metadate ER, Methylin*)
- Attention-deficit disorders, hyperkinetic syndrome, minimal brain dysfunction in children or adults with a behavioral syndrome characterized by the following symptoms: Moderate to severe distractibility, short attention span, hyperactivity, emotional lability, and impulsivity, not secondary to environmental factors or psychiatric disorders
- Unlabeled uses: Treatment of depression in the elderly, cancer and stroke patients; alleviation of neurobehavioral symptoms after traumatic brain injury; improvement in pain control and sedation in patients receiving opiates

Contraindications and cautions
- Contraindicated with hypersensitivity to methylphenidate; marked anxiety, tension, and agitation; glaucoma; motor tics, family history or diagnosis of Tourette syndrome; severe depression of endogenous or exogenous origin; normal fatigue states; concurrent use or use within 2 wk of MAOI.
- Use cautiously with seizure disorders; hypertension; drug dependence, alcoholism; emotional instability, psychosis; seizures; lactation, pregnancy; short gut syndrome, peritonitis, esophageal motility disorders (*Concerta*).

Available forms
Tablets—5, 10, 20 mg; chewable tablets— 2.5, 5, 10 mg; SR tablets ⊞—20 mg; ER tablets ⊞—10, 18, 20, 27, 36, 54 mg; ER capsules ⊞—20, 30 mg (*Metadate CD* ⊞); and 10, 20, 30, 40, 50, 60 mg (*Ritalin LA* ⊞); transdermal patch—1.1, 1.6, 2.2, 3.3 mg/hr; solution—1, 2 mg/mL

Dosages
Adults
Individualize dosage. Give orally in divided doses bid or tid, preferably 30–45 min before meals; dosage ranges from 10–60 mg/day PO.

If insomnia is a problem, drug should be taken before 6 PM. Timed-release tablets have a duration of 8 hr and may be used when timing and dosage are adjusted to the 8-hr daily regimen. ER forms: 18 mg PO daily in the morning; may be increased by 18 mg/day at 1-wk intervals to a maximum of 54 mg/day (*Concerta*); 10- to 20-mg/day increments to a maximum 60 mg/day (*Metadate CD, Ritalin LA*).

Pediatric patients 13–17 yr
Initially, 18 mg/day PO taken in the morning without regard to food; titrate to a maximum 72 mg/day PO. Do not exceed 2 mg/kg/day. Tablets must be swallowed whole and should not be cut, crushed, or chewed (*Concerta, Daytrana*). Or, 10–30 mg/day by transdermal patch; apply patch 2 hr before effect needed and remove after 9 hr.

Pediatric patients 6–12 yr
Start with small oral doses (5 mg PO before breakfast and lunch with gradual increments of 5–10 mg weekly). Daily dosage of more than 60 mg not recommended. Discontinue use after 1 mo if no improvement. Discontinue periodically to assess condition; usually discontinued after puberty. ER forms: Use adult dosage up to a maximum of 54 mg/day. Or, 10–30 mg/day by transdermal patch; apply patch 2 hr before effect needed and remove after 9 hr.

Pediatric patients younger than 6 yr
Not recommended.

Pharmacokinetics

Route	Onset	Peak	Duration
Oral	Varies	1–3 hr	3–6 hr
Oral (ER)	Varies	5–8 hr	3–12 hr
Transdermal	2 hr	3 hr	Up to 3 hr after removal

Metabolism: Hepatic; $T_{1/2}$: 1–3 hr (6.8 hr ER; 3–4 hr transdermal)
Distribution: Crosses placenta; may enter breast milk
Excretion: Urine

Adverse effects
- **CNS:** *Nervousness, insomnia,* dizziness, headache, dyskinesia, chorea, drowsiness, tics, **Tourette syndrome,** toxic psychosis, blurred vision, accommodation difficulties

Adverse effects in *italics* are most common; those in **bold** are life-threatening. ⊞ Do not crush.

- **CV:** *Increased or decreased pulse and BP; tachycardia,* angina, cardiac arrhythmias, palpitations
- **Dermatologic:** Rash, urticaria, fever, exfoliative dermatitis, erythema multiforme with necrotizing vasculitis and thrombocytopenic purpura, loss of scalp hair
- **GI:** *Anorexia, nausea, abdominal pain,* weight loss
- **Hematologic:** Leukopenia, anemia
- **Other:** Tolerance, psychological dependence, abnormal behavior with abuse, arthralgia

Interactions

✳ **Drug-drug** • Increased effects and toxicity of methylphenidate with MAOIs • Increased serum levels of phenytoin, TCAs, oral anticoagulants, SSRIs with methylphenidate; monitor for toxicity

✳ **Drug-lab test** • Methylphenidate may increase the urinary excretion of epinephrine

■ Nursing considerations
Assessment

- **History:** Hypersensitivity to methylphenidate; marked anxiety, tension, and agitation; glaucoma; motor tics, Tourette syndrome; severe depression; normal fatigue state; seizure disorders; hypertension; drug dependence, alcoholism, emotional instability; pregnancy, lactation
- **Physical:** Weight; T; skin color, lesions; orientation, affect, ophthalmologic examination (tonometry); P, BP, auscultation; R, adventitious sounds; bowel sounds, normal output; CBC with differential, platelet count, baseline ECG

Interventions

⊗ **Black box warning** Be aware that drug has potential for abuse; use caution with emotionally unstable patients.

- Ensure proper diagnosis before administering to children for behavioral syndromes; drug should not be used until other causes or concomitants of abnormal behavior (learning disability, EEG abnormalities, neurologic deficits) are ruled out.
- Ensure that patient does not have underlying cardiac problems before beginning therapy; serious cardiac effects have been reported. Baseline ECG is recommended.

- Apply transdermal patch to clean, dry area of the hip approximately 2 hr before effect needed. Remove after 9 hr. Alternate hips.
- Interrupt drug dosage periodically in children to determine if symptoms warrant continued drug therapy.
- Monitor growth of children on long-term methylphenidate therapy.
- Ensure that all timed-release tablets and capsules are swallowed whole, not chewed or crushed.
- Dispense the smallest feasible dose to minimize risk of overdose.
- Give before 6 PM to prevent insomnia.
- Monitor CBC and platelet counts periodically in patients on long-term therapy.
- Monitor BP frequently early in treatment.

Teaching points

- Take this drug exactly as prescribed. Timed-release tablets and capsules must be swallowed whole, not chewed or crushed. *Metadate CD* capsules may be opened and entire contents sprinkled on soft food—do not chew or crush granules. Transdermal patch should be applied to clean, dry area of the hip. Remove after 9 hours. Alternate hips.
- Chewable tablets must be taken with at least 8 ounces of water to reduce the risk of choking.
- Take drug before 6 PM to avoid nighttime sleep disturbance.
- Avoid alcohol and over-the-counter drugs, including nose drops, cold remedies; some over-the-counter drugs could cause dangerous effects.
- You may experience these side effects: Nervousness, restlessness, dizziness, insomnia, impaired thinking (may lessen over time; avoid driving or engaging in activities that require alertness); headache; loss of appetite; dry mouth.
- Avoid heating pads, electric blankets if wearing the transdermal patch; heat will alter drug's effects.
- Keep drug in secure place; do not share with others; upon removing the transdermal patch, fold patch so adhesive sides stick together and discard in a container with a lid.
- Report nervousness, insomnia, palpitations, vomiting, rash, fever, chest pain.

M

▽ **methylPREDNISolone**
(meth ill pred niss' oh lone)

methylPREDNISolone
Oral: Medrol

methylPREDNISolone acetate
IM injection: Depo-Medrol

methylPREDNISolone sodium succinate
IV, IM injection: A-Methapred, Solu-Medrol

PREGNANCY CATEGORY C

Drug classes
Corticosteroid
Glucocorticoid
Hormone

Therapeutic actions
Enters target cells and binds to intracellular corticosteroid receptors, initiating many complex reactions that are responsible for its anti-inflammatory and immunosuppressive effects.

Indications
- Short-term management of various inflammatory and allergic disorders, such as rheumatoid arthritis, collagen diseases (eg, SLE), dermatologic diseases (eg, pemphigus), status asthmaticus, and autoimmune disorders (eg, MS)
- Hematologic disorders: Thrombocytopenia purpura, erythroblastopenia
- Ulcerative colitis, acute exacerbations of MS, and palliation in some leukemias and lymphomas
- Trichinosis with neurologic or myocardial involvement
- Prevention of nausea and vomiting associated with chemotherapy
- Unlabeled uses: Septic shock, RDS, acute spinal cord injury, postherpetic neuralgia, nausea and vomiting of pregnancy.

Contraindications and cautions
- Contraindicated with infections, especially TB, fungal infections, amebiasis, vaccinia

and varicella, and antibiotic-resistant infections; lactation.
- Administration of live vaccines is contraindicated in patients receiving immunosuppressive doses.
- Use cautiously with kidney or liver disease, hypothyroidism, ulcerative colitis with impending perforation, diverticulitis, active or latent peptic ulcer, inflammatory bowel disease, heart failure, hypertension, thromboembolic disorders, osteoporosis, seizure disorders, diabetes mellitus, pregnancy.

Available forms
Tablets—2, 4, 8, 16, 24, 32 mg; powder for injection—40, 125, 500 mg/vial; 1, 2 g/vial; suspension for injection—20, 40, 80 mg/mL

Dosages
Adults
Individualize dosage, depending on severity and response. Give daily dose before 9 AM to minimize adrenal suppression. For maintenance, reduce initial dose in small increments at intervals until the lowest satisfactory clinical dose is reached. If long-term therapy is needed, consider alternate-day therapy with a short-acting corticosteroid. After long-term therapy, withdraw drug slowly to prevent adrenal insufficiency.
Oral
4–48 mg/day. For alternate-day therapy, give twice the usual dose every other morning.
IV, IM
10–40 mg IV administered over several min. Give subsequent doses IV or IM.
- *High-dose therapy:* 30 mg/kg IV infused over 10–30 min; may repeat every 4–6 hr but not longer than 72 hr.
- ⊗ *Warning* Rapid IV administration of large doses (more than 0.5–1 g in less than 10 min) has caused serious cardiac complications.

Methylprednisolone acetate
- *Rheumatoid arthritis, maintenance:* 40–120 mg IM weekly.
- *Adrenogenital syndrome:* 40 mg IM every 2 wk.
- *Dermatologic lesions:* 40–120 mg IM weekly for 1–4 wk.
- *Asthma and allergic rhinitis:* 80–120 mg IM.
- *Intralesional:* 20–60 mg.

- *Intra-articular dose depends on site of injection:* 4–10 mg (small); 10–40 mg (medium); 20–80 mg (large joints).

Pediatric patients
Individualize dosage on the basis of severity and response rather than by formulas of correct doses for age or weight. Carefully observe growth and development in infants and children on prolonged therapy. Minimum dose of methylprednisolone is 0.5 mg/kg per 24 hr.

Pharmacokinetics

Route	Onset	Peak	Duration
Oral	Varies	1–2 hr	1.2–1.5 days
IV	Rapid	Rapid	Unknown
IM	8–12 hr	Unknown	4–8 days

Metabolism: Hepatic; $T_{1/2}$: 78–188 min
Distribution: Crosses placenta; enters breast milk
Excretion: Urine

▼ IV FACTS

Preparation: No additional preparation is required.
Infusion: Inject directly into vein or into tubing of running IV; administer slowly, over at least 30 min, to reduce cardiac effects. Acetate form should not be given IV.
Incompatibilities: Do not combine with allopurinol, calcium gluconate, ciprofloxacin, docetaxel, etoposide, filgrastim, gemcitabine, glycopyrrolate, insulin, nafcillin, ondansetron, paclitaxel, penicillin G sodium, propofol, sargramostim, tetracycline, vinorelbine.

Adverse effects
Effects depend on dosage, route, and duration of therapy.

- **CNS:** *Vertigo, headache,* paresthesias, insomnia, seizures, psychosis, cataracts, increased IOP, glaucoma
- **CV:** Hypotension, **shock,** hypertension and heart failure secondary to fluid retention, thromboembolism, thrombophlebitis, fat embolism, cardiac arrhythmias
- **Electrolyte imbalance:** *Na+ and fluid retention,* hypokalemia, hypocalcemia
- **Endocrine:** Amenorrhea, irregular menses, growth retardation, decreased carbohydrate tolerance, diabetes mellitus, cushingoid state

(long-term effect), increased blood sugar, increased serum cholesterol, decreased T_3 and T_4 levels, HPA suppression with systemic therapy longer than 5 days

- **GI:** Peptic or esophageal ulcer, pancreatitis, abdominal distention, nausea, vomiting, *increased appetite, weight gain*
- **Hypersensitivity:** Anaphylactoid reactions
- **Musculoskeletal:** Muscle weakness, steroid myopathy, loss of muscle mass, osteoporosis, spontaneous fractures
- **Other:** *Immunosuppression; aggravation or masking of infections; impaired wound healing;* thin, fragile skin; petechiae, ecchymoses, purpura, striae; subcutaneous fat atrophy

Interactions
✳ **Drug-drug** • Increased therapeutic and toxic effects with erythromycin, azole antifungals, troleandomycin • Risk of severe deterioration of muscle strength when given to myasthenia gravis patients who are receiving ambenonium, edrophonium, neostigmine, pyridostigmine • Decreased steroid blood levels with barbiturates, phenytoin, rifampin • Decreased effectiveness of salicylates

✳ **Drug-lab test** • False-negative nitrobluetetrazolium test for bacterial infection • Suppression of skin test reactions

■ Nursing considerations
Assessment

- **History:** Infections; recent vaccinations; kidney or liver disease, hypothyroidism, ulcerative colitis, diverticulitis, active or latent peptic ulcer, inflammatory bowel disease, heart failure, hypertension, thromboembolic disorders, osteoporosis, seizure disorders, diabetes mellitus; pregnancy; lactation
- **Physical:** Weight, T, reflexes and grip strength, affect and orientation, P, BP, peripheral perfusion prominence of superficial veins, R and adventitious sounds, serum electrolytes, blood glucose

Interventions

- Use caution with the 24-mg tablets marketed as *Medrol;* these contain tartrazine, which may cause allergic reactions, especially in people who are allergic to aspirin.
- Give daily dose before 9 AM to mimic normal peak corticosteroid blood levels.

M

- Monitor glucose levels with prolonged therapy; dietary adjustments may be needed.
- Increase dosage when patient is subject to stress.

⊗ **Warning** Taper doses when discontinuing high-dose or long-term therapy to allow adrenal recovery.

⊗ **Warning** Do not give live-virus vaccines with immunosuppressive doses of corticosteroids.

⊗ **Warning** Some injectable products contain benzyl alcohol. Do not administer them to neonates or inject intrathecally.

Teaching points
- Do not stop taking the oral drug without consulting your health care provider.
- Avoid exposure to infections.
- Report unusual weight gain, swelling of the extremities, muscle weakness, black or tarry stools, fever, prolonged sore throat, colds or other infections, worsening of disorder.

▽**metoclopramide**

*(met oh kloe **pra'** mide)*

Apo-Metoclop (CAN), Metozolv ODT, Nu-Metoclopramide (CAN), Reglan

PREGNANCY CATEGORY B

Drug classes
Antiemetic
Dopaminergic blocker
GI stimulant

Therapeutic actions
Stimulates motility of upper GI tract without stimulating gastric, biliary, or pancreatic secretions; appears to sensitize tissues to action of acetylcholine; relaxes pyloric sphincter, which, when combined with effects on motility, accelerates gastric emptying and intestinal transit; little effect on gallbladder or colon motility; increases lower esophageal sphincter pressure; has sedative properties; induces release of prolactin.

Indications
- Relief of symptoms of acute and recurrent diabetic gastroparesis
- Short-term therapy (4–12 wk) for adults with symptomatic gastroesophageal reflux who fail to respond to conventional therapy

- Parenteral: Prevention of nausea and vomiting associated with emetogenic cancer chemotherapy
- Prophylaxis of postoperative nausea and vomiting when nasogastric suction is undesirable
- Single-dose parenteral use: Facilitation of small-bowel intubation when tube does not pass the pylorus with conventional maneuvers
- Single-dose parenteral use: Stimulation of gastric emptying and intestinal transit of barium when delayed emptying interferes with radiologic examination of the stomach or small intestine
- Unlabeled uses: Improvement of lactation (doses of 30–45 mg/day); treatment of nausea and vomiting of a variety of etiologies; adjunctive therapy for migraines, gastric bezoars, gastroparesis, hiccoughs, Tourette syndrome

Contraindications and cautions
- Contraindicated with allergy to metoclopramide; GI hemorrhage, mechanical obstruction or perforation; pheochromocytoma (may cause hypertensive crisis); epilepsy.
- Use cautiously with previously detected breast cancer (one-third of such tumors are prolactin dependent); lactation, pregnancy; fluid overload; renal impairment.

Available forms
Tablets—5, 10 mg; oral solution (syrup)—1 mg/mL; injection—5 mg/mL; orally disintegrating tablets—5, 10 mg

Dosages
Adults
- *Relief of symptoms of gastroparesis:* 10 mg PO 30 min before each meal and at bedtime for 2–8 wk. If symptoms are severe, initiate therapy with 10 mg IM or IV administration for up to 10 days until symptoms subside.
- *Symptomatic gastroesophageal reflux:* 10–15 mg PO up to four times/day 30 min before meals and at bedtime. If symptoms occur only at certain times or in relation to specific stimuli, single doses of 20 mg may be preferable; guide therapy by endoscopic results. Do not use longer than 12 wk.
- *Prevention of postoperative nausea and vomiting:* 10–20 mg IM at the end of surgery.

- *Prevention of chemotherapy-induced emesis:* Dilute and give by IV infusion over at least 15 min. Give first dose 30 min before chemotherapy; repeat every 2 hr for two doses, then every 3 hr for three doses. The initial two doses should be 2 mg/kg for highly emetogenic drugs (cisplatin, dacarbazine); 1 mg/kg may suffice for other chemotherapeutic drugs. If extrapyramidal symptoms occur, administer 50 mg of diphenhydramine IM.
- *Facilitation of small bowel intubation, gastric emptying:* 10 mg (2 mL) by direct IV injection over 1–2 min.

Pediatric patients

- *Facilitation of intubation, gastric emptying:*
Younger than 6 yr: 0.1 mg/kg by direct IV injection over 1–2 min.
6–14 yr: 2.5–5 mg by direct IV injection over 1–2 min.

Pharmacokinetics

Route	Onset	Peak	Duration
Oral	30–60 min	60–90 min	1–2 hr
IM	10–15 min	60–90 min	1–2 hr
IV	1–3 min	60–90 min	1–2 hr

Metabolism: Hepatic; $T_{1/2}$: 5–6 hr
Distribution: Crosses placenta; enters breast milk
Excretion: Urine

▼ IV FACTS

Preparation: Dilute dose in 50 mL of a parenteral solution (D_5W, sodium chloride injection, dextrose 5% in 0.45% sodium chloride, Ringer injection, or lactated Ringer injection). May be stored for up to 48 hr if protected from light or up to 24 hr under normal light.
Infusion: Give direct IV doses slowly (over 1–2 min); give infusions over at least 15 min.
Incompatibilities: Do not mix with solutions containing chloramphenicol, sodium bicarbonate, cisplatin, erythromycin.
Y-site incompatibilities: Do not give with allopurinol, furosemide, cefepime.

Adverse effects

- **CNS:** *Restlessness, drowsiness, fatigue, lassitude,* insomnia, *extrapyramidal reactions,* parkinsonism-like reactions, akathisia, dystonia, myoclonus, dizziness, anxiety
- **CV:** Transient hypertension
- **GI:** *Nausea, diarrhea*

Interactions

＊**Drug-drug** • Decreased absorption of digoxin from the stomach • Increased toxic and immunosuppressive effects of cyclosporine • Increased neuromuscular blocking effects with succinylcholine

■ Nursing considerations
Assessment

- **History:** Allergy to metoclopramide, GI hemorrhage, mechanical obstruction or perforation, depression, pheochromocytoma, epilepsy, lactation, previously detected breast cancer
- **Physical:** Orientation, reflexes, affect; P, BP; bowel sounds, normal output; EEG

Interventions

⊗ **Black box warning** Long-term treatment has been associated with permanent tardive dyskinesia; the risk increases with patients older than 60 yr, especially women. Use the smallest dose possible; do not exceed 3-mo therapy.
- Monitor BP carefully during IV administration.
- Monitor for extrapyramidal reactions, and consult physician if they occur.
- Monitor patients with diabetes, arrange for alteration in insulin dose or timing if diabetic control is compromised by alterations in timing of food absorption.
⊗ **Warning** Keep diphenhydramine injection readily available in case extrapyramidal reactions occur (50 mg IM).
⊗ **Warning** Have phentolamine readily available in case of hypertensive crisis (most likely to occur with undiagnosed pheochromocytoma).
- A Medication Guide must be dispensed with this drug.

Teaching points

- Take this drug exactly as prescribed.
- Do not use alcohol, sleep remedies, or sedatives; serious sedation could occur.
- You may experience these side effects: Drowsiness, dizziness (do not drive or perform other tasks that require alertness);

restlessness, anxiety, depression, headache, insomnia (reversible); nausea, diarrhea.

• Report involuntary movement of the face, eyes, or limbs, severe depression, severe diarrhea.

▽ **metolazone**
(me **tole'** *a zone)*

Zaroxolyn

PREGNANCY CATEGORY B

Drug class
Thiazide-like diuretic

Therapeutic actions
Inhibits reabsorption of sodium and chloride in distal renal tubule, increasing excretion of sodium, chloride, and water by the kidneys.

Indications
• Treatment of salt and water retention, including edema of HF and renal disease, nephrotic syndrome, and diminished renal function
• Hypertension, as monotherapy or in combination with other antihypertensives
• Unlabeled uses: Osteoporosis, diabetes insipidus

Contraindications and cautions
• Contraindicated with hypersensitivity to thiazides, hepatic coma, fluid or electrolyte imbalances, renal or liver disease, sulfonamide derivatives.
• Use cautiously with gout, SLE, glucose tolerance abnormalities, hyperparathyroidism, bipolar disorder, lactation, pregnancy.

Available forms
Tablets: 2.5, 5, 10 mg

Dosages
Adults
• *Hypertension:* 2.5–5 mg daily PO.
• *Edema of renal disease or HF:* 5–20 mg daily PO.
Pediatric patients
Not recommended.

Pharmacokinetics

Route	Onset	Peak	Duration
Oral	1 hr	8 hr	12–24 hr

Metabolism: Hepatic; $T_{1/2}$: 8–14 hr
Distribution: Crosses placenta; may enter breast milk
Excretion: Urine

Adverse effects
• **CNS:** *Dizziness, vertigo,* paresthesias, weakness, *headache,* drowsiness, *fatigue*
• **CV:** Orthostatic hypotension, venous thrombosis, volume depletion, cardiac arrhythmias, chest pain
• **Dermatologic:** Photosensitivity, rash, purpura, exfoliative dermatitis
• **GI:** *Nausea, anorexia, vomiting, dry mouth, diarrhea, constipation,* jaundice, hepatitis, pancreatitis
• **GU:** *Polyuria, nocturia, impotence,* decreased libido
• **Hematologic:** Leukopenia, thrombocytopenia, neutropenia, agranulocytosis, aplastic anemia, fluid and electrolyte imbalances
• **Other:** Muscle cramps and muscle spasms, fever, hives, gouty attacks, flushing

Interactions
✳ **Drug-drug** • Increased thiazide effects and chance of acute hyperglycemia with diazoxide • Decreased absorption with cholestyramine, colestipol • Increased risk of cardiac glycoside toxicity if hypokalemia occurs • Increased risk of lithium toxicity • Increased dosage of antidiabetics may be needed • Increased risk of severe hypokalemia with dofetilide; combination is contraindicated
✳ **Drug-lab test** • Decreased PBI levels without clinical signs of thyroid disturbances

■ Nursing considerations
Assessment
• **History:** Fluid or electrolyte imbalances, renal or liver disease, gout, SLE, glucose tolerance abnormalities, hyperparathyroidism, bipolar disorder, hepatic coma or precoma, lactation, pregnancy
• **Physical:** Skin color and lesions; orientation, reflexes, muscle strength; pulses, BP, orthostatic BP, perfusion, edema, baseline ECG; R, adventitious sounds; liver

evaluation, bowel sounds; CBC, serum electrolytes, blood glucose, LFTs, renal function tests, serum uric acid, urinalysis

Interventions
⊗ **Warning** Do not interchange *Zaroxolyn* with other formulations; they are not therapeutically equivalent.
⊗ **Warning** Withdraw drug 2–3 days before elective surgery; for emergency surgery, reduce dosage of preanesthetic or anesthetic.
• Give with food or milk if GI upset occurs.
• Measure and record body weight to monitor fluid changes.

Teaching points
• Take drug early in the day so sleep will not be disturbed by increased urination.
• Weigh yourself daily and record weights.
• Protect skin from the sun and bright lights.
• You may experience these side effects: Increased urination; dizziness, drowsiness, feeling faint (use caution; avoid driving or operating dangerous machinery); headache.
• Report rapid weight change, swelling in ankles or fingers, unusual bleeding or bruising, muscle cramps.

DANGEROUS DRUG

▷ **metoprolol**
(me toe' proe lole)

metoprolol
Apo-Metoprolol SR (CAN) ☉,
Gen-Metoprolol (CAN),
Lopressor, Novo-Metoprol (CAN),
Nu-Metop (CAN)

metoprolol succinate
Toprol-XL ☉

metoprolol tartrate
Apo-Metoprolol (CAN),
Lopressor Injection,
PMS-Metoprolol-L (CAN)

PREGNANCY CATEGORY C

Drug classes
Antihypertensive
Beta₁-selective adrenergic blocker

Therapeutic actions
Competitively blocks beta-adrenergic receptors in the heart and juxtaglomerular apparatus, decreasing the influence of the sympathetic nervous system on these tissues and the excitability of the heart, decreasing cardiac output and the release of renin, and lowering BP; acts in the CNS to reduce sympathetic outflow and vasoconstrictor tone.

Indications
• Hypertension, alone or with other drugs, especially diuretics
• Immediate-release tablets and injection: Prevention of reinfarction in MI patients who are hemodynamically stable or within 3–10 days of the acute MI
• Long-term treatment of angina pectoris
• ER forms only: Treatment of stable, symptomatic heart failure of ischemic, hypertensive, or cardiomyopathic origin
• Unlabeled uses: Adult migraine, pediatric hypertension

Contraindications and cautions
• Contraindicated with sinus bradycardia (HR less than 45 beats/min), second- or third-degree heart block (PR interval more than 0.24 sec), cardiogenic shock, HF, second and third trimesters of pregnancy.
• Use cautiously with diabetes or thyrotoxicosis; asthma or COPD; pregnancy.

Available forms
Tablets—25, 50, 100 mg; ER tablets ☉—25, 50, 100, 200 mg; injection—1 mg/mL

Dosages
Adults
• *Hypertension:* Initially, 100 mg/day PO in single or divided doses; gradually increase dosage at weekly intervals. Usual maintenance dose is 100–450 mg/day.
• *Angina pectoris:* Initially, 100 mg/day PO in two divided doses; may be increased gradually, effective range, 100–400 mg/day.
• *MI, early treatment:* Three IV bolus doses of 5 mg each at 2-min intervals with careful monitoring. If these are tolerated, give 50 mg PO 15 min after the last IV dose and every 6 hr for 48 hr. Thereafter, give a maintenance dose of 100 mg PO bid. Reduce initial PO doses to 25 mg, or discontinue in patients who do not tolerate the IV doses.

- *MI, late treatment:* 100 mg PO bid as soon as possible after infarct, continuing for at least 3 mo and possibly for 1–3 yr.

ER tablets

- *Hypertension:* 25–100 mg/day PO as one dose; may increase at weekly intervals to a maximum of 400 mg/day.
- *Angina:* 100 mg/day PO as one dose.
- *HF:* 12.5–25 mg/day ER tablets for 2 wk; may then be increased by 25 mg every 2 wk to a maximum of 200 mg.

Pediatric patients

Safety and efficacy not established.

Pharmacokinetics

Route	Onset	Peak	Duration
Oral	15 min	90 min	Varies
IV	Immediate	60–90 min	15–19 hr

Metabolism: Hepatic; $T_{1/2}$: 3–4 hr
Distribution: Crosses placenta; enters breast milk
Excretion: Urine

▼ IV FACTS

Preparation: No additional preparation is required.
Infusion: Inject directly into vein or into tubing of running IV over 1 min. Inject as a bolus; monitor carefully; wait 2 min between doses; do not give if bradycardia is less than 45 beats/min, heart block, systolic pressure less than 100 mm Hg.
Incompatibilities: Do not mix with amino acids, amphotericin B complex, aztreonam, dopamine.

Adverse effects

- **Allergic:** Pharyngitis, erythematous rash, fever, sore throat, **laryngospasm**
- **CNS:** Dizziness, vertigo, tinnitus, fatigue, emotional depression, paresthesias, sleep disturbances, hallucinations, disorientation, memory loss, slurred speech
- **CV:** *Heart failure, cardiac arrhythmias,* peripheral vascular insufficiency, claudication, **stroke,** pulmonary edema, hypotension
- **Dermatologic:** Rash, pruritus, sweating, dry skin, worsening of psoriasis
- **EENT:** Eye irritation, dry eyes, conjunctivitis, blurred vision

- **GI:** *Gastric pain, flatulence, constipation, diarrhea, nausea, vomiting,* anorexia, ischemic colitis, renal and mesenteric arterial thrombosis, retroperitoneal fibrosis, hepatomegaly, acute pancreatitis
- **GU:** *Impotence, decreased libido,* dysuria, Peyronie disease, nocturia, frequent urination
- **Musculoskeletal:** Joint pain, arthralgia, muscle cramp
- **Respiratory: Bronchospasm,** dyspnea, cough, bronchial obstruction, nasal stuffiness, rhinitis, pharyngitis
- **Other:** *Decreased exercise tolerance, development of ANA,* hyperglycemia or hypoglycemia, elevated serum transaminase, alkaline phosphatase

Interactions

✳ **Drug-drug** • Increased effects of metoprolol with verapamil, cimetidine, methimazole, propylthiouracil • Increased effects of both drugs if metoprolol is taken with hydralazine • Increased serum levels and toxicity of IV lidocaine, if given concurrently • Increased risk of orthostatic hypotension with prazosin • Decreased antihypertensive effects if taken with NSAIDs, clonidine, rifampin • Decreased therapeutic effects with barbiturates • Hypertension followed by severe bradycardia if given concurrently with epinephrine

✳ **Drug-lab test** • Possible false results with glucose or insulin tolerance tests (oral)

■ Nursing considerations

Assessment

- **History:** Sinus bradycardia (HR less than 45 beats/min), second- or third-degree heart block (PR interval greater than 0.24 sec), cardiogenic shock, heart failure, systolic BP less than 100 mm Hg; diabetes or thyrotoxicosis; asthma or COPD; lactation, pregnancy
- **Physical:** Weight, skin condition, neurologic status, P, BP, ECG, respiratory status, renal and thyroid function tests, blood and urine glucose

Interventions

⊗ *Black box warning* Do not discontinue drug abruptly after long-term therapy (hypersensitivity to catecholamines may have developed, causing exacerbation of angina, MI, and ventricular arrhythmias). Taper drug gradually over 2 wk with monitoring.

Adverse effects in italics *are most common; those in* **bold** *are life-threatening.* ⬛ Do not crush.

⊗ **Black box warning** Patients with bronchospastic diseases should not, in general, receive beta blockers. Use only in patients who do not respond to or cannot tolerate other antihypertensives; use with caution.

- Ensure that patient swallows the ER tablets whole; do not cut, crush, or chew. *Toprol XL* tablets may be divided at the score; divided tablets should be swallowed whole, not crushed or chewed.
- Consult physician about withdrawing drug if patient is to undergo surgery (controversial).
- Give oral drug with food to facilitate absorption.
- Provide continual cardiac monitoring for patients receiving IV metoprolol.

Teaching points
- Do not stop taking this drug unless instructed to do so by your health care provider.
- Swallow the extended-release tablets whole; do not cut, crush, or chew. If using ER tablets, you can divide the tablets at the score; divided tablets must be swallowed whole, not crushed or chewed.
- You may experience these side effects: Dizziness, drowsiness, light-headedness, blurred vision (avoid driving or dangerous activities); nausea, loss of appetite (eat frequent small meals); nightmares, depression (discuss change of medication); sexual impotence.
- Report difficulty breathing, night cough, swelling of extremities, slow pulse, confusion, depression, rash, fever, sore throat.

▽**metronidazole**
*(me troe **ni' da** zole)*

Apo-Metronidazole (CAN), Flagyl, Flagyl 375, Flagyl ER, MetroCream, MetroGel, MetroGel-Vaginal, MetroLotion, NidaGel (CAN), Noritate, Protostat, Vandazole

PREGNANCY CATEGORY B

Drug classes
Amebicide
Antibacterial
Antibiotic
Antiprotozoal

Therapeutic actions
Bactericidal: Inhibits DNA synthesis in specific (obligate) anaerobes, causing cell death; antiprotozoal-trichomonacidal, amebicidal: Biochemical mechanism of action is not known.

Indications
- Acute infection with susceptible anaerobic bacteria
- Acute intestinal amebiasis
- Amebic liver abscess
- Trichomoniasis (acute and partners of patients with acute infection)
- Bacterial vaginosis
- Preoperative, intraoperative, postoperative prophylaxis for patients undergoing colorectal surgery
- Topical application: Treatment of inflammatory papules, pustules, and erythema of rosacea
- Unlabeled uses: Prophylaxis for patients undergoing gynecologic, abdominal surgery; hepatic encephalopathy; Crohn disease; antibiotic-associated pseudomembranous colitis; treatment of *Gardnerella vaginalis,* giardiasis (use recommended by the CDC); infected decubitus ulcers; perioral dermatitis

Contraindications and cautions.
- Contraindicated with hypersensitivity to metronidazole; pregnancy (do not use for trichomoniasis in first trimester).
- Use cautiously with CNS diseases, hepatic disease, candidiasis (moniliasis), blood dyscrasias, lactation.

Available forms
Tablets—250, 500 mg; ER tablets—750 mg; capsules—375 mg; injection—500 mg/100 mL; lotion, cream, gel—0.75%; cream, gel—1%; vaginal gel—0.75%

Dosages
Adults
Oral
- *Amebiasis:* 750 mg PO tid for 5–10 days. (In amebic dysentery, combine with iodoquinol 650 mg PO tid for 20 days.)
- *Antibiotic-associated pseudomembranous colitis:* 1–2 g/day PO in 3–4 divided doses for 7–10 days.
- *Gardnerella vaginalis:* 500 mg PO bid for 7 days.

M

- *Giardiasis:* 250 mg PO tid for 7 days.
- *Trichomoniasis:* 2 g PO in 1 day (1-day treatment) *or* 250 mg PO tid for 7 days.
- *Bacterial vaginosis:*
  Nonpregnant women: 750 mg PO daily for 7 days.
  Pregnant women: 750 mg PO once daily for 7 days; avoid treatment in the first trimester.

IV
- *Anaerobic bacterial infection:* 15 mg/kg IV infused over 1 hr; then 7.5 mg/kg infused over 1 hr every 6 hr for 7–10 days, not to exceed 4 g/day.
- *Prophylaxis:* 15 mg/kg infused IV over 30–60 min and completed about 1 hr before surgery. Then 7.5 mg/kg infused over 30–60 min at 6- to 12-hr intervals after initial dose during the day of surgery only.

Topical (MetroGel)
- *Treatment of inflammatory papules, pustules, and erythema of rosacea:* Apply and rub in a thin film twice daily, morning and evening, to entire affected areas after washing; results should be seen within 3 wk; treatment through 9 wk has been effective.

Vaginal (MetroGel-Vaginal)
- *Nonpregnant women:* 1 applicatorful intravaginally one to two times/day for 5 days.

Pediatric patients
- *Anaerobic bacterial infection:* Not recommended.
- *Amebiasis:* 35–50 mg/kg/day PO in three divided doses for 10 days.

Pharmacokinetics

Route	Onset	Peak
Oral	Varies	1–2 hr
IV	Rapid	1–2 hr

Metabolism: Hepatic; $T_{1/2}$: 6–8 hr
Distribution: Crosses placenta; enters breast milk
Excretion: Feces, urine

▼ IV FACTS

Preparation: Reconstitute by adding 4.4 mL of sterile water for injection, bacteriostatic water for injection, 0.9% sodium chloride injection, or bacteriostatic 0.9% sodium chloride injection to the vial and mix thoroughly. Resultant volume is 5 mL with a concentration of 100 mg/mL. Solution should be clear to pale yellow to yellow-green; do not use if cloudy or contains precipitates; use within 24 hr; protect from light. Add reconstituted solution to glass or plastic container containing 0.9% sodium chloride injection, 5% dextrose injection or lactated Ringer to a final concentration of 8 mg/mL or less before administering; discontinue other solutions while running metronidazole.

Infusion: Before administration, add 5 mEq sodium bicarbonate injection for each 500 mg used (if not using premixed bags); mix thoroughly. Do not refrigerate neutralized solution. Do not administer solution that has not been neutralized. Infuse over 1 hr.

Adverse effects

- **CNS:** *Headache, dizziness, ataxia,* vertigo, incoordination, insomnia, seizures, peripheral neuropathy, fatigue
- **GI:** *Unpleasant metallic taste, anorexia, nausea, vomiting, diarrhea,* GI upset, cramps
- **GU:** Dysuria, incontinence, *darkening of the urine*
- **Local:** Thrombophlebitis (IV); *redness, burning, dryness,* and *skin irritation* (topical)
- **Other:** Severe, disulfiram-like interaction with alcohol, candidiasis (superinfection)

Interactions

✳ **Drug-drug** ● Decreased effectiveness with barbiturates ● Disulfiram-like reaction (flushing, tachycardia, nausea, vomiting) with alcohol ● Psychosis if taken with disulfiram ● Increased bleeding tendencies with oral anticoagulants

✳ **Drug-lab test** ● False-low (or zero) values in AST, ALT, LDH, triglycerides, hexokinase glucose tests

■ Nursing considerations
Assessment

- **History:** CNS or hepatic disease, candidiasis (moniliasis), blood dyscrasias, pregnancy, lactation
- **Physical:** Reflexes; affect; skin lesions; color (with topical application); abdominal examination, liver palpation; urinalysis, CBC, LFTs

Interventions

⊗ *Black box warning* Avoid use unless needed. Metronidazole may be carcinogenic.

Adverse effects in *italics* are most common; those in **bold** are life-threatening. ⊂▣⊃ Do not crush.

- Administer oral doses with food.
- Apply topically (*MetroGel*) after cleansing the area. Advise patient that cosmetics may be used over the area after application.
- Reduce dosage in hepatic disease.

Teaching points
- Take full course of drug therapy; take the drug with food if GI upset occurs.
- Do not drink alcohol (beverages or preparations containing alcohol, cough syrups) for 24–72 hr of drug use; severe reactions may occur.
- Your urine may be a darker color than usual; this is expected.
- Refrain from sexual intercourse during treatment for trichomoniasis, unless partner wears a condom.
- Apply the topical preparation by cleansing the area and then rubbing a thin film into the affected area. Avoid contact with the eyes. Cosmetics may be applied to the area after medication is dry.
- You may experience these side effects: Dry mouth with strange metallic taste (frequent mouth care, sucking sugarless candies may help); nausea, vomiting, diarrhea (eat frequent small meals).
- Report severe GI upset, dizziness, unusual fatigue or weakness, fever, chills.

▽ **metyrosine**

See Appendix R, *Less commonly used drugs*.

DANGEROUS DRUG

▽ **mexiletine hydrochloride**

(*mex ill' i teen*)

Mexitil, Novo-Mexiletine (CAN)

PREGNANCY CATEGORY C

Drug class
Antiarrhythmic

Therapeutic actions
Type I antiarrhythmic: Decreases automaticity of ventricular cells by membrane stabilization.

Indications
- Treatment of documented life-threatening ventricular arrhythmias (use with lesser arrhythmias is not recommended)
- Unlabeled uses: Prophylactic use to decrease arrhythmias in acute phase of acute MI (mortality may not be affected); reduction of pain, dysesthesia, and paresthesia associated with diabetic neuropathy

Contraindications and cautions
- Contraindicated with allergy to mexiletine, cardiogenic shock, hypotension, second- or third-degree heart block (without artificial pacemaker), lactation.
- Use cautiously with hepatic disease, seizure disorders, hypotension, severe HF, pregnancy.

Available forms
Capsules—150, 200, 250 mg

Dosages
Adults
200 mg every 8 hr PO. Increase in 50- to 100-mg increments every 2–3 days until desired antiarrhythmic effect is obtained. Maximum dose, 1,200 mg/day PO. Rapid control, 400 mg loading dose, then 200 mg every 8 hr PO.
- *Transferring from other antiarrhythmics: Lidocaine:* Stop the lidocaine with the first dose of mexiletine; leave IV line open until adequate arrhythmia suppression is ensured. *Quinidine sulfate:* Initial dose of 200 mg 6–12 hr PO after the last dose of quinidine. *Procainamide:* Initial dose of 200 mg 3–6 hr PO after the last dose of procainamide. *Disopyramide:* 200 mg 6–12 hr PO after the last dose of disopyramide.

Pediatric patients
Safety and efficacy not established.

Pharmacokinetics

Route	Onset	Peak
Oral	0.5–2 hr	2–3 hr

Metabolism: Hepatic; $T_{1/2}$: 10–12 hr
Distribution: Crosses placenta; enters breast milk
Excretion: Urine

Adverse effects
- **CNS:** *Dizziness, light-headedness, headache,* fatigue, drowsiness, *tremors, coordination*

difficulties, visual disturbances, numbness, nervousness, *sleep difficulties*
- **CV:** *Cardiac arrhythmias, chest pain*
- **GI:** *Nausea, vomiting, heartburn,* abdominal pain, diarrhea, liver injury
- **Hematologic:** Positive ANA, thrombocytopenia, leukopenia
- **Respiratory:** *Dyspnea*
- **Other:** *Rash*

Interactions
✳ **Drug-drug** ● Decreased mexiletine levels with hydantoins and rifampin ● Increased theophylline levels and toxicity with mexiletine ● Increased mexiletine levels with propafenone

■ Nursing considerations
Assessment
- **History:** Allergy to mexiletine, HF, cardiogenic shock, hypotension, second- or third-degree heart block, hepatic disease, seizure disorders, lactation, pregnancy
- **Physical:** Weight; orientation, reflexes; P, BP, auscultation, ECG, edema; R, adventitious sounds; bowel sounds, liver evaluation; urinalysis, urine pH, CBC, electrolytes, LFTs, renal function tests

Interventions
⊗ **Black box warning** Reserve use for life-threatening arrhythmias; may have serious proarrhythmic effects.
- Monitor patient response carefully, especially when beginning therapy.
- Reduce dosage with hepatic failure.
⊗ **Warning** Monitor for safe and effective serum levels (0.5–2 mcg/mL).

Teaching points
- Take with food to reduce GI problems.
- Frequent monitoring of cardiac rhythm is needed.
- Do not stop taking this drug without consulting your health care provider.
- Return for regular follow-up visits to check your heart rhythm and to have blood tests.
- Do not change your diet. Maintain acidity level in urine. Discuss dietary change with your health care provider.
- You may experience these side effects: Drowsiness, dizziness, numbness, visual disturbances (avoid driving or working with dangerous machinery); nausea, vomiting,

heartburn (eat frequent small meals); diarrhea; headache; sleep disturbances.
- Report fever, chills, sore throat, excessive GI discomfort, chest pain, excessive tremors, numbness, lack of coordination, headache, sleep disturbances.

▽ micafungin sodium
*(mick ah **fun**' gin)*

Mycamine

PREGNANCY CATEGORY C

Drug classes
Antifungal
Echinocandin

Therapeutic actions
Inhibits the synthesis of components needed for the production of fungal cell walls, leading to cell death.

Indications
- Treatment of patients with esophageal candidiasis
- Prevention of *Candida* infections in patients undergoing hematopoietic stem cell transplantation
- Treatment of candidemia, acute disseminated candidiasis, *Candida* peritonitis and abscesses

Contraindications and cautions
- Contraindicated with known hypersensitivity to micafungin.
- Use cautiously with liver impairment, renal impairment, pregnancy, lactation.

Available forms
Powder for injection—50, 100 mg

Dosages
Adults
- *Treatment of esophageal candidiasis:* 150 mg/day by IV infusion over 1 hr for 10–30 days.
- *Prophylaxis of* Candida *infection:* 50 mg/day by IV infusion over 1 hr for about 19 days.
- *Treatment of* Candida *infections:* 100 mg/day IV infused over 1 hr for 10–47 days based on infection being treated.

Pharmacokinetics

Route	Onset	Peak
IV	Rapid	End of infusion

Metabolism: $T_{1/2}$: 14–17 hr
Distribution: May cross placenta; may pass into breast milk
Excretion: Feces, urine

▼ IV FACTS

Preparation: Reconstitute with 5 mL 0.9% sodium chloride without bacteriostatic agent to yield 10 mg/mL using sterile technique. Swirl to mix; do not shake vigorously. Solution should be clear with no particulate matter. Protect reconstituted solution from light. Further dilute in 100 mL 0.9% sodium chloride injection. Discard any unused solution. Store diluted solution at room temperature for up to 24 hr; diluted solution protected from light, is stable for 24 hr.
Infusion: Infuse over 1 hr; flush the tubing of any running IV with 0.9% sodium chloride injection before infusing micafungin.
Incompatibilites: Do not mix in solution with any other drug; has been shown to form precipitates with many commonly used drugs.

Adverse effects

- **CNS:** Delirium, *headache,* dizziness, somnolence
- **CV:** Arrhythmias, changes in BP, cyanosis
- **GI:** Nausea, abdominal pain, vomiting, elevated liver enzymes
- **Hematologic:** Leukopenia, neutropenia, thrombocytopenia, anemia, lymphopenia, **hemolytic anemia**
- **Other: Potentially serious hypersensitivity reaction,** rash, *phlebitis*

Interactions

✴ **Drug-drug** • Concentrations of sirolimus and nifedipine may increase when used with micafungin; monitor for toxicity

■ Nursing considerations
Assessment

- **History:** Hypersensitivity to micafungin, hepatic impairment, renal impairment, pregnancy, lactation
- **Physical:** Orientation, reflexes; abdominal examination; skin color, lesions; LFTs, renal function tests, CBC with differential

Interventions

- Establish baseline liver function, renal function, and CBC before beginning therapy.
- Use sterile technique in preparing solution for IV infusion, there are no bacteriostatic agents in the preparation.
- Monitor injection site for any sign of reaction or the development of phlebitis.
- Maintain life support equipment on hand when beginning therapy, potentially serious hypersensitivity reactions have been reported.
- Advise the use of contraceptives during therapy.
- If the patient is breast-feeding during therapy, suggest another method of feeding the infant.
- Provide comfort measures and possible analgesics for headache and pain.
- Encourage frequent small meals if GI effects are uncomfortable.

Teaching points

- You will receive *Mycamine* as a 1-hour IV infusion each day. If you are being treated for an infection, this will last 10–47 days depending on your response. If prevention of the infection is the goal of therapy, treatment will last for about 19 days.
- If you experience shortness of breath or difficulty breathing, consult your health care provider immediately.
- It is not known how this drug could affect a breast-feeding baby. If you are breast-feeding, another method of feeding the infant should be selected.
- It is not known how this drug could affect a fetus, if you are pregnant or decide to become pregnant while on this drug, consult your health care provider. Use of contraceptive measures is advised.
- You will need to have periodic blood tests to evaluate the effects of this drug on your body.
- You may experience these side effects: Headache (consult your health care provider, medication may be available to help); nausea, diarrhea (eating frequent small meals may help); dizziness (do not drive a car or operate hazardous machinery if this occurs).
- Report redness, pain or swelling at the IV site; changes in the color of urine or stool, rash, yellowing of the skin or eyes, difficulty breathing, increased bleeding or bruising.

M

▷ **miconazole nitrate**
*(mi **kon'** a zole)*

Topical: Breeze Mist Antifungal,
Fungoid Tincture, Lotrimin AF,
Micatin, Neosporin AF, Tetterine, Ting,
Triple Paste AF, Zeasorb-AF

Vaginal suppositories, topical:
Micozole (CAN), Monistat 1,
Monistat 1 Combination Pack,
Monistat 1 Vaginal Ovule, Monistat 3,
Monistat 3 Combination Pack,
Monistat 3 Vaginal Ovule (CAN),
Monistat 7, Monistat 7 Combination
Pack, Monistat/Day or Night
Buccal tablet: Oravig ⓞⓝⓒ

PREGNANCY CATEGORY B (TOPICAL)

PREGNANCY CATEGORY C (BUCCAL)

Drug class
Antifungal

Therapeutic actions
Fungicidal: Alters fungal cell membrane permeability, causing cell death; also may alter fungal cell DNA and RNA metabolism or cause accumulation of toxic peroxides intracellularly.

Indications
• Vaginal suppositories: Local treatment of vulvovaginal candidiasis (moniliasis)
• Topical administration: Tinea pedis, tinea cruris, tinea corporis caused by *Trichophyton rubrum, Trichophyton mentagrophytes, Epidermophyton floccosum;* cutaneous candidiasis (moniliasis), tinea versicolor
• Buccal tablets: Treatment of oropharyngeal candidiasis in adults and children 16 yr and older

Contraindications and cautions
• Contraindicated with allergy to miconazole or components, including milk protein concentrate (*Oravig*) used in preparation.
• Use cautiously with pregnancy, lactation.

Available forms
Vaginal suppositories—100, 200, 1,200 mg;
topical cream—2%; vaginal cream—2%;
topical powder—2%; topical spray—1%, 2%;

topical ointment—2%; spray powder or liquid—2%; solution—2%; buccal tablets ⓞⓝⓒ—50 mg

Dosages
Adults
Vaginal suppositories
• *Monistat 3:* Insert 1 suppository intravaginally once daily at bedtime for 3 days. *Monistat 7:* One applicator cream or 1 suppository in the vagina daily at bedtime for 7 days. Repeat course if needed. Alternatively, one 1,200-mg suppository at bedtime for 1 dose.
Topical
• *Cream and lotion:* Cover affected areas bid, morning and evening. Powder: Spray or sprinkle powder liberally over affected area in the morning and evening.
Buccal tablets
Apply 1 tablet (50 mg) to gum region once daily for 14 days.
Pediatric patients
Topical
2 yr and older: Use adult dosage.
Younger than 2 yr: Not recommended.

Pharmacokinetics

Route	Onset	Peak
Topical	Rapid	Unknown
Vaginal	Unknown	Unknown

Metabolism: Hepatic; $T_{1/2}$: 21–24 hr
Distribution: Crosses placenta; may enter breast milk
Excretion: Feces, urine

Adverse effects
Vaginal suppositories
• **Local:** *Irritation,* sensitization or vulvovaginal burning, pelvic cramps
• **Other:** Rash, headache
Topical application
• **Local:** *Irritation, burning, maceration,* allergic contact dermatitis
Buccal tablets
• **CNS:** Headache
• **GI:** Nausea, vomiting, diarrhea, abdominal pain, dysqeusa

■ **Nursing considerations**
Assessment
• **History:** Allergy to miconazole or components used in preparation; lactation, pregnancy

- **Physical:** Skin color, lesions, area around lesions; T; orientation, affect; culture of area involved

Interventions

- Culture fungus involved before therapy.
- Insert vaginal suppositories high into the vagina; have patient remain recumbent for 10–15 min after insertion; provide sanitary napkin to protect clothing from stains.
- Apply buccal tablet to gum area once daily; ensure that patient does not cut, crush, or chew tablet.
- Monitor response; if none is noted, arrange for further cultures to determine causative organism.
- Apply lotion to intertriginous areas if topical application is required; if cream is used, apply sparingly to avoid maceration of the area.
- Ensure patient receives the full course of therapy to eradicate the fungus and to prevent recurrence.

⊗ **Warning** Discontinue topical or vaginal administration if rash or sensitivity occurs.

Teaching points

- Take the full course of drug therapy even if symptoms improve. Continue during menstrual period even if vaginal route is being used. Long-term use will be needed; beneficial effects may not be seen for several weeks.
- Place buccal tablet in gum region once daily; do not cut, crush, or chew tablet.
- Insert vaginal suppositories high into the vagina.
- Use hygiene measures to prevent reinfection or spread of infection.
- This drug is for the fungus being treated; do not self-medicate other problems with this drug.
- Refrain from sexual intercourse, or advise partner to use a condom to avoid reinfection; with vaginal form of drug, use a sanitary napkin to prevent staining of clothing.
- Avoid pregnancy while using buccal tablets; contraceptive use is advised.
- You may experience these side effects: Irritation, burning, stinging.
- Report local irritation, burning (topical application); rash, irritation, pelvic pain (vaginal use).

▽**midazolam hydrochloride**
(mid ay' zoh lam)

Apo-Midazolam (CAN)

PREGNANCY CATEGORY D

CONTROLLED SUBSTANCE C-IV

Drug classes

Benzodiazepine (short-acting)
CNS depressant

Therapeutic actions

Exact mechanisms of action not understood; acts mainly at the limbic system and reticular formation; potentiates the effects of GABA, an inhibitory neurotransmitter; anxiolytic and amnesia effects occur at doses below those needed to cause sedation, ataxia; has little effect on cortical function.

Indications

- IV or IM: Sedation, anxiolysis, and amnesia prior to diagnostic, therapeutic, or endoscopic procedures or surgery
- Induction of general anesthesia
- Continuous sedation of intubated and mechanically ventilated patients as a component of anesthesia or during treatment in the critical care setting
- Unlabeled use: Treatment of epileptic seizure or refractory status epilepticus

Contraindications and cautions

- Contraindicated with hypersensitivity to benzodiazepines, allergy to cherries (syrup), psychoses, acute narrow-angle glaucoma, shock, coma, acute alcoholic intoxication, pregnancy (cleft lip or palate, inguinal hernia, cardiac defects, microcephaly, pyloric stenosis have been reported when used in first trimester; neonatal withdrawal syndrome reported in infants) and in neonates.
- Use cautiously in elderly or debilitated patients; in patients being treated for open-angle glaucoma; with impaired liver or renal function, lactation.

Available forms

Injection—5 mg/mL, 1 mg/mL, syrup—2 mg/mL

Dosages

⊗ **Black box warning** M i d a z o l a m
should only be administered by a person trained
in general anesthesia and with equipment for
maintaining airway and resuscitation on hand;
respiratory depression and respiratory arrest can
occur. Administer IV with continuous monitoring of respiratory and CV function. Individualize dosage; use lower dosage in the elderly and
debilitated patients. Adjust dosage according to
use of other premedication.

⊗ **Warning** Rapid injection should be avoided
in neonates, especially when given with fentanyl.

⊗ **Warning** Midazolam syrup has been associated with respiratory depression and arrest,
especially when given with opioids.

Adults

- *Preoperative sedation, anxiety, amnesia:*
  Younger than 60 yr: 70–80 mcg/kg IM
  1 hr before surgery (usual dose, 5 mg).
  Older than 60 yr or debilitated: 20–
  50 mcg/kg IM 1 hr before surgery (usual
  dose, 1–3 mg).
- *Conscious sedation for short procedures:*
  Younger than 60 yr: 1–2.5 mg IV initially, maintenance dose of 25% of initial dose;
  total dose, 5 mg.
  Older than 60 yr: 1–1.5 mg IV initially,
  maintenance dose of 25% initial dose; total
  dose, 3.5 mg.
- *Induction of anesthesia:*
  Younger than 55 yr: 300–350 mcg/kg IV
  (up to a total of 600 mcg/kg).
  Older than 55 yr: 150–300 mcg/kg IV as
  initial dose.
  Debilitated adults: 200–250 mcg/kg IV as
  initial dose.
- *Sedation in critical care areas:* 10–50
  mcg/kg (0.5–4 mg usual dose) as a loading dose; may repeat every 10–15 min until desired effect is seen; continuous infusion of 20–100 mcg/kg/hr to sustain effect.

Pediatric patients

- *Preoperative sedation, anxiety, amnesia:*
  6 mo–16 yr: 0.1–0.15 mg/kg IM; do not
  exceed 10 mg/dose.
- *Conscious sedation for short procedures:*
  Older than 12 yr: 1–2.5 mg IV initially,
  maintenance dose of 25% of initial dose.
- *Conscious sedation for short procedures*
  prior to anesthesia:
  6–12 yr: 25–50 mcg/kg IV initially. Up to
  400 mcg/kg may be used; do not exceed
  10 mg/dose.

6 mo–5 yr: 50–100 mcg/kg IV. Do not exceed 6 mg total dose.

- *Sedation in critical care areas for intubated patients only:* 50–200 mcg/kg IV as
  a loading dose, then continuous infusion of
  60–120 mcg/kg/hr.
  Neonates older than 32 wk gestation:
  60 mcg/kg/hr IV.
  Neonates younger than 32 wk gestation:
  30 mcg/kg/hr IV.

▼ IV FACTS

Preparation: Do not mix with other solutions; do not mix in plastic bags or tubing;
may be used undiluted or diluted in D_5W, 0.9%
normal saline, or lactated Ringer.

Infusion: Inject slowly into large vein over
2 min, monitoring patient response.

Y-site incompatibilities: Albumin, ampicillin, ceftazidime, cefuroxime, clonidine, dexamethasone, foscarnet, furosemide, hydrocortisone, methotrexate, nafcillin, omeprazole,
sodium bicarbonate.

Pharmacokinetics

Route	Onset	Peak	Duration
IM	15 min	30 min	2–6 hr
IV	3–5 min	Less than 30 min	2–6 hr

Metabolism: Hepatic metabolism; $T_{1/2}$:
1.8–6.8 hr

Distribution: Crosses placenta; enters breast
milk

Excretion: Urine

Adverse effects

- **CNS:** Transient and mild drowsiness (initially), sedation, depression, lethargy, apathy, fatigue, light-headedness, disorientation, restlessness, confusion, crying, delirium,
  headache, slurred speech, dysarthria, stupor,
  rigidity, tremor, dystonia, vertigo, euphoria,
  nervousness, difficulty in concentration, vivid
  dreams, psychomotor retardation, extrapyramidal symptoms, mild paradoxic excitatory reactions (during first 2 wk of treatment), visual and auditory disturbances,
  diplopia, nystagmus, depressed hearing,
  nasal congestion
- **CV:** Bradycardia, tachycardia, CV collapse,
  hypertension, hypotension, palpitations,
  edema

Adverse effects in italics are most common; those in bold are life-threatening. ⬛ Do not crush.

- **Dependence:** Drug dependence with withdrawal syndrome when drug is discontinued (more common with abrupt discontinuation of higher dosage used for longer than 4 mo)
- **Dermatologic:** Urticaria, pruritus, skin rash, dermatitis
- **GI:** Constipation, diarrhea, dry mouth, salivation, nausea, anorexia, vomiting, difficulty in swallowing, gastric disorders, elevations of blood enzymes: LDH, alkaline phosphatase, AST, ALT, hepatic impairment, jaundice
- **GU:** Incontinence, urine retention, changes in libido, menstrual irregularities
- **Hematologic:** Decreased Hct, blood dyscrasias
- **Other:** Phlebitis and thrombosis at IV injection sites, hiccups, fever, diaphoresis, paresthesias, muscular disturbances, gynecomastia; pain, burning, and redness after IM injection

Interactions
✳ **Drug-drug** • Risk of increased CNS depression if combined with alcohol, antihistamines, opioids, other sedatives; protease inhibitors, decrease midazolam dose by up to 50% if any of these combinations are used • Decreased effectiveness if given with carbamazepine, phenytoin, rifampin, rifabutin, phenobarbital; monitor patient's response carefully
✳ **Drug-food** • Decreased metabolism and increased effects of midazolam with grapefruit juice; avoid this combination

■ Nursing considerations
Assessment
- **History:** Hypersensitivity to benzodiazepines; psychoses, acute narrow-angle glaucoma, shock, coma, acute alcoholic intoxication with depression of vital signs; elderly or debilitated; impaired liver or renal function; pregnancy, lactation
- **Physical:** Weight; skin color, lesions; orientation, affect, reflexes, sensory nerve function, ophthalmologic examination; P, BP; R, adventitious sounds; bowel sounds, normal output, liver evaluation; normal output; LFTs, renal function tests, CBC

Interventions
⊗ **Warning** Do not administer intra-arterially, which may produce arteriospasm or gangrene.

- Do not use small veins (dorsum of hand or wrist) for IV injection.
- Administer IM injections deep into muscle.
- Monitor IV injection site for extravasation.
- Arrange to reduce dosage of midazolam if patient is also being given opioid analgesics; reduce dosage by at least 50% and monitor patient closely.
- Monitor level of consciousness before, during, and for at least 2–6 hr after administration of midazolam.
- Carefully monitor P, BP, and respirations carefully during administration.

⊗ **Warning** Keep resuscitative facilities readily available; have flumazenil available as antidote if overdose should occur.

- Keep patient in bed for 3 hr; do not permit ambulatory patients to operate a vehicle following an injection.
- Arrange to monitor liver and renal function and CBC at intervals during long-term therapy.
- Establish safety precautions if CNS changes occur (use side rails, accompany ambulating patient).
- Provide comfort measures and reassurance for patients receiving diazepam for tetanus.
- Arrange to taper dosage gradually after long-term therapy.
- Provide patient with written information regarding recovery and follow-up care. Midazolam is a potent amnesiac and memory may be altered.

Teaching points
- This drug will help you to relax and will make you go to sleep; this drug is a potent amnesiac and you will not remember what has happened to you.
- Avoid using alcohol or sleep-inducing or over-the-counter drugs before receiving this drug. If you feel that you need one of these preparations, consult your health care provider.
- You may experience these side effects: Drowsiness, dizziness (these may become less pronounced after a few days; avoid driving a car or engaging in other dangerous activities if these occur); GI upset; dreams, difficulty concentrating, fatigue, nervousness, crying (it may help to know that these are effects of the drug; consult your health care provider if these become bothersome).

M

- Report severe dizziness, weakness, drowsiness that persists, rash or skin lesions, visual or hearing disturbances, difficulty voiding.

▷ midodrine

See Appendix R, *Less commonly used drugs.*

▷ mifepristone (RU-486)

(miff eh **prist'** *own)*

Korlym, Mifeprex

PREGNANCY CATEGORY X

Drug class
Abortifacient

Therapeutic actions
Acts as an antagonist of progesterone sites in the endometrium, allowing prostaglandins to stimulate uterine contractions, causing implanted trophoblast to separate from the placental wall; may also decrease placental viability and accelerate degenerative changes resulting in sloughing of the endometrium.

Indications
- Termination of pregnancy through 49 days gestational age; most effective when combined with a prostaglandin (*Mifeprix*)
- ▰ **NEW INDICATION:** Control of hyperglycemia secondary to hypercortisolism in adults with endogenous Cushing syndrome who have type 2 diabetes or glucose intolerance and have failed or are not candidates for surgery (*Korlym*)
- Unlabeled uses: Postcoital contraception, endometriosis, unresectable meningioma, fetal death, or nonviable early pregnancy

Contraindications and cautions
- Contraindicated with allergy to prostaglandin preparations; acute PID; active cardiac, hepatic, pulmonary, renal disease; undiagnosed adrenal mass; hemorrhagic disorder, anticoagulation; ectopic pregnancy; and in patients with an IUD in place.
- Use cautiously with history of asthma; anemia, jaundice, diabetes, epilepsy, scarred uterus, cervicitis, infected endocervical lesions, acute vaginitis.

Available forms
Tablets—200, 300 mg

Dosages
Adults
- *Termination of pregnancy:* Day 1: 600 mg (3 tablets) PO taken as a single dose. Day 3: If termination of pregnancy cannot be confirmed, 400 mcg (2 tablets) misoprostol (*Cytotec*). Day 14: Evaluation for termination of pregnancy; if unsuccessful, surgical intervention is suggested at this time. (*Mifeprex*)
- *Control of hyperglycemia with Cushing syndrome:* 300 mg/day PO with a meal; may be titrated to a maximum 1,200 mg/day. (*Korlym*)

Pharmacokinetics

Route	Onset	Peak
Oral	Rapid	1–3 hr

Metabolism: Tissue; $T_{1/2}$: 18 hr
Distribution: Crosses placenta; may enter breast milk
Excretion: Feces, urine

Adverse effects
- **CNS:** *Headache,* dizziness
- **GI:** *Vomiting, diarrhea, nausea, abdominal pain*
- **GU:** Heavy uterine bleeding, endometritis, uterine or vaginal pain
- **Other: Potentially serious to fatal infection,** loss of pregnancy

Interactions
✳ **Drug-drug** • Contraindicated in combination with simvastatin, lovastatin, cyclosporine, dihydrate ergotamine, ergotamine, fentanyl, pimozide, quinidine, sirolimus, tacrolimus; increased risk of severe adverse effects • Contraindicated with systemic corticosteroids; autaconizes effects

■ Nursing considerations

CLINICAL ALERT!
Name confusion has occurred between mifepristone and misoprostol and between *Mifeprex* and *Mirapex* (pramipexole); use extreme caution.

Assessment
- **History:** Allergy to prostaglandin preparations; acute PID; active cardiac, hepatic, pulmonary, renal disease; history of asthma; hypotension; hypertension; CV, adrenal, renal, or hepatic disease; anemia; jaundice; diabetes; epilepsy; scarred uterus; cervicitis, infected endocervical lesions, acute vaginitis
- **Physical:** T; BP, P, auscultation; bowel sounds, liver evaluation; vaginal discharge, pelvic examination, uterine tone; LFTs, renal function tests, WBC count, urinalysis, CBC

Interventions
⊗ **Black box warning** Serious or fatal infection may develop after abortion. Monitor patient for sustained fever, prolonged heavy bleeding, severe abdominal pain. Urge patient to seek emergency medical help if these occur.
⊗ **Black box warning** Ensure patient is not pregnant before treatment and recheck if therapy is interrupted for 14 days or more when using *Korlym*; any pregnancy would be terminated by drug's effects.
- Provide appropriate referrals and counseling for abortion.
- Alert patient that menses usually begins within 5 days of treatment and lasts for 1–2 wk.
- Arrange to follow drug within 48 hr with a prostaglandin (*Cytotec*) as appropriate.
⊗ **Warning** Ensure that abortion is complete or that other measures are used to complete the abortion if drug effects are not sufficient.
- Prepare for dilation and curettage if heavy bleeding does not resolve.
- Provide analgesic and antiemetic as needed to increase comfort.
- Ensure patient follow-up; serious to fatal infections have been reported.
- Have patient using *Korlym* swallow tablet whole. Tablet should not be cut, crushed, or chewed.
- Monitor serum glucose and potassium levels carefully when treating hyperglycemia.

Teaching points
Teaching about mifepristone should be incorporated into the total teaching plan for the patient undergoing an abortion; specific information that should be included follows:
- Menses begin within 5 days of treatment and will last 1–2 weeks.
- If you are taking this drug to control your blood sugar, take it once a day with a meal.

Swallow the tablet whole; do not cut, crush, or chew it.
- If you are taking this drug to control your blood sugar, you will need to use contraceptives and ensure that you are not pregnant.
- This drug will cause termination of pregnancy.
- You may experience these side effects: Nausea, vomiting, diarrhea (medication may be ordered); uterine or vaginal pain, headache (an analgesic may be ordered).
- Be aware that another pregnancy could occur before normal menses begin; start contraception as soon as termination of pregnancy is confirmed and sexual intercourse is resumed.
- Report immediately sustained fever, severe abdominal pain, prolonged heavy bleeding, dizziness on arising, persistent malaise, uncontrolled blood sugar.

DANGEROUS DRUG
▷ **miglitol**
(*mig' lah tall*)
Glyset
PREGNANCY CATEGORY B

Drug classes
Alpha-glucosidase inhibitor
Antidiabetic

Therapeutic actions
An alpha-glucosidase inhibitor that delays the digestion of ingested carbohydrates, leading to a smaller increase in blood glucose following meals and a decrease in glycosylated Hgb; does not enhance insulin secretion and so its effects are additive to those of the sulfonylureas in controlling blood glucose.

Indications
- Adjunct to diet and exercise to lower blood glucose in patients with type 2 diabetes mellitus whose hyperglycemia cannot be managed by diet and exercise alone
- Combination therapy with a sulfonylurea to enhance glycemic control in those patients with type 2 diabetes who do not receive adequate control with diet and either drug

Contraindications and cautions

- Contraindicated with hypersensitivity to the drug; diabetic ketoacidosis; cirrhosis; inflammatory bowel disease; intestinal obstruction or predisposition to intestinal obstruction; colon ulceration; type 1 diabetes; conditions that would deteriorate with increased gas in the bowel.
- Use cautiously with renal impairment, pregnancy, lactation.

Available forms

Tablets—25, 50, 100 mg

Dosages

Adults

- *Monotherapy:* Initial dose, 25 mg PO tid at the first bite of each meal; may start at 25 mg PO daily if severe GI effects are seen. After 4–8 wk, start maintenance, 50 mg PO tid at first bite of each meal. Maximum dose, 100 mg PO tid.
- *Combination with a sulfonylurea:* Blood glucose may be much lower; monitor closely and adjust dosages of each drug accordingly.

Pediatric patients

Safety and efficacy not established.

Pharmacokinetics

Route	Onset	Peak
Oral	Rapid	2–3 hr

Metabolism: Not metabolized; $T_{1/2}$: 2 hr
Distribution: Very little
Excretion: Urine

Adverse effects

- **Dermatologic:** Rash
- **Endocrine:** *Hypoglycemia* (taken in combination with other antidiabetic drugs)
- **GI:** Abdominal pain, flatulence, diarrhea, anorexia, nausea, vomiting

Interactions

✳ **Drug-drug** • Decreased bioavailability and effectiveness of propranolol, ranitidine • Miglitol is less effective if taken with digestive enzymes or charcoal; avoid combining

✳ **Drug-alternative therapy** • Increased risk of hypoglycemia if taken with juniper berries, ginseng, garlic, fenugreek, coriander, dandelion root, celery

■ Nursing considerations

Assessment

- **History:** Hypersensitivity to the drug; diabetic ketoacidosis; cirrhosis; inflammatory bowel disease; intestinal obstruction or predisposition to intestinal obstruction; type 1 diabetes; conditions that would deteriorate with increased gas in the bowel; renal impairment; pregnancy; lactation
- **Physical:** Skin color, lesions; T; orientation, reflexes, peripheral sensation; R, adventitious sounds; liver evaluation, bowel sounds; urinalysis, BUN, blood glucose, renal function tests

Interventions

- Give drug tid with the first bite of each meal.
- Monitor serum glucose levels often to determine effectiveness of drug and dosage.
- Tell patient abdominal pain and flatulence are likely.
- Arrange for consult with dietitian to establish weight loss program and dietary control as appropriate. Plan thorough diabetic teaching program to include disease, dietary control, exercise, signs and symptoms of hypoglycemia and hyperglycemia, avoidance of infection, and hygiene.

Teaching points

- Do not discontinue this medication without consulting your health care provider.
- Take this drug three times a day with the first bite of each meal.
- Monitor blood for glucose as prescribed.
- Continue diet and exercise program established for control of diabetes.
- You may experience these side effects: Abdominal pain, flatulence, bloating.
- Report fever, sore throat, unusual bleeding or bruising, severe abdominal pain.

▽ **miglustat**

See Appendix R, *Less commonly used drugs.*

▽ **milnacipran**

See Appendix R, *Less commonly used drugs.*

DANGEROUS DRUG

▷**milrinone lactate**
(*mill' ri none*)

PREGNANCY CATEGORY C

Drug class
Inotropic

Therapeutic actions
Increases force of contraction of ventricles (positive inotropic effect); causes vasodilation by a direct relaxant effect on vascular smooth muscle.

Indications
• Heart failure: Short-term IV management of patients with acute decompensated heart failure

Contraindications and cautions
• Contraindicated with allergy to milrinone or bisulfites; severe aortic or pulmonic valvular disease.
• Use cautiously in the elderly, and with pregnancy, lactation.

Available forms
Injection—1 mg/mL; premixed injection—0.2 mg/mL

Dosages
Adults
Loading dose, 50 mcg/kg IV bolus, given over 10 min. Maintenance infusion, 0.375–0.75 mcg/kg/min. Do not exceed a total of 1.13 mg/kg/day.
Pediatric patients
Not recommended.
Patients with renal impairment
Do not exceed 1.13 mg/kg/day. For patients with renal impairment, refer to this table:

CrCl (mL/min)	Infusion Rate (mcg/kg/min)
5	0.2
10	0.23
20	0.28
30	0.33
40	0.38
50	0.43

Pharmacokinetics

Route	Onset	Peak	Duration
IV	Immediate	5–15 min	8 hr

Metabolism: Hepatic; T$_{1/2}$: 2.3–2.5 hr
Distribution: Crosses placenta; may enter breast milk
Excretion: Urine

▼ IV FACTS

Preparation: Add diluent of 0.45% or 0.9% sodium chloride injection, USP or 5% dextrose injection, USP. Add 180 mL per 20-mg vial to prepare solution of 100 mcg/mL; 113 mL per 20-mg vial to prepare a solution of 150 mcg/mL; add 80 mL diluent to 20-mg vial to prepare solution of 200 mcg/mL. Or, premixed infusion may be used without further dilution.
Infusion: Administer while carefully monitoring patient's hemodynamic and clinical response; see manufacturer's insert for detailed guidelines.
Incompatibility: Do not mix directly with other drugs. Furosemide should not be administered through same IV line because precipitate may form.

Adverse effects
• **CNS:** Headache
• **CV:** *Ventricular arrhythmias,* hypotension, supraventricular arrhythmias, chest pain, angina, **death**
• **Hematologic:** Thrombocytopenia, hypokalemia

Interactions
✳ **Drug-drug** • Precipitate formation in solution if given in the same IV line with furosemide; avoid this combination

■ **Nursing considerations**
Assessment
• **History:** Allergy to milrinone or bisulfites, severe aortic or pulmonic valvular disease, lactation, pregnancy
• **Physical:** Weight, orientation, P, BP, cardiac auscultation, peripheral pulses and perfusion, R, adventitious sounds, serum electrolyte levels, platelet count, ECG, renal function tests

M

Interventions

- Monitor cardiac rhythm continually.
- Monitor BP and P and reduce dose if marked decreases occur.
- Monitor I & O and electrolyte levels.

Teaching points

- You will need frequent monitoring of your blood pressure, pulse, and heart activity during therapy.
- You may experience increased voiding; appropriate bathroom arrangements will be made.
- Report pain at IV injection site, numbness or tingling, shortness of breath, chest pain.

▽ **minocycline hydrochloride**

(mi noe sye' kleen)

Apo-Minocycline (CAN), Arestin, Cleervue-M, Dynacin, Gen-Minocycline (CAN), Minocin, Myrac, ratio-Minocycline (CAN), Solodyn

PREGNANCY CATEGORY D

Drug classes

Antibiotic
Tetracycline

Therapeutic actions

Bacteriostatic: Inhibits protein synthesis of susceptible bacteria, causing cell death.

Indications

- Infections caused by rickettsiae; *Mycoplasma pneumoniae*; agents of psittacosis, ornithosis, lymphogranuloma venereum and granuloma inguinale; *Borrelia recurrentis; Haemophilus ducreyi; Pasteurella pestis; Pasteurella tularensis; Bartonella bacilliformis; Bacteroides; Vibrio comma; Vibrio fetus; Brucella; Escherichia coli; Enterobacter aerogenes; Shigella; Acinetobacter calcoaceticus; Haemophilus influenzae; Klebsiella; Diplococcus pneumoniae; Staphylococcus aureus, Streptococcus pneumoniae*
- When penicillin is contraindicated, infections caused by *Neisseria gonorrhoeae, Tre-*

ponema pallidum, Treponema pertenue, Listeria monocytogenes, Clostridium, Bacillus anthracis, Fosobacterium fusiforme, Actinomyces israelii

- As an adjunct to amebicides in acute intestinal amebiasis
- Oral tetracyclines are indicated for treatment of severe acne, uncomplicated urethral, endocervical, or rectal infections in adults caused by *Chlamydia trachomatis*
- Treatment of inflammatory lesions of nonnodule, moderate to severe acne vulgaris in patients 12 yr and older (ER tablets)
- Oral minocycline is indicated in treatment of asymptomatic carriers of *N. meningitidis* (not useful for treating the infection); infections caused by *Mycobacterium marinum;* uncomplicated urethral, endocervical, or rectal infections caused by *Ureaplasma urealyticum;* uncomplicated gonococcal urethritis in men due to *N. gonorrhoeae*
- *Arestin:* Adjunct to scaling and root planing to reduce pocket depth in patients with adult periodontitis
- Unlabeled uses: Alternative to sulfonamides in the treatment of nocardiosis; treatment of early rheumatoid arthritis, gallbladder infection caused by *Escherichia coli*

Contraindications and cautions

- Contraindicated with allergy to tetracyclines.
- Use cautiously with renal or hepatic impairment, pregnancy, lactation, asthma.

Available forms

Capsules—50, 75, 100 mg; pellet-filled capsules—50, 100 mg; oral suspension—50 mg/5 mL; tablets—50, 75, 100 mg; sustained release microsphere—1 mg; ER tablets—45, 55, 65, 80, 90, 105, 115, 135 mg; injection—100 mg/vial

Dosages

Adults

200 mg initially, followed by 100 mg every 12 hr PO. May be given as 100–200 mg initially and then 50 mg qid PO.

- *Syphilis:* Usual PO dose for 10–15 days.
- *Urethral, endocervical, rectal infections:* 100 mg every 12 hr PO for 7 days.
- *Gonococcal urethritis in men:* 100 mg bid PO for 5 days.

- *Gonorrhea:* 200 mg PO followed by 100 mg every 12 hr for 4 days; get post-therapy cultures within 2–3 days.
- *Meningococcal carrier state:* 100 mg every 12 hr PO for 5 days.
- *Adult periodontitis:* Unit dose cartridge discharged in subgingival area.
- *Moderate to severe acne vulgaris (12 yr and older):* 1 mg/kg/day PO for up to 12 wk (ER tablets).

IV

200 mg followed by 100 mg every 12 hr. Do not exceed 400 mg/day. Switch to oral form as soon as possible.

Pediatric patients older than 8 yr

4 mg/kg PO followed by 2 mg/kg every 12 hr PO.

ER tablets

Once daily based on patient weight:
45–59 kg: 45 mg PO.
60–90 kg: 90 mg PO.
91–136 kg: 135 mg PO.

IV

4 mg/kg IV followed by 2 mg/kg every 12 hr. Switch to oral form as soon as possible.

Geriatric patients or patients with renal failure

Decrease recommended dosage; increase dosing interval with renal impairment. Do not exceed 200 mg *Minocin* in 24 hr in patients with renal impairment.

Pharmacokinetics

Route	Onset	Peak
Oral	Rapid	2–3 hr

Metabolism: Hepatic; T$_{1/2}$: 11–24 hr
Distribution: Crosses placenta; enters breast milk
Excretion: Feces, urine

▼ IV FACTS

Preparation: Reconstitute with 5 mL sterile water for injection and immediately dilute with 500–1,000 mL sodium chloride injection, dextrose, dextrose and sodium chloride injection, Ringer injection, or lactated Ringer. Administer immediately. Stable 24 hr at room temperature. Discard unused portion.
Infusion: Avoid rapid administration.
Incompatibilities: Do not mix in solution with other drugs, calcium, or whole blood.

Adverse effects

- **Dental:** *Discoloring and inadequate calcification of primary teeth of fetus if used by pregnant women; discoloring and inadequate calcification of permanent teeth if used during period of dental development*
- **Dermatologic:** *Phototoxic reactions, rash,* exfoliative dermatitis (more frequent and severe with this tetracycline than with others)
- **GI:** Fatty liver, **liver failure,** *anorexia, nausea, vomiting, diarrhea, glossitis,* dysphagia, enterocolitis, esophageal ulcer, dyspepsia
- **Hematologic:** Hemolytic anemia, thrombocytopenia, neutropenia, eosinophilia, leukocytosis, leukopenia
- **Local:** Local irritation at injection site
- **Other:** Superinfections, nephrogenic diabetes insipidus syndrome, exacerbation of autoimmune syndromes

Interactions

✴ **Drug-drug** ● Decreased absorption of minocycline with antacids, iron, alkali ● Increased digoxin toxicity ● Decreased activity of penicillin ● Decreased efficacy of hormonal contraceptives
✴ **Drug-food** ● Decreased absorption of minocycline if taken with food, dairy products

■ Nursing considerations
Assessment

- **History:** Allergy to tetracyclines, renal or hepatic impairment, pregnancy, lactation, autoimmune disease
- **Physical:** Skin status, orientation and reflexes, R and adventitious sounds, GI function and liver evaluation, urinalysis and BUN, LFTs, renal function tests; culture of infected area

Interventions

- Administer oral medication without regard to food or meals; if GI upset occurs, give with meals.
- Reserve IV use for situations in which oral use is not possible. Switch from IV to oral route as soon as possible.

Teaching points

- Take drug throughout the day for best results.
- Take with meals if GI upset occurs.

- *Arestin:* After treatment, avoid eating hard, crunchy, or sticky foods for 1 week and postpone brushing for 12 hours.
- This drug may cause hormonal contraceptives to be ineffective; use a second form of contraception while taking this drug.
- You may experience these side effects: Sensitivity to sunlight (wear protective clothing, use sunscreen); diarrhea, nausea (take with meals; eat frequent small meals).
- Report rash, itching; difficulty breathing; dark urine or light-colored stools; severe cramps, watery diarrhea.

▷minoxidil
(mi nox' i dill)

Topical: Rogaine, Rogaine Extra Strength

PREGNANCY CATEGORY C

Drug classes
Antihypertensive
Vasodilator

Therapeutic actions
Acts directly on vascular smooth muscle to cause vasodilation, reducing elevated systolic and diastolic BP; does not interfere with CV reflexes; does not usually cause orthostatic hypotension but does cause reflex tachycardia and renin release, leading to sodium and water retention; mechanism in stimulating hair growth is not known, possibly related to arterial dilation.

Indications
- Severe hypertension that is symptomatic or associated with target organ damage and is not manageable with maximum therapeutic doses of a diuretic plus two other antihypertensive drugs; use in milder hypertension not recommended
- Topical use (when compounded as a 1%–5% lotion or 1% ointment): Alopecia areata and male pattern alopecia

Contraindications and cautions
- Contraindicated with hypersensitivity to minoxidil or any component of the topical preparation (topical); pheochromocytoma (may stimulate release of catecholamines

from tumor); acute MI; dissecting aortic aneurysm; lactation.
- Use cautiously with malignant hypertension, HF (use diuretic), angina pectoris (use a beta blocker), pregnancy.

Available forms
Tablets—2.5, 10 mg; topical 2%, 5%

Dosages
Adults and patients 12 yr and older
Oral
- *Monotherapy:* Initial dosage is 5 mg/day PO as a single dose. Daily dosage can be increased to 10, 20, then 40 mg in single or divided doses. Effective range is usually 10–40 mg/day PO. Maximum dosage is 100 mg/day. If supine diastolic BP has been reduced less than 30 mm Hg, administer the drug only once a day. If reduced more than 30 mm Hg, divide the daily dose into two equal parts. Dosage adjustment should normally be at least at 3-day intervals; in emergencies, every 6 hr with careful monitoring is possible.
- *Concomitant therapy with diuretics:* Use minoxidil with a diuretic in patients relying on renal function for maintaining salt and water balance; the following diuretic dosages have been used when starting minoxidil therapy: Hydrochlorothiazide, 50 mg bid; chlorthalidone, 50–100 mg daily; furosemide, 40 mg bid. If excessive salt and water retention result in weight gain more than 5 lb, change diuretic therapy to furosemide; if patient already takes furosemide, increase dosage.
- *Concomitant therapy with beta-adrenergic blockers or other sympatholytics:* The following dosages are recommended when starting minoxidil therapy: Propranolol, 80–160 mg/day; other beta blockers, dosage equivalent to the above; methyldopa 250–750 mg bid (start methyldopa at least 24 hr before minoxidil); clonidine, 0.1–0.2 mg bid.

Topical
Apply 1 mL to the total affected areas of the scalp twice daily. The total daily dosage should not exceed 2 mL. Twice-daily application for longer than 4 mo may be required before evidence of hair regrowth is observed. Once hair growth is realized, twice daily application is necessary for continued and additional hair regrowth. Balding process reported to return

to untreated state 3–4 mo after cessation of the drug.

Pediatric patients younger than 12 yr

Experience is limited, particularly in infants; use recommendations as a guide; careful adjustment is necessary. Initial dosage is 0.2 mg/kg/day PO as a single dose. May increase by 50%–100% increments until optimum BP control is achieved. Effective range is usually 0.25–1 mg/kg/day; maximum dose is 50 mg daily. Experience in children is limited; monitor carefully.

Geriatric patients or patients with impaired renal function

Smaller doses may be required; closely supervise to prevent cardiac failure or exacerbation of renal failure.

Pharmacokinetics

Route	Onset	Peak	Duration
Oral	30 min	2–3 hr	75 hr

Metabolism: Hepatic; $T_{1/2}$: 4.2 hr
Distribution: Crosses placenta; enters breast milk
Excretion: Urine

Adverse effects

- **CNS:** Fatigue, headache
- **CV:** Tachycardia (unless given with beta-adrenergic blocker or other sympatholytic drug), pericardial effusion and tamponade; *changes in direction and magnitude of T-waves;* cardiac necrotic lesions (reported in patients with known ischemic heart disease, but risk of minoxidil-associated cardiac damage cannot be excluded)
- **Dermatologic:** *Temporary edema, hypertrichosis* (elongation, thickening, and enhanced pigmentation of fine body hair occurring within 3–6 wk of starting therapy; usually first noticed on temples, between eyebrows and extending to other parts of face, back, arms, legs, scalp); rashes including bullous eruptions; **Stevens-Johnson syndrome;** darkening of the skin
- **GI:** Nausea, vomiting
- **Hematologic:** Initial decrease in Hct, Hgb, RBC count
- **Local:** *Irritant dermatitis, allergic contact dermatitis, eczema, pruritus, dry skin or scalp, flaking, alopecia* (topical use)

- **Respiratory:** *Bronchitis, upper respiratory infection, sinusitis* (topical use)

■ Nursing considerations
Assessment
- **History:** Hypersensitivity to minoxidil or any component of the topical preparation; pheochromocytoma; acute MI, dissecting aortic aneurysm; malignant hypertension; heart failure; angina pectoris; lactation, pregnancy
- **Physical:** Skin color, lesions, hair, scalp; P, BP, orthostatic BP, supine BP, perfusion, edema, auscultation; bowel sounds, normal output; CBC with differential, renal function tests, urinalysis, ECG

Interventions
- Apply topical preparation to affected area; if you use your fingers, wash hands thoroughly afterward.
- Do not apply other topical drugs, including topical corticosteroids, retinoids, and petrolatum or agents known to enhance cutaneous drug absorption.
- Do not apply topical preparation to open lesions or breaks in the skin, which could increase risk of systemic absorption.

⊗ *Warning* Arrange to withdraw oral drug gradually, especially from children; rapid withdrawal may cause a sudden increase in BP (rebound hypertension has been reported in children, even with gradual withdrawal; use caution and monitor BP closely when withdrawing from children).

⊗ **Black box warning** Arrange for echocardiographic evaluation of possible pericardial effusion if using oral drug; more vigorous diuretic therapy, dialysis, other treatment (including minoxidil withdrawal) may be required.

⊗ **Black box warning** There is an increased risk of exacerbation of angina, malignant hypertension; when first administering drug, hospitalize patient and monitor closely. Use with a beta blocker and/or diuretic to decrease risk.

Teaching points
Oral
- Take this drug exactly as prescribed. Take all other medications that have been prescribed. Do not discontinue any drug or reduce the

dosage without consulting your health care provider.

- You may experience these side effects: Enhanced growth and darkening of fine body and face hair (do not discontinue medication without consulting your health care provider); GI upset (eat frequent small meals).
- Report increased heart rate of 20 beats or more per minute over normal (your normal heart rate is ___ beats per minute); rapid weight gain of more than 5 pounds; unusual swelling of the extremities, face, or abdomen; difficulty breathing, especially when lying down; new or aggravated symptoms of angina (chest, arm, or shoulder pain); severe indigestion; dizziness, lightheadedness, or fainting.

Topical

- Apply the prescribed amount to the affected area twice a day. If using your fingers, wash hands thoroughly after application. It may take 4 months or longer for any noticeable hair regrowth to appear. Response to this drug is very individual. If no response is seen within 4 months, consult your health care provider about efficacy of continued use.
- Do not apply more frequent or larger applications. This will not speed up or increase hair growth but may increase side effects.
- If one or two daily applications are missed, restart twice-daily applications, and return to usual schedule. Do not attempt to make up missed applications.
- Do not apply any other topical medication to the area while you are using this drug.
- Do not apply to any sunburned, broken skin or open lesions; this increases the risk of systemic effects. Do not apply to any part of the body other than the scalp.
- Twice-daily use of the drug will be needed to retain or continue the hair regrowth.

▽ **mirabegron**
(meer' ah beg' ron)

Myrbetriq

PREGNANCY CATEGORY C

Drug class

Beta-adrenergic agonist

Therapeutic actions

Relatively selective agonist of beta$_3$ adrenergic receptors. Stimulating these receptors relaxes the detrusor smooth muscle during the storage phase of bladder filling, which increases bladder capacity.

Indications

- Treatment of overactive bladder with symptoms of urge urinary incontinence, urgency, and frequency

Contraindications and cautions

- Contraindicated with history of serious hypersensitivity to components of drug, severe uncontrolled hypertension, lactation.
- Use cautiously with bladder outlet obstruction, hypertension, pregnancy.

Available forms

ER tablets—25, 50 mg

Dosages

Adults
25 mg/day PO; may increase to 50 mg/day PO after 8 wk if needed.
Patients with severe renal or moderate hepatic impairment
Do not exceed 25 mg/day.
Patients with end-stage renal disease or severe hepatic impairment
Not recommended.

Pharmacokinetics

Route	Onset	Peak
Oral	Rapid	3.5 hr

Metabolism: Hepatic; T$_{1/2}$: 50 hr
Distribution: May cross placenta; may enter breast milk
Excretion: Urine, feces

Adverse effects

- **CNS:** *Headache,* dizziness
- **CV:** *Hypertension,* tachycardia
- **Dermatologic:** Rash
- **GI:** Nausea, diarrhea, constipation, abdominal pain, dry mouth
- **GU:** *UTI,* urinary retention
- **Musculoskeletal:** Arthralgia, back pain
- **Respiratory:** *Nasopharyngitis*
- **Other:** Fatigue

Adverse effects in *italics* are most common; those in **bold** are life-threatening. ⊞⊡⊞ Do not crush.

Interactions

❋ **Drug-drug** ● Risk of increased serum levels and toxicity of drugs metabolized by the CYP2D6 system (metoprolol, desipramine, thioridazine, flecainide, propafenone); monitor patient and adjust dosage as needed ● Risk of increased digoxin level and toxicity if combined; use lowest digoxin dose possible, monitor serum levels regularly ● Risk of urinary retention if combined with anticholinergics for overactive bladder; avoid this combination

■ Nursing considerations

Assessment

● **History:** Allergy to components of the drug, hypertension, bladder outlet obstruction, hypertension, pregnancy, lactation
● **Physical:** P, BP; orientation; R; abdominal exam; bladder exam; **LFT,** renal function tests

Interventions

● Ensure diagnosis of overactive bladder; rule out infection and obstructions.
● Tablets must be swallowed whole with a full glass of water; ensure that patient does not cut, crush, or chew tablets.
● Monitor BP before and periodically during treatment.
● Assess patient for possible urinary retention after beginning treatment.
● Advise breast-feeding patients to choose another method of feeding the baby while taking this drug.

Teaching points

● Take this drug once a day with a full glass of water. Do not cut, crush, or chew the tablets; they must be swallowed whole.
● If you miss a dose, begin taking the drug again the next day. Do not take two doses on the same day.
● It is not known how this drug could affect a developing fetus; if you are pregnant or are thinking about becoming pregnant while taking this drug, discuss this with your health care provider.
● Find another method of feeding the baby if you are currently breast-feeding; it is not known how this drug could affect a breast-feeding baby.
● You may experience these side effects: Dizziness, headache (use care if driving or operating dangerous machinery until you know how this drug affects you); high blood pressure (report increasing headache; check your blood pressure periodically if you have a history of high blood pressure); urinary tract infection (report changes in urine or urination to your health care provider); urinary retention (this is more likely if mirabegron is combined with other drugs to treat irritable bladder; mirabegron should not be combined with these drugs).
● Report difficulty urinating, rash, persistent headache, fever, change in color or odor of urine.

▽ mirtazapine

*(mer **tab'** zah peen)*

Gen-Mirtazapine (CAN), Novo-Mirtazapine OD (CAN), Remeron, Remeron SolTab ⓪ⓝⓔ, Sandoz-Mirtazapine (CAN)

PREGNANCY CATEGORY C

M

Drug class

Antidepressant (tetracyclic)

Therapeutic actions

Mechanism of action unknown; appears to act similarly to TCAs, which inhibit the presynaptic reuptake of the neurotransmitters norepinephrine and serotonin; anticholinergic at CNS and peripheral receptors; sedating; relation of these effects to clinical efficacy is unknown.

Indications

● Treatment of major depressive disorder
● Unlabeled uses: Chronic urticaria, hot flashes, drug-induced hyperhidrosis, pruritus, prevention of migraines in adults

Contraindications and cautions

● Contraindicated with hypersensitivity to any tricyclic or tetracyclic drug; concomitant therapy with an MAOI; pregnancy (limb reduction abnormalities reported); lactation.
● Use cautiously with ECT; pre-existing CV disorders (eg, severe coronary heart disease, progressive HF, angina pectoris, paroxysmal tachycardia [possible increased risk of serious CVS toxicity with TCAs]); angle-closure

glaucoma, increased IOP; urine retention, ureteral or urethral spasm; seizure disorders (TCAs lower the seizure threshold); hyperthyroidism (predisposes to CVS toxicity, including cardiac arrhythmias); impaired hepatic, renal function; psychiatric patients (schizophrenic or paranoid patients may exhibit a worsening of psychosis with TCAs); bipolar disorder (may shift to hypomanic or manic phase); elective surgery (TCAs should be discontinued as long as possible before surgery).

Available forms

Tablets—7.5, 15, 30, 45 mg; orally disintegrating tablet ⊙ᴿᴰ—15, 30, 45 mg

Dosages

Adults

Initial dose, 15 mg PO daily, as a single dose in evening. May be increased up to 45 mg/day as needed. Change dose only at intervals greater than 1–2 wk. Continue treatment for up to 6 mo for acute episodes.

• *Switching from MAOI:* Allow at least 14 days between discontinuation of MAOI and beginning of mirtazapine therapy. Allow 14 days after stopping mirtazapine before starting MAOI.

Pediatric patients

Not recommended in patients younger than 18 yr.

Geriatric patients and patients with renal or hepatic impairment

Give lower doses to patients older than 60 yr; use with caution.

Pharmacokinetics

Route	Onset	Peak	Duration
Oral	Slow	2–4 hr	2–4 wk

Metabolism: Hepatic; $T_{1/2}$: 20–40 hr
Distribution: Crosses placenta; enters breast milk
Excretion: Feces, urine

Adverse effects

• **CNS:** *Sedation and anticholinergic (atropine-like) effects, confusion* (especially in elderly), *disturbed concentration,* hallucinations, disorientation, decreased memory, feelings of unreality, delusions, anxiety, nervousness, restlessness, agitation, panic, insomnia, nightmares, hypomania, mania, exacerbation of psychosis, drowsiness, weakness, fatigue, headache, numbness, agitation (less likely with this drug than with other antidepressants)

• **CV:** Orthostatic hypotension, hypertension, syncope, tachycardia, palpitations, **MI,** arrhythmias, **heart block,** precipitation of heart failure, **stroke**

• **Endocrine:** Elevated or depressed blood sugar; elevated prolactin levels; inappropriate ADH secretion

• **GI:** *Dry mouth, constipation,* paralytic ileus, *nausea* (less likely with this drug than with other antidepressants), *increased appetite, weight gain,* vomiting, anorexia, epigastric distress, diarrhea, flatulence, dysphagia, peculiar taste, increased salivation, stomatitis, glossitis, parotid swelling, abdominal cramps, black tongue, liver enzyme elevations

• **GU:** Urine retention, delayed micturition, dilation of urinary tract, gynecomastia, testicular swelling in men; breast enlargement, menstrual irregularity, galactorrhea in women; increased or decreased libido; impotence

• **Hematologic: Agranulocytosis,** *neutropenia*

• **Hypersensitivity:** Rash, pruritus, vasculitis, petechiae, photosensitization, edema

Interactions

✴ **Drug-drug** ⊗ *Warning* Risk of serious, sometimes fatal reactions if combined with MAOIs; do not use this combination or within 14 days of MAOI therapy • Possible increased risk of serotonin syndrome if combined with SSRIs; monitor patient.

■ Nursing considerations

Assessment

• **History:** Hypersensitivity to any antidepressant; concomitant therapy with MAOI; recent MI; myelography within previous 24 hr or scheduled within 48 hr; lactation; ECT; pre-existing CV disorders; angle-closure glaucoma, increased IOP; urine retention, ureteral or urethral spasm; seizure disorders; hyperthyroidism; impaired hepatic, renal function; psychiatric problems; bipolar disorder; elective surgery; pregnancy, lactation

• **Physical:** Body weight; T; skin color, lesions; orientation, affect, reflexes, vision and hearing; P, BP, orthostatic BP, perfusion; bowel sounds, normal output, liver evaluation; urine flow, normal output; usual sexual function, frequency of menses, breast and scrotal examination; LFTs, urinalysis, CBC, renal function tests; ECG

Interventions

⊗ **Black box warning** Ensure that depressed and potentially suicidal patients have access only to limited quantities of the drug; increased risk of suicidality in children, adolescents, and young adults. Observe patient for clinical worsening of depressive disorders, suicidality, unusual changes in behavior, especially when starting drug or changing dosage.

- Administer orally disintegrating tablets to patients who have difficulty swallowing: Open blister pack and have patient place tablet on tongue. Do not split tablet or allow patient to chew tablet.
- Expect clinical response in 3–7 days up to 3 wk (latter is more usual).
- Arrange for CBC if patient develops fever, sore throat, or other sign of infection during therapy.
- Establish safety precautions if CNS changes occur (raise side rails, accompany patient when ambulating).

Teaching points

- Take this drug exactly as prescribed; do not stop taking the drug abruptly or without consulting your health care provider.
- Place orally disintegrating tablet on tongue; it can be swallowed without water. Open blister pack with dry hands and use tablet immediately; do not cut, break, or chew tablet.
- Avoid using alcohol, other sleep-inducing drugs, or over-the-counter drugs while using this drug.
- Avoid prolonged exposure to sunlight or sunlamps; use a sunscreen or protective garments if long exposure to sunlight is unavoidable.
- You may experience these side effects: Headache, dizziness, drowsiness, weakness, blurred vision (reversible; avoid driving or performing tasks that require alertness); nausea, vomiting, loss of appetite, dry mouth (eat frequent small meals; use frequent mouth care, suck on sugarless candies); nightmares, inability to concentrate, confusion; changes in sexual function.
- Report fever, flulike symptoms, any infection, dry mouth, difficulty urinating, excessive sedation, suicidal thoughts.

▽ **misoprostol**
*(mye soe **prost'** ole)*

Apo-Misoprostol (CAN), Cytotec

PREGNANCY CATEGORY X

Drug class
Prostaglandin

Therapeutic actions
A synthetic prostaglandin E_1 analogue; inhibits gastric acid secretion and increases bicarbonate and mucus production, protecting the lining of the stomach.

Indications

- Prevention of NSAID (including aspirin)-induced gastric ulcers in patients at high risk of complications from a gastric ulcer (the elderly; patients with concomitant debilitating disease, history of ulcers)
- With mifepristone as an abortifacient (see mifepristone)
- Unlabeled uses: Appears effective in treating but not preventing duodenal ulcers in patients unresponsive to histamine-2 antagonists; cervical ripening and labor induction; postpartum hemorrhage; chronic idiopathic constipation

Contraindications and cautions

- Contraindicated with history of allergy to prostaglandins; pregnancy (abortifacient; advise women of childbearing age in written and oral form of use, have a negative serum pregnancy test within 2 wk prior to therapy, provide contraceptives, and begin therapy on the second or third day of the next normal menstrual period); lactation.
- Use cautiously in the elderly, and with renal impairment, duodenal ulcers.

Available forms
Tablets—100, 200 mcg

Dosages

Adults

200 mcg four times daily PO with food. If this dose cannot be tolerated, 100 mcg can be used. Take misoprostol for the duration of the NSAID therapy. Take the last dose of the day at bedtime.

Pediatric patients

Safety and efficacy in patients younger than 18 yr not established.

Geriatric patients or patients with renal impairment

Dosage adjustment is usually not needed, but dosage can be reduced if 200-mcg PO dose cannot be tolerated.

Pharmacokinetics

Route	Onset	Peak
Oral	Rapid	12–15 min

Metabolism: Hepatic; T$_{1/2}$: 20–40 min
Distribution: Crosses placenta; may enter breast milk
Excretion: Urine

Adverse effects

- **GI:** *Nausea, diarrhea, abdominal pain, flatulence,* vomiting, dyspepsia, constipation
- **GU:** *Miscarriage,* excessive bleeding, *spotting, cramping,* hypermenorrhea, menstrual disorders, dysmenorrhea
- **Other:** Headache

■ Nursing considerations

 CLINICAL ALERT!
Name confusion has occurred between misoprostol and mifepristone; use extreme caution.

Assessment

- **History:** Allergy to prostaglandins; pregnancy, lactation; renal impairment, duodenal ulcer
- **Physical:** Abdominal examination, normal bowel function, urinary output

Interventions

- Give to patients at high risk for developing NSAID-induced gastric ulcers; give for the full term of the NSAID use.
- ⊗ **Black box warning** Arrange for serum pregnancy test for any woman of child-bearing age; women must have a negative test within 2 wk of beginning therapy; drug can act as an abortifacient.
- Arrange for oral and written explanation of the risks to pregnancy; appropriate contraceptive measures must be taken; begin therapy on the second or third day of a normal menstrual period.

Teaching points

- Take this drug four times a day, with meals and at bedtime. Continue to take your NSAID while taking this drug. Take the drug exactly as prescribed. Do not give this drug to anyone else.
- This drug can cause miscarriage and is often associated with dangerous bleeding. Do not take if pregnant; do not become pregnant while taking this medication. If pregnancy occurs, discontinue drug, and consult your health care provider immediately.
- You may experience these side effects: Abdominal pain, nausea, diarrhea, flatulence (take with meals); menstrual cramping, abnormal menstrual periods, spotting, even in postmenopausal women (request analgesics); headache.
- Report severe diarrhea, spotting or menstrual pain, severe menstrual bleeding, pregnancy.

DANGEROUS DRUG

▽mitomycin (mitomycin-C, MTC)

*(mye toe **mye**' sin)*

PREGNANCY CATEGORY D

Drug classes

Antibiotic
Antineoplastic

Therapeutic actions

Cytotoxic: Inhibits DNA synthesis and cellular RNA and protein synthesis in susceptible cells, causing cell death.

Indications

- Disseminated adenocarcinoma of the stomach or pancreas; part of combination therapy or as palliative measure when other modalities fail

• Unlabeled uses: Intravesical route—superficial bladder cancer; ophthalmic route—may be useful adjunct to surgery in primary or recurrent pterygia; intra-arterial route—hepatocellular cancer; topical route—otolaryngologic procedures; other unlabeled uses include colorectal cancer; breast cancer; squamous cell carcinoma of the head, neck, lungs, and cervix; tracheal stenosis

Contraindications and cautions

• Contraindicated with allergy to mitomycin; thrombocytopenia, coagulation disorders, or increase in bleeding tendencies; severe impaired renal function (creatinine level above 1.7 mg/dL); myelosuppression; pregnancy; lactation.

• Use cautiously with renal impairment.

Available forms

Powder for injection—5-, 20-, 40-mg vials

Dosages

Adults

After hematologic recovery from previous chemotherapy, use the following schedule at 6- to 8-wk intervals: 20 mg/m^2 IV as a single dose. Re-evaluate patient for hematologic response between courses of therapy; adjust dosage accordingly:

Leukocytes (mm^3)	Platelets (mm^3)	% of Prior Dose to Be Given
More than 4,000	More than 100,000	100
3,000–3,999	75,000–99,999	100
2,000–2,999	25,000–74,999	70
Less than 2,000	Less than 25,000	50

Do not repeat dosage until leukocyte count has returned to 4,000/mm^3 and platelet count to 100,000/mm^3.

Pharmacokinetics

Route	Onset	Peak
IV	Slow	Unknown

Metabolism: Hepatic; T$_{1/2}$: 17 min
Distribution: Crosses placenta; may enter breast milk
Excretion: Urine

▼ IV FACTS

Preparation: Reconstitute 5- to 20-mg vial with 10 or 40 mL of sterile water for injection, respectively; reconstitute 40-mg vial with 80 mL sterile water. Shake vial to improve dissolution. If product does not dissolve immediately, allow to stand at room temperature until solution is obtained. This solution is stable for 14 days if refrigerated, 7 days at room temperature; further dilution in various IV fluids reduces stability—check manufacturer's insert.

Infusion: Infuse slowly over 5–10 min; monitor injection site to avoid local reaction.
Incompatibility: Do not mix with bleomycin.

Adverse effects

• **CNS:** Headache, blurred vision, confusion, drowsiness, syncope, fatigue
• **GI:** *Anorexia, nausea, vomiting,* diarrhea, hematemesis, stomatitis
• **GU:** Renal toxicity, **hemolytic uremic syndrome**
• **Hematologic: Bone marrow toxicity,** microangiopathic hemolytic anemia (a syndrome of anemia, thrombocytopenia, renal failure, hypertension)
• **Respiratory: Pulmonary toxicity, acute respiratory distress syndrome**
• **Other:** *Fever,* cancer in preclinical studies, *cellulitis at injection site, alopecia*

■ Nursing considerations

Assessment

• **History:** Allergy to mitomycin; thrombocytopenia, coagulation disorders or increase in bleeding tendencies; impaired renal function; myelosuppression; pregnancy; lactation
• **Physical:** T; skin color, lesions; weight; hair; local injection site; orientation, reflexes; R, adventitious sounds; mucous membranes; CBC, clotting tests, renal function tests

Interventions

• Do not give IM or subcutaneously due to severe local reaction and tissue necrosis.
⊗ **Warning** Monitor injection site for extravasation: If patient reports burning or stinging, discontinue infusion immediately and restart in another vein.
⊗ **Black box warning** Monitor patient response frequently at beginning of therapy (CBC, renal function tests, pulmonary examination) because of the risk of bone marrow

suppression and hemolytic uremic syndrome with renal failure. Adverse effects may require a decreased dose or discontinuation of drug; consult with physician.

Teaching points
- Prepare a calendar with return dates for drug therapy; this drug can only be given IV.
- Take precautions to avoid pregnancy while using this drug; using barrier contraceptives is advised.
- Have regular medical follow-up visits, including blood tests to monitor drug's effects.
- You may experience these side effects: Rash, skin lesions, loss of hair (head should be covered at extremes of temperature; skin care may help); loss of appetite, nausea, mouth sores (frequent mouth care, eat frequent small meals; maintain good nutrition; consult a dietitian; request an antiemetic); drowsiness, dizziness, syncope, headache (use caution driving or operating dangerous machinery; take special precautions to prevent injuries).
- Report difficulty breathing, sudden weight gain, swelling, burning or pain at injection site, unusual bleeding or bruising.

▷ **mitotane**

See Appendix R, *Less commonly used drugs.*

DANGEROUS DRUG

▷ **mitoxantrone hydrochloride**

*(mye toe **zan'** trone)*

Novantrone

PREGNANCY CATEGORY D

Drug classes
Antineoplastic
MS drug

Therapeutic actions
Cytotoxic; cell-cycle nonspecific, appears to be DNA reactive, RNA reactive, and potent inhibitor of topoisomerase II, causing the death of both proliferating and nonproliferating cells.

Indications
- As part of combination therapy in the treatment of acute nonlymphocytic leukemia in adults, including myelogenous, promyelocytic, monocytic, and erythroid acute leukemias
- Treatment of pain in patients with advanced prostatic cancer, in combination with steroids
- Treatment of chronic progressive, progressive relapsing, or worsening relapsing-remitting MS
- Unlabeled uses: Treatment of breast cancer, refractory lymphomas, autologous bone marrow transplantation

Contraindications and cautions
- Contraindicated with hypersensitivity to mitoxantrone, pregnancy.
- Use cautiously with bone marrow suppression, HF, lactation.

Available forms
Injection—2 mg/mL

Dosages
Adults
- *Combination therapy:* For induction, 12 mg/m^2 IV per day on days 1–3, with 100 mg/m^2 of cytarabine for 7 days given as a continuous infusion on days 1–7. If remission does not occur, a second series can be used, with mitoxantrone given for 2 days and cytarabine for 5 days.
- *Consolidation therapy:* Mitoxantrone 12 mg/m^2 IV for days 1 and 2, and cytarabine 100 mg/m^2 given as a continuous 24-hr infusion on days 1–5; first course given 6 wk after induction therapy if needed. Second course is generally administered 4 wk after first course. Severe myelosuppression may occur.
- *Hormone-refractory prostate cancer:* 12–14 mg/m^2 as short IV infusion every 21 days.
- *MS:* 12 mg/m^2 IV over 5–15 min every 3 mo; do not exceed cumulative lifetime dose of 140 mg/m^2.

Pediatric patients
Safety and efficacy not established.

Pharmacokinetics

Route	Onset	Duration
IV	Rapid	2–3 days

Adverse effects in italics *are most common; those in* **bold** *are life-threatening.* ▥ Do not crush.

Metabolism: Hepatic; $T_{1/2}$: 1–9 days
Distribution: Crosses placenta; may enter breast milk
Excretion: Feces, urine

▼ IV FACTS

Preparation: Dilute solution to at least 50 mL in either 0.9% sodium chloride or D_5W; may be further diluted in D_5W, normal saline, or dextrose 5% in normal saline if needed. Inject this solution into tubing of a freely running IV of 0.9% sodium chloride injection or 5% dextrose injection over period of at least 3 min. Use immediately after dilution and discard any leftover solution immediately. Wear gloves and goggles and avoid any contact with skin or mucous membranes.
Infusion: Inject slowly over at least 3 min.
Incompatibilities: Do not mix in solution with heparin; a precipitate may form. Do not mix in solution with any other drug; studies are not yet available regarding the safety of such mixtures.

Adverse effects

• **CNS:** Headache, seizures
• **CV: Heart failure,** potentially fatal; arrhythmias; chest pain
• **GI:** *Nausea, vomiting, diarrhea,* abdominal pain, mucositis, GI bleeding, jaundice
• **Hematologic: Bone marrow depression,** *infections of all kinds, hyperuricemia*
• **Respiratory:** *Cough,* dyspnea
• **Other:** *Fever, alopecia, cancer in laboratory animals*

■ Nursing considerations
Assessment

• **History:** Hypersensitivity to mitoxantrone, bone marrow depression, HF, pregnancy, lactation
• **Physical:** Neurologic status; T; P, BP, auscultation, peripheral perfusion; R, adventitious sounds; abdominal examination, mucous membranes; LFTs, CBC with differential

Interventions

⊗ *Black box warning* Follow CBC and LFTs carefully before and frequently during therapy; dose adjustment may be needed if myelosuppression becomes severe.

• Monitor patient for hyperuricemia, which frequently occurs as a result of rapid tumor lysis; monitor serum uric acid levels and arrange for appropriate treatment as needed.
⊗ *Warning* Handle drug with great care; the use of gloves, gowns, and goggles is recommended; if drug comes in contact with skin, wash immediately with warm water; clean spills with calcium hypochlorite solution.
⊗ *Black box warning* Monitor IV site for signs of extravasation; if extravasation occurs, stop administration and restart at another site immediately.
⊗ *Black box warning* Left ventricular ejection fraction (LVEF) should be evaluated before each dose when treating MS. Yearly evaluations should be done after finishing treatment to detect late cardiac toxic effects; decreased LVEF and frank HF can occur.
⊗ *Black box warning* Monitor BP, P, cardiac output regularly during administration; supportive care for heart failure should be started at the first sign of failure.
• Protect patient from exposure to infection; monitor occurrence of infection at any site and arrange for appropriate treatment.

Teaching points

• This drug will need to be given IV for 3 days in conjunction with cytarabine therapy; mark calendar with days of treatment. Regular blood tests will be needed to evaluate the effects of this treatment (antineoplastic).
• This drug will be given IV every 3 months when being used to treat MS.
• Using barrier contraceptives is advised; fetal harm may occur if you are pregnant while taking this drug.
• You may experience these side effects: Nausea, vomiting (may be severe; antiemetics may be helpful; eat frequent small meals); increased susceptibility to infection (avoid crowds and exposure to disease); loss of hair (obtain a wig; it is important to keep your head covered in extremes of temperature); blue-green color of the urine (may last for 24 hours after treatment is finished; the whites of the eyes may also be tinted blue for a time; this finding is expected and will pass).
• Report severe nausea and vomiting; fever, chills, sore throat; unusual bleeding or bruising; fluid retention or swelling; severe joint pain.

M

modafinil
(moe daff' in ill)

Alertec (CAN), Provigil

PREGNANCY CATEGORY C

CONTROLLED SUBSTANCE C-IV

Drug classes
CNS stimulant
Narcolepsy drug

Therapeutic actions
A CNS stimulant that helps to improve vigilance and decrease excessive daytime sleepiness associated with narcolepsy and other sleep disorders; may act through dopaminergic mechanisms; exact mechanism of action is not known. Not associated with the cardiac and other systemic stimulatory effects of amphetamines.

Indications
• Treatment of narcolepsy with excessive daytime sleepiness
• Improvement in wakefulness in patients with shift-work sleep disorder (SWSD)
• Improvement in wakefulness in patients with obstructive sleep apnea/hypopnea syndrome (OSAHS)
• Unlabeled uses: Treatment of fatigue associated with MS, Parkinson disease, brain injury

Contraindications and cautions
• Contraindicated with hypersensitivity to modafinil, left ventricular hypertrophy, ischemic ECG changes, mitral valve prolapse.
• Use cautiously with impaired renal or hepatic function, epilepsy, emotional instability, psychosis, depression, mania, pregnancy, lactation.

Available forms
Tablets—100, 200 mg

Dosages
Adults
• *Narcolepsy, OSAHS:* 200 mg PO daily given as a single dose. Up to 400 mg/day as a single dose may be used.
• *SWSD:* 200 mg/day PO taken 1 hr before start of shift.

Pediatric patients
Safety and efficacy not established in patients younger than 16 yr.
Geriatric patients or patients with hepatic impairment
In elderly patients, elimination may be reduced; monitor response and consider use of lower dose. With severe hepatic impairment, reduce dosage to 50%.

Pharmacokinetics

Route	Onset	Peak
Oral	Gradual	2–4 hr

Metabolism: Hepatic; $T_{1/2}$: 15 hr
Distribution: Crosses placenta; may enter breast milk
Excretion: Urine

Adverse effects
• **CNS:** *Insomnia, headache, nervousness, anxiety,* fatigue
• **Dermatologic:** Rashes, **Stevens-Johnson syndrome**
• **GI:** Dry mouth, choking, nausea, diarrhea, anorexia

Interactions
✳ **Drug-drug** • Increased plasma levels of triazolam when used concurrently; triazolam dosage may need reduction • Possible decreased effectiveness of hormonal contraceptives; suggest the use of barrier contraceptives • Risk of increased levels and effects of warfarin, phenytoin, and TCAs; monitor patient and decrease dosage as appropriate

■ Nursing considerations
Assessment
• **History:** Hypersensitivity to modafinil, left ventricular hypertrophy, mitral valve prolapse, ischemic ECG changes, epilepsy, pregnancy, lactation, drug dependence, emotional instability
• **Physical:** Body weight; T; skin color, lesions; orientation, affect, reflexes; P, BP, auscultation; R, adventitious sounds; bowel sounds, normal output; LFTs, renal function tests, baseline ECG

Interventions
• Ensure proper diagnosis before administering to rule out underlying medical problems.

⊗ **Warning** Arrange to dispense the least feasible amount of drug at any one time to minimize risk of overdose.

• Administer drug once a day in the morning.
• Arrange to monitor liver function tests periodically in patients on long-term therapy.
• Establish safety precautions if CNS changes occur (use side rails, accompany patient when ambulating).

Teaching points
• Take this drug exactly as prescribed; if taking to improve wakefulness with shift work, take 1 hour before the start of your shift.
• Avoid pregnancy while using this drug; using barrier contraceptives is advised.
• You may experience these side effects: Insomnia, nervousness, restlessness, dizziness, impaired thinking (these effects may become less pronounced after a few days; avoid driving a car or engaging in activities that require alertness if these effects occur, notify your health care provider if they are pronounced or bothersome), headache.
• Report insomnia, abnormal body movements, rash, severe diarrhea, pale-colored stools, yellowing of the skin or eyes.

▷ moexipril
(mo ex' ah pril)

Univasc

PREGNANCY CATEGORY C
(FIRST TRIMESTER)

PREGNANCY CATEGORY D
(SECOND AND THIRD TRIMESTERS)

Drug classes
ACE inhibitor
Antihypertensive

Therapeutic actions
Renin, synthesized by the kidneys, is released into the circulation where it acts on a plasma precursor to produce angiotensin I, which is converted by ACE to angiotensin II, a potent vasoconstrictor that also causes release of aldosterone from the adrenals. Both of these actions increase BP; moexipril blocks the conversion of angiotensin I to angiotensin II, leading to decreased BP, decreased aldosterone

secretion, a small increase in serum potassium levels, and sodium and fluid loss; increased prostaglandin synthesis may also be involved in the antihypertensive action.

Indications
• Treatment of hypertension, alone or in combination with other antihypertensives such as thiazide-type diuretics

Contraindications and cautions
• Contraindicated with allergy to ACE inhibitors, impaired renal function, HF, salt or volume depletion, history of ACE inhibitor-induced angioedema, lactation, pregnancy.
• Use cautiously with hepatic impairment and in elderly patients.

Available forms
Tablets—7.5, 15 mg

Dosages
Adults
• *Patients not receiving diuretics:* Initially, 7.5 mg PO daily, given 1 hr before a meal; for maintenance, 7.5–30 mg PO daily or in one to two divided doses 1 hr before meals.
• *Patients receiving diuretics:* Discontinue diuretic for 2 or 3 days before beginning moexipril; follow dosage listed above, if BP is not controlled, diuretic therapy may be added. If diuretic cannot be stopped, start moexipril therapy with 3.75 mg and monitor for symptomatic hypotension.
Pediatric patients
Safety and efficacy not established.
Geriatric patients and patients with renal impairment
Excretion is reduced in renal failure; use with caution. If creatinine clearance 40 mL/min or less, start with 3.75 mg PO daily, adjust up to a maximum of 15 mg/day.

Pharmacokinetics

Route	Onset	Peak	Duration
Oral	1.5 hr	3–4 hr	24 hr

Metabolism: $T_{1/2}$: 2–9 hr
Distribution: Crosses placenta; enters breast milk
Excretion: Urine

M

Adverse effects

- **CV:** *Tachycardia,* angina pectoris, **MI,** hypotension in salt- or volume-depleted patients
- **GI:** *Gastric irritation, aphthous ulcers, peptic ulcers, diarrhea, dysgeusia,* cholestatic jaundice, hepatocellular injury, anorexia, constipation
- **GU:** *Proteinuria,* renal insufficiency, renal failure, polyuria, oliguria, urinary frequency
- **Hematologic:** Neutropenia, agranulocytosis, thrombocytopenia, hemolytic anemia, **pancytopenia**
- **Skin:** *Rash, pruritus, flushing,* scalded mouth sensation, exfoliative dermatitis, photosensitivity, alopecia
- **Other:** *Cough,* malaise, dry mouth, lymphadenopathy, *flulike symptoms, dizziness,* angioedema

Interactions

✳ **Drug-drug** • Increased risk of hyperkalemia with potassium supplements, potassium-sparing diuretics, salt substitutes • Risk of excessive hypotension with diuretics • Risk of abnormal response with lithium

✳ **Drug-lab test** • False-positive test for urine acetone

■ Nursing considerations

Assessment

- **History:** Allergy to ACE inhibitors, impaired renal or hepatic function, HF, salt or volume depletion, pregnancy, lactation
- **Physical:** Skin color, lesions, turgor; T; P, BP, peripheral perfusion; mucous membranes, bowel sounds, liver evaluation; urinalysis, LFTs, renal function tests, CBC and differential

Interventions

⊗ *Warning* Alert the surgeon and mark patient's chart with notice that moexipril is being taken; the angiotensin II formation subsequent to compensatory renin release during surgery will be blocked; hypotension may be reversed with volume expansion.

⊗ **Black box warning** Do not administer during pregnancy; drug may cause serious fetal injury or death.

- Monitor patient closely for a fall in BP secondary to reduction in fluid volume from excessive perspiration and dehydration, vomiting, or diarrhea; excessive hypotension may occur. Monitor potassium levels carefully in patients receiving potassium supplements, using potassium-sparing diuretics or salt substitutes.
- Reduce dosage in patients with impaired renal function.
- Monitor for excessive hypotension with any diuretic therapy.

Teaching points

- Do not stop taking this drug without consulting your health care provider. Take tablet 1 hr before meals.
- This drug is associated with fetal defects; using barrier contraceptives is advised to prevent pregnancy.
- Be careful in any situation that may lead to a drop in blood pressure (diarrhea, sweating, vomiting, dehydration); if light-headedness or dizziness occurs, consult your health care provider.
- You may experience these side effects: GI upset, diarrhea, loss of appetite, change in taste perception; mouth sores (frequent mouth care may help); rash; fast heart rate; dizziness, light-headedness (transient; change position slowly and limit activities to those that do not require alertness and precision).
- Report mouth sores; sore throat, fever, chills; swelling of the hands or feet; irregular heartbeat, chest pains; swelling of the face, eyes, lips, tongue; difficulty breathing; leg cramps.

▷ montelukast sodium
(mon tell oo' kast)

Singulair

PREGNANCY CATEGORY B

Drug classes

Antiasthmatic
Leukotriene receptor antagonist

Therapeutic actions

Selectively and competitively blocks the receptor that inhibits leukotriene formation, thus blocking many of the signs and symptoms of asthma—neutrophil and eosinophil migration, neutrophil and monocyte aggregation, leukocyte adhesion, increased capillary permeability, and smooth muscle contraction. These actions contribute to inflammation, edema, mucus secretion, and bronchoconstriction associated with the signs and symptoms of asthma.

Indications

- Prophylaxis and chronic treatment of asthma in adults and children 12 mo and older
- Relief of symptoms of seasonal allergic rhinitis in adults and children 2 yr and older
- Relief of symptoms of perennial allergic rhinitis in adults and children 6 mo and older
- Prevention of exercise-induced bronchoconstriction in patients 15 yr and older
- Unlabeled uses: Chronic urticaria, atopic dermatitis, NSAID-induced urticaria

Contraindications and cautions

- Contraindicated with hypersensitivity to montelukast or any of its components; acute asthma attacks; status asthmaticus.
- Use cautiously with pregnancy and lactation.

Available forms

Tablets—10 mg; chewable tablets—4, 5 mg; granules—4 mg/packet

Dosages

Adults and patients 15 yr and older
One 10-mg tablet PO daily, taken in the evening. For exercise-induced bronchoconstriction, dose taken 2 hr before exercise and not repeated for at least 24 hr.
Pediatric patients
6 mo–23 mo (perennial allergic rhinitis): 1 packet (4 mg) PO per day.
6–23 mo (asthma only): 4-mg granules PO daily, taken in the evening.
2–5 yr: One 4-mg chewable tablet PO daily, taken in the evening.
6–14 yr: One 5-mg chewable tablet PO daily, taken in the evening.

Pharmacokinetics

Route	Onset	Peak
Oral	Rapid	2–4 hr

Metabolism: Hepatic; $T_{1/2}$: 2.7–5.5 hr
Distribution: Crosses placenta and enters breast milk
Excretion: Feces, urine

Adverse effects

- **CNS:** Headache, dizziness, fatigue, neuropsychiatric events

- **GI:** Nausea, diarrhea, abdominal pain, dental pain, liver impairment
- **Respiratory:** Influenza, cold, nasal congestion, URI, cough, sinusitis
- **Other:** Generalized pain, fever, rash, fatigue, otitis media

Interactions

✳ **Drug-drug** ● Decreased effects and bioavailability if taken with phenobarbital; monitor patient and adjust dosage as needed

■ Nursing considerations

Assessment

- **History:** Hypersensitivity to montelukast or any of its components, acute asthma attacks, status asthmaticus, pregnancy, lactation
- **Physical:** T; orientation, reflexes; R, adventitious sounds; GI evaluation

Interventions

- Administer in the evening without regard to food.
- Ensure that drug is taken continually for optimal effect.
- Do not administer for acute asthma attack or acute bronchospasm.
- Be aware of the risk of neuropsychiatric events, including behavior and mood changes; monitor patient accordingly.
- Avoid the use of aspirin or NSAIDs in patients with known sensitivities while they are using this drug.
⊗ *Warning* Ensure that patient has a readily available rescue medication for acute asthma attacks or situations when a short-acting inhaled drug is needed.

Teaching points

- Take this drug regularly as prescribed; do not stop taking this drug during symptom-free periods; do not stop taking this drug without consulting your health care provider. Continue taking any other drugs for treating your asthma that have been prescribed for you. Notify your health care provider if your asthma becomes worse.
- Do not take this drug for an acute asthma attack or acute bronchospasm; this drug is not a bronchodilator, and routine emergency procedures should be followed during acute attacks.
- If taking this drug to prevent exercise-induced bronchoconstriction, take it at least

2 hours before exercising, and do not take another dose for at least 24 hours.

- Avoid using aspirin or NSAIDs if you have a known sensitivity to these drugs. Montelukast will not prevent reactions.
- You may experience these side effects: Dizziness (use caution when driving or performing activities that require alertness); nausea, vomiting (eat frequent small meals, take drug with food); headache (analgesics may be available).
- Report fever, acute asthma attacks, flulike symptoms, lethargy, changes in behavior or mood.

DANGEROUS DRUG

▷**morphine sulfate**
(*mor' feen*)

Timed-release: Avinza ⒹⓃⒸ, Kadian ⒹⓃⒸ, MS Contin ⒹⓃⒸ, Oramorph SR ⒹⓃⒸ, ratio-Morphine SR (CAN) ⒹⓃⒸ
Oral solution: MSIR, Roxanol, Roxanol T
Rectal suppositories: RMS
Injection: Astramorph PF, Duramorph, Morphine HP Injection (CAN), MOS Sulfate (CAN), PMS Morphine (CAN)
Preservative-free concentrate for microinfusion devices for intraspinal use: Infumorph, Morphine LP Injection (CAN), Morphine LP Epidural (CAN)
Liposome injection: DepoDur

PREGNANCY CATEGORY C

CONTROLLED SUBSTANCE C-II

Drug class
Opioid agonist analgesic

Therapeutic actions
Principal opium alkaloid; acts as agonist at specific opioid receptors in the CNS to produce analgesia, euphoria, sedation; the receptors mediating these effects are thought to be the same as those mediating the effects of endogenous opioids (enkephalins, endorphins).

Indications
- Relief of moderate to severe acute and chronic pain
- Preoperative medication to sedate and allay apprehension, facilitate induction of anesthesia, and reduce anesthetic dosage
- Analgesic adjunct during anesthesia
- Component of most preparations that are oral alcoholic solutions used for chronic severe pain, especially in terminal cancer patients
- Intraspinal use with microinfusion devices for the relief of intractable pain
- Treatment of pain following major surgery, ER liposome injection for single-dose administration by epidural route at the lumbar level
- Unlabeled use: Relief of pain associated with MI

Contraindications and cautions
- Contraindicated with hypersensitivity to opioids; during labor or delivery of a premature infant (may cross immature blood–brain barrier more readily); after biliary tract surgery or surgical anastomosis; with pregnancy, labor (respiratory depression in neonate; may prolong labor).
- Use cautiously with head injury and increased intracranial pressure; acute asthma, COPD, cor pulmonale, pre-existing respiratory depression, hypoxia, hypercapnia (may decrease respiratory drive and increase airway resistance); lactation (wait 4–6 hr after administration to nurse the baby); acute abdominal conditions; CV disease, supraventricular tachycardias; myxedema, seizure disorders, acute alcoholism, delirium tremens; cerebral arteriosclerosis; ulcerative colitis; fever; kyphoscoliosis; Addison disease; prostatic hypertrophy, urethral stricture, recent GI or GU surgery, toxic psychosis, renal or hepatic impairment.

Available forms
Injection—0.5, 1, 2, 4, 5, 8, 10, 15, 25, 50 mg/mL; tablets—15, 30 mg; CR tablets ⒹⓃⒸ —15, 30, 60, 100, 200 mg; ER tablets ⒹⓃⒸ —15, 30, 60, 100, 200 mg; soluble tablets—10, 15, 30 mg; oral solution—20 mg/mL; 10, 20, 100 mg/5 mL; concentrated oral solution—20 mg/mL, 100 mg/5 mL; suppositories—5, 10, 20, 30 mg; SR capsules ⒹⓃⒸ —20, 30, 50, 60, 100 mg; ER capsules ⒹⓃⒸ: 10, 20, 30, 50, 60, 80, 90, 100, 120 mg; liposome injection—10 mg/mL

Dosages
Adults
Oral
One-third to one-sixth as effective as parenteral administration because of first-pass metabolism; 5–30 mg every 4 hr PO. CR, ER, and SR: 30 mg every 8–12 hr PO or as directed by physician; *Kadian:* 20–100 mg PO daily–24-hr release system; *MS Contin:* 200 mg PO every 12 hr; *Avinza:* 30 mg PO daily; if opioid naïve, increase by 30 mg (or lower) increments every 4 days.

IM or subcutaneous
10 mg (range, 5–20 mg) every 4 hr or as directed by physician.

IV
10 mg every 4 hr. Usual individual range is 5–15 mg; usual daily dose is 12–120 mg.

Rectal
10–20 mg every 4 hr or as directed by physician.

Epidural
Initial injection of 5 mg in the lumbar region may provide pain relief for up to 24 hr. If adequate pain relief is not achieved within 1 hr, incremental doses of 1–2 mg may be given at intervals sufficient to assess effectiveness, up to 10 mg/24 hr. For continuous infusion, initial dose of 2–4 mg/24 hr is recommended. Further doses of 1–2 mg may be given if pain relief is not achieved initially.

Liposome injection
10–15 mg by lumbar epidural injection using a catheter or needle prior to major surgery or after clamping the umbilical cord during cesarean section.

Intrathecal
Dosage is usually one-tenth that of epidural dosage; a single injection of 0.2–1 mg may provide satisfactory pain relief for up to 24 hr. Do not inject more than 2 mL of the 5-mg/10 mL ampule or more than 1 mL of the 10-mg/10 mL ampule. Use only in the lumbar area. Repeated intrathecal injections are not recommended; use other routes if pain recurs. For epidural or intrathecal dosing, use preservative-free morphine preparations only.

Pediatric patients
Do not use in premature infants.

IM, subcutaneous
0.1–0.2 mg/kg (up to 15 mg per dose) every 4 hr or as directed by physician.

IV
0.05 to 0.1 mg/kg (up to 10 mg per dose) administered slowly.

Geriatric patients or impaired adults
Use caution. Respiratory depression may occur in the elderly, the very ill, those with respiratory problems. Reduced dosage may be needed.

Epidural
Use extreme caution; injection of less than 5 mg in the lumbar region may provide adequate pain relief for up to 24 hr.

Intrathecal
Use lower dosages than those recommended above for adults.

Pharmacokinetics

Route	Onset	Peak	Duration
Oral	Varies	60 min	5–7 hr
Rectal	Rapid	20–60 min	5–7 hr
Subcut.	Rapid	50–90 min	5–7 hr
IM	Rapid	30–60 min	5–6 hr
IV	Immediate	20 min	5–6 hr

Metabolism: Hepatic; T$_{1/2}$: 1.5–2 hr
Distribution: Crosses placenta; enters breast milk
Excretion: Bile, urine

▼ IV FACTS

Preparation: No further preparation needed for direct injection; dilute for infusion to a concentration of 0.1–1 mg/mL in D$_5$W.

Infusion: Inject slowly directly IV or into tubing of running IV, each 15 mg over 4–5 min; monitor by controlled infusion device to maintain pain control.

Incompatibilities: Do not mix with aminophylline, amobarbital, chlorothiazide, heparin, meperidine, phenobarbital, phenytoin, sodium bicarbonate, sodium iodide, thiopental.

Y-site incompatibilities: Do not give with minocycline, tetracycline.

Adverse effects
- **CNS:** *Light-headedness, dizziness, sedation,* euphoria, dysphoria, delirium, insomnia, agitation, anxiety, fear, hallucinations, disorientation, drowsiness, lethargy, impaired mental and physical performance, coma, mood changes, weakness, headache, tremor, seizures, miosis, visual disturbances, suppression of cough reflex
- **CV:** Facial flushing, peripheral circulatory collapse, tachycardia, bradycardia,

M

arrhythmia, palpitations, chest wall rigidity, hypertension, hypotension, orthostatic hypotension, syncope
- **Dermatologic:** Pruritus, urticaria, **laryngospasm, bronchospasm,** edema
- **GI:** *Nausea, vomiting,* dry mouth, anorexia, constipation, biliary tract spasm; increased colonic motility in patients with chronic ulcerative colitis
- **GU:** Ureteral spasm, spasm of vesical sphincters, urine retention or hesitancy, oliguria, antidiuretic effect, reduced libido or potency
- **Local:** Tissue irritation and induration (subcutaneous injection)
- **Major hazards: Respiratory depression, apnea, circulatory depression, respiratory arrest, shock, cardiac arrest**
- **Other:** *Sweating,* physical tolerance and dependence, psychological dependence

Interactions

✱ **Drug-drug** • Increased likelihood of respiratory depression, hypotension, profound sedation or coma in patients receiving barbiturate general anesthetics • Risk of toxicity if combined with alcohol (ER forms especially likely)

✱ **Drug-lab test** • Elevated biliary tract pressure (an effect of opioids) may cause increases in plasma amylase, lipase; determinations of these levels may be unreliable for 24 hr

■ Nursing considerations
Assessment

- **History:** Hypersensitivity to opioids; diarrhea caused by poisoning; labor or delivery of a preterm infant; biliary tract surgery or surgical anastomosis; head injury and increased intracranial pressure; acute asthma, COPD, cor pulmonale, pre-existing respiratory depression; acute abdominal conditions; CV disease, supraventricular tachycardias, myxedema, seizure disorders, acute alcoholism, delirium tremens; cerebral arteriosclerosis; ulcerative colitis; fever; kyphoscoliosis; Addison disease; prostatic hypertrophy, urethral stricture, recent GI or GU surgery, toxic psychosis, renal or hepatic impairment; pregnancy; lactation
- **Physical:** T; skin color, texture, lesions; orientation, reflexes, bilateral grip strength, affect; P, auscultation, BP, orthostatic BP, perfusion; R, adventitious sounds; bowel sounds, normal output; urinary frequency, voiding

pattern, normal output; ECG; EEG; LFTs, renal and thyroid function tests

Interventions

⊗ ***Black box warning*** Caution patient not to chew or crush CR, ER, or SR preparations and ensure appropriate use of these forms.
- Be aware that *Kadian* and *Avinza* capsules can be opened and the contents sprinkled on applesauce. *Kadian* capsules may be opened and the contents sprinkled over 10 mL of water and flushed through a prewetted #16 French gastrostomy tube.

⊗ ***Black box warning*** Do not substitute *Infumorph* for *Duramorph;* concentrations differ significantly and serious overdose can occur.

⊗ ***Black box warning*** Make sure patient is observed for at least 24 hr in a fully equipped and staffed environment if morphine is given by epidural or intrathecal route because of risk of serious adverse effects.

⊗ ***Warning*** Dilute and administer slowly IV to minimize likelihood of adverse effects.
- Tell patient to lie down during IV administration.

⊗ ***Warning*** Keep opioid antagonist and facilities for assisted or controlled respiration readily available during IV administration.

⊗ ***Warning*** Use caution when injecting IM or subcutaneously into chilled areas or in patients with hypotension or in shock; impaired perfusion may delay absorption; with repeated doses, an excessive amount may be absorbed when circulation is restored.
- Reassure patients that they are unlikely to become addicted; most patients who receive opiates for medical reasons do not develop dependence syndromes.

⊗ ***Black box warning*** Liposome preparation is for lumbar epidural injection only; it should not be given intrathecally, IV, or IM.

Teaching points

- Take this drug exactly as prescribed. Avoid alcohol, antihistamines, sedatives, tranquilizers, and over-the-counter drugs.
- Swallow controlled-release, extended-release, or sustained-release preparations (*MS Contin, Oramorph SR*) whole; do not cut, crush, or chew. *Kadian* and *Avinza* capsules may be opened and the contents sprinkled on applesauce.

- Do not take leftover medication for other disorders, and do not let anyone else take your prescription. Store this drug in a secure place.
- You may experience these side effects: Nausea, loss of appetite (take with food, lie quietly); constipation (use laxative); dizziness, sedation, drowsiness, impaired visual acuity (avoid driving or performing tasks that require alertness and visual acuity).
- Report severe nausea, vomiting, constipation, shortness of breath or difficulty breathing, rash.

▷ moxifloxacin hydrochloride
(mocks ee flox' a sin)

Avelox, Avelox ABC Pack, Avelox IV, Moxeza, Vigamox

PREGNANCY CATEGORY C

Drug classes
Antibiotic
Fluoroquinolone

Therapeutic actions
Bactericidal; interferes with DNA replication, repair, transcription, and recombination in susceptible gram-negative and gram-positive bacteria, preventing cell reproduction and leading to cell death.

Indications
- Treatment of adults with community-acquired pneumonia caused by susceptible strains of *Streptococcus pneumoniae* (including multidrug resistant strains), *Haemophilus influenzae, Mycoplasma pneumoniae, Chlamydia pneumoniae, Moraxella catarrhalis, Staphylococcus aureus, Klebsiella pneumoniae*
- Treatment of bacterial sinusitis caused by *S. pneumoniae, H. influenzae, M. catarrhalis*
- Treatment of acute bacterial exacerbation of chronic bronchitis caused by *S. pneumoniae, H. influenzae, H. parainfluenzae, K. pneumoniae, S. aureus, M. catarrhalis*
- Treatment of uncomplicated skin and skin structure infections caused by *S. aureus* or *Streptococcus pyogenes*

- Treatment of complicated skin and skin structure infections and complicated intra-abdominal infections caused by methicillin–susceptible *S. aureus, E. coli, K. pneumoniae, Enterobacter cloacae*
- Treatment of bacterial conjunctivitis caused by susceptible strains of bacteria (ophthalmic solution)
- ▪■ NEW INDICATION: Unlabeled use: Hospital-acquired pneumonia, infective endocarditis in adults

Contraindications and cautions
- Contraindicated with allergy to fluoroquinolones, prolonged QT interval, hypokalemia, pregnancy, lactation, history of myasthenia gravis.
- Use cautiously with hepatic impairment, seizures.

Available forms
Tablets—400 mg; injection—400 mg in 250 mL; ophthalmic solution—0.5 %

Dosages: systemic
Adults
- *Pneumonia:* 400 mg PO or IV daily for 7–14 days.
- *Sinusitis:* 400 mg PO or IV daily for 10 days.
- *Acute exacerbation of chronic bronchitis:* 400 mg PO or IV daily for 5 days.
- *Uncomplicated skin and skin structure infections:* 400 mg PO daily for 7 days.
- *Complicated skin and skin structure infections:* 400 mg PO or IV daily for 7–21 days.
- *Complicated intra-abdominal infections:* 400 mg PO or IV for 5–14 days.

Pediatric patients
Not recommended in patients younger than 18 yr.

Dosages: ophthalmic
Adults and pediatric patients
- *Treatment of bacterial conjunctivitis:* 1 drop in affected eye(s) 2–3 times/day for 7 days.

Pharmacokinetics

Route	Onset	Peak
Oral	Varies	1–3 hr
IV	Rapid	Minutes

M

Metabolism: Hepatic; T$_{1/2}$: 12–13.5 hr
Distribution: Crosses placenta; enters breast milk
Excretion: Feces, urine

▼ IV FACTS

Preparation: Supplied in premixed 250-mL bags; do not refrigerate; single use only, discard any excess.
Infusion: Infuse over 60 min by direct infusion or into Y-site of running IV.
Compatibilities: Compatible with 0.9% sodium chloride injection, 1M sodium chloride injection, 5% or 10% dextrose injection, sterile water for injection, lactated Ringer for injection.

Adverse effects

- **CNS:** *Headache,* dizziness, *insomnia,* fatigue, somnolence, depression, nervousness, anxiety, paresthesia
- **CV:** Palpitations, tachycardia, hypertension, hypotension, **prolonged QT interval**
- **GI:** *Nausea,* vomiting, dry mouth, *diarrhea,* anorexia, gastritis, stomatitis
- **Hematologic:** Altered PT, thrombocytopenia, eosinophilia
- **Respiratory:** Asthma, cough, dyspnea, pharyngitis, rhinitis
- **Other:** Fever, rash, sweating, photosensitivity, tendonitis, tendon rupture

Interactions

✴ **Drug-drug** ⊗ *Warning* Risk of severe cardiac arrhythmias if combined with any other drug known to prolong the QTc interval (quinidine, procainamide, amiodarone, sotalol, phenothiazines); avoid these combinations.

- Decreased absorption and therapeutic effectiveness of moxifloxacin if taken with sucralfate, metal medications (antacids), multivitamins, didanosine chewable; moxifloxacin should be taken 4 hr before or at least 8 hr after any of these drugs ● Increased risk of seizures if fluoroquinolones are combined with NSAIDs; monitor patient closely

■ Nursing considerations
Assessment

- **History:** Allergy to fluoroquinolones, prolonged QTc interval, hypokalemia, hepatic impairment, seizures, lactation, pregnancy, history of myasthenia gravis

- **Physical:** Skin color, lesions; T; orientation, reflexes, affect; R, adventitious sounds; P, BP; mucous membranes, bowel sounds; LFTs, ECG, CBC

Interventions

- Arrange for culture and sensitivity tests before beginning therapy.
- Continue therapy as indicated for condition being treated.
- Administer oral drug 4 hr before or at least 8 hr after antacids or other anion-containing drugs.
- Do not change dosage when switching from IV to oral dose.
- ⊗ *Warning* Discontinue drug at any sign of hypersensitivity (rash, photophobia) or with severe diarrhea.
- ⊗ *Black box warning* Risk of tendonitis and tendon rupture increases, especially in patients older than age 60 yr, patients taking corticosteroids, and those who have received a kidney, heart, or lung transplant.
- ⊗ *Black box warning* There is a risk of exacerbated weakness in patients with myasthenia gravis; avoid use in patients with a history of myasthenia gravis.
- ⊗ *Warning* Discontinue drug and monitor ECG if palpitations or dizziness occurs.
- Monitor clinical response; if no improvement is seen or a relapse occurs, repeat culture and sensitivity tests.
- Review proper administration of ophthalmic solution.

Teaching points

- Take oral drug once a day for the period prescribed. If antacids are being taken, take drug 4 hours before or at least 8 hours after the antacid.
- If you are using of ophthalmic solution, use for 7 days.
- You may experience these side effects: Nausea, vomiting, abdominal pain (eat frequent small meals); diarrhea or constipation (consult your health care provider); drowsiness, blurring of vision, dizziness (observe caution if driving or using dangerous equipment); sensitivity to the sun (avoid exposure, use a sunscreen).
- Report rash, visual changes, severe GI problems, weakness, tremors, palpitations, sensitivity to light, pain or inflammation in tendons.

Adverse effects in *italics* are most common; those in **bold** are life-threatening. ▨ Do not crush.

▽ muromonab-CD3
(mew ro' mon ab)

Orthoclone OKT3

PREGNANCY CATEGORY C

Drug classes
Immunosuppressant
Monoclonal antibody

Therapeutic actions
A murine monoclonal antibody to the antigen of human T cells; functions as an immunosuppressant by blocking T cells.

Indications
- Acute allograft rejection in renal transplant patients
- Treatment of steroid-resistant acute allograft rejection in cardiac and hepatic transplant patients

Contraindications and cautions
- Contraindicated with allergy to muromonab or any murine product; fluid overload as evidenced by chest X-ray; more than 3% weight gain in 1 wk; history of seizures.
- Use cautiously with fever (use antipyretics to decrease fever before therapy); previous administration of muromonab-CD3 (antibodies frequently develop, risks serious reactions on repeat administration); pregnancy.

Available forms
Injection—5 mg/5 mL

Dosages
Give only as an IV bolus in less than 1 min. Do not infuse or give by any other route.
Adults
5 mg/day IV for 10–14 days. Begin treatment once acute renal rejection is diagnosed. It is strongly recommended that methylprednisolone sodium succinate 8 mg/kg IV be given 1–4 hr prior to muromonab-CD3.
Pediatric patients weighing 30 kg or less
Initially, 2.5 mg/day IV for 10–14 days.
Pediatric patients weighing more than 30 kg
5 mg/day IV for 10–14 days. May increase 2.5 mg/day increments if needed.

Pharmacokinetics

Route	Onset	Peak	Duration
IV	Minutes	2–7 days	7 days

Metabolism: Tissue; $T_{1/2}$: 47–100 hr
Distribution: Crosses placenta
Excretion: Unknown

▼ IV FACTS
Preparation: Draw solution into a syringe through a low protein-binding 0.2- or 0.22-mcm filter. Discard filter and attach needle for IV bolus injection. Solution may develop fine translucent particles that do not affect its potency. Refrigerate solution; do not freeze or shake. Use immediately; discard unused portions.

Infusion: Administer as an IV bolus over less than 1 min. Do not give as an IV infusion or with other drug solutions. Flush line with saline before and after IV injection.

Incompatibilities: Do not mix with any other drug solution; do not infuse simultaneously with any other drug. If sequential infusions are required, flush line with saline before and after administering muromonab.

Adverse effects
- **CNS:** Malaise, *tremors,* coma, seizures, headache
- **GI:** *Vomiting, nausea, diarrhea*
- **Respiratory: Acute pulmonary edema,** *dyspnea, chest pain,* wheezing
- **Other:** Lymphomas, *increased susceptibility to infection, fever, chills,* **cytokine-release syndrome** ("flu" to shock)

Interactions
✳ **Drug-drug** • Reduce dosage of other immunosuppressive drugs; severe immunosuppression can lead to increased susceptibility to infection and increased risk of lymphomas; other immunosuppressives can be restarted about 3 days prior to cessation of muromonab • Risk of encephalopathy and CNS effects with indomethacin

■ Nursing considerations
Assessment
- **History:** Allergy to muromonab or any murine product; fluid overload; fever; previous administration of muromonab-CD3; pregnancy; lactation

M

- **Physical:** T, weight; P, BP; R, adventitious sounds; chest X-ray, CBC

Interventions

- Obtain chest X-ray within 24 hr of therapy to ensure chest is clear.
- Arrange for antipyretics (acetaminophen) if patient is febrile before therapy.
- Monitor WBC levels and circulating T cells periodically during therapy.
- ⊗ **Black box warning** Monitor patient very closely after first dose; acetaminophen PRN should be ordered to cover febrile reactions; cooling blanket may be needed in severe cases. Equipment for intubation and respiratory support should be readily available for severe pulmonary reactions; anaphylactoid reactions may occur with any dose.

Teaching points

- There is often a severe reaction to the first dose, including high fever and chills, difficulty breathing, and chest congestion (you will be closely watched, and comfort measures will be given).
- Avoid infection; people may wear masks and rubber gloves when caring for you; visitors may be limited.
- Report chest pain, difficulty breathing, nausea, chills.

▽**mycophenolate**
*(my coe **fen' oh** late)*

**mycophenolate
mofetil**
CellCept

**mycophenolate
sodium**
Myfortic ▭

PREGNANCY CATEGORY D

Drug class
Immunosuppressant

Therapeutic actions
Immunosuppressant: Inhibits T-lymphocyte activation; exact mechanism of action unknown, but binds to intracellular protein, which may prevent the generation of nuclear factor of activated T cells, and suppresses the immune activation and response of T cells; inhibits proliferative responses of T and B cells.

Indications

- Prophylaxis of organ rejection in patients receiving allogeneic renal, hepatic, and heart transplants; intended to be used concomitantly with corticosteroids and cyclosporine; *Myfortic* used for renal transplants only
- Unlabeled uses: Refractory uveitis as 2 g/day alone or in combination therapy; second-line agent for Churg-Strauss syndrome; combined with prednisolone for diffuse proliferative lupus nephritis

Contraindications and cautions

- Contraindicated with allergy to mycophenolate, pregnancy, lactation.
- Use cautiously with impaired renal function.

Available forms
Capsules—250 mg; tablets—500 mg; DR tablets ▭—180, 360 mg (*Myfortic*); powder for oral suspension—200 mg/mL; powder for injection—500 mg/vial

Dosages
Adults

- *Renal transplantation:* 1 g bid PO or IV (administered over at least 2 hr) starting as soon as possible after transplant; 720 mg PO bid on an empty stomach (*Myfortic*).
- *Cardiac transplantation:* 1.5 g PO bid or IV (IV over at least 2 hr).
- *Hepatic transplantation:* 1 g IV bid or 1.5 g PO bid (over at least 2 hr).

Pediatric patients

- *Renal transplantation:* 600 mg/m^2 oral suspension PO bid (up to a maximum daily dose of 2 g/10 mL oral suspension); 400 mg/m^2 PO bid to a maximum 720 mg bid (*Myfortic*).

Geriatric patients
Maximum recommended dose is 720 mg PO bid (DR tablets) (*Myfortic*).

Patients with severe renal or hepatic impairment
Avoid doses of more than 1 g bid. Monitor patient carefully for adverse response.

Patients with cardiac dysfunction
1.5 g bid.

Adverse effects in *italics* are most common; those in **bold** are life-threatening. ▭ Do not crush.

Pharmacokinetics

Route	Onset	Peak
Oral	Varies	45–60 min

Metabolism: Hepatic; $T_{1/2}$: 17.9 hr
Distribution: Crosses placenta; enters breast milk
Excretion: Urine

▼ IV FACTS

Preparation: Reconstitute and dilute to 6 mg/mL with 5% dextrose injection. Reconstitute each 500-mg vial with 14 mL 5% dextrose injection. Gently shake. Solution should be slightly yellow without precipitates. For a 1-g dose, dilute contents of two reconstituted vials into 140 mL of D_5W; for a 1.5-g dose, dilute contents of three reconstituted vials into 210 mL of D_5W. Use caution to avoid contact with solution. If contact occurs, wash with soap and water.

Infusion: Infuse over at least 2 hr. Begin as soon as possible following transplant and continue for 14 days or less.

Incompatibilities: Do not mix with any other drugs or infusion admixtures.

Adverse effects

- **CNS:** *Tremor, headache, insomnia,* paresthesias
- **CV:** Chest pain, *hypertension,* peripheral edema
- **GI: Hepatotoxicity,** *constipation, diarrhea, nausea, vomiting,* anorexia
- **GU:** *Renal impairment,* nephrotoxicity, *UTI,* oliguria
- **Hematologic:** Leukopenia, *anemia,* hyperkalemia, hypokalemia, hyperglycemia, red blood cell aplasia
- **Other:** Abdominal pain, fever, asthenia, back pain, ascites, neoplasms, *infection*

Interactions

✻ **Drug-drug** • Decreased levels and effectiveness with cholestyramine, antacids • Decreased levels and effectiveness of theophylline, phenytoin

■ Nursing considerations
Assessment

- **History:** Allergy to mycophenolate; pregnancy, lactation; renal function

- **Physical:** T; skin color, lesions; BP, peripheral perfusion; liver evaluation, bowel sounds, gum evaluation; LFTs, renal function tests, CBC

Interventions

⊗ *Warning* Monitor renal and liver function before and periodically during therapy; marked decreases in function may require dosage change or discontinuation of therapy.

- Use caution; do not confuse *Myfortic* and *CellCept.*

- Prepare oral suspension by tapping closed bottle several times, adding 47 mL water to bottle, and shaking closed bottle for 1 min. Add another 47 mL water; shake for 1 min.

- Ensure that DR forms are swallowed whole; do not cut, crush, or allow patient to chew tablets.

⊗ *Black box warning* Protect patient from exposure to infections and maintain sterile technique for invasive procedures; risk for serious to life-threatening infection exists.

⊗ *Black box warning* Monitor patient for possible lymphoma development related to drug action.

- Risk of pure red blood cell aplasia; monitor patient accordingly.

Teaching points

- Avoid infection while using this drug; avoid crowds or people with infections. Notify your health care provider immediately if you injure yourself.

- Avoid sun exposure; use sunscreen if you cannot avoid exposure.

- Have periodic blood tests to monitor your response to the drug and its effects.

- Do not discontinue this drug without consulting your health care provider. Do not cut, crush, or chew delayed-release tablets; swallow tablets whole.

- This drug should not be taken during pregnancy. If you think you are pregnant or you want to become pregnant, consult your health care provider. Use of contraceptive measures is advised.

- You may experience these side effects: Nausea, vomiting (take drug with food); diarrhea; headache (request analgesics).

- Report unusual bleeding or bruising, fever, sore throat, mouth sores, tiredness.

▷**nabilone**
(nab' bah lone)

Cesamet

PREGNANCY CATEGORY C

CONTROLLED SUBSTANCE C-II

Drug classes
Antiemetic
Cannabinoid

Therapeutic actions
A synthetic cannabinoid that interacts with the cannabinoid receptor systems in the CNS, causing an antiemetic effect as well as effects on mental state, dry mouth, and hypotension.

Indications
Treatment of nausea and vomiting associated with chemotherapy in patients who have had inadequate response to conventional antiemetic therapies

Contraindications and cautions
• Contraindicated with hypersensitivity to any component of the drug.
• Use cautiously with pregnancy, lactation; current or previous psychiatric disorder; current therapy with sedatives, hypnotics, or psychoactive drugs; history of substance abuse, hypertension, heart disease.

Available forms
Capsules—1 mg

Dosages
Adults
1–2 mg PO bid. Initial dose given 1–3 hr before chemotherapy begins. Maximum recommended dose, 6 mg/day PO, divided and given tid. May be given daily during each chemotherapy cycle and for 48 hr after last dose in cycle, if needed. Patient should be under close supervision because of risk of altered mental state.
Pediatric patients younger than 18 yr
Safety and efficacy not established.

Pharmacokinetics

Route	Onset	Peak
Oral	Rapid	2 hr

Metabolism: Hepatic; $T_{1/2}$: 2–35 hr (active metabolites)
Distribution: May cross placenta; may enter breast milk
Excretion: Feces, urine

Adverse effects
• **CNS:** *Drowsiness, vertigo, euphoria, ataxia,* headache, *difficulty concentrating,* sleep disturbance, disorientation, depersonalization, vision disturbances
• **CV:** *Orthostatic hypotension,* hypotension, tachycardia, palpitations, hypertension, arrhythmia
• **Dependence:** Risk of psychological dependence
• **GI:** *Dry mouth,* nausea, anorexia, increased appetite, diarrhea, constipation
• **Other:** Fatigue, malaise

Interactions
✳ **Drug-drug** • Risk of additive hypertension, tachycardia, cardiac toxicity if combined with amphetamines, cocaine, sympathomimetics; use caution • Risk of tachycardia, drowsiness if combined with atropine, scopolamine, antihistamines, anticholinergics; use caution • Risk of tachycardia, hypertension, drowsiness if combined with amitriptyline, amoxapine, desipramine, TCAs; use caution • Risk of additive CNS depression if combined with barbiturates, benzodiazepines, ethanol, lithium, opioids, buspirone, antihistamines, muscle relaxants, other CNS depressants; use caution

■ Nursing considerations
Assessment
• **History:** Allergy to any component of the drug; pregnancy, lactation; current or previous psychiatric disorders; concurrent therapy with sedatives, hypnotics, or psychoactive drugs; history of substance abuse, hypertension, heart disease
• **Physical:** Orientation, affect, reflexes; BP, standing BP, P; abdominal examination

Interventions
• Limit prescriptions to the minimum amount needed for a single chemotherapy cycle because of abuse potential.
• Warn patient about drug's profound effects on mental state and abuse potential before starting therapy. Patient should receive full information about potential drug effects;

Adverse effects in *italics* are most common; those in **bold** are life-threatening. ⊂⊃ Do not crush.

they can persist 48–72 hr after stopping drug.

• Warn patient about potential effects on mood and behavior to prevent panic if these occur.

• Patient should be supervised by a responsible adult while taking this drug; monitor patient during first round of chemotherapy to determine effects and their duration to establish guidelines for supervision. Supervision should begin again whenever dosage changes.

• Provide safety measures if dizziness and light-headedness occur.

⊗ **Warning** Discontinue drug if psychotic reaction occurs; observe patient closely until evaluated and counseled. Patient should participate in decision about further use of drug, perhaps at a lower dosage.

Teaching points

• This drug is called a cannabinoid. It works in the brain much like marijuana. It has many of the associated mental changes and dependency issues that occur with marijuana. It is advisable to be with a responsible adult when beginning therapy or changing dosages in case disorientation should occur.

• Take this drug exactly as prescribed. Take the first dose of the cycle 1–3 hours before chemotherapy starts. Take the drug every day during the chemotherapy cycle; you may need the drug for 1–2 days after the cycle to maintain relief of nausea and vomiting.

• If you miss a dose of the daily medication, take the dose as soon as you remember; then return to your usual routine. Do not double the dose.

• Be aware that the effects of this drug may continue 2–3 days after you stop taking it.

• It is not known how this drug could affect a breast-feeding infant. If you are breast-feeding, consult your health care provider.

• It is not known how this drug could affect a fetus. If you are pregnant or you decide to become pregnant while taking this drug, consult your health care provider.

• This drug interacts with many other drugs, and the interaction could cause serious side effects. Tell any health care provider who is taking care of you that you are taking this drug.

• Do not drink alcohol while taking this drug.

• You may experience these side effects: Dizziness, drowsiness, anxiety, disorientation, dry mouth. Do not drive a car or operate dangerous machinery while taking this drug, and avoid making any important decisions. For dry mouth, practice frequent mouth care; sucking on sugarless candies may help.

• Report chest pain, rapid heartbeat, depression, feelings of panic, hallucinations.

▽**nabumetone**
(nah byoo' meh tone)

Apo-Nabumetone (CAN),
Gen-Nabumetone (CAN)

PREGNANCY CATEGORY C
(FIRST AND SECOND TRIMESTERS)

PREGNANCY CATEGORY D
(THIRD TRIMESTER)

Drug classes
Analgesic (nonopioid)
NSAID

Therapeutic actions
Analgesic, anti-inflammatory, and antipyretic activities largely related to inhibition of prostaglandin synthesis; exact mechanisms of action are not known.

Indications

• Acute and long-term treatment of signs and symptoms of rheumatoid arthritis and osteoarthritis

Contraindications and cautions

• Contraindicated with significant renal impairment, allergy to NSAIDs, pregnancy, lactation, postoperative coronary arterny bypass graft

• Use cautiously with hepatic, CV, and GI conditions.

Available forms
Tablets—500, 750 mg

Dosages
Adults
1,000 mg PO as a single dose with or without food. 1,500–2,000 mg/day have been used. May be given in divided doses.
Pediatric patients
Safety and efficacy not established.

Patients with renal impairment
Maximum starting dose should not exceed 750 mg daily for moderate insufficiency, 500 mg for severe insufficiency.

Pharmacokinetics

Route	Onset	Peak
Oral	30 min	30–60 min

Metabolism: Hepatic; $T_{1/2}$: 22.5–30 hr
Distribution: Crosses placenta; enters breast milk
Excretion: Urine

Adverse effects

- **CNS:** *Headache, dizziness, somnolence, insomnia,* fatigue, tiredness, dizziness, tinnitus, ophthalmic effects
- **Dermatologic:** *Rash,* pruritus, sweating, dry mucous membranes, stomatitis
- **GI:** *Nausea, dyspepsia, GI pain,* diarrhea, vomiting, *constipation,* flatulence
- **GU:** Dysuria, **renal impairment**
- **Hematologic:** Bleeding, platelet inhibition with higher doses, neutropenia, eosinophilia, leukopenia, pancytopenia, thrombocytopenia, agranulocytosis, granulocytopenia, aplastic anemia, decreased Hgb or Hct, bone marrow depression, menorrhagia
- **Respiratory:** Dyspnea, hemoptysis, pharyngitis, **bronchospasm**, rhinitis
- **Other:** Peripheral edema, anaphylactoid reactions to **fatal anaphylactic shock**

Interactions

✴ **Drug-drug** • Increased risk of bleeding if combined with warfarin, aspirin

■ Nursing considerations

Assessment
- **History:** Renal impairment; impaired hearing; allergies; hepatic, CV, and GI conditions; lactation; pregnancy
- **Physical:** Skin color and lesions; orientation, reflexes, ophthalmic and audiometric evaluation, peripheral sensation; P, edema; R, adventitious sounds; liver evaluation; CBC, clotting times, LFTs, renal function tests; serum electrolytes, stool guaiac

Interventions
⊗ **Black box warning** Be aware that patient may be at increased risk for CV events or GI bleeding; monitor accordingly.

⊗ **Black box warning** Drug is not for use for the treatment of perioperative pain following coronary artery bypass graft surgery.
- Administer drug with food or after meals if GI upset occurs.
- Arrange for periodic ophthalmologic examinations during long-term therapy.
⊗ **Warning** If overdose occurs, institute emergency procedures—gastric lavage, induction of emesis, supportive therapy.

Teaching points
- Take drug with food or meals if GI upset occurs; take only the prescribed dosage.
- Dizziness, drowsiness can occur (avoid driving or using dangerous machinery).
- Report sore throat, fever, rash, itching, weight gain, swelling in ankles or fingers; changes in vision; black, tarry stools, chest pain.

▽ **nadolol**
(nay doe' lol)

Corgard

PREGNANCY CATEGORY C

Drug classes
Antianginal
Antihypertensive
Beta-adrenergic blocker (nonselective)

Therapeutic actions
Competitively blocks beta-adrenergic receptors in the heart and juxtaglomerular apparatus, decreasing the influence of the sympathetic nervous system on these tissues and decreasing the excitability of the heart, cardiac output, oxygen consumption, renin release, and BP.

Indications
- Hypertension, alone or with other drugs, especially diuretics
- Long-term management of angina pectoris
- Unlabeled use: Migraines

Contraindications and cautions
- Contraindicated with sinus bradycardia (HR less than 45 beats/min), second- or third-degree heart block (PR interval greater than 0.24 sec), cardiogenic shock, HF, asthma, COPD, lactation.

- Use cautiously with diabetes or thyrotoxicosis, pregnancy.

Available forms
Tablets—20, 40, 80, 120, 160 mg

Dosages
Adults
- *Hypertension:* Initially, 40 mg PO daily; gradually increase dosage in 40- to 80-mg increments until optimum response is achieved. Usual maintenance dose is 40–80 mg/day; up to 320 mg daily may be needed. To discontinue, reduce dosage gradually over a 1- to 2-wk period.
- *Angina:* Initially, 40 mg PO daily; gradually increase dosage in 40- to 80-mg increments at 3- to 7-day intervals until optimum response is achieved or heart rate markedly decreases. Usual maintenance dose is 40–80 mg daily; up to 240 mg/day may be needed. Safety and efficacy of larger doses not established. To discontinue, reduce dosage gradually over 1- to 2-wk period.

Pediatric patients
Safety and efficacy not established.

Geriatric patients or patients with renal failure

CrCl (mL/min/1.73 m^2)	Dosage Intervals (hr)
More than 50	24
31–50	24–36
10–30	24–48
Less than 10	40–60

Pharmacokinetics

Route	Onset	Peak	Duration
Oral	Varies	3–4 hr	17–24 hr

Metabolism: T$_{1/2}$: 20–24 hr
Distribution: Crosses placenta; enters breast milk
Excretion: Urine

Adverse effects
- **Allergic reactions:** Pharyngitis, erythematous rash, fever, sore throat, **laryngospasm,** respiratory distress
- **CNS:** Dizziness, vertigo, tinnitus, fatigue, emotional depression, paresthesias, sleep disturbances, hallucinations, disorientation, memory loss, slurred speech
- **CV:** *Heart failure, cardiac arrhythmias,* peripheral vascular insufficiency, claudica-

tion, **stroke, pulmonary edema,** hypotension
- **Dermatologic:** Rash, pruritus, sweating, dry skin
- **EENT:** Eye irritation, dry eyes, conjunctivitis, blurred vision
- **GI:** *Gastric pain, flatulence, constipation, diarrhea, nausea, vomiting,* anorexia, ischemic colitis, renal and mesenteric arterial thrombosis, retroperitoneal fibrosis, hepatomegaly, acute pancreatitis
- **GU:** *Impotence, decreased libido,* Peyronie disease, dysuria, nocturia, urinary frequency
- **Musculoskeletal:** Joint pain, arthralgia, muscle cramp
- **Respiratory:** Bronchospasm, dyspnea, cough, bronchial obstruction, nasal stuffiness, rhinitis, pharyngitis (less likely than with propranolol)
- **Other:** *Decreased exercise tolerance, development of antinuclear antibodies,* hyperglycemia or hypoglycemia, elevated serum transaminase

Interactions
✳ **Drug-drug** • Increased effects with verapamil • Increased serum levels and toxicity of IV lidocaine, theophylline • Increased risk of orthostatic hypotension with alpha-adrenergic blockers • Increased risk of peripheral ischemia with ergotamine, dihydroergotamine • Decreased antihypertensive effects with NSAIDs, clonidine • Hypertension followed by severe bradycardia with epinephrine
✳ **Drug-lab test** • Possible false results with glucose or insulin tolerance tests

■ Nursing considerations
Assessment
- **History:** Sinus bradycardia, second- or third-degree heart block, cardiogenic shock, heart failure; asthma, COPD; diabetes or thyrotoxicosis; pregnancy; lactation
- **Physical:** Weight, skin condition, neurologic status, P, BP, ECG, respiratory status, renal and thyroid function tests, blood and urine glucose

Interventions
⊗ **Black box warning** Do not discontinue drug abruptly after long-term therapy (hypersensitivity to catecholamines may have developed, causing exacerbation of angina, MI,

and ventricular arrhythmias). Taper drug gradually over 2 wk with monitoring.

• Consult physician about withdrawing drug if patient is to undergo surgery (controversial).

Teaching points

• Do not stop taking unless instructed to do so by your health care provider; drug must be stopped gradually to prevent serious adverse effects.
• Avoid driving or dangerous activities if dizziness, disorientation occur.
• Report difficulty breathing, night cough, swelling of extremities, slow pulse, confusion, depression, rash, fever, sore throat.

▽ nafarelin acetate

(naf´ a re lin)

Synarel

PREGNANCY CATEGORY X

Drug class

Gonadotropin-releasing hormone (GnRH)

Therapeutic actions

A potent agonistic analogue of GnRH, which is released from the hypothalamus to stimulate LH and FSH release from the pituitary; these hormones are responsible for regulating reproductive status. Repeated dosing abolishes the stimulatory effect on the pituitary gland, leading to decreased secretion of gonadal steroids by about 4 wk; consequently, tissues and functions that depend on gonadal steroids for their maintenance become quiescent.

Indications

• Treatment of endometriosis, including pain relief and reduction of endometriotic lesions
• Treatment of central precocious puberty in children of both genders

Contraindications and cautions

• Contraindicated with known sensitivity to GnRH, GnRH-agonist analogues, excipients in the product; undiagnosed abnormal vaginal bleeding; pregnancy; lactation (potential androgenic effects on the fetus).
• Use cautiously with rhinitis.

Available forms

Nasal solution—2 mg/mL (200 mcg/spray)

Dosages

Adults

• *Endometriosis:* 400 mcg/day. One spray (200 mcg) into one nostril in the morning and 1 spray into the other nostril in the evening. Start treatment between days 2 and 4 of the menstrual cycle. 800-mcg dose may be administered as 1 spray into each nostril in the morning (a total of 2 sprays) and again in the evening for patients with persistent regular menstruation after 2 months of treatment. Treatment for 6 mo is recommended. Retreatment is not recommended because safety has not been established.

Pediatric patients

• *Central precocious puberty:* 1,600 mcg/day. Two sprays (400 mcg) in each nostril in the morning and 2 sprays in each nostril in the evening; may be increased to 1,800 mcg/day. If 1,800 mcg are needed, give 3 sprays into alternating nostrils three times/day. Continue until resumption of puberty is desired.

Pharmacokinetics

Route	Onset	Peak
Nasal	Rapid	4 wk

Metabolism: $T_{1/2}$: 2–4 hr
Distribution: Crosses placenta; may enter breast milk
Excretion: Urine

Adverse effects

• **CNS:** Dizziness, headache, sleep disorders, fatigue
• **Endocrine:** *Androgenic effects* (acne, edema, mild hirsutism, decrease in breast size, deepening of the voice, oily skin or hair, weight gain, clitoral hypertrophy or testicular atrophy), *hypoestrogenic effects* (flushing, sweating, vaginitis, nervousness, emotional lability)
• **GI:** Hepatic impairment
• **GU:** Fluid retention, vaginal dryness, ovarian cysts
• **Local:** *Nasal irritation*
• **Other:** Rash, pruritus; with prolonged therapy, bone density loss has been noted

Adverse effects in *italics* are most common; those in **bold** are life-threatening. ▣▣▣ Do not crush.

■ Nursing considerations
Assessment
- **History:** Sensitivity to GnRH, GnRH-agonist analogues, excipients in the product; undiagnosed abnormal genital bleeding; pregnancy; lactation; rhinitis
- **Physical:** Weight; hair distribution pattern; skin color, texture, lesions; breast examination; nasal mucosa; orientation, affect, reflexes; P, auscultation, BP, peripheral edema; liver evaluation; bone density studies in long-term therapy

Interventions
- Ensure that patient is not pregnant before therapy; begin therapy for endometriosis during menstrual period, days 2–4; advise the use of barrier contraceptives.
- Store drug upright; protect from exposure to light.
- Arrange for bone age and growth velocity studies before therapy and periodically thereafter if retreatment is suggested because of return of endometriosis.
- Ensure patient has enough of the drug to prevent interruption of therapy.
- Caution patient that androgenic effects may not be reversible when the drug is withdrawn.
- Monitor nasal mucosa for signs of erosion during course of therapy.
- If a topical decongestant needs to be used, wait at least 2 hr after dosing with nafarelin.

Teaching points
- Use this drug without interruption; be sure that you have enough on hand to prevent interruption. Store the drug upright. Protect the bottle from exposure to light. Clear nasal passages by gently blowing your nose before administering drug.
- Regular menstruation should cease within 4–6 weeks of therapy. Breakthrough bleeding or ovulation may still occur.
- Consult your health care provider if you need a topical nasal decongestant; a decongestant should be used at least 2 hours after nafarelin use.
- This drug is contraindicated during pregnancy; use a nonhormonal form of birth control during therapy. If you become pregnant, discontinue the drug and consult your health care provider immediately.

- You may experience these side effects: Masculinizing effects (acne, hair growth, deepening of voice, oily skin or hair; may not be reversible); low estrogen effects (flushing, sweating, vaginal irritation, nervousness); nasal irritation.
- Report abnormal growth of facial hair, deepening of the voice, unusual bleeding or bruising, fever, chills, sore throat, vaginal itching or irritation, nasal irritation or burning.

DANGEROUS DRUG

▽**nalbuphine hydrochloride**
(*nal' byoo feen*)

Nubain

PREGNANCY CATEGORY B

PREGNANCY CATEGORY D
(PROLONGED USE OR WITH HIGH DOSES AT TERM)

Drug class
Opioid agonist-antagonist analgesic

Therapeutic actions
Nalbuphine acts as an agonist at specific opioid receptors in the CNS to produce analgesia and sedation but also acts to cause hallucinations and is an antagonist at mu receptors.

Indications
- Relief of moderate to severe pain
- Preoperative analgesia, as a supplement to surgical anesthesia, and for obstetric analgesia during labor and delivery
- Unlabeled use: Prevention and treatment of intrathecal morphine–induced pruritus after cesarean section

Contraindications and cautions
- Contraindicated with hypersensitivity to nalbuphine, sulfites.
- Use cautiously with emotionally unstable patients or those with a history of opioid abuse, pregnancy prior to labor (neonatal withdrawal may occur if mothers used drug during pregnancy), labor or delivery (use with caution during delivery of premature infants, who are especially sensitive to respiratory depressant effects of opioids),

bronchial asthma, COPD, respiratory depression, anoxia, increased intracranial pressure, acute MI when nausea and vomiting are present, biliary tract surgery (may cause spasm of the sphincter of Oddi), lactation.

Available forms

Injection—10 mg/mL, 20 mg/mL

Dosages

Adults

Usual dose is 10 mg for a 70-kg person IM, IV, or subcutaneously every 3–6 hr as needed. Individualize dosage. In nontolerant patients, the recommended single maximum dose is 20 mg, with a maximum total daily dose of 160 mg. Patients dependent on opioids may experience withdrawal symptoms with administration of nalbuphine; control by small increments of morphine by slow IV administration until relief occurs. If the previous opioid was morphine, meperidine, codeine, or another opioid with similar duration of activity, administer one-fourth the anticipated nalbuphine dose initially, and observe for signs of withdrawal. If no untoward symptoms occur, progressively increase doses until analgesia is obtained.

- *Supplement to anesthesia:* Induction—0.3–3 mg/kg IV over 10–15 min; maintenance—0.25–0.5 mg/kg IV.

Pediatric patients younger than 18 yr

Not recommended.

Patients with renal or hepatic impairment

Reduce dosage.

Pharmacokinetics

Route	Onset	Peak	Duration
IV	2–3 min	15–20 min	3–6 hr
Subcut., IM	Less than 15 min	30–60 min	3–6 hr

Metabolism: Hepatic; $T_{1/2}$: 5 hr
Distribution: Crosses placenta; enters breast milk
Excretion: Urine

▼ IV FACTS

Preparation: No additional preparation is required.

Infusion: Administer by direct injection or into the tubing of a running IV.

Y-site incompatibilities: Do not give with nafcillin, ketorolac.

Adverse effects

- **CNS:** *Sedation, clamminess, sweating, headache,* nervousness, restlessness, depression, crying, confusion, faintness, hostility, unusual dreams, hallucinations, euphoria, dysphoria, unreality, *dizziness, vertigo,* floating feeling, feeling of heaviness, numbness, tingling, flushing, warmth, blurred vision
- **CV:** Hypotension, hypertension, bradycardia, tachycardia
- **Dermatologic:** Pruritus, burning, urticaria
- **GI:** Nausea, vomiting, cramps, dyspepsia, bitter taste, *dry mouth*
- **GU:** Urinary urgency
- **Respiratory:** Respiratory depression, dyspnea, asthma

Interactions

❋ **Drug-drug** • Potentiation of effects with barbiturate anesthetics or other CNS depressants

■ Nursing considerations

Assessment

- **History:** Hypersensitivity to nalbuphine, sulfites; lactation; emotional instability or history of opioid abuse; pregnancy; bronchial asthma, COPD, respiratory depression; anoxia; increased intracranial pressure; MI; biliary tract surgery
- **Physical:** Orientation, reflexes, bilateral grip strength, affect; pupil size, vision; pulse, auscultation, BP; R, adventitious sounds; bowel sounds, normal output; urine output; LFTs, renal function tests

Interventions

⊗ *Warning* Taper dosage when discontinuing after prolonged use to avoid withdrawal symptoms.

⊗ *Warning* Keep opioid antagonist and facilities for assisted or controlled respiration available in case of respiratory depression.

- Reassure patient about addiction liability; most patients who receive opiates for medical reasons do not develop dependence syndromes.

Teaching points

- This drug must be given by injection.
- You may experience these side effects: Dizziness, sedation, drowsiness, impaired visual acuity (avoid driving, performing tasks that require alertness), nausea, loss of appetite (lying quietly, eating frequent small meals may help).
- Report severe nausea, vomiting, palpitations, shortness of breath, or difficulty breathing.

▽naloxone hydrochloride

(nal ox' one)

PREGNANCY CATEGORY C

Drug classes

Diagnostic agent
Opioid antagonist

Therapeutic actions

Pure opioid antagonist; reverses the effects of opioids, including respiratory depression, sedation, hypotension; can reverse the psychotomimetic and dysphoric effects of opioid agonist-antagonists, such as pentazocine.

Indications

- Complete or partial reversal of opioid depression, including respiratory depression induced by opioids, including natural and synthetic narcotics, propoxyphene, methadone, nalbuphine, butorphanol, pentazocine
- Diagnosis of suspected acute opioid overdose
- Unlabeled uses: Dementia of Alzheimer type, tardive dyskinesia

Contraindications and cautions

- Contraindicated with allergy to opioid antagonists.
- Use cautiously with opioid addiction, CV disorders, pregnancy, lactation.

Available forms

Injection—0.4 mg/mL, 1 mg/mL

Dosages

IV administration is recommended in emergencies when rapid onset of action is required.

Adults

- *Opioid overdose:* Initial dose of 0.4–2 mg, IV. Additional doses may be repeated at 2- to 3-min intervals. If no response after 10 mg, question the diagnosis. IM or subcutaneous routes may be used if IV route is unavailable.
- *Postoperative opioid depression:* Titrate dose to patient's response. Initial dose of 0.1–0.2 mg IV at 2- to 3-min intervals until desired degree of reversal. Repeat doses may be needed within 1- to 2-hr intervals, depending on amount and type of opioid. Supplemental IM doses produce a longer-lasting effect.

Pediatric patients 1 mo and older

- *Opioid overdose:* Initial dose is 0.01 mg/kg IV. Subsequent dose of 0.1 mg/kg may be administered if needed. May be given IM or subcutaneously in divided doses.
- *Postoperative opioid depression:* For the initial reversal of respiratory depression, inject in increments of 0.005–0.01 mg IV at 2- to 3-min intervals to the desired degree of reversal.

Pediatric patients younger than 1 mo

- *Opioid-induced depression:* 0.01 mg/kg IV, IM, or subcutaneously; repeat as needed, following adult recommendations.

Pharmacokinetics

Route	Onset	Duration
IV	2 min	4–6 hr
IM, Subcut.	3–5 min	4–6 hr

Metabolism: Hepatic; $T_{1/2}$: 30–81 min
Distribution: Crosses placenta; may enter breast milk
Excretion: Urine

▼ IV FACTS

Preparation: Dilute in normal saline or 5% dextrose solutions for IV infusions. The addition of 2 mg in 500 mL of solution provides a concentration of 0.004 mg/mL; titrate rate by response. Use diluted mixture within 24 hr. After that time, discard any remaining solution.
Infusion: Inject directly, or titrate rate of infusion based on response.
Incompatibilities: Do not mix naloxone with preparations containing bisulfite, metabisulfite, high–molecular-weight anions, alkaline pH solutions.

Adverse effects
- **Acute opioid abstinence syndrome:** *Nausea, vomiting, sweating, tachycardia, increased BP, tremulousness*
- **CNS:** Reversal of analgesia and excitement (postoperative use)
- **CV:** *Hypotension, hypertension,* ventricular tachycardia and **fibrillation, pulmonary edema** (postoperative use)

■ Nursing considerations
Assessment
- **History:** Allergy to opioid antagonists; opioid addiction; CV disorders; lactation
- **Physical:** Sweating; reflexes, pupil size; P, BP; R, adventitious sounds

Interventions
- Monitor patient continuously after use of naloxone; repeat doses may be needed, depending on duration of opioid and time of last dose.
- ⊗ **Warning** Maintain open airway and provide artificial ventilation, cardiac massage, vasopressor drugs if needed to counteract acute opioid overdose.

Teaching points
- This drug must be given by injection.
- Report sweating, feelings of tremulousness.

▷ naltrexone hydrochloride
(nal trex' one)

ReVia, Vivitrol

PREGNANCY CATEGORY C

Drug class
Opioid antagonist

Therapeutic actions
Pure opiate antagonist; markedly attenuates or completely, reversibly blocks the subjective effects of IV opioids, including those with mixed opioid agonist-antagonist properties.

Indications
- Adjunct to treatment of alcohol or opioid dependence as part of a comprehensive treatment program

- Prevention of relapse to opioid dependence following opioid detoxification
- Unlabeled uses: Eating disorders, pathologic gambling, IBs, PTSD, pruritus, smoking cessation

Contraindications and cautions
- Contraindicated with allergy to opioid antagonists, acute hepatitis, liver failure, any patient who has failed the naloxone challenge.
- Use cautiously with opioid addiction (may produce withdrawal symptoms; do not administer unless patient has been opioid-free for 7–10 days); opioid withdrawal; lactation; depression, suicidal tendencies; pregnancy.

Available forms
Tablets— 50 mg; injection—380 mg/vial

Dosages
⊗ **Warning** Give naloxone challenge before use except in patients already showing clinical signs of opioid withdrawal.
Adults
IV challenge test
Draw 2 ampules of naloxone, 2 mL (0.8 mg) into a syringe. Inject 0.5 mL (0.2 mg). Leave needle in vein, and observe for 30 sec. If no signs of withdrawal occur, inject remaining 1.5 mL (0.6 mg), and observe for 20 min for signs and symptoms of withdrawal (stuffiness or running nose, tearing, yawning, sweating, tremor, vomiting, piloerection, feeling of temperature change, joint or bone and muscle pain, abdominal cramps, skin crawling).
Subcutaneous challenge
Administer 2 mL (0.8 mg) naloxone, and observe for signs and symptoms of withdrawal for 20 min. If any of the signs and symptoms of withdrawal occur or if there is any doubt that the patient is opioid free, do not administer naltrexone. Confirmatory rechallenge can be done within 24 hr. Inject 4 mL IV, and observe for signs and symptoms of withdrawal. Repeat until no signs and symptoms are seen and patient is no longer at risk.
Naltrexone
- *Alcoholism:* 50 mg/day PO or 380 mg IM into upper outer quadrant of gluteal muscle once every 4 wk (*Vivitrol*). Alternate buttock with each administration.

- *Opioid dependence:* Initial dose of 25 mg PO. Observe for 1 hr; if no signs or symptoms are seen, complete dose with 25 mg. Usual maintenance dose is 50 mg/24 hr PO. Flexible dosing schedule can be used with 100 mg every other day or 150 mg every third day.

Pediatric patients

Safety has not been established in patients younger than 18 yr.

Pharmacokinetics

Route	Onset	Peak	Duration
Oral	15–30 min	60 min	24–72 hr

Metabolism: Hepatic; $T_{1/2}$: 3.9–12.9 hr
Distribution: Crosses placenta; enters breast milk
Excretion: Urine

Adverse effects

- **CNS:** *Difficulty sleeping, anxiety, nervousness, headache, low energy,* increased energy, irritability, dizziness, blurred vision, burning, light sensitivity
- **CV:** Phlebitis, edema, increased BP, nonspecific ECG changes
- **Dermatologic:** *Rash,* oily skin, pruritus, acne
- **GI: Hepatocellular injury,** *abdominal pain or cramps, nausea, vomiting,* loss of appetite, diarrhea, constipation
- **GU:** *Delayed ejaculation, decreased potency,* increased frequency of or discomfort with voiding
- **Respiratory:** Nasal congestion, rhinorrhea, sneezing, sore throat, excess mucus or phlegm, sinus trouble, epistaxis, injection site reaction
- **Other:** *Chills, increased thirst,* increased appetite, weight change, yawning, swollen glands, *joint and muscle pain,* injection site reaction

Interactions

✷ **Drug-drug** • Decreased effectiveness of opioid analgesics or other opioid-containing preparations

■ Nursing considerations

Assessment

- **History:** Allergy to opioid antagonists; opioid addiction; opioid withdrawal; acute hepatitis, liver failure; lactation; depression, suicidal tendencies; pregnancy

- **Physical:** Sweating; skin lesions, color; reflexes, affect, orientation, muscle strength; P, BP, edema, baseline ECG; R, adventitious sounds; liver evaluation; urine screen for opioids, LFTs

Interventions

⊗ *Warning* Do not use until patient has been opioid free for 7–10 days; check urine opioid levels.

⊗ *Warning* Do not administer until patient has passed a naloxone challenge.

- Administer IM injection in the gluteal region, alternating buttocks.
- Initiate treatment slowly, and monitor until patient has been given naltrexone in the full daily dose with no signs and symptoms of withdrawal.

⊗ **Black box warning** Obtain periodic liver function tests during therapy; discontinue therapy at sign of increasing hepatic impairment (risk of hepatocellular injury).

- Do not use opioid drugs for analgesia, cough, and cold; do not use opioid antidiarrheal preparations; patient will not respond; use a nonopioid preparation.
- Ensure that patient is actively participating in a comprehensive treatment program.

Teaching points

- This drug will help facilitate abstinence from alcohol or opioids.
- This drug blocks the effects of opioids and other opiates.
- Wear or carry a medical ID tag to alert emergency medical personnel that you are taking this drug.
- Small doses of heroin or other opiate drugs will not have an effect. Self-administration of large doses of heroin or other opioids can overcome the blockade effect but may cause death, serious injury, or coma.
- You may experience these side effects: Drowsiness, dizziness, blurred vision, anxiety (avoid driving or operating dangerous machinery); diarrhea, nausea, vomiting (take drug with food to decrease these effects); decreased sexual function.
- Report unusual bleeding or bruising; dark, tarry stools; yellowing of eyes or skin; running nose; tearing; sweating; chills; joint or muscle pain.

▷naproxen
(na prox' en)

naproxen
Apo-Naproxen (CAN), Apo-
Naproxen EC (CAN), Apo-Naproxen
SR (CAN), EC-Naprosyn,
Gen-Naproxen EC (CAN), Naprelan ⓓⓝⓒ,
Naprosyn, Novo-Naprox (CAN),
Novo-Naprox-EC (CAN)

naproxen sodium
Aleve, Anaprox, Anaprox DS ⓓⓝⓒ,
Apo-Napro-Na (CAN), Apo-Napro-Na
DS (CAN) ⓓⓝⓒ, Mediproxen,
Midol Extended Relief,
Novo Naprox Sodium (CAN),
Novo Naprox Sodium DS (CAN) ⓓⓝⓒ,
Novo Naprox SR (CAN)

PREGNANCY CATEGORY C

Drug classes
Analgesic (nonopioid)
NSAID

Therapeutic actions
Analgesic, anti-inflammatory, and antipyretic activities largely related to inhibition of
prostaglandin synthesis; exact mechanisms of
action are not known.

Indications
- Mild to moderate pain
- Treatment of primary dysmenorrhea, rheumatoid arthritis, osteoarthritis, ankylosing
spondylitis, tendinitis, bursitis, acute gout
- OTC use: Temporary relief of minor aches
and pains associated with the common cold,
headache, toothache, muscular aches, backache, minor pain of arthritis, pain of menstrual cramps, reduction of fever
- Treatment of juvenile arthritis (*naproxen*)

Contraindications and cautions
- Contraindicated with allergy to naproxen,
salicylates, other NSAIDs; pregnancy; lactation, perioperative coronary artery bypass
graft.
- Use cautiously with asthma, chronic urticaria, CV dysfunction, hypertension, GI
bleeding, peptic ulcer, impaired hepatic or
renal function.

Available forms
Tablets—250, 375, 500 mg; 220, 275, 412.5,
500 mg (as naproxen sodium); DR tablets ⓓⓝⓒ—
375, 500 mg; CR tablets ⓓⓝⓒ—375, 500 mg;
suspension—125 mg/5 mL

Dosages
Do not exceed 1,500 mg/day (1,650 mg/day
naproxen sodium).
Adults
- *Rheumatoid arthritis or osteoarthritis,
ankylosing spondylitis:*
DR (EC-Naprosyn) ⓓⓝⓒ
375–500 mg PO bid.
CR (Naprelan) ⓓⓝⓒ
750–1,000 mg PO daily as a single dose.
Naproxen sodium
275–550 mg bid PO. May increase to 1.65
g/day for a limited period.
Naproxen tablets
250–500 mg PO bid.
Naproxen suspension
250 mg (10 mL), 375 mg (15 mL), 500 mg
(20 mL) PO bid.
- *Acute gout:*
CR (Naprelan) ⓓⓝⓒ
1,000–1,500 mg PO daily as a single dose.
Naproxen sodium
825 mg PO followed by 275 mg every 8 hr until attack subsides.
Naproxen
750 mg PO, followed by 250 mg every 8 hr until attack subsides.
- *Mild to moderate pain:*
CR (Naprelan) ⓓⓝⓒ
1,000 mg PO daily as a single dose.
Naproxen sodium
550 mg PO followed by 275 mg every 6–8 hr.
Naproxen
500 mg PO followed by 500 mg every 12 hr or
250 mg every 6–8 hr.
OTC
200 mg PO every 8–12 hr with a full glass of
liquid while symptoms persist. Do not exceed
600 mg in 24 hr.
Pediatric patients
- *Juvenile arthritis:*
Naproxen
10 mg/kg/day PO given in two divided doses.
Naproxen sodium
Safety and efficacy not established.
OTC
Do not give to children younger than 12 yr
unless under advice of physician.

Adverse effects in *italics* are most common; those in **bold** are life-threatening. ⓓⓝⓒ Do not crush.

Geriatric patients
Do not give more than 200 mg every 12 hr PO.

Pharmacokinetics

Drug	Onset	Peak	Duration
Naproxen	1 hr	2–4 hr	7 hr or less
Naproxen sodium	1 hr	1–2 hr	7 hr or less

Metabolism: Hepatic; $T_{1/2}$: 12–15 hr
Distribution: Crosses placenta; enters breast milk
Excretion: Urine

Adverse effects

- **CNS:** *Headache, dizziness, somnolence, insomnia,* fatigue, tiredness, dizziness, tinnitus, ophthalmic effects
- **Dermatologic:** *Rash,* pruritus, sweating, dry mucous membranes, stomatitis
- **GI:** *Nausea, dyspepsia, GI pain,* diarrhea, vomiting, *constipation,* flatulence
- **GU:** Dysuria, renal impairment, including renal failure, interstitial nephritis, hematuria
- **Hematologic:** Bleeding, platelet inhibition with higher doses, neutropenia, eosinophilia, leukopenia, pancytopenia, thrombocytopenia, agranulocytosis, granulocytopenia, aplastic anemia, decreased Hgb or Hct, menorrhagia
- **Respiratory:** Dyspnea, hemoptysis, pharyngitis, **bronchospasm,** rhinitis
- **Other:** Peripheral edema, **anaphylactoid reactions** to **anaphylactic shock**

Interactions

✴ **Drug-drug** • Increased serum lithium levels and risk of toxicity with naproxen
✴ **Drug-lab test** • Falsely increased values for urinary 17-ketogenic steroids; discontinue naproxen therapy for 72 hr before adrenal function tests • Inaccurate measurement of urinary 5-HIAA

■ Nursing considerations
Assessment

- **History:** Allergy to naproxen, salicylates, other NSAIDs; asthma, chronic urticaria, CV dysfunction; hypertension; GI bleeding; peptic ulcer; impaired hepatic or renal function; pregnancy; lactation
- **Physical:** Skin color and lesions; orientation, reflexes, ophthalmologic and audiometric evaluation, peripheral sensation; P, BP, edema; R, adventitious sounds; liver evaluation; CBC, clotting times, LFTs, renal function tests; serum electrolytes; stool guaiac

Interventions

⊗ *Black box warning* Be aware that patient may be at increased risk for CV events, GI bleeding; monitor accordingly.
⊗ *Black box warning* Contraindicated for treatment of perioperative pain following coronary artery bypass graft surgery; serious complications can occur.

- Give with food or after meals if GI upset occurs. Do not cut, crush, or allow patient to chew DR or CR forms.
- Arrange for periodic ophthalmologic examination during long-term therapy.

⊗ *Warning* If overdose occurs, institute emergency procedures—gastric lavage, induction of emesis, supportive therapy.

Teaching points

- Take drug with food or meals if GI upset occurs; take only the prescribed dosage. Do not cut, crush, or chew extended-release forms.
- Dizziness, drowsiness can occur (avoid driving or using dangerous machinery).
- Report sore throat; fever; rash; itching; weight gain; swelling in ankles or fingers; changes in vision; black, tarry stools; chest pain.

▽ **naratriptan**
*(nar ah **trip'** tan)*

Amerge

PREGNANCY CATEGORY C

Drug classes
Antimigraine drug (triptan)
Serotonin selective agonist

Therapeutic actions
Binds to serotonin receptors to cause vascular constrictive effects on cranial blood vessels, causing the relief of migraine in selective patients; migraine is believed to be caused by vasodilation of cranial blood vessels in these patients.

Indications
- Treatment of acute migraine attacks with or without aura

Contraindications and cautions

• Contraindicated with allergy to any triptan, active CAD, uncontrolled hypertension, cerebrovascular disease or peripheral vascular syndromes, severe renal or hepatic impairment.

• Use cautiously in the elderly; with lactation, pregnancy.

Available forms

Tablets—1, 2.5 mg

Dosages

Adults

Single dose of 1 mg PO or 2.5 mg PO; may be repeated in 4 hr if needed. Do not exceed 5 mg/24 hr.

Pediatric patients

Safety and efficacy not established.

Patients with renal or hepatic impairment

Contraindicated in severe renal impairment (creatinine clearance less than 15 mL/min) or severe hepatic impairment (Child-Pugh grade C). In mild or moderate renal or hepatic impairment, start with lowest dose and do not exceed 2.5 mg/24 hr.

Pharmacokinetics

Route	Onset	Peak
Oral	Slow	2–3 hr

Metabolism: Hepatic; $T_{1/2}$: 6 hr
Distribution: Crosses placenta; enters breast milk
Excretion: Urine

Adverse effects

• **CNS:** *Dizziness,* headache, anxiety, fatigue, drowsiness, paresthesias, corneal defects
• **CV:** BP alterations, tightness or pressure in chest
• **Other:** *Neck, throat, or jaw discomfort;* generalized pain, nausea

Interactions

✳ **Drug-drug** • Prolonged vasoactive reactions when taken concurrently with ergot-containing drugs; avoid this combination • Increased blood levels and prolonged effects if combined with hormonal contraceptives; monitor patient and adjust dosage as appropriate • Increased risk of serotonin syndrome if combined with SSRIs or selective norepinephrine reuptake inhibitors

■ Nursing considerations

Assessment

• **History:** Allergy to any triptan, active CAD, uncontrolled hypertension, severe renal or hepatic impairment, pregnancy, lactation
• **Physical:** Orientation, reflexes, peripheral sensation; P, BP; LFTs, renal function tests

Interventions

• Administer to relieve acute migraine, not as a prophylactic measure; administer with food.
• Establish safety measures if CNS or visual disturbances occur.
• Provide appropriate analgesics as needed for pain related to therapy.
• Recommend the use of barrier contraceptives to women of childbearing age; serious birth defects could occur.
• Control environment (lighting, temperature) as appropriate to help relieve migraine.
⊗ *Warning* Monitor BP of patients with possible coronary artery disease; discontinue naratriptan at any sign of angina or prolonged high BP.

Teaching points

• Take drug to relieve migraine; do not use as a means of prevention. Take drug with food.
• Dosage may be repeated in 4 hours if headache returns or has not been relieved. Do not take more than 5 milligrams in one 24-hour period.
• This drug should not be taken during pregnancy; if you suspect that you are pregnant, stop taking the drug, and contact your health care provider.
• Continue to do anything that usually helps you during a migraine—adjust lighting, control noise, and so forth.
⊗ *Warning* Contact your health care provider immediately if you experience chest pain or pressure that is severe or does not go away.
• You may experience these side effects: Dizziness, drowsiness (avoid driving or using dangerous machinery while taking this drug); numbness, tingling, feelings of tightness or pressure.
• Report severe pain or discomfort, visual changes, palpitations, unrelieved headache.

▽natalizumab
(nah tah liz' yoo mab)

Tysabri

PREGNANCY CATEGORY C

Drug classes
Monoclonal antibody
MS drug

Therapeutic actions
Monoclonal antibody specific for the alpha-4 subunit on the surface of all leukocytes except neutrophils. Binding with this subunit inhibits adhesion of leukocytes to their counter-receptors, including those on vascular endothelium. Preventing leukocyte adhesion inhibits migration of leukocytes into inflamed tissue and may inhibit recruitment and inflammatory activity of activated immune cells. The exact mechanism of action in MS (thought to be an autoimmune disorder) is not known, but natalizumab may prevent migration of leukocytes into the brain and reduce plaque formation.

Indications
• Monotherapy for patients with relapsing MS to delay physical disability and decrease the frequency of exacerbations.
• Treatment of Crohn disease in patients who have not responded to or are unable to tolerate other therapies.

Contraindications and cautions
• Contraindicated with allergy to any component of the preparation, progressive multifocal leukoencephalopathy (PML) or history of it, lactation.
• Use caution with immune supression, pregnancy.

Available forms
Single-use vials—300 mg/15 mL (20 mg/mL)

Dosages
Adults
300 mg by IV infusion over 1 hr every 4 wk.
Pediatric patients
Safety and efficacy not established.

Pharmacokinetics

Route	Onset	Peak
IV	Slow	7–8 days

Metabolism: Tissue; $T_{1/2}$: 11–15 days
Distribution: May cross placenta; may enter breast milk
Excretion: Tissue

▼ IV FACTS
Preparation: Withdraw 15 mL of natalizumab from vial using a sterile syringe and needle. Inject drug into 100 mL 0.9% sodium chloride injection. Gently invert to mix completely. Do not shake. Inspect solution; it should be clear and free of particulates. Use immediately, or refrigerate and use within 8 hr. Do not freeze. If refrigerated, warm to room temperature before infusion.
Infusion: Infuse over approximately 1 hr. After infusion, flush with 0.9% sodium chloride solution. Observe patient during and for 1 hr after infusion to detect hypersensitivity reactions. Do not give as an IV push or bolus.
Incompatibilities: Do not mix with any other drug or IV solution.

Adverse effects
• **CNS:** *Headache, depression,* dizziness, suicidal ideation, tremor, rigors, **PML**
• **GI:** *Gastroenteritis, abdominal discomfort, diarrhea,* **abnormal liver function,** tooth infections
• **GU:** Irregular menses, dysmenorrhea, amenorrhea, urinary urgency, urinary frequency, UTI
• **Hematologic:** *Increased levels of circulating lymphocytes, monocytes, eosinophils, basophils, nucleated RBCs*
• **Respiratory:** *Lower respiratory tract infections,* tonsillitis
• **Skin:** *Rash,* pruritus, dermatitis
• **Other:** *Infection, fatigue, arthralgia,* **anaphylactic reactions,** infusion reaction (headache, dizziness, fatigue, urticaria, pruritus, rigors, hypersensitivity reactions), weight changes

Interactions
✳ **Drug-drug** • Increased risk of infection if combined with corticosteroids or other immune suppressants including tumor necrosis factor α (TNF-α) inhibitors; avoid this combination

■ Nursing considerations

Assessment

- **History:** Allergy to any component of the preparation; pregnancy, lactation; immune suppression, PML
- **Physical:** T; skin color, lesions; orientation, reflexes; R, adventitious sounds; LFTs; anti-JC virus antibody status

Interventions

⊗ **Black box warning** Be aware that drug increases the risk of PML, which can be fatal. Natalizumab is available only through the TOUCH prescribing program; patients should be monitored closely for signs of PML, and drug should be stopped immediately if they occur. Drug is available only to prescribers and patients who have entered the TOUCH program and understand the risks of the drug and need to monitor closely. Risk increases with number of infusions, with treatment for longer than 2 yr, with prior use of immunosuppressants, or with presence of anti-JC virus antibodies. Determine anti-JC virus antibody status before use. There is a risk of immune reconstitution inflammatory syndrome (a severe immune reaction) in patients who developed PML and discontinued the drug.

- Withhold drug at any sign of PML (change in eyesight, thought disturbances, loss of balance or strength); an MRI will be ordered to evaluate the patient.
- Make sure patient is not immune-suppressed or taking immunosuppressants or TNF-α inhibitors.
- Refrigerate vials. Product contains no preservatives; do not use after expiration date. Protect from light. Do not freeze.
- Monitor patient during infusion and for 1 hr afterward for hypersensitivity reaction (headache, dizziness, urticaria, pruritus, rigors). Discontinue drug immediately at first sign of hypersensitivity reaction. Provide supportive care if reaction occurs after infusion.
- Do not administer drug to patient who has had a hypersensitivity reaction to it.
- Urge women of childbearing age to use barrier contraceptive; effects of this drug on a fetus are not known.
- If woman is breast-feeding, suggest another method of feeding the infant during therapy.

Teaching points

- You must enroll in the TOUCH Prescribing Program before you can receive this drug; the program includes careful monitoring and education about the risk of a serious, viral, brain lesion from using this drug.
- This drug is given by IV infusion every 4 weeks. The infusion will take about 1 hour, and you will need to be monitored for another hour. Keep a calendar to remind you of the dates for each infusion.
- This drug should not be taken during pregnancy or when breast-feeding unless absolutely necessary; use a barrier contraceptive, effects of the drug on a fetus or breast-feeding infant are not known.
- This drug increases your risk of infection. Contact your health care provider if fever or other signs of infection occur.
- You may experience these side effects: Headache (medication may be available to help); respiratory infection, urinary tract infection (avoid crowded areas and people with infections, and wash your hands often); upset stomach, GI discomfort (small, frequent meals may help).
- Report fever, hives, rash, depression, any sign of infection; changes in thinking, balance, strength, or eyesight that last for several days.

DANGEROUS DRUG

▷ **nateglinide**
*(nah **teg**' lah nyde)*

Starlix

PREGNANCY CATEGORY C

Drug classes

Antidiabetic
Meglitinide

Therapeutic actions

Closes potassium channels in the beta cells of the pancreas, which causes the opening of calcium channels and a resultant increase in insulin release; highly selective for pancreatic potassium channels with little effect on the vasculature. Glucose-lowering abilities depend on the existence of functioning beta cells in the pancreas.

Indications

- Adjunct to diet and exercise to lower blood glucose in patients with type 2 diabetes

mellitus whose hyperglycemia cannot be managed by diet and exercise alone
- Combination therapy with metformin or a thiazolidinedione for glycemic control in those patients with type 2 diabetes who do not receive adequate control with diet and either drug

Contraindications and cautions
- Contraindicated with hypersensitivity to the drug, diabetic ketoacidosis, type 1 diabetes, pregnancy, lactation.
- Use cautiously with hepatic impairment.

Available forms
Tablets—60, 120 mg

Dosages
Adults
120 mg PO tid taken 1–30 min before meals; 60 mg PO tid may be tried if patient is near HbA$_{1c}$ goal.
Pediatric patients
Safety and efficacy not established.

Pharmacokinetics

Route	Onset	Peak	Duration
Oral	Rapid	1 hr	4 hr

Metabolism: Hepatic; T$_{1/2}$: 1.5 hr
Distribution: Crosses placenta; may enter breast milk
Excretion: Feces, urine

Adverse effects
- **CNS:** *Headache,* paresthesias, dizziness
- **Endocrine:** Hypoglycemia (low risk)
- **GI:** Nausea, diarrhea, constipation, vomiting, dyspepsia
- **Respiratory:** *URI,* sinusitis, rhinitis, bronchitis

Interactions
✳ **Drug-drug** • Increased risk of hypoglycemia if taken with salicylates, NSAIDs, beta blockers, MAOIs; monitor patient closely

■ Nursing considerations
Assessment
- **History:** Hypersensitivity to the drug, diabetic ketoacidosis, type 1 diabetes, renal or hepatic impairment, pregnancy, lactation
- **Physical:** Skin color, lesions; T; orientation, reflexes, peripheral sensation; R, adventi-

tious sounds; liver evaluation, bowel sounds; blood glucose, LFTs, renal function tests

Interventions
- Administer drug three times a day 1–30 min before meals; if a patient skips or adds a meal, the dosage should be skipped or added appropriately.
- Monitor serum glucose levels and HbA$_{1c}$ levels frequently to determine effectiveness of drug and dosage being used.
- Arrange for consult with dietitian to establish weight loss program and dietary control as appropriate.
- Arrange for thorough diabetic teaching program to include disease, dietary control, exercise, signs and symptoms of hypoglycemia and hyperglycemia, avoidance of infection, and hygiene.

Teaching points
- Do not discontinue this medication without consulting your health care provider.
- Take this drug 1–30 minutes before meals (three times a day); if you skip a meal, skip the dosage; if you add a meal, take your dosage before that meal also.
- Monitor blood for glucose as prescribed.
- Return for regular follow-up visits to monitor your response to the drug and possible need for dosage adjustment.
- Continue diet and exercise program established for control of diabetes.
- Know the signs and symptoms of hypoglycemia and hyperglycemia and appropriate treatment as indicated; report the incidence of either to your health care provider.
- You may experience these side effects: Headache, increased upper respiratory infections, nausea.
- Report fever, sore throat, unusual bleeding or bruising; severe abdominal pain.

▽ **nebivolol**
*(nah **bev'** ah loll)*

Bystolic

PREGNANCY CATEGORY C

Drug classes
Antihypertensive
Beta-adrenergic blocker

N

Therapeutic actions

Decreases heart rate and contractility, suppresses renin release, and vasodilates and decreases peripheral vascular resistance, all leading to decreased blood pressure and decreased cardiac output and oxygen consumption.

Indications

- Treatment of hypertension, as monotherapy or with other antihypertensives

Contraindications and cautions

- Contraindicated with hypersensitivity to any component of the drug, severe bradycardia, heart block, cardiogenic shock, decompensated HF, sick sinus syndrome (unless a pacemaker is in place), severe hepatic impairment (Child-Pugh greater than grade B), lactation.
- Use cautiously with bronchospastic diseases, surgery, diabetes, hypoglycemia, thyroid dysfunction, renal impairment, hepatic impairment, history of anaphylactic reactions, pheochromocytoma, pregnancy.

Available forms

Tablets—2.5, 5, 10, 20 mg

Dosages

Adults
Starting dose: 5 mg/day PO; may be increased at 2-wk intervals to a maximum of 40 mg/day PO based on patient response.
Pediatric patients
Safety and efficacy not established.
Patients with severe renal impairment
If creatinine clearance is less than 30 mL/min, starting dose 2.5 mg/day PO; titrate slowly and monitor patient closely.
Patients with hepatic impairment
In moderate impairment, starting dose of 2.5 mg/day PO; titrate slowly and monitor patient closely. In severe impairment, drug not recommended.

Pharmacokinetics

Route	Onset	Peak
Oral	Rapid	1.5–4 hr

Metabolism: Hepatic; $T_{1/2}$: Not reported
Distribution: May cross placenta; may enter breast milk
Excretion: Urine, feces

Adverse effects

- **CNS:** *Headache,* dizziness, insomnia
- **CV:** Chest pain, bradycardia, arrhythmias, peripheral edema, hypotension
- **GI:** Nausea, diarrhea
- **Respiratory:** Dyspnea
- **Other:** Fatigue

Interactions

✳ **Drug-drug** • Risk of decreased HR and impaired conduction if combined with calcium antagonists (particularly verapamil, diltiazem), antiarrhythmics, cardiac glycosides; monitor patient closely because dosage adjustments may be needed • Risk of severe suppression of sympathetic activity if combined with other beta blockers, catecholamine-depleting drugs; avoid this combination or, if it must be used, monitor patient closely • Risk of unexpected BP response if combined with CYP2D6 inhibitors or inducers (quinidine, propafenone, fluoxetine, paroxetine); monitor patient response very closely and adjust dosage as needed • Risk of serious side effects when discontinuing combined use of clonidine and nebivolol; taper nebivolol and discontinue for several days before gradually tapering clonidine

■ Nursing considerations

Assessment

- **History:** Hypersensitivity to any component of drug, sinus bradycardia, heart block, HF, cardiogenic shock, renal impairment, liver impairment, diabetes, bronchospastic disorders, thyroid dysfunction, pregnancy, lactation, anaphylactic reactions
- **Physical:** Orientation, affect, reflexes; P, BP, heart sounds, peripheral perfusion; R, adventitious sounds; ECG, renal function tests, LFTs, thyroid levels, blood glucose

Interventions

⊗ *Warning* Do not stop this drug abruptly after long-term therapy; hypersensitivity to catecholamines can exacerbate angina, MI, ventricular arrhythmia. Taper drug gradually over 2 wk while monitoring patient.
- Consult surgeon about withdrawing drug if patient is to have surgery (withdrawal is controversial).
- Establish safety precautions if CNS changes occur (dizziness, altered thought process).

Teaching points

- This drug may be used with other antihypertensives; follow your drug regimen carefully.
- Take this drug once a day, with or without food. Try to take it at about the same time each day.
- If you miss a dose, take the next dose as soon as you remember. Do not make up or double doses; do not take more than one dose each day.
- Do not run out of tablets, and do not stop taking this drug suddenly. If it is decided that you need to stop this drug, the dose will be tapered slowly over 1 to 2 weeks to prevent possible side effects.
- If you have diabetes, be aware that this drug may block the signs or symptoms of hypoglycemia and hyperglycemia. You will need to monitor yourself carefully while taking this drug.
- Do not drive or operate dangerous machinery until you know how this drug affects you; it may cause dizziness and loss of alertness.
- It is not known how this drug could affect an unborn fetus. You should use contraception while you are taking this drug. If you become pregnant while taking this drug, consult your health care provider.
- It is not known how this drug could affect a breast-feeding infant. Because of the risk of serious side effects in an infant, you should choose another method of feeding the infant while taking this drug.
- You may experience these side effects: Dizziness, insomnia (do not drive a car or engage in activities that require alertness if these effects occur); headache (consult your health care provider about medication to relieve headache).
- Report difficulty breathing, increasing shortness of breath, swelling in the ankles or legs, sudden weight gain, or a very slow heart rate.

▽nefazodone

See Appendix R, *Less commonly used drugs*.

▽nelarabine

See Appendix R, *Less commonly used drugs*.

▽nelfinavir mesylate

(nell fin' a veer)

Viracept

PREGNANCY CATEGORY B

Drug classes
Antiviral
Protease inhibitor

Therapeutic actions
Inhibitor of the HIV-1 protease; prevents viral cleavage resulting in the production of immature, noninfectious virus. Though no controlled trials of the effectiveness of nelfinavir exist, studies may indicate effectiveness in combination with nucleoside analogues.

Indications
- Treatment of HIV infection when antiretroviral therapy is warranted in combination with nucleoside analogues or other antiretroviral drugs
- Unlabeled use: Postexposure prophylaxis following exposure to HIV

Contraindications and cautions
- Contraindicated with life-threatening allergy to any component, concurrent use of drugs dependent on CYP3A for clearance (amiodarone, quinidine, ergot derivatives, pimozide, midazolam, triazolam, lovastatin, simvastatin).
- Use cautiously with renal and hepatic impairment, hemophilia, pregnancy, lactation.

Available forms
Tablets—250, 625 mg

Dosages
Adults and patients older than 13 yr
750 mg PO tid or 1,250 mg PO bid in combination with other antiretroviral drugs; do not exceed 2,500 mg/day.
Pediatric patients 2–13 yr
45–55 mg/kg PO bid or 25–35 mg/kg PO tid.
Pediatric patients younger than 2 yr
Not recommended.

Pharmacokinetics

Route	Onset	Peak
Oral	Slow	2–4 hr

Metabolism: Hepatic; T$_{1/2}$: 3.5–5 hr
Distribution: May cross placenta; may enter breast milk
Excretion: Feces

Adverse effects

- **CNS:** Anxiety, depression, insomnia, myalgia, dizziness, paresthesias, **seizures,** suicide ideation
- **Dermatologic:** Dermatitis, folliculitis, fungal dermatitis, rash, sweating, urticaria
- **GI:** *Diarrhea, nausea, GI pain,* anorexia, vomiting, dyspepsia, liver enzyme elevations
- **Respiratory:** Dyspnea, pharyngitis, rhinitis, sinusitis
- **Other:** Eye disorders, sexual dysfunction

Interactions

✳ **Drug-drug** ⊗ *Warning* Risk of severe toxic effects and life-threatening arrhythmias with rifampin, triazolam, midazolam, amiodarone, quinidine, ergot derivatives, pimozide, lovastatin, simvastatin; avoid these combinations • Decreased effectiveness with rifabutin, phenobarbital, phenytoin, dexamethasone, carbamazepine • Possible loss of effectiveness of hormonal contraceptives with nelfinavir; recommend using barrier contraceptives

✳ **Drug-food** • Decreased metabolism and risk of toxic effects if combined with grapefruit juice; avoid this combination

✳ **Drug-alternative therapy** • Decreased effectiveness of nelfinavir if combined with St. John's Wort

■ Nursing considerations

CLINICAL ALERT!
Name confusion has occurred between *Viracept* (nelfinavir) and *Viramune* (nevirapine); use caution.

Assessment

- **History:** Life-threatening allergy to any component; impaired hepatic or renal function; pregnancy, lactation; hemophilia; concurrent drug, herbal therapy use
- **Physical:** T; affect, reflexes, peripheral sensation; R, adventitious sounds; bowel sounds, liver evaluation; LFTs, renal function tests

Interventions

- Administer with meals or a light snack.
- Monitor patient for signs of opportunistic infections that will need to be treated appropriately.
- Arrange for loperamide to control diarrhea if it occurs.
- Recommend that patient use barrier contraceptives while using this drug.

Teaching points

- Take drug exactly as prescribed; take missed doses as soon as possible and return to normal schedule; do not take double doses.
- Take with meals or a light snack; do not drink grapefruit juice while using this drug.
- These drugs are not a cure for AIDS or AIDS-related complex; opportunistic infections may occur and regular medical care should be sought to deal with the disease.
- The long-term effects of this drug are not yet known.
- This drug combination does not reduce the risk of transmission of HIV to others by sexual contact or blood contamination; use appropriate precautions.
- Use barrier contraceptives; this drug may block the effectiveness of hormonal contraceptives.
- Avoid St. John's Wort while taking this drug.
- You may experience these side effects: Nausea, loss of appetite, diarrhea (eat frequent small meals; medication is available to control diarrhea); dizziness, loss of feeling (take appropriate precautions).
- Report extreme fatigue, lethargy, severe headache, severe nausea, vomiting, difficulty breathing, rash, changes in color of urine or stool.

---

 neomycin sulfate
(nee o mye' sin)

Mycifradin, Neo-fradin, Neo-Tabs

PREGNANCY CATEGORY D

Drug class
Aminoglycoside

Therapeutic actions
Bactericidal: Inhibits protein synthesis in susceptible strains of bacteria; functional integrity

of bacterial cell membrane appears to be disrupted, causing cell death. Due to poor PO absorption, oral neomycin is used to suppress GI bacterial flora.

Indications
• Preoperative suppression of GI bacterial flora
• Adjunct treatment in hepatic coma to reduce ammonia-forming bacteria in the GI tract

Contraindications and cautions
• Contraindicated with allergy to aminoglycosides, intestinal obstruction, pregnancy, lactation.
• Use cautiously in the elderly or in patients with diminished hearing, decreased renal function, dehydration, neuromuscular disorders (myasthenia gravis, parkinsonism, infant botulism).

Available forms
Tablets—500 mg; oral solution—125 mg/5 mL

Dosages
Adults
• *Preoperative preparation for elective colorectal surgery:* See manufacturer's recommendations for a complex 3-day regimen that includes oral erythromycin, bisacodyl, magnesium sulfate, enemas, and dietary restrictions.
• *Hepatic coma:* 4–12 g/day PO in divided doses for 5–6 days, as adjunct to protein-free diet and supportive therapy, including transfusions, as needed.
Pediatric patients
• *Hepatic coma:* 50–100 mg/kg/day PO in divided doses for 5–6 days, as adjunct to protein-free diet and supportive therapy including transfusions, as needed.
Geriatric patients or patients with renal failure
Reduce dosage and carefully monitor serum drug levels and renal function tests throughout treatment. If this is not possible, reduce frequency of administration.

Pharmacokinetics

Route	Onset	Peak
Oral	Varies	1–4 hr

Metabolism: $T_{1/2}$: 3 hr
Distribution: Crosses placenta; enters breast milk
Excretion: Feces, urine

Adverse effects
Although limited absorption occurs across the intact GI mucosa, the risk of absorption from ulcerated area requires consideration of all side effects with oral and parenteral therapy.
• **CNS:** Ototoxicity—*tinnitus, dizziness,* vertigo, deafness (partially reversible to irreversible), vestibular paralysis, confusion, disorientation, depression, lethargy, nystagmus, visual disturbances, headache, *numbness, tingling,* tremor, paresthesias, muscle twitching, **seizures**
• **CV:** Palpitations, hypotension, hypertension
• **GI:** Hepatic toxicity, *nausea, vomiting, anorexia,* weight loss, stomatitis, increased salivation
• **GU:** Nephrotoxicity
• **Hematologic:** *Leukemoid reaction,* agranulocytosis, granulocytosis, leukopenia, leukocytosis, thrombocytopenia, eosinophilia, pancytopenia, anemia, hemolytic anemia, increased or decreased reticulocyte count, electrolyte disturbances
• **Hypersensitivity:** Hypersensitivity reactions—*purpura, rash,* urticaria, exfoliative dermatitis, itching
• **Local:** *Pain, irritation*
• **Other:** Fever, apnea, splenomegaly, joint pain, *superinfection*

Interactions
✳ **Drug-drug** • Increased ototoxic, nephrotoxic, neurotoxic effects with other aminoglycosides, potent diuretics • Increased neuromuscular blockade and muscular paralysis with anesthetics, nondepolarizing neuromuscular blocking drugs, succinylcholine, citrate-anticoagulated blood • Potential inactivation of both drugs if mixed with beta-lactam–type antibiotics • Increased bactericidal effect with penicillins, cephalosporins, carbenicillin, ticarcillin • Decreased absorption and therapeutic effects of digoxin

✳ **Drug-lab test** • Falsely low serum aminoglycoside levels with penicillin or cephalosporin therapy; these antibiotics can inactivate aminoglycosides after the blood sample is drawn

■ Nursing considerations

Assessment

- **History:** Allergy to aminoglycosides; intestinal obstruction, diminished hearing, decreased renal function, dehydration, neuromuscular disorders; pregnancy, lactation
- **Physical:** Renal function, eighth cranial nerve function, state of hydration, CBC, skin color and lesions, orientation and affect, reflexes, bilateral grip strength, body weight, bowel sounds

Interventions

- Ensure that the patient is well hydrated.

Teaching points

- Report hearing changes, dizziness, severe diarrhea.

▷ **neostigmine**
(nee oh stig' meen)
neostigmine bromide

**neostigmine
methylsulfate**
Prostigmin

PREGNANCY CATEGORY C

Drug classes

Antidote
Antimyasthenic
Cholinesterase inhibitor
Parasympathomimetic
Urinary tract drug

Therapeutic actions

Increases the concentration of acetylcholine at the sites of cholinergic transmission, and prolongs and exaggerates the effects of acetylcholine by reversibly inhibiting the enzyme acetylcholinesterase, causing parasympathomimetic effects and facilitating transmission at the skeletal neuromuscular junction; also has direct cholinomimetic activity on skeletal muscle; may have direct cholinomimetic activity on neurons in autonomic ganglia and the CNS.

Indications

- Prevention and treatment of postoperative distention and urinary retention
- Symptomatic control of myasthenia gravis

- Antidote for nondepolarizing neuromuscular junction blockers (tubocurarine or pancuronium) after surgery

Contraindications and cautions

- Contraindicated with hypersensitivity to anticholinesterases; adverse reactions to bromides (neostigmine bromide); intestinal or urogenital tract obstruction, peritonitis; pregnancy (may stimulate uterus and induce premature labor); lactation.
- Use cautiously with asthma, peptic ulcer, bradycardia, cardiac arrhythmias, recent coronary occlusion, vagotonia, hyperthyroidism, epilepsy.

Available forms

Injection—1:1,000 (1 mg/mL), 1:2,000 (0.5 mg/mL); tablets—15 mg

Dosages

Adults

- *Prevention of postoperative distention and urinary retention:* 0.25 mg neostigmine methylsulfate subcutaneously or IM as soon as possible after operation. Repeat every 4–6 hr for 2–3 days.
- *Treatment of postoperative distention:* 1 mL of the 1:2,000 solution (0.5 mg) neostigmine methylsulfate subcutaneously or IM, as required.
- *Treatment of urinary retention:* 1 mL of the 1:2,000 solution (0.5 mg) neostigmine methylsulfate subcutaneously or IM. If urination does not occur within 1 hr, catheterize the patient. After the bladder is emptied, continue 0.5-mg injections every 3 hr for at least five injections.
- *Symptomatic control of myasthenia gravis:* 1 mL of the 1:2,000 solution (0.5 mg) subcutaneously or IM. Individualize subsequent doses. Should be used with atropine to counteract adverse muscarinic effects. Tablets—15–375 mg/day PO; average daily dose is 150 mg.
- *Antidote for nondepolarizing neuromuscular blockers:* Give atropine sulfate 0.6–1.2 mg IV several min before slow IV injection of neostigmine 0.5–2 mg. Repeat as required. Total dose should usually not exceed 5 mg.

Pediatric patients

- *Prevention, treatment of postoperative distention and urinary retention:* Safety and efficacy not established.

Adverse effects in *italics* are most common; those in **bold** are life-threatening. ⚞⚟ Do not crush.

- *Symptomatic control of myasthenia gravis:* 0.01–0.04 mg/kg per dose IM, IV, or subcutaneously every 2–3 hr as needed. Tablets— 2 mg/kg/day PO every 3–4 hr as needed.
- *As antidote for nondepolarizing neuromuscular blocker:* Give 0.008–0.025 mg/kg atropine sulfate IV several min before slow IV injection of neostigmine 0.025–0.08 mg/ kg.

Pharmacokinetics

Route	Onset	Peak	Duration
Subcut., IM	20–30 min	20–30 min	2.5–4 hr
IV	10–30 min	20–30 min	2.5–4 hr
Oral	20–30 min	20–30 min	2–4 hr

Metabolism: Hepatic; $T_{1/2}$: 47–60 min
Distribution: May cross placenta or enter breast milk
Excretion: Urine

▼ IV FACTS

Preparation: No further preparation is required.
Infusion: Inject slowly directly into vein or into tubing of running IV, each 0.5 mg over 1 min.

Adverse effects

- **CNS:** Seizures, dysarthria, dysphonia, drowsiness, dizziness, headache, loss of consciousness
- **CV:** *Cardiac arrhythmias,* **cardiac arrest,** decreased cardiac output leading to hypotension, syncope
- **Dermatologic:** Diaphoresis, flushing, rash, urticaria, anaphylaxis
- **EENT:** *Lacrimation, miosis,* spasm of accommodation, diplopia, conjunctival hyperemia
- **GI:** *Salivation, dysphagia, nausea, vomiting, increased peristalsis, abdominal cramps,* flatulence, diarrhea
- **GU:** *Urinary frequency and incontinence,* urinary urgency
- **Local:** Thrombophlebitis after IV use
- **Peripheral:** Skeletal muscle weakness, fasciculations, muscle cramps, arthralgia
- **Respiratory:** *Increased pharyngeal and tracheobronchial secretions,* **laryngospasm, bronchospasm,** bronchiolar constriction, dyspnea, respiratory muscle paralysis, central respiratory paralysis

Interactions

٭ Drug-drug • Prolonged neuromuscular blockade of succinylcholine • Decreased effects and possible muscular depression with corticosteroids • Increased neuromuscular blocking effect due to aminoglycoside antibiotics

■ Nursing considerations

Assessment

- **History:** Hypersensitivity to anticholinesterases; adverse reactions to bromides; intestinal or urogenital tract obstruction, peritonitis; asthma, peptic ulcer, cardiac arrhythmias, recent coronary occlusion, vagotonia, hyperthyroidism, epilepsy; lactation, pregnancy
- **Physical:** Skin color, texture, lesions; reflexes, bilateral grip strength; P, auscultation, BP; R, adventitious sounds; salivation, bowel sounds, normal output; frequency, voiding pattern, normal output; EEG, thyroid tests

Interventions

- Administer IV slowly.
- Overdose with anticholinesterase drugs can cause muscle weakness (cholinergic crisis) that is difficult to differentiate from myasthenic weakness. The administration of atropine may mask the parasympathetic effects of anticholinesterase overdose and further confound the diagnosis.
- ⊗ **Warning** Keep atropine sulfate readily available as an antidote and antagonist in case of cholinergic crisis or hypersensitivity reaction.
- ⊗ **Warning** Discontinue drug, and consult physician if excessive salivation, emesis, frequent urination, or diarrhea occurs.
- Decrease dosage if excessive sweating or nausea occurs.

Teaching points

- Take this drug exactly as prescribed; patient and a significant other should receive extensive teaching about the effects of the drug, the signs and symptoms of myasthenia gravis, the fact that muscle weakness may be related both to drug overdose and to exacerbation of the disease, and that it is important to report muscle weakness promptly to your health care provider so that proper evaluation can be made.

- You may experience these side effects: Blurred vision, difficulty with far vision, difficulty with dark adaptation (use caution while driving, especially at night, or performing hazardous tasks in reduced light); increased urinary frequency, abdominal cramps; sweating (avoid hot or excessively humid environments).
- Report muscle weakness, nausea, vomiting, diarrhea, severe abdominal pain, excessive sweating, excessive salivation, frequent urination, urinary urgency, irregular heartbeat, difficulty breathing.

▽ **nesiritide (hBNP)**

See Appendix R, *Less commonly used drugs.*

▽ **nevirapine**
(neh veer' ah pine)

Viramune, Viramune XR ᴄᴀɴ

PREGNANCY CATEGORY B

Drug classes
Antiviral
Non-nucleoside reverse transcriptase inhibitor

Therapeutic actions
Antiretroviral activity; binds directly to HIV-1 reverse transcriptase and blocks the replication of HIV by changing the structure of the HIV enzyme.

Indications
- Treatment of HIV-1 infection in combination with other antiretroviral drugs

Contraindications and cautions
- Contraindicated with allergy to nevirapine; lactation; moderate to severe hepatic impairment.
- Use cautiously with renal or hepatic impairment, rash, pregnancy.

Available forms
Tablets—200 mg; ER tablets ᴄᴀɴ—400 mg; oral suspension—50 mg/5 mL

Dosages
Adults
200 mg PO daily for 14 days; if no rash appears, then 200 mg PO bid, or 400 mg ER tablet once

daily with other antivirals. Daily dose should not exceed 400 mg/day. If dosing is interrupted for more than 7 days, restart with 14-day immediate-release tablet regimen and if no rash occurs, ER tablet may be used for once-a-day dosing.
Pediatric patients 15 days and older
150 mg/m² PO once daily for 14 days, then 150 mg/m² PO bid; maximum dose, 400 mg/day.

Pharmacokinetics

Route	Onset	Peak
Oral	Rapid	4 hr

Metabolism: Hepatic; $T_{1/2}$: 45 hr, then 25–30 hr
Distribution: Crosses placenta; enters breast milk
Excretion: Urine

Adverse effects
- **CNS:** *Headache*
- **Dermatologic: Stevens-Johnson syndrome, rash, toxic epidermal necrolysis**
- **GI:** *Nausea, vomiting, diarrhea,* dry mouth, **hepatic impairment including hepatitis, hepatic necrosis**
- **Other:** Infection, chills, fever, fat redistribution

Interactions
✴ **Drug-drug** • Avoid concurrent use with protease inhibitors, hormonal contraceptives (metabolism is increased and effectiveness decreased)
- Decreased ketoconazole, itraconazole, clarithromycin, rifampin levels and effects; avoid this combination

✴ **Drug-alternative therapy** • Decreased effectiveness if combined with St. John's Wort

■ Nursing considerations

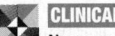 **CLINICAL ALERT!**
Name confusion has occurred between *Viramune* (nevirapine) and *Viracept* (nelfinavir); use caution.

Assessment
- **History:** Allergy to nevirapine, renal or hepatic impairment, pregnancy, lactation, rash

Adverse effects in italics are most common; those in bold are life-threatening. ᴄᴀɴ Do not crush.

- **Physical:** T; orientation, reflexes; peripheral perfusion; urinary output; skin color, perfusion, hydration; LFTs, renal function tests

Interventions
- Administer in combination with nucleoside analogues.
- ⊗ *Black box warning* Monitor renal and hepatic function tests before and during treatment. Discontinue drug at any sign of hepatic impairment; severe to life-threatening hepatotoxicity is possible. Monitor patient closely; greatest risk of hepatotoxicity occurs at 6–18 wk of therapy.
- ⊗ *Black box warning* Do not administer if severe rash occurs, especially accompanied by fever, blistering, lesion, swelling, general malaise; discontinue if rash recurs on rechallenge. Severe to life-threatening reactions are possible; risk is greatest 6–18 wk into therapy.
- Shake suspension gently before use. Rinse oral dosing cup and administer rinse to patient.
- Do not switch to ER form until patient is stabilized on immediate-release form (14 days). Ensure that ER tablet is swallowed whole; tablet is not to be cut, crushed, or chewed.

Teaching points
- Take this drug exactly as prescribed; do not take double doses if you miss a dose. Take your other HIV drugs as prescribed.
- If you are using the suspension form, shake gently before use. Dosing syringe is recommended to ensure the correct dose.
- If you are switched to the extended-release form after being stabilized on the drug, do not cut, crush, or chew tablet; it must be swallowed whole.
- Use some method of barrier birth control (not hormonal contraceptives) while using this medication. Severe birth defects can occur, and this drug causes loss of effectiveness of hormonal contraceptives.
- Do not use St. John's Wort while taking this drug.
- This drug does not cure HIV infection. Follow routine preventive measures and continue any other medication that has been prescribed.
- You may experience these side effects: Nausea, vomiting, loss of appetite, diarrhea, headache, fever, redistribution of body fat.

- Report rash, any lesions or blistering, changes in color of stool or urine, fever, muscle or joint pain.

▽niacin
(nye' ah sin)

Niacor, Niaspan, Slo-Niacin

PREGNANCY CATEGORY C

Drug classes
Antihyperlipidemic
Vitamin

Therapeutic actions
May partially inhibit the release of free fatty acids from adipose tissue and increase lipoprotein activity, which could increase the rate of triglyceride removal from plasma; these actions reduce the total LDL and triglycerides and increase HDL. Niacin also decreases serum levels of apo B and lipoprotein A.

Indications
- Adjunct to diet for treatment of adults with very high serum triglyceride levels (types IV and V hyperlipidemia) who present a risk of pancreatitis and who do not respond adequately to dietary control
- Adjunct for treatment of adults with hypercholesterolemia
- Treatment of pellagra, niacin deficiency
- Reduction of risk of nonfatal MI in patients with a history of MI and hyperlipidemia
- In combination with a bile acid–binding resin to slow the progression of atherosclerotic disease in patients with known CAD and hyperlipidemia

Contraindications and cautions
- Contraindicated with hepatic impairment, active peptic ulcer disease, arterial bleeding, lactation.
- Use cautiously with history of jaundice, hepatobiliary disease, peptic ulcer, high alcohol consumption, renal impairment, unstable angina, gout, recent surgery, pregnancy.

Available forms
ER tablets ᴼᵀᶜ—500, 750, 1,000 mg; tablets—50, 100, 250, 500 mg; OTC CR tablets ᴼᵀᶜ—250, 500, 750 mg; OTC CR capsules ᴼᵀᶜ—250, 400 mg; OTC SR capsules ᴼᵀᶜ—125, 500 mg

Dosages

Adults and pediatric patients older than 16 yr

Dyslipidemia: Initially, 100 mg PO tid, increased to 1,000 mg PO tid (immediate-release form); 500 mg/day PO at bedtime for 4 wk, then 1,000 mg/day PO at bedtime for another 4 wk (extended-release form); titrate to patient response and tolerance. Maximum dosage is 2,000 mg/day; 1,000–2,000 mg/day PO (sustained-release form).

CAD, post MI: 500 mg/day PO at bedtime, titrated at 4-wk intervals to maximum of 1,000–2,000 mg/day.

Pellagra: 50–100 mg PO tid to maximum of 500 mg/day.

Pediatric patients 16 yr and younger

Dyslipidemia: 100–250 mg/day PO in three divided doses with meals; may be increased at 2- to 3-wk intervals to maximum of 10 mg/kg/day (immediate-release form).

Pellagra: 50–100 mg PO tid.

Pharmacokinetics

Route	Onset	Peak
Oral	Rapid	45 min

Metabolism: Hepatic; $T_{1/2}$: Unknown
Distribution: Crosses placenta, enters breast milk
Excretion: Urine

Adverse effects

- **CNS:** *Headache,* anxiety
- **CV:** Arrhythmias, hypotension
- **Dermatologic:** *Flushing,* acanthosis nigricans, dry skin, *rash*
- **GI:** *GI upset,* peptic ulcer, abnormal liver function tests, *diarrhea, nausea, vomiting*
- **Hematologic:** Hyperuricemia
- **Other:** Glucose intolerance

Interactions

✳ **Drug-drug** • Increased risk of rhabdomyolysis and possible increased risk of stroke with HMG-CoA inhibitors • Increased effectiveness of antihypertensives, vasoactive drugs • Increased risk of bleeding with anticoagulants; monitor PT and platelet counts and adjust dosage accordingly • Decreased absorption with bile acid sequestrants; separate doses by at least 4–6 hr

■ Nursing considerations

Assessment

- **History:** Hepatic impairment, active peptic ulcer disease, arterial bleeding, lactation, hepatobiliary disease, peptic ulcer, high alcohol consumption, renal impairment, unstable angina, gout, recent surgery, pregnancy
- **Physical:** Skin lesions, color, T; orientation, affect, reflexes; P, auscultation, baseline ECG, BP; liver evaluation; lipid studies, LFTs

Interventions

- Administer drug at bedtime to minimize effects of flushing.
- When flushing is persistent, recommend 325 mg aspirin taken 30 min before each scheduled dose of niacin.
- ⊗ *Warning* Do not substitute ER products for immediate-release products at equivalent doses. Severe hepatic toxicity has occurred.
- Ensure that patient swallows ER products whole; do not cut, crush, or allow patient to chew ER tablets or capsules.
- Avoid ingestion of hot liquids or alcohol around the time of niacin administration to minimize flushing.
- Consult with a dietitian regarding a low-cholesterol diet.
- Arrange for regular follow-up during long-term therapy.

Teaching points

- Take drug at bedtime. The dose will change each week until the desired response is achieved. Do not cut, crush, or chew extended-release forms.
- Take your bile acid sequestrant (if appropriate) 4–6 hours apart from niacin; avoid alcohol while using this medication.
- Maintain your diet and exercise program for lowering lipid level.
- You may experience these side effects: Nausea, heartburn, loss of appetite (eat frequent small meals); headache (may lessen over time; if bothersome, consult your health care provider); rash, flushing (take drug at bedtime). You may take an aspirin or nonsteroidal anti-inflammatory drug 30 minutes before each dose to reduce GI distress and flushing.
- Report unusual bleeding or bruising, palpitations, fainting, rash, fever.

Adverse effects in *italics* are most common; those in **bold** are life-threatening. ⬛ Do not crush.

▷ **niCARdipine hydrochloride**
(nye kar' de peen)

Cardene, Cardene SR

PREGNANCY CATEGORY C

Drug classes
Antianginal
Antihypertensive
Calcium channel blocker

Therapeutic actions
Inhibits the movement of calcium ions across the membranes of cardiac and arterial muscle cells; calcium is involved in the generation of the action potential in specialized automatic and conducting cells in the heart, in arterial smooth muscle, and in excitation-contraction coupling in cardiac muscle cells. Inhibition of calcium flow results in the depression of impulse formation in specialized cardiac pacemaker cells, in slowing of the velocity of conduction of the cardiac impulse, in the depression of myocardial contractility, and in the dilation of coronary arteries and arterioles and peripheral arterioles; these effects lead to decreased cardiac work, decreased cardiac energy consumption, and increased delivery of oxygen to myocardial cells.

Indications
- Immediate-release only: Chronic stable (effort-related) angina. Use alone or with beta blockers
- Immediate-release and SR: Management of essential hypertension alone or with other antihypertensives
- IV: Short-term treatment of hypertension when oral use is not feasible

Contraindications and cautions
- Contraindicated with allergy to nicardipine, pregnancy, lactation, advanced aortic stenosis.
- Use cautiously with impaired hepatic or renal function, sick sinus syndrome, heart block (second- or third-degree), HF.

Available forms
Capsules—20, 30 mg; ER capsules—30, 45, 60 mg; injection—2.5 mg/mL; premixed bags—20 mg/200 mL, 40 mg/200 mL

Dosages
Adults
Oral
- *Angina:* Immediate-release only—individualize dosage. Usual initial dose is 20 mg tid PO. Range, 20–40 mg tid PO. Allow at least 3 days before increasing dosage to ensure steady-state plasma levels.
- *Hypertension:* Immediate-release—initial dose, 20 mg tid PO. Range, 20–40 mg tid. The maximum BP-lowering effect occurs in 1–2 hr. Adjust dosage based on BP response, allow at least 3 days before increasing dosage. SR—initial dose is 30 mg bid PO. Range, 30–60 mg bid.

IV
- *Hypertension:* For gradual reduction, begin infusion at 5 mg/hr. Increase by 2.5 mg/hr every 15 min to maximum of 15 mg/hr. For rapid reduction, begin infusion at 5 mg/hr. Increase by 2.5 mg/hr every 5 min to maximum of 15 mg/hr. Once BP is controlled, reduce to 3 mg/hr.

Pediatric patients
Safety and efficacy not established.
Patients with renal or hepatic impairment
For patients with renal impairment, adjust dosage beginning with 20 mg tid PO (immediate-release) or 30 mg bid PO (SR). For patients with hepatic impairment, starting dose 20 mg bid PO (immediate-release) with individual adjustment.

Pharmacokinetics

Route	Onset	Peak
Oral	20 min	0.5–2 hr

Metabolism: Hepatic; $T_{1/2}$: 2–4 hr
Distribution: Crosses placenta; enters breast milk
Excretion: Urine

▼ IV FACTS
Preparation: Dilute each ampule with 240 mL of solution to a concentration of 0.1 mg/mL; store at room temperature; protect from light; stable for 24 hr.
Infusion: Slow IV infusion; begin with 5 mg/hr. Increase by 2.5 mg/hr every 5 min (rapid control) or 15 min (slow control) to maximum of 15 mg/hr. When BP is controlled, use maintenance rate of 3 mg/hr (rapid control).

Compatibilities: Compatible with dextrose 5% injection, dextrose 5% and sodium chloride 0.45% or 0.9% injection; dextrose 5% with potassium; 0.45% or 0.9% sodium chloride.
Incompatibilities: Do not mix with 5% sodium bicarbonate or lactated Ringer.

Adverse effects
• **CNS:** *Dizziness, light-headedness, headache, asthenia,* fatigue
• **CV:** *Peripheral edema, angina,* hypotension, arrhythmias, *bradycardia, AV block,* **asystole**
• **Dermatologic:** *Flushing,* rash
• **GI:** *Nausea,* hepatic injury

Interactions
✷ **Drug-drug** • Increased serum levels and toxicity of cyclosporine

■ Nursing considerations
Assessment
• **History:** Allergy to nicardipine, impaired hepatic or renal function, sick sinus syndrome, heart block (second- or third-degree), pregnancy, lactation, aortic stenosis
• **Physical:** Skin lesions, color, edema; P, BP, baseline ECG, peripheral perfusion, auscultation; R, adventitious sounds; liver evaluation, normal GI output; LFTs, renal function tests, urinalysis

Interventions
• Monitor the patient carefully (BP, cardiac rhythm, and output) while drug is being titrated to therapeutic dose; dosage may be increased more rapidly in hospitalized patients under close supervision.
⊗ *Warning* Monitor BP very carefully with concurrent doses of nitrates.
• Monitor cardiac rhythm regularly during stabilization of dosage and long-term therapy.
• Provide small frequent meals if GI upset occurs.

Teaching points
• Take exactly as prescribed; do not exceed the prescribed daily dose.
• You may experience these side effects: Nausea, vomiting (eat frequent small meals); headache (monitor lighting, noise, and temperature; request medication if severe).
• Report irregular heartbeat, shortness of breath, swelling of the hands or feet, pronounced dizziness, constipation.

▽**nicotine**
(*nik' oh teen*)

Nicoderm CQ, Nicoderm Transdermal System, Nicotrol, Nicotrol Inhaler, Nicotrol NS

PREGNANCY CATEGORY D

Drug class
Smoking deterrent

Therapeutic actions
Nicotine acts at nicotinic receptors in the peripheral and CNS; produces behavioral stimulation and depression, cardiac acceleration, peripheral vasoconstriction, and elevated BP.

Indications
• Temporary aid to the cigarette smoker seeking to give up smoking while in a behavioral modification program under medical supervision
• Unlabeled use: Improvement of symptoms of Tourette syndrome

Contraindications and cautions
• Contraindicated with allergy to nicotine, arrhythmias, angina pectoris, pregnancy, lactation, and during the post-MI period. Inhaler is contraindicated with asthma, COPD.
• Use cautiously with hyperthyroidism, pheochromocytoma, type 2 diabetes (releases catecholamines from the adrenal medulla), hypertension, peptic ulcer disease.

Available forms
Transdermal system—7, 14, 21 mg/day; 5, 10, 15 mg/16 hr (*Nicotrol*); nasal spray—0.5 mg/actuation (10 mg/mL); inhaler—4 mg/ actuation

Dosages
Adults
Topical
Apply system, 5–21 mg, once every 24 hr. Dosage is based on response and stage of withdrawal. *Nicoderm:* 21 mg/day for first 6 wk; 14 mg/day for next 2 wk; 7 mg/day for next 2 wk. *Nicotrol:* 15 mg/day for first 6 wk; 10 mg/day for next 2 wk; 5 mg/day for last 2 wk.

Nasal spray
1 spray in each nostril as needed, one to two doses each hour, up to five doses/hr and 40 doses/day.

Nasal inhaler
1 spray in each nostril, one to two doses/hr to a maximum five doses/hr or 40 doses/day. Dosage is individualized; in studies, best results were achieved by continuous, frequent puffing over 20 min. Do not use longer than 6 mo. Patients are treated for 12 wk, then weaned off the daily dose over next 6–12 wk.

Pediatric patients
Safety and efficacy in children and adolescents who smoke have not been established.

Pharmacokinetics

Route	Onset	Peak	Duration
Dermal	1–2 hr	4–6 min	4–24 hr
Nasal	Rapid	15 min	NA

Metabolism: Hepatic; $T_{1/2}$: 1–4 hr
Distribution: Crosses placenta; enters breast milk
Excretion: Urine

Adverse effects
- **CNS:** *Headache, insomnia,* abnormal dreams, dizziness, light-headedness, sweating
- **GI:** Diarrhea, constipation, nausea, dyspepsia, abdominal pain, dry mouth
- **Local:** *Erythema, burning, pruritus* at site of patch; local edema
- **Respiratory:** Cough, pharyngitis, sinusitis
- **Other:** Backache, chest pain, asthenia, dysmenorrhea, flulike symptoms

Interactions
✳ **Drug-drug** • Increased circulating levels of cortisol, catecholamines with nicotine use; smoking dosage of adrenergic agonists, adrenergic blockers may need to be adjusted according to nicotine, smoking status of patient
• Smoking increases metabolism and lowers blood levels of caffeine, theophylline, imipramine, pentazocine; decreases effects of furosemide, propranolol

■ Nursing considerations
Assessment
- **History:** Allergy to nicotine; nonsmoker; post-MI, arrhythmias, angina pectoris; hyperthyroidism, pheochromocytoma, type 2 diabetes; hypertension, peptic ulcer disease; pregnancy; lactation
- **Physical:** Orientation, affect; P, auscultation, BP; oral mucous membranes, abdominal examination; thyroid function tests

Interventions
- Protect systems from heat; slight discoloration of system is not significant.
- Apply system to nonhairy, clean, dry skin site on upper body or upper outer arm; use only when the pouch is intact; use immediately after removal from pouch; use each system only once. Remove old system before applying a new system.
- Wash hands thoroughly after application; do not touch eyes.
- Wrap used system in foil pouch of newly applied system; fold over and dispose of immediately to prevent access by pets or children.
- Apply new system after 24 hr; do not reuse same site for at least 1 wk. *Nicotrol:* Apply a new system each day after waking, and remove at bedtime.
- ⊗ *Warning* Handle nasal spray carefully; if it comes in contact with skin, flush immediately; dispose of bottle with cap in place.
- Ensure that patient has stopped smoking; if the patient is unable to stop smoking within the first 4 wk of therapy, drug therapy should be stopped.
- Encourage patients who have been unsuccessful at any dose to take a "therapy holiday" before trying again; counseling should explore factors contributing to their failure and other means of success.

Teaching points
- Protect systems from heat; slight discoloration of system is not significant.
- Apply system to nonhairy, clean, dry skin site on upper body or upper outer arm; use only when the pouch is intact; use immediately after removal from pouch; use each system only once. Remove old system before applying a new system.
- Wash hands thoroughly after application; do not touch eyes. Wrap used system in foil pouch of newly applied system; fold over and dispose of immediately to prevent access by pets or children.

N

- Apply new system after 24 hours; do not reuse same site for at least 1 week. *Nicotrol:* Apply a new system each day after waking, and remove at bedtime.
- Tilt head back to administer spray; do not sniff, swallow, or inhale while spray is administered. If spray comes in contact with skin, flush immediately; discard bottle with cap in place.
- Store reusable mouthpiece for inhaler in plastic case; wash with soap and water. Throw inhaler cartridge away out of reach of children and pets.
- Abstain from smoking.
- You may experience these side effects: Dizziness, headache, light-headedness (use caution driving or performing tasks that require alertness); nausea, vomiting, constipation or diarrhea (frequent small meals, regular mouth care may help); skin redness, swelling at application site (good skin care, switching sites daily may help).
- Report nausea and vomiting, diarrhea, cold sweat, chest pain, palpitations, burning or swelling at application site.

▽**nicotine polacrilex (nicotine resin complex)** (*nik' oh teen*)

Commit, Nicorette, Nicorette Lozenges, Nicotine Gum

PREGNANCY CATEGORY C

Drug class
Smoking deterrent

Therapeutic actions
Acts as an agonist at nicotinic receptors in the peripheral and CNS; produces behavioral stimulation and depression, cardiac acceleration, peripheral vasoconstriction, and elevated BP.

Indications
- Temporary aid to the cigarette smoker seeking to give up smoking while in a behavior modification program under medical supervision

Contraindications and cautions
- Contraindicated with allergy to nicotine or resin used, arrhythmias, angina pectoris, active TMJ disease, pregnancy, lactation, and during the post-MI period.
- Use cautiously with hyperthyroidism, pheochromocytoma, type 2 diabetes (releases catecholamines from the adrenal medulla), hypertension, peptic ulcer disease.

Available forms
Chewing gum—2 or 4 mg/square; lozenge—2, 4 mg

Dosages
Adults
Chewing gum
If patient smokes less than 25 cigarettes/day, start with 2 mg; if more than 25 cigarettes/day, start with 4 mg. Have patient chew one piece of gum whenever the urge to smoke occurs. Have the patient chew each piece slowly until it tingles, then place it between the cheek and gums; when tingle is gone, have patient chew gum again and repeat the process. Gum usually lasts for about 30 min to promote even, slow, buccal absorption of nicotine. Patients often require 10 pieces daily during the first month. Do not exceed 24 pieces daily. Therapy may be effective for up to 3 mo; 4–6 mo for complete cessation has been used. Should not be used for longer than 4 mo.
Lozenge
Start with 2 mg if patient first smokes more than 30 min after waking up; 4 mg if patient starts smoking within 30 min of waking. Patient must place lozenge in mouth, let dissolve over 20–30 min, and avoid eating or drinking anything other than water for 15 min before use. In week 1–6, use 1 lozenge every 1–2 hr; in week 7–9, use 1 lozenge every 2–4 hr; in week 10–12, use 1 lozenge every 4–8 hr. Do not exceed 5 lozenges in 6 hr or 20 daily.
Pediatric patients
Safety and efficacy in children and adolescents who smoke have not been established.

Pharmacokinetics

Route	Onset	Peak
Oral	Slow	15–30 min

Metabolism: Hepatic; $T_{1/2}$: 30–120 min
Distribution: Crosses placenta; enters breast milk
Excretion: Urine

Adverse effects in *italics* are most common; those in **bold** are life-threatening. ▨▨ Do not crush.

Adverse effects
- **CNS:** Dizziness, light-headedness
- **GI:** *Mouth or throat soreness; hiccoughs, nausea, vomiting,* nonspecific GI distress, excessive salivation
- **Local:** Mechanical effects of chewing gum—traumatic injury to oral mucosa or teeth, *jaw ache,* eructation secondary to air swallowing

Interactions
✳ **Drug-drug** • Increased circulating levels of cortisol, catecholamines with nicotine use, smoking—dosage of adrenergic agonists, adrenergic blockers may need to be adjusted according to nicotine, smoking status of patient
• Smoking increases metabolism and lowers blood levels of caffeine, theophylline, imipramine, pentazocine; decreases effects of furosemide, propranolol

■ Nursing considerations
Assessment
- **History:** Allergy to nicotine or resin used; nonsmoker; post-MI period; arrhythmias; angina pectoris; active TMJ disease; hyperthyroidism, pheochromocytoma, type 2 diabetes; hypertension, peptic ulcer disease; pregnancy; lactation
- **Physical:** Jaw strength, symmetry; orientation, affect; P, auscultation, BP; oral mucous membranes, abdominal examination; thyroid function tests

Interventions
- Review mechanics of chewing gum with patient; patient must chew the gum slowly and intermittently to promote even, slow absorption of nicotine; discard chewed gum in wrapper to prevent access by children or pets.
- Have patient place lozenge in mouth and allow to dissolve in mouth over 20–30 min; do not allow patient to eat or drink for 15 min before use.
- Arrange to withdraw or taper use of gum or lozenges in abstainers at 3 mo; effectiveness after that time has not been established, and patients may be using gum as substitute source for nicotine dependence.

Teaching points
- Chew one piece of gum every time you have the desire to smoke. Chew each piece slowly

until it tingles. Then place the gum between the cheek and gums. When the tingle is gone, chew again and repeat the process. Do not chew more than 24 pieces of gum each day. Discard chewed gum in wrapper to prevent access by children or pets.
- Place lozenge in mouth and allow to dissolve over 20–30 minutes; do not eat or drink for 15 minutes before use. Do not use more than 5 lozenges in 6 hours or 20 in 1 day. If you remove a lozenge, wrap it up carefully to prevent access by children or pets.
- Do not consume liquids within 15 minutes before or while chewing gum or using lozenge; they may interfere with nicotine absorption.
- Abstain from smoking.
- Do not offer to nonsmokers; serious reactions can occur if used by nonsmokers.
- You may experience these side effects: Dizziness, headache, light-headedness (use caution driving or performing tasks that require alertness); nausea, vomiting, increased burping; jaw muscle ache (modify chewing technique).
- Report nausea and vomiting, increased salivation, diarrhea, cold sweat, headache, disturbances in hearing or vision, chest pain, palpitations.

▷ NIFEdipine
(nye fed' i peen)

Adalat CC, Adalat XL (CAN), Afeditab CR⦿, Apo-Nifed (CAN), Apo-Nifed AP (CAN), Nifediac CC, Nifedical XL, Procardia, Procardia XL

PREGNANCY CATEGORY C

Drug classes
Antianginal
Antihypertensive
Calcium channel blocker

Therapeutic actions
Inhibits the movement of calcium ions across the membranes of cardiac and arterial muscle cells; inhibition of transmembrane calcium flow results in the depression of impulse formation in specialized cardiac pacemaker cells, in slowing of the velocity of conduction of the cardiac impulse, in the depression of myocardial contractility, and in the dilation

of coronary arteries and arterioles and peripheral arterioles; these effects lead to decreased cardiac work, decreased cardiac energy consumption, and increased delivery of oxygen to myocardial cells.

Indications

- Angina pectoris due to coronary artery spasm (Prinzmetal variant angina)
- Chronic stable angina (effort-associated angina)
- ER preparation only: Treatment of hypertension
- Orphan drug use: Treatment of interstitial cystitis
- Unlabeled uses: Anal fissures, ureteral stones, topical use to improve wound healing, prevention of migraine, Raynaud phenomenon

Contraindications and cautions

- Contraindicated with allergy to nifedipine.
- Use cautiously with lactation, pregnancy, HF, aortic stenosis.

Available forms

ER tablets ⓒⓡ—30, 60, 90 mg; capsules—10, 20 mg

Dosages
Adults
Initial dose, 10 mg tid PO. Maintenance range, 10–20 mg tid. Higher doses (20–30 mg tid–qid) may be required, depending on patient response. Adjust over 7–14 days. More than 180 mg/day is not recommended.
ERⓒⓡ
30–60 mg PO once daily. Adjust over 7–14 days. Usual maximum dose is 90–120 mg/day.

Pharmacokinetics

Route	Onset	Peak
Oral	20 min	30 min
ER	20 min	2.5–6 hr

Metabolism: Hepatic; $T_{1/2}$: 2–5 hr
Distribution: Crosses placenta; enters breast milk
Excretion: Feces, urine

Adverse effects

- **CNS:** *Dizziness, light-headedness, headache, asthenia, fatigue, nervousness,* sleep disturbances, blurred vision, *weakness, tremor, mood changes*

- **CV:** *Peripheral edema, angina,* hypotension, arrhythmias, *AV block,* asystole
- **Dermatologic:** *Flushing, rash,* dermatitis, pruritus, urticaria
- **GI:** *Nausea, diarrhea, constipation,* cramps, flatulence, hepatic injury
- **Other:** *Nasal congestion, cough,* fever, chills, shortness of breath, muscle cramps, joint stiffness, sexual difficulties

Interactions

✴ **Drug-drug** ● Increased effects with cimetidine
✴ **Drug-food** ● Risk of increased toxic effects; avoid use with grapefruit juice

■ Nursing considerations
Assessment
- **History:** Allergy to nifedipine, pregnancy, lactation
- **Physical:** Skin lesions, color, edema; orientation, reflexes; P, BP, baseline ECG, peripheral perfusion, auscultation; R, adventitious sounds; liver evaluation, normal GI output; LFTs

Interventions
⊗ *Warning* Monitor patient carefully (BP, cardiac rhythm, and output) while drug is being adjusted to therapeutic dose; the dosage may be increased more rapidly in hospitalized patients under close supervision. Do not exceed 30 mg/dose increases.
- Ensure that patients do not chew or divide ER tablets.
- Taper dosage of beta blockers before nifedipine therapy.
- Protect drug from light and moisture.

Teaching points
- Do not chew, cut, or crush extended-release tablets. Swallow whole.
- Avoid grapefruit juice while taking this drug; it can cause increased toxicity.
- You may experience these side effects: Nausea, vomiting (eat frequent small meals); dizziness, light-headedness, vertigo (avoid driving and operating dangerous machinery; take special precautions to avoid falling); muscle cramps, joint stiffness, sweating, sexual difficulties (reversible).
- Report irregular heartbeat, shortness of breath, swelling of the hands or feet, pronounced dizziness, constipation.

▽nilotinib

See Appendix R, *Less commonly used drugs.*

▽nimodipine

See Appendix R, *Less commonly used drugs.*

▽nisoldipine
(nye sole' di peen)

Sular ⓞⓂⒸ

PREGNANCY CATEGORY C

Drug classes
Antihypertensive
Calcium channel blocker

Therapeutic actions
Inhibits the movement of calcium ions across the membranes of cardiac and arterial muscle cells; inhibits transmembrane calcium flow, which results in the depression of impulse formation in specialized cardiac pacemaker cells, slowing of the velocity of conduction of the cardiac impulse, depression of myocardial contractility, and dilation of coronary arteries and arterioles and peripheral arterioles; these effects in turn lead to decreased cardiac work, decreased cardiac energy consumption.

Indications
- Essential hypertension, alone or in combination with other antihypertensives

Contraindications and cautions
- Contraindicated with allergy to nisoldipine, impaired hepatic function, sick sinus syndrome, HF, heart block (second- or third-degree).
- Use cautiously with MI or severe CAD (increased severity of disease has occurred), lactation, pregnancy.

Available forms
ER tablets ⓞⓂⒸ—8.5, 17, 20, 25.5, 30, 34, 40 mg

Dosages
Adults
Initial dose of 17 mg PO daily; increase in weekly increments of 8.5 mg/wk until BP is controlled. Usual maintenance dose is 17–34 mg PO daily. Maximum dose, 34 mg/day.
Pediatric patients
Safety and efficacy not established.
Geriatric patients or patients with hepatic impairment
Monitor BP very carefully. Reduced starting doses (no more than 8.5 mg) and reduced maintenance doses are recommended.

Pharmacokinetics

Route	Onset	Peak	Duration
Oral	Slow	6–12 hr	24 hr

Metabolism: Hepatic; $T_{1/2}$: 7–12 hr
Distribution: Crosses placenta; may enter breast milk
Excretion: Urine

Adverse effects
- **CNS:** *Dizziness, light-headedness, headache, asthenia, fatigue,* lethargy
- **CV:** *Peripheral edema,* arrhythmias, **MI, increased angina**
- **Dermatologic:** *Flushing, rash*
- **GI:** *Nausea,* abdominal discomfort

Interactions
✳ **Drug-drug** ● Possible increased serum levels and toxicity of cyclosporine ● Possible increased serum levels and toxicity with cimetidine ● Increased risk of toxic cardiac effects with quinidine

✳ **Drug-food** ● Decreased metabolism and increased risk of toxic effects if combined with grapefruit juice; avoid this combination ● Excessive drug concentration if taken with a high-fat meal; avoid this combination

■ Nursing considerations
Assessment
- **History:** Allergy to nisoldipine, impaired hepatic function, sick sinus syndrome, heart block (second- or third-degree), lactation, HF, CAD, pregnancy
- **Physical:** Skin lesions, color, edema; P, BP; baseline ECG, peripheral perfusion, auscultation, R, adventitious sounds; liver evaluation, GI normal output; LFTs, renal function tests, urinalysis

Interventions
⊗ *Warning* Monitor patient carefully (BP, cardiac rhythm and output, angina, or MI in

N

patients with CAD) while drug is being adjusted to therapeutic dose; dosage may be increased more rapidly in hospitalized patients under close supervision.

- Monitor BP very carefully if patient is on concurrent doses of nitrates or other antihypertensives.
- Monitor cardiac rhythm regularly during stabilization of dosage and periodically during long-term therapy.
- Administer drug without regard to meals. Do not cut, crush, or allow patient to chew tablets.

Teaching points

- Take this drug with meals if upset stomach occurs; do not take with high-fat meals or grapefruit juice. Do not drink grapefruit juice while using this drug.
- Swallow tablet whole; do not chew, cut, or crush.
- You may experience these side effects: Nausea, vomiting (eat frequent small meals); headache (monitor lighting, noise, and temperature; request medication if severe).
- Report irregular heartbeat, shortness of breath, swelling of the hands or feet, pronounced dizziness, constipation, chest pain.

▽ nitazoxanide

See Appendix R, *Less commonly used drugs.*

▽ nitrofurantoin
(nye troe fyoor an' toyn)

nitrofurantoin
Apo-Nitrofurantoin (CAN),
Furadantin, Novo-Furantoin (CAN)

nitrofurantoin macrocrystals
Macrobid, Macrodantin

PREGNANCY CATEGORY B

Drug classes
Antibacterial
Urinary tract anti-infective

Therapeutic actions
Bacteriostatic in low concentrations, possibly by interfering with bacterial carbohydrate metabolism; bactericidal in high concentrations,

possibly by disrupting bacterial cell wall formation, causing cell death.

Indications

- Treatment of UTIs, including acute cystitis, caused by susceptible strains of *Escherichia coli, Staphylococcus aureus, Klebsiella, Enterobacter, Proteus*
- Prophylaxis or long-term suppression of UTIs

Contraindications and cautions

- Contraindicated with allergy to nitrofurantoin, renal impairment, pregnancy, lactation.
- Use cautiously in patients with G6PD deficiency, anemia, diabetes.

Available forms
Capsules—25, 50, 100 mg; dual-release capsules—100 mg; oral suspension—25 mg/5 mL

Dosages
Adults
50–100 mg PO qid for 10–14 days or 100 mg bid for 7 days (*Macrobid*). Do not exceed 400 mg/day.
- *Long-term suppressive therapy:* 50–100 mg PO at bedtime.

Pediatric patients
5–7 mg/kg/day in four divided doses PO. Not recommended in children younger than 1 mo.
- *Long-term suppressive therapy:* As low as 1 mg/kg/day PO in one to two doses.

Patients with renal impairment
Contraindicated with CrCl less than 60 mL/min.

Pharmacokinetics

Route	Onset	Peak
Oral	Rapid	30 min

Metabolism: Hepatic; $T_{1/2}$: 20–60 min
Distribution: Crosses placenta; enters breast milk
Excretion: Urine

Adverse effects

- **CNS:** Peripheral neuropathy, headache, dizziness, nystagmus, drowsiness, vertigo
- **Dermatologic:** Exfoliative dermatitis, **Stevens-Johnson syndrome,** alopecia, pruritus, urticaria, angioedema
- **GI:** *Nausea, abdominal cramps, vomiting, diarrhea, anorexia,* parotitis, pancreatitis, **hepatotoxicity**

Adverse effects in *italics* are most common; those in **bold** are life-threatening. ▨ Do not crush.

- **Hematologic:** Hemolytic anemia in G6PD deficiency; granulocytopenia, agranulocytosis, leukopenia, thrombocytopenia, eosinophilia, megaloblastic anemia
- **Respiratory: Pulmonary hypersensitivity**
- **Other:** Superinfections of the GU tract; hypotension; muscular aches; *brown-rust urine*

Interactions

✱ **Drug-lab test** • False elevations of urine glucose, bilirubin, alkaline phosphatase, BUN, urinary creatinine • False-positive urine glucose when using Benedict or Fehling reagent

■ Nursing considerations

Assessment

- **History:** Allergy to nitrofurantoin, renal impairment, G6PD deficiency, anemia, diabetes, pregnancy, lactation
- **Physical:** Skin color, lesions; orientation, reflexes; R, adventitious sounds; liver evaluation; CBC; LFTs, renal function tests; serum electrolytes; blood, urine glucose, urinalysis

Interventions

- Arrange for culture and sensitivity tests before and during therapy.
- Give with food or milk to prevent GI upset.
- Continue drug for at least 3 days after a sterile urine specimen is obtained.
- Monitor clinical response; if no improvement is seen or a relapse occurs, send urine for repeat culture and sensitivity.
- ⊗ *Warning* Monitor pulmonary function carefully; reactions can occur within hours or weeks of nitrofurantoin therapy.
- Arrange for periodic CBC and liver function tests during long-term therapy.

Teaching points

- Take drug with food or milk. Complete the full course of drug therapy to ensure a resolution of the infection. Take this drug at regular intervals around-the-clock; consult your nurse or pharmacist to set up a convenient schedule.
- You may experience these side effects: Nausea, vomiting, abdominal pain (eat frequent small meals); diarrhea; drowsiness, blurring of vision, dizziness (observe caution driving

or using dangerous equipment); brown or yellow-rust urine (expected effect).

- Report fever, chills, cough, chest pain, difficulty breathing, rash, numbness or tingling of the fingers or toes.

▽ nitroglycerin
(nye troe gli' ser in)

Intravenous: generic
Ointment: Rectiv
Spray: Nitrolingual Pumpspray
Sublingual: Gen-Nitroglycerin (CAN), Nitrostat
Sustained-release: Nitro-Time ⒹⓃⒸ
Topical: Nitro-Bid
Transdermal: Minitran, Nitrek, Nitro-Dur
Translingual: Nitrolingual

PREGNANCY CATEGORY C

Drug classes
Antianginal
Nitrate

Therapeutic actions
Relaxes vascular smooth muscle with a resultant decrease in venous return and decrease in arterial BP, which reduces left ventricular workload and decreases myocardial oxygen consumption.

Indications
- Sublingual, translingual preparations: Acute angina
- Oral SR, sublingual, topical, transdermal, translingual preparations: Prophylaxis of angina
- IV: Angina unresponsive to recommended doses of organic nitrates or beta blockers
- IV: Perioperative hypertension
- IV: HF associated with acute MI
- IV: To produce controlled hypotension during surgery
- Topical ointment: Treatment of moderate to severe pain associated with anal fissure (*Rectiv*)
- Unlabeled uses: Reduction of cardiac workload in acute MI and in HF (sublingual, topical) adjunctive treatment of Raynaud disease (topical)

Contraindications and cautions

- Contraindicated with allergy to nitrates, severe anemia, early MI, head trauma, cerebral hemorrhage, hypertrophic cardiomyopathy, pregnancy, lactation.
- Use cautiously with hepatic or renal disease, hypotension or hypovolemia, increased intracranial pressure, constrictive pericarditis, pericardial tamponade, low ventricular filling pressure or low PCWP.

Available forms

Injection for solution (requires dilution)—5 mg/mL; injection (premixed)—100, 200, 400 mcg/mL; sublingual tablets—0.3, 0.4, 0.6 mg; ER buccal tablets—2.3 mg; translingual spray—0.4 mg/spray; oral SR capsules—2.5, 6.5, 9 mg; transdermal—0.1, 0.2, 0.3, 0.4, 0.6, 0.8 mg/hr; topical ointment—0.4%, 2%

Dosages

Adults

IV

Initial dose, 5 mcg/min delivered through an infusion pump. Increase by 5-mcg/min increments every 3–5 min as needed. If no response at 20 mcg/min, increase increments to 10–20 mcg/min. Once a partial BP response is obtained, reduce dose and lengthen dosage intervals; continually monitor response and titrate carefully.

Sublingual

- *Acute attack:* Dissolve one tablet under tongue or in buccal pouch at first sign of anginal attack; repeat every 5 min until relief is obtained. Do not take more than three tablets/15 min. If pain continues or increases, patient should call physician or go to hospital.
- *Prophylaxis:* Use 5–10 min before activities that might precipitate an attack.

Buccal

Place tablet between the lip and gum and allow it to dissolve over 3–5 min. Do not chew or swallow the tablet. Initial dose is 1 mg every 5 hr while awake. Maintenance dose is 2 mg tid.

SR (oral) ⊖⊖⊖

Initial dose, 2.5–9 mg every 12 hr. Increase to every 8 hr as needed and tolerated. Doses as high as 26 mg given qid have been used.

Topical

Initial dose, one-half inch every 8 hr. Increase by one-half inch to achieve desired results. Usual dose is 1–2 inches every 8 hr; up to 4–5 inches every 4 hr have been used. 1 inch = 15 mg nitroglycerin.

Transdermal

Apply one patch each day. Adjust to higher doses by using patches that deliver more drug or by applying more than one patch. Apply patch to arm; remove at bedtime.

Translingual

Spray preparation delivers 0.4 mg/metered dose. At onset of attack, spray one to two metered doses into oral mucosa; no more than three doses/15 min should be used. If pain persists, seek medical attention. May be used prophylactically 5–10 min before activity that might precipitate an attack.

Rectal topical ointment

Apply 1 inch of ointment intra-anally every 12 hr for 3 wk (*Rectiv*).

Pediatric patients

Safety and efficacy not established.

Pharmacokinetics

Route	Onset	Duration
IV	1–2 min	3–5 min
Sublingual	1–3 min	30–60 min
Translingual spray	2 min	30–60 min
Oral, SR	20–45 min	8–12 hr
Topical ointment	30–60 min	4–8 hr
Transdermal	30–60 min	24 hr

Metabolism: Hepatic; $T_{1/2}$: 1–4 min
Distribution: Crosses placenta; enters breast milk
Excretion: Urine

▼ IV FACTS

Preparation: Dilute in 5% dextrose injection or 0.9% sodium chloride injection. Do not mix with other drugs; check the manufacturer's instructions carefully because products vary considerably in concentration and volume per vial. Use only with glass IV bottles and the administration sets provided. Protect from light and extremes of temperature.
Infusion: Do not give by IV push; regulate rate based on patient response and BP.
Incompatibilities: Do not mix in solution with other drugs.

Adverse effects

- **CNS:** Headache, apprehension, restlessness, weakness, vertigo, dizziness, faintness

- **CV:** Tachycardia, retrosternal discomfort, palpitations, **hypotension,** syncope, collapse, orthostatic hypotension, angina
- **Dermatologic:** Rash, exfoliative dermatitis, cutaneous vasodilation with flushing, pallor, perspiration, cold sweat, contact dermatitis—transdermal preparations, topical allergic reactions—topical nitroglycerin ointment
- **GI:** Nausea, vomiting, incontinence of urine and feces, abdominal pain
- **Local:** Local burning sensation at the point of dissolution (sublingual)
- **Other:** Ethanol intoxication with high-dose IV use (alcohol in diluent)

Interactions

✷ **Drug-drug** • Increased risk of hypertension and decreased antianginal effect with ergot alkaloids • Decreased pharmacologic effects of heparin • Risk of severe hypotension and adverse CV events with sildenafil, tadalafil, vardenafil; avoid this combination

✷ **Drug-lab test** • False report of decreased serum cholesterol if done by the Zlatkis-Zak color reaction

■ Nursing considerations

CLINICAL ALERT!
Name confusion has occurred between *NitroBid* (nitroglycerin) and *Nicotrol* (nicotine); between nitroglycerin and nitroprusside; use caution.

Assessment

- **History:** Allergy to nitrates, severe anemia, early MI, head trauma, cerebral hemorrhage, hypertrophic cardiomyopathy, hepatic or renal disease, xerostania, hypotension or hypovolemia, increased intracranial pressure, constrictive pericarditis, pericardial tamponade, low ventricular filling pressure or low PCWP, pregnancy, lactation
- **Physical:** Skin color, T, lesions; orientation, reflexes, affect; P, BP, orthostatic BP, baseline ECG, peripheral perfusion; R, adventitious sounds; liver evaluation, normal output; LFTs, renal function tests (IV); CBC, Hgb

Interventions

- Give sublingual preparations under the tongue or in the buccal pouch. Encourage patient

not to swallow. Ask patient if the tablet "fizzles" or burns. Always check the expiration date on the bottle; store at room temperature, protected from light. Discard unused drug 6 mo after bottle is opened (conventional tablets); stabilized tablets (*Nitrostat*) are less subject to loss of potency.

- Give SR preparations with water; warn the patient not to chew the tablets or capsules; do not crush these preparations.
- Administer topical ointment by applying the ointment over a 6″ × 6″ area in a thin, uniform layer using the applicator. Cover area with plastic wrap held in place by adhesive tape. Rotate sites of application to decrease the chance of inflammation and sensitization; close tube tightly when finished.
- Be aware that *Rectiv* rectal topical ointment is not for oral, vaginal, or opthalmic use; for topical use only.
- Administer transdermal systems to skin site free of hair and not subject to much movement. Shave areas that have a lot of hair. Do not apply to distal extremities. Change sites slightly to decrease the chance of local irritation and sensitization. Remove transdermal system before attempting defibrillation or cardioversion. Remove old system before applying a new one.
- Administer the translingual spray directly onto the oral mucosa; preparation is not to be inhaled or swallowed.

⊗ *Warning* Arrange to withdraw drug gradually; 4–6 wk is the recommended withdrawal period for the transdermal preparations.

Teaching points

- For sublingual tablets, place tablet under your tongue or in your cheek; do not chew or swallow the tablet; the tablet should burn or "fizzle" under the tongue. Take the nitroglycerin before chest pain begins, when you anticipate that your activities or situation may precipitate an attack. Sit or lie down before taking nitroglycerin. You may repeat your dose every 5 minutes for a total of three tablets. If the pain is still not relieved, contact emergency medical services. Do not buy large quantities; this drug does not store well. Keep the drug in a dark, dry place, in a dark-colored glass bottle with a tight lid; do not combine with other drugs.

N

- For buccal tablets, place tablet between your lip and gum and allow it to dissolve over 3–5 minutes. Do not chew or swallow the tablet.
- Do not chew or crush the timed-release preparations; take on an empty stomach.
- Spread a thin layer of topical ointment on the skin using the applicator. Do not rub or massage the area. Cover with plastic wrap held in place with adhesive tape. Wash your hands after application. Keep the tube tightly closed. Rotate the sites frequently to prevent local irritation.
- If using *Rectiv* for anal pain, apply 1 inch of ointment intra-anally every 12 hr for 3 wk.
- To use transdermal systems, you may need to shave an area for application. Apply to a slightly different area each day. Remove the old system before you apply a new one. Use care if changing brands; each system has a different concentration. Remove the old system before applying a new system.
- Spray translingual spray directly onto oral mucous membranes; do not inhale or swallow. Use 5–10 minutes before activities that you anticipate will precipitate an attack.
- You may experience these side effects: Dizziness, light-headedness (may be transient; change positions slowly); headache (lie down in a cool environment and rest; over-the-counter preparations may not help); flushing of the neck or face (transient).
- Report blurred vision, persistent or severe headache, rash, more frequent or more severe angina attacks, fainting.

▽ **nitroprusside sodium**
(nye troe **pruss'** *ide)*

Nipride (CAN), Nitropress

PREGNANCY CATEGORY C

Drug classes
Antihypertensive
Vasodilator

Therapeutic actions
Acts directly on vascular smooth muscle to cause vasodilation (arterial and venous) and reduce BP. Mechanism involves interference with calcium influx and intracellular activation of calcium. CV reflexes are not inhibited and reflex tachycardia, increased renin release occur.

Indications
- Hypertensive crises for immediate reduction of BP
- Production of controlled hypotension during anesthesia to reduce bleeding in surgical procedures
- Acute HF
- Unlabeled uses: Acute MI, with dopamine; left ventricular failure, with oxygen, morphine, loop diuretic

Contraindications and cautions
- Contraindicated with treatment of compensatory hypertension; to produce controlled hypotension during surgery with known inadequate cerebral circulation; emergency use in moribund patients; acute HF with peripheral vascular disease.
- Use cautiously with hepatic, renal insufficiency (drug decomposes to cyanide, which is metabolized by the liver and kidneys to thiocyanate ion); hypothyroidism (thiocyanate inhibits the uptake and binding of iodine); pregnancy; lactation.

Available forms
Powder for injection—50 mg/vial

Dosages
Administer only by continuous IV infusion with sterile D_5W.
Adults and pediatric patients
In patients not receiving antihypertensive medication, the average dose is 3 mcg/kg/min (range 0.3–10 mcg/kg/min). At this rate, diastolic BP is usually lowered by 30%–40% below pretreatment diastolic levels. Use smaller doses in patients on antihypertensive medication. Do not exceed infusion rate of 10 mcg/kg/min. If this rate of infusion does not reduce BP within 10 min, discontinue administration.
Geriatric patients or patients with renal impairment
Use with caution and in initial low dosage. The elderly may be more sensitive to the hypotensive effects.

Pharmacokinetics

Route	Onset	Duration
IV	1–2 min	1–10 min

Adverse effects in *italics* are most common; those in **bold** are life-threatening. ⬛⬛ Do not crush.

Metabolism: Hepatic; $T_{1/2}$: 2 min
Distribution: Crosses placenta; may enter breast milk
Excretion: Urine

▼ IV FACTS

Preparation: Dissolve contents of 50-mg vial in 2–3 mL of D₅W. Dilute the prepared stock solution in 250–1,000 mL of D₅W, and promptly wrap container in aluminum foil or other opaque material to protect from light; the administration set tubing does not need to be covered. Observe solution for color changes. Freshly prepared solution has a faint brown tint; discard it if highly colored (blue, green, or dark red). If properly protected from light, reconstituted solution is stable for 24 hr. Do not use the infusion fluid for administration of any other drugs. Do not infuse undiluted solution.
Infusion: Infuse slowly to reduce likelihood of adverse effects; use an infusion pump, micro-drip regulator, or similar device to allow precise control of flow rate; carefully monitor BP and regulate dose based on response.
Incompatibilities: Do not mix in solution with any other drugs.

Adverse effects

- **CNS:** *Apprehension, headache, restlessness, muscle twitching,* dizziness
- **CV:** *Retrosternal pressure, palpitations, hypotension,* bradycardia, tachycardia, ECG changes
- **Cyanide toxicity:** Increasing tolerance to drug and metabolic acidosis are early signs, followed by dyspnea, headache, vomiting, dizziness, ataxia, loss of consciousness, imperceptible pulse, absent reflexes, widely dilated pupils, pink skin color, distant heart sounds, shallow breathing (seen in overdose)
- **Dermatologic:** *Diaphoresis,* flushing
- **Endocrine:** Hypothyroidism
- **GI:** *Nausea, vomiting, abdominal pain*
- **Hematologic:** Methemoglobinemia, antiplatelet effects
- **Local:** Irritation at injection site

■ Nursing considerations
Assessment

- **History:** Hepatic or renal insufficiency, hypothyroidism, pregnancy, lactation
- **Physical:** Reflexes, affect, orientation, pupil size; BP, P, orthostatic BP, supine BP, perfu-

sion, edema, auscultation; R, adventitious sounds; LFTs, renal and thyroid function tests, blood acid–base balance

Interventions

- Monitor injection site carefully to prevent extravasation.
- ⊗ *Black box warning* Do not let BP drop too rapidly; do not lower systolic BP below 160 mm Hg. Monitor BP closely.
- ⊗ *Warning* Provide amyl nitrate inhalation, materials to make 3% sodium nitrite solution, sodium thiosulfate on standby in case of overdose of nitroprusside and depletion of the patient's body stores of sulfur occur, leading to cyanide toxicity.
- ⊗ *Black box warning* Monitor blood acid-base balance (metabolic acidosis is early sign of cyanide toxicity), serum thiocyanate levels daily during prolonged therapy, especially in patients with renal impairment.

Teaching points

- Anticipate frequent monitoring of blood pressure, blood tests, checks of IV dosage and rate.
- Report pain at injection site, chest pain.

N

▽ **nizatidine**
(nigh za' ti deen)

Apo-Nizatidine (CAN), Axid, Axid AR, Axid Pulvules, Gen-Nizatidine (CAN), PMS-Nizatidine (CAN)

PREGNANCY CATEGORY B

Drug class
Histamine-2 (H₂) antagonist

Therapeutic actions
Inhibits the action of histamine at the H₂ receptors of the parietal cells of the stomach, inhibiting basal gastric acid secretion and gastric acid secretion that is stimulated by food, caffeine, insulin, histamine, cholinergic agonists, gastrin, and pentagastrin. Total pepsin output also is reduced.

Indications

- Short-term and maintenance treatment of duodenal ulcer
- Short-term treatment of benign gastric ulcer
- GERD

- OTC: Prevention of heartburn, acid indigestion, and sour stomach brought on by eating
- Unlabeled uses: Prevention of olanzapine-related weight gain; prevention of NSAID-related ulcers

Contraindications and cautions
- Contraindicated with allergy to nizatidine, lactation.
- Use cautiously with impaired renal or hepatic function, pregnancy.

Available forms
Capsules—150, 300 mg; OTC tablets—75 mg; oral solution—15 mg/mL

Dosages
Adults
- *Active duodenal ulcer:* 300 mg PO daily at bedtime. 150 mg PO bid may be used. Most ulcers heal in 4 wk.
- *Maintenance of healed duodenal ulcer:* 150 mg PO daily at bedtime.
- *GERD:* 150 mg PO bid.
- *Benign gastric ulcer:* 150 mg PO bid or 300 mg daily at bedtime.
- *Prevention of heartburn, acid indigestion:* 75 mg PO 30–60 min before food or beverages that cause the problem, taken with water.
Pediatric patients
Safety and efficacy not established.
Geriatric patients or patients with renal impairment
For creatinine clearance 20–50 mL/min, use 150 mg/day PO for active ulcer; 150 mg every other day for maintenance. For creatinine clearance less than 20 mL/min, use 150 mg PO every other day for active ulcer; 150 mg PO every 3 days for maintenance.

Pharmacokinetics

Route	Onset	Peak
Oral	Varies	0.5–3 hr

Metabolism: Hepatic; $T_{1/2}$: 1–2 hr
Distribution: Crosses placenta; enters breast milk
Excretion: Urine

Adverse effects
- **CNS:** *Dizziness, somnolence, headache, confusion, hallucinations,* peripheral neuropathy; symptoms of brainstem dysfunction (dysarthria, ataxia, diplopia)

- **CV:** Cardiac arrhythmias, **cardiac arrest**
- **GI:** *Diarrhea,* hepatitis, pancreatitis, hepatic fibrosis
- **Hematologic:** Neutropenia, agranulocytosis, increases in plasma creatinine, serum transaminase
- **Other:** *Impotence,* gynecomastia, rash, arthralgia, myalgia

Interactions
✳ **Drug-drug** • Increased serum salicylate levels with aspirin
✳ **Drug-lab test** • False-positive tests for urobilinogen

■ Nursing considerations
Assessment
- **History:** Allergy to nizatidine, impaired renal or hepatic function, pregnancy, lactation
- **Physical:** Skin lesions; orientation, affect; P, baseline ECG; liver evaluation, abdominal examination, normal output; CBC, LFTs, renal function tests

Interventions
- Administer drug at bedtime.
- Decrease doses in renal and hepatic impairment.
- Switch to oral solution if swallowing is difficult.
- Arrange for regular follow-up, including blood tests to evaluate effects.

Teaching points
- Use oral solution if prescribed; may be stored at room temperature.
- Take over-the-counter drug 30–60 minutes before the food or beverage that causes the problem; take with water.
- Take drug at bedtime. Therapy may continue for 4–6 weeks or longer.
- Take antacids exactly as prescribed, being careful of the times of administration. Do not take over-the-counter drugs, and avoid alcohol. Many over-the-counter drugs contain ingredients that might interfere with this drug's effectiveness.
- Tell all health care providers, including dentists, that you are taking this drug. Dosage and timing of all your medications must be coordinated. If anything about the drugs that you are taking changes, consult your health care providers.

- Have regular medical follow-up visits to evaluate drug response.
- Report sore throat, fever, unusual bruising or bleeding, tarry stools, confusion, hallucinations, dizziness, muscle or joint pain.

DANGEROUS DRUG

▷**norepinephrine bitartrate (levarterenol)**
(nor ep i nef' rin)

Levophed

PREGNANCY CATEGORY C

Drug classes
Alpha-adrenergic agonist
Beta$_1$-adrenergic agonist
Cardiac stimulant
Sympathomimetic
Vasopressor

Therapeutic actions
Vasopressor and cardiac stimulant; effects are mediated by alpha$_1$- or beta$_1$-adrenergic receptors in target organs; potent vasoconstrictor (alpha effect) acting in arterial and venous beds; potent positive inotropic agent (beta$_1$ effect), increasing the force of myocardial contraction and increasing coronary blood flow.

Indications
- Restoration of BP in controlling certain acute hypotensive states (pheochromocytomomy, sympathectomy, poliomyelitis, spinal anesthesia, MI, septicemia, blood transfusion, and drug reactions)
- Adjunct in the treatment of cardiac arrest and profound hypotension

Contraindications and cautions
- Contraindicated with hypovolemia (not a substitute for restoration of fluids, plasma, electrolytes, and should not be used when there are blood volume deficits except as an emergency measure to maintain coronary and cerebral perfusion until blood volume replacement can be effected; if administered continuously to maintain BP when there is hypovolemia, perfusion of vital organs may be severely compromised and tissue hypoxia may result); general anesthesia with halogenated hydrocarbons or cyclopropane; pro-

found hypoxia or hypercarbia; mesenteric or peripheral vascular thrombosis (risk of extending the infarct).
- Use cautiously with pregnancy, lactation.

Available forms
Injection—1 mg/mL (as base)

Dosages
Individualize infusion rate based on response.
Adults
- *Restoration of BP in acute hypotensive states:* Add 4 mL of the solution (1 mg/mL) to 1,000 mL of 5% dextrose solution for a concentration of 4 mcg base/mL. Initially, give 8–12 mcg base per min. Adjust dose gradually to maintain desired BP (usually 80–100 mm Hg systolic). Average maintenance dose is 2–4 mcg base/min. Occasionally enormous daily doses are needed (68 mg base/day). Continue the infusion until adequate BP and tissue perfusion are maintained without therapy. Treatment may be required up to 6 days (vascular collapse due to acute MI). Reduce infusion gradually.
- *Adjunct in cardiac arrest:* Administer IV during cardiac resuscitation to restore and maintain BP after effective heartbeat and ventilation established. Dosages are similar to those used in acute hypotensive states.
Pediatric patients
Safety and efficacy not established.

Pharmacokinetics

Route	Onset	Duration
IV	Rapid	1–2 min

Metabolism: Neural; T$_{1/2}$: Unknown
Distribution: Crosses placenta
Excretion: Urine

▼**IV FACTS**

Preparation: Dilute drug in 5% dextrose solution in distilled water or 5% dextrose in saline solution; these dextrose solutions protect against oxidation. Do not administer in saline solution alone.
Infusion: Infusion rate is determined by response with constant BP monitoring; check manufacturer's insert for detailed guidelines.
Incompatibilities: Do not mix with blood products, aminophylline, amobarbital, lidocaine, pentobarbital, phenobarbital, phenytoin, secobarbital, sodium bicarbonate, thiopental.

Adverse effects
- **CNS:** *Headache*
- **CV:** *Bradycardia,* hypertension

Interactions
✳ **Drug-drug** • Increased hypertensive effects with TCAs (imipramine), reserpine, methyldopa • Decreased vasopressor effects with phenothiazines

■ Nursing considerations
Assessment
- **History:** Hypovolemia, general anesthesia with halogenated hydrocarbons or cyclopropane, profound hypoxia or hypercarbia, mesenteric or peripheral vascular thrombosis, lactation, pregnancy
- **Physical:** Weight; skin color, T, turgor; P, BP; R, adventitious sounds; urine output; serum electrolytes, ECG

Interventions
- Give whole blood or plasma separately, if indicated.
- Administer IV infusions into a large vein, preferably the antecubital fossa, to prevent extravasation.
- Do not infuse into femoral vein in elderly patients or those suffering from occlusive vascular disease (atherosclerosis, arteriosclerosis, diabetic endarteritis, Buerger disease); occlusive vascular disease is more likely to occur in lower extremity.
- Avoid catheter tie-in technique, if possible, because stasis around tubing may lead to high local concentrations of drug.
- Monitor BP every 2 min from the start of infusion until desired BP is achieved, then monitor every 5 min if infusion is continued.
- Monitor infusion site for extravasation.

⊗ **Black box warning** Provide phentolamine on standby in case extravasation occurs (5–10 mg phentolamine in 10–15 mL saline should be used to infiltrate the affected area).

⊗ *Warning* Do not use drug solutions that are pink or brown; drug solutions should be clear and colorless.

Teaching points
Because norepinephrine is used only in acute emergency situations, patient teaching will depend on patient's awareness and will relate mainly to patient's status and to monitoring being done, rather than specifically to therapy with norepinephrine.

▷ **norethindrone acetate**
*(nor eth **in'** drone)*

Aygestin

PREGNANCY CATEGORY X

Drug classes
Hormone
Progestin

Therapeutic actions
Progesterone derivative. Progesterone transforms proliferative endometrium into secretory endometrium; inhibits the secretion of pituitary gonadotropins, which prevents follicular maturation and ovulation; and inhibits spontaneous uterine contraction. Progestins have varying profiles of estrogenic, antiestrogenic, anabolic, and androgenic activity.

Indications
- Treatment of amenorrhea, abnormal uterine bleeding due to hormonal imbalance
- Treatment of endometriosis
- Base: Component of some hormonal contraceptive preparations

Contraindications and cautions
- Contraindicated with allergy to progestins; thrombophlebitis, thromboembolic disorders, cerebral hemorrhage or history of these conditions; hepatic disease; carcinoma of the breast or genital organs; undiagnosed vaginal bleeding; missed abortion; pregnancy; lactation.
- Use cautiously with epilepsy, migraine, asthma, cardiac dysfunction, or renal impairment.

Available forms
Tablets—5 mg

Dosages
Administer orally only.
Adults
- *Amenorrhea; abnormal uterine bleeding:* 2.5–10 mg PO for 5–10 days during second half of theoretical menstrual cycle.
- *Endometriosis:* 5 mg/day PO for 2 wk. Increase in increments of 2.5 mg/day every 2 wk

until 15 mg/day is reached. May be maintained for 6–9 mo or until breakthrough bleeding demands temporary termination.

Pharmacokinetics

Route	Onset
Oral	Varies

Metabolism: Hepatic; $T_{1/2}$: 8 hr
Distribution: Crosses placenta; enters breast milk
Excretion: Feces, urine

Adverse effects

- **CNS:** Sudden, partial, or complete loss of vision; proptosis; diplopia; migraine; precipitation of acute intermittent porphyria; mental depression; pyrexia; insomnia; somnolence
- **CV:** Thrombophlebitis, cerebrovascular disorders, retinal thrombosis, **pulmonary embolism,** thromboembolic and thrombotic disease, increased BP
- **Dermatologic:** *Rash with or without pruritus, acne,* melasma or chloasma, alopecia, hirsutism, photosensitivity
- **GI:** Cholestatic jaundice, nausea
- **GU:** *Breakthrough bleeding, spotting, change in menstrual flow, amenorrhea,* changes in cervical erosion and cervical secretions, breast tenderness and secretion
- **Other:** Decreased glucose tolerance, *fluid retention, edema, increase in weight*

Interactions

✳ **Drug-lab test** ● Inaccurate tests of hepatic and endocrine function

■ Nursing considerations
Assessment

- **History:** Allergy to progestins; thrombophlebitis, thromboembolic disorders, cerebral hemorrhage; hepatic disease; carcinoma of the breast or genital organs; undiagnosed vaginal bleeding; missed abortion; pregnancy; lactation; epilepsy, migraine; asthma; cardiac dysfunction, or renal impairment
- **Physical:** Skin color, lesions, turgor; hair; breasts; pelvic examination; orientation, affect; ophthalmologic examination; P, auscultation, peripheral perfusion, edema; R, adventitious sounds; liver evaluation; LFTs, renal function tests, glucose tolerance, Papanicolaou (Pap) test

Interventions

- Arrange for pretreatment and periodic (at least annual) history and physical, including BP, breasts, abdomen, pelvic organs, and a Pap test.
- Warn patient prior to therapy to prevent pregnancy and to obtain frequent medical follow-up care.
- ⊗ **Warning** Use caution when administering drug to ensure preparation ordered is the one being used; norethindrone acetate is approximately twice as potent as norethindrone.
- ⊗ **Warning** Discontinue medication and consult physician if sudden, partial, or complete loss of vision occurs; if papilledema or retinal vascular lesions are present, discontinue drug.
- ⊗ **Warning** Discontinue medication and consult physician at sign of thromboembolic disease—leg pain, swelling, peripheral perfusion changes, shortness of breath.

Teaching points

- Take drugs in accordance with a marked calendar.
- Avoid pregnancy; serious fetal abnormalities or fetal death could occur.
- You may experience these side effects: Sensitivity to light (avoid exposure to the sun; use sunscreen and protective clothing); dizziness, sleeplessness, depression (use caution driving or performing tasks that require alertness); skin rash, color changes, loss of hair; fever; nausea.
- Report pain or swelling and warmth in the calves, acute chest pain or shortness of breath, sudden severe headache or vomiting, dizziness or fainting, numbness or tingling in the arm or leg.

▷ norfloxacin
(nor flox' a sin)

Apo-Norflox (CAN), CO-Norfloxacin (CAN), Noroxin

PREGNANCY CATEGORY C

Drug classes

Antibiotic
Fluoroquinolone
Urinary tract anti-infective

Therapeutic actions

Bactericidal; interferes with DNA replication in susceptible gram-negative bacteria, leading to cell death.

Indications

- For the treatment of adults with UTIs caused by susceptible bacteria, including *Escherichia coli, Proteus mirabilis, Klebsiella pneumoniae, Enterobacter cloacae, Proteus vulgaris, Providencia rettgeri, Morganella morganii, Proteus aeruginosa, Citrobacter freundii, Staphylococcus aureus, S. epidermidis,* group D streptococci
- Uncomplicated urethral and cervical gonorrhea caused by *Neisseria gonorrhoeae*
- Prostatitis caused by *E. coli*
- Unlabeled uses: GI infections, traveler's diarrhea

Contraindications and cautions

- Contraindicated with allergy to norfloxacin, nalidixic acid, or cinoxacin; lactation; history of tendinitis or tendon rupture; history of myasthenia gravis.
- Use cautiously in patients with renal impairment, seizures, pregnancy.

Available forms

Tablets—400 mg

Dosages

Adults

- *Uncomplicated UTIs:* 400 mg every 12 hr PO for 7–10 days. Maximum dose, 800 mg/day.
- *Uncomplicated cystitis due to* E. coli, K. pneumonia, *or* P. mirabilis: 400 mg every 12 hr PO for 3 days.
- *Complicated UTI:* 400 mg PO every 12 hr for 10–21 days.
- *Uncomplicated gonorrhea:* 800 mg PO as a single dose.
- *Prostatitis:* 400 mg every 12 hr PO for 28 days.

Pediatric patients

Not recommended; produced lesions of joint cartilage in immature experimental animals.

Geriatric patients or patients with impaired renal function

For creatinine clearance of 30 mL/min or less use 400 mg/day, PO for 7–10 days.

Pharmacokinetics

Route	Onset	Peak
Oral	Varies	2–3 hr

Metabolism: Hepatic; $T_{1/2}$: 3–4.5 hr
Distribution: Crosses placenta; enters breast milk
Excretion: Urine

Adverse effects

- **CNS:** *Headache,* dizziness, insomnia, fatigue, somnolence, depression, blurred vision
- **CV:** Prolonged QT interval
- **GI:** *Nausea,* vomiting, dry mouth, diarrhea, abdominal pain, dyspepsia, flatulence, constipation, heartburn
- **Hematologic:** Elevated BUN, AST, ALT, serum creatinine and alkaline phosphatase; decreased WBC count, neutrophil count, Hct
- **Other:** Fever, rash, photosensitivity, tendinitis, tendon rupture

Interactions

✳ **Drug-drug** • Decreased therapeutic effect with iron salts, sucralfate • Decreased absorption with antacids • Increased serum levels and toxic effects of theophyllines, cyclosporine • Increased risk of QT prolongation with other drugs that prolong QT interval

✳ **Drug-alternative therapy** • Increased risk of severe photosensitivity reactions if combined with St. John's Wort therapy

■ Nursing considerations

CLINICAL ALERT!
Name confusion has occurred between *Noroxin* (norfloxacin) and *Neurontin* (gabapentin); use caution.

Assessment

- **History:** Allergy to norfloxacin, nalidixic acid, or cinoxacin; renal impairment; seizures; pregnancy; lactation; myasthenia gravis
- **Physical:** Skin color, lesions; T; orientation, reflexes, affect; mucous membranes, bowel sounds; LFTs, renal function tests

Interventions

⊗ *Black box warning* Risk of tendonitis and tendon rupture is increased, especially in patients older than 60 yr; patients who have

Adverse effects in *italics* are most common; those in **bold** are life-threatening. ⊂⊅ Do not crush.

undergone kidney, heart, or lung transplant; and those taking corticosteroids.

⊗ **Black box warning** There is risk of severe muscle weakness if used in patients with myasthenia gravis; do not use in patients with a history of myasthenia gravis.

• Arrange for culture and sensitivity tests before therapy.
• Administer drug 1 hr before or 2 hr after meals or ingestion of milk or dairy products. Give with a glass of water.
• Ensure that patient is well hydrated.
• Administer antacids, multivitamins, and other products containing iron or zinc at least 2 hr after dosing.
• Monitor clinical response; if no improvement is seen or a relapse occurs, send urine for repeat culture and sensitivity.

Teaching points

• Take drug on an empty stomach, 1 hour before or 2 hours after meals, milk, or dairy products. If an antacid is needed, do not take it within 2 hours of the norfloxacin dose.
• Drink plenty of fluids.
• You may experience these side effects: Nausea, vomiting, abdominal pain (eat frequent small meals); diarrhea or constipation; drowsiness, blurring of vision, dizziness (observe caution driving or using dangerous equipment).
• Report rash, visual changes, severe GI problems, weakness, tremors, tendon pain, severe diarrhea.

▽ norgestrel
*(nor **jess'** trel)*

PREGNANCY CATEGORY X

Drug classes
Hormonal contraceptive
Hormone
Progestin

Therapeutic actions
Progestational agent; the endogenous female progestin, progesterone, transforms proliferative endometrium into secretory endometrium; inhibits the secretion of pituitary gonadotropins, which prevents follicular maturation and ovulation; and inhibits spontaneous uterine contractions. The primary mechanism by which norgestrel prevents conception is not known, but progestin-only hormonal contraceptives alter the cervical mucus, exert a progestational effect on the endometrium that interferes with implantation, and in some patients, suppress ovulation.

Indications
• Prevention of pregnancy using hormonal contraceptives; somewhat less efficacious (3 pregnancies per 100 woman years) than the combined estrogen/progestin hormonal contraceptives (about 1 pregnancy per 100 woman years, depending on formulation)

Contraindications and cautions
• Contraindicated with allergy to progestins, tartrazine; thrombophlebitis, thromboembolic disorders, cerebral hemorrhage, or history of these conditions; CAD; hepatic disease; carcinoma of the breast or genital organs, undiagnosed vaginal bleeding, missed abortion; as a diagnostic test for pregnancy; pregnancy (fetal abnormalities—masculinization of the female fetus, congenital heart defects, and limb reduction defects); lactation.
• Use cautiously with epilepsy, migraine, asthma, cardiac dysfunction, or renal impairment.

Available forms
Tablets—0.075 mg

Dosages
Adults
Administer daily, starting on the first day of menstruation. Take one tablet, PO, at the same time each day, every day of the year. Missed dose: one tablet—take as soon as remembered, then take the next tablet at regular time; two consecutive tablets—take one of the missed tablets, discard the other, and take daily tablet at usual time; three consecutive tablets—discontinue immediately and use additional form of birth control until menses or pregnancy is ruled out.

Pharmacokinetics

Route	Onset
Oral	Varies

N

Metabolism: Hepatic; T$_{1/2}$: Unknown
Distribution: Crosses placenta; enters breast milk
Excretion: Urine

Adverse effects

- **CNS:** Neuro-ocular lesions, mental depression, migraine, *changes in corneal curvature,* contact lens intolerance
- **CV:** *Thrombophlebitis, thrombosis,* **pulmonary embolism,** coronary thrombosis, **MI,** cerebral thrombosis, Raynaud disease, arterial thromboembolism, renal artery thrombosis, **cerebral hemorrhage,** hypertension
- **Dermatologic:** Rash with or without pruritus, acne, melasma
- **GI:** Gallbladder disease, liver tumors, hepatic lesions, *nausea, vomiting,* abdominal cramps, bloating, cholestatic jaundice
- **GU:** *Breakthrough bleeding, spotting, change in menstrual flow, amenorrhea,* changes in cervical erosion and cervical secretions, endocervical hyperplasia, vaginal candidiasis
- **Other:** *Breast tenderness and secretion, enlargement;* fluid retention, edema, increase or decrease in weight

Interactions

✳ **Drug-drug** • Decreased effectiveness of hormonal contraceptives with barbiturates, hydantoins, carbamazepine, rifampin, griseofulvin, penicillins, tetracyclines; use alternate form of birth control if these drugs are needed

✳ **Drug-alternative therapy** • Decreased effectiveness if taken with St. John's Wort

■ Nursing considerations
Assessment

- **History:** Allergy to progestins, tartrazine; thrombophlebitis, thromboembolic disorders, cerebral hemorrhage; CAD; hepatic disease; carcinoma of the breast or genital organs, undiagnosed vaginal bleeding, missed abortion; epilepsy, migraine, asthma, cardiac dysfunction, or renal impairment; pregnancy; lactation
- **Physical:** Skin color, lesions, turgor; hair; breasts; pelvic examination; orientation, affect; ophthalmologic examination; P, auscultation, peripheral perfusion, edema; R, adventitious sounds; liver evaluation; LFTs,

renal function tests, glucose tolerance, Papanicolaou (Pap) test, pregnancy test

Interventions

- Arrange for pretreatment and periodic (at least annual) history and physical, including BP, breasts, abdomen, pelvic organs, and a Pap test.
- Start no earlier than 4 wk postpartum for postpartum use.
- ⊗ **Warning** Discontinue medication and consult physician if sudden, partial, or complete loss of vision occurs; if papilledema or retinal vascular lesions are present on examination, discontinue.
- ⊗ **Warning** Discontinue drug and consult physician at any sign of thromboembolic disease—leg pain, swelling, peripheral perfusion changes, shortness of breath.

Teaching points

- Take exactly as prescribed at intervals not exceeding 24 hours. Take at bedtime or with a meal to establish a routine; medication must be taken daily for prevention of pregnancy; if you miss one tablet, take as soon as remembered, then take the next tablet at regular time. If you miss two consecutive tablets, take one of the missed tablets, discard the other, and take daily tablet at usual time. If you miss three consecutive tablets, discontinue immediately, and use another method of birth control until your cycle starts again. It is a good idea to use an additional method of birth control if any tablets are missed.
- Discontinue drug and consult your health care provider if you decide to become pregnant. It may be suggested that you use a nonhormonal form of birth control for a few months before becoming pregnant.
- Do not take this drug during pregnancy; serious fetal abnormalities have been reported. If you think that you are pregnant, consult your health care provider immediately.
- Tell all health care providers, including dentists, that you take this drug. If other medications are prescribed, they may decrease the effectiveness of hormonal contraceptives and an additional method of birth control may be needed.
- You may experience these side effects: Sensitivity to light (avoid exposure to the sun;

use sunscreen and protective clothing); dizziness, sleeplessness, depression (use caution driving or performing tasks that require alertness); rash, skin color changes, loss of hair; fever; nausea; breakthrough bleeding or spotting (transient); intolerance to contact lenses due to corneal changes.

- Report pain or swelling and warmth in the calves, acute chest pain or shortness of breath, sudden severe headache or vomiting, dizziness or fainting, visual disturbances, numbness or tingling in the arm or leg, breakthrough bleeding or spotting that lasts into the second month of therapy.

▷ nortriptyline hydrochloride
*(nor **trip'** ti leen)*

Apo-Nortriptyline (CAN), Aventyl, Gen-Nortriptyline (CAN), Pamelor, ratio-Nortriptyline (CAN)

PREGNANCY CATEGORY D

Drug class
TCA (secondary amine)

Therapeutic actions
Mechanism of action unknown; the TCAs are structurally related to the phenothiazine antipsychotic drugs (eg, chlorpromazine), but inhibit the presynaptic reuptake of the neurotransmitters norepinephrine and serotonin; anticholinergic at CNS and peripheral receptors; sedating; the relationship of these effects to clinical efficacy is unknown.

Indications
- Relief of symptoms of depression (endogenous depression most responsive)
- Unlabeled uses: Treatment of panic disorders (25–75 mg/day), premenstrual depression (50–125 mg/day), dermatologic disorders (75 mg/day), chronic pain, headache prophylaxis

Contraindications and cautions
- Contraindicated with hypersensitivity to any tricyclic drug, concomitant therapy with an MAOI, within 2 wk of MAOI use, recent MI, myelography within previous 24 hr or sched-

uled within 48 hr, pregnancy (limb reduction abnormalities), lactation.
- Use cautiously with EST (increased hazard with TCAs); pre-existing CV disorders (possibly increased risk of serious CVS toxicity); angle-closure glaucoma, increased IOP; urinary retention, ureteral or urethral spasm (anticholinergic effects may exacerbate these conditions); seizure disorders; hyperthyroidism (predisposes to CVS toxicity, including cardiac arrhythmias); impaired hepatic, renal function; psychiatric patients (schizophrenic or paranoid patients may exhibit a worsening of psychosis); bipolar disorder (may shift to hypomanic or manic phase); elective surgery (discontinued as long as possible before surgery).

Available forms
Capsules—10, 25, 50, 75 mg; solution—10 mg/5 mL

Dosages
Adults
25 mg tid–qid PO. Begin with low dosage and gradually increase as required and tolerated. Doses of more than 150 mg/day are not recommended.
Pediatric patients 12 yr and older
30–50 mg/day PO in divided doses.
Pediatric patients younger than 12 yr
Not recommended.
Geriatric patients
30–50 mg/day PO in divided doses.

Pharmacokinetics

Route	Onset	Peak	Duration
Oral	Varies	2–4 hr	2–4 wk

Metabolism: Hepatic; T$_{1/2}$: 18–28 hr
Distribution: Crosses placenta; enters breast milk
Excretion: Urine

Adverse effects
- **CNS:** *Sedation and anticholinergic (atropine-like) effects* (dry mouth, blurred vision, disturbance of accommodation for near vision, mydriasis, increased IOP), *confusion* (especially in elderly), *disturbed concentration,* hallucinations, disorientation, decreased memory, feelings of unreality, delusions, anxiety, nervousness, restlessness,

agitation, panic, insomnia, nightmares, hypomania, mania, exacerbation of psychosis, drowsiness, weakness, fatigue, headache, numbness, tingling, paresthesias of extremities, incoordination, motor hyperactivity, akathisia, ataxia, tremors, peripheral neuropathy, extrapyramidal symptoms, **seizures,** speech blockage, dysarthria

• **CV:** *Orthostatic hypotension,* hypertension, syncope, tachycardia, palpitations, MI, arrhythmias, heart block, precipitation of heart failure, **stroke**

• **Endocrine:** Elevated or depressed blood sugar; elevated prolactin levels; inappropriate ADH secretion

• **GI:** *Dry mouth, constipation,* paralytic ileus, *nausea,* vomiting, anorexia, epigastric distress, diarrhea, flatulence, dysphagia, peculiar taste, increased salivation, stomatitis, glossitis, parotid swelling, abdominal cramps, black tongue, hepatitis; elevated transaminase, altered alkaline phosphatase

• **GU:** Urinary retention, delayed micturition, dilation of the urinary tract, gynecomastia, testicular swelling; breast enlargement, menstrual irregularity and galactorrhea; increased or decreased libido; impotence

• **Hematologic:** Bone marrow depression, including agranulocytosis; eosinophilia; purpura; thrombocytopenia; leukopenia

• **Hypersensitivity:** Rash, pruritus, vasculitis, petechiae, photosensitization, edema (generalized, facial, tongue), drug fever

• **Withdrawal:** Symptoms with abrupt discontinuation of prolonged therapy: Nausea, headache, vertigo, nightmares, malaise

• **Other:** Nasal congestion, excessive appetite, weight gain or loss; sweating, alopecia, lacrimation, hyperthermia, flushing, chills

Interactions

✳ **Drug-drug** • Increased TCA levels and pharmacologic (especially anticholinergic) effects with cimetidine, fluoxetine • Altered response, including arrhythmias and hypertension with sympathomimetics • Risk of severe hypertension with clonidine • Hyperpyretic crises, severe seizures, hypertensive episodes, and deaths when MAOIs are given with TCAs

Note: MAOIs and TCAs have been used successfully in some patients resistant to therapy with single agents; however, case reports indicate that the combination can cause serious and potentially fatal adverse effects.

■ Nursing considerations
Assessment

• **History:** Hypersensitivity to any tricyclic drug; concomitant therapy with an MAOI; recent MI; myelography within previous 24 hr or scheduled within 48 hr; pregnancy; lactation; EST; pre-existing CV disorders; angle-closure glaucoma, increased IOP; urinary retention, ureteral or urethral spasm; seizure disorders; hyperthyroidism; impaired hepatic, renal function; psychiatric disorders; bipolar disorder; elective surgery

• **Physical:** Weight; T; skin color, lesions; orientation, affect, reflexes, vision and hearing; P, BP, orthostatic BP, perfusion; bowel sounds, normal output, liver evaluation; urine flow, normal output; usual sexual function, frequency of menses, breast and scrotal examination; LFTs, urinalysis, CBC, ECG

Interventions

⊗ **Black box warning** Limit access to drug by depressed and potentially suicidal patients; risk of suicidality in children and adolescents and young adults. Monitor accordingly.

• When doses larger than 100 mg/day are given, plasma levels of nortriptyline should be monitored and maintained in the range of 50–150 ng/mL.

• Give major portion of dose at bedtime if drowsiness or severe anticholinergic effects occur.

• Reduce dosage if minor side effects develop; discontinue if serious side effects occur.

• Arrange for CBC if patient develops fever, sore throat, or other sign of infection.

Teaching points

• Take drug exactly as prescribed; do not stop taking this drug abruptly or without consulting your health care provider.

• Avoid alcohol, other sleep-inducing, or over-the-counter drugs.

• Avoid prolonged exposure to sunlight or sunlamps; use a sunscreen or protective garments if possible.

• You may experience these side effects: Headache, dizziness, drowsiness, weakness, blurred vision (reversible; use safety measures if severe; avoid driving or performing tasks that require alertness); nausea, vomiting, loss of appetite, dry mouth (eat frequent small meals, perform frequent mouth care, suck on sugarless candy); nightmares, inability to concentrate, confusion; changes in sexual function.

- Report dry mouth, difficulty in urination, excessive sedation, thoughts of suicide.

▷ **nystatin**
(nye stat' in)

Oral: Candistatin
(CAN), Mycostatin, Nilstat,
ratio-Nystatin (CAN)
Vaginal preparations: Mycostatin
Topical application: Mycostatin

PREGNANCY CATEGORY C

Drug class
Antifungal

Therapeutic actions
Fungicidal and fungistatic: Binds to sterols in the cell membrane of the fungus with a resultant change in membrane permeability, allowing leakage of intracellular components and causing cell death.

Indications
- Oral: Treatment of oropharyngeal candidiasis
- Vaginal: Local treatment of vaginal candidiasis (moniliasis)
- Topical applications: Treatment of cutaneous or mucocutaneous mycotic infections caused by *Candida albicans* and other *Candida* species

Contraindications and cautions
- Contraindicated with allergy to nystatin or components used in preparation.
- Use cautiously with pregnancy, lactation.

Available forms
Tablets—500,000 units; suspension—100,000 units/mL; vaginal tablets—100,000 units; topical cream, ointment, powder—100,000 units/g

Dosages
Adults
Vaginal preparations
1 tablet (100,000 units) or 1 applicator of cream (100,000 units) daily–bid for 2 wk.
Topical
- *Vaginal preparations:* Apply to affected area two to three times daily until healing is complete.
- *Topical foot powder:* For fungal infections of the feet, dust powder on feet and in shoes and socks.

Adults and pediatric patients except infants
Oral
- *Tablets:* 500,000–1,000,000 units tid. Continue for at least 48 hr after clinical cure.
- *Suspension:* 400,000–600,000 units four times/day for 14 days and for at least 48 hr after symptoms subside.

Pharmacokinetics
No general systemic absorption
Excretion: Feces, unchanged (oral use)

Adverse effects
Oral
- **GI:** *Nausea, vomiting, diarrhea, GI distress*
Vaginal
- **Local:** *Irritation, vulvovaginal burning*
Topical
- **Local:** *Local irritation*

■ Nursing considerations
Assessment
- **History:** Allergy to nystatin or components used in preparation, pregnancy, lactation
- **Physical:** Skin color, lesions, area around lesions; bowel sounds; culture of area involved

Interventions
- Culture fungus before therapy.
- Have patient retain oral suspension in mouth as long as possible before swallowing. Paint suspension on each side of the mouth. Continue local treatment for at least 48 hr after clinical improvement is noted.
- Prepare nystatin in the form of frozen flavored popsicles to improve oral retention of the drug for local application.

- Insert vaginal suppositories high into the vagina. Have patient remain recumbent for 10–15 min after insertion. Provide sanitary napkin to protect clothing from stains.
- Clean affected area before topical application, unless otherwise indicated.
- Monitor response to drug therapy. If no response is noted, arrange for further cultures to determine causative organism.
- Ensure that patient receives the full course of therapy to eradicate the fungus and to prevent recurrence.
- Discontinue topical or vaginal administration if rash or sensitivity occurs.

Teaching points

- Take the full course of drug therapy even if symptoms improve. Continue during menstrual period if vaginal route is being used. Long-term use of the drug may be needed; beneficial effects may not be seen for several weeks. Vaginal suppositories should be inserted high into the vagina.
- Use appropriate hygiene measures to prevent reinfection or spread of infection.
- This drug is for the fungus being treated; do not self-medicate other problems.
- Refrain from sexual intercourse or advise partner to use a condom to avoid reinfection; use a sanitary napkin to prevent staining of clothing with vaginal use.
- You may experience these side effects: Nausea, vomiting, diarrhea (oral use); irritation, burning, stinging (local use).
- Report worsening of condition; local irritation, burning (topical application); rash, irritation, pelvic pain (vaginal use); nausea, GI distress (oral administration).

▷octreotide acetate
*(ok **tree**' oh tide)*

Sandostatin, Sandostatin LAR Depot

PREGNANCY CATEGORY B

Drug classes
Antidiarrheal
Hormone

Therapeutic actions
Mimics the natural hormone somatostatin; suppresses secretion of serotonin, gastrin, vasoactive intestinal peptide, insulin, glucagon, secretin, motilin, and pancreatic polypeptide; also suppresses growth hormone and decreases splanchnic blood flow.

Indications
- Symptomatic treatment of patients with metastatic carcinoid tumors to suppress or inhibit the associated severe diarrhea and flushing episodes
- Treatment of the profuse watery diarrhea associated with vasoactive intestinal polypeptide tumors (VIPomas)
- Reduction of growth hormone blood levels in patients with acromegaly not responsive to other treatment
- Unlabeled uses: GI fistula, variceal bleeding, diarrheal states, pancreatic fistulas, IBS, dumping syndrome

Contraindications and cautions
- Contraindicated with hypersensitivity to octreotide or any of its components.
- Use cautiously with renal impairment, thyroid disease, diabetes mellitus, pregnancy, lactation.

Available forms
Injection—0.05, 0.1, 0.2, 0.5, 1 mg/mL; depot injection—10, 20, 30 mg/5 mL

Dosages
Adults
Subcutaneous injection is the route of choice. Initial dose is 50 mcg subcutaneously two to three times daily; the number of injections is increased based on response, usually bid–tid. IV bolus injections have been used in emergency situations—not recommended. Depot injection: Do not administer IV or subcutaneously; inject intragluteally at 4-wk intervals. Patients should be stabilized on subcutaneous octreotide for at least 2 wk before switching to long-acting depot.
- *Carcinoid tumors:* First 2 wk of therapy: 100–600 mcg/day subcutaneously in two to four divided doses (mean daily dosage, 300 mcg).
- *VIPomas:* 200–300 mcg subcutaneously in two to four divided doses during initial 2 wk of therapy to control symptoms. Range, 150–750 mcg subcutaneously; doses above 450 mcg are usually not required. Depot injection: 20 mg IM every 4 wk.

- *Acromegaly:* 50 mcg tid subcutaneously, adjusted up to 100–500 mcg tid. Withdraw for 4 wk once yearly. Depot injection: 20 mg IM intragluteally once every 4 wk; after 2–3 mo, re-evaluate patient to adjust dosage as needed.

Pediatric patients
Safety and efficacy for depot injection not established.

- *GI tumors:* 1–10 mcg/kg/day subcutaneously.

Geriatric patients or patients with renal impairment
Half-life may be prolonged; adjust dosage.

Pharmacokinetics

Route	Onset	Peak
Subcut.	Rapid	15 min

Metabolism: Hepatic; $T_{1/2}$: 1.5 hr
Distribution: May cross placenta; may enter breast milk
Excretion: Urine

Adverse effects

- **CNS:** Anxiety, *headache, dizziness, light-headedness,* fatigue, seizures, depression, drowsiness, vertigo, hyperesthesia, irritability, forgetfulness, malaise, nervousness, visual disturbances
- **CV:** Shortness of breath, hypertension, thrombophlebitis, ischemia, heart failure, palpitations, *bradycardia*
- **Dermatologic:** *Flushing,* edema, hair loss, thinning of skin, skin flaking, bruising, pruritus, rash
- **Endocrine:** *Hyperglycemia, hypoglycemia,* galactorrhea, clinical hypothyroidism
- **GI:** *Nausea, vomiting, diarrhea, abdominal pain, loose stools,* fat malabsorption, constipation, flatulence, hepatitis, rectal spasm, GI bleeding, heartburn, cholelithiasis, dry mouth, burning mouth
- **Local:** *Injection site pain*
- **Musculoskeletal:** Asthenia, weakness, leg cramps, muscle pain, joint pain, backache
- **Respiratory:** Rhinorrhea

■ Nursing considerations

CLINICAL ALERT!
Name confusion has occurred between *Sandostatin* (octreotide) and *Sandimmune* (cyclosporine); use caution.

Assessment

- **History:** Hypersensitivity to octreotide or any of its components; renal impairment; thyroid disease, diabetes mellitus; lactation
- **Physical:** Skin lesions, hair; reflexes, affect; BP, P, orthostatic BP; abdominal examination, liver evaluation, mucous membranes; renal and thyroid function tests, blood glucose, electrolytes

Interventions

- Administer by subcutaneous injection; avoid multiple injections in the same site within short periods.
- Administer depot injection by deep IM intragluteal injection; avoid deltoid injections. Administer LAR depot immediately after mixing.
- ⊗ **Warning** Monitor patients with renal function impairment closely; reduced dosage may be necessary.
- Store ampules in the refrigerator; may be at room temperature on day of use. Do not use if particulates or discoloration are observed.
- Monitor patient closely for endocrine reactions—blood glucose alterations, thyroid hormone changes, growth hormone level.
- Arrange for baseline and periodic gallbladder ultrasound to detect cholelithiasis.
- Monitor blood glucose, especially at start of therapy, to detect hypoglycemia or hyperglycemia. Patients with diabetes will require close monitoring.
- Arrange to withdraw the drug for 4 wk (8 wk for depot injection) once yearly when treating acromegaly.

Teaching points

- This drug must be injected. You and a significant other can be instructed in the procedure of subcutaneous injections. Review technique and process periodically. Do not use the same site for repeated injections; rotate injection sites. Dispose of needles and syringes properly. Dosage will be adjusted based on your response. Depot injection must be given IM once every 4 weeks.
- Arrange for periodic medical examinations, including blood tests and gallbladder tests.
- You may experience these side effects: Headache, dizziness, light-headedness, fatigue (avoid driving or performing tasks that

require alertness); nausea, diarrhea, abdominal pain (eat frequent small meals; maintain nutrition); flushing, dry skin, flaking of skin (skin care may prevent breakdown); pain at the injection site.
- Report sweating, dizziness, severe abdominal pain, fatigue, fever, chills, infection, or severe pain at injection sites.

▽ ofatumumab

See Appendix R, *Less commonly used drugs.*

▽ ofloxacin
(oh flox' a sin)

Floxin, Floxin Otic, Ocuflox

PREGNANCY CATEGORY C

Drug classes
Antibiotic
Fluoroquinolone

Therapeutic actions
Bactericidal; interferes with DNA replication in susceptible gram-positive and gram-negative bacteria, preventing cell reproduction.

Indications
- Acute bacterial exacerbations of COPD, community-acquired pneumonia caused by *Haemophilus influenzae, Streptococcus pneumoniae*
- Acute, uncomplicated urethral and cervical gonorrhea due to *Neisseria gonorrhoeae,* nongonococcal urethritis, and cervicitis due to *Chlamydia trachomatis,* mixed infections due to both
- Uncomplicated skin and soft tissue infections due to *Staphylococcus aureus, Streptococcus pyogenes, Proteus mirabilis*
- Uncomplicated UTIs caused by *Citrobacter diversus, Enterobacter aerogenes, Escherichia coli, Klebsiella pneumoniae, Pseudomonas aeruginosa,* and *P. mirabilis* caused by *C. trachomatis* and *N. gonorrhoeae*
- Complicated UTIs caused by *C. diversus, E. coli, K. pneumoniae, P. aeruginosa, P. mirabilis*
- Oral: Primary treatment of PID; complicated UTIs due to susceptible bacteria,

including *E. coli, K. pneumoniae, P. mirabilis, C. diversus,* or *P. aeruginosa*
- Prostatitis due to *E. coli*
- Ophthalmic solution: Treatment of ocular infections caused by susceptible organisms
- Orphan drug use: Treatment of bacterial corneal ulcers
- Otic: Otitis externa (patients 6 mo and older), chronic suppurative otitis media (patients 12 yr and older), acute otitis media (patients 1 yr and older); once daily treatment of swimmer's ear (otitis externa) caused by *E. coli, P. aeruginosa, S. aureus* (adults and children 6 mo and older)

Contraindications and cautions
- Contraindicated with allergy to fluoroquinolones, lactation, prolonged QT interval, history of myasthenia gravis.
- Use cautiously with renal impairment, seizures, pregnancy.

Available forms
Ophthalmic solution—3 mg/mL (0.3%); tablets—200, 300, 400 mg; otic solution—0.3%

Dosages
Adults
- *Uncomplicated UTIs:* 200 mg every 12 hr PO for 3–7 days.
- *Complicated UTIs:* 200 mg bid PO for 10 days.
- *Bacterial exacerbations of COPD, community-acquired pneumonia:* 400 mg every 12 hr PO for 10 days.
- *Mild to moderate skin infections:* 400 mg every 12 hr PO for 10 days.
- *Prostatitis:* 300 mg every 12 hr PO for 6 wk.
- *Acute, uncomplicated gonorrhea:* 400 mg PO as a single dose.
- *Cervicitis, urethritis:* 300 mg every 12 hr PO for 7 days.
- *Ocular infections:* 1–2 drops per eye as indicated.
- *Otic infections:* 10 drops in affected ear tid for 10–14 days.
- *Swimmer's ear:* 10 drops (1.5 mg) in affected ear, once daily for 7 days.
- *Chronic suppurative otitis media:* 10 drops in affected ear bid for 14 days.

Adverse effects in *italics* are most common; those in **bold** are life-threatening. ▭▭ Do not crush.

Pediatric patients younger than 18 yr
Systemic
Not recommended; produced lesions of joint cartilage in immature experimental animals.
Otic
1 yr–younger than 12 yr:
- *Swimmer's ear, acute otitis media with tympanostomy tubes:* 5 drops in affected ear bid for 10 days.
12 yr and older:
- *Swimmer's ear:* 10 drops in affected ear bid for 10 days.
- *Chronic otitis media:* 10 drops in affected ear bid for 14 days.
6 mo–13 yr:
- *Swimmer's ear:* 5 drops (0.75 mg) in affected ear once daily for 7 days.

Geriatric patients or patients with impaired renal function
For creatinine clearance 20–50 mL/min, use a 24-hr interval; for creatinine clearance less than 20 mL/min, use a 24-hr interval and half the recommended dose.

Pharmacokinetics

Route	Onset	Peak	Duration
Oral	Varies	1–2 hr	9 hr

Metabolism: Hepatic; $T_{1/2}$: 5–10 hr
Distribution: Crosses placenta; enters breast milk
Excretion: Bile, urine

Adverse effects
- **CNS:** *Headache,* dizziness, *insomnia,* fatigue, somnolence, depression, blurred vision
- **CV:** QT-interval prolongation
- **GI:** *Nausea,* vomiting, dry mouth, *diarrhea,* abdominal pain
- **Hematologic:** Elevated BUN, AST, ALT, serum creatinine and alkaline phosphatase; decreased WBC count, neutrophil count, Hct
- **Other:** Fever, rash, *photosensitivity;* ocular burning, tendinitis, tendon rupture

Interactions
✳ Drug-drug • Decreased therapeutic effect with iron salts, zinc, sucralfate • Decreased absorption with antacids • Increased risk of prolonged QT interval if combined with other drugs that prolong QT interval, antiarrhythmics

✳ Drug-alternative therapy • Increased risk of severe photosensitivity reactions if combined with St. John's Wort

■ Nursing considerations
Assessment
- **History:** Allergy to fluoroquinolones, renal impairment, seizures, lactation, pregnancy
- **Physical:** Skin color, lesions; T; orientation, reflexes, affect; mucous membranes, bowel sounds; LFTs, renal function tests

Interventions
⊗ **Black box warning** Fluoroquinolones are associated with increased risk of tendinitis and tendon rupture; risk is higher in patients older than 60 yr, women, and patients with kidney, heart, or lung transplants.

⊗ **Black box warning** There is risk of exacerbation of muscle weakness, sometimes severe, in patients with myasthenia gravis; do not administer to patients with history of myasthenia gravis.

- Arrange for culture and sensitivity tests before beginning therapy.
- Continue therapy for 2 days after the signs of infection have disappeared.
- Administer oral drug 1 hr before or 2 hr after meals with a glass of water.
- Ensure that patient is well hydrated.
- Administer antacids at least 2 hr before or after dosing.
- Monitor clinical response; if no improvement is seen or a relapse occurs, repeat culture and sensitivity tests.

Teaching points
- Take oral drug on an empty stomach, 1 hour before or 2 hours after meals. If an antacid is needed, do not take it within 2 hours of ofloxacin dose.
- Use eye or ear drops as instructed; keep tip away from surfaces; wash hands before administering.
- Avoid St. John's Wort while taking this drug.
- Drink plenty of fluids.
- Avoid prolonged exposure to sunlight.
- You may experience these side effects: Nausea, vomiting, abdominal pain (eat frequent small meals); diarrhea or constipation; drowsiness, blurring of vision, dizziness (use caution if driving or using dangerous equipment).

- Report rash, visual changes, severe GI problems, weakness, tremors, tendon pain.

▷olanzapine
(oh lan' za peen)

Zyprexa, Zyprexa IntraMuscular, Zyprexa Relprevv, Zyprexa Zydis

PREGNANCY CATEGORY C

Drug classes
Antipsychotic
Dopaminergic blocker

Therapeutic actions
Mechanism of action not fully understood; blocks dopamine receptors in the brain, depresses the RAS; blocks serotonin receptor sites; anticholinergic, antihistaminic (H_1), and alpha-adrenergic blocking activity may contribute to some of its therapeutic (and adverse) actions; produces fewer extrapyramidal effects than most antipsychotics.

Indications
- Treatment of schizophrenia
- Treatment of acute mixed or manic episodes associated with bipolar 1 disorder and maintenance of bipolar 1 disorder as monotherapy, or combined with lithium or valproate
- Treatment of agitation associated with schizophrenia and bipolar 1 mania (injection)
- Treatment of treatment-resistant depression and depression associated with bipolar 1 disorder, in combination with fluoxetine
- Unlabeled uses: Delusional parasitosis, stuttering

Contraindications and cautions
- Contraindicated with allergy to olanzapine, myeloproliferative disorders, severe CNS depression, comatose states, lactation.
- Use cautiously in elderly or debilitated patients or with CV or cerebrovascular disease, dehydration, seizure disorders, Alzheimer disease, prostate enlargement, narrow-angle glaucoma, history of paralytic ileus or breast cancer, pregnancy, phenylketonuria (if using orally disintegrating tablets, contain phenylalanine).

Available forms
Tablets—2.5, 5, 7.5, 10, 15, 20 mg; orally disintegrating tablets—5, 10, 15, 20 mg; powder for injection—10 mg; powder for suspension—210, 300, 405 mg/vial

Dosages
Adults
- *Schizophrenia:* Initially, 5–10 mg PO daily, increase to 10 mg PO daily within several days; may be increased by 5 mg/day at 1-wk intervals to achieve desired effect. Do not exceed 20 mg/day.
- *Bipolar mania:* 10–15 mg/day PO; adjust at 5-mg intervals as needed, not less than every 24 hr. Maximum dose, 20 mg/day. For maintenance, 5–20 mg/day PO. The initial dose is 10 mg of olanzapine when combined with lithium or valproate.
- *Agitation:* 10 mg IM; range 5–10 mg IM; dose may be repeated in 2 hr if needed; safety of giving more than 30 mg/24 hr not established.
- *Long-acting injection (Zyprexa Relprevv):* 150, 210, or 300 mg IM every 2 wk or 300 or 405 mg IM every 4 wk; establish dosage based on patient response.
- *Treatment-resistant depression:* 5 mg/day PO with fluoxetine 20 mg/day PO; adjust dosage as needed to range of 5–12.5 mg/day olanzapine with 20–50 mg/day PO fluoxetine.

Pediatric patients 13–17 yr
- *Schizophrenia, bipolar disorder:* Initially, 2.5–5 mg/day PO; titrate to target dose of 10 mg/day.

Pediatric patients younger than 13 yr
Safety and efficacy not established.

Geriatric patients
5 mg IM.

Debilitated patients
Start with initial dose of 5 mg; 2.5 mg IM. For long-acting injection (*Zyprexa Relprevv*), start with 150 mg IM every 4 wk.

Pharmacokinetics

Route	Onset	Peak	Duration
Oral	Varies	6 hr	Weeks
IM	Rapid	15–45 min	Weeks

Metabolism: Hepatic; $T_{1/2}$: 30 hr
Distribution: Crosses placenta; enters breast milk
Excretion: Feces, urine

Adverse effects in *italics* are most common; those in **bold** are life-threatening. ⚠ Do not crush.

Adverse effects

- **CNS:** *Somnolence, dizziness,* nervousness, headache, akathisia, personality disorders, tardive dyskinesia, **neuroleptic malignant syndrome**
- **CV:** *Orthostatic hypotension,* peripheral edema, tachycardia
- **GI:** *Constipation,* abdominal pain
- **Respiratory:** Cough, pharyngitis
- **Other:** *Fever,* weight gain, joint pain, development of diabetes mellitus, increased lipid levels

Interactions

✳ **Drug-drug** ● Increased risk of orthostatic hypotension with antihypertensives, alcohol, benzodiazepines; avoid use of alcohol and use caution with antihypertensives ● Increased risk of seizures with anticholinergics, CNS drugs ● May decrease effectiveness of levodopa, dopamine agonists ● Decreased effectiveness with rifampin, omeprazole, carbamazepine, smoking ● Increased risk of toxicity with fluvoxamine

■ Nursing considerations

 CLINICAL ALERT!
Name confusion has occurred between *Zyprexa* (olanzapine) and *Zyrtec* (cetirizine); use caution.

Assessment

- **History:** Allergy to olanzapine, myeloproliferative disorders, severe CNS depression, comatose states, history of seizure disorders, lactation, CV or cerebrovascular disease, dehydration, Alzheimer disease, prostate enlargement, narrow-angle glaucoma, history of paralytic ileus or breast cancer, elderly or debilitated, pregnancy
- **Physical:** T, weight; reflexes, orientation, IOP, ophthalmologic examination; P, BP, orthostatic BP, ECG; R, adventitious sounds; bowel sounds, normal output, liver evaluation; prostate palpation, normal urine output; CBC, urinalysis, LFTs, renal function tests

Interventions

- Do not dispense more than 1-wk supply at a time.
- Peel back foil on blister pack of disintegrating tablets; do not push through foil; use dry hands to remove tablet and place in mouth.

- Prepare solution for immediate-release IM injection using 2.1 mL sterile water for injection. Resulting solution contains 5 mg/mL. Solution should be clear yellow. Use within 1 hr of reconstitution. Discard any unused portion.
- Use special care to distinguish short-term IM form from long-term form (*Zyprexa Relprevv*).
- Dilute *Zyprexa Relprevv* only with the diluent provided. Ensure that patient is enrolled in *Zyprexa Relprevv* Patient Care Program. Monitor patient for at least 3 hr after injection.
- Monitor for the many possible drug interactions before beginning therapy.

⊗ **Black box warning** Risk of death is increased when drug is used to treat elderly patients with dementia-related psychosis; drug is not approved for this use.

⊗ **Black box warning** There is risk of severe sedation, including coma and delirium, after each injection of *Zyprexa Relprevv*. Patient must be observed for at least 3 hr after each injection, with ready access to emergency services. Because of risk, drug is available only through *Zyprexa Relprevv* Patient Care Program.

- Ensure that long-term injection (*Zyprexa Relprevv*) is given IM; long-term form is not to be used IV or subcutaneously.
- Encourage patient to void before taking the drug to help decrease anticholinergic effects of urinary retention.
- Monitor for elevations of temperature and differentiate between infection and neuroleptic malignant syndrome.
- Monitor adolescents carefully because of increased risk of sedation, weight gain, and lipid abnormalities.
- Monitor for orthostatic hypotension and provide appropriate safety measures as needed.
- Monitor patient regularly for signs and symptoms of diabetes mellitus; monitor lipid and triglyceride levels.
- Be aware that infants born to mothers who take antipsychotics during the last trimester of pregnancy may exhibit extrapyramidal effects.

Teaching points

- Take this drug exactly as prescribed; do not change dose without consulting your health care provider.

0

- Peel back foil on blister pack of disintegrating tablets; do not push through foil; use dry hands to remove tablet, place entire tablet in mouth.
- This drug cannot be taken during pregnancy. If you think you are pregnant or wish to become pregnant, contact your health care provider. Infants born to mothers taking antipsychotics in the third trimester may exhibit shaking.
- You may experience these side effects: Drowsiness, dizziness, sedation, seizures (avoid driving, operating machinery, or performing tasks that require concentration); dizziness, faintness on arising (change positions slowly, use caution); increased salivation (if bothersome, contact your health care provider); constipation (consult your health care provider for appropriate relief measures); fast heart rate (rest and take your time if this occurs); weight gain (monitor weight and discuss with health care provider).
- Report lethargy, weakness, fever, sore throat, malaise, mouth ulcers, and flulike symptoms.

▽ **olmesartan medoxomil**

(ol ma sar' tan)

Benicar

PREGNANCY CATEGORY C
(FIRST TRIMESTER)

PREGNANCY CATEGORY D
(SECOND AND THIRD TRIMESTERS)

Drug classes

Angiotensin II receptor antagonist (ARB)
Antihypertensive

Therapeutic actions

Selectively blocks the binding of angiotensin II to specific tissue receptors found in the vascular smooth muscle and adrenal gland; this action blocks the vasoconstricting effect of the renin-angiotensin system as well as the release of aldosterone leading to decreased BP; may prevent the vessel remodeling associated with the development of atherosclerosis.

Indications

- Treatment of hypertension, alone or in combination with other antihypertensives
- Unlabeled use: Prevention of migraines

Contraindications and cautions

- Contraindicated with hypersensitivity to any component of the drug, pregnancy (use during the second or third trimester can cause injury or death to the fetus), lactation.
- Use cautiously with renal impairment, hypovolemia, salt depletion.

Available forms

Tablets—5, 20, 40 mg

Dosages

Adults
20 mg/day PO as a once-daily dose; may titrate to 40 mg/day if needed after 2 wk.

Pediatric patients 6–16 yr
- *Weighing 35 kg or more:* 20 mg/day PO initially; then titrate to maximum dose of 40 mg/day PO.
- *Weighing 20 to less than 35 kg:* 10 mg/day PO initially; then titrate to maximum dose of 20 mg/day PO.

Pediatric patients younger than 6 yr
Safety and efficacy not established.

Pharmacokinetics

Route	Onset	Peak
Oral	Varies	1–2 hr

Metabolism: Hydrolyzed in GI tract; $T_{1/2}$: 13 hr
Distribution: Crosses placenta; enters breast milk
Excretion: Feces, urine

Adverse effects

- **CNS:** *Headache,* dizziness, syncope, muscle weakness
- **CV:** Hypotension, tachycardia
- **Dermatologic:** Rash, inflammation, urticaria, pruritus, alopecia, dry skin
- **GI:** *Diarrhea, abdominal pain, nausea,* constipation, dry mouth, dental pain
- **Hematologic:** Increased CK, hyperglycemia, hypertriglyceridemia
- **Respiratory:** *URI symptoms, bronchitis, cough,* sinusitis, rhinitis, pharyngitis
- **Other:** *Back pain, flulike symptoms,* fatigue, hematuria, arthritis, **angioedema**

Adverse effects in *italics* are most common; those in **bold** are life-threatening. ▭▭ Do not crush.

■ Nursing considerations

Assessment

- **History:** Hypersensitivity to any component of the drug, pregnancy, lactation, hepatic or renal impairment, hypovolemia, salt depletion, angioedema
- **Physical:** Skin lesions, turgor; body T; reflexes, affect; BP; R, respiratory auscultation; LFTs, renal function tests, serum electrolytes

Interventions

- Administer without regard to meals.
- If child is unable to swallow tablets, ask pharmacist to prepare a suspension form.
- ⊗ **Black box warning** Ensure that patient is not pregnant before beginning therapy. Suggest the use of barrier birth control while using olmesartan; fetal injury and deaths have been reported.
- Find an alternate method of feeding the infant if given to a breast-feeding mother. Depression of the renin-angiotensin system in infants is potentially very dangerous.
- ⊗ **Warning** Alert the surgeon and mark the patient's chart with notice that olmesartan is being taken. The blockage of the renin-angiotensin system following surgery can produce problems. Hypotension may be reversed with volume expansion.
- Monitor patient closely in any situation that may lead to a decrease in BP secondary to reduction in fluid volume—excessive perspiration, dehydration, vomiting, diarrhea; excessive hypotension can occur.

Teaching points

- Take drug without regard to meals. Do not stop taking this drug without consulting your health care provider.
- Use a barrier method of birth control while using this drug; if you become pregnant or desire to become pregnant, consult your health care provider.
- Take special precautions to maintain your fluid intake and provide safety precautions in any situation that might cause a loss of fluid volume—excessive perspiration, dehydration, vomiting, diarrhea; excessive hypotension can occur.
- You may experience these side effects: Dizziness (avoid driving a car or performing hazardous tasks); headache (medications may be available to help); nausea, vomiting,

diarrhea (proper nutrition is important, consult a dietitian to maintain nutrition); symptoms of upper respiratory tract, cough (do not self-medicate, consult your health care provider if this becomes uncomfortable).
- Report fever, chills, dizziness, pregnancy, swelling.

▽ olsalazine sodium

See Appendix R, *Less commonly used drugs.*

▽ omalizumab

See Appendix R, *Less commonly used drugs.*

▽ omega-3-acid ethyl esters

*(oh may gah-three-**ass'** id)*

Lovaza

PREGNANCY CATEGORY C

Drug classes

Lipid-lowering drug
Omega-3 fatty acid

Therapeutic actions

Inhibits liver enzyme systems leading to a decrease in the synthesis of triglycerides in the liver, lowering serum triglyceride levels.

Indications

- As an adjunct to diet to reduce very high (greater than 500 mg/dL) triglyceride levels in adult patients

Contraindications and cautions

- Contraindicated with known allergy to any component of the capsule.
- Use caution with known sensitivity to fish products, pregnancy, lactation.

Available forms

Capsules—1 g

Dosages

Adults

4 g/day PO taken as a single dose (4 capsules) or divided into two doses—2 capsules PO bid.

Pediatric patients
Safety and efficacy not established.

Pharmacokinetics

Route	Onset	Peak
Oral	Rapid	Unknown

Metabolism: $T_{1/2}$: Unknown
Distribution: May cross placenta; may pass into breast milk
Excretion: Tissues

Adverse effects
- **CV:** Angina
- **GI:** Taste perversion, dyspepsia, *eructation*
- **Other:** Pain, back pain, rash, flulike symptoms, *infection*

Interactions
✳ **Drug-drug** • Potential risk for increased bleeding if combined with anticoagulants; monitor patient closely and adjust anticoagulant dosage if needed

■ Nursing considerations

CLINICAL ALERT!
Name confusion has occurred between *Omacor* (the former trade name of omega-3-acid ethyl esters) and *Amicar* (amino caproic acid). Although the name of omega-3-acid esters has been changed to *Lovaza*, confusion may still occur; use caution.

Assessment
- **History:** Allergy to any component of the tablet, sensitivity to fish products, pregnancy, lactation
- **Physical:** T; abdominal examination; skin color, lesions; triglyceride levels

Interventions
- Reserve use for patients with very high triglyceride levels; obtain baseline level and periodically monitor levels.
- Assess patient for any potential underlying causes for elevated triglycerides.
- Ensure that patient continues diet and exercise program to control lipids.
- Suggest the use of contraceptive measures; it is not known if this drug could affect a fetus.
- Suggest another method of breast-feeding the infant if a woman is breast-feeding; it is not known if this drug enters breast milk.

- Encourage frequent small meals if GI effects are uncomfortable.

Teaching points
- Take this drug in one dose of four capsules, or you can take two doses of two capsules each. You can take this drug with meals.
- If you miss a dose of the daily medication, take it as soon as you remember and then return to your normal schedule. Do not make up doses. Do not take more than four capsules in one day.
- You should continue your dietary and exercise program to control your lipid levels.
- You may be asked to have periodic blood tests to evaluate the effects of this drug on your body.
- It is not known how this drug could affect a breast-feeding infant. If you are breast-feeding, another method of feeding the infant should be selected.
- It is not known how this drug could affect a fetus, if you are pregnant or decide to become pregnant while on this drug, consult your health care provider; use of contraceptive measures is advised while you are on this drug.
- You may experience these side effects: Taste changes, GI upset, frequent burping (this may stop after you have used the drug for awhile; frequent small meals may help); rash, fever, flulike symptoms (consult your health care provider; analgesics may be available to help).
- Report chest pain, severe headache, swelling, difficulty breathing.

▽ **omeprazole**
*(oh **me'** pray zol)*

Losec (CAN) ⓓⓝⓖ, Prilosec ⓓⓝⓖ,
Prilosec OTC ⓓⓝⓖ, Zegerid
(with sodium bicarbonate) ⓓⓝⓖ

PREGNANCY CATEGORY C

Drug classes
Antisecretory drug
Proton pump inhibitor

Therapeutic actions
Gastric acid-pump inhibitor: Suppresses gastric acid secretion by specific inhibition of the

hydrogen-potassium ATPase enzyme system at the secretory surface of the gastric parietal cells; blocks the final step of acid production.

Indications

- Short-term treatment of active duodenal ulcer
- Treatment of heartburn or symptoms of GERD
- Short-term treatment of active benign gastric ulcer
- GERD, severe erosive esophagitis, poorly responsive symptomatic GERD
- Long-term therapy: Treatment of pathologic hypersecretory conditions (Zollinger-Ellison syndrome, multiple adenomas, systemic mastocytosis)
- Eradication of *Helicobacter pylori* with amoxicillin or metronidazole and clarithromycin
- *Prilosec OTC:* Treatment of frequent heartburn (2 or more days per week)
- *Zegerid* oral suspension: Reduction of risk of upper GI bleeding in critically ill patients; includes sodium bicarbonate
- Unlabeled use: Posterior laryngitis

Contraindications and cautions

- Contraindicated with hypersensitivity to omeprazole or its components.
- Use cautiously because of possible increased risk of *Clostridium difficile* infection.
- Use cautiously with pregnancy, lactation.

Available forms

DR capsules ⒪Ⓝⓒ—10, 20, 40 mg; DR tablets ⒪ⓣⓒ—20 mg (OTC); powder for oral suspension—20, 40 mg/packet (*Zegerid*); capsules ⒪Ⓝⓒ—20, 40 mg (*Zegerid*)

Dosages
Adults

- *Active duodenal ulcer:* 20 mg PO daily for 2–8 wk. Should not be used for maintenance therapy.
- *Active gastric ulcer:* 40 mg PO daily for 4–8 wk.
- *Severe erosive esophagitis or poorly responsive GERD:* 20 mg PO daily for 4–8 wk. Do not use as maintenance therapy. An additional 4–8 wk course can be considered if needed.
- *Pathologic hypersecretory conditions:* Individualize dosage. Initial dose is 60 mg PO

daily. Doses up to 120 mg tid have been used. Administer daily amounts greater than 80 mg in divided doses.

- *Frequent heartburn (2 or more days per week):* 20 mg (*Prilosec OTC* tablet) PO once daily before eating in the morning for 14 days. May repeat the 14-day course every 4 mo.
- *Upper GI bleeding in critically ill patients:* 40 mg PO followed by 40 mg PO in 6–8 hr on day 1; then 40 mg/day for up to 14 days (*Zegerid*).

Pediatric patients 2 yr and older

- *GERD or other acid-related disorder:* 5 mg daily if patient weighs 5–10 kg; 10 mg if patient weighs 11 to less than 20 kg; 20 mg if 20 kg or more.

Pediatric patients younger than 2 yr
Safety and efficacy not established.

Pharmacokinetics

Route	Onset	Peak
Oral	Varies	0.5–3.5 hr

Metabolism: Hepatic; $T_{1/2}$: 0.5–1 hr
Distribution: Crosses placenta; may enter breast milk
Excretion: Bile, urine

Adverse effects

- **CNS:** *Headache, dizziness,* asthenia, vertigo, insomnia, apathy, anxiety, paresthesias, dream abnormalities
- **Dermatologic:** Rash, inflammation, urticaria, pruritus, alopecia, dry skin
- **GI:** *Diarrhea, abdominal pain, nausea, vomiting,* constipation, dry mouth, tongue atrophy
- **Respiratory:** *URI symptoms,* cough, epistaxis
- **Other:** Cancer in preclinical studies, back pain, fever, decreased bone density, bone fractures

Interactions

✳ **Drug-drug** ⊗ **Warning** Increased serum levels and potential increase in toxicity of benzodiazepines, phenytoin, warfarin; if these combinations are used, monitor patient closely ● Administration with clopidogrel can lead to therapeutic failure of clopidogrel; avoid this combination ● Decreased absorption with sucralfate; give these drugs at least 30 min apart

■ Nursing considerations
Assessment
- **History:** Hypersensitivity to omeprazole or any of its components, pregnancy, lactation
- **Physical:** Skin lesions; T; reflexes, affect; urinary output, abdominal examination; respiratory auscultation

Interventions
- Administer before meals. Caution patient to swallow capsules whole—not to open, chew, or crush them. If using oral suspension, empty packet into a small cup containing 2 tbsp of water. Stir and have patient drink immediately; fill cup with water and have patient drink this water. Do not use any other diluent.
- Be aware that patient may be at increased risk for hip, wrist, and spine fracture; weigh benefits and risks before use.
- ⊗ *Warning* Arrange for further evaluation of patient after 8 wk of therapy for GERD; not intended for maintenance therapy. Symptomatic improvement does not rule out gastric cancer, which did occur in preclinical studies.
- Administer antacids with, if needed.
- If patient cannot swallow *Prilosec* capsules, contents of capsule may be added to or sprinkled on 1 tablespoon applesauce. Mix capsule contents into applesauce and have patient swallow immediately without chewing pellets. Follow with a glass of water.
- *Zegerid* capsules should not be opened and contents should not be sprinkled on applesauce. Use suspension if swallowing is difficult.

Teaching points
- Take the drug before meals. Swallow the capsules whole; do not chew, open, or crush them. If using the oral suspension, empty packet into a small cup containing 2 tablespoons of water. Stir and drink immediately; fill cup with water and drink the water. Do not use any other liquid or food to dissolve the packet. This drug will need to be taken for up to 8 weeks (short-term therapy) or for a prolonged period (more than 5 years in some cases).
- If you take *Prilosec* capsules and cannot swallow them whole, capsule contents may be added to or sprinkled on 1 tablespoon of applesauce. Mix with applesauce, swallow immediately without chewing pellets, and follow with a glass of water. *Zegerid*

capsules should not be opened or added to food.
- Have regular medical follow-up visits.
- You may experience these side effects: Dizziness (avoid driving or performing hazardous tasks); headache (request medications); nausea, vomiting, diarrhea (maintain proper nutrition); symptoms of URI, cough (do not self-medicate; consult your health care provider if uncomfortable).
- Report severe headache, worsening of symptoms, fever, chills, severe diarrhea.

▽ ondansetron hydrochloride
*(on **dan'** sah tron)*

Zofran, Zofran ODT, Zuplenz

PREGNANCY CATEGORY B

Drug class
Antiemetic

Therapeutic actions
Blocks specific receptor sites (5-HT_3), which are associated with nausea and vomiting in the chemoreceptor trigger zone, centrally and at specific sites peripherally. It is not known whether its antiemetic actions are from actions at the central, peripheral, or combined sites.

Indications
- Parenteral and oral: Prevention of nausea and vomiting associated with emetogenic cancer chemotherapy in patients older than 6 mo
- Prevention of postoperative nausea and vomiting—to prevent further episodes or, when postoperative nausea and vomiting must be avoided (oral), prophylactically (parenteral) in patients older than 1 mo
- Prevention of nausea and vomiting associated with radiotherapy
- Unlabeled use: Treatment of nausea and vomiting associated with acetaminophen poisoning, prostacyclin therapy

Contraindications and cautions
- Contraindicated with allergy to ondansetron, congenital prolonged QT interval
- Use cautiously with pregnancy, lactation, hepatic impairment.

Available forms

Tablets—4, 8, 24 mg; orally disintegrating tablets—4, 8 mg; oral solution—4 mg/5 mL; oral soluble film—4, 8 mg; injection—2 mg/mL, 32 mg/50 mL

Dosages
Adults
Parenteral
- *Prevention of chemotherapy-induced nausea and vomiting:* Three 0.15 mg/kg doses IV: First dose is given over 15 min, beginning 30 min before chemotherapy; subsequent doses are given at 4 and 8 hr, or a single 32-mg dose is infused over 15 min beginning 30 min before the start of the chemotherapy.

Oral
- *Prevention of nausea and vomiting associated with cancer chemotherapy:* 8 mg PO 30 min prior to chemotherapy, then 8 mg 8 hr later; give 8 mg every 12 hr for 1–2 days after completion of chemotherapy. For highly emetogenic chemotherapy, give 24 mg PO 30 min before starting chemotherapy.
- *Prevention of nausea and vomiting associated with radiotherapy:* 8 mg PO tid. For total-body radiotherapy, administer 1–2 hr before radiation each day. For single high-dose radiotherapy to abdomen, give 1–2 hr before radiotherapy, then every 8 hr for 1–2 days after completion of therapy. For daily fractionated radiotherapy to abdomen, give 1–2 hr before therapy, then every 8 hr for each day therapy is given.

Parenteral or oral
- *Prevention of postoperative nausea and vomiting:* 4 mg undiluted IV, preferably over 2–5 min, or as a single IM dose immediately before induction of anesthesia or 16 mg PO 1 hr before anesthesia.

Pediatric patients
- *Prevention of chemotherapy-induced nausea and vomiting:*

Parenteral
6 mo–18 yr: Three doses of 0.15 mg/kg IV over 15 min given 30 min before the start of the chemotherapy, then 4 and 8 hr later.

Oral
12 yr and older: Same as adult.
4–11 yr: 4 mg PO 30 min prior to chemotherapy, 4 mg at 4 and 8 hr, then 4 mg PO tid for 1–2 days after completion of chemotherapy.

Younger than 4 yr: Safety and efficacy not established.
- *Prevention of postoperative nausea and vomiting:*
  1 mo–12 yr: 0.1 mg/kg IV if patient weighs less than 40 kg or a single dose of 4 mg IV if more than 40 kg, preferably given 2–5 min before or following induction of anesthesia. Infuse over at least 30 sec.

Patients with hepatic impairment
Maximum daily dose of 8 mg IV or PO.

Pharmacokinetics

Route	Onset	Peak
Oral	30–60 min	1.7–2.2 hr
IV	Immediate	Immediate

Metabolism: Hepatic; $T_{1/2}$: 3.5–6 hr
Distribution: Crosses placenta; may enter breast milk
Excretion: Urine

▼ IV FACTS

Preparation: Dilute in 50 mL of 5% dextrose injection or 0.9% sodium chloride injection; stable for 48 hr at room temperature after dilution.

Infusion: Infuse slowly over 15 min diluted or 2–5 min undiluted.

Compatibilities: May be diluted with 0.9% sodium chloride injection, 5% dextrose injection, 5% dextrose and 0.9% sodium chloride injection; 5% dextrose and 0.45% sodium chloride injection; 3% sodium chloride injection.

Incompatibilities: Do not mix with alkaline solutions.

Adverse effects
- **CNS:** *Headache, dizziness,* drowsiness, shivers, malaise, fatigue, weakness, *myalgia*
- **CV:** Chest pain, hypotension, **prolong QT interval,** arrhythmias
- **Dermatologic:** Pruritus
- **GI:** Abdominal pain, constipation, liver impairment, *diarrhea*
- **GU:** Urinary retention
- **Local:** Pain at injection site

Interactions
✻ **Drug-drug** • Increased risk of prolonged QT interval and potentially serious arrhythmias if combined with other drugs that prolong QT interval

✳ **Drug-food** • Increased extent of absorption if taken orally with food

■ Nursing considerations
Assessment
- **History:** Allergy to ondansetron, pregnancy, lactation, nausea and vomiting
- **Physical:** Skin color and texture; orientation, reflexes, bilateral grip strength, affect; P, BP; abdominal examination; urinary output; ECG

Interventions
- Ensure that the timing of drug doses corresponds to that of the chemotherapy or radiation.
- Use ECG monitoring in patients with electrolyte abnormalities, HF, or bradyarrhythmias and in patients taking drugs that prolong the QT interval; these patients are at increased risk for prolonged QT interval and serious arrhythmias.
- Administer oral drug for 1–2 days following completion of chemotherapy or radiation.
- For *Zofran ODT,* peel foil backing of one blister and remove tablet gently. Do not push tablet through the foil backing. Immediately place tablet on tongue, where it will dissolve in seconds, and have patient swallow it with saliva.
- For *Zuplenz,* with dry hands, fold pouch along dotted line to expose tear notch; while still folded, tear pouch along edge and remove film. Place film on top of the tongue; it will dissolve in 4–20 sec. Have patient swallow with or without liquid.

Teaching points
- Take oral drug for 1–2 days following chemotherapy or radiation therapy to maximize prevention of nausea and vomiting. Take the drug every 8 hours around-the-clock for best results.
- For *Zofran ODT,* peel foil backing of one blister and remove tablet gently. Do not push tablet through the foil backing. Immediately place tablet on tongue, where it will dissolve in seconds, and swallow with saliva.
- If you are using *Zuplenz*: With dry hands, fold pouch along dotted line to expose tear notch; while still folded, carefully tear pouch open along edge and remove the film. Place the film on top of your tongue; it will dissolve in 4–20 second. Swallow after it dissolves; you may swallow with liquid. Wash your hands when done.
- You may experience these side effects: Weakness, dizziness (change position slowly to avoid injury); dizziness, drowsiness (do not drive or perform tasks that require alertness).
- Report continued nausea and vomiting, pain at injection site, chest pain, palpitations.

DANGEROUS DRUG

▷ **opium preparations**
(oh' pee um)

Camphorated tincture: Paregoric

Deodorized tincture: Opium Tincture, Deodorized

PREGNANCY CATEGORY C

CONTROLLED SUBSTANCE C-III
(PAREGORIC)

CONTROLLED SUBSTANCE C-II
(OPIUM TINCTURE, DEODORIZED)

Drug classes
Antidiarrheal
Opioid agonist analgesic

Therapeutic actions
Activity is primarily due to morphine content; acts as agonist at specific opioid receptors in the CNS to produce analgesia, euphoria, sedation; the receptors mediating these effects are thought to be the same as those mediating the effects of endogenous opioids (enkephalins, endorphins); inhibits peristalsis and diarrhea by producing spasm of GI tract smooth muscle.

Indications
- Antidiarrheal
- Unlabeled uses: Neonatal abstinence syndrome, management of short-bowel syndrome

Contraindications and cautions
- Contraindicated with hypersensitivity to opioids, diarrhea caused by poisoning (before toxins are eliminated), pregnancy, labor or delivery (opioids given to mother can cause respiratory depression of neonate; premature infants are at special risk; may prolong

---

Adverse effects in *italics* are most common; those in **bold** are life-threatening. ▣▣▣ Do not crush.

labor), bronchial asthma, COPD, cor pulmonale, respiratory depression, anoxia, kyphoscoliosis, acute alcoholism, increased intracranial pressure, lactation.

- Use cautiously with acute abdominal conditions, CV disease, supraventricular tachycardias, myxedema, seizure disorders, delirium tremens, cerebral arteriosclerosis, ulcerative colitis, fever, Addison disease, prostatic hypertrophy, urethral stricture, recent GI or GU surgery, toxic psychosis, renal or hepatic impairment.

Available forms

Liquid—2 mg morphine equivalent/5 mL (*Paregoric*); 10 mg/mL (*Opium Tincture, Deodorized*)

Dosages

⊗ *Warning* Caution: ***Opium Tincture, Deodorized,*** contains 25 times more morphine than ***Paregoric.*** Do not confuse dosage; severe toxicity can occur.

Adults

Paregoric

5–10 mL PO daily–qid (5 mL is equivalent to 2 mg morphine).

Opium Tincture, Deodorized

0.6 mL qid. Maximum, 6 mL/day.

Pediatric patients

Contraindicated in premature infants.

Paregoric

0.25–0.5 mL/kg PO daily–qid.

Geriatric patients or impaired adults

⊗ *Warning* Use caution; respiratory depression may occur in the elderly, the very ill, those with respiratory problems. Reduced dosage may be necessary.

Pharmacokinetics

Route	Onset	Peak	Duration
Oral	Varies	0.5–1 hr	3–7 hr

Metabolism: Hepatic; $T_{1/2}$: 1.5–2 hr
Distribution: Crosses placenta; enters breast milk
Excretion: Urine

Adverse effects

- **CNS:** *Light-headedness, dizziness, sedation,* euphoria, dysphoria, delirium, insomnia, agitation, anxiety, fear, hallucinations, disorientation, drowsiness, lethargy, impaired mental and physical performance, coma, mood changes, weakness, headache, tremor, seizures, miosis, visual disturbances

- **CV:** Facial flushing, peripheral circulatory collapse, tachycardia, bradycardia, arrhythmia, palpitations, chest wall rigidity, hypertension, hypotension, orthostatic hypotension, syncope, circulatory depression, **shock, cardiac arrest**

- **Dermatologic:** Pruritus, urticaria, edema, hemorrhagic urticaria (rare)

- **GI:** *Nausea, vomiting, sweating,* dry mouth, anorexia, constipation, biliary tract spasm; increased colonic motility with chronic ulcerative colitis

- **GU:** Ureteral spasm, spasm of vesical sphincters, urinary retention or hesitancy, oliguria, antidiuretic effect, reduced libido or potency

- **Respiratory:** Suppression of cough reflex, respiratory depression, apnea, **respiratory arrest, laryngospasm, bronchospasm**

- **Other:** Physical tolerance and dependence, psychological dependence

Interactions

✷ **Drug-drug** ● Increased likelihood of respiratory depression, hypotension, profound sedation or coma with barbiturate general anesthetics

✷ **Drug-lab test** ● Elevated biliary tract pressure may cause increases in plasma amylase, lipase determinations 24 hr after administration

■ Nursing considerations

CLINICAL ALERT!
Name confusion has occurred between *Paregoric* (camphorated tincture of opium) and *Opium Tincture, Deodorized;* use caution.

Assessment

- **History:** Hypersensitivity to opioids, diarrhea caused by poisoning, bronchial asthma, COPD, cor pulmonale, respiratory depression, kyphoscoliosis, acute alcoholism, increased intracranial pressure, acute abdominal conditions, CV disease, supraventricular tachycardias, myxedema, seizure disorders, delirium tremens, cerebral arteriosclerosis, ulcerative colitis, fever, Addison disease, prostatic hypertrophy, urethral stricture, recent GI or GU surgery, toxic psychosis, renal or hepatic impairment, pregnancy, lactation

- **Physical:** T; skin color, texture, lesions; orientation, reflexes, bilateral grip strength, affect, pupil size; P, auscultation, BP, orthostatic BP, perfusion; R, adventitious sounds; bowel sounds, normal output; frequency and pattern of voiding, normal output; LFTs, renal and thyroid function tests

Interventions
- Give to lactating women 4–6 hr before the next feeding to minimize the amount in milk.
- Reassure patient that addiction is unlikely; most patients who receive opiates for medical reasons do not develop dependence syndromes.

Teaching points
- Take this drug exactly as prescribed.
- Do not take leftover medication for other disorders, and do not let anyone else take the prescription.
- If you are breast-feeding, take drug 4–6 hours before the next scheduled feeding.
- You may experience these side effects: Nausea, loss of appetite (take with food and lie quietly; eat frequent small meals); constipation (use a laxative); dizziness, sedation, drowsiness, impaired visual acuity (avoid driving, performing other tasks that require alertness, visual acuity).
- Report severe nausea, vomiting, constipation, shortness of breath, or difficulty breathing.

▽ **oprelvekin**

See Appendix R, *Less commonly used drugs.*

▽ **orlistat**
(ore' lah stat)

Alli, Xenical

PREGNANCY CATEGORY X

Drug classes
Lipase inhibitor
Weight loss drug

Therapeutic actions
Synthetic derivative of lipostatin, a naturally occurring lipase inhibitor or so-called fat blocker. Binds to gastric and pancreatic lipase to prevent the digestion of fats. When taken with fat-containing foods, the fat passes through the intestines unchanged and is not absorbed.

Indications
- Treatment of obesity as part of weight loss program that includes diet and exercise
- ■ NEW INDICATION: Reduction of risk of weight regain after prior weight loss

Contraindications and cautions
- Contraindicated with hypersensitivity to orlistat, pregnancy, lactation, chronic malabsorption syndrome, cholestasis, history of renal calculi.
- Use cautiously with impaired hepatic function, biliary obstruction, pancreatic disease.

Available forms
Capsules—60 (*Alli*), 120 mg (*Xenical*)

Dosages
Adults
120 mg tid PO with each main meal containing fat. For OTC use, 60 mg PO with each meal containing fat, not exceeding 3 capsules/day.
Pediatric patients 12 yr and older
120 mg PO tid with fat-containing meals; OTC not for use in children.
Pediatric patients younger than 12 yr
Safety and efficacy not established.

Pharmacokinetics
Not absorbed systemically

Adverse effects
- **Dermatologic:** *Rash, dry skin*
- **GI:** *Dry mouth,* nausea, flatulence, *loose stools,* oily stools, fecal incontinence or urgency, **severe liver injury,** cholelithiasis
- **Other:** Vitamin deficiency of fat-soluble vitamins (A, D, E, K), increased urinary oxalate level

Interactions
❋ **Drug-drug** • Decreased absorption of fat-soluble vitamins • Additive lipid-lowering effects with pravastatin; monitor patient response • Increased risk of bleeding related to decreased vitamin K; when taking with oral anticoagulants, monitor patient closely • Decreased cyclosporine level if combined; administer

cyclosporine 3 hr after orlistat; do not administer at the same time • Altered thyroid function if combined with levothyroxine; administer at least 4 hr apart

■ **Nursing considerations**
Assessment
• **History:** Hypersensitivity to orlistat, impaired hepatic or pancreatic function, pregnancy, biliary obstruction, lactation, LFTs, renal function tests
• **Physical:** Weight, T, skin rash, lesions; liver evaluation; LFTs

Interventions
• Rule out organic causes of obesity before beginning drug.
• Be aware that patient may be at increased risk for severe liver injury; monitor liver enzymes before and periodically during therapy.
• Ensure that patient is participating in a weight-loss diet and exercise program.
• Administer with meals.
• Arrange for administration of fat-soluble vitamins. Do not administer with orlistat; separate doses.
• Monitor patient for possible cholelithiasis and increasing urinary oxylate level, which could lead to renal failure.
• Provide sugarless candies and frequent mouth care if dry mouth is a problem.
• Ensure ready access to bathroom facilities if diarrhea occurs.
⊗ **Warning** Counsel patient about the use of barrier contraceptives while using this drug; pregnancy should be avoided because of the possible risk to the fetus.

Teaching points
• Take this drug with meals that contain fat. Do not take the drug if you do not eat a meal. This drug is not a substitute for a reduced-calorie diet.
• You may need to take a vitamin supplement while you are using this drug. Take the supplement at least 2 hours before or after taking orlistat.
• Do not take this drug during pregnancy. If you think that you are pregnant or you wish to become pregnant, consult your health care provider. This drug can cause serious fetal damage.
• You may experience these side effects: Dry mouth (suck sugarless candies and perform frequent mouth care), nausea, loose stools, flatulence (stay close to the bathroom; this may pass in time).
• Report rash, glossy tongue, vision changes, bruising, right upper quadrant pain, changes in stool or urine color, severe flank pain.

▷ **orphenadrine citrate**
(or fen' a dreen)

Banflex, Flexon, Norflex

PREGNANCY CATEGORY C

Drug class
Skeletal muscle relaxant (centrally acting)

Therapeutic actions
Precise mechanisms not known; acts in the CNS; does not directly relax tense skeletal muscles; does not directly affect the motor end-plate or motor nerves.

Indications
• Relief of discomfort associated with acute, painful musculoskeletal conditions; as an adjunct to rest, physical therapy, and other measures
• Unlabeled use: 100 mg at bedtime for the treatment of leg cramps

Contraindications and cautions
• Contraindicated with hypersensitivity to orphenadrine, glaucoma, pyloric or duodenal obstruction, stenosing peptic ulcers, achalasia, cardiospasm (megaesophagus), prostatic hypertrophy, bladder neck obstruction, myasthenia gravis, lactation.
• Use cautiously with cardiac decompensation, coronary insufficiency, cardiac arrhythmias, hepatic or renal impairment, pregnancy, allergy to sulfites with some products.

Available forms
SR tablets ⓐⓝⓒ—100 mg; injection—30 mg/mL; tablets—100 mg

Dosages
Adults
60 mg IV or IM. May repeat every 12 hr. Inject IV over 5 min. Alternatively, give 100 mg PO every morning and evening.

Pediatric patients
Safety and efficacy not established; not recommended.

Geriatric patients
Use caution and regulate dosage carefully; patients older than 60 yr frequently develop increased sensitivity to adverse CNS effects of anticholinergic drugs.

Pharmacokinetics

Route	Onset	Peak	Duration
IM, IV	Rapid	2 hr	4–6 hr
Oral	Rapid	2 hr	4–6 hr

Metabolism: Hepatic; $T_{1/2}$: 14 hr
Distribution: Crosses placenta; enters breast milk
Excretion: Feces, urine

▼ IV FACTS

Preparation: No further preparation is required.
Infusion: Administer slowly IV, each 60 mg over 5 min.

Adverse effects

- **CNS:** *Weakness, headache, dizziness, confusion* (especially in elderly), hallucinations, drowsiness, memory loss, psychosis, agitation, nervousness, delusions, delirium, paranoia, euphoria, depression, paresthesia, blurred vision, pupil dilation, increased intraocular tension
- **CV:** *Tachycardia,* palpitation, transient syncope, hypotension, orthostatic hypotension
- **Dermatologic:** Urticaria, other dermatoses
- **GI:** *Dry mouth, gastric irritation, vomiting, nausea, constipation,* dilation of the colon, paralytic ileus
- **GU:** *Urinary hesitancy and retention,* dysuria, difficulty achieving or maintaining an erection
- **Other:** *Flushing, decreased sweating,* elevated temperature, muscle weakness, cramping

Interactions

* **Drug-drug** • Additive anticholinergic effects with other anticholinergic drugs • Additive adverse CNS effects with phenothiazines • Possible masking of the development of persistent extrapyramidal symptoms, tardive dyskinesia in long-term therapy with phenothiazines, haloperidol

■ Nursing considerations
Assessment

- **History:** Hypersensitivity to orphenadrine, glaucoma, pyloric or duodenal obstruction, stenosing peptic ulcers, achalasia, cardiospasm, prostatic hypertrophy, bladder neck obstruction, myasthenia gravis, cardiac dysfunction, hepatic or renal impairment, lactation, pregnancy
- **Physical:** Weight; T; skin color, lesions; orientation, affect, reflexes, bilateral grip strength, vision examination with tonometry; P, BP, orthostatic BP, auscultation; bowel sounds, normal output, liver evaluation; prostate palpation, normal output, voiding pattern; urinalysis, CBC with differential, LFTs, renal function tests, ECG

Interventions

- Ensure that patient is supine during IV injection and for at least 15 min thereafter; assist patient from the supine position after treatment.
- Ensure that patients swallow SR tablets whole, and do not cut, crush, or chew them.
- ⊗ **Warning** Decrease or discontinue drug temporarily if dry mouth is so severe that swallowing or speaking becomes difficult.
- ⊗ **Warning** Give with caution, reduce dosage in hot weather; drug interferes with sweating and body's ability to thermoregulate in hot environments.
- Arrange for analgesics if headache occurs (adjunct for relief of muscle spasm).

Teaching points

- Swallow sustained-release tablets whole; do not cut, crush, or chew them.
- Do not consume alcohol while using this drug.
- You may experience these side effects: Drowsiness, dizziness, blurred vision (avoid driving or engaging in activities that require alertness and visual acuity); dry mouth (suck on sugarless candies or ice chips); nausea (eat frequent small meals); difficulty urinating (empty your bladder just before taking the medication); constipation (increase fluid and fiber intake and exercise regularly); headache (request medication).

Adverse effects in *italics* are most common; those in **bold** are life-threatening. ⊞ Do not crush.

- Report dry mouth, difficult urination, constipation, headache, or GI upset that persists; rash or itching; rapid heart rate or palpitations; mental confusion; eye pain; fever; sore throat; bruising.

▽ oseltamivir phosphate
*(oz el **tam**' ah ver)*

Tamiflu

PREGNANCY CATEGORY C

Drug classes
Antiviral
Neuraminidase inhibitor

Therapeutic actions
Selectively inhibits influenza virus neuraminidase; by blocking the actions of this enzyme, there is decreased viral release from infected cells, increased formation of viral aggregates, and decreased spread of the virus.

Indications
- Treatment of uncomplicated acute illness due to influenza virus (A or B) in adults and children who have been symptomatic for 2 days or less
- Prevention of naturally occurring influenza A and B in adults and children in close contact with the flu
- Unlabeled use: Treatment and prevention of H1N1 influenza A (swine flu)

Contraindications and cautions
- Contraindicated with allergy to any component of the drug.
- Use cautiously with pregnancy, lactation, asthma, COPD.

Available forms
Capsules—30, 45, 75 mg; powder for oral suspension—12 mg/mL

Dosages
Adults and patients 13 yr and older
- *Treatment:* 75 mg PO bid for 5 days, starting within 2 days of the onset of symptoms.
- *Prevention:* 75 mg/day PO for at least 10 days; begin treatment within 2 days of exposure.

Pediatric patients 1–12 yr
- *Treatment:* 30–75 mg PO bid for 5 days based on weight—use suspension.
- *Prevention:* If patient weighs 15 kg or less, 30 mg/day PO; if 15–23 kg, 45 mg/day PO; if 23–40 kg, 60 mg/day PO; if more than 40 kg, 75 mg/day PO. Continue for 10 days.

Pediatric patients 6–11 mo
- *Treatment:* 25 mg PO bid.
- *Prevention:* 25 mg/day PO for 10 days.

Pediatric patients 3–5 mo
- *Treatment:* 20 mg PO bid.
- *Prevention:* 20 mg/day PO for 10 days.

Pediatric patients younger than 3 mo
- *Treatment:* 12 mg PO bid.
- *Prevention:* Not recommended.

Patients with renal impairment
For creatinine clearance of 30 mL/min or less, use 75 mg/day PO for 5 days, 75 mg PO every other day for prophylaxis.

Pharmacokinetics

Route	Onset	Peak
Oral	Varies	2.5–6 hr

Metabolism: Hepatic; $T_{1/2}$: 6–10 hr
Distribution: Crosses placenta; may enter breast milk
Excretion: Urine

Adverse effects
- **CNS:** *Headache*, dizziness
- **GI:** *Nausea*, vomiting, *diarrhea, anorexia*
- **Respiratory:** Cough, *rhinitis*, bronchitis
- **Other:** Risk of self-injury and delirium, particularly in children

■ Nursing considerations
Assessment
- **History:** Allergy to any components of the drug, COPD, asthma, pregnancy, lactation
- **Physical:** T; orientation, reflexes; R, adventitious sounds; bowel sounds

Interventions
- Administer within 2 days of the onset of flu symptoms.
- Encourage patient to complete full 5-day course of therapy; advise patient that treatment does not decrease the risk of transmission of the flu to others.
- Start dosage for prevention within 2 days of exposure and continue for at least 10 days.

- Prepare solution by adding 23 mL of water to bottle containing powder; shake well for 15 sec. Shake solution well before each dose. The reconstituted oral suspension should be used within 10 days of preparation.
- Monitor children for self-injury, delirium.

Teaching points
- Take the full course of therapy as prescribed; be advised that this drug does not decrease the risk of transmitting the virus to others.
- Shake solution well before each use; store in refrigerator.
- You may experience these side effects: Nausea, vomiting, loss of appetite, diarrhea; headache, dizziness (use caution if driving an automobile or operating dangerous machinery).
- Report severe diarrhea, severe nausea, worsening of respiratory symptoms.

▽ oxacillin sodium
(ox a sill' in)

PREGNANCY CATEGORY B

Drug classes
Antibiotic
Penicillinase-resistant penicillin

Therapeutic actions
Bactericidal: Inhibits cell wall synthesis of sensitive organisms, causing cell death.

Indications
- Infections due to penicillinase-producing staphylococci; may be used to initiate treatment when a staphylococci infection is suspected
- Unlabeled use: Catheter-related bloodstream infections

Contraindications and cautions
- Contraindicated with allergies to penicillins, cephalosporins, or other allergens.
- Use cautiously with renal disorders, pregnancy, lactation (may cause diarrhea or candidiasis in infants).

Available forms
Powder for injection—500 mg; 1, 2 g

Dosages
Maximum recommended dosage is 6 g/day.

Adults and pediatric patients weighing 40 kg or more
250–500 mg every 4–6 hr IV. Up to 1 g every 4–6 hr in severe infections.
Pediatric patients weighing less than 40 kg
Neonates weighing less than 2 kg: 25–50 mg/kg every 12 hr IV.
Neonates weighing 2 kg or more: 25–50 mg/kg every 8 hr IV.
Children weighing less than 40 kg: 50–100 mg/kg/day IV in equally divided doses every 4–6 hr.

Pharmacokinetics

Route	Onset	Peak	Duration
IM	Rapid	30–60 min	4–6 hr
IV	Rapid	15 min	Length of infusion

Metabolism: Hepatic; $T_{1/2}$: 0.5–1 hr
Distribution: Crosses placenta; enters breast milk
Excretion: Bile, urine

▼ IV FACTS

Preparation: Dilute for direct IV administration to a maximum concentration of 1 g/10 mL using sodium chloride injection or sterile water for injection. For IV infusion: Reconstituted solution may be diluted with compatible IV solution: 0.9% sodium chloride injection, 5% dextrose in water or in normal saline, 10% D-fructose in water or in normal saline, lactated Ringer solution, lactated potassic saline injections, 10% invert sugar in water or in normal saline, 10% invert sugar plus 0.3% potassium chloride in water, Travert 10% Electrolyte 1, 2, or 3. 0.5–40 mg/mL solutions are stable for up to 12 hr at room temperature. Discard after that time.
Infusion: Give by direct administration slowly to avoid vein irritation, each 1 g over 10 min; infusion—up to 6 hr.
Incompatibilities: Do not mix in the same IV solution as other antibiotics.

Adverse effects
- **CNS:** Lethargy, hallucinations, **seizures**
- **GI:** *Glossitis, stomatitis, gastritis, sore mouth,* "furry" or black "hairy" tongue, *nausea, vomiting, diarrhea,* abdominal pain, bloody diarrhea, enterocolitis, pseudomembranous colitis, nonspecific hepatitis

Adverse effects in *italics* are most common; those in **bold** are life-threatening. ▭ Do not crush.

- **GU:** Nephritis—oliguria, proteinuria, hematuria, casts, azotemia, pyuria
- **Hematologic:** Anemia, thrombocytopenia, leukopenia, neutropenia, prolonged bleeding time (more common than with other penicillinase-resistant penicillins)
- **Hypersensitivity:** *Rash, fever, wheezing,* **anaphylaxis**
- **Local:** *Pain, phlebitis,* thrombosis at injection site
- **Other:** *Superinfections,* sodium overload leading to heart failure

Interactions

✳ **Drug-drug** • Decreased effectiveness with tetracyclines • Inactivation of aminoglycosides in parenteral solutions with oxacillin

✳ **Drug-lab test** • False-positive Coombs test with IV oxacillin

■ Nursing considerations

Assessment

- **History:** Allergies to penicillins, cephalosporins, or other allergens; renal disorders; pregnancy; lactation
- **Physical:** Culture infection; skin color, lesions; R, adventitious sounds; bowel sounds: CBC, LFTs, renal function tests, serum electrolytes, Hct, urinalysis

Interventions

⊗ *Warning* Patients taking this drug are at increased risk for infections by multiple drug-resistant organisms; weigh risks and benefits before use.

- Culture infection before treatment; reculture if response is not as expected.
- Continue therapy for at least 2 days after infection has disappeared, usually 7–10 days.
- Reconstitute for IM use to a dilution of 250 mg/1.5 mL using sterile water for injection or sodium chloride injection. Discard after 3 days at room temperature or after 7 days if refrigerated.
- Reconstituted oral solution is stable 3 days at room temperature, 14 days refrigerated.

⊗ *Warning* Keep epinephrine, IV fluids, vasopressors, bronchodilators, oxygen, and emergency equipment readily available in case of serious hypersensitivity reaction.

Teaching points

- You may experience these side effects: Upset stomach, nausea, diarrhea (eat frequent small meals), mouth sores (perform frequent mouth care), pain at the injection site.
- Report difficulty breathing, rashes, severe diarrhea, severe pain at injection site, mouth sores.
- Finish entire course of therapy as prescribed.

▽ oxaliplatin

See Appendix R, *Less commonly used drugs.*

▽ oxandrolone

(ox an' droh lone)

Oxandrin

PREGNANCY CATEGORY X

CONTROLLED SUBSTANCE C-III

Drug classes

Anabolic steroid
Hormone

Therapeutic actions

Testosterone analogue with androgenic and anabolic activity; promotes body tissue-building processes; reverses catabolic or tissue-depleting processes; increases Hgb and red cell mass.

Indications

- Relief of bone pain accompanying osteoporosis
- Adjunctive therapy to promote weight gain after weight loss following extensive surgery, chronic infections, trauma
- Offset protein catabolism associated with prolonged use of corticosteroids
- Orphan drug uses: Short stature associated with Turner syndrome, HIV wasting syndrome, and HIV-associated muscle weakness, Duchenne and Becker muscular dystrophies; constitutional delay of growth and puberty
- Unlabeled use: Alcoholic hepatitis

Contraindications and cautions

- Contraindicated with known sensitivity to anabolic steroids; prostate, breast cancer; BPH; pituitary insufficiency; MI (contraindicated because of effects on cholesterol); nephrosis; liver disease; hypercalcemia; pregnancy, lactation.

- Use cautiously with HF; cardiac, renal, or liver disease; epilepsy; migraines; diabetes.

Available forms
Tablets—2.5 mg, 10 mg

Dosages
Adults
2.5 mg PO bid–qid; up to 20 mg has been used to achieve the desired effect; 2–4 wk needed to evaluate response.
Pediatric patients
Give a total daily dose of 0.1 mg/kg or less or 0.045 mg/lb or less PO; may be repeated intermittently.

Pharmacokinetics

Route	Onset
Oral	Slow

Metabolism: Hepatic; $T_{1/2}$: 9 hr
Distribution: Crosses placenta; may enter breast milk
Excretion: Urine

Adverse effects
- **CNS:** *Excitation, insomnia,* chills, toxic confusion
- **Endocrine:** *Virilization: Prepubertal males*—phallic enlargement, hirsutism, increased skin pigmentation; *postpubertal males*—inhibition of testicular function, gynecomastia, testicular atrophy, priapism, baldness, epididymitis, change in libido; *females*—hirsutism, hoarseness, deepening of the voice, clitoral enlargement, menstrual irregularities, baldness; decreased glucose tolerance
- **GI:** Hepatotoxicity, peliosis, **hepatitis** with **liver failure or intra-abdominal hemorrhage; liver cell tumors,** sometimes malignant, *nausea, vomiting, diarrhea, abdominal fullness, loss of appetite, burning of tongue*
- **GU:** Possible increased risk of prostatic hypertrophy, carcinoma in geriatric patients
- **Hematologic:** *Blood lipid changes;* iron deficiency anemia, hypercalcemia, altered serum cholesterol levels; *retention of sodium, chloride, water;* potassium, phosphates and calcium
- **Other:** *Acne,* premature closure of the epiphyses, edema

Interactions
✴ **Drug-drug** • Potentiation of oral anticoagulants with anabolic steroids • Decreased need for insulin, oral hypoglycemia drugs with anabolic steroids. • Increased effects of warfarin; monitor PT/INR carefully
✴ **Drug-lab test** • Altered glucose tolerance tests • Decrease in thyroid function tests (may persist for 2–3 wk after stopping therapy) • Increased creatinine, creatinine clearance, which may last for 2 wk after therapy

■ **Nursing considerations**
Assessment
- **History:** Sensitivity to anabolic steroids; prostate or breast cancer; BPH; pituitary insufficiency; MI; nephrosis; liver disease; hypercalcemia; pregnancy; lactation; HF; renal, cardiac, or liver disease, epilepsy, diabetes, migraines
- **Physical:** Skin color, texture; hair distribution pattern; affect, orientation; abdominal examination, liver evaluation; serum electrolytes and cholesterol levels, glucose tolerance tests, thyroid function tests, long-bone X-ray (in children)

Interventions
- Administer with food if GI upset or nausea occurs.
⊗ *Warning* Monitor effect on children with long-bone x-rays every 3–6 mo; discontinue drug well before the bone age reaches the norm for the patient's chronologic age because effects may continue for 6 mo after therapy.
- Ensure that women of childbearing age are not pregnant and understand the need to use contraceptives to prevent pregnancy.
- Monitor patient for edema; arrange for diuretic therapy.
⊗ **Black box warning** Monitor liver function and serum electrolytes periodically, and consult with physician for corrective measures; risk of peliosis hepatitis, liver cell tumors.
⊗ **Black box warning** Measure cholesterol levels periodically in patients who are at high risk for CAD; lipid level may increase.
- Monitor diabetic patients closely because glucose tolerance may change. Adjustments may be needed in insulin, oral hypoglycemic dosage, and diet.

Teaching points

- Take drug with food if nausea or GI upset occurs.
- Diabetic patients need to monitor urine or blood sugar closely because glucose tolerance may change; report any abnormalities to your health care provider for corrective action.
- These drugs do not enhance athletic ability but do have serious effects. They should not be used for increasing muscle strength.
- Periodic blood tests will be needed to monitor drug effects on your body.
- This drug cannot be taken during pregnancy; serious adverse effects can occur. Using barrier contraceptives is advised.
- You may experience these side effects: Nausea, vomiting, diarrhea, burning of the tongue (eat frequent small meals); body hair growth, baldness, deepening of the voice, decrease in libido, impotence (most reversible); excitation, confusion, insomnia (avoid driving, performing tasks that require alertness); swelling of the ankles, fingers (request medication).
- Report ankle swelling, skin color changes, severe nausea, vomiting, hoarseness, body hair growth, deepening of the voice, acne, menstrual irregularities.

▽ oxaprozin
(oks a pro' zin)

oxaprozin
Apo-Oxaprozin (CAN), Daypro

oxaprozin potassium
Daypro ALTA

PREGNANCY CATEGORY C

Drug classes
Analgesic (nonopioid)
Antipyretic
NSAID

Therapeutic actions
Inhibits prostaglandin synthetase to cause antipyretic and anti-inflammatory effects; the exact mechanism of action is not known.

Indications
- Acute or long-term use in the management of signs and symptoms of osteoarthritis, rheumatoid arthritis, and juvenile rheumatoid arthritis

Contraindications and cautions
- Contraindicated with known hypersensitivity to NSAIDs, or components of drug, significant renal impairment, lactation, treatment of perioperative pain following CABG surgery.
- Use cautiously with impaired hearing, allergies, hepatic, CV, and GI conditions, pregnancy.

Available forms
Caplets, tablets—600 mg; tablets—678 mg (*Daypro ALTA* equivalent to 600 mg oxaprozin)

Dosages
Adjust to the lowest effective dose to minimize side effects. Maximum daily dose, 1,800 mg or 26 mg/kg, whichever is lower. Maximum dose for *Daypro ALTA* is 1,200 mg/day.

Adults
- *Osteoarthritis:* 1,200 mg PO once daily; use initial dose of 600 mg with low body weight or milder disease.
- *Rheumatoid arthritis:* 1,200 mg PO once daily.

Pediatric patients 6–16 yr
- *Juvenile rheumatoid arthritis (non-ALTA product only):* 600–1,200 mg/day PO based on body weight.

Patients with severe renal impairment
Initially, 600 mg/day PO. If, insufficient relief, cautiously increase dosage to 1,200 mg/day with close patient monitoring.

Pharmacokinetics

Route	Onset	Peak	Duration
Oral	Varies	3–5 hr	24–36 hr
Daypro ALTA	Unknown	2 hr	Unknown

Metabolism: Hepatic; $T_{1/2}$: 42–50 hr
Distribution: Crosses placenta; enters breast milk
Excretion: Feces, urine

Adverse effects
- **CNS:** Dizziness, somnolence, insomnia, fatigue, tiredness, dizziness, tinnitus, ophthalmic effects
- **Dermatologic:** Rash, pruritus, sweating, dry mucous membranes, stomatitis
- **GI:** *Nausea, dyspepsia,* GI pain, *diarrhea,* vomiting, *constipation,* flatulence

O

- **GU:** Dysuria, renal impairment
- **Hematologic:** Bleeding, platelet inhibition with higher doses
- **Other:** Peripheral edema, **anaphylactoid reactions** to **anaphylactic shock**

■ Nursing considerations
Assessment
- **History:** Renal impairment; impaired hearing; allergies; hepatic, CV, and GI conditions; lactation, pregnancy
- **Physical:** Skin color and lesions; orientation, reflexes, ophthalmologic and audiometric evaluation, peripheral sensation; P, edema; R, adventitious sounds; liver evaluation; CBC, clotting times, LFTs, renal function tests; serum electrolytes, stool guaiac

Interventions
⊗ **Black box warning** Be aware that patient may be at increased risk for CV events, GI bleeding; monitor accordingly.

⊗ **Black box warning** Drug is contraindicated for treatment of perioperative pain associated with CABG surgery.
- Administer drug with food or after meals if GI upset occurs.
- Arrange for periodic ophthalmologic examination during long-term therapy.

⊗ **Warning** If overdose occurs, institute emergency procedures—gastric lavage, induction of emesis, supportive therapy.

Teaching points
- Take drug with food or meals if GI upset occurs.
- Dizziness, drowsiness can occur (avoid driving or using dangerous machinery).
- Report sore throat, fever, rash, itching, weight gain, swelling in ankles or fingers, changes in vision, black tarry stools.

▽ **oxazepam**
(ox a' ze pam)

Apo-Oxazepam (CAN)

PREGNANCY CATEGORY D

CONTROLLED SUBSTANCE C-IV

Drug classes
Anxiolytic
Benzodiazepine

Therapeutic actions
Exact mechanisms not understood; acts mainly at subcortical levels of the CNS, leaving the cortex relatively unaffected; main sites of action may be the limbic system and reticular formation; benzodiazepines potentiate the effects of GABA, an inhibitory neurotransmitter; anxiolytic effects occur at doses well below those needed to cause sedation, ataxia.

Indications
- Management of anxiety disorders or for short-term relief of symptoms of anxiety; anxiety associated with depression also is responsive
- Management of anxiety, tension, agitation, and irritability in older patients
- Alcoholics with acute tremulousness, inebriation, or anxiety associated with alcohol withdrawal
- Unlabeled use: Irritable bowel syndrome

Contraindications and cautions
- Contraindicated with hypersensitivity to benzodiazepines, tartrazine (in the tablets); psychoses; acute narrow-angle glaucoma; shock; coma; acute alcoholic intoxication with depression of vital signs; pregnancy (risk of congenital malformations, neonatal withdrawal syndrome); labor and delivery ("floppy infant" syndrome); lactation (may cause infants to become lethargic and lose weight).
- Use cautiously with impaired liver or renal function, debilitation.

Available forms
Capsules—10, 15, 30 mg

Dosages
Increase dosage gradually to avoid adverse effects.
Adults
10–15 mg PO or up to 30 mg PO tid–qid, depending on severity of symptoms of anxiety. The higher dosage range is recommended in alcoholics.
Pediatric patients 6–12 yr
Dosage not established.
Geriatric patients or patients with debilitating disease
Initially, 10 mg PO tid. Gradually increase to 15 mg PO tid–qid if needed and tolerated. Do not exceed 60 mg/day.

Pharmacokinetics

Route	Onset	Peak
Oral	Slow	2–4 hr

Metabolism: Hepatic; $T_{1/2}$: 5–10 hr
Distribution: Crosses placenta; enters breast milk
Excretion: Urine

Adverse effects

- **CNS:** *Transient, mild drowsiness* (initially), *sedation, depression, lethargy, apathy, fatigue, light-headedness, disorientation,* restlessness, confusion, crying, delirium, headache, slurred speech, dysarthria, stupor, rigidity, tremor, dystonia, vertigo, euphoria, nervousness, difficulty in concentration, vivid dreams, transient amnesia, psychomotor retardation, extrapyramidal symptoms, mild paradoxic excitatory reactions during first 2 wk of treatment, visual and auditory disturbances, diplopia, nystagmus, depressed hearing
- **CV:** Bradycardia, tachycardia, **CV collapse,** hypertension and hypotension, palpitations, edema
- **Dermatologic:** Urticaria, pruritus, rash, dermatitis
- **GI:** *Constipation, diarrhea, dry mouth,* salivation, nausea, anorexia, vomiting, difficulty in swallowing, gastric disorders
- **GU:** *Incontinence, urinary retention,* changes in libido, menstrual irregularities
- **Hematologic:** Elevations of blood enzymes, hepatic impairment, blood dyscrasias: **Agranulocytosis,** leukopenia
- **Other:** *Nasal congestion, hiccups, fever, diaphoresis,* paresthesias, muscular disturbances, gynecomastia, drug dependence with withdrawal syndrome when drug is discontinued (more common with abrupt discontinuation of higher dosage used for longer than 4 mo)

Interactions

✻ **Drug-drug** • Increased CNS depression with alcohol or other CNS depressants • Decreased sedation when given to heavy smokers of cigarettes or if taken concurrently with theophyllines

■ Nursing considerations

Assessment

- **History:** Hypersensitivity to benzodiazepines, tartrazine; psychoses; acute narrow-angle glaucoma; shock; coma; acute alco-

holic intoxication; pregnancy; labor and delivery; lactation; impaired liver or renal function, debilitation
- **Physical:** Skin color, lesions; T; orientation, reflexes, affect, ophthalmologic examination; P, BP; R, adventitious sounds; liver evaluation, abdominal examination, bowel sounds, normal output; CBC, LFTs, renal function tests

Interventions

⊗ **Warning** Taper dosage gradually after long-term therapy, especially in patients with epilepsy.

Teaching points

- Take this drug exactly as prescribed; do not stop taking drug (during long-term therapy) without consulting health care provider.
- You may experience these side effects: Drowsiness, dizziness (may lessen; avoid driving or engaging in other dangerous activities); GI upset (take with food); depression, dreams, emotional upset, crying.
- Report severe dizziness, weakness, drowsiness that persists, palpitations, swelling of the extremities, visual changes, difficulty voiding, rash or skin lesion.

▷ **oxcarbazepine**

(oks car baz' e peen)

Apo–Oxcarbazepine (CAN), Trileptal

PREGNANCY CATEGORY C

Drug class

Antiepileptic

Therapeutic actions

Mechanism of action not understood; antiepileptic activity may be related to its ability to block voltage-sensitive sodium channels, increase potassium conductance, and affect high-voltage activated calcium channels, leading to enhanced membrane stability.

Indications

- As monotherapy or adjunct therapy in the treatment of partial seizures in adults and children 4 yr and older
- Adjunct therapy for children 2 yr and older with epilepsy

- Unlabeled uses: Alternative treatment of bipolar disorder, diabetic neuropathy, alcohol withdrawal

Contraindications and cautions
- Contraindicated with hypersensitivity to carbamazepine or oxcarbazepine; lactation.
- Use cautiously in the elderly and with hyponatremia, renal or hepatic impairment, pregnancy.

Available forms
Tablets—150, 300, 600 mg; suspension—60 mg/mL

Dosages
Adults
- *Adjunctive therapy:* 300 mg PO bid, may be increased to a total of 600 mg PO bid if clinically needed.
- *Conversion to monotherapy:* 300 mg PO bid started while reducing the dose of other antiepileptics; other drugs should be reduced over 3–6 wk while increasing oxcarbazepine over 2–4 wk to maximum of 2,400 mg/day (in divided doses).
- *Starting as monotherapy:* Start with 300 mg PO bid and increase by 300 mg/day every third day until the desired dose of 1,200 mg/day is reached. Some patients may benefit from doses as high as 2,400 mg/day but should be carefully monitored.

Pediatric patients 2–16 yr
- *Adjunctive therapy*
  4–16 yr: 8–10 mg/kg/day PO given in two equally divided doses not to exceed 600 mg/day. Achieve the target dose over 2 wk. Suggested target dosages follow:

Weight (kg)	Dosage (mg/day)
20–29	900
29.1–39	1,200
More than 39	1,800

  2–4 yr and more than 20 kg: 8–10 mg/kg/day PO not to exceed 600 mg/day.
  2–4 yr and less than 20 kg: 16–20 mg/kg/day PO not to exceed 600 mg/day.
- *Monotherapy for partial seizures in epileptic children 4–16 yr:* 8–10 mg/kg/day PO in two divided doses. If the patient is taking another antiepileptic, slowly withdraw that drug over 3–6 wk. Then, increase the oxcarbazepine in 10 mg/kg/day increments at

weekly intervals to the desired level. If the patient is not taking another antiepileptic, increase the dose by 5 mg/kg/day every third day to the recommended dosage. Recommended dosages by weight:

Weight (kg)	Dosage (mg/day)
20	600–900
25–30	900–1,200
35–40	900–1,500
45	1,200–1,500
50–55	1,200–1,800
60–65	1,200–2,100
70 or more	1,500–2,100

Geriatric patients or patients with renal impairment
Use caution, drug may cause confusion, agitation. For creatinine clearance less than 30 mL/min, initiate dosage at one-half the usual starting dose for the indication; increase slowly until desired clinical response is seen; monitor patient carefully.

Pharmacokinetics

Route	Onset	Peak
Oral	Slow	4–5 hr

Metabolism: Hepatic; $T_{1/2}$: 2 hr, then 9 hr
Distribution: Crosses placenta; enters breast milk
Excretion: Feces, urine

Adverse effects
- **CNS:** *Dizziness, drowsiness, unsteadiness,* disturbance of coordination, confusion, headache, fatigue, visual hallucinations, depression with agitation, behavioral changes in children, suicidal ideation
- **CV:** *Hypotension, hypertension, bradycardia, tachycardia,* atrial fibrillation
- **GI:** *Nausea, vomiting,* gastric distress, abdominal pain, diarrhea, increased liver enzymes
- **GU:** *Impaired fertility,* hematuria, dysuria, priapism, renal calculi
- **Metabolic and nutritional:** Respiratory acidosis, hyperkalemia, *hyponatremia,* thirst
- **Respiratory: Pulmonary edema,** pleural effusion, hypoventilation, *hypoxia,* dyspnea, **bronchospasm**
- **Other:** Fever, hypovolemia, sweating, rigors, acne, alopecia, anaphylactic reactions, angioedema, rash

Adverse effects in *italics* are most common; those in **bold** are life-threatening. ⬛ Do not crush.

Interactions

✷ **Drug-drug** • Possible decreased oxcarbazepine effectiveness if combined with phenytoin, carbamazepine, phenobarbital, valproic acid, verapamil; if these combinations are used, monitor patient closely • Decreased effectiveness of felodipine if combined with oxcarbazepine • Decreased effectiveness of hormonal contraceptives if combined with oxcarbazepine; suggest the use of barrier contraceptives if this combination is used • Increased serum levels and risk of toxicity of phenytoin, phenobarbital; if this combination is used, monitor patient closely for signs of toxicity and arrange to decrease drug dosage as needed • Possible increased sedation if combined with alcohol; avoid this combination

■ Nursing considerations

Assessment

- **History:** Hypersensitivity to carbamazepine or oxcarbazepine; hyponatremia; serious dermatologic reactions; renal or hepatic impairment; pregnancy, lactation
- **Physical:** T; skin color, lesions; orientation, affect, reflexes; P, BP, perfusion; ECG; R, adventitious sounds; bowel sounds, normal output; normal urinary output, voiding pattern; LFTs, renal function tests; serum sodium

Interventions

⊗ *Warning* Monitor serum sodium prior to and periodically during therapy with oxcarbazepine; serious hyponatremia can occur. Signs and symptoms of hyponatremia include nausea, malaise, headache, lethargy, confusion, and decreased sensation.

- Investigate if patient has a history of hypersensitivity to carbamazepine. Stop drug if signs or symptoms of hypersensitivity occur.
- Give drug with food or milk to prevent GI upset. Arrange for patient to have small, frequent meals if GI upset occurs.

⊗ *Warning* Arrange to reduce dosage or discontinue oxcarbazepine, or substitute other antiepileptic, gradually. Abrupt discontinuation of antiepileptic may precipitate status epilepticus.

- Monitor patient carefully when converting to monotherapy from combined therapy or when adding oxcarbazepine to an established regimen.

- Monitor patient for changes in behavior, depression, suicidality.
- Ensure ready access to bathroom facilities if GI effects occur.
- Establish safety precautions if CNS changes occur (use side rails, accompany patient when ambulating).
- Arrange for appropriate counseling for women of childbearing age who wish to become pregnant; using barrier contraceptives is recommended while using this drug.
- Offer support and encouragement for dealing with epilepsy and adverse drug effects; arrange for consultation with support groups for patients with epilepsy as needed.

Teaching points

- Take this drug exactly as prescribed.
- Do not discontinue this drug abruptly or change dosage, except on the advice of your health care provider.
- Avoid the use of alcohol, sleep-inducing, or over-the-counter drugs while you are using this drug; these could cause dangerous effects. If you think that you need one of these preparations, consult your health care provider.
- Use only barrier contraceptives; if you wish to become pregnant while you are taking this drug, you should consult your health care provider. Hormonal contraceptives may be ineffective.
- Blood tests to measure your blood sodium levels will be needed periodically while you are using this drug.
- Wear or carry a medical alert tag at all times so that any emergency medical personnel taking care of you will know that you have epilepsy and are taking antiepileptic medication.
- You may experience these side effects: Drowsiness, dizziness, blurred vision (avoid driving a car or performing other tasks requiring alertness or visual acuity if this occurs); GI upset (take the drug with food or milk and eat frequent small meals).
- Report bruising, unusual bleeding, abdominal pain, yellowing of the skin or eyes, pale-colored feces, darkened urine, impotence, severe central nervous system disturbances, edema, fever, chills, thirst, pregnancy, thoughts of suicide, rash or skin reaction.

▷ oxybutynin chloride
(ox i byoo' ti nin)

Anturol, Apo-Oxybutynin (CAN),
Ditropan XL ⚫, Gelnique,
Gen-Oxybutynin (CAN),
Oxytrol, PMS-Oxybutynin (CAN)

PREGNANCY CATEGORY B

Drug classes
Anticholinergic
Urinary antispasmodic

Therapeutic actions
Acts directly to relax smooth muscle and inhibits the effects of acetylcholine at muscarinic receptors; reported to be less potent an anticholinergic than atropine but more potent as antispasmodic and devoid of antinicotinic activity at skeletal neuromuscular junctions or autonomic ganglia.

Indications
- Relief of symptoms of bladder instability associated with voiding in patients with uninhibited neurogenic and reflex neurogenic bladder
- ER tablets: Treatment of signs and symptoms of overactive bladder (incontinence, urgency, frequency); treatment of pediatric patients 6 yr and older with symptoms of detrusor overactivity associated with a neurologic condition, such as spina bifida (*Ditropan XL*)

Contraindications and cautions
- Contraindicated with allergy to oxybutynin, pyloric or duodenal obstruction, obstructive intestinal lesions or ileus, intestinal atony, megacolon, colitis, obstructive uropathies, glaucoma, myasthenia gravis, CV instability in acute hemorrhage, urinary retention.
- Use cautiously with hepatic, renal impairment; pregnancy; lactation.

Available forms
Tablets—5 mg; syrup—5 mg/5 mL; ER tablets ⚫—5, 10, 15 mg; transdermal patch—3.9 mg/day; topical gel—100 mg/g, 3%

Dosages
Adults
5 mg PO bid or tid. Maximum dose is 5 mg qid. ER tablets—5 mg PO daily, up to a maximum of 30 mg/day; transdermal patch—1 patch applied to dry, intact skin on the abdomen, hip, or buttock every 3–4 days (twice weekly); topical gel—apply 1 sachet (1 g) to thigh, abdomen, or upper arm once every 24 hr.
Pediatric patients older than 5 yr
5 mg PO bid. Maximum dose is 5 mg tid.
Pediatric patients older than 6 yr
ER tablets: 5 mg PO daily. Dosage may be adjusted in 5-mg increments up to maximum of 20 mg/day.
Impaired geriatric patients
2.5 mg PO bid or tid.

Pharmacokinetics

Route	Onset	Peak	Duration
Oral	30–60 min	3–6 hr	6–10 hr
Transdermal	24–48 hr	Varies	96 hr

Metabolism: Hepatic; $T_{1/2}$: 2–3 hr (oral)
Distribution: Crosses placenta; may enter breast milk
Excretion: Urine

Adverse effects
- **CNS:** *Drowsiness, dizziness, blurred vision,* dilation of the pupil, cycloplegia, increased ocular tension, weakness, headache
- **CV:** Tachycardia, palpitations, hypertension
- **GI:** *Dry mouth, nausea,* vomiting, constipation, bloated feeling
- **GU:** *Urinary hesitancy,* retention, impotence
- **Hypersensitivity:** Allergic reactions including urticaria, dermal effect
- **Other:** *Decreased sweating,* heat prostration in high environmental temperatures secondary to loss of sweating

Interactions
✳ **Drug-drug** • Decreased effectiveness of phenothiazines with oxybutynin • Decreased effectiveness of haloperidol and development of tardive dyskinesia • Increased toxicity if combined with amantadine, nitrofurantoin • Increased cholinergic adverse effects if combined with anticholinergics

---

Adverse effects in *italics* are most common; those in **bold** are life-threatening. ⚫ Do not crush.

■ **Nursing considerations**

Assessment

- **History:** Allergy to oxybutynin, intestinal obstructions or lesions, intestinal atony, obstructive uropathies, glaucoma, myasthenia gravis, CV instability in acute hemorrhage, hepatic or renal impairment, pregnancy, lactation
- **Physical:** Skin color, lesions; T; orientation, affect, reflexes; ophthalmologic examination, ocular pressure measurement; P, rhythm, BP; bowel sounds, liver evaluation; LFTs, renal function tests, cystometry

Interventions

- Arrange for cystometry and other diagnostic tests before and during treatment.
- Arrange for ophthalmologic examination before therapy and periodically during therapy.
- Do not cut, crush, or allow patient to chew ER tablets.
- Apply gel to thigh, abdomen, or upper arm once daily; rotate sites.

Teaching points

- Take this drug as prescribed; do not cut, crush, or chew ER tablets.
- If using the transdermal patch, apply to dry, intact skin on the abdomen, hip, or buttock every 3–4 days (twice weekly). Remove the old system before applying a new one. Select a new site for application of each new system.
- If using the topical gel, apply 1 mL to thigh, abdomen, or upper arm once every 24 hours. Rotate application sites.
- Periodic bladder examinations will be needed during this treatment to evaluate therapeutic response.
- You may experience these side effects: Dry mouth (suck on sugarless candies and use frequent mouth care); GI upset; blurred vision; drowsiness (avoid driving or performing tasks that require alertness); decreased sweating (avoid high temperatures; serious complications can occur because you will be heat intolerant).
- Report blurred vision, fever, rash, nausea, vomiting.

DANGEROUS DRUG

▷ **oxycodone hydrochloride**
(ox i koe' done)

M-oxy, Oxecta ⓞⓝⓒ, OxyContin ⓞⓝⓒ, OxyFAST, OxyIR, Roxicodone, Roxicodone Intensol, Supeudol (CAN)

PREGNANCY CATEGORY B

CONTROLLED SUBSTANCE C-II

Drug class

Opioid agonist analgesic

Therapeutic actions

Acts as agonist at specific opioid receptors in the CNS to produce analgesia, euphoria, sedation; the receptors mediating these effects are thought to be the same as those mediating the effects of endogenous opioids (enkephalins, endorphins).

Indications

- Relief of moderate to moderately severe pain
- CR tablets: Management of moderate to severe pain when a continuous, around-the-clock analgesic is needed for an extended period of time

Contraindications and cautions

- Contraindicated with hypersensitivity to opioids; diarrhea caused by poisoning (before toxins are eliminated); pregnancy (readily crosses placenta; neonatal withdrawal); labor or delivery (opioids given to the mother can cause respiratory depression in neonate; premature infants are at special risk; may prolong labor); bronchial asthma, COPD, cor pulmonale, respiratory depression, anoxia; kyphoscoliosis; acute alcoholism, increased intracranial pressure, lactation.
- Use cautiously with acute abdominal conditions, CV disease, supraventricular tachycardias, myxedema, seizure disorders, delirium tremens, cerebral arteriosclerosis, ulcerative colitis, fever, Addison disease, prostatic hypertrophy, urethral stricture, recent GI or GU surgery, toxic psychosis, renal or hepatic impairment.

Available forms

Immediate-release capsules—5 mg; immediate-release tablets—5, 10, 15, 20, 30 mg; CR tablets ⓒⓡⓓ—10, 15, 20, 30, 40, 60, 80 mg; oral solution—5 mg/5 mL; solution concentrate—20 mg/mL; tablets in aversion technology ⓒⓡⓓ—5, 7.5 mg

Dosages

Individualize dosage.

Adults

- *Immediate-release tablets:* 5–15 mg PO every 4–6 hr; opioid-naïve patients, 10–30 mg PO every 4 hr. Use lowest dosage that achieves adequate pain relief. For chronic pain, administer on a regular schedule every 4–6 hr. Discontinue gradually.
- *Immediate-release capsules:* 5 mg PO every 6 hr.
- *Immediate-release tablets in aversion technology:* 5–15 mg PO every 4 hr as needed.
- *Oral solution:* 10–30 mg PO every 4 hr as needed. For chronic pain, give regularly every 4–6 hr at lowest dosage needed to relieve pain.
- *CR tablets:* Initially, 10 mg PO every 12 hr for patients taking nonopioid analgesics and requiring around-the-clock therapy for an extended period of time. Adjust dosage every 1–2 days as needed by increasing dose by 25% to 50%.
- *Breakthrough pain:* Immediate-release (*OxyIR*): 5 mg PO every 4 hr.

Pediatric patients

CR is not recommended for pediatric patients. Regular and immediate-release dosage should be individualized based on patient's age and size.

Geriatric patients or impaired adults

Use caution. Respiratory depression may occur in the elderly, the very ill, or those with respiratory problems.

Pharmacokinetics

Route	Onset	Peak	Duration
Oral	15–30 min	1 hr	4–6 hr

Metabolism: Hepatic; $T_{1/2}$: 2–3 hr
Distribution: Crosses placenta; enters breast milk
Excretion: Urine

Adverse effects

- **CNS:** *Light-headedness, dizziness, sedation,* euphoria, dysphoria, delirium, insomnia, agitation, anxiety, fear, hallucinations, disorientation, drowsiness, lethargy, impaired mental and physical performance, coma, mood changes, weakness, headache, tremor, seizures, miosis, visual disturbances
- **CV:** Facial flushing, peripheral circulatory collapse, tachycardia, bradycardia, arrhythmia, palpitations, chest wall rigidity, hypertension, hypotension, orthostatic hypotension, syncope, circulatory depression, **shock, cardiac arrest**
- **Dermatologic:** Pruritus, urticaria, edema, hemorrhagic urticaria (rare)
- **GI:** *Nausea, vomiting, sweating* (more common in ambulatory patients and those without severe pain), dry mouth, anorexia, constipation, biliary tract spasm; increased colonic motility in patients with chronic ulcerative colitis
- **GU:** Ureteral spasm, spasm of vesical sphincters, urinary retention or hesitancy, oliguria, antidiuretic effect, reduced libido or potency
- **Respiratory:** Suppression of cough reflex, respiratory depression, apnea, **respiratory arrest, laryngospasm, bronchospasm**
- **Other:** Physical tolerance and dependence, psychological dependence

Interactions

✴ **Drug-drug** • Increased likelihood of respiratory depression, hypotension, profound sedation or coma in patients receiving barbiturate general anesthetics, protease inhibitors, other opioids or CNS depressants

✴ **Drug-lab test** • Elevated biliary tract pressure may cause increases in plasma amylase, lipase; determinations for 24 hr after administration

■ Nursing considerations
Assessment

- **History:** Hypersensitivity to opioids, diarrhea caused by poisoning, pregnancy, labor or delivery, bronchial asthma, COPD, cor pulmonale, respiratory depression, kyphoscoliosis, acute alcoholism, increased intracranial pressure, acute abdominal conditions, CV disease, myxedema, seizure disorders, cerebral arteriosclerosis, ulcerative colitis, fever, Addison disease, prostatic hypertrophy, urethral stricture, recent GI or

GU surgery, toxic psychosis, renal or hepatic impairment, lactation

- **Physical:** T; skin color, texture, lesions; orientation, reflexes, bilateral grip strength; affect, pupil size; P, auscultation, BP, orthostatic BP, perfusion; R, adventitious sounds; bowel sounds, normal output; frequency and pattern of voiding, normal output; ECG; EEG; LFTs, renal and thyroid function tests

Interventions

- Administer to breast-feeding women 4–6 hr before the next feeding to minimize amount in milk.
- Do not crush, break, or allow patient to chew CR preparations or immediate-release tablets in aversion technology (*Oxecta*).
- Administer immediate-release preparations to cover breakthrough pain.
- Do not administer tablets in aversion therapy in nasogastric tubes or feeding tubes; tubes will clog (*Oxecta*).

⊗ **Black box warning** *OxyFAST* and *Roxicodone Intensol* are highly concentrated preparations. Use extreme care.

⊗ **Black box warning** Be aware that this drug has abuse potential, and monitor patients accordingly.

⊗ **Black box warning** Concomitant use with CYP3A4 inhibitors may result in increased drug effects and potentially fatal respiratory depression; avoid this combination.

⊗ **Warning** Keep opioid antagonist and facilities for assisted or controlled respiration readily available during parenteral administration.

- Reassure patient that addiction is unlikely; most patients who receive opiates for medical reasons do not develop dependence syndromes.

Teaching points

- Take drug exactly as prescribed. Do not crush, break, or chew controlled-release preparations or tablets in aversion technology (*Oxecta*).
- Do not take any leftover medication for other disorders, and do not let anyone else take the prescription.
- Use another method of feeding your baby if you and breast-feeding.
- You may experience these side effects: Nausea, loss of appetite (take with food; lie quietly; eat frequent small meals); constipation (use a laxative); dizziness, sedation, drowsiness, impaired visual acuity (avoid driving, performing other tasks that require alertness, visual acuity).
- Report severe nausea, vomiting, constipation, shortness of breath, or difficulty breathing.

▽ **oxymetazoline**
(ox i met az' oh leen)

Afrin No Drip 12-Hour, Afrin Severe Congestion with Menthol, Afrin 12-Hour Original, Afrin 12-Hour Original Pump Mist, Dristan 12 Hr Nasal, Duramist Plus, Genasal, Nasal Relief, Neo-Synephrine 12 Hour Extra Moisturizing, Nostrilla 12-Hour Nasal, Vicks Sinex 12-Hour Long Acting

PREGNANCY CATEGORY C

Drug class
Nasal decongestant

Therapeutic actions
Acts directly on alpha receptors to produce vasoconstriction of arterioles in nasal passages, which produces a decongestant response; no effect on beta receptors.

Indications
- Topical: Symptomatic relief of nasal and nasopharyngeal mucosal congestion due to colds, hay fever, or other respiratory allergies

Contraindications and cautions
- Contraindicated with allergy to oxymetazoline, angle-closure glaucoma, anesthesia with cyclopropane or halothane, thyrotoxicosis, diabetes, hypertension, CV disorders, women in labor whose BP exceeds 130/80.
- Use cautiously with angina, arrhythmias, prostatic hypertrophy, unstable vasomotor syndrome, lactation.

Available forms
Nasal spray or solution—0.05%

Dosages
Adults and pediatric patients older than 6 yr
Two to three sprays of 0.05% solution in each nostril bid morning and evening or every 10–12 hr for up to 3 days. Do not exceed two doses in 24 hr.

Pharmacokinetics

Route	Onset	Duration
Nasal	5–10 min	6–10 hr

Metabolism: Hepatic; $T_{1/2}$: Unknown
Distribution: Crosses placenta; may enter breast milk
Excretion: Urine

Adverse effects

Systemic effects are less likely with topical administration than with systemic administration, but because systemic absorption can take place, the systemic effects should be considered:

- **CNS:** *Fear, anxiety, tenseness, restlessness, headache, light-headedness, dizziness,* drowsiness, tremor, insomnia, hallucinations, psychological disturbances, seizures, CNS depression, weakness, blurred vision, ocular irritation, tearing, photophobia, symptoms of paranoid schizophrenia
- **CV:** Arrhythmias, hypertension resulting in intracranial hemorrhage, **CV collapse** with hypotension, palpitations, tachycardia, precordial pain in patients with ischemic heart disease
- **GI:** *Nausea,* vomiting, anorexia
- **GU:** Constriction of renal blood vessels, *dysuria, vesical sphincter spasm* resulting in difficult and painful urination, urinary retention with prostatism
- **Local:** *Rebound congestion* with topical nasal application
- **Other:** *Pallor,* respiratory difficulty, orofacial dystonia, sweating

Interactions

✳ Drug-drug • Severe hypertension with MAOIs, TCAs • Additive effects and increased risk of toxicity if taken with urinary alkalinizers • Decreased vasopressor response with reserpine, methyldopa, urinary acidifiers

■ Nursing considerations
Assessment

- **History:** Allergy to oxymetazoline; angle-closure glaucoma; anesthesia with cyclopropane or halothane; thyrotoxicosis, diabetes, hypertension, CV disorders; prostatic hypertrophy, unstable vasomotor syndrome; lactation, pregnancy
- **Physical:** Skin color, T; orientation, reflexes, peripheral sensation, vision; P, BP, auscultation, peripheral perfusion; R, adventitious sounds; urinary output pattern, bladder percussion, prostate palpation; nasal mucous membrane evaluation

Interventions

⊗ *Warning* Monitor CV effects carefully; patients with hypertension may experience changes in BP because of the additional vasoconstriction. If a nasal decongestant is needed, pseudoephedrine is the drug of choice.

Teaching points

- Do not exceed recommended dose. Use proper administration technique for topical nasal application. Avoid prolonged use because underlying medical problems can be disguised. Do not use longer than 3 days.
- Rebound congestion may occur when this drug is stopped; drink plenty of fluids, use a humidifier, and avoid smoke-filled areas to help decrease problems.
- You may experience these side effects: Dizziness, tremor, weakness, restlessness, light-headedness (avoid driving or operating dangerous equipment); urinary retention (void before taking drug).
- Report nervousness, palpitations, sleeplessness, sweating.

▽ **oxymetholone**
(ox i meth' oh lone)

Anadrol-50

PREGNANCY CATEGORY X

CONTROLLED SUBSTANCE C-III

Drug classes

Anabolic steroid
Hormone

Therapeutic actions

Testosterone analogue with androgenic and anabolic activity; promotes body tissue-building processes and reverses catabolic or tissue-depleting processes; increases Hgb and red cell mass.

Indications

- Anemias caused by deficient red cell production
- Acquired or congenital aplastic anemia

- Myelofibrosis and hypoplastic anemias due to myelotoxic drugs
- Unlabeled use: HIV-associated wasting

Contraindications and cautions

- Contraindicated with known sensitivity to oxymetholone or anabolic steroids, prostate or breast cancer, BPH, pituitary insufficiency, MI, nephrosis, liver disease, hypercalcemia, pregnancy, lactation.
- Use cautiously with diabetes; seizure disorders; migraines; hepatic, cardiac, or renal disease; HF.

Available forms

Tablets—50 mg

Dosages

Adults and pediatric patients

1–5 mg/kg/day PO. Usual effective dose is 1–2 mg/kg/day. Give for a minimum trial of 3–6 mo. Following remission, patients may be maintained without the drug or on a lower daily dose. Continuous therapy is usually needed in cases of congenital aplastic anemia.

Pediatric patients

Use with extreme caution due to risk of serious disruption of growth and development; weigh benefits and risks.

Pharmacokinetics

Route	Onset
Oral	Rapid

Metabolism: Hepatic; $T_{1/2}$: 9 hr
Distribution: Crosses placenta; enters breast milk
Excretion: Urine

Adverse effects

- **CNS:** *Excitation, insomnia,* chills, toxic confusion
- **Endocrine:** *Virilization: Prepubertal males*—phallic enlargement, hirsutism, increased skin pigmentation; *postpubertal males*—inhibition of testicular function, gynecomastia, testicular atrophy, priapism, baldness, epididymitis, change in libido; *females*—hirsutism, hoarseness, deepening of the voice, clitoral enlargement, menstrual irregularities, baldness; decreased glucose tolerance

- **GI:** Hepatotoxicity, peliosis, **hepatitis with liver failure or intra-abdominal hemorrhage; liver cell tumors,** sometimes malignant and fatal, *nausea, vomiting, diarrhea, abdominal fullness, loss of appetite, burning of tongue*
- **GU:** Possible increased risk of prostatic hypertrophy, carcinoma in geriatric patients
- **Hematologic:** *Blood lipid changes:* Decreased HDL and sometimes increased LDL; iron deficiency anemia; hypercalcemia; altered serum cholesterol levels; *retention of sodium, chloride, water,* potassium, phosphates, and calcium
- **Other:** *Acne,* premature closure of the epiphyses, edema

Interactions

✳ **Drug-drug** ● Potentiation of oral anticoagulants with anabolic steroids ● Decreased need for insulin, oral hypoglycemia drugs
✳ **Drug-lab test** ● Altered glucose tolerance tests ● Decrease in thyroid function tests, which may persist for 2–3 wk after therapy ● Increased creatinine, decreased creatinine clearance, which may last for 2 wk after therapy

■ Nursing considerations

Assessment

- **History:** Known sensitivity to oxymetholone or anabolic steroids; prostate or breast cancer; BPH; pituitary insufficiency; MI; nephrosis; liver disease; hypercalcemia; pregnancy; lactation, HF; cardiac, renal, or hepatic disease; migraines; seizures; diabetes
- **Physical:** Skin color, texture; hair distribution pattern; affect, orientation; abdominal examination, liver evaluation; serum electrolytes and cholesterol levels, glucose tolerance tests, thyroid function tests, long-bone X-ray (in children)

Interventions

- Administer with food if GI upset or nausea occurs.
⊗ *Warning* Monitor effect on children with long-bone x-rays every 3–6 mo; discontinue drug well before the bone age reaches the norm for the patient's chronologic age because effects may continue for 6 mo after therapy.
- Monitor for edema; arrange for diuretic therapy as needed.

⊗ **Black box warning** Monitor liver function and serum electrolytes during therapy, and consult with physician for corrective measures; peliosis hepatis, liver cell tumors can occur.

⊗ **Black box warning** Measure cholesterol levels in patients who are at high risk for CAD; lipid levels may increase.

- Caution patients that this drug cannot be used during pregnancy; advise patient to use barrier contraceptives.
- Monitor patients with diabetes closely because glucose tolerance may change. Adjust insulin, oral hypoglycemic dosage, and diet.

Teaching points

- Take with food if nausea or GI upset occurs.
- Patients with diabetes need to monitor urine sugar closely because glucose tolerance may change; report any abnormalities to your health care provider so corrective action can be taken.
- This drug cannot be taken during pregnancy; use barrier contraceptives while using this drug.
- These drugs do not enhance athletic ability but do have serious effects and should not be used for increasing muscle strength.
- You may experience these side effects: Nausea, vomiting, diarrhea, burning of the tongue (eat frequent small meals); body hair growth, baldness, deepening of the voice, decrease in libido, impotence (most reversible); excitation, confusion, insomnia (avoid driving, performing tasks that require alertness); swelling of the ankles, fingers (request medication).
- Report ankle swelling, skin color changes, severe nausea, vomiting, hoarseness, body hair growth, deepening of the voice, acne, menstrual irregularities in women.

DANGEROUS DRUG

▷ **oxymorphone hydrochloride**

(ox i mor' fone)

Opana, Opana ER ⊞

PREGNANCY CATEGORY C

CONTROLLED SUBSTANCE C-II

Drug class
Opioid agonist analgesic

Therapeutic actions
Acts as agonist at specific opioid receptors in the CNS to produce analgesia, euphoria, sedation; the receptors mediating these effects are thought to be the same as those mediating the effects of endogenous opioids (enkephalins, endorphins).

Indications
- Relief of moderate to moderately severe acute pain (immediate-release form)
- Parenterally (injection only) for preoperative medication, support of anesthesia, obstetric analgesia
- Relief of moderate to severe pain in patients who need around-the-clock opioid treatment for extended time (ER form)
- Relief of anxiety in patients with pulmonary edema associated with left ventricular dysfunction (parenteral)
- Relief of moderate to severe pain

Contraindications and cautions
- Contraindicated with hypersensitivity to opioids, diarrhea caused by poisoning (before toxins are eliminated), pregnancy (readily crosses placenta; neonatal withdrawal), labor or delivery (opioids given to the mother can cause respiratory depression of neonate; premature infants are at special risk; may prolong labor), bronchial asthma, COPD, cor pulmonale, respiratory depression, anoxia, kyphoscoliosis, acute alcoholism, increased intracranial pressure, lactation.
- Use cautiously with acute abdominal conditions, CV disease, supraventricular tachycardias, myxedema, seizure disorders, delirium tremens, cerebral arteriosclerosis, ulcerative colitis, fever, Addison disease, prostatic hypertrophy, urethral stricture, recent GI or GU surgery, toxic psychosis, renal or hepatic impairment.

Available forms
Injection—1 mg/mL; tablets—5, 10 mg; ER tablets ⊞—5, 10, 20, 30, 40 mg

Dosages
Adults
Oral
For immediate-release form, 10–20 mg PO every 4–6 hr. For ER tablets, 5 mg PO every 12 hr; may be increased in 5- to 10-mg increments every 3–7 days to cover pain.

IV
Initially, 0.5 mg IV.
Subcutaneous or IM
Initially, 1–1.5 IM or subcutaneously mg every 4–6 hr as needed. For analgesia during labor, 0.5–1 mg IM.
Pediatric patients
Safety and efficacy not established for children younger than 18 yr.
Geriatric patients or impaired adults
Use caution; respiratory depression may occur in the elderly, the very ill, and those with respiratory problems. Start at low end of dosage range and titrate slowly.
Patients with renal impairment
For creatinine clearance of less than 50 mL/min, use ER tablets at lowest possible dose.

Pharmacokinetics

Route	Onset	Peak	Duration
Oral (ER)	15–30 min	60 min	8–10 hr
Oral (immedi-ate-release)	5–10 min	1 hr	3–6 hr
IV	5–10 min	15–60 min	3–6 hr
IM, Subcut.	10–15 min	30–60 min	3–6 hr

Metabolism: Hepatic; $T_{1/2}$: 7–9 hr
Distribution: Crosses placenta; enters breast milk
Excretion: Urine

▼ IV FACTS

Preparation: No further preparation needed.
Infusion: Inject slowly over 5 min directly into vein or into tubing of running IV.

Adverse effects

- **CNS:** *Light-headedness, dizziness, sedation,* euphoria, dysphoria, delirium, insomnia, agitation, anxiety, fear, hallucinations, disorientation, drowsiness, lethargy, impaired mental and physical performance, coma, mood changes, weakness, headache, tremor, seizures, miosis, visual disturbances
- **CV:** Facial flushing, peripheral circulatory collapse, tachycardia, bradycardia, arrhythmia, palpitations, chest wall rigidity, hypertension, hypotension, orthostatic hypotension, syncope, circulatory depression, **shock, cardiac arrest**
- **Dermatologic:** Pruritus, urticaria, edema, hemorrhagic urticaria (rare)

- **GI:** *Nausea, vomiting, sweating* (more common in ambulatory patients and those without severe pain), dry mouth, anorexia, constipation, biliary tract spasm; increased colonic motility in patients with chronic ulcerative colitis
- **GU:** Ureteral spasm, spasm of vesical sphincters, urinary retention or hesitancy, oliguria, antidiuretic effect, reduced libido or potency
- **Local:** Pain at injection site, tissue irritation and induration (subcutaneous injection)
- **Respiratory:** Suppression of cough reflex, respiratory depression, apnea, **respiratory arrest, laryngospasm, bronchospasm**
- **Other:** Physical tolerance and dependence, psychological dependence

Interactions

✳ **Drug-drug** • Increased likelihood of respiratory depression, hypotension, profound sedation or coma in patients receiving barbiturate general anesthetics or other CNS depressants • Risk of severe increase in serum drug level and potentially fatal overdose if combined with alcohol; avoid this combination • Risk of withdrawal or reduced analgesic effects if given with agonist/antagonist opioids • Risk of depression, apnea, seizures if used with cimetidine • Risk of severe constipation, urinary retention with anticholinergics

✳ **Drug-lab test** • Elevated biliary tract pressure may cause increases in plasma amylase, lipase; determinations for 24 hr after administration of opioids

■ Nursing considerations
Assessment

- **History:** Hypersensitivity to opioids, diarrhea caused by poisoning, pregnancy, labor or delivery, bronchial asthma, COPD, cor pulmonale, respiratory depression, kyphoscoliosis, acute alcoholism, increased intracranial pressure, acute abdominal conditions, CV disease, myxedema, seizure disorders, delirium tremens, cerebral arteriosclerosis, ulcerative colitis, fever, Addison disease, prostatic hypertrophy, urethral stricture, recent GI or GU surgery, toxic psychosis, renal or hepatic impairment
- **Physical:** T; skin color, texture, lesions; orientation, reflexes, bilateral grip strength, affect, pupil size; P, auscultation, BP, orthostatic BP, perfusion; R, adventitious

sounds; bowel sounds, normal output; frequency and pattern of voiding, normal output; ECG; EEG; LFTs, renal and thyroid function tests

Interventions

⊗ **Black box warning** Make sure that patient swallows ER tablets whole. Cutting, crushing, or chewing them could cause rapid release and fatal overdose.

⊗ **Black box warning** Note that ER form has abuse potential; monitor patient accordingly. Drug is indicated only for around-the-clock use over an extended time. Drug is not to be given PRN.

⊗ **Black box warning** Patient must not consume alcohol in any form while taking oxycodone to avoid risk of serious increase in serum drug level and potentially fatal overdose.

⊗ *Warning* Keep opioid antagonist and facilities for assisted or controlled respiration readily available during parenteral administration.

⊗ *Warning* Use caution when injecting subcutaneously into chilled areas of the body or in patients with hypotension or in shock; impaired perfusion may delay absorption; with repeated doses, an excessive amount may be absorbed when circulation is restored.

• Reassure patient that addiction is unlikely; most patients who receive opiates for medical reasons do not develop dependence syndromes.

• Give to breast-feeding women 4–6 hr before the next feeding to minimize amount in milk; use is generally not advised in breast-feeding women because of risk of respiratory depression in the infant.

• Administer drug at least 1 hr before or 2 hr after a meal.

Teaching points

• Take this drug exactly as prescribed. If taking ER tablets, swallow them whole and take with enough water to ensure complete swallowing; do not cut, crush, or chew them. Take at least 1 hour before or 2 hours after eating.

• Do not consume alcohol or take medications that contain alcohol while taking oxycodone; doing so increases the risk of serious or fatal reactions.

• Do not take leftover medication for other disorders, and do not let anyone else take the prescription.

• Do not stop taking this drug suddenly; it must be tapered.

• You may experience these side effects: Nausea, loss of appetite (take drug with food and lie quietly; eat frequent small meals); constipation (use a laxative); dizziness, sedation, drowsiness, impaired visual acuity (avoid driving, performing other tasks that require alertness, visual acuity).

• Report severe nausea, vomiting, constipation, shortness of breath or difficulty breathing.

DANGEROUS DRUG

▷ **oxytocin**

(*ox i toe' sin*)

Pitocin

PREGNANCY CATEGORY X

Drug classes

Hormone
Oxytocic

Therapeutic actions

Synthetic form of an endogenous hormone produced in the hypothalamus and stored in the posterior pituitary; stimulates the uterus, especially the gravid uterus just before parturition, and causes myoepithelium of the lacteal glands to contract, which results in milk ejection in lactating women.

Indications

• Antepartum: To initiate or improve uterine contractions to achieve early vaginal delivery; stimulation or reinforcement of labor in select cases of uterine inertia; management of inevitable or incomplete abortion; second trimester abortion

• Postpartum: To produce uterine contractions during the third stage of labor and to control postpartum bleeding or hemorrhage

• Lactation deficiency

• Unlabeled uses: To evaluate fetal distress (oxytocin challenge test), treatment of breast engorgement

Contraindications and cautions

• Contraindicated with significant cephalopelvic disproportion, unfavorable fetal positions or presentations, obstetric emergencies that favor surgical intervention, prolonged use in severe toxemia, uterine

---

Adverse effects in *italics* are most common; those in **bold** are life-threatening. ⊞ Do not crush.

inertia, hypertonic uterine patterns, induction or augmentation of labor when vaginal delivery is contraindicated, previous cesarean section, pregnancy.
• Use cautiously with renal impairment.

Available forms
Injection—10 units/mL

Dosages
Adjust dosage based on uterine response.
Adults
• *Induction or stimulation of labor:* Initial dose of no more than 0.5–2 milliunits/min (0.0005–0.002 units/min) by IV infusion through an infusion pump. Increase the dose in increments of no more than 1–2 milliunits/min at 30- to 60-min intervals until a contraction pattern similar to normal labor is established. Rates exceeding 9–10 milliunits/min are rarely required. Discontinue in event of uterine hyperactivity, fetal distress.
• *Control of postpartum uterine bleeding:*
IV
Add 10–40 units to 1,000 mL of a nonhydrating diluent; infuse IV at a rate to control uterine atony. Do not exceed 40 units/1,000 mL
IM
Administer 10 units IM after delivery of the placenta.
• *Treatment of incomplete or inevitable abortion:* IV infusion of 10 units of oxytocin with 500 mL physiologic saline solution or 5% dextrose in physiologic saline infused at a rate of 10–20 milliunits (20–40 drops)/min. Do not exceed 30 units in 12 hr because of risk of water intoxication.

Pharmacokinetics

Route	Onset	Duration
IV	Immediate	60 min
IM	3–5 min	2–3 hr

Metabolism: Hepatic; $T_{1/2}$: 1–6 min
Distribution: Crosses placenta; enters breast milk
Excretion: Urine

▼ IV FACTS
Preparation: Add 1 mL (10 units) to 1,000 mL of 0.9% aqueous sodium chloride or other IV fluid; the resulting solution will contain 10 milliunits/mL (0.01 units/mL).
Infusion: Infuse via constant infusion pump to ensure accurate control of rate; rate determined by uterine response; begin with 1–2 mL/min and increase at 15- to 60-min intervals.
Compatibilities: Compatible at a concentration of 5 units/L in dextrose–Ringer combinations; dextrose–lactated Ringer combinations; dextrose–saline combinations; dextrose 2%, 5%, and 10% in water; fructose 10% in water; Ringer injection; lactated Ringer injection; sodium chloride 0.45% and 0.9% injection; and 1/6M sodium lactate.
Incompatibilities: Do not combine in solution with fibrinolysin or heparin.

Adverse effects
• **CV:** *Cardiac arrhythmias,* PVCs, hypertension, subarachnoid hemorrhage
• **Fetal effects:** *Fetal bradycardia,* neonatal jaundice, low Apgar scores
• **GI:** *Nausea, vomiting*
• **GU:** Postpartum hemorrhage, uterine rupture, pelvic hematoma, *uterine hypertonicity,* spasm, tetanic contraction, rupture of the uterus with excessive dosage or hypersensitivity
• **Hypersensitivity: Anaphylactic reaction**
• **Other:** Maternal and fetal deaths when used to induce labor or in first or second stages of labor; **afibrinogenemia; severe water intoxication** with seizures and coma, **maternal death** (associated with slow oxytocin infusion over 24 hr; oxytocin has antidiuretic effects)

■ Nursing considerations
Assessment
• **History:** Significant cephalopelvic disproportion, unfavorable fetal positions or presentations, severe toxemia, uterine inertia, hypertonic uterine patterns, previous cesarean section
• **Physical:** Fetal heart rate (continuous monitoring is recommended); fetal positions; fetal-pelvic proportions; uterine tone; timing and rate of contractions; breast examination; orientation, reflexes; P, BP, edema; R, adventitious sounds; CBC, bleeding studies, urinary output

O

Interventions

⊗ **Black box warning** Reserve for medical use, not elective induction.

• Ensure fetal position and size and absence of complications that are contraindicated with oxytocin before therapy.

⊗ **Warning** Ensure continuous observation of patient receiving IV oxytocin for induction or stimulation of labor; fetal monitoring is preferred. A physician should be immediately available to deal with complications if they arise.

• Regulate rate of oxytocin delivery to establish uterine contractions that are similar to normal labor; monitor rate and strength of contractions; discontinue drug and notify physician at any sign of uterine hyperactivity or spasm.

⊗ **Warning** Monitor maternal BP during oxytocin administration; discontinue drug and notify physician with any sign of hypertensive emergency.

• Monitor neonate for jaundice.

Teaching points

• The patient receiving parenteral oxytocin is usually receiving it as part of an immediate medical situation, and the drug teaching should be incorporated into the teaching about delivery. The patient needs to know the name of the drug and what she can expect after it is administered.

DANGEROUS DRUG

▷ **paclitaxel**

*(pak leh **tax' ell**)*

Abraxane

PREGNANCY CATEGORY D

Drug classes

Antimitotic
Antineoplastic

Therapeutic actions

Inhibits the normal dynamic reorganization of the microtubule network that is essential for dividing cells; leads to cell death in rapidly dividing cells.

Indications

• Treatment of metastatic carcinoma of the ovary as first-line therapy, in combination with cisplatin

• *Abraxane, generic:* Treatment of breast cancer after failure of combination therapy or relapse within 6 mo of adjuvant therapy

• First-line treatment of non–small-cell lung cancer, in combination with cisplatin

• Second-line treatment of AIDS-related Kaposi sarcoma

■▪ **NEW INDICATION:** Adjuvant treatment sequential to doxorubicin-containing therapy for node-positive breast cancer

• Unlabeled uses: Treatment of advanced head and neck cancer, previously untreated extensive-stage small-cell lung cancer, adenocarcinoma of the upper GI tract, hormone-refractory prostate cancer, leukemias

Contraindications and cautions

• Contraindicated with hypersensitivity to paclitaxel or drug formulated with polyoxyethylated castor oil, bone marrow depression, severe neurologic toxicity, lactation, pregnancy.

• Use cautiously with cardiac conduction defects, severe hepatic impairment.

Available forms

Injection—6 mg/mL; powder for injection—100 mg

Dosages

Adults

• *Ovarian cancer:* In previously untreated patients, 135 mg/m^2 IV over 24 hr *or* 175 mg/m^2 IV over 3 hr every 3 wk followed by 75 mg/m^2 IV cisplatin. In previously treated patients, 135 mg/m^2 *or* 175 mg/m^2 IV over 3 hr every 3 wk. Do not repeat the IV until the neutrophil count is at least 1,500 cells/mm^3 and platelet count is at least 100,000 cells/mm^3.

• *Breast cancer:* 175 mg/m^2 IV over 3 hr every 3 wk for four courses after failure of chemotherapy; 175 mg/m^2 IV over 3 hr every 3 wk after initial chemotherapy failure or relapse within 6 mo; or 260 mg/m^2 IV over 30 min every 3 wk (*Abraxane*). If neutrophil count is less than 500 cells/mm^3 for a wk or longer, reduce dose to 220 mg/m^2; with severe neutropenia, reduce dose to 180 mg/m^2.

• *Breast cancer adjuvant treatment:* 175 mg/m^2 IV over 3 hr every 3 wk for four courses, with doxorubicin-containing therapy.

Adverse effects in *italics* are most common; those in **bold** are life-threatening. ⬛⬛⬛ Do not crush.

- *AIDS-related Kaposi sarcoma:* 135 mg/m^2 IV over 3 hr every 3 wk *or* 100 mg/m^2 IV over 3 hr every 2 wk. Do not administer if neutrophil count is less than 1,000 cells/mm^3.
- *Non–small-cell-lung cancer:* 135 mg/m^2 IV over 24 hr followed by 75 mg/m^2 cisplatin IV every 3 wk. Reduce dose by 20% if neutrophil count is less than 500 cells/mm^3 for a week or longer.

Pediatric patients
Safety and efficacy not established.

Pharmacokinetics

Route	Onset	Duration
IV	Rapid	6–12 hr

Metabolism: Hepatic; T$_{1/2}$: 13–20 hr
Distribution: Crosses placenta; enters breast milk
Excretion: Bile

▼ IV FACTS

Preparation: Use extreme caution when handling drug; dilute before infusion in 0.9% sodium chloride, 5% dextrose injection, 5% dextrose and 0.9% sodium chloride injection, 5% dextrose in Ringer injection to a concentration of 0.3–1.2 mg/mL; stable at room temperature for 27 hr. Refrigerate unopened vials; avoid use of PVC infusion bags and tubing.
Infusion: Administer over 3 hr or 24 hr through an in-line filter not greater than 0.22 mcg. Do not use a filter with *Abraxane.*
Y-site compatibility: May be given with fluconazole.

Adverse effects

- **CNS:** Peripheral sensory neuropathy, mild to severe
- **CV:** Bradycardia, hypotension, severe CV events
- **GI:** *Nausea, vomiting,* mucositis, anorexia, elevated liver enzymes
- **Hematologic: Bone marrow depression, infection**
- **Other: Hypersensitivity reactions,** *myalgia, arthralgia, alopecia*

Interactions

✱Drug-drug • Increased myelosuppression with cisplatin and other antineoplastics
• Increased paclitaxel effects with ketoconazole, verapamil, diazepam, quinidine, dexamethasone, cyclosporine, teniposide, etoposide, vincristine, testosterone

■ Nursing considerations
Assessment

- **History:** Hypersensitivity to paclitaxel, castor oil; bone marrow depression; cardiac conduction defects; severe hepatic impairment; pregnancy; lactation
- **Physical:** Neurologic status, T; P, BP, peripheral perfusion; skin color, texture, hair distribution; abdominal examination, mucous membranes; LFTs, renal function tests, CBC

Interventions

⊗ *Black box warning* Do not administer drug unless blood counts are within acceptable parameters.

⊗ *Black box warning* Do not substitute *Abraxane* for any other paclitaxel formulation.

⊗ *Warning* Handle drug with great care; gloves are recommended. If drug comes in contact with skin, wash immediately with soap and water.

⊗ *Black box warning* Premedicate with one of the following drugs to prevent severe hypersensitivity reactions: Oral dexamethasone 20 mg, 12 hr and 6 hr before paclitaxel, 10 mg if AIDS-related Kaposi sarcoma; diphenhydramine 50 mg IV 30–60 min before paclitaxel; and cimetidine 300 mg IV or ranitidine 50 mg IV 30–60 min before paclitaxel.

- Monitor BP and pulse during administration.
- Monitor infusion site for possible extravasation.
- Obtain blood counts before and at least monthly during treatment.
- Monitor patient's neurologic status frequently during treatment.
- Advise patient to avoid pregnancy; serious fetal harm can occur; advise using barrier contraceptives.

Teaching points

- This drug must be given over a 30-minute, 3-hour, or 24-hour period once every 3 weeks. Mark a calendar noting drug days.
- Have regular blood tests and neurologic examinations while receiving this drug.

P

- Avoid pregnancy while you are taking this drug, serious fetal harm can occur; using barrier contraceptives is advised.
- You may experience these side effects: Nausea and vomiting (if severe, request antiemetics; frequent small meals also may help); weakness, lethargy (frequent rest periods will help); increased susceptibility to infection (avoid crowds and exposure to diseases); numbness and tingling in the fingers or toes (avoid injury to these areas; use care with tasks requiring precision); loss of hair (obtain a wig or other head covering; keep the head covered at extremes of temperature).
- Report severe nausea and vomiting; fever, chills, sore throat; unusual bleeding or bruising; numbness or tingling in your fingers or toes; chest pain.

▷ palifermin

See Appendix R, *Less commonly used drugs*.

▷ paliperidone
*(pal ah **peer'** ah dohn)*

Invega⊕, Invega Sustenna

PREGNANCY CATEGORY C

Drug classes
Atypical antipsychotic
Benzisoxazole

Therapeutic actions
Mechanism of action not completely understood; is the major active metabolite of risperidone. Blocks dopamine and serotonin receptors in the brain and depresses the RAS. Antihistaminic and alpha-adrenergic blocking activity may contribute to some therapeutic and adverse effects.

Indications
- Treatment of schizophrenia; acute and long-term maintenance treatment of schizophrenia; as monotherapy or as adjunct to mood stabilizers or antidepressants in patients 12 yr and older
- Acute treatment of schizoaffective disorder as monotherapy or with antidepressant or mood stabilizers (oral only)

Contraindications and cautions
- Contraindicated with hypersensitivity to any component of the drug or to risperidone, lactation, and in elderly patients with dementia-related psychosis.
- Use cautiously with prolonged QT interval and with other drugs that prolong QT interval; pregnancy; history of arrhythmias, GI disorders, seizures, hypotension; diabetes mellitus; CV disease; renal impairment; risk of aspiration; and in elderly patients.

Available forms
ER tablets⊕—1.5, 3, 6, 9 mg; injection—39/0.25 mL, 78 mg/0.25 mL, 117 mg/0.75 mL, 156 mg/mL, 234 mg/1.5 mL

Dosages
Adults
- *Schizophrenia and schizoaffective disorder:* 6 mg/day PO in the morning; may be adjusted to a maximum 12 mg/day PO if warranted and tolerated by the patient. Increases of 3 mg/day at intervals of at least 5 days are suggested.
- *Schizophrenia:* Parenteral—234 mg IM, followed by 156 mg IM in 1 wk, both injections in the deltoid. 117 mg IM 1 wk later in gluteal or deltoid site. Maintenance dose—39–234 mg IM once per month in deltoid or gluteal site.

Pediatric patients 12–17 yr
- *Treatment of schizophrenia:*
  Weighing 51 kg and more: Initially, 3 mg/day PO; range, 3–12 mg/day.
  Weighing less than 51 kg: Initially 3 mg/day PO; range, 3–6 mg/day.

Patients with renal impairment
In mild renal impairment (creatinine clearance 50–80 mL/min), maximum dosage 6 mg/day; or 156 mg IM, followed by 117 mg IM in 1 wk (both in deltoids), then monthly injections of 78 mg IM in deltoid or gluteal site. In severe renal impairment (creatinine clearance 10–50 mL/min), maximum dosage 3 mg/day. IM route not recommended.

Pharmacokinetics

Route	Onset	Peak
Oral	Gradual	24 hr

Metabolism: Hepatic; $T_{1/2}$: 23 hr
Distribution: Crosses placenta; enters breast milk
Excretion: Urine

Adverse effects

- **CNS:** *Headache, dizziness, akathisia, somnolence,* dystonia, *extrapyramidal disorders,* hypertonia, tremor, *parkinsonism,* anxiety, blurred vision, tardive dyskinesia
- **CV:** *Tachycardia,* arrhythmia, palpitations, hypotension, *orthostatic hypotension,* prolonged QT interval
- **GI:** Dyspepsia, nausea, dry mouth, salivary hypersecretion
- **Respiratory:** Cough
- **Other:** Fever, fatigue, pain, **increased mortality in geriatric patients with dementia-related psychosis, neuroleptic malignant syndrome,** hyperglycemia, hyperprolactinemia, dyslipidemia, weight gain

Interactions

⁎ Drug-drug • Risk of increased CNS depression if combined with alcohol and other central-acting depressants; use caution if this combination cannot be avoided • Potential for decreased effectiveness of levodopa or dopamine agonist; monitor patient closely and adjust dosage as needed • Risk of severe orthostatic hypotension if combined with other drugs that cause orthostatic hypotension; monitor patient closely and adjust dosage as needed • Increased risk of prolonged QT interval if used with other drugs that prolong QT interval; monitor ECG before and periodically during therapy

■ Nursing considerations

Assessment

- **History:** Hypersensitivity to any component of paliperidone or risperidone; pregnancy; lactation; dementia-related psychosis in elderly patients; suicide risk; prolonged QT interval or use of other drugs known to prolong it; history of arrhythmias, GI disorders, hypotension, or seizures; diabetes mellitus; CV disease; renal impairment; risk of aspiration
- **Physical:** Weight; orientation, affect, reflexes; BP, standing BP, P; renal function tests; blood glucose; ECG, lipid panel

Interventions

⊗ **Black box warning** Avoid use in elderly patients with dementia-related psychosis; increased risk of CV death. Drug is not approved for this use.

- Limit amount of drug dispensed to patients with suicidal ideation.

- Do not cut, crush, or allow patient to chew tablets; give with adequate liquids to ensure swallowing.
- Advise patient that the tablet matrix is insoluble and that it is normal to see tablets in the stool.
- Monitor patient's body temperature, and rule out infection if fever occurs; risk of neuroleptic malignant hyperthermia.
- Monitor patient regularly for hyperglycemia.
- Advise patient to avoid excessive heat and dehydration, which could aggravate orthostatic hypotension.
- Advise patient to use contraception while on this drug; advise breast-feeding women to find another method of feeding the infant while taking this drug.

Teaching points

- Take this drug in the morning; swallow tablet whole with a full glass of water. Do not cut, crush, or chew the tablet. If you miss a dose, do not double the following dose; instead, take a dose as soon as you remember and continue with your usual dose the following morning.
- Do not be concerned if you see tablets in your stool. This drug is in a matrix system that allows slow release throughout the day; the matrix will pass in your stool.
- This drug enters breast milk and could have effects on a breast-feeding infant; if you are breast-feeding, you should find another method of feeding the infant while you are on this drug.
- It is not known how this drug could affect a fetus. If you are pregnant or decide to become pregnant while on this drug, consult with your health care provider; use of contraception is advised.
- This drug interacts with some other drugs and could cause serious side effects; tell any health care provider who is taking care of you that you are on this drug.
- Avoid drinking alcoholic beverages while on this drug.
- You may experience these side effects: Impaired judgment, thinking, or motor skills, (do not drive a car or operate any dangerous machinery while on this drug, and avoid making any important decisions until you are sure how this drug is affecting you), low blood pressure on standing (stand up slowly, make sure you are steady before moving, avoid excessive heat exposure and dehydration).

P

- Report fever; suicidal thoughts; severe dizziness; increased thirst, hunger, or urination; anxiety; rapid or irregular heartbeat.

▷ palivizumab
(pa live ah zoo' mab)

Synagis

PREGNANCY CATEGORY C

Drug classes
Antiviral
Monoclonal antibody

Therapeutic actions
A murine and human monoclonal antibody produced by recombinant DNA technology specific to an antigenic site of the RSV; has neutralizing effects on the RSV.

Indications
- Prevention of serious lower respiratory tract disease caused by RSV in pediatric patients at high risk for RSV disease

Contraindications and cautions
- Contraindicated with allergy to palivizumab or any murine product.
- Use cautiously with fever (antipyretics should be used to decrease fever before beginning therapy); previous administration of palivizumab (antibodies frequently develop, causing a risk of serious reactions on repeat administration); pregnancy, history of bleeding disorders.

Available forms
Injection—50 mg/0.5 mL, 100 mg/mL

Dosages
Administer IM only.
Pediatric patients
15 mg/kg IM as a single injection, once a month during RSV season, with first dose given before start of RSV season. Give injection preferably in anterolateral aspect of thigh; do not use gluteal muscle because of risk of damaging sciatic nerve. For cardiopulmonary bypass patients, administer a dose as soon as possible following procedure, even if less than 1 month since previous dose.

Pharmacokinetics

Route	Onset	Peak
IM	Slow	2–7 days

Metabolism: Tissue; $T_{1/2}$: 18 days
Excretion: Unknown

Adverse effects
- **CNS:** Malaise
- **GI:** Nausea, vomiting, gastroenteritis
- **Respiratory:** URI, pharyngitis, otitis media
- **Other:** Increased susceptibility to infection; **risk of severe anaphylactoid reaction,** especially with repeated administrations, *fever, chills*

Interactions
✳ Drug-drug ⊗ *Warning* Reduce dosage of other immunosuppressive agents; severe immunosuppression can lead to increased susceptibility to infection and increased risk of lymphomas.

■ Nursing considerations
Assessment
- **History:** Allergy to palivizumab or any murine product; previous administration of palivizumab; bleeding disorders
- **Physical:** T, body weight; P, BP; R, adventitious sounds; CBC

Interventions
- Monitor WBC levels and circulating T cells periodically during therapy.
- Monitor patient for signs and symptoms of hypersensitivity reactions (rare but potentially serious).
- Monitor for any sign of RSV infection; do not use during acute RSV infection, use only for prophylaxis.
- Protect patient from exposure to infections and maintain sterile technique for invasive procedures.
- Arrange for nutritional consult if nausea and vomiting are persistent.

Teaching points
- Protect your child from exposure to infection while he or she is using this drug; people may wear masks and rubber gloves when caring for your child; visitors may have to be limited.
- Report fever, fussiness, other infections; difficulty breathing.

▷palonosetron hydrochloride

*(pal on **os'** e tron)*

Aloxi

PREGNANCY CATEGORY B

Drug classes
Antiemetic
Selective serotonin receptor antagonist

Therapeutic actions
Selectively binds to serotonin receptors in the CTZ, blocking the nausea and vomiting caused by the release of serotonin by mucosal cells during chemotherapy, radiotherapy, or surgical invasion, an action that stimulates the CTZ and causes nausea and vomiting.

Indications
• Prevention of acute and delayed nausea and vomiting associated with initial and repeat courses of moderately and highly emetogenic chemotherapy
• Prevention of postoperative nausea and vomiting for up to 24 hr after surgery (IV)

Contraindications and cautions
• Contraindicated with allergy to palonosetron or any of its components.
• Use cautiously with known prolonged QT interval or high risk for prolongation of QT interval (hypokalemia, hypomagnesemia, diuretic use, antiarrhythmic use) pregnancy, lactation.

Available forms
Injection—0.25 mg/5 mL; capsules—0.5 mg

Dosages
Adults
• *Chemotherapy-induced nausea and vomiting:* 0.25 mg IV as a single dose over 30 sec, given 30 min before the start of chemotherapy, or 0.5 mg PO 1 hr before start of chemotherapy.
• *Postoperative nausea and vomiting:* 0.075 mg IV as a single dose over 10 sec, given immediately before induction of anesthesia.
Pediatric patients
Safety and efficacy not established.

Pharmacokinetics

Route	Onset	Peak
IV	Immediate	End of infusion
Oral	Rapid	5 hr

Metabolism: Hepatic; T$_{1/2}$: 40 hr
Distribution: May cross placenta; may enter breast milk
Excretion: Feces, urine

▼ IV FACTS
Preparation: No further preparation is needed; solution should be clear and free of particulate matter before use. Store at room temperature; protect from light.
Infusion: Infuse over 30 sec (chemotherapy-induced nausea and vomiting) or over 10 sec (postoperative nausea and vomiting); flush the infusion line with normal saline before and after administration.
Compatibilities: Do not mix in solution with any other drugs.

Adverse effects
• **CNS:** *Headache,* somnolence, drowsiness, sedation, paresthesia, anxiety, insomnia
• **CV:** Tachycardia, bradycardia, hypotension, other arrhythmias, vein distention
• **GI:** Diarrhea, *constipation,* abdominal pain, dyspepsia, dry mouth, hiccups, flatulence
• **Other:** Fever, pruritus, flulike symptoms, fatigue

■ Nursing considerations
Assessment
• **History:** Allergy to palonosetron, pregnancy, lactation, electrolyte abnormality, risk for prolonged QT interval
• **Physical:** Orientation, reflexes, affect; skin evaluation; cardiac rhythm, P, BP; bowel sounds; T, serum electrolytes

Interventions
• Provide mouth care and sugarless candies to suck to help alleviate nausea and dry mouth.
• Establish safety precautions (side rails, assistance with ambulation, proper lighting) if CNS or visual effects occur.
• Provide appropriate analgesics for headache.

P

Teaching points

- This drug is given IV or orally just before you receive your chemotherapy or before surgery. It will help decrease nausea and vomiting.
- You may experience these side effects: Lack of sleep, drowsiness (use caution if driving or performing tasks that require alertness); constipation; headache (appropriate medication will be provided).
- Report severe headache, fever, numbness or tingling, severe constipation, dizziness.

▷ **pamidronate disodium**

*(pah **mih'** dro nate)*

Aredia

PREGNANCY CATEGORY D

Drug classes
Bisphosphonate
Calcium regulator

Therapeutic actions
Slows normal and abnormal bone resorption without inhibiting bone formation and mineralization.

Indications
- Treatment of hypercalcemia associated with malignancy
- Treatment of moderate to severe Paget disease
- Treatment of osteolytic lesions in breast cancer patients receiving chemotherapy and hormonal therapy
- Treatment of osteolytic bone lesions of multiple myeloma
- Unlabeled uses: Postmenopausal osteoporosis, hyperparathyroidism, prostatic carcinoma, immobilization-related hypercalcemia to prevent fractures and bone pain, osteoporosis with spinal cord injury

Contraindications and cautions
- Contraindicated with allergy to pamidronate disodium or bisphosphonates.
- Use cautiously with renal failure, enterocolitis, pregnancy, lactation.

Available forms
Powder for injection—30, 90 mg; injection—3, 6, 9 mg/mL

Dosages
Adults
- *Hypercalcemia:* 60–90 mg IV given over 2–24 hr as a single dose. Do not exceed 90 mg in a single dose.
- *Paget disease:* 30 mg/day IV as a 4-hr infusion on 3 consecutive days for a total dose of 90 mg. Do not exceed 90 mg in a single dose.
- *Osteolytic bone lesions:* 90 mg IV as a 2-hr infusion every 3–4 wk. For bone lesions caused by multiple myeloma, give as 4-hr infusion once monthly. Do not exceed 90 mg in single dose.

Pediatric patients
Safety and efficacy not established.

Patients with renal impairment
Do not exceed single dose of 90 mg.

Pharmacokinetics

Route	Onset	Duration
IV	Rapid	72 hr

Metabolism: Not metabolized
Distribution: Crosses placenta; may enter breast milk
Excretion: Urine

▼ IV FACTS

Preparation: Reconstitute by adding 10 mL sterile water for injection to each vial; allow drug to dissolve. For treatment of malignancy-associated hypercalcemia, may be further diluted in 1,000 mL sterile 0.45% or 0.9% sodium chloride or 5% dextrose injection; stable for 24 hr at room temperature.
Infusion: Infuse over 2–24 hr (90-mg dose); over 4 hr (30–60-mg dose).
Incompatibilities: Do not mix with calcium-containing infusions, such as Ringer; give in a single IV infusion and keep line separate from all other drugs.

Adverse effects
- **CNS:** Headache, insomnia
- **GI:** *Nausea, diarrhea*
- **Musculoskeletal:** *Increased or recurrent bone pain* at pagetic sites, focal osteomalacia, osteonecrosis of the jaw (cancer patients)
- **Other:** Fever, fatigue

■ Nursing considerations
Assessment
- **History:** Allergy to pamidronate disodium or any bisphosphonates, renal failure, enterocolitis, lactation

- **Physical:** Skin lesions, color, T; muscle tone, bone pain; bowel sounds; urinalysis, serum calcium; serum electrolytes, CBC with differential, serum creatinine

Interventions

- Provide saline hydration before administration.
- Monitor serum calcium levels before, during, and after therapy. Consider retreatment if hypercalcemia recurs, but allow at least 7 days between treatments.
- Do not give foods high in calcium, vitamins with mineral supplements, or antacids high in metals within 2 hr of dosing.
- Advise a dental examination and completion of any needed preventive care before beginning therapy in cancer patients. Avoid any dental work during therapy.
- Maintain adequate nutrition, particularly intake of calcium and vitamin D.
- Monitor patients with renal impairment carefully; arrange for reduction of dosage if glomerular filtration rate is reduced.

⊗ **Warning** Keep calcium readily available in case hypocalcemic tetany develops.

Teaching points

- Do not take foods high in calcium, antacids, or vitamins with minerals within 2 hours of receiving this drug.
- You should have a dental examination and complete any needed dental care before beginning therapy if you are being treated for cancer.
- You may experience these side effects: Nausea, diarrhea, recurrent bone pain.
- Report twitching, muscle spasms, dark urine, severe diarrhea.

▽ **pancrelipase**
(pan kre ly' pase)

Creon Delayed-Release Capsules ⓞⓣⓒ,
Pancreaze Delayed-Release
Capsules ⓞⓣⓒ, Pertyze ⓞⓣⓒ, Ultresa ⓞⓣⓒ,
Viokace ⓞⓣⓒ

PREGNANCY CATEGORY C

Drug class

Digestive enzyme

Therapeutic actions

Replacement of pancreatic enzymes: Helps to digest and absorb fat, proteins, and carbohydrates.

Indications

- Replacement therapy in patients with deficient exocrine pancreatic secretions, cystic fibrosis, chronic pancreatitis, postpancreatectomy, ductal obstructions, pancreatic insufficiency, steatorrhea or malabsorption syndrome, and postgastrectomy
- Presumptive test for pancreatic function

Contraindications and cautions

- Contraindicated with allergy to any component, pork products; acute pancreatitis; acute exacerbations of chronic pancreatitis.
- Use cautiously with pregnancy, lactation, gout, renal impairment, hyperuricemia.

Available forms (in lipase units)

DR capsules ⓞⓣⓒ—3,000, 4,200, 6,000, 8,000, 10,500, 12,000, 13,800, 16,000, 16,800, 20,700, 21,000, 23,000, 24,000; tablets ⓞⓣⓒ—10,440, 12,880

Dosages

Adults

Capsules and tablets
4,000–20,000 units PO with each meal and with snacks, usually 1–3 capsules or tablets before or with meals and snacks. May be increased to 8 capsules or tablets in severe cases. 500 units/kg/meal to maximum of 2,500 units/kg/meal (*Viokace*). Patients with pancreatectomy or obstruction, 72,000 lipase units/meal while consuming 100 g fat/day (*Creon*).

Pediatric patients 4 yr and older
500 lipase units/kg/meal to a maximum of 2,500 units/kg/meal.

Pediatric patients 1 to younger than 4 yr
1,000 units/kg/meal to maximum of 2,500 units/kg/meal or 10,000 units/kg/day.

Pediatric patients up to 1 yr
3,000 units lipase PO per 120 mL of formula or per breast-feeding session; 2,000–4,000 units per feeding (*Pancreaze*).

Pharmacokinetics

Generally no systemic absorption.

Adverse effects

- **GI:** *Nausea, abdominal cramps, diarrhea*
- **GU:** Hyperuricosuria, hyperuricemia with extremely high doses
- **Hypersensitivity:** Asthma with inhalation of fine-powder concentrates in sensitized individuals

■ Nursing considerations

Assessment

- **History:** Allergy to any component, pork products; pregnancy, lactation; gout, renal impairment
- **Physical:** R, adventitious sounds; abdominal examination, bowel sounds; pancreatic function tests, renal function tests, uric acid levels

Interventions

- Administer before or with meals and snacks.
- Do not mix capsules directly into infant formula or breast milk; drug administration should be followed by breast milk or formula.
- ⊗ *Warning* Dosages above recommended range may result in colonic strictures, especially in patients with cystic fibrosis.
- Be aware that *Creon* and *Viokace* are not interchangeable with other pancrelipase preperations. Be aware that most products are not interchangeable.
- Do not crush or let patient chew the enteric-coated capsules; drug will not survive acid environment of the stomach.

Teaching points

- Take drug before or with meals and snacks.
- Do not crush or chew the enteric-coated capsules; swallow whole. *Ultresa* capsules may be opened and the contents sprinkled on food if swallowing capsule is difficult. Do not mix contents of capsules directly with infant formula or breast milk; give capsules before formula or a breast-feeding session.
- You may experience these side effects: Abdominal discomfort, diarrhea.
- Report joint pain, swelling, soreness; difficulty breathing; GI upset.

▽ **panitumumab**

See Appendix R, *Less commonly used drugs*.

▽ **pantoprazole**
(pan toe' pray zol)

Panto IV (CAN), Pantoloc (CAN), Protonix ⊂ᴰᴺᴳ⊃, Protonix IV

PREGNANCY CATEGORY B

Drug classes

Antisecretory drug
Proton pump inhibitor

Therapeutic actions

Gastric acid-pump inhibitor: Suppresses gastric acid secretion by specific inhibition of the hydrogen-potassium ATPase enzyme system at the secretory surface of the gastric parietal cells; blocks the final step of acid production.

Indications

- Oral: Short-term (8 wk or less) and long-term treatment of GERD
- Maintenance healing of erosive esophagitis
- Long-term treatment of pathologic hypersecretory conditions
- IV: Short-term (7–10 days) treatment of GERD in patients unable to continue oral therapy
- IV: Treatment of pathologic hypersecretory conditions associated with Zollinger-Ellison syndrome and other neoplastic conditions
- Unlabeled uses: Treatment of duodenal ulcer, prevention of GI bleeding in patients receiving antiplatelet drugs

Contraindications and cautions

- Contraindicated with hypersensitivity to any proton pump inhibitor or any drug components.
- Use cautiously because of possible increased risk of *Clostridium difficile* infection.
- Use cautiously with pregnancy, lactation.

Available forms

DR tablet ⊂ᴰᴺᴳ⊃—20, 40 mg; granules for oral suspension—40 mg/packet; powder for injection—40 mg/vial

Dosages

Adults

40 mg PO daily for short-term treatment and maintenance healing of erosive esophagitis for 8 wk or less. The 8-wk course may be repeated if healing has not occurred. Give continually for

---

Adverse effects in *italics* are most common; those in **bold** are life-threatening. ⊂ᴰᴺᴳ⊃ Do not crush.

hypersecretory disorders: 40 mg/day IV bid, up to 240 mg/day (2-yr duration) or 40 mg/day IV for 7–10 days. For severe hypersecretory syndromes, 40 mg every 12 hr (up to 240 mg/day) PO or IV (6-day duration) has been used.

Pediatric patients 5 yr and older
- *Short-term treatment of GERD: 15 kg to less than 40 kg:* 20 mg/day PO for up to 8 wk. *40 kg or more:* 40 mg/day PO for up to 8 wk.

Patients with hepatic impairment
Use caution and monitor patient closely.

Pharmacokinetics

Route	Onset	Peak
Oral	1 hr	3–5 hr
IV	Rapid	3–5 hr

Metabolism: Hepatic; $T_{1/2}$: 1.5 hr
Distribution: Crosses placenta; may enter breast milk
Excretion: Bile, urine

▼ IV FACTS

Preparation: Reconstitute with 10 mL 0.9% sodium chloride; may then be further diluted with 100 mL 5% dextrose injection, 0.9% sodium chloride injection or lactated Ringer, final concentration 0.4 mg/mL; reconstituted solution can be stored 2 hr, dilution up to 12 hr at room temperature. Avoid use of spiked IV system adapters with vials.
Infusion: Infuse over at least 15 min using in-line filter.
Incompatibilities: Do not mix with or administer through the same line as other IV solutions.

Adverse effects

- **CNS:** *Headache, dizziness,* asthenia, vertigo, insomnia, apathy, anxiety, paresthesias, dream abnormalities
- **Dermatologic:** Rash, inflammation, urticaria, pruritus, alopecia, dry skin
- **GI:** *Diarrhea, abdominal pain, nausea, vomiting,* constipation, dry mouth, tongue atrophy, *C. difficile* diarrhea
- **Respiratory:** *URI symptoms,* cough, epistaxis, pneumonia
- **Other:** Cancer in preclinical studies, back pain, fever, vitamin B_{12} deficiency, loss of bone density, bone fractures, decreased magnesium levels, thrombophlebitis with IV use

Interactions

✳ **Drug-drug** ● Possible decreased serum levels of atazanavir, nelfinavir; avoid this combination ● Possible increased methotrexate level; monitor patient closely ● Possible increased warfarin level; monitor INR closely

■ Nursing considerations
Assessment

- **History:** Hypersensitivity to any proton pump inhibitor or any drug components, pregnancy, lactation
- **Physical:** Skin lesions; T; reflexes, affect; urinary output, abdominal examination; respiratory auscultation

Interventions

- Administer once or twice a day. Caution patient to swallow tablets whole; not to cut, chew, or crush.
⊗ *Warning* Arrange for further evaluation of patient after 4 wk of therapy for gastroesophageal reflux disorders. Symptomatic improvement does not rule out gastric cancer; gastric cancer did occur in preclinical studies.
⊗ *Warning* Patient may be at risk for loss of bone density and fractures; monitor accordingly and weigh risks and benefits.
- Maintain supportive treatment as appropriate for underlying problem.
- Evaluate patients with persistent diarrhea for possible *C. difficile* infection.
- Switch patients on IV therapy to oral dosage as soon as possible.
- Provide additional comfort measures to alleviate discomfort from GI effects and headache.

Teaching points

- Take the drug once or twice a day. Swallow the tablets whole—do not chew, cut, or crush them.
- Arrange to have regular medical follow-up care while you are using this drug.
- Maintain all of the usual activities and restrictions that apply to your condition. If this becomes difficult, consult your health care provider.
- You may experience these side effects: Dizziness (avoid driving a car or performing hazardous tasks); headache (consult your health care provider if these become bothersome; medications may be available to help); nausea, vomiting, diarrhea (proper nutrition is important; consult a dietitian to maintain nutrition; stay near a bathroom); symptoms of upper respiratory tract infection, cough (this is a drug effect;

do not self-medicate; consult your health care provider if this becomes uncomfortable).
- Report severe headache, worsening of symptoms, fever, chills, blurred vision, periorbital pain, severe diarrhea.

▷ paricalcitol

See Appendix R, *Less commonly used drugs.*

▷ paroxetine
(pah rox' a teen)

paroxetine hydrochloride

Apo-Paroxetine (CAN), CO Paroxetine (CAN), Gen-Paroxetine (CAN), Novo-Paroxetine (CAN), Paxil, Paxil CR ⊙ᴺᴰ, ratio-Paroxetine (CAN)

paroxetine mesylate

Pexeva

PREGNANCY CATEGORY D

Drug classes

Antidepressant
SSRI

Therapeutic actions

Potentiates serotonergic activity in the CNS, resulting in antidepressant effect.

Indications

- Treatment of major depressive disorder
- Treatment of OCD
- Treatment of panic disorders
- Treatment of social anxiety disorder (social phobia)
- Treatment of generalized anxiety disorder
- Treatment of PTSD
- Treatment of PMDD
- Unlabeled uses: Treatment of hot flashes, diabetic neuropathy, traumatic brain injury, pruritus, stuttering; smoking cessation; prevention of migraines

Contraindications and cautions

- Contraindicated with use of MAOI, thioridazine, pimozide, linezolid, methylene blue.

- Use cautiously in the elderly; with renal or hepatic impairment, pregnancy, lactation, suicidal patients.

Available forms

Tablets—10, 20, 30, 40 mg; CR tablets ⊙ᴺᴰ—12.5, 25, 37.5 mg; suspension—10 mg/5 mL

Dosages
Adults

- *Depression:* 20 mg/day PO as a single daily dose. Range, 20–50 mg/day. Or 25–62.5 mg/day CR tablet.
- *OCD:* 20 mg/day PO as a single dose, may increase in 10-mg/day increments; do not exceed 60 mg/day.
- *Panic disorder:* 10 mg/day PO; increase in increments of 10 mg/wk; usual range, 10–60 mg/day. Or 12.5–75 mg/day PO CR tablet; do not exceed 75 mg/day.
- *Social anxiety disorder:* 20 mg/day PO as a single dose in the morning. Or, 12.5 mg/day PO CR form. May increase up to 60 mg/day or 37.5 mg/day PO CR form.
- *Generalized anxiety disorder:* 20 mg/day PO as a single daily dose. Range, 20–50 mg/day.
- *PMDD:* 12.5 mg/day PO as a single dose in the morning. Range, 12.5–25 mg/day. May be given daily or just during the luteal phase of the cycle.
- *PTSD:* 20 mg/day PO as a single dose. Range, 20–50 mg/day PO.
- *Switching to or from an MAOI:* At least 14 days should elapse between discontinuation of MAOI and initiation of paroxetine therapy; similarly, allow 14 days between discontinuing paroxetine and beginning MAOI.

Pediatric patients
Safety and efficacy not established.

Geriatric patients or patients with renal or hepatic impairment
10 mg/day PO; do not exceed 40 mg/day. Or 12.5 mg/day CR tablet; do not exceed 50 mg/day.

Pharmacokinetics

Route	Onset
Oral	Slow

Metabolism: Hepatic; $T_{1/2}$: 24 hr
Distribution: Crosses placenta; enters breast milk
Excretion: Urine

Adverse effects

- **CNS:** *Somnolence, dizziness, insomnia, tremor, nervousness, headache,* anxiety, paresthesia, blurred vision
- **CV:** Palpitations, vasodilation, orthostatic hypotension, hypertension
- **Dermatologic:** *Sweating,* rash, redness
- **GI:** *Nausea, dry mouth, constipation, diarrhea,* anorexia, flatulence, vomiting
- **GU:** *Ejaculatory disorders, male genital disorders,* urinary frequency
- **Respiratory:** Yawns, pharyngitis, cough
- **Other:** *Asthenia*

Interactions

✳ **Drug-drug** ● Increased paroxetine levels and toxicity with cimetidine, MAOIs ● Decreased therapeutic effects of phenytoin, digoxin ● Decreased effectiveness of paroxetine with phenobarbital, phenytoin, fosamprenavir, ritonavir ● Increased serum levels and possible toxicity of procyclidine, tryptophan, pimozide, TCAs, resperidone, antiarrhythmics, warfarin ● Risk of serotonin syndrome (hypertension, hyperthermia, mental status changes) if used with other SSRIs or other serotonergic agents

✳ **Drug-alternative therapy** ● Increased sedative-hypnotic effects with St. John's Wort

■ Nursing considerations

Assessment

- **History:** Hypersensitivity to paroxetine, renal or hepatic impairment, seizure disorder, pregnancy, lactation
- **Physical:** Orientation, reflexes; P, BP, perfusion; R, adventitious sounds; bowel sounds, normal output; urinary output; liver evaluation; LFTs, renal function tests

Interventions

⊗ **Black box warning** Be alert for increased suicidality in children, adolescents, and young adults; monitor accordingly.

- Administer once a day in the morning.
- Shake suspension well before using.
- Ensure that patient swallows CR tablets whole; do not cut, crush, or chew.
- Limit amount of drug given to potentially suicidal patients.
- Abruptly discontinuing the drug may result in discontinuation symptoms (agitation, palpitations); consider tapering.
- Advise patient to avoid using if pregnant or lactating.

Teaching points

- Take this drug exactly as directed and as long as directed. Shake suspension well before using. Swallow controlled-release tablets whole; do not cut, crush, or chew.
- Abruptly stopping the drug without tapering the dose may cause symptoms including agitation and palpitations.
- This drug should not be taken during pregnancy or when breast-feeding; using barrier contraceptives is advised.
- You may experience these side effects: Drowsiness, dizziness, tremor (use caution and avoid driving or performing other tasks that require alertness); GI upset (frequent small meals, frequent mouth care may help); alterations in sexual function.
- Report severe nausea, vomiting; palpitations; blurred vision; excessive sweating; thoughts of suicide.

▷ **pazopanib**

See Appendix R, *Less commonly used drugs.*

▷ **pegaptanib**

See Appendix R, *Less commonly used drugs.*

▷ **pegaspargase**

See Appendix R, *Less commonly used drugs.*

▷ **pegfilgrastim (G-CSF conjugate)**

(peg fill grass' stim)

Neulasta

PREGNANCY CATEGORY C

Drug classes

Colony-stimulating factor
Hematopoietic agent

Therapeutic actions

Covalent conjugate of the human granulocyte colony-stimulating factor (filgrastim) produced by recombinant DNA technology; has a longer duration of action than filgrastim; increases the production of neutrophils within the bone marrow with little effect on the production of other hematopoietic cells.

Indications

- To decrease the incidence of infection in patients with nonmyeloid malignancies receiving myelosuppressive anticancer drugs associated with a significant incidence of severe febrile neutropenia

Contraindications and cautions

- Contraindicated with hypersensitivity to *Escherichia coli* products, filgrastim.
- Use cautiously with sickle cell disease, pregnancy, lactation.

Available forms

Injection—6 mg/0.6 mL in prefilled syringes

Dosages

Adults and children weighing more than 45 kg
6 mg subcutaneously as a single dose once per chemotherapy cycle. Do not give in the period 14 days before and 24 hr after administration of cytotoxic chemotherapy.
Pediatric patients
Safety and efficacy not established.

Pharmacokinetics

Route	Peak	Duration
Subcut.	8 hr	Varies

Metabolism: Unknown; $T_{1/2}$: 15–80 hr
Distribution: Crosses placenta; may enter breast milk
Excretion: Unknown

Adverse effects

- **CNS:** *Headache, generalized weakness, fatigue, dizziness, insomnia*
- **Dermatologic:** *Alopecia,* rash, *mucositis*
- **GI:** *Nausea, vomiting, stomatitis, anorexia, diarrhea, constipation, taste perversion, dyspepsia, abdominal pain*
- **Respiratory: Acute respiratory distress syndrome**
- **Other: Splenic rupture,** aggravation of sickle cell disease, *fever, arthralgia, peripheral edema, myalgia, bone pain, granulocytopenic allergic reactions* (anaphylaxis, rash, urticaria), *increased LDH, alkaline phosphatase, uric acid*

Interactions

＊**Drug-drug** • Risk of increased effects if combined with lithium; if this combina-

tion is used, monitor neutrophil counts frequently

■ Nursing considerations

✦ CLINICAL ALERT!
Name confusion has been reported between *Neulasta* (pegfilgrastim) and *Neumega* (oprelvekin); use caution.

Assessment

- **History:** Hypersensitivity to *E. coli* products, filgrastim; sickle cell disease; pregnancy, lactation
- **Physical:** Skin color, lesions, hair; T; orientation, affect; abdominal examination, status of mucous membranes; CBC, platelets

Interventions

- Obtain CBC and platelet count prior to and twice weekly during therapy.
- ⊗ *Warning* Administer no earlier than 24 hr after cytotoxic chemotherapy and not in the period of 14 days before the administration of chemotherapy.
- Give one injection with each course of chemotherapy.
- Store in refrigerator; allow to warm to room temperature before use; if syringe is at room temperature for 48 hr or longer, discard. Use each syringe for one dose.
- Do not shake syringe before use. Protect syringe from light. Make sure the syringe is free of particulate matter and that the solution is not discolored before using.
- Monitor patient for any sign of infection and arrange for appropriate treatment.
- Protect patient from exposure to infection.
- Provide appropriate comfort and supportive measures for headache, bone pain, or GI discomfort.
- Arrange for patient to obtain wig or other head covering if alopecia occurs; cover head at extremes of temperature.
- Arrange for small frequent meals if nausea and vomiting are a problem.
- Offer support and encouragement to deal with pain, discomfort, and hair loss.

Teaching points

- This drug will be given by subcutaneous injection once with each cycle of your chemotherapy.

Adverse effects in *italics* are most common; those in **bold** are life-threatening. ▣▣▣ Do not crush.

- Avoid exposure to infection while you are receiving this drug (avoid crowds and people with known infections).
- Keep appointments for frequent blood tests to evaluate effects of drug on your blood count.
- You may experience these side effects: Bone pain (analgesia may be ordered), nausea and vomiting (eat frequent small meals), loss of hair (you may want to arrange for appropriate head covering; it is very important to cover head in extreme temperatures).
- Report fever, chills, severe bone pain, sore throat, weakness, pain or swelling at injection site.

▷ peginesatide
(peg in es' ah tyde)

Omontys

PREGNANCY CATEGORY C

Drug class
Erythropoiesis-stimulating agent

Therapeutic actions
Binds to and activates human erythropoietin receptors and stimulates RBC production in the bone marrow.

Indications
- Treatment of anemia due to chronic kidney disease in adults on dialysis

Contraindications and cautions
- Contraindicated with patients not on dialysis, patients receiving treatment for cancer; uncontrolled hypertension.
- Use cautiously with CV disease, pregnancy, lactation.

Available forms
Single-use vials—2, 3, 4, 5, 6 mg/0.5 mL; prefilled syringes—1, 2, 3, 4, 5, 6 mg/0.5 mL; multiple-use vials—10, 20 mg/2 mL

Dosages
Adults
0.04 mg/kg subcutaneously or IV once per mo. Adjust dosage based on hemoglobin levels, no more frequently than every 4 wk. When switching from other erythropoiesis-stimulating

agents, base monthly dose on total weekly injection doses at time of conversion.
Pediatric patients
Not recommended.

Pharmacokinetics

Route	Onset	Peak
Subcut, IV	Slow	48 hr

Metabolism: Serum; $T_{1/2}$: 25–32 hr
Distribution: Crosses placenta; may enter breast milk
Excretion: Urine

▼ IV FACTS

Preparation: Use as provided; solution should be colorless to light yellow and free of particulate matter. Protect from light. For single-use vials, discard any unused portion. Multiple-use vials should be refrigerated and discarded after 28 days.
Injection: Inject dose directly into vein.
Incompatibilities: Do not dilute in other solutions. Do not administer with other drug solutions.

Adverse effects
- **CNS: Stroke,** headache, fatigue, dizziness
- **CV: MI, thromboembolic events, hypertension**
- **GI:** *Nausea, diarrhea,* vomiting
- **Respiratory:** *Cough, dyspnea*
- **Other:** *Arteriovenous fistula–site complications*

■ Nursing considerations
Assessment
- **History:** Chronic kidney disease, dialysis schedule, CV disease
- **Physical:** BP; P, R; adventitious sounds; orientation; iron stores, renal function tests, hemoglobin levels

Interventions
⊗ *Black box warning* Risk of death and serious CV events, including MI, stroke, and thromboembolic events; risk of rapid tumor progression or recurrence as hemoglobin level exceeds 11 g/dL. Target hemoglobin level to no greater than 11g/dL. Ensure appropriate use of drug; use lowest dose possible to get therapeutic effects.

- Drug is for use only in adults with chronic kidney disease on dialysis. Not for use with other anemias, patients being treated for cancer, or patients not on dialysis. Drug is not a substitute for emergency RBC transfusion.
- Monitor iron stores and provide iron as needed; monitor hemoglobin level and stop drug or decrease dosage as level approaches 11 g/dL.
- Monitor BP regularly because of risk of severe hypertension; ensure proper use of antihypertensives as needed.
- Monitor injection site for possible reactions.

Teaching points
- This drug is given once a month to increase your red blood cell count. It will be given either subcutaneously or IV.
- If you are going to be giving the drug at home, learn proper administration and disposal of needles and syringes. Some vials and syringes are for single use and some are for multiple use. Dispose of any unused portion of single-use vials or syringes immediately; dispose of multiple-use vials within 28 days.
- Protect the drug from light. Store multiple-use vials in the refrigerator. Mark a calendar with injection days.
- You will need regular blood tests to monitor your hemoglobin level.
- Your blood pressure will be monitored closely; if you are prescribed antihypertensive medications, it is important that you take them as prescribed.
- You may be asked to take iron supplements while using this drug.
- Be aware that there is an increased risk of heart attack, stroke, and blood clots while using this drug.
- You may experience these side effects: nausea, diarrhea (small frequent meals may help, consult with your health care provider if diarrhea is a problem); headache (analgesics may be available to help); dizziness (avoid driving a car or operating machinery until you know how this drug will affect you).
- Report chest pain, changes in strength, numbness or tingling, pain in the calf or leg, difficulty breathing, sudden changes in vision or balance, difficulty speaking, fainting.

▽ peginterferon alfa-2a

See Appendix R, *Less commonly used drugs*.

▽ peginterferon alfa-2b

See Appendix R, *Less commonly used drugs*.

▽ pegloticase

See Appendix R, *Less commonly used drugs*.

▽ pegvisomant

See Appendix R, *Less commonly used drugs*.

▽ pemetrexed

See Appendix R, *Less commonly used drugs*.

▽ penbutolol sulfate
*(pen **byoo**' toe lole)*

Levatol

PREGNANCY CATEGORY C

Drug classes
Antihypertensive
Beta-adrenergic blocker

Therapeutic actions
Competitively blocks beta-adrenergic receptors in the heart and juxtaglomerular apparatus, reducing the influence of the sympathetic nervous system on these tissues; decreasing the excitability of the heart, cardiac output, and release of renin; and lowering BP.

Indications
- Treatment of mild to moderate hypertension, alone or as part of combination therapy

Contraindications and cautions
- Contraindicated with sinus bradycardia, bronchial asthma, second- or third-degree heart block, cardiogenic shock, HF, lactation.
- Use cautiously with renal failure, diabetes or thyrotoxicosis, asthma, COPD, impaired hepatic function, pregnancy.

Available forms
Tablets—20 mg

Dosages
Adults
Usual starting dose, maintenance dose, and dose used in combination with other

antihypertensives: 20 mg PO daily. Doses of 40–80 mg daily have been used but with no additional antihypertensive effect.

Pediatric patients
Safety and efficacy not established.

Pharmacokinetics

Route	Onset	Peak	Duration
Oral	Varies	2–3 hr	20 hr

Metabolism: Hepatic; $T_{1/2}$: 5 hr
Distribution: Crosses placenta; enters breast milk
Excretion: Urine

Adverse effects

- **Allergic reactions:** Pharyngitis, erythematous rash, fever, sore throat, **laryngospasm,** respiratory distress
- **CNS:** Dizziness, vertigo, tinnitus, fatigue, emotional depression, paresthesias, sleep disturbances, hallucinations, disorientation, memory loss, slurred speech
- **CV:** *Bradycardia, HF, cardiac arrhythmias, sinoatrial or AV nodal block, tachycardia,* peripheral vascular insufficiency, claudication, **stroke, pulmonary edema,** hypotension
- **Dermatologic:** Rash, pruritus, sweating, dry skin
- **EENT:** Eye irritation, dry eyes, conjunctivitis, blurred vision
- **GI:** *Gastric pain, flatulence, constipation, diarrhea, nausea, vomiting,* anorexia, ischemic colitis, mesenteric arterial thrombosis, retroperitoneal fibrosis, hepatomegaly, acute hepatitis
- **GU:** *Impotence, decreased libido,* Peyronie disease, dysuria, nocturia, frequent urination, renal arterial thrombosis
- **Musculoskeletal:** Joint pain, arthralgia, muscle cramp
- **Respiratory: Bronchospasm,** dyspnea, cough, bronchial obstruction, nasal stuffiness, rhinitis, pharyngitis (less likely than with propranolol)
- **Other:** *Decreased exercise tolerance, development of ANA,* hyperglycemia or hypoglycemia, elevated serum transaminase, alkaline phosphatase, and LDH

Interactions

✳ **Drug-drug** • Increased effects and adverse effects with verapamil, other calcium channel blockers • Decreased effects with epinephrine • Increased risk of peripheral ischemia, even gangrene, with ergot alkaloids (dihydroergotamine, ergotamine) • Prolonged hypoglycemic effects of insulin • Increased first-dose response to prazosin • Paradoxic hypertension when clonidine is given with beta blockers; increased rebound hypertension when clonidine is discontinued in patients on beta blockers • Decreased hypertensive effect if given with NSAIDs (piroxicam, indomethacin, ibuprofen) • Decreased bronchodilator effects of theophylline and decreased bronchial and cardiac effects of sympathomimetics with penbutolol

✳ **Drug-lab test** • Possible false results with glucose or insulin tolerance tests

■ Nursing considerations
Assessment

- **History:** Sinus bradycardia, heart block, cardiogenic shock, HF, renal failure, diabetes or thyrotoxicosis, asthma or COPD, impaired hepatic function, lactation, pregnancy
- **Physical:** Weight, skin condition, neurologic status, P, BP, ECG, respiratory status, renal and thyroid function tests, blood and urine glucose

Interventions

- Give drug once a day. Monitor response and maintain at lowest possible dose.
- ⊗ **Warning** Do not discontinue drug abruptly after long-term therapy (hypersensitivity to catecholamines may have developed, causing exacerbation of angina, MI, and ventricular arrhythmias; taper drug gradually over 2 wk with monitoring).
- Consult surgeon about withdrawing drug if patient is to undergo surgery (withdrawal is controversial).

Teaching points

- Do not stop taking this drug unless instructed to do so by your health care provider.
- Avoid driving or dangerous activities if dizziness or drowsiness occurs.
- Report difficulty breathing, night cough, swelling of extremities, slow pulse, confusion, depression, rash, fever, sore throat.

▽ **penicillamine**

See Appendix R, *Less commonly used drugs.*

▷ penicillin G benzathine
(pen i sill' in)

Bicillin L-A, Permapen

PREGNANCY CATEGORY B

Drug classes
Antibiotic
Penicillin antibiotic

Therapeutic actions
Bactericidal: Inhibits synthesis of cell wall of sensitive organisms, causing cell death.

Indications
• Severe infections caused by sensitive organisms (streptococci)
• URI caused by sensitive streptococci
• Treatment of syphilis, bejel, congenital syphilis, pinta, yaws
• Prophylaxis of rheumatic fever and chorea

Contraindications and cautions
• Contraindicated with allergies to penicillins, cephalosporins, or other allergens.
• Use cautiously with renal disorders, pregnancy, lactation (may cause diarrhea or candidiasis in the infant).

Available forms
Injection—600,000, 1.2 million, 2.4 million units/dose

Dosages
Adults
• *Streptococcal infections (including otitis media, URIs of mild to moderate severity):* 1.2 million units IM as a single dose.
• *Early syphilis:* 2.4 million units IM as a single dose.
• *Syphilis lasting longer than 1 yr:* 7.2 million units given as 2.4 million units IM weekly for 3 wk.
• *Yaws, bejel, pinta:* 1.2 million units IM as a single dose.
• *Erysipeloid:* 1.2 million units IM as a single dose.
• *Prophylaxis of rheumatic fever or chorea:* 1.2 million units IM every month; alternatively, 600,000 units every 2 wk.

Pediatric patients
• *Streptococcal infections (including otitis media, URIs of mild to moderate severity):* Children weighing less than 60 lb: 300,000–600,000 units IM as a single injection. Older children: 900,000 units IM as a single injection.
• *Congenital syphilis: Children younger than 2 yr:* 50,000 units/kg body weight IM. *Children 2 to 12 yr:* Adjust dosage based on adult schedule.

Pharmacokinetics

Route	Onset	Peak	Duration
IM	Slow	12–24 hr	Days

Metabolism: Hepatic; $T_{1/2}$: 30–60 min
Distribution: Crosses placenta; enters breast milk
Excretion: Urine

Adverse effects
• **CNS:** Lethargy, hallucinations, seizures
• **GI:** *Glossitis, stomatitis, gastritis, sore mouth,* furry tongue, black "hairy" tongue, *nausea, vomiting, diarrhea,* abdominal pain, bloody diarrhea, enterocolitis, pseudomembranous colitis, nonspecific hepatitis
• **GU:** Nephritis
• **Hematologic:** Anemia, thrombocytopenia, leukopenia, neutropenia, prolonged bleeding time (more common than with other penicillinase-resistant penicillins)
• **Hypersensitivity:** *Rash, fever, wheezing,* **anaphylaxis**
• **Local:** *Pain, phlebitis,* thrombosis at injection site, Jarisch-Herxheimer reaction when used to treat syphilis
• **Other:** *Superinfections,* sodium overload, leading to heart failure

Interactions
✻ **Drug-drug** • Decreased effectiveness of penicillin G benzathine with tetracyclines • Inactivation of parenteral aminoglycosides (amikacin, gentamicin, kanamycin, neomycin, tobramycin); separate administration times

■ Nursing considerations
Assessment
• **History:** Allergies to penicillins, cephalosporins, other allergens; renal disorders; pregnancy, lactation

---

- **Physical:** Culture infection; skin color, lesions; R, adventitious sounds; bowel sounds: CBC, LFTs, renal function tests, serum electrolytes, Hct, urinalysis

Interventions

⊗ **Black box warning** Drug is not for IV use. Do not inject or admix with other IV solutions. Inadvertent IV administration has caused cardiorespiratory arrest and death.
- Culture infection before beginning treatment; reculture if response is not as expected.
- Give by IM route only.
- Continue therapy for at least 2 days after infection has disappeared, usually 7–10 days.
- Give IM injection in upper outer quadrant of the buttock. In infants and small children, the midlateral aspect of the thigh may be preferred.

Teaching points

- You will need to receive a full course of drug therapy.
- You may experience these side effects: Nausea, vomiting, diarrhea, mouth sores, pain at injection sites.
- Report difficulty breathing, rashes, severe diarrhea, severe pain at injection site, mouth sores, unusual bleeding or bruising.

▽**penicillin G potassium**
(pen i sill' in)

penicillin G potassium (aqueous)
Pfizerpen

penicillin G sodium
PREGNANCY CATEGORY B

Drug classes
Antibiotic
Penicillin antibiotic

Therapeutic actions
Bactericidal: Inhibits synthesis of cell wall of sensitive organisms, causing cell death.

Indications
- Treatment of severe infections caused by sensitive organisms—streptococci, pneumococci, staphylococci, *Neisseria gonorrhoeae, Treponema pallidum,* meningococci, *Actinomyces israelii, Clostridium perfringens* and *tetani, Leptotrichia buccalis* (Vincent disease), *Spirillum minus* or *Streptobacillus moniliformis, Listeria monocytogenes, Fusobacterium fusiformisans, Pasteurella multocida, Erysipelothrix insidiosa, Escherichia coli, Enterobacter aerogenes, Alcaligenes faecalis, Salmonella, Shigella, Proteus mirabilis, Corynebacterium diphtheriae, Bacillus anthracis*
- Treatment of syphilis, gonococcal infections
- Unlabeled use: Treatment of Lyme disease

Contraindications and cautions
- Contraindicated with allergy to penicillins, cephalosporins, imipenem, beta-lactamase inhibitors, other allergens.
- Use cautiously with renal disease, pregnancy, lactation (may cause diarrhea or candidiasis in the infant).

Available forms
Injection—1, 2, 3 million units/50 mL; powder for injection—5, 20 million units/vial

Dosages
Adults
- *Meningococcal meningitis:* 1–2 million units every 2 hr IM or by continuous IV infusion of 20–30 million units/day.
- *Actinomycosis:* 1–6 million units/day IM in divided doses every 4–6 hr for 6 wk or IV for cervicofacial cases; 10–20 million units/day IV for thoracic and abdominal diseases.
- *Clostridial infections:* 20 million units/day in divided doses every 4–6 hr IM or IV with antitoxin therapy.
- *Fusospirochetal infections (Vincent disease):* 5–10 million units/day IM or IV in divided doses every 4–6 hr.
- *Rat-bite fever:* 12–20 million units/day IM or IV in divided doses every 4–6 hr for 3–4 wk.
- *Listeria infections:* 15–20 million units/day IM or IV in divided doses every 4–6 hr for 2 or 4 wk (meningitis or endocarditis, respectively).
- *Pasteurella infections:* 4–6 million units/day IM or IV in divided doses every 4–6 hr for 2 wk.
- *Erysipeloid endocarditis:* 12–20 million units/day IM or IV in divided doses every 4–6 hr for 4–6 wk.

- *Diphtheria (adjunctive therapy with antitoxin to prevent carrier state):* 2–3 million units/day IM or IV in divided doses every 4–6 hr for 10–12 days.
- *Anthrax:* Minimum of 5 million units/day IM or IV in divided doses.
- *Serious streptococcal infections:* 5–24 million units/day in divided doses every 4–6 hr.
- *Syphilis:* 18–24 million units/day IV every 4–6 hr for 10–14 days followed by benzathine penicillin G 2.4 million units IM weekly for 3 wk.
- *Gonorrhea:* 10 million units/day IV every 4–6 hr until improvement occurs.

Pediatric patients
- *Meningitis:* 250,000 units/kg/day IM or IV in divided doses every 4 hr for 7–14 days.
- *Streptococcal infections:* 150,000 units/kg/day IV or IM every 4–6 hr.
  Infants older than 7 days: 75,000 units/kg/day IV in divided doses every 8 hr.
- *Meningitis:* 200,000–300,000 units/kg/day IV every 6 hr.
  Infants younger than 7 days: 50,000 units/kg/day IV in divided doses every 12 hr.
- *Group B streptococcus:* 100,000 units/kg/day IV.

Pharmacokinetics

Route	Onset	Peak
IM, IV	Rapid	15–30 min

Metabolism: Hepatic; $T_{1/2}$: 30–60 min
Distribution: Crosses placenta; enters breast milk
Excretion: Urine

▼ IV FACTS
Preparation: Prepare solution using sterile water for injection, isotonic sodium chloride injection, or 5% dextrose injection. Loosen powder in vial; reconstitute with vial held horizontally. Shake vigorously. Do not use with carbohydrate solutions at alkaline pH; do not refrigerate powder; sterile solution is stable for 1 wk refrigerated. IV solutions are stable at 24 hr at room temperature. Discard solution after 24 hr.
Infusion: Administer doses of 10–20 million units by slow infusion.
Incompatibilities: Do not mix with aminoglycosides, amphotericin B, bleomycin, chlorpromazine, cytarabine, hydroxyzine, methylprednisolone, prochlorperazine, promethazine.

Adverse effects
- **CNS:** Lethargy, hallucinations, seizures
- **GI:** *Glossitis, stomatitis, gastritis, sore mouth,* furry tongue, black "hairy" tongue, *nausea, vomiting, diarrhea,* abdominal pain, bloody diarrhea, enterocolitis, pseudomembranous colitis, nonspecific hepatitis
- **GU:** Nephritis—oliguria, proteinuria, hematuria, casts, azotemia, pyuria
- **Hematologic:** Anemia, thrombocytopenia, leukopenia, neutropenia, prolonged bleeding time
- **Hypersensitivity reactions:** *Rash, fever, wheezing,* anaphylaxis
- **Local:** *Pain, phlebitis,* thrombosis at injection site, Jarisch-Herxheimer reaction when used to treat syphilis
- **Other:** *Superinfections;* sodium overload, leading to HF

Interactions
✳ **Drug-drug** • Decreased effectiveness of penicillin G with tetracyclines • Inactivation of parenteral aminoglycosides (amikacin, gentamicin, kanamycin, neomycin, streptomycin, tobramycin); separate dosing times of combination is needed
✳ **Drug-lab test** • False-positive Coombs test (IV)

■ Nursing considerations
Assessment
- **History:** Allergy to penicillins, cephalosporins, imipenem, beta-lactamase inhibitors, other allergens, renal disease, lactation, pregnancy
- **Physical:** Culture infection; skin rashes, lesions; R, adventitious sounds; bowel sounds, normal output; CBC, LFTs, renal function tests, serum electrolytes, Hct, urinalysis; skin test with benzylpenicilloyl-polylysine if hypersensitivity reactions to penicillin have occurred

Interventions
- Culture infection before beginning treatment; reculture if response is not as expected.
- Use the smallest volume possible for IM injection to avoid pain and discomfort.
- Continue treatment for 48–72 hr after the patient is asymptomatic.
- ⊗ *Warning* Monitor serum electrolytes and cardiac status if penicillin G is given by IV infusion. Sodium or potassium preparations have been associated with severe electrolyte imbalances.

Adverse effects in *italics* are most common; those in **bold** are life-threatening. ⦿ Do not crush.

- Explain the reason for parenteral administration; offer support and encouragement to deal with therapy.
⊗ **Warning** Keep epinephrine, IV fluids, vasopressors, bronchodilators, oxygen, and emergency equipment readily available in case of serious hypersensitivity reaction.
- Arrange for corticosteroids or antihistamines for skin reactions.

Teaching points
- This drug must be given by injection for severe infections.
- You may experience these side effects: Upset stomach, nausea, vomiting (eat frequent small meals); sore mouth (frequent mouth care may help); diarrhea; pain or discomfort at the injection site.
- Report unusual bleeding, sore throat, rash, hives, fever, severe diarrhea, difficulty breathing.

▷**penicillin G procaine**
(penicillin G procaine,
aqueous, APPG)
(pen i sill' in)

Wycillin

PREGNANCY CATEGORY B

Drug classes
Antibiotic
Penicillin (long-acting, parenteral)

Therapeutic actions
Bactericidal: Inhibits cell wall synthesis of sensitive organisms, causing cell death.

Indications
- Treatment of moderately severe infections caused by sensitive organisms—streptococci, pneumococci, staphylococci, meningococci, *Actinomyces israelii, Clostridium perfringens* and *tetani, Leptotrichia buccalis* (Vincent disease), *Spirillum minus, Streptobacillus moniliformis, Listeria monocytogenes, Pasteurella multocida, Erysipelothrix insidiosa, Escherichia coli, Enterobacter aerogenes, Alcaligenes faecalis, Salmonella, Shigella, Proteus mirabilis, Corynebacterium diphtheriae, Bacillus anthracis*
- Treatment of specific STDs

Contraindications and cautions
- Contraindicated with allergies to penicillins, cephalosporins, procaine, or other allergens.
- Use cautiously with renal disorders, pregnancy, lactation (may cause diarrhea or candidiasis in the infant).

Available forms
Injection—600,000 units/dose, 1,200,000 units/dose

Dosages
Adults
- *Moderately severe infections caused by sensitive strains of streptococci, pneumococci, staphylococci:* Minimum of 600,000–1 million units/day IM for a minimum of 10 days.
- *Bacterial endocarditis (group A streptococci):* 600,000–1 million units/day IM.
- *Fusospirochetal infections:* 600,000–1 million units/day IM.
- *Rat-bite fever:* 600,000–1 million units/day IM.
- *Erysipeloid:* 600,000–1 million units/day IM.
- *Diphtheria:* 300,000–600,000 units/day IM with antitoxin.
- *Diphtheria carrier state:* 300,000 units/day IM for 10 days.
- *Anthrax:* 600,000–1 million units/day IM.
- *Syphilis (negative spinal fluid):* 600,000 units/day IM for 8 days.
- *Late syphilis:* 600,000 units/day IM for 10–15 days.
- *Neurosyphilis:* 2.4 million units/day IM with 500 mg probenecid PO qid for 10–14 days, followed by 2.4 million units IM benzathine penicillin G following completion of treatment regimen.

Pediatric patients
- *Congenital syphilis in patients weighing less than 32 kg:* 50,000 units/kg per day IM for 10 days.
- *Syphilis in children older than 12 yr:* 600,000 units/day IM for 8 days.
- *Group A streptococcal and staphylococcal pneumonia in patients weighing less than 27 kg:* 300,000 units/day/IM.

Pharmacokinetics

Route	Onset	Peak	Duration
IM	Varies	4 hr	15–20 hr

P

Metabolism: Hepatic; T$_{1/2}$: 30–60 min
Distribution: Crosses placenta; enters breast milk
Excretion: Urine

Adverse effects

- **CNS:** Lethargy, hallucinations, seizures
- **GI:** *Glossitis, stomatitis, gastritis, sore mouth,* furry tongue, black "hairy" tongue, *nausea, vomiting, diarrhea,* abdominal pain, bloody diarrhea, enterocolitis, pseudomembranous colitis, nonspecific hepatitis
- **GU:** Nephritis—oliguria, proteinuria, hematuria, casts, azotemia, pyuria
- **Hematologic:** Anemia, thrombocytopenia, leukopenia, neutropenia, prolonged bleeding time
- **Hypersensitivity:** *Rash, fever, wheezing,* **anaphylaxis**
- **Local:** *Pain, phlebitis,* thrombosis at injection site, Jarisch-Herxheimer reaction when used to treat syphilis
- **Other:** *Superinfections;* sodium overload, leading to HF

Interactions

✷ **Drug-drug** • Decreased effectiveness of penicillin G procaine with tetracyclines • Inactivation of parenteral aminoglycosides (amikacin, gentamicin, kanamycin, neomycin, streptomycin, tobramycin); separate dosing times if combination is needed

■ Nursing considerations
Assessment

- **History:** Allergies to penicillins, cephalosporins, procaine, other allergens, renal disorders, pregnancy, lactation
- **Physical:** Culture infection; skin color, lesions; R, adventitious sounds; bowel sounds; CBC, LFTs, renal function tests, serum electrolytes, Hct, urinalysis

Interventions

- Culture infection before beginning treatment; reculture if response is not as expected.
- Administer by IM route only.
- Continue therapy for at least 2 days after infection has disappeared, usually 7–10 days.
- Administer IM injection in upper outer quadrant of the buttock. In infants and small children, the midlateral aspect of the thigh may be preferred.

Teaching points

- This drug can be given only by IM injection.
- You may experience these side effects: Nausea, vomiting, diarrhea, mouth sores, pain at injection sites.
- Report difficulty breathing, rashes, severe diarrhea, severe pain at injection site, mouth sores, unusual bleeding or bruising.

▽ **penicillin V**
(penicillin V potassium)
(pen i sill' in)

Apo-Pen-VK (CAN),
Nu-Pen-VK (CAN)

PREGNANCY CATEGORY B

Drug classes
Antibiotic
Penicillin (acid stable)

Therapeutic actions
Bactericidal: Inhibits cell wall synthesis of sensitive organisms, causing cell death.

Indications

- Mild to moderately severe infections caused by sensitive organisms—streptococci, pneumococci, staphylococci, fusospirochetes
- Unlabeled uses: Prophylactic treatment of children with sickle cell anemia, actinomycosis, Lyme disease, postexposure anthrax prophylaxis

Contraindications and cautions

- Contraindicated with allergies to penicillins, cephalosporins, or other allergens.
- Use cautiously with renal disorders, pregnancy, lactation (may cause diarrhea or candidiasis in the infant).

Available forms
Tablets—250, 300, 500 mg; powder for oral solution—125, 250, 300 mg/5 mL

Dosages
Adults and patients older than 12 yr

- *Fusospirochetal infections:* 250–500 mg every 6–8 hr PO.
- *Streptococcal infections (including otitis media, URIs of mild to moderate severity,*

scarlet fever, erysipelas): 125–250 mg every 6–8 hr PO for 10 days.

- *Pneumococcal infections:* 250–500 mg every 6 hr PO until afebrile for 48 hr.
- *Staphylococcal infections of skin and soft tissues:* 250–500 mg every 6–8 hr PO.
- *Prevention of recurrence of rheumatic fever/chorea:* 125–250 mg twice daily.
- *Lyme disease:* 500 mg PO qid for 10–20 days.
- *Mild, uncomplicated cutaneous anthrax:* 200–500 mg PO qid.

Adults and patients older than 9 yr
- *Anthrax prophylaxis:* 7.5 mg/kg PO qid.

Pediatric patients younger than 12 yr
15–62.5 mg/kg/day PO given every 6–8 hr. Calculate doses according to weight.
- *Sickle cell anemia as prophylaxis of* S. pneumoniae *septicemia:* 250 mg PO bid; 3 mo–5 yr: 125 mg PO bid.
- *Mild, uncomplicated cutaneous anthrax in children older than 2 yr:* 25–50 mg/kg PO daily in two or four divided doses.

Pediatric patients younger than 9 yr
- *Anthrax prophylaxis:* 50 mg/kg/day PO in four divided doses.

Pharmacokinetics

Route	Onset	Peak
Oral	Varies	60 min

Metabolism: Hepatic; $T_{1/2}$: 30 min
Distribution: Crosses placenta; enters breast milk
Excretion: Urine

Adverse effects

- **CNS:** Lethargy, hallucinations, seizures
- **GI:** *Glossitis, stomatitis, gastritis, sore mouth,* furry tongue, black "hairy" tongue, *nausea, vomiting, diarrhea,* abdominal pain, bloody diarrhea, enterocolitis, pseudomembranous colitis, nonspecific hepatitis
- **GU:** Nephritis—oliguria, proteinuria, hematuria, casts, azotemia, pyuria
- **Hematologic:** Anemia, thrombocytopenia, leukopenia, neutropenia, prolonged bleeding time
- **Hypersensitivity reactions:** *Rash, fever, wheezing,* **anaphylaxis** (sometimes fatal)
- **Other:** *Superinfections;* sodium overload leading to HF; potassium poisoning— hyper-reflexia, coma, cardiac arrhythmias, **cardiac arrest** (potassium preparations)

Interactions

✳ **Drug-drug** • Decreased effectiveness with tetracyclines

■ Nursing considerations

Assessment

- **History:** Allergies to penicillins, cephalosporins, or other allergens; renal disorders; pregnancy; lactation
- **Physical:** Culture infection; skin color, lesions; R, adventitious sounds; bowel sounds; CBC, LFTs, renal function tests, serum electrolytes, Hct, urinalysis

Interventions

- Culture infection before beginning treatment; reculture if response is not as expected.
- Continue therapy for at least 2 days after infection has disappeared, usually 7–10 days.
- Do not administer oral drug with milk, fruit juices, or soft drinks; a full glass of water is preferred; this oral penicillin is less affected by food than other penicillins.

Teaching points

- Refrigerate suspension after reconstitution; stable for up to a maximum of 14 days.
- Avoid self-treating other infections with this antibiotic because it is specific for the infection being treated. Complete the full course of drug therapy.
- Take drug with water; do not take with milk, fruit juice, or soft drinks.
- You may experience these side effects: Nausea, vomiting, diarrhea, mouth sores.
- Report difficulty breathing, rashes, severe diarrhea, mouth sores, unusual bleeding, or bruising.

▽**pentamidine isethionate**
(pen ta' ma deen ess thye' oh nate)

Parenteral: Pentacarinat, Pentam 300
Inhalation: NebuPent

PREGNANCY CATEGORY C

Drug class
Antiprotozoal

Therapeutic actions

Antiprotozoal activity in susceptible *Pneumocystis jiroveci* pneumonia infections; mechanism of action is not fully understood, but the drug interferes with nuclear metabolism and inhibits the synthesis of DNA, RNA, phospholipids, and proteins, which lead to cell death.

Indications

- Treatment of *P. jiroveci* pneumonia, especially in patients who do not respond to therapy with the less toxic trimethoprim-sulfamethoxazole combination (injection)
- Inhalation: Prevention of *P. jiroveci* pneumonia in high-risk, HIV-infected patients
- Unlabeled use (injection): Treatment of trypanosomiasis, visceral leishmaniasis

Contraindications and cautions

If the diagnosis of *P. jiroveci* pneumonia has been confirmed, there are no absolute contraindications to the use of this drug.

- Contraindicated with history of anaphylactic reaction to inhaled or parenteral pentamidine isethionate (inhalation therapy), lactation.
- Use cautiously with hypotension, hypertension, hypoglycemia, hyperglycemia, hypocalcemia, leukopenia, thrombocytopenia, anemia, asthma, QT-interval prolongation, hepatic or renal impairment, pregnancy.

Available forms

Injection—300 mg/vial; powder for injection—300 mg; aerosol—300 mg

Dosages

Adults and pediatric patients

Parenteral

4 mg/kg once a day for 14–21 days by deep IM injection or IV infusion over 60–120 min.

Inhalation

300 mg once every 4 wk administered through the *Respirgard II* nebulizer.

Pharmacokinetics

Route	Onset
IM	Slow
Inhalation	Rapid

Metabolism: $T_{1/2}$: 6.4–9.4 hr
Distribution: Crosses placenta; enters breast milk
Excretion: Urine

▼ IV FACTS

Preparation: Prepare solution by dissolving contents of 1 vial in 3–5 mL of sterile water for injection or 5% dextrose injection; do not use saline for reconstitution. Dilute the calculated dose further in 50–250 mL of 5% dextrose solution; solutions of 1 and 2.5 mg/mL in 5% dextrose are stable at room temperature for up to 24 hr. Protect from light.
Infusion: Infuse the diluted solution over 60–120 min.
Y-site incompatibility: Do not mix with foscarnet or fluconazole.

Adverse effects

Parenteral

- **CV:** *Hypotension,* tachycardia
- **GI:** *Nausea, anorexia*
- **GU:** *Elevated serum creatinine,* **acute renal failure**
- **Hematologic:** *Leukopenia, hypoglycemia,* thrombocytopenia, hypocalcemia, elevated LFTs
- **Local:** *Pain, abscess at injection site*
- **Other:** **Stevens-Johnson syndrome,** *fever, rash,* **severe hypotension,** hypoglycemia, and cardiac arrhythmias

Inhalation

- **CNS:** *Fatigue, dizziness,* headache, tremors, confusion, anxiety, memory loss, seizures, insomnia, drowsiness
- **CV:** Tachycardia, hypotension, hypertension, palpitations, syncope, vasodilation
- **GI:** *Metallic taste in mouth, anorexia, nausea, vomiting,* gingivitis, dyspepsia, oral ulcer, gastritis, hypersalivation, dry mouth, melena, colitis, abdominal pain
- **Respiratory:** *Shortness of breath, cough, pharyngitis, congestion,* **bronchospasm,** rhinitis, laryngitis, **laryngospasm,** hyperventilation, pneumothorax
- **Other:** *Rash, night sweats, chills*

■ Nursing considerations

Assessment

- **History:** History of anaphylactic reaction to inhaled or parenteral pentamidine isethionate, hypotension, hypertension, hypoglycemia, hyperglycemia, hypocalcemia, leukopenia, thrombocytopenia, anemia, hepatic or renal impairment, pregnancy, lactation
- **Physical:** Skin lesions, color; T; reflexes, affect (inhalation); BP, P, baseline ECG; BUN,

serum creatinine, blood glucose, CBC, platelet count, LFTs, serum calcium

Interventions

- Culture before use to ensure appropriate use of drug.
- Follow safe-handling procedures; this drug is a known biohazard agent.

⊗ **Warning** Monitor patient closely during administration; fatalities have been reported.

- Arrange for these tests to be performed before, during, and after therapy: Daily BUN, daily serum creatinine, daily blood glucose; regular CBC, platelet counts, LFTs, serum calcium; periodic ECG.

⊗ **Warning** Position patient in supine position before parenteral administration to protect patient if BP changes.

- Reconstitute for inhalation: Dissolve contents of 1 vial in 6 mL of sterile water for injection. Use only sterile water. Saline cannot be used, precipitates will form. Place entire solution in nebulizer reservoir. Solution is stable for 48 hr in original vial at room temperature if protected from light. Do not mix with other drugs.
- Administer inhalation using the *Respirgard II* nebulizer. Deliver the dose using a flow rate of 5–7 L/min and an air or oxygen source set at 40–50 PSI until the chamber is empty (30–45 min).
- For IM use: Prepare IM solution by dissolving contents of 1-g vial in 3 mL of sterile water for injection; protect from light. Discard any unused portions. Inject deeply into large muscle group. Inspect injection site regularly; rotate injection sites.
- Instruct patient and significant other in the reconstitution of inhalation solutions and administration for outpatient use.

Teaching points

- Parenteral drug can be given only IV or IM and must be given every day. Inhalation drug must be given using the *Respirgard II* nebulizer. Prepare the solution as instructed by your health care provider, using only sterile water for injection. Protect the medication from exposure to light. Use freshly reconstituted solution. The drug must be used once every 4 weeks. Prepare a calendar with drug days marked as a reminder. Do not mix any other drugs in the nebulizer.

- Have frequent blood tests and blood pressure checks because this drug may cause many changes in your body.
- You may feel weak and dizzy with sudden position changes; take care to change position slowly.
- If using the inhalation, metallic taste and GI upset may occur. Frequent small meals and mouth care may help.
- Report pain at injection site, confusion, hallucinations, unusual bleeding or bruising, weakness, fatigue.

DANGEROUS DRUG

▷ pentazocine
(pen taz' oh seen)

pentazocine hydrochloride with naloxone hydrochloride, 0.5 mg

pentazocine lactate
Parenteral: Talwin

PREGNANCY CATEGORY C

CONTROLLED SUBSTANCE C-IV

Drug class
Opioid agonist-antagonist analgesic

Therapeutic actions
Pentazocine acts as an agonist at specific (kappa) opioid receptors in the CNS to produce analgesia, sedation; acts as an agonist at sigma opioid receptors to cause dysphoria, hallucinations; acts at mu opioid receptors to antagonize the analgesic and euphoric activities of some other opioid analgesics. Has lower abuse potential than morphine, other pure opioid agonists; the oral preparation contains the opioid antagonist naloxone, which has poor bioavailability when given orally and does not interfere with the analgesic effects of pentazocine but serves as a deterrent to the unintended IV injection of solutions made from the oral tablets.

Indications
- Relief of moderate to severe pain
- Preanesthetic medication and as supplement to surgical anesthesia

Contraindications and cautions

- Contraindicated with hypersensitivity to opioids, sulfites (oral and parenteral), naloxone (oral form); pregnancy (neonatal withdrawal); lactation.
- Use cautiously with physical dependence on an opioid analgesic (can precipitate a withdrawal syndrome); bronchial asthma, COPD, cor pulmonale, respiratory depression, anoxia, increased intracranial pressure; acute MI with hypertension, left ventricular failure or nausea and vomiting; renal or hepatic impairment; labor or delivery (opioids given to the mother can cause neonatal respiratory depression; premature infants are especially at risk; may prolong labor).

Available forms

Injection—30 mg/mL; tablets—50 mg with naloxane 0.5 mg

Dosages
Adults
Oral

Initially, 50 mg every 3–4 hr. Increase to 100 mg if needed. Do not exceed a total dose of 600 mg/24 hr.

Parenteral

30 mg IM, subcutaneously, or IV. May repeat every 3–4 hr. Doses exceeding 30 mg IV or 60 mg IM or subcutaneously are not recommended. Do not exceed 360 mg/24 hr. Give subcutaneously only when necessary; repeat injections should be given IM.

- *Patients in labor:* A single 30-mg IM dose is most common. A 20-mg IV dose given 2–3 times at 2- to 3-hr intervals relieves pain when contractions become regular.

Pediatric patients younger than 12 yr

Not recommended.

Geriatric patients or impaired adults

Use caution; respiratory depression may occur in the very ill, and those with respiratory problems. Dosage may need to be reduced. Avoid long-term use for pain due to risk of falls, fractures, confusion, dependency, and withdrawal.

Pharmacokinetics

Route	Onset	Peak	Duration
Oral, IM, Subcut.	15–30 min	1–3 hr	3 hr
IV	2–3 min	15 min	3 hr

Metabolism: Hepatic; $T_{1/2}$: 2–3 hr
Distribution: Crosses placenta; enters breast milk
Excretion: Feces, urine

▼ IV FACTS

Preparation: No further preparation is required.
Infusion: Inject directly into vein or into tubing of actively running IV; infuse slowly, each 5 mg over 1 min.
Incompatibilities: Do not mix in same syringe as barbiturates; precipitate will form.

Adverse effects

- **CNS:** *Light-headedness, dizziness, sedation, euphoria,* dysphoria, delirium, insomnia, agitation, anxiety, fear, hallucinations, disorientation, drowsiness, lethargy, impaired mental and physical performance, coma, mood changes, weakness, headache, tremor, seizures, miosis, visual disturbances
- **CV:** Facial flushing, peripheral circulatory collapse, tachycardia, bradycardia, arrhythmia, palpitations, chest wall rigidity, hypertension, hypotension, orthostatic hypotension, syncope, circulatory depression, **shock, cardiac arrest**
- **Dermatologic:** Pruritus, urticaria, edema
- **GI:** *Nausea, vomiting, sweating* (more common in ambulatory patients and those without severe pain), dry mouth, anorexia, constipation, biliary tract spasm; increased colonic motility in patients with chronic ulcerative colitis
- **GU:** Ureteral spasm, spasm of vesical sphincters, urinary retention or hesitancy, oliguria, antidiuretic effect, reduced libido or potency
- **Local:** Pain at injection site, tissue irritation and induration (subcutaneous injection)
- **Respiratory:** Suppression of cough reflex, respiratory depression, apnea, respiratory arrest, **laryngospasm, bronchospasm**
- **Other:** Physical tolerance and dependence, psychological dependence (**the oral form has been especially abused in combination with tripelennamine—"Ts and Blues"—with serious and fatal consequences;** addition of naloxone to oral formulation may decrease this abuse)

Interactions
✳ **Drug-drug** • Increased likelihood of respiratory depression, hypotension, profound sedation, or coma with barbiturate general anesthetics
• Precipitation of withdrawal syndrome in patients previously given other opioid analgesics, including morphine, methadone (note that this applies to the parenteral preparation without naloxone and to the oral preparation that includes naloxone)

■ Nursing considerations
Assessment
• **History:** Hypersensitivity to opioids, naloxone (oral form), sulfites (oral and parenteral); physical dependence on an opioid analgesic; pregnancy; labor or delivery; lactation; respiratory disease; anoxia; increased intracranial pressure; acute MI; renal or hepatic impairment
• **Physical:** T; skin color, texture, lesions; orientation, reflexes, bilateral grip strength, affect, pupil size; P, auscultation, BP, orthostatic BP, perfusion; R, adventitious sounds; bowel sounds, normal output; frequency and pattern of voiding, normal output; LFTs, renal function tests, CBC with differential

Interventions
⊗ **Black box warning** Be aware that pentazocine/naloxone combination is for oral use only; drug can be lethal if injected.
• Do not mix parenteral pentazocine in same syringe as barbiturates; precipitate will form.
⊗ *Warning* Keep opioid antagonist, equipment for assisted or controlled respiration readily available during parenteral administration.
⊗ *Warning* Use caution when injecting subcutaneously into chilled areas of the body or in patients with hypotension or in shock; impaired perfusion may delay absorption; with repeated doses, an excessive amount may be absorbed when circulation is restored.
⊗ *Warning* Withdraw drug gradually if it has been given for 4 or 5 days, especially to emotionally unstable patients or those with a history of drug abuse; a withdrawal syndrome sometimes occurs in these circumstances.
• Reassure patient that addiction is unlikely; most patients who receive opiates for medical reasons do not develop dependence syndromes.

Teaching points
• Take drug exactly as prescribed.
• Avoid alcohol, antihistamines, sedatives, tranquilizers, and over-the-counter drugs while taking this drug.
• Do not take any leftover medication for other disorders, and do not let anyone else take the prescription.
• You may experience these side effects: Nausea, loss of appetite (take drug with food, lie quietly, eat frequent small meals); constipation (a laxative may help); dizziness, sedation, drowsiness, impaired visual acuity (avoid driving or performing other tasks that require alertness, visual acuity).
• Report severe nausea, vomiting, constipation, shortness of breath or difficulty breathing.

▷**pentetate calcium trisodium (Ca-DTPA), pentetate zinc trisodium (Zn-DTPA)**
See Appendix R, *Less commonly used drugs*.

DANGEROUS DRUG
▷**pentobarbital, pentobarbital sodium**
(pen toe bar' bi tal)
Nembutal
PREGNANCY CATEGORY D
CONTROLLED SUBSTANCE C-II

Drug classes
Antiepileptic
Barbiturate
Hypnotic
Sedative or hypnotic

Therapeutic actions
General CNS depressant; barbiturates inhibit impulse conduction in the ascending RAS, depress the cerebral cortex, alter cerebellar function, depress motor output, and can produce excitation, sedation, hypnosis, anesthesia, and deep coma; at anesthetic doses, has antiseizure activity.

Indications
• Sedative/hypnotic
• Preanesthetic in pediatric patients

- Antiepileptic, in anesthetic doses, for emergency control of certain acute seizure episodes (eg, status epilepticus, eclampsia, meningitis, tetanus, toxic reactions to strychnine or local anesthetics)

Contraindications and cautions

- Contraindicated with hypersensitivity to barbiturates, manifest or latent porphyria, marked liver impairment, nephritis, severe respiratory distress, previous addiction to sedative-hypnotic drugs, pregnancy (fetal damage, neonatal withdrawal syndrome), lactation.
- Use cautiously with acute or chronic pain (paradoxical excitement or masking of important symptoms), seizure disorders (abrupt discontinuation of daily doses can result in status epilepticus), fever, hyperthyroidism, diabetes mellitus, severe anemia, pulmonary or cardiac disease, status asthmaticus, shock, uremia.

Available forms

Injection—50 mg/mL

Dosages

Adults

Use only when prompt action is imperative.
IV: Give by slow IV injection, not to exceed 50 mg/min. Initial dose is 100 mg in a 70-kg adult. Wait at least 1 min for full effect. Base dosage on response. Additional small increments may be given up to a total of 200–500 mg. Minimize dosage in seizure states to avoid compounding the depression that may follow seizures.
IM: Inject deeply into a muscle mass. Usual adult dose is 150–200 mg. Do not exceed a volume of 5 mL at any site due to tissue irritation.

Pediatric patients

Use caution; barbiturates may produce irritability, aggression, inappropriate tearfulness.
IV: Reduce initial adult dosage on basis of age, weight, and patient's condition.
IM: Dosage frequently ranges from 25–80 mg or 2–6 mg/kg. Do not exceed 100 mg.

Geriatric patients or patients with debilitating disease

Reduce dosage and monitor closely. May produce excitement, depression, or confusion.

Pharmacokinetics

Route	Onset	Duration
IM, IV	Rapid	2–3 hr

Metabolism: Hepatic; $T_{1/2}$: 15–50 hr
Distribution: Crosses placenta; enters breast milk
Excretion: Urine

▼ IV FACTS

Preparation: No further preparation is required.
Infusion: Infuse slowly, each 50 mg over 1 min; monitor patient response to dosage.
Incompatibilities: Do not combine with chlorpheniramine, codeine, ephedrine, erythromycin, hydrocortisone, insulin, norepinephrine, penicillin G, potassium, phenytoin, vancomycin.

Adverse effects

- **CNS:** *Somnolence, agitation, confusion, hyperkinesia, ataxia, vertigo, CNS depression, nightmares, lethargy, residual sedation (hangover), paradoxic excitement, nervousness, psychiatric disturbance, hallucinations, insomnia, anxiety, dizziness, thinking abnormality*
- **CV:** *Bradycardia, hypotension, syncope*
- **GI:** *Nausea, vomiting, constipation, diarrhea, epigastric pain*
- **Hypersensitivity:** Rashes, angioneurotic edema, serum sickness, morbiliform rash, urticaria; rarely, exfoliative dermatitis, **Stevens-Johnson syndrome**
- **Local:** *Pain, tissue necrosis at injection site*; gangrene; arterial spasm with inadvertent intra-arterial injection; thrombophlebitis; permanent neurologic deficit if injected near a nerve
- **Respiratory:** *Hypoventilation, apnea, respiratory depression*, **laryngospasm, bronchospasm, circulatory collapse**
- **Other:** Tolerance, psychological and physical dependence; **withdrawal syndrome**

Interactions

✳ **Drug-drug** • Increased CNS depression with alcohol or other CNS depressants • Decreased effects of these drugs: Oral anticoagulants, corticosteroids, hormonal contraceptives and estrogens, beta-adrenergic blockers (especially propranolol, metoprolol), theophylline, metronidazole, doxycycline, phenylbutazones, quinidine

■ Nursing considerations

Assessment

- **History:** Hypersensitivity to barbiturates, manifest or latent porphyria, marked liver impairment, nephritis, severe respiratory distress, previous addiction to sedative-hypnotic drugs, acute or chronic pain, seizure disorders, pregnancy, lactation, fever, hyperthyroidism, diabetes mellitus, severe anemia, pulmonary or cardiac disease, shock, uremia
- **Physical:** Weight; T; skin color, lesions, injection site; orientation, affect, reflexes; P, BP, orthostatic BP; R, adventitious sounds; bowel sounds, normal output, liver evaluation; LFTs, renal function tests, blood and urine glucose, BUN

Interventions

⊗ **Warning** Do not administer intra-arterially; may produce arteriospasm, thrombosis, or gangrene.

- Administer IV doses slowly.
- Administer IM doses deep in a muscle mass.

⊗ **Warning** Do not use parenteral form if solution is discolored or contains a precipitate.

⊗ **Warning** Monitor injection sites carefully for irritation and extravasation (IV use); solutions are alkaline and very irritating to the tissues.

- Monitor P, BP, and respiration carefully during IV administration.

⊗ **Warning** Taper dosage gradually after repeated use, especially in patients with epilepsy.

Teaching points

- This drug will make you drowsy and less anxious.
- Do not try to get up after you have received this drug (request assistance to sit up or move about).

▽ pentosan polysulfate sodium

See Appendix R, *Less commonly used drugs*.

▽ pentostatin (2′ deoxycoformycin [DCF])

See Appendix R, *Less commonly used drugs*.

▽ pentoxifylline
*(pen tox **ib'** fi leen)*

Apo-Pentoxifilline SR (CAN) ⊞,
Nu-Pentoxifylline SR (CAN) ⊞,
ratio-Pentoxifylline (CAN), Trental ⊞

PREGNANCY CATEGORY C

Drug classes
Hemorrheologic drug
Xanthine

Therapeutic actions
Reduces RBC aggregation and local hyperviscosity, decreases platelet aggregation, decreases fibrinogen concentration in the blood; precise mechanism of action is not known.

Indications
- Intermittent claudication, to improve function and symptoms
- Unlabeled uses: Cerebrovascular insufficiency to improve psychopathologic symptoms, diabetic vascular disease, aphthous stomatitis

Contraindications and cautions
- Contraindicated with allergy to pentoxifylline or methylxanthines (eg, caffeine, theophylline; drug is a dimethylxanthine derivative); recent cerebral or retinal hemorrhage.
- Use cautiously with pregnancy, lactation.

Available forms
ER tablets ⊞—400 mg

Dosages

Adults
400 mg tid PO with meals. Decrease to 400 mg bid if adverse side effects occur. Continue for at least 8 wk.

Pediatric patients
Safety and efficacy not established.

Patients with renal impairment
If creatinine clearance is more than 50 mL/min, give usual dosage every 8–12 hr; if creatinine clearance is 10–50 mL/min, give usual dosage every 12–24 hr; if creatinine clearance is less than 10 mL/min, give usual dosage every 24 hr.

Pharmacokinetics

Route	Onset	Peak
Oral	Varies	60 min

P

Metabolism: Hepatic; $T_{1/2}$: 0.4–1.6 hr
Distribution: Crosses placenta; enters breast milk
Excretion: Urine

Adverse effects

- **CNS:** *Dizziness, headache,* tremor, anxiety, confusion
- **CV:** Angina, chest pain, arrhythmia, hypotension, dyspnea
- **Dermatologic:** Brittle fingernails, pruritus, rash, urticaria
- **GI:** *Dyspepsia, nausea,* vomiting
- **Hematologic:** Pancytopenia, purpura, thrombocytopenia

Interactions

✳ **Drug-drug** • Increased therapeutic and toxic effects of theophylline when combined; monitor closely and adjust dosage as needed
• Increased risk of bleeding in patients receiving oral anticoagulants; monitor patient closely, with frequent PT, if combination is used

■ Nursing considerations
Assessment

- **History:** Allergy to pentoxifylline or methylxanthines, pregnancy, lactation
- **Physical:** Skin color, T; orientation, reflexes; P, BP, peripheral perfusion; CBC

Interventions

- Monitor patient for angina and arrhythmias.
- Administer drug with meals.
- Caution patient to swallow tablets whole and not to cut, crush, or chew them.

Teaching points

- Take drug with meals. Swallow tablets whole; do not cut, crush, or chew.
- This drug helps the signs and symptoms of claudication, but additional therapy is sometimes needed.
- Dizziness may occur as a result of therapy; avoid driving and operating dangerous machinery; take precautions to prevent injury.
- Report chest pain, flushing, loss of consciousness, twitching, numbness, and tingling.

▷ **perampanel**
(*per am' pah nel*)

Fycompa

PREGNANCY CATEGORY C

CONTROLLED SUBSTANCE - TBA?

Drug classes
Antiepileptic
Glutamate receptor antagonist

Therapeutic actions
Noncompetitive glutamate receptor antagonist; glutamate is a primary excitatory neurotransmitter; precise mechanism of antiepileptic effect is not understood.

Indications
- Adjunct treatment of partial-onset seizures with or without secondary generalized seizures in patients 12 yr and older with epilepsy

Contraindications and cautions
- Contraindicated with known allergy to components of drug, severe hepatic or renal impairment, concurrent use of strong CYP3A inducers.
- Use cautiously with mild to moderate hepatic impairment, concurrent use of other antiepileptics, pregnancy, lactation.

Available forms
Tablets—2, 4, 6, 8, 10, 12 mg

Dosages
Adults and children 12 yr and older
Starting dose, 2 mg/day PO at bedtime, 4 mg/day PO at bedtime if also taking other enzyme-inducing antiepileptics. May increase by maximum 2 mg/day at weekly intervals to maximum dose of 12 mg/day PO at bedtime.
Patients with mild to moderate hepatic impairment
Maximum daily dose is 6 mg/day PO at bedtime for mild impairment, 4 mg/day PO at bedtime for moderate impairment.
Patients with severe hepatic or renal impairment, patients on dialysis
Not recommended.

Pharmacokinetics

Route	Onset	Peak
Oral	Rapid	0.5–2.5 hr

Metabolism: Hepatic; T$_{1/2}$: 105 hr
Distribution: May cross placenta; may enter breast milk
Excretion: Feces, urine

Adverse effects

- **CNS: Suicidality, serious psychiatric and behavioral reactions,** *dizziness, gait disturbances, somnolence, fatigue, balance disorders, vertigo, ataxia, irritability*
- **GI:** *Nausea, weight gain,* vomiting, diarrhea
- **Respiratory:** Cough, URI
- **Other:** *Falls,* back pain, musculoskeletal pain

Interactions

✳ **Drug-drug** ● Increased toxicity if combined with alcohol or other CNS depressants ● Potential loss of effectiveness of hormonal contraceptives; suggest use of alternative form of contraception ● Decreased effectiveness of perampanel if combined with carbamazepine, phenytoin, oxcarbazepine; increase starting dose of perampanel and monitor patient closely ● Loss of effectiveness if combined with rifampin; avoid this combination

✳ **Drug-alternative therapy** ● Loss of effectiveness if combined with St. John's Wort, rifampin; avoid this combination

■ Nursing considerations
Assessment

- **History:** Hypersensitivity to components of drug, hepatic or renal disease, pregnancy, lactation
- **Physical:** Orientation, affect, reflexes, gait, behavioral profile, LFTs, renal function tests

Interventions

⊗ **Black box warning** Risk of serious to life-threatening psychiatric and behavioral adverse reactions, including aggression, hostility, anger, and homicidal ideation and threats. Monitor patient closely, especially when starting drug or changing dosage. Reduce dosage if symptoms occur; discontinue if symptoms are severe or worsening.

- Taper gradually after long-term use; there is risk of seizures with rapid dosage reduction.
- Increase dosage carefully and monitor patient closely with dosage change.

- Monitor patient for signs and symptoms of suicidality.
- Advise women of childbearing age to avoid pregnancy; effects on the fetus are unknown.
- Protect patient from falls; serious injury could occur.
- Advise patient to avoid driving and operating dangerous machinery if neurologic effects occur.

Teaching points

- Take drug once a day at bedtime. If you forget a dose, consult your health care provider. Do not double up doses.
- Do not stop taking drug suddenly; make sure you have a supply on hand. Suddenly stopping drug can cause seizures.
- It is not known if drug could cause harm to a fetus if taken during pregnancy. This drug may make hormonal contraceptives ineffective; use of barrier contraceptives is advised. If you are pregnant or thinking about becoming pregnant, discuss this with your health care provider.
- This drug may appear in breast milk; if you are breast-feeding, you will need to find another method of feeding the baby.
- This drug is a controlled substance and can lead to addiction or dependence; make sure you secure the drug to prevent abuse or misuse.
- Do not drink alcohol while taking this drug because increased sedation and dizziness may occur.
- Avoid St. John's Wort while taking this drug.
- This drug can cause increased thoughts of suicide; report thoughts of suicide or worsening depression.
- This drug can cause changes in behavior, including aggression and hostility. Alert your significant others that this can occur and encourage them to report any changes to your health care provider.
- This drug can cause falls that could result in serious injury due to changes in balance or stability. Take precautions to ensure safety.
- You may experience these side effects: Dizziness, sleepiness, slowed thinking (do not drive or operate hazardous machinery if these effects occur); back pain, muscle aches and pains (medication may be available to help; consult your health care provider).
- Report changes in behavior, thoughts of suicide, falls, severe dizziness, trouble walking.

▷ perindopril erbumine
(pur in' doh pril)

Aceon, APO-Perindopril (CAN)

PREGNANCY CATEGORY C
(FIRST TRIMESTER)

PREGNANCY CATEGORY D
(SECOND AND THIRD TRIMESTERS)

Drug classes
ACE inhibitor
Antihypertensive

Therapeutic actions
Renin, synthesized by the kidneys, is released into the circulation where it acts on a plasma precursor to produce angiotensin I, which is converted by ACE to angiotensin II—a potent vasoconstrictor that also causes release of aldosterone from the adrenals. Perindopril blocks the conversion of angiotensin I to angiotensin II, leading to decreased BP, decreased aldosterone secretion, a small increase in serum potassium levels, and sodium and fluid loss.

Indications
- Treatment of hypertension, alone or in combination with other antihypertensive
- Treatment of patients with stable coronary artery disease to reduce the risk of CV mortality and nonfatal MI

Contraindications and cautions
- Contraindicated with allergy to any ACE inhibitor, pregnancy, history of ACE inhibitors–associated angioedema.
- Use cautiously with impaired renal function, HF, salt or volume depletion, lactation.

Available forms
Tablets—2, 4, 8 mg

Dosages
Adults
- *Hypertension:* 4 mg PO daily; may be titrated to a maximum of 16 mg/day.
- *CV disease:* 4 mg/day PO for 2 wk; increase to a maintenance dose of 8 mg/day PO.

Pediatric patients
Safety and efficacy not established.

Geriatric patients
Maximum daily dosage should not exceed 8 mg/day.

Geriatric patients older than 70 yr with stable CV disease
2 mg/day PO for first wk; increase to 4 mg/day PO for second wk. Maintenance dose is 8 mg/day PO.

Patients with renal impairment
For creatinine clearance greater than 30 mL/min, give initial dose of 2 mg/day PO. Maximum dose, 8 mg/day. For creatinine clearance of 30 mL/min or less, do not administer drug.

Pharmacokinetics

Route	Onset	Peak
Oral	1 hr	3–7 hr

Metabolism: Hepatic; $T_{1/2}$: 30–120 hr
Distribution: Crosses placenta; enters breast milk
Excretion: Urine

Adverse effects
- **CNS:** *Headache, dizziness, insomnia, fatigue,* paresthesias
- **CV:** *Orthostatic hypotension,* tachycardia, angina pectoris, MI, Raynaud syndrome, HF (severe hypotension in salt- or volume-depleted patients)
- **GI:** *Gastric irritation, nausea, diarrhea,* aphthous ulcers, peptic ulcers, dysgeusia, cholestatic jaundice, hepatocellular injury, anorexia, constipation
- **GU:** *Proteinuria,* renal insufficiency, renal failure, polyuria, oliguria, frequency of urination
- **Hematologic:** Neutropenia, agranulocytosis, thrombocytopenia, hemolytic anemia, **pancytopenia,** hyperkalemia
- **Other:** *Angioedema* (particularly of the face, extremities, lips, tongue, larynx; death has been reported with **airway obstruction**—greater risk in black patients); *cough,* muscle cramps, impotence

Interactions
✳ **Drug-drug** • Decreased antihypertensive effects if taken with indomethacin, NSAIDs
• Risk of hyperkalemia if combined with potassium-sparing diuretics, potassium supplements, other drugs causing hyperkalemia
• Risk of increased lithium levels if taken with

lithium compounds • Increased risk of renal toxicity with NSAIDs; monitor patient closely • Risk of nitritoid reaction if given with injectable gold

■ **Nursing considerations**

Assessment
- **History:** Allergy to any ACE inhibitor; impaired renal function; HF; salt or volume depletion; pregnancy, lactation ACE inhibitor–associated angioedema
- **Physical:** Skin color, lesions, turgor; T; P, BP; peripheral perfusion; mucous membranes, bowel sounds, liver evaluation; urinalysis, LFTs, renal function tests, CBC and differential

Interventions

⊗ *Warning* Keep epinephrine readily available in case of angioedema of the face or neck region; if patient has difficulty breathing, consult with physician and administer epinephrine as appropriate.

⊗ *Warning* Alert surgeon and mark the patient's chart with notice that perindopril is being taken. The angiotensin II formation subsequent to compensatory renin release during surgery will be blocked. Hypotension may be reversed with volume expansion.

- Monitor patients on diuretic therapy for excessive hypotension; the diuretic can be stopped 2–3 days before beginning therapy with perindopril and reintroduced slowly, monitoring patient response.
- Monitor patient closely in any situation that may lead to a fall in BP secondary to reduction in fluid volume—excessive perspiration and dehydration, vomiting, diarrhea—as excessive hypotension may occur.
- Arrange for reduced dosage in patients with impaired renal function.

⊗ **Black box warning** Caution patient that this drug can cause serious fetal injury; advise using barrier contraceptives.

Teaching points
- Take this drug once a day; it may be taken with meals. Do not stop taking the medication without consulting your health care provider.
- Use caution with any condition that may lead to a drop in blood pressure—diarrhea, sweating, vomiting, dehydration. If light-headedness or dizziness should occur, consult your health care provider.

- Do not use potassium supplements or salt substitutes containing potassium while taking this drug.
- Avoid the use of over-the-counter medications while you are on this drug—especially avoid cough, cold, or allergy medications that may contain ingredients that will interact with this drug. If you feel that you need one of these preparations, consult your health care provider.
- Avoid pregnancy while using this drug; serious fetal injury could occur. Using barrier contraceptives is advised; if pregnancy should occur, stop drug and notify your health care provider.
- You may experience these side effects: GI upset, loss of appetite, change in taste perception (these may be limited effects that will pass; taking the drug with meals may help); mouth sores (frequent mouth care may help); rash; fast heart rate; dizziness, light-headedness (this usually passes after the first few days of therapy; if it occurs, change position slowly and limit your activities to ones that do not require alertness and precision); headache, fatigue, sleeplessness.
- Report mouth sores, sore throat, fever, chills, swelling of the hands, feet, irregular heartbeat, chest pains, swelling of the face, eyes, lips, tongue, difficulty breathing.

▷**pertuzumab**

See Appendix R, *Less commonly used drugs.*

▷**phenazopyridine hydrochloride (phenylazodiaminopyridine hydrochloride)**

*(fen az oh **peer'** i deen)*

Azo-Standard, Baridium, Geridium, Phenazo (CAN), Prodium, Pyridium, Pyridium Plus, Urogesic, UTI Relief

PREGNANCY CATEGORY B

Drug class
Urinary analgesic

Therapeutic actions
An azo dye that is excreted in the urine and exerts a direct topical analgesic effect on urinary

tract mucosa; exact mechanism of action is not understood.

Indications

- Symptomatic relief of pain, urgency, burning, frequency, and discomfort related to irritation of the lower urinary tract mucosa caused by infection, trauma, surgery, endoscopic procedures, passage of sounds or catheters

Contraindications and cautions

- Contraindicated with allergy to phenazopyridine, renal insufficiency.
- Use cautiously with pregnancy, lactation.

Available forms

Tablets—95, 97.2, 97.5, 100, 200 mg

Dosages

Adults

100–200 mg PO tid after meals. Do not exceed 2 days if used with antibacterial agent.

Pediatric patients 6–12 yr

12 mg/kg/day divided into three doses PO for no longer than 2 days.

Geriatric patients and patients with renal impairment

Do not give to patients with renal insufficiency. A yellowish tinge to skin or sclera may indicate drug accumulation due to impaired renal excretion; discontinue therapy if yellowing of skin or eyes occurs.

Pharmacokinetics

Route	Onset
Oral	Rapid

Metabolism: Hepatic; $T_{1/2}$: Unknown
Distribution: Crosses placenta; may enter breast milk
Excretion: Urine

Adverse effects

- **CNS:** *Headache*
- **Dermatologic:** *Rash,* yellowish tinge to skin or sclera, pruritus
- **GI:** *GI disturbances*
- **Hematologic:** Methemoglobinemia, hemolytic anemia
- **Other:** Renal and hepatic toxicity, *yellow-orange discoloration of urine*

Interactions

✳ **Drug-lab test** • Interference with colorimetric laboratory test procedures

■ Nursing considerations

Assessment

- **History:** Allergy to phenazopyridine, renal insufficiency, pregnancy
- **Physical:** Skin color, lesions; urinary output; normal GI output, bowel sounds, liver palpation; urinalysis, LFTs, renal function tests, CBC

Interventions

- Give after meals to avoid GI upset.
- Warn patient drug may stain contact lenses.
- Do not give longer than 2 days if being given with antibacterial agent for treatment of UTI.
- Alert patient that urine may turn reddish-orange and may stain fabric.
- ⊗ *Warning* Discontinue drug if skin or sclera become yellowish, a sign of drug accumulation.

Teaching points

- Take drug after meals to avoid GI upset.
- Urine may be reddish-orange (normal effect; urine may stain fabric). Contact lenses may be permanently stained.
- Report yellowish staining of skin or eyes, headache, unusual bleeding or bruising, fever, sore throat.

▽**phenelzine sulfate**
(fen' el zeen)

Nardil

PREGNANCY CATEGORY C

Drug classes

Antidepressant
MAOI

Therapeutic actions

Irreversibly inhibits MAO, an enzyme that breaks down biogenic amines, such as epinephrine, norepinephrine, and serotonin, thus allowing these biogenic amines to accumulate in neuronal storage sites. According to the biogenic amine hypothesis, this accumulation of amines is responsible for the clinical efficacy of MAOIs as antidepressants.

Indications

- Treatment of patients with depression characterized as atypical, nonendogenous, or neurotic; patients who are unresponsive to other antidepressive therapy; and patients in whom other antidepressive therapy is contraindicated
- Unlabeled uses: Treatment of bulimia, PTSD, chronic migraine not responsive to standard treatment, social anxiety disorders

Contraindications and cautions

- Contraindicated with hypersensitivity to any MAOI, pheochromocytoma, HF, history of liver disease or abnormal LFTs, severe renal impairment, confirmed or suspected cerebrovascular defect, CV disease, hypertension, history of headache, suicidal ideation.
- Use cautiously with seizure disorders; hyperthyroidism; impaired hepatic, renal function; psychiatric patients (agitated or schizophrenic patients may show excessive stimulation; bipolar patients may shift to hypomanic or manic phase); patients scheduled for elective surgery; pregnancy; lactation.

Available forms

Tablets—15 mg

Dosages

Adults
Initially, 15 mg PO tid. Increase dosage to at least 60 mg/day at a rapid pace consistent with patient tolerance. Many patients require therapy at 60 mg/day for at least 4 wk before response. Some patients may require 90 mg/day. After maximum benefit is achieved, reduce dosage slowly over several weeks. Maintenance may be 15 mg/day or every other day.
Pediatric patients younger than 16 yr
Not recommended.
Geriatric patients
Elderly patients are more prone to develop adverse effects; adjust dosage accordingly.

Pharmacokinetics

Route	Onset	Peak	Duration
Oral	Slow	1 hr	48–96 hr

Metabolism: Hepatic; $T_{1/2}$: 12 hr
Distribution: Crosses placenta; enters breast milk
Excretion: Urine

Adverse effects

- **CNS:** *Dizziness, vertigo, headache, overactivity, hyper-reflexia, tremors, muscle twitching, mania, hypomania, jitteriness, confusion, memory impairment, insomnia, weakness, fatigue, drowsiness, restlessness, overstimulation, increased anxiety, agitation, blurred vision, sweating,* akathisia, ataxia, coma, euphoria, neuritis, repetitious babbling, chills, glaucoma, nystagmus, suicidal thoughts
- **CV: Hypertensive crises** (sometimes fatal, sometimes with intracranial bleeding, usually attributable to ingestion of contraindicated food or drink containing tyramine; see drug-food interactions below; symptoms include some or all of the following: Occipital headache, which may radiate frontally; palpitations; neck stiffness or soreness; nausea; vomiting; sweating; dilated pupils; photophobia; tachycardia or bradycardia; chest pain); *orthostatic hypotension, sometimes associated with falling; disturbed cardiac rate and rhythm,* palpitations, tachycardia
- **Dermatologic:** Minor skin reactions, spider telangiectases, photosensitivity
- **GI:** *Constipation, diarrhea, nausea, abdominal pain, edema, dry mouth, anorexia, weight changes*
- **GU:** Dysuria, incontinence, urinary retention, sexual disturbances
- **Other:** Hematologic changes, black tongue, hypernatremia

Interactions

✳ **Drug-drug** ⊗ *Warning* Hypertensive crisis, coma, severe seizures with TCAs (eg, imipramine, desipramine). Note: MAOIs and TCAs have been used successfully in some patients resistant to therapy with single agents; however, case reports indicate that the combination can cause serious and potentially fatal side effects.

- Increased sympathomimetic effects (hypertensive crisis) with sympathomimetic drugs (norepinephrine, epinephrine, dopamine, dobutamine, levodopa, ephedrine, carbamazepine),

P

amphetamines, other anorexiants, local anesthetic solutions containing sympathomimetic • Additive hypoglycemic effect with insulin, oral sulfonylureas • Increased hypotensive effects with beta blockers, anesthetics, thiazide diuretics • Increased risk of adverse interaction with meperidine, dextromethorphan • Risk of serotonin syndrome if combined with SSRIs or other serotonergic agents

✳ **Drug-food** ⊗ *Warning* Tyramine (and other pressor amines) contained in foods are normally broken down by MAO enzymes in the GI tract; in the presence of MAOIs, these vasopressors may be absorbed in high concentrations; in addition, tyramine releases accumulated norepinephrine from nerve terminals; thus, hypertensive crisis may occur when the following foods that contain tyramine or other vasopressors are ingested by a patient on an MAOI: Dairy products (blue, Camembert, cheddar, mozzarella, parmesan, Romano, Roquefort, and Stilton cheeses; sour cream; yogurt); meats, fish (liver, pickled herring, fermented sausages—bologna, pepperoni, salami; caviar; dried fish; other fermented or spoiled meat or fish); undistilled beverages (imported beer, ale; red wine, especially Chianti; sherry; coffee, tea, colas and other beverages containing caffeine; chocolate drinks); fruits and vegetables (avocado, fava beans, figs, raisins, bananas); yeast extracts; soy sauce; chocolate

✳ **Drug-alternative therapy** • May cause headaches, manic episodes if combined with ginseng therapy

■ **Nursing considerations**
Assessment
• **History:** Hypersensitivity to any MAOI; pheochromocytoma; HF; abnormal LFTs; severe renal impairment; cerebrovascular defect; CV disease, hypertension; history of headache; seizure disorders; hyperthyroidism; impaired hepatic, renal function; psychiatric disorder; elective surgery; pregnancy, lactation; suicidal ideation
• **Physical:** Weight; T; skin color, lesions; orientation, affect, reflexes, vision; P, BP, orthostatic BP, auscultation, perfusion; bowel sounds, normal output, liver evaluation; urine flow, normal output; thyroid palpation; LFTs, renal and thyroid function tests, urinalysis, CBC, ECG, EEG

Interventions
⊗ **Black box warning** Be aware of an increased risk of suicidality in children, adolescents, and young adults; monitor patients accordingly.
• Limit amount of drug that is available to suicidal patients.
• Monitor BP and orthostatic BP carefully; arrange for more gradual increase in dosage in patients who show tendency for hypotension.

⊗ *Warning* Have periodic LFTs during therapy; discontinue drug at first sign of hepatic impairment or jaundice.

⊗ *Warning* Discontinue drug and monitor BP carefully if patient reports unusual or severe headache.

⊗ *Warning* Keep phentolamine or another alpha-adrenergic blocking drug readily available in case hypertensive crisis occurs.
• Provide a diet that is low in tyramine-containing foods.

Teaching points
• Take drug exactly as prescribed. Do not stop taking this drug abruptly or without consulting your health care provider.
• Avoid ingestion of tyramine-containing foods while you are taking this drug and for 2 weeks afterward (patient and significant other should receive a list of such foods).
• Avoid alcohol; other sleep-inducing drugs; all over-the-counter drugs, including nose drops, cold and hay fever remedies, and appetite suppressants. Many of these contain substances that could cause serious or even life-threatening problems. Avoid ginseng while taking this drug.
• You may experience these side effects: Dizziness, weakness or fainting when arising from a horizontal or sitting position (transient; change position slowly); drowsiness, blurred vision (reversible; if severe, avoid driving or performing tasks that require alertness); nausea, vomiting, loss of appetite (frequent small meals, frequent mouth care may help); memory changes, irritability, emotional changes, nervousness (reversible).
• Report headache, rash, darkening of the urine, pale stools, yellowing of the eyes or skin, fever, chills, sore throat, thoughts of suicide, and any other unusual symptoms.

DANGEROUS DRUG

▷**phenobarbital**
(fee noe bar' bi tal)

phenobarbital
Oral preparations: Bellatal,
Solfoton

phenobarbital sodium
Parenteral: Luminal Sodium,
PMS-Phenobarbital (CAN)

PREGNANCY CATEGORY D

CONTROLLED SUBSTANCE C-IV

Drug classes
Antiepileptic
Barbiturate (long-acting)
Hypnotic
Sedative

Therapeutic actions
General CNS depressant; barbiturates inhibit impulse conduction in the ascending RAS, depress the cerebral cortex, alter cerebellar function, depress motor output, and can produce excitation, sedation, hypnosis, anesthesia, and deep coma; at subhypnotic doses, has antiseizure activity, making it suitable for long-term use as an antiepileptic.

Indications
- Oral or parenteral: Sedative
- Oral or parenteral: Hypnotic, treatment of insomnia for up to 2 wk
- Oral: Long-term treatment of generalized tonic-clonic and cortical focal seizures
- Oral: Emergency control of certain acute seizures (eg, those associated with status epilepticus, eclampsia, meningitis, tetanus, and toxic reactions to strychnine or local anesthetics)
- Parenteral: Preanesthetic
- Parenteral: Treatment of generalized tonic-clonic and cortical focal seizures
- Parenteral: Emergency control of acute seizures (tetanus, eclampsia, epilepticus)

Contraindications and cautions
- Contraindicated with hypersensitivity to barbiturates, manifest or latent porphyria, marked liver impairment, nephritis, severe respiratory distress, previous addiction to sedative-hypnotic drugs (may be ineffective and may contribute to further addiction), pregnancy (fetal damage, neonatal withdrawal syndrome).
- Use cautiously with acute or chronic pain (drug may cause paradoxic excitement or mask important symptoms); seizure disorders (abrupt discontinuation of daily doses can result in status epilepticus); lactation (secreted in breast milk; drowsiness in breast-feeding infants); fever, hyperthyroidism, diabetes mellitus, severe anemia, pulmonary or cardiac disease, status asthmaticus, shock, uremia, impaired liver or renal function, debilitation.

Available forms
Tablets—15, 16, 30, 32.4, 60, 64.8, 90, 97.2, 100 mg; capsules—16 mg; elixir— 20 mg/5 mL; injection— 65, 130 mg/mL

Dosages
Adults
Oral
- *Sedation:* 30–120 mg/day PO in two to three divided doses. No more than 400 mg per 24 hr.
- *Hypnotic:* 100–320 mg PO at bedtime.
- *Antiepileptic:* 60–300 mg/day PO.

IM or IV
- *Sedation:* 30–120 mg/day IM or IV in two to three divided doses.
- *Preoperative sedation:* 100–200 mg IM, 60–90 min before surgery.
- *Hypnotic:* 100–320 mg IM or IV.
- *Acute seizures:* 200–320 mg IM or IV repeated in 6 hr if needed.

Pediatric patients
Oral
- *Sedation:* 6 mg/kg/day PO in divided doses.
- *Hypnotic:* Determine dosage using age and weight charts.
- *Antiepileptic:* 3–6 mg/kg/day PO.

IM or IV
- *Preoperative sedation:* 1–3 mg/kg IM or IV 60–90 min before surgery.
- *Antiepileptic:* 4–6 mg/kg/day for 7–10 days to a blood level of 10–15 mcg/mL or 10–15 mg/kg/day IV or IM.
- *Status epilepticus:* 15–20 mg/kg IV over 10–15 min.

Geriatric patients or patients with debilitating disease or renal or hepatic impairment
Reduce dosage and monitor closely—may produce excitement, depression, or confusion.

P

Pharmacokinetics

Route	Onset	Duration
Oral	30–60 min	10–16 hr
IM, Subcut.	10–30 min	4–6 hr
IV	5 min	4–6 hr

Metabolism: Hepatic; $T_{1/2}$: 79 hr; 110 hr (children)

Distribution: Crosses placenta; enters breast milk

Excretion: Urine

▼ IV FACTS

Preparation: No further preparation is needed.

Infusion: Infuse very slowly, each 60 mg over 1 min, directly IV or into tubing or running IV; inject partial dose and observe for response before continuing. It may require at least 15 min to achieve peak levels in brain tissue. Avoid overdosing by observing effects before continued dosing.

Incompatibilities: Do not combine with chlorpromazine, ephedrine, hydralazine, hydrocortisone, hydroxyzine, insulin, levorphanol, meperidine, morphine, norepinephrine, pentazocine, procaine, promethazine, streptomycin, vancomycin.

Adverse effects

- **CNS:** *Somnolence, agitation, confusion, hyperkinesia, ataxia, vertigo, CNS depression, nightmares, lethargy, residual sedation (hangover), paradoxic excitement, nervousness, psychiatric disturbance, hallucinations, insomnia, anxiety, dizziness, thinking abnormality*
- **CV:** *Bradycardia, hypotension, syncope*
- **GI:** *Nausea, vomiting, constipation, diarrhea, epigastric pain*
- **Hypersensitivity:** Rashes, angioneurotic edema, serum sickness, morbiliform rash, urticaria; rarely, exfoliative dermatitis, **Stevens-Johnson syndrome**
- **Local:** *Pain, tissue necrosis at injection site,* gangrene; arterial spasm with inadvertent intra-arterial injection; thrombophlebitis; permanent neurologic deficit if injected near a nerve
- **Respiratory: Hypoventilation, apnea, respiratory depression, laryngospasm, bronchospasm, circulatory collapse**

- **Other:** Tolerance, psychological and physical dependence, **withdrawal syndrome**

Interactions

✳ Drug-drug • Increased serum levels and therapeutic and toxic effects with valproic acid • Increased CNS depression with alcohol • Increased risk of neuromuscular excitation and hypotension with barbiturate anesthetic • Decreased effects of the following drugs: theophyllines, oral anticoagulants, beta blockers, doxycycline, corticosteroids, hormonal contraceptives and estrogens, metronidazole, phenylbutazones, quinidine, felodipine, fenoprofen

■ Nursing considerations
Assessment

- **History:** Hypersensitivity to barbiturates, manifest or latent porphyria, marked liver impairment, nephritis, severe respiratory distress, previous addiction to sedative-hypnotic drugs, pregnancy, acute or chronic pain, seizure disorders, lactation, fever, hyperthyroidism, diabetes mellitus, severe anemia, cardiac disease, shock, uremia, impaired liver or renal function, debilitation
- **Physical:** Weight; T; skin color, lesions; orientation, affect, reflexes; P, BP, orthostatic BP; R, adventitious sounds; bowel sounds, normal output, liver evaluation; LFTs, renal function tests, blood and urine glucose, BUN

Interventions

⊗ **Black box warning** Risk of suicidal ideation is increased; monitor patient accordingly.

- Monitor patient responses, blood levels (as appropriate) if any interacting drugs listed above are given with phenobarbital; suggest alternative means of contraception to women using hormonal contraceptives.

⊗ **Warning** Do not give intra-arterially; may produce arteriospasm, thrombosis, or gangrene.

- Administer IV doses slowly at no more than 60 mg/min.
- Administer IM doses deep in a large muscle mass (gluteus maximus, vastus lateralis) or other areas where there is little risk of encountering a nerve trunk or major artery.

⊗ **Warning** Monitor injection sites carefully for irritation, extravasation (IV use). Solutions

---

Adverse effects in *italics* are most common; those in **bold** are life-threatening. ⬛ Do not crush.

are alkaline and very irritating to the tissues. Inject 0.5% procaine at affected site if extravasation occurs; apply heat to area.

- Monitor P, BP, and respiration carefully during IV administration.
- Arrange for periodic lab tests of hematopoietic, renal, and hepatic systems during long-term therapy.

⊗ **Warning** Taper dosage gradually after repeated use, especially in patients with epilepsy. When changing from one antiepileptic to another, taper dosage of the drug being discontinued while increasing the dosage of the replacement drug.

Teaching points
- This drug will make you drowsy and less anxious; do not try to get up after you have received this drug (request assistance to sit up or move around).
- Take this drug exactly as prescribed; this drug is habit forming; its effectiveness in facilitating sleep disappears after a short time.
- Do not take this drug longer than 2 weeks (for insomnia), and do not increase the dosage without consulting your health care provider.
- Do not reduce the dosage or discontinue this drug (when used for epilepsy); abrupt discontinuation could result in a serious increase in seizures.
- Wear a medical alert tag so that emergency medical personnel will know you have epilepsy and are taking this medication.
- Avoid pregnancy while taking this drug; use a means of contraception other than hormonal contraceptives.
- You may experience these side effects: Drowsiness, dizziness, hangover, impaired thinking (may lessen after a few days; avoid driving or engaging in dangerous activities); GI upset (take drug with food); dreams, nightmares, difficulty concentrating, fatigue, nervousness (reversible).
- Report severe dizziness, weakness, drowsiness that persists, rash or skin lesions, fever, sore throat, mouth sores, easy bruising or bleeding, nosebleed, petechiae, pregnancy, thoughts of suicide.

▽**phentolamine mesylate**

*(fen **tole**′ a meen)*

OraVerse, Regitine (CAN), Rogitine (CAN)

PREGNANCY CATEGORY C

Drug classes
Alpha-adrenergic blocker
Diagnostic agent

Therapeutic actions
Competitively blocks postsynaptic alpha$_1$-adrenergic receptors, decreasing sympathetic tone on the vasculature, dilating blood vessels, and lowering arterial BP (no longer used to treat essential hypertension because it also blocks presynaptic alpha$_2$-adrenergic receptors that are believed to mediate a feedback inhibition of further norepinephrine release; this accentuates the reflex tachycardia caused by the lowering of BP); use of phentolamine injection as a test for pheochromocytoma depends on the premise that a greater BP reduction will occur with pheochromocytoma than with other etiologies of hypertension.

Indications
- Pheochromocytoma: Prevention or control of hypertensive episodes that may result from stress or manipulation during preoperative preparation and surgical excision
- Pharmacologic test for pheochromocytoma (urinary assays of catecholamines, other biochemical tests have largely supplanted the phentolamine test)
- Prevention and treatment of dermal necrosis and sloughing following IV administration or extravasation of norepinephrine or dopamine
- Reversal of soft-tissue anesthesia (*OraVerse*)
- Unlabeled use: Treatment of hypertensive crises secondary to interactions between MAOIs and sympathomimetic amines, or secondary to rebound hypertension on withdrawal of clonidine, propranolol, or other antihypertensives

Contraindications and cautions
- Contraindicated with hypersensitivity to phentolamine or related drugs, evidence of CAD (MI, angina, coronary insufficiency).
- Use cautiously with pregnancy, lactation.

Available forms

Powder for injection—5 mg; injection—0.4 mg/1.7 mL

Dosages

Adults

- *Prevention or control of hypertensive episodes in pheochromocytoma:* For use in preoperative reduction of elevated BP, inject 5 mg IV or IM 1–2 hr before surgery. Repeat if necessary. Administer 5 mg IV during surgery as indicated to control paroxysms of hypertension, tachycardia, respiratory depression, seizures, or other effects of epinephrine toxicity.
- *Prevention of tissue necrosis and sloughing following extravasation of IV dopamine:* Infiltrate 10–15 mL of 0.9% sodium chloride injection containing 5–10 mg of phentolamine mesylate.
- *Prevention of tissue necrosis and sloughing following extravasation of IV norepinephrine:* 10 mg phentolamine added to each liter of IV fluids containing norepinephrine.
- *Diagnosis of pheochromocytoma:* See the manufacturer's recommendations. This test should be used only to confirm evidence and after the risks have been carefully considered. Usual dose, 5 mg IM or IV.
- *Reversal of soft-tissue anesthesia:* 0.2–0.8 mg, based on amount of local anesthetic administered, injected into anesthetized area (*OraVerse*).

Pediatric patients

- *Prevention or control of hypertensive episodes in pheochromocytoma:* For use in preoperative reduction of elevated BP, inject 1 mg IV or IM 1–2 hr before surgery. Repeat if necessary. Administer 1 mg IV during surgery as indicated to control paroxysms of hypertension, tachycardia, respiratory depression, seizures.
- *Prevention of tissue necrosis and sloughing following extravasation of IV dopamine:* Use 0.1–0.2 mg/kg up to maximum of 10 mg.
- *Reversal of soft-tissue anesthesia:* 6 yr and older weighing more than 30 kg, use adult dose with a maximum dose of 0.4 mg; 6 yr and older weighing 15–30 kg, maximum dose of 0.2 mg; younger than 6 yr, safety and efficacy not established (*OraVerse*).

Pharmacokinetics

Route	Onset	Peak	Duration
IM	Rapid	20 min	30–45 min
IV	Immediate	2 min	15–30 min

Metabolism: Unknown; $T_{1/2}$: 19 min
Distribution: Unknown
Excretion: Urine

▼ IV FACTS

Preparation: Reconstitute by adding 1 mL of sterile water for injection to the vial, producing a solution of 5 mg/mL.
Infusion: Inject slowly directly into vein or into tubing of actively running IV, each 5 mg over 1 min.

Adverse effects

- **CNS:** *Weakness, dizziness*
- **CV:** *Acute and prolonged hypotensive episodes,* orthostatic hypotension, **MI,** cerebrovascular spasm, cerebrovascular occlusion, *tachycardia, arrhythmias*
- **GI:** *Nausea,* vomiting, diarrhea
- **Other:** Flushing, nasal stuffiness

Interactions

✳ **Drug-drug** • Decreased vasoconstrictor and hypertensive effects of epinephrine, ephedrine

■ Nursing considerations

Assessment

- **History:** Hypersensitivity to phentolamine or related drugs, evidence of CAD, pregnancy
- **Physical:** Orientation, affect, reflexes; ophthalmologic examination; P, BP, orthostatic BP, supine BP, perfusion, edema, auscultation; bowel sounds, normal output

Interventions

- Administer *OraVerse* following the dental procedure, using same locations as local anesthetic.
- Ensure that patients change positions slowly.
- Monitor BP response and HR carefully.

Teaching points

- Report dizziness, palpitations.

DANGEROUS DRUG

▷ **phenylephrine hydrochloride**
(fen ill ef' rin)

Parenteral: Neo-Synephrine
Oral: AH-chew D, Sudafed PE
Oral drops: Little Colds
Decongestant for Infants & Children,
PediaCare Children's Decongestant

**Topical OTC nasal
decongestants:** Little Noses
Gentle Formula, Neo-Synephrine,
Rhinall, Vicks Sinex Ultra Fine Mist

Strips: Sudafed PE Quick-Dissolve,
Thin Strips Decongestant; Triaminic
Thin Strips Cold

**Ophthalmic preparations
(0.12% solutions are OTC):**
AK-Dilate, Mydfrin, Neo-Synephrine

PREGNANCY CATEGORY C

Drug classes
Alpha-adrenergic agonist
Nasal decongestant
Ophthalmic vasoconstrictor or mydriatic
Sympathomimetic amine
Vasopressor

Therapeutic actions
Powerful postsynaptic alpha-adrenergic receptor stimulant that causes vasoconstriction and increased systolic and diastolic BP with little effect on the beta receptors of the heart. Topical application causes vasoconstriction of the mucous membranes, which in turn relieves pressure and promotes drainage of the nasal passages. Topical ophthalmic application causes contraction of the dilator muscles of the pupil (mydriasis), vasoconstriction, and increased outflow of aqueous humor.

Indications
Parenteral
• Treatment of vascular failure in shock, shocklike states, drug-induced hypotension, or hypersensitivity
• To overcome paroxysmal supraventricular tachycardia
• To prolong spinal anesthesia
• Vasoconstrictor in regional anesthesia

• To maintain an adequate level of BP during spinal and inhalation anesthesia
Nasal solution and oral
• Symptomatic relief of nasal and nasopharyngeal mucosal congestion due to the common cold, sinusitis, hay fever, or other respiratory allergies
• Adjunctive therapy of middle ear infections by decreasing congestion around the eustachian ostia
Ophthalmic solution
• 10% solution: Decongestant and vasoconstrictor and for pupil dilation in uveitis, wideangle glaucoma, and surgery
• 2.5% solution: Decongestant and vasoconstrictor and for pupil dilation in uveitis, openangle glaucoma in conjunction with miotics, refraction, ophthalmoscopic examination, diagnostic procedures, and before intraocular surgery
• 0.12% solution: Decongestant to provide temporary relief of minor eye irritations caused by hay fever, colds, dust, wind, smog, or hard contact lenses

Contraindications and cautions
• Contraindicated with hypersensitivity to phenylephrine or sulfites; severe hypertension, ventricular tachycardia; narrow-angle glaucoma.
• Use cautiously with thyrotoxicosis, diabetes, hypertension, CV disorders; prostatic hypertrophy, unstable vasomotor syndrome, bronchial asthma, lactation, pregnancy.

Available forms
Chewable tablets—10 mg; tablets—10 mg; oral drops—2.5 mg/mL, 7.5 mg/5 mL; strips—1.25, 2.5, 10 mg; nasal solution—0.125%, 0.25%, 0.5%, 1%; ophthalmic solution—0.12%, 2.5%, 10%; injection—10 mg/mL

Dosages
Parenteral preparations may be given IM, subcutaneously, by slow IV injection, or as a continuous IV infusion of dilute solutions; for supraventricular tachycardia and emergency use, give by direct IV injection.
Adults
Parenteral
• *Mild to moderate hypotension (adjust dosage on basis of BP response):* 1–10 mg subcutaneously or IM; do not exceed an initial dose of 5 mg. A 5-mg IM dose should raise

BP for 1–2 hr. Or for IV use, 0.1–0.5 mg IV. Initial dose should not exceed 0.5 mg. Do not repeat more often than every 10–15 min. 0.5 mg IV should raise the pressure for 15 min.

- *Severe hypotension and shock:* For continuous infusion, add 10 mg to 500 mL of dextrose injection or sodium chloride injection. Start infusion at 100–180 mcg/min (based on a drop factor of 20 drops/mL; this would be 100–180 drops/min). When BP is stabilized, maintain at 40–60 mcg/min. If prompt vasopressor response is not obtained, add 10-mg increments to infusion bottle.

- *Spinal anesthesia:* 2–3 mg subcutaneously or IM 3–4 min before injection of spinal anesthetic.

- *Hypotensive emergencies during anesthesia:* Give 0.2 mg IV. Do not exceed 0.5 mg/dose.

- *Prolongation of spinal anesthesia:* Addition of 2–5 mg to the anesthetic solution increases the duration of motor block by as much as 50%.

- *Vasoconstrictor for regional anesthesia:* 1:20,000 concentration (add 1 mg of phenylephrine to every 20 mL of local anesthetic solution).

- *Paroxysmal supraventricular tachycardia:* Rapid IV injection (within 20–30 sec) is recommended. Do not exceed an initial dose of 0.5 mg. Subsequent doses should not exceed the preceding dose by more than 0.1–0.2 mg and should never exceed 1 mg. Use only after other treatments have failed.

Nasal solution

- *Nasal congestion:* 2–3 sprays or drops of the 0.25% or 0.5% solution in each nostril every 3–4 hr. In severe cases, the 0.5% or 1% solution may be needed; 10 mg PO bid–qid.

Ophthalmic solution

- *Vasoconstriction and pupil dilation:* 1 drop of 2.5% or 10% solution on the upper limbus. May be repeated in 1 hr. Precede instillation with a local anesthetic to prevent tearing and dilution of the drug solution.

- *Uveitis to prevent posterior synechiae:* 1 drop of the 2.5% or 10% solution on the surface of the cornea with atropine. May be repeated as necessary; not to exceed three times.

- *Glaucoma:* 1 drop of 2.5% or 10% solution on the upper surface of the cornea repeated as often as necessary and in conjunction with miotics in patients with wide-angle glaucoma.

- *Intraocular surgery:* 2.5% or 10% solution may be instilled in the eye 30–60 min before the operation.

- *Refraction:* 1 drop of a cycloplegic drug followed in 5 min by 1 drop of phenylephrine 2.5% solution and in 10 min by another drop of the cycloplegic.

- *Ophthalmoscopic examination:* 1 drop of 2.5% phenylephrine solution in each eye. Mydriasis is produced in 15–30 min and lasts for 4–6 hr.

- *Minor eye irritation:* 1–2 drops of the 0.12% solution in eye bid–qid as needed.

Oral

- *Nasal congestion:* 1 to 2 tablets every 4 hr. Strips: 1 strip every 4 hr; do not exceed 6 strips in 24 hr. Place 1 strip on tongue and let dissolve. Liquid: 10 mL every 6 hr.

Pediatric patients
Parenteral

- *Hypotension during spinal anesthesia:* 0.5–1 mg/25 lb subcutaneously or IM.

Nasal solution

- *Nasal congestion:*
  2–5 yr: 2–3 drops of 0.125% solution in each nostril every 4 hr, prn.
  Older than 6 yr: 2–3 sprays of the 0.25% solution in each nostril no more than every 4 hr.

Ophthalmic solution

- *Refraction:* 1 drop of atropine sulfate 1% in each eye. Follow in 10–15 min with 1 drop of phenylephrine 2.5% solution and in 5–10 min with a second drop of atropine. Eyes will be ready for refraction in 1–2 hr.

Oral

- *Nasal congestion:*
  Children 2–5 yr: 1 dropperful (5 mL or 2.5 mg) of 0.25% oral drops every 4 hr; do not exceed 6 mL (15 mg)/day.
  Children 6–11 yr: 1 tablet every 4 hr.

Geriatric patients
These patients are more likely to experience adverse reactions; use with caution.

Pharmacokinetics

Route	Onset	Duration
IV	Immediate	15–20 min
IM, Subcut.	10–15 min	30–120 min

Topical form is generally not absorbed systemically.

Adverse effects in *italics* are most common; those in **bold** are life-threatening. ⬛ Do not crush.

Metabolism: Hepatic and tissue; $T_{1/2}$: 2–3 hr
Distribution: Crosses placenta; enters breast milk
Excretion: Urine

▼ IV FACTS

Preparation: Inject directly for emergency use as a 1 mg/mL solution; dilute phenylephrine 1 mg/L is compatible with dextrose-Ringer combinations; dextrose-lactated Ringer combinations; dextrose-saline combinations; dextrose 2.5%, 5%, and 10% in water; Ringer injection; lactated Ringer injection; 0.45% and 0.9% sodium chloride injection; 1/6 M sodium lactate injection.
Infusion: Give single dose over 20–30 sec to 1 min. Determine actual rate of continuous infusion using an infusion pump by patient response. For infusion, add 10 mg phenylephrine to 500 mg of diluent.

Adverse effects

Adverse effects are less likely with topical administration.
Systemic administration
- **CNS:** *Fear, anxiety, tenseness, restlessness, headache, light-headedness, dizziness,* drowsiness, tremor, insomnia, hallucinations, psychological disturbances, seizures, CNS depression, weakness, blurred vision, ocular irritation, tearing, photophobia, symptoms of paranoid schizophrenia
- **CV: Cardiac arrhythmias**
- **GI:** *Nausea,* vomiting, anorexia
- **GU:** Constriction of renal blood vessels and *decreased urine formation* (initial parenteral administration), *dysuria, vesical sphincter spasm* resulting in difficult and painful urination, urinary retention in males with prostatism
- **Local:** Necrosis and sloughing if extravasation occurs with IV use
- **Other:** *Pallor,* respiratory difficulty, orofacial dystonia, sweating
Nasal solution
- **EENT:** *Blurred vision,* ocular irritation, tearing, photophobia
- **Local:** *Rebound congestion, local burning and stinging,* sneezing, dryness, contact dermatitis
Ophthalmic solutions
- **CNS:** *Headache, browache, blurred vision,* photophobia, difficulty with night vision, *pig-*

mentary (adrenochrome) deposits in the cornea, conjunctiva, or lids if applied to damaged cornea
- **Local:** *Transitory stinging on initial instillation*
- **Other:** Rebound miosis, decreased mydriatic response in older patients; significant BP elevation in compromised elderly patients with cardiac problems

Interactions

✳ **Drug-drug** ⊗ *Warning* Severe headache, hypertension, hyperpyrexia, possibly resulting in hypertensive crisis with MAOIs (isocarboxazid, phenelzine, tranylcypromine). Do not administer sympathomimetic amines to patients on MAOIs.
• Increased sympathomimetic effects with TCAs (eg, imipramine) • Decreased antihypertensive effect of methyldopa • Potential for serious arrhythmias with halogenated hydrocarbon anesthetics • Increased pressor effect with oxytocic drugs; use with extreme caution

■ Nursing considerations

Assessment
- **History:** Hypersensitivity to phenylephrine; severe hypertension, ventricular tachycardia; narrow-angle glaucoma; thyrotoxicosis; diabetes; CV disorders; prostatic hypertrophy; unstable vasomotor syndrome; pregnancy; lactation; sulfite sensitivity
- **Physical:** Skin color, T; orientation, reflexes, affect, peripheral sensation, vision, pupils; BP, P, auscultation, peripheral perfusion; R, adventitious sounds; urinary output, bladder percussion, prostate palpation; ECG

Interventions
⊗ *Warning* Protect parenteral solution from light; do not administer unless solution is clear; discard unused portion.
⊗ *Warning* Keep an alpha-adrenergic blocking agent readily available in case of severe reaction or overdose.
⊗ *Warning* Infiltrate area of extravasation with phentolamine (5–10 mg in 10–15 mL of saline), using a fine hypodermic needle; usually effective if area is infiltrated within 12 hr of extravasation.
- Monitor P, BP continuously during parenteral administration.
- Ensure than patient is hydrated during therapy.

- Do not administer ophthalmic solution that has turned brown or contains precipitates; prevent prolonged exposure to air and light.
- Administer ophthalmic solution as follows: Have patient lie down or tilt head backward and look at ceiling. Hold dropper above eye; drop medicine inside lower lid while patient is looking up. Do not touch dropper to eye, fingers, or any surface. Have patient keep eye open and avoid blinking for at least 30 sec. Apply gentle pressure with fingers to inside corner of the eye for about 1 min. Caution patient not to close eyes tightly and not to blink more often than usual.
- Do not administer other eye drops for at least 5 min after phenylephrine.
- Do not administer nasal decongestant for longer than 3–5 days.
- Do not administer ophthalmic solution for longer than 72 hr.
- Monitor BP and cardiac response regularly in patients with any CV disorders.
- Use topical anesthetics if ophthalmic preparations are painful and burning.
- Monitor CV effects carefully; patients with hypertension who take this drug may experience changes in BP because of the additional vasoconstriction. If a nasal decongestant is needed, pseudoephedrine is the drug of choice.

Teaching points
- Do not exceed recommended dose. Demonstrate proper use of topical nasal and ophthalmic preparations to your health care provider.
- Avoid prolonged use, because underlying medical problems can be disguised. Usual limit is 3–5 days for nasal decongestant, 72 hours for ophthalmic preparations.
- You may experience these side effects: Dizziness, drowsiness, fatigue, apprehension (use caution if driving or performing tasks that require alertness); *nasal solution*—burning or stinging when first used (transient); *ophthalmic solution*—slight stinging when first used (usually transient); blurring of vision.
- Report nervousness, palpitations, sleeplessness, sweating; *ophthalmic solution*—severe eye pain, vision changes, floating spots, eye redness or sensitivity to light, headache.

▷ **phenytoin (diphenylhydantoin, phenytoin sodium)**
(fen' i toe in)

Dilantin-125, Dilantin Infatab, Dilantin Injection, Phenytek

PREGNANCY CATEGORY D

Drug classes
Antiarrhythmic, group 1b
Antiepileptic
Hydantoin

Therapeutic actions
Has antiepileptic activity without causing general CNS depression; stabilizes neuronal membranes and prevents hyperexcitability caused by excessive stimulation; limits the spread of seizure activity from an active focus; also effective in treating cardiac arrhythmias, especially those induced by cardiac glycosides; antiarrhythmic properties are very similar to those of lidocaine; both are class IB antiarrhythmics.

Indications
- Control of generalized tonic-clonic and partial seizures
- Prevention and treatment of seizures occurring during or following neurosurgery
- Parenteral administration: Control of status epilepticus of the generalized tonic-clonic type
- Unlabeled uses: Antiarrhythmic, particularly in arrhythmias induced by cardiac glycosides (IV preparations); treatment of trigeminal neuralgia (tic douloureux); rectal administration

Contraindications and cautions
- Contraindicated with hypersensitivity to hydantoins, sinus bradycardia, sinoatrial block, Stokes-Adams syndrome, pregnancy (data suggest an association between antiepileptic use and an elevated incidence of birth defects; however, do not discontinue antiepileptic therapy in pregnant women who are receiving such therapy to prevent major seizures; stopping drug is likely to precipitate status epilepticus, with attendant hypoxia and risk to both mother and fetus), lactation.
- Use cautiously with acute intermittent porphyria, hypotension, severe myocardial insufficiency, diabetes mellitus, hyperglycemia.

Adverse effects in *italics* are most common; those in **bold** are life-threatening. ⊞ Do not crush.

Available forms
Chewable tablets—50 mg; oral suspension—
125 mg/5 mL; ER capsules—30, 100, 200,
300 mg; injection—50 mg/mL

Dosages
Adults
Phenytoin sodium, parenteral
- *Status epilepticus:* 10–15 mg/kg by slow IV.
  For maintenance, 100 mg PO or IV every
  6–8 hr. Higher doses may be required. Do not
  exceed an infusion rate of 50 mg/min. Follow each IV injection with an injection of sterile saline through the same needle or IV
  catheter to avoid local venous irritation by
  the alkaline solution. Continuous IV infusion
  is not recommended.
- *Neurosurgery (prophylaxis):* 100–200 mg
  IM every 4 hr during surgery and the postoperative period (IM route is not recommended
  because of erratic absorption, pain, and muscle damage at the injection site).
- *IM therapy in a patient previously stabilized on oral dosage:* Increase dosage by 50%
  over oral dosage. When returning to oral
  dosage, decrease dose by 50% of the original
  oral dose for 1 wk to prevent excessive plasma levels due to continued absorption from
  IM tissue sites. Avoid IM route of administration if possible due to erratic absorption and
  pain and muscle damage at injection site.

Phenytoin and phenytoin sodium, oral
Individualize dosage. Determine serum levels
for optimal dosage adjustments. The clinically effective serum level is usually between
10 and 20 mcg/mL.
- *Loading dose (hospitalized patients without renal or liver disease):* Initially, 1 g of
  phenytoin capsules (phenytoin sodium,
  prompt) is divided into three doses (400 mg,
  300 mg, 300 mg) and given PO every 2 hr.
  Normal maintenance dosage is then instituted 24 hr after the loading dose with frequent serum determinations.
- *No previous treatment:* Start with 100 mg
  tid PO. Satisfactory maintenance dosage is
  usually 300–400 mg/day. An increase to
  600 mg/day may be needed.
- *Single daily dosage (phenytoin sodium, extended):* If seizure control is established with
  divided doses of three 100-mg extended phenytoin sodium capsules PO per day, once-a-day
  dosage with 300 mg PO may be considered. Do

not use prompt phenytoin capsules, suspension, or chewable tablets for once-daily dosing.
Pediatric patients
Phenytoin sodium, parenteral
- *Status epilepticus:* Administer phenytoin IV.
  Determine dosage according to weight in proportion to dose for a 70-kg adult (see adult
  dosage earlier on this page; see Appendix I,
  Calculating pediatric dosages). Pediatric
  dosage may be calculated on the basis of 250
  mg/m^2 IV. Dosage for infants and children
  also may be calculated on the basis of 10–15
  mg/kg, given in divided doses of 5–10 mg/kg
  IV. For neonates, 15–20 mg/kg IV in divided
  doses of 5–10 mg/kg is recommended.

Phenytoin and phenytoin sodium, oral
Children not previously treated: Initially,
5 mg/kg/day in two to three equally divided doses. Subsequent dosage should be individualized
to a maximum of 300 mg/day. Daily maintenance dosage is 4–8 mg/kg. Children older than
6 yr may require the minimum adult dose of
300 mg/day.
Geriatric patients and patients with hepatic impairment
Use caution and monitor for early signs of toxicity; phenytoin is metabolized in the liver.

Pharmacokinetics

Route	Onset	Peak	Duration
Oral	Slow	2–12 hr	6–12 hr
IV	1–2 hr	Rapid	12–24 hr

Metabolism: Hepatic; $T_{1/2}$: 10–22 hr
Distribution: Crosses placenta; enters breast
milk
Excretion: Urine

▼ IV FACTS
Preparation: Administration by IV infusion
is not recommended because of low solubility
of drug and likelihood of precipitation; however, this may be feasible if proper precautions are
observed. Use suitable vehicle of 0.9% sodium
chloride or lactated Ringer injection, appropriate concentration (less than 6.7 mg/mL);
prepare immediately before administration, and
use an in-line filter.

⊗ *Black box warning* Drug must be
administered slowly; for adults, do not exceed
50 mg/min; for neonates, do not exceed 1–3
mg/kg min.

Infusion: Infuse slowly in small increments, each 25–50 mg over 1–5 min; infuse flush immediately after drug to reduce the risk of damage to vein and tissues.

Incompatibilities: Do not combine with other medications in solution.

Y-site incompatibility: Do not give with amphotericin B, ciprofloxacin, clarithromycin, diltiazem, enalaprilat, fentanyl, gatifloxacin, heparin, heparin with hydrocortisone, hydromorphone, linezolid, methadone, morphine, potassium, propofol, sufentanil, theophylline, vitamin B complex with C.

Adverse effects

Some adverse effects are related to plasma concentrations, as follows:

Plasma Concentration	Adverse Effects
5–10 mcg/mL	Some therapeutic effects
10–20 mcg/mL	Usual therapeutic range
More than 20 mcg/mL	Far-lateral nystagmus risk
More than 30 mcg/mL	Ataxia is usually seen
More than 40 mcg/mL	Significantly diminished mental capacity

- **CNS:** *Nystagmus, ataxia, dysarthria, slurred speech, mental confusion, dizziness, drowsiness, insomnia, transient nervousness, motor twitchings, fatigue, irritability, depression, numbness, tremor, headache,* photophobia, diplopia, conjunctivitis, suicidal ideation
- **CV: CV collapse,** hypotension (when administered rapidly IV; not to exceed 50 mg/min)
- **Dermatologic:** Dermatologic reactions, scarlatiniform, morbilliform, maculopapular, urticarial and nonspecific rashes; serious and sometimes fatal dermatologic reactions— **bullous, exfoliative, or purpuric dermatitis, lupus erythematosus, and Stevens-Johnson syndrome,** toxic epidermal necrolysis, hirsutism, alopecia, coarsening of the facial features, enlargement of the lips, Peyronie disease
- **GI:** *Nausea,* vomiting, diarrhea, constipation, *gingival hyperplasia,* toxic hepatitis, **liver damage,** sometimes fatal; hypersensitivity reactions with hepatic involvement, including hepatocellular degeneration and fatal hepatocellular necrosis
- **GU:** Nephrosis
- **Hematologic: Hematopoietic complications,** sometimes fatal: thrombocytopenia, leukopenia, **granulocytopenia, agranulocytosis,** pancytopenia; macrocytosis and megaloblastic anemia that usually respond to folic acid therapy; eosinophilia, monocytosis, leukocytosis, simple anemia, hemolytic anemia, **aplastic anemia,** hyperglycemia
- **IV use complications:** Hypotension, transient hyperkinesia, drowsiness, nystagmus, circumoral tingling, vertigo, nausea, CV collapse, CNS depression
- **Respiratory:** Pulmonary fibrosis, acute pneumonitis
- **Other:** Lymph node hyperplasia, sometimes progressing to **frank malignant lymphoma,** monoclonal gammopathy and multiple myeloma (prolonged therapy), polyarthropathy, osteomalacia, weight gain, chest pain, periarteritis nodosa

Interactions

✷ **Drug-drug** ● Increased pharmacologic effects with allopurinol, benzodiazepines, chloramphenicol, cimetidine, disulfiram, ethanol (acute ingestion), isoniazid, metronidazole, miconazole, omeprazole, phenacemide, phenylbutazone, sulfonamides, trimethoprim ● Complex interactions and effects when phenytoin and valproic acid are given together; phenytoin toxicity with apparently normal serum phenytoin levels; decreased plasma levels of valproic acid; breakthrough seizures when the two drugs are given together ● Decreased pharmacologic effects with antineoplastics, diazoxide, ethanol (chronic ingestion), folic acid, loxapine, nitrofurantoin, pyridoxine, sucralfate, rifampin, theophylline (applies only to oral hydantoins, absorption of which is decreased) ● Increased pharmacologic effects and toxicity with amiodarone, chloramphenicol, fluconazole, isoniazid ● Increased pharmacologic effect of primidone ● Increased hepatotoxicity with acetaminophen ● Decreased pharmacologic effects of amiodarone, cardiac glycosides, corticosteroids, cyclosporine, disopyramide, doxycycline, estrogens, furosemide, haloperidol, levodopa, methadone, metyrapone, mexiletine, phenothiazide, sulfonylureas, hormonal contraceptives, quinidine, atracurium, pancuronium, vecuronium, carbamazepine, diazoxide ● Severe hypotension and bradycardia when IV phenytoin is given with dopamine

✷ **Drug-lab test** ● Interference with the metyrapone and the 1-mg dexamethasone tests for at least 7 days

✳ **Drug-food** • Enteral tube feedings may delay absorption of drug. Provide a 2-hr window between *Dilantin* doses and tube feedings

■ Nursing considerations
Assessment

- **History:** Hypersensitivity to hydantoins, sinus bradycardia, AV heart block, Stokes-Adams syndrome, acute intermittent porphyria, hypotension, severe myocardial insufficiency, diabetes mellitus, hyperglycemia, pregnancy, lactation
- **Physical:** T; skin color, lesions; lymph node palpation; orientation, affect, reflexes, vision examination; P, BP; R, adventitious sounds; bowel sounds, normal output, liver evaluation; periodontal examination; LFTs, urinalysis, CBC and differential, blood proteins, blood and urine glucose, EEG, ECG

Interventions

- Use only clear parenteral solutions; a faint yellow color may develop, but this has no effect on potency. If the solution is refrigerated or frozen, a precipitate might form, but it will dissolve if the solution is allowed to stand at room temperature. Do not use solutions that have haziness or a precipitate.

⊗ **Black box warning** Administer IV slowly to prevent severe hypotension and venous irritation; the margin of safety between full therapeutic and toxic doses is small. Continually monitor patient's cardiac rhythm and check BP frequently and regularly during IV infusion. Suggest use of fosphenytoin sodium if IV route is needed.

- Monitor injection sites carefully; drug solutions are very alkaline and irritating.

⊗ **Warning** Monitor for therapeutic serum levels of 10–20 mcg/mL.

- Give oral drug with or without food in a consistent manner. Give with food if patient complains of GI upset.
- Recommend that the oral phenytoin prescription be filled with the same brand each time; differences in bioavailability have been documented.
- Suggest that adult patients who are controlled with 300-mg extended phenytoin capsules try once-a-day dosage to increase compliance and convenience.

⊗ **Warning** Reduce dosage, discontinue phenytoin, or substitute other antiepileptic gradually; abrupt discontinuation may precipitate status epilepticus.

- Phenytoin is ineffective in controlling absence (petit mal) seizures. Patients with combined seizures will need other medication for their absence seizures.

⊗ **Warning** Discontinue drug if rash, depression of blood count, enlarged lymph nodes, hypersensitivity reaction, signs of liver damage, or Peyronie disease (induration of the corpora cavernosa of the penis) occurs. Institute another antiepileptic promptly.

- Monitor hepatic function periodically during long-term therapy; monitor blood counts and urinalysis monthly.
- Monitor blood or urine sugar of patients with diabetes mellitus regularly. Adjustment of dosage of hypoglycemic patients may be needed because antiepileptic may inhibit insulin release and induce hyperglycemia.
- Monitor patient for suicidality, thoughts of suicide; patient may be at increased risk.

⊗ **Warning** Have lymph node enlargement occurring during therapy evaluated carefully. Lymphadenopathy that simulates Hodgkin lymphoma has occurred. Lymph node hyperplasia may progress to lymphoma.

- Monitor blood proteins to detect early malfunction of the immune system (eg, multiple myeloma).
- Arrange instruction in proper oral hygiene technique for long-term patients to prevent development of gum hyperplasia.

Teaching points

- Take this drug exactly as prescribed, with food to reduce GI upset, or without food—but maintain consistency in the manner in which you take it. Be especially careful not to miss a dose if you are on once-a-day therapy.
- Do not discontinue this drug abruptly or change dosage, except on the advice of your health care provider.
- Maintain good oral hygiene (regular brushing and flossing) to prevent gum disease; arrange frequent dental checkups to prevent serious gum disease.
- Arrange for frequent checkups to monitor your response to this drug.
- Monitor your blood or urine sugar regularly, and report any abnormality to your health care provider if you have diabetes.
- This drug is not recommended for use during pregnancy. It is advisable to use some form of contraception other than hormonal contraceptives.

P

- Wear or carry a medical alert tag so that any emergency medical personnel will know that you have epilepsy and are taking antiepileptic medication.
- You may experience these side effects: Drowsiness, dizziness, confusion, blurred vision (avoid driving or performing other tasks requiring alertness or visual acuity; alcohol may intensify these effects); GI upset (take drug with food, eat frequent small meals).
- Report rash, severe nausea or vomiting, drowsiness, slurred speech, impaired coordination (ataxia), swollen glands, bleeding, swollen or tender gums, yellowish discoloration of the skin or eyes, joint pain, unexplained fever, sore throat, unusual bleeding or bruising, persistent headache, malaise, any indication of an infection or bleeding tendency, abnormal erection, pregnancy, thoughts of suicide.

▽pilocarpine hydrochloride

See Appendix R, *Less commonly used drugs.*

▽pimozide

See Appendix R, *Less commonly used drugs.*

▽pindolol
(*pin' doe lole*)

Apo-Pindol (CAN), Gen-Pindolol (CAN), Nu-Pindol (CAN), Visken

PREGNANCY CATEGORY B

Drug classes
Antihypertensive
Beta-adrenergic blocker (nonselective)

Therapeutic actions
Competitively blocks beta-adrenergic receptors but also has some intrinsic sympathomimetic activity; however, the mechanism by which it lowers BP is unclear, because it only slightly decreases resting cardiac output and inconsistently affects plasma renin levels.

Indications
- Management of hypertension, alone or with other drugs, especially diuretics

- Unlabeled uses: Treatment of fibromyalgia; prevention of migraine; traumatic brain injury

Contraindications and cautions
- Contraindicated with sinus bradycardia, second- or third-degree heart block, cardiogenic shock, HF, bronchial asthma, severe COPD, pregnancy (embryotoxic in preclinical studies), lactation.
- Use cautiously with diabetes, thyrotoxicosis.

Available forms
Tablets—5, 10 mg

Dosages
Adults
Initially, 5 mg PO bid. Adjust dosage as needed in increments of 10 mg/day at 3- to 4-wk intervals to a maximum of 60 mg/day. Usual maintenance dose is 5 mg tid.
Pediatric patients
Safety and efficacy not established.

Pharmacokinetics

Route	Onset
Oral	Varies

Metabolism: Hepatic; $T_{1/2}$: 3–4 hr
Distribution: Crosses placenta; enters breast milk
Excretion: Urine

Adverse effects
- **Allergic reactions:** Pharyngitis, erythematous rash, fever, sore throat, **laryngospasm,** respiratory distress
- **CNS:** *Dizziness,* vertigo, tinnitus, *fatigue,* emotional depression, paresthesias, sleep disturbances, hallucinations, disorientation, memory loss, slurred speech
- **CV:** *Bradycardia, **HF**, cardiac arrhythmias, sinoatrial or AV nodal block, tachycardia,* peripheral vascular insufficiency, claudication, **stroke,** pulmonary edema, hypotension
- **Dermatologic:** Rash, pruritus, sweating, dry skin
- **EENT:** Eye irritation, dry eyes, conjunctivitis, blurred vision
- **GI:** *Gastric pain, flatulence, constipation, diarrhea, nausea, vomiting,* anorexia, ischemic colitis, renal and mesenteric arterial thrombosis, retroperitoneal fibrosis, hepatomegaly, **acute pancreatitis**

Adverse effects in *italics* are most common; those in **bold** are life-threatening. ⊞ Do not crush.

- **GU:** *Impotence, decreased libido,* Peyronie disease, dysuria, nocturia, urinary frequency
- **Musculoskeletal:** Joint pain, arthralgia, muscle cramp
- **Respiratory: Bronchospasm,** dyspnea, cough, bronchial obstruction, nasal stuffiness, rhinitis, pharyngitis (less likely than with propranolol)
- **Other:** *Decreased exercise tolerance, development of ANAs,* hyperglycemia or hypoglycemia, elevated serum transaminase, alkaline phosphatase, and LDH

Interactions

✳ **Drug-drug** • Increased effects with verapamil • Decreased effects with indomethacin, ibuprofen, naproxen, piroxicam, sulindac • Prolonged hypoglycemic effects of insulin • Peripheral ischemia possible if pindolol combined with ergot alkaloids • Increased risk of prolonged QT interval and potentially serious arrhythmia if combined with thioridazine; avoid this combination • Initial hypertensive episode followed by bradycardia with epinephrine • Increased first-dose response to prazosin • Increased serum levels and toxic effects with lidocaine • Paradoxic hypertension when clonidine is given with beta blockers; increased rebound hypertension when clonidine is discontinued in patients on beta blockers • Decreased bronchodilator effects of theophyllines

✳ **Drug-lab test** • Possible false results with glucose or insulin tolerance tests

■ Nursing considerations

CLINICAL ALERT!
Name confusion has occurred between pindolol and *Plendil* (felodipine); use caution.

Assessment

- **History:** Sinus bradycardia, second- or third-degree heart block, cardiogenic shock, HF, diabetes, thyrotoxicosis, asthma, pregnancy, lactation
- **Physical:** Weight, skin condition, neurologic status, P, BP, ECG, respiratory status, renal and thyroid function, blood and urine glucose

Interventions

⊗ *Warning* Do not discontinue drug abruptly after long-term therapy (hypersensitivity to catecholamines may have developed, causing exacerbation of angina, MI, and ventricular arrhythmias). Taper drug gradually over 2 wk with monitoring.
- Consult with surgeon about withdrawing drug if patient is to undergo surgery (withdrawal is controversial).

Teaching points

- Do not stop taking this drug unless instructed to do so by your health care provider. The drug cannot be stopped suddenly; it needs to be tapered down.
- Avoid driving or dangerous activities if you are drowsy or dizzy.
- Report difficulty breathing, night cough, swelling of extremities, slow pulse, confusion, depression, rash, fever, sore throat.

DANGEROUS DRUG

▷ pioglitazone
(pie oh glit' ah zohn)

Actos, Apo-Pioglitazone (CAN), ratio-Pioglitazone (CAN)

PREGNANCY CATEGORY C

Drug classes
Antidiabetic
Thiazolidinedione

Therapeutic actions
Resensitizes tissues to insulin; stimulates insulin receptor sites to lower blood glucose and improve the action of insulin; decreases hepatic gluconeogenesis and increases insulin-dependent muscle glucose uptake.

Indications

- Monotherapy as an adjunct to diet and exercise to improve glucose control in patients with type 2 diabetes
- As part of combination with a sulfonylurea, metformin, or insulin when diet, exercise plus a single agent alone do not result in adequate glycemic control in type 2 diabetes
- Unlabeled uses: Polycystic ovary syndrome; prevention of stent restenosis

Contraindications and cautions

- Contraindicated with allergy to any thiazolidinedione, type 1 diabetes, ketoacidosis, New York Heart Association Class III or IV HF, lactation, bladder cancer or history of bladder cancer.

• Use cautiously with advanced heart disease, liver failure, pregnancy.

Available forms

Tablets—15, 30, 45 mg

Dosages

Adults

15–30 mg daily as a single oral dose; if adequate response is not seen, dosage may be increased to a maximum 45 mg daily PO.

• *Combination therapy with sulfonylurea or metformin:* 15–30 mg daily PO added to the established dose of the other agent; if hypoglycemia occurs, reduce the dose of the other agent.

• *Combination therapy with insulin:* Initiate pioglitazone at 15 or 30 mg PO while maintaining insulin dose. Decrease insulin dose by 10%–25% if hypoglycemic or if glucose is less than 100 mg/dL.

Pediatric patients

Safety and efficacy not established.

Patients with hepatic impairment

Use caution and monitor patient closely. Do not administer if ALT exceeds 2.5 times the upper limit of normal.

Pharmacokinetics

Route	Onset	Peak
Oral	Rapid	2–4 hr

Metabolism: Hepatic; $T_{1/2}$: 3–7 hr
Distribution: Crosses placenta; enters breast milk
Excretion: Feces, urine

Adverse effects

• **CNS:** *Headache, pain, myalgia*
• **CV:** Fluid retention, **HF**
• **Endocrine: Hypoglycemia, hyperglycemia,** *aggravated diabetes*
• **GI:** Diarrhea, liver injury
• **Respiratory:** Sinusitis, URI, rhinitis
• **Other:** *Infections, fatigue,* tooth disorders, **bladder cancer**

Interactions

✳ **Drug-drug** • Decreased effectiveness of hormonal contraceptives, which may result in ovulation and risk of pregnancy; suggest the use of an alternative method of birth control or consider a higher dose of the contraceptive • Increased serum pioglitazone level with CYP2C8 inhibitors (gemfibrozil), monitor glucose level closely • Decreased effectiveness with rifampin

✳ **Drug-alternative therapy** • Increased risk of hypoglycemia if taken with juniper berries, ginseng, garlic, fenugreek, coriander, dandelion root, celery

■ Nursing considerations

> **CLINICAL ALERT!**
> Name confusion has occurred between *Actos* (pioglitazone) and *Actonel* (risedronate); use caution.

Assessment

• **History:** Allergy to any thiazolidinedione, type 1 diabetes, ketoacidosis, serious hepatic impairment, advanced heart disease, pregnancy, lactation
• **Physical:** T; orientation, reflexes, peripheral sensation; R, adventitious sounds; liver evaluation; LFTs, blood glucose, CBC

Interventions

• Monitor baseline LFTs before beginning therapy and periodically during therapy.
• Monitor urine or blood glucose levels frequently to determine effectiveness of drug and dosage being used.

⊗ *Black box warning* Thiazolidinediones cause or worsen HF in some patients, and pioglitazone is not recommended for patients with symptomatic heart failure (contraindicated in New York Heart Association Classes III and IV HF). After starting or increasing pioglitazone, watch carefully for signs or symptoms of HF. If they develop, manage HF according to current standards of care. Pioglitazone may be reduced or discontinued.

⊗ *Warning* There is an increased risk of bladder cancer when drug is used for longer than 1 year; monitor patient accordingly.

• Administer without regard to meals.
• Arrange for consultation with dietitian to establish weight loss program and dietary control as appropriate.
• Arrange for thorough diabetic teaching program to include disease, dietary control, exercise, signs and symptoms of hypoglycemia and hyperglycemia, avoidance of infection, hygiene.

Teaching points

• Do not discontinue this medication without consulting your health care provider;

continue with your diet and exercise program for diabetes control.

- Take this drug without regard to meals. If a dose is missed, it may be taken at the next scheduled time. If dose is missed for an entire day, do not take a double dose the next day.
- Monitor blood very closely for glucose, as prescribed, while adjusting to drug.
- Use barrier contraceptives if currently using hormonal contraceptives; these contraceptives may be ineffective if combined with pioglitazone.
- Report fever, sore throat, unusual bleeding or bruising, rash, dark urine, light-colored stools, hypoglycemic or hyperglycemic reactions, swelling, difficulty breathing.

▽ **piroxicam**

(peer ox' i kam)

Apo-Piroxicam (CAN), Feldene, Gen-Piroxicam (CAN)

PREGNANCY CATEGORY C

Drug class
NSAID (oxicam derivative)

Therapeutic actions
Anti-inflammatory, analgesic, and antipyretic activities related to inhibition of prostaglandin synthesis; exact mechanisms of action are not known.

Indications
- Relief of the signs and symptoms of acute and chronic rheumatoid arthritis and osteoarthritis
- Unlabeled uses: Dysmenorrhea, juvenile rheumatoid arthritis

Contraindications and cautions
- Contraindicated with hypersensitivity to piroxicam or any other NSAID, for perioperative pain in CABG surgery, lactation.
- Use cautiously in the elderly and with renal, hepatic, CV, GI conditions; pregnancy; HF.

Available forms
Capsules—10, 20 mg

Dosages
Adults
Single daily dose of 20 mg PO. Dose may be divided. Steady-state blood levels are not achieved

for 7–12 days. Therapeutic response occurs early but progresses over several wk; do not evaluate for 2 wk.
Pediatric patients
Safety and efficacy not established.

Pharmacokinetics

Route	Onset	Peak
Oral	1 hr	3–5 hr

Metabolism: Hepatic; $T_{1/2}$: 50 hr
Distribution: Crosses placenta; enters breast milk
Excretion: Urine

Adverse effects
- **CNS:** *Headache, dizziness, somnolence, insomnia,* fatigue, tiredness, dizziness, tinnitus, ophthalmologic effects
- **Dermatologic:** *Rash,* pruritus, sweating, dry mucous membranes, stomatitis
- **GI:** *Nausea, dyspepsia, GI pain,* diarrhea, vomiting, *constipation,* flatulence
- **GU:** Dysuria, renal impairment
- **Hematologic:** Bleeding, platelet inhibition with higher doses, neutropenia, eosinophilia, leukopenia, **pancytopenia,** aplastic anemia, thrombocytopenia, **agranulocytosis,** granulocytopenia, decreased Hgb or Hct, bone marrow depression, mennorhagia
- **Respiratory:** Dyspnea, hemoptysis, pharyngitis, **bronchospasm,** rhinitis
- **Other:** Peripheral edema, **anaphylactoid reactions to anaphylactic shock**

Interactions
✳ **Drug-drug** ● Increased serum lithium levels and risk of toxicity ● Decreased antihypertensive effects of beta blockers ● Decreased therapeutic effects with cholestyramine ● Increased risk of bleeding with other anticoagulants

■ **Nursing considerations**
Assessment
- **History:** Allergies; renal, hepatic, CV, GI conditions; history of ulcers; pregnancy; lactation
- **Physical:** Skin color and lesions; orientation, reflexes, ophthalmologic and audiometric evaluation, peripheral sensation; P, edema; R, adventitious sounds; liver evaluation; CBC, clotting times, LFTs, renal function tests; serum electrolytes, stool guaiac

P

Interventions

⊗ **Black box warning** Be aware that patient may be at increased risk for CV event, GI bleeding; monitor accordingly.

⊗ **Black box warning** Contraindicated for treatment of perioperative pain following coronary artery bypass graft surgery.

• Give drug with food or milk if GI upset occurs.

• Arrange for periodic ophthalmologic examination during long-term therapy.

⊗ **Warning** If overdose occurs, institute emergency procedures (gastric lavage, induction of emesis, supportive therapy).

Teaching points

• Take drug with food or meals if GI upset occurs.

• You may experience these side effects: Dizziness, drowsiness (avoid driving or using dangerous machinery).

• Report sore throat, fever, rash, itching, weight gain, swelling in ankles or fingers, changes in vision, black, tarry stools.

▷ **pitavastatin**
(pih ta' vah sta' tin)

Livalo

PREGNANCY CATEGORY X

Drug classes

Antihyperlipidemic
HMG-CoA reductase inhibitor

Therapeutic actions

Inhibits HMG-CoA reductase, the enzyme that catalyzes the first step in the cholesterol synthesis pathway, resulting in a decrease in serum cholesterol, serum LDLs (associated with increased risk of CAD), and increased serum HDLs (associated with decreased CAD risk); increases hepatic LDL recapture sites and enhances reuptake and catabolism of LDL; lowers triglyceride levels.

Indications

• As adjunctive therapy to exercise and diet to reduce elevated total cholesterol, LDLs, apolipoprotein B, and triglycerides and increase HDL in patients with primary hyperlipidemia and mixed dyslipidemia

Contraindications and cautions

• Contraindicated with hypersensitivity to components of drug, active liver disease, concurrent use of cyclosporine, unexplained persistent serum transaminase elevations, pregnancy, lactation.

• Use cautiously with advanced age, renal impairment, hypothyroidism, concurrent use of fibrates.

Available forms

Tablets—1, 2, 4 mg

Dosages

Adults
Starting dosage, 2 mg/day PO; may increase to a maximum of 4 mg/day.

Pediatric patients
Safety and efficacy not established.

Patients with moderate to end-stage renal impairment on hemodialysis
1 mg/day PO; maximum dosage is 2 mg/day.

Pharmacokinetics

Route	Onset	Peak
Oral	Rapid	1 hr

Metabolism: Hepatic; $T_{1/2}$: 12 hr
Distribution: Crosses placenta; enters breast milk
Excretion: Feces

Adverse effects

• **CNS:** Headache

• **GI:** Liver enzyme abnormalities, diarrhea, constipation

• **Respiratory:** Nasal pharyngitis

• **Other: Rhabdomyolysis,** *back pain,* myalgia, flulike symptoms, rash

Interactions

✴ **Drug-drug** • Increased serum levels and risk of toxicity with cyclosporine, lopinavir/ritonavir; avoid these combinations • Increased serum levels and risk of toxic effects with erythromycin; limit dosage to 1 mg/day if this combination is used • Increased serum levels and risk of toxic effects with rifampin; limit dosage to 2 mg/day if this combination is used • Potential increased risk of myopathy if taken with fibrates, niacin; if this combination is used, monitor patient closely and use caution • Increased risk of liver damage if taken with large amounts of alcohol; monitor patient closely

■ **Nursing considerations**
Assessment
- **History:** Hypersensitivity to components of drug, active liver disease, renal impairment, hypothyroidism, history of other drugs being used
- **Physical:** Weight; reflexes; R; LFTs, lipid profile, CK levels

Interventions
- Obtain LFTs before beginning therapy, at 12 wk following start of therapy or with dosage elevations, then semiannually.
- Administer at any time of day, without regard to food.
- Ensure that patient continues a diet and exercise program.
- Suggest the use of contraceptive measures for women of childbearing age.
- Advise breast-feeding patient to select another method of feeding the infant.
- Advise patient to promptly notify health care provider if unexplained muscle pain, tenderness, or weakness occurs.

Teaching points
- Take this drug once a day without regard to food, exactly as prescribed.
- Continue the diet and exercise program prescribed for lowering your lipid levels.
- If you miss a dose, take the next dose as soon as you remember. Do not take more than the prescribed amount each day.
- This drug could harm a fetus; the use of contraceptive measures is recommended. If you become pregnant or wish to become pregnant, consult your health care provider.
- It is not known how this drug affects a breast-feeding baby. Because of the potential for serious adverse effects in an infant, you should use another method of feeding the baby while you are taking this drug.
- You will need periodic blood tests to monitor your lipid levels and your liver.
- You may experience these side effects: Headache, muscle aches, runny nose.
- Report unexplained muscle pain, tenderness, or weakness; fever; changes in color of urine or stool.

▷**plasma kallikrein inhibitor**

See Appendix R, *Less commonly used drugs*.

▷**plasma protein fraction**

Plasmanate, Plasma-Plex, Protenate

PREGNANCY CATEGORY C

Drug classes
Blood product
Plasma protein

Therapeutic actions
Maintains plasma colloid osmotic pressure and carries intermediate metabolites in the transport and exchange of tissue products; important in the maintenance of normal blood volume.

Indications
- Supportive treatment of shock due to burns, trauma, surgery, and infections
- Hypoproteinemia–nephrotic syndrome, hepatic cirrhosis, toxemia of pregnancy, postoperative patients, tuberculous patients, acute respiratory distress syndrome (ARDS), renal dialysis
- Acute liver failure
- Sequestration of protein-rich fluids
- Hyperbilirubinemia and erythroblastosis fetalis as an adjunct to exchange transfusions

Contraindications and cautions
- Contraindicated with allergy to albumin, severe anemia, cardiac failure, normal or increased intravascular volume, current use of cardiopulmonary bypass.
- Use cautiously with hepatic or renal failure, pregnancy.

Available forms
Injection—5%

Dosages
Administer by IV infusion only. Contains 130–160 mEq sodium/L. Do not give more than 250 g in 48 hr; if it seems that more is required, patient probably needs whole blood or plasma.

P

Adults
- *Hypovolemic shock:* 250–500 mL IV as an initial dose. Do not exceed 10 mL/min. Adjust dosage based on patient response. Do not exceed 5–8 mL/min as plasma volume approaches normal.
- *Hypoproteinemia:* Daily doses of 1,000–1,500 mL IV are appropriate. Do not exceed 5–8 mL/min. Adjust infusion rate based on patient response.

Pediatric patients
Safety and efficacy not established, may be useful in initial therapy of shock due to dehydration or infection.

Pharmacokinetics

Route	Duration
IV	Stays in the intravascular space

Metabolism: $T_{1/2}$: Unknown
Excretion: Unknown

▼ IV FACTS

Preparation: No further preparation required; discard within 4 hr of entering a bottle; store at room temperature; do not use if there is sediment in the bottle. Do not freeze.
Infusion: Regulate based on patient response. Do not exceed 10 mL/min.
Compatibilities: Administer in combination with or through the same administration set as the usual IV solutions of saline or carbohydrates.
Incompatibilities: Do not use with alcohol or protein hydrolysates; precipitates may form.

Adverse effects
- **CV:** *Hypotension,* **HF, pulmonary edema following rapid infusion**
- **Hypersensitivity:** Fever, chills, changes in BP, flushing, nausea, vomiting, changes in respiration, rashes

■ Nursing considerations
Assessment
- **History:** Allergy to albumin, severe anemia, cardiac failure, normal or increased intravascular volume, current use of cardiopulmonary bypass, renal or hepatic failure, pregnancy
- **Physical:** Skin color, lesions; T; P, BP, peripheral perfusion; R, adventitious sounds; LFTs, renal function tests, Hct, serum electrolytes

Interventions
- Administer by IV infusion only, without regard to blood group or type.
- Consider the need for whole blood based on the patient's clinical condition; this infusion only provides symptomatic relief of the patient's hypoproteinemia.
- Monitor BP during infusion; discontinue if hypotension occurs.
- Monitor patient for hyperproteinemia (dyspnea, fluid in lungs, abnormal hypertension, increased CVP).

⊗ **Warning** Stop infusion if headache, flushing, fever, or changes in BP occur. Arrange to treat reaction with antihistamines. If a plasma protein is still needed, try material from a different lot number.
- Monitor patient's clinical response and adjust infusion rate accordingly.

Teaching points
- Rate will be adjusted based on your response, so constant monitoring is needed.
- Report headache, nausea, vomiting, difficulty breathing, back pain.

▽ plerixafor
See Appendix R, *Less commonly used drugs.*

▽ polidocanol
See Appendix R, *Less commonly used drugs.*

▽ poly-L-lactic acid
See Appendix R, *Less commonly used drugs.*

DANGEROUS DRUG
▽ polymyxin B sulfate
*(pol i **mix'** in)*

PREGNANCY CATEGORY C

Drug class
Antibiotic

Therapeutic actions
Bactericidal: Has surfactant (detergent) activity that allows it to penetrate and disrupt the cell membranes of susceptible gram-negative bacteria, causing cell death; not effective against *Proteus* species.

Adverse effects in *italics* are most common; those in **bold** are life-threatening. ⬛ Do not crush.

Indications

- Acute infections caused by susceptible strains of *Pseudomonas aeruginosa, Haemophilus influenzae, Escherichia coli, Aerobacter aerogenes, Klebsiella pneumoniae* when less toxic drugs are ineffective or contraindicated
- Intrathecal: Meningeal infections caused by *P. aeruginosa*

Contraindications and cautions

- Contraindicated with allergy to polymyxins (polymyxin B, colistin, colistimethate).
- Use cautiously with renal disease, pregnancy, lactation.

Available forms

Injection—500,000 units/vial

Dosages

Adults

IV

15,000–25,000 units/kg/day IV may be given every 12 hr. Do not exceed 25,000 units/kg/day.

IM

25,000–30,000 units/kg/day IM divided and given at 4- to 6-hr intervals.

Intrathecal

50,000 units once daily for 3–4 days; then 50,000 units every other day for at least 2 wk after cultures of CSF are negative, and glucose content is normal.

Pediatric patients

IV

Infants: Up to 40,000 units/kg/day IV.
Older than 2 yr: Use adult dosage.

IM

Infants: Up to 40,000 units/kg/day IM; doses as high as 45,000 units/kg/day have been used in cases of sepsis caused by *P. aeruginosa.*
Older than 2 yr: Use adult dosage.

Intrathecal

Younger than 2 yr: 20,000 units once daily for 3–4 days or 25,000 units once every other day. Continue with 25,000 units once every other day for at least 2 wk after cultures of CSF are negative and glucose content is normal.
Older than 2 yr: Use adult dosage.

Patients with renal failure

Reduce dosage from the recommended dose, and follow renal function tests during therapy (IM). Adjust dosage downward from 15,000 units/kg with IV use.

Pharmacokinetics

Route	Onset	Peak
IV	Rapid	Unknown
IM	Gradual	2 hr

Metabolism: $T_{1/2}$: 4.3–6 hr
Distribution: Does not cross placenta
Excretion: Urine

▼ IV FACTS

Preparation: Dissolve 500,000 units in 300–500 mL of D_5W. Dissolve 500,000 units in 2 mL sterile distilled water or sodium chloride injection, or 1% procaine hydrochloride solution; refrigerate and discard any unused portion after 72 hr.
Infusion: Administer by continuous IV drip using an infusion pump. Usually given over 60–90 min; do not infuse over less than 30 min.
Incompatibilities: Do not mix with amphotericin B, chloramphenicol, heparin, magnesium sulfate, tetracycline.

Adverse effects

- **CNS:** Neurotoxicity—*facial flushing, dizziness, ataxia, drowsiness,* paresthesias
- **Dermatologic:** Rash, urticaria
- **GU:** Nephrotoxicity
- **Local:** *Pain at IM injection site; thrombophlebitis at IV injection sites*
- **Respiratory:** Apnea (high dosage)
- **Other:** Drug fever, superinfections

Interactions

✳ **Drug-drug** • Increased neuromuscular blockade, apnea, and muscular paralysis when given with nondepolarizing neuromuscular blocking drugs • Increased risk of respiratory paralysis and renal impairment when given with aminoglycosides

■ Nursing considerations
Assessment

- **History:** Allergy to polymyxins, renal disease, lactation
- **Physical:** Site of infection, skin color, lesions; orientation, reflexes, speech; R; urinary output; urinalysis, serum creatinine, renal function tests

Interventions

⊗ *Black box warning* Monitor the patient's renal function carefully; nephrotoxicity

P

can occur. Avoid concurrent use of other nephrotoxic drugs. Be aware that neurotoxicity can result in respiratory paralysis; monitor accordingly.

• Store drug solutions in refrigerator, and discard any unused portion after 72 hr.

⊗ **Black box warning** Be aware that IM and intrathecal administration is for hospitalized patients only.

• For intrathecal use: Dissolve 500,000 units in 10 mL sterile physiologic saline for a concentration of 50,000 units/mL.

• Culture infection before beginning therapy.
• Monitor renal function tests during therapy.
• Monitor for superinfection.
• Do not use IM route routinely; severe pain occurs at injection site.

Teaching points

• You may experience these side effects: Vertigo, dizziness, drowsiness, slurring of speech (avoid driving or using hazardous equipment); numbness, tingling of the tongue, extremities (decrease the dosage); superinfections (frequent hygiene measures will help; request medications); burning, stinging, blurring of vision (ophthalmic; transient).

• Report difficulty breathing, rash or skin lesions, pain at injection site or IV site, change in urinary voiding patterns, fever, flulike symptoms, changes in vision, severe stinging or itching (ophthalmic).

▷ **poractant alfa (DDPC, natural lung surfactant; porcine origin)**

(poor ak' tant)

Curosurf

PREGNANCY CATEGORY NR

Drug class
Lung surfactant

Therapeutic actions
A natural porcine compound containing lipids and apoproteins that reduce surface tension and allow expansion of the alveoli; replaces the surfactant missing in the lungs of neonates suffering from RDS.

Indications

• Rescue treatment of infants who have developed RDS
• Unlabeled uses: Severe meconium aspiration syndrome; respiratory failure caused by group B streptococcal infection in neonates

Contraindications and cautions

• Because poractant is used as an emergency drug in acute respiratory situations, the benefits usually outweigh any possible risks.
• Use cautiously with any known family history of allergy to porcine products.

Available forms
Suspension for intratracheal instillation: 1.5, 3 mL

Dosages
⊗ **Warning** Accurate determination of birth weight is essential for determining appropriate dosage. Poractant is instilled into the trachea using a catheter inserted into the endotracheal tube.

Administer entire contents of vial (2.5 mL/kg birth weight) intratracheally, giving one-half of the dose into each bronchi. Administer the first dose as soon as possible after the diagnosis of RDS is made and when the patient is on the ventilator. Up to 2 subsequent doses of 1.25 mL/kg birth weight at 12-hr intervals may be needed. Maximum total dose is 5 mL/kg (sum of initial and 2 repeat doses).

Pharmacokinetics

Route	Onset	Peak
Intratracheal	Immediate	3 hr

Metabolism: Normal surfactant metabolic pathways; $T_{1/2}$: 25 hr
Distribution: Lung tissue
Excretion: Unknown

Adverse effects

• **CNS:** Seizures
• **CV: Patent ductus arteriosus, intraventricular hemorrhage,** *hypotension, bradycardia, flushing*
• **Hematologic:** *Hyperbilirubinemia, thrombocytopenia*
• **Respiratory: Pneumothorax,** *pulmonary air leak,* pulmonary hemorrhage (more often seen with infants weighing less than 700 g), *apnea,* pneumomediastinum,

emphysema, endotracheal tube blockage, oxygen desaturation
- **Other:** *Sepsis, nonpulmonary infections*

■ **Nursing considerations**
Assessment
- **History:** Time of birth, exact birth weight
- **Physical:** T, color; R, adventitious sounds, oximeter, endotracheal tube position and patency, chest movement; ECG, P, BP, peripheral perfusion, arterial pressure (desirable); oxygen saturation, blood gases, CBC; muscular activity, facial expression, reflexes

Interventions
- Arrange for appropriate assessment and monitoring of critically ill infant.
- Monitor ECG and transcutaneous oxygen saturation continually during administration.
- Ensure that endotracheal tube is in the correct position, with bilateral chest movement and lung sounds.
- Arrange for staff to preview teaching videotape, available from the manufacturer, before regular use to cover all of the technical aspects of administration.
- Suction the infant immediately before administration, but do not suction for 2 hr after administration unless clinically necessary.
- Warm vial to room temperature before using, up to 24 hr. No other warming methods should be used. Gently turn vial upside down to obtain uniform suspension. Do not shake vial.
- Store drug in refrigerator. Protect from light. Enter drug vial only once. Discard remaining drug after use.
- Insert 5 French catheter into the endotracheal tube; do not instill into the main stream bronchus.
- Instill dose slowly; inject one-fourth of dose over 2–3 sec; remove catheter and reattach infant to ventilator for at least 30 sec or until stable; repeat procedure administering one-fourth of dose at a time.
- Do not suction infant for 1 hr after completion of full dose; do not flush catheter.
- Continually monitor patient color, lung sounds, ECG, oximeter and blood gas readings during administration and for at least 30 min following administration.
- Maintain appropriate interventions for critically ill infant.
- Offer support and encouragement to parents.

Teaching points
- Parents of the critically ill infant will need a comprehensive teaching and support program. Details of drug effects and administration are best incorporated into the comprehensive program.

▷**porfimer sodium**

See Appendix R, *Less commonly used drugs.*

▷**posaconazole**
*(pahs ah **kon'** ah zall)*

Noxafil

PREGNANCY CATEGORY C

Drug class
Antifungal (triazole)

Therapeutic actions
Inhibits the synthesis of ergosterol, a key component of the fungal cell membrane; this inhibition leads to inability of the fungus to form the fungal cell wall and results in cell death.

Indications
- Prophylaxis of invasive *Aspergillus* and *Candida* infections in patients 13 yr and older who are at risk of developing these infections because they are immunosuppressed because of prolonged neutropenia from antineoplastic chemotherapy, graft-versus-host disease secondary to bone marrow transplants, or hematologic malignancies
- Treatment of oropharyngeal candidiasis including cases refractory to itraconazole or fluconazole

Contraindications and cautions
- Contraindicated with hypersensitivity to any component of the drug and with concurrent use of ergot alkaloids, drugs that are CYP3A4 substrates (pimozide, quinidine), sirolimus, simvastatin.
- Use cautiously with liver impairment, concurrent use of cyclosporine, prolonged QT interval, pregnancy, lactation.

Available forms
Oral suspension—40 mg/mL

P

Dosages

Adults and children 13 yr and older
Prevention: 200 mg (5 mL) PO tid. Give with a full meal or liquid nutritional supplement.
Treatment: Loading dose of 100 mg (2.5 mL) PO bid on day 1; then 100 mg/day PO for 13 days. For refractory infection, 400 mg (10 mL) PO bid, with duration based on patient response.
Patients with hepatic impairment
Use cautiously and monitor closely.

Pharmacokinetics

Route	Onset	Peak
Oral	Rapid	3–5 hr

Metabolism: Hepatic; $T_{1/2}$: 20–66 hr
Distribution: May cross placenta; may pass into breast milk
Excretion: Feces

Adverse effects

- **CNS:** *Headache, dizziness, insomnia,* anxiety
- **CV:** *Hypotension, hypertension, tachycardia,* prolonged QT interval
- **GI:** *Diarrhea, nausea, vomiting, abdominal pain, constipation, mucositis, dyspepsia, anorexia, liver enzyme changes*
- **Hematologic:** *Anemia, neutropenia, hypokalemia, hypomagnesemia, hyperglycemia,* hypocalcemia, **thrombocytopenia**
- **Respiratory:** *Cough, dyspnea, epistaxis*
- **Other:** *Rash, fever, fatigue,* weakness, infections

Interactions

✴ **Drug-drug** ● Decreased serum levels and loss of effectiveness if combined with rifabutin, phenytoin, cimetidine, esomeprazole; avoid these combinations ● Potential for increased serum levels and increased risk of toxicity of cyclosporine, sirolimus, tacrolimus, rifabutin, midazolam, phenytoin if combined with posaconazole; monitor patient closely and reduce dosages as appropriate ● Increased serum levels of ergots and risk of ergotism; this combination is contraindicated ● Increased serum levels of pimozide, quinidine, leading to risk of prolonged QT interval and potentially fatal arrhythmias; avoid this combination ● Increased serum levels of vincristine, vinblastine, and potential neurotoxicity; reduce dosage of these drugs and monitor patient closely ● Potential for increased

levels of statins, leading to possible rhabdomyolysis; reduce dosage of statins if used concurrently ● Potential for increased levels of calcium channel blockers, sirolimus; reduce dosage and monitor patient closely

■ Nursing considerations

Assessment

- **History:** Hypersensitivity to any component of the drug; concurrent use of ergot alkaloids drugs that are CYP3A4 substrates (pimozide, quinidine), sirolimus, simvastatin; liver impairment; concurrent use of cyclosporine; prolonged QT interval; pregnancy, lactation
- **Physical:** T; orientation; reflexes; skin; BP; R, adventitious sounds; abdominal examinations; LFTs, culture of infected area, CBC, serum electrolytes, ECG

Interventions

- Culture infected area prior to starting drug; drug can be started before results are known, but appropriate adjustments in treatment should be made when culture results are evaluated.
- Give with a full meal or nutritional supplement. If patient is not able to eat a full meal or tolerate oral nutritional supplement, consider a different antifungal agent, or monitor carefully for breakthrough fungal infections.
- Correct serum electrolyte levels before beginning therapy.
- Shake bottle well before use. Use the measuring spoon provided for accuracy.
- Periodically monitor LFTs to make sure hepatotoxicity does not occur.
- Obtain a baseline ECG and monitor any patient at risk for proarrhythmias or prolonged QT interval.
- Suggest the use of contraceptive measures while using this drug; the potential effects on a fetus are not known.
- Advise nursing mothers to use another method of feeding the infant while on this drug.
- Provide supportive measures for GI effects as needed.

Teaching points

- This drug must be taken three times a day (prevention) or twice a day (treatment) with a full meal or nutritional supplement (*Ensure* for example). If you are unable to eat, contact your health care provider.

Adverse effects in italics *are most common; those in* **bold** *are life-threatening.* ⚠ Do not crush.

- Store the bottle at room temperature, and shake it well before each use. To measure your dose accurately, use the spoon that comes with the bottle.
- Tell your health care provider about any other drugs you take; this drug can interact with many other drugs, and appropriate precautions will need to be taken.
- It is very important to maintain your fluid and food intake, which will help healing. Notify your health care provider if nausea or vomiting prevents this.
- You may need blood tests to evaluate the effects of the drug on your body.
- It is not known how this drug could affect a fetus. If you are pregnant or decide to become pregnant while on this drug, consult your health care provider; use of contraceptive measures is advised.
- It is not known how this drug could affect a breast-feeding infant. If you are breast-feeding, you should select another method of feeding.
- You may experience these side effects: Headache, nausea, diarrhea (consult your health care provider; medications may be available to help).
- Report severe diarrhea or vomiting, fever that persists, changes in color of stool or urine, palpitations.

DANGEROUS DRUG

▷**potassium salts**
(*po tass' ee um*)

potassium acetate

potassium chloride
Oral: Apo-K (CAN), Cena-K, Effer-K, Gen-K, Kaon-Cl, Kaylixir, K-Dur 10, K-Dur 20, K-Lor, K-Tab, Klor-Con⊙⊞, Klor-Con 8, Klor-Con 10⊙⊞, Klor-Con M 10⊙⊞, Klor-Con M 15⊙⊞, Klor-Con M 20⊙⊞, Klorvess, Klotrix⊙⊞, K+ 10, Micro-K Extencaps⊙⊞, Potasalan, Ten K
Injection: Potassium Chloride

potassium gluconate
Kaon, K-G Elixir, Tri-K

PREGNANCY CATEGORY C

Drug class
Electrolyte

Therapeutic actions
Principal intracellular cation of most body tissues, participates in a number of physiologic processes—maintaining intracellular tonicity; transmission of nerve impulses; contraction of cardiac, skeletal, and smooth muscle; maintenance of normal renal function; also plays a role in carbohydrate metabolism and various enzymatic reactions.

Indications
- Prevention and correction of potassium deficiency; when associated with alkalosis, use potassium chloride; when associated with acidosis, use potassium acetate, bicarbonate, citrate, or gluconate
- IV: Treatment of cardiac arrhythmias due to cardiac glycosides

Contraindications and cautions
- Contraindicated with allergy to tartrazine, aspirin (tartrazine is found in some preparations marketed as *Kaon-Cl, Klor-Con*); therapy with potassium-sparing diuretics or aldosterone-inhibiting agents; severe renal impairment with oliguria, anuria, azotemia; untreated Addison disease; hyperkalemia; adynamia episodica hereditaria; acute dehydration; heat cramps; GI disorders that delay passage in the GI tract.
- Use cautiously with cardiac disorders, especially if treated with cardiac glycosides, pregnancy, lactation.

Available forms
Liquids—20, 40 mEq/15 mL; powders—15, 20, 25 mEq/packet; effervescent tablets—20, 25, 50 mEq; CR tablets⊙⊞—8, 10, 15, 20 mEq; CR capsules⊙⊞—8, 10 mEq; tablets—99, 500, 595 mg; injection—2, 10, 20, 30, 40, 60, 90 mEq

Dosages
Individualize dosage based on patient response using serial ECG and electrolyte determinations in severe cases.
Adults
Oral
- *Prevention of hypokalemia:* 16–24 mEq/day PO.
- *Treatment of potassium depletion:* 40–100 mEq/day PO.

P

IV

⊗ **Warning** Do not administer undiluted.
Dilute in dextrose solution to 40–80 mEq/L.
Use the following as a guide to administration:

Serum Potassium	Maximum Infusion Rate	Maximum Concentration	Maximum 24-hr Dose
More than 2.5 mEq/L	10 mEq/hr	40 mEq/L	200 mEq
Less than 2 mEq/L	40 mEq/hr	80 mEq/L	400 mEq

Pediatric patients
• *Replacement:* 1–4 mEq/kg/day PO or 0.5–1 mEq/kg/hr IV for 1–2 hr.

Geriatric patients or patients with renal impairment
Carefully monitor serum potassium concentration and reduce dosage appropriately.

Pharmacokinetics

Route	Onset	Peak
Oral	Slow	1–2 hr
IV	Rapid	End of infusion

Metabolism: Cellular; $T_{1/2}$: Unknown
Distribution: Crosses placenta; enters breast milk
Excretion: Urine

▼ IV FACTS

Preparation: Do not administer undiluted potassium IV; dilute in dextrose solution to 40–80 mEq/L; in critical states, potassium chloride can be administered in saline.
Infusion: Adjust dosage based on patient response at a maximum of 40–80 mEq/L; do not exceed 10–40 mEq/hr.
Incompatibility: Do not mix with amphotericin B.
Y-site incompatibilities: Do not give with amphotericin B, azithromycin, diazepam, ergotamine, phenytoin.

Adverse effects

• **Dermatologic:** Rash
• **GI:** *Nausea, vomiting, diarrhea, abdominal discomfort,* GI obstruction, GI bleeding, GI ulceration or perforation
• **Hematologic:** Hyperkalemia—increased serum potassium, ECG changes (peaking of T waves, loss of P waves, depression of ST segment, prolongation of QTc interval)
• **Local:** Tissue sloughing, local necrosis, local phlebitis, and venospasm with injection

Interactions

✳ **Drug-drug** • Increased risk of hyperkalemia with potassium-sparing diuretics, salt substitutes using potassium

■ Nursing considerations

Assessment

• **History:** Allergy to tartrazine, aspirin; severe renal impairment; untreated Addison disease; hyperkalemia; adynamia episodica hereditaria; acute dehydration; heat cramps; GI disorders that cause delay in passage in the GI tract; cardiac disorders; lactation
• **Physical:** Skin color, lesions, turgor; injection sites; P, baseline ECG; bowel sounds, abdominal examination; urinary output; serum electrolytes, serum bicarbonate

Interventions

• Arrange for serial serum potassium levels before and during therapy.
• Administer liquid form to any patient with delayed GI emptying.
• Administer oral drug after meals or with food and a full glass of water to decrease GI upset.
• Caution patient not to chew or crush tablets; have patient swallow tablet whole.
• Mix or dissolve oral liquids, soluble powders, and effervescent tablets completely in 3–8 oz of cold water, juice, or other suitable beverage, and have patient drink it slowly.
• Arrange for further dilution or dose reduction if GI effects are severe.
• Agitate prepared IV solution to prevent "layering" of potassium; do not add potassium to an IV bag in the hanging position.
• Monitor IV injection sites regularly for necrosis, tissue sloughing, and phlebitis.
• Monitor cardiac rhythm carefully during IV administration.
• Caution patient that expended wax matrix capsules will be found in the stool.
• Caution patient not to use salt substitutes.

Teaching points

• Take drug after meals or with food and a full glass of water to decrease GI upset. Do not chew or crush tablets, swallow tablets whole.

Adverse effects in *italics* are most common; those in **bold** are life-threatening. ⬛ Do not crush.

Mix or dissolve oral liquids, soluble powders, and effervescent tablets completely in 3–8 ounces of cold water, juice, or other suitable beverage, and drink it slowly. Take the drug as prescribed; do not take more than prescribed.

- Do not use salt substitutes.
- You may find wax matrix capsules in the stool. The wax matrix is not absorbed in the GI tract.
- Have periodic blood tests and medical evaluation.
- You may experience these side effects: Nausea, vomiting, diarrhea (taking the drugs with meals, diluting them further may help).
- Report tingling of the hands and feet, unusual tiredness or weakness, feeling of heaviness in the legs, severe nausea, vomiting, abdominal pain, black or tarry stools, pain at IV injection site.

▽ pralatrexate

See Appendix R, *Less commonly used drugs*.

▽ pralidoxime chloride (2-PAM)

(*pra li dox' eem*)

Protopam Chloride

PREGNANCY CATEGORY C

Drug class
Antidote

Therapeutic actions
Reactivates cholinesterase (mainly outside the CNS) inactivated by phosphorylation due to organophosphate pesticide or related compound. Relieves respiratory muscle paralysis related to organophosphate toxicity.

Indications
- Antidote in poisoning due to organophosphate pesticides and chemicals with anticholinesterase activity
- IM use as an adjunct to atropine in poisoning by nerve agents having anticholinesterase activity (autoinjector)
- Control of overdose by anticholinesterase drugs used to treat myasthenia gravis

Contraindications and cautions
- Contraindicated with concomitant use of theophylline, morphine, aminophylline, and succinylcholine and allergy to any component of drug.
- Use cautiously with impaired renal function, myasthenia gravis, pregnancy, lactation.

Available forms
Injection—1 g

Dosages
Adults
- *Organophosphate poisoning:* In absence of cyanosis, give atropine 2–4 mg IV. If cyanosis is present, give 2–4 mg atropine IM while improving ventilation; repeat every 5–10 min until signs of atropine toxicity appear. Maintain atropinization for at least 48 hr. *Give pralidoxime concomitantly:* Inject an initial dose of 1–2 g pralidoxime IV, preferably as a 15- to 30-min infusion in 100 mL of saline. After 1 hr, give a second dose of 1–2 g IV if muscle weakness is not relieved. Give additional doses cautiously every 10–12 hr. If IV administration is not feasible or if pulmonary edema is present, give IM or subcutaneously.
- *Anticholinesterase (eg, neostigmine, pyridostigmine, ambenonium) overdose:* 1–2 g IV followed by increments of 250 mg every 5 min.
- *Exposure to nerve agents:* Administer atropine and pralidoxime as soon as possible after exposure. Use the autoinjectors, giving the atropine first; repeat both atropine and pralidoxime after 15 min. If symptoms exist after an additional 15 min, repeat injections. If symptoms persist after third set of injections, seek medical help.

Pediatric patients 16 yr and younger
- *Nerve gas exposure, or ganphospate poisoning IV:* Loading dose of 20–50 mg/kg (do not exceed 2,000 mg/dose) IV over 15–30 min, followed by continuous IV infusion of 10–20 mg/kg/hr.
- *Intermittent IV:* 20–50 mg/kg (do not exceed 2,000 mg/dose) over 15–30 min. Give second dose of 20–50 mg/kg if muscle weakness is not relieved in 1 hr. Repeat dosing may be done every 10–12 hr as needed.
- *IM:* 40 kg and over, 1,800 mg per course of treatment. Less than 40 kg, 15 mg/kg IM

P

every 15 min, if needed, to a total of three doses (45 mg/kg).

Pharmacokinetics

Route	Onset	Peak
IV	Rapid	5–15 min
IM	Rapid	10–20 min

Metabolism: Hepatic; $T_{1/2}$: 0.8–2.7 hr
Distribution: May cross placenta; may enter breast milk
Excretion: Urine

▼ IV FACTS

Preparation: Dilute 1–2 g pralidoxime in 100 mL saline.
Infusion: Administer over 15–30 min.

Adverse effects

- **CNS:** *Dizziness, blurred vision, diplopia, headache,* drowsiness, nausea, impaired accommodation
- **CV:** Tachycardia
- **Hematologic:** *Transient AST, ALT, CPK elevations*
- **Local:** *Mild to moderate pain at the injection site* 40–60 min after IM injection
- **Respiratory:** Hyperventilation
- **Other:** Muscular weakness

■ Nursing considerations

Assessment

- **History:** Allergy to any component of drug, impaired renal function, myasthenia gravis, lactation, pregnancy
- **Physical:** Reflexes, orientation, vision examination, muscle strength; P, auscultation, baseline ECG; liver evaluation; LFTs, renal function tests

Interventions

- Remove secretions, maintain patent airway, and provide artificial ventilation as needed for acute organophosphate poisoning; then begin drug therapy.
- Institute treatment as soon as possible after exposure to the poison.
- ⊗ **Warning** Remove clothing; thoroughly wash hair and skin with sodium bicarbonate or alcohol as soon as possible after dermal exposure to organophosphate poisoning.

- Use IV sodium thiopental or diazepam if seizures interfere with respiration after organophosphate poisoning.
- ⊗ **Warning** Administer by slow IV infusion; tachycardia, laryngospasm, muscle rigidity have occurred with rapid injection. Do not exceed injection rate of 200 mg/min.

Teaching points

- Discomfort may be experienced at IM injection site. If you receive the autoinjector, you need to understand the indications and proper use of the mechanism, review the signs and symptoms of poisoning.
- Report blurred or double vision, dizziness, nausea.

▽ pramipexole dihydrochloride

*(pram ah **pex'** ole)*

Mirapex, Mirapex ER ⊡ᴺᴄ

PREGNANCY CATEGORY C

Drug classes

Antiparkinsonian
Dopamine receptor agonist

Therapeutic actions

Stimulates dopamine receptors in the striatum, leading to decrease in parkinsonian symptoms thought to be related to low dopamine levels.

Indications

- Treatment of the signs and symptoms of idiopathic Parkinson disease
- Treatment of moderate to severe primary restless legs syndrome (*Mirapex*)
- Unlabeled use: Treatment of fibromyalgia

Contraindications and cautions

- Contraindicated with hypersensitivity to pramipexole.
- Use cautiously with symptomatic hypotension, impaired renal function, pregnancy, lactation.

Available forms

Tablets—0.125, 0.25, 0.5, 0.75, 1, 1.5 mg; ER tablets ⊡ᴺᴄ—0.375, 0.75, 1.5, 2.25, 3, 3.75, 4.5 mg

Dosages
Adults
- *Parkinson disease:* Increase dosage gradually from a starting dose of 0.125 mg PO tid for 1 wk; wk 2—0.25 mg PO tid; wk 3—0.5 mg PO tid; wk 4—0.75 mg PO tid; wk 5—1 mg PO tid; wk 6—1.25 mg PO tid; wk 7—1.5 mg PO tid. Once levels are established, ER tablets may be used for once-a-day dosing. If used in combination with levodopa, consider levodopa dose reduction.
- *Restless legs syndrome:* Initially, 0.125 mg/day PO taken 2–3 hr before bedtime; dose may be increased every 4–7 days, if needed, to 0.25 mg/day and maximum of 0.5 mg/day.

Pediatric patients
Safety and efficacy not established.

Patients with renal impairment

CrCl (mL/min)	Starting Dose	Maximum Dose
More than 60	0.125 mg PO tid	1.5 mg PO tid
35–59	0.125 mg PO bid	1.5 mg PO bid
15–34	0.125 mg PO daily	1.5 mg PO daily
Less than 15	Safety and efficacy not established; data not available	

Pharmacokinetics

Route	Onset	Peak
Oral	Varies	2 hr

Metabolism: Hepatic; $T_{1/2}$: 2–6 hr
Distribution: May cross placenta; may enter breast milk
Excretion: Urine

Adverse effects
- **CNS:** *Headache, dizziness, insomnia,* **somnolence,** hallucinations, confusion, amnesia, extrapyramidal syndrome
- **CV:** Orthostatic hypotension, hypertension, arrhythmia, palpitations, hypotension, tachycardia
- **GI:** *Nausea, constipation,* anorexia, dysphagia
- **Other:** Peripheral edema, decreased weight, *asthenia,* fever

Interactions
✻ **Drug-drug** • Increase in levodopa levels and effects if combined • Increase in levels with cimetidine, ranitidine, diltiazem, triamterene, verapamil, quinidine, quinine, and drugs eliminated via renal secretion • Decreased effectiveness with dopamine antagonists

■ Nursing considerations
Assessment
- **History:** Hypersensitivity to pramipexole, symptomatic hypotension, impaired renal function, pregnancy, lactation
- **Physical:** Reflexes, affect; T, BP, P, peripheral perfusion; abdominal examination, normal output; auscultation; R; urinary output, renal function tests

Interventions
⊗ **Warning** Administer with extreme caution to patients with a history of hypotension, hallucinations, confusion, or dyskinesias.
⊗ **Warning** Alert patient that sudden onset of sleep can occur. Patient should avoid driving, alcohol, and sedating medications.
- Administer with food if GI upset becomes a problem.
- Ensure that ER tablets are swallowed whole; ER tablets should not be cut, crushed, or chewed.
⊗ **Warning** Do not discontinue abruptly; taper gradually over at least 1 wk.
- Monitor patient while adjusting drug to establish therapeutic dosage. Dosage of levodopa and carbidopa may need to be reduced accordingly to balance therapeutic effects.
- Provide safety precautions as needed if hallucinations occur (more common with elderly).

Teaching points
- For Parkinson disease, take this drug exactly as prescribed, three times per day, with breakfast, lunch, and dinner. Continue to take your levodopa and carbidopa if prescribed. The dosage of levodopa may need to be decreased after a few days of therapy. The dosage of pramipexole will be slowly increased over a 7-week period. Write your dose down and follow this pattern. You may be switched to an extended-release tablet to allow once-a-day dosing. Swallow this tablet whole; do not cut, crush, or chew it.
- For restless legs syndrome, take the dose daily 2–3 hours before bedtime. Dosage may be increased as needed.
- Do not stop taking this drug without consulting your health care provider; serious side effects could occur. The drug should be tapered over at least 1 week.

- Avoid becoming pregnant while using this drug; using barrier contraceptives is advised. If you think you are pregnant, notify your health care provider.
- You may experience these side effects: Dizziness, light-headedness, insomnia (avoid driving or operating dangerous machinery); nausea (take drug with meals); edema; weight loss; low blood pressure (change positions slowly; use caution in extremes of heat or exertion); hallucinations (safety precautions may be needed); falling asleep while engaged in activities of daily living (use caution to avoid injury; avoid alcohol or other sedating drugs).
- Report severe nausea, severe swelling, sweating, hallucinations, dizziness, fainting.

DANGEROUS DRUG

▷**pramlintide acetate**
(*pram' lin tyde*)

Symlin

PREGNANCY CATEGORY C

Drug classes
Amylinomimetic
Antidiabetic

Therapeutic actions
A synthetic analogue of human amylin, a hormone produced by the beta cells in the pancreas that helps to control glucose levels in the postprandial period; modulates gastric emptying, causes a feeling of fullness or satiety, prevents the postprandial rise in serum glucagon levels all leading to lower serum glucose levels.

Indications
- Adjunct treatment in patients with type 1 diabetes who use mealtime insulin and who have failed to achieve desired glucose control despite optimal insulin therapy
- Adjunct treatment in type 2 diabetes patients who use mealtime insulin and who have failed to achieve desired glucose control despite optimal insulin therapy with or without a concurrent sulfonylurea or metformin

Contraindications and cautions
- Contraindicated with known hypersensitivity to pramlintide or any of its components, gastroparesis, hypoglycemia unawareness.
- Use cautiously with pregnancy, lactation.

Available forms
Solution for injection—0.6 mg/mL

Dosages
Adults
- *Type 2 diabetes:* Initially, 60 mcg by subcutaneous injection immediately prior to major meals. Dose may be increased to 120 mcg if needed and tolerated. Dosage of oral drugs and insulins will need to be reduced, usually by 50% based on patient response.
- *Type 1 diabetes:* Initially, 15 mcg by subcutaneous injection immediately before major meals, titrate at 15 mcg increments to a maintenance dose of 30 or 60 mcg as tolerated. Dosage of insulins will need to be reduced by 50% and the patient must be monitored closely to achieve optimal glucose control.

Pharmacokinetics

Route	Onset	Peak
Subcut.	Rapid	21 min

Metabolism: Renal; $T_{1/2}$: 48 min
Distribution: May cross placenta; may pass into breast milk
Excretion: Urine

Adverse effects
- **CNS:** Dizziness, headache, fatigue
- **GI:** *Nausea,* anorexia, *vomiting,* abdominal pain
- **Respiratory:** Cough, pharyngitis
- **Other: Hypoglycemia,** injection site reaction

Interactions
✴ **Drug-drug** • Risk of delayed absorption of oral medications because of effects on gastric emptying; if rapid effect is needed, take oral medication 1 hr prior to or 2 hr after pramlintide • Risk of combined effects on gastric emptying if combined with anticholinergic drugs or drugs that slow intestinal absorption of nutrients; avoid this combination

■ Nursing considerations
Assessment
- **History:** Hypersensitivity to pramlintide or any of its components, gastroparesis, hypoglycemia unawareness, pregnancy, lactation
- **Physical:** Orientation, reflexes, affect; abdominal examination; injection site; blood glucose levels

Interventions

⊗ **Black box warning** Be aware that severe hypoglycemia has been associated with combined use of insulin, pramlintide; usually seen within 3 hr of pramlintide injection. Monitor accordingly.

- Inject subcutaneously before each major meal of the day; inject it into a site that is more than 2 inches away from the site of insulin injection.
- Do not combine in syringe with insulin.
- Maintain other antidiabetic drugs, diet and exercise regimen for control of diabetes.
- Administer oral medications at least 1 hr before or 2 hr after administering pramlintide.
- Monitor serum glucose levels and HbA$_{1c}$ levels frequently to evaluate effectiveness of drug on controlling glucose levels.
- Arrange for thorough diabetic teaching program to include disease, dietary control, exercise, signs and symptoms of hypoglycemia and hyperglycemia, avoidance of infection and hygiene.

Teaching points

- This drug is given subcutaneously. Use sterile technique. Dispose of syringes appropriately.
- Do not use any solution that appears cloudy; do not combine this drug in syringe with insulin.
- Inject it into a site on your thigh or abdomen. Rotate injection sites periodically; inject into a site that is at least 2 inches away from the site of your insulin injection.
- Store unopened vials in the refrigerator. Opened bottles may be kept at room temperature. Throw away any out-of-date bottles.
- Inject this drug before any major meal that you are eating; do not use if you are not going to be eating; if you forget a dose, do not inject after you have eaten.
- Be aware that alcohol consumption can change your blood glucose levels and may alter your response to this drug.
- Do not take this drug if you are not able to eat or if you plan to skip a meal or if your blood sugar is too low.
- Do not change the dosage of this drug without consulting your health care provider.
- It is not known how this drug affects a pregnancy. If you think you are pregnant or would

like to become pregnant, consult your health care provider.
- It is not known how this drug could affect a breast-feeding infant. If you are breast-feeding, consult your health care provider.
- You will need to regularly monitor your blood glucose levels. Your health care provider may change the dose of pramlintide or your other antidiabetic drugs, based on your blood glucose response.
- It is important that you follow the diet, exercise, and drug guidelines related to your disease.
- Review the signs and symptoms of hypoglycemia; be prepared to treat hypoglycemia with fast-acting sugar or glucagon.
- Do not drive a car or operate potentially dangerous machinery until you are aware of how pramlintide will affect your blood sugar. Low blood sugar can cause dizziness and changes in thinking.
- This drug affects how fast your stomach empties, which may affect other drugs you may be taking. Consult your health care provider about the need to change the timing of drug administration.
- You may experience these side effects: Injection site reactions (proper injection and rotation of injection sites should help; if problems occur, consult your health care provider); hypoglycemia (use fast-acting sugars or glucagons if this occurs; proper use and eating of meals should prevent this effect); nausea (this usually passes after a few days).
- Report hypoglycemic reactions; redness, pain or swelling at injection sites; stomach pain; vomiting.

DANGEROUS DRUG

▽ **prasugrel**
(*pra' soo grel*)

Effient

PREGNANCY CATEGORY B

Drug class
Platelet inhibitor

Therapeutic actions
Inhibits platelet activation and aggregation by irreversibly binding to the P2Y$_{12}$ class of ADP receptors on platelets.

Indications

- To reduce the risk of thrombotic cardiovascular events (including stent thrombosis) in patients with acute coronary syndrome who are to be managed with percutaneous coronary intervention, including patients with unstable angina or non-ST-elevation MI and patients with ST-elevation MI who will be managed with primary or delayed percutaneous coronary intervention

Contraindications and cautions

- Contraindicated with hypersensitivity to components of drug, active pathologic bleeding, history of TIA or stroke, patients likely to undergo CABG surgery.
- Use cautiously with age 75 yr and older, body weight less than 60 kg, bleeding tendency, use of drugs that increase risk of bleeding, pregnancy, lactation.

Available forms

Tablets—5, 10 mg

Dosages

Adults
Loading dose: 60 mg PO as single dose, then 10 mg/day PO without regard to food; use 5 mg/day in patients weighing less than 60 kg. Patient should also be receiving aspirin (75–325 mg/day).

Pediatric patients
Safety and efficacy not established.

Geriatric patients
Not recommended in patients 75 yr or older except in high-risk situations in which benefit outweighs risk.

Pharmacokinetics

Route	Onset	Peak
Oral	Rapid	30 min

Metabolism: Hepatic; $T_{1/2}$: 2–15 hr
Distribution: May cross placenta; may enter breast milk
Excretion: Urine, feces

Adverse effects

- **CNS:** *Headache,* dizziness
- **CV:** *Hypertension,* hypotension, peripheral edema, atrial fibrillation, bradycardia
- **GI:** Nausea, diarrhea
- **Hematologic:** *Hypercholesterolemia, hyperlipidemia,* leukopenia

- **Respiratory:** Dyspnea, cough
- **Other: Bleeding, thrombotic thrombocytopenic purpura,** rash, fever, fatigue, pain, **risk of thrombotic episodes if stopped prematurely**

Interactions

✴ **Drug-drug** • Increased risk of bleeding if combined with warfarin or prolonged use of NSAIDs; monitor patient closely and adjust dosage as appropriate

■ Nursing considerations

Assessment

- **History:** Hypersensitivity to components of drug, active pathologic bleeding, history of TIA or stroke, planned or anticipated CABG surgery, pregnancy, lactation, age, body weight under 60 kg, bleeding tendency, use of drugs that increase the risk of bleeding
- **Physical:** Weight; T; skin—color, lesions; orientation, affect; P, BP, periphery evaluation for edema; R, adventitious sounds

Interventions

⊗ **Black box warning** There is a risk of serious to fatal bleeding with drug administration; do not use with active bleeding or history of TIA or stroke. Risk increases in patients older than 75 yr, patients weighing less than 60 kg, patients with bleeding tendency, and patients taking warfarin or NSAIDs. Do not use in patients who are likely candidates for CABG surgery; if patients taking drug require CABG, stop prasugrel at least 7 days before surgery. Suspect bleeding in patient who becomes hypotensive and has undergone invasive procedures. If possible, control bleeding without discontinuing prasugrel; premature discontinuation increases risk of thrombotic episodes.

- Administer loading dose and then give once a day without regard to food.
- Patient should also be taking aspirin once a day. Check with health care provider.
- Advise patient to use contraceptive measures because it is not known if drug affects a fetus.
- Advise breast-feeding patient to select another method of feeding the infant; it is not known if drug enters breast milk.
- Limit invasive procedures; be aware that patient may experience prolonged bleeding if undergoing invasive procedures.

Adverse effects in *italics* are most common; those in **bold** are life-threatening. ⊞ Do not crush.

- Protect patient from injury; risk of bruising and bleeding is increased.
- Do not discontinue drug prematurely because of increased risk of thrombotic events.
- Alert surgeons that patient is taking drug; if possible, drug should be discontinued at least 7 days before surgery.

Teaching points
- Take this drug exactly as prescribed, once a day without regard to food.
- If you forget a dose, take the next dose at the regular time. Do not attempt to make up or double doses unless you have been instructed to do so by your health care provider.
- Do not run out of this drug or stop taking this drug for any reason. If you stop taking the drug, immediately contact your health care provider because serious events could occur.
- Keep a list of all drugs you are taking, including over-the-counter drugs and herbal therapies, so your health care provider can adjust dosages as needed.
- Inform all your health care providers, including your dentist and surgeons, that you are taking this drug. Because this drug makes you bleed longer, appropriate measures will be needed if invasive procedures are planned.
- You should carry or wear a Medical Alert card to alert people who may care for you during an emergency that you are taking this drug.
- It is not known if this drug affects a fetus; the use of contraceptive measures is advised.
- It is not known if this drug enters breast milk. If you are breast-feeding, you should use another method of feeding the infant.
- You may experience these side effects: Increased bleeding and bruising (take extra precautions to avoid injury; be aware that if you are injured, it will take longer to stop bleeding), nausea, diarrhea (small, frequent meals may help; consult your health care provider if this becomes too uncomfortable); rash, fatigue.
- Rarely, a serious disorder called thrombotic thrombocytopenic purpura can occur. Notify your health care provider immediately if you experience fever, weakness, purple skin patches, yellowing of the skin or eyes, extreme paleness, mental changes.
- Report excessive bruising or bruising from no known cause, uncontrollable bleeding, pink or brown urine, red or tarlike stools, coughing up blood or clots, vomiting blood, or vomit that looks like coffee grounds.

▽ pravastatin sodium
(prah va sta' tin)

Apo-Pravastatin (CAN), CO Pravastatin (CAN), Gen-Pravastatin (CAN), Novo-Pravastatin (CAN), Nu-Pravastatin (CAN), PMS-Pravastatin (CAN), Pravachol, ratio-Pravastatin (CAN)

PREGNANCY CATEGORY X

Drug classes
Antihyperlipidemic
HMG-CoA reductase inhibitor

Therapeutic actions
Inhibits the enzyme HMG-CoA that catalyzes the first step in the cholesterol synthesis pathway, resulting in a decrease in serum cholesterol, serum LDLs (associated with increased risk of CAD), and either an increase or no change in serum HDLs (associated with decreased risk of CAD).

Indications
- Prevention of first MI and reduction of death from CV disease in patients with hypercholesterolemia at risk of first MI
- Adjunct to diet in the treatment of elevated total cholesterol and LDL cholesterol with primary hypercholesterolemia (types IIa and IIb) in patients unresponsive to dietary restriction of saturated fat and cholesterol and other nonpharmacologic measures
- Slow the progression of coronary atherosclerosis in patients with clinically evident CAD to reduce the risk of acute coronary events in hypercholesterolemia patients
- Reduce the risk of stroke or TIA in patients with history of MI and normal cholesterol levels
- Reduce the risk of recurrent MI and death from heart disease in patients with history of MI and normal cholesterol levels
- Treatment of children 8 yr and older with heterozygous familial hypercholesterolemia as an adjunct to diet and exercise

Contraindications and cautions

- Contraindicated with allergy to pravastatin, fungal byproducts, active liver disease, unexplained elevated serum transaminases, pregnancy, lactation.
- Use cautiously with impaired hepatic function, cataracts, alcoholism.

Available forms

Tablets—10, 20, 40, 80 mg

Dosages

Adults

Initially, 40 mg/day PO given once daily. Adjust dosage every 4 wk based on response. Maximum daily dose is 80 mg. Maintenance doses range from 40–80 mg/day in a single bedtime dose.

- *Concomitant immunosuppressive therapy:* 10 mg PO daily at bedtime to a maximum of 20 mg/day.

Pediatric patients 14–18 yr

40 mg/day PO.

Pediatric patients 8–13 yr

20 mg/day PO.

Geriatric patients and patients with renal or hepatic impairment

10 mg PO once daily at bedtime; may increase up to 20 mg/day.

Pharmacokinetics

Route	Onset	Peak
Oral	Slow	60–90 min

Metabolism: Hepatic; $T_{1/2}$: 1.8 hr
Distribution: Crosses placenta; enters breast milk
Excretion: Feces, urine

Adverse effects

- **CNS:** *Headache, blurred vision,* dizziness, insomnia, fatigue, muscle cramps, cataracts
- **GI:** *Flatulence, abdominal pain, cramps, constipation, nausea, vomiting,* heartburn
- **Hematologic:** Elevations of CK, alkaline phosphatase, and transaminases

Interactions

✳ **Drug-drug** • Possible severe myopathy or rhabdomyolysis with cyclosporine, erythromycin, gemfibrozil, niacin • Possible increased digoxin, warfarin levels if combined; monitor patient and decrease dosage as needed • Increased pravastatin levels with itraconazole; avoid this combination • Decreased pravastatin levels if combined with bile acid sequestrants; space at least 4 hr apart

■ Nursing considerations

Assessment

- **History:** Allergy to pravastatin, fungal byproducts; impaired hepatic function; cataracts; pregnancy; lactation
- **Physical:** Orientation, affect, ophthalmologic examination; liver evaluation; lipid studies, LFTs, CK levels

Interventions

- Ensure that patient is on a cholesterol-lowering diet before and during therapy.
- Caution patient that this drug cannot be used during pregnancy; advise patient to use barrier contraceptives.
- Suggest another method of feeding the infant if patient is breast-feeding.
- Administer drug at bedtime; highest rates of cholesterol synthesis occur between midnight and 5 AM.
- Arrange for periodic ophthalmologic examination to check for cataract development; monitor liver function.

Teaching points

- Take drug at bedtime.
- Continue your cholesterol-lowering diet and exercise program.
- This drug cannot be taken during pregnancy; using barrier contraceptives is advised.
- This drug cannot be taken while breast-feeding; another method of feeding the infant will be needed.
- Have periodic ophthalmic examinations while you are using this drug.
- You may experience these side effects: Nausea (eat frequent small meals); headache, muscle and joint aches and pains (may lessen); sensitivity to sunlight (use sunblock and wear protective clothing).
- Report severe GI upset, changes in vision, unusual bleeding or bruising, dark urine or light-colored stools, muscle pain or weakness.

▽ **praziquantel**

See Appendix R, *Less commonly used drugs.*

Adverse effects in *italics* are most common; those in **bold** are life-threatening. ⊂ﬆ⊃ Do not crush.

▷ prazosin hydrochloride
(pra' zoe sin)

Apo-Prazo (CAN), Minipress, Novo-Prazin (CAN)

PREGNANCY CATEGORY C

Drug classes
Alpha-adrenergic blocker
Antihypertensive

Therapeutic actions
Selectively blocks postsynaptic alpha$_1$-adrenergic receptors, decreasing sympathetic tone on the vasculature, dilating arterioles and veins, and lowering supine and standing BP; unlike conventional alpha-adrenergic blocking agents (eg, phentolamine), it does not block alpha$_2$ presynaptic receptors, so it does not cause reflex tachycardia.

Indications
- Treatment of hypertension, alone or in combination with other agents
- Unlabeled uses: Management of Raynaud vasospasm, pediatric hypertension

Contraindications and cautions
- Contraindicated with hypersensitivity to prazosin, lactation.
- Use cautiously with HF, angina pectoris, renal failure, pregnancy.

Available forms
Capsules—1, 2, 5 mg

Dosages
⊗ *Warning* First dose may cause syncope with sudden loss of consciousness. First dose should be limited to 1 mg PO and given at bedtime.
Adults
Initial dosage is 1 mg PO bid–tid. Increase dosage to a total of 20 mg/day given in divided doses. When increasing dosage, give the first dose of each increment at bedtime. Maintenance dosages most commonly range from 6–15 mg/day given in divided doses.
- *Concomitant therapy:* When adding a diuretic or other antihypertensive drug, reduce dosage to 1–2 mg PO tid and then re-adjust.

Pediatric patients
Safety and efficacy not established.

Pharmacokinetics
Route	Onset	Peak
Oral	Varies	1–3 hr

Metabolism: Hepatic; T$_{1/2}$: 2–3 hr
Distribution: Crosses placenta; may enter breast milk
Excretion: Bile, feces, and urine

Adverse effects
- **CNS:** *Dizziness, headache, drowsiness, lack of energy, weakness,* nervousness, vertigo, depression, paresthesia
- **CV:** *Palpitations,* sodium and water retention, increased plasma volume, edema, dyspnea, syncope, tachycardia, orthostatic hypotension
- **Dermatologic:** Rash, pruritus, alopecia, lichen planus
- **EENT:** Blurred vision, reddened sclera, epistaxis, tinnitus, dry mouth, nasal congestion
- **GI:** *Nausea,* vomiting, diarrhea, constipation, abdominal discomfort or pain
- **GU:** Urinary frequency, incontinence, impotence, priapism
- **Other:** Diaphoresis, lupus erythematosus

Interactions
✳ **Drug-drug** • Severity and duration of hypotension following first dose of prazosin may be greater in patients receiving beta-adrenergic blocking drugs (eg, propranolol), verapamil; first dose of prazosin should be only 0.5 mg or less • Increased risk of hypotension with phosphodiesterase-5 inhibitors (sildenafil, tadalafil, vardenafil)

■ Nursing considerations
Assessment
- **History:** Hypersensitivity to prazosin, HF, angina pectoris, renal failure, lactation, pregnancy
- **Physical:** Weight; skin color, lesions; orientation, affect, reflexes; ophthalmologic examination; P, BP, orthostatic BP, supine BP, perfusion, edema, auscultation; R, adventitious sounds; status of nasal mucous membranes; bowel sounds, normal output; voiding pattern, normal output; renal function tests, urinalysis

Interventions

- Administer, or have patient take, first dose just before bedtime to lessen likelihood of first dose effect (syncope), believed due to excessive orthostatic hypotension.
- Have patient lie down and treat patient supportively if syncope occurs; condition is self-limited.
- Monitor for orthostatic hypotension, which is most marked in the morning and is accentuated by hot weather, alcohol, and exercise.
- Monitor edema and weight in patients with incipient cardiac decompensation, and add a thiazide diuretic to the drug regimen if sodium and fluid retention or signs of impending heart failure occur.

Teaching points

- Take this drug exactly as prescribed. Take the first dose just before bedtime. Do not drive or operate machinery for 4 hours after the first dose.
- You may experience these side effects: Dizziness, weakness (more likely when changing position, in the early morning, after exercise, in hot weather, and with alcohol; some tolerance may occur; avoid driving or engaging in tasks that require alertness; change position slowly, and use caution when climbing stairs; lie down for a while if dizziness persists); GI upset (eat frequent small meals); impotence; dry mouth (sucking on sugarless candies, ice chips may help); stuffy nose. Most effects are transient.
- Report frequent dizziness or faintness.

▷ **prednisoLONE**

*(pred **niss' ** ob lone)*

prednisolone
Oral: Prelone

prednisolone acetate
Ophthalmic solution: Pred Forte, Pred Mild, ratio-Prednisolone (CAN)

prednisolone sodium phosphate
Oral: Hydrocortone, Orapred, Orapred ODT, Pediapred

PREGNANCY CATEGORY C

Drug classes

Anti-inflammatory
Corticosteroid (intermediate-acting)
Glucocorticoid
Hormone

Therapeutic actions

Enters target cells and binds to intracellular corticosteroid receptors, thereby initiating many complex reactions that are responsible for its anti-inflammatory and immunosuppressive effects.

Indications

Systemic

- Hypercalcemia associated with cancer
- Short-term management of various inflammatory and allergic disorders, such as rheumatoid arthritis, collagen diseases (eg, SLE), dermatologic diseases (eg, pemphigus), status asthmaticus, and autoimmune disorders
- Hematologic disorders: Thrombocytopenia purpura, erythroblastopenia
- Ulcerative colitis, acute exacerbations of MS and palliation in some leukemias and lymphomas
- Trichinosis with neurologic or myocardial involvement
- Prednisolone has weaker mineralocorticoid activity than hydrocortisone and is not used as physiologic replacement therapy

Ophthalmic

- Inflammation of the lid, conjunctiva, cornea, and globe

Contraindications and cautions

- Contraindicated with infections (especially TB, fungal infections, amebiasis, vaccinia and varicella, and antibiotic-resistant infections), lactation, idiopathic thrombocytopenic purpura.
- Use cautiously with renal or liver disease, hypothyroidism, ulcerative colitis with impending perforation, diverticulitis, active or latent peptic ulcer, inflammatory bowel disease, heart failure, hypertension, thromboembolic disorders, osteoporosis, seizure disorders, diabetes mellitus, pregnancy.

Ophthalmic preparations

- Contraindicated with acute superficial herpes simplex keratitis; fungal infections of ocular structures; vaccinia, varicella, and other viral diseases of the cornea and conjunctiva; ocular TB.

Adverse effects in *italics* are most common; those in **bold** are life-threatening. ▭ Do not crush.

Available forms

Tablets—5 mg; rapidly dissolving tablets—10, 15, 30 mg; oral syrup—15 mg/5 mL, 5 mg/5 mL; ophthalmic suspension—0.12%, 1%; oral suspension—5, 15 mg/5 mL

Dosages
Adults

Individualize dosage, depending on severity of condition and patient's response. Administer daily dose before 9 AM to minimize adrenal suppression. If long-term therapy is needed, consider alternate-day therapy. After long-term therapy, withdraw drug slowly to avoid adrenal insufficiency. For maintenance therapy, reduce initial dose in small increments at intervals until the lowest dose that maintains satisfactory clinical response is reached.

Oral

Prednisolone: 5–60 mg/day PO.

• *Acute exacerbations of MS:* 200 mg/day PO for 1 wk, followed by 80 mg every other day for 1 mo (prednisolone sodium phosphate).

Adults and pediatric patients
Ophthalmic

Prednisolone acetate: 2 drops qid. For *Pred Mild* or *Pred Forte,* 1–2 drops every hr during the day and every 2 hr at night. With favorable results, 1 drop every 4 hr, than 1 drop three to four times/day to control symptoms.

Prednisolone sodium phosphate: 1–2 drops up to every hr during the day and every 2 hr during the night. After a favorable response, reduce to 1 drop every 4 hr. Later, further reduction to 1 drop 3–4 times daily may suffice.

Pediatric patients

Individualize dosage depending on severity of condition and patient's response rather than by strict adherence to formulas that correct adult doses for age or weight. Carefully observe growth and development in infants and children on prolonged therapy.

Oral suspension

0.14–2 mg/kg/day PO in three to four divided doses.

• *Nephrotic syndrome (prednisolone sodium phosphate):* 60 mg/m²/day PO in three divided doses for 4 wk. Then single doses for 4 wk. Alternatively, 40 mg/m²/day PO.

Pharmacokinetics

Route	Onset	Peak	Duration
Oral	Varies	1–2 hr	1–1.5 days

Metabolism: Hepatic; $T_{1/2}$: 3.5 hr
Distribution: Crosses placenta; enters breast milk
Excretion: Urine

Adverse effects

Effects depend on dose, route, and duration of therapy. The following are primarily associated with systemic absorption.

• **CNS:** *Vertigo, headache,* paresthesias, insomnia, seizures, psychosis, cataracts, increased IOP, glaucoma (long-term therapy), *euphoria, depression*
• **CV:** Hypotension, **shock,** hypertension and HF secondary to fluid retention, thromboembolism, thrombophlebitis, fat embolism, cardiac arrhythmias
• **Electrolyte imbalance:** *Na+ and fluid retention,* hypokalemia, hypocalcemia
• **Endocrine:** Amenorrhea, irregular menses, growth retardation, decreased carbohydrate tolerance, diabetes mellitus, cushingoid state (long-term effect), increased blood sugar, increased serum cholesterol, decreased T_3 and T_4 levels, HPA suppression with systemic therapy longer than 5 days
• **GI:** Peptic or esophageal ulcer, pancreatitis, abdominal distention, nausea, vomiting, *increased appetite, weight gain* (long-term therapy)
• **Hypersensitivity:** Hypersensitivity or anaphylactoid reactions
• **Musculoskeletal:** Muscle weakness, steroid myopathy, loss of muscle mass, osteoporosis, spontaneous fractures (long-term therapy)
• **Other:** *Immunosuppression, aggravation, or masking of infections; impaired wound healing;* thin, fragile skin; petechiae, ecchymoses, purpura, striae; subcutaneous fat atrophy

Ophthalmic solutions

• **Local:** Infections, especially fungal; glaucoma, cataracts with long-term therapy
• **Other:** Systemic absorption and adverse effects (see above) with prolonged use

Interactions

✳ **Drug-drug** • Increased therapeutic and toxic effects of prednisolone with ketoconazole
• Increased therapeutic and toxic effects of estrogens, including hormonal contraceptives
• Risk of severe deterioration of muscle strength in myasthenia gravis patients who also are receiving ambenonium, edrophonium,

neostigmine, pyridostigmine • Decreased steroid blood levels with barbiturates, phenytoin, rifampin, cyclosporine • Decreased effectiveness of salicylates

✳ **Drug-lab test** • False-negative nitroblue tetrazolium test for bacterial infection • Suppression of skin test reactions

■ **Nursing considerations**
Assessment
• **History:** Infections; renal or liver disease; hypothyroidism; ulcerative colitis with impending perforation; diverticulitis; active or latent peptic ulcer; inflammatory bowel disease; HF; hypertension; thromboembolic disorders; osteoporosis; seizure disorders; diabetes mellitus; pregnancy; lactation. Ophthalmic: Acute superficial herpes simplex keratitis; fungal infections of ocular structures; vaccinia, varicella, and other viral diseases of the cornea and conjunctiva; ocular TB
• **Physical:** Weight, T, reflexes and grip strength, affect and orientation, P, BP, peripheral perfusion, prominence of superficial veins, R, adventitious sounds, serum electrolytes, blood glucose

Interventions
• Administer once-a-day doses before 9 AM to mimic normal peak corticosteroid blood levels.
• Increase dosage when patient is subject to stress.
• Have patient place orally disintegrating tablet in mouth, let dissolve, and then swallow.
⊗ **Warning** Taper doses when discontinuing high-dose or long-term therapy to avoid adrenal insufficiency.
⊗ **Warning** Do not give live virus vaccines with immunosuppressive doses of corticosteroids.

Teaching points
Systemic
• Take once-daily doses before 9 AM; if using orally dissolving tablet, place in mouth, let dissolve, and then swallow.
• Do not stop taking the drug without consulting your health care provider.
• Avoid exposure to infections.
• Report unusual weight gain, swelling of the extremities, muscle weakness, black or tarry stools, fever, prolonged sore throat, colds or other infections, worsening of the disorder for which the drug is being taken.

Ophthalmic preparations
• Learn the proper administration technique: Shake suspension well before each use. Lie down or tilt head backward, and look at ceiling. Pull lower eyelid down to form a pocket. Drop suspension inside lower eyelid while looking up. After instilling eye drops, release lower lid, but do not blink for at least 30 seconds; apply gentle pressure to the inside corner of the eye for 1 minute. Do not close eyes tightly, and try not to blink more often than usual. Do not touch dropper to eye, fingers, or any surface. Wait at least 5 minutes before using any other eye preparations.
• Eyes may be sensitive to bright light; sunglasses may help.
• Report worsening of the condition, pain, itching, swelling of the eye, failure of the condition to improve after 1 week.

▽ **predniSONE**
(pred' ni sone)

Apo-Prednisone (CAN), Novo-Prednisone (CAN), Prednisone Intensol Concentrate, Winpred (CAN)

PREGNANCY CATEGORY C

Drug classes
Corticosteroid (intermediate-acting)
Glucocorticoid
Hormone

Therapeutic actions
Enters target cells and binds to intracellular corticosteroid receptors, initiating many complex reactions that are responsible for its anti-inflammatory and immunosuppressive effects.

Indications
• Replacement therapy in adrenal cortical insufficiency
• Hypercalcemia associated with cancer
• Short-term management of various inflammatory and allergic disorders, such as rheumatoid arthritis, collagen diseases (eg, SLE), dermatologic diseases (eg, pemphigus), status asthmaticus, and autoimmune disorders
• Hematologic disorders: Thrombocytopenia purpura, erythroblastopenia
• Ulcerative colitis, acute exacerbations of MS and palliation in some leukemias and lymphomas

- Trichinosis with neurologic or myocardial involvement

Contraindications and cautions

- Contraindicated with infections, especially tuberculosis, fungal infections, amebiasis, vaccinia and varicella, and antibiotic-resistant infections; lactation.
- Use cautiously with renal or liver disease, hypothyroidism, ulcerative colitis with impending perforation, diverticulitis, active or latent peptic ulcer, inflammatory bowel disease, heart failure, hypertension, thromboembolic disorders, osteoporosis, seizure disorders, diabetes mellitus, hepatic disease, pregnancy (monitor infants for adrenal insufficiency).

Available forms

Tablets—1, 2.5, 5, 10, 20, 50 mg; oral solution—5 mg/5 mL, 5 mg/mL

Dosages

Adults

Individualize dosage depending on severity of condition and patient's response. Administer daily dose before 9 AM to minimize adrenal suppression. If long-term therapy is needed, consider alternate-day therapy. After long-term therapy, withdraw drug slowly to avoid adrenal insufficiency. Initial dose, 5–60 mg/day PO. For maintenance therapy, reduce initial dose in small increments at intervals until lowest dose that maintains satisfactory clinical response is reached. For acute exacerbations of MS, 200 mg/day PO for 1 wk, then 80 mg PO every other day for 1 month.

Pediatric patients

- *Physiologic replacement:* 0.05–2 mg/kg/day PO or 4–5 mg/m^2/day PO in equal divided doses every 12 hr.
- *Other indications:* Individualize dosage depending on severity of condition and the patient's response rather than by strict adherence to formulas that correct adult doses for age or body weight. Carefully observe growth and development in infants and children on prolonged therapy.

Pharmacokinetics

Route	Onset	Peak	Duration
Oral	Varies	1–2 hr	1–1.5 days

Metabolism: Hepatic; T$_{1/2}$: 3.5 hr
Distribution: Crosses placenta; enters breast milk
Excretion: Urine

Adverse effects

- **CNS:** *Vertigo, headache,* paresthesias, insomnia, seizures, psychosis, cataracts, increased IOP, glaucoma (long-term therapy), *euphoria, depression*
- **CV:** Hypotension, **shock,** hypertension and HF secondary to fluid retention, thromboembolism, thrombophlebitis, fat embolism, cardiac arrhythmias
- **Electrolyte imbalance:** *Sodium and fluid retention,* hypokalemia, hypocalcemia
- **Endocrine:** Amenorrhea, irregular menses, growth retardation, decreased carbohydrate tolerance, diabetes mellitus, cushingoid state (long-term effect), increased blood sugar, increased serum cholesterol, decreased T$_3$ and T$_4$ levels, HPA suppression with systemic therapy longer than 5 days
- **GI:** Peptic or esophageal ulcer, pancreatitis, abdominal distention, nausea, vomiting, *increased appetite, weight gain* (long-term therapy)
- **Hypersensitivity:** Hypersensitivity or anaphylactoid reactions
- **Musculoskeletal:** Muscle weakness, steroid myopathy, loss of muscle mass, osteoporosis, spontaneous fractures (long-term therapy)
- **Other:** *Immunosuppression, aggravation or masking of infections; impaired wound healing;* thin, fragile skin; petechiae, ecchymoses, purpura, striae; subcutaneous fat atrophy

Interactions

✳ **Drug-drug** • Increased therapeutic and toxic effects with ketoconazole • Increased therapeutic and toxic effects of estrogens, including hormonal contraceptives • Risk of severe deterioration of muscle strength in myasthenia gravis patients who also are receiving ambenonium, edrophonium, neostigmine, pyridostigmine • Decreased steroid blood levels with barbiturates, phenytoin, rifampin • Decreased effectiveness of salicylates

✳ **Drug-lab test** • False-negative nitroblue tetrazolium test for bacterial infection • Suppression of skin test reactions

■ Nursing considerations

Assessment
- **History:** Infections, renal or liver disease, hypothyroidism, ulcerative colitis with impending perforation, diverticulitis, active or latent peptic ulcer, inflammatory bowel disease, HF, hypertension, thromboembolic disorders, osteoporosis, seizure disorders, diabetes mellitus, hepatic disease, lactation
- **Physical:** Weight, T, reflexes and grip strength, affect and orientation, P, BP, peripheral perfusion, prominence of superficial veins, R, adventitious sounds, serum electrolytes, blood glucose

Interventions
- Administer once-a-day doses before 9 AM to mimic normal peak corticosteroid blood levels.
- Increase dosage when patient is subject to stress.
- ⊗ *Warning* Taper doses when discontinuing high-dose or long-term therapy to avoid adrenal insufficiency.
- ⊗ *Warning* Do not give live virus vaccines with immunosuppressive doses of corticosteroids.

Teaching points
- Do not stop taking the drug without consulting your health care provider; take once-daily doses at about 9 AM.
- Avoid exposure to infections.
- Report unusual weight gain, swelling of the extremities, muscle weakness, black or tarry stools, fever, prolonged sore throat, colds or other infections, worsening of the disorder for which the drug is being taken.

▽ pregabalin
(pray gab' ah lin)

Lyrica

PREGNANCY CATEGORY C

CONTROLLED SUBSTANCE V

Drug classes
Analgesic
Antiepileptic
Calcium channel modulator

Therapeutic actions
Binds to alpha₂-delta sites on the nerves in the CNS, which reduces the calcium influx into the cell and decreases the release of neurotransmitters into the synaptic cleft, resulting in less stimulation of the nerve; in lab studies, it also increases the transport and density of GABA, which is known to suppress nerve activity.

Indications
- Management of acute pain associated with diabetic peripheral neuropathy
- Management of post-herpetic neuralgia
- Adjunct therapy of adult patients with partial onset seizures
- Management of fibromyalgia
- ◼ **NEW INDICATION:** Management of neuropathic pain due to spinal cord injuries
- Unlabeled use: Treatment of generalized anxiety disorders

Contraindications and cautions
- Contraindicated with known hypersensitivity to pregabalin or any component of the drug, lactation.
- Use cautiously with diabetes, HF, pregnancy.

Available forms
Capsules—25, 50, 75, 100, 150, 200, 225, 300 mg; oral solution—20 mg/mL

Dosages
Adults
- *Neuropathic pain associated with diabetic neuropathy:* 100 mg PO tid. Maximum, 300 mg/day.
- *Postherpetic neuralgia:* 75–150 mg PO bid or 50–100 mg PO tid as needed to control pain; may be adjusted up to a maximum dose of 600 mg/day.
- *Epilepsy:* 150–600 mg/day PO, divided into two to three doses.
- *Fibromyalgia:* 75 mg PO bid. May be increased within 1 wk to 150 mg PO bid. Maximum dose, 450 mg/day.
- *Neuropathic pain associated with spinal cord injuries:* Initially, 75 mg PO bid; increase to 150 mg PO bid within 1 wk. If relief is not sufficient within 2–3 wk, may increase to 300 mg PO bid.

Pediatric patients
Safety and efficacy not established.

Patients with renal impairment

If creatinine clearance is 60 mL/min or greater, 150–600 mg/day PO in two to three divided doses; if creatinine clearance is 30–60 mL/min, 75–300 mg/day PO in two to three divided doses; if creatinine clearance is 15–30 mL/min, 25–150 mg/day PO in one dose or divided into two doses; if creatinine clearance is less than 15 mL/min, 25–75 mg/day as one dose.

Pharmacokinetics

Route	Onset	Peak
Oral	Rapid	1.5 hr

Metabolism: None; T$_{1/2}$: 6.3 hr
Distribution: May cross placenta; may pass into breast milk
Excretion: Urine

Adverse effects

- **CNS:** *Dizziness, somnolence, neuropathy,* ataxia, vertigo, confusion, euphoria, incoordination, vision abnormalities, tremors, thinking abnormalities, suicidal ideation
- **GI:** *Dry mouth, constipation,* flatulence
- **Other:** *Peripheral edema, weight gain,* hypoglycemia, back pain, chest pain, *infection, creatine kinase elevations,* loss of fertility (male), **angioedema, thrombocytopenia**

Interactions

✳ **Drug-drug** • Increased risk of sedation and dizziness if combined with CNS depressants, alcohol • Increased incidence of weight gain if combined with pioglitazone, rosiglitazone; monitor patient weight and blood glucose if this combination is used

■ Nursing considerations
Assessment

- **History:** Lactation, pregnancy, diabetes, heart failure, allergy to pregabalin
- **Physical:** Weight; orientation, reflexes, affect, vision; renal function tests, blood glucose level

Interventions

⊗ **Black box warning** Risk of suicidal ideation is increased; monitor patient accordingly.

- Do not administer this drug after a fatty or large meal, absorption can be affected.
- Do not stop taking this drug suddenly; dosage should be adjusted to avoid adverse effects.

- Provide safety measures if dizziness, somnolence, changes in thinking occur.
- Monitor weight gain and fluid retention; adjust treatment for diabetes, HF accordingly.
- Encourage women of childbearing age to use barrier contraceptives while on this drug because the effects of the drug on a fetus are not known.
- Advise breast-feeding women to find another method of feeding the infant; it is not known if this drug can affect a breast-feeding infant.
- Advise men who plan to father a child that in animal studies, this drug affected fertility and was related to birth defects in the offspring of male animals taking the drug. The decision to take the drug may be affected by this information.

Teaching points

- Take this drug exactly as prescribed. Do not increase the dose without consulting your health care provider.
- Do not stop taking this drug suddenly; serious adverse effects could occur.
- Do not share this drug with anyone else. Carefully dispose of any unused or outdated drug.
- Do not take this drug with or immediately after a high fat or heavy meal. This could interfere with the absorption and effectiveness of the drug.
- It is not known how this drug would affect a pregnancy. If you think you are pregnant or would like to become pregnant, consult your health care provider. You should use contraceptive measures while taking this drug.
- This drug should not be taken while breast-feeding. If you are breast-feeding, you should use another method of feeding the infant while taking this drug.
- Do not drink alcohol while you are using this drug.
- If you are a man who wants to father a child, discuss this with your health care provider; this drug caused animals to be less fertile and caused some birth defects in the offspring of males taking this drug.
- You may experience these side effects: Dizziness, sleepiness, changes in thinking and alertness (do not drive a car, operate potentially dangerous equipment, or make important legal decisions if this occurs); dry mouth (sucking on sugarless candies, frequent mouth care may help).

P

- Report rash; changes in vision; weight gain; swelling in feet, legs, face, or tongue; increased bleeding; fever; sudden pain; weakness; or thoughts of suicide.

▽ **primidone**
(pri' mi done)

Apo-Primidone (CAN), Mysoline

PREGNANCY CATEGORY D

Drug classes
Anticonvulsant
Antiepileptic

Therapeutic actions
Mechanism of action not understood; primidone and its two metabolites, phenobarbital and phenylethylmalonamide, all have antiepileptic activity.

Indications
- Control of tonic-clonic, psychomotor, or focal epileptic seizures, either alone or with other antiepileptics; may control tonic-clonic seizures refractory to other antiepileptics
- Unlabeled use: Treatment of benign familial tremor (essential tremor)—750 mg/day

Contraindications and cautions
- Contraindicated with hypersensitivity to phenobarbital and primidone, porphyria, lactation (somnolence and drowsiness may occur in breast-feeding newborns).
- Use cautiously with pregnancy (association between use of antiepileptics and an elevated incidence of birth defects; however, do not discontinue antiepileptic therapy in pregnant women who are receiving such therapy to prevent major seizures; discontinuing medication is likely to precipitate status epilepticus, with attendant hypoxia and risk to both mother and fetus; to prevent neonatal hemorrhage, primidone should be given with prophylactic vitamin K_1 therapy for 1 mo before and during delivery).

Available forms
Tablets—50, 250 mg

Dosages
Adults
- *Regimen for patients who have received no previous therapy:* Days 1–3, 100–125 mg PO at bedtime; days 4–6, 100–125 mg PO bid; days 7–9, 100–125 mg PO tid; day 10–maintenance, 250 mg tid. The usual maintenance dosage is 250 mg tid–qid. If required, increase dosage to 250 mg five to six times daily, but do not exceed dosage of 500 mg qid (2 g/day).
- *Regimen for patients already receiving other antiepileptics:* Start primidone at 100–125 mg PO at bedtime. Gradually increase to maintenance level as the other drug is gradually decreased. Continue this regimen until satisfactory dosage level is achieved for the combination, or the other medication is completely withdrawn. When use of primidone alone is desired, the transition should not be completed in less than 2 wk.

Pediatric patients
- *Regimen for patients who have received no previous therapy:*
  Younger than 8 yr: Days 1–3, 50 mg PO at bedtime; days 4–6, 50 mg PO bid; days 7–9, 100 mg PO bid; day 10–maintenance, 125–250 mg PO tid. The usual maintenance dosage is 125–250 mg PO tid or 10–25 mg/kg/day PO in divided doses.
  Older than 8 yr: Use adult dosage.

Pharmacokinetics

Route	Onset	Peak
Oral	Varies	3–7 hr

Metabolism: Hepatic; $T_{1/2}$: 10–12 hr
Distribution: Crosses placenta; enters breast milk
Excretion: Urine

Adverse effects
- **CNS:** *Ataxia, vertigo, fatigue, hyperirritability,* emotional disturbances, nystagmus, diplopia, drowsiness, personality deterioration with mood changes and paranoia, suicidal ideation, tolerance
- **GI:** *Nausea, anorexia,* vomiting
- **GU:** Sexual impotence
- **Hematologic:** Megaloblastic anemia that responds to folic acid therapy, thrombocytopenia
- **Other:** Morbilliform skin eruptions

Interactions
✱ Drug-drug • Toxicity with phenytoins • Increased CNS effects, impaired hand-eye coordination, and death may occur with acute alcohol ingestion • Decreased serum

concentrations of primidone and increased serum concentrations of carbamazepine if taken concurrently • Decreased serum concentrations with acetazolamide • Increased levels with isoniazid, nicotinamide, succinimides

■ **Nursing considerations**
Assessment
• **History:** Hypersensitivity to phenobarbital, porphyria, pregnancy, lactation, suicidal ideation
• **Physical:** Skin color, lesions; orientation, affect, reflexes, vision examination; bowel sounds, normal output; CBC and SMA-12, EEG

Interventions
⊗ **Black box warning** Risk of suicidal ideation is increased. Monitor patient accordingly.

⊗ **Warning** Reduce dosage, discontinue primidone, or substitute other antiepileptic gradually; abrupt discontinuation may precipitate status epilepticus.
• Arrange for patient to have CBC and SMA-12 test every 6 mo during therapy.
• Arrange for folic acid therapy if megaloblastic anemia occurs; primidone does not need to be discontinued.
• Obtain counseling for women of childbearing age who wish to become pregnant.
⊗ **Warning** Evaluate for therapeutic serum levels—5–12 mcg/mL for primidone.

Teaching points
• Take this drug exactly as prescribed; do not discontinue this drug abruptly or change dosage, except on the advice of your health care provider.
• Arrange for frequent checkups, including blood tests, to monitor your response to this drug. Keep all appointments for checkups.
• Use contraception at all times. If you wish to become pregnant while you are taking this drug, you should consult your health care provider.
• Wear a medical alert tag at all times so that emergency medical personnel will know that you have epilepsy and are taking antiepileptic medication.
• You may experience these side effects: Drowsiness, dizziness, muscular incoordination (transient; avoid driving or performing other tasks requiring alertness); vision changes

(avoid performing tasks that require visual acuity); GI upset (take drug with food or milk, eat frequent small meals).
• Report rash, joint pain, unexplained fever, pregnancy, thoughts of suicide.

▽ **probenecid**
(proe ben' e sid)

Benuryl (CAN), Probalan

PREGNANCY CATEGORY B

Drug classes
Antigout drug
Uricosuric drug

Therapeutic actions
Inhibits the renal tubular reabsorption of urate, increasing the urinary excretion of uric acid, decreasing serum uric acid levels, retarding urate deposition, and promoting resorption of urate deposits; also inhibits the renal tubular reabsorption of most penicillins and cephalosporins.

Indications
• Treatment of hyperuricemia associated with gout and gouty arthritis (adults)
• Adjuvant to therapy with penicillins or cephalosporins, for elevation and prolongation of plasma levels of the antibiotic

Contraindications and cautions
• Contraindicated with allergy to probenecid, blood dyscrasias, uric acid kidney stones, acute gouty attack.
• Use cautiously with peptic ulcer, acute intermittent porphyria, G6PD deficiency, chronic renal insufficiency, in patients with sulfa allergy, lactation, pregnancy.

Available forms
Tablets—0.5 g

Dosages
Adults
• *Gout:* 0.25 g PO bid for 1 wk; then 0.5 g PO bid. Maximum 2–3 g/day. For maintenance, continue dosage that maintains the normal serum uric acid levels. When no attacks occur for 6 mo or longer, decrease the daily dosage by 0.5 g every 6 mo.

- *Penicillin or cephalosporin therapy:* 2 g/day PO in divided doses.
- *Gonorrhea treatment:* Single 1-g dose PO 30 min before penicillin administration.

Pediatric patients
- *Penicillin or cephalosporin therapy: Younger than 2 yr:* Do not use.
  2–14 yr: 25 mg/kg PO initial dose, then 40 mg/kg/day divided in four doses.
  Children 50 kg or greater: Use adult dosage.
- *Gonorrhea treatment in children less than 45 kg:* 23 mg/kg PO in one single dose 30 min before penicillin administration.

Geriatric patients or patients with renal impairment
1 g/day PO may be adequate. Daily dosage may be increased by 0.5 g every 4 wk. Probenecid may not be effective in chronic renal insufficiency when GFR less than 30 mL/min.

Pharmacokinetics

Route	Onset	Peak
Oral	Varies	2–4 hr

Metabolism: Hepatic; $T_{1/2}$: 4–17 hr
Distribution: Crosses placenta; may enter breast milk
Excretion: Urine

Adverse effects
- **CNS:** *Headache*
- **GI:** *Nausea, vomiting, anorexia,* sore gums
- **GU:** *Urinary frequency,* exacerbation of gout and uric acid stones
- **Hematologic:** Anemia, hemolytic anemia
- **Hypersensitivity:** Reactions including **anaphylaxis,** dermatitis, pruritus, fever
- **Other:** Blushing, dizziness

Interactions
✳ **Drug-drug** ● Decreased effectiveness with salicylates ● Decreased renal excretion and increased serum levels of methotrexate, dyphylline ● Increased pharmacologic effects of thiopental, acyclovir, allopurinol, benzodiazepines, clofibrate, dapsone, NSAIDs, sulfonamides, zidovudine, rifampin

✳ **Drug-lab test** ● False-positive test for urine glucose if using Benedict test, *Clinitest* (use *Clinistix*) ● Falsely high determination of theophylline levels ● Inhibited excretion of urinary 17-ketosteroids, phenolsulfonphthalein, sulfobromophthalein

■ Nursing considerations
Assessment
- **History:** Allergy to probenecid, blood dyscrasias, uric acid kidney stones, acute gouty attack, peptic ulcer, acute intermittent porphyria, G6PD deficiency, chronic renal insufficiency, pregnancy, lactation
- **Physical:** Skin lesions, color; reflexes; gait; liver evaluation, normal output, gums; urinary output; CBC, LFTs, renal function tests, urinalysis

Interventions
- Administer drug with meals or antacids if GI upset occurs.
- Encourage patient to drink 2.5 to 3 L/day of fluids to decrease the risk of renal stone development.
- Check urine alkalinity; urates crystallize in acid urine; sodium bicarbonate or potassium citrate may be ordered to alkalinize urine.
- Arrange for regular medical follow-up and blood tests.
- Double-check any analgesics ordered for pain; salicylates should be avoided.

Teaching points
- Take the drug with meals or antacids if GI upset occurs.
- You may experience these side effects: Headache (monitor lighting, temperature, noise; consult your health care provider if severe); dizziness (change position slowly; avoid driving or operating dangerous machinery); exacerbation of gouty attack or renal stones (drink plenty of fluids—2.5–3 liters per day); nausea, vomiting, loss of appetite (take drug with meals or request antacids).
- Report flank pain, dark urine or blood in urine, acute gout attack, unusual fatigue or lethargy, unusual bleeding or bruising.

▷ **procarbazine hydrochloride**

See Appendix R, *Less commonly used drugs.*

Adverse effects in *italics* are most common; those in **bold** are life-threatening. ⬚ Do not crush.

▷ prochlorperazine
(proe klor per' a zeen)

prochlorperazine

prochlorperazine edisylate

prochlorperazine maleate
Procomp

PREGNANCY CATEGORY C

Drug classes
Antiemetic
Antipsychotic
Anxiolytic
Dopaminergic blocker
Phenothiazine (piperazine)

Therapeutic actions
Mechanism of action not fully understood: Antipsychotics block postsynaptic dopamine receptors in the brain, but this may not be necessary and sufficient for antipsychotic activity; depresses the RAS, including the parts of the brain involved with wakefulness and emesis; anticholinergic, antihistaminic (H_1), and alpha-adrenergic blocking activity also may contribute to some of its therapeutic (and adverse) actions.

Indications
- Management of manifestations of psychotic disorders
- Control of severe nausea and vomiting
- Short-term treatment of nonpsychotic anxiety (not drug of choice)

Contraindications and cautions
- Contraindicated with hypersensitivity to phenothiazines, coma or severe CNS depression, bone marrow depression, blood dyscrasia, circulatory collapse, subcortical brain damage, Parkinson disease, liver damage, cerebral arteriosclerosis, coronary disease, congenital long-QT syndrome, severe hypotension or hypertension, history of cardiac arrhythmias.
- Use cautiously with elderly patients, respiratory disorders, glaucoma, prostatic hypertrophy, epilepsy, breast cancer (elevations in prolactin may stimulate a prolactin-dependent tumor), thyrotoxicosis, peptic

ulcer, decreased renal function, myelography within previous 24 hr or scheduled within 48 hr, exposure to heat or phosphorous insecticides, pregnancy, lactation, children younger than 12 yr, especially those with chickenpox, CNS infections (children are especially susceptible to dystonias that may confound the diagnosis of Reye syndrome).

Available forms
Tablets—5, 10, 25 mg; suppositories—25 mg; injection—5 mg/mL

Dosages
Adults
- *Psychotic disturbances:* Initially, 5–10 mg PO tid or qid. Gradually increase dosage every 2–3 days as needed up to 50–75 mg/day for mild or moderate disturbances, 100–150 mg/day for more severe disturbances. For immediate control of severely disturbed adults, 10–20 mg IM repeated every 2–4 hr (every hour for resistant cases); switch to oral therapy as soon as possible.
- *Antiemetic:* For control of severe nausea and vomiting, 5–10 mg PO tid–qid; 15 mg (SR) on arising; 25 mg rectally bid; or 5–10 mg IM initially, repeated every 3–4 hr up to 40 mg/day.
- *Nausea, vomiting related to surgery:* 5–10 mg IM 1–2 hr before anesthesia or during and after surgery (may repeat once in 30 min); 5–10 mg IV 15 min before anesthesia or during and after surgery (may repeat once); or as IV infusion, 20 mg/L of isotonic solution added to infusion 15–30 min before anesthesia.
- *Nonpsychotic anxiety:* 5 mg PO tid or qid. Do not give more than 20 mg/day or for longer than 12 wk.

Pediatric patients
Do not use in pediatric surgery.
Less than 9 kg or younger than 2 yr: Generally not recommended.
Psychotic disturbances: 2–12 yr: 2.5 mg PO or rectally bid–tid. Do not give more than 10 mg on first day. Increase dosage according to patient response; total daily dose usually does not exceed 20 mg (2–5 yr) or 25 mg (6–12 yr).
Younger than 12 yr: 0.132 mg/kg by deep IM injection. Switch to oral dosage as soon as possible (usually after one dose).
- *Antiemetic for control of severe nausea and vomiting:*

P.

Oral or rectal
More than 20 lb or older than 2 yr:
9.1–13.2 kg: 2.5 mg daily–bid, not to exceed 7.5 mg/day.
13.6–17.7 kg: 2.5 mg bid–tid, not to exceed 10 mg/day.
18.2–38.6 kg: 2.5 mg tid or 5 mg bid, not to exceed 15 mg/day.

IM
2 yr and older weighing at least 9.1 kg: 0.132 mg/kg IM (usually only one dose).

Pharmacokinetics

Route	Onset	Duration
Oral	30–40 min	3–4 hr
SR	30–40 min	10–12 hr
Rectal	60–90 min	3–4 hr
IM	10–20 min	3–4 hr
IV	Immediate	3–4 hr

Metabolism: Hepatic; $T_{1/2}$: Unknown
Distribution: Crosses placenta; enters breast milk
Excretion: Urine

▼ IV FACTS

Preparation: Dilute 20 mg in not less than 1 L of isotonic solution.
Infusion: Inject 5–10 mg directly IV 15–30 min before induction (may be repeated once), or infuse dilute solution 15–30 min before induction; do not exceed 5 mg/mL/min.

Adverse effects

- **Autonomic:** Dry mouth, salivation, nasal congestion, nausea, vomiting, anorexia, fever, pallor, flushed facies, sweating, constipation, paralytic ileus, urinary retention, incontinence, polyuria, enuresis, priapism, ejaculation inhibition, male impotence
- **CNS:** *Drowsiness, dizziness,* insomnia, vertigo, headache, weakness, tremor, ataxia, slurring, cerebral edema, seizures, exacerbation of psychotic symptoms, extrapyramidal syndromes—*pseudoparkinsonism; dystonias; akathisia,* tardive dyskinesia, potentially irreversible; **NMS**
- **CV:** Hypotension, orthostatic hypotension, hypertension, tachycardia, bradycardia, cardiac arrest, **HF,** cardiomegaly, **refractory arrhythmias,** pulmonary edema

- **EENT:** Glaucoma, *photophobia, blurred vision,* miosis, mydriasis, deposits in the cornea and lens (opacities), pigmentary retinopathy
- **Endocrine:** Lactation, breast engorgement, galactorrhea; SIADH; amenorrhea, menstrual irregularities; gynecomastia; changes in libido; hyperglycemia or hypoglycemia; glycosuria; hyponatremia; pituitary tumor with hyperprolactinemia; inhibition of ovulation, infertility, pseudopregnancy; reduced urinary levels of gonadotropins, estrogens, progestins
- **Hematologic:** Eosinophilia, leukopenia, leukocytosis, anemia; **aplastic anemia; hemolytic anemia;** thrombocytopenic or nonthrombocytopenic purpura; pancytopenia
- **Hypersensitivity:** Jaundice, urticaria, angioneurotic edema, laryngeal edema, photosensitivity, eczema, asthma, anaphylactoid reactions, exfoliative dermatitis
- **Respiratory: Bronchospasm, laryngospasm,** dyspnea; suppression of cough reflex and potential for aspiration
- **Other:** *Urine discolored pink to red-brown*

Interactions

✳ **Drug-drug** • Additive CNS depression with alcohol • Additive anticholinergic effects and possibly decreased antipsychotic efficacy with anticholinergic drugs • Increased chance of severe neuromuscular excitation and hypotension with barbiturate anesthetics (methohexital, phenobarbital, thiopental)

✳ **Drug-lab test** • False-positive pregnancy tests (less likely if serum test is used) • Increase in PBI, not attributable to an increase in thyroxine • False-positive PKU test results

■ Nursing considerations
Assessment

- **History:** Coma or severe CNS depression; bone marrow depression; circulatory collapse; subcortical brain damage; Parkinson disease; liver damage; cerebral arteriosclerosis; coronary disease; severe hypotension or hypertension; respiratory disorders; allergy to phenothiazines; glaucoma, prostatic hypertrophy; epilepsy; breast cancer; thyrotoxicosis; peptic ulcer, decreased renal function; myelography within previous 24 hr or scheduled within 48 hr; exposure to heat or phosphorous insecticides; pregnancy; lactation; age younger than 12 yr

- **Physical:** Weight; T; reflexes, orientation, IOP; P, BP, orthostatic BP; R, adventitious sounds; bowel sounds and normal output; liver evaluation; urinary output, prostate size; CBC; urinalysis; LFTs, renal and thyroid function tests

Interventions

⊗ **Black box warning** There is an increased risk of death if used to treat dementia-related psychosis in elderly patients; not approved for this use.

- Do not administer subcutaneously because of local irritation.
- Give IM injections deeply into the upper outer quadrant of the buttock.
- Avoid skin contact with oral solution; contact dermatitis may occur.

⊗ **Warning** Discontinue drug if serum creatinine or BUN become abnormal or if WBC count is depressed.

- Elderly patients may be more sensitive to antidopaminergic and anticholinergic effects; monitor accordingly.
- Monitor elderly patients for dehydration, and institute remedial measures promptly; sedation and decreased sensation of thirst related to CNS effects of drug can lead to severe dehydration.
- Consult physician regarding appropriate warning of patient or patient's guardian about tardive dyskinesias.
- Consult physician about dosage reduction, use of anticholinergic antiparkinsonians (controversial) if extrapyramidal effects occur.

Teaching points

- Take drug exactly as prescribed.
- Maintain fluid intake, and use precautions against heatstroke in hot weather.
- Avoid exposure to ultraviolet or sunlight to prevent photosensitivity. Use sunscreen and protective clothing.
- Avoid driving or engaging in other dangerous activities if dizziness, drowsiness, or vision changes occur.
- Report sore throat, fever, unusual bleeding or bruising, rash, weakness, tremors, impaired vision, dark urine (expect pink or reddish-brown urine), pale stools, yellowing of the skin or eyes.

▽ **progesterone**
(proe jess' ter own)

Progesterone in oil (parenteral):
Progesterone aqueous
Progesterone
Crinone, Prometrium
Vaginal insert: Endometrin

PREGNANCY CATEGORY B

PREGNANCY CATEGORY D (INJECTION)

Drug classes

Hormone
Progestin

Therapeutic actions

Endogenous female progestational substance; transforms proliferative endometrium into secretory endometrium; inhibits the secretion of pituitary gonadotropins, which prevents follicular maturation and ovulation; inhibits spontaneous uterine contractions; may have some estrogenic, anabolic, or androgenic activity.

Indications

- Treatment of primary and secondary amenorrhea
- Treatment of abnormal uterine bleeding
- Prevention of endometrial hyperplasia
- Treatment of endometrial hyperplasia in non-hysterectomized women who are receiving conjugated estrogens
- Vaginal: To support embryo implantation and early pregnancy by supplementation of corpus luteal function as part of an assisted reproductive technology treatment program for infertile women
- Gel: Infertility, as part of assisted reproductive technology for infertile women
- Unlabeled uses: Treatment of PMS, prevention of premature labor and habitual abortion in the first trimester, treatment of menorrhagia (intrauterine system)

Contraindications and cautions

- Contraindicated with allergy to progestins, allergy to peanuts (oral), thrombophlebitis, thromboembolic disorders, cerebral hemorrhage or history of these conditions, hepatic

P

disease, carcinoma of the breast or genital organs, undiagnosed vaginal bleeding, missed abortion, diagnostic test for pregnancy, pregnancy (fetal abnormalities, including masculinization of the female fetus have occurred), PID, venereal disease, postpartum endometritis, pelvic surgery, uterine or cervical carcinoma (intrauterine system).

• Use cautiously with epilepsy, migraine, asthma, cardiac dysfunction, renal impairment, lactation (oral).

Available forms

Injection—50 mg/mL; vaginal gel—45 mg (4%), 90 mg (8%); capsules—100, 200 mg; vaginal insert—100 mg

Dosages

Administer parenteral preparation by IM route only.

Adults

• *Amenorrhea:* 5–10 mg/day IM for 6–8 consecutive days. Expect withdrawal bleeding 48–72 hr after the last injection. Or use 400 mg PO in the evening for 10 days. Spontaneous normal cycles may follow.

• *Secondary amenorrhea:* Using 4% gel, 45 mg every other day to maximum of 6 doses. For women who do not respond, trial of 8% gel every other day to maximum of 6 doses.

• *Uterine bleeding:* 5–10 mg/day IM for six doses. Bleeding should cease within 6 days. If estrogen is being given, begin progesterone after 2 wk of estrogen therapy. Discontinue injections when menstrual flow begins.

• *Endometrial hyperplasia:* 200 mg/day PO in the evening for 12 days per 28-day cycle in combination with a daily conjugated estrogen.

• *Infertility:* 90 mg vaginally daily in women requiring progesterone supplementation; 90 mg vaginally bid for replacement— continue for 10–12 wk into pregnancy if it occurs.

• *Support for implantation:* 100 mg inserted vaginally two to three times daily starting at oocyte retrieval and continuing for up to 10 wk.

Pharmacokinetics

Route	Onset	Peak	Duration
Oral	Varies	1–2 hr	Unknown
IM	Varies	Unknown	Unknown
Vaginal gel	Slow	Unknown	25–50 hr

Adverse effects in italics are most common; those in bold are life-threatening. ⊕ *Do not crush.*

Metabolism: Hepatic; $T_{1/2}$: 8–9 hr on steady-state
Distribution: Crosses placenta; enters breast milk
Excretion: Urine, bile

Adverse effects
Parenteral and oral

• **CNS:** Sudden, partial, or complete loss of vision, proptosis, diplopia, migraine, precipitation of acute intermittent porphyria, mental depression, pyrexia, insomnia, *somnolence, dizziness, headache*

• **CV:** Thrombophlebitis, cerebrovascular disorders, retinal thrombosis, **pulmonary embolism**

• **Dermatologic:** Rash with or without pruritus, acne, melasma or chloasma, alopecia, hirsutism, *photosensitivity*

• **GI:** Cholestatic jaundice, nausea, *abdominal cramping, constipation*

• **GU:** *Breakthrough bleeding, spotting, change in menstrual flow, amenorrhea, changes in cervical erosion and cervical secretions, breast tenderness* and secretion, transient increase in sodium and chloride excretion

• **Other:** Fluid retention, edema, *change in weight,* effects similar to those seen with hormonal contraceptives, breast pain

Oral contraceptives

• **CV:** Increased BP, **thromboembolic and thrombotic disease**

• **Endocrine:** Decreased glucose tolerance

• **GI:** Hepatic adenoma

Vaginal gel

• **CNS:** *Somnolence, headache,* nervousness, depression

• **GI:** *Constipation,* nausea, diarrhea

• **Other:** *Breast enlargement,* nocturia, perineal pain

Interactions

✳ **Drug-lab test** • Inaccurate tests of hepatic and endocrine function

✳ **Drug-food** • Decreased metabolism and risk of toxic effects if combined with grapefruit juice; avoid this combination

■ Nursing considerations
Assessment

• **History:** Allergy to progestins, allergy to peanuts (oral), thrombophlebitis, thromboembolic disorders, cerebral hemorrhage, hepatic disease, carcinoma of the breast or genital organs, undiagnosed vaginal bleeding, missed abortion, epilepsy, migraine, asthma, cardiac dysfunction, renal impairment, PID, venereal disease, postpartum endometritis, pelvic surgery, uterine or cervical carcinoma, pregnancy, lactation

- **Physical:** Skin color, lesions, turgor; hair; breasts; pelvic examination; orientation, affect; ophthalmologic examination; P, auscultation, peripheral perfusion, edema; R, adventitious sounds; liver evaluation; LFTs, renal function tests, glucose tolerance; Papanicolaou (Pap) test

Interventions

- Arrange for pretreatment and periodic (at least annual) history and physical examination, including BP, breasts, abdomen, pelvic organs, and a Pap test.
- Arrange for insertion of intrauterine system during or immediately after menstrual period to ensure that the patient is not pregnant; arrange to have patient re-examined after first month menses to ensure that system has not been expelled.

⊗ **Black box warning** Do not use progestins for the prevention of CV disease. Drug is not effective for this use; risk of CV disease may actually be increased.

⊗ *Warning* Caution patient before therapy of the need to prevent pregnancy during treatment and to obtain frequent medical follow-up.

- Administer parenteral preparations by IM injection only.

⊗ *Warning* Discontinue medication and consult physician if sudden partial or complete loss of vision occurs; discontinue if papilledema or retinal vascular lesions are present on examination.

⊗ *Warning* Discontinue drug and consult physician at the first sign of thromboembolic disease—leg pain, swelling, peripheral perfusion changes, shortness of breath.

Teaching points

- This drug can be given IM; it will be given daily for the specified number of days, or inserted vaginally and can remain for 1 year (as appropriate), or inserted vaginally using the applicator system one to two times per day; or given orally for 10 days.

- If used for fertility program, continue vaginal gel or insert 10–12 weeks into pregnancy until placental autonomy is achieved.
- Do not drink grapefruit juice while using this drug.
- This drug should not be taken during pregnancy (except vaginal gel); serious fetal abnormalities have been reported. If you may be pregnant, consult your health care provider immediately.
- Perform a monthly breast self-examination while using this drug.
- You may experience these side effects: Sensitivity to light (avoid exposure to the sun; use sunscreen and protective clothing); dizziness, sleeplessness, depression (use caution if driving or performing tasks that require alertness); rash, skin color changes, loss of hair; fever; nausea.
- Report pain or swelling and warmth in the calves, acute chest pain or shortness of breath, sudden severe headache or vomiting, dizziness or fainting, visual disturbances, numbness or tingling in the arm or leg.

Vaginal gel or insert

- Report severe headache, abnormal vaginal bleeding or discharge, acute calf or chest pain, fever.

DANGEROUS DRUG

▽ **promethazine hydrochloride**

(*proe meth' a zeen*)

Phenadoz, Phenergan, Promethegan

PREGNANCY CATEGORY C

Drug classes

Antiemetic
Antihistamine
Anti–motion-sickness drug
Dopaminergic blocker
Phenothiazine
Sedative-hypnotic

Therapeutic actions

Selectively blocks histamine-1 receptors, diminishing the effects of histamine on cells of the upper respiratory tract and eyes and decreasing the sneezing, mucus production, itching, and tearing that accompany allergic reactions in sensitized people exposed to antigens;

blocks cholinergic receptors in the vomiting center that are believed to mediate the nausea and vomiting caused by gastric irritation, by input from the vestibular apparatus (motion sickness, nausea associated with vestibular neuritis), and by input from the chemoreceptor trigger zone (drug- and radiation-induced emesis); depresses the RAS, including the parts of the brain involved with wakefulness.

Indications

• Symptomatic relief of perennial and seasonal allergic rhinitis, vasomotor rhinitis, allergic conjunctivitis; mild, uncomplicated urticaria and angioedema; amelioration of allergic reactions to blood or plasma; dermatographism, adjunctive therapy (with epinephrine and other measures) in anaphylactic reactions
• Treatment and prevention of motion sickness; prevention and control of nausea and vomiting associated with anesthesia and surgery
• Preoperative, postoperative, or obstetric sedation
• Adjunct to analgesics to control postoperative pain
• Adjunctive IV therapy with reduced amounts of meperidine or other opioid analgesics in special surgical situations, such as repeated bronchoscopy, ophthalmic surgery, or in poor-risk patients
• Unlabeled use: Treatment of nausea and vomiting in pregnancy

Contraindications and cautions

• Contraindicated with hypersensitivity to antihistamines or phenothiazines, coma or severe CNS depression, bone marrow depression, vomiting of unknown cause, concomitant therapy with MAOIs, lactation (lactation may be inhibited).
• Use cautiously with lower respiratory tract disorders (may cause thickening of secretions and impair expectoration), glaucoma, prostatic hypertrophy, CV disease or hypertension, breast cancer, thyrotoxicosis, pregnancy (jaundice and extrapyramidal effects in infants; drug may inhibit platelet aggregation in neonate if taken by mother within 2 wk of delivery), children (antihistamine overdose may cause hallucinations, seizures, and death), a child with a history of sleep apnea, a family history of SIDS, or Reye syndrome (may mask the symptoms of Reye

syndrome and contribute to its development), the elderly (more likely to cause dizziness, sedation, syncope, toxic confusional states, hypotension, and extrapyramidal effects).

Available forms

Tablets—12.5, 25, 50 mg; syrup—6.25 mg/5 mL; suppositories—12.5, 25, 50 mg; injection—25, 50 mg/mL

Dosages
Adults

• *Allergy:* Average dose is 25 mg PO or by rectal suppository, preferably at bedtime. If needed, 12.5 mg PO before meals and at bedtime; 25 mg IM or IV for serious reactions. May repeat within 2 hr if needed.
• *Motion sickness:* 25 mg PO bid. Initial dose should be scheduled 30–60 min before travel; repeat in 8–12 hr if needed. Thereafter, give 25 mg on arising and before evening meal.
• *Nausea and vomiting:* 25 mg PO; repeat doses of 12.5–25 mg as needed, every 4–6 hr. Give rectally or parenterally if oral dosage is not tolerated. 12.5–25 mg IM or IV, not to be repeated more frequently than every 4–6 hr.
• *Sedation:* 25–50 mg PO, IM, or IV.
• *Preoperative use:* 50 mg PO the night before, or 50 mg with an appropriately reduced dose of meperidine and the required amount of belladonna alkaloid.
• *Postoperative sedation and adjunctive use with analgesics:* 25–50 mg PO, IM, or IV.
• *Labor:* 50 mg IM or IV in early stages. When labor is established, 25–75 mg with a reduced dose of opioid. May repeat once or twice at 4-hr intervals. Maximum dose within 24 hr is 100 mg.

Pediatric patients older than 2 yr

• *Allergy:* 25 mg PO at bedtime or 6.25–12.5 mg tid.
• *Motion sickness:* 12.5–25 mg PO or rectally bid.
• *Nausea and vomiting:* 0.5 mg/lb of body weight IM every 4–6 hr as needed.
• *Sedation:* 12.5–25 mg PO or 12.5–25 mg PO or rectally at bedtime.
• *Preoperative use:* 0.5 mg/lb of body weight PO in combination with an appropriately reduced dose of opioid or barbiturate and the required amount of an atropine-like drug.

Adverse effects in *italics* are most common; those in **bold** are life-threatening. ▣ Do not crush.

- *Postoperative sedation and adjunctive use with analgesics:* 0.5 mg/lb up to 12.5–25 mg PO, IM, IV, or rectally.

Pharmacokinetics

Route	Onset	Duration
Oral	20 min	12 hr
IM	20 min	12 hr
IV	3–5 min	12 hr

Metabolism: Hepatic; T$_{1/2}$: 9–16 hr
Distribution: Crosses placenta; enters breast milk
Excretion: Urine

▼ IV FACTS

Preparation: Dilute to a concentration no greater than 25 mg/mL.
Infusion: Infuse no faster than 25 mg/min.
Incompatibilities: Do not combine with aminophylline, chloramphenicol, heparin, hydrocortisone, pentobarbital, thiopental.
Y-site incompatibilities: Do not give with foscarnet, heparin, hydrocortisone, potassium chloride.

Adverse effects

- **CNS:** *Dizziness, drowsiness, poor coordination, confusion, restlessness, excitation,* seizures, tremors, headache, blurred vision, diplopia, vertigo, tinnitus
- **CV:** Hypotension, palpitations, bradycardia, tachycardia, extrasystoles
- **Dermatologic:** Urticaria, rash, photosensitivity, chills
- **GI:** *Epigastric distress,* nausea, vomiting, diarrhea, constipation
- **GU:** *Urinary frequency, dysuria,* urinary retention, decreased libido, impotence
- **Hematologic:** Hemolytic anemia, hypoplastic anemia, thrombocytopenia, leukopenia, **agranulocytosis, pancytopenia**
- **Respiratory:** *Thickening of bronchial secretions;* chest tightness; dry mouth, nose, and throat; respiratory depression; suppression of cough reflex; potential for aspiration
- **Other:** Tingling, heaviness and wetness of the hands

Interactions

✳ **Drug-drug** • Additive anticholinergic effects with anticholinergic drugs • Increased frequency and severity of neuromuscular excitation and hypotension with methohexital, phenobarbital anesthetic, thiopental • Enhanced CNS depression with alcohol

■ Nursing considerations
Assessment

- **History:** Hypersensitivity to antihistamines or phenothiazines, severe CNS depression, bone marrow depression, vomiting of unknown cause, concomitant therapy with MAOIs, lactation, lower respiratory tract disorders, glaucoma, prostatic hypertrophy, CV disease or hypertension, breast cancer, thyrotoxicosis, pregnancy, history of sleep apnea or a family history of SIDS, child with Reye syndrome
- **Physical:** Weight; T; reflexes, orientation, IOP; P, BP, orthostatic BP; R, adventitious sounds; bowel sounds and normal output, liver evaluation; urinary output, prostate size; CBC; urinalysis; LFTs, renal and thyroid function tests

Interventions

⊗ **Black box warning** Do not give to children younger than 2 yr because of risk of fatal respiratory depression; use lowest effective dose and caution in children 2 yr and older.

- Give IM injections deep into muscle.
- Do not administer subcutaneously; tissue necrosis may occur.

⊗ **Black box warning** Do not administer intra-arterially; arteriospasm and gangrene of the limb may result. Do not administer subcutaneously into an artery or under the skin; drug may leach into tissue and cause serious injury. If IV route is used, limit drug concentration and rate of administration and ensure open IV line.

⊗ **Warning** Reduce dosage of barbiturates given concurrently with promethazine by at least one-half; arrange for dosage reduction of opioid analgesics given concomitantly by one-fourth to one-half.

Teaching points

- Take drug exactly as prescribed.
- Avoid using alcohol.
- Avoid driving or engaging in other dangerous activities if dizziness, drowsiness, or vision changes occur.
- Avoid prolonged exposure to sun, or use a sunscreen or covering garments.

P

- Maintain fluid intake, and use precautions against heatstroke in hot weather.
- Report sore throat, fever, unusual bleeding or bruising, rash, weakness, tremors, impaired vision, dark urine, pale stools, yellowing of the skin or eyes.

DANGEROUS DRUG

▷ **propafenone hydrochloride**

(*proe paf′ a non*)

Apo-Propafenone (CAN), Gen-Propafenone (CAN), Rythmol, Rythmol SR◉

PREGNANCY CATEGORY C

Drug class
Antiarrhythmic

Therapeutic actions
Class IC antiarrhythmic: Local anesthetic effects with a direct membrane stabilizing action on the myocardial membranes; refractory period is prolonged with a reduction of spontaneous automaticity and depressed trigger activity.

Indications
- Treatment of documented life-threatening ventricular arrhythmias; reserve use for those patients in whom the benefits outweigh the risks
- To prolong the time to recurrence of symptomatic atrial fibrillation in patients with structural heart disease (ER capsules)
- Unlabeled use: Treatment of supraventricular tachycardias, including atrial fibrillation associated with Wolff-Parkinson-White syndrome

Contraindications and cautions
- Contraindicated with hypersensitivity to propafenone, uncontrolled HF, cardiogenic shock, cardiac conduction disturbances in the absence of an artificial pacemaker, bradycardia, marked hypotension, bronchospastic disorders, manifest electrolyte imbalance, pregnancy (teratogenic in preclinical studies), lactation.
- Use cautiously with hepatic, renal impairment; elevated ANA.

Available forms
Tablets—150, 225, 300 mg; ER capsules◉—225, 325, 425 mg

Dosages
Adults
Adjust on the basis of response and tolerance. Initiate with 150 mg PO every 8 hr (450 mg/day). Dosage may be increased at a minimum of 3- to 4-day intervals to 225 mg PO every 8 hr (675 mg/day) and if necessary, to 300 mg PO every 8 hr (900 mg/day). Do not exceed 900 mg/day. Decrease dosage with significant widening of the QRS complex or with AV block; ER capsules—initially, 225 mg PO every 12 hr titrate at 5-day intervals to maximum 425 mg every 12 hr.
Pediatric patients
Safety and efficacy not established.
Geriatric patients
Use with caution; increase dose more gradually during the initial phase of treatment.

Pharmacokinetics

Route	Onset	Peak
Oral	Varies	3.5 hr
ER	Unknown	3–8 hr

Metabolism: Hepatic; $T_{1/2}$: 2–10 hr
Distribution: Crosses placenta; enters breast milk
Excretion: Urine

Adverse effects
- **CNS:** *Dizziness, headache, weakness, fatigue, blurred vision,* abnormal dreams, speech or vision disturbances, **coma,** confusion, depression, memory loss, numbness, paresthesias, psychosis/mania, seizures, tinnitus, vertigo
- **CV:** *First-degree AV block, intraventricular conduction disturbances,* **HF,** atrial flutter, AV dissociation, **cardiac arrest,** sick sinus syndrome, sinus pause, sinus arrest, supraventricular tachycardia, *bradycardia, angina*
- **Dermatologic:** Alopecia, pruritus
- **GI:** *Unusual taste, nausea, vomiting, constipation,* dyspepsia, cholestasis, gastroenteritis, hepatitis
- **Hematologic: Agranulocytosis,** anemia, granulocytopenia, leukopenia, purpura, thrombocytopenia, positive ANA

Adverse effects in *italics* are most common; those in **bold** are life-threatening. ◉ Do not crush.

- **Musculoskeletal:** Muscle weakness, leg cramps, muscle pain

Interactions

✳ **Drug-drug** • Increased serum levels of propafenone and risk of increased toxicity with quinidine, cimetidine, ritonavir, SSRIs • Increased serum levels of digoxin, warfarin, cyclosporine, beta blockers, theophylline

■ Nursing considerations
Assessment

- **History:** Hypersensitivity to propafenone, uncontrolled HF, cardiogenic shock, cardiac conduction disturbances in the absence of an artificial pacemaker, bradycardia, marked hypotension, bronchospastic disorders, manifest electrolyte imbalance, hepatic or renal impairment, pregnancy, lactation
- **Physical:** Reflexes, affect; BP, P, ECG, peripheral perfusion, auscultation; abdomen, normal function; LFTs, renal function tests; CBC, Hct, electrolytes; ANA

Interventions

⊗ *Warning* Monitor patient response carefully, especially when beginning therapy. Increase dosage at minimum of 3- to 4-day intervals only.

- Ensure that ER capsules are not cut, crushed, or chewed.
- Reduce dosage with renal or hepatic impairment and with marked previous myocardial damage.
- Increase dosage slowly in patients with myocardial dysfunction; renal or hepatic impairment.

⊗ **Black box warning** Arrange for periodic ECG monitoring to monitor effects on cardiac conduction; risk of serious proarrhythmias.

Teaching points

- Take the drug every 8 hours around-the-clock; determine a schedule that will interrupt sleep the least. Do not cut, crush, or chew capsules; swallow them whole.
- Frequent monitoring of ECG will be needed to adjust dosage or determine effects of drug on cardiac conduction.
- Do not stop taking this drug for any reason without consulting your health care provider.
- Avoid pregnancy while using this drug; use of barrier contraceptives is advised.

- You may experience these side effects: Dizziness, headache (avoid driving or performing hazardous tasks); headache, weakness (request medications; rest periods may help); nausea, vomiting, unusual taste (maintain proper nutrition; take drug with meals); constipation.
- Report swelling of the extremities, difficulty breathing, fainting, palpitations, vision changes, chest pain.

▽ **propantheline bromide**

See Appendix R, *Less commonly used drugs.*

DANGEROUS DRUG

▽ **propranolol hydrochloride**
(*proe pran' oh lol*)

Apo-Propranolol (CAN), Inderal, Inderal LA, InnoPran XL

PREGNANCY CATEGORY C

Drug classes
Antianginal
Antiarrhythmic
Antihypertensive
Beta-adrenergic blocker (nonselective)

Therapeutic actions
Competitively blocks beta-adrenergic receptors in the heart and juxtoglomerular apparatus, decreasing the influence of the sympathetic nervous system on these tissues, the excitability of the heart, cardiac workload and oxygen consumption, and the release of renin and lowering BP; has membrane-stabilizing (local anesthetic) effects that contribute to its antiarrhythmic action; acts in the CNS to reduce sympathetic outflow and vasoconstrictor tone. The mechanism by which it prevents migraine headaches is unknown.

Indications
- Hypertension alone or with other drugs, especially diuretics
- Angina pectoris caused by coronary atherosclerosis (not ER products)
- Idiopathic hypertrophic subaortic stenosis to manage associated stress-induced angina, palpitations, and syncope

- Atrial fibrillation; to control rapid ventricular rate (not ER products)
- To reduce CV mortality in clinically stable patients 5–21 days after MI (not ER products)
- Pheochromocytoma, an adjunctive therapy after treatment with an alpha-adrenergic blocker to manage tachycardia before or during surgery or if the pheochromocytoma is inoperable (not ER products)
- Prophylaxis for migraine headache
- Treatment of essential tremor, familial or hereditary (not ER products)
- Unlabeled uses: Migraine prevention in children and adolescents; smoking cessation; traumatic brain injury

Contraindications and cautions

- Contraindicated with allergy to beta-blocking agents, sinus bradycardia, second- or third-degree heart block, cardiogenic shock, HF, bronchial asthma, bronchospasm, COPD, pregnancy (neonatal bradycardia, hypoglycemia, and apnea, and low birth weight with long-term use during pregnancy), lactation.
- Use cautiously with hypoglycemia and diabetes, thyrotoxicosis, hepatic impairment, Raynaud disease.

Available forms

ER capsules—60, 80, 120, 160 mg; tablets—10, 20, 40, 60, 80 mg; injection—1 mg/mL; oral solution—4, 8 mg/mL

Dosages
Adults
Oral

- *Hypertension:* 40 mg regular propranolol bid PO or 80 mg PO SR or ER daily initially; usual maintenance dose, 120–240 mg/day PO given bid or tid or 120–160 mg SR or ER daily (maximum dose, 640 mg/day).
- *Angina:* 80–320 mg/day PO divided bid, tid, or qid or 80 mg PO SR or ER daily initially; gradually increase SR or ER dosage at 3- to 7-day intervals; usual maintenance dose, 160 mg/day PO (maximum dose, 320 mg/day).
- *IHSS:* 20–40 mg PO tid or qid or 80–160 mg PO SR or ER daily.
- *Arrhythmias:* 10–30 mg PO tid or qid.
- *Post-MI:* 120 mg/day PO divided tid. After 1 mo, may titrate to 180–240 mg/day tid or qid (maximum dose, 240 mg/day).

- *Pheochromocytoma:* Preoperatively, 60 mg/day PO for 3 days in divided doses; inoperable tumor, 30 mg/day in divided doses.
- *Migraine:* 80 mg/day PO daily (SR or ER) or in divided doses; usual maintenance dose, 160–240 mg/day.
- *Essential tremor:* 40 mg PO bid; usual maintenance dose, 120 mg/day (maximum dose, 320 mg/day).

Parenteral
⊗ **Warning** IV dose is markedly less than oral because of first-pass effect with oral propranolol.

- *Life-threatening arrhythmias:* 1–3 mg IV with careful monitoring, not to exceed 1 mg/min; may give second dose in 2 min, but then do not repeat for 4 hr.

Pediatric patients
Safety and efficacy not established.

Pharmacokinetics

Route	Onset	Peak	Duration
Oral	20–30 min	60–90 min	6–12 hr
IV	Immediate	1 min	4–6 hr

Metabolism: Hepatic; $T_{1/2}$: 3–5 hr; 8–11 hr (SR form)
Distribution: Crosses placenta; enters breast milk
Excretion: Urine

▼ IV FACTS
Preparation: No further preparation is needed.
Infusion: Inject directly IV or into tubing of running IV; do not exceed 1 mg/min.

Adverse effects

- **Allergic reactions:** Pharyngitis, erythematous rash, fever, sore throat, **laryngospasm,** respiratory distress
- **CNS:** Dizziness, vertigo, tinnitus, *fatigue,* emotional depression, paresthesias, sleep disturbances, hallucinations, disorientation, memory loss, slurred speech
- **CV:** *Bradycardia,* **HF,** *cardiac arrhythmias, sinoatrial or AV nodal block,* peripheral vascular insufficiency, claudication, **stroke, pulmonary edema,** hypotension
- **Dermatologic:** Rash, pruritus, sweating, dry skin
- **EENT:** Eye irritation, dry eyes, conjunctivitis, blurred vision

- **GI:** *Gastric pain, flatulence, constipation, diarrhea, nausea, vomiting,* anorexia, ischemic colitis, renal and mesenteric arterial thrombosis, retroperitoneal fibrosis, hepatomegaly, acute pancreatitis
- **GU:** *Impotence, decreased libido,* Peyronie disease, dysuria, nocturia, frequency
- **Musculoskeletal:** Joint pain, arthralgia, muscle cramp
- **Respiratory: Bronchospasm,** dyspnea, cough, bronchial obstruction, nasal stuffiness, rhinitis, pharyngitis
- **Other:** *Decreased exercise tolerance, development of ANAs,* hyperglycemia or hypoglycemia, elevated serum transaminase, alkaline phosphatase, and LDH

Interactions

✴ **Drug-drug** • Increased effects with verapamil • Decreased effects with indomethacin, ibuprofen, piroxicam, sulindac, barbiturates • Prolonged hypoglycemic effects of insulin • Initial hypertensive episode followed by bradycardia with epinephrine • Increased first-dose response to prazosin • Increased serum levels and toxic effects with lidocaine, cimetidine • Increased serum levels of propranolol and phenothiazines, hydralazine if the two drugs are taken concurrently • Paradoxic hypertension when clonidine is given with beta blockers; increased rebound hypertension when clonidine is discontinued in patients on beta blockers • Decreased serum levels and therapeutic effects with methimazole, propylthiouracil • Decreased bronchodilator effects of theophyllines • Decreased antihypertensive effects with NSAIDs (ie, ibuprofen, indomethacin, piroxicam, sulindac), rifampin

✴ **Drug-lab test** • Interference with glucose or insulin tolerance tests, glaucoma screening tests

■ Nursing considerations

Assessment

- **History:** Allergy to beta-blocking agents, sinus bradycardia, second- or third-degree heart block, cardiogenic shock, HF, bronchial asthma, bronchospasm, COPD, hypoglycemia and diabetes, thyrotoxicosis, hepatic impairment, pregnancy, lactation, peripheral vascular disease
- **Physical:** Weight, skin color, lesions, edema, T; reflexes, affect, vision, hearing, orientation; BP, P, ECG, peripheral perfusion; R, auscultation; bowel sounds, normal output, liver eval-

uation; bladder palpation; LFTs, thyroid function tests; blood and urine glucose

Interventions

⊗ **Black box warning** Do not discontinue drug abruptly after long-term therapy (hypersensitivity to catecholamines may have developed, causing exacerbation of angina, MI, and ventricular arrhythmias). Taper drug gradually over 2 wk with monitoring.

⊗ **Warning** Ensure that alpha-adrenergic blocker has been given before giving propranolol when treating patients with pheochromocytoma; endogenous catecholamines secreted by the tumor can cause severe hypertension if vascular beta receptors are blocked without concomitant alpha blockade.

- Consult with surgeon about withdrawing drug if patient is to undergo surgery (withdrawal is controversial).
- Provide continuous cardiac and regular BP monitoring with IV form. Change to oral form as soon as possible.
- Give oral drug with food to facilitate absorption.

Teaching points

- Take this drug with meals. Do not discontinue the medication abruptly; abrupt discontinuation can cause worsening of your disorder.
- If you have diabetes, the normal signs of hypoglycemia (tachycardia) may be blocked by this drug; monitor your blood or urine glucose carefully; eat regular meals, and take your diabetic medication regularly.
- You may experience these side effects: Dizziness, drowsiness, light-headedness, blurred vision (avoid driving or performing hazardous tasks); nausea, loss of appetite (eat frequent small meals); nightmares, depression (request change of your medication); sexual impotence.
- Report difficulty breathing, night cough, swelling of extremities, slow pulse, confusion, depression, rash, fever, sore throat.

▽ **propylthiouracil (PTU)**
(proe pill thye ob yoor' a sill)

Propyl-Thyracil (CAN)

PREGNANCY CATEGORY D

Drug class

Antithyroid drug

Therapeutic actions

Inhibits the synthesis of thyroid hormones; partially inhibits the peripheral conversion of T_4 to T_3, the more potent form of thyroid hormone.

Indications

- Hyperthyroidism
- Unlabeled use: Reduces mortality associated with alcoholic liver disease

Contraindications and cautions

- Contraindicated with allergy to antithyroid drugs, pregnancy (can induce hypothyroidism or cretinism in the fetus; use only if absolutely necessary and when mother has been informed about potential harm to the fetus; if antithyroid drug is needed, this is the drug of choice).
- Use cautiously with lactation (if antithyroid drug is needed, this is the drug of choice).

Available forms

Tablets—50 mg, 100 mg (CAN)

Dosages

Administered usually in three equal doses every 8 hr.

Adults

- Initially, 300 mg/day PO in divided doses every 8 hr, up to 400–900 mg/day in severe cases. For maintenance, 100–150 mg/day in divided doses every 8 hr.

Pediatric patients

Reserve use for children allergic to or intolerant of other therapies.

6 yr and older: 50 mg/day PO with careful titration if needed. Give in divided doses every 8 hr. Monitor TSH and T_4 levels carefully.

Pharmacokinetics

Route	Onset
Oral	Varies

Metabolism: Hepatic; $T_{1/2}$: 1–2 hr
Distribution: Crosses placenta; enters breast milk
Excretion: Urine

Adverse effects

- **CNS:** *Paresthesias, neuritis, vertigo, drowsiness,* neuropathies, depression, headache
- **CV:** Vasculitis, periarteritis
- **Dermatologic:** *Skin rash, urticaria,* pruritus, skin pigmentation, exfoliative dermatitis, lupus-like syndrome, loss of hair

- **GI:** *Nausea, vomiting, epigastric distress,* loss of taste, jaundice, hepatitis, **severe liver injury**
- **GU:** Nephritis
- **Hematologic: Agranulocytosis,** granulocytopenia, thrombocytopenia, hypoprothrombinemia, bleeding, aplastic anemia
- **Other:** Arthralgia, myalgia, edema, lymphadenopathy, drug fever

Interactions

✳ **Drug-drug** • Increased risk of bleeding with oral anticoagulants • Alterations in theophylline, metoprolol, propranolol, cardiac glycoside clearance, serum levels and effects as patient moves from hyperthyroid state to euthyroid state

■ Nursing considerations

CLINICAL ALERT!
Name confusion has occurred between propylthiouracil and *Purinethol* (mercaptopurine). Serious adverse effects can occur; use extreme caution.

Assessment

- **History:** Allergy to antithyroid drugs, pregnancy, lactation
- **Physical:** Skin color, lesions, pigmentation; orientation, reflexes, affect; liver evaluation; CBC, differential, PT, LFTs, renal function tests, thyroid function tests

Interventions

⊗ **Black box warning** Drug has been associated with severe liver injury, which may be fatal. Monitor patient carefully for signs and symptoms of liver adverse effects, especially during first 6 months of therapy. Do not use in children unless they are allergic to or intolerant of other therapies; risk of liver toxicity is higher in children.

⊗ **Black box warning** Propylthioyracil may be treatment of choice when an antithyroid drug is needed during or just prior to the first trimester of pregnancy, because of risk of fetal abnormalities associated with methimazole.

- Administer drug in three equally divided doses at 8-hr intervals; schedule to maintain the patient's sleep pattern.
- Arrange for regular, periodic blood tests to monitor bone marrow depression and bleeding tendencies.

Adverse effects in *italics* are most common; those in **bold** are life-threatening. ▨ Do not crush.

⊗ *Warning* Advise medical personnel doing surgical procedures that this patient is using this drug and is at greater risk for bleeding problems.

Teaching points

- Take this drug around-the-clock at 8-hour intervals.
- This drug must be taken for a prolonged period to achieve the desired effects.
- You may experience these side effects: Dizziness, weakness, vertigo, drowsiness (use caution if operating a car or dangerous machinery); nausea, vomiting, loss of appetite (eat frequent small meals); rash, itching.
- Report fever, sore throat, unusual bleeding or bruising, headache, general malaise, changes in color of urine or stool.

▽ protamine sulfate
(proe' ta meen)

PREGNANCY CATEGORY C

Drug class
Heparin antagonist

Therapeutic actions
Strongly basic proteins found in salmon sperm; protamines form stable salts with heparin, which results in the immediate loss of anticoagulant activity; administered when heparin has not been given; protamine has weak anticoagulant activity.

Indications
- Treatment of heparin overdose

Contraindications and cautions
- Contraindicated with allergy to protamine sulfate or fish products.
- Use cautiously with pregnancy, lactation.

Available forms
Injection—10 mg/mL

Dosages
Dosage is determined by the amount of heparin in the body and the time that has elapsed since the heparin was given; the longer the interval, the smaller the dose required.
Adults and pediatric patients
1 mg IV neutralizes not less than 100 heparin units.

Pharmacokinetics

Route	Onset	Duration
IV	5 min	2 hr

Metabolism: Degraded in body; $T_{1/2}$: Unknown
Distribution: Crosses placenta; may enter breast milk
Excretion: Unknown

▼ IV FACTS

Preparation: Administer injection undiluted; if dilution is needed, use 5% dextrose in water or saline; refrigerate any diluted solution. Do not store diluted solution; no preservatives are added. Stable at room temperature for 72 hr.

Infusion: Administer very slowly IV over at least 10 min; do not exceed 50 mg in any 10-min period; do not give more than 100 mg over a 2-hr period. Guide dosing with coagulation studies.

Incompatibilities: Do not mix in lines with incompatible antibiotics, including many penicillins and cephalosporins.

Adverse effects
- **CV:** *Hypotension,* bradycardia
- **GI:** *Nausea, vomiting*
- **Hypersensitivity:** Anaphylactoid reactions—dyspnea, flushing, hypotension, bradycardia, **anaphylaxis**

■ Nursing considerations
Assessment
- **History:** Allergy to protamine sulfate or fish products, pregnancy, lactation
- **Physical:** Skin color, T; orientation, reflexes; P, BP, auscultation, peripheral perfusion; R, adventitious sounds; plasma thrombin time

Interventions
⊗ *Warning* Keep emergency equipment for resuscitation and treatment of shock readily available in case of anaphylactoid reaction.
⊗ *Warning* Monitor coagulation studies to adjust dosage, and screen for heparin rebound and response to drug.

Teaching points
- Report shortness of breath, difficulty breathing, flushing, feeling of warmth, dizziness, lack of orientation, numbness, tingling.

▷ protein C concentrate

See Appendix R, *Less commonly used drugs.*

▷ protriptyline hydrochloride

*(proe **trip'** ti leen)*

Vivactil

PREGNANCY CATEGORY C

Drug class
TCA (secondary amine)

Therapeutic actions
Mechanism of action unknown; the TCAs are structurally related to the phenothiazine antipsychotic drugs (eg, chlorpromazine), but in contrast to the phenothiazines, TCAs inhibit the presynaptic reuptake of the neurotransmitters norepinephrine and serotonin; anticholinergic at CNS and peripheral receptors; the relation of these effects to clinical efficacy is unknown.

Indications
- Relief of symptoms of depression (endogenous depression most responsive; unlike other TCAs, protriptyline is "activating" and may be useful in withdrawn and anergic patients)
- Unlabeled uses: Treatment of obstructive sleep apnea, prevention of migraine

Contraindications and cautions
- Contraindicated with hypersensitivity to any tricyclic drug, concomitant therapy with an MAOI, recent MI, myelography within previous 24 hr or scheduled within 48 hr, pregnancy (limb reduction abnormalities), lactation.
- Use cautiously with ECT; pre-existing CV disorders (eg, severe coronary heart disease, progressive HF, angina pectoris, paroxysmal tachycardia); angle-closure glaucoma, increased IOP, urinary retention, ureteral or urethral spasm; seizure disorders (TCAs lower the seizure threshold); hyperthyroidism (predisposes to CVS toxicity, including cardiac arrhythmias); impaired hepatic, renal function; psychiatric patients (schizophrenic or paranoid patients may exhibit a worsening of psychosis); patients with bipolar disorder (may shift to hypomanic or manic phase); elective surgery (TCAs should be discontinued as long as possible before surgery).

Available forms
Tablets—5, 10 mg

Dosages
Adults
15–40 mg/day PO in three to four divided doses initially. May gradually increase to 60 mg/day if necessary. Do not exceed 60 mg/day. Make increases in dosage in the morning dose.
Pediatric patients
Not recommended; may increase risk of suicidal ideation.
Geriatric patients and adolescents
Initially, 5 mg tid PO. Increase gradually if needed. Monitor CV system closely if dose exceeds 20 mg/day.

Pharmacokinetics

Route	Onset	Peak
Oral	Slow	8–12 hr

Metabolism: Hepatic; $T_{1/2}$: 67–89 hr
Distribution: Crosses placenta; enters breast milk
Excretion: Urine

Adverse effects
- **CNS:** *Sedation and anticholinergic (atropine-like) effects*—dry mouth, blurred vision, disturbance of accommodation for near vision, mydriasis, increased IOP, *confusion* (especially in elderly), *disturbed concentration,* hallucinations, disorientation, decreased memory, feelings of unreality, delusions, anxiety, nervousness, restlessness, agitation, panic, insomnia, nightmares, hypomania, mania, exacerbation of psychosis, drowsiness, weakness, fatigue, headache, numbness, tingling, paresthesias of extremities, uncoordination, motor hyperactivity, akathisia, ataxia, tremors, peripheral neuropathy, extrapyramidal symptoms, *seizures,* speech blockage, dysarthria, tinnitus, altered EEG
- **CV:** *Orthostatic hypotension,* hypertension, syncope, tachycardia, palpitations, **MI,** arrhythmias, heart block, precipitation of HF, **stroke**
- **Endocrine:** Elevated or depressed blood sugar; elevated prolactin levels; inappropriate ADH secretion

Adverse effects in *italics* are most common; those in **bold** are life-threatening. ▣▣▣ Do not crush.

- **GI:** *Dry mouth, constipation,* paralytic ileus, *nausea,* vomiting, anorexia, epigastric distress, diarrhea, flatulence, dysphagia, peculiar taste, increased salivation, stomatitis, glossitis, parotid swelling, abdominal cramps, black tongue
- **GU:** Urinary retention, delayed micturition, dilation of the urinary tract, gynecomastia, testicular swelling; breast enlargement, menstrual irregularity and galactorrhea; increased or decreased libido; impotence
- **Hematologic:** Bone marrow depression, including agranulocytosis; eosinophilia; purpura; thrombocytopenia; leukopenia
- **Hypersensitivity:** Skin rash, pruritus, vasculitis, petechiae, photosensitization, edema (generalized or of face and tongue), drug fever
- **Withdrawal:** Symptoms with abrupt discontinuation of prolonged therapy: Nausea, headache, vertigo, nightmares, malaise
- **Other:** Nasal congestion, excessive appetite, weight change, sweating, alopecia, lacrimation, hyperthermia, flushing, chills

Interactions
✷ **Drug-drug •** Increased TCA levels and pharmacologic effects with cimetidine, fluoxetine, ranitidine • Altered response, including arrhythmias and hypertension with sympathomimetics
• Risk of severe hypertension with clonidine
• Hyperpyretic crises, severe seizures, hypertensive episodes, and deaths with MAOIs • Increased CNS effects with alcohol; avoid this combination
• Increased risk of seizures with tramadol

■ **Nursing considerations**
Assessment
- **History:** Hypersensitivity to any tricyclic drug; concomitant therapy with an MAOI; recent MI; myelography within previous 24 hr or scheduled within 48 hr; pregnancy; lactation; ECT; pre-existing CV disorders; angle-closure glaucoma, increased IOP, urinary retention, ureteral or urethral spasm; seizure disorders; hyperthyroidism; impaired hepatic, renal function; psychiatric disorder; bipolar disorders; elective surgery
- **Physical:** Weight; T; skin color, lesions; orientation, affect, reflexes, vision and hearing; P, BP, orthostatic BP, perfusion; bowel sounds, normal output, liver evaluation; urine flow, normal output; usual sexual function, frequency of menses, breast and scrotal examination; LFTs, urinalysis, CBC, ECG

Interventions
⊗ **Black box warning** Limit drug access for depressed and potentially suicidal patients; increased risk of suicidality in children, adolescents, and young adults; monitor accordingly.
⊗ **Warning** Reduce dosage if minor side effects develop; discontinue if serious side effects occur.
- Arrange for CBC if patient develops fever, sore throat, or other sign of infection.

Teaching points
- Take drug exactly as prescribed; do not stop taking this drug abruptly or without consulting your health care provider.
- Avoid alcohol and other sleep-inducing or over-the-counter drugs.
- Avoid prolonged exposure to sunlight or sunlamps; use a sunscreen or protective garments.
- You may experience these side effects: Headache, dizziness, drowsiness, weakness, blurred vision (reversible; take safety measures if severe; avoid driving or performing tasks that require alertness); nausea, vomiting, loss of appetite, dry mouth (frequent small meals, frequent mouth care, and sucking on sugarless candies may help); nightmares, inability to concentrate, confusion; changes in sexual function; fetal abnormalities (avoid pregnancy, use contraceptive measures).
- Report dry mouth, difficulty in urination, excessive sedation, thoughts of suicide.

▽ **pseudoephedrine**
(soo dow e fed' rin)

pseudoephedrine hydrochloride (d-isoephedrine hydrochloride)
Congest Aid, Efidac/24 ⓞⓣⓒ, Eltor (CAN), Genaphed, Sudafed, Unifed

pseudoephedrine sulfate
ElixSure Children's Congestion

PREGNANCY CATEGORY C

Drug classes
Nasal decongestant
Sympathomimetic amine

P

Therapeutic actions

Effects are mediated by alpha-adrenergic receptors; causes vasoconstriction in mucous membranes of nasal passages, resulting in their shrinkage, which promotes drainage and improves ventilation.

Indications

- Temporary relief of nasal congestion caused by the common cold, hay fever, other respiratory allergies
- Nasal congestion associated with sinusitis
- Promotes nasal or sinus drainage
- Relief of eustachian tube congestion

Contraindications and cautions

- Contraindicated with MAOI therapy, allergy or idiosyncrasy to sympathomimetic amines, severe hypertension, and CAD.
- Use cautiously with hyperthyroidism, diabetes mellitus, arteriosclerosis, ischemic heart disease, increased IOP, prostatic hypertrophy, lactation, pregnancy.

Available forms

Tablets—30, 60 mg; CR tablets ⊚—240 mg; ER tablets ⊚—120 mg; chewable tablets—15 mg; capsules—30, 60 mg; drops—7.5 mg/0.8 mL; syrup—15 mg/5 mL; suspension—50 mg/5 mL

Dosages

Adults and children older than 12 yr

60 mg every 4–6 hr PO (ER, 120 mg PO every 12 hr; 240 mg/day CR); do not exceed 240 mg in 24 hr.

Pediatric patients 6–12 yr

30 mg every 4–6 hr PO; do not exceed 120 mg in 24 hr. Do not administer ER forms to children younger than 12 yr.

Pediatric patients 2–5 yr

15 mg as syrup every 4–6 hr PO; do not exceed 60 mg in 24 hr.

Pediatric patients 2 yr and younger

Consult physician.

Geriatric patients

These patients are more likely to experience adverse reactions; use with caution.

Pharmacokinetics

Route	Onset	Duration
Oral	30 min	4–6 hr

Metabolism: Hepatic; $T_{1/2}$: 7 hr
Distribution: Crosses placenta; enters breast milk
Excretion: Urine

Adverse effects

- **CNS:** *Fear, anxiety, tenseness, restlessness, headache, light-headedness, dizziness, drowsiness, tremors,* insomnia, hallucinations, psychological disturbances, prolonged psychosis, **seizures,** CNS depression, weakness, blurred vision, ocular irritation, tearing, photophobia, orofacial dystonia
- **CV:** *Hypertension, arrhythmias,* CV collapse with hypotension, palpitations, tachycardia, precordial pain
- **Dermatologic:** *Pallor,* sweating
- **GI:** *Nausea, vomiting,* anorexia
- **GU:** Dysuria, urinary retention in BPH

Interactions

✻ **Drug-drug** • Increased hypertension with MAOIs • Increased duration of action with urinary alkalinizers (potassium citrate, sodium citrate, sodium lactate, tromethamine, sodium acetate, sodium bicarbonate) • Decreased therapeutic effects and increased elimination of pseudoephedrine with urinary acidifiers (ammonium chloride, sodium acid phosphate, potassium phosphate) • Decreased antihypertensive effects of methyldopa

■ Nursing considerations

Assessment

- **History:** Allergy or idiosyncrasy to sympathomimetic amines, severe hypertension and CAD, hyperthyroidism, diabetes mellitus, arteriosclerosis, increased IOP, prostatic hypertrophy, pregnancy, lactation
- **Physical:** Skin color, T; reflexes, affect, orientation, peripheral sensation, vision; BP, P, auscultation; R, adventitious sounds; urinary output, bladder percussion, prostate palpation

Interventions

⊗ **Warning** Administer cautiously to patients with CV disease, diabetes mellitus, hyperthyroidism, increased IOP, hypertension, and to patients older than 60 yr who may have increased sensitivity to sympathomimetic amines.

- Avoid prolonged use; underlying medical problems may be causing the congestion.

Adverse effects in *italics* are most common; those in **bold** are life-threatening. ⊚ Do not crush.

- Do not cut, crush, or allow patient to chew ER tablets.
- Monitor CV effect carefully; hypertensive patients who take this drug may experience changes in BP because of the additional vasoconstriction. However, if a nasal decongestant is needed, pseudoephedrine is the drug of choice.

Teaching points

- Do not exceed the recommended daily dose; serious overdose can occur. Use caution when using more than one over-the-counter preparation because many of these drugs contain pseudoephedrine, and unintentional overdose may occur.
- Do not cut, crush, or chew ER tablets.
- Avoid prolonged use because underlying medical problems can be disguised.
- You may experience these side effects: Dizziness, restlessness, light-headedness, tremors, weakness (avoid driving or performing hazardous tasks).
- Report palpitations, nervousness, sleeplessness, sweating.

▽ pyrantel pamoate
(pi ran' tel)

Combantrin (CAN), Pin-Rid, Pin-X, Reese's Pinworm

PREGNANCY CATEGORY C

Drug class
Anthelmintic

Therapeutic actions
A depolarizing neuromuscular blocking agent that causes spastic paralysis of *Enterobius vermicularis* and *Ascaris lumbricoides*. Also effective against *Ancyclostoma duodenale* (hookworm).

Indications
- Treatment of enterobiasis (pinworm infection)
- Treatment of ascariasis (roundworm infection)
- Unlabeled use: Hairworm

Contraindications and cautions
- Contraindicated with allergy to pyrantel pamoate.

- Use cautiously with pregnancy, lactation, hepatic disease.

Available forms
Capsules—180 mg; tablets—180 mg; oral suspension—50 mg/mL, 144 mg/mL; chewable tablets—720.5 mg

Dosages
Adults and pediatric patients older than 2 yr
11 mg/kg (5 mg/lb) PO as a single oral dose. Maximum total dose of 1 g.
Pediatric patients younger than 2 yr
Safety and efficacy not established.
Patients with hepatic impairment
Do not use unless benefit clearly outweighs risks.

Pharmacokinetics

Route	Onset	Peak
Oral	Slow	1–3 hr

Metabolism: Hepatic; T$_{1/2}$: 47–100 hr
Distribution: Crosses placenta; may enter breast milk
Excretion: Feces, urine

Adverse effects
- **CNS:** Headache, dizziness, drowsiness, insomnia
- **Dermatologic:** Rash
- **GI:** *Anorexia, nausea, vomiting, abdominal cramps, diarrhea,* gastralgia, tenesmus, transient elevation of AST

Interactions
✻ **Drug-drug** • Pyrantel and piperazine are antagonistic in *Ascaris;* avoid concomitant use
- Increases theophylline concentrations; monitor patient closely

■ Nursing considerations
Assessment
- **History:** Allergy to pyrantel pamoate, pregnancy, lactation, hepatic impairment
- **Physical:** Skin color, lesions; orientation, affect; bowel sounds; AST levels

Interventions
- Culture for ova and parasites.
- Administer drug with fruit juice or milk; ensure that entire dose is taken at once. Shake suspension well before each dose.

- Treat all family members (pinworm infestations).
- Disinfect toilet facilities after patient use (pinworms).
- Launder bed linens, towels, nightclothes, and undergarments (pinworms) daily.

Teaching points
- Take the entire dose at once. Drug may be taken with fruit juice or milk. Shake suspension well before each use.
- Pinworms are easily transmitted; all family members should be treated for complete eradication. Do not repeat treatment unless otherwise indicated.
- Strict handwashing and hygiene measures are important. Launder undergarments, bed linens, nightclothes daily; disinfect toilet facilities daily and bathroom floors periodically (pinworm).
- You may experience these side effects: Nausea, abdominal pain, diarrhea (eat frequent small meals); drowsiness, dizziness, insomnia (avoid driving and using dangerous machinery).
- Report rash, joint pain, severe GI upset, severe headache, dizziness.

▽**pyrazinamide**
(peer a zin' a myde)

PREGNANCY CATEGORY C

Drug class
Antituberculotic

Therapeutic actions
Bacteriostatic or bacteriocidal against *Mycobacterium tuberculosis;* mechanism of action is unknown.

Indications
- Initial treatment of active TB in adults and children when combined with other antituberculotics
- Treatment of active TB after treatment failure with primary drugs
- Treatment of drug-resistant TB as part of an individualized regimen

Contraindications and cautions
- Contraindicated with allergy to pyrazinamide, acute hepatic disease, lactation, acute gout.
- Use cautiously with diabetes mellitus, acute intermittent porphyria, pregnancy.

Available forms
Tablets—500 mg

Dosages
Adults and pediatric patients
15–30 mg/kg/day PO, given once a day; do not exceed 2 g/day. Always use with up to four other antituberculotics; administer for the first 2 mo of a 6-mo treatment program. 50–70 mg/kg PO twice weekly may increase compliance and is being studied as an alternative dosing schedule. Patients with HIV infection may require a longer course of therapy.

Pharmacokinetics

Route	Onset	Peak
Oral	Rapid	2 hr

Metabolism: Hepatic; $T_{1/2}$: 9–10 hr
Distribution: Crosses placenta; enters breast milk
Excretion: Urine

Adverse effects
- **Dermatologic:** Rashes, photosensitivity
- **GI:** *Hepatotoxicity, nausea, vomiting,* diarrhea, anorexia
- **Hematologic:** Sideroblastic anemia, thrombocytopenia, adverse effects on clotting mechanism or vascular integrity
- **Other:** Active gout

Interactions
✳ **Drug-lab test** ● False readings on *Acetest, Ketostix* urine tests

■ **Nursing considerations**
Assessment
- **History:** Allergy to pyrazinamide, acute hepatic disease, gout, diabetes mellitus, acute intermittent porphyria, pregnancy, lactation
- **Physical:** Skin color, lesions; joint status; T; liver evaluation; LFTs, serum and urine uric acid levels, blood and urine glucose, CBC

Interventions
- Administer only in conjunction with other antituberculotics.
- Administer once a day.
- Arrange for follow-up of LFTs (AST, ALT) prior to and every 2–4 wk during therapy.

⊗ *Warning* Discontinue drug if liver damage or hyperuricemia in conjunction with acute gouty arthritis occurs.

Teaching points
- Take this drug once a day; it will need to be taken with your other tuberculosis drugs.
- Take this drug regularly; avoid missing doses. Do not discontinue this drug without first consulting your health care provider.
- Have regular, periodic medical checkups, including blood tests to evaluate the drug effects.
- You may experience these side effects: Loss of appetite, nausea, vomiting (take drug with food); rash, sensitivity to sunlight (avoid exposure to the sun).
- Report fever, malaise, loss of appetite, nausea, vomiting, darkened urine, yellowing of skin and eyes, severe pain in great toe, instep, ankle, heel, knee, or wrist.

▷ pyridostigmine bromide
(peer id oh stig' meen)

Mestinon, Regonol

PREGNANCY CATEGORY C

Drug classes
Antidote
Antimyasthenic
Cholinesterase inhibitor

Therapeutic actions
Increases the concentration of acetylcholine at the sites of cholinergic transmission and prolongs and exaggerates the effects of acetylcholine by reversibly inhibiting the enzyme acetylcholinesterase, thus facilitating transmission at the skeletal neuromuscular junction.

Indications
- Treatment of myasthenia gravis
- Parenteral: Antidote for nondepolarizing neuromuscular junction blockers (eg, tubocurarine) after surgery
- To increase survival after exposure to sarin "nerve gas" poisoning in conjunction with protective measures
- Unlabeled use: Postpoliomyelitis syndrome

Contraindications and cautions
- Contraindicated with hypersensitivity to anticholinesterases; adverse reactions to bromides; intestinal or urogenital tract obstruction, peritonitis, lactation.
- Use cautiously with asthma, peptic ulcer, bradycardia, cardiac arrhythmias, recent coronary occlusion, vagotonia, hyperthyroidism, epilepsy, pregnancy (given IV near term, drug may stimulate uterus and induce premature labor).

Available forms
Tablets—60 mg ER tablets ⊞—180 mg; syrup—60 mg/5 mL; injection—5 mg/mL

Dosages
Adults
Oral
- *Symptomatic control of myasthenia gravis:* Average dose is 600 mg PO given over 24 hr; range, 60–1,500 mg, spaced to provide maximum relief. ER tablets, average dose is 180–540 mg PO daily or bid. Individualize dosage, allowing at least 6 hr between doses. Optimum control may require supplementation with the more rapidly acting syrup or regular tablets.
- *Military personnel who face the threat of sarin nerve gas:* 30 mg PO every 8 hr starting several hr before exposure; stop drug if exposure occurs.

Parenteral
- *To supplement oral dosage preoperatively and postoperatively, during labor, during myasthenic crisis, etc:* Give ⅓₀ the oral dose IM or very slowly IV. May be given 1 hr before second stage of labor is complete (enables patient to have adequate strength and protects neonate in immediate postnatal period).
- *Antidote for nondepolarizing neuromuscular blockers:* Give atropine sulfate 0.6–1.2 mg IV immediately before slow IV injection of pyridostigmine 0.1–0.25 mg/kg. 10–20 mg pyridostigmine usually suffices. Full recovery usually occurs within 15 min but may take 30 min.

Pediatric patients
Oral
- *Symptomatic control of myasthenia gravis:* 7 mg/kg/day PO divided into five or six doses for children older than 30 days; 5 mg/kg/day PO divided into five or six doses for children 29 days or younger.

P

Parenteral

- Neonates who have myasthenic mothers and who have difficulty swallowing, sucking, breathing: 0.05–0.15 mg/kg IM. Change to syrup as soon as possible.

Pharmacokinetics

Route	Onset	Duration
Oral	20–30 min	3–6 hr
IM	15 min	2–4 hr
IV	5 min	2–4 hr

Metabolism: Hepatic and tissue; $T_{1/2}$: 1.9–3.7 hr
Distribution: Crosses placenta; enters breast milk
Excretion: Urine

▼ IV FACTS

Preparation: No further preparation is required.
Infusion: Infuse very slowly, each 0.5 mg over 1 min for myasthenia gravis, each 5 mg over 1 min as a muscle relaxant agonist, directly into vein or into tubing of actively running IV of $D_{25}W$, 0.9% sodium chloride, lactated Ringer solution, or $D_{25}W$ and lactated Ringer solution.

Adverse effects

- **CNS:** Seizures, dizziness, dysarthria, dysphonia, drowsiness, headache, loss of consciousness
- **CV:** *Bradycardia, cardiac arrhythmias,* AV block and nodal rhythm, **cardiac arrest,** decreased cardiac output leading to hypotension, syncope
- **Dermatologic:** Diaphoresis, flushing, skin rash, urticaria
- **EENT:** *Lacrimation, miosis,* spasm of accommodation, diplopia, conjunctival hyperemia
- **GI:** *Salivation, dysphagia, nausea, vomiting, increased peristalsis, abdominal cramps,* flatulence, diarrhea
- **GU:** *Urinary frequency and incontinence,* urinary urgency
- **Local:** Thrombophlebitis after IV use
- **Peripheral:** Skeletal muscle weakness, fasciculations, muscle cramps, arthralgia
- **Respiratory:** *Increased pharyngeal and tracheobronchial secretions,* **laryngospasm, bronchospasm,** bronchiolar constriction, dyspnea, respiratory muscle

paralysis, central respiratory paralysis, **anaphylaxis**

Interactions

✳ **Drug-drug** • Decreased effectiveness with profound muscular depression with corticosteroids • Increased and prolonged neuromuscular blockade with succinylcholine

■ Nursing considerations

Assessment

- **History:** Hypersensitivity to anticholinesterases, adverse reactions to bromides, intestinal or urogenital tract obstruction, peritonitis, lactation, asthma, peptic ulcer, cardiac arrhythmias, recent coronary occlusion, vagotonia, hyperthyroidism, epilepsy, pregnancy
- **Physical:** Bowel sounds, normal output; urinary frequency, voiding pattern, normal output; R, adventitious sounds; P, auscultation, BP; reflexes, bilateral grip strength, ECG; thyroid function tests; skin color, texture, lesions

Interventions

- Administer IV slowly.
- Overdose with anticholinesterase drugs can cause muscle weakness (cholinergic crisis) that is difficult to differentiate from myasthenic weakness; administration of atropine may mask the parasympathetic effects of anticholinesterase overdose and further confound the diagnosis.
- ⊗ **Warning** Keep atropine sulfate readily available as an antidote and antagonist to pyridostigmine in case of cholinergic crisis or unusual sensitivity to pyridostigmine.
- ⊗ **Warning** Discontinue drug and consult physician if excessive salivation, emesis, frequent urination, or diarrhea occurs.
- Have patient swallow ER tablets whole; do not cut, crush, or allow patient to chew ER tablets.
- Decrease dosage of drug if excessive sweating or nausea occurs.

Teaching points

- Take drug exactly as prescribed. Your health care provider should teach you and your significant other about drug effects, signs and symptoms of myasthenia gravis, the fact that muscle weakness may be related both to drug overdose and to exacerbation of the disease, and the importance of reporting muscle weakness promptly to the nurse or physician for proper evaluation.

- Do not cut, crush, or chew ER tablets.
- You may experience these side effects: Blurred vision, difficulty with far vision, difficulty with dark adaptation (use caution while driving, especially at night, or performing hazardous tasks in reduced light); increased urinary frequency, abdominal cramps; sweating (avoid hot or excessively humid environments).
- Report muscle weakness, nausea, vomiting, diarrhea, severe abdominal pain, excessive sweating, excessive salivation, frequent urination, urinary urgency, irregular heartbeat, difficulty breathing.

▷quazepam

(kwa' ze pam)

Doral

PREGNANCY CATEGORY X

CONTROLLED SUBSTANCE C-IV

Drug classes
Benzodiazepine
Sedative-hypnotic

Therapeutic actions
Exact mechanisms of action not understood; acts mainly at subcortical levels of the CNS, leaving the cortex relatively unaffected; main sites of action may be the limbic system and mesencephalic reticular formation; benzodiazepines potentiate the effects of GABA, an inhibitory neurotransmitter.

Indications
- Insomnia characterized by difficulty in falling asleep, frequent nocturnal awakenings, or early morning awakening

Contraindications and cautions
- Contraindicated with hypersensitivity to benzodiazepines, established or suspected sleep apnea, psychoses, acute narrow-angle glaucoma, shock, coma, acute alcoholic intoxication with depression of vital signs, pregnancy (congenital malformations, neonatal withdrawal syndrome), labor and delivery ("floppy infant" syndrome), lactation (infants become lethargic and lose weight).

- Use cautiously with elderly patients, impaired liver or renal function, debilitation, depression, suicidal tendencies.

Available forms
Tablets—15 mg

Dosages
Adults
Initially, 15 mg PO at bedtime. May reduce to 7.5 mg at bedtime in some patients.
Pediatric patients
Not for use in patients younger than 18 yr.
Geriatric patients or patients with debilitating disease
Initially, 7.5 mg PO; if not effective after 1 or 2 nights, increase to 15 mg. In some patients, the dosage may later be reduced to 7.5 mg.

Pharmacokinetics

Route	Onset	Peak
Oral	Varies	2 hr

Metabolism: Hepatic; $T_{1/2}$: 41 hr
Distribution: Crosses placenta; enters breast milk
Excretion: Urine

Adverse effects
- **CNS:** *Transient, mild drowsiness initially;* sedation; depression; lethargy; apathy; fatigue; light-headedness; disorientation; restlessness; confusion; crying; delirium; *headache;* slurred speech; dysarthria; stupor; rigidity; tremor; dystonia; vertigo; euphoria; nervousness; difficulty in concentration; vivid dreams; psychomotor retardation; extrapyramidal symptoms; mild paradoxic excitatory reactions during first 2 wk of treatment (especially in psychiatric patients, aggressive children, and with high dosage); visual and auditory disturbances; diplopia; nystagmus; depressed hearing; nasal congestion; complex sleep-related behaviors
- **CV:** *Bradycardia, tachycardia,* **CV collapse,** hypertension and hypotension, palpitations, edema
- **Dependence:** *Drug dependence with withdrawal syndrome* when drug is discontinued (more common with abrupt discontinuation of higher dosage used for longer than 4 mo)

Q

- **Dermatologic:** Pruritus, skin rash, dermatitis
- **GI:** *Constipation, diarrhea, dry mouth,* salivation, nausea, anorexia, vomiting, difficulty in swallowing, gastric disorders, elevations of blood enzymes, hepatic impairment, jaundice
- **GU:** Incontinence, changes in libido, urinary retention, menstrual irregularities
- **Hematologic:** Decreased Hct (primarily with long-term therapy), blood dyscrasias (agranulocytosis, leukopenia, neutropenia)
- **Other: Anaphylaxis, angioedema,** hiccups, fever, diaphoresis, paresthesias, muscular disturbances, gynecomastia

Interactions

✳ **Drug-drug** • Increased CNS depression with alcohol anticonvulsants, antihistamines, psychotropic medications • Increased pharmacologic effects with cimetidine, disulfiram, hormonal contraceptives • Decreased sedative effects with theophylline, aminophylline • Decreased sedative effects with smoking • Risk of serious to fatal respiratory depression if combined with methadone, avoid this combination

■ Nursing considerations
Assessment

- **History:** Hypersensitivity to benzodiazepines, psychoses, acute narrow-angle glaucoma, shock, coma, acute alcoholic intoxication, pregnancy, labor and delivery, lactation, impaired liver or renal function, debilitation, depression, suicidal tendencies
- **Physical:** Skin color, lesions; T; orientation, reflexes, affect, ophthalmologic examination; P, BP; R, adventitious sounds; liver evaluation, abdominal examination, bowel sounds, normal output; CBC, LFTs, renal function tests

Interventions

⊗ **Warning** Ensure that patient is not pregnant before use; recommend the use of barrier contraceptives.
- Monitor liver and renal function and CBC during long-term therapy.

⊗ **Warning** Taper dosage gradually after long-term therapy, especially in patients with epilepsy, to prevent refractory seizures.

Teaching points

- Take drug exactly as prescribed.
- Do not stop taking this drug (in long-term therapy) without consulting your health care provider.
- This drug should not be used during pregnancy; using barrier contraceptives is advised.
- You may experience these side effects: Drowsiness, dizziness (may lessen; avoid driving or engaging in other dangerous activities); allergic reaction; GI upset (take with water); depression, dreams, complex sleep disorders, emotional upset, crying; nocturnal sleep may be disturbed for several nights after discontinuing the drug.
- Report severe dizziness, weakness, drowsiness that persists, complex sleep-related behaviors, rash or skin lesions, palpitations, swelling of the extremities, visual changes, difficulty voiding, allergic reaction.

▽**quetiapine fumarate**
*(kwe **tie'** ah peen)*

Seroquel, Seroquel XR⊙

PREGNANCY CATEGORY C

Drug classes
Antipsychotic
Dibenzothiazepine

Therapeutic actions
Mechanism of action not fully understood: Blocks dopamine and serotonin receptors in the brain; also acts as a receptor antagonist at histamine and adrenergic receptor sites (which may contribute to the adverse effects of orthostatic hypotension and somnolence).

Indications

- Treatment of schizophrenia in patients older than 13 yr
- Adjunctive treatment of major depressive disorder in children (ER forms only)
- Short-term treatment of acute manic or mixed episodes associated with bipolar I disorder, as monotherapy or in combination with lithium or divalproex
- Acute treatment of depressive episodes associated with bipolar I disorder
- Maintenance treatment of bipolar disorder as an adjunct to lithium or divalproex

---

*Adverse effects in italics are most common; those in **bold** are life-threatening. ⊙ Do not crush.*

- Unlabeled uses: Alcohol dependence, OCD, Tourette syndrome

Contraindications and cautions

- Contraindicated with coma or severe CNS depression, allergy to quetiapine, lactation.
- Use cautiously with CV disease, hypotension, hepatic impairment, seizures, exposure to extreme heat, autonomic instability, tardive dyskinesia, dehydration, thyroid disease, pregnancy, elderly patients with dementia-related psychosis.

Available forms

Tablets—25, 50, 100, 200, 300, 400 mg; ER tablets ⊕—50, 150, 200, 300, 400 mg

Dosages
Adults

- *Schizophrenia:* 25 mg PO bid. Increase in increments of 25–50 mg bid–tid on days 2 and 3; dosage range by day 4: 300–400 mg/day in two to three divided doses. Further increases can be made at no less than 2-day intervals. Maximum dose, 800 mg/day. When patient is stabilized on divided doses, may be switched to ER form at the total equivalent dose taken once per day. For ER tablets, 300 mg PO once daily in the evening; range, 400–800 mg/day.
- *Manic episodes:* 100 mg/day PO divided bid on day 1; increase to 400 mg/day PO in bid divided doses by day 4 using 100-mg/day increments. Range, 400–800 mg/day given in divided doses. ER forms: 300 mg/day PO on day 1,600 mg on day 2; may be adjusted to 800 mg on day 3 if needed.
- *Depressive episodes (ER form):* 50 mg PO on day 1, then 100 mg PO on day 2 given daily at bedtime; increase to desired dose of 300 mg/day by day 4.
- *Major depressive disorder* (ER form): Initially, 50 mg PO at bedtime; on day 3, increase to 150 mg PO in the evening. Range is 150–300 mg/day. Give with other antidepressants.

Pediatric patients 10–17 yr

- *Acute treatment of manic episodes:* 50 mg PO on day 1, 100 mg PO on day 2, 200 mg PO on day 3, 300 mg PO on day 4, 400 mg PO on day 5. Maximum dose is 600 mg/day.

Pediatric patients 13–17 yr

- *Schizophrenia:* Give in divided dose twice a day. Total dose: day 1, 50 mg PO; day 2, 100 mg; day 3, 200 mg; day 4, 300 mg; day 5, 400 mg. Usual range is 400–800 mg/day.

Geriatric or debilitated patients or patients with hepatic impairment

Use lower doses starting with 25 mg/day PO and increase dosage more gradually than in other patients. For schizophrenia, when stabilized on 200 mg/day PO, patient may be switched to ER tablets.

Pharmacokinetics

Route	Onset	Peak	Duration
Oral	Slow	1.5 hr	Unknown

Metabolism: Hepatic; $T_{1/2}$: 6 hr
Distribution: Crosses placenta; enters breast milk
Excretion: Feces, urine

Adverse effects

- **Autonomic:** Dry mouth, salivation, nasal congestion, nausea, vomiting, anorexia, fever, pallor, flushed facies, sweating, constipation
- **CNS:** *Drowsiness,* insomnia, vertigo, *headache,* weakness, tremor, tardive dyskinesias, **NMS,** suicidal ideation, agitation
- **CV:** Hypotension, *orthostatic hypotension,* syncope
- **Hematologic:** Increased ALT, total cholesterol and triglycerides
- **Other:** Risk of development of diabetes mellitus, weight gain, hyperglycemia

Interactions

✳ **Drug-drug** • CNS effects potentiated by alcohol, CNS depressants • Effects decreased with phenytoin, thioridazine, carbamazepine, phenobarbital, rifampin, glucocorticoids; monitor patient closely and adjust dosages appropriately when these drugs are added to or discontinued from regimen • Increased effects of antihypertensives, lorazepam • Decreased effects of levodopa, dopamine antagonists • Potential for heatstroke and intolerance with drugs that affect temperature regulation (anticholinergics); use extreme caution and monitor patient closely • Increased risk of prolonged QT interval if combined with other drugs that prolong QT interval; use with caution

■ **Nursing considerations**

Assessment

- **History:** Coma or severe CNS depression, allergy to quetiapine, lactation, pregnancy, CV disease, hypotension, hepatic impairment, seizures, exposure to extreme heat, autonomic instability, tardive dyskinesia, dehydration, thyroid disease, suicidal tendencies
- **Physical:** Body weight, T; reflexes, orientation, IOP; P, BP, orthostatic BP; R, adventitious sounds; CBC, urinalysis, LFTs, renal and thyroid function tests, lipid profile

Interventions

⊗ **Black box warning** Do not use this drug to treat elderly patients with dementia-related psychosis; it causes increased risk of CV mortality, including stroke, MI.

⊗ **Black box warning** Increased risk of suicidality in children, adolescents, and young adults; not approved for use in children. Monitor patients accordingly.

⊗ **Warning** Administer small quantity to any patient with suicidal ideation.

- Make sure patient does not cut, crush, or chew ER tablets; they must be swallowed whole.
- Administer ER tablet once daily in the evening.
- Monitor elderly patients for dehydration and institute remedial measures promptly; sedation and decreased sensation of thirst related to CNS effects of drug can lead to severe dehydration.
- Monitor patient closely in any setting that would promote overheating.
- Regularly monitor patient for signs and symptoms of diabetes mellitus.
- Consult physician about dosage reduction and use of anticholinergic antiparkinsonians (controversial) if extrapyramidal effects occur.

Teaching points

- Take this drug exactly as prescribed.
- Take extended-release tablet once daily in the evening. Do not cut, crush, or chew tablets; they must be swallowed whole.
- This drug should not be used during pregnancy; using barrier contraceptives is advised.
- Maintain fluid intake and use precautions against heatstroke in hot weather.

- You may experience these side effects: Dizziness, drowsiness, fainting (avoid driving or engaging in other dangerous activities); dry mouth, nausea, loss of appetite (frequent mouth care, frequent small meals, and increased fluid intake may help), weight gain.
- Report sore throat, fever, unusual bleeding or bruising, rash, weakness, tremors, dark-colored urine, pale stools, yellowing of the skin or eyes, suicidal thoughts.

▽**quinapril hydrochloride**

(kwin' ah pril)

Accupril

PREGNANCY CATEGORY C
(FIRST TRIMESTER)

PREGNANCY CATEGORY D
(SECOND AND THIRD TRIMESTERS)

Drug classes

ACE inhibitor
Antihypertensive

Therapeutic actions

Quinapril blocks ACE from converting angiotensin I to angiotensin II, a powerful vasoconstrictor, leading to decreased BP, decreased aldosterone secretion, a small increase in serum potassium levels, and sodium and fluid loss; increased prostaglandin synthesis also may be involved in the antihypertensive action.

Indications

- Treatment of hypertension alone or in combination with thiazide-type diuretics
- Adjunctive therapy in the management of HF with cardiac glycosides, diuretics, and beta-adrenergic blockers
- Unlabeled use: Pediatric hypertension

Contraindications and cautions

- Contraindicated with allergy to quinapril or other ACE inhibitors, pregnancy, angioedema.
- Use cautiously with impaired renal function, unilateral or bilateral renal artery stenosis, salt or volume depletion, lactation.

Available forms
Tablets—5, 10, 20, 40 mg

Dosages
Adults
- *Hypertension:* Initial dose, 10 or 20 mg PO daily. Maintenance dose, 20–80 mg/day PO as a single dose or two divided doses. Patients on diuretics should discontinue the diuretic 2–3 days before beginning quinapril therapy. If BP is not controlled, add diuretic slowly. If diuretic cannot be discontinued, begin quinapril therapy with 5 mg and monitor carefully for hypotension.
- *HF:* Initial dose, 5 mg PO bid. Dose may be increased as needed to relieve symptoms; usual range, 10–20 mg PO bid; increase doses at weekly intervals until effective dose is reached.

Pediatric patients
Safety and efficacy not established.

Geriatric patients or patients with renal impairment
Initial dose: 10 mg PO if creatinine clearance greater than 60 mL/min, 5 mg PO if creatinine clearance 30–60 mL/min, 2.5 mg PO if creatinine clearance 10–30 mL/min.

Pharmacokinetics

Route	Onset	Peak	Duration
Oral	1 hr	1 hr	24 hr

Metabolism: Hepatic; $T_{1/2}$: 2 hr
Distribution: Crosses placenta; enters breast milk
Excretion: Urine

Adverse effects
- **CV:** Angina pectoris, orthostatic hypotension in salt- or volume-depleted patients, palpitations, *dizziness, headache*
- **Dermatologic:** Rash, pruritus, diaphoresis, flushing, photosensitivity
- **GI:** Elevated LFTs, pancreatitis
- **Respiratory:** *Cough*
- **Other:** Angioedema, arthralgia

Interactions
✳ **Drug-drug** ● Increased lithium levels ● Decreased tetracycline absorption. Separate drugs by 1–2 hr ● Risk of hyperkalemia if combined with potassium-sparing diuretics

■ Nursing considerations
Assessment
- **History:** Allergy to quinapril, other ACE inhibitors; impaired renal function; HF; salt or volume depletion; lactation, pregnancy
- **Physical:** Skin color, lesions, turgor; T; P, BP, peripheral perfusion; mucous membranes, bowel sounds, liver evaluation; urinalysis, LFTs, renal function tests, CBC and differential

Interventions
⊗ *Warning* Alert surgeon and mark the patient's chart with notice that quinapril is being taken; the angiotensin II formation subsequent to compensatory renin release during surgery will be blocked; hypotension may be reversed with volume expansion.

⊗ **Black box warning** Caution patient that this drug should not be used during pregnancy; advise patient to use barrier contraceptives.

- Monitor patient closely in any situation that may lead to a fall in BP secondary to reduction in fluid volume (excessive perspiration and dehydration, vomiting, diarrhea) because excessive hypotension may occur.

Teaching points
- Do not stop taking the medication without consulting your health care provider.
- Be careful in any situation that may lead to a drop in blood pressure (diarrhea, sweating, vomiting, dehydration); if light-headedness or dizziness occurs, consult your health care provider.
- This drug should not be used during pregnancy; using barrier contraceptives is advised.
- You may experience these side effects: GI upset, loss of appetite (transient); light-headedness (usually transient; change position slowly and limit activities to those that do not require alertness and precision); dry cough (not harmful).
- Report mouth sores; sore throat, fever, chills; swelling of the hands, feet; irregular heartbeat, chest pains; swelling of the face, eyes, lips, tongue; difficulty breathing; persistent cough.

Q

DANGEROUS DRUG

▷quinidine
(qwin' i deen)

quinidine gluconate ⓒⓝⓖ

quinidine sulfate ⓒⓝⓖ

PREGNANCY CATEGORY C

Drug class
Antiarrhythmic

Therapeutic actions
Type IA antiarrhythmic: Decreases automaticity in ventricles, decreases height and rate of rise of action potential, decreases conduction velocity, increases fibrillation threshold.

Indications
- Treatment of atrial arrhythmias, paroxysmal or chronic ventricular tachycardia without heart block
- Maintenance therapy after electrocardioversion of atrial fibrillation or atrial flutter
- Treatment of life-threatening *Plasmodium falciparum* infections when IV therapy (quinidine gluconate) is indicated

Contraindications and cautions
- Contraindicated with allergy or idiosyncrasy to quinidine, second- or third-degree heart block, myasthenia gravis, pregnancy (neonatal thrombocytopenia), lactation, thrombocytopenic purpura, in patients with diseases that might be adversely affected by an anticholinergic agent.
- Use cautiously with renal disease, especially renal tubular acidosis, HF, hepatic insufficiency.

Available forms
Tablets—200, 300 mg; SR tablets ⓒⓝⓖ—300, 324 mg; injection—80 mg/mL

Dosages
Quinidine gluconate contains 62% anhydrous quinidine alkaloid. Quinidine sulfate contains 83% anhydrous quinidine alkaloid.
Adults
Administer a test dose of 200 mg PO or 200 mg IV to test for idiosyncratic reaction. Maintenance therapy, 200–300 mg tid or qid PO or 300–600 mg every 8 hr or every 12 hr if SR form is used.

- *Paroxysmal supraventricular arrhythmias:* 400–600 mg (sulfate) PO every 2–3 hr until paroxysm is terminated.
- *Conversion of atrial flutter/fibrillation:* 648 mg (gluconate) PO every 8 hr; may increase after three to four doses if needed. Or 324 mg (gluconate) PO every 8 hr for 2 days, then 648 mg PO every 8 hr for 2 days. Or 5–10 mg/kg (gluconate) IV. For ER tablets, 300 mg (sulfate) PO every 8–12 hr; may increase dosage cautiously if serum levels are in therapeutic range. For immediate-release tablets, 400 mg (sulfate) PO every 6 hr; may increase dosage after four to five doses if conversion has not occurred.
- *Reduction of relapse:* 324 mg (gluconate) PO every 8–12 hr. For ER tablets, 300 mg (sulfate) PO every 8–12 hr. For immediate-release tablets, 200 mg (sulfate) PO every 6 hr.
- *P. falciparum* malaria: 24 mg/kg quinidine gluconate IV in 250 mL normal saline infused over 4 hr; then 12 mg/kg infused over 4 hr every 8 hr for 7 days (patients who are able can switch to same dosage of quinidine sulfate orally). Or, 10 mg/kg quinidine gluconate in 5 mL/Kg normal saline as a loading dose; then a maintenance infusion of 20 mcg/kg/min. Patient may switch to same oral dosage of quinidine sulfate every 8 hr for 72 hr or until parasitemia is decreased to 1% or less.
Pediatric patients
- *P. falciparum* malaria: 10 mg/kg quinidine gluconate in 5 mL/kg normal saline IV over 1–2 hr, then 20 mcg/kg/min IV maintenance dose. When patient can tolerate oral dosing, convert maintenance dosage to same amount of quinidine base, as quinidine sulfate orally every 8 hr.
Patients with hepatic or renal impairment
Reduce dosage and monitor patient closely.

Pharmacokinetics

Route	Onset	Duration
Oral	1–3 hr	6–8 hr
IV	Rapid	6–8 hr

Metabolism: Hepatic; $T_{1/2}$: 6–7 hr
Distribution: Crosses placenta; enters breast milk
Excretion: Feces, urine

▼ IV FACTS

Preparation: Dilute 800 mg quinidine gluconate in 50 mL 5% dextrose injection. Minimize tubing length; quinidine absorbs PVC. Drug may be stored for up to 24 hr at room temperature or 48 hr refrigerated.

Infusion: Inject slowly at rate of 0.25 mg/kg/min.

Y-site incompatibility: Do not inject with furosemide.

Adverse effects

- **CNS:** Vision changes (photophobia, blurring, loss of night vision, diplopia), *lightheadedness*
- **CV: Cardiac arrhythmias,** cardiac conduction disturbances, including heart block, hypotension
- **GI:** *Nausea*, vomiting, *diarrhea,* liver toxicity
- **Hematologic:** Hemolytic anemia, hypoprothrombinemia, thrombocytopenic purpura, agranulocytosis, lupus erythematosus-like syndrome (resolves after withdrawal)
- **Hypersensitivity:** Rash, flushing, urticaria, angioedema, respiratory arrest
- **Other:** *Cinchonism* (tinnitus, headache, nausea, dizziness, fever, tremor, visual disturbances)

Interactions

❋ **Drug-drug** • Increased effects and increased risk of toxicity with cimetidine, amiodarone, verapamil • Increased cardiac depressant effects with sodium bicarbonate • Decreased levels with phenobarbital, hydantoins, rifampin, sucralfate • Increased neuromuscular blocking effects of depolarizing and nondepolarizing neuromuscular blocking agents, succinylcholine • Increased digoxin levels and toxicity • Increased effect of oral anticoagulants and bleeding • Increased effects of TCAs

❋ **Drug-food** • Decreased metabolism and increased risk of toxic effects if combined with grapefruit juice; avoid this combination

❋ **Drug-lab test** • Quinidine serum levels are inaccurate if the patient is also taking triamterene

■ Nursing considerations
Assessment

- **History:** Allergy or idiosyncrasy to quinidine, second- or third-degree heart block, myasthenia gravis, renal disease, HF, hepatic insufficiency, pregnancy, lactation

- **Physical:** Skin color, lesions; orientation, cranial nerves, bilateral grip strength, reflexes; P, BP, auscultation, ECG, edema; bowel sounds, liver evaluation; urinalysis, LFTs, renal function tests; CBC

Interventions

- Monitor response carefully, especially when beginning therapy.
- Reduce dosage in patients with hepatic or renal failure.
- Reduce dosage with digoxin; monitor digoxin levels closely.
- Adjust dosage if phenobarbital, hydantoin, or rifampin is added or discontinued.
- Check to see that patients with atrial flutter or fibrillation have been digitalized before starting quinidine.
- Differentiate the SR form from the regular form. Make sure SR form is not cut, crushed, or chewed.
- Monitor cardiac rhythm carefully, and frequently monitor BP if given IV.
- Arrange for periodic ECG monitoring when on long-term therapy.
- Monitor blood counts, liver function tests frequently during long-term therapy.

⊗ *Warning* Evaluate for safe and effective serum drug levels: 2–6 mcg/mL.

Teaching points

- Take this drug exactly as prescribed. Do not chew the sustained-release tablets. If GI upset occurs, take drug with food. Do not drink grapefruit juice while using this drug.
- You will need frequent cardiac rhythm monitoring and blood tests.
- Wear a Medical Alert tag stating that you are using this drug.
- Return for regular follow-up visits to check your heart rhythm and blood counts.
- You may experience these side effects: Nausea, loss of appetite, vomiting (eat frequent small meals); dizziness, light-headedness, vision changes (do not drive or operate dangerous machinery); rash (use skin care).
- Report sore mouth, throat, or gums, fever, chills, cold or flulike symptoms, ringing in the ears, severe vision disturbances, headache, unusual bleeding or bruising.

▽ **quinine sulfate**

See Appendix R, *Less commonly used drugs.*

▷ rabeprazole sodium
(rah beb' pray zol)

AcipHex⊙ℕ⊙, Parlet (CAN)

PREGNANCY CATEGORY B

Drug classes
Antisecretory drug
Proton pump inhibitor

Therapeutic actions
Gastric acid-pump inhibitor: Suppresses gastric acid secretion by specific inhibition of the hydrogen and potassium ATPase enzyme system at the secretory surface of the gastric parietal cells; blocks the final step of acid production.

Indications
- Healing and maintenance of erosive or ulcerative GERD; 4–8 wk therapy; may use additional 8 wk as needed
- Short-term treatment of GERD in children 12 yr and older
- Treatment of daytime and nighttime heartburn and other symptoms of GERD
- Healing of duodenal ulcers as short-term treatment of less than 4 wk
- Treatment of pathologic hypersecretory conditions (eg, Zollinger-Ellison syndrome, multiple adenomas, systemic mastocytosis)
- Eradication of *Helicobacter pylori* in combination with amoxicillin and clarithromycin
- Unlabeled use: Prevention of GI bleeding in patients taking antiplatelet drugs

Contraindications and cautions
- Contraindicated with hypersensitivity to any proton pump inhibitor or any drug components.
- Use cautiously because of possible increased risk of *Clostridium difficile* diarrhea.
- Use cautiously with pregnancy, lactation.

Available forms
DR tablet⊙ℕ⊙——10 (CAN), 20 mg

Dosages
Adults
- *Healing of GERD:* 20 mg PO daily for 4–8 wk.
- *Maintenance of GERD:* 20 mg daily PO.

- *Healing of duodenal ulcer:* 20 mg PO daily for up to 4 wk.
- *Pathologic hypersecretory conditions:* 60 mg PO daily to bid for as long as clinically indicated.
- H. pylori *eradication:* 20 mg PO bid with amoxicillin 1,000 mg PO bid and clarithromycin 500 mg PO bid with meals for 7 days.

Pediatric patients 12 yr and older
- *Treatment of GERD:* 20 mg/day PO for up to 8 wk.

Patients with hepatic impairment
Use extreme caution with severe hepatic impairment.

Pharmacokinetics

Route	Onset	Peak
Oral	1 hr	3–5 hr

Metabolism: Hepatic; $T_{1/2}$: 1.5 hr
Distribution: Crosses placenta; may enter breast milk
Excretion: Feces, urine

Adverse effects
- **CNS:** *Headache, dizziness,* asthenia, vertigo, insomnia, apathy, anxiety, paresthesias, dream abnormalities
- **Dermatologic:** Rash, inflammation, urticaria, pruritus, alopecia, dry skin
- **GI:** *Diarrhea,* possible increased risk of *C. difficile* diarrhea, *abdominal pain, nausea, vomiting,* constipation, dry mouth, tongue atrophy
- **Respiratory:** *URI symptoms,* cough, epistaxis
- **Other:** Cancer in preclinical studies, back pain, fever, increased risk of long-bone fractures, decreased magnesium levels with long-term use

Interactions
✳ **Drug-drug** ● Increased toxic effects of warfarin, digoxin; monitor patient closely and arrange for dosage adjustment as needed ● Decreased effectiveness of azole antifungals; monitor patient closely

■ Nursing considerations
Assessment
- **History:** Hypersensitivity to any proton pump inhibitor or any drug components, pregnancy, lactation

Adverse effects in italics *are most common; those in* **bold** *are life-threatening.* ⊙ℕ⊙ Do not crush.

- **Physical:** Skin lesions; body T; reflexes, affect; urinary output, abdominal examination; respiratory auscultation

Interventions

- Administer once a day. Caution patient to swallow tablets whole, not to cut, crush, or chew.
- Symptomatic improvement does not rule out gastric cancer.
- If administering antacids, they may be administered concomitantly with rabeprazole.
- Maintain supportive treatment as appropriate for underlying problem.
- Provide additional comfort measures to alleviate discomfort such as from GI effects or headache.

Teaching points

- Take the drug once a day. Swallow the tablets whole—do not chew, cut, or crush. This drug will need to be taken for up to 4 weeks (in short-term therapy) or for a prolonged period depending on the condition being treated.
- Arrange to have regular medical follow-up while you are using this drug.
- Maintain all of the usual activities and restrictions that apply to your condition. If this becomes difficult, consult your health care provider.
- You may experience these side effects: Dizziness (avoid driving a car or performing hazardous tasks); headache (consult your health care provider if these become bothersome; medications may be available to help); nausea, vomiting, diarrhea (proper nutrition is important, consult a dietitian to maintain nutrition; ensure ready access to bathroom facilities); symptoms of upper respiratory tract infection, cough (it may help to know that this is a drug effect, do not self-medicate, consult your health care provider if this becomes uncomfortable).
- Report severe headache, worsening of symptoms, fever, chills.

▷**raloxifene hydrochloride**
(rah lox' i feen)

Evista

PREGNANCY CATEGORY X

Drug class

Selective estrogen receptor modulator

Therapeutic actions

Increases bone mineral density without stimulating endometrium in women; modulates effects of endogenous estrogen at specific receptor sites.

Indications

- Prevention and treatment of osteoporosis in postmenopausal women
- Reduction of risk of invasive breast cancer in postmenopausal women with osteoporosis and a high risk of invasive breast cancer
- Unlabeled uses: Uterine leiomyoma, pubertal gynecomastia, prevention of bone loss in men with prostate cancer

Contraindications and cautions

- Contraindicated with allergy to raloxifene, pregnancy, lactation, active or history of DVT, pulmonary embolism, or retinal vein thrombosis.
- Use cautiously with history of smoking, venous thrombosis.

Available forms

Tablets—60 mg

Dosages
Adults
60 mg PO daily.

Pharmacokinetics

Route	Onset	Peak
Oral	Varies	4–7 hr

Metabolism: Hepatic; T$_{1/2}$: 27.7 hr
Distribution: Crosses placenta; enters breast milk
Excretion: Feces

Adverse effects

- **CNS:** Depression, insomnia, vertigo, neuralgia, hypoesthesia
- **CV: Venous thromboembolism**
- **Dermatologic:** *Hot flashes, skin rash*
- **GI:** *Nausea, vomiting,* food distaste
- **GU:** Vaginal bleeding, vaginal discharge
- **Other:** Peripheral edema, flulike syndrome, rhinitis, sinusitis, bronchitis

Interactions
✳ **Drug-drug** • Decreased effectiveness of oral anticoagulants; monitor PT or INR closely • Decreased raloxifene absorption if taken with cholestyramine; avoid this combination

■ Nursing considerations
Assessment
- **History:** Allergy to raloxifene, pregnancy, lactation, smoking, history of venous thrombosis
- **Physical:** Skin lesions, color, turgor; pelvic examination; orientation, affect, reflexes; peripheral pulses, edema; LFTs, CBC and differential, bone density

Interventions
- Administer daily without regard to food.
- Arrange for periodic blood counts during therapy.

⊗ **Black box warning** Drug increases risk of deep vein thromboses and pulmonary emboli; monitor patient accordingly.

⊗ **Black box warning** Drug increases risk of stroke and CV events in women with documented CAD; weigh benefits against risks before using drug with these women.

⊗ **Warning** Counsel patient about the need to use contraceptive measures to avoid pregnancy while taking this drug; inform patient that serious fetal harm could occur.

- Provide comfort measures to help patient deal with drug effects: Hot flashes (control environmental temperature); headache, depression (monitor light and noise); vaginal bleeding (use good hygiene).

Teaching points
- Take this drug as prescribed.
- This drug can cause serious fetal harm and must not be taken during pregnancy. Contraceptive measures should be used while you are taking this drug. If you become pregnant or would like to become pregnant, consult your health care provider immediately.
- You may experience these side effects: Bone pain; hot flashes (staying in cool places may help); nausea, vomiting (eat frequent small meals); weight gain; dizziness, headache, light-headedness (use caution if driving or performing tasks that require alertness).
- Report marked weakness, sleepiness, mental confusion, pain or swelling of the legs, shortness of breath, blurred vision, numbness or tingling.

raltegravir
*(rahl **teb'** gra veer)*

Isentress

PREGNANCY CATEGORY C

Drug classes
Antiretroviral
Integrase inhibitor

Therapeutic action
Inhibits the virus-specific enzyme integrase, an encoded enzyme needed for viral replication. Blocking this enzyme prevents formation of HIV-1 provirus and leads to decreased viral load and increased active CD4 cells.

Indications
- In combination with other antiretrovirals for the treatment of HIV-1 infection in adults

Contraindications and cautions
- Contraindicated with hypersensitivity to any component of drug, treatment-naïve adults, children, lactation.
- Use cautiously with patients taking strong inducers of uridine disphosphate glucuronsyltransferase 1A1, patients at risk for rhabdomyolysis or myopathy, pregnant patients.

Available forms
Tablets—400 mg; chewable tablets—25, 100 mg

Dosages
Adults
400 mg PO bid taken with other antivirals and without regard to food. If given with rifampin, 800 mg PO bid without regard to food.
Pediatric patients
- *12 yr and older:* 400 mg PO bid.
- *6 to younger than 12 yr:* 25 kg or more, 400 mg PO bid or up to 300 mg PO bid chewable tablets; less than 25 kg, chewable tablets weight-based to maximum 300 mg bid.
- *2 to younger than 6 yr:* Chewable tablets, based on weight: less than 10 kg, not recommended; 10 to less than 14 kg, 75 mg

Adverse effects in *italics* are most common; those in **bold** are life-threatening. ⬛ Do not crush.

PO bid; 14 to less than 20 kg, 100 mg PO bid; 20 to less than 28 kg, 150 mg PO bid; 28 to less than 40 kg, 200 mg PO bid; 40 kg or more, 300 mg PO bid.

Pharmacokinetics

Route	Onset	Peak
Oral	Rapid	3 hr

Metabolism: Hepatic; $T_{1/2}$: 9 hr
Distribution: May cross placenta; may enter breast milk
Excretion: Feces, urine

Adverse effects

- **CNS:** *Headache,* dizziness, insomnia
- **GI:** *Nausea, diarrhea,* abdominal pain, vomiting
- **Other:** *Fever,* rhabdomyolysis, immune reconstitution syndrome

Interactions

❋ **Drug-drug** • Decreased serum levels of raltegravir if combined with rifampin; monitor patient and adjust dosage if this combination must be used

❋ **Drug-drug** • Potential for loss of effectiveness if combined with St. John's Wort; avoid this combination

■ Nursing considerations

Assessment

- **History:** Hypersensitivity to raltegravir or any of its components; risk for myopathy or rhabdomyolysis, pregnancy, lactation
- **Physical:** T; orientation; abdominal examination, LFTs, HIV testing

Interventions

- Make sure patient is taking other antiviral drugs when taking this drug.
- Administer without regard to food. For children, calculate weight-based doses for chewable tablets.
- Encourage women of childbearing age to use barrier contraceptives while on this drug because drug effects on fetus are not known.
- Advise women who are breast-feeding to find another method of feeding the infant; potential effects on the infant are not known.
- Explain that drug does not cure disease and that there is still a risk of transmitting HIV to others.

- Maintain all other therapies related to the HIV infection.

Teaching points

- This drug does not cure HIV. It works with other antiviral drugs to decrease the amount of virus in your body.
- To prevent the spread of HIV, take precautions to avoid exposing others to your blood and body fluids, and use condoms during sex.
- If you miss a dose, take it as soon as you remember and resume your regular schedule. If you don't remember until it's almost time to take the next dose, skip the missed dose and continue your usual schedule. Do not take two tablets at the same time to make up for a skipped dose. Do not take more than two doses each day.
- Do not let your prescription run out. If you stop taking this drug temporarily, the virus could become resistant to antiviral drugs, decreasing the effectiveness of antiviral treatment and increasing your viral load.
- You will need regular health care, including blood tests, to monitor the effects of this drug on your body.
- It is not known how this drug could affect a fetus. If you are pregnant or decide to become pregnant while on this drug, consult your health care provider.
- It is not known how this drug could affect a breast-feeding infant. If you are breast-feeding, you should select another feeding method.
- You may experience these side effects: Headache (consult your health care provider, medication may be available to help); nausea (small, frequent meals may help); diarrhea (it may lessen with time, but alert your health care provider if it becomes severe).
- Report signs of infection; unexplained muscle pain, tenderness, or weakness; severe diarrhea; headache that will not go away.

▽**ramelteon**
*(rah **mell'** tee on)*

Rozerem

PREGNANCY CATEGORY C

Drug classes
Melatonin receptor agonist
Sedative-hypnotic

R

Therapeutic actions

Agonist at melatonin receptor sites believed to contribute to sleep promotion and thought to be involved in the maintenance of circadian rhythm underlying the normal sleep-wake cycle.

Indications

- Treatment of insomnia characterized by difficulty with sleep onset

Contraindications and cautions

- Contraindicated with known hypersensitivity to any component of the drug, severe hepatic impairment, concurrent use of fluvoxamine, lactation, severe sleep apnea, severe COPD.
- Use cautiously with moderate hepatic impairment, pregnancy.

Available forms

Tablets—8 mg

Dosages

Adults

8 mg PO taken within 30 min of going to bed.

Pediatric patients

Safety and efficacy not established.

Patients with hepatic impairment

- *Severe hepatic impairment:* Not recommended.
- *Moderate hepatic impairment:* Use with caution.
- *Concurrent use of CYP1A2 inhibitors (such as ciprofloxacin):* Use with caution.

Pharmacokinetics

Route	Onset	Peak
Oral	Rapid	0.5–1.5 hr

Metabolism: Hepatic; $T_{1/2}$: 2-5 hr
Distribution: May cross placenta; may pass into breast milk
Excretion: Feces, urine

Adverse effects

- **CNS:** Dizziness, somnolence, depression, insomnia, *headache,* complex sleep disorders
- **GI:** Nausea, diarrhea
- **GU:** Decreased testosterone levels (decreased libido, fertility issues), increased prolactin levels (galactorrhea, amenorrhea, problems with fertility)
- **Respiratory:** URIs

- **Other:** Influenza, arthralgia, myalgia, decreased cortisol levels, **anaphylaxis, angioedema**

Interactions

❋ **Drug-drug** ● Risk of severe increase in serum levels and toxicity of ramelteon if combined with fluvoxamine; avoid this combination ● Increased serum levels and risk of adverse effects if combined with potent CYP inhibitors (ketoconazole, fluconazole, itraconazole, clarithromycin, nefazodone, ritonavir, nelfinavir); monitor patient and adjust dosages as needed

■ Nursing considerations

Assessment

- **History:** Hypersensitivity to any component of the drug, hepatic impairment, concurrent use of fluvoxamine, lactation, severe sleep apnea, severe COPD, pregnancy
- **Physical:** Orientation, reflexes, affect; R, adventitious sounds; abdominal examination; chest examination

Interventions

- Administer drug 30 min before patient is going to bed; encourage no other activities after the patient takes the drug.
- Monitor patients using drug for suicidal ideation.
- Do not administer this drug after a fatty or large meal, absorption can be affected.
- Encourage women of childbearing age to use barrier contraceptives while on this drug; effects of the drug on a fetus are not known.
- Advise women who are breast-feeding to find another method of feeding the infant; it is not known if this drug can affect a nursing infant.

Teaching points

- Take this drug exactly as prescribed, 30 minutes before going to bed. Do not use it longer than advised by your health care provider.
- Do not take this drug unless you are about to get into bed and are able to get 8 or more hours of sleep before you need to be alert again; after taking the drug, limit activities to those involved with getting ready for bed.
- Do not take this drug with or immediately after a high-fat or heavy meal. This could interfere with the absorption and effectiveness of the drug.

Adverse effects in *italics* are most common; those in **bold** are life-threatening. ⬚ Do not crush.

- Do not combine this drug with other sleep drugs, including over-the-counter products.
- It is not known how this drug would affect a pregnancy. If you think you are pregnant or would like to become pregnant, consult your health care provider.
- This drug should not be taken while breast-feeding. If you are breast-feeding, another method of feeding the infant should be used while you are taking this drug.
- Consult your health care provider if you experience worsening of your insomnia or if you develop any new behavioral signs or symptoms, such as complex sleep-related behaviors.
- You may experience these side effects: Allergic reaction, swelling, changes in thinking, alertness (do not drive a car, operate potentially dangerous equipment, or make important legal decisions the day after you take this drug); headache (consult your health care provider for potential pain medications if this occurs); unpleasant taste, nausea (frequent mouth care, frequent small meals may help); cessation of your period (women), enlargement of breasts, fertility problems.
- Report depression, thoughts of suicide or disturbing thoughts, cessation of menses or breast enlargement or engorgement in women, decreased libido, problems with fertility.

▷**ramipril**
(ra mi' pril)

Altace

PREGNANCY CATEGORY C
(FIRST TRIMESTER)

PREGNANCY CATEGORY D
(SECOND AND THIRD TRIMESTERS)

Drug classes
ACE inhibitor
Antihypertensive

Therapeutic actions
Ramipril blocks ACE from converting angiotensin I to angiotensin II, a powerful vasoconstrictor, leading to decreased BP, decreased aldosterone secretion, a small increase in serum potassium levels, and sodium and fluid loss;

increased prostaglandin synthesis also may be involved in the antihypertensive action.

Indications
- Treatment of hypertension alone or in combination with thiazide-type diuretics
- Treatment of HF in stable patients in the first few days after MI
- To decrease the risk of MI, stroke, death from CV disease in patients 55 yr and older who are at risk for developing CAD

Contraindications and cautions
- Contraindicated with allergy to ramipril, pregnancy (embryocidal in preclinical studies).
- Use cautiously with impaired renal function, HF, salt or volume depletion, lactation.

Available forms
Capsules—1.25, 2.5, 5, 10 mg; tablets—1.25, 2.5, 5, 10 mg

Dosages
Adults
- *Hypertension:* Initial dose, 2.5 mg PO daily. Adjust dosage according to BP response, usually 2.5–20 mg/day as a single dose or in two equally divided doses. If BP is not controlled, a diuretic may be added.
- *HF:* Initial dose, 2.5 mg PO bid; if patient becomes hypotensive, 1.25 mg PO bid may be used while adjusting up to target dose of 5 mg PO bid; increase dose every 3 wk until target dose is reached. Discontinue diuretic 2–3 days before beginning therapy; if not possible, administer initial dose of 1.25 mg.
- *Decrease risk of CV events:* Initial dose, 2.5 mg PO once daily for 1 wk, then 5 mg PO once daily for next 3 wk; for maintenance, 10 mg PO daily.

Pediatric patients
Safety and efficacy not established.
Geriatric patients
Greater sensitivity to drug effects is possible.
Patients with renal impairment
Excretion is reduced in renal failure. Use smaller initial dose: 25% of normally used dose is suggested; for hypertension, 1.25 mg PO daily in patients with creatinine clearance less than 40 mL/min; dosage may be titrated upward until pressure is controlled or a maximum of 5 mg/day.

R

Pharmacokinetics

Route	Onset	Peak	Duration
Oral	1–2 hr	1–4 hr	24 hr

Metabolism: Hepatic; $T_{1/2}$: 13–17 hr
Distribution: Crosses placenta; enters breast milk
Excretion: Feces, urine

Adverse effects

- **CV:** *Tachycardia,* angina pectoris, **HF,** MI, Raynaud syndrome, hypotension in salt- or volume-depleted patients, syncope
- **Dermatologic:** *Rash,* pemphigoid-like reaction, *pruritus,* photosensitivity, erythema multiforme, **Stevens-Johnson syndrome**
- **GI:** *Gastric irritation, aphthous ulcers, dysgeusia,* cholestatic jaundice, hepatocellular injury, anorexia, constipation, pancreatitis, nausea, vomiting
- **GU:** *Proteinuria,* renal insufficiency, renal failure, polyuria, oliguria, urinary frequency
- **Hematologic:** Neutropenia, **agranulocytosis,** thrombocytopenia, hemolytic anemia, **pancytopenia,** hyperkalemia
- **Other:** *Cough,* malaise, dry mouth, **angioedema**

Interactions

✳ **Drug-drug** • Exacerbation of cough if taken with capsaicin • Increased serum levels and increased toxicity with lithium; monitor patient closely

✳ **Drug-food** • Rate of absorption is reduced with food

✳ **Drug-lab test** • False-positive test for urine acetone

■ Nursing considerations

Assessment

- **History:** Allergy to ramipril, impaired renal function, HF, salt or volume depletion, pregnancy, lactation
- **Physical:** Skin color, lesions, turgor; T; P; BP, peripheral perfusion; mucous membranes, bowel sounds, liver evaluation; urinalysis, LFTs, renal function tests, CBC and differential

Interventions

⊗ **Black box warning** Do not use during pregnancy; risk of fetal harm. Advise use of a contraceptive.

- Discontinue diuretic for 2–3 days before beginning therapy, if possible, to avoid severe hypotensive effect.
- Open capsules and sprinkle contents over a small amount of applesauce or mix in applesauce or water if patient has difficulty swallowing capsules. Mixture is stable for 24 hr at room temperature and 48 hr if refrigerated.

⊗ *Warning* Alert surgeon and mark chart that ramipril is being used; the angiotensin II formation subsequent to compensatory renin release during surgery will be blocked; hypotension may be reversed with volume expansion.

- Monitor patient closely for falling BP secondary to reduction in fluid volume (excessive perspiration and dehydration, vomiting, diarrhea) because excessive hypotension may occur.
- Reduce dosage in patients with impaired renal function.

Teaching points

- Do not stop taking without consulting your health care provider.
- Be careful in any situation that may lead to a drop in blood pressure (diarrhea, sweating, vomiting, dehydration); if dizziness or light-headedness occurs, consult your health care provider.
- Avoid becoming pregnant while taking this drug; use of a contraceptive is advised.
- You may experience these side effects: GI upset, loss of appetite, change in taste perception (transient); mouth sores (frequent mouth care may help); rash; fast heart rate; dizziness, light-headedness (transient; change position slowly, and limit your activities to those that do not require alertness and precision).
- Report mouth sores; sore throat, fever, chills; swelling of the hands, feet; irregular heartbeat, chest pains; swelling of the face, eyes, lips, tongue; difficulty breathing.

▽ **ranibizumab**

See Appendix R, *Less commonly used drugs.*

Adverse effects in *italics* are most common; those in **bold** are life-threatening. ▭ Do not crush.

▽**ranitidine hydrochloride**
(ra *nye' te deen*)

Apo-Ranitidine (CAN), CO Ranitidine (CAN), Gen-Ranitidine (CAN), Novo-Ranidine, (CAN), Nu-Ranit (CAN), PMS-Ranitidine (CAN), ratio-Ranitidine (CAN), Zantac, Zantac EFFERdose, Zantac 75, Zantac 150

PREGNANCY CATEGORY B

Drug classes
Gastric acid secretion inhibitor
Histamine-2 (H$_2$) antagonist

Therapeutic actions
Competitively inhibits the action of histamine at the H$_2$ receptors of the parietal cells of the stomach, inhibiting basal gastric acid secretion and gastric acid secretion that is stimulated by food, insulin, histamine, cholinergic agonists, gastrin, and pentagastrin.

Indications
- Short-term treatment of active duodenal ulcer
- Maintenance therapy for duodenal ulcer at reduced dosage
- Short-term treatment and maintenance therapy of active, benign gastric ulcer
- Short-term treatment of GERD
- Pathologic hypersecretory conditions (eg, Zollinger-Ellison syndrome) (adults only)
- Treatment and maintenance of healing of erosive esophagitis
- Treatment of heartburn, acid indigestion, sour stomach

Contraindications and cautions
- Contraindicated with allergy to ranitidine, lactation.
- Use cautiously with impaired renal or hepatic function, pregnancy.

Available forms
Tablets—75, 150, 300 mg; capsules—150, 300 mg; effervescent tablets—25 mg; syrup—15 mg/mL; oral solution—15 mg/mL; injection—25 mg/mL

Dosages
Adults
- *Active duodenal ulcer:* 150 mg bid PO for 4–8 wk. Alternatively, 300 mg PO once daily at bedtime or 50 mg IM or IV every 6–8 hr *or* by intermittent IV infusion, diluted to 100 mL and infused over 15–20 min. Do not exceed 400 mg/day.
- *Maintenance therapy, duodenal ulcer:* 150 mg PO at bedtime.
- *Maintenance therapy, gastric ulcer:* 150 mg PO at bedtime.
- *Active erosive esophagitis or gastric ulcer:* 150 mg bid PO *or* 50 mg IM or IV every 6–8 hr.
- *Pathologic hypersecretory syndrome:* 150 mg bid PO. Individualize the dose with patient's response. Do not exceed 6 g/ day.
- *GERD maintenance, esophagitis, benign gastric ulcer:* 150 mg bid PO.
- *Treatment of heartburn, acid indigestion:* 75 mg PO as needed.

Pediatric patients 1 mo–16 yr
Injection: 2–4 mg/kg/day IV or IM every 6–8 hr to a maximum of 50 mg every 6–8 hr.
Oral: 2–4 mg/kg PO bid for treatment; once a day for maintenance. Maximum dosage, 300 mg/day for treatment, 150 mg/day for maintenance.

Geriatric patients or patients with impaired renal function
For creatinine clearance less than 50 mL/min, accumulation may occur; use lowest dose possible, 150 mg every 24 hr PO or 50 mg IM or IV every 18–24 hr. Dosing may be increased to every 12 hr if patient tolerates it and blood levels are monitored.

Pharmacokinetics

Route	Onset	Peak	Duration
Oral	Varies	1–3 hr	8–12 hr
IM	Rapid	15 min	8–12 hr
IV	Immediate	5–10 min	8–12 hr

Metabolism: Hepatic; T$_{1/2}$: 2–3 hr
Distribution: Crosses placenta; enters breast milk
Excretion: Urine

▼**IV FACTS**

Preparation: For IV injection, dilute 50 mg in 0.9% sodium chloride injection, 5% or 10% dextrose injection, lactated Ringer solution,

R

5% sodium bicarbonate injection to a volume of 20 mL; solution is stable for 48 hr at room temperature. For intermittent IV, use as follows: Dilute 50 mg in 100 mL of 5% dextrose injection or other compatible solution.

Infusion: Inject over 5 min or more; for intermittent infusion, infuse over 15–20 min; continuous infusion, 6.25 mg/hr.

Incompatibility: Do not mix with amphotericin B.

Adverse effects

- **CNS:** *Headache,* malaise, dizziness, somnolence, insomnia, vertigo
- **CV:** Tachycardia, bradycardia, PVCs (rapid IV administration)
- **Dermatologic:** *Rash,* alopecia
- **GI:** *Constipation, diarrhea, nausea, vomiting, abdominal pain,* hepatitis, increased ALT levels
- **GU:** Gynecomastia, impotence or decreased libido
- **Hematologic:** Leukopenia, granulocytopenia, thrombocytopenia, pancytopenia
- **Local:** *Pain at IM site, local burning or itching at IV site*
- **Other:** Arthralgias

Interactions

✳ **Drug-drug** • Increased effects of warfarin, TCAs; monitor patient closely and adjust dosage as needed

■ Nursing considerations

CLINICAL ALERT!
Name confusion has occurred between *Zantac* (ranitidine), *Zyrtec* (cetirizine), and *Xanax* (alprazolam); use caution.

Assessment

- **History:** Allergy to ranitidine, impaired renal or hepatic function, lactation, pregnancy
- **Physical:** Skin lesions; orientation, affect; pulse, baseline ECG; liver evaluation, abdominal examination, normal output; CBC, LFTs, renal function tests

Interventions

- Administer oral drug with meals and at bedtime.
- Decrease doses in renal and liver failure.
- Provide concurrent antacid therapy to relieve pain.

- Administer IM dose undiluted, deep into large muscle group.
- Arrange for regular follow-up, including blood tests, to evaluate effects.

Teaching points

- Take drug with meals and at bedtime. Therapy may continue for 4–6 weeks or longer.
- If you also are using an antacid, take it exactly as prescribed, being careful of the times of administration.
- Have regular medical follow-up care to evaluate your response.
- You may experience these side effects: Constipation or diarrhea (request aid from your health care provider); nausea, vomiting (take drug with meals); enlargement of breasts, impotence or decreased libido (reversible); headache (adjust lights and temperature and avoid noise).
- Report sore throat, fever, unusual bruising or bleeding, tarry stools, confusion, hallucinations, dizziness, severe headache, muscle or joint pain.

 ranolazine
*(ran **oh'** lah zeen)*

Ranexa ⓒⒶⓃ

PREGNANCY CATEGORY C

Drug classes

Antianginal
Piperazineacetamide

Therapeutic actions

Antianginal, anti-ischemic. Mechanism of action is not known. Prolongs the QT interval; does not decrease HR or BP; decreases myocardial workload.

Indications

- Treatment of chronic angina

Contraindications and cautions

- Contraindicated with hypersensitivity to any component of the drug; preexisting QT prolongation, concurrent use of QT-interval prolonging drugs; hepatic impairment; concurrent use of potent or moderately potent CYP3A inhibitors, including diltiazem; lactation.

• Use cautiously with severe renal impairment, history of ventricular tachycardia, pregnancy.

Available forms

ER tablets ⓒⓜⒸ—500, 1,000 mg

Dosages

Adults
500 mg PO bid; may be increased to maximum of 1,000 mg bid.

Pediatric patients
Safety and efficacy not established.

Patients with hepatic impairment
Not recommended with mild, moderate, or severe hepatic impairment.

Pharmacokinetics

Route	Onset	Peak
Oral	Rapid	2–5 hr

Metabolism: Hepatic; $T_{1/2}$: 7 hr
Distribution: May cross placenta; may pass into breast milk
Excretion: Urine, feces

Adverse effects

• **CNS:** *Dizziness, headache,* tinnitus, vertigo
• **CV:** Palpitations, peripheral edema, **prolonged QT interval**
• **GI:** *Nausea, constipation,* dry mouth, vomiting, abdominal pain
• **Respiratory:** Dyspnea

Interactions

✳ **Drug-drug** • Risk of increased serum level and toxicity of ranolazine if combined with ketoconazole, diltiazem, verapamil, rifampin, macrolide antibiotics, HIV protease inhibitors; dosage adjustment will be needed; do not exceed 500 mg bid for ranolazine • Risk of increased serum digoxin level if taken concurrently; digoxin dosage may need to be decreased • Monitor patients receiving TCAs; antipsychotics or other drugs known to prolong QT interval concurrently; may need lower doses of these drugs

✳ **Drug-food** • Risk of toxic effects if combined with grapefruit juice; avoid drinking grapefruit juice while on ranolazine

■ Nursing considerations

Assessment

• **History:** Allergy to any component of the tablet, preexisting QT-interval prolongation, concurrent use of QT-interval prolonging

drugs, hepatic impairment, concurrent use of potent or moderately potent CYP3A inhibitors, renal failure, pregnancy, lactation.

• **Physical:** Orientation, reflexes; BP; respiratory evaluation; baseline ECG, LFTs, and renal function tests

Interventions

• Obtain baseline ECG, LFTs, and renal function tests before starting therapy.
• Ensure that patient swallows tablets whole; do not cut, crush, or let patient chew the tablets.
• Ensure that patient continues to use other prescribed antianginal medications.
• Advise patient to avoid grapefruit juice and grapefruit products while using this drug.
• Suggest use of contraceptive measures while taking this drug; potential effects on a fetus are not known.
• Advise breast-feeding patients that another method of feeding the infant will be needed while taking this drug.
• Provide safety measures if dizziness and light-headedness occur.

Teaching points

• Take this drug twice a day. Swallow the tablet whole; do not cut, crush, or chew it.
• If you miss a dose of the daily medication, take it as soon as you remember and then return to your usual routine. Do not take more than two doses in one day.
• Do not take this drug for an acute anginal attack; this drug helps chronic chest pain. Continue to use your other angina drugs as prescribed.
• You may be asked to have periodic ECGs and blood tests to monitor the effects of this drug on your body.
• Do not consume grapefruit juice or grapefruit products while taking this drug.
• It is not known how this drug could affect a breast-feeding infant. If you are breast-feeding, you should select another method of feeding the infant.
• It is not known how this drug could affect a fetus. If you are pregnant or decide to become pregnant while on this drug, consult your health care provider.
• You may experience these side effects: Dizziness, light-headedness (if this occurs, avoid driving a car or operating dangerous machinery); headache, constipation (consult

R

your health care provider because medications may be available to help).
• Report palpitations, fainting spells, severe constipation.

▽rasagiline
(raz ab' gab leen)

Azilect

PREGNANCY CATEGORY C

Drug classes
Antiparkinsonian
MAO type B inhibitor

Therapeutic actions
Inhibits MAO type B (found mostly in the CNS), leading to increased levels of dopamine at the synapse particularly in areas of the brain responsible for controlling movement and coordination; much less effect in the periphery leads to fewer peripheral adverse effects.

Indications
• Treatment of signs and symptoms of idiopathic Parkinson disease as initial monotherapy and as adjunct therapy with levodopa

Contraindications and cautions
• Contraindicated with known hypersensitivity to any component of the drug; concurrent use of meperdine, tramadol, methadone, propoxyphene, dextromethorphan, sympathomimetic amines, MAOIs, SSRIs, TCAs; elective surgery; pheochromocytomas; diets rich in tyramine; severe hepatic insufficiency.
• Use cautiously with mild hepatic insufficiency, pregnancy, lactation, use of other CYP1A2 inhibitors.

Available forms
Tablets—0.5, 1 mg

Dosages
Adults
Initial monotherapy: 1 mg/day PO.
Adjunct therapy with levodopa: 0.5 mg/day PO; if response is insufficient, may increase to 1 mg/day PO. In some patients, levodopa dose may need to be decreased. Monitor patient response closely.

Patients with hepatic impairment
In mild hepatic impairment, 0.5 mg/day PO; not recommended in moderate to severe hepatic impairment.
Patients taking CYP1A2 inhibitors (such as ciprofloxacin)
0.5 mg/day PO.
Pediatric patients
Safety and efficacy not established.

Pharmacokinetics

Route	Onset	Peak
Oral	Rapid	1 hr

Metabolism: Hepatic; $T_{1/2}$: 3 hr
Distribution: May cross placenta; may pass into breast milk
Excretion: Urine

Adverse effects
• **CNS:** *Headache,* conjunctivitis, depression, paresthesia, vertigo
• **CV:** *Hypotension*
• **GI:** *Dyspepsia, dry mouth,* gastroenteritis
• **Respiratory:** Rhinitis
• **Other:** *Arthralgia,* flulike symptoms, fever, arthritis, malaise, neck pain, weight loss, bruising, **melanoma**

Interactions
✴ **Drug-drug** ⊗ *Warning* Risk of severe reaction if combined with meperidine or other analgesics including tramadol, methadone; avoid these combinations. • Risk of psychosis or bizarre behavior when combined with dextromethorphan, mirtazapine, cyclobenzaprine; avoid these combinations • Risk of hypertensive crisis if combined with sympathomimetic amines, MAOIs; avoid these combinations • Risk of hyperpyrexia when combined with some antidepressants (SSRIs, TCAs); monitor patient closely if these combinations are used • Risk of increased rasagiline levels in patients taking other CYP1A2 inhibitors, such as ciprofloxacin; reduce dose of rasagiline if this combination is used
✴ **Drug-alternative therapy** ⊗ *Warning* Risk of serious reaction if combined with St. John's Wort; avoid this combination.
✴ **Drug-food** ⊗ *Warning* Risk of hypertensive crisis with ingestion of tyramine-rich foods or beverages or dietary supplements containing amines.

Adverse effects in *italics* are most common; those in **bold** are life-threatening. ⚏ Do not crush.

■ Nursing considerations

Assessment

- **History:** Allergy to any component of the drug; concurrent use of meperidine, tramadol, methadone, dextromethorphan, symp-athomimetic amines, MAOIs, SSRIs, TCAs, other CYP1A2 inhibitors; elective surgery; pheochromocytomas; diets rich in tyramine; hepatic insufficiency; pregnancy; lactation
- **Physical:** T; skin evaluation, lesions; orientation, reflexes, grip strength, gait; BP; LFTs

Interventions

- Obtain LFTs and skin evaluation, preferably by a dermatologist, before and periodically during therapy.
- Ensure that patient has a list of tyramine-containing foods and understands the importance of avoiding them; hypertensive crisis could occur. However, studies indicate less of a risk than originally thought.
- Ensure that patient continues to use other medications for Parkinson disease as prescribed.
- Instruct patient and a significant other in the warning signs of a hypertensive crisis.
- Advise patient to avoid use of any other medications, including OTC products and herbal therapies, without consulting a health care provider.
- Provide safety measures if dizziness and light-headedness occur.

Teaching points

- Take this drug once a day as prescribed.
- If you miss a dose of the daily medication, take it as soon as you remember and then return to your usual routine. Do not take more than one dose in one day.
- Inspect your skin regularly for lesions, moles, and other changes. Melanoma occurs more often in patients with Parkinson disease. Consult a dermatologist for a baseline report and periodically during therapy.
- If you also take levodopa, you may experience a worsening of your tremor and a drop in blood pressure when you stand. Notify your health care provider if this occurs; a dosage adjustment may be possible.
- You will need to avoid large amounts of food rich in tyramine while taking this drug and for 2 weeks after finishing it. Tyramine-containing foods and beverages include aged or smoked meats or fish, aged cheeses, con-

centrated yeast extract, and beers and wines that have not been pasteurized.
- It is not known how this drug could affect a fetus. If you are pregnant or decide to become pregnant while on this drug, consult your health care provider.
- It is not known how this drug could affect a breast-feeding infant. If you are breast-feeding, consult your health care provider.
- This drug interacts with many other drugs and could cause serious side effects; do not take any other drug, including over-the-counter drugs and herbal therapies, until you have checked with your health care provider.
- You may experience these side effects: Vertigo, light-headedness (avoid driving a car or operating dangerous machinery); headache (consult your health care provider; medications may be available to help); dry mouth, upset stomach (frequent mouth care, sugar-free candies may help).
- Report severe headache, dizziness, blurred vision, difficulty thinking, changes in your skin, chest pain, worsening of your condition.

▽rasburicase

See Appendix R, *Less commonly used drugs*.

▽raxibacumab

See Appendix R, *Less commonly used drugs*.

▽regorafenib

See Appendix R, *Less commonly used drugs*.

DANGEROUS DRUG

▽repaglinide
(re pag' lah nyde)

GlucoNorm (CAN), Prandin

PREGNANCY CATEGORY C

Drug classes
Antidiabetic
Meglitinide

Therapeutic actions
Closes potassium channels in the beta cells of the pancreas, which causes the opening of calcium channels and a resultant increase in

insulin release; highly selective for beta cells in the pancreas. Glucose-lowering abilities depend on the existence of functioning beta cells in the pancreas.

Indications
- Adjunct to diet and exercise to lower blood glucose in patients with type 2 diabetes mellitus whose hyperglycemia cannot be managed by diet and exercise alone
- Combination therapy with metformin or thiazolidinediones to lower blood glucose in patients whose hyperglycemia cannot be controlled by diet and exercise plus monotherapy with any of the following agents alone: Metformin, sulfonylureas, or thiazolidinediones

Contraindications and cautions
- Contraindicated with hypersensitivity to the drug, diabetic ketoacidosis, type 1 diabetes, lactation.
- Use cautiously with renal or hepatic impairment, pregnancy.

Available forms
Tablets—0.5, 1, 2 mg

Dosages
Adults
0.5–4 mg PO taken tid or qid 15–30 min (usually within 15 min) before meals; determine dosage based on patient response; maximum dose is 16 mg/day. Monitor patient regularly and adjust dosage as needed, waiting 1 wk between dose adjustments to assess patient response.
Pediatric patients
Safety and efficacy not established.
Patients with renal or hepatic impairment
For severe renal impairment, use starting dose of 0.5 mg PO and titrate carefully. Use cautiously with hepatic impairment; monitor closely.

Pharmacokinetics

Route	Onset	Peak
Oral	Rapid	1 hr

Metabolism: Hepatic; $T_{1/2}$: 1 hr
Distribution: May cross placenta; may enter breast milk
Excretion: Feces, urine

Adverse effects
- **CNS:** *Headache*, paresthesias

- **Endocrine:** *Hypoglycemia*
- **GI:** *Nausea, diarrhea,* constipation, vomiting, dyspepsia
- **Respiratory:** *URI*, sinusitis, rhinitis, bronchitis

Interactions
✴ **Drug-drug** ⊗ *Warning* Risk of severe hypoglycemia if combined with both gemfibrozil and itraconazole; avoid this combination.
- Risk of hypoglycemia if combined with gemfibrozil; use caution; monitor patient closely
✴ **Drug-alternative therapy** • Increased risk of hypoglycemia if taken with juniper berries, ginseng, garlic, fenugreek, coriander, dandelion root, celery

■ Nursing considerations
Assessment
- **History:** Hypersensitivity to the drug, diabetic ketoacidosis, type 1 diabetes, renal or hepatic impairment, pregnancy, lactation
- **Physical:** Skin color, lesions; T; orientation, reflexes, peripheral sensation; R, adventitious sounds; liver evaluation, bowel sounds; blood glucose, LFTs, renal function tests

Interventions
- Administer drug before meals; if a patient skips or adds a meal, the dosage should be skipped or added appropriately.
- Monitor urine or serum glucose levels frequently to determine effectiveness of drug and dosage being used.
- Arrange for consult with dietitian to establish weight loss program and dietary control as appropriate.
- Arrange for thorough diabetic teaching program to include disease, dietary control, exercise, signs and symptoms of hypoglycemia and hyperglycemia, avoidance of infection, hygiene.

Teaching points
- Do not discontinue this medication without consulting your health care provider.
- Take this drug before meals (three to four times a day); if you skip a meal, skip the dose; if you add a meal, take a dose before that meal also.
- Monitor blood for glucose as prescribed.
- Return for regular follow-up and monitoring of your response to the drug and possible need for dosage adjustment.
- Continue diet and exercise program established for control of diabetes.

- Know the signs and symptoms of hypoglycemia and hyperglycemia and appropriate treatment as indicated; report the occurrence of either to your health care provider.
- You may experience these side effects: Headache, increased upper respiratory infections, nausea.
- Report fever, sore throat, unusual bleeding or bruising, severe abdominal pain.

▽ **ribavirin**

(rye ba vye' rin)

Copegus, Rebetol, Ribasphere, Virazole

PREGNANCY CATEGORY X

Drug class

Antiviral

Therapeutic actions

Antiviral activity against RSV, influenza virus, hepatitis C virus, and HSV; mechanism of action is not known.

Indications

- Treatment of carefully selected hospitalized infants and children with severe RSV infection of lower respiratory tract (aerosol only)
- Treatment of chronic hepatitis C in combination with peginterferon alfa-2a (*Pegasys*) or interferon alfa-2b (*Intron A*) in patients 3 yr or older with compensated liver disease untreated with or refractory to alfa interferon therapy
- With *Pegasys*, treatment of adults with hepatitis C who have compensated liver disease and no previous alfa interferon therapy
- Orphan drug use: Treatment of hemorrhagic fever with renal syndrome
- Unlabeled uses for aerosol: Treatment of some influenza types A and B infections, herpes simplex virus
- Unlabeled use for oral preparation: Treatment of some viral diseases, including Crimean-Congo hemorrhagic fever

Contraindications and cautions

- Contraindicated with allergy to drug product, COPD, pregnancy or male whose female partner is pregnant (causes fetal damage), lactation, thalassemia, sickle-cell anemia, severe renal impairment.

- Use cautiously with renal impairment, respiratory dysfunction.

Available forms

Capsules—200 mg; oral solution—40 mg/mL; powder for aerosol reconstitution—6 g/100 mL vial; tablets—200, 400, 600 mg

Dosages

Adults

- *Chronic hepatitis C, Genotype 1, 4:*
  75 kg or less: Two 200-mg capsules PO in the AM, three 200-mg capsules PO in the PM with *Intron A,* 3 million international units subcutaneously three times per wk; or with 180 mcg *Pegasys* subcutaneously per wk for 24–48 wk.
  More than 75 kg: Three 200-mg capsules PO in AM, three 200-mg capsules PO in PM with 3 million international units *Intron A,* subcutaneously three times per wk; or with 180 mcg *Pegasys* subcutaneously per wk for 24–48 wk.
- *Chronic hepatitis C, Genotype 2, 3:* Two 200-mg tablets PO in AM, two 200-mg tablets PO in PM with 180 mcg peg-interferon subcutaneously once per wk for 24 wk.

Pediatric patients

Aerosol

For use only with small-particle aerosol generator. Check operating instructions carefully. Dilute aerosol powder to 20 mg/mL and deliver for 12–18 hr/day for at least 3 but not more than 7 days.

Oral

15 mg/kg/day PO in divided doses AM and PM. Children 25–62 kg who cannot swallow tablets may use oral solution. Give with interferon alfa-2b (*Intron A*), 3 million international units/m², subcutaneously three times per wk.

Patients with anemia as manifested by decrease in Hgb

No cardiac disease, Hgb less than 10 g/dL: Decrease to 600 mg PO daily (one 200-mg capsule in AM; two 200-mg capsules in PM); 12 mg/kg/day PO for children; reduce to 8 mg/kg/day PO if needed.

No cardiac disease, Hgb less than 8.5 g/dL: Discontinue ribavirin.

Cardiac disease, Hgb decreased by 2 g/dL or more during any 4-wk period of treatment: Decrease to 600 mg PO daily (one 200-mg capsule in AM; two 200-mg capsules in PM);

R

12 mg/kg/day PO for children, reduce to 8 mg/kg/day PO if needed.
Cardiac history, Hgb less than 12 g/dL after 4 wk of decreased dose: Discontinue ribavirin.
Patients with hepatitis C and HIV coinfection: 800 mg/day PO ribavirin with 180 mcg *Pegasys* by subcutaneous injection once each wk for 48 wk.
Patients with renal impairment: Do not use if creatinine clearance is less than 50 mL/min.

Pharmacokinetics

Route	Onset	Peak
Aerosol	Slow	60–90 min

Metabolism: Cellular; $T_{1/2}$: 9.5 hr (aerosol), 298 hr (oral)
Distribution: Crosses placenta; enters breast milk
Excretion: Feces, urine

Adverse effects

- **CNS:** Depression, suicidal behavior, nervousness
- **CV: Cardiac arrest,** hypotension
- **Dermatologic:** Rash
- **Hematologic:** Anemia
- **Respiratory:** *Deteriorating respiratory function,* pneumothorax, apnea, bacterial pneumonia
- **Other:** Conjunctivitis, testicular lesions

Interactions

❋ **Drug-drug** ● Decreased levels of ribavirin when given with antacids; avoid with nucleoside reverse transcriptase inhibitors

■ Nursing considerations
Assessment

- **History:** Allergy to drug product, COPD, pregnancy, lactation, renal impairment
- **Physical:** Skin rashes, lesions; P, BP, auscultation; R, adventitious sounds; Hct

Interventions

- Ensure proper use of small-particle aerosol generator; check operating instructions carefully.
- Ensure that water used as diluent contains no other substance.
- Replace solution in the unit every 24 hr.
- Store reconstituted solution at room temperature for up to 24 hr.

- For patients on mechanical ventilators, clean and check tubing to prevent accumulation of drug and malfunction of the machine.
- ⊗ **Black box warning** Inhaled form of drug is not for use in adults; testicular lesions, birth defects can occur.
- ⊗ **Black box warning** Ribavirin monotherapy is not effective for the treatment of chronic hepatitis C and should not be used alone for this indication.
- ⊗ **Black box warning** Use of this drug makes patients at high risk for hemolytic anemia, which could lead to MI; do not use in patients with significant or unstable CV disease.
- ⊗ **Black box warning** Monitor respiratory status frequently; pulmonary deterioration and death have occurred during and shortly after treatment with inhalation product.
- ⊗ **Black box warning** Risk of significant fetal defects exists. Caution women to avoid pregnancy while using this drug; use of barrier contraceptives is advised; male partners of pregnant women should not take this drug.
- ⊗ *Warning* Use extreme caution in adults with history of depression or psychiatric disorders.
- Monitor BP and P frequently.

Teaching points

- Explain the use of small-particle aerosol generator to patient or family.
- Take capsules or tablets in morning and evening; mark calendar with days to inject *Intron A* or *Pegasys* as appropriate.
- Avoid pregnancy while taking this drug; using barrier contraceptives is advised; male partners of pregnant women should avoid intercourse.
- Report depression, suicidal ideation, difficulty breathing, muscle pain, dizziness, confusion, shortness of breath (pediatric patients).

▽ **rifabutin**

See Appendix R, *Less commonly used drugs.*

▽ **rifampin**
(rif' am pin)

Rifadin, Rofact (CAN)

PREGNANCY CATEGORY C

Drug classes
Antibiotic
Antituberculotic (first-line)

Adverse effects in *italics* are most common; those in **bold** are life-threatening. ⬛ Do not crush.

Therapeutic actions

Inhibits DNA-dependent RNA polymerase activity in susceptible bacterial cells.

Indications

- Treatment of pulmonary TB in conjunction with at least one other effective antituberculotic
- *Neisseria meningitidis* carriers, for asymptomatic carriers to eliminate meningococci from nasopharynx; not for treatment of meningitis
- Unlabeled uses: Infections caused by *Staphylococcus aureus* and *Staphylococcus epidermidis,* usually in combination therapy; gram-negative bacteremia in infancy; *Legionella pneumophila* infections not responsive to erythromycin; leprosy (in combination with dapsone); prophylaxis of meningitis caused by *Haemophilus influenzae,* catheter-related bloodstream infections (adults); cholestatic pruritus (adults)

Contraindications and cautions

- Contraindicated with allergy to any rifamycin, acute hepatic disease, lactation.
- Use cautiously with pregnancy (teratogenic effects have been reported in preclinical studies; safest antituberculous regimen for use in pregnancy is considered to be rifampin, isoniazid, and ethambutol).

Available forms

Capsules—150, 300 mg; powder for injection—600 mg

Dosages

Adults

- *Pulmonary TB:* 10 mg/kg/day; not to exceed 600 mg in a single daily dose PO or IV (used in conjunction with other antituberculotics). Continue therapy until bacterial conversion and maximal improvement occur.
- *Meningococcal carriers:* 600 mg PO or IV once daily for 4 consecutive days or 600 mg every 12 hr for 2 days.

Pediatric patients

- *Pulmonary TB:*
  10–20 mg/kg/day PO or IV not to exceed 600 mg/day.
- *Meningococcal carriers:*
  Younger than 1 mo: 5 mg/kg PO or IV every 12 hr for 2 days.

Older than 1 mo: 10 mg/kg PO or IV every 12 hr for 2 days, do not exceed 600 mg/dose.

Patients with renal impairment

For creatinine clearance less than 50 mL/min or for patients on dialysis, give 50% to 100% of usual dose.

Pharmacokinetics

Route	Onset	Peak
Oral	Varies	1–4 hr
IV	Rapid	End of infusion

Metabolism: Hepatic; $T_{1/2}$: 3–5.1 hr
Distribution: Crosses placenta; enters breast milk
Excretion: Bile, urine

▼ IV FACTS

Preparation: Reconstitute by transferring 10 mL sterile water for injection to vial containing 600 mg rifampin; swirl gently. Resultant fluid contains 60 mg/mL; stable at room temperature for 24 hr. Further mix with 100–500 mL of dextrose 5% or sterile saline.
Infusion: Infuse over 30–180 min, depending on volume.
Y-site: Do not administer with diltiazem.

Adverse effects

- **CNS:** *Headache, drowsiness, fatigue, dizziness,* inability to concentrate, mental confusion, generalized numbness, ataxia, muscle weakness, visual disturbances, exudative conjunctivitis
- **Dermatologic:** *Rash,* pruritus, urticaria, pemphigoid reaction, flushing, *reddish-orange discoloration of body fluids—tears, saliva, urine, sweat, sputum*
- **GI:** *Heartburn, epigastric distress,* anorexia, nausea, vomiting, gas, cramps, diarrhea, pseudomembranous colitis, pancreatitis, *elevations of liver enzymes,* hepatitis
- **GU:** Hemoglobinuria, hematuria, renal insufficiency, **acute renal failure,** menstrual disturbances
- **Hematologic:** *Eosinophilia, thrombocytopenia, transient leukopenia,* hemolytic anemia, decreased Hgb, hemolysis
- **Other:** Pain in extremities, osteomalacia, myopathy, fever, *flulike symptoms*

R

Interactions

❋ **Drug-drug** • Increased incidence of rifampin-related hepatitis with isoniazid
• Decreased concentrations of itraconazole
• Decreased effectiveness of metoprolol, propranolol, antiarrhythmics, benzodiazepine, buspirone, cyclosporine, digoxin, doxycycline, fluoroquinolones, nifedipine, zolpidem, quinidine, corticosteroids, hormonal contraceptives, methadone, oral anticoagulants, oral sulfonylureas, theophyllines, phenytoin, cyclosporine, ketoconazole, verapamil

❋ **Drug-lab test** • Rifampin inhibits standard assays for serum folate and vitamin B_{12}

■ Nursing considerations

Assessment

• **History:** Allergy to any rifamycin, acute hepatic disease, pregnancy, lactation
• **Physical:** Skin color, lesions; T; gait, muscle strength; orientation, reflexes, ophthalmologic examination; liver evaluation; CBC, LFTs, renal function tests, urinalysis

Interventions

• Administer on an empty stomach, 1 hr before or 2 hr after meals.
• Administer in a single daily dose.
• Consult pharmacist for rifampin suspension for patients unable to swallow capsules.
• Prepare patient for the reddish-orange coloring of body fluids (urine, sweat, sputum, tears, feces, saliva); soft contact lenses may be permanently stained; advise patients not to wear them during therapy.
⊗ **Warning** Arrange for follow-up visits for liver and renal function tests, CBC, and ophthalmologic examinations.

Teaching points

• Take drug as directed. Take on an empty stomach, 1 hour before or 2 hours after meals.
• Take this drug regularly; avoid missing any doses; do not discontinue this drug without consulting your health care provider.
• Have periodic medical checkups, including eye examinations and blood tests, to evaluate the drug effects.
• You may experience these side effects: Reddish-orange coloring of body fluids (tears, sweat, saliva, urine, feces, sputum; stain will wash out of clothing, but soft contact lenses may be permanently stained; do not wear

them); nausea, vomiting, epigastric distress; skin rashes or lesions; numbness, tingling, drowsiness, fatigue (use caution if driving or operating dangerous machinery; use precautions to avoid injury).
• Report fever, chills, muscle and bone pain, excessive tiredness or weakness, loss of appetite, nausea, vomiting, yellowing of skin or eyes, unusual bleeding or bruising, skin rash or itching.

▽ **rifapentine**
*(rif ab **pin'** ten)*

Priftin

PREGNANCY CATEGORY C

Drug classes

Antibiotic
Antituberculotic

Therapeutic actions

Inhibits DNA-dependent RNA polymerase activity in susceptible strains of *Mycobacterium tuberculosis,* causing cell death.

Indications

• Treatment of pulmonary TB in conjunction with at least one other effective antituberculotic
• Orphan drug use: Prophylaxis and treatment of *Mycobacterium avium* complex in patients with AIDS

Contraindications and cautions

• Contraindicated with allergy to any rifamycin, acute hepatic disease.
• Use cautiously with pregnancy (teratogenic effects have been reported in preclinical studies), lactation, hepatic impairment.

Available forms

Tablets—150 mg

Dosages

Adults

• *TB, intensive phase:* 600 mg PO twice weekly with an interval of at least 72 hr between doses; continue for 2 mo. Always give rifapentine in combination with other antituberculotics.

Adverse effects in *italics* are most common; those in **bold** are life-threatening. ⊞ Do not crush.

• *Continuation phase:* 600 mg PO once a wk for 4 mo in combination with other agents to which the organism is susceptible.

Pediatric patients
Safety and efficacy not established in patients younger than 12 yr.

Geriatric patients
Start at low end of dosing range; monitor patient closely.

Pharmacokinetics

Route	Onset	Peak
Oral	Slow	5–6 hr

Metabolism: Hepatic; $T_{1/2}$: 13–19 hr
Distribution: May cross placenta; may enter breast milk
Excretion: Feces, urine

Adverse effects

• **CNS:** *Headache, dizziness*
• **Dermatologic:** Pruritus, acne
• **GI:** Nausea, vomiting, diarrhea, cramps
• **GU:** *Pyuria, proteinuria, hematuria*
• **Hematologic:** *Hyperuricemia,* liver enzyme elevations
• **Other:** Pain, arthralgia, *reddish discoloration of body fluids*

Interactions

✳ **Drug-drug** • Decreased effectiveness of protease inhibitors; use extreme caution if this combination is needed; try to avoid this combination • Decreased effectiveness of rifampin if taken with p-aminosalicylic acid, ketoconazole—give the drugs at least 8–12 hr apart • Decreased effectiveness of metoprolol, propranolol, quinidine, corticosteroids, hormonal contraceptives, methadone, oral anticoagulants, oral sulfonylureas, theophyllines, phenytoin, cyclosporine, ketoconazole, verapamil if taken concurrently with rifapentine; monitor patient carefully and adjust dosage as needed

✳ **Drug-lab test** • Rifapentine inhibits standard assays for serum folate and vitamin B_{12}

■ Nursing considerations

Assessment

• **History:** Allergy to any rifamycin, acute hepatic disease, pregnancy, lactation
• **Physical:** Skin color, lesions; T; gait, muscle strength; orientation, reflexes, CBC, LFTs, renal function tests, urinalysis

Interventions

• Administer on an empty stomach, 1 hr before 2 hr after meals; if GI upset is severe, drug may be taken with food.
• Always use in combination with other antituberculotics.
• Prepare patient for the reddish-orange coloring of body fluids (urine, sweat, sputum, tears, feces, saliva); soft contact lenses may be permanently stained, patients should be advised not to wear them during drug therapy.
• Recommend the use of barrier contraceptives while using this drug; hormonal contraceptives may be ineffective.
• Provide small, frequent meals if GI upset occurs.
• Provide skin care if dermatologic effects occur.

Teaching points

• Take drug along with any other prescribed antituberculotics. Take on an empty stomach—1 hour before or 2 hours after meals. If your stomach is very upset by the drug, it may be taken with food.
• Take this drug regularly; avoid missing any doses; do not discontinue this drug without consulting your health care provider. Make sure doses are at least 72 hours apart.
• Avoid pregnancy while taking this drug, using barrier contraceptives is advised.
• Arrange to have periodic medical checkups, which will include blood tests to evaluate the drug effects.
• You may experience these side effects: Reddish-orange coloring of body fluids (tears, sweat, saliva, urine, feces, sputum; this is an expected occurrence and is not dangerous, do not be alarmed—stain will wash out of clothing but soft contact lenses may be permanently stained, do not wear them when on this drug); nausea, vomiting, epigastric distress (consult your health care provider if any of these become too uncomfortable); skin rashes or lesions (consult your health care provider for appropriate skin care).
• Report fever, chills, muscle and bone pain, excessive tiredness or weakness, loss of appetite, yellowing of skin or eyes, unusual bleeding or bruising, skin rash or itching.

R

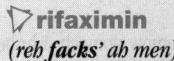

▽ **rifaximin**
(reh facks' ah men)

Xifaxan ⓞⓝⓒ

PREGNANCY CATEGORY C

Drug classes
Antibiotic
Antidiarrheal

Therapeutic actions
A structural analogue of rifampin; binds to bacterial DNA-dependent RNA polymerase and inhibits bacterial RNA synthesis. Ninety-seven percent passes through the GI tract unchanged; affects *Escherichia coli* in the GI tract; cause of most traveler's diarrhea.

Indications
- Treatment of patients 12 yr or older with traveler's diarrhea caused by noninvasive strains of *E. coli*
- Reduction of recurrence of hepatic encephalopathy in patients with advanced liver disease
- Unlabeled uses: IBS, *Clostridium difficile*–associated diarrhea

Contraindications and cautions
- Contraindicated with allergy to rifaximin, rifampin, or any component of the drug; diarrhea complicated by fever or blood in the stool or caused by pathogens other than *E. coli*; lactation.
- Use cautiously with pregnancy.

Available forms
Tablets ⓞⓝⓒ—200, 550 mg

Dosages
Adults and patients 12 yr and older
- *Traveler's diarrhea:* 200 mg PO tid for 3 days.
Adults
- *Hepatic encephalopathy:* 550 mg PO bid.
Pediatric patients younger than 12 yr
Safety and efficacy not established.

Pharmacokinetics

Route	
Oral	Not absorbed systemically

Metabolism: None; T$_{1/2}$: 5.4–6.2 hr
Distribution: May cross placenta; may enter breast milk
Excretion: Feces

Adverse effects
- **CNS:** Headache, dizziness, fatigue, insomnia
- **GI:** Diarrhea, flatulence, nausea, ascites, abdominal pain, rectal tenesmus, defecation urgency, constipation, vomiting, **pseudomembranous colitis**
- **Respiratory:** Rhinitis, cough, dyspnea, pharyngitis, bronchitis
- **Skin:** Allergic dermatitis, rash, urticaria, pruritus
- **Other:** *Fever,* angioneurotic edema, peripheral edema

■ Nursing considerations
Assessment
- **History:** Allergy to rifaximin, rifampin or any component of the drug, diarrhea complicated by fever or blood in the stool or caused by pathogens other than *E. coli;* lactation, pregnancy
- **Physical:** Skin lesions; orientation, reflexes; abdominal examination

Interventions
- Administer three times a day for traveler's diarrhea and twice a day for hepatic encephalopathy prophylaxis, with or without food; ensure that the tablet is swallowed whole.
- ⊗ *Warning* Do not administer if the patient has diarrhea complicated by fever or blood in the stool.
- Administer only to patients with traveler's diarrhea caused by *E. coli;* this drug is not effective for systemic bacterial infections because it is not absorbed.
- Encourage the use of barrier contraceptives during treatment with this drug; it is not known if this drug crosses the placenta.
- Find another method of feeding the infant if patient is breast-feeding; it is not known if this enters breast milk.
- Discontinue drug if diarrhea persists for longer than 24–48 hr or worsens.
- Maintain other measures appropriate for traveler's diarrhea—avoidance of local water, pushing fluids to maintain hydration.
- Maintain other measures for treatment of advanced liver disease.

Teaching points

- Take this drug three times a day, with or without food, for the treatment of traveler's diarrhea or two times a day for advanced liver disease.
- Swallow the tablet whole; do not cut, crush, or chew the tablets.
- If you forget a dose, take it as soon as you remember and return to your usual regimen. Do not make up doses and do not take more than three doses in 24 hours.
- Do not use this drug to treat any infection other than traveler's diarrhea or your liver disease; it is not absorbed into the bloodstream and is not effective in treating other infections.
- Stop taking the drug and notify your health care provider if a fever develops or blood in the diarrhea occurs, or if the diarrhea persists or worsens after 24–48 hours.
- Avoid pregnancy while taking this drug; if you suspect that you are pregnant, consult your health care provider.
- You should find another method of feeding the infant if you are breast-feeding; it is not known if this drug enters breast milk.
- You may experience these side effects: Dizziness (if this occurs, do not drive a car or operate heavy machine until you know how you will be affected), flatulence, abdominal pain, nausea (try to maintain your hydration drinking bottled water or beverages).
- Report bloody diarrhea, fever, worsening diarrhea.

▽ **rilonacept**

See Appendix R, *Less commonly used drugs.*

▽ **rilpivirine**
(rill pah vye' rin)

Edurant

PREGNANCY CATEGORY B

Drug classes

Antiviral
Nonnucleoside reverse transcriptase inhibitor

Therapeutic actions

Binds directly to reverse transcriptase and blocks both RNA- and DNA-dependent polymerase activity, leading to inability for viral replication, a decrease in viral load, and subsequent increase; increases number of healthy CD4 cells, does not inhibit DNA polymerase.

Indications

- Treatment of HIV infection in treatment-naïve adults, in combination with at least two other antiretrovirals

Contraindications and cautions

- Contraindicated with history of serious hypersensitivity reactions to rilpivirine, concurrent use of CYP3A4/5 inducers or inhibitors, use of other nonnucleoside reverse transcriptase inhibitors, lactation.
- Use cautiously with prolonged QT interval, depressive disorders, pregnancy.

Available forms

Tablets-25 mg

Dosages
Adults

25 mg/day PO with food. If also taking didanosine, didanosine should be taken at least 2 hr before or 4 hr after rilpivirine.
Pediatric patients

Safety and efficacy not established.

Pharmacokinetics

Route	Onset	Peak
Oral	Moderate	4-5 hr

Metabolism: Hepatic; $T_{1/2}$: 50 hr
Distribution: May cross placenta; may enter breast milk
Excretion: Feces

Adverse effects

- **CNS:** *Depression, insomnia, abnormal dreams, headache,* **suicidality**
- **GI:** Nausea, vomiting, elevated liver enzymes
- **Other:** *Fatigue, fat redistribution, rash,* increased cholesterol levels

Interactions

✳ **Drug-drug** • Decreased serum concentration and therapeutic effects if combined with antacids or drugs that alter stomach

R

acidity; give antacids, H₂ receptor blockers, proton pump inhibitors at least 2 hr before or 4 hr after rilpivirine • Risk of increased toxicity if combined with clarithromycin, troleandomycin, erythromycin, atazanavir, fosamprenavir, indinavir, nelfinavir, tipranavir, saquinavir, other nonnucleoside reverse transcriptase inhibitors; monitor patient closely • Possible loss of effectiveness with carbamazepine, oxcarbazepine, phenobarbital, phenytoin, rifabutin, rifampin, rifapentine, dexamethasone; avoid these combinations • Possible increased risk of prolonged QT interval if taken with drugs that prolong QT interval; monitor patient accordingly

＊Drug-alternative therapy • Loss of effectiveness if taken with St. John's Wort; avoid this combination

■ Nursing considerations

Assessment
- **History:** Hypersensitivity to components of drug, pregnancy, lactation, all other drugs being taken, depressive disorders
- **Physical:** Neurologic exam; orientation; skin evaluation; T; CD4 level, viral load

Interventions
- Review all drugs being taken to assess for possible interactions before beginning therapy.
- Ensure that patient is treatment-naïve.
- Ensure that patient is also taking other drugs for HIV treatment.
- Have patient take drug once a day with food. If patient is also taking drugs that lower stomach acidity, those drugs should be taken at least 2 hr before or 4 hr after rilpivirine.
- Do not stop drug suddenly; increased risk of increased viral load may occur if drug is stopped.
- Encourage breast-feeding mothers to find another method of feeding the baby.
- Evaluate patient immediately and arrange for appropriate intervention if severe depression, thoughts of suicide occur.

Teaching points
- Take this drug once a day with a meal; if you are taking drugs to decrease the acid in your stomach, they should be taken at least 2 hours before of 4 hours after this drug.
- If you miss a dose and it is within 12 hours before the next dose is due, take that dose

with a meal and take your next dose at the regularly scheduled time. If it is more than 12 hours, skip that dose and take the usual dose at the usual time.
- Tell your health care provider about all drugs, over-the-counter products, and herbs you might be using; this drug interacts with many other drugs and dosage adjustment may be needed. Do not use St. John's Wort while taking this drug.
- Do not run out of this drug; if you are running low, it is important to get more tablets. Suddenly stopping this drug can result in an increased viral load.
- This drug does not cure HIV or AIDS. Be alert for opportunistic infections; use appropriate precautions to prevent transmitting the disease to others.
- It is not known how this drug could affect a developing fetus; if you become pregnant or wish to become pregnant, discuss this with your health care provider.
- It is not known if this drug appears in breast milk; if you are breast-feeding, you should use a different method of feeding the baby.
- You may experience these side effects: GI upset, nausea (small, frequent meals may help); headache (consult your health care provider for an appropriate pain medication); redistribution of body fat to the core; depression, thoughts of suicide (contact your health care provider immediately if you notice changes in mood or behavior).
- Report fever, signs of infection, thoughts of suicide, changes in your prescribed drugs or other drugs you are taking.

▽ **riluzole**

See Appendix R, *Less commonly used drugs*.

▽ **rimantadine hydrochloride**
(*ri **man'** ta deen*)

Flumadine

PREGNANCY CATEGORY C

Drug class
Antiviral

Therapeutic actions

Synthetic antiviral agent that inhibits viral replication, possibly by preventing the uncoating of the virus.

Indications

- Prophylaxis and treatment of illness caused by influenza A virus in adults
- Prophylaxis against influenza A virus in children
- Unlabeled uses: Treatment and prophylaxis of H1N1 (swine flu) infection, treatment of influenza A in children

Contraindications and cautions

- Contraindicated with allergy to amantadine, rimantadine; lactation.
- Use cautiously with seizures, liver or renal disease, pregnancy.

Available forms

Tablets—100 mg

Dosages

Adults and patients older than 10 yr
- *Prophylaxis:* 100 mg/day PO bid.
- *Treatment:* Same dose as above; start treatment as soon after exposure as possible, continuing for 7 days from initial onset of symptoms.

Pediatric patients 1–9 yr
- *Prophylaxis:* 5 mg/kg PO once daily. Maximum dose, 150 mg.

Geriatric patients in nursing homes and patients with severe renal or hepatic impairment
Dose of 100 mg PO daily is recommended.

Pharmacokinetics

Route	Onset	Peak
Oral	Slow	6 hr

Metabolism: $T_{1/2}$: 25.4–32 hr
Distribution: May cross placenta; may enter breast milk
Excretion: Urine

Adverse effects

- **CNS:** *Light-headedness, dizziness, insomnia,* confusion, irritability, ataxia, psychosis, depression, hallucinations, seizures
- **CV: HF,** orthostatic hypotension, dyspnea
- **GI:** *Nausea,* anorexia, constipation, dry mouth

Interactions

✳ **Drug-drug** • Decreased effectiveness with acetaminophen, aspirin • Increased serum levels and effects with cimetidine • Intranasal influenza virus vaccine may interfere with rimantadine; do not vaccinate for 48 hr after rimantadine therapy is complete; do not administer rimantadine for 2 wk after intranasal influenza vaccine administration.

■ Nursing considerations

Assessment
- **History:** Allergy to amantadine, rimantadine; seizures; liver or renal disease, pregnancy, lactation
- **Physical:** Orientation, vision, speech, reflexes; BP, orthostatic BP, P, auscultation, perfusion, edema; R, adventitious sounds; urinary output; BUN, creatinine clearance

Interventions
- Administer full course of drug to achieve the beneficial antiviral effects. Initiate therapy for treatment within 48 hr of onset of symptoms and continue for 7 days.

Teaching points
- You may experience these side effects: Drowsiness, blurred vision (use caution in driving or using dangerous equipment); dizziness, light-headedness (avoid sudden position changes); irritability or mood changes (common; if severe, request a drug change).
- Report swelling of the fingers or ankles, shortness of breath, difficulty urinating, tremors, slurred speech, difficulty walking.

▽**risedronate sodium**
*(rah **sed'** dro nate)*

Actonel, Atelvia ⒸⒶⓃ

PREGNANCY CATEGORY C

Drug class

Bisphosphonate

Therapeutic actions

Affects osteoclast activity by reducing the enzymatic and transport processes that lead to resorption of the bone and by inhibiting the osteoclast proton pump, leading to a rate of

R

bone turnover near normal in patients with Paget disease.

Indications

- Treatment of Paget disease of bone
- Treatment and prevention of osteoporosis in postmenopausal women
- Treatment and prevention of glucocorticoid-induced osteoporosis
- To increase bone mass in men with osteoporosis

Contraindications and cautions

- Contraindicated with allergy to bisphosphonates; severe renal disease, hypocalcemia, inability to stand or sit upright for at least 30 min, esophageal abnormalities that delay esophageal emptying.
- Use cautiously with renal impairment, pregnancy, lactation, upper GI problems, oral surgery.

Available forms

Tablets—5, 30, 35, 75 (CAN), 150 mg; DR tablets ⬛—35 mg

Dosages

Adults

- *Treatment and prevention of postmenopausal osteoporosis:* 5 mg PO once daily taken in an upright position with 6–8 oz of water at least 30 min before or after any other beverage or food. For postmenopausal osteoporosis, may switch to 35-mg tablet or 35-mg DR tablet taken PO once per wk or 75 mg PO taken on 2 consecutive days each mo (total of 2 tablets per mo) or one 150-mg tablet PO per mo.
- *Treatment or prevention of glucocorticoid osteoporosis:* 5 mg/day PO.
- *Paget disease:* 30 mg PO once daily for 2 mo taken in an upright position with 6–8 oz of plain water at least 30 min before or after any other beverage or food; may retreat after at least a 2-mo post-treatment period if indicated.
- *To increase bone mass in men with osteoporosis:* 35 mg PO once/wk.

Pediatric patients

Safety and efficacy not established.

Patients with renal impairment

Not recommended with creatinine clearance less than 30 mL/min; no dosage adjustment

is needed if creatinine clearance greater than 30 mL/min.

Pharmacokinetics

Route	Onset	Peak
Oral	Rapid	1 hr

Metabolism: Not metabolized; $T_{1/2}$: Initial half-life: 1.5 hr; terminal half-life: 48 hr
Distribution: May cross placenta; may enter breast milk
Excretion: Urine

Adverse effects

- **CNS:** *Headache,* paresthesia, *dizziness*
- **CV:** Chest pain, edema, hypertension
- **EENT:** Glaucoma, conjunctivitis, cataract
- **GI:** *Nausea, diarrhea, dyspepsia,* abdominal pain, *anorexia*
- **Skeletal:** *Increased or recurrent bone pain,* osteonecrosis of the jaw
- **Other:** *Arthralgia,* bone pain, leg cramps, *rash*

Interactions

✴ **Drug-drug** • Absorption of risedronate decreased by calcium, aspirin, aluminum, magnesium; avoid these drugs for 2 hr before to 2 hr after taking risedronate

■ Nursing considerations

Assessment

- **History:** Allergy to bisphosphonates, renal failure, hypocalcemia, pregnancy, lactation, esophageal abnormalities, upper GI problems, recent oral surgery
- **Physical:** Muscle tone, bone pain; bowel sounds; eye examination; urinalysis, serum calcium; orientation, affect

Interventions

⊗ *Warning* Administer with a full glass of plain (not mineral) water, at least 30 min before or after any other beverage, food, or medication; have patient remain in an upright position for at least 30 min to decrease the incidence of GI effects. Patients taking weekly dose should mark calendar as a reminder. Ensure that patient swallows DR tablet whole. DR tablet is only approved for treatment of osteoporosis in postmenopausal women.

- Monitor serum calcium levels before, during, and after therapy.

⊗ **Warning** Osteonecrosis of the jaw has occurred in patients taking bisphosphonates. Patients undergoing invasive dental procedures should discuss risks with health care provider; discontinuing the bisphosphonate may reduce the risk.

⊗ **Warning** Ensure at least a 2-mo rest period after 2-mo course of treatment if retreatment is required for Paget disease.

- Ensure adequate vitamin D and calcium intake.
- Provide comfort measures if bone pain returns.

Teaching points
- Take this drug with a full glass of water (plain water, not mineral water), at least 30 minutes before or after any other beverage, foods, or medication; remain in an upright position for at least 30 minutes to decrease the GI side effects of the drug. If taking a once-weekly dose, mark a calendar as a reminder. If using delayed-release tablet, swallow whole; do not cut, crush, or chew tablet.
- Inform dentist that you are taking this drug before any dental surgery.
- Maintain adequate vitamin D and calcium intake while you are using this drug.
- You may experience these side effects: Nausea, diarrhea; bone pain, headache (analgesics may be available to help); rash (appropriate skin care will be suggested).
- Report twitching, muscle spasms, dark-colored urine, edema, bone pain, rash, difficulty swallowing.

▽**risperidone**
(ris **peer'** i dohn)

Risperdal, Risperdal Consta, Risperdal M-TAB

PREGNANCY CATEGORY C

Drug classes
Antipsychotic
Benzisoxazole

Therapeutic actions
Mechanism of action not fully understood: Blocks dopamine and serotonin receptors in the brain, depresses the RAS; anticholinergic, antihistaminic, and alpha-adrenergic blocking activity may contribute to some of its therapeutic and adverse actions.

Indications
- Treatment of schizophrenia
- Delaying relapse in long-term treatment of schizophrenia
- Short-term treatment of acute manic or mixed episodes associated with bipolar 1 disorder; alone or in combination with lithium or valproate (oral only)
- Long-acting injection used as monotherapy or as adjunct to lithium or valproate for maintenance treatment of bipolar 1 disorder (*Risperdal Consta*)
- Treatment of irritability (aggression, self-injury, temper tantrums, quickly changing moods) associated with autistic disorders in children and adolescents (5–16 yr)
- Unlabeled uses: Treatment of OCD refractory to SSRIs; treatment of tics in Tourette syndrome; stuttering

Contraindications and cautions
- Contraindicated with hypersensitivity to risperidone, lactation.
- Use cautiously with CV disease, pregnancy, renal or hepatic impairment, hypotension.

Available forms
Tablets—0.25, 0.5, 1, 2, 3, 4 mg; oral solution—1 mg/mL; orally disintegrating tablets—0.25, 0.5, 1, 2, 3, 4 mg; powder for injection—12.5, 25, 37.5, 50 mg

Dosages
Adults
Schizophrenia
- *Initial treatment:* 1 mg PO bid or 2 mg PO once daily; then gradually increase with daily dosage increments of 1 mg bid on the second and third days to a target dose of 3 mg PO bid by the third day. Range, 4–8 mg/day or 25 mg IM every 2 wk; do not exceed 50 mg IM every 2 wk.
- *Reinitiation of treatment:* Follow initial dosage guidelines, using extreme care due to increased risk of severe adverse effects with reexposure.
- *Switching from other antipsychotics:* Minimize the overlap period and discontinue other antipsychotic before beginning risperidone therapy.

- *Delaying relapse time in long-term treat-ment:* 2–8 mg/day PO.

Bipolar 1 disorder

- *Long-term maintenance:* 25–50 mg IM every 2 wk.

Bipolar mania

- 2–3 mg/day PO as a once daily dose; range 1–6 mg/day.

Pediatric patients with irritability associated with autistic disorder (5–16 yr)

Initially, 0.25 mg/day PO for patients weigh-ing less than 20 kg or 0.5 mg/day for patients 20 kg or more. After at least 4 days, may in-crease to 0.5 mg/day for patients less than 20 kg or 1 mg/day for patients 20 kg or more. Maintain dosage for at least 14 days; may then increase in increments of 0.25 mg/day (less than 20 kg) or 0.5 mg/day (20 kg or more) at 2-wk intervals. Dose may be divided; give at bedtime if somolence occurs.

Pediatric patients

- *Schizophrenia (13–17 yr):* Initially, 0.5 mg/day PO; adjust in increments of 0.5–1 mg/day at intervals of at least 24 hr. Usual dose, 3 mg/day; dose may be split and giv-en bid if drowsiness is a problem.
- *Bipolar mania (10–17 yr):* Initially, 0.5 mg/day PO; adjust in increments of 0.5–1 mg/day at intervals of at least 24 hr. Usual dose, 2.5 mg/day; dose may be split and giv-en bid if drowsiness is a problem.

Geriatric patients or patients with renal or hepatic impairment

Initial dose of 0.5 mg PO bid or 25 mg IM every 2 wk; monitor patient for adverse effects and response.

Pharmacokinetics

Route	Onset	Peak	Duration
Oral	Varies	3–17 hr	Weeks
IM	Slow	3 wk	6 wk

Metabolism: Hepatic; $T_{1/2}$: 20 hr
Distribution: Crosses placenta; enters breast milk
Excretion: Feces, urine

Adverse effects

- **CNS:** *Insomnia, anxiety, agitation, head-ache,* somnolence, aggression, dizziness, tardive dyskinesias
- **CV:** Orthostatic hypotension, **arrhythmias**

- **Dermatologic:** Rash, dry skin, seborrhea, photosensitivity
- **GI:** *Nausea, vomiting, constipation,* ab-dominal discomfort, dry mouth, increased saliva
- **Respiratory:** Rhinitis, coughing, sinusi-tis, pharyngitis, dyspnea
- **Other:** Chest pain, arthralgia, back pain, fever, **NMS,** diabetes mellitus, hyperglycemia

Interactions

✱ **Drug-drug** • Increased therapeutic and toxic effects with clozapine • Decreased thera-peutic effect with carbamazepine • Decreased effectiveness of levodopa • Increased toxic ef-fects with alcohol

■ Nursing considerations

 CLINICAL ALERT!
Name confusion has occurred between *Risperdal* (risperidone) and *Requip* (ropini-role); use caution.

Assessment

- **History:** Allergy to risperidone, lactation, CV disease, pregnancy, renal or hepatic im-pairment, hypotension
- **Physical:** T, weight; reflexes, orientation; P, BP, orthostatic BP; R, adventitious sounds; bowel sounds, normal output, liver evalua-tion; CBC, urinalysis, LFTs, renal function tests

Interventions

⊗ **Black box warning** Do not use drug to treat geriatric patients with dementia-relat-ed psychosis; it increases risk of CV mortality; drug is not approved for this use.

⊗ **Warning** Maintain seizure precautions, especially when initiating therapy and in-creasing dosage.

⊗ **Warning** Administer oral solution directly from calibrated pipette or mix oral solution with 3–4 oz of water, coffee, orange juice, or low-fat milk. Do not mix with cola or tea.

- Open blister units of orally disintegrating tablets individually; do not push tablet through the foil. Use dry hands to remove tablet—immediately place on tongue. Do not allow patient to chew tablet.

⊗ **Warning** Monitor patient regularly for signs and symptoms of diabetes mellitus.

- Monitor T. If fever occurs, rule out underlying infection, and consult physician for appropriate comfort measures.
- Advise patient to use contraception during drug therapy.

⊗ *Warning* Follow guidelines for discontinuation or reinstitution of the drug carefully.

Teaching points
- Dosage will be increased gradually to achieve most effective dose. Do not take more than your prescribed dosage. Do not make up missed doses; contact your health care provider if this occurs. Do not stop taking this drug suddenly; gradual reduction of dosage is needed to prevent side effects.
- Mix oral solution in 3–4 ounces of water, coffee, orange juice, or low-fat milk. Do not mix with cola or tea.
- Remove orally disintegrating tablet with dry hands. Do not push tablet through foil. Immediately place tablet on tongue; do not split or chew tablet. The tablet will disintegrate within seconds and you can then swallow.
- If receiving IM doses, mark your calendar for every-2-week injections.
- This drug should not be taken during pregnancy. If you think you are pregnant or wish to become pregnant, consult your health care provider.
- Avoid alcohol while taking this drug.
- You may experience these side effects: Drowsiness, dizziness, sedation, seizures (avoid driving, operating machinery, or performing tasks that require concentration); dizziness, faintness on arising (change positions slowly; use caution); increased salivation (reversible); constipation; sensitivity to the sun (use a sunscreen or protective clothing).
- Report lethargy, weakness, fever, sore throat, malaise, mouth ulcers, palpitations, increased thirst, increased urination, increased hunger.

▽**ritonavir**
*(ri **ton'** ah veer)*

Norvir

PREGNANCY CATEGORY B

Drug class
Antiretroviral

Therapeutic actions
Antiviral activity; inhibits HIV protease activity, leading to decrease in production of HIV particles.

Indications
- Treatment of HIV infection in combination with other antiretrovirals

Contraindications and cautions
- Contraindicated with allergy to ritonavir, use of certain drugs (see Interactions).
- Use cautiously with pregnancy, hepatic impairment, lactation.

Available forms
Capsules—100 mg; tablets—100 mg; oral solution—80 mg/mL

Dosages
Adults
600 mg PO bid with food; 100–400 mg/day PO when used as a pharmacokinetic booster with other proteuse inhibitors.
Pediatric patients
Start at 250 mg/m^2 PO bid and increase by 50 mg/m^2 twice daily at 2–3 day intervals, to maximum of 400 mg/m^2 PO bid; do not exceed 600 mg bid. Use in combination with other antiretrovirals.

Pharmacokinetics

Route	Onset	Peak
Oral	Rapid	2–4 hr

Metabolism: Hepatic; $T_{1/2}$: 3–5 hr
Distribution: May cross placenta; may enter breast milk
Excretion: Feces, urine

Adverse effects
- **CNS:** *Asthenia, peripheral and circumoral paresthesias,* anxiety, dreams, headache, dizziness, hallucinations, personality changes
- **CV:** Hemorrhage, hypotension, syncope, tachycardia, increased PR interval, increased QT interval
- **Dermatologic:** Acne, dry skin, contact dermatitis, rash
- **GI:** *Nausea, vomiting, diarrhea, anorexia, abdominal pain, taste perversion,* dry mouth, hepatitis, hepatic impairment, dehydration

R

- **GU:** Dysuria, hematuria, nocturia, pyelonephritis
- **Respiratory:** Apnea, dyspnea, cough, rhinitis
- **Other:** Hypothermia, chills, back pain, chest pain, edema, cachexia

Interactions

✳ Drug-drug

⊗ **Black box warning** Potentially large increase in serum concentration of alfuzosin, amiodarone, astemizole, bepridil, bupropion, clozapine, ergotamine, flecainide, meperidine, pimozide, piroxicam, propafenone, quinidine, rifabutin, terfenadine, voriconazole; potential for serious arrhythmias, seizures, and fatal reactions; do not administer ritonavir with any of these drugs.

⊗ **Black box warning** Potentially large increases in serum concentration of these sedatives and hypnotics: alprazolam, clonazepam, diazepam, estazolam, flurazepam, midazolam, triazolam, zolpidem; extreme sedation and respiratory depression could occur; do not administer ritonavir with any of these drugs. ● Risk of prolonged QT interval; do not give with other drugs that prolong QT interval

✳ Drug-food ● Absorption increased by presence of food; taking drug with food is strongly recommended ● Decreased metabolism and risk of toxic effects if combined with grapefruit juice; avoid this combination

✳ Drug-alternative therapy ● Decreased effectiveness if taken with St. John's Wort

■ Nursing considerations

✦ CLINICAL ALERT!
Name confusion has been reported between *Retrovir* (zidovudine) and ritonavir; use caution.

Assessment

- **History:** Allergy to ritonavir, hepatic impairment, pregnancy, lactation
- **Physical:** T; orientation, reflexes; BP, P, peripheral perfusion; R, adventitious sounds; bowel sounds; skin color, perfusion; LFTs

Interventions

- Capsules and oral solution should be stored in refrigerator; solution can be left at room temperature if used within 30 days; protect from light and extreme heat.

- Administer with meals or food to increase absorption.

⊗ **Black box warning** Carefully screen drug history to avoid potentially dangerous or life-threatening drug interactions.

Teaching points

- Take this drug with meals or food. Store capsules in refrigerator; tablets and solution can be left at room temperature if used within 30 days. Taste of solution may be improved if mixed with chocolate milk, *Ensure,* or *Advera* 1 hour before taking. Do not drink grapefruit juice while using this drug.
- Take the full course of therapy as prescribed; do not take double doses if one is missed; do not change dosage without consulting your health care provider. Always take in combination with your other HIV drugs.
- This drug does not cure HIV infection; long-term effects are not yet known; continue to take precautions as the risk of transmission is not reduced by this drug.
- Do not take any other drugs, prescription or over-the-counter, without consulting your health care provider; this drug interacts with many other drugs and serious problems can occur.
- You may experience these side effects: Nausea, vomiting, loss of appetite, diarrhea, abdominal pain, headache, dizziness, numbness, tingling.
- Report severe diarrhea, severe nausea, personality changes, changes in color of urine or stool, fever, chills.

▽ rituximab

See Appendix R, *Less commonly used drugs.*

▽ rivaroxaban
(riv' a rox' a ban)

Xarelto

PREGNANCY CATEGORY C

Drug classes
Anticoagulant
Factor Xa inhibitor

Therapeutic actions

Factor Xa inhibitor that selectively blocks the active site of factor Xa and does not require a cofactor for activity; factor Xa plays a central role in the blood coagulation cascade.

Indications

- Prophylaxis of DVT, which may lead to pulmonary embolism in patients undergoing knee or hip replacement surgery
- Reduction of risk of stroke in patients with nonvalvular atrial fibrillation (AF)
- Treatment of deep vein thrombosis (DVT) and pulmonary embolism
- Reduction of the risk of recurrent DVT and pulmonary embolism following initial treatment

Contraindications and cautions

- Contraindicated with known hypersensitivity to components of the drug; active pathologic bleeding, severe renal impairment, moderate to severe hepatic impairment.
- Use cautiously with invasive procedures, surgery, pregnancy, lactation.

Available forms

Tablets—10, 15, 20 mg

Dosages

Adults
- *Prophylaxis of DVT:* 10 mg/day PO without regard to food. Start dosing within 6–10 hr of surgery; continue for 35 days after hip replacement, 12 days after knee replacement.
- *Nonvalvular AF:* 20 mg/day PO with evening meal.

Pediatric patients
Safety and efficacy not established.

Patients with renal impairment
For creatinine clearance of more than 15 mL/ min but less than 50 mL/min, monitor patient closely for signs of bleeding; maximum dose, 15 mg/day for AF. Avoid use if creatinine clearance is less than 15 mL/min.

Patients with hepatic impairment
Avoid use in patients with moderate to severe hepatic impairment (Child-Pugh score B or C) or with hepatic disease associated with coagulopathy.

Pharmacokinetics

Route	Onset	Peak
Oral	Rapid	2–4 hr

Metabolism: Hepatic; $T_{1/2}$: 5–9 hr
Distribution: May cross placenta; may enter breast milk
Excretion: Urine and feces

Adverse effects

- **Dermatological:** Pruritus, blisters
- **GI:** Elevated liver enzymes
- **GU:** Dysuria
- **Other: bleeding, hemorrhage,** muscle spasm, pain in extremities

Interactions

✳ **Drug-drug** • Potential for increased effectiveness if combined with P-gp and CYP3A4 inhibitors (ketoconazole, ritonavir, clarithromycin, erythromycin); avoid this combination; if combination cannot be avoided, lower rivaroxaban dosage and monitor patient closely • Decreased effectiveness if combined with P-gp and CYP3A4 inducers (rifampin, carbamazepine, phenytoin; avoid these combinations; if combination cannot be avoided, increase rivaroxaban dosage and monitor patient closely • Increased risk of bleeding if combined with other drugs that increase bleeding (NSAIDs, aspirin, platelet inhibitors, warfarin, clopidogrel); if these combinations are used, monitor patient closely for potential bleeding problems

✳ **Drug-alternative therapy** • Decreased effectiveness if combined with St. John's Wort; avoid this combination

■ Nursing considerations

⊗ *Black box warning* Risk of epidural or spinal hematomas with related neurologic impairment and possible paralysis if used in patients receiving neuraxial anesthesia or undergoing spinal puncture. Carefully consider benefits and risks of using neuraxial intervention in patients who are anticoagulated or who will be anticoagulated. If rivaroxaban is used, monitor patients frequently for signs of neurologic impairment; be prepared for rapid treatment if necessary.

⊗ *Black box warning* Discontinuing rivaroxaban increases risk of thromboembolic events. If drug must be stopped for reasons other than pathologic bleeding, consider administering another anticoagulant.

Assessment
- **History:** History of hypersensitivity to components of the drug; pathologic bleeding, pregnancy, lactation, planned invasive procedures, renal impairment, hepatic impairment
- **Physical:** Skin evaluation, renal function tests, LFTs, aPPT, PT

Interventions
- Begin drug administration within 6–10 hr of surgery. For knee or hip replacement. Administer drug for stroke prevention in patients with AF once daily in the evening.
- Administer at approximately the same time each day; do not double up missed doses.
- Provide safety measures if bleeding becomes an issue.
- Counsel pregnant and breast-feeding women regarding the risk of bleeding while taking this drug and its possible effects on the neonate; use of contraceptive measures is advised.
- Do not interrupt drug unless absolutely necessary (surgery, bleeding). Risk of stroke increases when anticoagulants are stopped. If drug must be stopped for any reason other than bleeding, start another anticoagulant.

Teaching points
- Take this drug once a day at approximately the same time each day; you can take it with or without food. If taking this drug and have atrial fibrillation, take it once a day in the evening.
- If you forget a dose, take it as soon as you remember; then begin your usual dosage the next day. Do not make up skipped doses and do not take more than one dose each day.
- Do not stop taking this drug without consulting your health care provider; make sure you do not run out of this drug.
- Tell your health care provider about OTC drugs, herbs, or other drugs you may be taking that may affect bleeding. You may need a dosage change while you are taking this drug.
- It is not known how this drug could affect a fetus. If you are pregnant or thinking about becoming pregnant, discuss this with your health care provider; use of contraceptive measures is advised.
- It is not known how this drug could affect a breast-feeding infant. If you are breast-feeding, you should use another method of feeding the infant.
- This drug will increase your risk of bleeding. Tell all health care professionals caring for you that you are taking this drug; it is especially important to do so before procedures that could cause bleeding, such as dental work or surgery. Do not take this drug with other anticoagulants unless instructed by your health care provider.
- You may experience these effects: Increased risk of bleeding (use a soft-bristled tooth brush and an electric razor; avoid contact sports), rash, muscle aches and pains.
- Report unusual bruising, pink or brown urine, red or black stool, coughing up blood, vomiting blood, nose bleeds, bleeding that takes a long time to stop, heavier than normal menstrual flow, headache, dizziness, weakness.

▽ rivastigmine tartrate
*(riv ah **stig'** meen)*

Exelon, Exelon Oral Solution, Exelon Patch

PREGNANCY CATEGORY B

Drug classes
Alzheimer disease drug
Cholinesterase inhibitor

Therapeutic actions
Centrally acting, selective, long-acting reversible cholinesterase inhibitor; causes elevated acetylcholine levels in the cortex, which slows the neuronal degradation that occurs in Alzheimer disease.

Indications
- Treatment of mild to moderate dementia of the Alzheimer type
- Treatment of mild to moderate dementia associated with Parkinson disease
- Unlabeled use: Treatment of behavioral effects of Lewy-body dementia

Contraindications and cautions

- Contraindicated with hypersensitivity to rivastigmine.
- Use cautiously with sick sinus syndrome, GI bleeding, seizures, asthma, COPD, pregnancy, lactation.

Available forms

Capsules—1.5, 3, 4.5, 6 mg; oral solution with dosing syringe—2 mg/mL; transdermal patch—4.6 mg/24 hr, 9.5 mg/24 hr

Dosages
Adults

- *Alzheimer disease:* Initial dosage, 1.5 mg PO bid with food. If tolerated, may adjust to higher doses at 1.5-mg intervals every 2 wks. Usual range, 6–12 mg/day; should not exceed 12 mg/day. If dose is not tolerated, stop drug for several doses and then restart at the same or a lower level. For transdermal patch, initially one 4.6-mg/24 hr patch once/day; after 4 or more wk, may be increased to one 9.5-mg/24 hr patch.
- *Parkinson dementia:* 3–12 mg/day PO in divided doses bid. Initial dose, 1.5 mg PO bid; increase every 4 wk based on patient tolerance. For transdermal patch, initially one 4.6-mg/24 hr patch once/day; after 4 or more wk, may be increased to one 9.5-mg/24 hr patch.

Pediatric patients
Safety and efficacy not established.

Pharmacokinetics

Route	Onset	Peak	Duration
Oral	Varies	1.4–2.6 hr	12 hr
Transdermal	1 hr	8–16 hr	24 hr

Metabolism: Hepatic; $T_{1/2}$: 1.5–3 hr
Distribution: Crosses placenta; may enter breast milk
Excretion: Urine

Adverse effects

- **CNS:** *Insomnia, fatigue,* dizziness, confusion, ataxia, insomnia, somnolence, tremor, agitation, depression, anxiety, abnormal thinking, syncope
- **CV:** Bradycardia
- **GI:** *Nausea, vomiting, diarrhea, dyspepsia, anorexia, abdominal pain,* flatulence, constipation
- **Other:** Weight loss

Interactions

✳ **Drug-drug** • Increased effects and risk of toxicity if theophylline, cholinesterase inhibitors taken concurrently • Decreased effects of anticholinergics taken concurrently • Increased risk of GI bleeding if taken with NSAIDs

■ Nursing considerations
Assessment

- **History:** Allergy to rivastigmine; pregnancy; lactation; sick sinus syndrome; GI bleeding; seizures; asthma; COPD
- **Physical:** Orientation, affect, reflexes; BP, P; abdominal examination; LFTs, renal function tests

Interventions

- Establish baseline functional profile to follow evaluation of drug effectiveness.
- Administer with food in the morning and evening to decrease GI discomfort.
- Mix solution with water, fruit juice, or soda to improve compliance. Dosage of capsules and solution is interchangeable.
- Apply patch to clean, dry skin once daily. Rotate application sites, and remove old patch before applying new one.
- Monitor patient for weight loss, diarrhea, arrhythmias before use and periodically with prolonged use.
- Provide small, frequent meals if GI upset is severe.
- Provide patient safety measures if CNS effects occur.
- ⊗ *Warning* Notify surgeons that patient is on rivastigmine; exaggerated muscle relaxation may occur if succinylcholine-type drugs are used.

Teaching points

- Take drug exactly as prescribed, take with food to decrease GI upset. Solution may be swallowed directly from the syringe or mixed in a small glass of water, cold fruit juice, or soda. In cold fruit juice or soda, mixture is stable up to 4 hours at room temperature.
- Patch should be applied to clean, dry skin. Rotate sites, and remove old patch before applying a new one.
- This drug does not cure the disease but may slow down the degeneration associated with the disease.

R

- Dosage changes may be needed to achieve the best drug levels.
- You may experience these side effects: Nausea, vomiting (eat frequent small meals) insomnia, fatigue, confusion (use caution if driving or performing tasks that require alertness).
- Report severe nausea, vomiting, changes in stool or urine color, diarrhea, changes in neurologic functioning, palpitations.

▷rizatriptan
(rih zah trip' tan)

Maxalt, Maxalt-MLT

PREGNANCY CATEGORY C

Drug classes
Antimigraine drug
Serotonin selective agonist

Therapeutic actions
Binds to serotonin receptors to cause vascular constrictive effects on cranial blood vessels, causing the relief of migraine in select patients whose migraines are caused by vasodilation.

Indications
- Treatment of acute migraine attacks with or without aura

Contraindications and cautions
- Contraindicated with allergy to rizatriptan, active CAD, Prinzmetal angina, uncontrolled hypertension; recent (within 24 hr) treatment with another 5-HT agonist or an ergotamine-containing or ergot type medication; hemiplegic or basilar migraine.
- Use cautiously with hepatic impairment, dialysis, pregnancy, lactation.

Available forms
Tablets—5, 10 mg; orally disintegrating tablets—5, 10 mg

Dosages
Adults
5 or 10 mg PO at onset of headache; may repeat in 2 hr if needed. Wait 2 hr between doses. Maximum dose, 30 mg/day.

Pediatric patients 6–17 yr
40 kg or more: 10 mg PO per attack.
30 kg or less: 5 mg PO per attack.
Patients with hepatic or renal impairment
Use lowest possible dose, monitor patient closely.

Pharmacokinetics

Route	Onset	Peak
Oral	Rapid	1 hr

Metabolism: Hepatic; $T_{1/2}$: 2 hr
Distribution: May cross placenta; may enter breast milk
Excretion: Feces, urine

Adverse effects
- **CNS:** *Dizziness, vertigo, weakness, somnolence, paresthesias*
- **CV:** BP increase, palpitations, chest pain
- **GI:** Dry mouth, nausea
- **Other:** *Chest, jaw, or throat pressure*

Interactions
✳ **Drug-drug** ⊗ *Warning* Prolonged vasoactive reactions when taken concurrently with ergot-containing drugs; do not use within 24 hr of each other or other serotonin agonist.
- Risk of severe effects if taken with or within 2 wk of discontinuation of an MAOI ● Risk of increased serum levels and toxic effects with propanolol; recommend 5-mg dose no more than three doses per 24-hr period
✳ **Drug-food** ● Food will delay peak onset by 1 hr

■ Nursing considerations
Assessment
- **History:** Allergy to rizatriptan, active CAD, Prinzmetal angina, uncontrolled hypertension, hepatic impairment, dialysis, pregnancy, lactation
- **Physical:** Skin color and lesions; orientation, reflexes, peripheral sensation; P, BP; LFTs, renal function tests

Interventions
- Administer to relieve acute migraine, not as a prophylactic measure.
- Have patient place orally disintegrating tablet on tongue and swallow with or without water.
- Establish safety measures if CNS or visual disturbances occur.

- Control environment as appropriate to help relieve migraine (lighting, temperature, noise).
⊗ *Warning* Monitor BP of patients with possible CAD; discontinue at any sign of angina, prolonged high BP, or other adverse signs.

Teaching points

- Take drug exactly as prescribed, at the onset of headache or aura; dosage may be repeated in 2 hours if needed. Place orally disintegrating tablet on tongue and allow to dissolve before eating or drinking.
- This drug should not be taken during pregnancy; if you suspect that you are pregnant, consult your health care provider and stop using drug.
- Continue to do anything that normally helps you during a migraine, such as controlling lighting or noise.
- Contact your health care provider immediately if you experience chest pain or pressure that is severe or does not go away.
- You may experience these side effects: Dizziness, drowsiness (avoid driving or the use of dangerous machinery while using this drug); numbness, tingling, feelings of tightness or pressure.
- Report feelings of heat, flushing, tiredness, feelings of sickness, chest pain.

▽ roflumilast
(roe flu' ma last)

Daliresp

PREGNANCY CATEGORY C

Drug class
Phosphodiesterase-4 (PDE4) inhibitor

Therapeutic actions
Selectively inhibits PDE4 activity, leading to an accumulation of intracellular cyclic AMP in lung cells. How this helps the COPD patient is not clearly understood.

Indications
- Reduction of exacerbation risk in patients with severe COPD associated with chronic bronchitis and a history of exacerbation

Contraindications and cautions
- Contraindicated with known hypersensitivity to components of the drug, moderate to severe liver impairment, acute bronchospasm, pregnancy, lactation.
- Use cautiously with a history of depression or suicide attempts.

Available forms
Tablets—500 mcg

Dosages
Adults
500 mcg/day PO with or without food.
Pediatric patients younger than 18 yr
Safety and efficacy not established.
Patients with hepatic impairment
Contraindicated for patients with moderate to severe liver impairment (Child-Pugh class B or C).

Pharmacokinetics

Route	Onset	Peak
Oral	Rapid	0.5–2 hr

Metabolism: Hepatic: $T_{1/2}$: 17–30 hr
Distribution: May cross placenta; may enter breast milk
Excretion: Urine

Adverse effects
- **CNS:** Headache, dizziness, *insomnia, depression,* **suicidality,** tremor, anxiety
- **GI:** *Diarrhea,* nausea, decreased appetite, vomiting, abdominal pain
- **Respiratory:** Rhinitis, sinusitis
- **Other:** *Weight loss,* back pain, flulike symptoms

Interactions
✳ **Drug-drug** • Decreased efficacy if combined with strong CYP450 inducers (rifampin, phenobarbital, carbamazepine, phenytoin); this combination it not recommended • Increased risk of toxicity if combined with cimetidine, erythromycin, fluvoxamine, ketoconazole, ethinyl estradiol

NURSING CONSIDERATIONS
Assessment
- **History:** Known hypersensitivity to components of the drug, lactation, pregnancy, hepatic impairment, acute bronchospasm, history of depression or suicide attempts

R

- **Physical:** Weight; orientation, affect, reflexes: R, adventitious sounds; GI exam; respiratory function evaluation, LFTs

Interventions

- Ensure that patient does not have acute bronchospasm; this drug is not a bronchodilator and is not for use in acute bronchospasm.
- Administer without regard to meals.
- Monitor patient's weight regularly. If significant weight loss occurs, consider discontinuing drug.
- Monitor patient for depression, behavioral changes, or suicidality. Carefully evaluate drug's benefits versus risks if signs and symptoms of severe depression occur.
- This drug should not be taken during pregnancy; suggest use of contraceptive measures.
- It is not known how this drug could affect a breast-feeding infant. Help breast-feeding patient find an alternative method of feeding the infant.
- Ensure that patient continues other therapies for treatment of COPD as indicated.

Teaching points

- Take this drug without regard to meals.
- If you miss a dose, take it as soon as you remember; then resume your usual daily schedule. If you remember close to your next dose, do not take the dose you missed. Do not take more than one dose each day.
- Monitor your weight; weigh yourself regularly in the same clothing and at about the same time each day. If you notice that you are losing weight consistently, contact your health care provider.
- Be aware that this drug can cause depression, thoughts of suicide, or insomnia. If you notice changes in behavior, thoughts of death or suicide, or inability to sleep, contact your health care provider.
- Pregnant women should not take this drug because it can have serious effects on the fetus or even cause fetal death. Use of a barrier contraceptive is advised. If you become pregnant, consult your health care provider immediately.
- If you are breast-feeding, you should use another method of feeding the infant while you are taking this drug; the drug could cause serious adverse effects in a infant.

- Make sure you tell your health care provider about all drugs, herbal supplements, or over-the-counter products you are using.
- This drug is not used to treat an acute bronchospasm. If you experience an acute bronchospasm, you need to use your rescue bronchodilator.
- Continue all other therapies prescribed for your COPD.
- Report significant weight loss, thoughts of suicide, changes in behavior, severe diarrhea.

▷ **romidepsin**

See Appendix R, *Less commonly used drugs*.

▷ **romiplostim**

See Appendix R, *Less commonly used drugs*.

▷ **ropinirole hydrochloride**
*(row **pin**' ah roll)*

Requip, Requip XL ⓓⓝ©

PREGNANCY CATEGORY C

Drug classes
Antiparkinsonian
Dopamine receptor agonist

Therapeutic actions
Acts as a non-ergot dopamine agonist acting directly on postsynaptic dopamine receptors of neurons in the brain, mimicking the effects of the neurotransmitter dopamine, which is thought to be deficient in parkinsonism.

Indications

- Treatment of idiopathic Parkinson disease in the early stages as well as in the late stages (immediate-release or ER)
- Treatment of moderate to severe primary restless legs syndrome (immediate-release only)

Contraindications and cautions

- Contraindicated with hypersensitivity to ropinirole, severe ischemic heart disease or peripheral vascular disease, lactation.

- Use cautiously with dyskinesia, orthostatic hypotension, hepatic or renal impairment, pregnancy, history of sleep disorders or somnolence.

Available forms
Tablets—0.25, 0.5, 1, 2, 3, 4, 5 mg; ER tablets⊚ —2, 4, 6, 8, 12 mg

Dosages
Adults
- *Parkinson disease:* Initially, 0.25 mg PO tid for 1st wk; 0.5 mg PO tid for 2nd wk; 0.75 mg PO tid for 3rd wk; 1 mg PO tid for 4th wk. May increase by 1.5 mg/day at 1-wk intervals to 9 mg/day, then by up to 3 mg/day at 1-wk intervals to a maximum dose of 24 mg/day. ER tablets: Initially, 2 mg/day PO; after 1–2 wk, may increase by 2 mg/day; titrate with weekly increases of 2 mg/day to a maximum of 24 mg/day. If used with levodopa, decrease levodopa dosage gradually; average dosage reduction is 31% with immediate-release ropinirole and 34% with ER forms.
- *Restless legs syndrome:* 0.25 mg/day PO, 1–3 hr before bed; after 2 days, increase to 0.5 mg/day PO; after 1 week to 1 mg/day PO. Week 3, increase to 1.5 mg/day; week 4—2 mg/day, week 5—2.5 mg/day; week 6—3 mg/day; week 7—4 mg/day PO if needed to control symptoms.
Pediatric patients
Safety and efficacy not established.
Geriatric patients
Elderly are at higher risk for development of hallucinations; monitor closely and adjust dosage more slowly.

Pharmacokinetics

Route	Onset	Peak	Duration
Oral	Varies	1–2 hr	8 hr
ER	Varies	6–10 hr	16 hr

Metabolism: Hepatic; $T_{1/2}$: 6 hr
Distribution: Crosses placenta; enters breast milk
Excretion: Urine

Adverse effects
- **CNS:** *Dizziness, somnolence, insomnia, hypokinesia or hyperkinesia,* syncope, asthenia, confusion, hallucinations (more common in the elderly), abnormal vision, tremor, anxiety, paresthesias, aggravated parkinsonism, worsening of impulse control symptoms (eg, gambling), falling asleep during daily activities
- **CV:** *Orthostatic hypotension,* edema
- **GI:** *Nausea, constipation*
- **Other:** Fatigue, infections, sweating, pharyngitis, pain, arthralgia

Interactions
✴ **Drug-drug** • Increased effects of levodopa; consider decreasing levodopa dose • Increased CNS depression with alcohol, CNS depressants • Monitor and adjust ropinirole dose if estrogen is added to or discontinued from regimen • Increased effects with ciprofloxacin • Increased risk of bleeding with warfarin

■ **Nursing considerations**

 CLINICAL ALERT!
Name confusion has occurred between *Requip* (ropinirole) and *Risperdal* (risperidone); use caution.

Assessment
- **History:** Hypersensitivity to ropinirole, severe ischemic heart disease or peripheral vascular disease, pregnancy, lactation, dyskinesia, orthostatic hypotension, hepatic or renal impairment
- **Physical:** Skin T, color, lesions; orientation, affect, reflexes, bilateral grip strength; vision examination including visual fields; P, BP, orthostatic BP, auscultation; liver evaluation; LFTs, renal function tests

Interventions
- Administer drug with food if GI upset becomes a problem. Ensure that patient does not cut, crush, or chew ER tablets.
- Monitor patient for orthostatic hypotension and establish safety precautions if needed (use side rails, accompany patient).
- ⊗ *Warning* Withdraw gradually over 1 wk to avoid serious side effects.
- Monitor patient carefully and adjust dosage more slowly if patient has hypotension or dyskinesias.
- Monitor elderly patients for the development of hallucinations; provide appropriate safety measures as needed.

R

⊗ **Warning** Start adjustment of drug over again if drug has been discontinued and is being restarted.

• Monitor hepatic and renal function periodically during therapy.

⊗ **Warning** Patients have reported falling asleep during daily activities as well as daytime somnolence; warn patient and monitor accordingly.

Teaching points
• Take this drug exactly as prescribed; take with food if GI upset occurs. Dosage will change gradually over several weeks. Do not cut, crush, or chew ER tablets.

• Do not discontinue this drug without consulting your health care provider; drug must be stopped gradually to prevent serious adverse effects.

• You may experience these side effects: Drowsiness, dizziness, confusion (avoid driving or engaging in activities that require alertness); nausea (take drug with meals; eat frequent small meals); dizziness or faintness when you get up (change position slowly, exercise caution when climbing stairs); headache, nasal stuffiness (consult your health care provider; there may be medications for these).

• Report fainting, light-headedness, dizziness; black, tarry stools; hallucinations; falling asleep during activities of daily living.

▽ **rosiglitazone**

See Appendix R, *Less commonly used drugs*.

▽ **rosuvastatin calcium**
*(row **sue'** va sta tin)*

Crestor

PREGNANCY CATEGORY X

Drug classes
Antihyperlipidemic drug
HMG-CoA reductase inhibitor (statin)

Therapeutic actions
A fungal metabolite that inhibits the enzyme (HMG-CoA) that catalyzes the first step in the cholesterol synthesis pathway, resulting in a decrease in serum cholesterol, serum LDLs (associated with increased risk of coronary artery disease) and either an increase or no change in serum HDLs (associated with decreased risk of coronary artery disease).

Indications
• As an adjunct to diet in the treatment of elevated total cholesterol and LDL cholesterol and triglyceride levels in patients with primary hypercholesterolemia (familial and nonfamilial), and in patients with mixed dyslipidemia

• Adjunct to diet to slow atherosclerosis progression in patients with elevated cholesterol

• As an adjunct to diet for the treatment of patients with elevated serum triglyceride levels

• To reduce LDL-C, total cholesterol, and ApoB in patients with homozygous familiar hypercholesterolemia as an adjunct to other lipid-lowering treatments or if such treatments are not available

• Treatment of patients with primary dysbetalipoproteinemia

• Treatment of children 10–17 yr (girls must be at least 1 yr postmenarchal) with heterozygous familial hypercholesterolemia when diet therapy fails

• Primary prevention of CV disease; to reduce risk of stroke, MI, and arterial revascularization procedures in patients with no clinically evident CAD but at increased risk due to age (50 and older in men, 60 and older in women), elevated C-reactive protein, and at least one other risk factor (hypertension, low HDL, smoking, family history)

Contraindications and cautions
• Contraindicated with allergy to any component of the product, active liver disease or persistent elevated serum transaminases, pregnancy, lactation.

• Use cautiously with impaired hepatic function, alcoholism, renal impairment, advanced age, hypothyroidism.

Available forms
Tablets—5, 10, 20, 40 mg

Dosages
Adults
• *Hypercholesteremia; mixed dyslipidemia; primary dysbetalipoproteinemia; hypertriglyceridemia; primary prevention of*

CAD; atherosclerosis: 5–40 mg daily PO. Usual starting dose is 10–20 mg daily with titration based on serum lipid levels, monitored every 2–4 wk until desired level is achieved.

- *Homozygous familial hypercholesterolemia:* 20 mg daily PO with a maximum 40 mg per day.
- *In combination with cyclosporine:* 5 mg daily PO.
- *In combination with other lipid-lowering drugs:* 10 mg daily PO.

Asian patients

Initiate therapy at 5 mg PO once daiy. Risk of serious side effects if dose increase is needed to control lipid levels.

Pediatric patients 10–17 yr

5–20 mg/day PO. Adjust dosage at intervals of 4 wk or more.

Patients with severe renal impairment

5 mg daily PO; do not exceed 10 mg per day.

Pharmacokinetics

Route	Onset	Peak
Oral	Slow	3–5 hr

Metabolism: Hepatic metabolism; $T_{1/2}$: 19 hr
Distribution: Crosses placenta; enters breast milk
Excretion: Feces

Adverse effects

- **CNS:** *Headache,* dizziness, insomnia, hypertonia, paresthesia, depression, anxiety, vertigo, neuralgia
- **CV:** Hypertension, angina pectoris, vasodilatation, palpitation, peripheral edema
- **GI:** *Nausea,* dyspepsia, *diarrhea,* constipation, gastroenteritis, vomiting, flatulence, periodontal abscess, gastritis, **liver failure**
- **Respiratory:** *Pharyngitis, rhinitis, sinusitis,* cough, dyspnea, pneumonia
- **Other:** Arthritis, arthralgia, **rhabdomyolysis, myopathy,** *flulike symptoms,* **myalgia**

Interactions

✴ **Drug-drug** ⊗ **Warning** Possible increased serum levels and risk of toxicity if taken with cyclosporine, gemfibrozil, lopinavir/ritonavir; adjust dosage accordingly and monitor patient; 10 mg/day is suggested maximum dosage.

- Increased risk of bleeding with coumarin anticoagulants; lower dose and monitor bleeding levels frequently to establish correct dosage
- Decreased absorption if taken with aluminum or magnesium hydroxide antacids; if this combination is used, take the antacid at least 2 hr after the rosuvastatin

■ Nursing considerations

Assessment

- **History:** Allergy to any component of the product, liver disease or persistent elevated serum transaminases, pregnancy, lactation, alcoholism, renal impairment, advanced age, hypothyroidism
- **Physical:** Orientation, affect, P, BP, R, adventitious sounds; liver evaluation; lipid studies, LFTs, renal function tests

Interventions

- Establish baseline serum lipid levels and liver function test results before beginning therapy.
- Arrange for proper consultation about need for diet and exercise changes.
- Administer drug at bedtime (highest rates of cholesterol synthesis occur between midnight and 5 AM).
- Arrange for regular follow-up during long-term therapy.
- Monitor patient closely for signs of muscle injury, especially at higher doses, in Asian patients, and when used in combination with gemfibrozil or cyclosporine.
- Provide comfort measures to deal with headache, muscle cramps, or nausea.
- Advise women of childbearing age that this drug is contraindicated during pregnancy; advise the use of barrier contraceptives.
- Suggest an alternate means of feeding the infant to any breast-feeding mother who is prescribed this drug.
- Offer support and encouragement to deal with disease, diet, drug therapy, and follow-up care.

Teaching points

- Recommendations suggest taking drug at bedtime.
- Institute appropriate diet and exercise changes that need to be made.
- If you miss a dose, take the next dose as soon as you remember and begin again the next day. Do not take two doses in 1 day.

R

- Avoid pregnancy while taking this drug; using a barrier contraceptive is advised.
- If you are also taking antacids, take the antacid at least 2 hours after your rosuvastatin.
- Stop the drug and contact your health care provider immediately if you experience unexplained muscle pain, tenderness, or weakness with fever or malaise.
- You may experience these side effects: Nausea (eat frequent small meals); headache, flulike symptoms (analgesics may help).
- Report severe GI upset, unusual bleeding or bruising, dark urine or light-colored stools, unexplained muscle pain, tenderness, or weakness.

▽rotigotine
*(roe **tig** oh teen)*

Neupro

PREGNANCY CATEGORY C

Drug classes
Antiparkinsonian
Dopamine agonist

Therapeutic actions
Dopamine agonist; stimulates dopamine receptors within the caudate putamen in the brain, which relieves some of the signs and symptoms of Parkinson disease. Restless legs syndrome is thought to be related to inability to stimulate dopamine receptors in this area of the brain.

Indications
- Treatment of signs and symptoms of Parkinson disease
- Treatment of moderate to severe restless legs syndrome

Contraindications and cautions
- Contraindicated with history of serious hypersensitivity reactions to component of the drug or sulfites (components of the transdermal patch)
- Use cautiously with hypotension, lactation, pregnancy.

Available forms
Transdermal patch-1, 2, 3, 4, 6, 8 mg/24 hr

Dosages
Adults
- *Parkinson disease:* 2-mg/24-hr transdermal patch for early stage disease to 4-mg/24-hr transdermal patch for advanced disease; may increase to a maximum 6-mg/24-hr transdermal patch for early stage disease or 8-mg/24-hr transdermal patch for advanced disease.
- *Restless legs syndrome:* 1-mg/24-hr transdermal patch up to a maximum 3-mg/24-hr transdermal patch as needed

Pharmacokinetics

Route	Onset	Peak
Transdermal	Rapid	15–18 hr

Metabolism: Hepatic; T1/2: 3 hr, then 5–7 hr
Distribution: May cross placenta; enters breast milk
Excretion: Urine

Adverse effects
- **CNS:** *Somnolence, dizziness, insomnia, headache, dyskinesia, hallucinations, psychotic-like behavior*
- **CV:** *Edema, hypotension, orthostatic hypotension,* tachycardia
- **GI:** *Nausea, vomiting, anorexia*
- **Respiratory: Pulmonary fibrosis**
- **Other:** *Application-site reactions,* **melanoma, hyperpyrexia with rapid dosage reduction, severe allergic reaction**

Interactions
✳ **Drug-drug** • Possible decreased effectiveness if combined with dopamine antagonists, such as antipsychotics, metoclopramide

---

■ **Nursing considerations**
Assessment
- **History:** Hypersensitivity to components of drug, sulfite allergy, pregnancy, lactation
- **Physical:** T, P, BP, R; adventitious sounds; orientation, affect, reflexes; skin evaluation

Interventions
- Apply daily to clean, dry skin; press firmly in place for 30 sec. Do not apply to oily, irritated, or damaged skin or to areas that will be rubbed by tight clothing. Rotate application sites; do not use the same site more often than

every 14 days. Remove old patch before applying new patch.

- Arrange to taper dosage gradually after long-term use; risk of withdrawal reaction with rapid dosage reduction.
- Remove patch if patient is to have an MRI; arcing and burning can occur
- Encourage patient not to apply heat to applied patch.
- Be aware of risk of patient falling asleep during activities of daily living; patient could experience loss of impulse control, psychotic behavior, hallucinations, and orthostatic hypotension. Provide safety measures as needed.
- Advise women of childbearing age to avoid pregnancy; fetal harm has been reported in animal studies.

Teaching points

- Do not open patch until you are ready to apply it. Apply daily to clean, dry skin; press firmly in place for 30 seconds. Do not apply to oily, irritated, or damaged skin or to areas that will be rubbed by tight clothing. Rotate application sites; keep a chart and do not use the same site more often than every 14 days. Remove the old patch before applying new patch.
- Monitor your skin for signs of reaction to the patch; avoid sun exposure to irritated areas. Report severe reactions.
- If you forget or miss a dose, change the patch as soon as you remember and then return to the daily schedule at the normal time. If your patch loosens while you are swimming or bathing or if the edges of the patch lift up, tape them down with bandaging tape and replace the patch at the usual scheduled time.
- Do not stop taking this drug suddenly; make sure you have a supply on hand. Suddenly stopping the drug can cause serious effects.
- Tell all your health care providers that you are wearing this patch; the patch will need to be removed if you undergo an MRI.
- Do not apply heat to the patch.
- This drug could harm a fetus if taken during pregnancy. If you are pregnant or thinking about becoming pregnant, discuss this with your health care provider.
- Do not drive or operate hazardous machinery until you know how this drug affects you; falling asleep suddenly has been reported.
- This drug can lead to changes in behavior and hallucinations; report changes in be-

havior and avoid making important decisions until you know how this drug is affecting you.

- You may experience these side effects: Sleepiness, dizziness (do not drive or operate hazardous machinery if these effects occur; changing positions slowly may help); headache (medication may be available to help).
- Report severe skin reactions, fainting, difficulty breathing, swelling of the face or neck.

▽ rufinamide

See Appendix R, *Less commonly used drugs*.

▽ sacrosidase

See Appendix R, *Less commonly used drugs*.

▽ saliva substitute
(sa lye' vah)

Aquoral, Entertainer's Secret, Moi-Stir, Moi-Stir Swabsticks, MouthKote, Numoisyn, Salivart

PREGNANCY CATEGORY UNKNOWN

Drug class
Saliva substitute

Therapeutic actions
Contains electrolytes and carboxymethylcellulose as a thickening agent to serve as a substitute for saliva in dry mouth syndromes.

Indications
- Management of dry mouth and throat in xerostomia and hyposalivation caused by stroke, medications (including those that cause dysfunction of the salivary glands), radiation therapy, chemotherapy, Sjögren syndrome, Bell palsy, HIV/AIDS, lupus, aging, emotional factors, hoarse voice, scratchy throat, salivary gland disorders, other illnesses

Contraindications and cautions
- Contraindicated with hypersensitivity to carboxymethylcellulose, parabens, components of the preparation.
- Use cautiously with renal failure, HF, hypertension, pregnancy.

R

Available forms
Solution; lozenges; spray; swab sticks

Dosages
Adults
Spray for one-half second or apply to oral mucosa; maximum dose for lozenges, 16/day.
Pediatric patients
Safety and efficacy not established.

Pharmacokinetics
No general systemic absorption. Electrolytes may be absorbed and dealt with in normal electrolyte pathways.

Adverse effects
Other: Excessive absorption of electrolytes (elevated magnesium, sodium, potassium)

■ Nursing considerations
Assessment
- **History:** Allergy to carboxymethylcellulose, parabens, HF, hypertension, renal failure
- **Physical:** BP, P, auscultation, edema; renal function tests; mucosa evaluation

Interventions
- Give for dry mouth and throat.
- Have patient try to swish saliva substitute around mouth following application.
- Monitor patient while eating; swallowing may be impaired and additional therapy required.

Teaching points
- Apply the drug as instructed; swish it around in your mouth after application.
- Use as needed for dry mouth and throat.
- Take care when eating because swallowing may be difficult; additional therapy may be needed.
- Report swelling, headache, irregular heartbeat, leg cramps, failure to relieve discomfort of dry mouth and throat.

▽**salmeterol xinafoate**
(*sal **mee'** ter ol ze inn ah **foh'** ate*)

Serevent Diskus

PREGNANCY CATEGORY C

Drug classes
Antiasthmatic
Beta$_2$-selective adrenergic agonist

Therapeutic actions
Long-acting agonist that binds to beta$_2$ receptors in the lungs, causing bronchodilation; also inhibits the release of inflammatory mediators in the lungs, blocking swelling and inflammation.

Indications
- Maintenance therapy for asthma and prevention of bronchospasm in patients 4 yr and older with reversible obstructive airway disease including nocturnal asthma
- Long-term maintenance treatment of bronchospasm related to COPD
- Prevention of exercise-induced bronchospasm in patients 4 yr and older

Contraindications and cautions
- Contraindicated with hypersensitivity to salmeterol, acute asthma attack, worsening or deteriorating asthma (life-threatening), acute airway obstruction, treatment of asthma without concurrent use of a long-term asthma-control medication such as an inhaled corticosteroid.
- Use cautiously with pregnancy, lactation.

Available forms
Inhalation powder—50 mcg (*Diskus*)

Dosages
Adults and patients 12 yr and older
- *Asthma or bronchospasm:* 1 inhalation (50 mcg) bid at 12-hr intervals.
- *Exercise-induced asthma:* 1 inhalation 30 min or more before exertion.
- *COPD:* 1 inhalation (50 mcg) bid at 12-hr intervals.
Pediatric patients 4–12 yr
- *Asthma or bronchospasm:* 1 inhalation (50 mcg) bid, 12 hr apart.
- *Prevention of exercise-induced asthma:* 1 inhalation 30 min or more before exercising.

Pharmacokinetics

Route	Onset	Peak	Duration
Inhalation	13–20 min	3–4 hr	7.5–17 hr

Metabolism: Hepatic; $T_{1/2}$: Unknown
Distribution: May cross placenta; may enter breast milk
Excretion: Feces, urine

Adverse effects

- **CNS:** *Headache, tremor,* dizziness
- **CV:** *Tachycardia, palpitations,* hypertension
- **Respiratory:** Worsening of asthma, difficulty breathing, **bronchospasm; asthma related deaths (risk higher in black than white patients)**
- **Other:** Pain

Interactions

✴ Drug-drug • Risk of severe bronchospasm if combined with beta blockers; use a cardioselective beta blocker and monitor patient closely if this combination is used • Potential for worsened hypokalemia and ECG abnormalities if combined with diuretics; monitor patient very closely • Administer with extreme caution to patients being treated with MAOIs or TCAs, or within 2 wk of discontinuation of such agents because the action of salmeterol may be potentiated by these agents • Risk of severe toxicity if combined with antiviral protease inhibitors; avoid this combination

■ Nursing considerations
Assessment

- **History:** Allergy to salmeterol, pregnancy, acute asthma attack, worsening asthma, lactation
- **Physical:** R, adventitious sounds; P, BP, ECG; orientation, reflexes; LFTs

Interventions

⊗ **Black box warning** Ensure that drug is not used to treat acute asthma or with worsening or deteriorating asthma (risk of death).

⊗ **Black box warning** There is increased risk of asthma-related hospitalizations when used in children and adolescents. For patients who need a long-acting sympathomimetic and an inhaled corticosteroid, the use of a fixed-dose combination is strongly recommended.

⊗ **Black box warning** Do not use for asthma unless combined with a long-term asthma-control medication (risk of death); use only as an additional therapy in patients not controlled by other medications.

- Assess asthma patients regularly to determine when tapering off drug can begin.
- Instruct in the proper use of *Diskus.*
- Have patients who experience exercise-induced asthma use it 30–60 min before activity.
- Arrange for periodic evaluation of respiratory condition.

Teaching points

- Use only twice a day. If drug is to be used periodically for exercise-induced asthma, use 30–60 minutes before activity.
- To gain full therapeutic benefit in the treatment of reversible airway obstruction, administer twice a day (morning and evening).
- Do not use salmeterol as a substitute for oral or inhaled corticosteroids.
- This drug is not for treatment of acute asthma attacks. Never take this drug alone for treating asthma; it must be combined with other long-term asthma-control medications.
- Obtain periodic evaluations of your respiratory problem.
- You may experience these side effects: Headache (request analgesics); tremors (use care in performing dangerous tasks); fast heartbeat, palpitations (monitor activity; rest frequently).
- Report severe headache, irregular heartbeat, worsening of asthma, difficulty breathing.

▷ **salsalate
(salicylsalicylic acid)**
(sal' sa layt)

Amigesic, Argesic-SA, Artha-G, Disalcid, Marthritic, Salflex, Salsitab

PREGNANCY CATEGORY C

Drug classes

Analgesic (nonopioid)
Anti-inflammatory
Antirheumatic
NSAID
Salicylate

Therapeutic actions

Analgesic and antirheumatic effects are attributable to the ability to inhibit the synthesis of prostaglandins, important mediators of inflammation; antipyretic effects are not fully understood, but salicylates probably act in the thermoregulatory center of the hypothalamus to block the effects of endogenous pyrogen by inhibiting the synthesis of the prostaglandin intermediary; after absorption, this drug is hydrolyzed into two molecules of salicylic acid; insoluble in gastric secretions, it is not absorbed in the stomach, but in the small intestine; reported to cause fewer GI adverse effects than aspirin.

Indications

- Relief of mild to moderate pain
- Relief of symptoms of various inflammatory conditions—rheumatic disorders, rheumatoid arthritis, osteoarthritis

Contraindications and cautions

- Contraindicated with allergy to salicylates or NSAIDs, bleeding disorders, impaired hepatic or renal function, GI ulceration (less of a problem with salsalate than with other anti-inflammatories), lactation and perioperatively in patients undergoing coronary artery bypass graft surgery.
- Use cautiously in pregnancy; and in children and teenagers with influenza or chickenpox—use of salicylates in these patients may be associated with the development of Reye syndrome. This acute, life-threatening condition, characterized by vomiting, lethargy, and belligerence, may progress to delirium and coma and has a mortality rate of 20%–30%.

Available forms

Tablets—500, 750 mg

Dosages

Adults
3,000 mg/day PO given in divided doses.
Pediatric patients
Safety and efficacy not established.

Pharmacokinetics

Route	Onset	Peak	Duration
Oral	10–30 min	1–3 hr	3–16 hr

Metabolism: Hepatic; $T_{1/2}$: 2–3 hr (15–30 hr with large doses over extended periods)
Distribution: Crosses placenta; enters breast milk
Excretion: Urine

Adverse effects

- **Acute salicylate toxicity:** Respiratory alkalosis, hyperpnea, tachypnea, hemorrhage, excitement, confusion, asterixis, pulmonary edema, seizures, tetany, metabolic acidosis, fever, coma, **CV collapse, renal and respiratory failure**
- **CNS:** *Headache, dizziness, somnolence, insomnia,* fatigue, tiredness, dizziness, tinnitus, ophthalmologic effects
- **Dermatologic:** *Rash,* pruritus, sweating, dry mucous membranes, stomatitis
- **GI:** *Nausea, dyspepsia, GI pain,* diarrhea, vomiting, *constipation,* flatulence
- **GU:** Dysuria, renal impairment
- **Hematologic:** Bleeding, platelet inhibition with higher doses, neutropenia, eosinophilia, leukopenia, pancytopenia, thrombocytopenia, agranulocytosis, granulocytopenia, aplastic anemia, decreased Hgb or Hct, bone marrow depression, menorrhagia
- **Respiratory:** Dyspnea, hemoptysis, pharyngitis, **bronchospasm,** rhinitis
- **Salicylism:** Dizziness, tinnitus, difficulty hearing, nausea, vomiting, diarrhea, mental confusion, lassitude (dose-related)
- **Other:** Peripheral edema, **anaphylactoid reactions** to **anaphylactic shock**

Interactions

✳ **Drug-drug** • Increased risk of GI ulceration with corticosteroids and alcohol • Increased risk of salicylate toxicity with carbonic anhydrase inhibitors • Increased toxicity of carbonic anhydrase inhibitors, valproic acid • Decreased serum salicylate levels with corticosteroids, antacids, urine alkalinizers (sodium acetate, sodium bicarbonate, sodium citrate, sodium lactate, tromethamine) • Increased methotrexate levels and toxicity • Greater glucose-lowering effect of sulfonylureas, insulin with large doses of salicylates • Decreased uricosuric effect of probenecid, sulfinpyrazone • Decreased diuretic effect of spironolactone

✳ **Drug-lab test** • Salicylate competes with thyroid hormone for binding to plasma proteins, which may be reflected in a depressed plasma T_4 value • False-negative readings for urine glucose by glucose oxidase method and copper reduction method • Interference with urine 5-HIAA determinations by fluorescent methods but not by nitrosonaphthol colorimetric method • Interference with urinary ketone determination by ferric chloride method

• Falsely elevated urine VMA levels with most tests; false decrease in VMA using the Pisano method • Serum uric acid levels are elevated by salicylate levels less than 10 mg/dL and decreased by levels greater than 10 mg/dL

■ Nursing considerations
Assessment
• **History:** Allergy to salicylates or NSAIDs, bleeding disorders, impaired hepatic or renal function, GI ulceration, lactation, pregnancy
• **Physical:** Skin color and lesions; eighth cranial nerve function, orientation, reflexes, affect; P, BP, perfusion; R, adventitious sounds; liver evaluation and bowel sounds; CBC, urinalysis, stool guaiac, LFTs, renal function tests

Interventions
⊗ **Black box warning** Patient may be at increased risk for GI bleeding and CV events; monitor accordingly.
• Administer drug with food or after meals if GI upset occurs.
• Administer drug with a full glass of water to reduce risk of tablet or capsule lodging in the esophagus.
⊗ **Warning** Institute emergency procedures if overdose occurs: Gastric lavage, induction of emesis, activated charcoal, supportive therapy.
• Provide further comfort measures to reduce pain, fever, and inflammation.

Teaching points
• Take the drug with food or after meals if GI upset occurs.
• Do not take this drug with other salicylates.
• Report ringing in the ears, dizziness, confusion, abdominal pain, rapid or difficult breathing, nausea, vomiting.

▽ **sapropterin dihydrochloride**

See Appendix R, *Less commonly used drugs.*

▽ **saquinavir mesylate**
(sa kwen' a veer)

Invirase

PREGNANCY CATEGORY B

Drug classes
Antiretroviral
Protease inhibitor

Therapeutic actions
Protease inhibitor, which in combination with nucleoside analogues is effective in HIV infections with changes in surrogate markers.

Indications
• Treatment of HIV infection in combination with other antiretrovirals in patients older than 16 yr

Contraindications and cautions
• Contraindicated with life-threatening allergy to any component, severe hepatic impairment, congenital prolonged QT interval, complete AV block, hypokalemia, hypomagnesemia, concurrent use of saquinavir/ritonavir with rifompin.
• Use cautiously with pregnancy, lactation, hemophilia, diabetes.

Available forms
Capsules—200 mg; tablets—500 mg

Dosages
Adults and patients older than 16 yr
1,000 mg bid with ritonavir 100 mg bid given together within 2 hr after a meal or with lopinavir 400 mg/ritonavir 100 mg PO bid (tablets); 1,000 mg bid PO with lopinavir 400 mg ritonavir 100 mg PO bid (capsules).
Pediatric patients younger than 16 yr
Safety and efficacy not established.
Patients with hepatic impairment
Drug is contraindicated with severe hepatic impairment.

Pharmacokinetics

Route	Onset	Peak
Oral	Slow	Unknown

Metabolism: Hepatic; $T_{1/2}$: 3–6 hr

S .

Distribution: May cross placenta; may enter breast milk
Excretion: Feces

Adverse effects

- **CNS:** *Headache,* insomnia, myalgia, malaise, dizziness, paresthesia, fatigue
- **CV:** Prolonged QT interval, prolonged PR interval
- **GI:** *Nausea, GI pain, diarrhea,* anorexia, vomiting, dyspepsia
- **Metabolic:** Fat redistribution may occur (central obesity, buffalo hump, cushingoid appearance), hyperglycemia
- **Other:** *Asthenia,* elevated CPK, elevated triglycerides, cholesterol, myalgia

Interactions

✳ **Drug-drug** • Decreased effectiveness with rifampin, rifabutin, phenobarbital, phenytoin, dexamethasone, carbamazepine, nevirapine • Increased saquinavir plasma concentrations with clarithromycin, indinavir, ritonavir, nelfinavir, delavirdine, ketoconazole • Increased sildenafil concentrations when coadministered with saquinavir • Potential for serious to life-threatening reactions with docetaxel, ergot derivatives, midazolam, triazolam, antiarrhythmics, rifampin • Risk of serious hepatic toxicity if combined with HMG-CoA inhibitors (statins); avoid this combination and, if use is required, monitor LFTs regularly • Risk of severe prolonged QT interval if combined with other drugs that prolong QT interval; avoid this combination.

✳ **Drug-food** • Decreased metabolism and risk of toxic effects if combined with grapefruit juice, garlic capsules; avoid these combinations

✳ **Drug-alternative therapy** • Decreased effectiveness if combined with St. John's Wort

■ Nursing considerations

CLINICAL ALERT!
Name confusion has occurred between saquinavir and *Sinequan;* use caution.

Assessment

- **History:** Life-threatening allergy to any component; impaired hepatic function, pregnancy, lactation, diabetes, hemophilia
- **Physical:** T; affect, reflexes, peripheral sensation; bowel sounds, liver evaluation; LFTs, CPK levels, abdominal examination, baseline ECG

Interventions

⊗ ***Black box warning*** Capsules and tablets are not interchangeable; use tablets only when combined with ritonavir. If saquinavir is the only protease inhibitor in a treatment regimen, use capsules.

- Administer within 2 hr after a full meal.
- Monitor patient for signs of opportunistic infections that will need to be treated appropriately.
- Administer the drug concurrently with a nucleoside analogue.
- Offer support and encouragement to the patient to deal with the diagnosis as well as the effects of drug therapy and the high expense of treatment.

Teaching points

- Take drug as prescribed; take within 2 hours of a full meal; take concurrently with other prescribed medication. Do not drink grapefruit juice while using this drug. Do not use St. John's Wort while taking this drug.
- Store drug at room temperature; use by expiration date.
- These drugs are not a cure for AIDS or AIDS-related complex; opportunistic infections may occur and regular medical care should be sought to deal with the disease.
- The long-term effects of this drug are not yet known.
- This drug combination does not reduce the risk of transmission of HIV to others by sexual contact or blood contamination—use appropriate precautions.
- You may experience these side effects: Nausea, loss of appetite, change in taste (eat frequent small meals); dizziness, loss of feeling (take appropriate precautions).
- Report extreme fatigue, lethargy, severe headache, severe nausea, vomiting, difficulty breathing, rash, changes in color of urine or stool.

▽ **sargramostim**
(granulocyte macrophage colony–stimulating factor, GM-CSF)
*(sar **gram**' oh stim)*

Leukine

PREGNANCY CATEGORY C

Drug class
Colony-stimulating factor

Therapeutic actions
Human GM-CSF produced by recombinant DNA technology; increases the proliferation and differentiation of hematopoietic progenitor cells; can activate mature granulocytes and macrophages.

Indications
- Myeloid reconstitution after autologous bone marrow transplantation and allogenic bone marrow transplantation
- Treatment of neutropenia associated with bone marrow transplantation failure or engraftment delay
- Induction chemotherapy in AML to shorten neutrophil recovery time
- Acceleration of myeloid recovery in patients with non-Hodgkin lymphoma, acute lymphoblastic leukemia, and Hodgkin lymphoma undergoing autologous bone marrow transplantation
- Mobilization of hematopoietic progenitor cells for collection by leukapheresis and to accelerate myeloid reconstitution following peripheral blood progenitor cell (PBPC) transplantation
- Unlabeled uses: Treatment of myelodysplastic syndrome, decreases nadir of leukopenia related to myelosuppression of chemotherapy, corrects neutropenia in aplastic anemia patients, decreases transplant-associated organ system damage, promotes early grafting; stomatitis, melanoma, drug-induced neutropenia, Crohn disease, oral mucositis

Contraindications and cautions
- Contraindicated with hypersensitivity to yeast products; excessive leukemic myeloid blasts in bone marrow or peripheral blood; in neonates (benzyl alcohol is a constituent of *Leukine* liquid and bacteriostatic water for injection diluent and should not be administered to neonates because of association with fatal "gasping syndrome"); concomitant use with chemotherapy and radiation therapy or within 24 hr preceding or following chemotherapy or radiation therapy.
- Use cautiously with renal or hepatic failure, pregnancy, lactation.

Available forms
Powder for injection—250 mcg; solution for injection—500 mg/mL

Dosages
Adults
- *Myeloid reconstitution after autologous or allogenic bone marrow transplantation:* 250 mcg/m^2/day for 21 days as a 2-hr IV infusion beginning 2–4 hr after the autologous bone marrow infusion and not less than 24 hr after the last dose of chemotherapy and radiation therapy. Patient should not receive sargramostim until post-marrow infusion ANC is less than 500 cells/mm^3. Continue until ANC is greater than 1,500 cells/mm^3 for 3 consecutive days. If severe adverse reactions occur, decrease dose by 50% or stop drug. If patient has blast cells or disease progression, stop drug immediately.
- *Bone marrow transplantation failure or engraftment delay:* 250 mcg/m^2/day for 14 days as a 2-hr IV infusion; the dose can be repeated after 7 days off therapy if engraftment has not occurred. If engraftment still does not occur, third dose of 500 mcg/m^2/day may be administered for 14 days after another 7 days off therapy.
- *Neutrophil recovery following chemotherapy in AML:* 250 mcg/m^2/day IV over 4 hr starting on about day 11 or 4 days after chemotherapy induction. Continue until ANC is greater than 1,500 cells/mm^3 for 3 consecutive days, or a maximum of 42 days.
- *Mobilization of PBPC:* 250 mcg/m^2/day IV over 24 hr or subcutaneously once daily; continue throughout harvesting.
- *Post-PBPC transplant:* 250 mcg/m^2/day IV over 24 hr or subcutaneously once daily beginning immediately after infusion of progenitor cells; continue until ANC is greater than 1,500 cells/mm^3 for 3 consecutive days.

Pediatric patients
Safety and efficacy not established.

Pharmacokinetics

Route	Peak	Duration
IV	2 hr or more	6 hr
Subcut.	1–3 hr	6 hr

Metabolism: Unknown; $T_{1/2}$ (IV): 60 min; subcutaneous: 162 min

Distribution: May cross placenta; may enter breast milk
Excretion: Unknown

▼**IV FACTS**

Preparation: Reconstitute powder with 1 mL sterile water for injection or 1 mL bacteriostatic water for injection; gently swirl contents to avoid foaming. Do not shake, and avoid excessive agitation. Resulting solution should be clear, colorless, and isotonic. Do not reenter vial; discard any unused portion. Dilute in 0.9% sodium chloride injection; administer within 6 hr; refrigerate until ready to use.
Infusion: ⊗ *Warning* Infuse over 2 hr; do not use an in-line membrane filter; do not mix with any other medication in any other diluent (except if albumin is needed for final concentration; see package label).
Incompatibilities: Do not mix with any solution other than 0.9% sodium chloride. Do not add to any other medications.

Adverse effects

- **CNS:** Headache, *fever,* generalized weakness, fatigue, *malaise, asthenia*
- **CV:** Edema, **hemorrhage**
- **Dermatologic:** *Alopecia,* rash, mucositis
- **GI:** *Nausea, vomiting,* stomatitis, anorexia, *diarrhea,* constipation
- **Other:** *Bone pain,* generalized pain, sore throat, cough, arthralgia

Interactions

✷ **Drug-drug** • Drugs that may potentiate the myeloproliferative effects of sargramostim, such as lithium and corticosteroids, should be used with caution

■ **Nursing considerations**
Assessment

- **History:** Hypersensitivity to yeast products; pregnancy, lactation, excessive leukemic myeloid blasts in bone marrow or peripheral blood, renal or hepatic failure
- **Physical:** Skin color, lesions, hair; T; abdominal examination, status of mucous membranes; blood counts, platelets, body weight and hydration status

Interventions

- Obtain CBC and platelet count prior to and twice weekly during therapy.

⊗ *Warning* Administer no less than 24 hr after cytotoxic chemotherapy and within 2–4 hr of bone marrow infusion.
- Administer daily as a 2-hr infusion.
⊗ *Warning* Store in refrigerator; do not freeze or shake. Use powder within 6 hr of mixing. If using powder, use each vial for one dose; do not reenter vial. Discard any unused drug.
- Do not shake vial before use.

Teaching points

- This drug must be taken as long as needed.
- Avoid exposure to infection (avoid crowds, visitors with infections).
- This drug should not be taken during pregnancy; using barrier contraceptives is advised.
- Frequent blood tests will be needed to evaluate drug effects.
- You may experience these side effects: Nausea and vomiting (eat frequent small meals); loss of hair (obtain appropriate head covering; cover head in temperature extremes); fever (request medication).
- Report fever, chills, sore throat, weakness, pain or swelling at injection site, difficulty breathing, chills.

DANGEROUS DRUG

▷ **saxagliptin hydrochloride**
(sacks ah **glip'** *ten)*

Onglyza

PREGNANCY CATEGORY B

Drug classes
Antidiabetic drug
DPP4 (dipeptidyl peptidase-4) enzyme inhibitor

Therapeutic actions
Slows the inactivation of the incretin hormones, increasing these hormone levels and prolonging their activity. The incretin hormones stimulate insulin release in response to a meal and help regulate glucose homeostasis throughout the day. This increases and prolongs insulin release and reduces hepatic glucose production to help achieve glycemic control.

Indications
- As an adjunct to diet and exercise to improve glycemic control in adults with type 2 diabetes

Contraindications and cautions
- Contraindicated with history of serious hypersensitivity reactions to saxagliptin; type 1 diabetes, diabetic ketoacidosis.
- Use cautiously with moderate or severe renal impairment, concurrent use of strong CYP3A inhibitors, pregnancy, lactation.

Available forms
Tablets—2.5, 5 mg

Dosages
Adults
2.5–5 mg/day PO without regard to meals.
Pediatric patients
Safety and efficacy not established.
Patients with renal impairment
2.5 mg/day PO for moderate to severe renal impairment (CrCl 50 mL/min or less); administer following hemodialysis.

Pharmacokinetics
Route	Onset	Peak
Oral	Moderate	2 hr

Metabolism: Hepatic; $T_{1/2}$: 2.5–3 hr
Distribution: May cross placenta; enters breast milk
Excretion: Feces, urine

Adverse effects
- **CNS:** *Headache*, dizziness
- **GI:** Abdominal pain, gastroenteritis, vomiting
- **GU:** *UTI*
- **Respiratory:** *URI*, nasopharyngitis
- **Other:** Hypoglycemia

Interactions
＊ **Drug-drug** • Risk of increased plasma levels and toxicity if combined with strong CYP3A4/5 inhibitors (atazanavir, clarithromycin, ketoconazole, indinavir, itraconazole, nefazodone, nelfinavir, ritonavir, saquinavir, telithromycin); if this combination is used, limit saxagliptin dosage to 2.5 mg/day

＊ **Drug-alternative therapies** • Increased risk of hypoglycemia if taken with celery, coriander, dandelion root, fenugreek, garlic, ginseng, juniper berries

■ Nursing considerations
Assessment
- **History:** Hypersensitivity to component of drug, renal impairment, pregnancy, lactation
- **Physical:** R, adventitious sounds; renal function tests; blood glucose, HbA_{1c} levels

Interventions
- Monitor blood glucose and HbA_{1c} levels before and periodically during therapy.
- Monitor renal function tests before and periodically during therapy.
- Ensure that patient continues diet and exercise program for management of type 2 diabetes.
- If appropriate, ensure that patient continues use of other prescribed drugs to manage type 2 diabetes.
- Arrange for thorough diabetic teaching program, including diet, exercise, signs and symptoms of hypoglycemia and hyperglycemia, and safety measures to avoid infections and injuries.

Teaching points
- Take this drug once a day, with or without food.
- If you forget a dose, take it as soon as you remember; then begin your usual dosage the next day. Do not make up skipped doses and do not take more than one dose each day.
- Maintain your blood glucose level as directed by your health care provider.
- Continue the diet and exercise program designed for the treatment of your type 2 diabetes. Continue other drugs you may be using to treat your diabetes if instructed to do so by your health care provider.
- Arrange for periodic monitoring of your fasting blood glucose and glycosylated hemoglobin levels.
- Know that your health care provider will request periodic blood tests to monitor your kidney function.
- It is not known how this drug affects a fetus. If you are pregnant or thinking about becoming pregnant, discuss this with your health care provider.
- This drug does enter breast milk, but it is not known how this could affect a breast-feeding infant. If you are breast-feeding, discuss this with your health care provider.
- During times of stress (surgery, infection, injury), the needs of your body change.

S

Consult your health care provider immediately if you experience stress. The dosage of your antidiabetic drugs and the actual drugs that are needed may change.

- Report the use of herbal or over-the-counter therapies or other prescription drugs to your health care provider; many of these may change your glucose level and dosage adjustments will be needed,
- Report signs and symptoms of infection, uncontrolled glucose level, severe headache, increased stress, trauma.

▽**scopolamine hydrobromide (hyoscine HBr)**

(*skoe pol' a meen*)

Parenteral: Scopolamine HBr
Transdermal system:
Transderm-Scop, Transderm-V (CAN)
Ophthalmic solution: Isopto Hyoscine Ophthalmic

PREGNANCY CATEGORY C

Drug classes
Anticholinergic
Antiemetic
Anti–motion-sickness drug
Antimuscarinic
Antiparkinsonian
Antispasmodic
Belladonna alkaloid
Parasympatholytic

Therapeutic actions
Mechanism of action as anti–motion-sickness drug not understood; antiemetic action may be mediated by interference with cholinergic impulses to the vomiting center (CTZ); has sedative and amnesia-inducing properties; blocks effects of acetylcholine at muscarinic cholinergic receptors that mediate effects of parasympathetic postganglionic impulses, thus depressing salivary and bronchial secretions, inhibiting vagal influences on the heart, relaxing the GI and GU tracts, inhibiting gastric acid secretion, relaxing the pupil of the eye (mydriatic effect), and preventing accommodation for near vision (cycloplegic effect).

Indications
- Transdermal system: Prevention and control of nausea and vomiting associated with motion sickness and recovery from surgery
- Injection: Preanesthetic medication to control bronchial, nasal, pharyngeal, and salivary secretions; prevent bronchospasm and laryngospasm; block cardiac vagal inhibitory reflexes during induction of anesthesia and intubation; produce sedation
- Injection: Induction of obstetric amnesia with analgesics calming delirium
- Oral: Treatment of postencephalitic parkinsonism and paralysis agitans; relief of symptoms in spastic states; maniacal states; delirium tremens
- Ophthalmic solution: Diagnostically to produce mydriasis and cycloplegia
- Ophthalmic solution: Preoperative and postoperative states in the treatment of iridocyclitis
- Unlabeled uses: Sialorrhea (transdermal), postoperative and chemotherapy-induced nausea and vomiting (oral)

Contraindications and cautions
- Contraindicated with hypersensitivity to anticholinergic drugs; glaucoma; adhesions between iris and lens; stenosing peptic ulcer, pyloroduodenal obstruction, paralytic ileus, intestinal atony, severe ulcerative colitis, toxic megacolon, symptomatic prostatic hypertrophy, bladder neck obstruction; bronchial asthma, COPD, cardiac arrhythmias, tachycardia, myocardial ischemia; impaired metabolic, liver, or renal function (increased likelihood of adverse CNS effects); myasthenia gravis; pregnancy (causes respiratory depression in neonates, contributes to neonatal hemorrhage); lactation.
- Use cautiously with Down syndrome, brain damage, spasticity, hypertension, hyperthyroidism; glaucoma or tendency to glaucoma (ophthalmic solution).

Available forms
Injection—0.3, 0.4, 0.86, 1 mg/mL; transdermal system—1.5 mg; ophthalmic solution—0.25%

Adverse effects in *italics* are most common; those in **bold** are life-threatening. ⊂▣⊃ Do not crush.

Dosages
Adults
Transdermal system
- *Motion sickness:* Apply one transdermal system to the postauricular skin at least 4 hr before antiemetic effect is required or on the evening before scheduled surgery. Scopolamine 1 mg will be delivered over 3 days. If continued effect is needed, replace system every 3 days.
Parenteral
- *Obstetric amnesia, preoperative sedation:* 0.32–0.65 mg subcutaneously or IM. May give IV after dilution in sterile water for injection. May repeat if needed up to qid.
- *Sedation, tranquilization:* 0.6 mg subcutaneously or IM three or four times a day.
- *Antiemetic:* 0.6–1 mg subcutaneously.
Ophthalmic solution
- *Refraction:* Instill 1–2 drops into the eye or eyes 1 hr before refracting.
- *Uveitis:* Instill 1–2 drops into the eye or eyes up to four times a day.
Pediatric patients
Transdermal system
Do not use transdermal system in children.
Parenteral
0.006 mg/kg subcutaneously, IM or IV; maximum dose is 0.3 mg. 6 mo–3 yr: 0.1–0.15 mg IM or IV. 3 yr–6 yr: 0.2–0.3 mg IM or IV.
Antiemetic
0.006 mg/kg subcutaneously.
Geriatric patients
More likely to cause serious adverse reactions, especially CNS reactions; use lowest possible dose and monitor patient closely.

Pharmacokinetics

Route	Onset	Peak	Duration
IM, Subcut.	30 min	1 hr	4–6 hr
IV	10 min	1 hr	2–4 hr
Transdermal	4–5 hr	24 hr	72 hr
Ophthalmic	10–20 min	30–45 min	Days

Metabolism: Hepatic; $T_{1/2}$: 8 hr
Distribution: Crosses placenta; enters breast milk
Excretion: Urine

IV FACTS
Preparation: Dilute in sterile water for injection.
Infusion: Inject directly into vein or into tubing of actively running IV; inject slowly over 5–10 min.

Adverse effects
- **CNS:** *Pupil dilation, photophobia, blurred vision, headache, drowsiness,* dizziness, mental confusion, excitement, restlessness, hallucinations, delirium in the presence of pain, elevated intraocular pressure
- **CV:** Palpitations, tachycardia
- **GI:** *Dry mouth, constipation,* paralytic ileus, altered taste perception, nausea, vomiting, dysphagia, heartburn
- **GU:** *Urinary hesitancy and retention,* impotence
- **Hypersensitivity: Anaphylaxis,** urticaria, other dermatologic effects
- **Other:** Suppression of lactation, flushing, fever, *nasal congestion, decreased sweating*

Interactions
❋ Drug-drug ● Decreased antipsychotic effectiveness of haloperidol ● Decreased effectiveness of phenothiazines, but increased incidence of paralytic ileus ● Increased CNS depression with alcohol ● Added anticholinergic effects if combined with antihistamines or antidepressants

■ Nursing considerations
Assessment
- **History:** Hypersensitivity to anticholinergic drugs; glaucoma; adhesions between iris and lens; stenosing peptic ulcer, pyloroduodenal obstruction, intestinal atony, severe ulcerative colitis, symptomatic prostatic hypertrophy, bladder neck obstruction; bronchial asthma, COPD; cardiac arrhythmias, myocardial ischemia; impaired metabolic, liver, or renal function; myasthenia gravis; Down syndrome; brain damage, spasticity; hypertension; hyperthyroidism; pregnancy; lactation
- **Physical:** Skin color, lesions, texture; T; orientation, reflexes, bilateral grip strength; affect; ophthalmic examination; P, BP; R, adventitious sounds; bowel sounds, normal output; urinary output, prostate palpation; LFTs, renal function tests, ECG

Interventions

- Ensure adequate hydration; provide environmental control (temperature) to prevent hyperpyrexia.

Teaching points

- Take as prescribed, 30–60 minutes before meals. Avoid excessive dosage.
- Avoid hot environments. You will be heat intolerant, and dangerous reactions may occur.
- Avoid alcohol; serious sedation could occur.
- When using transdermal system, take care to wash hands thoroughly after handling patch and dispose of patch properly to avoid contact with children and pets. Remove the old patch before applying a new one. Do not cut the patch.
- You may experience these side effects: Dizziness, sedation, drowsiness (use caution driving or performing tasks that require alertness); constipation (ensure adequate fluid intake, proper diet); dry mouth (sugarless candies, frequent mouth care may help; may lessen); blurred vision, sensitivity to light (reversible, avoid tasks that require acute vision; wear sunglasses); impotence (reversible); difficulty urinating (empty bladder before taking drug).
- Report rash, flushing, eye pain, difficulty breathing, tremors, loss of coordination, irregular heartbeat, abdominal distention, hallucinations, severe or persistent dry mouth, difficulty urinating, constipation, sensitivity to light.

DANGEROUS DRUG

▷secobarbital sodium

*(see koe **bar'** bi tal)*

Seconal Sodium

PREGNANCY CATEGORY D

CONTROLLED SUBSTANCE C-II

Drug classes

Antiepileptic
Barbiturate (short-acting)
Sedative-hypnotic

Therapeutic actions

General CNS depressant; barbiturates inhibit impulse conduction in the ascending RAS, depress the cerebral cortex, alter cerebellar function, depress motor output, and can produce excitation (especially with subanesthetic doses with pain), sedation, hypnosis, anesthesia, and deep coma; at anesthetic doses, has antiepileptic activity.

Indications

- Intermittent use as a sedative, hypnotic, or preanesthetic medication

Contraindications and cautions

- Contraindicated with hypersensitivity to barbiturates; manifest or latent porphyria; marked liver impairment; nephritis; severe respiratory distress, respiratory disease with dyspnea, obstruction, or cor pulmonale; previous addiction to sedative-hypnotic drugs (drug may be ineffective, and use may contribute to further addiction); pregnancy (readily crosses placenta and has caused fetal damage, neonatal withdrawal syndrome).
- Use cautiously with acute or chronic pain (drug may cause paradoxical excitement or mask important symptoms); seizure disorders (abrupt discontinuation of daily doses can result in status epilepticus); lactation (has caused drowsiness in breast-feeding infants); fever, hyperthyroidism, diabetes mellitus, severe anemia, pulmonary or cardiac disease, status asthmaticus, shock, uremia; impaired liver or renal function, debilitation.

Available forms

Capsules—100 mg

Dosages
Adults
Adjust dosage on basis of age, weight, condition.
- *Preoperative sedation:* 200–300 mg PO 1–2 hr before surgery.
- *Bedtime hypnotic:* 100 mg PO at bedtime; do not use longer than 2 wk.

Pediatric patients
⊗ **Warning** Barbiturates may produce irritability, excitability, inappropriate tearfulness, and aggression.
- *Preoperative sedation:* 2–6 mg/kg PO 1–2 hr before surgery; maximum dose, 100 mg.

Geriatric patients or patients with debilitating disease
Reduce dosage and monitor closely. May produce excitement, depression, or confusion.
Patients with hepatic or renal impairment
Reduce dosage.

Pharmacokinetics

Route	Onset	Duration
Oral	10–15 min	3–4 hr

Metabolism: Hepatic; $T_{1/2}$: 15–40 hr
Distribution: Crosses placenta; enters breast milk
Excretion: Urine

Adverse effects

- **CNS:** *Somnolence, agitation, confusion, hyperkinesia, ataxia, vertigo, CNS depression, nightmares, lethargy, residual sedation (hangover), paradoxical excitement, nervousness, psychiatric disturbance, hallucinations, insomnia, anxiety, dizziness, thinking abnormality,* complex sleep disorders
- **CV:** *Bradycardia, hypotension, syncope*
- **GI:** *Nausea, vomiting, constipation, diarrhea, epigastric pain*
- **Hypersensitivity:** Rashes, angioneurotic edema, serum sickness, morbilliform rash, urticaria; rarely, exfoliative dermatitis, **Stevens-Johnson syndrome**
- **Respiratory:** *Hypoventilation, apnea, respiratory depression,* **laryngospasm, bronchospasm,** circulatory collapse
- **Other:** Tolerance, psychological and physical dependence; **anaphylaxis, angioedema, withdrawal syndrome**

Interactions

✳ **Drug-drug** • Increased CNS depression with alcohol, antihistamines, sedatives, hypnotics • Decreased effects of oral anticoagulants, corticosteroids, hormonal contraceptives and estrogens, metronidazole, metoprolol, propranolol, doxycycline, oxyphenbutazone, phenylbutazone, quinidine with barbiturates • Decreased theophylline serum levels and effectiveness secondary to increased clearance • Decreased bioavailability of verapamil

■ Nursing considerations
Assessment

- **History:** Hypersensitivity to barbiturates; manifest or latent porphyria; nephritis; severe respiratory distress; previous addiction to sedative-hypnotic drugs; pregnancy; acute or chronic pain; seizure disorders; lactation; fever, hyperthyroidism, diabetes mellitus, severe anemia, pulmonary or cardiac disease, shock, uremia; impaired liver or renal function, debilitation
- **Physical:** Weight; T; skin color, lesions; orientation, affect, reflexes; P, BP, orthostatic BP; R, adventitious sounds; bowel sounds, normal output, liver evaluation; LFTs, renal function tests, blood and urine glucose, BUN

Interventions

⊗ *Warning* Monitor patient for anaphylaxis, angioedema, blood levels with the above interacting drugs; suggest alternatives to hormonal contraceptives.
- Do not use as a bedtime hypnotic for longer than 2 wk.
- Stay with children who have received preoperative sedation.

⊗ *Warning* Taper dosage gradually after repeated use, especially in patients who have epilepsy, to avoid refractory seizures.

Teaching points

- Do not use this drug with alcohol.
- Do not increase the dose of this drug without consulting your health care provider because of the risk of psychological or physical dependence.
- Do not use this drug during pregnancy; use of barrier contraceptives is recommended.
- If you are breast-feeding, you should use another method of feeding the infant.
- Do not stand or sit up after you have received this drug (request assistance if you must sit up or move about).
- This drug will make you drowsy (or induce sleep) and make you less anxious. This drug may cause allergic reaction, swelling, complex sleep-related behaviors.

▷ **secretin**
See Appendix R, *Less commonly used drugs.*

▽ selegiline hydrochloride

(se leh' ge leen)

Apo-Selegiline (CAN), Eldepryl, Emsam, Gen-Selegiline (CAN), Zelapar

PREGNANCY CATEGORY C

Drug classes
Antidepressant
Antiparkinsonian
MAO type B inhibitor

Therapeutic actions
Mechanism of action not completely understood; inhibits MAO type B activity; may have other mechanisms of increasing dopaminergic activity.

Indications
- Adjunct in management of patients with Parkinson disease whose response to levodopa and carbidopa has decreased
- Treatment of major depressive disorder (Emsam)
- Unlabeled use: Alzheimer disease

Contraindications and cautions
- Contraindicated with hypersensitivity to any component of the drug, pregnancy, lactation; concurrent use of carbamazepine or oxcarbazine, other MAOIs, methadone, tramadol, meperidine, dextromethorphan.
- Use cautiously with geriatric patients.

Available forms
Capsules—5 mg; tablets—5 mg; orally disintegrating tablets—1.25 mg; transdermal system—6 mg/24 hr, 9 mg/24 hr, 12 mg/24 hr

Dosages
Adults
- Parkinson disease: 10 mg/day PO in divided doses of 5 mg each taken at breakfast and lunch. After 2–3 days, attempt to decrease dose of levodopa and carbidopa; reductions of 10%–30% are typical. If using orally disintegrating tablet, 1.25 mg/day PO in the morning before breakfast. Place tablet on top of tongue; avoid food or beverage for 5 min. May be increased after 6 wk to 2.5 mg/day. Patient should be under close

supervision because of risk of altered mental state.
- Depression: Apply one patch (Emsam) daily to dry, intact skin on upper torso, upper thigh, or outer surface of upper arm. Start with 6-mg/24-hr system and increase to maximum of 12 mg/24 hr if needed and tolerated.

Pediatric patients
Not recommended for children younger than 12 yr (transdermal) or 16 yr (orally disintegrating).

Geriatric patients
Usual dose of transdermal system, 6 mg/24 hr. Use with caution and carefully monitor for orthostatic BP changes.

Pharmacokinetics

Route	Onset	Peak
Oral	Rapid	30–120 min

Metabolism: Hepatic; $T_{1/2}$: 20.5 hr
Distribution: Crosses placenta; enters breast milk
Excretion: Urine

Adverse effects
- **CNS:** Headache, dizziness, light-headedness, confusion, hallucinations, dyskinesias, vivid dreams, increased tremor, loss of balance, restlessness, depression, drowsiness, disorientation, apathy, blurred vision, diplopia
- **CV:** Orthostatic hypotension, hypertension, arrhythmia, palpitations, hypotension, tachycardia
- **Dermatologic:** Increased sweating, diaphoresis, facial hair development, hair loss, hematoma, rash, photosensitivity; application-site reaction (transdermal)
- **GI:** Nausea, vomiting, abdominal pain, dry mouth, constipation, rectal bleeding, heartburn, diarrhea, anorexia
- **GU:** Slow urination, transient nocturia, prostatic hypertrophy, urinary hesitancy, urine retention
- **Other: Asthma**

Interactions
❋ **Drug-drug** • Severe adverse effects to fatalities if combined with meperidine, fluoxetine, methadone, tramadol, TCAS; avoid these combinations • Use extreme caution with opioid analgesics • Concurrent use of carbamazepine, oxcarbazepine is contraindicated • Allow 2 wk after discontinuing any CNS stimulant (eg,

Adverse effects in *italics* are most common; those in **bold** are life-threatening. ⬚ Do not crush.

amphetamine, methylphenidate) before beginning selegiline

✴ **Drug-food** • Avoid tyramine-rich foods and beverages starting on first day of therapy with 9- or 12-mg patch; continue to avoid for 2 wk after reduction to 6-mg patch or discontinuation of 9- or 12-mg patch

■ **Nursing considerations**

Assessment

- **History:** Hypersensitivity to any component of drug; pregnancy, lactation
- **Physical:** Skin color, lesions; orientation, affect, reflexes; BP, standing BP, P; abdominal examination; prostate examination (males)

Interventions

⊗ *Black box warning* Risk of suicidality in children, adolescents, and young adults is increased; monitor accordingly.

- Administer oral drug only as adjunct to levodopa and carbidopa in patients whose symptoms are deteriorating; administer twice daily with breakfast and lunch.
- Limit oral drug to 10 mg/day; larger doses may lead to loss of MAO type B specificity and increase risk of severe hypertensive reactions.
- Dispense least amount of drug possible, especially with depressed patients.
- Administer orally disintegrating tablet by placing on patient's tongue; do not allow food or beverages for 5 min.
- Apply dermal patch to dry, intact skin on upper torso, upper thigh, or outer upper arm. Replace every 24 hr; remove the old patch before applying a new one.
- Monitor the patient for improvement in Parkinson disease symptoms; if symptoms improve after 2–3 days, begin reducing dosage of levodopa and carbidopa.
- Provide safety measures if dizziness and lightheadedness occur.
- Provide small, frequent meals if GI upset is a problem.
- Provide ice, sugarless candies to suck and frequent mouth care if dry mouth is an issue.
- Maintain usual program for treatment of patients with Parkinson disease.

Teaching points

- Take the oral drug twice a day, with breakfast and lunch. Continue to take your levodopa and carbidopa; the dosage may be decreased in a few days. Do not exceed 10 milligrams per

day; serious effects could occur; maintain all of your usual activities and restrictions related to your Parkinson disease.

- If using orally disintegrating tablets, place on your tongue and allow to dissolve; do not eat or drink anything for 5 minutes; do this in the morning before breakfast.
- If using the patch, apply to your upper torso, upper thigh, or outer upper arm on dry, intact skin; replace the patch every 24 hours; always remove the old patch before applying a new one.
- It is not known how this drug could affect a fetus, if you are pregnant or decide to become pregnant while on this drug, consult your health care provider.
- It is not known how this drug could affect a breast-feeding infant. If you are breast-feeding; consult your health care provider.
- This drug interacts with some other drugs, and this interaction could cause serious side effects; tell any health care provider who is taking care of you that you are on this drug.
- You may experience these side effects: Dizziness, drowsiness, anxiety, disorientation (do not drive a car or operate any dangerous machinery while on this drug; avoid making any important decisions); dry mouth (frequent mouth care, sugarless candies may help); nausea, vomiting (it is important to try to maintain your fluid intake and nutrition, let your health care provider know if this becomes difficult).
- Report severe headache, mood changes, confusion, sleep disturbances, dizziness on rising, fainting.

▽**sertraline hydrochloride**

(sir' trah leen)

Apo-Sertraline (CAN), Novo-Sertraline (CAN), ratio-Sertraline (CAN), Zoloft

PREGNANCY CATEGORY C (FIRST TRIMESTER)

PREGNANCY CATEGORY D (THIRD TRIMESTER)

Drug classes

Antidepressant
SSRI

Therapeutic actions

Acts as an antidepressant by inhibiting CNS neuronal uptake of serotonin; blocks uptake of serotonin with little effect on norepinephrine, muscarinic, histaminergic, and alpha₁-adrenergic or dopaminergic receptors.

Indications

- Treatment of major depressive disorder
- Treatment of OCD
- Treatment of panic disorder with or without agoraphobia
- Treatment of PTSD; long-term use to prevent relapse and sustain symptom improvement
- Treatment of PMDD
- Treatment of social anxiety disorder (social phobia)
- Unlabeled uses: Nocturnal enuresis, hot flashes, cholestatic pruritus, migraine prevention, smoking cessation, traumatic brain injury

Contraindications and cautions

- Contraindicated with hypersensitivity to sertraline; concurrent use of MAOIs, pimozide, disulfiram (oral concentrate).
- Use cautiously with impaired hepatic or renal function, pregnancy, lactation, latex sensitivity if using dropper dispenser.

Available forms

Tablets—25, 50, 100, 150, 200 mg; oral concentrate—20 mg/mL

Dosages

Adults

- *Major depressive disorder and OCD:* Administer once a day, morning or evening. 50 mg PO daily; may be increased to up to 200 mg/day; dosage increases should not occur at intervals less than 1 wk.
- *Panic disorder and PTSD:* 25 mg PO daily. After 1 wk increase to 50 mg once daily. Dose may be increased to 200 mg/day as needed.
- *PMDD:* 50 mg/day PO daily or just during luteal phase of menstrual cycle. Range, 50–150 mg/day.
- *Social anxiety disorder:* 25 mg/day PO; increase to 50 mg/day after 1 wk. Range, 50–200 mg/day.

Pediatric patients

- *OCD:*

6–12 yr: 25 mg PO once daily. May be increased slowly as needed. Maximum, 200 mg/day.
13–17 yr: 50 mg PO once daily. May be increased slowly at intervals of at least 1 wk as needed, to maximum of 200 mg/day.

Patients with hepatic impairment

Give a lower or less frequent dose. Use response as dosage guide.

Pharmacokinetics

Route	Onset	Peak
Oral	Slow	4.5–8.4 hr

Metabolism: Hepatic; $T_{1/2}$: 26 hr (104–active metabolite)
Distribution: Crosses placenta; may enter breast milk
Excretion: Feces, urine

Adverse effects

- **CNS:** *Headache, nervousness, drowsiness, anxiety, tremor, dizziness, insomnia,* lightheadedness, agitation, sedation, abnormal gait, psychosis, seizures, *vision changes, fatigue,* **suicidality**
- **CV:** Hot flashes, palpitations, chest pain
- **Dermatologic:** *Sweating,* rash, pruritus, acne, contact dermatitis
- **GI:** *Nausea,* vomiting, *diarrhea, dry mouth,* anorexia, dyspepsia, constipation, taste changes, flatulence, gastroenteritis, dysphagia, gingivitis
- **GU:** *Painful menstruation,* sexual dysfunction, frequency, cystitis, impotence, urgency, vaginitis
- **Respiratory:** URIs, pharyngitis, cough, dyspnea, bronchitis, *rhinitis*
- **Other:** Fever, back pain, thirst, serotonin syndrome

Interactions

❋ **Drug-drug** ⊗ *Warning* Serious, sometimes fatal, reactions with MAOIs; allow at least 14 days to elapse between MAOI and sertraline use.

⊗ *Warning* Possible risk of increased QTc interval if combined with pimozide or other drugs known to prolong QT interval; do not use together.

- Increased serum levels of sertraline with cimetidine

✳ **Drug-food** • Increased rate of absorption with food

✳ **Drug-alternative therapy** • Increased risk of severe reaction if combined with St. John's Wort

■ **Nursing considerations**
Assessment

• **History:** Hypersensitivity to sertraline, impaired hepatic or renal function, lactation, pregnancy

• **Physical:** Weight; T; skin rash, lesions; reflexes, affect; bowel sounds, liver evaluation; P, peripheral perfusion; urinary output, LFTs, renal function tests

Interventions
⊗ **Black box warning** Risk of suicidality is increased in children, adolescents, and young adults; monitor accordingly. Drug is only approved to, treat OCD in children; it's not approved for any other indication in children.

• Use lower dose in elderly patients and with hepatic or renal impairment.

• Dilute oral concentrate in 4 oz water, ginger ale, lemon-lime soda, lemonade, or orange juice only; administer immediately after diluting.

⊗ **Warning** Establish suicide precautions for severely depressed patients. Limit number of tablets given at any time.

• Give drug once a day, morning or evening.

• Increase dosage at intervals of not less than 1 wk.

• Counsel patient to use nonhormonal contraceptives; pregnancy should be avoided due to risk to fetus.

Teaching points

• Take this drug once a day, at the same time, morning or evening; do not exceed the prescribed dose. It may take 4–6 weeks to see any improvement.

• Dilute concentrate immediately before use in 4 ounces of water, ginger ale, lemon-lime soda, lemonade, or orange juice only.

• Consult your health care provider if you think that you are pregnant or wish to become pregnant.

• You may experience these side effects: Dizziness, drowsiness, nervousness, insomnia (avoid driving or performing hazardous tasks); nausea, vomiting (eat frequent small

meals); dry mouth (suck sugarless candies; perform frequent mouth care); excessive sweating (monitor temperature; avoid overheating).

• Report rash, mania, seizures, edema, difficulty breathing, increased depression, thoughts of suicide.

▽ **sevelamer hydrochloride**

See Appendix R, *Less commonly used drugs.*

▽ **sildenafil citrate**
(sill den' ah fill)

Revatio, Viagra

PREGNANCY CATEGORY B

Drug classes
Impotence drug
Phosphodiesterase inhibitor

Therapeutic actions
Selectively inhibits cGMP-specific phosphodiesterase type 5. The mechanism of penile erection involves the release of nitric oxide into the corpus cavernosum of the penis during sexual stimulation. Nitrous oxide activates cGMP, which causes smooth muscle relaxation, allowing the flow of blood into the corpus cavernosum. Sildenafil prevents the breakdown of cGMP by phosphodiesterase, leading to increased cGMP levels and prolonged smooth muscle relaxation, promoting the flow of blood into the corpus cavernosum and decreasing pressure in the pulmonary bed.

Indications

• Treatment of ED in the presence of sexual stimulation (*Viagra*)

• Treatment of pulmonary arterial hypertension to improve exercise ability (*Revatio*)

• Unlabeled uses: Esophageal motility disorders, anal fissures, antidepressant/antipsychotic-induced sexual dysfunction, pulmonary hypertension in children, Raynaud phenomenon, sexual dysfunction in women

Contraindications and cautions

• Contraindicated with allergy to any component of the tablet, concomitant use of

S

nitrates; contraindicated for women or children if used for sexual dysfunction.
- Use cautiously with hepatic or renal impairment; with anatomic deformation of the penis; with known cardiac disease (effects of sexual activity need to be evaluated); concomitant use of protease inhibitors when used for pulmonary hypertension

Available forms

Tablets—20 mg (*Revatio*); 25, 50, 100 mg (*Viagra*); single use vial for injection—10 mg/12.5 mL (*Revatio*)

Dosages
Adults
ED: 50 mg PO taken 1 hr before anticipated sexual activity; range, 25–100 mg PO. May be taken 30 min–4 hr before sexual activity. Limit use to once per day (*Viagra*).
Pulmonary arterial hypertension: 20 mg PO tid, at least 4–6 hr apart and without regard to food (*Revatio*); or 10 mg by IV bolus tid (*Revatio*).
Pediatric patients
Not intended for use in children.
Geriatric patients
For patients older than 65 yr, start with 25 mg PO when used for erectile dysfunction.
Patients with renal or hepatic impairment
Patients with hepatic impairment or creatinine clearance less than 30 mL/min may have increased serum levels; start dose at 25 mg PO (*Viagra*); no dosage adjustment needed for *Revatio*.

Pharmacokinetics

Route	Onset	Peak
Oral	Rapid	30–120 min
IV	Rapid	Unknown

Metabolism: Hepatic; $T_{1/2}$: 4 hr
Distribution: Not intended for use in women, no clear studies on crossing the placenta or entering breast milk (*Viagra*)
Excretion: Feces, urine

▼ IV FACTS

Preparation: Use as provided; solution should be clear and colorless. Store at room temperature. Single use only.

Infusion: Administer as IV bolus into actively running line or by direct IV injection.

Adverse effects
- **CNS:** *Headache,* abnormal vision, dizziness, nasal congestion, ischemic optic neuropathy, sudden loss of hearing, temporary amnesia
- **CV:** *Flushing*
- **GI:** *Dyspepsia,* diarrhea
- **Other:** UTI, rash, priapism

Interactions
✳ **Drug-drug** ⊗ **Warning** Possible severe hypotension and serious cardiac events if combined with nitrates or alpha adrenergic blockers; this combination must be avoided.
- Increased risk of bleeding with warfarin; closely monitor patient of this combination is used • Possible increased sildenafil levels and effects if taken with cimetidine, amlodipine, erythromycin, protease inhibitors; monitor patient and reduce dosage as needed • Risk of toxic effects if combined with protease inhibitors when used to treat pulmonary hypertension; avoid this combination • Risk of orthostatic hypotension with alcohol; avoid this combination
✳ **Drug-food** • Decreased rate of absorption and onset of action if taken with a high-fat meal
- Decreased metabolism and risk of toxic effects if combined with grapefruit juice; avoid this combination

■ Nursing considerations
Assessment
- **History:** Allergy to any component of the tablet; hepatic or renal impairment; with anatomical deformation of the penis, known cardiac disease; concomitant use of nitrates
- **Physical:** Orientation, affect; skin color, lesions; P, BP, ECG, LFTs, renal function tests

Interventions
- Ensure diagnosis of pulmonary arterial hypertension (*Revatio*). Reserve IV use for patients unable to take oral form.
- Ensure diagnosis of ED and determine underlying causes and other appropriate treatment (*Viagra*).
- Advise patient that drug does not work in the absence of sexual stimulation. Limit use to once per day (*Viagra*).

Adverse effects in italics *are most common; those in* **bold** *are life-threatening.* ⬛ Do not crush.

- Remind patient that drug does not protect against STDs and appropriate measures should be taken.

⊗ *Warning* Advise patient to never take this drug with nitrates; serious and even fatal complications can occur.

⊗ *Warning* Advise patients receiving HIV medications that there is an increased risk of sildenafil-associated adverse drug reactions, including hypotension, visual changes, and priapism. Do not exceed 25 mg of sildenafil in 48 hr; use extreme caution if using *Revatio*.

⊗ *Warning* Advise patients not to take this drug within 4 hr of an alpha blocker.

Teaching points

- For erectile dysfunction, take this drug 30 minutes to 4 hours before anticipated sexual activity. The usual timing is 1 hour. The drug will have no effect in the absence of sexual stimulation.
- If taking this drug for pulmonary arterial hypertension take three times a day; make sure the doses are 4–6 hours apart.
- Onset of drug effects will be slowed if taken with a high-fat meal; plan accordingly. Avoid drinking grapefruit juice if using this drug.
- This drug will not protect you from sexually transmitted diseases; use appropriate precautions.
- Erections lasting longer than 4 hr have occurred when drug is used for erectile dysfunction. If this should occur, seek medical attention immediately to prevent tissue damage.
- Stop the drug and call your health care provider immediately if you experience sudden loss of vision.
- Do not take this drug if you are taking any nitrates; serious side effects and even death can occur.
- You may experience these side effects: Headache, dizziness, rash, flushing.
- Report difficult or painful urination, rash, dizziness, palpitations, loss of vision or hearing.

▽ silodosin
*(sill oh **do'** zin)*

Rapaflo

PREGNANCY CATEGORY B

Drug classes
Alpha$_1$-adrenergic blocker
BPH drug

Therapeutic actions
Blocks the smooth muscle alpha$_1$-adrenergic receptors in the prostate, prostatic capsule, prostatic urethra, and bladder neck, leading to bladder and prostate relaxation and improved urine flow in cases of BPH.

Indications
- Treatment of signs and symptoms of BPH

Contraindications and cautions
- Contraindicated with known hypersensitivity to any component of the drug, lactation, pregnancy, severe renal impairment, severe hepatic impairment, concurrent use of strong CP450 inhibitors.
- Use cautiously in patients with hypotension, prostate cancer, cataract surgery, moderate renal impairment.

Available forms
Capsules: 4, 8 mg

Dosages
Adults
8 mg/day PO once daily with a meal.
Pediatric patients
Safety and efficacy not established.
Patients with renal impairment
With severe renal impairment (creatinine clearance of 30 mL/min or less), drug is contraindicated; with moderate renal impairment (creatinine clearance of 30–50 mL/min), 4 mg/day PO once daily with a meal.
Patients with hepatic impairment
With severe hepatic impairment (Child-Pugh score of 10 or more), drug is contraindicated. With mild to moderate hepatic impairment, no dosage adjustment is needed.

S

Pharmacokinetics

Route	Onset	Peak
Oral	Rapid	2–3.5 hr

Metabolism: Hepatic; $T_{1/2}$: 5–20 hr
Distribution: May cross placenta; may enter breast milk (not indicated for use in women)
Excretion: Feces, urine

Adverse effects

- **CNS:** *Dizziness, headache,* insomnia
- **CV:** Orthostatic hypotension
- **GI:** Diarrhea, impaired hepatic function
- **GU:** *Retrograde ejaculation, abnormal ejaculate*
- **Respiratory:** Nasopharyngitis, nasal congestion, sinusitis
- **Other:** Pruritus, purpura, intraoperative floppy iris syndrome with cataract surgery

Interactions

✴ **Drug-drug** • Increased risk of elevated silodosin serum levels and toxicity if combined with strong CP450 inhibitors (ketoconazole, clarithromycin, itraconazole, ritonavir); this combination is contraindicated • Increased risk of hypotension if combined with other alpha blockers; if this combination is used, monitor patient closely and adjust dosages as needed • Risk of increased serum levels if combined with cyclosporine; avoid this combination

■ Nursing considerations

Assessment

- **History:** Known hypersensitivity to any component of the drug, lactation, pregnancy, renal impairment, hepatic impairment, concurrent use of strong CP450 inhibitors, hypotension, prostate cancer, cataract surgery
- **Physical:** Orientation, affect, reflexes; skin color, lesions; BP, orthostatic BP, status of nasal mucosa; prostate examination, voiding pattern, normal output; LFTs, renal function tests, PSA level

Interventions

- Ensure that patient does not have prostate cancer before beginning therapy.
- Administer drug once a day with a meal.
- If patient is to undergo cataract surgery, there is a risk of intraoperative floppy iris syndrome. Surgeon should be alerted to the use of the drug, even if the drug has been discontinued; the patient may require additional surgical intervention.
- Provide safety measures if CNS effects occur.
- Monitor patient carefully for orthostatic hypotension; dizziness and syncope may occur. Establish safety precautions as needed. (Use side rails and provide assistance with ambulation.)

Teaching points

- Take this drug exactly as prescribed, once a day with a meal.
- Tell your surgeon that you are taking or have taken this drug if you are considering cataract surgery.
- You may experience these side effects: Headache (medications may be available to help); dizziness, weakness, which may become less over time (this is more likely when you are changing positions, after exercise, in hot weather, and after consuming alcohol; do not drive or operate hazardous machinery if this occurs; change position slowly, use caution when climbing stairs, lie down if the dizziness becomes severe); abnormal ejaculation, ejaculate with little to no semen (this is reversible when the drug is discontinued).
- Report fainting, changes in the color of stool or urine, severe dizziness, worsening of symptoms, rash.

▽ **simethicone**
(sigh meth' ih kohn)

Flatulex, Gas-X, Genasyme Drops, Mylicon Drops, Ovol (CAN), Phazyme, Phazyme 95, Phazyme 125, Phazyme Quick Dissolve

PREGNANCY CATEGORY C

Drug class

Antiflatulent

Therapeutic actions

Defoaming action disperses and prevents the formation of mucus-surrounded gas pockets in the GI tract; changes the surface tension of gas bubbles in the stomach and small intestine, enabling the bubbles to coalesce, allowing gas to be more easily freed by belching or flatus.

Indications
- Relief of symptoms of pressure, bloating, and fullness from excess gas in the digestive tract; postoperative gaseous distention and pain, use in endoscopic examination; air swallowing; functional dyspepsia; spastic or irritable colon; diverticulosis
- Unlabeled use: Treatment of colic in infants

Contraindications and cautions
- Contraindicated with allergy to components of the product.

Available forms
Chewable tablets—80, 125 mg; capsules—125, 180 mg; drops—20 mg/0.3 mL, 40 mg/0.6 mL; strips—40, 62.5 mg

Dosages
Adults
40–360 mg PO as needed after meals and at bedtime. Do not exceed 500 mg/day.
Pediatric patients 2–12 yr weighing more than 11 kg
40 mg PO as needed after each meal and at bedtime.
Pediatric patients younger than 2 yr
20 mg PO as needed after each meal and at bedtime; up to 240 mg/day.

Pharmacokinetics
Not absorbed systemically; excreted unchanged in feces

Adverse effects
- **GI:** Nausea, vomiting, *diarrhea*, constipation, belching, passing of flatus

■ Nursing considerations
Assessment
- **History:** Hypersensitivity to simethicone
- **Physical:** Bowel sounds, normal output

Interventions
- Give as needed after each meal and at bedtime.
- Shake drops thoroughly before each use.
- Allow strips to dissolve on tongue.

- Add drops to 30 mL cool water, infant formula, or other liquid to ease administration to infants.
- Ensure chewable tablets are chewed thoroughly before swallowing.

Teaching points
- Take drug after each meal and at bedtime. Chew chewable tablets thoroughly before swallowing; shake drops bottle before administration. Allow strips to dissolve on tongue. Parents may want to add drops to 30 milliliters of cool water, infant formula, or other liquid to ease administration.
- You may experience increased belching and passing of flatus as gas disperses.
- Report extreme abdominal pain, worsening of condition being treated, vomiting.

▽ simvastatin
*(sim va **stah' tin**)*

Apo-Simvastatin (CAN), CO Simvastatin (CAN), Gen-Simvastatin (CAN), Novo-Simvastatin (CAN), PMS-Simvastatin (CAN), ratio-Simvastatin (CAN), Zocor

PREGNANCY CATEGORY X

Drug classes
Antihyperlipidemic
HMG-CoA reductase inhibitor

Therapeutic actions
Inhibits HMG-CoA reductase, the enzyme that catalyzes the first step in the cholesterol synthesis pathway, resulting in a decrease in serum cholesterol, serum LDLs, and either an increase or no change in serum HDLs.

Indications
- Adjunct to diet in the treatment of hyperlipidemia
- To reduce the risk of coronary disease, mortality, and CV events, including stroke, TIA, MI, and reduction in need for bypass surgery and angioplasty in patients with coronary heart disease and hypercholesterolemia
- Treatment of adolescents 10–17 yr with heterozygous familial hypercholesterolemia

Contraindications and cautions

- Contraindicated with allergy to simvastatin, fungal by-products; active liver disease or unexplained, persistent elevations of serum transaminases; concurrent use of HIV protease inhibitors, erythromycin, clarithromycin, telithromycin, nefazodone, gemfibrozil, cyclosporine, danazol; pregnancy, lactation.
- Use cautiously with impaired hepatic and renal function, cataracts, Asian-Americans (increased risk of myopathy).

Available forms

Tablets—5, 10, 20, 40, 80 mg

Dosages

Adults

- *Hyperlipidemia:* Initially, 10–20 mg PO; up to 40 mg PO daily in the evening. Usual range, 5–40 mg/day. Maximum dose, 40 mg/day. Adjust at 4-wk intervals.
- *Prevention of coronary events:* 10–20 mg PO once daily in the evening. Patients at high risk: Start at 40 mg/day.
- *Familial hypercholesterolemia:* 40 mg/day PO in the evening.
- *Combination therapy:* Do not combine with other statins; if used with fibrates or niacin, do not exceed 10 mg/day; regular dose if combined with bile acid sequestrants. Give at least 4 hr before simvastatin. Combined with cyclosporine, start with 5 mg/day; do not exceed 10 mg/day. If used with diltiazem or verapamil, dose should not exceed 10 mg/day. If used with amiodarone, amlodipine, ranolazine, dose should not exceed 20 mg/day.

Pediatric patients 10–17 yr

10 mg/day PO in the evening. Range, 10–40 mg/day based on response.

Patients with renal impairment

For severe impairment, starting dose is 5 mg/day PO; increase dose slowly, monitoring response. No dosage adjustment needed for mild to moderate impairment.

Pharmacokinetics

Route	Onset	Peak
Oral	Slow	1.3–4 hr

Metabolism: Hepatic; $T_{1/2}$: 3 hr
Distribution: Crosses placenta; enters breast milk
Excretion: Feces, urine

Adverse effects

- **CNS:** *Headache,* asthenia, sleep disturbances
- **GI:** *Flatulence, diarrhea, abdominal pain, cramps, constipation, nausea,* dyspepsia, heartburn, **liver failure**
- **Respiratory:** Sinusitis, pharyngitis
- **Other: Rhabdomyolysis, acute renal failure,** arthralgia, myalgia

Interactions

✳ **Drug-drug** ⊗ *Warning* Increased risk of myopathy and rhabdomyolysis with boceprevir, clarithromycin, erythromycin, HIV protease inhibitors, itraconazole, ketoconazole, nefazodone, telaprevir; avoid concomitant use or suspend therapy during treatment with clarithromycin, erythromycin, itraconazole, and ketoconazole.• Increased risk of myopathy and rhabdomyolysis with verapamil; do not exceed 10 mg simvastatin daily • Increased risk of myopathy and rhabdomyolysis with amiodarone, amlodipine, ranolazine; do not exceed 20 mg simvastatin daily • Increased risk of myopathy and rhabdomyolysis with cyclosporine, fibrates, niacin; monitor patient closely if use together cannot be avoided. Do not exceed 10 mg simvastatin daily • Digoxin levels may increase slightly; closely monitor plasma digoxin levels at the start of simvastatin therapy • Increased risk for hepatotoxicity with hepatotoxic drugs; avoid concurrent use • Simvastatin may slightly enhance anticoagulant effect of warfarin; monitor PT and INR at the start of therapy and during dose adjustment • Increased risk of myopathy with diltiazem; do not exceed 10 mg/day if this combination is used

✳ **Drug-food** • Decreased metabolism and risk of toxic effects if combined with grapefruit juice; avoid this combination

■ Nursing considerations

Assessment

- **History:** Allergy to simvastatin, fungal by-products; impaired hepatic function; pregnancy; lactation
- **Physical:** Orientation, affect; liver evaluation, abdominal examination; lipid studies, LFTs

Interventions

- Ensure that patient has tried a cholesterol-lowering diet regimen for 3–6 mo before beginning therapy.
- Give in the evening; highest rates of cholesterol synthesis are between midnight and 5 AM.
- Do not use 80-mg dose because of increased risk of muscle injury and rhabdomyolysis with high dose. If patient is already stabilized on this dose, monitor closely. If lipid levels cannot be maintained on 40-mg dose, consider switching to a different drug.
- Advise patient that this drug cannot be taken during pregnancy; advise patient to use barrier contraceptives.
- Arrange for regular follow-up during long-term therapy. Consider reducing dose if cholesterol falls below target.

Teaching points

- Take drug in the evening. Do not drink large quantities (more than 1 quart/day) of grapefruit juice while using this drug.
- Have periodic blood tests.
- This drug cannot be taken during pregnancy; using barrier contraceptives is recommended.
- Find another method of feeding the baby of you are breast-feeding; this drug should not be used while breast-feeding.
- You may experience these side effects: Nausea (eat frequent small meals); headache, muscle and joint aches and pains (may lessen); sensitivity to light (use a sunscreen and wear protective clothing).
- Report severe GI upset, changes in vision, unusual bleeding or bruising, dark urine or light-colored stools, fever, muscle pain, or soreness.

▷**sipuleucel-T**

See Appendix R, *Less commonly used drugs*.

▷**sirolimus**

See Appendix R, *Less commonly used drugs*.

DANGEROUS DRUG

▷**sitagliptin phosphate**
(*sit ah* **glip**′ *ten*)

Januvia

PREGNANCY CATEGORY B

Drug classes

Antidiabetic drug

DPP-4 (dipeptidyl peptidase-4) enzyme inhibitor

Therapeutic actions

Slows the inactivation of the incretin hormones, increasing these hormone levels and prolonging their activity. The incretin hormones stimulate insulin release in response to a meal and help to regulate glucose homeostasis throughout the day. This increases and prolongs insulin release and reduces hepatic glucose production to help achieve glycemic control.

Indications

- Adjunct to diet and exercise to improve glycemic control in patients with type 2 diabetes mellitus, as monotherapy or with other oral antidiabetics

Contraindications and cautions

- Contraindicated with history of serious hypersensitivity reactions to sitagliptin, type 1 diabetes, diabetic ketoacidosis.
- Use cautiously with renal insufficiency, concurrent use of other drugs known to cause hypoglycemia, pregnancy, lactation.

Available forms

Tablets—25, 50, 100 mg

Dosages

Adults

100 mg/day PO as monotherapy or combined with metformin, pioglitazone, rosiglitazone, or other oral drugs.

Pediatric patients

Safety and efficacy not established.

Patients with renal impairment

With creatinine clearance of 30–50 mL/min, 50 mg/day PO; with creatinine clearance less than 30 mL/min, 25 mg/day PO.

S

Pharmacokinetics

Route	Onset	Peak
Oral	Rapid	1–4 hr

Metabolism: Hepatic; $T_{1/2}$: 12.4 hr
Distribution: May cross placenta; may enter breast milk
Excretion: Urine

Adverse effects
- **CNS:** *Headache*
- **Respiratory:** *Nasopharyngitis, URIs*
- **Other:** Hypoglycemia

Interactions
✳ **Drug-drug** • Risk of hypoglycemia when combined with other drugs or herbal remedies known to cause hypoglycemia; monitor patient closely and adjust dosages as needed

■ Nursing considerations
Assessment
- **History:** Renal impairment, pregnancy, lactation
- **Physical:** R, adventitious sounds; blood sugar, HbA$_{1C}$, renal function tests

Interventions
- Monitor blood glucose levels and HbA$_{1C}$ before and periodically during therapy.
- Ensure that patient continues exercise and diet program for management of type 2 diabetes.
- Monitor baseline renal function tests before and periodically during therapy.
- Ensure that patient continues with appropriate use of other drugs to manage type 2 diabetes if indicated.
- Arrange for thorough diabetic teaching program to include diet, exercise, signs and symptoms of hypoglycemia and hyperglycemia, safety measures to avoid infections, injuries.

Teaching points
- This drug should be taken once a day, with or without food.
- If you forget a dose of the drug, take it as soon as you remember, then begin your usual dosage the next day. Do not make up skipped doses or take more than one dose each day.
- Monitor your blood glucose levels as directed by your health care provider.
- Continue the diet and exercise program designed for the treatment of your type 2 diabetes; continue any other drugs used to treat your diabetes if instructed to do so by your health care provider.
- Arrange for periodic monitoring of your fasting blood sugar and glycosylated hemoglobin levels.
- It is not known if this drug could affect a fetus. If you are pregnant or are thinking about becoming pregnant, consult your health care provider.
- It is not known how this drug could affect a breast-feeding infant; discuss the use of this drug during breast-feeding with your health care provider.
- During times of stress (surgery, infection, injury), your body's needs change. Consult your health care provider immediately if you experience times of stress; your dosage or drug choices may need to change.
- Report any other drug, herbal remedies, or over-the-counter medications you may be using to your health care provider; many of these are known to alter your glucose levels, and dosage adjustments may be needed.
- Report fever or signs of infection, uncontrolled glucose levels, severe headache, stress, or trauma.

▽ sodium bicarbonate
(soe' dee um)

Parenteral: Neut
Prescription and OTC preparations: Bell/ans

**PREGNANCY CATEGORY C
(PARENTERAL)**

**PREGNANCY CATEGORY UNKNOWN
(ORAL)**

Drug classes
Antacid
Electrolyte
Systemic alkalinizer
Urinary alkalinizer

Therapeutic actions
Increases plasma bicarbonate; buffers excess hydrogen ion concentration; raises blood pH; reverses the clinical manifestations of acidosis; increases the excretion of free base in the urine, effectively raising the urinary pH; neutralizes or reduces gastric acidity, resulting in

an increase in the gastric pH, which inhibits the proteolytic activity of pepsin.

Indications

- Treatment of metabolic acidosis, with measures to control the cause of the acidosis
- Adjunctive treatment in severe diarrhea with accompanying loss of bicarbonate
- Treatment of certain drug intoxications, hemolytic reactions that require alkalinization of the urine; prevention of methotrexate nephrotoxicity by alkalinization of the urine
- Minimization of uric acid crystalluria in gout, with uricosuric agents
- Minimization of sulfonamide crystalluria
- Oral: Symptomatic relief of upset stomach from hyperacidity associated with peptic ulcer, gastritis, peptic esophagitis, gastric hyperacidity, hiatal hernia
- Oral: Prophylaxis of GI bleeding, stress ulcers, aspiration pneumonia
- To reduce the incidence of chemical phlebitis and patient discomfort due to vein irritation at or near the infusion site by raising the pH of IV acid solutions

Contraindications and cautions

- Contraindicated with allergy to components of preparations; low serum chloride (secondary to vomiting, continuous GI suction, diuretics associated with hypochloremic alkalosis); metabolic and respiratory alkalosis; hypocalcemia (alkalosis may precipitate tetany).
- Use cautiously with impaired renal function, HF, edematous or sodium-retaining states, oliguria or anuria, potassium depletion (may predispose to metabolic alkalosis), pregnancy, lactation.

Available forms

Injection—0.5, 0.6, 0.9, 1.0 mEq/mL; neutralizing additive solution—0.48, 0.5 mEq/mL; tablets—325, 650 mg

Dosages
Adults
- *Urinary alkalinization:* Initially, 3,900 mg PO; then 1,300–2,600 mg every 4 hr.
- *Antacid:* 300 mg–2 g daily to qid PO, usually 1–3 hr after meals and at bedtime.

- *Elderly patients:* 1 or 2 tablets PO every 4 hr; maximum, 12 tablets/24 hr for maximum of 2 wk.
- *Younger than 60 yr:* 1–4 tablets PO every 4 hr; maximum, 24 tablets/24 hr for maximum of 2 wk.

- *Adjunct to advanced CV life support during CPR:* Although no longer routinely recommended, inject IV either 300–500 mL of a 5% solution or 200–300 mEq of a 7.5% or 8.4% solution as rapidly as possible. Base further doses on subsequent blood gas values. Alternatively for adults, 1 mEq/kg dose, IV, then repeat 0.5 mEq/kg every 10 min.
- *Severe metabolic acidosis:* Dose depends on blood carbon dioxide content, pH, and patient's clinical condition. Generally, administer 90–180 mEq/L IV during first hr, then adjust PRN.

Adults and adolescents
- *Less urgent metabolic acidosis:* 2–5 mEq/kg as a 4–8 hr IV infusion. May be added to IV fluids, with rate and dosage determined by arterial blood gases and estimation of base deficit.

Pediatric patients
- *Cardiac arrest:*
  2 yr and older: 1 to 2 mEq/kg (1 mL/kg of an 8.4% solution) by slow IV.
  Younger than 2 yr: Use 4.2% solution. Don't exceed 8 mEq/kg daily.
- *Metabolic acidosis:*
  Younger children: Use caution, and base dosage on blood gases and calculation of base deficit.
  Older children: Follow adult recommendation.
- *Urinary alkalinization:* 84–840 mg/kg PO daily.

Geriatric patients or patients with renal impairment
Reduce dosage and carefully monitor base deficit, serum electrolytes, and clinical response.

Pharmacokinetics

Route	Onset	Peak	Duration
Oral	Rapid	30 min	1–3 hr
IV	Immediate	Rapid	Unknown

Metabolism: $T_{1/2}$: Unknown
Distribution: Crosses placenta; enters breast milk
Excretion: Urine

S

▼ IV FACTS

Preparation: Direct IV push requires no further preparation; continuous infusion may be diluted in saline, dextrose, and dextrose and saline solutions.

Infusion: Administer by IV direct injection slowly; continuous infusion should be regulated with close monitoring of electrolytes and response, 2–5 mEq/kg over 4–8 hr.

Incompatibilities: Avoid solutions containing calcium; precipitation may occur.

Y-site incompatibilities: Do not give with inamrinone, verapamil, calcium. Norepinephrine and dobutamine are also incompatible.

Adverse effects

- **GI:** Gastric rupture following ingestion
- **Hematologic:** *Systemic alkalosis* (headache, nausea, irritability, weakness, tetany, confusion), hypokalemia secondary to intracellular shifting of potassium, hypernatremia
- **Local:** Chemical cellulitis, tissue necrosis, ulceration and sloughing at the site of infiltration (parenteral)

Interactions

✳ **Drug-drug** • Increased pharmacologic effects of anorexiants, flecainide, quinidine, sympathomimetics with oral sodium bicarbonate • Increased half-lives and duration of effects of amphetamines, ephedrine, pseudoephedrine due to alkalinization of urine • Decreased pharmacologic effects of lithium, salicylates, sulfonylureas, methotrexate, doxycycline, and other tetracyclines

■ Nursing considerations

Assessment

- **History:** Allergy to components of preparations, low serum chloride, metabolic and respiratory alkalosis, hypocalcemia, impaired renal function, HF, edematous or sodium-retaining states, oliguria or anuria, potassium depletion, pregnancy
- **Physical:** Skin color, turgor; injection sites; P, rhythm, peripheral edema; bowel sounds, abdominal examination; urinary output; serum electrolytes, serum bicarbonate, arterial blood gases, urinalysis, renal function tests

Interventions

⊗ **Warning** Monitor arterial blood gases, and calculate base deficit when administering parenteral sodium bicarbonate. Adjust dosage based on response. Administer slowly, and do not attempt complete correction within the first 24 hr; risk of systemic alkalosis is increased.

- Give parenteral preparations by IV route.

⊗ **Warning** Check serum potassium levels before IV administration; risk of metabolic acidosis is increased in states of hypokalemia, requiring reduction of sodium bicarbonate. Monitor IV injection sites carefully; if infiltration occurs, promptly elevate the site, apply warm soaks, and if needed, arrange for the local injection of lidocaine or hyaluronidase to prevent sloughing.

- Have patient chew oral tablets thoroughly before swallowing, and follow them with a full glass of water.
- Do not give oral sodium bicarbonate within 1–2 hr of other oral drugs to reduce risk of drug interactions.
- Monitor cardiac rhythm carefully during IV administration.

Teaching points

- Chew oral tablets thoroughly, and follow with a full glass of water. Do not take within 1–2 hours of any other drugs to decrease risk of drug interactions.
- Have periodic blood tests and medical evaluations.
- Report irritability, headache, tremors, confusion, swelling of extremities, difficulty breathing, black or tarry stools, pain at IV injection site (parenteral form).

▷ sodium ferric gluconate complex

See Appendix R, *Less commonly used drugs*.

Adverse effects in *italics* are most common; those in **bold** are life-threatening. ▣ Do not crush.

▽sodium fluoride
(soe' dee um)

ACT, Fluor-A-Day (CAN), Fluorigard, Fluorinse, Fluoritab, Flura, Flura-Drops, Flura-Loz, Gel Kam, Gel-Tin, Karidium, Karigel, Karigel-N, Luride, MouthKote F/R, Pharmaflur, Pharmaflur df, Pharmaflur 1.1, Phos-Flur, PreviDent 5000 Plus, Stop, Thera-Flur-N Gel-Drops

PREGNANCY CATEGORY C

Drug classes
Mineral
Trace element

Therapeutic actions
Acts systemically before tooth eruption and topically after tooth eruption to increase tooth resistance to acid dissolution and promote remineralization of teeth and inhibit caries formation by microbes.

Indications
• Prevention of dental caries
• Unlabeled use: Prevention of osteoporosis

Contraindications and cautions
• Contraindicated in areas where fluoride content of drinking water exceeds 0.7 parts per million (ppm), with low-sodium or sodium-free diets, hypersensitivity to fluoride. Do not use in children younger than 3 yr when the fluoride content of drinking water is 0.3 ppm or more. Do not use 1 mg/5 mL (as a supplement) in children younger than 6 yr.
• Use cautiously with pregnancy, lactation.

Available forms
Chewable tablets—0.25, 0.5, 1 mg; tablets—1 mg; drops—0.125, 0.25, 0.5 mg/mL; lozenges—1 mg; solution—0.2 mg/mL; rinse—0.02%, 0.04%, 0.09%, 0.2%; gel—0.1%, 0.5%, 1.2%, 1.23%

Dosages
Adults
Rinse or topical rinse
10 mL once daily or weekly; swish around teeth and spit out.

Gel or cream
Apply thin ribbon to toothbrush or mouth tray for 1 min; brush, rinse, and spit out.
Pediatric patients
Oral
• Fluoride content of drinking water less than 0.3 ppm:
  6 mo–3 yr: 0.25 mg PO daily.
  3–6 yr: 0.5 mg PO daily.
  6–16 yr: 1 mg PO daily.
• Fluoride content of drinking water 0.3–0.6 ppm:
  6 mo–3 yr: None.
  3–6 yr: 0.25 mg PO daily.
  6–16 yr: 0.5 mg PO daily.
• Fluoride content of drinking water more than 0.6 ppm: None.
Rinse or topical rinse
6–12 yr: 5–10 mL/day.
Older than 12 yr: 10 mL/day; have patient swish around teeth for 1 min and spit out.
Gel
Apply 4–6 drops on applicator. Put applicator over teeth and bite down for 6 min. Have patient spit out excess gel.

Pharmacokinetics

Route	Onset
Oral	Unknown

Metabolism: $T_{1/2}$: Unknown
Distribution: Crosses placenta; enters breast milk
Excretion: Feces, sweat, urine

Adverse effects
• **Dermatologic:** Eczema, atopic dermatitis, urticaria, rash
• **Other:** Gastric distress, headache, weakness, staining of teeth (with stannous fluoride rinse)

Interactions
✳ **Drug-food** • Milk, dairy products may decrease absorption; avoid simultaneous use

■ Nursing considerations
Assessment
• **History:** Fluoride content of drinking water; low-sodium or sodium-free diets; hypersensitivity to fluoride; pregnancy, lactation
• **Physical:** Skin color, turgor; state of teeth and gums

S

Interventions

- Do not give within 1 hr of milk or dairy products.
- Tablets may be chewed, swallowed whole, or added to drinking water or juice.
- Give drops undiluted, or with fluids or food.
- Ensure that patient has brushed and flossed teeth before using rinse and that patient expectorates fluid; it should not be swallowed.
- Ensure that patients using cream or gel rinse thoroughly and spit out fluid. Do not allow patient to eat, drink, or rinse mouth for 30 min after application.
- Monitor teeth, and arrange for dental consultation if mottling of teeth occurs.
- ⊗ *Warning* Monitor patient for signs of overdose (salivation, nausea, abdominal pain, vomiting, diarrhea, irritability, seizures, respiratory arrest); forced diuresis, gastric lavage, or supportive measures may be required.

Teaching points

- Take this drug as prescribed; chew tablets, swallow whole, or add to drinking water or fruit juice.
- Dilute drops in fluids or food, or take undiluted.
- Brush and floss before using rinse; swish around mouth and spit out liquid; do not eat, drink, or rinse out mouth for 30 minutes after use. If using cream or gel, apply thin ribbon to toothbrush, brush, rinse thoroughly and spit.
- Avoid using milk or dairy products and this drug within 1 hour of each other.
- Arrange to have regular dental examinations.
- Report increased salivation, nausea, abdominal pain, diarrhea, irritability, mottling of teeth.

▷ sodium oxybate
(soe' dee um)

Xyrem

PREGNANCY CATEGORY B

CONTROLLED SUBSTANCE C-III

Drug classes

Anticataplectic
CNS depressant

Therapeutic actions

CNS depressant, its mechanism of action in affecting cataplexy is not understood.

Indications

- Treatment of excessive daytime sleepiness and cataplexy in patients with narcolepsy
- Unlabeled uses: Fibromyalgia pain, fatigue

Contraindications and cautions

- Contraindicated with hypersensitivity to any component of the drug, succinic semialdehyde dehydrogenase deficiency, concomitant treatment with sedative-hypnotics.
- Use cautiously with respiratory dysfunction, depression, pregnancy, lactation.

Available forms

Solution—500 mg/mL

Dosages
Adults

4.5 g/day PO divided into two equal doses of 2.25 g. Administer drug at bedtime and again 2.5–4 hr later. Doses may be increased no more than every 1–2 wk to a maximum of 9 g/day in increments of 1.5 g/day (0.75 g/dose). Usual range, 6–9 g night.
Pediatric patients younger than 16 yr
Safety and efficacy not established.
Patients with hepatic impairment
Reduce initial dose by half, and adjust dosage to effect while watching closely for adverse reactions.

Pharmacokinetics

Route	Onset	Peak
Oral	Varies	0.5–1.25 hr

Metabolism: Hepatic; $T_{1/2}$: 0.5–1 hr
Distribution: Crosses placenta; may enter breast milk
Excretion: Lungs, urine

Adverse effects

- **CNS:** *Headache, dizziness, somnolence,* sleepwalking, nervousness, confusion, depression, abnormal dreams, asthenia, muscle weakness, loss of consciousness, insomnia
- **GI:** *Diarrhea, nausea, vomiting,* abdominal pain, dyspepsia
- **GU:** Urinary incontinence

- **Respiratory:** *URI symptoms, pharyngitis,* sinusitis, rhinitis, **respiratory depression**
- **Other:** *Flulike symptoms,* accidental injury, back pain, infections

Interactions
✳ **Drug-drug** ● Risk for serious CNS depression if combined with any sedative-hypnotic drug, including alcohol; avoid this combination

■ Nursing considerations
Assessment
- **History:** Hypersensitivity to any component of the drug, succinic semialdehyde dehydrogenase deficiency, concomitant treatment with sedative-hypnotic agents, respiratory dysfunction, depression, pregnancy, lactation
- **Physical:** T; reflexes, affect, orientation; R, respiratory auscultation; LFTs

Interventions
⊗ **Black box warning** Counsel patient that this drug is also known as GHB, a drug known for abuse. The patient will be asked to view an educational program, agree to the safety measures to ensure that only the patient has access to the drug, and agree to return for follow-up at least every 3 mo.
- Dilute each dose with 60 mL water in the child-resistant dosing cups. Prepare both the bedtime dose and the repeat dose at the same time.
- Encourage patient to refrain from eating for at least 2 hr before going to bed and taking the drug.
⊗ **Warning** Administer first dose of the day when the patient is in bed. Patient should stay in bed after taking the dose. The second dose should be given 2½–4 hr later, with the patient sitting up in bed. After taking the second dose, the patient should lie in bed.
- Encourage patient to avoid driving or performing tasks that require alertness for at least 6 hr after taking the drug.
- Do not administer any sedative or hypnotic drugs to a patient who is taking sodium oxybate.
- Provide safety precautions for storage and dispensing of the drug.

Teaching points
- Prepare two doses of the drug in the evening before going to bed. Add 60 milliliters

(4 measuring tablespoons) water to the dose of the drug. Place the doses in the child-resistant dosing cups provided with the drug. Take the first dose when you first go to bed. Place the second dose in easy reach from your bed, but out of the reach of children or pets. Set your alarm to take the second dose 2½–4 hours later. Sit up in bed and take the dose. Lie back down and go back to sleep.
- Avoid eating for at least 2 hours before going to bed. Food will interfere with the actions of this drug.
- Take special precautions to ensure the safety of this drug. It is a controlled substance and cannot be shared with or given to any other person. The drug should be locked up and secured from other people and from children. Keep the drug in the original bottle. When the bottle is empty, remove the label, wash out the bottle and throw the bottle away.
- You may experience these side effects: Dizziness (avoid driving a car or performing hazardous tasks for at least 6 hours after taking the drug); headache (medications may be available to help); nausea, vomiting, diarrhea (proper nutrition is important, consult a dietitian to maintain nutrition); symptoms of upper respiratory tract infection, cough (do not self-medicate; consult your health care provider if this becomes uncomfortable); urinary incontinence or bed-wetting (consult your health care provider if this occurs).
- Report fever, difficulty breathing, bed-wetting, confusion, depression, pregnancy.

▽ **sodium phenylacetate/sodium benzoate**

See Appendix R, *Less commonly used drugs.*

▽ **sodium polystyrene sulfonate**
(soe' dee um)

Kalexate, Kayexalate, Kionex, SPS

PREGNANCY CATEGORY C

Drug class
Potassium-removing resin

Therapeutic actions

An ion exchange resin that releases sodium ions in exchange for potassium ions as it passes along the intestine after oral administration or is retained in the colon after enema, thus reducing elevated serum potassium levels; action is limited and unpredictable.

Indications

• Treatment of hyperkalemia

Contraindications and cautions

• Contraindicated with allergy to any component of the drug, obstructive bowel, severe hypertension, severe HF, marked edema (risk of sodium overload); for rectal administration in neonates, neonates with reduced gastric motility.

• Use cautiously with severe hyperkalemia; may need other definitive measures.

Available forms

Suspension—15 g/60 mL; powder 4.1 mEq/g

Dosages

Adults

Oral

15–60 g/day PO, best given as 15 g daily to qid. Powder may be given as suspension with water or syrup (20–100 mL). May be introduced into stomach via nasogastric tube.

Enema

30–50 g every 6 hr given in appropriate vehicle and retained for 30–60 min or as long as possible.

Pediatric patients

Give lower doses, using the exchange ratio of 1 mEq potassium/g resin as the basis for calculation.

Pharmacokinetics

Route	Onset
Oral	2–12 hr
Rectal	Very long

Excretion: Feces

Adverse effects

• **GI:** *Constipation,* fecal impaction, *gastric irritation, anorexia, nausea, vomiting*
• **Hematologic:** *Hypokalemia,* electrolyte abnormalities (particularly decreases in calcium and magnesium)

Interactions

✳ **Drug-drug** • Risk of metabolic alkalosis with nonabsorbable cation-donating antacids (eg, magnesium hydroxide, aluminum carbonate)

■ Nursing considerations

Assessment

• **History:** Severe hypertension, severe HF; marked edema
• **Physical:** Orientation, reflexes; P, auscultation, BP, baseline ECG, peripheral edema; bowel sounds, abdominal examination; serum electrolytes

Interventions

• Administer resin through plastic stomach tube, or mixed with a diet appropriate for renal failure.
• Give powder form of resin in an oral suspension with a syrup base to increase palatability.
• Administer as an enema after first giving a cleansing enema; insert a soft, large (French 28) rubber tube into the rectum for a distance of about 20 cm; with the tip well into the sigmoid colon, tape into place. Suspend the resin in 100 mL sorbitol or 20% dextrose in water at body temperature, introduce by gravity, keeping the particles in suspension by stirring. Flush with 50–100 mL fluid and clamp the tube, leaving it in place. If back leakage occurs, elevate hips or have patient assume the knee-chest position. Retain suspension for at least 30 min (several hours is preferable), then irrigate the colon with a non–sodium-containing solution at body temperature; 2 quarts of solution may be necessary to remove the resin. Drain the return constantly through a Y-tube connection.

⊗ *Warning* Prepare fresh suspensions for each dose. Do not store beyond 24 hr. Do not heat suspensions; this may alter the exchange properties.

• Monitor patient and consider use of other measures (IV calcium, sodium bicarbonate, or glucose and insulin) in cases of severe hyperkalemia, with rapid tissue breakdown: burns, renal failure.
• Monitor serum electrolytes (potassium, sodium, calcium, magnesium) regularly, and arrange to counteract disturbances.

Adverse effects in *italics* are most common; those in **bold** are life-threatening. ⬛ᴰᴺ Do not crush.

- If clinically significant constipation occurs, discontinue treatment until normal bowel function resumes. Do not use magnesium-containing laxatives or sorbitol.

Teaching points

- This drug is often used in emergencies. Drug instruction should be incorporated within general emergency instructions.
- Frequent blood tests will be needed to monitor drug effect.
- You may experience these side effects: GI upset, constipation.
- Report confusion, irregular heartbeats, constipation, severe GI upset.

▽**solifenacin succinate**
(*sole ah fen' ah sin suck' sin ate*)

VESIcare ᴼᴿᶜ

PREGNANCY CATEGORY C

Drug classes

Muscarinic receptor antagonist
Urinary antispasmodic

Therapeutic actions

Counteracts smooth muscle spasm of the urinary tract by relaxing the detrusor and other smooth muscles through action at the muscarinic parasympathetic receptors.

Indications

- Treatment of overactive bladder with symptoms of urge urinary incontinence, urgency, and urinary frequency

Contraindications and cautions

- Contraindicated with allergy to drug or any component of the drug, severe hepatic impairment, urine retention, gastric retention, uncontrolled narrow-angle glaucoma, lactation.
- Use cautiously with presence of bladder outflow obstruction, GI obstructive disorders, decreased GI motility, controlled narrow-angle glaucoma, reduced renal or hepatic function, congenital or acquired QT prolongation, pregnancy.

Available forms

Tablets ᴼᴿᶜ—5, 10 mg

Dosages

Adults
5 mg/day PO, swallowed whole with water. May be increased to 10 mg/day if desired effect is not seen.

Pediatric patients
Safety and efficacy not established.

Patients with severe renal or moderate hepatic impairment
Do not exceed 5 mg/day PO.

Patients with severe hepatic impairment
Not recommended.

Pharmacokinetics

Route	Onset	Peak
Oral	Slow	3–8 hr

Metabolism: Hepatic; $T_{1/2}$: 45–68 hr
Distribution: May cross placenta, may enter breast milk
Excretion: Feces, urine

Adverse effects

- **CNS:** Dizziness, blurred vision, dry eyes
- **CV:** Prolonged QT interval
- **GI:** *Dry mouth, constipation,* nausea, dyspepsia, upper abdominal pain, vomiting
- **GU:** Urinary retention
- **Respiratory:** Cough
- **Other:** Fatigue, lower limb edema

Interactions

✳ **Drug-drug** ⊗ *Warning* There is a risk of prolonged QT interval and potential serious cardiac arrhythmias if combined with other drugs that prolong QT interval; monitor patient closely.

- Risk of increased serum levels and toxic effects if combined with ketoconazole; if this combination is used, monitor patient and consider lowering dose of solifenacin; maximum dose of 5 mg daily with ketoconazole or other potent CYP3A4 inhibitors
- Risk of arrhythmias and toxic effects with potassium chloride; do not administer with solid forms of potassium chloride

■ Nursing considerations
Assessment

- **History:** Allergy to drug or any component of the drug, urinary retention, gastric retention, uncontrolled narrow-angle glaucoma, lactation, bladder outflow obstruction, GI

S

obstructive disorders, decreased GI motility, reduced renal or hepatic function, congenital or acquired QT prolongation, pregnancy
- **Physical:** Orientation, affect, reflexes, ophthalmic examination, ocular pressure measurement; P; bowel sounds, oral mucous membranes; baseline ECG, LFTs, renal function tests, bladder residual volume

Interventions

- Arrange for definitive treatment of underlying medical conditions that may be causing overactive bladder.
- Ensure that patient does not cut, crush, or chew tablets.
- Provide sugarless candies for patient to suck and frequent mouth care if dry mouth is a serious problem.
- Provide frequent small meals if GI upset occurs.
- Establish bowel program if constipation is a problem.
- Arrange for ophthalmic examination before beginning therapy and periodically during therapy.
- Establish safety precautions if CNS effects occur.
- Measure post-void residual urine volume if patient has difficulty voiding.

Teaching points

- Take drug once a day with water. Swallow whole, do not cut, crush or chew tablet. Take with or without food.
- Be aware that this drug is meant to relieve the symptoms you are experiencing; other medications may be used to treat the cause of the symptoms.
- You may not be able to sweat normally while on this drug; use caution in any situation that could lead to overheating.
- Consult your health care provider if you become pregnant or want to become pregnant; it is not known if this drug affects the fetus.
- If you are breast-feeding, another method of feeding the infant should be used while you are on this drug.
- Discontinue drug and seek immediate medical attention if you experience edema of the tongue or throat, or difficulty breathing.
- You may experience these side effects: Dry mouth, GI upset (sucking on sugarless candies and frequent mouth care may help); drowsiness, blurred vision (avoid driving or

performing tasks that require alertness while on this drug); constipation (medication may be available to help).
- Report inability to void, fever, blurring of vision, severe constipation.

▽ **somatropin**
*(soe ma **troe'** pin)*

Genotropin, Genotropin Miniquick, Humatrope, HumatroPen, Norditropin, Nutropin, Nutropin AQ, Nutropin AQ Pen, Omnitrope, Saizen, Serostim, Tev-Tropin, Zorbtive

PREGNANCY CATEGORY C

PREGNANCY CATEGORY B
(GENOTROPIN, OMNITROPE, SAIZEN, SEROSTIM), ZORBTIVE)

Drug class

Hormone

Therapeutic actions

Hormone of recombinant DNA origin; contains the identical amino acid sequence of pituitary-derived human growth hormone; therapeutically equivalent to endogenous growth hormone; stimulates skeletal (linear) growth, growth of internal organs, protein synthesis, many other metabolic processes required for normal growth.

Indications

- All but *Serostim:* Long-term treatment of children with growth failure due to lack of adequate endogenous growth hormone secretion
- *Nutropin* and *Nutropin AQ:* Treatment of children with growth failure related to chronic renal failure, chronic renal insufficiency, up to the time of renal transplantation
- *Genotropin, Norditropin, Nutropin, Nutropin AQ,* and *Humatrope, HumatroPen:* Treatment of girls suffering from Turner syndrome
- *Serostim:* Treatment of AIDS wasting and cachexia to increase lean body mass and improve physical endurance

- *Genotropin:* Long-term treatment of children with growth failure due to Prader-Willi syndrome (PWS)
- *Genotropin:* Long-term treatment of growth failure in children of small gestational age (SGA) who do not catch up by 2 yr
- *Genotropin, Norditropin, Nutropin, Nutropin AQ, Humatrope, Omnitrope, Saizen:* Growth hormone deficiency (GHD) in adults
- *Humatrope, HumatroPen:* Treatment of short stature or growth failure in children with short staturehomeobox (SHOX)-containing gene deficiency whose epiphyses have not closed.
- *Humatrope, Norditropin:* Treatment of short stature in children of SGA who do not present with catch-up growth by 2–4 yr
- *Humatrope, Nutropin, Nutropin AQ, Humatropen, Genotropin:* Long-term treatment of idiopathic short stature in pediatric patients whose epiphyses are not closed and for whom diagnostic evaluation excludes other causes treatable by other means
- *Norditropin:* Treatment of short stature in children with Noonan syndrome or Turner syndrome
- *Norditropin:* Treatment of adults with severe GHD
- *Saizen, Genotropin, Humatrope, Humatropen, Norditropin, Nutropin, Nutropin AQ, Omnitrope:* Replacement of endogenous growth hormone in adults with GHD who have GHD alone or in combination with multiple hormone deficiencies as a result of pituitary disease, hypothalamic disease, surgery, radiation therapy, or trauma or who had GHD as a child and who have had continued GHD established as an adult
- *Zorbtive:* Treatment of short bowel syndrome in patients receiving specialized nutritional support

Contraindications and cautions

- Contraindicated with known sensitivity to somatropin, benzyl alcohol, glycerin (*Humatrope*), closed epiphyses, underlying cranial lesions, neoplasms, diabetic retinopathy, acute illness secondary to complications of open-heart surgery, abdominal surgeries, accidental trauma.
- Use cautiously with pregnancy, lactation.

Available forms

Powder for injection—varies for each brand; prefilled injection pen—5, 10, 15 mg/1.5 mL; 10, 20 mg/2 mL; 30 mg/3 mL

Dosages

Individualize dosage based on response.

Adults

Serostim

Weighing less than 35 kg: 0.1 mg/kg subcutaneously daily at bedtime.

Weighing 35–45 kg: 4 mg subcutaneously daily at bedtime.

Weighing 45–55 kg: 5 mg subcutaneously daily at bedtime.

Weighing more than 55 kg: 6 mg subcutaneously daily at bedtime.

Humatrope, HumatroPen

Up to 0.006 mg/kg/day subcutaneously; may increase to 0.0125 mg/kg/day.

Nutropin, Nutropin AQ

Up to 0.006 mg/kg/day subcutaneously up to 0.025 mg/kg/day in patients younger than 35 yr and 0.0125 mg/kg/day in patients older than 35 yr. Increase dose in increments of 0.1–0.2 mg/day.

Norditropin

Up to 0.004 mg/kg/day subcutaneously; may be increased to 0.016 mg/kg/day after 6 wk if needed.

Saizen

Up to 0.005 mg/kg/day by subcutaneous injection; may be increased up to 0.01 mg/kg/day after 4 wk depending on response and tolerance. Titration should be based on age and gender adjusted serum growth factor levels.

Omnitrope, Genotropin

0.04 mg/kg/wk subcutaneously divided into seven daily injections; increase at 4- to 8-wk intervals to a maximum of 0.08 mg/kg/wk.

Zorbtive

0.1 mg/kg/day subcutaneously for a maximum of 8 mg/day. Administer daily for 4 wk.

Pediatric patients

Humatrope, HumatroPen

0.18–0.3 mg/kg/wk subcutaneously divided into doses given six or seven times/wk for GHD.

- *Turner syndrome:* Up to 0.375 mg/kg/wk subcutaneously divided into equal doses given six to seven times/wk.
- *Short stature with SHOX:* 0.35 mg/kg by subcutaneous injection each week, divided into equal daily doses.

S

- *Idiopathic short stature:* Up to 0.37 mg/kg/wk divided into six or seven subcutaneous injections.

Nutropin or Nutropin AQ

- *GHD:* Up to 0.3 mg/kg/wk subcutaneously up to 0.7 mg/kg/wk in divided daily injections.
- *Chronic renal insufficiency:* 0.35 mg/kg/wk subcutaneously divided into daily doses.
- *Turner syndrome:* Up to 0.375 mg/kg/wk subcutaneously divided into equal doses given either daily or on 3 alternate days.
- *Idiopathic short stature:* Up to 0.3 mg/kg/wk divided into daily subcutaneous injections.

Omnitrope

0.16–0.24 mg/kg/wk subcutaneously divided into daily doses given six to seven times/wk.

Saizen

0.06 mg/kg subcutaneously or IM three times/wk.

Norditropin

0.024–0.034 mg/kg subcutaneously, six to seven times/wk.

- *Noonan syndrome:* Up to 0.066 mg/kg/day subcutaneously.
- *Turner syndrome:* Up to 0.067 mg/kg/day subcutaneously.

Tev-Tropin

Up to 0.1 mg/kg subcutaneously three times per wk.

Genotropin

0.24 mg/kg/wk subcutaneously for PWS divided into six to seven doses; 0.16–0.24 mg/kg/wk subcutaneously for GHD divided into six to seven doses; 0.48 mg/kg/wk for SGA; 0.33 mg/kg/wk divided into six or seven subcutaneous injections for Turner syndrome; 0.47 mg/kg/wk divided into six or seven subcutaneous injections for idiopathic short stature.

Pharmacokinetics

Route	Onset	Peak
IM, Subcut.	Varies	3–7.5 hr

Metabolism: Hepatic; T$_{1/2}$: 1.7–4.2 hr
Distribution: Crosses placenta; enters breast milk
Excretion: Feces, urine

Adverse effects

- **Endocrine:** Hypothyroidism, insulin resistance
- **Hematologic:** *Development of antibodies to growth hormone, leukemia*

- **Other:** Swelling, joint pain, muscle pain, carpal tunnel syndrome, increased growth of preexisting nevi, headache, injection site pain

Interactions

✳ **Drug-drug** • Use caution in combination with drugs metabolized by CYP450 liver enzymes

■ Nursing considerations

Assessment

- **History:** Known sensitivity to somatropin, closed epiphyses, underlying cranial lesions
- **Physical:** Height; weight; thyroid function tests, glucose tolerance tests, growth hormone levels

Interventions

- Administer drug IM or subcutaneously as appropriate.
- Divide total dose into smaller increments given six to seven times/wk for smaller patients unable to tolerate injections.
- Reconstitute drug following manufacturer's instructions; do not shake; do not inject if solution is cloudy or contains particles.
- Refrigerate vials; reconstituted vials should be used within 7 days; do not freeze drug. Cloudiness may develop after refrigeration; if cloudiness persists after drug has come to room temperature, do not use.
- Arrange for tests of glucose tolerance, thyroid function, and growth hormone antibodies. Arrange for treatment as indicated.

Teaching points

- This drug must be given IM or subcutaneously. It can be given in six to seven smaller doses if needed. Dispose of syringes properly.
- You may experience these side effects: Sudden growth, increased appetite; decreased thyroid function (fatigue, malaise, hair loss, dry skin—request hormone).
- Report lack of growth, increased hunger, thirst, increased and frequent voiding, fatigue, dry skin, intolerance to cold.

▽ **sorafenib tosylate**

See Appendix R, *Less commonly used drugs.*

Adverse effects in *italics* are most common; those in **bold** are life-threatening. ▄▄▄ Do not crush.

▷ sotalol hydrochloride
(sob' tal lole)

Apo-Sotalol (CAN), Betapace, Betapace AF, Gen-Sotalol (CAN), PMS-Sotalol (CAN), ratio-Sotalol (CAN), Sorine

PREGNANCY CATEGORY B

Drug classes
Antiarrhythmic, classes II and III
Beta-adrenergic blocker

Therapeutic actions
Blocks beta-adrenergic receptors of the sympathetic nervous system in the heart and juxtaglomerular apparatus (kidneys), thus decreasing the excitability of the heart, decreasing cardiac output and oxygen consumption.

Indications
- Treatment of life-threatening ventricular arrhythmias; because of proarrhythmic effects, use for less than life-threatening arrhythmias, even symptomatic ones, is not recommended
- *Betapace AF:* Maintenance of normal sinus rhythm—to delay the time to recurrence of atrial fibrillation or flutter in patients with symptomatic atrial fibrillation or flutter who are currently in sinus rhythm

Contraindications and cautions
- Contraindicated with bronchial asthma (*Betapace*), sinus bradycardia (HR less than 45 beats/min), second- or third-degree heart block (PR interval greater than 0.24 sec), cardiogenic shock, uncontrolled HF, lactation, congenital or acquired long QT syndromes, hypokalemia and hypomagnesemia.
- Use cautiously with diabetes or thyrotoxicosis, hepatic or renal impairment, sick sinus syndrome, recent MI, pregnancy, lactation.

Available forms
Tablets—80, 120, 160, 240 mg; injection—15 mg/mL

Dosages
Adults
Initial dose, 80 mg PO bid. Adjust gradually, every 3 days, until appropriate response occurs; may require 240–320 mg/day (*Betapace*); up to 120 mg bid (*Betapace AF*). Use IV dose as a substitute for oral therapy when patient is unable to take drug orally. Initially, 75 mg IV over 5 hours twice a day; may be increased in increments of 75 mg/day every 3 days. Range: 225–300 mg once or twice a day for ventricular arrhythmias; 112.5 mg once or twice a day for AF. Monitor QT interval. Switch to oral form as soon as possible. Converting between oral and IV doses: 80 mg oral–75 mg IV; 120 mg oral–112.5 mg IV; 160 mg oral–150 mg IV

Pediatric patients older than 2 yr with normal renal function
30 mg/m² PO tid. Can titrate to a maximum of 60 mg/m² PO tid. Allow 36 hr between increments.

Pediatric patients younger than 2 yr
See manufacturer's instructions.

Geriatric patients or patients with renal impairment

Betapace
For creatinine clearance less than 10 mL/min, individualize dose based on response. See table below for dosing intervals.

CrCl (mL/min)	Dosing Intervals
More than 60	12 hr
30–59	24 hr
10–29	36–48 hr

Betapace AF
Betapace AF is contraindicated for creatinine clearance less than 40 mL/min. See table below for dosing intervals.

CrCl (mL/min)	Dosing Intervals
More than 60	12 hr
40–59	24 hr

Pharmacokinetics

Route	Onset	Peak
Oral	Varies	3–4 hr

Metabolism: $T_{1/2}$: 12 hr
Distribution: Crosses placenta; enters breast milk
Excretion: Urine

▼ IV FACTS
Preparation: Dilute before infusing in normal saline, D_5W, or lactated Ringer. Prepare a volume of 100–250 mL.
Infusion: Infuse using a volumetric infusion pump to deliver a constant rate over 5 hr.

S

Adverse effects

- **Allergic reactions:** Pharyngitis, erythematous rash, fever, sore throat, **laryngospasm, respiratory distress**
- **CNS:** Dizziness, vertigo, tinnitus, fatigue, emotional depression, paresthesias, sleep disturbances, hallucinations, disorientation, memory loss, slurred speech
- **CV:** *HF, cardiac arrhythmias, SA or AV nodal block,* peripheral vascular insufficiency, claudication, **stroke, pulmonary edema,** hypotension
- **Dermatologic:** Rash, pruritus, sweating, dry skin
- **EENT:** Eye irritation, dry eyes, conjunctivitis, blurred vision
- **GI:** *Gastric pain, flatulence, constipation, diarrhea, nausea, vomiting,* anorexia
- **GU:** *Impotence, decreased libido,* Peyronie disease, dysuria, nocturia, frequent urination
- **Musculoskeletal:** Joint pain, arthralgia, muscle cramp
- **Respiratory: Bronchospasm,** dyspnea, cough, bronchial obstruction, nasal stuffiness, rhinitis
- **Other:** *Decreased exercise tolerance, development of antinuclear antibodies,* hyperglycemia or hypoglycemia, elevated serum transaminase

Interactions

✳ **Drug-drug** • Possible increased effects with verapamil • Increased risk of orthostatic hypotension with prazosin • Possible increased BP lowering effects with aspirin, bismuth subsalicylate, magnesium salicylate, sulfinpyrazone, hormonal contraceptives • Decreased antihypertensive effects with NSAIDs, clonidine • Possible increased hypoglycemic effect of insulin • Risk of potentially fatal arrhythmias if combined with drugs that increase QTc interval (classes I and III antiarrhythmics, phenothiazines, TCAs, bepridil, certain oral macrolides, certain quinolone antibiotics) • Possible reduction of efficacy when given with antacids containing aluminum oxide and magnesium hydroxide

✳ **Drug-lab test** • Possible false results with glucose or insulin tolerance tests (oral)

■ Nursing considerations

Assessment

- **History:** Sinus bradycardia; second- or third-degree heart block; cardiogenic shock, HF; asthma, COPD; pregnancy, lactation; diabetes or thyrotoxicosis; prolonged QTc interval, bronchial asthma
- **Physical:** Weight; skin condition; neurologic status; P, BP, ECG; respiratory status, renal and thyroid function tests, blood and urine glucose

Interventions

- Administer this drug on an empty stomach.
⊗ ***Black box warning*** Do not give drug for ventricular arrhythmias unless the patient is unresponsive to other antiarrhythmics and has a life-threatening ventricular arrhythmia. Monitor patient response carefully; proarrhythmic effect can be pronounced. Do not initiate sotalol therapy if baseline QT interval is greater than 450 msec. If QT interval increases to 500 msec or longer during therapy, reduce dosage, extend infusion time, or discontinue drug.
- Maintain patient on continuous cardiac monitoring for at least 3 days when initiating or reinitiating therapy.
⊗ **Warning** Do not discontinue drug abruptly after long-term therapy. Taper drug gradually over 2 wk with monitoring (abrupt withdrawal may cause serious beta-adrenergic rebound effects).
- Discontinue other antiarrhythmics gradually, allowing for two to three plasma half-lives of the drug before starting sotalol. After discontinuing amiodarone, do not start sotalol until QTc interval is normalized.
- Reserve IV use for patients unable to take drug orally. Monitor QT interval carefully. Switch to oral form as soon as feasible. Convert from IV to oral form; dosages are not the same.
- Consult with physician about withdrawing drug if patient is to undergo surgery (withdrawal is controversial).

Teaching points

- Take drug on an empty stomach. You will be monitored closely as the drug is started.
- Do not stop taking unless told to do so by your health care provider.
- Avoid driving or dangerous activities if dizziness or weakness occurs.
- You may experience these side effects: Dizziness, light-headedness, loss of appetite, nightmares, depression, sexual impotence.

Adverse effects in *italics* are most common; those in **bold** are life-threatening. ▨ Do not crush.

- Report difficulty breathing, night cough, swelling of extremities, slow pulse, confusion, depression, rash, fever, sore throat.

▽ **spironolactone**
*(speer on oh **lak' tone**)*

Aldactone, Novo-Spiroton (CAN)

PREGNANCY CATEGORY C

PREGNANCY CATEGORY D
(GESTATIONAL HYPERTENSION)

Drug classes
Aldosterone antagonist
Potassium-sparing diuretic

Therapeutic actions
Competitively blocks the effects of aldosterone in the renal tubule, causing loss of sodium and water and retention of potassium.

Indications
- Diagnosis and maintenance of primary hyperaldosteronism
- Adjunctive therapy in edema associated with HF, nephrotic syndrome, hepatic cirrhosis when other therapies are inadequate or inappropriate
- Treatment of hypokalemia or prevention of hypokalemia in patients who would be at high risk if hypokalemia occurred (eg, patients receiving cardiac glycosides), patients with cardiac arrhythmias
- Essential hypertension, usually in combination with other drugs
- Adjunctive therapy for treatment of severe heart failure (NYHA class III to IV) to increase survival and decrease need for hospitalization
- Unlabeled uses: Treatment of hirsutism because of its antiandrogenic properties, palliation of symptoms of PMS, treatment of familial male precocious puberty, short-term treatment of acne vulgaris, pediatric hypertension

Contraindications and cautions
- Contraindicated with allergy to spironolactone, hyperkalemia, renal disease, anuria, amiloride or triamterene use.
- Use cautiously with pregnancy, lactation.

Available forms
Tablets—25, 50, 100 mg

Dosages
Adults
- *Edema:* Initially, 100 mg/day PO (range, 25–200 mg/day). When given as the sole agent, continue at least 5 days; then adjust dosage or add another diuretic or both.
- *Diagnosis of hyperaldosteronism:* 400 mg/day PO for 3–4 wk (long test). Correction of hypokalemia and hypertension are presumptive evidence of primary hyperaldosteronism. 400 mg/day PO for 4 days (short test). If serum potassium increases but decreases when drug is stopped, presumptive diagnosis can be made.
- *Maintenance therapy for hyperaldosteronism:* 100–400 mg/day PO in preparation for surgery.
- *Essential hypertension:* 50–100 mg/day PO. Continue treatment for at least 2 wk before reevaluating. May be combined with other diuretics.
- *Hypokalemia:* 25–100 mg/day PO.
- *Severe heart failure:* 25 mg/day PO if potassium level is 5 mEq/L or less and creatinine level is 2.5 mg/dL or less. Dose may be increased to 50 mg/day if well tolerated or reduced to 25 mg every other day if not well tolerated.

Pediatric patients
- Safety and efficacy not established.

Pharmacokinetics

Route	Onset	Peak	Duration
Oral	24–48 hr	48–72 hr	48–72 hr

Metabolism: Hepatic; $T_{1/2}$: 20 hr
Distribution: Crosses placenta; enters breast milk
Excretion: Feces, urine

Adverse effects
- **CNS:** *Dizziness, headache, drowsiness,* fatigue, ataxia, confusion
- **Dermatologic:** *Rash,* urticaria
- **GI:** *Cramping, diarrhea,* dry mouth, thirst, vomiting
- **GU:** Impotence, irregular menses, amenorrhea, postmenopausal bleeding, renal dysfunction
- **Hematologic:** Hyperkalemia, hyponatremia, agranulocytosis

S

- **Other:** Carcinogenic in animals, *deepening of the voice, hirsutism, gynecomastia*

Interactions

✸ Drug-drug • Increased hyperkalemia with potassium supplements, ACE inhibitors, diets rich in potassium, potassium-sparing diuretics • Decreased diuretic effect with salicylates • Decreased hypoprothrombinemic effect of anticoagulants • Increased hypotensive effect with diuretics and other hypotensive drugs, especially ganglionic blockers

✸ Drug-food • Increased absorption when taken with food

✸ Drug-lab test • Interference with radioimmunoassay for digoxin; false increase in serum digoxin levels • Interference with fluorometric determinations of plasma and urinary cortisol

✸ Drug-alternative therapy • Decreased effectiveness if combined with licorice therapy

■ Nursing considerations

Assessment

- **History:** Allergy to spironolactone, hyperkalemia, renal disease, pregnancy, lactation
- **Physical:** Skin color, lesions, edema; orientation, reflexes, muscle strength; P, baseline ECG, BP; R, pattern, adventitious sounds; liver evaluation, bowel sounds; urinary output patterns, menstrual cycle; CBC, serum electrolytes, renal function tests, urinalysis

Interventions

⊗ **Black box warning** Drug has been shown to be a tumorigen with chronic toxicity in rats; avoid unnecessary use of this drug.

- Mark calendars of edema outpatients as reminders of alternate-day or 3- to 5-day/wk therapy.
- Give daily doses early so that increased urination does not interfere with sleep.
- Measure and record regular weight to monitor mobilization of edema fluid.
- Avoid giving food rich in potassium.
- Arrange for regular evaluation of serum electrolytes and BUN.

Teaching points

- Record alternate-day therapy on a calendar, or prepare dated envelopes. Take the drug early because of increased urination.

- Weigh yourself on a regular basis, at the same time and in the same clothing, and record the weight on your calendar.
- Avoid foods that are rich in potassium (fruits, *Sanka*); avoid licorice.
- You may experience these side effects: Increased volume and frequency of urination; dizziness, confusion, feeling faint on arising, drowsiness (avoid rapid position changes, hazardous activities such as driving, using alcohol); increased thirst (suck on sugarless candies; use frequent mouth care); changes in menstrual cycle, deepening of the voice, impotence, enlargement of the breasts can occur (reversible).
- Report weight change of more than 3 pounds in 1 day, swelling in your ankles or fingers, dizziness, trembling, numbness, fatigue, enlargement of breasts, deepening of voice, impotence, muscle weakness, or cramps.

▽ stavudine (d4T)
(stay vyoo' deen)

Zerit

PREGNANCY CATEGORY C

Drug classes
Antiviral
Nucleoside reverse transcriptase inhibitor

Therapeutic actions
Inhibits replication of some retroviruses, including HIV, HTLV III, LAV, and ARV.

Indications
- Treatment of HIV-1 infection in combination with other antiretroviral therapy

Contraindications and cautions
- Contraindicated with life-threatening allergy to any component, lactation.
- Use cautiously with compromised bone marrow, impaired renal or hepatic function, or risk factors for liver disease, pregnancy.

Available forms
Capsules—15, 20, 30, 40 mg; oral solution—1 mg/mL

Adverse effects in *italics* are most common; those in **bold** are life-threatening. ▨▨▨ Do not crush.

Dosages
Adults
Weighing 60 kg or more: 40 mg PO every 12 hr.
Weighing less than 60 kg: 30 mg PO every 12 hr.
Pediatric patients older than 13 days
Weighing 60 kg or more: 40 mg PO every 12 hr.
Weighing 30 kg to less than 60 kg: 30 mg PO every 12 hr.
Weighing less than 30 kg: 1 mg/kg/dose PO every 12 hr.
Pediatric patients, birth to 13 days
0.5 mg/kg/dose PO every 12 hr.
Patients with renal impairment

CrCl (mL/min)	Weighing 60 kg or more	Weighing less than 60 kg
More than 50	40 mg every 12 hr	30 mg every 12 hr
26–50	20 mg every 12 hr	15 mg every 12 hr
10–25	20 mg/day	15 mg/day

Patients with persistent peripheral neuropathy
Dose may be resumed at 50% of normal after temporary withdrawal.

Pharmacokinetics

Route	Onset	Peak
Oral	Varies	60–90 min

Metabolism: Unknown; $T_{1/2}$: 30–120 min
Distribution: Crosses placenta; may enter breast milk
Excretion: Urine

Adverse effects
- **CNS:** *Headache,* insomnia, myalgia, *asthenia,* malaise, dizziness, paresthesia, somnolence, motor weakness, peripheral neuropathy
- **GI:** *Nausea, GI pain, diarrhea,* anorexia, vomiting, dyspepsia, **hepatomegaly with steatosis, pancreatitis**
- **Hematologic:** *Agranulocytopenia,* severe anemia requiring transfusions
- **Other:** *Fever,* diaphoresis, dyspnea, *rash,* taste perversion, **lactic acidosis,** body fat redistribution, laboratory test abnormalities (AST, ALT, amylase)

Interactions
✴ **Drug-drug** ● Increased risk of fatal or nonfatal pancreatitis if combined with didanosine; monitor closely ● Increased risk of lactic acidosis, severe hepatomegaly when taken with zidovudine, doxorubicin, ribavirin ● Incresed risk of hepatotoxicity if taken with hydroxyurea; avoid this combination.

■ Nursing considerations
Assessment
- **History:** Life-threatening allergy to any component; compromised bone marrow; impaired renal or hepatic function; pregnancy, lactation
- **Physical:** Rashes, lesions, texture; T; affect, reflexes, peripheral sensation; bowel sounds, liver evaluation; LFTs, renal function tests, CBC and differential

Interventions
⊗ **Black box warning** Monitor patient closely for pancreatitis throughout therapy; fatal and nonfatal pancreatitis have occurred.
- Monitor hematologic indices every 2 wk during therapy.
⊗ **Warning** Monitor neurologic function. If neuropathy occurs, discontinue. Restart at 50% dose when neuropathy resolves.
- Give every 12 hr, around-the-clock; schedule dose so it will not interrupt sleep.
⊗ **Black box warning** Monitor LFTs; lactic acidosis and severe hepatomegaly may occur.

Teaching points
- Take drug once each day. Do not share this drug; take exactly as prescribed.
- Stavudine is not a cure for AIDS; opportunistic infections may occur; regular medical care should be sought to deal with the disease.
- Always take this drug in combination with other HIV drugs.
- Frequent blood tests are needed; results may indicate a need to decrease or discontinue drug temporarily.
- Stavudine does not reduce the risk of HIV transmission by sexual contact or blood contamination; use appropriate precautions.
- This drug should be used during pregnancy only if the potential benefit justifies the potential risk; using barrier contraceptives is advised.

- Avoid breast-feeding to reduce risk of transmission of HIV to the baby.
- You may experience these side effects: Nausea, loss of appetite, change in taste (eat frequent small meals); dizziness, loss of feeling (take precautions); headache, fever, muscle aches, redistribution of body fat.
- Report extreme fatigue, lethargy, severe headache, severe nausea, vomiting, difficulty breathing, rash, numbness or tingling in feet or hands.

▷streptomycin sulfate

See Appendix R, *Less commonly used drugs*.

▷streptozocin

See Appendix R, *Less commonly used drugs*.

▷succimer (DMSA)
(sux' i mer)

Chemet

PREGNANCY CATEGORY C

Drug classes
Antidote
Chelate

Therapeutic actions
Forms water-soluble chelates with lead, leading to increased urinary excretion of lead.

Indications
- Treatment of lead poisoning in children with blood levels greater than 45 mcg/dL (not for prophylactic use)
- Orphan drug use: Prevention of cystine kidney stones in patients with homozygous cystinuria
- Unlabeled use: Treatment of other heavy metal poisonings (mercury, arsenic)

Contraindications and cautions
- Contraindicated with allergy to succimer, pregnancy (teratogenic and embryotoxic), lactation.
- Use cautiously with impaired renal or hepatic function.

Available forms
Capsules—100 mg

Dosages
Pediatric patients
Starting dose of 10 mg/kg or 350 mg/m^2 every 8 hr PO for 5 days; reduce dosage to 10 mg/kg or 350 mg/m^2 every 12 hr PO for 2 wk (therapy runs for 19 days).

Pharmacokinetics

Route	Onset	Peak
Oral	Varies	1–2 hr

Metabolism: Hepatic; T$_{1/2}$: 2 days
Distribution: Crosses placenta; may enter breast milk
Excretion: Feces, urine

Adverse effects
- **CNS:** Drowsiness, dizziness, sleepiness, otitis media, watery eyes
- **Dermatologic:** Papular rash, herpetic rash, mucocutaneous eruptions, pruritus
- **GI:** *Nausea, vomiting,* diarrhea, severe transaminases, metallic taste in mouth, loss of appetite
- **GU:** Decreased urination, voiding difficulty
- **Hematologic:** Neutropenia, increased platelets, intermittent eosinophilia
- **Other:** *Back, stomach, flank, head, rib pain;* chills; fever; flulike symptoms

Interactions
✳ **Drug-drug** • High risk of toxicity with other chelating agents (EDTA)
✳ **Drug-lab test** • False-positive tests of urine ketones using *Ketostix* • False decrease in serum uric acid, CPK

■ Nursing considerations
Assessment
- **History:** Allergy to succimer; lactation, pregnancy; renal or hepatic impairment
- **Physical:** Weight; orientation, affect; liver evaluation; urinalysis; LFTs, renal function tests; serum lead levels

Interventions
- Test serum blood levels before therapy and monitor weekly.
- Monitor serum transaminase level prior to and weekly during treatment.

Adverse effects in *italics* are most common; those in **bold** are life-threatening. ⏣ Do not crush.

- Identify the source of lead and facilitate its removal; succimer is not prophylactic to prevent lead poisoning.
- Ensure that patient continues therapy for full 19 days.
- For children unable to swallow capsules: Separate capsules and give medicated beads on a small amount of soft food or by spoon followed by fruit drink.
- All patients undergoing treatment should be adequately hydrated.
- Monitor patient for signs and symptoms of infection; provide appropriate assessment and interventions.

Teaching points
- For children unable to swallow capsules: Separate capsules and give medicated beads on a small amount of soft food or by spoon followed by fruit drink.
- Ensure child maintains good fluid intake.
- You may experience these side effects: Nausea, vomiting, loss of appetite (eat frequent small meals); abdominal, back, rib, flank pain (request medication).
- Report rash, difficulty breathing, difficulty walking, tremors, signs and symptoms of infection.

▷ sucralfate
*(soo **kral´ fayt**)*

Apo-Sucralfate (CAN), Carafate, Sulcrate (CAN)

PREGNANCY CATEGORY B

Drug class
Antiulcer drug

Therapeutic actions
Forms an ulcer-adherent complex at duodenal ulcer sites, protecting the ulcer against acid, pepsin, and bile salts, thereby promoting ulcer healing; also inhibits pepsin activity in gastric juices.

Indications
- Short-term treatment of duodenal ulcers, up to 8 wk
- Maintenance therapy for duodenal ulcer at reduced dosage after healing

- Orphan drug use: Treatment of oral and esophageal ulcers due to radiation, chemotherapy, and sclerotherapy
- Unlabeled uses: Accelerates healing of gastric ulcers, long-term treatment of gastric ulcers, treatment of reflux and peptic esophagitis, treatment of NSAID or aspirin-induced GI symptoms and GI damage, prevention of stress ulcers in critically ill patients

Contraindications and cautions
- Contraindicated with allergy to sucralfate, chronic renal failure or dialysis (buildup of aluminum may occur with aluminum-containing products).
- Use cautiously with pregnancy, lactation.

Available forms
Tablets—1 g; suspension—1 g/10 mL

Dosages
Adults
- *Active duodenal ulcer:* 1 g PO qid on an empty stomach (1 hr before meals and at bedtime). Continue treatment for 4–8 wk.
- *Maintenance:* 1 g PO bid.
Pediatric patients
Safety and efficacy not established.

Pharmacokinetics

Route	Onset	Duration
Oral	30 min	5 hr

Minimal systemic absorption

Adverse effects
- **CNS:** Dizziness, sleeplessness, vertigo
- **Dermatologic:** Rash, pruritus
- **GI:** *Constipation,* diarrhea, nausea, indigestion, gastric discomfort, dry mouth
- **Other:** Back pain

Interactions
✳ **Drug-drug** ● Decreased serum levels and effectiveness of phenytoin, ciprofloxacin, norfloxacin, digoxin, ketoconazole, tetracycline, theophylline, penicillamine, warfarin, levothyroxine, quinidine; separate administration by 2 hr ● Risk of aluminum toxicity with aluminum-containing antacids

■ **Nursing considerations**

Assessment

- **History:** Allergy to sucralfate; chronic renal failure or dialysis; pregnancy, lactation
- **Physical:** Skin color, lesions; reflexes, orientation; mucous membranes, normal output

Interventions

- Give drug on an empty stomach, 1 hr before or 2 hr after meals and at bedtime.
- Monitor pain; use antacids to relieve pain.
- Administer antacids between doses of sucralfate, not within 30 min before or after sucralfate doses.

Teaching points

- Take the drug on an empty stomach, 1 hour before or 2 hours after meals and at bedtime.
- If you are also taking antacids for pain relief, do not take antacids 30 minutes before or after taking sucralfate.
- You may experience these side effects: Dizziness, vertigo (avoid driving or operating dangerous machinery); indigestion, nausea (eat frequent small meals); dry mouth (use frequent mouth care, suck on sugarless candies); constipation (request aid).
- Report severe gastric pain.

DANGEROUS DRUG

▷**sufentanil citrate**

(*soo fen' ta nil*)

Sufenta

PREGNANCY CATEGORY C

CONTROLLED SUBSTANCE C-II

Drug class

Opioid agonist analgesic

Therapeutic actions

Acts at specific opioid receptors, causing analgesia, respiratory depression, physical depression, euphoria.

Indications

- Analgesic adjunct to maintain balanced general anesthesia
- Primary anesthetic with 100% oxygen to induce and maintain anesthesia in major surgical procedures
- Epidural analgesia with bupivacaine during labor and delivery

Contraindications and cautions

- Contraindicated with known sensitivity to sufentanil, pregnancy.
- Use cautiously with obesity, hepatic disease, head injury, arrhythmias, lactation, severe debilitation, renal or pulmonary disease.

Available forms

Injection—50 mcg/mL

Dosages

Individualize dosage; monitor vital signs routinely.

Adults

- *Adjunct to general anesthesia:* 1–2 mcg/kg IV initially; 10–25 mcg for maintenance; not to exceed 1 mcg/kg/hr of expected surgical time.
- *With oxygen and skeletal muscle relaxant for anesthesia:* 8–30 mcg/kg IV initially; supplement with doses of 0.5–10 mcg/ kg IV; not to exceed 30 mcg/kg for the procedure.
- *Epidural analgesia:* 10–15 mcg via epidural administration with 10 mL bupivacaine 0.125%; may repeat twice at 1-hr or longer intervals (total of three doses).

Pediatric patients 2–12 yr

- *With oxygen and skeletal muscle relaxant for anesthesia:* 10–25 mcg/kg IV initially; supplement with doses of 25–50 mcg IV.

Pharmacokinetics

Route	Onset	Duration
IV	Immediate	5 min
Epidural	10 min	1.7 hr

Metabolism: Hepatic; $T_{1/2}$: 2.7 hr
Distribution: Crosses placenta; enters breast milk
Excretion: Urine

IV FACTS

Preparation: Protect vials from light.
Infusion: Give slowly over 1–2 min by direct injection or into running IV tubing.

Adverse effects

- **CNS:** *Sedation, clamminess, sweating, headache, vertigo, floating feeling, dizziness, lethargy, confusion, light-headedness,*

nervousness, unusual dreams, agitation, euphoria, hallucinations, delirium, insomnia, anxiety, fear, disorientation, impaired mental and physical performance, coma, mood changes, weakness, headache, tremor, seizures
- **CV:** Palpitations, change in BP, circulatory depression, **cardiac arrest, shock,** tachycardia, **bradycardia, arrhythmia**
- **Dermatologic:** Rash, hives, pruritus, flushing, warmth, sensitivity to cold
- **EENT:** Diplopia, blurred vision
- **GI:** *Nausea, vomiting,* dry mouth, anorexia, constipation, biliary tract spasm
- **GU:** Ureteral spasm, spasm of vesical sphincters, urinary retention or hesitancy, oliguria, antidiuretic effect, reduced libido or potency
- **Local:** Phlebitis following IV injection, pain at injection site
- **Respiratory:** Slow, shallow respiration, apnea, suppression of cough reflex, **laryngospasm, bronchospasm**
- **Other:** Physical tolerance and dependence; psychological dependence; skeletal muscle rigidity, possibly requiring neuromuscular blocker

Interactions

✳ **Drug-drug** • Potentiation of effects with general anesthetics, opiate agonists, tranquilizers, sedatives, hypnotics (barbiturates) • Increased risk of hypotension and bradycardia if given with beta blockers, calcium channel blockers

✳ **Drug-food** • Decreased metabolism and risk of toxic effects if combined with grapefruit juice; avoid this combination

✳ **Drug-lab test** • Elevated biliary tract pressure may cause increases in plasma amylase, lipase; determinations of these levels may be unreliable for 24 hr after administration of opioids

■ **Nursing considerations**

⭐ **CLINICAL ALERT!**
Name confusion has occurred between sufentanil and fentanyl; use extreme caution.

Assessment

- **History:** Hypersensitivity to sufentanil or opioids; physical dependence on an opioid analgesic; pregnancy, lactation; COPD; increased intracranial pressure; acute MI, biliary tract surgery; renal or hepatic impairment
- **Physical:** Orientation, reflexes, bilateral grip strength, affect; pupil size, vision; pulse, auscultation, BP; R, adventitious sounds; bowel sounds, normal output; LFTs, renal function tests

Interventions

- Give to breast-feeding women 4–6 hr before the next feeding to minimize the amount in milk.
- Ensure that patient avoids grapefruit juice while using this drug.
⊗ *Warning* Provide opioid antagonist, keep equipment for assisted or controlled respiration readily available during parenteral administration.

Teaching points

- Incorporate teaching about drug into preoperative or postoperative teaching program.
- You may experience these side effects: Dizziness, sedation, drowsiness, impaired visual acuity (ask for assistance to move); nausea, loss of appetite (lie quietly, eat frequent small meals); constipation (use a laxative).
- Report severe nausea, vomiting, palpitations, shortness of breath or difficulty breathing.

▷ **sulfADIAZINE**
*(sul fa **dye'** a zeen)*

PREGNANCY CATEGORY C

PREGNANCY CATEGORY D
(LABOR AND DELIVERY)

Drug classes
Antibiotic
Sulfonamide

Therapeutic actions
Bacteriostatic: Competitively antagonizes PABA, an essential component of folic acid synthesis in gram-negative and gram-positive bacteria; prevents cell replication.

Indications
- Treatment of acute infections caused by susceptible organisms: UTIs, chancroid, inclusion conjunctivitis, trachoma, nocardiosis, toxoplasmosis (with pyrimethamine), malaria (as adjunctive therapy for chloroquine-resistant strains of *Plasmodium falciparum*), acute otitis media (due to *Haemophilus influenzae* when used with

penicillin or erythromycin), *H. influenzae* meningitis (as adjunctive therapy with parenteral streptomycin), meningococcal meningitis, rheumatic fever

- Orphan drug use: With pyrimethamine for treatment of *Toxoplasma gondii* encephalitis in patients with AIDS

Contraindications and cautions

- Contraindicated with allergy to sulfonamides, sulfonylureas, thiazides; pregnancy (teratogenic; may cause kernicterus); lactation (risk of kernicterus, diarrhea, rash).
- Use cautiously with impaired renal or hepatic function, G6PD deficiency, porphyria.

Available forms

Tablets—500 mg

Dosages

Adults

Loading dose, 2–4 g PO. Maintenance, 2–4 g/day PO in three to six divided doses.

- Prevention of recurrent attacks of rheumatic fever (not for initial therapy of streptococcal infections):
Weight less than 30 kg: 0.5 g/day PO.
Weight more than 30 kg: 1 g/day PO.
- *Toxoplasmosis:* 1–1.5 g PO qid in combination with pyrimethamine for 3–4 wk.
- *For suppressive or maintenance therapy in HIV patients:* 0.5–1 g every 6 hr PO with oral pyrimethamine and leucovorin.

Pediatric patients

Younger than 2 mo: Not recommended except to treat congenital toxoplasmosis.
Older than 2 mo: Initial dose, 75 mg/kg PO. Maintenance, 150 mg/kg/day PO in four to six divided doses with a maximum dose of 6 g/day.

- *Toxoplasmosis:* 100–200 mg/kg PO daily in combination with pyrimethamine for 3–4 wk.
- For suppressive or maintenance therapy in HIV patients:
Infants and children: 85–120 mg/kg PO daily in two to four divided doses with oral pyrimethamine and leucovorin.
Adolescents: 0.5–1 g every 6 hr PO with oral pyrimethamine and leucovorin.

Pharmacokinetics

Route	Onset	Peak
Oral	Varies	3–6 hr

Metabolism: Hepatic; $T_{1/2}$: Unknown
Distribution: Crosses placenta; enters breast milk
Excretion: Urine

Adverse effects

- **CNS:** *Headache,* peripheral neuropathy, mental depression, seizures, ataxia, hallucinations, tinnitus, vertigo, insomnia, hearing loss, drowsiness, transient lesions of posterior spinal column, transverse myelitis
- **Dermatologic:** *Photosensitivity,* cyanosis, petechiae, alopecia
- **GI:** *Nausea, emesis, abdominal pains,* diarrhea, bloody diarrhea, anorexia, pancreatitis, stomatitis, impaired folic acid absorption, hepatitis, **hepatocellular necrosis**
- **GU:** *Crystalluria, hematuria,* proteinuria, nephrotic syndrome, toxic nephrosis with oliguria and anuria, oligospermia, infertility
- **Hematologic:** Hemolytic anemia, hypoprothrombinemia, methemoglobinemia, megaloblastic anemia
- **Hypersensitivity: Stevens-Johnson syndrome,** generalized skin eruptions, epidermal necrolysis, urticaria, serum sickness, pruritus, exfoliative dermatitis, anaphylactoid reactions, periorbital edema, conjunctival and scleral redness, photosensitization, arthralgia, allergic myocarditis, transient pulmonary changes with eosinophilia, decreased pulmonary function
- **Other:** Drug fever, chills, periarteritis nodosum

Interactions

✳ **Drug-drug** • Increased risk of hypoglycemia when tolbutamide, tolazamide, glyburide, glipizide, acetohexamide, chlorpropamide are taken concurrently • Increased risk of phenytoin toxicity with sulfonamides • Risk of hemorrhage when combined with oral anticoagulants • Increased risk of nephrotoxicity with cyclosporine and decreased cyclosporine effect

✳ **Drug-lab test** • False-positive urinary glucose tests using Benedict method

■ Nursing considerations

CLINICAL ALERT!
Name confusion has occurred between sulfadiazine and *Silvadine* (silver sulfadiazine); use caution.

Assessment

- **History:** Allergy to sulfonamides, sulfonyl-ureas, thiazides; pregnancy, lactation; impaired renal or hepatic function; G6PD deficiency
- **Physical:** T; skin color, lesions; culture of infected site; orientation, reflexes, affect, peripheral sensation; R, adventitious sounds; mucous membranes, bowel sounds, liver evaluation; LFTs, renal function tests, CBC and differential, urinalysis

Interventions

- Arrange for culture and sensitivity tests of infection before therapy; repeat cultures if response is not as expected.
- Administer drug on an empty stomach, 1 hr before or 2 hr after meals, with a full glass of water.
- ⊗ *Warning* Ensure adequate fluid intake; sulfadiazine is very insoluble and may cause crystalluria if high concentrations occur in the urine; alkalinization of the urine may be necessary.
- ⊗ *Warning* Discontinue drug immediately if hypersensitivity reaction occurs.

Teaching points

- Complete full course of therapy.
- Take the drug on an empty stomach, 1 hour before or 2 hours after meals, with a full glass of water.
- Drink 8 glasses of water per day.
- This drug is specific to this disease; do not self-treat any other infection.
- You may experience these side effects: Sensitivity to sunlight (use sunscreens; wear protective clothing); dizziness, drowsiness, difficulty walking, loss of sensation (avoid driving or performing tasks that require alertness); nausea, vomiting, diarrhea; loss of fertility.
- Report blood in the urine, rash, ringing in the ears, difficulty breathing, fever, sore throat, chills, pallor, jaundice.

▽**sulfasalazine**
*(sul fa **sal'** a zeen)*

Azulfidine, Azulfidine EN-Tabs⊕,
PMS-Sulfasalazine (CAN), PMS-
Sulfasalazine EC (CAN)⊕,
Salazopyrin EN-Tabs (CAN)⊕

PREGNANCY CATEGORY B

Drug classes

Anti-inflammatory
Antirheumatic
Sulfonamide

Therapeutic actions

Bacteriostatic: Competitively antagonizes PABA, an essential component of folic acid synthesis in susceptible gram-negative and gram-positive bacteria; one-third of the oral dose is absorbed from the small intestine; remaining two-thirds passes into the colon where it is split into 5-aminosalicylic acid and sulfapyridine; most of the sulfapyridine is absorbed; the 5-aminosalicylic acid acts locally as an anti-inflammatory agent.

Indications

- Treatment of ulcerative colitis
- Delayed-release: Treatment of rheumatoid arthritis (RA) in patients intolerant or unresponsive to other anti-inflammatories
- *Azulfidine EN-Tabs:* Treatment of children 6–16 yr with juvenile rheumatoid arthritis, (JRA) involving five joints, who have not responded adequately to salicylates or other NSAIDs
- Unlabeled uses: Crohn disease, ankylosing spondylitis, psoriatic arthritis, regional enteritis, granulomatous colitis

Contraindications and cautions

- Contraindicated with allergy to sulfonamides, sulfonylureas, thiazides, salicylates; lactation (risk of kernicterus, diarrhea, rash); intestinal or urinary obstruction; porphyria; and in pediatric patients younger than 2 yr.
- Use cautiously with impaired renal or hepatic function, G6PD deficiency, blood dyscrasias, pregnancy.

Available forms

Tablets—500 mg; DR tablets⊕—500 mg

Dosages

Administer around-the-clock; dosage intervals should not exceed 8 hr. Give after meals.
Adults

- *Ulcerative colitis:* Initial therapy, 3–4 g/day PO in evenly divided doses. Initial doses of 1–2 g/day PO may lessen adverse GI effects. Doses of more than 4 g/day increase risk of toxicity. Maintenance, 2 g/day PO in evenly spaced doses (500 mg qid).

- *Adult RA:* Initially, 0.5–1 g/day PO (DR tablet); may be increased to 2 g daily in two evenly divided doses.

Pediatric patients

- *Ulcerative colitis:* For children 6 yr or older, initial therapy, 40–60 mg/kg/24 hr PO in three to six divided doses. Maintenance therapy, 30 mg/kg/24 hr PO in four equally divided doses. Maximum dosage, 2 g/day.
- *JRA—polyarticular course:* For children 6 yr or older, 30–50 mg/kg PO daily in two evenly divided doses. Maximum, 2 g/day.

Pharmacokinetics

Route	Onset	Peak
Oral	Varies	1.5–6 hr, 6–24 hr metabolite

Metabolism: Hepatic; $T_{1/2}$: 5–10 hr
Distribution: Crosses placenta; enters breast milk
Excretion: Urine

Adverse effects

- **CNS:** *Headache,* peripheral neuropathy, mental depression, seizures, ataxia, hallucinations, tinnitus, vertigo, insomnia, hearing loss, drowsiness, transient lesions of posterior spinal column, transverse myelitis
- **Dermatologic:** Photosensitivity, cyanosis, petechiae, alopecia
- **GI:** *Nausea, emesis, abdominal pains,* diarrhea, bloody diarrhea, *anorexia,* pancreatitis, stomatitis, impaired folic acid absorption, hepatitis, **hepatocellular necrosis**
- **GU:** *Crystalluria, hematuria,* proteinuria, nephrotic syndrome, toxic nephrosis with oliguria and anuria, *oligospermia,* infertility
- **Hematologic: Agranulocytosis, aplastic anemia, thrombocytopenia,** leukopenia, hemolytic anemia, hypoprothrombinemia, methemoglobinemia, megaloblastic anemia
- **Hypersensitivity: Stevens-Johnson syndrome,** generalized skin eruptions, epidermal necrolysis, urticaria, serum sickness, pruritus, exfoliative dermatitis, anaphylactoid reactions, periorbital edema, conjunctival and scleral redness, photosensitization, arthralgia, allergic myocarditis, transient pulmonary changes with eosinophilia, decreased pulmonary function
- **Other:** Drug fever, chills, periarteritis nodosum

Interactions

✳ **Drug-drug** ● Decreased absorption of digoxin with lessened therapeutic effect; monitor patient, space doses at least 2 hr apart ● Increased risk of folate deficiency, monitor for signs of folate deficiency

■ Nursing considerations

Assessment

- **History:** Allergy to sulfonamides, sulfonylureas, thiazides, salicylates; pregnancy; lactation; impaired renal or hepatic function; G6PD deficiency; porphyria
- **Physical:** T; skin color, lesions; culture of infected site; orientation, reflexes, affect, peripheral sensation; R, adventitious sounds; mucous membranes, bowel sounds, liver evaluation; LFTs, renal function tests, CBC and differential, urinalysis

Interventions

- Administer drug after meals or with food to prevent GI upset. Administer it around-the-clock.
- Ensure that patient swallows DR tablets whole; tablets should not be cut, crushed, or chewed.
⊗ **Warning** Ensure adequate fluid intake; sulfasalazine is very insoluble and may cause crystalluria if high concentrations occur in the urine; alkalinization of the urine may be needed.
⊗ **Warning** Discontinue drug immediately if hypersensitivity reaction occurs.

Teaching points

- Complete full course of therapy. Swallow delayed-release tablets whole; do not cut, crush, or chew tablets.
- Take the drug with food or meals to decrease GI upset.
- Drink eight glasses of water per day.
- You may experience these side effects: Sensitivity to sunlight (use sunscreen, wear protective clothing); dizziness, drowsiness, difficulty walking, loss of sensation (avoid driving or performing tasks that require alertness); nausea, vomiting, diarrhea; loss of fertility; yellow-orange urine.
- Report blood in the urine, rash, ringing in the ears, difficulty breathing, fever, sore throat, chills.

Adverse effects in *italics* are most common; those in **bold** are life-threatening. ⊞ Do not crush.

▷ sulindac
*(sul **in**' dak)*

Apo-Sulin (CAN), Clinoril

PREGNANCY CATEGORY B
(FIRST AND SECOND TRIMESTERS)

PREGNANCY CATEGORY D
(THIRD TRIMESTER)

Drug classes
Analgesic
Antipyretic
NSAID

Therapeutic actions
Anti-inflammatory, analgesic, and antipyretic activities largely related to inhibition of prostaglandin synthesis; exact mechanisms of action are not known.

Indications
- Acute or long-term use to relieve signs and symptoms of osteoarthritis, rheumatoid arthritis, acute gouty arthritis
- Acute or long-term use in relief of signs and symptoms of ankylosing spondylitis, acute painful shoulder
- ■ **NEW INDICATION:** Unlabeled use: Treatment of juvenile rheumatoid arthritis

Contraindications and cautions
- Contraindicated for perioperative pain in coronary artery bypass graft (CABG) surgery and in late pregnancy, lactation.
- Use cautiously with patients for whom acute asthmatic attacks, urticaria, or rhinitis are precipitated by aspirin or other NSAIDs, renal, hepatic, CV, and GI conditions.

Available forms
Tablets—150, 200 mg

Dosages
Do not exceed 400 mg/day.
Adults
- *Rheumatoid arthritis or osteoarthritis, ankylosing spondylitis:* Initial dose of 150 mg bid PO; maximum dose, 400 mg/day. Individualize dosage.
- *Acute painful shoulder, acute gouty arthritis:* 200 mg bid PO; maximum dose, 400 mg/day. After adequate response,

reduce dosage. Acute painful shoulder usually requires 7–14 days of therapy; acute gouty arthritis, 7 days.
Pediatric patients
Safety and efficacy not established.
Patients with hepatic or renal impairment
Reduce dosage.

Pharmacokinetics

Route	Onset	Peak	Duration
Oral	Varies	2–4 hr	10–12 hr

Metabolism: Hepatic; $T_{1/2}$: 7.8 hr (parent drug), 16.4 hr (active metabolite)
Distribution: Crosses placenta; enters breast milk
Excretion: Feces, urine

Adverse effects
- **CNS:** *Headache, dizziness, somnolence, insomnia,* fatigue, tiredness, dizziness, tinnitus, ophthalmologic effects
- **CV: Heart failure,** CV events
- **Dermatologic:** *Rash,* pruritus, sweating, dry mucous membranes, stomatitis
- **GI:** *Nausea, dyspepsia, GI pain,* diarrhea, vomiting, *constipation,* flatulence, anorexia, GI ulceration
- **GU:** Dysuria, renal impairment, pancreatitis
- **Hematologic:** Bleeding, platelet inhibition with higher doses, neutropenia, eosinophilia, leukopenia, **pancytopenia,** thrombocytopenia, **agranulocytosis,** granulocytopenia, aplastic anemia, decreased Hgb or Hct, bone marrow depression, menorrhagia
- **Respiratory:** Dyspnea, hemoptysis, pharyngitis, **bronchospasm,** rhinitis
- **Other:** Peripheral edema, **anaphylactoid reactions** to **fatal anaphylactic shock**

Interactions
✳ **Drug-drug** • Increased serum lithium levels and risk of toxicity • Decreased antihypertensive effects of beta blockers • Decreased therapeutic effects of bumetanide, furosemide, ethacrynic acid • Decreased serum levels if combined with aspirin
✳ **Drug-food** • Decreased rate and extent of absorption when taken with food

S

■ Nursing considerations

Assessment

- **History:** Allergies; renal, hepatic, CV, and GI conditions; pregnancy; lactation
- **Physical:** Skin color and lesions; orientation, reflexes, ophthalmologic and audiometric evaluation, peripheral sensation; P, edema; R, adventitious sounds; liver evaluation; CBC, clotting times, LFTs, renal function tests; serum electrolytes, stool guaiac

Interventions

⊗ **Black box warning** Be aware that patient may be at increased risk for CV events, GI bleeding; monitor accordingly. Drug is contraindicated for treating perioperative pain in CABG surgery.

- Give with food or milk if GI upset occurs.
- Arrange for periodic ophthalmologic examination during long-term therapy.

⊗ **Warning** If overdose occurs, institute emergency procedures—gastric lavage, induction of emesis, supportive therapy.

Teaching points

- Take with food or meals if GI upset occurs.
- Take only the prescribed dosage.
- You may experience these side effects: Dizziness, drowsiness (avoid driving or using dangerous machinery).
- Report sore throat; fever; rash; itching; weight gain; swelling in ankles or fingers; changes in vision; black, tarry stools; right upper quadrant tenderness; fatigue.

▽ **sumatriptan succinate**

*(sue mah **trip' tan**)*

Alsuma, Apo-Sumatriptan (CAN), Gen-Sumatriptan (CAN), Imitrex, Novo-Sumatriptan (CAN), Novo-Sumatriptan DF (CAN), PMS-Sumatriptan (CAN), ratio-Sumatriptan (CAN), Sumavel DosePro

PREGNANCY CATEGORY C

Drug classes

Antimigraine drug (triptan)
Serotonin-selective agonist

Therapeutic actions

Binds to serotonin receptors to cause vascular constrictive effects on cranial blood vessels, causing the relief of migraine in selective patients.

Indications

- Treatment of acute migraine attacks with or without aura (oral, nasal, subcutaneously)
- Unlabeled use: Migraine headaches in children and adolescents

Contraindications and cautions

- Contraindicated with allergy to sumatriptan, cerebrovascular or peripheral vascular syndromes, severe hepatic impairment, MAOIs, uncontrolled hypertension, hemiplegic migraine, pregnancy, CAD
- Use cautiously with the elderly, lactation, renal function impairment.

Available forms

Tablets—25, 50, 100 mg; injection—4 mg/0.5 mL, 6 mg/0.5 mL; nasal spray—5 mg/0.1 mL, 20 mg/0.1 mL; needle-free injection system—4, 6 mg/0.5 mL

Dosages

Adults

Oral

25, 50, or 100 mg PO; additional doses may be repeated in 2 hr or more; up to a maximum of 200 mg/day.

Subcutaneous

6 mg subcutaneously, may be repeated in 1 hr. Maximum, 12 mg/24 hr. Needle-free autoinjector is available.

Intranasal

5, 10, or 20 mg spray into one nostril or 10 mg divided into two doses of 5 mg, one in each nostril, may be repeated after 2 hr. Maximum, 40 mg/24 hr.

Pediatric patients

Safety and efficacy not established.

Patients with hepatic impairment

Maximum single dose, 50 mg. Do not use in severe hepatic impairment.

Pharmacokinetics

Route	Onset	Peak
Subcut.	Varies	5–20 min
Oral	60–90 min	2–4 hr
Injection	Rapid	90 min

Metabolism: Hepatic; $T_{1/2}$: 115 min
Distribution: Crosses placenta; enters breast milk
Excretion: Urine, feces (tablets)

Adverse effects

- **CNS:** *Dizziness, vertigo,* headache, anxiety, malaise or fatigue, *weakness, myalgia*
- **CV:** *BP alterations, tightness or pressure in chest,* **shock**
- **GI:** Abdominal discomfort, dysphagia
- **Local:** *Injection site discomfort,* nose and throat discomfort (nasal spray)
- **Other:** *Tingling, warm/hot sensations, burning sensation, feeling of heaviness, pressure sensation, numbness, feeling of tightness,* feeling strange, cold sensation

Nasal spray

- **GI:** Bad taste in mouth, nausea

Interactions

✳ **Drug-drug** • Prolonged vasoactive reactions with ergot-containing drugs (should not be used within 24 hr of each other) • Increased serum levels and toxicity of sumatriptan with MAOIs; avoid this combination and for 2 wk after MAOI discontinuation • Increased risk of serotonin syndrome if combined with SSRTs, serotonin-norepinephrine reuptake inhibitors

✳ **Drug-alternative therapy** • Increased risk of severe reaction if combined with St. John's Wort therapy

■ Nursing considerations

Assessment

- **History:** Allergy to sumatriptan; active CAD; uncontrolled hypertension; hemiplegic migraine; pregnancy, lactation
- **Physical:** Skin color and lesions; orientation, reflexes, peripheral sensation; P, BP; LFTs, renal function tests

Interventions

- Administer to relieve acute migraine, not as a prophylactic measure.
- Administer as subcutaneous injection just below the skin as soon as possible after symptoms begin.
- Repeat injection only after 1 hr if relief is not obtained; only 2 injections may be given each 24 hr.
- Administer PO with fluids; may repeat in 2 hr if no relief.
- Repeat nasal spray after 2 hr if headache returns or does not respond.
- Monitor BP of patients with possible CAD; discontinue at any sign of angina, prolonged high BP.

Teaching points

- Learn to use the autoinjector; injection may be repeated only after 1 hour if relief is not obtained; do not administer more than two injections in 24 hours.
- Inject just below the skin as soon as possible after onset of migraine; this drug is for an acute attack only, not for use to prevent attacks. Dispose of needles and syringes appropriately.
- Administer nasal spray as a single dose; repeat if needed only after 2 hours.
- Take oral drug with fluids, may be repeated in 2 hours if no relief or return of headache.
- This drug should not be taken during pregnancy; if you suspect that you are pregnant, consult your health care provider and stop using drug.
- Contact your health care provider immediately if you experience severe or continuous chest pain or pressure or sudden severe abdominal pain.
- You may experience these side effects: Dizziness, drowsiness (avoid driving or the use of dangerous machinery); numbness, tingling, feelings of tightness or pressure.
- Report feelings of heat, flushing, tiredness, feelings of sickness, swelling of lips or eyelids.

▷**sunitinib**

See Appendix R, *Less commonly used drugs.*

S

▽ tacrolimus (FK 506)
(tack row' lim us)

Advagraf (CAN), Hecoria, Prograf, Protopic

PREGNANCY CATEGORY C

Drug classes
Immunomodulator
Immunosuppressant

Therapeutic actions
Immunosuppressant; inhibits T-lymphocyte activation; exact mechanism of action not known but binds to intracellular protein, which may prevent the generation of nuclear factor of activated T cells and suppress the immune activation and response of T cells.

Indications
- Prophylaxis for organ rejection in liver, kidney, and heart transplants in conjunction with adrenal corticosteroids
- Topical: Short-term and intermittent long-term treatment of moderate to severe atopic dermatitis when other therapies are not effective or contraindicated
- Unlabeled uses: Crohn disease, pyoderma gangrenosum, psoriasis, prevention and treatment of acute graft-versus-host disease following hematopoietic stem-cell transplantation, rheumotoid arthritis, uveitis

Contraindications and cautions
- Contraindicated with allergy to tacrolimus, hypersensitivity to HCO-60 polyoxyl 60 hydrogenated castor oil (IV form), pregnancy, lactation.
- Use cautiously with impaired renal function, hyperkalemia, malabsorption, impaired hepatic function.

Available forms
Capsules—0.5, 1, 5 mg; injection—5 mg/mL; ointment—0.03%, 0.1%

Dosages
Adults
Oral
- *Kidney transplant:* 0.2 mg/kg/day PO divided every 12 hr if given with azathioprine. Reduce dosage to 0.1 mg/kg/day PO in divided doses if given with mycopheuolate,

mofetil and/or interleukin-2 receptor antagonists.
- *Liver transplant:* 0.10–0.15 mg/kg/day PO divided every 12 hr; administer initial dose no sooner than 6 hr after transplant. If transferring from IV, give first dose 8–12 hr after discontinuing IV infusion. Adjust dosage based on clinical assessment of rejection tolerance of drug.
- *Heart transplant:* 0.075 mg/kg/day PO or IV in two divided doses given every 12 hr. Give first dose no sooner than 6 hr after transplant. If therapy starts with IV route, switch to oral route as soon as possible, 8–12 hr after discontinuing IV infusion.

Parenteral
For patients unable to take capsules, 0.03–0.05 mg/kg/day (liver or kidney transplant) or 0.01 mg/kg/day (heart transplant) as continuous IV infusion begun no sooner than 6 hr after transplant. Switch to oral drug as soon as possible.

Topical
Apply thin layer of 0.03% or 0.1% ointment to affected area bid. Rub in gently and completely. Stop drug when signs and symptoms resolve.

Pediatric patients
Children may require the larger dose; begin treatment at higher end of recommended adult dose.

Oral
- *Liver transplant:* 0.15–0.20 mg/kg/day in divided doses.

Parenteral
- *Liver transplant:* 0.03–0.05 mg/kg/day.

Topical
2–15 yr: Apply thin layer of 0.03% ointment bid. Rub in gently and completely. Stop drug when signs and symptoms resolve.
Younger than 2 yr: Not recommended.

Patients with hepatic or renal impairment
Start with lowest possible dose; delay therapy up to 48 hr in patients with postoperative oliguria.

Pharmacokinetics

Route	Onset	Peak
Oral	Varies	1.5–3.5 hr
IV	Rapid	1–2 hr

Metabolism: Hepatic; $T_{1/2}$: 11.7–18.8 hr (IV)
Distribution: Crosses placenta; enters breast milk
Excretion: Urine, feces

Adverse effects in *italics* are most common; those in **bold** are life-threatening. ⊂⊃ Do not crush.

▼ IV FACTS

Preparation: Wearing gloves, dilute IV solution immediately before use; use 0.9% sodium chloride injection or 5% dextrose injection to a concentration between 0.004 and 0.02 mg/mL Store in glass or polyethylene container between 5° and 25°C. Do not store in a PVC container; discard after 24 hr.

Infusion: Give by continuous IV infusion using an infusion pump.

Incompatibilities: Do not mix with solutions with a pH of 9 or greater (acyclovir, ganciclovir).

Adverse effects

- **CNS:** *Tremor, headache, insomnia,* paresthesias
- **CV:** Hypertension
- **GI: Hepatotoxicity,** *constipation, diarrhea, nausea, vomiting,* anorexia
- **GU:** *Renal impairment,* nephrotoxicity, UTI, oliguria
- **Hematologic:** Leukopenia, anemia, hyperkalemia, hypokalemia, hyperglycemia, hypomagnesemia
- **Other:** Abdominal pain, fever, asthenia, back pain, ascites, neoplasias, increased susceptibility to infection, lymphoma development, diabetes mellitus, hypercholesterolemia, **anaphylaxis**

Interactions

✳ **Drug-drug** • Increased risk of nephrotoxicity with other nephrotoxic agents (cyclosporine) • Risk of severe myopathy or rhabdomyolysis with any HMG-CoA inhibitor • Increased risk of toxicity with metoclopramide, nicardipine, cimetidine, clarithromycin, erythromycin, calcium channel blockers • Decreased therapeutic effect with carbamazepine, phenobarbital, phenytoin, rifamycins • Potentially severe hyperkalemia with potassium-sparing diuretics or potassium supplements

✳ **Drug-food** • Decreased metabolism and risk of toxic effects if combined with grapefruit juice; avoid this combination

✳ **Drug-alternative therapy** • Decreased therapeutic effect with St. John's Wort

■ Nursing considerations

Assessment

- **History:** Allergy to tacrolimus or polyoxyethylated castor oil; impaired renal function; malabsorption; lactation, pregnancy
- **Physical:** T; skin color, lesions; BP, peripheral perfusion; liver evaluation, bowel sounds, gum evaluation; LFTs, renal function tests, CBC, potassium, glucose

Interventions

⊗ **Black box warning** Protect patient from infection. Risk of infection, lymphoma is high; monitor closely.

- Use parenteral administration only if patient is unable to take the oral drug; transfer to oral drug as soon as possible.
- Apply thin layer of ointment to affected area; do not use occlusive dressings; do not apply to wet skin; encourage patient to avoid exposure to sunlight.

⊗ *Warning* Monitor renal function and LFTs before and periodically during therapy; marked decreases in function may require dosage changes or discontinuation.

- Monitor tacrolimus blood concentrations.
- Monitor liver function and hematologic tests to determine dosage.

Teaching points

- Avoid infections; avoid crowds and people with infections. Also avoid having vaccinations while taking this drug. Notify your health care provider at once if you injure yourself.
- Do not drink grapefruit juice while using this drug.
- Do not use St. John's Wort while taking this drug.
- This drug should not be taken during pregnancy. If you think that you are pregnant or you want to become pregnant, consult your health care provider.
- Arrange to have periodic blood tests to monitor drug response and effects.
- Be aware that transplant patients (particularly those of black or Hispanic heritage) are at increased risk for post-transplant new-onset diabetes. Report unusual thirst or increased frequency of urination.
- Do not discontinue without consulting your health care provider. Continue use of topical ointment for 1 week after resolution of the infection.
- If you are using the topical form, avoid sunlight, use sunscreen and protective clothing. Do not use occlusive dressings.

T

- You may experience these side effects: Nausea, vomiting (take drug with food); diarrhea; headache (request analgesics).
- Report unusual bleeding or bruising, fever, sore throat, mouth sores, tiredness.

▽tadalafil
(tah dal' ah fill)

Adcirca, Cialis

PREGNANCY CATEGORY B

Drug classes
Impotence drug
Phosphodiesterase-5 inhibitor

Therapeutic actions
Selectively inhibits cyclic guanosine monophosphate (cGMP) specific phosphodiesterase type 5. The mechanism of penile erection involves the release of nitric oxide into the corpus cavernosum of the penis during sexual stimulation. Nitrous oxide activates cGMP, which causes smooth muscle relaxation allowing the flow of blood into the corpus cavernosum. Tadalafil prevents the breakdown of cGMP by phosphodiesterase, leading to increased cGMP levels and prolonged smooth muscle relaxation, thus promoting the flow of blood into the corpus cavernosum, relaxation of pulmonary muscle cells, and vasodilation of the pulmonary vascular bed.

Indications
- Treatment of erectile dysfunction (ED) in the presence of sexual stimulation (*Cialis*)
- Once daily for treatment of ED in men who anticipate having sex more than twice weekly (*Cialis*)
- Treatment of pulmonary arterial hyertension, to improve exercise tolerance (*Adcirca*)
- Treatment of symptoms of BPH; combination therapy for men with both ED and BPH
- Unlabeled use: Raynaud phenomenon

Contraindications and cautions
- Contraindicated with allergy to any component of the tablet, concurrent use of nitrates.
- Use cautiously with hepatic or renal impairment; with anatomical deformation of the penis, with known cardiac disease (effects of sexual activity need to be evaluated), congenital prolonged QT interval, unstable angina; hypotension (systolic pressure less than 90 mm Hg); uncontrolled hypertension (BP higher than 170/110 mm Hg); concurrent use of alpha blockers; hereditary degenerative retinal disorders; MI in past 3 months; angina during intercourse; stroke in last 6 mo; NYNA class II or greater HF.

Available forms
Tablets—2.5, 5, 10, 20 mg (*Cialis*); 20 mg (*Adcirca*)

Dosages
Adults
ED: 10 mg PO taken before anticipated sexual activity; range 5–20 mg PO. Limit use to once per day.
For once-daily use: 2.5 mg/day PO without regard to timing of sexual activity. May be increased to 5 mg/day PO based on patient response.
Pulmonary arterial hypertension: 40 mg/day PO without regard to food, given as a once-daily dose. Do not divide.
Pediatric patients
Not intended for use in children.
Patients receiving itraconazole, ketoconazole, ritonavir other potent CYP3AY inhibitors being treated for ED
Do not exceed one 10-mg dose in 72-hr period.
Patients with renal impairment being treated for ED
For creatinine clearance 31–50 mL/min, initial dose not to exceed 5 mg PO daily or 10 mg PO every 48 hr.; no further adjustment needed for once-daily use. For creatinine clearance less than 30 mL/min, 5 mg PO every 72 hr; once-daily use not recommended (*Cialis*).
Patients with renal impairment being treated for pulmonary arterial hypertension
For creatinine clearance of 31–80 mL/min, starting dose is 20 mg/day PO; increase to 40 mg/day based on patient response. For creatinine clearance of less than 30 mL/min and patients on hemodialysis, avoid use.
Patients with hepatic impairment being treated for ED
For Child-Pugh class A or B, maximum dosage should not exceed 10 mg PO daily. Use caution with once-daily use; Child-Pugh class C not recommended (*Cialis*).

Adverse effects in *italics* are most common; those in **bold** are life-threatening. ▭ Do not crush.

Patients with hepatic impairment being treated for pulmonary arterial hypertension

For Child-Pugh class A or B, starting dose is 20 mg/day. Avoid use with severe hepatic cirrhosis.

Pharmacokinetics

Route	Onset	Peak
Oral	Rapid	0.5–6 hr

Metabolism: Hepatic; $T_{1/2}$: 17.5 hr
Distribution: May cross placenta; may enter breast milk
Excretion: Feces, urine

Adverse effects

- **CNS:** *Headache,* abnormal vision, changes in color vision, fatigue, ischemic optic neuropathy, sudden loss of hearing
- **CV:** *Flushing,* angina, chest pain, hypertension, hypotension, **MI,** palpitation, postural hypotension, tachycardia
- **GI:** *Dyspepsia,* diarrhea, abdominal pain, dry mouth, esophagitis, gastritis, GERD, nausea, abnormal liver function test results
- **GU:** Abnormal erection, spontaneous erection, priapism
- **Respiratory:** Rhinitis, sinusitis, dyspnea, epistaxis, pharyngitis, nasal congestion
- **Other:** Flulike symptoms, edema, pain, rash, sweating, **Stevens-Johnson syndrome,** myalgia

Interactions

✳ Drug-drug ⊗ *Warning* Possible severe hypotension and serious cardiac events if combined with nitrates; this combination is contraindicated. • Risk of hypotension if combined with other antihypertensives, particularly alpha blockers
• Possible increased tadalafil levels and effects if taken with ketoconazole, itraconazole, erythromycin; monitor patient and reduce dosage as needed • Increased tadalafil serum levels if combined with indinavir, ritonavir; if these drugs are being used, limit tadalafil dose to 10 mg in a 72-hr period • Reduced tadalafil levels and effectiveness if combined with rifampin
• Risk for increased cardiac effects, decreased BP, or flushing if combined with alcohol; warn patient of this possibility if patient uses alcohol

✳ Drug-food • Possible increased tadalafil levels if taken with grapefruit juice

■ Nursing considerations

Assessment

- **History:** Allergy to any component of the tablet; concurrent use of nitrates or alpha blockers; unstable angina, hypotension, uncontrolled hypertension; severe hepatic impairment; end-stage renal disease with dialysis; hereditary degenerative retinal disorders; anatomical deformation of the penis; cardiac disease; congenital prolonged QT interval
- **Physical:** Orientation, affect; skin color, lesions; R, adventitious sounds; P, BP, ECG, LFTs, renal function tests

Interventions

- Ensure diagnosis of ED and determine underlying causes and other appropriate treatment.
- Advise patient with ED that drug does not work without sexual stimulation. Limit use to once per day.
- Remind patient with ED that drug does not protect against STDs and appropriate measures should be taken.
- Ensure that patient with pulmonary arterial hypertension takes dose all at once, once a day.
- ⊗ *Warning* Tell patient to never take this drug with nitrates because serious, even fatal complications can occur.
- Warn patient of the risk of lowered BP or dizziness if drug is taken with alcohol.

Teaching points

- If you are taking this drug for erectile dysfunction, take the drug before anticipated sexual activity. The drug will stay in your body for up to 3 days. The drug will have no effect unless there is sexual stimulation. If you anticipate sexual activity more than twice per week, daily dosing should be considered.
- If you are taking this drug for erectile dysfunction, this drug will not protect you from sexually transmitted diseases; use appropriate precautions.
- If you are taking this drug for pulmonary arterial hypertension, this drug will help to increase your ability to exercise. Take the drug once a day; do not split the dose.
- Do not take this drug if you are taking nitrates, alpha blockers, or other drugs for treating erectile dysfunction; serious side effects and even death can occur.

T

- Many drugs may interact with tadalafil; always consult your health care provider before taking any drug, including over-the-counter drugs and herbal therapies. Dosage adjustments may be needed.
- Stop taking the drug and contact your health care provider if you experience sudden loss of vision.
- Combining this drug with alcohol could cause dizziness, loss of blood pressure, or increased flushing.
- You may experience these side effects: Headache, dizziness, upset stomach, runny nose, muscle pains. These side effects should go away within a couple of hours. If side effects persist, consult your health care provider.
- Report difficult or painful urination, vision changes, fainting, erection that persists for longer than 4 hours (if this occurs, seek medical assistance as soon as possible), sudden loss of vision or hearing.

▷talc, USP

See Appendix R, *Less commonly used drugs.*

▷taliglucerase

See Appendix R, *Less commonly used drugs.*

DANGEROUS DRUG

▷tamoxifen citrate
(ta mox' i fen)

Apo-Tamox (CAN), Gen-Tamoxifen (CAN), Tamofen (CAN)

PREGNANCY CATEGORY D

Drug classes
Antiestrogen
Antineoplastic

Therapeutic actions
Potent antiestrogenic effects: Competes with estrogen for binding sites in target tissues, such as the breast.

Indications
- Treatment of metastatic breast cancer in women and men; in premenopausal women with metastatic breast cancer, tamoxifen is

an alternative to oophorectomy or ovarian irradiation
- Treatment of node-positive breast cancer in postmenopausal women following total mastectomy or segmental mastectomy, axillary dissection, and breast irradiation
- Treatment of axillary node-negative breast cancer in women following total mastectomy or segmental mastectomy, axillary dissection, and breast irradiation
- Reduction in risk of invasive breast cancer in women with ductal carcinoma in situ (DCIS) following breast surgery and radiation
- Reduction in occurrence of contralateral breast cancer in patients receiving adjuvant tamoxifen therapy for breast cancer
- Reduction in incidence of breast cancer in women at high risk for breast cancer
- Unlabeled uses: Treatment of mastalgia; useful for decreasing size and pain of gynecomastia; treatment of McCune-Albright syndrome and precocious puberty in girls 2–10 yr; malignant carcinoid tumor, carcinoid syndrome; menstrual migraine; oligospermia; metastatic melanoma desmoid tumors

Contraindications and cautions
- Contraindicated with allergy to tamoxifen, pregnancy, lactation, women who require concomitant coumarin-type anticoagulation therapy, or in women with a history of DVT or PE.
- Use cautiously in women with a history of thromboembolic events.

Available forms
Tablets—10, 20 mg; oral solution—10 mg/5 mL

Dosages
Adults
- *Breast cancer:* 20–40 mg/day PO for 5 yr. Dosages of more than 20 mg/day should be given in divided doses, morning and evening.
- *Reduction in breast cancer incidence:* 20 mg/day PO for 5 yr.
- *DCIS:* 20 mg/day PO for 5 yr.

Pharmacokinetics

Route	Onset	Peak
Oral	Varies	4–7 hr

Metabolism: Hepatic; $T_{1/2}$: 7–14 days

Distribution: Crosses placenta; may enter breast milk
Excretion: Feces

Adverse effects

- **CNS:** Depression, light-headedness, dizziness, headache, corneal opacity, decreased visual acuity, retinopathy, **stroke**
- **Dermatologic: Stevens-Johnson syndrome,** *hot flashes, rash*
- **EENT:** pharyngitis
- **GI:** *Nausea, vomiting,* food distaste, alterations in liver enzymes
- **GU:** *Vaginal bleeding, vaginal discharge, menstrual irregularities,* pruritus vulvae, endometrial cancer, uterine sarcoma
- **Hematologic:** Hypercalcemia, especially with bone metastases, thrombocytopenia, leukopenia, anemia, **DVT**
- **Other:** Peripheral edema; increased bone and tumor pain and local disease (initially seen with a good tumor response, usually subsides); cancer in animal studies, **PE**

Interactions

✳ Drug-drug • Increased risk of bleeding with oral anticoagulants • Increased serum levels with bromocriptine • Increased risk of thromboembolic events if given with cytotoxic agents

✳ Drug-food • Decreased metabolism and risk of toxic effects if combined with grapefruit juice; avoid this combination

✳ Drug-lab test • Possible increase in calcium levels, elevated T_4 levels without hyperthyroidism

■ Nursing considerations
Assessment

- **History:** Allergy to tamoxifen, pregnancy, lactation, previous DVT or PE
- **Physical:** Skin lesions, color, turgor; pelvic examination; orientation, affect, reflexes; ophthalmologic examination; peripheral pulses, edema; LFTs, CBC and differential, estrogen receptor evaluation of tumor cells

Interventions

⊗ **Black box warning** Alert women with DCIS and those at high risk for breast cancer of risks for serious to potentially fatal drug effects, including stroke, embolic events, and uterine malignancies; discuss benefits versus risks.

- Give doses greater than 20 mg in divided doses. Administer bid, in the morning and the evening.
- Arrange for periodic blood counts.
- Arrange for initial ophthalmologic examination and periodic examinations if visual changes occur.
- Counsel patient to use contraception while taking this drug; inform patient that serious fetal harm could occur.
- Decrease dosage if adverse effects become severe.

Teaching points

- For doses greater than 20 milligrams, take the drug twice a day, in the morning and evening. Do not drink grapefruit juice while using this drug.
- This drug can cause serious fetal harm and must not be taken during pregnancy. Contraceptive measures should be used. If you become pregnant or you want to become pregnant, consult your health care provider immediately. Avoid breast-feeding during therapy.
- Have regular gynecologic examinations during therapy.
- You may experience these side effects: Bone pain; hot flashes (staying in cool places may help); nausea, vomiting (eat frequent small meals); weight gain; menstrual irregularities; dizziness, headache, light-headedness (use caution if driving or performing tasks that require alertness).
- Report marked weakness, sleepiness, mental confusion, pain or swelling of the legs, shortness of breath, blurred vision.

▷**tamsulosin hydrochloride**
*(tam soo **low'** sin)*

Flomax ⓒⓐⓝ

PREGNANCY CATEGORY B

Drug class

Alpha-adrenergic blocker (peripherally acting)

Therapeutic actions

Blocks the smooth muscle alpha$_1$-adrenergic receptors in the prostate, prostatic capsule, prostatic urethra, and bladder neck, leading to relaxation of the bladder and prostate and improving the flow of urine in cases of BPH, with little effect on systemic blood pressure.

Indications
- Treatment of the signs and symptoms of BPH
- Unlabeled use: Adjunct in managing ureteral stones

Contraindications and cautions
- Contraindicated with hypersensitivity to tamsulosin, prostate cancer, pregnancy, lactation.
- Use cautiously with hypotension, sulfa hypersensitivity.

Available forms
Capsules⊕—0.4 mg

Dosages
Adults
0.4 mg PO daily 30 min after the same meal each day; if response is not satisfactory in 2–4 wk, dosage may be increased to 0.8 mg PO daily 30 min after the same meal each day. If therapy is interrupted for any reason for several days, resume dosing at 0.4 mg PO daily.
Pediatric patients
Safety and efficacy not established.

Pharmacokinetics

Route	Onset	Peak
Oral	Varies	4–6 hr

Metabolism: Hepatic; $T_{1/2}$: 9–15 hr
Distribution: May cross placenta; enters breast milk
Excretion: Feces, urine

Adverse effects
- **CNS:** *Somnolence, insomnia,* headache, dizziness
- **CV:** *Orthostatic hypotension,* syncope
- **GI:** *Nausea,* dyspepsia
- **GU:** *Abnormal ejaculation, decreased libido*
- **Other:** Cough, sinusitis, rhinitis, *increased risk of intraoperative floppy iris syndrome with cataract surgery*

Interactions
❋ **Drug-drug** • Possible increased hypotensive effects with other alpha-adrenergic antagonists, sildenafil, tadalafil, vardenafil

- Risk of increased toxic effects with cimetidine

■ Nursing considerations

⬥ CLINICAL ALERT!
Name confusion has occurred between *Flomax* (tamsulosin) and *Fosamax* (alendronate); use caution.

Assessment
- **History:** Allergy to tamsulosin or sulfa drugs; pregnancy, lactation; prostatic cancer; hypotension
- **Physical:** Body weight; skin color, lesions; orientation, affect, reflexes; ophthalmologic examination; P, BP, orthostatic BP; R, adventitious sounds, status of nasal mucous membranes; voiding pattern, normal output, urinalysis

Interventions
- Ensure that patient does not have prostatic cancer before beginning treatment.
- Administer once a day, 30 min after the same meal each day.
- Resume therapy at 0.4 mg daily if therapy is interrupted for several days for any reason.
- Ensure that patient does not crush, chew, or open capsule. Capsule should be swallowed whole.
- Monitor patient carefully for orthostatic hypotension; chance of orthostatic hypotension, dizziness, and syncope is high with the first dose. Establish safety precautions as appropriate.
- Alert surgeon that patient is on this drug if patient is going to have cataract surgery; increased risk of intraoperative floppy iris syndrome may require additional surgical intervention

Teaching points
- Take this drug exactly as prescribed, once a day. Do not chew, crush, or open capsules; capsules must be swallowed whole. Use care when beginning therapy; the chance of dizziness or syncope is greatest at that time. Change position slowly to avoid increased dizziness. Take the drug 30 minutes after the same meal each day.
- This drug should not be combined with drugs used to treat erectile dysfunction.

Adverse effects in *italics* are most common; those in **bold** are life-threatening. ⊕ Do not crush.

- Tell your surgeon that you are taking this drug if you are considering cataract surgery.
- You may experience these side effects: Dizziness, weakness (more likely when you change position, in the early morning, after exercise, in hot weather, and when you have consumed alcohol; some tolerance may occur after you have taken the drug for a while; avoid driving or engaging in tasks that require alertness; change position slowly, use caution in climbing stairs, lie down if dizziness persists); GI upset (eat frequent small meals); impotence (discuss this with your health care provider); stuffy nose. Most of these effects will disappear gradually with continued therapy.
- Report frequent dizziness or fainting, worsening of symptoms.

▽**tapentadol**

*(tah **pen**' tah dohl)*

Nucynta Nucynta CR (CAN) ⓒⒶⓃ, Nucynta ER ⓒⒶⓃ

Pregnancy Category C

Controlled Substance C-II

Drug classes

Norepinephrine reuptake inhibitor
Opioid receptor analgesic (mu specific)

Therapeutic actions

Binds to and activates mu-opioid receptors in the CNS, inhibiting transmission of pain at the spinal cord, and affects activity in parts of the brain that control how pain is perceived; analgesic properties are enhanced by the blocking of norepinephrine reuptake at the nerve synapse, increasing concentration of norepinephrine in the synaptic cleft.

Indications

- Relief of moderate to severe pain in patients 18 yr and older (immediate-release)
- ◢■ NEW INDICATION: Management of moderate to severe chronic pain in adults when continual, round-the-clock opioid use is needed for an extended period (ER forms)

Contraindications and cautions

- Contraindicated with known hypersensitivity to any component of the drug, increased in-

tracranial pressure, impaired consciousness or coma, significant respiratory depression, acute or severe bronchial asthma, hypercapnia, paralytic ileus, within 14 days of MAOI use, pregnancy.
- Use cautiously with elderly or debilitated patients, asthma, COPD, severe obesity, sleep apnea syndrome, myxedema, CNS depression, lactation, pancreatic or biliary tract disease, hepatic or renal impairment, seizure disorders.

Available forms

Tablets–50, 75, 100 mg; ER tablets ⓒⒶⓃ—50, 100, 150, 200, 250 mg

Dosages

Adults
50–100 mg (immediate-release) PO every 4–6 hr. On first day; may give second dose within 1 hr if pain control is not adequate. Maximum dose, 700 mg/day on first day, 600 mg/day thereafter. ER forms—100–250 mg PO bid. Reduce initial dose by 50 mg in analgesic-naïve patients. Maximum dose, 500 mg/day.
Pediatric patients
Safety and efficacy not established.
Geriatric or debilitated patients
Use caution. Start with the smallest dose and evaluate response.
Patients with moderate hepatic impairment
Do not exceed three doses/day (immediate-releuseo) or 100 mg/day (ER forms).

Pharmacokinetics

Route	Onset	Peak
Oral	Rapid	1 hr

Metabolism: Hepatic; $T_{1/2}$: Unknown
Distribution: May cross placenta; may enter breast milk
Excretion: Urine

Adverse effects

- **CNS:** *Drowsiness, dizziness,* changes in thinking, *headache*
- **GI:** *Nausea, vomiting,* constipation
- **Respiratory:** Respiratory depression
- **Other:** Drug abuse

Interactions

❋ **Drug-drug** • Risk of increased CNS depression (which could lead to respiratory depression) if combined with general anesthetics, opioids, phenothiazines, sedatives, hypnotics, alcohol; if these combinations are used, monitor patient closely and adjust dosages as needed • Risk of potentially life-threatening serotonin syndrome if combined with SSRIs, TCAs, triptans, other norepinephrine reuptake inhibitors or with MAOIs; use within 14 days of MAOIs is contraindicated; if other combinations are used, patient should be strictly monitored and dosage adjustments made as needed • Alcohol ingestion from any source may cause drug to be released from ER formulation, resulting in toxic overdose; avoid all forms of alcohol

Drug-alternative therapy • Risk of serotonin syndrome if combined with St. John's Wort; advise patient to avoid this combination

■ **Nursing considerations**
Assessment
• **History:** Hypersensitivity to any component of the drug; acute or severe bronchial asthma, COPD, hypercapnia; MAOI use within 14 days; severe obesity, sleep apnea syndrome; myxedema, CNS depression, seizure disorders; increased intracranial pressure; pancreatic or biliary tract disease, alcohol ingestion; paralytic ileus; hepatic or renal impairment; pregnancy, lactation
• **Physical:** Orientation, affect, pain evaluation; R, adventitious sounds; bowel sounds; LFTs, renal function tests

Interventions
• Assess for pain before beginning therapy and periodically during therapy.
• Dispense the least amount of drug feasible; risk of abuse exists. Ensure patient swallows ER form whole and does not cut, crush, or chew it.
• Institute safety measures (use side rails, assist with ambulation); drug increases risk of dizziness and drowsiness.
• Provide frequent small meals if GI upset is a problem.

Teaching points
• Take this drug exactly as prescribed; do not increase dosage without consulting the health care provider. Swallow ER form whole. Do not cut, crush, or chew it.
• This drug may enter breast milk and could affect your infant if you are breast-feeding. Consider an alternate method of feeding your infant or an alternate pain medication.
• Be aware that alcohol may increase the sedation effects of this drug; avoid this combi-

nation. When taking ER form, avoid ingesting alcohol in any form, including over-the-counter or prescription drugs; serious to fatal overdose could occur.
• This drug may interact with many other medications. Tell your health care provider about every medication you are taking.
• Do not use St. John's Wort while you are taking this drug; serious side effects can occur.
• You may experience these side effects: Headache (medication may be available to help); nausea and vomiting (frequent small meals may help); dizziness and drowsiness (avoid driving a car or operating hazardous machinery until you know how this drug will affect you); constipation (there may be medication available to help).
• Report severe nausea and vomiting, shortness of breath, rash.

▽ **teduglutide**
See Appendix R, *Less commonly used drugs.*

telaprevir
(tel a' pre veer)

Incivek

PREGNANCY CATEGORY B

Drug classes
Antiviral
Protease inhibitor

Therapeutic actions
Antiviral; inhibits hepatitis C virus (HCV)–specific protease, which inhibits viral replication in the hepatitis C infected cell.

Indications
• Treatment of chronic HCV, genotype-1 infection in adults with compensated liver disease who are previously untreated or who have failed on interferon and ribavirin therapy; must be given in combination with peginterferon alfa and ribavirin

Contraindications and cautions
• Contraindicated with history of serious hypersensitivity to telaprevir, concurrent use of CYP3A4/5 inducers or inhibitors, moderate to severe hepatic impairment, solid

organ transplants, use of sildenafil or tadalafil for the treatment of pulmonary hypertension, pregnancy, lactation.

- Use cautiously with coinfection with HIV, hepatitis B; elderly patients.

Available forms
Tablets—375 mg

Dosages
Adults
750 mg PO tid (every 7–9 hr) with food for 12 wk; followed by 12–16 wk of peginterferon and ribavirin.
Pediatric patients
Safety and efficacy not established.

Pharmacokinetics

Route	Onset	Peak
Oral	Moderate	4–5 hr

Metabolism: Hepatic; $T_{1/2}$: 9–11 hr
Distribution: May cross placenta; may enter breast milk
Excretion: Feces, urine

Adverse effects
- **CNS:** Headache, insomnia
- **Dermatological:** *Rash, pruritus,* **Stevens-Johnson syndrome**
- **GI:** *Nausea, dysgeusia, vomiting, diarrhea, hemorrhoids, anorectal discomfort*
- **Hematological:** *Anemia,* neutropenia
- **Other:** *Fatigue*

Interactions
＊ **Drug-drug** • Increased toxicity with alfuzosin, atorvastatin, atazanavir, bosentan, budesonide, fluticasone, prednisone, calcium channel blockers, rifampin, dihydroergotamine, ergotamine, methylergonovine, cisapride, pimozide, triazolam, sildenafil, tadalafil, vardenafil, pimozide, alprazolam, midazolam, cyclosporine, sirolimus, tacrolimus; use of these drugs with telaprevir is contraindicated • Increased antiarrhythmic and digoxin levels; monitor patient closely • Increased colchicine level; dosage must be reduced; combination should not be used in patients with renal or hepatic impairment • Loss of effectiveness of hormonal contraceptives, zolpidem

＊ **Drug-alternative therapy** • Loss of effectiveness with St. John's Wort; avoid this combination

■ Nursing considerations
Assessment
- **History:** Hypersensitivity to components of drug, concurrent infection with HIV, hepatitis B; hepatic impairment, solid organ transplant, pregnancy, lactation
- **Physical:** Neurologic exam; skin evaluation; GI exam; CBC; HIV, hepatitis B, hepatitis C testing

Interventions
- Drug must be given with peginterferon alfa and ribavirin; consider all cautions and contraindications for those drugs.
- Rule out HIV and hepatitis B infection before beginning therapy.
- Ensure patient will receive 12–16 wk of peginterferon alfa and ribavirin after finishing 12 wk of combined therapy with telaprevir.
- Monitor CBC regularly; follow dosage adjustments if anemia becomes severe.
- Monitor patient for rash. Mild to moderate rash is expected, but discontinue telaprevir if rash becomes severe.
- Administer tid with food, allowing 7–9 hr between doses.
- Encourage small, frequent meals and comfort measures if GI upset and taste changes are severe.
- Rule out pregnancy because this drug combination can cause severe fetal abnormalities. Men taking this combination should not father a child. Two forms of contraception should be used and routine, monthly pregnancy tests should be performed.
- Patient should be advised that transmission of hepatitis C may still occur and to take appropriate precautions.

Teaching points
- You must take this drug with peginterferon alfa and ribavirin.
- Take this drug three times a day with food; allow 7 to 9 hours between doses. If you miss a dose and it is less than 2 hours before the next dose is due, skip that dose. If you miss a dose and it is more than 2 hours before the next dose is due, take the missed dose with food and resume the normal dosing schedule.
- Tell your health care provider about all drugs, over-the-counter products, and herbs you might be using; this drug interacts with

many other drugs and dosage adjustment may be needed. Avoid St. John's Wort while taking this drug.

- This combination of drugs can cause serious fetal abnormalities. Use two forms of contraception to ensure that pregnancy does not occur; a routine pregnancy test will be done monthly. Men should not father a child while taking these drugs and should suggest the use of two forms of contraception with their partner.
- This combination of drugs may appear into breast milk; if you are breast-feeding, you should use a different method of feeding the baby.
- Transmission of hepatitis C may still occur during therapy with this drug combination; take precautions to prevent transmission.
- You may be more susceptible to infection; avoid exposure to infection.
- You may experience these side effects: GI upset, nausea (small, frequent meals may help); fatigue, anemia (spacing activities throughout the day may help); headache (consult your health care provider for an appropriate pain medication); rectal discomfort (this should pass with time; consult your health care provider if this becomes uncomfortable).
- Report severe rash, extreme fatigue, changes in your drug regimen, pregnancy.

▽**telavancin**
(tell ah van' sin)

Vibativ

PREGNANCY CATEGORY C

Drug classes
Antibiotic
Lipoglycopeptide

Therapeutic actions
A lipoglycopeptide, a semisynthetic derivative of vancomycin, that inhibits bacterial cell-wall synthesis by interfering with the polymerization and cross-linking of peptidoglycan; binds to the bacterial membrane and disrupts membrane-barrier function, causing bacterial cell death.

Indications
- Treatment of complicated skin and skin-structure infections caused by susceptible strains

of gram-positive organisms (*Staphylococcus aureus* [including methicillin-susceptible and methicillin-resistant isolates], *Streptococcus pyogenes, Streptococcus agalactiae, Streptococcus anginosus, Enterococcus faecalis* [vancomycin-susceptible isolates only]); combination therapy may be indicated of gram-negative pathogens are documented or suspected

Contraindications and cautions
- Contraindicated in known hypersensitivity to components of the drug, lactation, pregnancy.
- Use cautiously with renal impairment, QTc-interval prolongation or risk of prolongation.

Available forms
Single-use vials—250, 750 mg

Dosages
Adults
10 mg/kg IV infused over 60 min once every 24 hr for 7–14 days.
Pediatric patients younger than 18 yr
Safety and efficacy not established.
Patients with renal impairment
For creatinine clearance of more than 50 mL/min, 10 mg/kg IV every 24 hr; for creatinine clearance of 30–50 mL/min, 7.5 mg/kg IV every 24 hr; for creatinine clearance of 10 to less than 30 mL/min, 10 mg/kg IV every 48 hr. No recommendations are available for creatinine clearance of less than 10 mL/min or for patients on hemodialysis.

Pharmacokinetics

Route	Onset	Peak
IV	Rapid	End of infusion

Metabolism: Unknown; $T_{1/2}$: 8–9.5 hr
Distribution: May cross placenta; may enter breast milk
Excretion: Urine

▼ IV FACTS
Preparation: Reconstitute with 5% dextrose injection, sterile water for injection, or 0.9% sodium chloride injection to a concentration of 15 mg/mL (15 mL added to 250-mg vial, 45 mL added to 750-mg vial). Mix thoroughly and ensure that contents have dissolved completely

and that solution contains no particulate matter. Use within 4 hr when kept at room temperature or within 72 hr if refrigerated.
Infusion: Infuse over 60 min.
Incompatibilities: Do not administer in the same line as other medications; if the line is used for other solutions, flush the line before administering telavancin.

Adverse effects
- **CNS:** dizziness
- **CV:** QTc-interval prolongation
- **GI:** *nausea, vomiting,* diarrhea, abdominal pain, *Clostridium difficile* diarrhea, decreased appetite, *taste disturbance*
- **GU: nephrotoxicity,** *foamy urine*
- **Other:** rash, pruritus, rigors, infusion-site pain and redness; infusion reactions (red man syndrome) with rapid infusion

Interactions
✳ Drug-drug • Increased risk of prolonged QTc interval if combined with other drugs known to cause QTc-interval prolongation; obtain baseline ECG and monitor patient accordingly • Increased risk of nephrotoxicity if combined with other nephrotoxic drugs; monitor patient accordingly
✳ Drug-lab test • Alterations in INR, PT, APPT, activated clotting time, and coagulation-based factor Xa tests with no effect on coagulation; take blood samples as close as possible before administration of next dose

■ Nursing considerations
Assessment
History: Known hypersensitivity to components of the drug, lactation, pregnancy, renal impairment, QTc-interval prolongation
Physical: Reflexes; skin color, lesions; abdominal exam; renal function tests; baseline ECG; culture and sensitivity of infected area

Interventions
⊗ **Black box warning** Drug poses fetal risk; women of childbearing age should have a serum pregnancy test before start of therapy. Avoid use in pregnancy and advise patient to use contraception.
- Obtain culture and sensitivity tests of the infected area before start of therapy. Ensure that the drug is used only to treat susceptible strains, to prevent development of drug-resistant bacteria.

- Ensure that drug infuses over at least 60 min; too rapid infusion can result in red man syndrome.
- Monitor patient for *C. difficile* diarrhea. If this occurs, drug may need to be stopped and antibiotics administered. Provide fluid and electrolyte support.
- Monitor renal function before and periodically during treatment; if renal toxicity occurs, a different antibiotic should be considered.
- Be aware of drug's effects on various coagulation tests; draw blood for these tests as close as possible before administration of next dose.

Teaching points
- This drug can only be given intravenously. It will be given over 1 hour, once a day for 7 to 14 days depending on your response to the drug. It is important not to skip doses.
- This drug should not be taken during pregnancy; it can have serious effects on the fetus. Women of childbearing age will need to have a serum pregnancy test before beginning therapy. Use of contraceptive measures is advised.
- If you are breast-feeding, you should use another method of feeding the infant while you are taking this drug because the drug could cause serious adverse effects in your infant.
- You will need to have blood tests to monitor the effects of this drug on your kidneys.
- You may experience these side effects: Dizziness (use caution when moving about, and change position slowly); nausea and vomiting; changes in taste (small, frequent meals may help; medication may be available to relieve these symptoms); rash; foamy urine (this is an effect of the drug and will go away when the drug is stopped).
- Report severe diarrhea, fever, irregular heartbeat, hives, rash, flushing, worsening of your infection.

▽**telbivudine**

See Appendix R, *Less commonly used drugs.*

▽**telithromycin**
*(tell ith roe **mye**´ sin)*

Ketek⬛ⓒ

PREGNANCY CATEGORY C

T

Drug classes
Antibiotic
Ketolide

Therapeutic actions
Bacteriostatic or bactericidal in susceptible bacteria; binds to sites on bacterial ribosomes, causing change in protein function, leading to cell death.

Indications
- Only for treatment of mild to moderately severe community-acquired pneumonia caused by *Streptococcus pneumoniae* (including multi-drug resistant strains), *Haemophilus influenzae, Moraxella catarrhalis, Chlamydophilia pneumoniae, Mycoplasma pneumoniae* in patients 18 yr and older
- ■ **NEW INDICATION:** Unlabeled use: Sinusitis

Contraindications and cautions
- Contraindicated with allergy to telithromycin, to any component of the drug, or any macrolide antibiotic or cisapride; congenital QT prolongation, proarrhythmic conditions (hypokalemia), significant bradycardia; concurrent use of pimozide, class Ia or III antiarrhythmics, simvastatin, lovastatin, atorvastatain; myasthenia gravis; history of hepatitis or jaundice.
- Use cautiously with renal or hepatic impairment, pregnancy, lactation.

Available forms
Tablets⊞—300, 400 mg

Dosages
Adults
Give 800 mg once daily PO for 7–10 days.
Pediatric patients
Safety and efficacy not established.
Patients with renal impairment
In patients with creatinine clearance less than 30 mL/min, including those on dialysis, give 600 mg PO once daily for 7–10 days after dialysis session is complete. In patients with creatinine clearance less than 30 mL/min and coexisting hepatic impairment, give 400 mg PO once daily for 7–10 days.

Pharmacokinetics

Route	Onset	Peak
Oral	Rapid	0.5–4 hr

Metabolism: Hepatic metabolism; T$_{1/2}$: 10 hr

Distribution: May cross placenta; passes into breast milk
Excretion: Feces, urine

Adverse effects
- **CNS:** Headache, dizziness, vertigo
- **CV: Prolonged QT interval, torsades de pointes**
- **GI:** *Diarrhea,* nausea, vomiting, taste alterations, loose stools, **pseudomembranous colitis,** hepatic impairment
- **Other:** *Superinfections,* hypersensitivity reactions ranging from rash to **anaphylaxis,** visual disturbances

Interactions
✴ **Drug-drug** ⊗ *Warning* Risk of increased serum levels and potentially serious adverse effects if combined with pimozide, simvastatin, lovastatin, atorvastatin, midazolam; avoid these combinations.
- Risk of increased exposure to metoprolol if given in combination, caution should be used • Risk of increased levels of digoxin; if this combination is used, monitor serum digoxin levels regularly and adjust dosage accordingly • Risk of decreased telithromycin levels and loss of therapeutic effect if combined with rifampin, phenytoin, carbamazepine, phenobarbital; suggest use of a different antibiotic if these drugs are used • Risk of increased GI effects of theophylline if taken together, separate doses by at least 1 hr if these two drugs are used

■ Nursing considerations
Assessment
- **History:** Known allergy to telithromycin, to any component of the drug, or to any macrolide antibiotic; congenital QT prolongation, proarrhythmic conditions, significant bradycardia; concurrent use of pimozide, class Ia or III antiarrhythmics, simvastatin, lovastatin, atorvastatin; myasthenia gravis; renal or hepatic impairment; pregnancy; lactation
- **Physical:** Site of infection, skin color, lesions; orientation, affect; baseline ECG, GI output, bowel sounds, liver evaluation; culture and sensitivity tests of infection, LFTs, renal function tests

Interventions
⊗ **Black box warning** Contraindicated for use in patients with myasthenia gravis; life-threatening respiratory failure may occur.

Adverse effects in *italics* are most common; those in **bold** are life-threatening. ⊞ Do not crush.

- Culture site of infection before beginning therapy; make sure drug is used only as indicated.
- Administer at about the same time each day, without regard to food.
- Make sure that the tablet is swallowed whole; do not cut, crush, or allow the patient to chew the tablet.
- Monitor liver function in patients on prolonged therapy.
- Institute appropriate hygiene measures and arrange treatment if superinfections occur.
- If GI upset occurs provide frequent, small meals; encourage patient to maintain fluid intake and nutrition.
- Establish safety measures (eg, accompany patient, side rails) if CNS changes occur.

Teaching points

- Take this drug at about the same time each day, without regard to food. Do not cut, crush or chew the tablets; they must be swallowed whole.
- If you miss a dose, take the next dose as soon as you remember and then again about that time the next day; do not take more than one dose per day.
- Avoid quickly looking between objects in the distance and objects nearby if you are having visual difficulties.
- Take the full, prescribed dose of *Ketek*. Do not use the drug after the expiration date and do not save tablets for future use.
- You may experience these side effects: Nausea, diarrhea, abdominal discomfort (eat frequent small meals), headache (analgesics may be available to help, consult with your health care provider), dizziness (do not drive a car or operate hazardous machinery if this occurs).
- Report persistent or bloody diarrhea, visual disturbances that interfere with your daily activities, fainting, yellow color to the eyes or skin.

▷**telmisartan**
*(tell mah **sar'** tan)*

Micardis

PREGNANCY CATEGORY C
(FIRST TRIMESTER)

PREGNANCY CATEGORY D
(SECOND AND THIRD TRIMESTERS)

Drug classes
Angiotensin II receptor antagonist
Antihypertensive

Therapeutic actions
Selectively blocks the binding of angiotensin II to specific tissue receptors found in the vascular smooth muscle and adrenal gland; this action blocks the vasoconstriction effect of the renin-angiotensin system, as well as the release of aldosterone, leading to decreased BP.

Indications
- Treatment of hypertension, alone or in combination with other antihypertensive
- CV risk reduction, including risk of MI, stroke, or death, in patients 55 yr and older at high risk for developing major CV events who are unable to take ACE inhibitors

Contraindications and cautions
- Contraindicated with hypersensitivity to telmisartan, pregnancy (use during the second or third trimester can cause injury or death to the fetus), lactation.
- Use cautiously with hepatic or biliary impairment, hypovolemia.

Available forms
Tablets—20, 40, 80 mg

Dosages
Adults
Usual starting dose, 40 mg PO daily. Adjust dosage based on patient response. Range, 20–80 mg/day. Maximum dose, 80 mg/day. If response is still not as expected, a diuretic may be added. For CV risk reduction, 80 mg PO once a day.
Pediatric patients
Safety and efficacy not established.

Pharmacokinetics

Route	Onset	Peak	Duration
Oral	Rapid	0.5–1 hr	24 hr

Metabolism: Hepatic; $T_{1/2}$: 24 hr
Distribution: May cross placenta; may enter breast milk
Excretion: Feces

Adverse effects
- **CNS:** *Light-headedness, headache, dizziness,* muscle weakness

T

- **CV:** Hypotension, palpitations
- **Dermatologic:** Rash, dermatitis, eczema, urticaria, pruritus
- **GI:** Constipation, flatulence, gastritis, vomiting, dry mouth, dental pain
- **GU:** Decreased renal function
- **Respiratory:** Asthma, dyspnea, epistaxis, cough
- **Other:** Back pain, gout

Interactions

✳ **Drug-drug** • Increased serum levels and risk of toxicity of digoxin if combined. Increased risk of hyperkalemia if combined with potassium-sparing diuretics

■ Nursing considerations
Assessment

- **History:** Hypersensitivity to telmisartan; pregnancy, lactation; hepatic or biliary impairment; hypovolemia; renal stenosis
- **Physical:** Skin lesions, turgor; T; orientation, reflexes, affect; BP; R, respiratory auscultation; LFTs

Interventions

- Administer without regard to meals.

⊗ **Black box warning** Ensure that patient is not pregnant before beginning therapy. Suggest the use of barrier birth control while using telmisartan; fetal injury and deaths have been reported.

- If giving to a breast-feeding patient, help the patient find an alternative method of feeding the infant. Depression of the renin-angiotensin system in infants is potentially very dangerous.

⊗ **Warning** Alert the surgeon and mark the patient's chart with notice that telmisartan is being taken. The blockage of the renin-angiotensin system following surgery can produce problems. Hypotension may be reversed with volume expansion.

- If BP control does not reach desired levels, diuretics or other antihypertensives may be added to telmisartan. Monitor patient's BP carefully.
- Monitor patient closely in any situation that may lead to a decrease in BP secondary to reduction in fluid volume—excessive perspiration, dehydration, vomiting, diarrhea—excessive hypotension can occur.

Teaching points

- Take drug without regard to meals. Do not stop taking this drug without consulting your health care provider.
- Use a barrier method of birth control while taking this drug; if you become pregnant or want to become pregnant, consult your health care provider.
- You may experience these side effects: Dizziness (avoid driving a car or performing hazardous tasks); headache (medications may be available to help); nausea, vomiting, diarrhea (proper nutrition is important, consult with your dietitian to maintain nutrition); symptoms of upper respiratory tract infection; cough (do not self-medicate, consult your health care provider if this becomes uncomfortable).
- Report fever, chills, dizziness, pregnancy.

▽ **temazepam**
(te maz' e pam)

Apo-Temazepam (CAN), CO Temazepam (CAN), Gen-Temazepam (CAN), Novo-Temazepam (CAN), PMS-Temazepam (CAN), ratio-Temazepam (CAN), Restoril

PREGNANCY CATEGORY X

CONTROLLED SUBSTANCE C-IV

Drug classes
Benzodiazepine
Sedative-hypnotic

Therapeutic actions
Exact mechanisms of action not understood; acts mainly at subcortical levels of the CNS, leaving the cortex relatively unaffected; main sites of action may be the limbic system and mesencephalic reticular formation; benzodiazepines potentiate the effects of GABA, an inhibitory neurotransmitter.

Indications
- Short-term treatment of insomnia (7–10 days)

Contraindications and cautions
- Contraindicated with hypersensitivity to benzodiazepines, psychoses, acute narrow-angle

glaucoma, shock, coma, acute alcoholic intoxication with depression of vital signs, pregnancy (risk of congenital malformations, neonatal withdrawal syndrome), labor and delivery ("floppy infant" syndrome), lactation (infants may become lethargic and lose weight).

- Use cautiously with impaired liver or renal function, debilitation, depression, suicidal tendencies.

Available forms
Capsules—7.5, 15, 22.5, 30 mg

Dosages
Adults
15–30 mg PO before bedtime; 7.5 mg may be sufficient for some patients.
Pediatric patients
Not for use in patients younger than 18 yr.
Geriatric or debilitated patients
Initially, 7.5 mg PO; adjust dosage, increasing if needed.

Pharmacokinetics

Route	Onset	Peak
Oral	Varies	1.2–1.6 hr

Metabolism: Hepatic; $T_{1/2}$: 8.8 hr
Distribution: Crosses placenta; enters breast milk
Excretion: Urine

Adverse effects

- **CNS:** *Transient, mild drowsiness initially; sedation, depression, lethargy, apathy, fatigue, light-headedness, disorientation, restlessness, confusion,* crying, delirium, headache, slurred speech, dysarthria, stupor, rigidity, tremor, dystonia, vertigo, euphoria, nervousness, difficulty concentrating, vivid dreams, psychomotor retardation, extrapyramidal symptoms, mild paradoxical excitatory reactions during first 2 wk of treatment (especially in psychiatric patients, aggressive children, and with high dosage), visual and auditory disturbances, diplopia, nystagmus, depressed hearing, nasal congestion, complex sleep-related behaviors
- **CV:** *Bradycardia, tachycardia,* **CV collapse,** hypertension and hypotension, palpitations, edema
- **Dependence:** *Drug dependence with withdrawal syndrome* when drug is discontinued

- **Dermatologic:** Urticaria, pruritus, rash, dermatitis
- **GI:** *Constipation, diarrhea,* dry mouth, salivation, nausea, anorexia, vomiting, difficulty in swallowing, gastric disorders, elevations of blood enzymes; hepatic impairment, jaundice
- **GU:** Incontinence, urinary retention, changes in libido, menstrual irregularities
- **Hematologic:** Decreased Hct (primarily with long-term therapy), blood dyscrasias
- **Other:** Hiccups, fever, diaphoresis, paresthesias, muscular disturbances, gynecomastia, **anaphylaxis, angioedema**

Interactions
✳ **Drug-drug** • Increased CNS depression with alcohol and other CNS depressants (eg, barbiturates, opioids) • Decreased sedative effects with theophylline, aminophylline, dyphylline

■ Nursing considerations
Assessment
- **History:** Hypersensitivity to benzodiazepines; psychoses; acute narrow-angle glaucoma; shock, coma; acute alcoholic intoxication; pregnancy, lactation; impaired liver or renal function, debilitation; depression, suicidal tendencies
- **Physical:** Skin color, lesions; T; orientation, reflexes, affect, ophthalmologic examination; P, BP; R, adventitious sounds; liver evaluation, abdominal examination, bowel sounds, normal output; CBC, LFTs, renal function tests

Interventions
⊗ **Warning** Taper dosage gradually after long-term therapy, especially in patients with epilepsy, to prevent refractory seizures.
- Caution patient to avoid pregnancy while taking this drug; advise patient to use barrier contraceptives.

Teaching points
- Take drug exactly as prescribed.
- During long-term therapy, do not stop taking this drug without consulting your health care provider.
- Do not drink alcohol or use other CNS depressants while on this drug.
- Avoid pregnancy while taking this drug; serious fetal harm could occur. Using contraceptive measures is advised.
- Nocturnal sleep may be disturbed for several nights after discontinuing the drug.

T

- You may experience these side effects: Drowsiness, dizziness (may lessen; avoid driving or engaging in other dangerous activities); swelling, allergic reaction; GI upset (take drug with water); depression, dreams, emotional upset, crying, complex sleep-related behaviors, swelling.
- Report severe dizziness, allergies, weakness, drowsiness that persists, rash or skin lesions, palpitations, swelling of extremities, visual changes, difficulty voiding, sleep disorders.

▽ temozolomide

See Appendix R, *Less commonly used drugs.*

▽ temsirolimus

See Appendix R, *Less commonly used drugs.*

DANGEROUS DRUG
▽ tenecteplase
*(teh **nek**' ti plaze)*

TNKase

PREGNANCY CATEGORY C

Drug class
Thrombolytic enzyme

Therapeutic actions
Enzyme that converts plasminogen to the enzyme plasmin (fibrinolysin), which degrades fibrin clots; lyses thrombi and emboli; is most active at the site of the clot and causes little systemic fibrinolysis.

Indications
- Reduction of mortality associated with acute MI

Contraindications and cautions
- Contraindicated with allergy to tenecteplase; active internal bleeding; history of stroke; intracranial or intraspinal surgery or trauma (within 2 mo); intracranial neoplasm, arteriovenous malformation, or aneurysm; known bleeding diathesis; severe uncontrolled hypertension.
- Use cautiously with recent major surgery, previous puncture of noncompressible vessels, cerebrovascular disease, recent GI or GU bleeding, recent trauma, hypertension, high likelihood

of left heart thrombus, acute pericarditis, subacute bacterial endocarditis, hemostatic defects (including those secondary to severe hepatic or renal disease), severe hepatic impairment, pregnancy, diabetic hemorrhagic retinopathy or other hemorrhagic ophthalmic conditions, septic thrombophlebitis or occluded AV cannula at seriously infected site, advanced age, patients currently receiving oral anticoagulants, recent use of GP IIb/IIIa inhibitors, any other condition in which bleeding constitutes a significant hazard or would be particularly difficult to manage because of its location.

Available forms
Powder for injection—50 mg

Dosages
Adults
⊗ **Warning** Do not exceed 50 mg/dose. Initiate treatment as soon as possible after onset of acute MI. Administer as IV bolus over 5 sec. Dose is based on weight:
Less than 60 kg: 30 mg IV.
60–69 kg: 35 mg IV.
70–79 kg: 40 mg IV.
80–89 kg: 45 mg IV.
90 kg or more: 50 mg IV.
Pediatric patients
Safety and efficacy not established.
Geriatric patients
Dosage adjustment is not recommended, but elderly patients have an increased risk of adverse effects. Monitor closely for early signs of bleeding.

Pharmacokinetics

Route	Onset	Peak
IV	Immediate	5–10 min

Metabolism: Hepatic; $T_{1/2}$: 90–130 min
Distribution: Crosses placenta; may enter breast milk
Excretion: Bile

▼ IV FACTS

Preparation: Reconstitute using the supplied 10-cc syringe with twinpack dual cannula device and 10 mL sterile water for injection. Do not shake. Slight foaming is normal and should dissipate if left standing for 10 min. Reconstituted solution is 5 mg/mL. Use immediately or may be refrigerated for up to 8 hr.

Infusion: Infuse as a bolus injection over 5 sec. Flush any dextrose-containing lines with saline before injecting and after administration. Discard any leftover solution.

Incompatibilities: Do not add other medications to infusion solution.

Adverse effects

- **CV:** Cardiac arrhythmias with coronary reperfusion, hypotension, AV block, **MI**, cardiogenic shock, cholesterol embolization (eg, livedo reticularis, "purple toe" syndrome, acute renal failure, pancreatitis, hypertension)
- **Hematologic: Bleeding,** particularly at venous or arterial access sites; GI bleeding; intracranial hemorrhage
- **Other:** Urticaria, nausea, vomiting, fever, allergic reactions

Interactions

✳ **Drug-drug** • Increased risk of hemorrhage if used with heparin or oral anticoagulants, aspirin, dipyridamole, ticlopidine, clopidogrel; monitor patient very closely if these combinations are used • Decreased effectiveness if combined with aminocaproic acid

✳ **Drug-lab test** • During tenecteplase therapy, results of coagulation tests or measures of fibrinolytic activity may be unreliable unless specific precautions are taken to prevent *in vitro* artifacts

■ Nursing considerations
Assessment

- **History:** Allergy to tenecteplase; active internal bleeding; recent (within 2 mo) stroke; intracranial or intraspinal surgery or neoplasm; recent major surgery, obstetric delivery, organ biopsy, or rupture of a noncompressible blood vessel; recent serious GI bleed; recent serious trauma, including CPR; SBE; hemostatic defects; cerebrovascular disease; early-onset, type 1 diabetes; severe uncontrolled hypertension; liver disease; pregnancy; lactation
- **Physical:** Skin color, T, lesions; orientation, reflexes; P, BP, peripheral perfusion, baseline ECG; R, adventitious sounds; liver evaluation, Hct, platelet count, thrombin time (TT), aPTT, PT/INR

Interventions

⊗ **Warning** Arrange to discontinue concurrent heparin and tenecteplase if serious bleeding occurs.
- Arrange for regular monitoring of coagulation studies.

⊗ **Warning** Apply pressure or pressure dressings or both to control superficial bleeding (at invaded or disturbed areas); avoid IM injections, invasive procedures, and excessive handling of the patient.
- Avoid any arterial invasive procedures during therapy.
- Arrange for typing and cross-matching of blood in case serious blood loss occurs and whole blood transfusions are required.
- Monitor patient for signs of bleeding; provide safety procedures to avoid injury.

Teaching points

- This drug can only be given IV and you will need to be closely monitored during drug treatment.
- You may experience these side effects: Tendency to bleed easily (use caution to avoid injury; use electric razor, a soft toothbrush; use caution with sharp objects), strict bed rest will help to decrease the risk of bleeding. If bleeding does occur, apply pressure to the site until bleeding stops.
- Report bruising or bleeding; blood in urine, stool, or with coughing; bleeding gums; changes in vision; difficulty breathing, chest pain.

▽**tenofovir disoproxil fumarate**

*(te **noe'** fo veer)*

Viread

PREGNANCY CATEGORY B

Drug classes
Antiviral
Nucleotide reverse transcriptase inhibitor

Therapeutic actions
Antiviral activity; inhibits HIV reverse transcriptase activity, leading to a blocking of HIV reproduction.

Indications

- Treatment of HIV-1 infection in combination with other antiretrovirals
- Treatment of chronic hepatitis B in adults

Contraindications and cautions

- Contraindicated with allergy to tenofovir or other components of the product; breast-feeding HIV patients
- Use cautiously in pregnancy, hepatic or renal impairment, lactation (hepatitis B).

Available forms

Tablets—150, 200, 250, 300 mg; power—40 mg/g

Dosages

Adults

300 mg/day PO without regard to food.

Pediatric patients 2 yr and older

- *HIV:* 38 mg/kg/day PO.
- *Chronic hepatitis B:* Not recommended.

Patients with renal impairment

Adjust dosage as follows:

CrCl (mL/min)	Dose (PO)
50 or more	300 mg every 24 hr
30–49	300 mg every 48 hr
10–29	300 mg twice a wk
Hemodialysis	300 mg every wk or after a total of about 12 hr of dialysis

Pharmacokinetics

Route	Onset	Peak
Oral	Rapid	45–75 min

Metabolism: Unknown; $T_{1/2}$: 17 hr
Distribution: May cross placenta; may enter breast milk
Excretion: Urine

Adverse effects

- **CNS:** *Headache, asthenia*
- **GI:** *Nausea, vomiting, diarrhea,* anorexia, abdominal pain, flatulence, **severe hepatomegaly with steatosis**
- **Metabolic: Lactic adicosis, sometimes severe**
- **Other:** *Rash*

Interactions

✳ Drug-drug • Increased concentration and toxicity of didanosine if used concurrently; decrease didanosine dose to 250 mg in patients weighing more than 60 kg • Increased teno-

fovir concentrations with atazanavir and lopinavir; monitor patient closely • Risk of decreased atazanavir levels if combined with tenofovir; administer 300 mg atazanavir with 100 mg ritonavir only; do not administer atazanavir alone • Avoid use with other combination drugs that include tenofovir.

✳ Drug-food • Increased bioavailability if combined with food; tenofovir can be taken without regard to meals

■ Nursing considerations

Assessment

- **History:** Allergy to tenofovir, renal or hepatic impairment, pregnancy, lactation
- **Physical:** T, orientation, reflexes, abdominal examination, LFTs, renal function tests

Interventions

- Administer with other antiretrovirals; do not use as monotherapy.

⊗ **Black box warning** Monitor hepatic function closely; risk of lactic acidosis and severe hepatic toxicity.

⊗ **Black box warning** Severe exacerbation of hepatitis B has occurred when anti–hepatitis B therapy is discontinued. Monitor patient for several months if drug is discontinued.

- Monitor patients with hepatic or renal problems for possible adverse effects.

⊗ **Warning** Withdraw drug and monitor patient if signs or symptoms of lactic acidosis or hepatotoxicity develop, including hepatomegaly and steatosis. These are more common in women, obesity, and prolonged tenofovir use.

- Encourage women of childbearing age to use barrier contraceptives while taking this drug because the effects of the drug on the fetus are not known.
- Advise women who are breast-feeding to find another method of feeding the infant.

Teaching points

- Take this drug once a day without regard to meals or food. Do not stop taking this drug until you have consulted your health care provider.
- Take the full course of therapy as prescribed; always take in combination with other antivirals; if you miss a dose, take it as soon as you remember and then take the next dose at the usual time. If it is almost time for the

Adverse effects in *italics* are most common; those in **bold** are life-threatening. ⬛ Do not crush.

next dose when you remember, just take the next dose. Do not take any double doses.

- This drug does not cure HIV infection; long-term effects are not yet known; continue to take precautions because the risk of transmission is not reduced by this drug.
- Avoid pregnancy while taking this drug; using barrier contraceptives is advised.
- Do not take any other drug, prescription or over-the-counter, without consulting your health care provider; this drug interacts with other drugs and serious problems can occur.
- You may experience these side effects: Nausea, vomiting, loss of appetite, diarrhea, abdominal pain, headache (try to maintain nutrition and fluid intake as much as possible; eat frequent small meals); redistribution of fat on the body (arms and legs may become thin, a "buffalo hump" may develop on the back of the neck, and fat may be distributed in the breasts and along the trunk).
- Report severe diarrhea, jaundice, changes in color of stool or urine, rapid respirations.

▽terazosin hydrochloride
(ter ay' zoe sin)

Apo-Terazocin (CAN), Hytrin, Novo-Terazocin (CAN), PMS-Terazocin (CAN), ratio-Terazocin (CAN), Teva-Terazosin (CAN)

PREGNANCY CATEGORY C

Drug classes
Alpha$_1$-adrenergic blocker
Antihypertensive
BPH drug

Therapeutic actions
Drug selectively blocks postsynaptic alpha$_1$-adrenergic receptors, decreasing peripheral vascular resistance, and lowering supine and standing BP; unlike conventional alpha-adrenergic blocking agents (eg, phentolamine), it does not also block alpha$_2$ presynaptic receptors, does not cause reflex tachycardia. Relaxes the smooth muscle by blocking alpha$_1$-adrenergic receptors in the bladder neck and prostate, thereby improving the symptoms of BPH.

Indications
- Treatment of symptomatic BPH
- Treatment of hypertension alone or in combination with other drugs
- Unlabeled uses: Symptomatic treatment of ureteral stones, pediatric hypertension

Contraindications and cautions
- Contraindicated with hypersensitivity to terazosin and during lactation.
- Use cautiously in patients taking other antihypertensives, pregnancy.

Available forms
Capsules—1, 2, 5, 10 mg

Dosages
Adults
Adjust dose and dosing interval (12 or 24 hr) individually.
- *Hypertension:* Initial dose, 1 mg PO at bedtime. Do not exceed 1 mg; strictly adhere to this regimen to avoid severe hypotensive reactions. Slowly increase dose to achieve desired BP response. Usual range, 1–5 mg PO daily. Up to 20 mg/day has been beneficial. Monitor BP 2–3 hr after dosing to determine maximum effect. If response is diminished after 24 hr, consider increasing dosage or use a twice daily regimen. If drug is not taken for several days, restart with initial 1-mg dose.
- *BPH:* Initial dose, 1 mg PO at bedtime. Increase to 2, 5, or 10 mg PO daily. 10 mg/day for 4–6 wk may be required to assess benefit. If drug is not taken for several days, restart with the initial dose.

Pediatric patients
Safety and efficacy not established.

Pharmacokinetics

Route	Onset	Peak
Oral	Varies	1 hr

Metabolism: Unknown; $T_{1/2}$: 12 hr
Distribution: Crosses placenta; may enter breast milk
Excretion: Feces, urine

Adverse effects
- **CNS:** *Dizziness, headache, drowsiness, lack of energy, weakness, somnolence,* nervousness, vertigo, depression, paresthesia
- **CV:** *Palpitations,* sodium and water retention, increased plasma volume, *edema,*

syncope, tachycardia, *orthostatic hypotension,* angina
- **Dermatologic:** Rash, pruritus, alopecia
- **EENT:** Blurred vision, reddened sclera, floppy iris syndrome during cataract surgery, epistaxis, tinnitus, dry mouth, nasal congestion
- **GI:** *Nausea,* vomiting, diarrhea, constipation, abdominal discomfort or pain
- **GU:** Urinary frequency, incontinence, impotence, priapism
- **Respiratory:** *Dyspnea, nasal congestion, sinusitis*
- **Other:** Diaphoresis, **allergic anaphylaxis**

Interactions

✴ **Drug-drug** • Risk of marked hypotension with drugs used to treat ED; use caution

■ Nursing considerations

Assessment
- **History:** Hypersensitivity to terazosin; HF; renal failure; pregnancy, lactation
- **Physical:** Weight; skin color, lesions; orientation, affect, reflexes; ophthalmologic examination; P, BP, orthostatic BP, supine BP, perfusion, edema, auscultation; R, adventitious sounds, status of nasal mucous membranes; bowel sounds, normal output; voiding pattern, urinary output; renal function tests, urinalysis

Interventions
⊗ *Warning* Administer or have patient take first dose just before bedtime to lessen likelihood of first dose effect, syncope due to excessive orthostatic hypotension.

⊗ *Warning* Have patient lie down, and treat supportively if syncope occurs; condition is self-limited.
- Monitor patient for orthostatic hypotension, which is most marked in the morning, and is accentuated by hot weather, alcohol, exercise.
- Monitor edema and weight in patients with incipient cardiac decompensation, and add a thiazide diuretic to the drug regimen if sodium and fluid retention, signs of impending HF, occur.

Teaching points
- Take this drug exactly as prescribed. Take the first dose just before bedtime. Do not drive or

operate machinery for 12 hours after the first dose.
- Use caution if you are using drugs to treat erectile dysfunction; dizziness, low blood pressure can occur.
- You may experience these side effects: Dizziness, weakness (more likely when changing position, in early morning, after exercise, in hot weather, and with alcohol use; some tolerance may occur after taking the drug for a while, but avoid driving or engaging in tasks that require alertness; change position slowly; use caution when climbing stairs; lie down for a while if dizziness persists); GI upset (eat frequent small meals); impotence; dry mouth (suck on sugarless candies or ice chips); stuffy nose. Most effects will gradually disappear.
- Report frequent dizziness or faintness.

▷ **terbinafine hydrochloride**
(ter bin' ah feen)
Apo-Terbinafine (CAN), CO Terbinafine (CAN), Gen Terbinafine (CAN), Lamisil, Lamisil AT, Lamisil Oral Granules, PMS-Terbinafine (CAN), Terbinex

PREGNANCY CATEGORY B

Drug classes
Allylamine
Antifungal

Therapeutic actions
A synthetic allylamine that is thought to block squalene oxidase, thus preventing the biosynthesis of ergosterol, an essential component of fungal cell walls.

Indications
- Treatment of tinea capitis in patients 4 yr and older (oral granules)
- Treatment of onychomycosis of the toenail or fingernail caused by dermatophytes
- Topical treatment of tinea versicolor, tinea pedis, tinea cruris, tinea corporis

Contraindications and cautions
- Contraindicated with allergy to any component of the product, hepatic failure, lactation.

- Use cautiously with hepatic impairment, renal impairment, immunodeficiency, pregnancy.

Available forms
Tablets—250 mg; oral granules—125, 187.5 mg; cream, gel, spray—1%

Dosages
Adults
- *Fingernail onychomycosis:* 250 mg/day PO for 6 wk.
- *Toenail onychomycosis:* 250 mg/day PO for 12 wk.
- *Tinea capitis:* 250 mg/day PO for 6 wk.

Pediatric patients
Tinea capitis
Weight less than 25 kg: 125 mg/day PO for 6 wk.
25–35 kg: 187.5 mg/day PO for 6 wk.
Weight more than 35 kg: 250 mg/day PO for 6 wk.

Adults and pediatric patients
Topical
- *Athlete's foot:* Apply cream, gel, or spray topically bid between toes for 1 wk; extend treatment an additional week of bottom or sides of foot are affected.
- *Ringworm or jock itch:* Apply cream, gel, or spray topically once daily for 1 wk.

Pharmacokinetics

Route	Onset	Peak
Oral	Moderate	2 hr

Metabolism: Hepatic metabolism, $T_{1/2}$: 36 hr
Distribution: May cross placenta; enters breast milk
Excretion: Urine

Adverse effects
- **CNS:** Headache, taste disturbance, visual disturbance
- **Dermatologic: Rash,** *pruritus,* urticaria
- **GI:** Diarrhea, abdominal pain, dyspepsia, nausea, flatulence, **hepatic failure,** liver enzyme abnormalities, taste disturbances

Interactions
✳ **Drug-drug** ● Decreased effectiveness of terbinafine if combined with rifampin, cyclosporine ● Increased serum levels and risk of toxicity if combined with cimetidine ● Increased serum levels of dextromethorphan and risk of toxicity if combined with terbinafine; monitor patient closely if this combination must be used

■ Nursing considerations

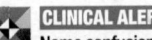 **CLINICAL ALERT!**
Name confusion has occurred between *Lamisil* (terbinafine) and *Lamictal* (lamotrigine) and *Lamisil AF* (tolnaftate) and *Lamisil AT* (terbinafine); use extreme caution.

Assessment
- **History:** Allergy to any component of the product, hepatic or renal impairment, immunodeficiency, pregnancy, lactation
- **Physical:** Skin evaluation; liver examination, bowel sounds; T; nail specimen culture, LFTs

Interventions
- Obtain nail culture or biopsy to confirm the diagnosis of onychomycosis before beginning therapy.
- Suggest waiting until after delivery instead of using this drug during pregnancy or lactation; effects on the fetus are not known.
- Suggest an alternative method of feeding the infant if this drug is prescribed for a breast-feeding mother.
- For oral granules, sprinkle entire packet of granules on a spoonful of nonacidic food, such as mashed potatoes. Have patient swallow entire spoonful without chewing.
- Monitor the patient regularly for any sign of hepatic impairment; liver failure can occur.
- Discontinue drug if a skin rash appears, or with hepatic failure.
- Provide appropriate analgesics for headache.

Teaching points
- Take this drug for the full recommended course of treatment.
- If using oral granules, sprinkle entire packet on a spoonful of nonacidic food, such as mashed potatoes. Then swallow entire spoonful without chewing.
- You may experience these side effects: Headache (medication will be arranged), diarrhea, abdominal pain, nausea (eat frequent small meals).
- Report persistent nausea, lack of appetite, yellowing of the eyes or skin, dark urine or pale stools.
- Report rash to your health care provider immediately.

T

▷terbutaline sulfate
(ter byoo' ta leen)

PREGNANCY CATEGORY B

Drug classes
Antiasthmatic
Beta$_2$-selective adrenergic agonist
Bronchodilator
Sympathomimetic
Tocolytic drug

Therapeutic actions
In low doses, acts relatively selectively at beta$_2$-adrenergic receptors to cause bronchodilation and relax the pregnant uterus; at higher doses, beta$_2$ selectivity is lost and the drug acts at beta$_1$ receptors to cause typical sympathomimetic cardiac effects.

Indications
- Prophylaxis and treatment of bronchial asthma and reversible bronchospasm that may occur with bronchitis and emphysema in patients 12 yr and older
- Unlabeled use: Tocolytic to prevent preterm labor

Contraindications and cautions
- Contraindicated with hypersensitivity to terbutaline; tachyarrhythmias, tachycardia caused by digoxin toxicity; general anesthesia with halogenated hydrocarbons or cyclopropane, which sensitize the myocardium to catecholamines; unstable vasomotor system disorders; labor and delivery (may inhibit labor; parenteral use of beta-adrenergic agonists can accelerate fetal heartbeat, cause hypoglycemia, hypokalemia, and pulmonary edema in the mother and hypoglycemia in the neonate); lactation.
- Use cautiously with diabetes, coronary insufficiency, CAD, history of stroke, COPD patients who have developed degenerative heart disease, hyperthyroidism, history of seizure disorders, psychoneurotic individuals, hypertension.

Available forms
Tablets—2.5, 5 mg; injection—1 mg/mL

Dosages
Adults and patients older than 15 yr
Oral
5 mg PO tid at 6-hr intervals during waking hours. If side effects are pronounced, reduce to 2.5 mg tid. Do not exceed 15 mg/day.
Parenteral
0.25 mg subcutaneously into lateral deltoid area. If no significant improvement in 15–30 min, give another 0.25-mg dose. Do not exceed 0.5 mg/4 hr. If patient fails to respond to second 0.25-mg dose within 15–30 min, other therapeutic measures should be considered.
Pediatric patients
Oral
12–15 yr: 2.5 mg PO tid. Do not exceed 7.5 mg/24 hr.
Younger than 12 yr: Not recommended.
Parenteral
Use adult dosing.
Geriatric patients
Patients older than 60 yr are more likely to experience side effects. Use with extreme caution.

Pharmacokinetics

Route	Onset	Peak	Duration
Subcut.	5–15 min	30–60 min	1.5–4 hr
Oral	30 min	2–3 hr	4–8 hr

Metabolism: Tissue; T$_{1/2}$: 2–4 hr
Distribution: May cross placenta; enters breast milk
Excretion: Urine

Adverse effects
- **CNS:** *Restlessness, apprehension, anxiety, fear,* CNS stimulation, hyperkinesia, insomnia, tremor, drowsiness, irritability, weakness, vertigo, headache, seizures
- **CV:** *Cardiac arrhythmias, palpitations,* anginal pain (less likely with bronchodilator doses of this drug than with bronchodilator doses of a nonselective beta agonist [isoproterenol]), changes in BP and ECG
- **GI:** *Nausea,* vomiting, heartburn, unusual or bad taste in mouth
- **Respiratory:** *Respiratory difficulties,* **pulmonary edema,** *coughing,* **bronchospasm**
- **Other:** Sweating, pallor, flushing, muscle cramps, elevated LFTs

Interactions
* **Drug-drug** • Increased likelihood of cardiac arrhythmias with halogenated hydrocarbon

anesthetics (halothane), cyclopropane • Risk of hypokalemia if combined with diuretics • Increased risk of hypokalemia and ECG changes with MAOIs and TCAs • Do not administer with other sympathomimetics, theophylline

■ **Nursing considerations**

> ★ **CLINICAL ALERT!**
> Due to similar packaging, terbutaline injection has been confused with methergine injection (methylergonovine maleate); use extreme caution.

Assessment
- **History:** Hypersensitivity to terbutaline; tachyarrhythmias; general anesthesia with halogenated hydrocarbons or cyclopropane; unstable vasomotor system disorders; hypertension; CAD; history of stroke; COPD patients who have developed degenerative heart disease; hyperthyroidism; history of seizure disorders; psychoneurotic individuals; pregnancy; labor and delivery; lactation
- **Physical:** Weight; skin color, T, turgor; orientation, reflexes; P, BP; R, adventitious sounds; blood and urine glucose; serum electrolytes; LFTs, thyroid function tests; ECG

Interventions
- Use minimal doses for minimal periods of time; drug tolerance can occur with prolonged use.
- ⊗ **Black box warning** Injectable terbutaline should not be used in pregnant women for prevention or prolonged treatment (beyond 48–72 hr) of preterm labor in the hospital or outpatient setting because of the potential for serious maternal heart problems and death.
- ⊗ **Warning** Keep a beta blocker (a cardioselective beta blocker, such as atenolol, should be used in patients with respiratory distress) readily available in case cardiac arrhythmias occur.
- Do not exceed recommended dosage.

Teaching points
- Do not exceed recommended dosage; adverse effects or loss of effectiveness may result. Read product instructions; consult your health care provider if you have any questions.
- You may experience these side effects: Weakness, dizziness, inability to sleep (use caution when driving or performing activities that require alertness); nausea, vomiting (eat frequent small meals); fast heart rate, anxiety.

- Report chest pain, dizziness, insomnia, weakness, tremor or irregular heartbeat, failure to respond to usual dosage.

▽ **teriparatide**

See Appendix R, *Less commonly used drugs.*

▽ **testosterone**
*(tess **toss'** ter ohn)*

testosterone

Transdermal patch: Androderm

Transdermal gel: AndroGel 1%, AndroGel 1.62%, Fortesta

Testim

Testosterone pellets: Testopel Pellets

Testosterone buccal: Striant

Testosterone spray: Axiron

testosterone cypionate (long-acting)
Depo-Testosterone

testosterone enanthate (long-acting)
Delatestryl

testosterone propionate
First-Testosterone, First-Testosterone MC

PREGNANCY CATEGORY X

CONTROLLED SUBSTANCE C-III

Drug classes
Androgen
Hormone

Therapeutic actions
Primary natural androgen; responsible for growth and development of male sex organs and the maintenance of secondary sex characteristics; administration of exogenous testosterone increases the retention of nitrogen, sodium, potassium, phosphorus; decreases urinary excretion of calcium; increases protein anabolism and decreases protein catabolism; stimulates the production of RBCs.

Indications
- Replacement therapy in hypogonadism—primary hypogonadism, hypogonadotropic hypogonadism, delayed puberty (men)
- Testosterone enanthate only: Inoperable breast cancer, metastatic mammary cancer, delayed puberty

Contraindications and cautions
- Contraindicated with known sensitivity to androgens; prostate or breast cancer in men; pregnancy; lactation; serious cardiac, hepatic, or renal disease. *Androderm* and *Striant* contraindicated for use in women.
- Use cautiously with MI.

Available forms
Transdermal system—2, 4 mg/24 hr; transdermal gel, 1%, 1.62% pellets—75 mg; testosterone enanthate injection—200 mg/mL; spray—30 mg per actation (*Axiron*), 10 mg per actuation (*Fortesta*); buccal system—30 mg; testosterone cypionate injection—100, 200 mg/mL; testosterone propionate ointment, cream—2%

Dosages
Adults
- *Carcinoma of the breast and metastatic mammary cancer:* 200–400 mg IM (testosterone enanthate) every 2–4 wk.
- *Male hypogonadism (replacement therapy):* 50–400 mg testosterone cypionate or testosterone enanthate every 2–4 wk given IM, or 150–450 mg testosterone enanthate pellets implanted subcutaneously every 3–6 mo.
- *Males with delayed puberty:* 50–200 mg IM (testosterone enanthate) every 2–4 wk for a limited duration (4–6 mo) or 150 mg pellets subcutaneously every 3–6 mo (testosterone pellets).
- *Primary hypogonadism, hypogonadotropic hypogonadism in males:* Testosterone patch, initially 4-mg/day system applied to non-scrotal skin; then 2.5-mg/day system (*Androderm*) (dosage may be adjusted based on patient response); testosterone gel—5 mg/day (preferably in the morning) applied to clean, dry, intact skin of the shoulders, upper arms, or abdomen (*AndroGel* or *Testim*); spray (*Fortesta*)—4 actuations (40 mg) applied to inner thighs in the morning, or spray (*Axiron*) 1 pump actuation (30 mg) to each axilla once a day; *AndroGel* 1.62%—2 ac-

tuations (40.5 mg) once daily in the morning to shoulders or upper arms; apply one buccal system (30 mg) to gum region bid (morning and evening), rotate sites, usual position is above incisor on either side of mouth (*Striant*).

Pharmacokinetics

Route	Onset	Duration
IM	Slow	1–3 days
IM cypionate	Slow	2–4 wk
IM enanthate	Slow	2–4 wk
Dermal	Rapid	24 hr
Buccal	Rapid	12 hr

Metabolism: Hepatic; $T_{1/2}$: 10–100 min; up to 8 days (cypionate)
Distribution: Crosses placenta; may enter breast milk
Excretion: Feces, urine

Adverse effects
- **CNS:** *Dizziness, headache, sleep disorders, fatigue,* tremor, sleeplessness, generalized paresthesia, sleep apnea syndrome, hot flashes, hypertension (topical gel)
- **Dermatologic:** *Rash,* dermatitis, anaphylactoid reactions, acne
- **Endocrine:** *Androgenic effects* (acne, edema, mild hirsutism, decrease in breast size, deepening of the voice, oily skin or hair, weight gain, clitoral hypertrophy or testicular atrophy), *hypoestrogenic effects* (flushing, sweating, vaginitis, nervousness, emotional lability), gynecomastia in males
- **GI:** *Nausea,* hepatic impairment; **hepatocellular carcinoma**
- **GU:** Fluid retention, decreased urinary output, changes in libido
- **Hematologic:** *Polycythemia; leukopenia;* hypercalcemia; altered serum cholesterol levels; retention of sodium, chloride, water, potassium, phosphates, and calcium
- **Respiratory:** dyspnea
- **Other:** Chills, premature closure of the epiphyses

Interactions
✳ **Drug-drug** • Risk of acute or severe alcohol intolerance if gel combined with methonidazole, disulfiram (gel contains alcohol); caution patient appropriately

✴ **Drug-food** • Decreased metabolism and risk of toxic effects if combined with grapefruit juice; avoid this combination

✴ **Drug-lab test** • Altered glucose tolerance tests • With no evidence of clinical thyroid dysfunction, decrease in thyroid function tests, which may persist for 2–3 wk after therapy • Increased creatinine, creatinine clearance, which may last for 2 wk after therapy

■ Nursing considerations
Assessment
- **History:** Known sensitivity to androgens, prostate or breast cancer in males, cardiac disease, renal disease, liver disease, pregnancy, lactation
- **Physical:** Skin color, lesions, texture; hair distribution pattern; injection site; affect, orientation; peripheral sensation; abdominal examination; liver evaluation; serum electrolytes, serum cholesterol levels, LFTs, glucose tolerance tests, thyroid function tests, long-bone X-ray (in children)

Interventions
- Apply dermal patch to clean, dry skin as directed. Do not use chemical depilatories. *Androderm* is to be applied to nonscrotal skin on back, abdomen, upper arms, or thighs. Remove the old patch before applying a new one.
- ⊗ **Black box warning** There is a risk of toxic effects (enlarged genitalia, greater-than-normal bone age) in children exposed to patients using transdermal form (*AndroGel, Testim*). Patient should wash hands after applying drug and cover treated area with clothing to reduce exposure.
- Apply buccal system to gum region above incisor on either side of mouth; rotate sites (*Striant*). Place rounded side of buccal system against gum and hold firmly in place for 30 sec to ensure adhesion. If system falls off during 12-hr period, remove old system and replace with new system.
- Inject testosterone deeply into gluteal muscle.
- Be aware that sprays are not interchangeable. Dosage and site of application vary between products.
- Shake vials well before use; crystals will redissolve.
- Do not administer frequently; these drugs are absorbed slowly; testosterone enanthate and

cypionate are long acting and provide therapeutic effects for about 4 wk.

- Monitor effect on children with long-bone X-rays every 3–6 mo during therapy; discontinue drug well before the bone age reaches the norm for the patient's chronologic age.
- Monitor patient for edema; arrange for diuretic therapy as needed.
- Monitor liver function and serum electrolytes periodically during therapy, and consult with physician for corrective measures as needed.
- Periodically measure cholesterol levels in patients who are at high risk for CAD.
- Monitor patients with diabetes closely because glucose tolerance may change; adjustments may be needed in insulin, oral hypoglycemic dosage, and diet.
- Periodically monitor urine and serum calcium during treatment of disseminated breast carcinoma and metastatic mammary cancer, and arrange for appropriate treatment or discontinuation of the drug.
- Monitor elderly men for prostatic hypertrophy and carcinoma.
- Advise female patients, especially pregnant patients, that they should avoid contact with application site of testosterone gel as well as transdermal patches.

⊗ **Warning** Discontinue drug and arrange for consultation if abnormal vaginal bleeding occurs.

Teaching points
- The injection forms of this drug can only be given by IM injection. Mark a calendar indicating days for injection. If using the dermal patch, apply the patch to dry, clean skin as directed. *Androderm* is to be applied to nonscrotal skin on your back, abdomen, thighs, or upper arms; rotate sites. Remove the old patch before applying a new one. *AndroGel* is to be applied to skin of the shoulders and upper arms. Do not shower or swim for at least 1 hour after application of gel. Wash hands after applying gel. Cover area with clothing if you are in contact with children because children can experience adverse effects if exposed to the gel. *Axiron* is sprayed under each arm once a day; *Fortesta* is sprayed on inner thighs once a day. Check with your health care provider to get exact details about your form of therapy.
- Apply buccal system to gum region above incisor on either side of mouth; rotate sites.

T

Check to make sure system remains in place after brushing teeth, using mouthwash, eating, and drinking.
- Avoid grapefruit juice while using this drug.
- This drug cannot be taken during pregnancy; serious fetal effects could occur. Women should use contraceptive measures.
- Patients with diabetes should monitor serum glucose closely because glucose tolerance may change; report any abnormalities to prescriber, so corrective action can be taken.
- You may experience these side effects: Body hair growth, baldness, deepening of the voice, loss of libido, impotence (reversible); excitation, confusion, insomnia (avoid driving or performing tasks that require alertness); swelling of the ankles, fingers (request medication).
- Report ankle swelling; nausea; vomiting; yellowing of skin or eyes; unusual bleeding or bruising; penile swelling or pain; hoarseness, body hair growth, deepening of the voice, acne, menstrual irregularities, pregnancy.

▽**tetrabenazine**
*(tet ra **ben'** ah zeen)*

Xenazine

PREGNANCY CATEGORY C

Drug classes
Anti-chorea drug
Monoamine depletor

Therapeutic actions
Inhibits monoamine transport systems, resulting in a decreased uptake of the monoamines dopamine, serotonin, norepinephrine, and histamine into synaptic vesicles and a depletion of monoamine stores; exact mechanism of action of effects on chorea are not understood.

Indications
- Treatment of chorea associated with Huntington disease

Contraindications and cautions
- Contraindicated with active suicidality, untreated or inadequately treated depression, impaired hepatic function, concurrent use of MAOIs or reserpine.

- Use cautiously with prolonged QT interval, pregnancy, lactation.

Available forms
Tablets—12.5, 25 mg

Dosages
Adults
12.5 mg/day PO in the morning; after 1 week, increase to 12.5 mg PO bid; may be slowly titrated as needed to a maximum dose of 100 mg/day in divided doses.
Pediatric patients
Safety and efficacy not established.

Pharmacokinetics

Route	Onset	Peak
Oral	Slow	2 hr

Metabolism: Hepatic; $T_{1/2}$: 4–8 hr, then 2–4 hr (active metabolite)
Distribution: May cross placenta; may enter breast milk
Excretion: Urine

Adverse effects
- **CNS:** *Sedation, insomnia, depression, anxiety,* irritability, obsessive reaction, *akathisia,* parkinsonism, dizziness, headache, unsteady gait
- **GI:** *Nausea,* vomiting, decreased appetite
- **Respiratory:** *URI,* shortness of breath, bronchitis
- **Other:** *Fatigue*

Interactions
✳ **Drug-drug** • Risk of increased serum levels and toxicity if given with any potent CYP2D6 inhibitor (fluoxetine, paroxetine, quinidine); dosage of tetrabenazine should be halved if combined with any of these drugs • Increased risk of prolonged QT interval if combined with any other drugs that prolong QT interval (antipsychotics, antiarrhythmics); avoid this combination • Increased sedation if combined with alcohol or other sedating drugs • Increased adverse reactions if combined with dopamine agonists; monitor patient carefully • Increased risk of serious adverse effects if taken with MAOIs, reserpine; avoid this combination; at least 20 days should elapse and chorea symptoms should return before switching a patient from these drugs to tetrabenazine

Adverse effects in *italics* are most common; those in **bold** are life-threatening. ⬛ Do not crush.

■ Nursing considerations

Assessment

- **History:** Active suicidality, untreated or inadequately treated depression; impaired hepatic function; concurrent use of MAOIs, reserpine; prolonged QT interval; pregnancy, lactation
- **Physical:** T; orientation, affect; R, adventitious sounds; CBC with platelet counts, peripheral blood smear, ECG, LFTs

Interventions

⊗ **Black box warning** There is an increased risk of depression and suicidality with drug administration; monitor patient accordingly.

- Tell patient and his family that there is a risk of increased suicidal ideation and increased depression while on this drug. Discuss signs to watch for and tell them whom to notify if these effects occur.
- Establish a baseline of patient's chorea symptoms to evaluate drug's effectiveness and to create guidelines for dosing.
- Inform patient that motor function changes, including Parkinson-like symptoms, and sedation and confusion may occur. Advise patient to avoid driving, operating dangerous machinery, or making important decisions until the effects of the drug on the patient are known.
- Advise the use of contraceptive measures while on this drug.
- Encourage breast-feeding mothers to find a different method of feeding the infant while taking this drug.

Teaching points

- Take this drug once a day in the morning initially. Your dosage will be adjusted over time to determine the dosage that is most effective for you; when your maintenance dosage is determined, you may need to take the drug two to three times a day.
- Be aware that this drug may increase signs and symptoms of depression and may lead to thoughts of suicide. You and a significant other should be aware of these signs (withdrawal, irritability, inability to sleep, aggression, anxiety) and should report them to your health care provider immediately if they occur.
- Always tell your health care provider about other drugs or alternative therapies that you might be using or that you might stop using. This drug can be affected by many other drugs, and your dosage may need to be adjusted.
- It is not known whether this drug affects fetus. If you wish to become pregnant, discuss this wish with your health care provider. If you should become pregnant while taking this drug, consult your health care provider.
- It is not known how this drug affects a breast-feeding infant. Because of the potential for adverse effects to the infant, another method of feeding the infant should be used while you are taking this drug.
- Be aware that alcohol or use of any other CNS depressants, such as sleeping aids, may increase the sedative effects of this drug; avoid these combinations.
- You may experience these side effects: Sedation, drowsiness, changes in level of alertness (do not drive a car or operate dangerous machinery and do not make important decisions until you know how this drug will affect you); changes in motor function with tremors, Parkinson-like symptoms. (This is an effect of the drug; if it becomes too uncomfortable, discuss this problem with your health care provider; your dosage may need to be adjusted.)
- Report tremors, restlessness, thoughts of suicide, increased depression, inability to stay alert, sudden behavioral changes.

▽ tetracycline hydrochloride

(tet ra sye' kleen)

Apo-Tetra (CAN), Nu-Tetra (CAN)

PREGNANCY CATEGORY D

Drug classes

Antibiotic
Tetracycline

Therapeutic actions

Bacteriostatic: Inhibits protein synthesis of susceptible bacteria, preventing cell replication.

Indications

Systemic administration

- Infections caused by rickettsiae; *Mycoplasma pneumoniae;* agents of psittacosis, ornithosis, lymphogranuloma venereum and granuloma inguinale; *Borrelia recurrentis,*

T

Haemophilus ducreyi, Yersinia pestis, Francisella tularensis, Bartonella bacilliformis, Bacteroides, Vibrio cholerae, Campylobacter fetus, Brucella, Escherichia coli, Enterobacter aerogenes, Shigella, Acinetobacter, Haemophilus influenzae, Klebsiella, trachoma

- When penicillin is contraindicated, infections caused by *Neisseria gonorrhoeae, Treponema pallidum, Treponema pertenue, Listeria monocytogenes, Clostridium, Bacillus anthracis, Fusobacterium fusiforme, Actinomyces*
- Adjunct to amebicides in acute intestinal amebiasis
- Uncomplicated urethral, endocervical, or rectal infections in adults caused by *Chlamydia trachomatis*
- Adjunctive therapy for severe acne

Contraindications and cautions
Systemic administration and dermatologic solution

- Contraindicated with allergy to any of the tetracyclines, pregnancy (toxic to the fetus), lactation, children younger than (causes damage to the teeth of infant).
- Use cautiously with hepatic or renal impairment.

Available forms
Capsules—250, 500 mg

Dosages
Adults
1–2 g/day PO in two to four equal doses. Up to 500 mg PO qid.
- *Brucellosis:* 500 mg PO four times daily for 3 wk with 1 g streptomycin bid IM the first wk and daily the second wk.
- *Syphilis:* 30–40 g PO in divided doses over 10–15 days (*Sumycin*); 500 mg PO four times daily for 15–30 days (all others).
- *Uncomplicated gonorrhea:* 500 mg every 6 hr PO for 7 days.
- *Gonococcal urethritis:* 500 mg every 6 hr for 7 days.
- *Uncomplicated urethral, endocervical, or rectal infections with chlamydia trachomatis:* 500 mg four times daily PO for at least 7 days.
- *Severe acne:* 1 g/day PO in divided doses; then 125–500 mg/day.

Pediatric patients older than 8 yr
25–50 mg/kg/day PO in four equal doses.

Pharmacokinetics

Route	Onset	Peak
Oral	Varies	2–4 hr

Metabolism: $T_{1/2}$: 6–12 hr
Distribution: Crosses placenta; enters breast milk
Excretion: Feces, urine

Adverse effects
Systemic administration

- **Dermatologic:** *Phototoxic reactions, rash,* exfoliative dermatitis
- **GI:** *Discoloring and inadequate calcification of primary teeth of fetus if used by pregnant women, discoloring and inadequate calcification of permanent teeth if used during period of dental development,* fatty liver, liver failure, *anorexia, nausea, vomiting, diarrhea, glossitis, dysphagia,* enterocolitis, esophageal ulcers, esophagitis
- **Hematologic:** Hemolytic anemia, thrombocytopenia, neutropenia, eosinophilia, leukocytosis, leukopenia
- **Hypersensitivity:** Reactions from urticaria to **anaphylaxis,** including intracranial hypertension
- **Other:** *Superinfections,* local irritation at parenteral injection sites

Interactions
✳ **Drug-drug** • Decreased absorption with calcium salts, magnesium salts, zinc salts, aluminum salts, bismuth salts, iron, urinary alkalinizers, food, dairy products, charcoal
- Decreased effectiveness of hormonal contraceptives, although rare, has been reported with a risk of breakthrough bleeding or pregnancy
- Decreased activity of penicillins

■ Nursing considerations
Assessment

- **History:** Systemic administration and dermatologic solution: Allergy to any of the tetracyclines; hepatic or renal impairment; pregnancy, lactation
- **Physical:** Systemic administration, topical dermatologic solution: Site of infection, skin color, lesions; R, adventitious sounds; bowel sounds, output, liver evaluation; urinalysis,

---

BUN, LFTs, renal function tests. Dermatologic ointment: Site of infection

Interventions

- Administer oral medication on an empty stomach, 1 hr before or 2–3 hr after meals. Do not give with antacids. If antacids must be used, give them 2 hr before or after the dose of tetracycline.
- Culture infection before beginning drug therapy; many resistant strains have been identified.
- Do not administer during pregnancy; drug is toxic to the fetus.
- ⊗ **Warning** Do not use outdated drugs; degraded drug is highly nephrotoxic and should not be used.
- ⊗ **Warning** Tetracycline is not the drug of choice for any type of staphylococcal infection.
- Arrange for regular renal function tests with long-term therapy.

Teaching points

- Take the drug throughout the day for best results. The drug should be taken on an empty stomach, 1 hour before or 2–3 hours after meals, with a full glass of water. Do not take the drug at the same time as food, dairy products, iron preparations, or antacids; separate by 2 hours.
- Finish your complete prescription; if any is left, discard it immediately. Never take an outdated tetracycline product.
- There have been reports of pregnancy occurring when taking tetracycline with hormonal contraceptives. To be certain of avoiding pregnancy, use an additional type of contraceptive.
- This drug should not be used during pregnancy; using barrier contraceptives is advised.
- You may experience these side effects: Stomach upset, nausea (reversible); superinfections in the mouth, vagina (frequent washing may help this problem; if severe, request medication); sensitivity of the skin to sunlight (use protective clothing and sunscreen).
- Report severe cramps, watery diarrhea, rash or itching, difficulty breathing, dark urine or light-colored stools, yellowing of the skin or eyes.

▽ tetrahydrozoline hydrochloride

*(tet rah hi **draz'** oh leen)*

Tyzine

OTC ophthalmic preparation:
Altazine Irritation Relief, Altazine Moisture Relief, Murine Plus, Opticlear, Optigene 3, Visine, Visine AC, Visine Advanced Relief, Visine Maximum Redness Relief, Visine Totally Multisymptom Relief

PREGNANCY CATEGORY C

Drug classes

Alpha agonist
Nasal decongestant
Ophthalmic decongestant
Ophthalmic vasoconstrictor and mydriatic

Therapeutic actions

Acts directly on alpha receptors to produce vasoconstriction of arterioles in nasal passages, which produces a decongestant response; no effect on beta receptors; dilates pupils; increases flow of aqueous humor, vasoconstricts in eyes.

Indications

- Intranasal: Symptomatic relief of nasal and nasopharyngeal mucosal congestion due to the common cold, hay fever, or other respiratory allergies
- Ophthalmic: Temporary relief of redness, burning, and irritation due to dryness of the eye or discomfort due to minor irritations or to exposure to wind or sun

Contraindications and cautions

- Contraindicated with allergy to tetrahydrozoline, angle-closure glaucoma, anesthesia with cyclopropane or halothane, women in labor whose BP exceeds 130/80 mm Hg, concurrent MAOI use.
- Use cautiously with angina, arrhythmias, prostatic hypertrophy, unstable vasomotor syndrome, lactation, thyrotoxicosis, diabetes, hypertension, CV disorders

Available forms

Nasal solution—0.05%, 0.1%; nasal spray—0.1%; ophthalmic solution—0.05%, 0.1%

T

Dosages
Adults
Nasal
2–4 drops of 0.1% solution in each nostril three to four times/day; *or* 3–4 sprays in each nostril every 4 hr as needed. Never use more frequently than every 3 hr.
Ophthalmic
Instill 1–2 drops into eye or eyes up to four times/day.
Pediatric patients
Nasal
2–6 yr: 2–3 drops of 0.05% solution in each nostril every 4–6 hr as needed, but not more frequently than every 3 hr.
6 yr and older: Use adult dosage.
Ophthalmic
Safety and efficacy not established.

Pharmacokinetics

Route	Onset	Duration
Nasal	5–10 min	6–10 hr

Ophthalmic: No general systemic absorption.

Metabolism: Hepatic; $T_{1/2}$: Unknown
Distribution: Crosses placenta; may enter breast milk
Excretion: Urine

Adverse effects
- **CNS:** *Anxiety, tenseness, restlessness, headache, light-headedness, dizziness,* drowsiness, tremor, insomnia, hallucinations, psychological disturbances, seizures, CNS depression, weakness, blurred vision, ocular irritation, tearing, photophobia
- **CV:** Arrhythmias, hypertension resulting in intracranial hemorrhage, **CV collapse with hypotension,** palpitations, tachycardia, precordial pain in patients with ischemic heart disease
- **GI:** *Nausea,* vomiting, anorexia
- **GU:** Constriction of renal blood vessels, *dysuria, vesical sphincter spasm,* resulting in difficult and painful urination, urinary retention in males with prostatism
- **Local:** *Rebound congestion* with topical nasal application, burning, stinging, sneezing, dryness
- **Other:** *Pallor,* respiratory difficulty, orofacial dystonia, sweating

Interactions
✴ **Drug-drug** • Severe hypertension when taken with MAOIs, TCAs • Additive effects increase risk of toxicity with urinary alkalinizers • Decreased vasopressor response with reserpine, methyldopa, urinary acidifiers

■ Nursing considerations
Assessment
- **History:** Allergy to tetrahydrozoline; narrow-angle glaucoma; anesthesia with cyclopropane or halothane; thyrotoxicosis, diabetes, hypertension, CV disorders; prostatic hypertrophy, unstable vasomotor syndrome; lactation; pregnancy
- **Physical:** Skin color, T; orientation, reflexes, peripheral sensation, vision; P, BP, auscultation, peripheral perfusion; R, adventitious sounds; urinary output pattern, bladder percussion, prostate palpation; nasal mucous membrane evaluation

Interventions
- Do not administer ophthalmic solution if it is cloudy or changes color.
- ⊗ **Warning** Monitor CV effects carefully; patients with hypertension who take this drug may experience changes in BP because of the additional vasoconstriction. If an oral nasal decongestant is needed, pseudoephedrine is the drug of choice.

Teaching points
- Do not exceed recommended dose. Demonstrate proper administration technique for topical nasal application and administration of eyedrops. Do not use nasal spray more frequently than every 3 hours. Remove contact lenses before using eyedrops. Avoid prolonged use because underlying medical problems can be disguised.
- Rebound congestion may occur when this drug is stopped; drink plenty of fluids, use a humidifier, avoid smoke-filled areas, limit use to 72 hours.
- You may experience these side effects: Dizziness, weakness, restlessness, light-headedness, tremor (avoid driving or operating dangerous equipment); urinary retention (empty bladder before taking drug).
- Report nervousness, palpitations, sleeplessness, sweating, blurred vision.

▽thalidomide

See Appendix R, *Less commonly used drugs.*

Adverse effects in *italics* are most common; those in **bold** are life-threatening. ⊝⊚ Do not crush.

▷theophylline

(thee off' i lin)
Elixir: Elixophyllin
Timed-release capsules:
Theo-24 ⒞ⓝⓒ
Timed-release tablets:
Theochron ⒞ⓝⓒ

PREGNANCY CATEGORY C

Drug classes
Bronchodilator
Xanthine

Therapeutic actions
Relaxes bronchial smooth muscle, causing bronchodilation and increasing vital capacity that has been impaired by bronchospasm and air trapping; actions may be mediated by inhibition of phosphodiesterase, which increases the concentration of cyclic adenosine monophosphate; in concentrations that may be higher than those reached clinically, it also inhibits the release of slow-reacting substance of anaphylaxis and histamine.

Indications
- Symptomatic relief or prevention of bronchial asthma and reversible bronchospasm associated with chronic bronchitis and emphysema
- Unlabeled use of 5 mg/kg loading dose, then 3–6 mg/kg/day in divided doses every 6 to 8 hr to maintain serum concentrations between 3 and 5 mcg/mL: Treatment of apnea and bradycardia of prematurity

Contraindications and cautions
- Contraindicated with hypersensitivity to any xanthines, peptic ulcer, active gastritis, pregnancy, underlying seizure disorders (unless receiving appropriate antiepileptic).
- Use cautiously with cardiac arrhythmias, acute myocardial injury, HF, cor pulmonale, severe hypertension, severe hypoxemia, renal or hepatic disease, hyperthyroidism, alcoholism, labor (may inhibit uterine contractions), lactation, status asthmaticus.

Available forms
CR tablets ⒞ⓝⓒ—100, 200, 300, 450, 600 mg; ER capsules ⒞ⓝⓒ—100, 200, 300, 400 mg; elixir—80 mg/15 mL; injection—0.8, 1.6, 2, 3.2, 4 mg/mL

Dosages
Maintain serum levels in the therapeutic range of 5–15 mcg/mL; base dosage on lean body mass.

Anhydrous Theophylline Content in Theophylline Derivatives (these products are more water soluble than anhydrous theophylline)

Drug	Anhydrous Theophylline Content
aminophylline anhydrous	85.7%
aminophylline hydrous	78.9%
theophylline monohydrate	90.7%

Adults and children weighing more than 45 kg without risk of impaired excretion
- *Elixophyllin:* Initially, 300 mg/day PO in divided doses every 6–8 hr. After 3 days, may be increased to 400 mg/day PO in divided doses every 6–8 hr. After 3 more days may be increased to 600 mg/day PO in divided doses every 6–8 hr if tolerated and needed.
- *ER capsule:* Initially, 300 mg/day PO in divided doses every 8–12 hr. After 3 days, may be increased to 400 mg/day PO in divided doses every 8–12 hr. After 3 more days, may be increased to 600 mg/day PO in divided doses every 8–12 hr if tolerated and needed.
- *Theo-24:* Initially, 300–400 mg/day PO once every 24 hr. After 3 days, may be increased to 400–600 mg/day PO once every 24 hr. After 3 more days, may be increased based on the-ophylline level to stay within safe range.

Adults and children with risk factors for impaired clearance, geriatric patients, patients for whom monitoring serum theophylline levels is not feasible
- *Elixophyllin: Children 1–15 yr:* Final dose should not exceed 16 mg/kg/day PO up to a maximum 400 mg/day. *Patients 16 yr and older and geriatric patients:* Final dose should not exceed 400 mg/day PO.
- *Theo-24: Children 12–15 yr:* Final dose should not exceed 16 mg/kg/day PO up to a maximum 400 mg/day. *Patients older than 16 yr and geriatric patients:* Final dose should not exceed 400 mg/day PO.
  Serum theophylline level 5–10 mcg/mL: Increase dose by about 25% at 3-day intervals until desired response or serum level occurs.

Serum theophylline level 10–14.9 mcg/mL: Maintain dosage; recheck at 6- to 12-mo intervals.

Serum theophylline level 15–19.9 mcg/mL: Consider a decrease in dose by 10% to provide a greater margin of safety.

Serum theophylline level 20–25 mcg/mL: Decrease dose by about 25%; recheck level in 3 days.

Serum theophylline level 25–30 mcg/mL: Skip next dose, and decrease subsequent doses by 25%; recheck level after 3 days.

Serum theophylline level greater than 30 mcg/mL: Skip next two doses and decrease later doses by 50%. Recheck level after 3 days.

• *Measurement of serum theophylline levels during chronic therapy:* Measure serum theophylline in blood sample drawn 1–2 hr after administration of immediate-release preparations, 5–9 hr after administration of most timed-release products.

Adults
Parenteral
A loading dose of 4.6 mg/kg IV over 30 min should produce a serum concentration at the lower end of the desired range. This is only done if patient has not had theophylline in the past 24 hr.

Check serum levels after 24 hr when changing IV doses.

• *Nonsmokers ages 16–60 yr:* 0.4 mg/kg/hr IV.
• *Patients with HF, liver function impairment, sepsis, organ failure:* 0.2 mg/kg/hr IV.
• *Geriatric patients:* 0.3 mg/kg/hr IV.
• *Dosage adjustment based on serum theophylline levels during long-term therapy:* Serum theophylline levels less than 10 mcg/mL are too low, levels of 10–15 mcg/mL are within normal limits, and levels greater than 20 mcg/mL are too high.

Pediatric patients
Oral
Premature infants younger than 24 days: 1 mg/kg PO every 12 hr.

Premature infants 24 days and older: 1.5 mg/kg PO every 12 hr.

Full-term infants and infants up to 26 wk: Total dose in mg = [(0.2 × age in weeks) + 5] × body weight in kilograms, divided into three equal doses PO every 8 hr.

Infants 26 wk and older: Total dose in mg = [(0.2 × age in weeks) + 5] × body weight in kilograms, divided into four equal doses PO every 6 hr.

Parenteral
Neonates 24 days and younger: 1 mg/kg IV every 12 hr.

Neonates older than 24 days: 1.5 mg/kg IV every 12 hr.

Infants: mg/hr IV = 0.008 × age in weeks + 0.21 IV.

Children 1–9 yr: 0.8 mg/kg/hr IV.

Children 9–12 yr: 0.7 mg/kg/hr IV.

Children 12–16 yr who smoke cigarettes or marijuana: 0.7 mg/kg/hr IV.

Children 12–16 yr who are nonsmokers: 0.5 mg/kg/hr IV.

Pediatric patients weighing less than 45 kg without risk of impaired clearance
Oral
Elixophyllin: Initially, 12–14 mg/kg/day PO up to a maximum 300 mg/day PO in divided doses every 4–6 hr. After 3 days, may be increased to 16 mg/kg/day PO up to a maximum 400 mg/day PO in divided doses every 4–6 hr. After 3 more days, may be increased to 20 mg/kg/day PO up to a maximum 600 mg/day PO in divided doses every 4–6 hr if tolerated and needed.

ER capsule: Initially, 12–14 mg/kg/day PO up to a maximum 300 mg/day PO in divided doses every 8–12 hr. After 3 days, may be increased to 16 mg/kg/day PO up to a maximum 400 mg/day PO in divided doses every 8–12 hr. After 3 more days, may be increased to 20 mg/kg/day PO up to a maximum 600 mg/day PO in divided doses every 8–12 hr if tolerated and needed.

Theo-24, Uniphyl: Initially, 12–14 mg/kg/day PO up to a maximum 300 mg/day PO once every 24 hr. After 3 days, may be increased to 16 mg/kg/day PO up to a maximum 400 mg/day PO once every 24 hr. After 3 more days, may be increased to 20 mg/kg/day PO up to a maximum 600 mg/day PO once every 24 hr if tolerated and needed.

Pharmacokinetics

Route	Onset	Peak
Oral	Varies	2 hr
IV	Immediate	End of infusion

Metabolism: Hepatic; $T_{1/2}$: 3–15 hr (nonsmokers) or 4–5 hr (smokers)
Distribution: Crosses placenta; enters breast milk
Excretion: Urine

Adverse effects in *italics* are most common; those in **bold** are life-threatening. ⊘ Do not crush.

▼ IV FACTS

Preparation: Prepare using sterile technique. Drug provided in 5% dextrose solution. Store at room temperature.

Infusion: Titrate based on patient response. Do not exceed 17 mg/hr. Monitor serum concentration.

Incompatibilities: Do not add any other drugs to solution.

Adverse effects

- **CNS:** *Irritability (especially children), restlessness,* dizziness, headache, seizures, muscle twitching, severe depression, stammering speech, abnormal behavior characterized by withdrawal, mutism, and unresponsiveness alternating with hyperactive periods
- **CV:** Palpitations, sinus tachycardia, ventricular tachycardia, **life-threatening ventricular arrhythmias,** circulatory failure
- **GI:** *Loss of appetite,* hematemesis, epigastric pain, gastroesophageal reflux during sleep
- **GU:** Proteinuria, increased excretion of renal tubular cells and RBCs; diuresis (dehydration), urinary retention in men with prostate enlargement
- **Respiratory:** Tachypnea, **respiratory arrest**
- **Serum theophylline levels less than 20 mcg/mL:** Adverse effects uncommon
- **Serum theophylline levels greater than 20–25 mcg/mL:** *Nausea, vomiting, diarrhea, headache, insomnia, irritability* (75% of patients)
- **Serum theophylline levels greater than 35 mcg/mL:** Hyperglycemia, hypotension, cardiac arrhythmias, tachycardia (greater than 10 mcg/mL in premature newborns); seizures, brain damage, **death**
- **Other:** Fever, flushing, hyperglycemia, SIADH, rash, increased AST

Interactions

✱ **Drug-drug** • Increased effects and toxicity with cimetidine, erythromycin, ciprofloxacin, norfloxacin, ofloxacin, hormonal contraceptives, ticlopidine, ranitidine • Possibly decreased effects with rifampin • Increased serum levels and risk of toxicity in hypothyroid patients, decreased levels in patients who are hyperthyroid; monitor patients on thioamides, thyroid hormones for changes in serum levels as patients become euthyroid • Increased cardiac toxicity with halothane • Decreased effects in patients who are cigarette smokers (1–2 packs/day); theophylline dosage may need to be increased 50%–100% • Decreased effects with barbiturates, charcoal • Decreased effects of phenytoins, benzodiazepines • Decreased effects of nondepolarizing neuromuscular blockers • Mutually antagonistic effects of beta blockers and theophylline preparations

✱ **Drug-food** • Theophylline elimination is increased by a low-carbohydrate, high-protein diet and by charcoal-broiled beef • Theophylline elimination is decreased by a high-carbohydrate, low-protein diet • Food may alter bioavailability, absorption of timed-release theophylline preparations; these may rapidly release their contents with food and cause toxicity. Timed-release forms should be taken on an empty stomach

✱ **Drug-lab test** • Interference with spectrophotometric determinations of serum theophylline levels by furosemide, probenecid, theobromine; coffee, tea, cola beverages, chocolate, acetaminophen cause falsely high values • Alteration in assays of uric acid, urinary catecholamines, plasma free fatty acids

✱ **Drug-alternative therapy** • Decreased effectiveness if taken with St. John's Wort

■ Nursing considerations
Assessment

- **History:** Hypersensitivity to any xanthines; peptic ulcer, active gastritis; status asthmaticus; cardiac arrhythmias, acute myocardial injury, HF, cor pulmonale; severe hypertension; severe hypoxemia; renal or hepatic disease; hyperthyroidism; pregnancy, lactation
- **Physical:** Skin color, texture, lesions; reflexes, bilateral grip strength, affect; P, auscultation, BP, perfusion; R, adventitious sounds; bowel sounds, normal output; frequency, voiding pattern, normal urinary output; ECG; EEG; LFTs, renal and thyroid function tests

Interventions

- Caution patient not to chew or crush enteric-coated timed-release preparations.
- Give liquid dosage forms in divided doses. Give with food if GI effects occur.
- Do not give timed-release preparations with food; these should be given on an empty stomach, 1 hr before or 2 hr after meals.

T

- Advise patients that this drug should not be used during pregnancy; using barrier contraceptives is recommended.

⊗ **Warning** Monitor results of serum theophylline level determinations carefully, and reduce dosage if serum levels exceed therapeutic range of 10–20 mcg/mL.

- Monitor carefully for clinical signs of adverse effects, particularly if serum theophylline levels are not available.

⊗ **Warning** Keep diazepam readily available to treat seizures.

Teaching points

- Take this drug exactly as prescribed. If a timed-release product is prescribed, take it on an empty stomach, 1 hour before or 2 hours after meals. Do not chew or crush timed-release preparations; it may be necessary for you to take this drug around-the-clock for adequate control of asthma attacks.
- Avoid excessive intake of coffee, tea, cocoa, cola beverages, and chocolate. These contain theophylline-related substances that may increase your side effects. Avoid St. John's Wort while taking this drug.
- Smoking cigarettes or other tobacco products may markedly influence the effects of theophylline. It is preferable not to smoke while you are taking this drug. Notify your health care provider if you change your smoking habits while you are taking this drug; it may be necessary to change your drug dosage.
- Have frequent blood tests to monitor drug effects and ensure safe and effective dosage.
- Do not use this drug during pregnancy; using barrier contraceptives is advised.
- You may experience these side effects: Nausea, loss of appetite (take drug with food if taking immediate-release or liquid dosage forms); difficulty sleeping, depression, emotional lability.
- Report nausea, vomiting, severe GI pain, restlessness, seizures, irregular heartbeat.

DANGEROUS DRUG

▽**thioguanine**
(TG, 6-Thioguanine)
(thye oh gwah' neen)

Lanvis (CAN), Tabloid

PREGNANCY CATEGORY D

Drug classes
Antimetabolite
Antineoplastic

Therapeutic actions
Tumor-inhibiting properties, probably due to interference with a number of steps in the synthesis and use of purine nucleotides, which are normally incorporated into DNA and RNA.

Indications
- Remission induction, consolidation, and maintenance therapy of acute nonlymphocytic leukemias—usually used in combination therapy
- Unlabeled uses: Crohn disease, psoriasis, chronic myelogenous leukemia, second-line treatment of ulcerative colitis

Contraindications and cautions
- Contraindicated with allergy to thioguanine, prior resistance to thioguanine or mercaptopurine, hematopoietic depression, pregnancy (potential mutagen and teratogen), lactation.
- Use cautiously with impaired hepatic or renal function.

Available forms
Tablets—40 mg

Dosages
Adults and pediatric patients 3 yr and older
Total dose may be given at one time. Initial dosage, 2 mg/kg/day PO daily for 4 wk. If no clinical improvement is seen and there are no toxic effects, increase dose to 3 mg/kg/day. If complete hematologic remission is obtained, institute maintenance therapy. If used as part of combination therapy, suggested dose is 75–200 mg/m².

Pharmacokinetics

Route	Onset	Peak
Oral	Slow	8 hr

Metabolism: Hepatic; $T_{1/2}$: 11 hr
Distribution: Crosses placenta; may enter breast milk
Excretion: Urine

Adverse effects
- **GI: Hepatotoxicity,** *nausea, vomiting, anorexia,* diarrhea, stomatitis

---

Adverse effects in *italics* are most common; those in **bold** are life-threatening. ▭▭ Do not crush.

- **Hematologic:** *Bone marrow suppression, immunosuppression, hyperuricemia* due to rapid lysis of malignant cells
- **Other:** Fever, weakness, cancer, chromosomal aberrations

■ **Nursing considerations**

Assessment

- **History:** Allergy to thioguanine, prior resistance to thioguanine; hematopoietic depression; impaired hepatic function; pregnancy, lactation
- **Physical:** Skin color; mucous membranes, liver evaluation, abdominal examination; CBC, differential, Hgb, platelet counts; LFTs; serum uric acid

Interventions

- Evaluate hematopoietic status before and frequently during therapy.
- ⊗ **Warning** Discontinue drug therapy if platelet count is less than 50,000 or polymorphonuclear granulocyte count is less than 1,000; consult physician for dosage adjustment.
- ⊗ **Warning** Arrange for discontinuation of this drug at any sign of hematologic or hepatic toxicity; consult physician.
- Ensure that patient is not pregnant before administration.
- ⊗ **Warning** Ensure that patient is well hydrated before and during therapy to minimize adverse effects of hyperuricemia; allopurinol and drugs to alkalinize the urine are sometimes prescribed.
- Administer as a single daily dose on an empty stomach.

Teaching points

- Drink adequate fluids while you are using this drug; drink at least 8–10 glasses of fluid each day.
- This drug may cause miscarriages and birth defects. Both men and women who receive this drug should be using a reliable form of contraception. Discuss with your health care provider how long you should wait to conceive a child after therapy ends.
- Have frequent, regular medical follow-up visits, including frequent blood tests to assess drug effects.
- You may experience these side effects: Mouth sores (use frequent mouth care); nausea, vomiting, loss of appetite (eat frequent small meals); increased susceptibility to infection (avoid crowds and infections).
- Report fever, chills, sore throat, unusual bleeding or bruising, yellow discoloration of the skin or eyes, abdominal pain, flank pain, joint pain, swelling of the feet or legs.

DANGEROUS DRUG

▷**thiotepa (triethylenethiophosphoramide, TESPA, TSPA)**

*(thye oh **tep**' ah)*

Thioplex

PREGNANCY CATEGORY D

Drug classes

Alkylating drug
Antineoplastic

Therapeutic actions

Cytotoxic: Disrupts the bonds of DNA, causing cell death; cell cycle nonspecific.

Indications

- Treatment of adenocarcinoma of the breast, ovary
- Superficial papillary carcinoma of the urinary bladder
- Controlling intracavitary effusions secondary to diffuse or localized neoplastic disease of various serosal cavities
- Treatment of lymphoma, including Hodgkin lymphoma (no longer a drug of choice)

Contraindications and cautions

- Contraindicated with allergy to thiotepa, hematopoietic depression, pregnancy, lactation.
- Use cautiously with impaired hepatic or renal function, concomitant therapy with other alkylating agents or irradiation.

Available forms

Powder for injection—15 mg

Dosages

Adults

IV

0.3–0.4 mg/kg by rapid IV infusion at 1- to 4-wk intervals.

Intratumor

Drug is diluted in sterile water to a concentration of 10 mg/mL, then 0.6–0.8 mg/kg is injected directly into the tumor after a local anesthetic is injected through the same needle. Maintenance doses of 0.6–0.8 mg/kg every 1–4 wk depending on patient's condition.

Intrcavitary

0.6–0.8 mg/kg every 1–4 wk through the same tube that is used to remove fluid from the cavity.

Intravesical

Dehydrate patient with papillary carcinoma of the bladder for 8–12 hr prior to treatment. Then instill 30–60 mg in 60 mL of sodium chloride injection into the bladder by catheter. Retain for 2 hr. If patient is unable to retain 60 mL, give the dose in 30 mL. Repeat once a week for 4 wk. Maintenance doses with 30–60 mg intravesically once monthly for up to 1 yr may be required.

Pharmacokinetics

Route	Onset
IV	Gradual

Metabolism: Hepatic; $T_{1/2}$: 2 hr
Distribution: Crosses placenta; may enter breast milk
Excretion: Urine

▼ IV FACTS

Preparation: Reconstitute powder with sterile water for injection. 1.5 mL of diluent gives a drug concentration of 5 mg/0.5 mL of solution. May be further diluted with sodium chloride injection, dextrose injection, dextrose and sodium chloride injection, Ringer injection, lactated Ringer injection. Store powder in the refrigerator; reconstituted solution is stable for 8 hr if refrigerated. Sterile water for injection produces a hypotonic solution; other diluents may produce a hypertonic solution that may cause mild to moderate discomfort on injection. ⊗ *Warning* Check solution before use; solution should be clear grossly opaque solutions or solutions with precipitates should not be used. Reconstituted solution that is nazy should be filtered through a 0.22-micron sterile filter such as *Acrodisc*.
Infusion: Administer IV dose directly and rapidly, 60 mg over 1 min. There is no need for slow IV drip or the use of large volumes of fluid.

Adverse effects

• **CNS:** *Dizziness*, headache, blurred vision
• **Dermatologic:** Hives, rash, weeping from subcutaneous lesions, contact dermatitis at injection site, alopecia
• **GI:** *Nausea, vomiting,* anorexia
• **GU:** *Amenorrhea, interference with spermatogenesis,* dysuria, urinary retention
• **Hematologic:** *Hematopoietic toxicity*
• **Other:** Febrile reactions, cancer, fatigue

■ Nursing considerations

Assessment

• **History:** Allergy to thiotepa; hematopoietic depression; impaired renal or hepatic function; concomitant therapy with other alkylating agents or irradiation; pregnancy, lactation
• **Physical:** Weight; skin color, lesions; T; orientation, reflexes; CBC, differential; urinalysis; LFTs, renal function tests

Interventions

• Ensure that patient is not pregnant before administration; advise the use of barrier contraceptives.
⊗ *Warning* Wear gloves to avoid skin reactions with accidental exposure. If skin comes into contact with thiotepa, washed area immediately with soap and water and rinse thorough with water.
• Arrange for blood tests to evaluate bone marrow function before therapy, weekly during therapy, and for at least 3 wk after therapy.
• Mix solution with 2% procaine hydrochloride, 1:1,000 epinephrine hydrochloride, or both for local use into single or multiple sites.
• Reduce dosage with renal or hepatic impairment and for bone marrow depression.

Teaching points

• This drug can only be given parenterally. Prepare a calendar of treatment days.
• This drug should not be taken during pregnancy; use birth control while you are being treated with this drug. If you become pregnant, consult your health care provider.
• Have regular medical follow-up visits, including blood tests, to assess drug effects.
• You may experience these side effects: Nausea, vomiting, loss of appetite (request an antiemetic; eat frequent small meals); dizziness, headache (use special safety precautions to prevent falls or injury); amenorrhea in women, change in sperm production.

- Report unusual bleeding or bruising, fever, chills, sore throat, stomach or flank pain, severe nausea and vomiting, skin rash or hives.

▷thiothixene
(thiothixene
hydrochloride)
(thye oh thix' een)

Navane

PREGNANCY CATEGORY C

Drug classes
Antipsychotic
Dopaminergic blocker
Thioxanthene

Therapeutic actions
Mechanism of action not fully understood: Blocks postsynaptic dopamine receptors in the brain, but this may not be necessary and sufficient for antipsychotic activity.

Indications
- Management of schizophrenia

Contraindications and cautions
- Contraindicated with coma or severe CNS depression, blood dyscrasia, circulatory collapse, subcortical brain damage, Parkinson disease, liver damage, cerebral arteriosclerosis, coronary disease, severe hypotension or hypertension, pregnancy, lactation.
- Use cautiously with respiratory disorders ("silent pneumonia"); glaucoma, prostatic hypertrophy; epilepsy or history of epilepsy (drug lowers seizure threshold); breast cancer; thyrotoxicosis (severe neurotoxicity); peptic ulcer, decreased renal function; myelography within previous 24 hr or scheduled within 48 hr; exposure to heat or phosphorous insecticides; children younger than 12 yr, especially those with chickenpox, CNS infections (children are especially susceptible to dystonias that may confound the diagnosis of Reye syndrome).

Available forms
Capsules—1, 2, 5, 10 mg

Dosages
Full clinical effects may require 6 wk–6 mo of therapy.
Adults
Initially, 2 mg PO tid (mild conditions) or 5 mg bid (more severe conditions). Increase dose as needed; the usual optimum dose is 20–30 mg/day. May increase to 60 mg/day, but further increases rarely increase beneficial response.
Pediatric patients
Not recommended for children younger than 12 yr.
Geriatric or debilitated patients
Use lower doses and increase more gradually.

Pharmacokinetics

Route	Onset	Duration
Oral	Slow	12 hr

Metabolism: Hepatic; $T_{1/2}$: 34 hr
Distribution: Crosses placenta; enters breast milk
Excretion: Bile, feces

Adverse effects
- **Autonomic:** *Dry mouth, salivation, nasal congestion, nausea,* vomiting, anorexia, fever, pallor, flushed facies, sweating, constipation, paralytic ileus, urinary retention, incontinence, polyuria, enuresis, priapism, ejaculation inhibition, male impotence
- **CNS:** *Drowsiness,* insomnia, vertigo, headache, weakness, tremor, ataxia, slurring, cerebral edema, seizures, exacerbation of psychotic symptoms, extrapyramidal syndromes—*pseudoparkinsonism; dystonias; akathisia,* tardive dyskinesias, potentially irreversible NMS; extrapyramidal symptoms, hyperthermia, **autonomic disturbances** (rare, but 20% fatal)
- **CV:** Hypotension, orthostatic hypotension, hypertension, tachycardia, bradycardia, cardiac arrest, **HF,** cardiomegaly, **refractory arrhythmias** (some fatal), pulmonary edema
- **EENT:** Glaucoma, *photophobia, blurred vision,* miosis, mydriasis, deposits in the cornea and lens (opacities), pigmentary retinopathy
- **Endocrine:** Lactation, breast engorgement, galactorrhea; SIADH; amenorrhea, menstrual irregularities; gynecomastia; changes in libido; hyperglycemia or hypoglycemia; glycosuria; hyponatremia; pituitary tumor with hyperprolactinemia; inhibition of ovulation,

T

infertility, pseudopregnancy; reduced urinary levels of gonadotropins, estrogens, progestins

- **Hematologic:** Eosinophilia, leukopenia, leukocytosis, anemia, **aplastic anemia,** hemolytic anemia, thrombocytopenic or **nonthrombocytopenic purpura, pancytopenia**
- **Hypersensitivity:** Jaundice, urticaria, angioneurotic edema, laryngeal edema, photosensitivity, eczema, asthma, anaphylactoid reactions, exfoliative dermatitis
- **Respiratory: Bronchospasm, laryngospasm,** dyspnea, suppression of cough reflex and potential for aspiration
- **Other:** *Urine discolored pink to red-brown*

Interactions

✳ **Drug-drug** ● Decreased effects with carbamazepine ● Possible increased CNS effects with CNS agents such as alcohol ● Risk of decreased blood pressure with antihypertensives

✳ **Drug-lab test** ● False-positive pregnancy tests (less likely if serum test is used) ● Increase in PBI not attributable to an increase in thyroxine

■ Nursing considerations

CLINICAL ALERT!
Name confusion has been reported between *Navane* (thiothixene) and *Norvasc* (amlodipine). Use caution.

Assessment

- **History:** Severe CNS depression; blood dyscrasia; circulatory collapse; subcortical brain damage; dementia-related psychosis; Parkinson disease; liver damage; cerebral arteriosclerosis; coronary disease, severe hypotension or hypertension; respiratory disorders; glaucoma; prostatic hypertrophy; epilepsy; breast cancer; thyrotoxicosis; peptic ulcer; decreased renal function; myelography within previous 24 hr or scheduled within 48 hr; exposure to heat, phosphorous insecticides; pregnancy, lactation; chickenpox; CNS infections
- **Physical:** Weight; T; reflexes, orientation, IOP; P, BP, orthostatic BP; R, adventitious sounds; bowel sounds and normal output, liver evaluation; urinary output, prostate size; CBC, urinalysis, LFTs, renal and thyroid function tests

Interventions

⊗ **Black box warning** Risk of death increases if antipsychotics are used to treat elderly patients with dementia-related psychosis; drug is not approved for this use.

⊗ **Warning** Discontinue drug if serum creatinine or BUN becomes abnormal or if WBC count is depressed.

- Notify patient that babies born to mothers who take this drug during the last trimester may exhibit abnormal muscle movements.
- Monitor elderly patients for dehydration, and institute remedial measures promptly; sedation and decreased sensation of thirst related to CNS effects can lead to severe dehydration.
- Consult physician regarding appropriate warning of patient or patient's guardian about tardive dyskinesias.
- Consult physician about dosage reduction, use of anticholinergic antiparkinsonians (controversial) if extrapyramidal effects occur.

Teaching points

- Take drug exactly as prescribed.
- Avoid driving or engaging in other dangerous activities if drowsiness, tremor, weakness, or vision changes occur.
- Avoid prolonged exposure to sun or use a sunscreen or covering garments.
- Maintain fluid intake, and use precautions against heatstroke in hot weather.
- Report sore throat, fever, unusual bleeding or bruising, rash, weakness, tremors, impaired vision, dark urine (pink or reddish-brown urine is to be expected), pale stools, yellowing of the skin or eyes.

▷**thyroid, desiccated**
(thye′ roid)

Armour Thyroid, Nature-Throid, NP Thyroid, Thyroid USP, Westhroid

PREGNANCY CATEGORY A

Drug class

Thyroid hormone preparation (contains T_3 and T_4 in their natural state and ratio)

Therapeutic actions

Increases the metabolic rate of body tissues, increasing oxygen consumption, respiratory and heart rate; rate of fat, protein, and carbohydrate metabolism; and growth and maturation; exact mechanism of action is not known.

Indications

- Replacement therapy in hypothyroidism
- Treatment of thyroid cancer
- Treatment or prevention of various types of euthyroid goiters
- Treatment of thyrotoxicosis with antithyroid drugs to prevent goitrogenesis and hypothyroidism and thyrotoxicosis during pregnancy
- Diagnostic use in suppression tests

Contraindications and cautions

- Contraindicated with allergy to active drug or excipients; thyrotoxicosis and acute MI uncomplicated by hypothyroidism; uncorrected adrenal insufficiency.
- Use cautiously with Addison disease (treatment of hypoadrenalism with corticosteroids should precede thyroid therapy), pregnancy, lactation, myxedema, allergy to pork products, CV disease, elderly patients.

Available forms

Tablets—15, 16.25, 30, 32.5, 48.75, 60, 65, 81.25, 90, 97.5, 113.75, 120, 130, 146.25, 162.5, 180, 195, 240, 260, 300, 325 mg

Dosages

Adults

- *Hypothyroidism:* Initially, 30 mg/day PO, increased by 15 mg/day every 2–3 wk. Usual maintenance dose is 60–120 mg PO daily.

Geriatric patients or patients with heart disease or longstanding hypothyroidism

Initially, 15 mg/day PO.

Pediatric patients

15 mg PO daily. May increase dosage at 2-wk intervals.

0–6 mo: 7.5–30 mg/day PO.
6–12 mo: 30–45 mg/day PO.
1–5 yr: 45–60 mg/day PO.
6–12 yr: 60–90 mg/day PO.
Older than 12 yr: 90 mg/day PO.

Pharmacokinetics

Route	Onset	Peak
Oral	Varies	4 hr

Metabolism: Liver, kidneys, and tissue; $T_{1/2}$: 1–2 days (T_{13}), 6–7 days (T_4)
Distribution: Does not readily cross placenta; minimally enters breast milk
Excretion: Feces, urine

Adverse effects

All adverse effects are rare at therapeutic doses.

- **Dermatologic:** Partial loss of hair in first few months of therapy in children
- **Endocrine:** Hyperthyroidism (palpitations, elevated pulse pressure, tachycardia, arrhythmias, angina pectoris, **cardiac arrest;** tremors, headache, nervousness, insomnia; nausea, diarrhea, changes in appetite; weight loss, menstrual irregularities, sweating, heat intolerance, fever)
- **Hypersensitivity:** Allergic skin reactions

Interactions

✳ **Drug-drug** • Decreased absorption with cholestyramine and antacids; give 4 hr apart from thyroid • Increased risk of bleeding with warfarin • Decreased effectiveness of cardiac glycosides with thyroid replacement • Alterations in theophylline clearance occur in hypothyroid patients; if thyroid state changes during therapy, monitor patient carefully • Possible decreased effects with estrogen products and hormonal contraceptives

■ Nursing considerations

Assessment

- **History:** Allergy to active drug or excipients or porcine products; thyrotoxicosis; acute MI uncomplicated by hypothyroidism; Addison disease; lactation
- **Physical:** Skin lesions, color, T, texture; muscle tone, orientation, reflexes; P, auscultation, baseline ECG, BP; R, adventitious sounds; thyroid function tests

Interventions

⊗ **Black box warning** Do not use to treat obesity. Large doses used in euthyroid patients may produce serious to life-threatening manifestations of toxicity.

- Avoid use elderly patients because of potential cardiac adverse events.
- Monitor response carefully when beginning therapy, and adjust dosage accordingly.
- Administer as a single daily dose before breakfast with a full glass of water.

- Arrange for regular, periodic blood tests of thyroid function.
- Monitor cardiac response throughout therapy. Reduce dose if angina occurs.

Teaching points

- Take as a single dose before breakfast with a full glass of water. Take drug 4 hours apart from antacids.
- This drug replaces a very important hormone and will need to be taken for life. Do not discontinue this drug without consulting your health care provider; serious problems can occur.
- Wear or carry a medical alert tag to alert emergency medical personnel that you are using this drug.
- Nausea and diarrhea may occur (dividing the dose may help).
- Have periodic blood tests and medical evaluations while you are using this drug. Keep your scheduled appointments.
- Report headache, chest pain, palpitations, fever, weight loss, sleeplessness, nervousness, irritability, unusual sweating, intolerance to heat, diarrhea.

▽tiagabine hydrochloride

(tye ag' ah bine)

Gabitril Filmtabs

PREGNANCY CATEGORY C

Drug class

Antiepileptic

Therapeutic actions

Increases GABA levels in the brain, which may result in antiseizure effects. GABA is the major inhibitory neurotransmitter in the CNS; tiagabine binds to GABA reuptake sites, preventing its reuptake, and increases levels in the presynaptic neurons and the glia.

Indications

- Adjunctive therapy in patients older than 12 yr with partial seizures
- Unlabeled uses: Bipolar disorders, PTSD; refractory seizures in children; insomnia.

Contraindications and cautions

- Contraindicated with hypersensitivity to tiagabine, hepatic disease or significant hepatic impairment.
- Use cautiously with pregnancy, lactation, and the elderly.

Available forms

Tablets—2, 4, 12, 16 mg

Dosages

Adults

4 mg PO daily for 1 wk; may be increased by 4–8 mg/wk until desired response is seen; maximum dose, 56 mg/day in two to four divided doses. Usual maintenance dose is 32–56 mg PO daily.

Pediatric patients 12–18 yr

4 mg PO daily for 1 wk; may be increased to 8 mg/day in two divided doses for 1 wk; then increased by 4–8 mg/wk up to a maximum of 32 mg/day PO in two to four divided doses.

Pediatric patients younger than 12 yr

Not recommended.

Pharmacokinetics

Route	Onset	Peak
Oral	Rapid	30–60 min

Metabolism: Hepatic; $T_{1/2}$: 7–9 hr
Distribution: Crosses placenta; may enter breast milk
Excretion: Feces, urine

Adverse effects

- **CNS:** *Dizziness, asthenia, somnolence,* nervousness, tremor, concentration difficulties
- **Dermatologic: Serious rash**
- **EENT:** Possible long-term ophthalmic effects
- **GI:** *GI upset, pain, nausea*
- **GU:** Irregular menses, secondary amenorrhea, dysuria, incontinence

Interactions

* **Drug-drug** • Decreased serum levels with carbamazepine, phenytoin, primidone; phenobarbital, adjustment in tiagabine dosage may be needed • Possible interaction with valproate; monitor patient closely • Increased CNS depression if combined with other CNS depressants (alcohol, hypnotics)

■ Nursing considerations

Assessment

- **History:** Hypersensitivity to tiagabine; hepatic disease or significant hepatic impairment; pregnancy, lactation
- **Physical:** Weight; skin color, lesions; orientation, eye examination, affect, reflexes; LFTs

Interventions

⊗ **Black box warning** Risk of suicidal ideation is increased; monitor patient accordingly.

- Give drug with food.
- Reduce dosage and adjust more slowly if patient is not on concomitant phenytoin, phenobarbital, or carbamazepine.
- Provide frequent skin care if dermatologic effects occur.

⊗ **Warning** Avoid abrupt discontinuation; serious side effects could occur.

- Establish safety precautions (use side rails, accompany patient) if CNS changes occur.
- Arrange for appropriate counseling for women of childbearing age who wish to become pregnant.

Teaching points

- Take this drug exactly as prescribed. If you miss a dose, take it as soon as you remember; do not double doses.
- Do not discontinue this drug abruptly or change dosage, except on the advice of your health care provider.
- Avoid the use of alcohol and sleep-inducing or over-the-counter drugs while you are using this drug; these preparations could cause dangerous effects. If you feel that you need one of these preparations, consult your health care provider.
- Use contraceptives at all times. If you want to become pregnant while you are taking this drug, consult your health care provider.
- Wear a medical alert bracelet at all times so that any emergency medical personnel will know that you have epilepsy and are taking antiepileptic medication.
- You may experience these side effects: Drowsiness (avoid driving or performing other tasks requiring alertness); GI upset (take the drug with food or milk; eat frequent small meals).
- Report bruising, yellowing of the skin or eyes, pale-colored feces, rash, pregnancy, vision changes, thoughts of suicide.

ticagrelor

(tye ka' grel or)

Brilinta

PREGNANCY CATEGORY C

Drug class

Antiplatelet

Therapeutic actions

Inhibits platelet activation and aggregation, reversibly interacting with platelet adenosine diphosphate receptors.

Indications

- Reduction of the rate of thrombotic CV event in patients with acute coronary syndrome

Contraindications and cautions

- Contraindicated with history of intracranial bleeding, active pathologic bleeding, severe hepatic impairment, pregnancy, lactation.
- Use cautiously with moderate hepatic impairment.

Available forms

Tablets—90 mg

Dosages

Adults

180 mg PO loading dose, then 90 mg PO bid. Should give with a loading dose of aspirin, 325 mg PO, then a daily maintenance dose of aspirin, 75–100 mg PO.

Pharmacokinetics

Route	Onset	Peak
Oral	Rapid	2.5 hr

Metabolism: Hepatic; $T_{1/2}$: 7–9 hr
Distribution: May cross placenta; enters breast milk
Excretion: Biliary secretion

Adverse effects

- **CNS:** Headache, dizziness, fatigue
- **CV:** Chest pain, atrial fibrillation, hypertension, bradycardia
- **GI:** Nausea, diarrhea
- **Respiratory:** *Dyspnea*
- **Other: Bleeding,** back pain

Interactions

✳ **Drug-drug** • Do not use with potent CYP3A4 inducers (rifampin, dexamethasone, phenytoin, carbamazepine, phenobarbital) or potent CYP3A4 inhibitors (ketoconazole, itraconazole, voriconazole, clarithromycin, nefazodone, ritonavir, saquinavir, nelfinavir, indinavir, atazanavir, telithromycin) • Risk of toxic effects of simvastatin and lovastatin; if this combination is used, avoid doses of either drug greater than 40 mg • Risk of digoxin toxicity if combined; monitor digoxin level with ticagrelor initiation or dosage change • Increased risk of bleeding if combined with other drugs that affect coagulation; monitor patient closely

■ Nursing considerations

Assessment

- **History:** History of intracranial bleeding, active pathologic bleeding, hepatic impairment, pregnancy, lactation
- **Physical:** T, P, BP, R; adventitious sounds; orientation

Interventions

⊗ **Black box warning** Significant to fatal bleeding episodes can occur. Do not use with active pathologic bleeding or history of intracranial hemorrhage. Do not initiate treatment if coronary artery bypass graft (CABG) surgery is planned (discontinue at least 5 days before surgery, if possible). Suspect bleeding in patients who are hypotensive and have recently undergone coronary angiography, percutaneous coronary intervention, CABG, or other surgical procedures. If possible, manage bleeding without discontinuing ticagrelor; stopping drug increases risk of CV events.

⊗ **Black box warning** Maintenance doses of aspirin above 100 mg reduce effectiveness of ticagrelor. Avoid aspirin doses above 100 mg PO; use doses of 75–100 mg/day.

- Monitor patient for signs and symptoms of bleeding,
- Administer with maintenance dose of aspirin, 75–100 mg/day PO.
- Do not stop drug except for pathologic bleeding because of increased risk of CV events. If drug must be stopped, consider starting an anticoagulant.
- Asses patient reporting dyspnea for underlying issues; dyspnea is common but is usually self-limited.

- Encourage women to avoid pregnancy; advise use of barrier contraceptives. Women who are breast-feeding should find another method of feeding the baby.

Teaching points

- Take this drug exactly as prescribed; do not change doses. Take with the prescribed aspirin; do not increase the aspirin dose.
- Do not stop taking this drug suddenly; make sure you have a supply on hand. Suddenly stopping the drug can cause serious effects.
- Tell your health care provider about all drugs, including over-the-counter products and herbs, you are using and any changes as they occur; many drug interactions can occur with this drug.
- It is not known how this drug could affect a developing fetus. Because this drug may make hormonal contraceptives ineffective, you should use barrier contraceptives. If you are pregnant or thinking about becoming pregnant, discuss this with your health care provider.
- It is not known if this drug appears in breast milk. If you are breast-feeding, you will need to find another method of feeding the baby.
- You will bleed longer and more easily than usual while taking this drug. Tell all your health care providers, including your dentist, that you are taking this drug, especially if any surgery is planned.
- You may experience shortness of breath. This is usually self-limited. Contact your health care provider if it becomes too uncomfortable.
- Report excessive bleeding, difficulty breathing, chest pain, numbness or tingling.

▽ **ticlopidine hydrochloride**

(tye klob' pih deen)

Apo-ticlopidine (CAN), Gen-Ticlopidine (CAN), Nu-Ticlopidine (CAN), Ticlid

PREGNANCY CATEGORY B

Drug class

Antiplatelet

Therapeutic actions

Interferes with platelet membrane function by inhibiting fibrinogen binding and platelet-platelet interactions; inhibits platelet aggregation and prolongs bleeding time; effect is irreversible for life of the platelet.

Indications

- Reduces risk of thrombotic stroke in patients who have experienced stroke precursors and in patients who have had a completed thrombotic stroke; reserve use for patients who are intolerant to aspirin therapy because side effects may be life-threatening
- Prevention of acute stent thrombosis in coronary arteries; used with antiplatelet doses of aspirin
- Unlabeled uses: Intermittent claudication, chronic arterial occlusion, subarachnoid hemorrhage, uremic patients with AV shunts or fistulas, open-heart surgery, coronary artery bypass grafts, primary glomerulonephritis, sickle cell disease

Contraindications and cautions

- Contraindicated with allergy to ticlopidine, neutropenia, thrombocytopenia, history of thrombotic thrombocytopenic purpura (TTP), hemostatic disorders, bleeding ulcer, intracranial bleeding, severe liver disease, lactation.
- Use cautiously with renal disorders, pregnancy, elevated cholesterol, recent trauma.

Available forms

Tablets—250 mg

Dosages

Adults
250 mg PO bid with food.
Pediatric patients
Safety and efficacy not established for patients younger than 18 yr.

Pharmacokinetics

Route	Onset	Peak
Oral	Rapid	2 hr

Metabolism: Hepatic; $T_{1/2}$: 12.6 hr, then 4–5 days
Distribution: Crosses placenta; enters breast milk
Excretion: Feces, urine

Adverse effects

- **CNS:** Dizziness
- **GI:** *Diarrhea, nausea, vomiting, abdominal pain,* flatulence, dyspepsia, anorexia
- **Hematologic: Neutropenia, TTP,** bleeding
- **Local:** *Pain, phlebitis,* thrombosis at injection site
- **Other:** *Rash,* purpura

Interactions

✳ **Drug-drug** • Decreased effectiveness of digoxin • Increased serum levels and effects of theophylline, aspirin, NSAIDs • Increased effects with cimetidine • Decreased absorption with antacids

✳ **Drug-food** • Increased availability with food

∎ Nursing considerations
Assessment

- **History:** Allergy to ticlopidine; neutropenia, thrombocytopenia; hemostatic disorders; bleeding ulcer, intracranial bleeding; severe liver disease; renal disorders; pregnancy, lactation, elevated cholesterol; recent trauma
- **Physical:** Skin color, lesions; orientation; bowel sounds, normal output; CBC, LFTs, renal function tests, serum cholesterol

Interventions

⊗ **Black box warning** Monitor WBC count before use and frequently while initiating therapy; if neutropenia is present or occurs, discontinue drug immediately.
- Administer with food or just after eating to minimize GI irritation and increase absorption.
- Monitor patient for any sign of excessive bleeding (eg, bruises, dark stools), and monitor bleeding times.
- Provide increased precautions against bleeding during invasive procedures; bleeding will be prolonged.

⊗ *Warning* Mark chart of patient receiving drug to alert medical personnel of increased risk of bleeding in cases of surgery or dental surgery.

Teaching points

- Take drug with meals or just after eating.
- You will need regular blood tests to monitor your response to this drug.

- It may take longer than normal to stop bleeding; avoid contact sports, use electrical razors; apply pressure for extended periods to bleeding sites.
- Notify dentist or surgeon that you are using this drug before invasive procedures.
- You may experience these side effects: Upset stomach, nausea, diarrhea, loss of appetite (eat frequent small meals).
- Report fever, chills, sore throat, rash, bruising, bleeding, dark stools or urine.

▷**tigecycline**
*(tye gah **sigh' klin**)*

Tygacil

PREGNANCY CATEGORY D

Drug classes
Antibiotic
Glycylcycline

Therapeutic actions
Inhibits protein translation on ribosomes in specific bacteria, leading to inhibition of bacterial cell growth and cell death; mechanism is not used by many resistant strains.

Indications
- Treatment of complicated skin and skin structure infections caused by susceptible strains of *Escherichia coli, Enterococcus faecalis* (vancomycin-susceptible strains only), *Staphylococcus aureus* (methicillin-susceptible and resistant strains), *Streptococcus agalactiae, Streptococcus anginosus, Streptococcus pyogenes, Bacteroides fragilis, Klebsiella pneumoniae, Enterobacter cloacae*
- Treatment of adults with community-acquired pneumonia caused by *Streptococcus pneumoniae, Haemophilus influenzae, Legionella pneumophila*
- Treatment of intra-abdominal infections caused by *Citrobacter freundii, Enterobacter cloacae, E. coli, Klebsiella oxytoca, Klebiella pneumoniae, Enteroccus faecalis* (vancomycin susceptible strains only), *S. anginosus, B. fragilis, Bacteroides thetaiotaomicron, Bacteroides uniformis, Bacteroides vulgatus, Clostridium perfringens, Peptostreptococcus micros*

- Unlabeled use: Hospital-acquired pneumonia

Contraindications and cautions
- Contraindicated with hypersensitivity to tigecycline or any of its components, pregnancy.
- Use cautiously with allergy to tetracycline antibiotics, lactation.

Available forms
Powder for reconstitution for injection—50 mg/5 mL vial

Dosages
Adults
100 mg IV, followed by 50 mg IV every 12 hr. *Tygacil* should be infused over 30–60 min. Therapy should continue for 5–14 days, based on patient response and bacterial progress.
- *Severe hepatic impairment (Child-Pugh C):* 100 mg IV, followed by 25 mg IV every 12 hr. Patient should be monitored closely.

Pharmacokinetics

Route	Onset	Peak
IV	Rapid	End of infusion

Metabolism: Minimal metabolism: $T_{1/2}$: 27–42 hr
Distribution: May cross placenta; may pass into breast milk
Excretion: Feces, urine

▼ IV FACTS
Preparation: Reconstitute with 5.3 mL 0.9% sodium chloride, 5% dextrose, or Ringer lactate to yield 10 mg/mL. Gently swirl vial until drug dissolves, withdraw 5 mL of solution and immediately add to 100 mL 0.9% sodium chloride or 5% dextrose in an IV bag for infusion. Add an additional 50 mg in 5 mL to the same 100-mL IV bag if making a 100-mg dose. Reconstituted solution should be orange to yellow in color. Solution should be clear with no particulate matter. If particulate matter or discoloration (green to black) is seen, discard solution. Reconstituted solution is stable for up to 6 hr at room temperature, 24 hr if refrigerated, or up to 48 hr if refrigerated in IV bag.
Infusion: Infuse over 30–60 min; flush the tubing of any running IV with 0.9% sodium chloride injection, 5% dextrose injection, or

Ringer lactate before and after infusing *Tygacil.*

Y-site incompatibilities: Amphotericin B, chlorpromazine, methyprednisolone, voriconazole, diazepam, esomeprazole, omeprazole.

Y-site compatibilities: Dobutamine, dopamine, lactated Ringer solution, lidocaine, potassium chloride, ranitidine, theophylline, morphine.

Adverse effects

- **CNS:** Dizziness, insomnia, *headache*
- **CV:** Phlebitis, peripheral edema
- **GI:** *Diarrhea,* **pseudomembranous colitis,** dyspepsia, *nausea, vomiting,* constipation, liver enzyme elevations
- **Respiratory:** Cough, dyspnea
- **Other:** Pruritus, rash, sweating, fever, pain, superinfections, photosensitivity

Interactions

❋ **Drug-drug** • Possible decreased effectiveness of oral contraceptives; suggest use of barrier contraceptives during treatment • Possible alteration in effects of warfarin if taken in combination; monitor patient closely and follow coagulation tests closely

■ Nursing considerations
Assessment

- **History:** Hypersensitivity to tigecycline or any of its components, pregnancy, allergy to tetracycline antibiotics, lactation
- **Physical:** T; orientation, reflexes; BP, peripheral pulses; abdominal examination; skin color, lesions; R, chest sounds; LFTs; culture and sensitivity of infected site

Interventions

- Perform culture and sensitivity tests to assure that this is the most appropriate antibiotic for the infection being treated.
- ⊗ *Warning* There is an increased risk of mortality with drug use. Monitor patient closely and weigh risks before starting drug.
- Advise the use of barrier contraceptives during therapy.
- Suggest another method of feeding the infant if patient is breast-feeding during therapy.
- Provide comfort measures and possible analgesics for headache and pain.
- Encourage frequent, small meals if GI effects are uncomfortable.

Teaching points

- You will receive *Tygacil* as an IV infusion over 30–60 minutes every 12 hours for 5–14 days.
- Tests will be run to make sure that this is the most appropriate antibiotic for your particular infection.
- It is not known how this drug could affect a fetus. If you are pregnant or decide to become pregnant while on this drug, consult your health care provider. Use of barrier contraceptives is advised; this drug may block the effects of hormone contraceptives.
- It is not known how this drug could affect a breast-feeding infant. If you are breast-feeding, another method of feeding the infant should be selected.
- You may experience these side effects: Nausea, vomiting, and diarrhea (these symptoms may lessen over time; if they become bothersome, talk to your health care provider about possible treatments); sensitivity to light (use a sunscreen and wear protective clothing and sunglasses if you have to be exposed to sunlight).
- Report bloody diarrhea, unrelenting diarrhea, rash, swelling of the extremities, discomfort at the injection site.

▽ tiludronate disodium

See Appendix R, *Less commonly used drugs.*

▽ timolol maleate
(tim' oh lol)

Apo-Timol (CAN), Apo-Timop (CAN), Betimol, Blocadren, Gen-Timolol (CAN), Istalol, PMS-Timolol (CAN), Timoptic, Timoptic Ocudose, Timoptic-XE

PREGNANCY CATEGORY C

Drug classes
Antiglaucoma drug
Antihypertensive
Beta-adrenergic blocker

Therapeutic actions
Competitively blocks beta-adrenergic receptors in the heart and juxtaglomerular apparatus, decreasing the influence of the sympathetic nervous system on these tissues and decreasing the excitability of the heart, decreasing cardiac output

and oxygen consumption, decreasing the release of renin, and lowering BP; reduces IOP by decreasing the production of aqueous humor and possibly by increasing aqueous humor outflow.

Indications

- Hypertension, used alone or in combination with other antihypertensives, especially thiazide-type diuretics
- Prevention of reinfarction in MI patients who are hemodynamically stable
- Prophylaxis of migraine
- Ophthalmic solution: Reduction of IOP in open-angle glaucoma, ocular hypertension

Contraindications and cautions

- Contraindicated with hypersensitivity to components of the drug, sinus bradycardia (HR less than 45 beats/min), second- or third-degree heart block (PR interval greater than 0.24 sec), cardiogenic shock, HF, asthma, COPD, pregnancy, lactation.
- Use cautiously with diabetes or thyrotoxicosis (timolol can mask the usual cardiac signs of hypoglycemia and thyrotoxicosis), with general anesthesia in major surgery.

Available forms

Tablets—5, 10, 20 mg; ophthalmic solution, gel—0.25%, 0.5%

Dosages
Adults
Oral

- *Hypertension:* Initially, 10 mg PO bid. Increase dosage at 1-wk intervals to a maximum of 60 mg/day PO divided into two doses, as needed. Usual maintenance dose is 20–40 mg/day given in two divided doses.
- *Prevention of reinfarction in MI (long-term prophylaxis in patients who survived the acute phase):* 10 mg bid PO within 1–4 wk of infarction.
- *Migraine:* 10 mg PO bid; during maintenance, the 20 mg/day may be given as a single dose. May be increased to a maximum of 30 mg/day in divided doses or decreased to 10 mg/day. Discontinue if satisfactory response is not obtained after 6–8 wk.

Ophthalmic
Initially, 1 drop of 0.25% solution bid into the affected eye or eyes. Adjust dosage on basis of response to 1 drop of 0.5% solution bid or 1 drop of 0.25% solution daily. When replacing other agents, make change gradually and individualize dosage. One drop in the affected eye each morning (*Istalol*).

Pediatric patients
Safety and efficacy not established.

Pharmacokinetics

Route	Onset	Peak
Oral	Varies	1–2 hr
Ophthal	Rapid	1–5 hr

Metabolism: Hepatic; $T_{1/2}$: 3–4 hr
Distribution: Crosses placenta; enters breast milk
Excretion: Urine

Adverse effects
Oral

- **Allergic reactions:** Pharyngitis, erythematous rash, fever, sore throat, **laryngospasm,** respiratory distress
- **CNS:** Dizziness, vertigo, tinnitus, fatigue, emotional depression, paresthesias, sleep disturbances, hallucinations, disorientation, memory loss
- **CV:** *HF, cardiac arrhythmias, sinoatrial or AV nodal block,* peripheral vascular insufficiency, claudication, **stroke, pulmonary edema,** hypotension, chest pain
- **Dermatologic:** Rash, pruritus, sweating, dry skin
- **EENT:** Eye irritation, dry eyes, conjunctivitis, blurred vision
- **GI:** *Gastric pain, flatulence, constipation, diarrhea, nausea, vomiting,* anorexia, ischemic colitis, renal and mesenteric arterial thrombosis, retroperitoneal fibrosis, hepatomegaly, acute pancreatitis
- **GU:** *Impotence, decreased libido,* Peyronie disease, dysuria, nocturia, frequent urination
- **Musculoskeletal:** Joint pain, arthralgia, muscle cramp
- **Respiratory: Bronchospasm,** dyspnea, cough, bronchial obstruction, nasal stuffiness, rhinitis, pharyngitis (less likely than with propranolol)
- **Other:** *Decreased exercise tolerance, development of ANA,* hyperglycemia or hypoglycemia, elevated serum transaminase

Ophthalmic

- **Local:** Ocular irritation, decreased corneal sensitivity, visual refractive changes, diplopia, ptosis, tearing

---

Adverse effects in *italics* are most common; those in **bold** are life-threatening. ⬛ Do not crush.

Interactions

✳ Drug-drug • Increased effects with verapamil • Increased risk of orthostatic hypotension with prazosin • Decreased antihypertensive effects with NSAIDs • Risk of rebound hypertension following clonidine withdrawal • Decreased elimination of theophyllines with resultant decrease in expected actions of both drugs when taken concurrently • Peripheral ischemia and possible gangrene with ergotamine, dihydroergotamine • Increased risk of hypoglycemia and masked signs of hypoglycemia with insulin • Hypertension followed by severe bradycardia with epinephrine • All of the above may occur with ophthalmic timolol; in addition, additive effects are possible with oral beta blockers

✳ Drug-lab test • Possible false results with glucose or insulin tolerance tests (oral)

■ Nursing considerations
Assessment

- **History:** Sinus bradycardia, second- or third-degree heart block, cardiogenic shock, HF, asthma, COPD, pregnancy, lactation, diabetes or thyrotoxicosis
- **Physical:** Weight, skin condition, neurologic status, P, BP, ECG, respiratory status, renal and thyroid function, blood and urine glucose

Interventions

⊗ Black box warning Do not discontinue the drug abruptly after long-term therapy (hypersensitivity to catecholamines may have developed, causing exacerbation of angina, MI, and ventricular arrhythmias). Taper drug gradually over 2 wk with monitoring.

- Consult with surgeon about withdrawal if patient is to undergo surgery (withdrawal is controversial).

Teaching points

- Do not stop taking this drug unless instructed to do so by your health care provider.
- Avoid driving or dangerous activities if dizziness or shaking occurs.
- If using ophthalmic form, administer eye drops properly to minimize systemic absorption.
- Report difficulty breathing, night cough, swelling of extremities, slow pulse, confusion, depression, rash, fever, sore throat.

▽**tinidazole**

*(teh **nid'** ah zol)*

Tindamax

PREGNANCY CATEGORY C

Drug classes
Antiprotozoal
Nitroimidazole

Therapeutic actions

Antiprotozoal; mechanism of action against *Giardia, Entamoeba* species is not known.

Indications

- Treatment of trichomoniasis caused by *Trichomonas vaginalis*
- Treatment of giardiasis caused by *Giardia duodenalis* or *G. lamblia* in patients 3 yr and older
- Treatment of amebiasis and amebic liver abscess caused by *Entamoeba histolytica* in patients 3 yr and older
- Treatment of bacterial vaginosis in nonpregnant adult women

Contraindications and cautions

- Contraindicated with allergy to tinidazole, any component of the drug, or other nitroimidazoles; the first trimester of pregnancy; lactation.
- Use cautiously with second or third trimester of pregnancy, history of blood dyscrasias, CNS disorders, hepatic impairment.

Available forms
Tablets—250, 500 mg

Dosages
Adults

- *Trichomoniasis, giardiasis:* Single dose of 2 g PO taken with food.
- *Amebiasis:* 2 g/day PO for 3 days, taken with food.
- *Amebic liver abscess:* 2 g/day PO for 3–5 days, taken with food.
- *Bacterial vaginosis:* 2 g/day PO for 2 days or 1 g/day PO for 5 days.

Pediatric patients older than 3 yr

- *Giardiasis:* Single dose of 50 mg/kg PO (up to 2 g) taken with food.
- *Amebiasis:* 50 mg/kg/day PO (up to 2 g/day) for 3 days, taken with food.

T

• *Amebic liver abscess:* 50 mg/kg/day PO (up to 2 g/day) for 3–5 days, taken with food.

Pharmacokinetics

Route	Onset	Peak
Oral	Rapid	1.6 hr

Metabolism: Hepatic metabolism; $T_{1/2}$: 12–14 hr
Distribution: Crosses placenta; passes into breast milk
Excretion: Feces, urine

Adverse effects

• **CNS:** Weakness, fatigue, malaise, dizziness, headache, drowsiness, **seizures,** peripheral neuropathy

• **GI:** Metallic taste, nausea, anorexia, dyspepsia, cramps, vomiting, constipation, diarrhea, stomatitis
• **GU:** Darkened urine
• **Other:** *Transient neutropenia, transient leukopenia,* superinfections (*Candida*); **severe hypersensitivity reactions,** including urticaria, pruritus, angioedema, Stevens-Johnson syndrome, erythema multiforme

Interactions

✳ Drug-drug ⊗ *Warning* Risk of severe adverse effects if combined with alcohol; advise patient to avoid intake of alcohol while on tinidazole and for 3 days after treatment.
• Possibility of increased effects of oral anticoagulants; monitor the patient and adjust dosage of oral anticoagulant appropriately for up to 8 days after stopping tinidazole therapy • Risk of psychotic reactions if combined with disulfiram; avoid this combination and avoid use within 2 wk of tinidazole therapy • Potential for increased serum levels of lithium if taken concurrently; monitor patient for any sign of lithium intoxication • Potential risk for increased serum levels of cyclosporine, tacrolimus, IV phenytoin, 5-FU if taken with tinidazole; monitor patients for potential toxicity and decrease dosage appropriately • Potential for decreased effectiveness of tinidazole if combined with cholestyramine or oxytetracycline • Potential for increased serum levels and risk of toxicity if combined with cimetidine, ketoconazole, other CYP3A4 inhibitors; monitor patient closely

■ Nursing considerations

Assessment

• **History:** Allergy to tinidazole or any component of the drug or to other nitroimidazoles, pregnancy, lactation, history of blood dyscrasias, CNS disorders, hepatic impairment
• **Physical:** Orientation, affect, reflexes; GI mucosa, output, bowel sounds, liver evaluation; CBC, LFTs, renal function tests

Interventions

⊗ **Black box warning** Avoid use unless clearly needed; tinidazole is carcinogenic in laboratory animals.
• Administer with food to decrease GI side effects.
• Institute appropriate hygiene measures and arrange treatment if superinfections occur.
• If GI upset occurs provide frequent small meals; encourage patient to maintain fluid intake and nutrition.
• Establish safety measures (eg, accompany patient, side rails) if CNS changes occur.
• Suggest another method of feeding the infant if patient is breast-feeding.
• Recommend the use of contraceptive measures while using this drug.

Teaching points

• Take this drug exactly as prescribed, complete the full course of the therapy and do not use this drug to treat any other infections.
• If you miss a dose, take the next dose as soon as you remember; do not take more than the prescribed dose each day.
• Take the drug with food to help decrease GI side effects.
• Be aware that your urine may become dark; this is a drug effect.
• Do not drink alcohol while taking this drug and for three days following completion of the treatment; serious adverse effects could occur.
• This drug should not be used during pregnancy or while breast-feeding; use of contraceptives is recommended while on this drug. If you are breast-feeding, you should select another method of feeding the infant.
• You may experience these side effects: Nausea, diarrhea, metallic taste (frequent small meals, frequent mouth care may help); headache (analgesics may be available to help, consult your health care provider); dizziness

(do not drive a car or operate hazardous machinery if this occurs).
- Report vaginal itching, white patches in the mouth, numbness or tingling of the extremities.

▷ tiopronin

See Appendix R, *Less commonly used drugs.*

▷ tiotropium bromide
(tye oh trob' pee um)

Spiriva

PREGNANCY CATEGORY C

Drug classes
Anticholinergic
Antimuscarinic
Bronchodilator

Therapeutic actions
Competitively antagonistic at muscarinic receptor sites; causes smooth muscle relaxation, leading to bronchodilation.

Indications
- Long-term once-daily maintenance treatment of bronchospasm associated with COPD, including chronic bronchitis and emphysema

Contraindications and cautions
- Contraindicated with allergy to atropine or its derivatives, ipratropium or any component of the product.
- Use cautiously with narrow-angle glaucoma, prostatic hyperplasia, bladder neck obstruction, moderate to severe renal impairment (creatinine clearance of 50 mL/min or less), pregnancy, lactation.

Available forms
Powder for inhalation—18 mcg supplied with *Handibaler* inhalation device

Dosages
Adults
Two inhalations of the contents of one capsule per day using the *Handibaler* inhalation device.
Pediatric patients
Safety and efficacy not established.

Pharmacokinetics

Route	Onset	Peak
Inhalation	Rapid	5 min

Metabolism: $T_{1/2}$: 5–6 days
Distribution: May cross placenta; may enter breast milk
Excretion: Urine, feces

Adverse effects
- **CNS:** *Blurred vision*
- **CV:** Edema
- **GI:** *Dry mouth,* constipation, abdominal pain, dyspepsia, vomiting
- **Respiratory:** Epistaxis, pharyngitis, rhinitis, *sinusitis, URI,* cough
- **Other:** Myalgia, rash, infections, *accidents,* candidiasis, UTI, flulike symptoms, arthritis

Interactions
✳ **Drug-drug** • Risk of increased adverse effects if combined with other anticholinergics; avoid this combination

■ Nursing considerations
Assessment
- **History:** Allergy to atropine or its derivatives, ipratropium, or any component of the product; narrow-angle glaucoma; prostatic hyperplasia, bladder neck obstruction, severe renal impairment; pregnancy, lactation
- **Physical:** Orientation, vision, IOP; skin evaluation; cardiac rhythm, bowel sounds; R, adventitious sounds

Interventions
- Do not use this drug for acute respiratory problems.
- Instruct patient in the proper use of the *Handibaler* inhalation device.
- Do not use any other drugs in the *Handibaler* inhalation device.
⊗ *Warning* Evaluate patient for glaucoma; discontinue drug at first sign of developing glaucoma—eye pain, blurred vision, visual halos with red eye and corneal edema.
- Have patient void before using medication if urinary retention is a problem.

Teaching points
- Administer this drug once daily using the provided *Handibaler* inhalation device. Do not use this device for any other drugs. Do not swallow capsules.

- Keep the capsule in the foil blister pack until ready to use; discard any capsules inadvertently opened and left exposed to the air.
- Follow the directions that come with the *Handihaler* for proper administration of the drug and cleaning of the device.
- Avoid getting the inhalation powder in your eyes; if this occurs, gently wash the eye.
- Use this drug for maintenance of your COPD. Do not use it if you have acute trouble breathing.
- Empty your bladder before using this drug if you have a problem with urinary retention.
- You may experience these side effects: Dry mouth (drink plenty of fluids; suck sugarless candies); constipation (consult your health care provider); blurred vision (avoid driving a car or operating hazardous machinery).
- Report eye pain, eye discomfort, blurred vision, visual halos or colored images along with red eye (consult your health care provider immediately), urinary retention, difficulty urinating.

▽**tipranavir**
(tip ran' ah veer)

Aptivus Ⓒᴬⁿ

PREGNANCY CATEGORY C

Drug classes
Antiviral drug
Protease inhibitor

Therapeutic actions
Inhibits virus specific processing of polyproteins, leading to the inability to produce mature virions and decreasing virus levels.

Indications
- Along with ritonavir, as combination treatment of patients infected with HIV, with evidence of viral replication who are treatment-experienced or have HIV-1 strains resistant to more than one protease inhibitor

Contraindications and cautions
- Contraindicated with known hypersensitivity tipranavir or any of its components, moderate to severe hepatic insufficiency (Child-Pugh class B or C); administration with other drugs that are CYP3A inducers or

that depend extensively on CYP3A for clearance.
- Use cautiously with diabetes mellitus, hyperglycemia, known allergy to sulfonamides, hemophilia, hepatits B or C infection, pregnancy, lactation.

Available forms
Capsules Ⓒᴬⁿ—250 mg; solution—100 mg/mL

Dosages
Adults
500 mg/day PO in combination with 200 mg ritonavir, taken with food.
Pediatric patients ages 2–18 yr
14 mg/kg with 6 mg/kg of ritonavir PO bid (375 mg/m² with 150 mg/m² ritonavir PO bid). Maximum dose, 500 mg with 200 mg ritonavir twice daily, taken with food.

Pharmacokinetics

Route	Onset	Peak
Oral	Slow	2.9 hr

Metabolism: Hepatic; $T_{1/2}$: 4.8–6 hr
Distribution: May cross placenta; may pass into breast milk
Excretion: Feces, urine

Adverse effects
- **CNS:** Depression, insomnia, headache
- **GI:** *Nausea,* vomiting, abdominal pain, *diarrhea,* potentially fatal liver impairment
- **Respiratory:** Cough, bronchitis
- **Other:** Skin rash, flulike symptoms, fever, malaise, increased cholesterol, triglycerides

Interactions
✳ **Drug-drug** • Potential for serious to life-threatening reactions if combined with amiodarone, flecainide, propafenone, quinidine, rifampin, dihydroergotamine, ergonovine, ergotamine, methylergonovine, lovastatin, simvastatin, pimozide, midazolam, triazolam; these combinations are contraindicated • Potential for decreased serum levels of didanosine if combined; space doses of didanosine and tipranavir and ritonavir by at least 2 hr • Potential for decreased serum levels of amprenavir, lopinavir, saquinavir if combined with tipranavir and ritonavir; avoid this combination • Potential for increased serum levels of itraconazole, ketoconazole, voriconazole if used in combination

with tipranavir and ritonavir; avoid high doses, monitor patient closely • Potential for adverse effects if combined with calcium channel blockers; use caution and monitor patient closely • Potential for increased levels of desipramine if used in combination; dosage reduction of desipramine and careful patient monitoring is recommended • Potential for disulfiram-like reaction if combined with disulfiram, metronidazole; monitor patient • Risk of increased levels of oral antidiabetic drugs, leading to potential for hypoglycemia; monitor glucose levels closely and adjust dosages as needed • Risk of increased tipranavir levels and atorvastatin levels if these two drugs are combined; start with lowest possible dose of atorvastatin and monitor patient closely • Risk of increased serum levels and toxic effects of cyclosporine, sirolimus, tacrolimus if used in combination; monitor serum levels closely and adjust dosages as needed • Possible decreased levels of meperidine, methadone if combined with tipranavir and ritonavir; monitor patient and adjust dosages as needed • Risk of decreased serum levels of hormonal contraceptives, leading to lack of effectiveness, and ethinyl estradiol; alternate forms of birth control should be used; monitor women on replacement therapy for low levels of estrogen • Risk of increased serum levels and adverse effects of sildenafil, tadalafil, vardenafil; use extreme caution, start at lowest possible doses and limit use to every 48 hr (sildenafil) or 72 hr (tadalafil, vardenafil) • Risk of increased serum levels of SSRIs; monitor patient and adjust dosage as needed • Potential for unpredictable effects of warfarin when used in combination; monitor bleeding times carefully and adjust dosages as needed

✳ **Drug-alternative therapy** • Potential for loss of effectiveness if combined with St. John's Wort; avoid this combination

■ Nursing considerations
Assessment:

- **History:** Hypersensitivity to tipranavir or any of its components, moderate to severe hepatic insufficiency, diabetes mellitus, hypergylcemia, known allergy to sulfonamides, hemophilia, hepatitis B or C infection, pregnancy, lactation
- **Physical** T; orientation; skin color, lesions; abdominal examination, LFTs, HIV testing, blood counts

Interventions
⊗ *Black box warning* Assess liver function before and periodically during therapy; increased risk of hepatotoxicity in patients with hepatitis. Administration of tipranavir with ritonavir has caused fatal and nonfatal intracranial hemorrhage; monitor patient carefully.

- Make sure that the patient also takes ritonavir when taking this drug.
- Make sure that the patient swallows capsules whole; do not cut, crush, or allow the patient to chew the capsules.
- Administer ritonavir and tipranavir with food.
- Before beginning therapy, assess the patient's drug regimen for numerous potential drug interactions.
- Withdraw drug and monitor patient if patient develops signs of lactic acidosis or hepatotoxicity, including hepatomegaly and steatosis.
- Encourage women of childbearing age to use barrier contraceptives while on this drug because the effects of the drug on a fetus are not known.
- Advise women who are breast-feeding to find another method of feeding the infant; potential effects on the infant are not known.
- Advise patient that this drug does not cure the disease and there is still a risk of transmitting the disease to others.
- Maintain all other therapies related to the HIV infection.

Teaching points
- This drug is not a cure for HIV. It works with ritonavir to decrease the number of viruses in your body.
- You should still take precautions to prevent the spread of HIV; do not share any personal items that may have blood or body fluids on them; use barrier contraceptives if having intercourse.
- Always take tipranavir with ritonavir; take these drugs with food.
- Do not cut, crush, or chew the capsules; swallow capsules whole.
- Store unopened bottles of these capsules in the refrigerator. Once opened, they may be stored in the refrigerator or at room temperature; use within 60 days of opening. Do not use this drug after the expiration date on the bottle. Do not refrigerate or freeze oral solution; use within 60 days of opening bottle.

T

- If you forget a dose of the drug, take that dose along with your ritonavir as soon as you remember, then take your next dose at the usual time. Do not take more than one dose each day.
- This drug interacts with many other drugs; make sure to tell all health care providers that you are taking this drug.
- You will need to have regular health care, including blood tests, to monitor the effects of this drug on your body.
- It is not known how this drug could affect a fetus; if you are pregnant or want to become pregnant while on this drug, consult your health care provider.
- It is not known how this drug could affect a breast-feeding infant. If you are breast-feeding, another method of feeding the infant should be selected while you are taking this drug.
- You may experience these side effects: Headache (consult your health care provider; medication may be available to help); nausea (eating frequent small meals may help); diarrhea (this may lessen with time; alert your health care provider if this becomes severe); liver injury (this could be serious; stop taking the drug and alert your health care provider if you experience yellowing of your skin or eyes, tea-colored urine, general tiredness, pale stools, pain or sensitivity on your right side).
- Report yellowing of the skin or eyes, general malaise and flulike symptoms, changes in the color of your urine or stool, right-sided pain or tenderness.

▽ tirofiban hydrochloride

(tye row fye' ban)

Aggrastat

PREGNANCY CATEGORY B

Drug classes
Antiplatelet
Glycoprotein IIb/IIIa inhibitor

Therapeutic actions
Inhibits platelet aggregation by binding to the platelet receptor glycoprotein IIb/IIIa, which prevents the binding of fibrinogen and other adhesive ligands to the platelet.

Indications
- Treatment of acute coronary syndrome in combination with heparin
- Prevention of cardiac ischemic complications in patients undergoing elective, emergency, or urgent percutaneous coronary intervention

Contraindications and cautions
- Contraindicated with allergy to any component of this product, bleeding diathesis, hemorrhagic stroke, active or abnormal bleeding or stroke within 30 days, uncontrolled or severe hypertension, major surgery within 4 wk, low platelet count, aortic aneurysm, aortic dissection, acute pericarditis, history of intracranial hemorrhage, intracranial neoplasm, aneurysm.
- Use cautiously with pregnancy, lactation, renal insufficiency, the elderly, platelet count less than 150,000/mm^3, dialysis.

Available forms
Injection—50 mcg/mL

Dosages
Adults
0.4 mcg/kg/min IV infusion over 30 min, then continue at rate of 0.1 mcg/kg/min IV.
Pediatric patients
Not recommended.
Patients with renal impairment
Use one-half the recommended adult dosage and monitor patient closely if creatinine clearance is less than 30 mL/min.

Pharmacokinetics

Route	Onset	Peak	Duration
IV	15 min	30 min	4–8 hr

Metabolism: Tissue; T$_{1/2}$: 2 hr
Distribution: Crosses placenta; may enter breast milk
Excretion: Feces, urine

▼ IV FACTS

Preparation: Premixed tirofiban is available in *IntraVia* containers at a concentration of 50 mcg/mL. To open, tear off dust cover; squeeze bag to ensure that no leaks occur—if fluid leaks out, discard solution as sterility has been compromised.

Infusion: Infuse loading dose of 0.4 mcg/kg/min over 30 min; continue infusion at rate of 0.1 mcg/kg/min.

Incompatibilities: Do not mix in solution with diazepam. May be given in same IV line as heparin, dopamine, lidocaine, potassium chloride, famotidine, furosemide, morphine, nitroglycerin, propranolol.

Adverse effects
- **CNS:** *Dizziness,* weakness, syncope, flushing
- **CV:** Bradycardia
- **GI:** Nausea, GI distress, constipation, diarrhea
- **Other:** *Bleeding, hypotension,* edema, pain

Interactions
✳ **Drug-drug** • Increased risk of bleeding when combined with aspirin, warfarin, NSAIDs, antiplatelet agents, heparin; monitor patient closely
✳ **Drug-alternative therapy** • Increased risk of bleeding if combined with chamomile, garlic, ginger, ginkgo and ginseng, turmeric, horse chestnut seed, green tea leaf, grape seed extract, feverfew, don quai; monitor patient closely

■ Nursing considerations

> **CLINICAL ALERT!**
> Name confusion has occurred with *Aggrastat* (tirofiban) and argatroban. Use extreme caution.

Assessment
- **History:** Allergy to any component of this product; bleeding diathesis; hemorrhagic stroke; active, abnormal bleeding or stroke within 30 days; uncontrolled or severe hypertension; major surgery within previous month; dialysis; low platelet count; aortic aneurysm; aortic dissection; pregnancy; lactation; renal impairment
- **Physical:** Skin color, T, lesions; orientation, reflexes, affect; P, BP, orthostatic BP, baseline ECG, peripheral perfusion; respiratory rate, adventitious sounds, aPTT, PT, active clotting time, CBC

Interventions
- Use tirofiban in conjunction with heparin.
- To minimize patient's blood loss, use as few arterial and venous punctures, IM injections, catheterizations, and intubations as possible.
- ⊗ **Warning** Avoid the use of noncompressible IV access sites to prevent excessive, uncontrollable bleeding.

- Arrange for baseline and periodic CBC, PT, aPTT, and active clotting time. Maintain aPTT between 50–70 sec; and active bleeding time between 300 and 350 sec.
- Properly care for femoral access site to minimize bleeding. Document aPTT of less than 45 sec, and stop heparin for 3–4 hr before pulling sheath.

Teaching points
- This drug is given to minimize blood clotting and cardiac damage. It must be given IV.
- You will be monitored closely and your blood will be tested periodically to monitor the effects of this drug on your body.
- You may experience these side effects: Dizziness, light-headedness, bleeding.
- Report light-headedness, palpitations, pain at IV site, bleeding.

---

 tizanidine
(tis an' i deen)

Apo-Tizanidine (CAN), Zanaflex

PREGNANCY CATEGORY C

Drug classes
Alpha$_2$-adrenergic agonist (centrally acting)
Antispasmodic
Sympatholytic (centrally acting)

Therapeutic actions
Centrally acting alpha$_2$-agonist; antispasmodic effect thought to be a result of indirect depression of polysynaptic reflexes by blocking the excitatory actions of spinal motor neurons.

Indications
- Acute and intermittent management of increased muscle tone associated with spasticity

Contraindications and cautions
- Contraindicated with hypersensitivity to tizanidine, concomitant use of fluroxamine, ciprofloxacin.
- Use cautiously with hepatic or renal impairment, hypotension, pregnancy, lactation.

Available forms
Tablets—2, 4 mg; capsules—2, 4, 6 mg

T

Dosages
Adults
4 mg/day PO, increased in 2- to 4-mg increments as needed over 2–4 wk. Usual maintenance dose is 8 mg PO every 6–8 hr; maximum dose, 36 mg/day in divided doses.
Pediatric patients
Safety and efficacy not established.
Patients with renal or hepatic impairment
Use lower doses. Monitor response with renal impairment; use extreme caution with hepatic impairment.

Pharmacokinetics

Route	Onset	Peak	Duration
Oral	30–60 min	1–2 hr	3–6 hr

Metabolism: Hepatic; $T_{1/2}$: 2.7–4.2 hr
Distribution: Crosses placenta; may enter breast milk
Excretion: Urine

Adverse effects
- **CNS:** *Drowsiness, sedation, dizziness, asthenia,* headache, hallucinations, somnolence
- **CV:** *Hypotension, orthostatic hypotension,* bradycardia
- **GI:** *Dry mouth, constipation,* anorexia, malaise, nausea, vomiting, parotid pain, parotitis, mild transient abnormalities in LFTs

Interactions
✴ **Drug-drug** • Potential risk of increased depression with alcohol, baclofen, other CNS depressants • Possible increased effects with hormonal contraceptives; monitor patient and decrease tizanidine dose • Do not use in combination with other alpha$_2$-adrenergic agonists • Increased risk of QT prolongation with other drugs that can prolong QT interval (antiarrhythmics, fluoroquinolones) • Risk of increased toxicity if used with CYP1A2 inhibitors; avoid this combination

■ Nursing considerations
Assessment
- **History:** Hypersensitivity to tizanidine, clonidine; hepatic or renal impairment; hypotension; pregnancy, lactation
- **Physical:** Mucous membranes—color, lesions; orientation, affect; P, BP, orthostatic BP; perfusion; liver evaluation; LFTs, renal function tests

Interventions
- Administer drug every 6–8 hr around-the-clock for best effects.
- Adjust drug dosage slowly, which helps to decrease side effects. Do not exceed three doses in 24 hr.
- Continue all supportive measures used for spinal cord–injured or neurologically damaged patients.
- Provide sugarless candies or ice chips, as appropriate, if dry mouth or altered taste occurs.
- Establish safety precautions if CNS or hypotensive changes occur (use side rails, accompany patient when ambulating).
- Attempt to lower dose if side effects become severe or intolerable.

Teaching points
- Take this drug exactly as prescribed. It is important that you not miss doses. Consult your health care provider to determine a schedule that will not interfere with rest.
- Continue all other supportive measures for your condition.
- You may experience these side effects: Drowsiness, dizziness, light-headedness, headache, weakness (use caution while driving or performing tasks that require alertness or physical dexterity); dry mouth (suck on sugarless candies or ice chips); GI upset (eat frequent small meals); dizziness, light-headedness when changing position (rise slowly, use caution when transferring).
- Report changes in urine or stool, severe dizziness or passing out, changes in vision, difficulty swallowing.

▷**tobramycin sulfate**
(toe bra mye' sin)

Parenteral: generic
Nebulizer solution: TOBI
Ophthalmic: Tobrex Ophthalmic, Tobrasol

PREGNANCY CATEGORY D
(INJECTION, INHALATION)

PREGNANCY CATEGORY B
(OPHTHALMIC)

Drug class
Aminoglycoside antibiotic

Therapeutic actions

Bactericidal: Inhibits protein synthesis in susceptible strains of gram-negative bacteria; mechanism of lethal action is not fully understood, but functional integrity of bacterial cell membrane appears to be disrupted.

Indications

- Parenteral: Serious infections caused by susceptible strains of *Pseudomonas aeruginosa*, *Proteus* species, *Providencia* species, *Escherichia coli*, *Klebsiella-Enterobacter-Serratia* group, *Citrobacter* species, and staphylococci (including *Staphylococcus aureus*)
- Staphylococcal infections when penicillin is contraindicated or when the bacteria are not susceptible
- Serious, life-threatening, gram-negative infections when susceptibility studies have not been completed (sometimes concurrent penicillin or cephalosporin therapy)
- Nebulizer solution: Management of cystic fibrosis patients with *P. aeruginosa*
- Ophthalmic: Treatment of superficial ocular infections due to susceptible strains of organisms

Contraindications and cautions

- Contraindicated with hypersensitivity to aminoglycosides; pregnancy, lactation.
- Use cautiously with patients who are elderly or who have diminished hearing, decreased renal function, dehydration, neuromuscular disorders (myasthenia gravis, parkinsonism, infant botulism), herpes, vaccinia, varicella, mycobacterial infections, fungal infections.

Available forms

Injection—0.8, 1.2, 10, 40 mg/mL, 80 mg/100 mL normal saline; nebulizer solution—300 mg/5 mL; ophthalmic solution—0.3%; ophthalmic ointment—3 mg/g

Dosages

IM or IV

Doses based on ideal body weight.

Adults

3 mg/kg/day in three equal doses every 8 hr. Up to 5 mg/kg/day in three to four equal doses can be used in life-threatening infections, but reduce to 3 mg/kg/day as soon as possible. Do not exceed 5 mg/kg/day unless serum levels are monitored.

Pediatric patients older than 1 wk

6–7.5 mg/kg/day in three to four equally divided doses.

Premature infants or neonates 1 wk and younger

Up to 4 mg/kg/day in two equal doses every 12 hr.

Geriatric patients or patients with renal failure

Reduce dosage, and carefully monitor serum drug levels and renal function tests throughout treatment. Reduced dosage nomogram is available; check manufacturer's information.

Adults and children 6 yr and older

Nebulizer solution

300 mg bid. Administer in 28-day cycles: 28 days on, 28 days of rest. Inhale over 10–15 min.

Ophthalmic solution

- *Mild to moderate infection:* One or two drops into conjunctival sac of affected eye or eyes every 4 hr.
- *Severe infection:* Two drops into conjunctival sac of affected eye or eyes hourly until improvement occurs.

Ophthalmic ointment

One-half-inch ribbon bid–tid.

- *Severe infection:* One-half inch every 3–4 hr.

Pharmacokinetics

Route	Onset	Peak
IM, IV	Rapid	30–90 min
Ophthalmologic	Rapid	Unknown
Inhalation	Rapid	20 min

Metabolism: Minimal hepatic; $T_{1/2}$: 2–3 hr
Distribution: Crosses placenta; enters breast milk
Excretion: Urine

▼ IV FACTS

Preparation: Use the 10- or 40-mg/mL vials and add required dose to 50–100 mL of 0.9% sodium chloride injection or 5% dextrose injection (less for children). Premixed solutions can be used without other dilution.

Infusion: Infuse over 20–60 min.

Incompatibilities: Do not premix with other drugs; administer other drugs separately.

T

Adverse effects

- **CNS:** Ototoxicity, vestibular paralysis, confusion, disorientation, depression, lethargy, nystagmus, visual disturbances, headache, *numbness, tingling,* tremor, paresthesias, muscle twitching, seizures, muscular weakness, neuromuscular blockade
- **CV:** Palpitations, hypotension, hypertension
- **EENT:** Localized ocular toxicity and hypersensitivity reactions; *lid itching, swelling;* conjunctival erythema; punctate keratitis
- **GI:** Hepatic toxicity, *nausea, vomiting, anorexia,* weight loss, stomatitis, increased salivation
- **GU:** *Nephrotoxicity*
- **Hematologic:** Agranulocytosis, *leukemoid reaction,* granulocytosis, leukopenia, leukocytosis, thrombocytopenia, eosinophilia, pancytopenia, anemia, hemolytic anemia, increased or decreased reticulocyte count, electrolyte disturbances
- **Hypersensitivity:** *Purpura, rash,* urticaria, exfoliative dermatitis, itching
- **Local:** *Pain, irritation, arachnoiditis at IM injection sites*
- **Other:** Fever, apnea, splenomegaly, joint pain, *superinfections*

Interactions

✳ **Drug-drug** ● Increased ototoxic, nephrotoxic, neurotoxic effects with other aminoglycosides, potent diuretics ● Increased neuromuscular blockade and muscular paralysis with anesthetics, nondepolarizing neuromuscular blocking drugs, succinylcholine ● Potential inactivation of both drugs if mixed with beta-lactam-type antibiotics ● Increased bactericidal effect with penicillins, cephalosporins

■ Nursing considerations
Assessment

- **History:** Allergy to aminoglycosides, diminished hearing, decreased renal function, dehydration, neuromuscular disorders, lactation, pregnancy, infections (ophthalmic solutions)
- **Physical:** Weight; renal function, eighth cranial nerve function; state of hydration; hepatic function, CBC; skin color and lesions; orientation and affect; reflexes; bilateral grip strength; bowel sounds

Interventions

⊗ **Black box warning** Injection may cause serious ototoxicity, nephrotoxicity, and neurotoxicity. Monitor patient closely for changes in renal and CNS function.

- Arrange culture and sensitivity tests of infection before beginning therapy.

⊗ **Warning** Limit duration of treatment to short term to reduce the risk of toxicity; usual duration of treatment is 7–14 days.

- Use ophthalmologic tobramycin only when indicated by sensitivity tests; use of ophthalmologic tobramycin may cause sensitization that will contraindicate the systemic use of tobramycin or other aminoglycosides in serious infections.
- Monitor total serum concentration of tobramycin if ophthalmologic solution or inhaled tobramycin is used concurrently with parenteral aminoglycosides.
- Administer IM dose by deep IM injection.
- Administer nebulizer solution for 28 days; followed by 28 days of rest; have patient in upright position, inhale over 10–15 min.
- Ensure that patient is well hydrated before and during therapy.

Teaching points
Parenteral

- Report hearing changes, dizziness, pain at injection site.

Ophthalmic solution

- Tilt head back; place medication into conjunctival sac, and close eye; apply light finger pressure on lacrimal sac for 1 minute.
- Solution may cause blurring of vision or stinging on administration.
- Report severe stinging, itching, or burning.

Nebulizer solution

- Inhale over 10–15 minutes while in an upright position.
- Mark calendar with 28 days of using drug followed by 28 days without using drug.
- Store drug in refrigerator; do not expose to intense light.

▽tocilizumab
(toe sib liz' oo mab)

Actemra

PREGNANCY CATEGORY C

Drug classes
Antirheumatic
Interleukin-6 receptor inhibitor
Monoclonal antibody

Therapeutic actions
Binds with interleukin receptors, inhibiting interleukin-6-mediated signaling to a variety of cells, including T cells, B cells, lymphocytes, monocytes, and fibroblasts. This action decreases the inflammatory processes that occur in rheumatoid arthritis. Also decreases rheumatoid factor, erythrocyte sedimentation rate, serum amyloid A, and neutrophil counts and increases hemoglobin level.

Indications
- Treatment of patients with moderately to severely active rheumatoid arthritis who have had an inadequate response to one or more tumor necrosis factor (TNF) antagonist therapies
- Treatment of active systemic juvenile idiopathic arthritis in patients 2 yr and older.
- Treatment of Still disease (systemic idiopathic juvenile arthritis) in patients 2 yr and older

Contraindications and cautions
- Contraindicated with history of serious allergy to components of the drug, pregnancy, lactation, active infection.
- Use cautiously with GI perforation or history of ulcers, bone marrow suppression, liver impairment, history of TB or hepatitis B.

Available forms
Single-use vials—80 mg/4 mL, 200 mg/10 mL, 400 mg/20 mL

Dosages
Adults
4 mg/kg by IV infusion over 1 hr, followed by an increase to 8 mg/kg based on clinical response; can repeat infusion once every 4 wk. Maximum dose, 800 mg/infusion.
Pediatric patients 2 yr and older
- *Weighing 30 kg or more:* 8 mg/kg IV every 2 wk.
- *Weighing less than 30 kg:* 12 mg/kg IV every 2 wk.

Pharmacokinetics

Route	Onset	Peak
IV	Moderate	End of infusion

Metabolism: Endogenous; T$_{1/2}$: 11 days
Distribution: May cross placenta; may enter breast milk
Excretion: Endogenous clearance

▼ **IV FACTS**

Preparation: Adults and children weighing 30 kg or more: Dilute to 100 mL using 0.9% sodium chloride injection. Children weighing less than 30 kg: Dilute to 50 mL using 0.9% sodium chloride injection. Withdraw a volume equal to the *Actemra* solution to be used. Slowly add drug to infusion bag, then mix gently, inverting the bag to avoid foaming; inspect for particulate matter or discoloration. Diluted solution may be stored at room temperature, protected from light, for up to 24 hr.
Infusion: Infuse over 60 min through an infusion set; do not administer by IV push or bolus.
Incompatibilities: Do not infuse through the same infusion line as other drugs; do not mix in solution with other drugs.

Adverse effects
- **CNS:** *headache,* dizziness, demyelinating disorders
- **CV:** *hypertension*
- **GI:** mouth ulcerations, upper abdominal pain, gastritis, GI perforation, lipid changes, *increased liver enzymes*
- **Respiratory:** URI, *nasopharyngitis*
- **Other: infections, potentially serious;** infusion reaction, bone marrow suppression, **anaphylaxis**

Interactions
✳ **Drug-drug** • Possible serious infections if combined with TNF antagonists, interleukin receptor antagonist or anti-CD20 monoclonal antibodies; these combinations are not recommended • Possible increased toxicity of drugs metabolized by CYP450 substrates (such as statins, omeprazole, warfarin, cyclosporine); dosage increases for these drugs may be needed to obtain their therapeutic effect during and for 6 months after tocilizumab is discontinued; monitor patient closely • Live vaccines should be avoided during drug therapy

■ Nursing considerations
Assessment
- **History:** Hypersensitivity to components of the drug; GI perforation; infections, including TB and hepatitis B; liver impairment; bone marrow suppression; pregnancy; lactation
- **Physical:** Orientation; temperature; R, adventitious sounds; GI exam; CBC, LFTs

T

Interventions

⊗ **Black box warning** Serious to life-threatening infections may occur with drug use, including TB and bacterial, invasive fungal, viral, and opportunistic infections. Perform TB test before start of therapy. Interrupt treatment if serious infection occurs; monitor patient for signs and symptoms of TB during therapy.

- Obtain CBC and LFTs before start of therapy. Do not initiate in patients with neutrophil count below 2,000/mm³, platelet count below 100,000/mm³, or ALT or AST level above 1.5 times the upper limit of normal.
- Monitor liver enzyme and lipid levels and neutrophil and platelet counts periodically during therapy. Dosage adjustments may be needed in response to changes in these parameters.
- Protect patient from infection; monitor patient for signs and symptoms of active infection.
- Continue other nonbiologic drugs used for treating arthritis, such as methotrexate, corticosteroids, and NSAIDs.
- Ensure that patient continues all other therapies for rheumatoid arthritis.

Teaching points

- This drug will need to be infused into a vein over 1 hour once every 2 (children) or 4 weeks. Mark your calendar for the days you will need to have these infusions.
- If you forget a date for a scheduled infusion, talk to your health care provider about a new schedule.
- Continue other drugs prescribed for your rheumatoid arthritis and any other therapies you have been using.
- Keep appointments for periodic blood tests to check your liver enzyme levels and blood counts, which might be affected by this drug. The dosage or timing of your drug may be changed based on the results of these tests.
- It is not known if this drug could affect a fetus but studies have shown that the drug adversely affects animal fetuses. If you are pregnant or thinking about becoming pregnant, discuss this with your health care provider; use of contraceptives is advised.
- This drug may appear in breast milk and may have serious effects on your infant. If you are breast-feeding, you should use another method of feeding the baby while taking this drug.
- Do not get live vaccines while taking this drug; tell your health care provider about other drugs you might be taking.
- You may experience these side effects: Upper respiratory infections, stuffy nose; lower white blood cell count (you will be more susceptible to infections; avoid crowds and people you know to be sick); low platelet count (you will be more prone to bleeding; avoid situations in which you could be easily injured and use a soft-bristled toothbrush); tears in the GI tract (this is very rare and occurs more frequently in people with a history of ulcers, but you should report fever, stomach pain, and change in bowel habits).
- Report signs and symptoms of infection (fever, chills, muscle aches, cough, skin sores, diarrhea, burning on urination), shortness of breath, rash, swelling of the lips or face, chest pain, dizziness, difficulty breathing, black or tarry stools, severe abdominal pain, excessive bruising or bleeding.

▷ tofacitinib

See Appendix R, *Less commonly used drugs.*

▷ TOLAZamide

See Appendix R, *Less commonly used drugs.*

▷ TOLBUTamide

See Appendix R, *Less commonly used drugs.*

▷ tolcapone
*(toll **kap**' own)*

Tasmar

PREGNANCY CATEGORY C

Drug classes

Antiparkinsonian
COMT inhibitor

Therapeutic actions

Selectively and reversibly inhibits COMT, an enzyme that eliminates biologically active catecholamines including dopa, dopamine, norepinephrine, epinephrine; when given with levodopa, tolcapone's inhibition of COMT is believed to increase the plasma concentrations and duration of action of levodopa.

Indications
- Adjunct with levodopa and carbidopa in the treatment of the signs and symptoms of idiopathic Parkinson disease

Contraindications and cautions
- Contraindicated with hypersensitivity to drug or its components, lactation, liver disease, patients with a history of nontraumatic rhabdomyolysis or hyperpyrexia and confusion.
- Use cautiously with hypertension, hypotension, or renal impairment; pregnancy.

Available forms
Tablets—100 mg

Dosages
Adults
Initial maintenance dosage, 100 mg PO tid. Maximum daily dose, 600 mg. 200 mg tid is more associated with liver enzyme elevation and is only recommended when benefit outweighs risk. However, 200 mg tid can be used if benefit is justified. If patient does not show a clinical benefit within 3 wk of treatment with 200 mg tid, tolcapone should be discontinued.
Pediatric patients
Safety and efficacy not established.
Patients with renal or hepatic impairment
Discontinue drug if liver enzyme values are greater than twice upper limit of normal. Patients with moderate to severe hepatic impairment should not exceed 100 mg PO tid; patients with liver enzyme values greater than the upper limit of normal at initiation should not receive this drug. Use caution in patients with renal impairment.

Pharmacokinetics

Route	Onset	Peak
Oral	Varies	2 hr

Metabolism: Hepatic; $T_{1/2}$: 2–3 hr
Distribution: Crosses placenta; enters breast milk
Excretion: Feces, urine

Adverse effects
- **CNS:** *Disorientation, confusion,* memory loss, *hallucinations,* psychoses, agitation, nervousness, delusions, delirium, paranoia, euphoria, excitement, *light-headedness, dizziness,* depression, drowsiness, weakness, giddiness, paresthesia, heaviness of the limbs, numbness of fingers
- **CV:** Hypotension, orthostatic hypotension
- **Dermatologic:** Rash, urticaria, other dermatoses
- **GI:** Acute suppurative parotitis, *nausea, vomiting,* diarrhea, epigastric distress, flatulence, **fulminant and possibly fatal liver failure**
- **Respiratory:** URIs, dyspnea, sinus congestion
- **Other:** Muscular weakness, muscular cramping

Interactions
✴ **Drug-drug** • Risk of serious reaction if combined with MAOIs; avoid this combination

■ Nursing considerations
Assessment
- **History:** Hypersensitivity to drug or its components; hypertension, hypotension; hepatic or renal impairment; pregnancy, lactation
- **Physical:** Weight; T; skin color, lesions; orientation, affect, reflexes, bilateral grip strength, visual examination; P, BP, orthostatic BP, auscultation; bowel sounds, normal output, liver evaluation; urinary output, voiding pattern, LFTs, renal function tests

Interventions
- Administer in conjunction with levodopa and carbidopa. Monitor patient response; customary levodopa dosage may need to be decreased.
- ⊗ **Black box warning** Risk of potentially fatal acute fulminant liver failure exists. Monitor LFTs before and every 2 wk during therapy; discontinue drug at any sign of liver damage; use drug for patients no longer responding to other therapies.
- Provide sugarless candies or ice chips to suck if dry mouth is a problem.
- Give with meals if GI upset occurs; give before meals to patients bothered by dry mouth; give after meals if drooling is a problem or if drug causes nausea.

⊗ **Warning** Avoid abrupt withdrawal of drug, which can lead to more serious complications. Taper drug slowly over 2 wk if possible.

• Advise patient to use barrier contraceptives; serious birth defects can occur while using this drug. Advise breast-feeding patients to use another means of feeding the infant because drug can enter breast milk and adversely affect the infant.

• Establish safety precautions if CNS, vision changes, hallucinations, or hypotension occurs (eg, use side rails, accompany patient when ambulating).

• Provide additional comfort measures appropriate to patient with parkinsonism.

Teaching points
• Take this drug exactly as prescribed. Take in conjunction with your levodopa and carbidopa. Do not stop this drug suddenly; it must be tapered over 2 weeks.

• Use barrier contraceptives while using this drug; serious birth defects can occur. Do not breast-feed while using this drug; the drug enters breast milk and can adversely affect the infant.

• You may experience these side effects: Drowsiness, dizziness, confusion, blurred vision (avoid driving a car or engaging in activities that require alertness and visual acuity if these occur; rise slowly when changing positions to help decrease dizziness); nausea (eat frequent small meals); dry mouth (suck sugarless candies or ice chips); hallucinations (it may help to know that this is a side effect of the drug; use care and have someone stay with you if this occurs); constipation (if maintaining adequate fluid intake and exercising regularly do not help, consult your health care provider).

• Report constipation, rapid or pounding heartbeat, confusion, eye pain, hallucinations, rash, changes in color of urine or stools, fever, chills, fatigue, yellowing of skin or eyes.

▷**tolmetin sodium**
(tole' met in)

PREGNANCY CATEGORY C

PREGNANCY CATEGORY D
(3RD TRIMESTER)

Drug class
NSAID

Therapeutic actions
Anti-inflammatory, analgesic, and antipyretic activities largely related to inhibition or prostaglandin synthesis; exact mechanisms of action are not known.

Indications
• Treatment of acute flares and long-term management of rheumatoid arthritis and osteoarthritis

• Treatment of juvenile rheumatoid arthritis in patients older than 2 yr

Contraindications and cautions
• Contraindicated with hypersensitivity to the drug or any of its components, in patients who have had reactions to aspirin or other NSAIDs; with lactation, treatment of perioperative pain in the setting of CABG surgery.

• Use cautiously with allergies; renal, hepatic, CV and GI conditions; coagulation defects; patients taking anticoagulants; pregnancy.

Available forms
Tablets—200, 600 mg; capsules—400 mg

Dosages
Adults
Do not exceed 1,800 mg/day. Doses exceeding 1.8 g daily have not been studied. Subsequent dosing adjustment based on response and tolerance after 1–2 wk.

• *Rheumatoid arthritis or osteoarthritis:* Initial dose, 400 mg PO tid (1,200 mg/day) preferably including dose on arising and at bedtime. Maintenance dose, 600–1,800 mg/day in three to four divided doses for rheumatoid arthritis; 600–1,600 mg/day in three to four divided doses for osteoarthritis.

Pediatric patients 2 yr and older
Initially, 20 mg/kg/day PO in three to four divided doses; when control has been achieved, the usual dose is 15–30 mg/kg/day. Do not exceed 30 mg/kg/day.

Pharmacokinetics

Route	Onset	Peak
Oral	Varies	30–60 min

Metabolism: Hepatic; $T_{1/2}$: 2–7 hr

Distribution: Crosses placenta; enters breast milk
Excretion: Urine

Adverse effects

- **CNS:** *Headache, dizziness, somnolence, insomnia,* fatigue, tiredness, dizziness, tinnitus, *ophthalmologic effects,* weakness
- **CV:** Hypertension, edema
- **Dermatologic:** *Rash,* pruritus, sweating, dry mucous membranes, stomatitis
- **GI:** *Nausea, dyspepsia, GI pain, diarrhea,* vomiting, constipation, flatulence, gastric ulcer, peptic ulcer
- **GU:** Dysuria, renal impairment, including renal failure, interstitial nephritis, hematuria
- **Hematologic:** Bleeding, platelet inhibition with higher doses, neutropenia, eosinophilia, *leukopenia,* pancytopenia, thrombocytopenia, agranulocytosis, granulocytopenia, aplastic anemia, decreased Hgb or Hct, bone marrow depression, *menorrhagia*
- **Respiratory:** Dyspnea, hemoptysis, pharyngitis, **bronchospasm,** rhinitis
- **Other:** Peripheral edema, **anaphylactoid reactions** to **fatal anaphylactic shock**

Interactions

⁕ **Drug-lab test** • False-positive tests for proteinuria using acid precipitation tests; no interference has been reported with dye-impregnated reagent strips

■ Nursing considerations

Assessment

- **History:** Allergies; renal, hepatic, CV, and GI conditions; pregnancy, lactation
- **Physical:** Skin color, lesions; orientation, reflexes, ophthalmologic and audiometric evaluation, peripheral sensation; P, edema; R, adventitious sounds; liver evaluation; CBC, clotting times, LFTs, renal function tests; serum electrolytes, stool guaiac

Interventions

- Administer with milk if GI upset occurs; do not give with food—bioavailability is decreased by up to 16%.
- Use antacids other than sodium bicarbonate if GI upset occurs.
- Arrange for periodic ophthalmologic examination during long-term therapy.

⊗ *Warning* If overdose occurs, institute emergency procedures—gastric lavage, induction of emesis, supportive therapy.

⊗ **Black box warning** Be aware that patient may be at increased risk for CV event, GI bleeding; monitor accordingly. Drug is not for use for perioperative pain in the setting of CABG surgery.

Teaching points

- Take drug on an empty stomach; may be taken with milk or antacids other than sodium bicarbonate if GI upset occurs.
- Take only the prescribed dosage.
- You may experience these side effects: Dizziness, drowsiness (avoid driving or using dangerous machinery).
- Report sore throat, fever, rash, itching, weight gain, swelling in ankles or fingers; changes in vision; black, tarry stools; chest pain.

▷ **tolterodine tartrate**
*(toll **tear'** oh deen)*

Detrol, Detrol LA ⒸⒶⓃ

PREGNANCY CATEGORY C

Drug class

Antimuscarinic

Therapeutic actions

Competitively blocks muscarinic receptor sites; bladder contraction is mediated by muscarinic receptors—blocking these receptors decreases bladder contraction.

Indications

- Treatment of overactive bladder in patients with symptoms of urinary frequency, urgency or incontinence

Contraindications and cautions

- Contraindicated with urinary retention, uncontrolled narrow-angle glaucoma, gastric retention, allergy to the drug or any of its components.
- Use cautiously with renal or hepatic impairment, pregnancy, lactation.

Available forms

Tablets—1, 2 mg; ER capsules ⒸⒶⓃ—2, 4 mg

T

Dosages

Adults

2 mg PO bid, may be lowered to 1 mg PO bid based on individual response; ER capsules— 4 mg PO taken once daily; may be lowered to 2 mg once daily based on response.

Pediatric patients

Safety and efficacy not established.

Patients with hepatic and renal impairment

Reduce dosage to 1 mg PO bid (2 mg daily ER capsules) and monitor patient.

Pharmacokinetics

Route	Onset	Duration
Oral	1–2 hr	6–8 hr

Metabolism: Hepatic; $T_{1/2}$: 1.9–3.7 hr
Distribution: Crosses placenta; enters breast milk
Excretion: Urine

Adverse effects

- **CNS:** *Blurred vision,* headache, dizziness, somnolence
- **Dermatologic:** Pruritus, rash, erythema, dry skin
- **GI:** *Nausea, vomiting, constipation, dyspepsia,* flatulence, *dry mouth,* abdominal pain
- **GU:** *Dysuria,* urinary retention; impotence, UTIs
- **Other:** Weight gain, pain, fatigue, acute myopia and secondary angle closure glaucoma (pain, visual changes, redness, increased IOP)

Interactions

＊**Drug-drug** • Risk of increased serum levels and toxicity if given with drugs that inhibit CYP2D6 (such as fluoxetine) or with potent CYP3A4 inhibitors (such as azole antifungals); reduce tolterodine dose to 1 mg PO bid (2 mg daily ER capsules)

■ Nursing considerations

Assessment

- **History:** Urinary retention, uncontrolled narrow-angle glaucoma, allergy to the drug or any of its components, renal or hepatic impairment, pregnancy, lactation
- **Physical:** Bowel sounds, normal output; normal urinary output, prostate palpation; IOP, vision; LFTs, renal function tests; skin color, lesions, texture; weight

Interventions

- Ensure that patient does not cut, crush, or chew ER forms.
- Provide frequent small meals if GI upset is severe.
- Provide frequent mouth hygiene or skin care if dry mouth or skin occurs.
- Arrange for safety precautions if blurred vision occurs.
- Monitor bowel function and arrange for bowel program if constipation occurs.

Teaching points

- Take drug exactly as prescribed. Do not cut, crush, or chew ER forms.
- You may experience these side effects: Constipation (ensure adequate fluid intake, proper diet; consult your health care provider if this becomes a problem); dry mouth (suck sugarless candies, practice frequent mouth care; this effect sometimes lessens over time); blurred vision (it may help to know that these are drug effects that will go away when you discontinue the drug; avoid tasks that require acute vision); difficulty in urination (it may help to empty the bladder immediately before taking each dose of drug).
- Report rash, flushing, eye pain, difficulty breathing, tremors, loss of coordination, irregular heartbeat, palpitations, headache, abdominal distention.

▽**tolvaptan**

See Appendix R, *Less commonly used drugs.*

▽**topiramate**
(toe pie' rah mate)

Gen-Topiramate (CAN), PMS-Topiramate (CAN), ratio-Topiramate (CAN), Topamax ⊙ℝℇ, Topamax Sprinkle, Topiragen

PREGNANCY CATEGORY D

Drug classes

Antiepileptic
Antimigraine

Therapeutic actions

Mechanism of action not understood; antiepileptic effects may be due to the actions of blocking sodium channels in neurons with sustained depolarization; increasing GABA activity at receptors, thus potentiating the effects of this inhibitory neurotransmitter; and blocking excitatory neurotransmitters at neuron receptor sites.

Indications

- Monotherapy for the treatment of patients 2 yr and older with partial onset or primary generalized tonic-clonic seizures
- Adjunctive therapy for partial-onset seizure treatment in adults and children 2–16 yr
- Adjunctive therapy for seizures associated with Lennox-Gastaut syndrome in adults and children older than 2 yr
- Adjunctive therapy for primary generalized tonic-clonic seizures in adults and children 2–16 yr
- Prophylaxis of migraine headaches in adults
- Unlabeled uses: Cluster headaches, infantile spasms, alcohol dependence, bulimia nervosa, weight loss, smoking cessation, restless legs syndrome, neuropathic pain, essential tumor, bipolar disorder

Contraindications and cautions

- Contraindicated with hypersensitivity to any component of the drug; pregnancy.
- Use cautiously with lactation, renal or hepatic impairment, renal stones, glaucoma.

Available forms

Tablets ⊙⊙—25, 50, 100, 200 mg; sprinkle capsules—15, 25 mg

Dosages
Adults 17 yr and older

- *Migraine prophylaxis:* Initially, 25 mg PO in the evening for 1 wk; week 2—25 mg PO bid, morning and evening; week 3—25 mg PO in the morning and 50 mg PO in the evening; week 4—50 mg PO morning and evening.
- *Seizure disorder:* 200–400 mg PO daily in two divided doses. Therapy should be initiated at a dose of 25–50 mg/day titrated up in increments of 25–50 mg/wk.
Patients 10 yr and older

- *Monotherapy for epilepsy:* 25 mg PO bid, titrating to maintenance dose of 200 mg PO bid over 6 wk. Week 1—25 mg PO bid; week 2—50 mg PO bid; week 3—75 mg PO bid;

week 4—100 mg PO bid; week 5—150 mg PO bid; week 6—200 mg PO bid.
Pediatric patients 2–16 yr

5–9 mg/kg/day PO in two divided doses. Therapy should be initiated at a nightly dose of 25 mg (or less, based on 1–3 mg/kg/day) for the first week. The dose may be titrated up by increments of 1–3 mg/kg/day (administered in two divided doses) at 1–2 wk intervals.
Patients with hepatic or renal impairment

For creatinine clearance less than 70 mL/min, use one-half the usual dose; allow increased time to reach desired level. For patients with hepatic impairment, adjust slowly; monitor patient carefully.

Pharmacokinetics

Route	Onset	Peak
Oral	Rapid	2 hr

Metabolism: Hepatic; $T_{1/2}$: 21 hr
Distribution: Crosses placenta; enters breast milk
Excretion: Urine
Removed by hemodialysis: Supplemental dose may be needed

Adverse effects

- **CNS:** *Ataxia, somnolence, dizziness, nystagmus,* nervousness, anxiety, tremor, speech impairment, *paresthesias,* confusion, depression
- **GI:** *Nausea, dyspepsia,* anorexia, taste perversion, vomiting
- **GU:** Dysmenorrhea, renal stones
- **Hematologic:** Leukopenia
- **Respiratory:** *URI,* pharyngitis, sinusitis
- **Other:** *Fatigue,* rash, acute myopia and secondary angle-closure glaucoma (pain, visual disturbances, pupil dilation, redness, increased IOP), weight loss

Interactions

✳ **Drug-drug** ● Increased CNS depression if taken with alcohol or CNS depressants; use extreme caution ● Increased risk of renal stone development with carbonic anhydrase inhibitors ● Decreased effects of hormonal contraceptives with topiramate; suggest use of barrier contraceptives instead ● Decreased serum levels if combined with phenytoin, carbamazepine, valproic acid

T

■ Nursing considerations

CLINICAL ALERT!

Name confusion has occurred between *Topamax* and *Toprol-XL* (metoprolol); use caution.

Assessment

- **History:** Hypersensitivity to any component of the drug; pregnancy, lactation; renal or hepatic impairment, renal stones
- **Physical:** Skin color, lesions; orientation, affect, reflexes, vision examination; R, adventitious sounds; LFTs, renal function tests

Interventions

⊗ *Warning* Reduce dosage; discontinue or substitute other antiepileptic gradually; abrupt discontinuation may precipitate status epilepticus.

⊗ **Black box warning** There is an increased risk of suicidality with drug administration; monitor patient accordingly.

⊗ *Warning* Stop the drug immediately and arrange for appropriate consultations at first sign of blurred vision, periorbital edema, or redness.

- Administer with food if GI upset occurs.
- Caution patient not to chew or break tablets because of bitter taste.
- Have patient swallow sprinkle capsules whole or by carefully opening capsule and sprinkling onto a soft food. Swallow this immediately; do not allow it to be chewed.
- Encourage patients with a history of renal stone development to maintain adequate fluid intake while using this drug.
- Suggest using barrier contraceptives to patients taking this drug. There is an increased risk of cleft palate in infants born to mothers taking this drug.
- Arrange for consultation with appropriate epilepsy support groups as needed.

Teaching points

- Take this drug exactly as prescribed. Do not break or chew tablets; they have a very bitter taste. Sprinkle capsule may also be swallowed whole. If using sprinkle capsules, open carefully and sprinkle onto soft food and swallow immediately; do not chew.
- Do not discontinue this drug abruptly or change dosage except on the advice of your health care provider.

- Arrange for frequent check-ups to monitor your response to this drug. It is very important that you keep all appointments for check-ups.
- Wear or carry medical identification at all times so that any emergency medical personnel will know that you have epilepsy and are taking antiepileptic medication.
- Avoid using alcohol while you are taking this drug; serious sedation could occur.
- Use of barrier contraceptives is advised; babies born to mothers taking this drug have an increased risk of cleft palate.
- You may experience these side effects: Drowsiness, dizziness, sleepiness (avoid driving or performing other tasks that require alertness; symptoms may occur initially but usually disappear with continued therapy); vision changes (avoid performing tasks that require visual acuity); GI upset (take drug with food; eat frequent small meals).
- Report fatigue, vision changes, speech problems, personality changes, thoughts of suicide.

▽ topotecan hydrochloride

See Appendix R, *Less commonly used drugs.*

DANGEROUS DRUG

▽ toremifene citrate

(tore em' ah feen)

Fareston

PREGNANCY CATEGORY D

Drug classes

Antineoplastic
Estrogen receptor modulator

Therapeutic actions

Binds to estrogen receptors, has antiestrogen effects, and inhibits growth of estrogen receptor–positive breast cancer cell lines.

Indications

- Treatment of advanced breast cancer in postmenopausal women with estrogen receptor positive disease or estrogen receptor unknown tumors

---

Adverse effects in *italics* are most common; those in **bold** are life-threatening. ⊜ Do not crush.

Contraindications and cautions

- Contraindicated with allergy to toremifene, history of thromboembolic disorder, pregnancy, lactation, prolonged QT interval, hypokalemia, hypomagnesemia.
- Use cautiously with history of hypercalcemia, hepatic impairment, preexisting endometrial hyperplasia.

Available forms

Tablets—60 mg

Dosages

Adults

60 mg PO daily; continue until disease progression occurs.

Pharmacokinetics

Route	Onset	Peak
Oral	Rapid	3 hr

Metabolism: Hepatic; $T_{1/2}$: 5–6 days
Distribution: Crosses placenta; enters breast milk
Excretion: Feces, urine

Adverse effects

- **CNS:** Depression, light-headedness, *dizziness,* headache, hallucinations, vertigo
- **CV:** Prolonged QT interval
- **Dermatologic:** *Hot flashes, skin rash*
- **GI:** *Nausea, vomiting,* food distaste
- **GU:** Vaginal bleeding, vaginal discharge
- **Other:** Peripheral edema, hypercalcemia, cataracts, sweating, thrombophlebitis, pulmonary embolism

Interactions

✳ Drug-drug ● Increased risk of bleeding if taken with oral anticoagulants; monitor the patient's INR ● Increased risk of hypercalcemia if taken with remifene or drugs that decrease renal calcium excretion; monitor patient accordingly ● Increased risk of serious cardiac arrhythmias if taken with other drugs that prolong QT interval; avoid this combination

■ Nursing considerations

Assessment

- **History:** Allergy to toremifene, pregnancy, lactation, hypercalcemia, hepatic impairment, thromboembolism history, and preexisting endometrial hyperplasia

- **Physical:** Skin lesions, color, turgor; pelvic examination; orientation, affect, reflexes; BP, peripheral pulses, edema; LFTs, serum electrolytes

Interventions

⊗ **Black box warning** There is risk of prolongation of the QT interval; obtain baseline and periodic ECG and avoid concurrent use of other drugs that prolong the QT interval.
- Administer daily without regard to food.
- Counsel patient about the need to use contraceptive measures while taking this drug; inform patient that serious fetal harm could occur.
- Provide comfort measures to help patient deal with drug effects: Hot flashes (control temperature of environment); headache, depression (monitor exposure to light and noise); vaginal bleeding (use hygiene measures).

Teaching points

- Take this drug as prescribed.
- This drug can cause serious fetal harm and must not be taken during pregnancy. Barrier contraceptives should be used while you are taking this drug. If you become pregnant or decide that you want to become pregnant, consult your health care provider immediately.
- A baseline ECG will be needed before starting this drug. Other drugs may cause serious problems if combined with this drug. Tell all health care providers you see that you are taking this drug.
- You may experience these side effects: Hot flashes (stay in cool places); nausea, vomiting (eat frequent small meals); weight gain; dizziness, headache, light-headedness (use caution if driving or performing tasks that require alertness).
- Report marked weakness, sleepiness, mental confusion, changes in color of urine or stool, rash, vision changes.

▽**torsemide**
(tor' seb myde)

Demadex

PREGNANCY CATEGORY B

Drug classes

Loop (high-ceiling) diuretic
Sulfonamide

Therapeutic actions

Inhibits the reabsorption of sodium and chloride from the proximal and distal renal tubules and the loop of Henle, leading to a natriuretic diuresis.

Indications

- Treatment of hypertension and edema associated with HF, hepatic cirrhosis, renal failure

Contraindications and cautions

- Contraindicated with allergy to torsemide; known hypersensitivity to sulfonylureas; anuria, severe renal failure; hepatic coma.
- Use cautiously with SLE, electrolyte depletion, gout, diabetes mellitus, lactation, pregnancy.

Available forms

Tablets—5, 10, 20, 100 mg; injection 10 mg/mL

Dosages

Adults

⊗ **Warning** Do not exceed 200 mg/day.

- *HF:* 10–20 mg PO or IV daily. Dose may be titrated upward by doubling the dose until desired results are seen. Do not exceed 200 mg/day.
- *Chronic renal failure:* 20 mg PO or IV daily. Dose may be titrated upward by doubling the dose until desired results are seen. Do not exceed 200 mg/day.
- *Hepatic failure:* 5–10 mg PO or IV daily. Do not exceed 40 mg/day.
- *Hypertension:* 5 mg PO daily. May be increased to 10 mg if response is not sufficient.

Pediatric patients

Safety and efficacy not established.

Pharmacokinetics

Route	Onset	Peak	Duration
Oral	60 min	60–120 min	6–8 hr
IV	10 min	60 min	6–8 hr

Metabolism: Hepatic; $T_{1/2}$: 3.5 hr
Distribution: Crosses placenta; may enter breast milk
Excretion: Urine

▼ IV FACTS

Preparation: May be given direct IV over 2 min or diluted in solution with D_5W, 0.9% sodium chloride, 0.45% sodium chloride. Discard unused solution after 24 hr.

Infusion: Give by direct injection slowly, over 1–2 min. Further diluted in solution, give slowly, each 200 mg over 2 min.

Adverse effects

- **CNS:** *Asterixis, dizziness,* vertigo, paresthesias, confusion, fatigue, nystagmus, *weakness, headache, drowsiness,* fatigue, blurred vision, tinnitus, irreversible hearing loss
- **CV:** *Orthostatic hypotension,* volume depletion, cardiac arrhythmias, thrombophlebitis
- **GI:** *Nausea, anorexia, vomiting, diarrhea,* gastric irritation and pain, dry mouth, acute pancreatitis, jaundice, polydipsia
- **GU:** *Polyuria, nocturia,* glycosuria, renal failure
- **Hematologic:** *Hypokalemia,* leukopenia, anemia, thrombocytopenia, hyperuricemia, hypoglycemia
- **Local:** *Pain, phlebitis at injection site*
- **Other:** Muscle cramps and muscle spasms, weakness, arthritic pain, fatigue, hives, photosensitivity, rash, pruritus, sweating, nipple tenderness, impotence

Interactions

✳ **Drug-drug** • Decreased diuresis and natriuresis with NSAIDs • Increased risk of cardiac glycoside toxicity (secondary to hypokalemia) • Increased risk of ototoxicity with aminoglycoside antibiotics, cisplatin, ethacrynic acid

■ Nursing considerations

Assessment

- **History:** Allergy to torsemide, sulfonylurea; electrolyte depletion; anuria; severe renal failure; hepatic coma; SLE; gout; diabetes mellitus; lactation, pregnancy
- **Physical:** Skin color, lesions; edema; orientation, reflexes, hearing; pulses, baseline ECG, BP, orthostatic BP, perfusion; R, pattern, adventitious sounds; liver evaluation, bowel sounds; urinary output patterns; CBC, serum electrolytes, blood sugar, LFTs, renal function tests, uric acid, urinalysis

Interventions

- Administer with food or milk to prevent GI upset.
- Mark calendars or other reminders of drug days if intermittent therapy is optimal for treating edema.

- Administer single daily doses early in the day so increased urination will not disturb sleep.
- Avoid IV use if oral use is at all possible.
- Measure and record regular weights to monitor fluid changes.
- Monitor serum electrolytes, hydration, and liver function during long-term therapy.
- Provide diet rich in potassium or give supplemental potassium.

Teaching points

- Record alternate-day or intermittent therapy on a calendar or dated envelopes.
- Take the drug early in the day so increased urination will not disturb sleep.
- Take the drug with food or meals to prevent GI upset.
- Weigh yourself on a regular basis, at the same time and in the same clothing, and record the weight on your calendar.
- You may experience these side effects: Increased volume and frequency of urination; dizziness, feeling faint on arising, drowsiness (avoid rapid position changes, driving a car and other hazardous activities, and alcohol consumption); sensitivity to sunlight (use sunglasses and sunscreen; wear protective clothing when outdoors); increased thirst (suck sugarless candies; practice frequent mouth care); loss of body potassium (a potassium-rich diet, or even a potassium supplement, will be needed).
- Report weight change of more than 3 pounds in 1 day; swelling in ankles or fingers; unusual bleeding or bruising; nausea, dizziness, trembling, numbness, fatigue; muscle weakness or cramps.

▽**tositumomab and
iodine I-131
tositumomab**

See Appendix R, *Less commonly used drugs.*

DANGEROUS DRUG

▽**tramadol
hydrochloride**
(tram' ah doll)

ConZip, Rybix ODT, Ryzolt ☐☐, Ultram,
Ultram ER ☐☐

PREGNANCY CATEGORY C

Drug classes

Analgesic (centrally acting)
Opioid analgesic

Therapeutic actions

Binds to mu-opioid receptors and inhibits the re-uptake of norepinephrine and serotonin; causes many effects similar to the opioids—dizziness, somnolence, nausea, constipation—but does not have the respiratory depressant effects.

Indications

- Relief of moderate to moderately severe pain
- Relief of moderate to severe chronic pain in adults who need around-the-clock treatment for extended periods (ER tablets)
- Unlabeled uses: Premature ejaculation; restless legs syndrome

Contraindications and cautions

- Contraindicated with allergy to tramadol or opioids or acute intoxication with alcohol, opioids, or psychoactive drugs.
- Use cautiously with pregnancy, lactation; seizures; concomitant use of CNS depressants, MAOIs, SSRIs, TCAs; renal impairment; history of seizures; hepatic impairment.

Available forms

Tablets—50 mg; ER tablets ☐☐—100, 200, 300 mg; ER capsules—100, 200, 300 mg; orally disintegrating tablets—50 mg

Dosages

Adults

Patients who require rapid analgesic effect: 50–100 mg PO every 4–6 hr; do not exceed 400 mg/day.

Patients with moderate to moderately severe chronic pain: Initiate at 25 mg/day PO in the morning, and titrate in 25-mg increments every 3 days to reach 100 mg/day PO. Then, increase in 50-mg increments every 3 days to reach 200 mg/day. After titration, 50–100 mg PO every 4–6 hr; do not exceed 400 mg/day. Alternatively, 100-mg ER tablet or capsule once daily PO, titrated by 100-mg increments every 2–3 days (*Ryzolx*) or every 5 days (*Ultram* ER, *ConZip*); do not exceed 300 mg/day. For orally disintegrating tablets, do not exceed 200 mg/day.

Pediatric patients

Safety and efficacy not established.

Geriatric patients or patients with hepatic or renal impairment

Older than 75 yr: Do not exceed 300 mg/day PO.
Patients with cirrhosis: 50 mg PO every 12 hr. ER tablets should not be used in severe hepatic impairment (Child-Pugh class C).
Patients with creatinine clearance less than 30 mL/min: 50–100 mg PO every 12 hr. Maximum 200 mg/day. ER tablets should not be used in patients with creatinine clearance less than 30 mL/min.

Pharmacokinetics

Route	Onset	Peak
Oral	1 hr	2 hr
Oral (ER)	Delayed	12 hr

Metabolism: Hepatic; $T_{1/2}$: 6–7 hr
Distribution: Crosses placenta; enters breast milk
Excretion: Urine

Adverse effects

- **CNS:** *Sedation, dizziness or vertigo, headache,* confusion, dreaming, sweating, anxiety, **seizures**
- **CV:** *Hypotension,* tachycardia, bradycardia, vasodilation, syncope, orthostatic hypotension
- **Dermatologic:** *Sweating,* pruritus, rash, pallor, urticaria
- **GI:** *Nausea, vomiting,* dry mouth, constipation, flatulence
- **Other:** Potential for abuse, **anaphylactoid reactions**

Interactions

✳ **Drug-drug** • Decreased effectiveness with carbamazepine • Increased risk of tramadol toxicity with MAOIs or SSRIs • Increased risk of respiratory depression if combined with other CNS depressants, alcohol

■ Nursing considerations
Assessment

- **History:** Hypersensitivity to tramadol; pregnancy; acute intoxication with alcohol, opioids, psychotropic drugs or other centrally acting analgesics; lactation; seizures; concomitant use of CNS depressants or MAOIs; renal or hepatic impairment; past or present history of opioid addiction
- **Physical:** Skin color, texture, lesions; orientation, reflexes, bilateral grip strength, affect;

P, auscultation, BP; bowel sounds, normal output; LFTs, renal function tests

Interventions

- Control environment (temperature, lighting) if sweating or CNS effects occur.
- Ensure that patient does not cut, crush, or chew ER tablets.
- Be aware there is an increased risk of seizures in patients with a history of seizures or who are taking other drugs that lower the seizure threshold.

⊗ **Warning** Patient may be at increased risk for suicidality. Risk increases with concurrent use of antidepressants or anxiolytics; monitor patient accordingly.

⊗ **Warning** Limit use in patients with past or present history of addiction to or dependence on opioids.

Teaching points

- Do not cut, crush, or chew ER tablets; swallow them whole. Dissolve orally disintegrating tablets in your mouth and swallow without water.
- You may experience these side effects: Dizziness, sedation, drowsiness, impaired visual acuity (avoid driving or performing tasks that require alertness); nausea, loss of appetite (lie quietly, eat frequent small meals).
- Report severe nausea, dizziness, severe constipation, thoughts of suicide.

▽ **trandolapril**
(tran dole' ah pril)

Mavik

PREGNANCY CATEGORY C
(FIRST TRIMESTER)

PREGNANCY CATEGORY D
(SECOND AND THIRD TRIMESTERS)

Drug classes
ACE inhibitor
Antihypertensive

Therapeutic actions

Blocks ACE from converting angiotensin I to angiotensin II, a powerful vasoconstrictor, leading to decreased BP, decreased aldosterone secretion, a small increase in serum potassium levels, and sodium and fluid loss; increased prostaglandin synthesis may also be involved in the antihypertensive action.

Indications
- Treatment of hypertension, alone or in combination with other antihypertensives
- Treatment of post-MI patients with evidence of left-ventricular dysfunction and symptoms of HF
- Unlabeled use: Diabetic nephropathy

Contraindications and cautions
- Contraindicated with allergy to ACE inhibitors, history of ACE-associated angioedema.
- Use cautiously with impaired renal function, HF, CAD, sodium or volume depletion, surgery, pregnancy, lactation, renal artery stenosis.

Available forms
Tablets—1, 2, 4 mg

Dosages
Adults
- *Hypertension:* African-American patients: 2 mg PO daily. All other patients: 1 mg PO daily. For maintenance, 2–4 mg/day. Maximum, 8 mg.
- *Patients on diuretics:* To prevent hypotension, stop diuretic 2–3 days before beginning trandolapril. Resume diuretic only if BP is not controlled. If diuretic cannot be discontinued, start at 0.5 mg PO daily and adjust upward as needed.
- *HF post-MI:* May start therapy 3 to 5 days after the MI. 1 mg/day PO; adjust to a target of 4 mg/day.

Pediatric patients
Safety and efficacy not established.

Patients with renal or hepatic impairment
0.5 mg PO daily, adjust at 1-wk intervals to control BP; usual range is 2–4 mg PO daily.

Pharmacokinetics

Route	Peak	Duration
Oral	3–4 hr	24 hr

Metabolism: $T_{1/2}$: 14–16 hr
Distribution: Crosses placenta; enters breast milk
Excretion: Feces, urine

Adverse effects
- **CNS:** Headache, fatigue
- **CV:** *Tachycardia,* angina pectoris, **MI,** HF, Raynaud syndrome, hypotension in sodium- or volume-depleted patients
- **Dermatologic:** *Rash*
- **GI:** *Diarrhea,* GI upset
- **GU:** Renal insufficiency, renal failure, polyuria, oliguria, urinary frequency, UTI
- **Other:** *Cough, dizziness,* malaise, dry mouth

Interactions
✳ Drug-drug • Excessive hypotension may occur with diuretics; monitor closely • Hyperkalemia may occur with potassium supplements, potassium-sparing diuretics, salt substitutes; monitor serum potassium levels
• Potential increase in lithium levels if taken concurrently; decreased lithium dose may be needed

■ Nursing considerations
Assessment
- **History:** Allergy to ACE inhibitors, impaired renal or hepatic function, CAD, HF, salt or volume depletion, surgery, pregnancy, lactation
- **Physical:** Skin color, lesions, turgor; T; P, BP, peripheral perfusion; mucous membranes, bowel sounds, liver evaluation; urinalysis, LFTs, renal function tests, CBC and differential

Interventions
⊗ Black box warning Ensure that patient is not pregnant before administering; advise patient to use barrier contraceptives. Fetal injury or death has occurred when this drug was used in the second or third trimester.
• Administer once a day at same time each day.
⊗ **Warning** Alert surgeon and mark the patient's chart with notice that trandolapril is being taken; angiotensin II formation subsequent to compensatory renin release during surgery will need to be blocked; hypotension may be reversed with volume expansion.
• Monitor patient closely in any situation that may lead to fall in BP secondary to reduction in fluid volume—excessive perspiration and dehydration, vomiting, diarrhea—as excessive hypotension may occur.
• Reduce dosage in patients with impaired renal or hepatic function.

T

⊗ **Warning** Discontinue immediately if laryngeal edema, angioedema, or jaundice occurs.

Teaching points

- Take drug once a day at generally the same time each day. Do not stop taking this medication without consulting your health care provider.
- This drug cannot be used during pregnancy; using barrier contraceptives is recommended.
- Be careful in situations that may lead to drop in blood pressure (diarrhea, sweating, vomiting, dehydration); if light-headedness or dizziness occurs, consult your health care provider.
- While taking this drug, avoid using over-the-counter medications, especially cough, cold, or allergy medications; they may contain ingredients that will interact with this drug. If you feel that you need one of these preparations, consult your health care provider.
- You may experience these side effects: GI upset, diarrhea (limited effects that will pass); dizziness, light-headedness (usually passes after first few days; change position slowly and limit your activities to those that do not require alertness and precision); cough (can be very irritating and does not respond to cough suppressants; notify health care provider if very uncomfortable).
- Report sore throat, fever, chills; swelling of the hands or feet; irregular heartbeat, chest pains; swelling of the face, eyes, lips, tongue; difficulty breathing; yellowing of skin.

▽**tranexamic acid**

See Appendix R, *Less commonly used drugs.*

▽**tranylcypromine sulfate**

*(tran ill **sip'** roe meen)*

Parnate

PREGNANCY CATEGORY C

Drug classes

Antidepressant
MAOI

Therapeutic actions

Irreversibly inhibits MAO, an enzyme that breaks down biogenic amines, such as epinephrine, norepinephrine, and serotonin, allowing these biogenic amines to accumulate in neuronal storage sites; according to the biogenic amine hypothesis, this accumulation of amines is responsible for the clinical efficacy of MAOIs as antidepressants.

Indications

- Treatment of adult outpatients with a major depressive episode without melancholia who have failed to respond to more commonly used antidepressants; efficacy in endogenous depression has not been established
- Unlabeled uses: Migraine headache, panic disorder, social anxiety disorder, bipolar depression, Alzheimer disease, Parkinson disease

Contraindications and cautions

- Contraindicated with hypersensitivity to any MAOI; pheochromocytoma, HF; history of liver disease or abnormal LFTs; severe renal impairment; confirmed or suspected cerebrovascular defect; CV disease, hypertension; history of headache (headache is an indicator of hypertensive reaction to drug); myelography within previous 24 hr or scheduled within 48 hr; lactation; patients scheduled for elective surgery (MAOIs should be discontinued 10 days before surgery).
- Use cautiously with seizure disorders; hyperthyroidism; impaired hepatic, renal function; psychiatric patients (agitated or schizophrenic patients may show excessive stimulation; bipolar patients may shift to hypomanic or manic phase); pregnancy or in women of childbearing age.

Available forms

Tablets—10 mg

Dosages

Adults

Usual effective dose is 30 mg/day PO in divided doses. If no improvement is seen within 2–3 wk, increase dosage in 10 mg/day increments every 1–3 wk. May be increased to a maximum of 60 mg/day.

Pediatric patients

Not recommended for patients younger than 16 yr.

Adverse effects in *italics* are most common; those in **bold** are life-threatening. ⬛ Do not crush.

Geriatric patients

Patients older than 60 yr are more prone to develop side effects; use with caution.

Pharmacokinetics

Route	Onset	Duration
Oral	Rapid	3–5 days

Metabolism: Hepatic; $T_{1/2}$: Unknown
Distribution: Crosses placenta; enters breast milk
Excretion: Urine

Adverse effects

- **CNS:** *Dizziness, vertigo, headache, overactivity, hyper-reflexia, tremors, muscle twitching, mania, hypomania, jitteriness, confusion, memory impairment, insomnia, weakness, fatigue, drowsiness, restlessness, overstimulation, increased anxiety, agitation, blurred vision, sweating,* akathisia, ataxia, coma, euphoria, neuritis, repetitious babbling, chills, glaucoma, nystagmus
- **CV: Hypertensive crises, sometimes fatal,** sometimes with intracranial bleeding, usually attributable to tyramine ingestion (see Drug–food interactions); symptoms include occipital headache, which may radiate frontally; palpitations; neck stiffness or soreness; nausea; vomiting; sweating (sometimes with fever, cold and clammy skin); dilated pupils; photophobia; tachycardia or bradycardia; chest pain; *orthostatic hypotension, sometimes associated with falling; disturbed cardiac rate and rhythm,* palpitations, tachycardia
- **Dermatologic:** Minor skin reactions, spider telangiectases, photosensitivity
- **GI:** *Constipation, diarrhea, nausea, abdominal pain, edema, dry mouth, anorexia, weight changes*
- **GU:** Dysuria, incontinence, urinary retention, sexual disturbances
- **Other:** Hematologic changes, black tongue, hypernatremia

Interactions

✳ **Drug-drug** ⊗ **Warning** Potentially dangerous hypotension with general anesthetics; avoid this combination.

- Increased sympathomimetic effects (hypertensive crisis) with sympathomimetic drugs (norepinephrine, epinephrine, dopamine, dobutamine, levodopa, ephedrine), amphetamines, other anorexiants, local anesthetic solutions containing sympathomimetics • Hypertensive crisis, coma, severe seizures with TCAs (eg, imipramine, desipramine) • Additive hypoglycemic effect with insulin, oral sulfonylureas (eg, tolbutamide) • Increased risk of adverse interactive actions with meperidine
- Reduce dose of barbiturates if given with MAOIs • Toxic levels of buspirone and bupropion if combined with MAOIs; separate use by 10 or 14 days, respectively • Increased hypertension effects with carbamazepine, levodopa
- Risk of hypotension with thiazide diuretics
- Serious, sometimes fatal, reactions with SSRIs; separate use by 5 wk with fluoxetine, 2 wk with sertraline and paroxetine

✳ **Drug-food** ⊗ **Warning** Tyramine (and other pressor amines) contained in foods are normally broken down by MAO enzymes in the GI tract; in the presence of MAOIs, these vasopressors may be absorbed in high concentrations; in addition, tyramine releases accumulated norepinephrine from nerve terminals; thus, hypertensive crisis may occur when the following foods that contain tyramine or other vasopressors are ingested by a patient on an MAOI: Dairy products (blue, Camembert, cheddar, mozzarella, Parmesan, Romano, Roquefort, Stilton cheeses; sour cream; yogurt); meats, fish (liver, pickled herring, fermented sausages [bologna, pepperoni, salami], caviar, dried fish, other fermented or spoiled meat or fish); undistilled beverages (imported beer, ale; red wine, especially Chianti; sherry; coffee, tea, colas containing caffeine; chocolate drinks); fruits, vegetables (avocado, fava beans, figs, raisins, bananas, yeast extracts, soy sauce, chocolate).

■ Nursing considerations

Assessment

- **History:** Hypersensitivity to any MAOI; pheochromocytoma; HF; abnormal LFTs; severe renal impairment; confirmed or suspected cerebrovascular defect; CV disease, hypertension; history of headache; myelography within previous 24 hr or scheduled within 48 hr; lactation; seizure disorders; hyperthyroidism; impaired hepatic, renal function; psychiatric disorders; scheduled elective surgery; pregnancy
- **Physical:** Weight; T; skin color, lesions; orientation, affect, reflexes, vision; P, BP, orthostatic BP, perfusion; bowel sounds, normal

T

output, liver evaluation; urine flow, normal output; LFTs, renal function tests, urinalysis, CBC, ECG, EEG

Interventions

⊗ **Black box warning** Limit amount of drug available to suicidal patients; possible increased risk of suicidality in children, adolescents, and young adults; monitor accordingly.

- Monitor BP and orthostatic BP carefully; arrange for more gradual increase in dosage initially in patients who show tendency for hypotension.

⊗ **Warning** Arrange for periodic LFTs during therapy; discontinue drug at first sign of hepatic impairment or jaundice.

- Monitor BP carefully (and if appropriate, discontinue drug) if patient reports unusual or severe headache.

⊗ **Warning** Keep phentolamine or another alpha-adrenergic blocking drug readily available in case of hypertensive crisis.

Teaching points

- Take drug exactly as prescribed. You should begin to improve within 2 days to 3 weeks after starting therapy.
- Do not stop taking drug abruptly or without consulting your health care provider.
- Avoid ingesting tyramine-containing foods or beverages while using this drug and for 10 days afterward (patient and significant other should receive a list of such foods and beverages; see Appendix B, *Important dietary guidelines for patient teaching*).
- You may experience these side effects: Dizziness, weakness or fainting when arising from a horizontal or sitting position (transient; change position slowly); drowsiness, blurred vision (reversible; safety measures may need to be taken if severe; avoid driving or performing tasks that require alertness); nausea, vomiting, loss of appetite (frequent small meals, frequent mouth care may help); nightmares, confusion, inability to concentrate, emotional changes; changes in sexual function.
- Report headache, rash, darkening of the urine, pale stools, yellowing of the eyes or skin, fever, chills, sore throat, or any other unusual symptoms, thoughts of suicide.

DANGEROUS DRUG

▽ **trastuzumab**

*(trass too **zoo'** mab)*

Herceptin

PREGNANCY CATEGORY D

Drug classes

Antineoplastic
Monoclonal antibody (anti-HER2)

Therapeutic actions

Humanized monoclonal antibody to the human epidermal growth factor receptor 2 (HER2) protein. This protein is often overexpressed in patients with aggressive, metastatic breast cancer.

Indications

- Treatment of metastatic breast cancer with tumors that overexpress HER2 protein as a first-line therapy in combination with paclitaxel and as a single agent in second- and third-line therapies
- Adjunct treatment of patients with HER2-overexpressing breast cancer in combination with doxorubicin, cyclophosphamide, and either docetaxol or paclitaxel; in combination with docetaxol and carboplatin; as a single agent following multimodality anthracycline-based therapy
- Part of combination therapy for treatment of metastatic gastric cancer when it is HER2 positive

Contraindications and cautions

- Contraindicated with allergy to trastuzumab or any component of the drug, breast cancers without HER2 overexpression.
- Use cautiously with known cardiac disease, bone marrow depression, lactation, pregnancy.

Available forms

Powder for injection—440 mg

Dosages
Adults

- *Metastatic HER2 overexpressing breast cancer:* Initially, 4 mg/kg IV once by IV infusion over 90 min. For maintenance, 2 mg/kg IV once weekly over at least 30 min as tolerated. Do not exceed 500 mg/dose.
- *Adjuvant treatment:* After completion of doxorubicin and cyclophosphamide therapy, give

---

Adverse effects in *italics* are most common; those in **bold** are life-threatening. ⬚⬚⬚ Do not crush.

trastuzumab weekly for 52 wk. Initial dose, 4 mg/kg over 90 min by IV infusion; maintenance dose, 2 mg/kg over 30 min by IV infusion weekly. Or, initial dose, 8 mg/kg over 90 min by IV infusion; then 6 mg/kg over 30–90 min by IV infusion every 3 wk. During the first 12 wk, give trastuzumab with paclitaxel.

• *Metastatic gastric cancer:* 8 mg/kg IV over 90 min; then 6 mg/kg IV over 30 min every 3 wk until disease progression.

Pharmacokinetics

Route	Onset	Duration
IV	Slow	Days

Metabolism: Tissue; $T_{1/2}$: 2–9 days
Distribution: Crosses placenta, may enter breast milk

▼ IV FACTS

Preparation: Reconstitute powder with diluent provided; dilute further in 250 mL 0.9% sodium chloride injection. Note that diluent contains benzyl alcohol. For patients sensitive to this preservative, may reconstituted drug with 20 mL sterile water for injection. Do not shake; foaming may prevent dissolution. Handle gently and allow to stand for 5 min after reconstitution. Solution should be colorless to pale yellow. Solution is stable for 28 days after reconstitution with diluent provided. Must write expiration date on vial (28 days after reconstitution).
Infusion: Infuse initial dose over 90 min; maintenance doses may be infused over 30–90 min.
Incompatibilities: Do not mix with any other drug solution or add any other drugs to the IV line.

Adverse effects

• **CNS:** Malaise, headache, tremor, insomnia, paresthesia
• **CV: Serious cardiac toxicity**
• **GI:** Vomiting, nausea, *diarrhea, abdominal pain*
• **Other:** *Anemia,* pain, edema, *increased susceptibility to infection, leukopenia, local reaction at infusion site, infusion reaction* (flushing, sweating, chills, fever), *fever, chills,* hypersensitivity reactions, myalgia, rash, pulmonary toxicity

■ Nursing considerations
Assessment

• **History:** Allergy to trastuzumab or any component of the product; known cardiac disease, bone marrow depression; pregnancy, lactation
• **Physical:** T; P, BP; R, adventitious sounds; baseline ECG; orientation, affect, CBC with differential, tumor testing for HER2 status

Interventions

⊗ *Black box warning* Monitor patient at time of infusion and provide comfort measures and analgesics as appropriate if infusion reaction occurs.

⊗ *Black box warning* Monitor cardiac status, especially if patient is receiving chemotherapy; do not give with anthracycline chemotherapy. Keep emergency equipment readily available if cardiac toxicity occurs; cardiomyopathy may occur.

⊗ *Black box warning* Monitor patient for possibly severe pulmonary toxicity, especially within 24 hours of infusion. Discontinue at signs or symptoms of respiratory involvement.

• Protect patient from exposure to infections and maintain sterile technique for invasive procedures.

Teaching points

• This drug is given IV to help fight your breast cancer or gastric cancer. It will be given once a week for breast cancer or once every 3 wk for gastric cancer. Mark a calendar with return dates for repeat infusion.
• Avoid infection while you are using this drug; stay away from crowded areas and people with known infections.
• You may experience these side effects: Discomfort, sweating, fever during infusion (comfort measures and analgesics may help); diarrhea, nausea, abdominal pain.
• Report chest pain, difficulty breathing, chills, fever, swelling.

▽ trazodone hydrochloride

See Appendix R, *Less commonly used drugs.*

T

▷treprostinil sodium
*(tra **pros'** tin ill)*

Remodulin, Tyvaso

PREGNANCY CATEGORY B

Drug classes
Endothelin receptor antagonist
Prostacyclin analogue (vasodilating drug)

Therapeutic actions
Specifically blocks receptor sites for endothelin (ET_A and ET_B) in the endothelium and vascular smooth muscles; these endothelins are elevated in plasma and lung tissue of patients with pulmonary arterial hypertension; also inhibits platelet aggregation.

Indications
• Treatment of pulmonary arterial hypertension in patients with NYNA class II–class IV symptoms, to improve exercise ability and to decrease the rate of clinical worsening
• To diminish the rate of deterioration in patients undergoing transition from epoprostenol (*Flolan*)

Contraindications and cautions
• Contraindicated with allergy to treprostinil or any component of the drug.
• Use cautiously in elderly patients and with hepatic or renal impairment, lactation, pregnancy.

Available forms
Multi-use vials—1, 2.5, 5, 10 mg/mL; solution for inhalation—0.6 mg/mL

Dosages
Adults
Administered by continuous subcutaneous or IV infusion. Subcutaneous route is preferred. Use IV route only in situations in which subcutaneous route is not tolerated because of severe site reactions or pain. Initially the rate is 1.25 nanograms/kg/min. If this initial dose cannot be tolerated, the infusion rate should be reduced to 0.625 nanograms/kg/min. Rate is increased in increments of no more than 1.25 nano-grams/kg/min/wk for the first 4 wk, then by 2.5 nanograms/kg/min/wk. Do not exceed 40 nanograms/kg/min. Dosage is based on clinical response and patient tolerance.

Abrupt withdrawal or significant decrease in dosage may result in worsening symptoms. See the manufacturer's instructions for infusion weight charts.
• *Transition from Flolan:* Base rate of change on individual patient response. Start *Remodulin* infusion at 10% of starting *Flolan* dose. Decrease *Flolan* to 80% starting dose and increase *Remodulin* dose to 30% starting *Flolan* dose. Decrease *Flolan* dose to 60% starting and increase *Remodulin* dose to 50% starting *Flolan* dose. Decrease *Flolan* dose to 40% starting dose and increase *Remodulin* dose to 70% starting *Flolan* dose. Decrease *Flolan* dose to 20% starting dose and increase *Remodulin* dose to 90% starting *Flolan* dose. Decrease *Flolan* dose to 5% starting dose and increase *Remodulin* dose to 110% starting *Flolan* dose. Discontinue *Flolan* and continue *Remodulin* dose at 110% of *Flolan* starting dose plus an additional 5%–10% as needed.
• *Inhalation:* Initially, 3 breaths (18 mcg), using *Tyvaso* Inhalation System, per treatment session; 4 sessions per day, approximately 4 hr apart during waking hours. Increase by additional 3 breaths per session at 1- to 2-wk intervals if needed and tolerated. Maintenance dose, 9 breaths (54 mcg) per session.

Pediatric patients
Safety and efficacy not established.
Patients with hepatic impairment
Decrease initial dose to 0.625 nanograms/kg/min and increase slowly.

Pharmacokinetics

Route	Onset	Peak
Subcut.	Gradual	10 hr

Metabolism: Hepatic; $T_{1/2}$: 2–4 hr
Distribution: Crosses placenta; may enter breast milk
Excretion: Feces, urine

Adverse effects
• **CNS:** *Headache,* dizziness
• **CV:** Edema, hypotension, dyspnea, chest pain
• **GI:** *Nausea, diarrhea,* vomiting
• **Skin:** Pruritus, *rash*
• **Other:** *Pain at injection site, local reaction at infusion site,* increased bleeding, *jaw pain*

Interactions

✳ **Drug-drug** • Potential for increased hypotensive effects if combined with other drugs that decrease BP; monitor patient carefully • Potential for increased bleeding tendencies if combined with drugs that alter blood clotting or inhibit platelets

■ Nursing considerations

Assessment

- **History:** Allergy to treprostinil or any component of the drug, hepatic or renal impairment, pregnancy, lactation, advanced age
- **Physical:** Skin color, lesions; injection site; orientation, BP; LFTs, renal function tests, CBC

Interventions

- Evaluate the patient for the ability to accept, place, and care for a subcutaneous catheter and to use a continuous infusion pump.
- Ensure that patient is re-evaluated weekly for possible adjustments in dosage.
- In rare situations in which IV infusion must be used, use only sterile water for injection or 0.9% sodium chloride to dilute product before administration.
- Inspect solution to make sure no particulate matter is present before use. Use vial within 14 days of opening.
- Monitor injection site for any sign of reaction of infection.
- When giving drug through inhalation route, administer only through the *Tyvaso* Inhalation System. Administer undiluted as supplied.

⊗ *Warning* Monitor patients who are discontinuing treprostinil; tapering of dose may be needed to avoid sudden worsening of disease.

- Provide analgesics as appropriate for patients who develop headache or injection site pain.
- Monitor patient's functional level to note improvement in exercise tolerance.
- Maintain other measures used to treat pulmonary arterial hypertension.

Teaching points

- This drug must be given by a continuous subcutaneous infusion pump. It may be needed for prolonged periods, possibly years. The pump is lightweight and attached to a catheter that goes into your skin. You will need to care

for the insertion site and set and monitor the pump. It is recommended to have a significant other who is also able to care for and maintain the site and the pump as a backup for you.

- If receiving this drug by inhalation, use undiluted only through the *Tyvaso* Inhalation System. Before first inhalation session, transfer contents of a single ampule into the medicine cup supplied by manufacturer. Each ampule contains enough medication fore 1 day of treatment. Between treatments, cap the inhalation device and stone upright. Any remaining solution can be stored up to 24 hours.
- Avoid contact of the solution with eyes or skin.
- This drug should not be taken during pregnancy; using a barrier contraceptive is advised.
- Keep a chart of your exercise tolerance to help monitor improvement in your condition.
- This drug should not be discontinued abruptly. It must be tapered. Notify your health care provider if anything happens to prevent you from getting your continuous infusion or inhalation of the drug.
- Continue your usual procedures for treating your pulmonary arterial hypertension.
- You will need to be followed closely to determine the correct dose of the drug that is best for your situation.
- You may experience these side effects: Headache (analgesics may help); stomach upset (taking with food); pain at the injection site (analgesics may also help, monitor the site for any sign of redness, heat, or swelling).
- Report swelling of the extremities, dizziness, chest pain, fever, changes in the appearance of the catheter insertion site.

DANGEROUS DRUG

▷**tretinoin
(retinoic acid)**
(*tret' i noyn*)

Atralin, Avita, Refissa, Renova, Retin-A, Retin-A Micro, Stieva-A (CAN), Tretin-X

PREGNANCY CATEGORY D

Drug classes

Antineoplastic
Retinoid (topical form)

Therapeutic actions

Induces cell differentiation and decreases proliferation of acute promyelocytic leukemia cells, leading to an initial maturation of the primitive promyelocytes, followed by a repopulation of the bone marrow and peripheral blood by normal hematopoietic cells in patients achieving complete remission; exact mechanism of action is not understood. Acne: decreased cohesiveness and increased turnover of follicular epithelial cells, decreasing comedones.

Indications

- Induction of remission in acute promyelocytic leukemia (APL)
- Topical treatment of acne vulgaris
- Adjunctive agent for use in mitigation of fine wrinkles, mottled hyperpigmentation, and tactile roughness in select patients (topical)
- Unlabeled uses: Hyperpigmentation of photoaged skin, postinflammatory hyperpigmentation, facial actinic keratoses (topical), acute promyelocytic leukemia (oral), emphysema (oral)

Contraindications and cautions

- Contraindicated with allergy to retinoids or parabens, suicidal tendencies, pregnancy, lactation.
- Use cautiously with liver disease, hypercholesterolemia, hypertriglyceridemia.

Available forms

Capsule ⓒⓝⓒ—10 mg; cream—0.02%, 0.025%, 0.05%, 0.1%; gel—0.01%, 0.025%, 0.035%, 0.04%, 0.05%, 0.1%

Dosages

Adults and children 1 yr and older
Oral
45 mg/m²/day PO administered in two or three evenly divided doses until complete remission is documented; discontinue therapy 30 days after complete remission is obtained or after 90 days, whichever comes first.
Adults
Topical
Apply once a day before bedtime. Cover entire affected area lightly, avoiding mucous membranes.
Pediatric patients
Not recommended for use in children younger than 1 yr.

Pharmacokinetics

Route	Onset	Peak
Oral	Slow	1–2 hr

Metabolism: Hepatic; $T_{1/2}$: 0.5–2 hr
Distribution: Crosses placenta; may enter breast milk
Excretion: Feces, urine

Adverse effects

- **CNS:** *Fever, headache,* **pseudotumor cerebri** (papilledema, headache, nausea, vomiting, visual disturbances), *earache, visual disturbances, malaise, sweating,* suicidal ideation
- **CV:** Arrhythmias, flushing, hypotension, heart failure, **MI, cardiac arrest**
- **Dermatologic:** *Skin fragility, dry skin, pruritus, rash,* thinning hair, peeling of palms and soles, skin infections, photosensitivity, nail brittleness, petechiae
- **GI:** *Hemorrhage, nausea, vomiting, abdominal pain,* anorexia, inflammatory bowel disease
- **GU:** Renal insufficiency, dysuria, frequency, enlarged prostate
- **Hematologic: Rapid and evolving leukocytosis,** *decreased liver function, elevated lipids, elevated liver enzymes*
- **Musculoskeletal:** Skeletal hyperostosis, arthralgia, *bone and joint pain* and stiffness
- **Respiratory: Retinoic acid-APL syndrome** (fever, dyspnea, weight gain, pulmonary infiltrates, pleural or pericardial effusion, hypotension may progress to death)

Interactions

✳ **Drug-drug** • Increased risk of high serum levels and toxicity with ketoconazole • Combination therapy with hydroxyurea may lead to massive cell lysis and bone marrow necrosis • Increased risk of skin irritability if topically used with keratolytic agents (sulfur, resorcinol, benzoyl peroxide, salicyclic acid); avoid this combination • Increased risk of pseudotumor cerebri or intracranial hypertension with tetracyclines; monitor patient closely

■ Nursing considerations
Assessment

- **History:** Allergy to retinoids or parabens; pregnancy, lactation; liver disease; hypercholesterolemia, hypertriglyceridemia; suicidal tendencies

- **Physical:** Skin color, lesions, turgor, texture; joints—range of motion; orientation, reflexes, affect, ophthalmologic examination; mucous membranes, bowel sounds; R, adventitious sounds, auscultation; serum triglycerides, HDL, sedimentation rate, CBC and differential, urinalysis, pregnancy test, chest X-ray

Interventions

⊗ *Black box warning* Ensure that patient is not pregnant before administering; arrange for a pregnancy test within 2 wk of beginning therapy. Advise patient to use two forms of contraception during treatment and for 1 mo after treatment is discontinued.

⊗ *Black box warning* There is a risk of rapid leukocytosis with oral use (40% of patients); notify physician immediately if WBC coont is more than 5×10^9/L.

⊗ *Black box warning* This drug should only be used under the supervision of an experienced practitioner or in an institution experienced with its use.

⊗ *Warning* Monitor patient for any suicidal tendencies. The risk of suicide should be explained, the Medication Guide brochure should be given, and the patient must sign the release affirming that he or she understands the potential risk.

- Oral tretinoin is for induction of remission only; arrange for consolidation or maintenance chemotherapy for acute promyelocytic leukemia after induction therapy.
- Arrange for baseline recording of serum lipids and triglyceride levels, LFTs, chest X-ray, CBC with differential and coagulation profile; monitor for changes frequently.

⊗ *Black box warning* Discontinue drug and notify physician if LFTs are greater than five times upper range of normal, pulmonary infiltrates appear, or patient has difficulty breathing; serious side effects can occur.

⊗ *Warning* Discontinue drug if signs of papilledema occur; consult a neurologist for further care.

⊗ *Black box warning* Monitor patient for retinoic acid-APL syndrome (fever, dyspnea, acute respiratory distress, weight gain, pulmonary infiltrates, pleural and pericardial effusion, multiorgan failure). Endotracheal intubation and mechanical ventilation may be required.

⊗ *Warning* Discontinue drug if visual disturbances occur, and arrange for an ophthalmologic examination.

⊗ *Warning* Discontinue drug if abdominal pain, rectal bleeding, or severe diarrhea occurs, and consult physician.

- Monitor triglycerides during therapy; if elevations occur, institute other measures to lower serum triglycerides—reduce weight, dietary fat; exercise; increase intake of insoluble fiber; decrease alcohol consumption.

⊗ *Warning* Keep high-dose steroids readily available in case of severe leukocytosis or liver damage.

- Administer drug with meals; do not crush capsules.
- Do not administer vitamin supplements that contain vitamin A.
- Maintain supportive care appropriate for patients with APL (eg, monitor for and treat infections, prophylaxis for bleeding).
- Topical form should be applied lightly to entire area before bed. Clean area thoroughly before use.

Teaching points

- Take the oral drug with meals; do not crush or cut capsules.
- Frequent blood tests will be needed to evaluate the drug's effects on your body.
- This drug has been associated with severe birth defects and miscarriages; it should not be used by pregnant women. Use contraceptives during treatment and for 1 month after treatment is discontinued. If you think you are pregnant, consult your health care provider immediately.
- You will not be permitted to donate blood while using this drug because of its possible effects on the fetus of a blood recipient.
- Avoid the use of vitamin supplements containing vitamin A; serious toxic effects may occur. Limit alcohol consumption. You may also need to limit your intake of fats and increase exercise to limit the drug's effects on blood triglyceride levels.
- At bedtime, clean affected area well and apply topical form lightly to entire area.
- Apply sunscreen every morning (SPF 15 or greater). Avoid direct sun and sunlamp exposure.
- You may experience these side effects: Dizziness, lethargy, headache, visual changes (avoid driving or performing tasks that

T

require alertness); sensitivity to the sun (avoid sunlamps, exposure to the sun; use sunscreens and protective clothing); diarrhea, abdominal pain, loss of appetite (take drug with meals); dry mouth (suck sugarless candies); eye irritation and redness, inability to wear contact lenses; dry skin, itching, redness.

- Report headache with nausea and vomiting, difficulty breathing, severe diarrhea or rectal bleeding, visual difficulties, suicidal ideas or feelings.

▷ triamcinolone
(trye am sin' oh lone)

triamcinolone acetonide

IM, intra-articular, or soft-tissue injection; intraocular injection; respiratory inhalant; dermatologic ointment, cream, lotion, aerosol: Kenalog, Nasacort AQ, Oracort (CAN), Triderm, Trie sence, Trivaris
Dental paste: Kenalog in Orabase

triamcinolone hexacetonide

Intra-articular, intralesional injection: Aristospan Intra-articular, Aristospan Intralesional

PREGNANCY CATEGORY C

Drug classes
Corticosteroid (intermediate-acting)
Glucocorticoid
Hormone

Therapeutic actions
Enters target cells and binds to cytoplasmic receptors, thereby initiating many complex reactions that are responsible for its anti-inflammatory and immunosuppressive effects.

Indications
- Systemic: Hypercalcemia associated with cancer
- Short-term management of inflammatory and allergic disorders such as rheumatoid arthritis, collagen diseases (eg, SLE), der-

matologic diseases (eg, pemphigus), status asthmaticus, and autoimmune disorders
- Adjunctive therapy for short-term treatment of acute gouty arthritis, bursitis, tenosynovitis, epicondylitis, rheumatoid arthritis, or synovitis of osteoarthritis
- Hematologic disorders: Thrombocytopenia purpura, erythroblastopenia
- Ulcerative colitis, acute exacerbations of MS, and palliation in some leukemias and lymphomas
- Trichinosis with neurologic or myocardial involvement
- Pulmonary emphysema with bronchial spasm or edema; diffuse interstitial pulmonary fibrosis; with diuretics in HF with edema and in cirrhosis with refractory ascites
- Postoperative dental inflammatory reactions
- Intra-articular, soft-tissue administration for conditions such as arthritis, psoriatic plaques
- Respiratory inhalant: Control of bronchial asthma requiring corticosteroids in conjunction with other therapy
- Prophylactic therapy in the maintenance treatment of asthma (bid use)
- Dermatologic preparations: To relieve inflammatory and pruritic manifestations of dermatoses that are steroid responsive
- Nasal spray: Treatment of seasonal and perennial allergic-rhinitis symptoms in patients 2 yr and older
- Dental paste: Treatment of oral lesions

Contraindications and cautions
- Contraindicated with infections, especially TB, fungal infections, amebiasis, vaccinia and varicella, and antibiotic-resistant infections; lactation.
- Use cautiously with pregnancy (teratogenic in preclinical studies), renal or liver disease, hypothyroidism, ulcerative colitis with impending perforation, diverticulitis, active or latent peptic ulcer, inflammatory bowel disease, heart failure, hypertension, thromboembolic disorders, osteoporosis, seizure disorders, diabetes mellitus.

Available forms
Injection—10, 25, 40 mg/mL; intraocular suspension—40 mg/mL; aerosol—100 mcg/actuation; topical ointment—0.025, 0.05, 0.1, 0.5%; cream—0.25, 0.1, 0.5%; lotion—0.025, 0.1%; nasal spray—55 mcg/actuation; dental

Adverse effects in *italics* are most common; those in **bold** are life-threatening. ⬛ Do not crush.

paste—0.1%; aerosal, foam, topical—0.2% spray

Dosages
Adults
Systemic
Individualize dosage, depending on the severity of the condition and the patient's response. Administer daily dose before 9 AM to minimize adrenal suppression. If long-term therapy is needed, consider alternate-day therapy. After long-term therapy, withdraw drug slowly to avoid adrenal insufficiency. For maintenance therapy, reduce initial dose in small increments at intervals until the lowest effective dose is reached.

IM (triamcinolone acetonide)
2.5–100 mg/day.

Respiratory inhalant (triamcinolone acetonide)
200 mcg released with each actuation delivers about 100 mcg to the patient. Two inhalations tid–qid, not to exceed 16 inhalations/day.

Nasal spray
Two sprays (220 mcg total dose) in each nostril daily—maximum of four sprays/day (two sprays in each nostril daily).

Intraocular
Initially, 4 mg (100 microliters of a 40 mg/mL solution) by intraocular injection; adjust dosage as needed over course of treatment. 1–4 mg injected intravitreally for visualization during vitrectomy.

Adults and pediatric patients
Intra-articular, intralesional
Dose will vary with joint or soft-tissue site to be injected.
- *Triamcinolone acetonide:* 2.5–15 mg.
- *Triamcinolone hexacetonide:* 2–20 mg intra-articular; up to 0.5 mg/square inch of affected area intralesional.

Topical dermatologic preparations
Apply sparingly to affected area bid–qid.

Pediatric patients
Systemic
Individualize dosage, depending on the severity of the condition and the patient's response rather than by formulas that correct adult doses for age or body weight. Carefully observe growth and development in infants and children on prolonged therapy.

Respiratory inhalant (triamcinolone acetonide)
200 mcg released with each actuation delivers about 100 mcg to the patient.
6–12 yr: One or two inhalations tid–qid, not to exceed 12 inhalations/day.

Nasal spray
6–12 yr: One spray in each nostril once per day (100–110 mcg dose), maximum dose two sprays/nostril/day.

Topical dermatologic preparations
Apply low-potency form sparingly to affected area bid–qid.

Dental paste
Adults: Press small dab (1/4 inch) to each lesion until thin film develops. May apply two to three times a day, preferably after meals.
Pediatric patients: Use not recommended.

Pharmacokinetics

Route	Onset	Peak	Duration
IM	24–48 hr	8–10 hr	1–6 wk

Metabolism: Hepatic; $T_{1/2}$: 2–5 hr
Distribution: Crosses placenta; enters breast milk
Excretion: Urine

Adverse effects
Effects depend on dose, route, and duration of therapy.
- **CNS:** *Vertigo, headache,* paresthesias, insomnia, seizures, psychosis, cataracts, increased IOP, glaucoma (long-term therapy)
- **CV:** Hypotension, shock, hypertension and heart failure secondary to fluid retention, thromboembolism, thrombophlebitis, fat embolism, cardiac arrhythmias
- **Electrolyte imbalance:** *Sodium and fluid retention,* hypokalemia, hypocalcemia
- **Endocrine:** Amenorrhea, irregular menses, growth retardation, decreased carbohydrate tolerance, diabetes mellitus, cushingoid state (long-term effect), hyperglycemia, increased serum cholesterol, decreased T_3 and T_4 levels, HPA suppression with systemic therapy longer than 5 days
- **GI:** Peptic or esophageal ulcer, pancreatitis, abdominal distention, nausea, vomiting, *increased appetite, weight gain* (long-term therapy)
- **Hypersensitivity:** Hypersensitivity or anaphylactoid reactions

- **Musculoskeletal:** Muscle weakness, steroid myopathy, loss of muscle mass, osteoporosis, spontaneous fractures (long-term therapy)
- **Other:** *Immunosuppression, aggravation, or masking of infections; impaired wound healing;* thin, fragile skin; petechiae, ecchymoses, purpura, striae; subcutaneous fat atrophy

Intra-articular
- **Local:** Osteonecrosis, tendon rupture, infection

Intralesional (face and head)
- **Local:** Blindness (rare)

Respiratory inhalants
- **Local:** Oral, laryngeal, and pharyngeal irritation; fungal infections

Topical dermatologic ointments, creams, sprays
- **Local:** Local burning, irritation, acneiform lesions, striae, skin atrophy

Interactions
✳ **Drug-drug** ● Risk of deterioration of muscle strength when given to myasthenia gravis patients who are also receiving ambenonium, edrophonium, neostigmine, pyridostigmine ● Decreased steroid blood levels with barbiturates, phenytoin, rifampin ● Decreased effectiveness of salicylates, oral antidiabetics
✳ **Drug-lab test** ● False-negative nitrobluetetrazolium test for bacterial infection ● Suppression of skin test reactions

■ Nursing considerations
Assessment
- **History:** Infections; renal or liver disease; hypothyroidism; ulcerative colitis with impending perforation; diverticulitis; active or latent peptic ulcer; inflammatory bowel disease; HF; hypertension; thromboembolic disorders; osteoporosis; seizure disorders; diabetes mellitus; pregnancy; lactation
- **Physical:** Weight, T; reflexes and grip strength, affect and orientation, P, BP, peripheral perfusion, prominence of superficial veins; R, adventitious sounds; serum electrolytes, blood glucose

Interventions
- Administer once-a-day doses before 9 AM to mimic normal peak corticosteroid blood levels.
- Increase dosage when patient is subject to stress.

⊗ **Warning** Taper doses when discontinuing high-dose or long-term therapy to allow adrenal recovery.
- Do not give live virus vaccines with immunosuppressive doses of corticosteroids.

⊗ **Warning** Taper systemic steroids carefully during transfer to inhalational steroids; deaths caused by adrenal insufficiency have occurred.
- Use caution when occlusive dressings or tight diapers cover affected area; these can increase systemic absorption when using topical preparations.
- Avoid prolonged use of topical preparations near the eyes, in genital and rectal areas, and in skin creases.

Teaching points
- If using dental paste, press a small dab onto lesion until a thin film develops; do not rub in. You may need to apply two to three times a day, after meals.
- Do not stop taking the drug without consulting your health care provider.
- Avoid exposure to infections.
- Report unusual weight gain, swelling of the extremities, muscle weakness, black or tarry stools, fever, prolonged sore throat, colds or other infections, worsening of your disorder.

Intra-articular administration
- Do not overuse joint after therapy, even if pain is gone.

Respiratory inhalant
- Do not use during an acute asthmatic attack or to manage status asthmaticus.
- Do not use with systemic fungal infections.
- Do not use more often than prescribed.
- Do not stop using this drug without consulting your health care provider.
- Administer inhalational bronchodilator drug first, if also receiving bronchodilator therapy; rinse mouth after use.

Nasal spray
- Do not spray in eyes.
- Prime pump before first use and again if not used for more than 2 weeks.

Intraocular
- Discuss use of any other drugs or herbs, signs of infection before administration.
- Report any changes in vision.

Topical dermatologic preparations
- Apply drug sparingly, avoid contact with eyes.

Adverse effects in *italics* are most common; those in **bold** are life-threatening. ⊜ Do not crush.

- Report irritation or infection at the site of application.

▽triamterene
(trye am' ter een)

Dyrenium

PREGNANCY CATEGORY C

Drug class
Potassium-sparing diuretic

Therapeutic actions
Inhibits sodium reabsorption in the renal distal tubule, causing loss of sodium and water and retention of potassium.

Indications
- Edema associated with HF, nephrotic syndrome, hepatic cirrhosis; steroid-induced edema, edema from secondary hyperaldosteronism (alone or with other diuretics for added diuretic or potassium-sparing effects), hypertension
- Unlabeled use: Pediatric hypertension

Contraindications and cautions
- Contraindicated with allergy to triamterene, hyperkalemia, renal disease (except nephrosis), liver disease, lactation.
- Use cautiously with diabetes mellitus, hyperuricemia, pregnancy.

Available forms
Capsules—50, 100 mg

Dosages
Adults
Edema: 100 mg bid PO if used alone after meals. Reduce dosage if added to other diuretic or antihypertensive therapy. Maintenance dosage should be individualized, may be as low as 100 mg every other day. Do not exceed 300 mg/day.
Hypertension: Start with 25 mg PO once daily; usual dose 50–100 mg/day.
Pediatric patients
Safety and efficacy not established.

Pharmacokinetics

Route	Onset	Peak	Duration
Oral	2–4 hr	3 hr	7–9 hr

Metabolism: Hepatic; T$_{1/2}$: 3 hr
Distribution: Crosses placenta; enters breast milk
Excretion: Urine

Adverse effects
- **CNS:** *Headache,* drowsiness, fatigue, *weakness*
- **Dermatologic:** Rash, photosensitivity
- **GI:** *Nausea, anorexia, vomiting, dry mouth,* diarrhea, jaundice, hepatic impairment
- **GU:** Renal stones, interstitial nephritis
- **Hematologic: Hyperkalemia**, blood dyscrasias, increased BUN, azotemia

Interactions
❋ **Drug-drug** • Increased hyperkalemia with potassium supplements, diets rich in potassium, ACE inhibitors, other potassium-sparing diuretics, salt substitutes • Increased serum levels and possible toxicity with cimetidine, indomethacin, lithium • Increased risk of amantadine toxicity
❋ **Drug-lab test** • Interference with fluorescent measurement of serum quinidine levels

■ Nursing considerations
Assessment
- **History:** Allergy to triamterene, hyperkalemia, renal or liver disease, diabetes mellitus, pregnancy, lactation
- **Physical:** Skin color, lesions, edema; orientation, reflexes, muscle strength; pulses, baseline ECG, BP; R, pattern, adventitious sounds; liver evaluation, bowel sounds; urinary output patterns; CBC, serum electrolytes, blood sugar, LFTs, renal function tests, urinalysis

Interventions
- Administer with food or milk if GI upset occurs.
- Mark calendars or provide other reminders of drug days for outpatients if alternate-day or 3- to 5-day/wk therapy is optimal for treating edema.
- Administer early in the day so that increased urination does not disturb sleep.
- Measure and record regular weights to monitor mobilization of edema fluid.
- Arrange for regular evaluation of serum electrolytes and BUN.

Teaching points

- Record alternate-day therapy on a calendar, or make dated envelopes. Take the drug early in the day as increased urination will occur. The drug may be taken with food or meals if GI upset occurs.
- Weigh yourself on a regular basis, at the same time and in the same clothing, and record the weight on your calendar.
- You may experience these side effects: Increased volume and frequency of urination; drowsiness (avoid rapid position changes; do not engage in hazardous activities such as driving a car; this problem is often made worse by the use of alcohol); avoid foods that are rich in potassium (eg, fruits, *Sanka*); sensitivity to sunlight and bright lights (wear sunglasses; use sunscreens and protective clothing).
- Report weight change of more than 3 pounds in 1 day, swelling in ankles or fingers, fever, sore throat, mouth sores, unusual bleeding or bruising, dizziness, trembling, numbness, fatigue.

▽triazolam
(trye ay' zoe lam)

Apo-Triazo (CAN), Gen-Triazolam (CAN), Halcion

PREGNANCY CATEGORY X

CONTROLLED SUBSTANCE C-IV

Drug classes
Benzodiazepine
Sedative-hypnotic

Therapeutic actions
Exact mechanisms of action not understood; acts mainly at subcortical levels of the CNS, leaving the cortex relatively unaffected; main sites of action may be the limbic system and mesencephalic reticular formation; benzodiazepines potentiate the effects of GABA, an inhibitory neurotransmitter.

Indications
- Insomnia characterized by difficulty falling asleep, frequent nocturnal awakenings, or early morning awakening (short-term use: 7–10 days)
- Acute or chronic medical situations requiring restful sleep

Contraindications and cautions
- Contraindicated with hypersensitivity to benzodiazepines; pregnancy (risk of congenital malformations, neonatal withdrawal syndrome); labor and delivery ("floppy infant" syndrome); lactation (infants may become lethargic and lose weight).
- Use cautiously with impaired liver or renal function, debilitation, depression, suicidal tendencies.

Available forms
Tablets—0.125, 0.25 mg

Dosages
Adults
0.125–0.25 mg PO before retiring. May be increased to 0.5 mg if needed. Do not exceed 0.5 mg/day.
Pediatric patients
Not for use in patients younger than 18 yr.
Geriatric or debilitated patients
Initially, 0.125–0.25 mg PO. Adjust as needed and tolerated. Do not exceed 0.25 mg/day.

Pharmacokinetics

Route	Onset	Peak
Oral	Varies	30 min–2 hr

Metabolism: Hepatic; $T_{1/2}$: 1.5–5.5 hr
Distribution: Crosses placenta; enters breast milk
Excretion: Urine

Adverse effects
- **CNS:** *Transient, mild drowsiness initially; sedation, depression, lethargy,* apathy, fatigue, *light-headedness, disorientation, restlessness, confusion,* crying, delirium, headache, slurred speech, dysarthria, stupor, rigidity, tremor, dystonia, vertigo, euphoria, nervousness, difficulty in concentration, vivid dreams, psychomotor retardation, extrapyramidal symptoms; *mild paradoxical excitatory reactions during first 2 wk of treatment* (especially in psychiatric patients, aggressive children, and with high dosage), visual and auditory disturbances, diplopia, nystagmus, depressed hearing, nasal congestion, retrograde amnesia, "traveler's amnesia," complex sleep-related behaviors
- **CV:** *Bradycardia, tachycardia,* CV collapse, hypertension and hypotension, palpitations, edema

- **Dependence:** *Drug dependence with withdrawal syndrome* when drug is discontinued (more common with abrupt discontinuation of higher dosage used for longer than 4 mo)
- **Dermatologic:** Urticaria, pruritus, rash, dermatitis
- **GI:** *Constipation, diarrhea,* dry mouth, salivation, nausea, anorexia, vomiting, difficulty in swallowing, gastric disorders, elevations of blood enzymes—hepatic impairment, jaundice
- **GU:** *Incontinence, changes in libido, urine retention,* menstrual irregularities
- **Hematologic:** Anemia, blood dyscrasias
- **Other:** Hiccups, fever, diaphoresis, paresthesias, muscular disturbances, gynecomastia, **anaphylaxis, angioedema**

Interactions
✴ **Drug-drug** ⊗ *Warning* Potentially serious to fatal reactions with ketoconazole, itraconazole or other CYP3A inhibitors; avoid this combination.
- Increased CNS depression and sedation with alcohol, cimetidine, omeprazole, disulfiram, hormonal contraceptives • Decreased sedative effects with theophylline, aminophylline, dyphylline
✴ **Drug-food** • Decreased metabolism and risk of toxic effects if combined with grapefruit juice; avoid this combination

■ Nursing considerations
Assessment
- **History:** Hypersensitivity to benzodiazepines; pregnancy, lactation; impaired liver or renal function; debilitation; depression, suicidal tendencies
- **Physical:** Skin color, lesions; T; orientation, reflexes, affect, ophthalmologic examination; P, BP; R, adventitious sounds; liver evaluation, abdominal examination, bowel sounds, normal output; CBC, LFTs, renal function tests

Interventions
- Arrange for periodic blood counts, urinalyses, and blood chemistry analyses with protracted treatment.
- Caution women of childbearing age to avoid pregnancy; using barrier contraceptives is advised.

⊗ *Warning* Taper dosage gradually after long-term therapy, especially in patients with epilepsy.

Teaching points
- Take drug exactly as prescribed. Do not drink grapefruit juice while using this drug.
- Do not stop taking drug without consulting your health care provider.
- Avoid alcohol and sleep-inducing and over-the-counter drugs.
- Avoid pregnancy while taking this drug; using contraceptives is advised; serious fetal harm could occur.
- Use for longer than 7–10 days is not recommended. Continued problems of insomnia require medical reevaluation. Taking drug for longer than 10 days may result in dependence and addiction.
- You may experience these side effects: Drowsiness, dizziness (may lessen; avoid driving or engaging in hazardous activities); allergic reaction, swelling; GI upset (take drug with food); depression, dreams, emotional upset, crying; sleep disturbance for several nights after discontinuing the drug, complex sleep-related behaviors.
- Report severe dizziness, allergies, weakness, drowsiness that persists, rash or skin lesions, palpitations, swelling of extremities, visual changes, difficulty voiding, sleep disorders.

▽ trientine hydrochloride
See Appendix R, *Less commonly used drugs.*

▽ trihexyphenidyl hydrochloride
(trye hex ee fen' i dill)

Apo-Trihex (CAN)

PREGNANCY CATEGORY C

Drug class
Antiparkinsonian (anticholinergic type)

Therapeutic actions
Has anticholinergic activity in the CNS that is believed to help normalize the hypothesized imbalance of cholinergic and dopaminergic neurotransmission created by the loss of

dopaminergic neurons in the basal ganglia of the brain of parkinsonism patients; reduces severity of rigidity and reduces to a lesser extent the akinesia and tremor that characterize parkinsonism; less effective overall than levodopa; peripheral anticholinergic effects suppress secondary symptoms of parkinsonism, such as drooling.

Indications
- Adjunct in the treatment of parkinsonism (postencephalitic, arteriosclerotic, and idiopathic)
- Adjuvant therapy with levodopa for the treatment of Parkinson disease
- Control of drug-induced extrapyramidal disorders

Contraindications and cautions
- Contraindicated with hypersensitivity to trihexyphenidyl; glaucoma, especially angle-closure glaucoma; pyloric or duodenal obstruction, stenosing peptic ulcers, achalasia (megaesophagus); myasthenia gravis; lactation.
- Use cautiously with cardiac arrhythmias, hypertension, hypotension, hepatic or renal impairment, alcoholism, chronic illness, people who work in hot environment, pregnancy, prostatic hypertrophy or bladder neck obstructions.

Available forms
Tablets—2, 5 mg; elixir—2 mg/5 mL

Dosages
Adults
Tablets
- *Parkinsonism:* 1 mg PO the first day. Increase by 2-mg increments at 3- to 5-day intervals until a total of 6–10 mg is given daily. Postencephalitic patients may require 12–15 mg/day PO. Tolerated best if daily dose is divided into three (or four) doses administered at mealtimes (and bedtime).
- *Concomitant use with levodopa:* Usual dose of each may need to be reduced; however, trihexyphenidyl has been shown to decrease bioavailability of levodopa. Adjust dosage on basis of response. 3–6 mg/day PO of trihexyphenidyl is usually adequate.
- *Concomitant use with other anticholinergics:* Gradually substitute trihexyphenidyl for all or part of the other anticholinergic and reduce dosage of the other anticholinergic gradually.

- *Drug-induced extrapyramidal symptoms:* Initially, 1 mg PO. Dose of tranquilizer may need to be reduced temporarily to expedite control of extrapyramidal symptoms. Adjust dosage of both drugs subsequently to maintain ataractic effect without extrapyramidal reactions. Usual dose 5–15 mg daily. If reactions are not controlled in a few hours, progressively increase subsequent doses until control is achieved.

Pediatric patients
Safety and efficacy not established.

Geriatric patients
Patients older than 60 yr often develop increased sensitivity to the CNS effects of anticholinergic drugs.

Pharmacokinetics

Route	Onset	Peak	Duration
Oral	1 hr	2–3 hr	6–12 hr

Metabolism: Hepatic; $T_{1/2}$: 5.6–10.2 hr
Distribution: Crosses placenta; enters breast milk
Excretion: Urine

Adverse effects
- **CNS** (some CNS effects are characteristic of centrally acting anticholinergics): *Disorientation, confusion,* memory loss, hallucinations, psychoses, agitation, nervousness, delusions, delirium, paranoia, euphoria, excitement, *light-headedness, dizziness,* depression, drowsiness, weakness, giddiness, paresthesia, heaviness of the limbs, numbness of fingers, *blurred vision, mydriasis,* diplopia, increased intraocular tension, angle-closure glaucoma
- **CV:** Tachycardia, palpitations, hypotension, orthostatic hypotension
- **Dermatologic:** Rash, urticaria, other dermatoses
- **GI:** *Dry mouth, constipation,* dilation of the colon, paralytic ileus, acute suppurative parotitis, nausea, vomiting, epigastric distress
- **GU:** *Urinary retention,* urinary hesitancy, dysuria, difficulty achieving or maintaining an erection
- **Other:** Muscular weakness, muscular cramping, *flushing, decreased sweating,* elevated temperature

Interactions
✳ Drug-drug • Additive adverse CNS effects; toxic psychosis with phenothiazines • Possible

masking of the development of persistent extrapyramidal symptoms, tardive dyskinesia, in patients on long-term therapy with antipsychotics, such as phenothiazines, haloperidol
• Decreased therapeutic efficacy of antipsychotics (phenothiazines, haloperidol)

■ **Nursing considerations**
Assessment
• **History:** Hypersensitivity to trihexyphenidyl; glaucoma; pyloric or duodenal obstruction, stenosing peptic ulcers; achalasia; prostatic hypertrophy or bladder neck obstructions; myasthenia gravis, tachycardia, cardiac arrhythmias; hypertension, hypotension; hepatic or renal impairment; alcoholism; chronic illness; work environment; pregnancy, lactation
• **Physical:** Weight, T; skin color, lesions; orientation, affect, reflexes, bilateral grip strength, visual examination, including tonometry; P, BP, orthostatic BP, auscultation; bowel sounds, normal output, liver evaluation; urinary output, voiding pattern, prostate palpation; LFTs, renal function tests

Interventions
⊗ *Warning* Decrease dosage or discontinue drug temporarily if dry mouth is so severe that swallowing or speaking becomes difficult.
• Give with caution and arrange dosage reduction in hot weather; drug interferes with sweating and ability of body to maintain body heat equilibrium; anhidrosis and fatal hyperthermia have occurred.
• Ensure that patient voids before receiving each dose if urinary retention is a problem.

Teaching points
• Take this drug exactly as prescribed.
• Use caution in hot weather (this drug makes you more susceptible to heat prostration).
• You may experience these side effects: Drowsiness, dizziness, confusion, blurred vision (avoid driving or engaging in activities that require alertness and visual acuity); nausea (eat frequent small meals); dry mouth (suck sugarless candies or ice chips); painful or difficult urination (emptying the bladder immediately before each dose may help); constipation (if maintaining adequate fluid intake and exercising regularly do not help, consult your health care provider).

• Report difficult or painful urination, constipation, rapid or pounding heartbeat, confusion, eye pain, or rash.

▽**trimethobenzamide hydrochloride**
*(trye meth oh **ben'** za myde)*

Oral preparations: Tigan
Parenteral preparations: Tigan

PREGNANCY CATEGORY C

Drug class
Antiemetic (anticholinergic)

Therapeutic actions
Mechanism of action not understood; antiemetic action may be mediated through the CTZ; impulses to the vomiting center do not appear to be affected.

Indications
• Control of postoperative nausea and vomiting and nausea associated with gastroenteritis

Contraindications and cautions
• Contraindicated with allergy to trimethobenzamide, benzocaine, or similar local anesthetics; uncomplicated vomiting in children (drug may contribute to development of Reye syndrome or unfavorably influence its outcome; extrapyramidal effects of drugs may obscure diagnosis of Reye syndrome); pregnancy.
• Use cautiously with lactation; acute febrile illness, appendicitis, encephalitis, gastroenteritis, dehydration, electrolyte imbalance, especially when these occur in children, the elderly, or debilitated; narrow-angle glaucoma; stenosing peptic ulcer; symptomatic prostatic hypertrophy; bronchial asthma; bladder neck obstruction; pyloroduodenal obstruction; cardiac arrhythmias; recent use of CNS-acting drugs (phenothiazine, barbiturates, belladonna alkaloids).

Available forms
Capsules—300 mg; injection—100 mg/mL

T

Dosages

Adults

Oral

- *Nausea and vomiting:* 300 mg three to four times a day PO.
- *Postoperative nausea/vomiting or for treatment of gastroenteritis:* 300 mg three to four times a day PO.

Parenteral

200 mg IM tid–qid.

Pediatric patients

Not recommended.

Geriatric patients

More likely to cause serious adverse reactions in elderly patients; use with caution.

Pharmacokinetics

Route	Onset	Duration
Oral	10–40 min	3–4 hr
IM	15 min	2–3 hr

Metabolism: Hepatic; T$_{1/2}$: 7–9 hr
Distribution: Crosses placenta; enters breast milk
Excretion: Urine

Adverse effects

- **CNS:** Parkinson-like symptoms, coma, seizures, opisthotonus, depression, disorientation, *dizziness, drowsiness, headache, blurred vision*
- **CV:** Hypotension
- **GI:** Diarrhea
- **Hematologic:** Blood dyscrasias, jaundice
- **Hypersensitivity:** Allergic-type skin reactions
- **Local:** *Pain with burning, redness, and swelling following IM injections*

■ Nursing considerations

Assessment

- **History:** Allergy to trimethobenzamide, benzocaine, or similar local anesthetics; uncomplicated vomiting in children; pregnancy, lactation; acute febrile illness, encephalitis, gastroenteritis, dehydration, electrolyte imbalance; narrow-angle glaucoma; stenosing peptic ulcer; symptomatic prostatic hypertrophy; bronchial asthma; bladder neck obstruction; pyloroduodenal obstruction; cardiac arrhythmias
- **Physical:** Skin color, lesions, texture; T; orientation, reflexes, affect; vision examination;

P, BP; R, adventitious sounds; bowel sounds; prostate palpation; CBC, serum electrolytes

Interventions

- Administer IM injections deep into upper outer quadrant of the gluteal region.
- Ensure adequate hydration.

Teaching points

- Take as prescribed. Avoid excessive dosage.
- Avoid alcohol while taking this drug; serious sedation could occur.
- You may experience these side effects: Dizziness, sedation, drowsiness (use caution if driving or performing tasks that require alertness); diarrhea; blurred vision (reversible).
- Report difficulty breathing, tremors, loss of coordination, sore muscles or muscle spasms, unusual bleeding or bruising, sore throat, visual disturbances, irregular heartbeat, yellowing of the skin or eyes.

▷ trimethoprim (TMP)

(trye meth' oh prim)

Primsol, Trimpex

PREGNANCY CATEGORY C

Drug class

Antibacterial

Therapeutic actions

Inhibits folic acid reduction to tetrahydrofolate in susceptible bacteria; the bacterial enzyme involved in this reaction is more readily inhibited than the mammalian enzyme.

Indications

- Uncomplicated UTIs caused by susceptible strains of *Escherichia coli, Proteus mirabilis, Klebsiella pneumoniae, Enterobacter* species, and coagulase-negative *Staphylococcus* species, including *S. saprophyticus*
- Treatment of acute otitis media due to susceptible strains of *Streptococcus pneumoniae* and *Haemophilus influenzae* in children
- Unlabeled uses: With dapsone for treatment of initial episodes of *Pneumocystis jiroveci (carinii)* pneumonia in patients who cannot tolerate co-trimoxazole; treatment and prevention of traveler's diarrhea

Contraindications and cautions

- Contraindicated with allergy to trimethoprim, pregnancy (teratogenic in preclinical studies), megaloblastic anemia due to folate deficiency.
- Use cautiously with hepatic or renal impairment, lactation.

Available forms

Tablets—100, mg; solution—50 mg/5 mL

Dosages

Adults and children 12 yr and older
100 mg PO every 12 hr or 200 mg every 24 hr for 10 days for acute uncomplicated UTIs.

Pediatric patients
- *Otitis media:* 10 mg/kg/day PO in divided doses every 12 hr for 10 days.

Geriatric patients or patients with renal impairment
For creatinine clearance of 15–30 mL/min, 50 mg PO every 12 hr; for creatinine clearance less than 15 mL/min, not recommended.

Pharmacokinetics

Route	Onset	Peak
Oral	Varies	1–4 hr

Metabolism: Hepatic; T₁/₂: 8–10 hr
Metabolism: Hepatic; $T_{1/2}$: 8–10 hr
Distribution: Crosses placenta; enters breast milk
Excretion: Urine

Adverse effects

- **Dermatologic:** *Rash, pruritus,* exfoliative dermatitis
- **GI:** *Epigastric distress,* nausea, vomiting, glossitis
- **Hematologic:** Thrombocytopenia, leukopenia, neutropenia, megaloblastic anemia, methemoglobinemia, elevated serum transaminase and bilirubin, increased BUN and serum creatinine levels, hyperkalemia, hyponatremia
- **Other:** Fever

Interactions

✳ Drug-drug • Increased phenytoin effects if taken concomitantly; increases phenytoin half-life by 51%

■ Nursing considerations

Assessment

- **History:** Allergy to trimethoprim, megaloblastic anemia due to folate deficiency, renal or hepatic impairment, pregnancy, lactation
- **Physical:** Skin color, lesions; T; status of mucous membranes; CBC; LFTs, renal function tests

Interventions

- Perform culture and sensitivity tests before beginning drug therapy.
- Protect the 200-mg tablets from exposure to light.
- Arrange for regular, periodic blood counts during therapy.
- ⊗ **Warning** Discontinue drug and consult physician if any significant reduction in any formed blood element occurs.

Teaching points

- Take the full course of the drug; take all the tablets prescribed.
- Have periodic medical checkups, including blood tests.
- You may experience these side effects: Epigastric distress, nausea, vomiting (eat frequent small meals); rash (consult your health care provider for appropriate skin care).
- Report fever, sore throat, unusual bleeding or bruising, dizziness, headaches, rash.

▽ trimipramine maleate
*(trye **mi'** pra meen)*

Apo-Trimip (CAN), Surmontil

PREGNANCY CATEGORY C

Drug classes

Antidepressant
TCA (tertiary amine)

Therapeutic actions

Mechanism of action unknown; the TCAs are structurally related to the phenothiazine antipsychotics (eg, chlorpromazine); TCAs inhibit the presynaptic reuptake of the neurotransmitters norepinephrine and serotonin; anticholinergic at CNS and peripheral receptors; the relation of these effects to clinical efficacy is unknown.

T

Indications

- Relief of symptoms of depression (endogenous depression most responsive); sedative effects of tertiary amine TCAs may be helpful in patients whose depression is associated with anxiety and sleep disturbance
- Unlabeled use: Duodenal ulcers

Contraindications and cautions

- Contraindicated with hypersensitivity to any tricyclic drug, concomitant therapy with an MAOI, recent MI, myelography within previous 24 hr or scheduled within 48 hr, pregnancy (limb reduction abnormalities may occur), lactation.
- Use cautiously with EST; pre-existing CV disorders (eg, severe CAD, progressive HF, angina pectoris, paroxysmal tachycardia); angle-closure glaucoma, increased IOP; urinary retention, ureteral or urethral spasm (anticholinergic effects of TCAs may exacerbate these conditions); seizure disorders (TCAs lower the seizure threshold); hyperthyroidism (predisposes to CVS toxicity, including cardiac arrhythmias); impaired hepatic, renal function; psychiatric patients (schizophrenic or paranoid patients may exhibit a worsening of psychosis); patients with bipolar disorder (may shift to hypomanic or manic phase); elective surgery (TCAs should be discontinued as long as possible before surgery).

Available forms

Capsules—25, 50, 100 mg

Dosages

Adults

- *Hospitalized patients:* Initially, 100 mg/day PO in divided doses. Gradually increase to 200 mg/day as required. If no improvement in 2–3 wk, increase to a maximum dose of 250–300 mg/day.
- *Outpatients:* Initially, 75 mg/day PO in divided doses. May increase to 150 mg/day. Do not exceed 200 mg/day. Total daily dosage may be administered at bedtime. Maintenance dose is 50–150 mg/day given as a single dose at bedtime. After satisfactory response, reduce to lowest effective dosage. Continue therapy for 3 mo or longer to lessen possibility of relapse.

Pediatric patients 12 yr and older

50 mg/day PO with gradual increases up to 100 mg/day.

Pediatric patients younger than 12 yr

Not recommended.

Geriatric patients

50 mg/day PO with gradual increases up to 100 mg/day PO.

Pharmacokinetics

Route	Onset	Peak
Oral	Varies	2 hr

Metabolism: Hepatic; T$_{1/2}$: 7–30 hr
Distribution: Crosses placenta; enters breast milk
Excretion: Feces, urine

Adverse effects

- **CNS:** *Sedation and anticholinergic (atropine-like) effects; confusion* (especially in elderly), *disturbed concentration,* hallucinations, disorientation, decreased memory, feelings of unreality, delusions, anxiety, nervousness, restlessness, agitation, panic, insomnia, nightmares, hypomania, mania, exacerbation of psychosis, drowsiness, weakness, fatigue, headache, numbness, tingling, paresthesias of extremities, incoordination, motor hyperactivity, akathisia, ataxia, tremors, peripheral neuropathy, extrapyramidal symptoms, *seizures,* speech blockage, dysarthria, tinnitus, altered EEG, suicidal ideation
- **CV:** *Orthostatic hypotension,* hypertension, syncope, tachycardia, palpitations, **MI,** arrhythmias, heart block, **precipitation of HF, stroke**
- **Endocrine:** Hypoglycemia or hyperglycemia, elevated prolactin levels, SIADH secretion
- **GI:** *Dry mouth, constipation,* paralytic ileus, *nausea,* vomiting, anorexia, epigastric distress, diarrhea, flatulence, dysphagia, peculiar taste in mouth, increased salivation, stomatitis, glossitis, parotid swelling, abdominal cramps, black tongue, hepatitis, jaundice (rare), elevated transaminase, altered alkaline phosphatase
- **GU:** Urinary retention, delayed micturition, dilation of the urinary tract, gynecomastia, testicular swelling; breast enlargement, menstrual irregularity and galactorrhea; increased or decreased libido; impotence
- **Hematologic:** Bone marrow depression including agranulocytosis; eosinophilia, purpura, thrombocytopenia, leukopenia

Adverse effects in *italics* are most common; those in **bold** are life-threatening. ▣ Do not crush.

- **Hypersensitivity:** Rash, pruritus, vasculitis, petechiae, photosensitization, edema (generalized, facial, tongue), drug fever
- **Withdrawal:** Symptoms with abrupt discontinuation of prolonged therapy: Nausea, headache, vertigo, nightmares, malaise
- **Other:** Nasal congestion, excessive appetite, weight gain or loss, sweating, alopecia, lacrimation, hyperthermia, flushing, chills

Interactions

✴ **Drug-drug** • Increased TCA levels and pharmacologic (especially anticholinergic) effects with cimetidine, fluoxetine, ranitidine • Risk of arrhythmias and hypertension with sympathomimetics • Risk of severe hypertension with clonidine • Risk of life-threatening cardiac arrhythmias if combined with fluoroquinolone antibiotics; avoid this combination • Hyperpyretic crises, severe seizures, hypertensive episodes and deaths with MAOIs. *Note:* MAOIs and TCAs have been used successfully in some patients resistant to therapy with single agents; however, case reports indicate that the combination can cause serious and potentially fatal adverse effects • Increased adverse effects if combined with alcohol

■ Nursing considerations
Assessment

- **History:** Hypersensitivity to any tricyclic drug; concomitant therapy with an MAOI; recent MI; myelography within previous 24 hr or scheduled within 48 hr; pregnancy; lactation; EST; preexisting CV disorders; angleclosure glaucoma, increased IOP; urinary retention, ureteral or urethral spasm; seizure disorders; hyperthyroidism; impaired hepatic, renal function; psychiatric disorders; bipolar disorder; elective surgery
- **Physical:** Weight; T; skin color, lesions; orientation, affect, reflexes, vision and hearing; P, BP, orthostatic BP, perfusion; bowel sounds, normal output; liver evaluation; urine flow, normal output; usual sexual function, frequency of menses, breast and scrotal examination; LFTs, urinalysis; CBC, ECG

Interventions

⊗ **Black box warning** Ensure that depressed and potentially suicidal patients have access to limited quantities of the drug. Monitor patients for suicidal ideation, especially when beginning therapy or changing doses; high risk

of suicidality in children, adolescents, and young adults.

- Administer major portion of dose at bedtime if drowsiness or severe anticholinergic effects occur.

⊗ *Warning* Reduce dosage if minor side effects develop; discontinue if serious side effects occur.

- Arrange for CBC if patient develops fever, sore throat, or other sign of infection.

Teaching points

- Take drug exactly as prescribed.
- Do not stop taking this drug abruptly or without consulting your health care provider.
- Avoid alcohol, other sleep-inducing drugs, and over-the-counter drugs.
- Avoid prolonged exposure to sunlight or sunlamps; use a sunscreen or protective garments.
- You may experience these side effects: Headache, dizziness, drowsiness, weakness, blurred vision (reversible; safety measures may need to be taken if severe; avoid driving or performing tasks that require alertness); nausea, vomiting, loss of appetite, dry mouth (eat frequent small meals; practice frequent mouth care; suck sugarless candies); nightmares, inability to concentrate, confusion; changes in sexual function.
- Report dry mouth, difficulty in urination, excessive sedation, suicidal thoughts.

DANGEROUS DRUG

▷ **triptorelin pamoate**
(trip toe rell' in)

Trelstar Depot, Trelstar LA, Trelstar Mixject

PREGNANCY CATEGORY X

Drug classes
Antineoplastic
Hormone
LHRH analogue

Therapeutic actions
An analogue of LHRH; causes a decrease in FSH and LH levels, leading to a suppression of ovarian and testicular hormone production, which causes decreased levels of estrogens (in women) and testosterone (in men); after continuous

use, a sustained decrease in FSH and LH levels occurs.

Indications

- Palliative treatment of advanced prostate cancer
- Unlabeled uses: Central precocious puberty, ovarian cancer, pancreatic carcinoma, endometriosis, hyperandrogenism, in vitro fertilization, uterine leiomyomata

Contraindications and cautions

- Contraindicated with pregnancy, lactation, hypersensitivity to LHRH or any component.
- Use cautiously with urinary tract obstructions, metastatic vertebral lesions.

Available forms

Injectable suspension—3.75 mg, 11.25 mg, 22.5 mg

Dosages
Adults

- *Palliative treatment:* 3.75 mg depot injection IM once monthly into buttock, or 11.25 mg injection IM every 12 wk into buttock, or 22.5 mg IM every 24 wk into buttock.

Pediatric patients
Safety and efficacy not established.

Pharmacokinetics

Route	Onset	Peak
IM	Slow	1–3 hr

Metabolism: Hepatic; $T_{1/2}$: 2.8–4 hr
Distribution: Crosses placenta; may enter breast milk
Excretion: Bile, urine

Adverse effects

- **CNS:** Insomnia, dizziness, lethargy, anxiety, depression, *headache*
- **CV:** HF, edema, hypertension, arrhythmia, chest pain, CV events
- **GI:** Nausea, anorexia
- **GU:** *Hot flashes, sexual dysfunction, decreased erections, lower urinary tract symptoms*
- **Other:** *Bone pain,* rash, sweating, cancer, **anaphylaxis, angioedema,** injection-site pain

Interactions

✳ **Drug-drug •** Do not administer with drugs that increase prolactin production—antipsychotics, metoclopramide; risk of severe hyperprolactinemia

■ Nursing considerations
Assessment

- **History:** Pregnancy, lactation, hypersensitivity to LHRH or other LHRH drugs
- **Physical:** Skin T, lesions; reflexes, affect; BP, P; urinary output; serum testosterone levels, PSA levels

Interventions

- Reconstitute with 2 mL sterile water for injection. Shake well (suspension will appear milky). Withdraw the entire contents of the vial into the syringe and inject immediately into buttock; alternate injection sites.
- Monitor testosterone and PSA levels prior to and periodically during therapy.
- Ensure repeat injection every 4, 12 or 24 wk. It is important to keep as close to this schedule as possible.
- Be aware that patient may be at increased risk for CV events; monitor accordingly.
- Offer appropriate comfort measures (eg, temperature control, analgesics) to help patient cope with hot flashes, urinary retention, and bone pain. Most likely to occur at initiation of therapy.

Teaching points

- This drug must be injected every 4, 12, or 24 weeks.
- Your cancer symptoms may worsen during and for the first few weeks after treatment; this should resolve within 3–4 weeks.
- You may experience these side effects: Hot flashes (staying in a cool place may help you to cope with this effect); sexual dysfunction, such as regression of sex organs, impaired fertility, decreased erections (it may help to know that these are drug effects; if these become worrisome, consult your health care provider); bone pain, urinary retention, blood in the urine (these effects usually resolve within the first week of treatment; analgesics may be ordered to help you cope with the pain).
- Report chest pain, rapid heartbeat, numbness or tingling, breast pain, difficulty breathing, unresolved nausea and vomiting, signs of infection at the injection site.

Adverse effects in *italics* are most common; those in **bold** are life-threatening. ⬛ Do not crush.

▽trospium chloride
(troz' pee um)

Sanctura, Sanctura XR ⓒ

PREGNANCY CATEGORY C

Drug classes
Antimuscarinic
Antispasmodic

Therapeutic actions
Competitively blocks muscarinic receptor sites; bladder contraction is mediated by muscarinic receptors—blocking these receptors decreases bladder contraction, relieving bladder spasm.

Indications
- Treatment of urinary incontinence, urgency, and frequency caused by overactive bladder

Contraindications and cautions
- Contraindicated with allergy to trospium or any component of the drug; presence of or risk for urinary retention, gastric retention, uncontrolled narrow-angle glaucoma.
- Use cautiously with renal or hepatic impairment, ulcerative colitis, intestinal atony, myasthenia gravis, bladder or gastric outlet obstruction, pregnancy, lactation.

Available forms
Tablets—20 mg; ER capsules ⓒ —60 mg

Dosages
Adults younger than 75 yr
20 mg PO bid taken on an empty stomach, at least 1 hr before meals. Alternatively, 60 mg ER tablet PO once/day.
Adults 75 yr and older
Monitor patient response and adjust dosage down to 20 mg/day PO.
Pediatric patients
Safety and efficacy not established.
Patients with renal impairment
For creatinine clearance less than 30 mL/min, 20 mg/day PO given at bedtime. ER tablets are not recommended.

Pharmacokinetics

Route	Onset	Peak
Oral	Slow	5–6 hr

Metabolism: Hepatic metabolism; $T_{1/2}$: 20 hr
Distribution: May cross placenta; passes into breast milk
Excretion: Feces, urine

Adverse effects
- **CNS:** *Headache,* dry eyes, dizziness, blurred vision
- **GI:** *Dry mouth, constipation,* abdominal pain, dyspepsia, flatulence, vomiting
- **GU:** Urinary retention
- **Other:** *Fatigue,* decreased sweating

Interactions
✳ **Drug-drug** • Increased risk of adverse effects if combined with any other anticholinergic drugs; if this combination is used, monitor patient carefully and adjust dosages accordingly • Potential for altered excretion of other drugs eliminated by tubular secretion (digoxin, morphine, metformin, tenfovir, procainamide, pancuronium, vancomycin); if any of these drugs are given concurrently, monitor patient carefully for increased adverse effects or decreased therapeutic effects of both drugs and adjust dosages accordingly

■ Nursing considerations
Assessment
- **History:** Allergy to trospium or any component of the drug; presence of or risk for urinary retention, gastric retention, uncontrolled narrow-angle glaucoma, renal or hepatic impairment, ulcerative colitis, intestinal atony, myasthenia gravis, bladder or gastric outlet obstruction; pregnancy, lactation
- **Physical:** Orientation, affect, vision, IOP; GI output, bowel sounds, liver evaluation; normal urinary output, prostate palpation; LFTs, renal function tests

Interventions
- Administer drug on an empty stomach, at least 1 hr before meal. Ensure that patient does not cut, crush, or chew ER form.
- Provide frequent small meals if GI upset is severe.

T

- Establish safety measures (eg, accompany patient, use side rails) if vision changes occur.
- Provide frequent mouth hygiene and sugarless candies if dry mouth is a problem.
- Monitor bowel function and arrange for appropriate bowel program if constipation occurs.

Teaching points
- Take this drug twice a day on an empty stomach, at least 1 hour before your next meal. Do not cut, crush, or chew ER form.
- If you miss a dose, take the next dose as soon as you remember and then again about that time the next day; do not take more than two doses per day.
- Know that you may be at higher risk for developing heat-related problems—sweating may be decreased so your body will not be able to cool off. Avoid excessive heat if at all possible; if you are in a hot environment drink plenty of fluids.
- You may experience these side effects: Dry mouth (sucking on sugarless candies and frequent mouth care may help); GI upset, nausea (frequent small meals may help); headache (analgesics may be available to help, consult with your health care provider); dizziness (do not drive a car or operate hazardous machinery if this occurs); urinary retention (emptying your bladder before taking the medicine may help); constipation (if this becomes a problem, consult your health care provider for appropriate remedies).
- Report inability to urinate, abdominal pain, severe constipation, fever.

▷ urofollitropin, purified

See Appendix R, *Less commonly used drugs*.

▷ ursodiol
(ursodeoxycholic acid)
(ur soe dye' ole)

Actigall, URSO 250,
URSO DS (CAN), URSO Forte

PREGNANCY CATEGORY B

Drug class
Gallstone-solubilizing drug

Therapeutic actions
A naturally occurring bile acid that suppresses hepatic synthesis of cholesterol and inhibits intestinal absorption of cholesterol, leading to a decreased cholesterol concentration in the bile and a bile that is cholesterol solubilizing and not cholesterol precipitating.

Indications
- Treatment of select patients with radiolucent, noncalcified gallstones less than 20 mm in diameter in gallbladders for whom elective surgery is contraindicated
- Prevention of gallstone formation in obese patients experiencing rapid weight loss
- Treatment of primary biliary cirrhosis (tablets only)
- Unlabeled uses: Cholestasis-associated pruritus, primary sclerosing cholangitis

Contraindications and cautions
- Contraindicated with allergy to bile salts, calcified stones, radiopaque stones or radiolucent bile pigment stones, unremitting acute cholecystitis, cholangitis, biliary obstruction, gallstone pancreatitis, biliary GI fistula (cholecystectomy required), pregnancy.
- Use cautiously with lactation, hepatic impairment.

Available forms
Capsules—300 mg; tablets—250, 500 mg

Dosages
Adults
- *Solubilization of gallstones:* 8–10 mg/kg/day PO given in two to three divided doses. Resolution of the gallstones requires months of therapy; condition needs to be monitored with ultrasound at 6-mo and 1-yr intervals.
- *Treatment of biliary cirrhosis:* 13–15 mg/kg/day PO administered in two to four divided doses with food; readjust dosage based on patient response.
- *Prevention of gallstones:* 300 mg PO bid or 8–10 mg/kg/day PO in two to three divided doses.

Pediatric patients
Safety and efficacy not established.

Adverse effects in *italics* are most common; those in **bold** are life-threatening. ⬛ Do not crush.

Pharmacokinetics

Route	Onset	Peak
Oral	Varies	Days

Metabolism: Hepatic; $T_{1/2}$: Unknown
Distribution: Crosses placenta; may enter breast milk
Excretion: Feces

Adverse effects

- **CNS:** Headache, fatigue, anxiety, depression, sleep disorder
- **Dermatologic:** Pruritus, rash, urticaria, dry skin, sweating, hair thinning
- **GI:** *Diarrhea*, cramps, heartburn, constipation, nausea, vomiting, anorexia, epigastric distress, dyspepsia, flatulence, abdominal pain
- **Respiratory:** Rhinitis, cough
- **Other:** Back pain, arthralgia, myalgia

Interactions

✳ **Drug-drug** • Absorption decreased if taken with bile acid sequestering agents (cholestyramine, colestipol), aluminum-based antacids

■ Nursing considerations
Assessment

- **History:** Allergy to bile salts, hepatic impairment, calcified stones, radiopaque stones or radiolucent bile pigment stones, unremitting acute cholecystitis, cholangitis, biliary obstruction, gallstone pancreatitis, biliary-GI fistula, pregnancy, lactation
- **Physical:** Liver evaluation, abdominal examination; affect, orientation; skin color, lesions; LFTs, hepatic and biliary radiologic studies, biliary ultrasound

Interventions

- Assess patient carefully for suitability of ursodiol therapy. Alternative therapy should be reviewed before using ursodiol.
- Give drug in two to three divided doses.
- Do not administer drug with aluminum-based antacids. If such drugs are needed, administer 2–3 hr after ursodiol.
- Schedule patients for periodic oral cholecystograms or ultrasonograms to evaluate drug effectiveness at 6-mo intervals until resolution, then every 3 mo to monitor stone formation. Stones recur within 5 yr in more than 50% of patients. If gallstones appear to have

dissolved, continue treatment for 3 mo and perform follow-up ultrasound.
- Monitor LFTs periodically. Carefully assess patient if any change in liver function occurs.

Teaching points

- Take drug two to four times a day. Take the drug as long as prescribed. It may be needed for a long time.
- This drug may dissolve your gallstones; it does not "cure" the problem that caused the stones, and in many cases, the stones can recur. Medical follow-up care is important.
- Arrange to receive periodic X-rays or ultrasound tests of your gallbladder; you also will need periodic blood tests to evaluate your response to this drug. Keep follow-up appointments.
- Do not take with any aluminum-based antacids.
- You may experience these side effects: Diarrhea; rash (skin care may help); headache, fatigue (request analgesics).
- Report gallstone attacks (abdominal pain, nausea, vomiting), yellowing of the skin or eyes.

▽ustekinumab

See Appendix R, *Less commonly used drugs.*

▽valacyclovir hydrochloride
*(val ah **sye'** kloe veer)*

Valtrex

PREGNANCY CATEGORY B

Drug class
Antiviral

Therapeutic actions
Antiviral activity; inhibits viral DNA replication and deactivates viral DNA polymerase.

Indications
Adults
- Treatment of herpes zoster (shingles)
- Episodic treatment of first-episode or recurrent genital herpes in immunocompetent patients

U

- Suppression of recurrent episodes of genital herpes in HIV patients
- Reduction of risk of heterosexual transmission of genital herpes to healthy partners when combined with safe sex practices
- Treatment of cold sores (herpes labialis) in healthy adults and adolescents
- Unlabeled use: Prevention of cytomegalovirus in patients with renal transplantation

Pediatric patients
- Treatment of cold sores in patients 12 yr and older
- Treatment of chickenpox in immunocompetent patients 2 to younger than 18 yr; initiate therapy within 24 hr of onset of rash

Contraindications and cautions
- Contraindicated with allergy to valacyclovir or acyclovir.
- Use cautiously with pregnancy, renal impairment, thrombotic thrombocytopenic purpura, lactation.

Available forms
Tablets—500 mg, 1 g

Dosages
Adults
- *Herpes zoster:* 1 g tid PO for 7 days; most effective if started within 48 hr of onset of symptoms (rash).
- *Genital herpes:* 1 g PO bid for 7–10 days for initial episode.
- *Episodic treatment of recurrent genital herpes:* 500 mg PO bid for 3 days or 1 g/day for 5 days.
- *Cold sores:* 2 g PO bid for one day, given 12 hr apart.
- *Suppression of recurrent episodes of genital herpes:* 1 g PO daily; patients with history of less than nine episodes in 1 yr may respond to 500 mg PO daily.
- *Suppression of recurrent episodes in HIV-infected patients:* 500 mg PO bid for 5–10 days.
- *Reduction of risk of transmission:* 500 mg/day PO for the source partner. For HIV-positive patients, 500 mg PO bid.

Pediatric patients
- *Chickenpox:* Children 2–18 yr: 20 mg/kg PO tid for 5 days. Maximum dose, 1 g tid.
- *Cold sores:* Children 12 yr and older: 2 g PO every 12 hr for one day.

Patients with renal impairment
Dosage (PO) adjustment variations by indication and CrCl

Indication	CrCl 30–49	CrCl 10–29	CrCl less than 10
Herpes zoster	1 g every 12 hr	1 g every 24 hr	500 mg every 24 hr
Genital herpes			
–initial treatment	1 g every 12 hr	1 g every 24 hr	500 mg every 24 hr
–recurrent episodes	500 mg every 12 hr	500 mg every 24 hr	500 mg every 24 hr
–suppressive therapy	1 g every 24 hr	500 mg every 24 hr	500 mg every 24 hr
–suppressive therapy for 9 or fewer episodes	500 mg every 24 hr	500 mg every 48 hr	500 mg every 48 hr

Pharmacokinetics

Route	Onset	Peak
Oral	Rapid	3 hr

Metabolism: Not metabolized; $T_{1/2}$: 2.5–3.3 hr
Distribution: Crosses placenta; enters breast milk
Excretion: Feces, urine

Adverse effects
- **CNS:** Headache, dizziness
- **GI:** *Nausea, vomiting,* diarrhea, anorexia, **abdominal pain**
- **GU:** Acute renal failure
- **Other:** Rash

Interactions
⁂ **Drug-drug** • Decreased rate of effectiveness with probenecid, cimetidine

■ Nursing considerations

> **CLINICAL ALERT!**
> Name confusion has occurred with *Valtrex* (valacyclovir) and *Valcyte* (valganciclovir); use caution.

Assessment
- **History:** Allergy to valacyclovir, acyclovir; renal disease; lactation; thrombotic thrombocytopenic purpura; pregnancy
- **Physical:** Orientation; urinary output; abdominal examination, normal output; BUN, creatinine clearance

Interventions

- Begin treatment within 48–72 hr of onset of symptoms of shingles or within 24 hr of onset of chickenpox rash in children.
- Administer without regard to meals; administer with meals to decrease GI upset, if needed.
- Provide appropriate analgesics for headache and discomfort of shingles.
- Advise continued use of safe sex practices.

Teaching points

- Take this drug without regard to meals; if GI upset is a problem, take with meals.
- Take the full course of therapy as prescribed.
- Avoid contact with lesions and avoid intercourse when lesions or symptoms are present to avoid infecting others.
- Start therapy at first sign of an episode when treating recurrent herpes.
- You may experience these side effects: Nausea, vomiting, loss of appetite, diarrhea, headache, dizziness.
- Report severe diarrhea, nausea, headache, worsening of the shingles.

▷**valganciclovir hydrochloride**

*(val gan **sigh' kloe** veer)*

Valcyte ꞉

PREGNANCY CATEGORY C

Drug class

Antiviral

Therapeutic actions

Antiviral activity; inhibits viral DNA replication in cytomegalovirus (CMV).

Indications

- Treatment of CMV retinitis in patients with AIDS
- Prevention of CMV infection in high-risk kidney-pancreas, kidney, and heart transplant patients
- Prevention of CMV infection in pediatric patients with kidney or heart transplant at high risk for CMV infection

Contraindications and cautions

- Contraindicated with hypersensitivity to valganciclovir, ganciclovir, or acyclovir; lactation; liver transplant patients.
- Use cautiously in the elderly; with cytopenia, history of cytopenic reactions, impaired renal function, bone marrow suppression, hemodialysis, pregnancy.

Available forms

Tablets ꞉—450 mg; oral solution—50 mg/mL

Dosages

Adults

900 mg PO bid for 21 days; maintenance, 900 mg PO daily.

- *Prevention of CMV:* 900 mg PO daily initiated within 10 days of transplantation and continued for 100 days after transplantation

Pediatric patients 4 mo–16 yr

Dose in mg = 7 × BSA × CrCl PO. Maximum dose, 900 mg/day. May use oral solution or tablets.

Patients with renal impairment

Do not administer to patients on hemodialysis. For patients with renal impairment, see the following table:

CrCl (mL/min)	Initial Dose	Maintenance Dose
60 or more	900 mg PO bid	900 mg/day PO
40–59	450 mg PO bid	450 mg/day PO
25–39	450 mg PO daily	450 mg PO every other day
10–24	450 mg PO every 2 days	450 mg PO twice weekly

Pharmacokinetics

Route	Onset	Peak
Oral	Slow	1–3 hr

Metabolism: Hepatic transformation to ganciclovir; $T_{1/2}$: 4 hr
Distribution: Crosses placenta; may enter breast milk
Excretion: Urine

Adverse effects

- **CNS:** *Headache, insomnia,* neuropathy, paresthesias, confusion, hallucinations, tremor
- **GI:** *Nausea, vomiting,* anorexia, *diarrhea,* abdominal pain

V

- **Hematologic:** *Neutropenia, anemia,* thrombocytopenia
- **Other:** *Fever,* retinal detachment, graft rejection

Interactions

✷ **Drug-drug** ⊗ *Warning* Use with extreme caution with cytotoxic drugs because the accumulation effect could cause severe bone marrow depression and other GI and dermatologic problems.

- Increased risk of didanosine toxicity if combined; monitor patient for need to lower didanosine dose.

⊗ *Warning* Extreme drowsiness and risk of bone marrow depression if taken with zidovudine; avoid this combination.

- Increased valganciclovir effects if taken with probenecid • Increased risk of seizures if taken concurrently with imipenem-cilastatin

■ Nursing considerations

CLINICAL ALERT!
Name confusion has occurred with *Valcyte* **(valganciclovir) and** *Valtrex* **(valacyclovir); use caution.**

Assessment

- **History:** Hypersensitivity to valganciclovir, ganciclovir, or acyclovir; cytopenia; history of cytopenic reactions; impaired renal function; pregnancy; lactation
- **Physical:** T, orientation, reflexes, urinary output, CBC, BUN, creatinine clearance

Interventions

- Administer drug with food to maximize absorption and to decrease GI upset.

⊗ *Warning* Do not exceed the recommended dosage or frequency; note that valganciclovir cannot be substituted for ganciclovir capsules on a one-to-one basis.

- Arrange for decreased dosage in patients with impaired renal function.

⊗ **Black box warning** Arrange for CBC before beginning therapy and at least weekly thereafter. Consult with physician and arrange for reduced dosage if WBC count or platelets fall. Toxicity includes granulocytopenia, anemia, and thrombocytopenia.

⊗ *Warning* Consult with pharmacy for proper disposal of unused tablets. Precautions are required for disposal of nucleoside analogues. Do not cut, crush, or allow patient to chew tablets. Avoid handling broken tablets.

- Arrange for periodic ophthalmic examinations during therapy. Drug is not a cure of the disease and deterioration may occur.
- Provide comfort measures for patients who develop fever, rash, or headache.
- Advise patients that valganciclovir can decrease sperm production in men and cause birth defects in the fetus. Advise the patient to use some form of contraception during valganciclovir therapy. Men receiving valganciclovir therapy should use some form of barrier contraception during and for at least 90 days after therapy.

⊗ **Black box warning** Advise patient that valganciclovir has caused cancer and fetal damage in animals and that risk is possible in humans.

- Maintain support therapy and program for AIDS patients who are receiving this drug as part of their overall treatment plan.

Teaching points

- Take this drug with food to help the absorption of the drug and possibly decrease GI upset. Swallow tablets whole. Do not cut, crush, or chew them.
- Drink 2 to 3 liters of water each day while taking this drug, unless otherwise instructed by your health care provider.
- Make appointments for frequent blood tests that will need to be done to determine the effects of the drug on your blood count and to determine the appropriate dosage needed. It is important that you keep appointments for these tests.
- Arrange for periodic eye examinations (every 4–6 weeks) during therapy to evaluate progress of the disease. This drug is not a cure for your retinitis.
- If you are also receiving zidovudine, the two drugs cannot be given concomitantly; severe adverse effects may occur.
- If you think you are pregnant or want to become pregnant, consult your health care provider. Use contraception during drug therapy. Male patients should use barrier contraceptives during drug therapy and for at least 90 days after therapy.
- You may experience these side effects: Decreased blood count leading to susceptibility to infection (frequent blood tests will be needed; avoid crowds and exposure to disease as

much as possible); birth defects and decreased sperm production (drug cannot be taken during pregnancy); sedation, dizziness, confusion (avoid driving or operating dangerous machinery if these effects occur).

- Report bruising, bleeding, infection, extreme fatigue, edema.

▷valproic acid
(val proe' ik)

valproic acid
Apo-Valproic Acid (CAN), Gen-Valproic (CAN), PMS-Valproic Acid (CAN), ratio-Valproic (CAN), Stavzor
Capsules: Depakene ⓄⓉⒸ

sodium valproate
Syrup: Depakene

valproate acid
Injection: Depacon
Capsules: Stavzor ⓄⓉⒸ

divalproex sodium
Tablets, enteric coated: Depakote ⓄⓉⒸ, Depakote ER ⓄⓉⒸ, Depakote Sprinkle, Divalproex, Epival (CAN)

PREGNANCY CATEGORY D

Drug class
Anticonvulsant

Therapeutic actions
Mechanism of action not understood: Antiepileptic activity may be related to the metabolism of the inhibitory neurotransmitter, GABA; divalproex sodium is a compound containing equal proportions of valproic acid and sodium valproate.

Indications
- *Valproic acid:* Sole and adjunctive therapy in simple (petit mal) and complex absence seizures; acute treatment of manic episodes associated with bipolar disorder; prophylaxis of migraine headaches; adjunctive therapy for multiple seizure disorders

- *Depakote ER:* Treatment of epilepsy in children 10 yr and older; treatment of acute manic or mixed episodes associated with bipolar disorder, with or without psychotic features
- *Depakote ER:* Treatment of bipolar mania
- *Depakote, Depakote ER:* Prophylaxis for migraine headaches
- *Divalproex, sodium valproate injection:* Treatment of complex partial seizures as monotherapy or with other antiepileptics
- Unlabeled uses: Adjunct in symptom management of schizophrenia, treatment of aggressive outbursts in children with ADHD, organic brain syndrome, status epilepticus in children

Contraindications and cautions
- Contraindicated with hypersensitivity to valproic acid, hepatic disease, or significant hepatic impairment.
- Use cautiously with children younger than 18 mo; children younger than 2 yr, especially with multiple antiepileptics, congenital metabolic disorders, severe seizures accompanied by severe mental retardation, organic brain disorders (higher risk of developing fatal hepatotoxicity); pregnancy (fetal neural tube defects; do not discontinue to prevent major seizures; discontinuing such medication is likely to precipitate status epilepticus, hypoxia and risk to both mother and fetus); lactation.

Available forms
Capsules—250 mg; DR capsules ⓄⓉⒸ—125, 250, 500 mg; syrup—250 mg/5 mL; DR tablets ⓄⓉⒸ—125, 250, 500 mg; sprinkle capsules—125 mg; injection—100 mg/mL; ER tablets ⓄⓉⒸ—125, 250, 500 mg

Dosages
Adults
Dosage is expressed as valproic acid equivalents. Initial dose is 10–15 mg/kg/day PO, increasing at 1-wk intervals by 5–10 mg/kg/day PO until seizures are controlled or side effects preclude further increases. Maximum recommended dosage is 60 mg/kg/day PO. If total dose exceeds 250 mg/day, give in divided doses.
- *Acute mania or bipolar disorder:* Initially, 25 mg/kg/day PO once daily. Dose should be increased rapidly to achieve the lowest therapeutic dose. Maximum dose 60 mg/kg/day PO (*Depakote ER* only).

V

- *Bipolar mania:* 750 mg PO daily in divided doses; do not exceed 60 mg/kg/day PO (*Divalproex DR* tablets only).
- *Migraine:* 250 mg PO bid; up to 1,000 mg/day has been used (*Divalproex DR* tablets and *Stavzor* capsules); 500 mg ER tablet PO once a day.

Pediatric patients 10 yr and older
10–15 mg/kg/day PO.

Pediatric patients 10 yr and younger
Use extreme caution. Fatal hepatotoxicity has occurred. Children younger than 2 yr are especially susceptible. Monitor all children carefully.

Pharmacokinetics

Route	Onset	Peak
Oral	Varies	1–4 hr
IV	Rapid	1 hr

Metabolism: Hepatic; $T_{1/2}$: 6–16 hr
Distribution: Crosses placenta; enters breast milk
Excretion: Urine

▼ IV FACTS

Preparation: Dilute vial in 5% dextrose injection, 0.9% sodium chloride injection or lactated Ringer injection. Stable for 24 hr at room temperature. Discard unused portions.
Infusion: Administer over 60 min, not more than 20 mg/min. Do not use more than 14 days; switch to oral products as soon as possible.

Adverse effects

- **CNS:** *Sedation,* tremor (may be dose-related), emotional upset, depression, psychosis, aggression, hyperactivity, behavioral deterioration, weakness, suicidality
- **Dermatologic:** Transient increases in hair loss, rash, petechiae
- **GI:** *Nausea, vomiting, indigestion,* diarrhea, abdominal cramps, constipation, anorexia with weight loss, increased appetite with weight gain, **life-threatening pancreatitis, hepatic failure**; elevated liver enzyme, serum bilirubin
- **GU:** Irregular menses, secondary amenorrhea
- **Hematologic:** Altered bleeding time; thrombocytopenia; bruising; hematoma formation;

frank hemorrhage; relative lymphocytosis; hypofibrinogenemia; leukopenia, eosinophilia, anemia, bone marrow suppression

Interactions

✳ Drug-drug ● Increased serum phenobarbital, primidone, ethosuximide, diazepam, zidovudine levels ● Complex interactions with phenytoin; breakthrough seizures have occurred with the combination of valproic acid and phenytoin ● Increased serum levels and toxicity with salicylates, cimetidine, chlorpromazine, erythromycin, felbamate ● Decreased effects with carbamazepine, rifampin, lamotrigine ● Decreased serum levels with charcoal ● Increased sedation with alcohol, other CNS depressants
✳ Drug-lab test ● False interpretation of urine ketone test

■ Nursing considerations

 CLINICAL ALERT!
Confusion has occurred between DR *Depakote* and *Depakote ER.* Dosage is very different and serious adverse effects can occur; use extreme caution.

Assessment

- **History:** Hypersensitivity to valproic acid; hepatic impairment; pregnancy, lactation
- **Physical:** Weight; skin color, lesions; orientation, affect, reflexes; bowel sounds, normal output; CBC and differential, bleeding time tests, LFTs, serum ammonia level, exocrine pancreatic function tests, EEG

Interventions

- Give drug with food if GI upset occurs; substitution of the enteric-coated formulation also may be of benefit; have patient swallow ER tablet whole; do not cut, crush, or chew.
⊗ Black box warning Be aware that patient may be at increased risk for suicidal ideation and suicidality; monitor accordingly.
⊗ Warning Reduce dosage, discontinue, or substitute other antiepileptics gradually; abrupt discontinuation of all antiepileptics may precipitate absence seizures.
⊗ Black box warning Arrange for frequent LFTs; discontinue drug immediately with suspected or apparent significant hepatic impairment; continue LFTs to determine if hepatic

---

Adverse effects in *italics* are most common; those in **bold** are life-threatening. ⬛ Do not crush.

impairment progresses in spite of drug discontinuation.

⊗ *Warning* Arrange for patient to have platelet counts, bleeding time determination before therapy, periodically during therapy, and prior to surgery. Monitor patient carefully for clotting defects (bruising, blood-tinged toothbrush). Discontinue if there is evidence of hemorrhage, bruising, or disorder of hemostasis.

• Monitor ammonia levels, and discontinue if there is clinically significant elevation in level.

• Monitor serum levels of valproic acid and other antiepileptics given concomitantly, especially during the first few weeks of therapy. Adjust dosage on the basis of these data and clinical response.

Black box warning Arrange for counseling for women of childbearing age who wish to become pregnant; drug may be teratogenic. Drug is not recommended for women of childbearing age because of the risk of lower cognitive test scores in children when drug is taken during pregnancy compared with other antiseizure medication.

Black box warning Discontinue the drug at any sign of pancreatitis; life-threatening pancreatitis has occurred.

⊗ *Warning* Evaluate for therapeutic serum levels—usually 50–100 mcg/mL.

Teaching points

• Take this drug exactly as prescribed. Do not chew tablets or capsules before swallowing them. Swallow them whole to prevent local irritation of mouth and throat. *Depakote Sprinkle* tablets may be opened and sprinkled on applesauce or pudding.

• Do not discontinue this drug abruptly or change dosage, except on the advice of your health care provider.

• Avoid alcohol and sleep-inducing and over-the-counter drugs. These could cause dangerous effects.

• Have frequent checkups, including blood tests, to monitor your drug response. Keep all appointments for checkups.

• Use contraceptive techniques at all times. If you want to become pregnant, consult your health care provider.

• Wear a medical ID tag to alert emergency medical personnel that you have epilepsy and are taking antiepileptic medication.

• If you have diabetes, this drug may interfere with urine tests for ketones.

• You may experience these side effects: Drowsiness (avoid driving or performing other tasks requiring alertness; take at bedtime); GI upset (take with food or milk, eat frequent small meals; if problem persists, substitute enteric-coated drug); transient increase in hair loss.

• Report bruising, pink stain on the toothbrush, yellowing of the skin or eyes, pale feces, rash, pregnancy, abdominal pain with nausea, vomiting, anorexia, thoughts of suicide.

▽ valsartan

(val sar' tan)

Diovan

PREGNANCY CATEGORY C
(FIRST TRIMESTER)

PREGNANCY CATEGORY D
(SECOND AND THIRD TRIMESTERS)

Drug classes
Angiotensin II receptor blocker
Antihypertensive

Therapeutic actions
Selectively blocks the binding of angiotensin II to specific tissue receptors found in the vascular smooth muscle and adrenal gland; this action blocks the vasoconstricting effect of the renin–angiotensin system as well as the release of aldosterone, leading to decreased BP; may prevent the vessel remodeling associated with the development of atherosclerosis.

Indications
• Treatment of hypertension, alone or in combination with other antihypertensives
• Treatment of HF in patients who are intolerant of ACE inhibitors
• Reduction in CV mortality in stable patients with left ventricular failure or left ventricular dysfunction following MI

Contraindications and cautions
• Contraindicated with hypersensitivity to valsartan, pregnancy (use during second or third trimester can cause injury or even death to fetus), lactation.

V

- Use cautiously with hepatic or renal impairment, hypovolemia.

Available forms
Tablets—40, 80, 160, 320 mg

Dosages
Adults
- *Hypertension:* 80 mg PO daily; range 80–320 mg/day.
- *HF:* Starting dose is 40 mg PO bid, titration to 80 mg and 160 mg PO bid should be done to the highest dose, as tolerated by the patient. Maximum daily dose is 320 mg daily given in divided doses. May be given in combination with other antihypertensives. Consider dosage reduction if used with diuretics.
- *Post-MI left ventricular dysfunction:* Start as early as 12 hr post-MI; 20 mg PO bid, may increase after 7 days to 40 mg PO bid; titrate to 160 mg PO bid if tolerated.

Pediatric patients 6–16 yr
- *Hypertension:* Starting dosage, 1.3 mg/kg PO once daily (up to 40 mg). Target dosage, 1.3–2.7 mg/kg PO once daily (40–160 mg/day.

Patients with severe hepatic or renal impairment
Exercise caution and monitor patient frequently.

Pharmacokinetics

Route	Onset	Peak
Oral	Varies	2–4 hr

Metabolism: Hepatic; $T_{1/2}$: 6 hr
Distribution: Crosses placenta; enters breast milk
Excretion: Feces, urine

Adverse effects
- **CNS:** *Headache, dizziness,* syncope, muscle weakness
- **CV:** Hypotension
- **Dermatologic:** Rash, inflammation, urticaria, pruritus, alopecia, dry skin
- **GI:** *Diarrhea, abdominal pain, nausea,* constipation, dry mouth, dental pain
- **Respiratory:** *URI symptoms, cough,* sinus disorders
- **Other:** Back pain, fever, gout, hyperkalemia

■ Nursing considerations
Assessment
- **History:** Hypersensitivity to valsartan; pregnancy, lactation; hepatic or renal impairment; hypovolemia
- **Physical:** Skin lesions, turgor; T; reflexes, affect; BP; R, respiratory auscultation; LFTs, renal function tests

Interventions
- Administer without regard to meals.

⊗ **Black box warning** Ensure that patient is not pregnant before beginning therapy; suggest use of barrier birth control while using drug; fetal injury and deaths have been reported.

- A breast-feeding patient should find an alternative method of feeding the infant. Depression of renin-angiotensin system in infants is potentially very dangerous.

⊗ **Warning** Alert surgeon and mark the patient's chart that valsartan is being given. Blockage of renin-angiotensin system following surgery can produce problems. Hypotension may be reversed with volume expansion.

- Monitor patient closely in any situation that may lead to decrease in BP secondary to reduction in fluid volume—excessive perspiration, dehydration, vomiting, diarrhea—because excessive hypotension can occur.

Teaching points
- Take this drug without regard to meals. Do not stop taking drug without consulting your health care provider.
- Use a barrier method of birth control while using this drug; if you become pregnant or want to become pregnant, consult your health care provider. If you are breast-feeding, you should use another method of feeding the infant while taking this drug.
- You may experience these side effects: Dizziness (avoid driving or performing hazardous tasks); headache (medications may be available to help); nausea, vomiting, diarrhea (proper nutrition is important; consult a dietitian); symptoms of upper respiratory tract infection, cough (do not self-medicate; consult your health care provider if this becomes uncomfortable).
- Report fever, chills, dizziness, pregnancy.

▷**vancomycin hydrochloride**

(van koe mye' sin)

Vancocin

PREGNANCY CATEGORY C

PREGNANCY CATEGORY B
(PULVULES)

Drug class
Antibiotic

Therapeutic actions
Bactericidal: Inhibits cell wall synthesis of susceptible organisms, causing cell death.

Indications
- Parenteral: Potentially life-threatening staphylococcal infections not treatable with other less toxic antibiotics
- Parenteral: Treatment of staphylococcal or streptococcal endocarditis
- Oral: Staphylococcal enterocolitis and antibiotic-associated pseudomembranous colitis caused by *Clostridium difficile*

Contraindications and cautions
- Contraindicated with allergy to vancomycin.
- Use cautiously with hearing loss, renal impairment, pregnancy, lactation.

Available forms
Capsules—125, 250 mg; injection—500 mg, 750 mg; 1, 5, 10 g

Dosages
Adults
500 mg–2 g/day PO in three or four divided doses for 7–10 days; 500 mg IV every 6 hr or 1 g IV every 12 hr.
- *Pseudomembranous colitis caused by* C. difficile: 125 mg PO four times a day for 10 days.

Pediatric patients
40 mg/kg/day PO in three to four divided doses for 7–10 days. 10 mg/kg/dose IV every 6 hr. Do not exceed 2 g/day.

Premature and full-term neonates
Use with caution because of incompletely developed renal function. Initial dose of 15 mg/kg IV, followed by 10 mg/kg IV every 12 hr in first week of life and every 8 hr thereafter up to age of 1 mo.

- *Pseudomembranous colitis caused by* C. difficile: 40 mg/kg/day in four divided doses PO for 7–10 days. Do not exceed 2 g/day.

Geriatric patients or patients with renal failure
Monitor dosage and serum levels very carefully. Dosage nomogram is available for determining the dose according to creatinine clearance (see manufacturer's insert).

Pharmacokinetics

Route	Onset	Peak
Oral	Varies	Varies
IV	Rapid	End of infusion

Metabolism: $T_{1/2}$: 4–6 hr
Distribution: Crosses placenta; may enter breast milk
Excretion: Urine

▼ IV FACTS

Preparation: Not for IM administration. Reconstitute with 10 mL sterile water for injection; 500 mg/mL concentration results. Dilute reconstituted solution with 100–200 mL of 0.9% sodium chloride injection or D_5W for intermittent infusion. For continuous infusion (use only if intermittent therapy is not possible), add 2–4 (1–2 g) vials reconstituted solution to sufficiently large volume of 0.9% sodium chloride injection or D_5W to permit slow IV drip of the total daily dose over 24 hr. Refrigerate reconstituted solution; stable over 14 days. Further diluted solution is stable for 24 hr.
Infusion: For intermittent infusion, infuse every 6 hr over at least 60 min, no faster than 1,000 mg/hr, to avoid irritation, flushing, hypotension, throbbing back and neck pain. Give continuously slowly over 24 hr.
Incompatibilities: Do not mix with amobarbital, chloramphenicol, dexamethasone, heparin, barbiturates, warfarin.
Y-site incompatibility: Do not give with foscarnet.

Adverse effects
- **CNS:** Ototoxicity
- **CV:** Hypotension (IV administration)
- **Dermatologic:** *Urticaria,* macular rashes
- **GI:** *Nausea*
- **GU:** *Nephrotoxicity*
- **Hematologic:** Eosinophilia, neutropenia

V

- **Other:** Superinfections; "red neck" or "red man syndrome" (sudden and profound fall in BP, fever, chills, paresthesias, erythema of the neck and back)

Interactions

✳ **Drug-drug** • Increased neuromuscular blockade with atracurium, pancuronium, tubocurarine, vecuronium • Increased risk of ototoxicity or nephrotoxicity when administered with other ototoxic or nephrotoxic drugs (aminoglycosides, amphotericin B, bacitracin, cisplatin)

■ Nursing considerations

Assessment

- **History:** Allergy to vancomycin, hearing loss, renal impairment, pregnancy, lactation
- **Physical:** Site of infection, skin color, lesions; orientation, reflexes, auditory function; BP, perfusion; R, adventitious sounds; CBC, LFTs, renal function tests, auditory tests

Interventions

⊗ **Warning** Drug may increase risk of development of multiple drug-resistant organisms; ensure appropriate use of drug.

⊗ **Warning** Observe the patient very closely when giving parenteral solution, particularly the first doses; "red man" syndrome can occur (see adverse effects); slow administration decreases the risk of adverse effects.

- Culture site of infection before beginning therapy.
- Monitor renal function tests with prolonged therapy.

⊗ **Warning** Evaluate for safe serum levels; concentrations of 60–80 mcg/mL are toxic.

Teaching points

- This drug is available only in the IV and oral forms.
- Do not stop taking this drug without notifying your health care provider.
- Take the full prescribed course of this drug.
- You may experience these side effects: Nausea (eat frequent small meals); changes in hearing; superinfections in the mouth, vagina (frequent hygiene measures will help).
- Report ringing in the ears, loss of hearing, difficulty voiding, rash, flushing.

▷ **vardenafil hydrochloride**
(var den' ah fill)

Levitra, Staxyn

PREGNANCY CATEGORY B

Drug classes

Impotence drug
Phosphodiesterase type 5 inhibitor

Therapeutic actions

Selectively inhibits cyclic guanosine monophosphate (cGMP) specific phosphodiesterase type 5. The mechanism of penile erection involves the release of nitric oxide into the corpus cavernosum of the penis during sexual stimulation. Nitrous oxide activates cGMP, which causes smooth muscle relaxation allowing the flow of blood into the corpus cavernosum. Vardenafil prevents the breakdown of cGMP by phosphodiesterase, leading to increased cGMP levels and prolonged smooth muscle relaxation promoting the flow of blood into the corpus cavernosum.

Indications

- Treatment of ED occurring in the presence of sexual stimulation
- Unlabeled use: Raynaud phenomenon

Contraindications and cautions

- Contraindicated with allergy to any component of the tablet, concurrent use of nitrates or alpha blockers.
- Contraindicated for women or children.
- Use cautiously with hepatic or renal impairment; with anatomic deformation of the penis, with known cardiac disease (effects of sexual activity need to be evaluated), congenital prolonged QT interval, unstable angina; hypotension (systolic pressure less than 90 mm Hg); uncontrolled hypertension (greater than 170/110 mm Hg), severe hepatic impairment; end-stage renal disease with dialysis; hereditary degenerative retinal disorders.

Available forms

Tablets—2.5, 5, 10, 20 mg; orally disintegrating tablets—10 mg

Dosages

Adults
5–10 mg PO taken 1 hr before anticipated sexual activity; range 5–20 mg PO. Limit use to once per day.

Pediatric patients
Not intended for use in children.

Geriatric patients and those with moderate hepatic impairment
Starting dose of 5 mg PO is suggested.

Pharmacokinetics

Route	Onset	Peak
Oral	Rapid	30–120 min

Metabolism: Hepatic, $T_{1/2}$: 4–5 hr
Distribution: Not intended for use in women, no clear studies on crossing the placenta or entering breast milk
Excretion: Feces

Adverse effects

- **CNS:** *Headache,* abnormal vision, dizziness, hypertonia, insomnia, somnolence, vertigo, ischemic optic neuropathy, sudden hearing loss
- **CV:** *Flushing,* angina, chest pain, hypertension, hypotension, **MI,** palpitation, postural hypotension, tachycardia
- **GI:** *Dyspepsia,* diarrhea, abdominal pain, dry mouth, esophagitis, gastritic, GERD
- **GU:** Abnormal ejaculation, priapism
- **Respiratory:** Rhinitis, sinusitis, dyspnea, epistaxis, pharyngitis
- **Other:** Flulike symptoms, edema, pain, rash, sweating

Interactions

✳ **Drug-drug** ⊗ *Warning* Possible severe hypotension and serious cardiac events if combined with nitrates, alpha blockers; this combination must be avoided.

• Possible increased vardenafil levels and effects if taken with ketoconazole, itraconazole, erythromycin; monitor patient and reduce dosage as needed, usually to 2.5 mg/day PO • Increased vardenafil serum level if combined with indinavir, ritonavir; if these drugs are being used, limit vardenafil dose to 2.5 mg in a 24-hr period

■ Nursing considerations

Assessment
- **History:** Allergy to any component of the tablet, concurrent use of nitrates or alpha block-

ers; unstable angina, hypotension, uncontrolled hypertension; severe hepatic impairment; end-stage renal disease with dialysis; hereditary degenerative retinal disorders; anatomical deformation of the penis; cardiac disease, congenital prolonged QT interval
- **Physical:** Orientation, affect; skin color, lesions; R, adventitious sounds; P, BP, ECG, LFTs, renal function tests; hearing, vision examinations

Interventions
- Ensure diagnosis of ED and determine underlying causes and other appropriate treatment.
- Advise patient that drug does not work without sexual stimulation. Limit use to once per day.
- Teach patient to contact health care provider about any loss of vision or hearing.
- Remind patient that drug does not protect against STDs and appropriate measures should be taken.

⊗ *Warning* Advise patient to never take this drug with nitrates or alpha blockers; serious and even fatal complications can occur.

Teaching points
- Take this drug 60 minutes before anticipated sexual activity. The drug will have no effect unless there is sexual stimulation.
- This drug will not protect you from sexually transmitted diseases; use appropriate precautions.
- Do not take this drug if you are taking any nitrates or alpha blockers; serious side effects or death can occur.
- Many drugs may interact with vardenafil; always consult your health care provider before taking any drug, including over-the-counter drugs and herbal therapies; dosage adjustments may be needed.
- You may experience these side effects: Headache, dizziness, upset stomach, runny nose; these side effects should go away within a couple of hours. If side effects persist, consult your health care provider.
- Stop drug and consult your health care provider immediately if you experience sudden loss of vision or hearing.
- Report difficult or painful urination, vision changes, fainting, erection that persists for longer than 4 hours, sudden loss of vision.

V

▷varenicline tartrate
(var en' ah klin)

Chantix

PREGNANCY CATEGORY C

Drug classes
Nicotine receptor agonist
Smoking deterrent

Therapeutic actions
Selectively binds with specific neuronal nicotinic acetylcholine receptors; acts as an agonist at these sites while preventing nicotine binding to these receptors. This mechanism is thought to aid in smoking cessation.

Indications
• Aid to smoking cessation treatment

Contraindications and cautions
• Contraindicated with hypersensitivity to any component of the drug, lactation.
• Use cautiously with pregnancy, history of CV disease.

Available forms
Capsules—0.5, 1 mg

Dosages
Adults
Patient should pick a date to stop smoking and begin drug therapy 1 wk before that date; or patient can begin drug and quit smoking between days 8 and 35 of treatment.
Days 1–3, 0.5 mg/day PO; days 4–7, 0.5 mg PO bid; day 8 until the end of treatment, 1 mg PO bid. Drug should be taken after eating with a full glass of water. Treatment should last 12 wk; patients who successfully quit smoking in that time may benefit from another 12 wk to increase the likelihood of long-term abstinence. Patients who fail to quit smoking during the 12 wk or who relapse after treatment can be treated again when factors leading to failed attempt have been identified and addressed.
Pediatric patients
Not recommended for children younger than 18 yr.
Patients with severe renal impairment
Initially, 0.5 mg/day PO; titrate to 0.5 mg PO bid. If on dialysis, 0.5 mg/day.

Pharmacokinetics

Route	Onset	Peak
Oral	Rapid	3–4 hr

Metabolism: Minimal; $T_{1/2}$: 24 hr
Distribution: May cross placenta; may enter breast milk
Excretion: Unchanged in urine

Adverse effects
• **CNS:** *Headache, insomnia, abnormal dreams,* somnolence, lethargy, dysgeusia, behavioral changes, suicidal ideation, agitation, depression
• **CV:** Angina; **MI, stroke,** TIA, peripheral vascular disease
• **Dermatologic:** Rash
• **GI:** *Nausea,* cbdominal pain, *flatulence,* dyspepsia, *vomiting, constipation,* dry mouth, GERD, increased appetite, anorexia
• **Respiratory:** Rhinorrhea, dyspnea, URIs
• **Other:** Fatigue, malaise, asthenia

Interactions
✳ **Drug-drug** • Increased risk of adverse effects if combined with nicotine transdermal systems and cimetidine; avoid these combinations

■ Nursing considerations
Assessment
• **History:** Hypersensitivity to any component of drug; lactation, pregnancy; smoking history
• **Physical:** Orientation, affect, reflexes; R, breath sounds; abdominal examination

Interventions
⊗ **Black box warning** There is a risk of serious mental health events, including changes in behavior, depressed mood, hostility, and suicidal thoughts, with drug administration; monitor patient accordingly.
• Instruct patient to pick a day to quit smoking; drug therapy should begin 1 wk before that date, or patient can start drug and quit between days 8 and 35 of treatment.
• Administer drug after patient has eaten, with a full glass of water.
• Provide patient with educational materials and support for smoking cessation.
• Encourage patient to continue efforts at smoking cessation even if a lapse occurs.

Adverse effects in *italics* are most common; those in **bold** are life-threatening. ⓒⓡⓢ Do not crush.

- Provide safety measures if insomnia, lethargy occur.
- Be aware that patient with a history of CV disease may be at increased risk for potentially serious CV events; monitor patient closely and advise patient to immediately report new or worsening signs and symptoms of CV disease.
- Suggest use of contraceptive measures; help patient select another method of feeding the infant if she is breast-feeding during drug therapy.
- Consider a second 12-wk course of therapy if patient is successful at smoking cessation to improve the chances of continued abstinence.
- Monitor patient for behavioral changes and suicidal ideation; stop drug and get medical attention if these effects occur.

Teaching points

- This drug reacts with nicotine receptors in your brain to decrease your desire for nicotine and will alter your reaction to nicotine when you do smoke, making it less desirable. You should have support for your efforts to stop smoking.
- You will take *Chantix* after eating with a full glass of water. The dose will need to be adjusted.
- Select a day to stop smoking. Begin taking *Chantix* 1 week before that day. Days 1–3 of that week, you will take 0.5 mg (white tablet) once each day. Days 4–7, you will take 0.5 mg twice a day, once in the morning and once in the evening. From day 8 until you are finished with treatment, you will take 1 mg (blue tablet) twice a day, once in the morning and once in the evening. The course of treatment is usually 12 weeks. If you have good success, you may have another 12-week course to help increase the chances of long-term success.
- If you forget a dose of the drug, take it as soon as you remember; if you remember close to the time for your next dose, just take that dose. Do not double the dose.
- If you have a relapse, keep taking the drug and continue to try to stop smoking.
- It is not known if this drug could affect a fetus. If you are pregnant or are thinking about becoming pregnant, consult your health care provider before using this drug; you should not smoke when you are pregnant.
- It is not known how this drug could affect a breast-feeding infant. If you are breast-

feeding, use another method of feeding the infant during drug treatment.
- Stop drug and seek medical help if agitation, depression, or thoughts of suicide occur.
- You may experience these side effects: nausea, insomnia (when starting therapy; they should pass as your body adjusts to the drug; if they should become severe, contact your health care provider).
- Report severe constipation, severe vomiting, failure to quit smoking, behavioral changes, thoughts of suicide, new or worsening signs and symptoms of cardiovascular disease.

▽velaglucerase

See Appendix R, *Less commonly used drugs*.

▽vemurafenib

See Appendix R, *Less commonly used drugs*.

▽venlafaxine hydrochloride
*(vin lah **facks'** in)*

Effexor XR ⊙ⓝ⊙

PREGNANCY CATEGORY C

Drug classes
Antidepressant
Anxiolytic

Therapeutic actions
Potentiates the neurotransmitter activity in the CNS; inhibits serotonin, norepinephrine, and dopamine reuptake leading to prolonged stimulation at neuroreceptors.

Indications
- Treatment of major depressive disorder
- Treatment of generalized anxiety disorder (ER capsules only)
- Treatment of social anxiety disorder (ER only)
- Treatment of panic disorder, with or without agoraphobia (ER capsules only)
- Unlabeled uses: PMDD, hot flushes, autism, pain, binge-eating disorder, diabetic neuropathy, migraine prevention

V

Contraindications and cautions

- Contraindicated with allergy to venlafaxine, use of MAOIs within last 14 days.
- Use cautiously with pregnancy, lactation, patients whose underlying medical condition might be compromised by increased heart rate (hyperthyroidism, HF, recent MI).

Available forms

Tablets—25, 37.5, 50, 75, 100 mg; ER capsules⊕ —37.5, 75, 150 mg; ER tablets⊕ — 37.5, 75, 150, 225 mg

Dosages
Adults

- *Depression:* Starting dose, 75 mg/day PO in two to three divided doses taken with food. May be increased at intervals of no less than 4 days up to 225 mg/ day PO to achieve desired effect; maximum dose 375 mg/day PO in three divided doses. ER forms: 37.5 mg/day PO may; increase to 75 mg/day PO in 4–7 days. Maximum dose, 225 mg/day.
- *Transfer to or from MAOI:* At least 14 days should elapse from the discontinuation of the MAOI and the starting of venlafaxine; allow at least 7 days to elapse from the stopping of venlafaxine to the starting of an MAOI.
- *Generalized anxiety disorder/social anxiety:* 75–225 mg/day PO should be taken on a daily basis, not as needed (ER only).
- *Panic disorder:* 37.5 mg/day PO for 7 days, then increase based on patient response to 75 mg/day for 7 days, and then 75 mg/day weekly increases to a maximum of 225 mg/day (ER only).

Pediatric patients

Safety and efficacy not established.

Patients with renal or hepatic impairment

For patients with creatinine clearance of 10–70 mL/min, reduce dosage by 25%–50%. For patients on dialysis, reduce dosage by 50% (give after dialysis completion on dialysis days). For patients with hepatic impairment, reduce total daily dose by 50%, and increase very slowly to achieve desired effect.

Pharmacokinetics

Route	Onset	Duration
Oral	2–3 hr	48 hr
Oral (ER)	5.5 hr	9 hr

Metabolism: Hepatic; $T_{1/2}$: 1.3–2 hr
Distribution: Crosses placenta; may enter breast milk
Excretion: Urine

Adverse effects

- **CNS:** *Somnolence, dizziness, insomnia, nervousness,* anxiety, tremor, dreams, suicidal ideation, abnormal dreams
- **CV:** Vasodilation, hypertension, tachycardia
- **Dermatologic:** *Sweating,* rash, pruritus
- **GI:** *Nausea, constipation, anorexia,* diarrhea, vomiting, dyspepsia, *dry mouth,* flatulence
- **GU:** *Abnormal ejaculation,* impotence, urinary frequency
- **Other:** *Headache, asthenia,* infection, chills, chest pain

Interactions

✳ **Drug-drug** • Increased serum levels and risk of toxicity, including serious to fatal reactions, with MAOIs (within last 14 days), cimetidine • Serotonin syndrome may occur if combined with trazodone • Increased sedation with alcohol
✳ **Drug-alternative therapy** • Increased sedation and hypnotic effects with St. John's Wort

■ Nursing considerations
Assessment

- **History:** Allergy to venlafaxine; use of MAOIs within last 14 days; pregnancy, lactation
- **Physical:** Skin color, T, lesions; reflexes, gait, sensation, cranial nerve evaluation; mucous membranes, abdominal examination, normal output; P, BP, peripheral perfusion

Interventions

- Limit amount of drug available; increased risk of successful suicide attempts with this antidepressant.
- Give with food to decrease GI effects. Ensure that patient swallows ER capsules whole; do not allow patient to cut, crush, or chew them.
- Advise patient to use contraceptives.

⊗ *Black box warning* Monitor patients for suicidal ideation, especially when beginning therapy or changing dosage; high risk in children, adolescents, and young adults.

Teaching points

- Take with food to decrease GI upset. Do not cut, crush, or chew capsules; swallow capsules whole.
- Avoid alcohol while using this drug.
- This drug cannot be taken during pregnancy; use controceptives. If you become pregnant, consult your health care provider.
- You may experience these side effects: Loss of appetite, nausea, vomiting, dry mouth (use frequent mouth care; eat frequent small meals; suck sugarless candies); constipation (request bowel program); dizziness, drowsiness, tremor (avoid driving or operating dangerous machinery).
- Report rash, hives, increased depression, thoughts of suicide, pregnancy.

DANGEROUS DRUG

▷verapamil hydrochloride
(ver ap' a mill)

Apo-Verap (CAN), Apo-Verap SR ᴏᴺᴄ (CAN), Calan, Calan SR ᴏᴺᴄ, Covera-HS, Gen-Verapamil (CAN), Gen-Verapamil SR ᴏᴺᴄ (CAN), Isoptin SR ᴏᴺᴄ, Nu-Verap (CAN), Verelan ᴏᴺᴄ, Verelan PM ᴏᴺᴄ

PREGNANCY CATEGORY C

Drug classes
Antianginal
Antiarrhythmic
Antihypertensive
Calcium channel blocker

Therapeutic actions
Inhibits the movement of calcium ions across the membranes of cardiac and arterial muscle cells; calcium is involved in the generation of the action potential in specialized automatic and conducting cells in the heart, in arterial smooth muscle, and in excitation-contraction coupling in cardiac muscle cells; inhibition of transmembrane calcium flow results in the depression of impulse formation in specialized cardiac pacemaker cells, slowing of the velocity of conduction of the cardiac impulse, the depression of myocardial contractility, and the dilation of coronary arteries and arterioles and peripheral arterioles; these effects lead to de-

creased cardiac work, decreased cardiac energy consumption, and in patients with vasospastic (Printzmetal) angina, increased delivery of oxygen to myocardial cells.

Indications
- Angina pectoris due to coronary artery spasm (Printzmetal variant angina)
- Effort-associated angina
- Chronic stable angina
- Unstable, crescendo, preinfarction angina
- Essential hypertension
- Treatment of chronic atrial fibrillation or flutter with digoxin
- Parenteral: Treatment of supraventricular tachyarrhythmias
- Parenteral: Temporary control of rapid ventricular rate in atrial flutter or atrial fibrillation
- Unlabeled uses: Prevention of migraine, tardive dyskinesia, cluster headache, hypertrophic cardiomyopathy

Contraindications and cautions
- Contraindicated with allergy to verapamil; sick sinus syndrome, except with ventricular pacemaker; heart block (second- or third-degree); hypotension; pregnancy, lactation.
- Use cautiously with idiopathic hypertrophic subaortic stenosis, cardiogenic shock, severe HF, impaired renal or hepatic function, and in patients with atrial flutter or atrial fibrillation and an accessory to bypass tract.

Available forms
Tablets—40, 80, 120 mg; SR tablets ᴏᴺᴄ—120, 180, 240 mg; ER tablets ᴏᴺᴄ—120, 180, 240 mg; injection—2.5 mg/mL; ER capsules ᴏᴺᴄ—100, 120, 180, 200, 240, 300, 360 mg

Dosages
Adults
Oral
Immediate-release
- *Angina:* 80–120 mg PO tid. Doses of 40 mg PO tid may be used. Maintenance 240–480 mg daily.
- *Arrhythmias:* 240–480 mg/day PO in divided doses.
- *In digitalized adults:* 240–320 mg/day PO.
- *Hypertension:* 40–80 mg PO tid.
ER
- *Capsules:* 120–240 mg/day PO in the morning. Titrate dose to a maximum 480 mg/day.

V

- *Tablets:* 120–180 mg/day PO in the morning. Titrate to maximum 240 mg every 12 hr.

SR
- 120–180 mg/day PO. Titrate up to a maximum 480 mg PO in the morning.

Parenteral

IV use only. Initial dose, 5–10 mg over 2 min; may repeat dose of 10 mg 30 min after first dose if initial response is inadequate.

Pediatric patients

IV

1 yr and younger: Initial dose, 0.1–0.2 mg/kg IV over 2 min.

1–15 yr: Initial dose, 0.1–0.3 mg/kg IV over 2 min. Do not exceed 5 mg. Repeat above dose 30 min after initial dose if response is not adequate. Repeat dose should not exceed 10 mg.

Geriatric patients or patients with renal impairment

Reduce dosage, and monitor patient response carefully. Give IV doses over 3 min to reduce risk of serious side effects. Administer IV doses very slowly, over 2 min.

Pharmacokinetics

Route	Onset	Peak	Duration
Oral	30 min	1–2.2 hr	3–7 hr
IV	1–5 min	3–5 min	2 hr

Metabolism: Hepatic; $T_{1/2}$: 3–7 hr
Distribution: Crosses placenta; enters breast milk
Excretion: Urine

IV FACTS

Preparation: No further preparation required.
Infusion: Infuse very slowly over 2–3 min.
Y-site incompatibilities: Do not give with albumin, ampicillin, nafcillin, oxacillin, sodium bicarbonate, amphotericin B, hydralazine, aminophylline.

Adverse effects

- **CNS:** *Dizziness,* vertigo, emotional depression, sleepiness, *headache*
- **CV:** *Peripheral edema, hypotension,* arrhythmias, bradycardia; AV heart block
- **GI:** *Nausea, constipation*
- **Other:** Muscle fatigue, diaphoresis, rash

Interactions

✳ Drug-drug ⊗ *Warning* Risk of serious cardiac effects with IV beta blockers; do not give these drugs within 48 hr before or 24 hr after IV verapamil.

- Increased cardiac depression with beta blockers • Additive effects of verapamil and digoxin to slow AV conduction • Increased serum levels of digoxin, carbamazepine, prazosin, quinidine • Increased respiratory depression with atracurium, pancuronium, tubocurarine, vecuronium • Decreased effects with calcium, rifampin • Increased risk of hypotension if combined with other antihypertensives

✳ Drug-food • Decreased metabolism and risk of toxic effects if combined with grapefruit juice; avoid this combination

■ Nursing considerations

Assessment

- **History:** Allergy to verapamil; sick sinus syndrome; heart block; IHSS; cardiogenic shock, severe HF; hypotension; impaired hepatic or renal function; pregnancy, lactation
- **Physical:** Skin color, edema; orientation, reflexes; P, BP, baseline ECG, peripheral perfusion, auscultation; R, adventitious sounds; liver evaluation, normal output; LFTs, renal function tests, urinalysis

Interventions

⊗ *Warning* Monitor patient carefully (BP, cardiac rhythm, and output) while drug is being titrated to therapeutic dose. Dosage may be increased more rapidly in hospitalized patients under close supervision.

- Ensure that patient swallows SR or ER tablets whole; patient should not cut, crush, or chew them.
- Monitor BP very carefully with concurrent doses of antihypertensives.
- Monitor cardiac rhythm regularly during stabilization of dosage and periodically during long-term therapy.
- Administer SR or ER form in the morning with food to decrease GI upset.
- Protect IV solution from light.
- Monitor patients with renal or hepatic impairment carefully for possible drug accumulation and adverse reactions.

Teaching points

- Take extended- or sustained-release form in the morning with food; swallow it whole; do not cut, crush, or chew it. Do not drink grapefruit juice while using this drug.
- You may experience these side effects: Nausea, vomiting (eat frequent small meals); headache (adjust lighting, noise, and temperature;

request medication); dizziness, sleepiness (avoid driving or operating dangerous equipment); emotional depression (reversible); constipation (request aid).

- Report irregular heartbeat, shortness of breath, swelling of the hands or feet, pronounced dizziness, nausea, constipation.

▷ verteporfin

See Appendix R, *Less commonly used drugs.*

▷ vigabatrin

See Appendix R, *Less commonly used drugs.*

▷ vilazodone hydrochloride
(vil az' ah dohn)

Viibryd

PREGNANCY CATEGORY C

Drug classes
Antidepressant
SSRI

Therapeutic actions
Acts as an antagonist at central serotonin receptor sites and as an SSRI; this action is thought to account for its antidepressive effect.

Indications
- Treatment of adults with major depressive disorder

Contraindications and cautions
- Contraindicated with history of serious hypersensitivity reactions to vilazodone; concurrent use of MAOIs, lactation.
- Use cautiously with seizure disorders, bipolar disorders, pregnancy.

Available forms
Tablets—10, 20, 40 mg

Dosages
Adults
Initially, 10 mg/day PO for 7 days, followed by 20 mg/day PO for 7 days; then increase to main-

tenance dosage of 40 mg/day PO taken with food.
Pediatric patients
Safety and efficacy not established.

Pharmacokinetics

Route	Onset	Peak
Oral	Intermediate	4–5 hr

Metabolism: Hepatic; T$_{1/2}$; 25 hr
Distribution: May cross placenta; may enter breast milk
Excretion: Urine

Adverse effects
- **CNS:** *Dizziness,* somnolence, paresthesia, tremor, *insomnia,* restlessness, abnormal dreams, suicidality, activation of mania, **seizures**
- **CV:** Palpitations
- **GI:** *Nausea, diarrhea, dry mouth, vomiting,* dyspepsia, flatulence, gastroenteritis
- **GU:** Delayed ejaculation, erectile dysfunction, decreased libido
- **Other: Neuroleptic malignant syndrome,** bleeding disorders

Interactions
✷ **Drug-drug** ⊗ *Warning* Possible fatal reactions with MAOIs; do not administer concurrently or within 2 wk of MAOIs • Increased risk of bleeding with drugs that affect blood clotting, such as NSAIDs, aspirin, warfarin; monitor patient carefully if this combination is used • Potential for serious adverse effects if combined with strong CYP3A4 inhibitors (ketoconazole, diltiazem); if this combination is used, decrease vilazodone dosage to 20 mg/day • Increased risk of serotonin syndrome if combined with other drugs that increase serotonin levels • Increased risk of CNS effects if taken with alcohol; avoid this combination

■ Nursing considerations
Assessment
- **History:** Serious hypersensitivity reactions to vilazodone; concurrent use of MAOIs, history of seizure disorders, bipolar disorders, pregnancy, lactation
- **Physical:** T; orientation, reflexes; P; abdominal exam, renal and liver function tests

V

Interventions

⊗ **Black box warning** There is a high risk of suicidality in children, adolescents, and young adults; establish suicide precautions for severely depressed patients and limit quantity of drug dispensed. Vilazodone is not approved for use in children.

• Administer drug in the morning with food.

⊗ **Warning** Taper drug when discontinuing, to avoid withdrawal effects.

• Provide safety measures if CNS effects occur.

• Monitor patient for signs and symptoms of mania/hypomania at the start of therapy.

• Alert patient that full therapeutic effects may not be seen for up to 4 wk.

Teaching points

• You should take this drug once a day in the morning with food.

• If you forget a dose, take it as soon as you remember; then resume your usual daily schedule. Do not make up skipped doses and do not take more than one dose each day.

• Avoid consuming alcohol while taking this drug; serious effects could occur.

• You may experience increased bleeding if you are also taking nonsteroidal anti-inflammatory drugs or other drugs that increase bleeding risk. Report any increase in bleeding episodes.

• You should not stop this drug suddenly. If the drug is to be discontinued, your health care provider will taper the dosage. Make sure you always have the drug on hand.

• It is not known how this drug could affect a fetus; serious adverse effects have occurred with other drugs in this class. If you are pregnant or thinking about becoming pregnant, discuss this with your health care provider.

• This drug may enter breast milk, but it is not known how this could affect a breast-feeding infant. If you are breast-feeding, you should use another method of feeding the infant.

• You may experience these side effects: Dizziness, sleepiness, drowsiness, changes in mental functioning (avoid driving or operating hazardous machinery if this occurs); nausea, vomiting, weight loss (small, frequent meals may help); sexual dysfunction (if this becomes a problem, discuss with your health care provider).

• Report fever, seizures, mania, thoughts of suicide.

DANGEROUS DRUG

▷vinBLAStine sulfate (VLB)

(vin blas' teen)

Velban

PREGNANCY CATEGORY D

Drug classes

Antineoplastic
Mitotic inhibitor

Therapeutic actions

Inhibits microtubule formation in the mitotic spindle, leading to cell-cycle arrest in dividing cells in metaphase.

Indications

• Palliative treatment for lymphocytic lymphoma, histiocytic lymphoma, generalized Hodgkin lymphoma (stages III and IV), mycosis fungoides, advanced testicular carcinoma, Kaposi sarcoma, Letterer-Siwe disease

• Treatment of choriocarcinoma, breast cancer unresponsive to other therapies

• Hodgkin lymphoma (advanced) alone or in combination therapies

• Advanced testicular germinal-cell cancers alone or in combination therapy

Contraindications and cautions

• Contraindicated with allergy to vinblastine, leukopenia (unless leukopenia is the result of the disease being treated); acute infection; pregnancy; lactation.

• Use cautiously with liver disease.

Available forms

Powder for injection—10 mg; injection—1 mg/mL

Dosages

⊗ **Warning** Do not administer more than once a wk because of leukopenic response.

Adults

Initial dose, 3.7 mg/m² as a single IV dose, followed at weekly intervals by increasing doses at 1.8 mg/m² increments; a conservative regimen follows:

Adverse effects in *italics* are most common; those in **bold** are life-threatening. ⊕ Do not crush.

Week	Dose (mg/m² IV)
First wk	3.7
Second wk	5.5
Third wk	7.4
Fourth wk	9.25
Fifth wk	11.1

Use these increments until a maximum dose of 18.5 mg/m² is reached; do not increase dose after WBC count is reduced to 3,000/mm³.

• *Maintenance therapy:* When dose produces WBC count of 3,000/mm³, use a dose one increment smaller for weekly maintenance. Do not give another dose until WBC count is 4,000/mm³ even if 7 days have passed. Duration of therapy depends on disease and response; up to 2 yr may be needed.

Pediatric patients
Initial dose, 2.5 mg/m² as a single IV dose, followed at weekly intervals by increasing doses at 1.25 mg/m² increments; a conservative regimen follows:

Week	Pediatric Dose (mg/m² IV)
First wk	2.5
Second wk	3.75
Third wk	5
Fourth wk	6.25
Fifth wk	7.5

Use these increments until a maximum dose of 12.5 mg/m² is reached; do not increase dose after WBC count is reduced to 3,000/mm³.

Patients with hepatic impairment
For serum bilirubin exceeding 3 mg/dL, decrease dose by 50%.

Pharmacokinetics

Route	Onset
IV	Slow

Metabolism: Hepatic; $T_{1/2}$: 3.7 min, then 1.6 hr, then 24.8 hr
Distribution: Crosses placenta; enters breast milk
Excretion: Bile

▼ IV FACTS

Preparation: Add 10 mL of sodium chloride injection preserved with phenol or benzyl alcohol to the vial for a concentration of 1 mg/mL. Refrigerate drug; opened vials are stable for 28 days when refrigerated.

Infusion: Inject into tubing of a running IV or directly into the vein over 1 min or as a prolonged infusion over up to 96 hr. Rinse syringe and needle with venous blood prior to withdrawing needle from vein (to minimize extravasation). Do not inject into an extremity with poor circulation or repeatedly into the same vein.
Y-site incompatibility: Do not give with furosemide.

Adverse effects

• **CNS:** Numbness, paresthesias, peripheral neuritis, mental depression, loss of deep tendon reflexes, *headache,* seizures, malaise, *weakness,* dizziness
• **CV:** Hypertension
• **Dermatologic:** *Alopecia,* vesiculation of the skin
• **GI:** *Nausea, vomiting,* pharyngitis, vesiculation of the mouth, ileus, *diarrhea,* constipation, *anorexia,* abdominal pain, rectal bleeding, hemorrhagic enterocolitis
• **GU:** Aspermia
• **Hematologic:** *Leukopenia,* anemia, thrombocytopenia
• **Local:** *Local cellulitis,* phlebitis, sloughing if extravasation occurs
• **Other:** Pain in tumor site

Interactions

❉ **Drug-drug** • Decreased serum concentrations of phenytoins • Risk of toxicity if combined with erythromycin
❉ **Drug-food** • Decreased metabolism and risk of toxic effects if combined with grapefruit juice; avoid this combination

■ Nursing considerations

CLINICAL ALERT!
Confusion has occurred between vinblastine and vincristine; use extreme caution if giving either drug.

Assessment

• **History:** Allergy to vinblastine, leukopenia, acute infection, liver disease, pregnancy, lactation
• **Physical:** Weight; hair; T; reflexes, gait, sensation, orientation, affect; mucous membranes, abdominal examination, rectal examination; CBC, LFTs, serum albumin

Interventions

- Ensure that patient is not pregnant before administering; advise patients to use contraceptive measures.

⊗ **Black box warning** Do not administer IM or subcutaneously due to severe local reaction and tissue necrosis. Fatal if given intrathecally. Use extreme caution.

⊗ **Black box warning** Watch for irritation and infiltration; extravasation causes tissue damage and necrosis. If it occurs, discontinue injection immediately, and give remainder of dose in another vein. Consult physician to arrange for hyaluronidase injection into local area, after which apply moderate heat to disperse drug and minimize pain.

⊗ **Warning** Avoid contact with the eyes; if contact occurs, immediately wash thoroughly with water.

- Consult physician if antiemetic is needed for severe nausea and vomiting.
- Check CBC before each dose; leukopenia nadir occurs at 5–10 days, recovery at 7–14 days post infusion.

Teaching points

- Prepare a calendar for dates to return for treatment and drug therapy. Avoid grapefruit juice while you are using this drug.
- This drug should not be used during pregnancy. Use birth control. If you become pregnant, consult your health care provider.
- Have regular blood tests to monitor the drug's effects.
- You may experience these side effects: Loss of appetite, nausea, vomiting, mouth sores (use frequent mouth care; eat frequent small meals; maintain nutrition; request an antiemetic); constipation (a bowel program may be ordered); malaise, weakness, dizziness, numbness and tingling (avoid injury); loss of hair, rash (obtain a wig; keep the head covered in extremes of temperature).
- Report severe nausea, vomiting, pain or burning at injection site, abdominal pain, rectal bleeding, fever, chills, acute infection.

DANGEROUS DRUG

▷ **vinCRIStine sulfate (LCR, VCR)**

(*vin **kris'** teen*)

Oncovin, Vincasar PFS

vincristine sulfate liposome injection
Marqibo

PREGNANCY CATEGORY D

Drug classes
Antineoplastic
Mitotic inhibitor

Therapeutic actions
Mitotic inhibitor: Arrests mitotic division at the stage of metaphase by inhibiting microtubular formation; exact mechanism of action unknown.

Indications
- Acute leukemia
- Hodgkin lymphoma, non-Hodgkin lymphoma, rhabdomyosarcoma, neuroblastoma, Wilms tumor as part of combination therapy
- Unlabeled uses: Kaposi sarcoma, breast cancer, bladder cancer, CNS tumors, multiple myeloma, chronic lymphocytic leukemia, idiopathic thrombocytopenic purpura
- ◼ **NEW INDICATION:** Treatment of adults with Philadelphia chromosome-negative acute lymphoblastic leukemia (ALL) who have relapsed after treatment with two or more regimens of antileukemia therapy

Contraindications and cautions
- Contraindicated with allergy to vincristine, leukopenia, acute infection, pregnancy, lactation, demyelinating form of Charcot-Marie-Tooth syndrome.
- Use cautiously with neuromuscular disease, diabetes insipidus, hepatic impairment.

Available forms
Injection—1 mg/mL; liposomal injection—5 mg/31 mL

Dosages
Adults
1.4 mg/m^2 IV at weekly intervals.

- *Philadelphia chromosome–negative ALL:* 2.25 mg/m² IV over 1 hr every 7 days *(Marqibo).*

Pediatric patients

1–2 mg/m² IV weekly. Maximum dose, 2 mg/dose.

- *Weight less than 10 kg or body surface area less than 1 m²:* 0.05 mg/kg IV once per wk.
- *Weight more than 10 kg:* 1–2 mg/m² IV once per wk.

Geriatric patients or patients with hepatic impairment

For serum bilirubin exceeding 3 mg/dL, reduce dosage by 50%.

Pharmacokinetics

Route	Onset	Peak
IV	Varies	15–30 min

Metabolism: Hepatic; T₁/₂: 5 min, then 2.3 hr, then 85 hr

Distribution: Crosses placenta; enters breast milk

Excretion: Feces, urine

▼ IV FACTS

Preparation: No further preparation required; drug should be refrigerated.

Infusion: Inject solution directly into vein or into the tubing of a running IV infusion.

Y-site incompatibility: Do not give with furosemide.

Adverse effects

- **CNS:** *Ataxia, cranial nerve manifestations;* foot drop, headache, seizures, bladder neuropathy, *paresthesias,* sensory impairment, *neuritic pain, muscle wasting,* SIADH, optic atrophy, transient cortical blindness, ptosis, diplopia, photophobia
- **GI:** *Constipation,* oral ulcerations, abdominal cramps, vomiting, diarrhea, intestinal necrosis
- **GU:** Acute uric acid nephropathy, polyuria, dysuria, urinary retention
- **Hematologic:** Leukopenia
- **Local:** Local irritation, cellulitis if extravasation occurs
- **Other:** *Weight loss, loss of hair,* fever, death with serious overdose

Interactions

✳ **Drug-drug** • Decreased serum levels and therapeutic effects of digoxin • If L-asparaginase is administered first, the hepatic clearance of vincristine may be reduced. Give vincristine 12–24 hr before L-asparaginase to minimize toxicity

✳ **Drug-food** • Decreased metabolism and risk of toxic effects if combined with grapefruit juice; avoid this combination

■ Nursing considerations

CLINICAL ALERT!
Confusion has occurred between vincristine and vinblastine; use extreme caution if giving either drug.

Assessment

- **History:** Allergy to vincristine, leukopenia, acute infection, neuromuscular disease, diabetes insipidus, hepatic impairment, pregnancy, lactation
- **Physical:** Weight; hair; T; reflexes, gait, sensation, cranial nerve evaluation, ophthalmic examination; mucous membranes, abdominal examination; CBC, serum sodium, LFTs, urinalysis

Interventions

- Ensure that patient is not pregnant before administering; using barrier contraceptives is advised.
- Tell patient to avoid grapefruit juice while being treated with this drug.

⊗ *Black box warning* Do not administer IM or subcutaneously due to severe local reaction and tissue necrosis. Do not give intrathecally; drug is fatal if given intrathecally. Use extreme caution.

⊗ *Black box warning* Watch for irritation and infiltration; extravasation causes tissue damage and necrosis. If extravasation occurs, discontinue injection immediately and give remainder of dose in another vein. Consult with physician to arrange for hyaluronidase injection into local area, and apply heat to disperse the drug and to minimize pain.

- Arrange for wig or suitable head covering if hair loss occurs; ensure that patient's head is covered in extremes of temperature.
- Monitor urine output and serum sodium; if SIADH occurs, consult with physician, and

V

arrange for fluid restriction and perhaps a potent diuretic. Dispose of excretions properly.
- Consider stimulant laxative to prevent or treat constipation.

Teaching points
- Prepare a calendar of dates to return for treatment and additional therapy.
- Avoid grapefruit juice while you are using this drug.
- This drug cannot be taken during pregnancy; use birth control. If you become pregnant, consult your health care provider.
- Have regular blood tests to monitor the drug's effects.
- You may experience these side effects: Loss of appetite, nausea, vomiting, mouth sores (frequent mouth care, frequent small meals may help; maintain nutrition; request an antiemetic); constipation (bowel program may be ordered); sensitivity to light (wear sunglasses; avoid bright lights); numbness, tingling, change in style of walking (reversible; may persist for up to 6 weeks); hair loss (transient; obtain a wig or other suitable head covering; keep the head covered at extremes of temperature).
- Report change in frequency of voiding; swelling of ankles, fingers, and so forth; changes in vision; severe constipation, abdominal pain.

DANGEROUS DRUG

▽ vinorelbine tartrate
(vin oh rel' been)

Navelbine

PREGNANCY CATEGORY D

Drug classes
Antineoplastic
Mitotic inhibitor

Therapeutic actions
Inhibits microtubule formation in the mitotic spindle, leading to cell-cycle arrest in dividing cells in metaphase.

Indications
- First-line treatment of ambulatory patients with unresectable advanced non–small-cell lung cancer

- Treatment of stage IV non–small-cell lung cancer alone or with cisplatin
- Treatment of stage III non–small-cell lung cancer with cisplatin
- Unlabeled uses: Breast cancer, ovarian cancer, Hodgkin lymphoma, desmoid tumors and fibromatosis, advanced Kaposi sarcoma, non-Hodgkin lymphoma

Contraindications and cautions
- Contraindicated with allergy to vinca alkaloids, pretreatment granulocyte counts of 1,000 cells/mm^3 or less, pregnancy, lactation.
- Use cautiously with liver disease.

Available forms
Injection—10 mg/mL

Dosages
Adults
⊗ **Warning** Do not administer more than once a wk because of leukopenic response.
- *Monotherapy:* Initial dose, 30 mg/m^2 as single IV dose; repeat once a wk until progression of disease or toxicity limits use.
- *With cisplatin:* 25 mg/m^2 IV every 7 days in combination with cisplatin 100 mg/m^2 IV given every 4 wk, or 30 mg/m^2 IV with cisplatin 120 mg/m^2 IV given on days 1 and 29, then every 6 wk.
Pediatric patients
Safety and efficacy not established.
Patients with hepatic impairment
If total serum bilirubin concentration is 2.1–3 mg/dL, reduce dose to 50% of starting dose; if greater than 3 mg/dL, reduce to 25% of starting dose.

Pharmacokinetics

Route	Onset
IV	Slow

Metabolism: Hepatic; T$_{1/2}$: 22–66 hr
Distribution: Crosses placenta; enters breast milk
Excretion: Bile, feces

▼ IV FACTS

Preparation: Dilute for 50- or 10-mg solution. Supplied as single-use vials only. Discard after withdrawing solution.
Infusion: Inject into tubing of a running IV or directly into the vein over 6–10 min. Rinse

---

syringe and needle with venous blood prior to withdrawing needle from vein (to minimize extravasation). Do not inject into an extremity with poor circulation or repeatedly into the same vein. Follow with 150–250 mL saline or dextrose to decrease phlebitis. If administered via IV piggyback, should be done via central access.

Adverse effects

- **CNS:** Numbness, paresthesias (less common than with other vinca alkaloids); headache, weakness, dizziness
- **CV:** Chest pain
- **Dermatologic:** Alopecia, vesiculation of the skin
- **GI:** Nausea, vomiting, pharyngitis, vesiculation of the mouth, ileus, diarrhea, constipation, anorexia, abdominal pain, *increased liver enzymes*
- **Hematologic: Granulocytopenia, leukopenia, anemia, thrombocytopenia**
- **Local:** Local cellulitis, phlebitis, sloughing with extravasation
- **Other:** Myalgia, arthralgia, fatigue

Interactions

✳ Drug-drug • Acute pulmonary reactions with mitomycin • Increased risk of granulocytopenia with cisplatin • Risk of neuropathies if combined or given sequentially with paclitaxel; monitor patient closely

■ Nursing considerations
Assessment

- **History:** Allergy to vinca alkaloids, leukopenia, acute infection, liver disease, pregnancy, lactation
- **Physical:** Weight; hair; T; reflexes, gait, sensation, orientation, affect; mucous membranes, abdominal examination; CBC, LFTs, serum albumin

Interventions

- Ensure that patient is not pregnant before use; advise patient to use barrier contraceptives.

⊗ **Black box warning** Do not administer IM or subcutaneously—severe local reaction and tissue necrosis occur. Fatal if given intrathecally. Use extreme caution.

⊗ **Black box warning** Watch for irritation and infiltration; extravasation can cause tissue damage and necrosis. If extravasation should occur, discontinue injection immediately and consult physician to arrange for hyaluronidase

injection into local area, after which apply moderate heat to disperse drug and minimize pain.

⊗ **Warning** Avoid contact with the eyes; if contact occurs, immediately wash thoroughly with water.

- Consult physician if antiemetic is needed for severe nausea and vomiting.

⊗ **Black box warning** Check CBC before each dose; severe granulocytosis is possible. Granulocyte count should be 1,000 cells/m^3 prior to treatment. Leukopenia/granulocytopenia nadir occurs at 7–10 days, recovery at 14–21 days. Adjust or delay dose as appropriate.

Teaching points

- Prepare a calendar for dates to return for treatment and additional therapy.
- This drug should not be used during pregnancy. Use birth control. If you become pregnant, consult your health care provider.
- Have regular blood tests to monitor the drug's effects.
- You may experience these side effects: Loss of appetite, nausea, vomiting, mouth sores (frequent mouth care, frequent small meals may help; maintain nutrition; request an antiemetic); constipation (bowel program may be ordered); malaise, weakness, dizziness, numbness and tingling (avoid injury); loss of hair, rash (obtain a wig; keep the head covered in extremes of temperature).
- Report severe nausea, vomiting, pain or burning at injection site, abdominal pain, rectal bleeding, fever, chills, acute infection.

▽vismodegib

See Appendix R, *Less commonly used drugs.*

▽voriconazole
*(vor ah **kon'** ah zole)*

Vfend

PREGNANCY CATEGORY D

Drug class
Triazole antifungal

Therapeutic actions
Inhibits fungal ergosterol biosynthesis leading to cell membrane rupture and cell death in susceptible fungi.

Indications

- Treatment of invasive aspergillosis
- Treatment of serious fungal infections caused by *Scedosporium apiospermum, Pseudallescheria boydii,* and *Fusarium* species in patients intolerant of or refractory to other therapy
- Treatment of esophageal candidiasis
- Treatment of candidemia in nonneutropenic patients with disseminated skin infections and abdominal, kidney, bladder wall, and wound infections

Contraindications and cautions

- Contraindicated with hypersensitivity to voriconazole, treatment with other drugs that could prolong the QTc interval, severe hepatic impairment, galactose intolerance, and in patients taking the following drugs: Ergot alkaloids, sirolimus, rifabutin, rifampin, carbamazepine, long-acting barbiturates, or other CYP3A4 substrates.
- Use cautiously with known allergies to other azoles; pregnancy; lactation.

Available forms

Tablets—50, 200 mg; powder for injection—200 mg to be reconstituted to 10 mg/mL; powder for oral suspension—40 mg/mL

Dosages

Adults

Loading dose of 6 mg/kg IV every 12 hr for two doses, then 3–4 mg/kg IV every 12 hr or 200 mg PO every 12 hr. Switch to oral dose as soon as patient is able:

Weight less than 40 kg: 100 mg PO every 12 hr; may increase to 150 mg PO every 12 hr if needed.

Weight of 40 kg or more: 200 mg PO every 12 hr; may increase to 300 mg PO every 12 hr if needed.

- *Esophageal candidiasis:* 200–300 mg PO every 12 hr (reduce to 100–150 mg PO every 12 hr if weight is less than 40 kg) for 14 days or for at least 7 days following symptom resolution.

Pediatric patients younger than 12 yr

Safety and efficacy not established.

Pharmacokinetics

Route	Peak	Duration
Oral	1–2 hr	96 hr
IV	Onset of infusion	96 hr

Metabolism: Hepatic; $T_{1/2}$: 24 hr
Distribution: Crosses placenta; may enter breast milk
Excretion: Urine

▼ IV FACTS

Preparation: Reconstitute powder with 19 mL of water for injection, resulting solution contains 10 mg/mL. Shake the vial until powder is dissolved. Further dilute *Vfend* to obtain a concentration of 5 mg/mL using 0.9% sodium chloride, lactated Ringer solution, 5% dextrose and lactated Ringer solution, 5% dextrose and 0.45% sodium chloride, 5% dextrose, 5% dextrose and 20 mEq potassium chloride, 0.45% sodium chloride, 5% dextrose and 0.9% sodium chloride. Do not use if solution is not clear or if it contains particulate matter. Use immediately after reconstitution. Discard any unused solution.

Infusion: Infuse over 1–2 hr at no more than 3 mg/kg/hr.

Incompatibilities: Do not infuse with parenteral nutrition, blood products, electrolyte supplements, any alkaline solution, other drug infusions.

Adverse effects

- **CNS:** *Headache, visual disturbance,* hallucinations, dizziness
- **CV:** Tachycardia, BP changes, vasodilation, chest pain, *peripheral edema,* prolonged QTc interval
- **GI:** *Nausea, vomiting, diarrhea,* dry mouth, abnormal LFTs, *abdominal pain*
- **Hematologic:** Anemia, thrombocytopenia, leukopenia
- **Other:** *Fever,* chills, *rash,* pruritus, **anaphylactic reaction, Stevens-Johnson syndrome**

Interactions

✴ **Drug-drug** ⊗ *Warning* Decreased serum levels and effectiveness of voriconazole if combined with rifampin, rifabutin, carbamazepine, phenobarbital, mephobarbital; avoid these combinations.

⊗ *Warning* Increased serum levels of sirolimus, pimozide, quinidine, ergot alkaloids if taken with voriconazole; avoid these combinations.

⊗ *Warning* Increased plasma concentration of ergot alkaloids, which may lead to ergotism; avoid this combination.

• Possible alterations in serum levels and effectiveness of warfarin, tacrolimus, statins, oral anticoagulants, benzodiazepine, calcium channel blockers, sulfonylureas, vincristine, vinblastine, when taken with voriconazole; patients should be monitored closely and appropriate dosage adjustments made • Altered serum levels and risk of adverse effects from both drugs when voriconazole is taken concomitantly with phenytoin, omeprazole, protease inhibitors; patients should be monitored frequently and appropriate dosage adjustments made • Increased plasma levels of cyclosporine; reduce cyclosporine dose to one-half of the starting dose and monitor cyclosporine blood levels frequently; after voriconazole therapy ends, increase cyclosporine dose as needed ✳ **Drug alternative therapy** • Risk of increased serum levels and toxicity if combined with St. John's Wort; this combination is contraindicated

■ **Nursing considerations**
Assessment
• **History:** Hypersensitivity to *Escherichia coli* products, filgrastim, sickle cell disease, pregnancy, lactation
• **Physical:** Skin color, lesions, hair; T; orientation, affect; abdominal examination, status of mucous membranes; LFTs, renal function tests, CBC, platelets

Interventions
• Obtain baseline liver function before beginning therapy and repeat during the course of therapy. Stop drug at first sign of significant liver toxicity.
⊗ *Warning* Check patient's medications carefully before beginning drug therapy; voriconazole is associated with many drug interactions.
• Oral tablets contain lactose. Do not give to patients with galactose intolerance, Lapp lactase deficiency, or glucose-galactose malabsorption.

• Administer oral drug on an empty stomach, at least 1 hr before or 2 hr after meals.
• Monitor vision changes. Advise patient not to drive at night or perform potentially hazardous tasks because of possible visual disturbances.
• Protect patient from exposure to strong sunlight while using this drug.
• Women of childbearing age should be advised to use barrier contraceptives while using this drug because of the risk of fetal death or abnormalities.
• Provide appropriate comfort and supportive measures for headache or GI discomfort.
• Arrange for frequent small meals if nausea and vomiting are a problem.

Teaching points
• This drug will be started by IV infusion and then you will switch to an oral form.
• Take the drug on an empty stomach 1 hour before or 2 hours after a meal.
• Avoid exposure to strong sunlight while you are using this drug.
• Do not use St. John's Wort while taking this drug.
• If you are a women of childbearing age, you should use barrier contraceptives while taking this drug; it has been associated with fetal abnormalities.
• Tell any other health care provider that you see that you are taking this drug; it has been associated with many drug interactions when taken with other drugs. Adjustments may be needed.
• You may experience these side effects: Nausea and vomiting (eat frequent small meals); headache, fever (analgesics may be available that will help); visual changes (do not drive at night, avoid performing potentially hazardous tasks while on this drug).
• Report fever, chills, changes in color of stool or urine, visual disturbances.

▽**vorinostat**

See Appendix R, *Less commonly used drugs.*

V

DANGEROUS DRUG

▽warfarin sodium
(war' far in)

Apo-Warfarin (CAN), Coumadin,
Gen-Warfarin (CAN), Jantoven

PREGNANCY CATEGORY X

Drug classes
Coumarin derivative
Oral anticoagulant

Therapeutic actions
Interferes with the hepatic synthesis of vitamin K–dependent clotting factors (factors II-prothrombin, VII, IX, and X), resulting in their eventual depletion and prolongation of clotting times.

Indications
- Venous thrombosis and its extension, treatment, and prophylaxis
- Treatment of thromboembolic complications of atrial fibrillation (AF) with embolization, and cardiac valve replacement
- PE treatment and prophylaxis
- Prophylaxis of systemic embolization after acute MI

Contraindications and cautions
- Contraindicated with allergy to warfarin; SBE; hemorrhagic disorders; TB; hepatic diseases; GI ulcers; renal disease; indwelling catheters, spinal puncture; aneurysm; diabetes; visceral carcinoma; uncontrolled hypertension; severe trauma (including recent or contemplated CNS, eye surgery; recent placement of IUD); threatened abortion, menometrorrhagia; pregnancy (fetal damage and death); lactation (suggest using heparin if anticoagulation is required).
- Use cautiously with HF; diarrhea; fever; thyrotoxicosis; senile, psychotic, or depressed patients.

Available forms
Tablets—1, 2, 2.5, 3, 4, 5, 6, 7.5, 10 mg; powder for injection—5 mg, reconstitutes to 2 mg/mL

Dosages
Dosage and administration must be individualized for each patient according to patient's prothrombin time (PT) and INR response.

Target of therapy is INR of 2–3 for AF, DVT, and PE or 2.5–3.5 for mechanical heart valve. IV use is reserved for situations in which oral warfarin is not feasible. Dosages are the same for oral and IV forms.

Adults
Initially, 2–5 mg/day PO. Adjust dosage according to PT response. For maintenance, 2–10 mg/day PO based on INR.

Geriatric patients
Lower doses are usually needed; begin with smaller doses than those recommended for adults, and closely monitor PT ratio or INR.

Pharmacokinetics

Route	Peak	Duration
Oral	1.5–3 days	2–5 days

Metabolism: Hepatic; $T_{1/2}$: 1–2.5 days
Distribution: Crosses placenta; enters breast milk
Excretion: Feces, urine

▼ IV FACTS
Preparation: Reconstitute vial with 2.7 mL of sterile water. Protect from light. Use within 4 hr of reconstitution.
Infusion: Inject slowly over 1–2 min; switch to oral preparation as soon as possible.

Adverse effects
- **Dermatologic:** *Alopecia, urticaria, dermatitis*
- **GI:** *Nausea,* vomiting, anorexia, abdominal cramping, diarrhea, retroperitoneal hematoma, hepatitis, jaundice, mouth ulcers
- **GU:** Priapism, nephropathy, red-orange urine
- **Hematologic:** Granulocytosis, leukopenia, eosinophilia; **hemorrhage**—GI or urinary tract bleeding (hematuria, dark stools; paralytic ileus, intestinal obstruction from hemorrhage into GI tract); petechiae and purpura, bleeding from mucous membranes; hemorrhagic infarction, vasculitis, skin necrosis; adrenal hemorrhage and resultant adrenal insufficiency; compressive neuropathy secondary to hemorrhage near a nerve
- **Other:** Fever, "purple toes" syndrome

Interactions
✳ **Drug-drug** • Increased bleeding tendencies with salicylates, chloral hydrate, clofibrate,

Adverse effects in *italics* are most common; those in **bold** are life-threatening. ⬛ Do not crush.

disulfiram, chloramphenicol, metronidazole, cimetidine, ranitidine, co-trimoxazole, sulfin-pyrazone, quinidine, quinine, thyroid drugs, glucagon, danazol, erythromycin, androgens, amiodarone, cefotetan, cefazolin, cefoxitin, cef-triaxone, meclofenamate, mefenamic acid, famotidine, nizatidine, nalidixic acid, aceta-minophen, allopurinol, quinolones, azole an-tifungals, fluvastatin, simvastatin, lovastatin, NSAIDs, alcohol ● Decreased anticoagulation ef-fect may occur with barbiturates, griseofulvin, rifampin, phenytoin, carbamazepine, vitamin K, vitamin E, cholestyramine ● Altered effects with methimazole, propylthiouracil ● Increased activity and toxicity of phenytoin when taken with oral anticoagulants

✳ **Drug-lab test** ● Red-orange discoloration of alkaline urine may interfere with some lab tests

✳ **Drug-alternative therapy** ● Increased risk of bleeding if combined with angelica, cat's claw, chamomile, chondroitin, feverfew, garlic, ginkgobiloba, goldenseal, grape seed extract, green leaf tea, horse chestnut seed, psyllium, fish oil, vitamin E, and tumeric

■ **Nursing considerations**

Assessment

● **History:** Allergy to warfarin; SBE; hemor-rhagic disorders; TB; hepatic diseases; GI ul-cers; renal disease; indwelling catheters, spinal puncture; aneurysm; diabetes; visceral carci-noma; uncontrolled hypertension; severe trau-ma; threatened abortion, menometrorrhagia; pregnancy; lactation; HF; diarrhea; fever; thy-rotoxicosis; senility, psychosis, or depression

● **Physical:** Skin lesions, color, T; orientation, reflexes, affect; P, BP, peripheral perfusion, baseline ECG; R, adventitious sounds; liver evaluation, bowel sounds, normal output; CBC, urinalysis, guaiac stools, PT, LFTs, re-nal function tests

Interventions

● Genetic testing can help to determine reason-able dosage. Decreased clearance occurs with CYP2C9*2 and CYP2C9*3 variant alleles and VKORC1 mutation.

● Do not use drug if patient is pregnant (hep-arin is anticoagulant of choice); advise pa-tient to use contraceptives.

● Monitor PT ratio or INR regularly to adjust dosage.

● Administer IV form to patients stabilized on *Coumadin* who are not able to take oral drug. Dosages are the same. Return to oral form as soon as feasible.

● Do not change brand names once stabilized; bioavailability may be a problem.

⊗ *Black box warning* Evaluate patient regularly for signs of blood loss (petechiae, bleeding gums, bruises, dark stools, dark urine). Maintain INR ratio of 2–3, 2.5–3.5 with me-chanical prosthetic valves or recurrent systemic emboli; risk of serious to fatal bleeding exists.

● Do not give patient any IM injections.

⊗ *Warning* Double check all drugs ordered for potential drug interactions; dosages of both drugs may need to be adjusted.

● Use caution when discontinuing other drugs; warfarin dosage may need to be adjusted; carefully monitor PT values.

● Keep vitamin K readily available in case of overdose.

● Arrange for frequent follow-up, including blood tests to evaluate drug effects.

⊗ *Warning* Evaluate for therapeutic effects: INR within therapeutic range.

Teaching points

● Many factors may change your body's response to this drug—fever, change of diet, change of environment, other medications. Do not drink alcohol while taking this drug. Your dosage may have to be changed repeatedly. Write down changes that are prescribed.

● Do not start or stop taking any medication without consulting your health care provider. Other drugs can affect your anticoagulant; starting or stopping another drug can cause excessive bleeding or interfere with the de-sired drug effects.

● Carry or wear a medical ID tag to alert emer-gency medical personnel that you are taking this drug.

● Avoid situations in which you could be eas-ily injured (contact sports, shaving with a straight razor).

● Have periodic blood tests to check on the drug action. These tests are important.

● Use contraception; do not become pregnant while taking this drug.

● You may experience these side effects: Stom-ach bloating, cramps (transient); loss of hair, rash; orange-red discoloration to the urine (if upsetting, add vinegar to your urine and the color should disappear).

W

- Report unusual bleeding (from brushing your teeth, excessive bleeding from injuries, excessive bruising), black or bloody stools, cloudy or dark urine, sore throat, fever, chills, severe headaches, dizziness, suspected pregnancy.

▷ **zafirlukast**
(zah fur' luh kast)

Accolate

PREGNANCY CATEGORY B

Drug classes
Antiasthmatic
Leukotriene receptor antagonist

Therapeutic actions
Selectively and competitively blocks receptor for leukotriene D_4 and E_4, components of SRS-A, thus blocking airway edema, smooth muscle constriction, and cellular activity associated with inflammatory process that contribute to signs and symptoms of asthma.

Indications
- Prophylaxis and long-term treatment of bronchial asthma in adults and children 5 yr and older
- Unlabeled use: Chronic urticaria

Contraindications and cautions
- Contraindicated with hypersensitivity to zafirlukast or any of its components, acute asthma attacks, status asthmaticus, hepatic impairment including hepatic cirrhosis.
- Use cautiously in patients who previously required corticosteroid therapy to control asthma; with renal impairment; as oral steroid use is decreased; pregnancy; lactation.

Available forms
Tablets—10, 20 mg

Dosages
Adults and patients 12 yr and older
20 mg PO bid on an empty stomach 1 hr before or 2 hr after eating.
Pediatric patients 5–11 yr
10 mg PO bid on an empty stomach.

Pharmacokinetics

Route	Onset	Peak
Oral	Rapid	3 hr

Metabolism: Hepatic; $T_{1/2}$: 10 hr
Distribution: Crosses placenta; enters breast milk
Excretion: Feces, urine

Adverse effects
- **CNS:** *Headache,* dizziness, myalgia, behavior and mood changes
- **GI:** Nausea, diarrhea, abdominal pain, vomiting, liver enzyme elevation, **hepatotoxicity**
- **Other:** Generalized pain, fever, accidental injury, infection; **Churg-Strauss syndrome** (eosinophilia, vasculitic rash, pulmonary and cardiac complications) when oral steroid dose is reduced

Interactions
✴ **Drug-drug** • Increased risk of bleeding with warfarin; these patients should have INR done regularly and warfarin dose decreased accordingly • Potential for increased effects and toxicity of calcium channel blockers, cyclosporine • Decreased effectiveness with erythromycin, theophylline • Possible severe reaction when oral steroid dose is reduced while on zafirlukast; monitor patients very closely

✴ **Drug-food** • Bioavailability decreased markedly by presence of food; administer at least 1 hr before or 2 hr after meals

■ Nursing considerations
Assessment
- **History:** Hypersensitivity to zafirlukast; impaired renal or hepatic function; pregnancy, lactation; acute asthma or bronchospasm
- **Physical:** T; orientation, reflexes; R, adventitious sounds; GI evaluation; LFTs, renal function tests

Interventions
- Administer on an empty stomach 1 hr before or 2 hr after meals.
- Ensure that drug is taken continually for optimal effect.
- Monitor LFTs; risk of hepatotoxicity.
- ⊗ **Warning** Do not administer for acute asthma attack or acute bronchospasm.
- ⊗ **Warning** There is a risk of neuropsychiatric events, mood and behavior changes with

Adverse effects in *italics* are most common; those in **bold** are life-threatening. ⊞ Do not crush.

drug administration. Monitor patient accordingly; discontinue drug if these occur.

Teaching points
- Take this drug on an empty stomach, 1 hour before or 2 hours after meals.
- Take this drug regularly as prescribed; do not stop taking it during symptom-free periods; do not stop taking it without consulting your health care provider.
- Do not take this drug for acute asthma attack or acute bronchospasm; this drug is not a bronchodilator; routine emergency procedures should be followed during acute attacks.
- Avoid use of over-the-counter medications while using this drug; many of them contain products that can interfere with drug or cause serious side effects. If you think that you need one of these products, consult your health care provider.
- You may experience these side effects: Dizziness (use caution when driving or performing activities that require alertness); nausea, vomiting (eat frequent small meals); headache (analgesics may be helpful).
- Report fever, acute asthma attacks, severe headache.

▽ **zaleplon**
(zal' ah plon)

Sonata

PREGNANCY CATEGORY C

CONTROLLED SUBSTANCE C-IV

Drug class
Sedative-hypnotic (nonbenzodiazepine)

Therapeutic actions
Interacts with GABA-B$_2$ receptor complex to cause suppression of neurons leading to sedation and hypnosis.

Indications
- Short-term treatment of insomnia

Contraindications and cautions
- Contraindicated with hypersensitivity to zaleplon, lactation.
- Use cautiously with impaired hepatic or respiratory function, depressed patients, pregnancy, labor and delivery.

Available forms
Capsules—5, 10 mg

Dosages
Adults
10 mg PO at bedtime. Patient must remain in bed for 4 hr after taking the drug. Do not exceed 20 mg/day.
Pediatric patients
Safety and efficacy not established.
Geriatric patients or debilitated patients
5 mg PO at bedtime. Do not exceed 10 mg/day.
Patients with hepatic impairment
Mild to moderate impairment: 5 mg/day
Severe impairment: Not recommended.

Pharmacokinetics

Route	Onset	Peak
Oral	Rapid	1 hr

Metabolism: Hepatic; T$_{1/2}$: 1 hr
Distribution: Crosses placenta; may enter breast milk
Excretion: Urine

Adverse effects
- **CNS:** *Headache,* depression, drowsiness, somnolence, dizziness, abnormal vision, lack of coordination, *short-term memory impairment,* complex sleep-related behaviors
- **GI:** Diarrhea, nausea
- **Hypersensitivity:** Generalized allergic reactions; pruritus, rash; **anaphylaxis; angioedema**

Interactions
✴ **Drug-drug** • Increased sedation with alcohol or other CNS depressants; avoid this combination • Risk of increased serum levels and toxicity with cimetidine and other CYP3A4 inhibitors • Decreased levels and loss of therapeutic effect if combined with rifampin

■ Nursing considerations
Assessment
- **History:** Hypersensitivity to zaleplon, impaired hepatic or respiratory function, pregnancy, labor or delivery, lactation, depression
- **Physical:** T, orientation, affect, reflexes, vision examination; P, BP; bowel sounds, normal output, liver evaluation; LFTs

Z

Interventions

- Do not prescribe or dispense more than 1 month's supply at a time.
- ⊗ **Warning** Limit amount of drug dispensed to depressed patients.
- Administer to patient at bedtime; onset of action is rapid and sleep usually occurs within 20 min; encourage patient to remain in bed for 4 hr after taking drug to ensure patient safety.
- Help patients with prolonged insomnia to seek the cause of their problem and not to rely on drugs for sleep (eg, ingestion of stimulants such as caffeine shortly before bedtime, fear).
- Institute appropriate additional measures for rest and sleep (eg, back rub, quiet environment, warm milk, reading).

Teaching points

- Take this drug exactly as prescribed. Do not exceed prescribed dosage. Long-term use is not recommended. Time your drug dose to allow you to go to bed immediately after taking the drug. Drug effects will be felt for 4 hours; after that time you may safely become active again.
- You may experience these side effects: Drowsiness, allergic reactions, swelling, dizziness, blurred vision (avoid driving a car or performing tasks requiring alertness or visual acuity if these occur); diarrhea (ensure ready access to bathroom facilities), sleep disorders.
- Report rash, sore throat, fever, bruising, allergic reaction, swelling, complex sleep-related behaviors.

▽ **zanamivir**
(zan am' ah ver)

Relenza

PREGNANCY CATEGORY C

Drug classes

Antiviral
Neuroaminidase inhibitor

Therapeutic actions

Selectively inhibits influenza virus neuroaminidase; by blocking the actions of this enzyme, there is decreased viral release from infected cells, increased formation of viral aggregates, and decreased spread of the virus.

Indications

- Prevention and treatment of uncomplicated acute illness due to influenza virus in adults and children 7 yr and older who have been symptomatic for no more than 2 days
- Prevention of influenza in patients 5 yr and older
- Unlabeled use: Treatment of H1N1 infection

Contraindications and cautions

- Contraindicated with allergy to any component of the drug.
- Use cautiously with pregnancy, lactation, asthma, COPD, or severe medical conditions.

Available forms

Powder blister for inhalation—5 mg

Dosages

Adults and children 7 yr and older
Treatment: Two inhalations (one 5-mg blister per inhalation administered with a *Diskhaler* device, for a total of 10 mg) bid at 12-hr intervals for 5 days. Should be started within 2 days of onset of flu symptoms; give two doses on the first treatment day, at least 2 hr apart; subsequent doses should be separated by 12 hr.

Adults and children 5 yr and older
Prevention in community outbreak: Two inhalations (10 mg) per day for 28 days. Dose should be given at about the same time each day.
Prevention in household exposure: Two inhalations (10 mg) per day for 10 days. Dose should be given at about the same time each day.

Pharmacokinetics

Route	Onset	Peak
Inhalation	Rapid	1–2 hr

Metabolism: Hepatic; $T_{1/2}$: 2.5–5 hr
Distribution: Crosses placenta; may enter breast milk
Excretion: Feces, urine

Adverse effects

- **CNS:** *Headache*, dizziness
- **GI:** *Nausea*, vomiting, *diarrhea, anorexia*
- **Respiratory:** Cough; *rhinitis;* bronchitis; ear, nose, and throat infections; **bronchospasm; serious respiratory effects**
- **Other:** Flulike symptoms, bacterial infections

Adverse effects in *italics* are most common; those in **bold** are life-threatening. ⬚ Do not crush.

■ Nursing considerations

Assessment
- **History:** Allergy to any components of the drug; COPD, asthma; pregnancy, lactation
- **Physical:** T; orientation, reflexes; R, adventitious sounds; bowel sounds

Interventions
- Administer using a *Diskhaler* delivery system. Demonstrate use of system to patient.
- Encourage patient to complete full course of therapy; advise patient that risk of transmission of flu to others is not decreased.
- Administer bronchodilators before using zanamivir if they are due at the same time as zanamivir dose.

⊗ *Warning* Caution patients with asthma or COPD of the risk of bronchospasm; a fast-acting inhaled bronchodilator should be on hand in case bronchospasm occurs; zanamivir should be discontinued and physician consulted promptly if respiratory symptoms worsen.

Teaching points
- Take this drug every 12 hours, at the same time each day, for as many days as prescribed. Use the *Diskhaler* delivery system provided.
- Take the full course of therapy as prescribed; this drug does not decrease the risk of transmitting the virus to others.
- If a bronchodilator is being used to treat a respiratory problem, the bronchodilator should be used before this drug.
- You may experience these side effects: Nausea, vomiting, loss of appetite, diarrhea; headache, dizziness (use caution if driving or operating dangerous machinery).
- Report severe diarrhea, severe nausea, worsening of respiratory symptoms.

▽**ziconotide**

See Appendix R, *Less commonly used drugs.*

▽**zidovudine**
(azidothymidine, AZT, Compound S)
(zid o vew' den)

Retrovir

PREGNANCY CATEGORY C

Drug class
Antiviral

Therapeutic actions
Thymidine analogue isolated from the sperm of herring; drug is activated to a triphosphate form that inhibits replication of some retroviruses, including HIV, HTLV III, alpha retrovirus, lymphadenopathy-associated virus.

Indications
- Management of certain adult patients with symptomatic HIV infection in combination with other antiretrovirals
- Prevention of maternal–fetal HIV transmission

Contraindications and cautions
- Contraindicated with life-threatening allergy to any component, lactation.
- Use cautiously with compromised bone marrow, impaired renal or hepatic function, pregnancy.

Available forms
Capsules—100 mg; tablets—300 mg; syrup—50 mg/5 mL; injection—10 mg/mL

Dosages
Adults
Oral
- *Symptomatic HIV infection:* 600 mg PO daily in divided doses as either 200 mg tid or 300 mg bid. Monitor hematologic indices every 2 wk. If significant anemia (Hgb less than 7.5 g/dL, reduction of more than 25%) or reduction of granulocytes more than 50% below baseline occurs, dose interruption is necessary until evidence of bone marrow recovery is seen. If less severe bone marrow depression occurs, a dosage reduction may be adequate.
- *Prevention of maternal–fetal transmission:* 100 mg PO five times/day until the start of labor.
IV
1 mg/kg IV 5–6 times/day infused over 1 hr. During labor and delivery 2 mg/kg IV loading dose; then 1 mg/kg/hr until umbilical cord is clamped.
Pediatric patients 6 wk–12 yr
4 to less than 9 kg: 24 mg/kg/day PO in two to three divided doses.
9 to less than 30 kg: 18 mg/kg/day PO in two to three divided doses.

Z

30 kg and over: 600 mg/day PO in two to three divided doses.

Infants born to HIV-infected mothers

2 mg/kg PO every 6 hr starting within 12 hr of birth to 6 wk of age or 1.5 mg/kg IV over 30 min every 6 hr.

Pharmacokinetics

Route	Onset	Peak
Oral	Varies	30–90 min
IV	Rapid	End of infusion

Metabolism: Hepatic; $T_{1/2}$: 30–60 min
Distribution: Crosses placenta; enters breast milk
Excretion: Urine

▼ IV FACTS

Preparation: Remove desired dose from vial, and dilute in D_5W to a concentration no greater than 4 mg/mL. Discard after 24 hr. Protect from light.
Infusion: Administer over 60 min; avoid rapid infusion. For a pregnant patient, when labor starts, given to the mother as a single 2 mg/kg dose infused over 1 hr followed by 1 mg/kg/hr given by continuous IV infusion until the umbilical cord is clamped.
Incompatibilities: Do not mix with blood or blood products.

Adverse effects

- **CNS:** *Headache,* insomnia, myalgia, *asthenia,* malaise, dizziness, paresthesias, somnolence
- **GI:** *Nausea, GI pain, diarrhea,* anorexia, vomiting, dyspepsia, lactic acidosis with severe hepatomegaly
- **Hematologic:** *Agranulocytopenia,* severe anemia requiring transfusions
- **Other:** *Fever,* diaphoresis, dyspnea, *rash,* taste perversion

Interactions

✳ Drug-drug • Increased risk of hematologic toxicity if combined with nephrotoxic, cytotoxic, or bone marrow suppressing drugs, ganciclovir, interferon alfa, probenecid, methadone, phenytoin • Increased risk of neurotoxicity when used with acyclovir • Severe drowsiness and lethargy with cyclosporine

✳ Drug-alternative therapy • Decreased effectiveness if taken with St. John's Wort

■ Nursing considerations

 CLINICAL ALERT!
Name confusion has occurred between *Retrovir* (zidovudine) and ritonavir; use caution.

Assessment

- **History:** Life-threatening allergy to any component, compromised bone marrow, impaired renal or hepatic function, pregnancy, lactation
- **Physical:** Skin rashes, lesions, texture; T; affect, reflexes, peripheral sensation; bowel sounds, liver evaluation; LFTs, renal function tests, CBC and differential

Interventions

⊗ **Black box warning** Monitor hematologic indices every 2 wk; hematologic toxicity has occurred.
- Give the drug around-the-clock; rest periods may be needed during the day due to interrupted sleep.

⊗ **Black box warning** Monitor LFTs; lactic acidosis with severe hepatomegaly is possible.
⊗ **Black box warning** Patient is at increased risk for symptomatic myopathy; monitor accordingly.

Teaching points

- Take drug every 4 hours, around-the-clock. Use an alarm clock to wake you up at night; rest periods during the day may be needed. Do not share this drug; take exactly as prescribed. Take this drug with your other HIV medications.
- Zidovudine is not a cure for AIDS or AIDS-related complex; opportunistic infections may occur; obtain continuous medical care.
- Arrange for frequent blood tests; results of blood counts may indicate dosage needs to be decreased or drug discontinued temporarily.
- Zidovudine does not reduce the risk of transmission of HIV to others by sexual contact or blood contamination; use precautions.
- You may experience these side effects: Nausea, loss of appetite, change in taste (eat frequent small meals); dizziness, loss of feeling (use precautions); headache, fever, muscle aches.

Adverse effects in *italics* are most common; those in **bold** are life-threatening. ⬛ Do not crush.

- Report extreme fatigue, lethargy, severe headache, severe nausea, vomiting, difficulty breathing, rash.

▽zileuton
*(zye **loot**' on)*

Zyflo, Zyflo CR ⓞⓣⓒ

PREGNANCY CATEGORY C

Drug classes
Antiasthmatic
Leukotriene synthesis inhibitor

Therapeutic actions
Inhibits the enzyme that catalyzes the formation of leukotrienes from arachidonic acid, thus blocking many of the signs and symptoms of asthma (neutrophil and eosinophil migration, neutrophil and monocyte aggregation, leukocyte adhesion, increased capillary permeability, and smooth muscle contraction). These actions contribute to inflammation, edema, mucus secretion and bronchoconstriction caused by cold air challenge in patients with asthma.

Indications
- Prophylaxis and long-term treatment of asthma in adults and children 12 yr and older

Contraindications and cautions
- Contraindicated with hypersensitivity to zileuton or any of its components, acute asthma attacks, status asthmaticus, pregnancy and lactation, severe hepatic impairment.
- Use cautiously with hepatic impairment.

Available forms
CR tablets ⓞⓣⓒ—600 mg; tablets—600 mg

Dosages
Adults and patients 12 yr and older
CR tablets, 1,200 mg (2 tablets) PO bid within 1 hr after morning and evening meals for a total daily dose of 2,400 mg. Tablets, 600 mg PO four times daily for a total daily dose of 2,400 mg.
Patients with hepatic impairment
Use caution; contraindicated if liver enzymes (AST, ALT) three or more times normal.

Pharmacokinetics

Route	Onset	Peak
Oral	Rapid	1.7 hr

Metabolism: Hepatic; $T_{1/2}$: 2.5 hr
Distribution: Crosses placenta; may enter breast milk
Excretion: Unknown

Adverse effects
- **CNS:** *Headache,* dizziness, myalgia, behavior and mood changes
- **GI:** Nausea, diarrhea, abdominal pain, dyspepsia, vomiting, **elevation of liver enzymes**
- **Other:** Generalized pain, fever, myalgia, sinusitis, rash

Interactions
✳ **Drug-drug** • Increased effects of propranolol, theophylline, warfarin; monitor patient and decrease dose as appropriate
✳ **Drug-food** • Bioavailability decreased markedly by the presence of food; administer at least 1 hr before or 2 hr after meals

■ Nursing considerations
Assessment
- **History:** Hypersensitivity to zileuton, impaired hepatic function, lactation, pregnancy, acute asthma or bronchospasm
- **Physical:** T; orientation, reflexes; R, adventitious sounds; GI evaluation; LFTs

Interventions
⊗ *Warning* Obtain baseline LFTs before beginning therapy; monitor liver enzymes on a regular basis during therapy; discontinue drug and consult prescriber if enzymes rise more than three times normal.
⊗ *Warning* There is a risk of neuropsychiatric events, including mood and behavior changes with drug administration. Monitor accordingly; discontinue drug if these occur.
- Administer CR tablets within 1 hour after morning and evening meals. Do not cut, crush, or let patient chew CR tablets.
- Ensure that drug is taken continually for optimal effect.
⊗ *Warning* Do not administer for acute asthma attack or acute bronchospasm.

Teaching points
- Take this drug regularly as prescribed; do not stop taking this drug during symptom-free

Z

periods; do not stop taking this drug without consulting your health care provider. Continue taking any other antiasthmatics that have been prescribed for you.

- Do not cut, crush, or chew CR tablets; swallow them whole. Take CR tablets within 1 hour after morning and evening meals.

- Do not take this drug for an acute asthma attack or acute bronchospasm; this drug is not a bronchodilator; routine emergency procedures should be followed during acute attacks.

- Avoid the use of over-the-counter drugs while you are using this medication; many of them contain products that can interfere with or cause serious side effects when used with this drug. If you feel that you need one of these products, consult your health care provider.

- You may experience these side effects: Dizziness (use caution when driving or performing activities that require alertness); nausea, vomiting (eat frequent small meals; take drug with food); headache (analgesics may be helpful).

- Report fever, acute asthma attacks, flulike symptoms, lethargy, pruritus, changes in color or of urine or stool.

▽ziprasidone
(zih praz' i done)

Geodon

PREGNANCY CATEGORY C

Drug classes
Atypical antipsychotic
Benzisoxazole

Therapeutic actions
Mechanism of action not fully understood; blocks dopamine and serotonin receptors in the brain, depresses the reticular activating system; effective in suppressing many of the negative aspects of schizophrenia (blunted affect, social withdrawal, lack of motivation, anger).

Indications
- Treatment of schizophrenia and to delay the time and rate of relapse
- Oral: Treatment of acute bipolar mania including manic or mixed episodes associated

with bipolar disorder with or without psychotic features; maintenance treatment, used with lithium and valproate
- IM: Rapid control of agitated behavior and psychotic symptoms in patients with acute schizophrenia exacerbations
- Unlabeled uses: Autism, Tourette syndrome

Contraindications and cautions
- Contraindicated with allergy to ziprasidone, prolonged QTc interval, history of severe cardiac disease.
- Use cautiously with renal or hepatic impairment, CV disease, pregnancy, lactation.

Available forms
Capsules—20, 40, 60, 80 mg; powder for injection—20 mg/mL

Dosages
Adults
- *Schizophrenia:* Initially, 20 mg PO bid with food. Adjust as needed. Effective range, 20–100 mg PO bid.
- *Rapid control of agitated behavior:* 10–20 mg IM; doses of 10 mg may be repeated every 2 hr; doses of 20 mg may be repeated in 4 hr. Maximum dose, 40 mg/day.
- *Bipolar mania:* 40 mg PO bid with food. May be increased to 60 or 80 mg PO bid with food.

Pediatric patients
Safety and efficacy not established.

Pharmacokinetics

Route	Onset	Peak	Duration
Oral	Varies	1 hr	6–8 hr

Metabolism: Hepatic; T$_{1/2}$: 3 hr
Distribution: Crosses placenta; may enter breast milk
Excretion: Urine

Adverse effects
- **CNS:** *Somnolence, drowsiness, sedation, headache,* extrapyramidal reactions
- **CV: Arrhythmias,** hypotension, ECG changes, hypertension, prolonged QTc interval
- **GI:** *Nausea, dyspepsia, constipation,* abdominal discomfort, dry mouth
- **GU:** Polyuria
- **Other:** *Fever,* weight gain (not as likely as with other antipsychotics), rash, risk of development of diabetes mellitus

Adverse effects in *italics* are most common; those in **bold** are life-threatening. ⬛ Do not crush.

Interactions
✳ **Drug-drug** ⊗ *Warning* Increased risk of severe cardiac arrhythmias if taken with other drugs that prolong the QTc interval.
• Additive hypotension when given with antihypertensives
✳ **Drug-alternative therapy** • Possibility of increased toxicity if taken with St. John's Wort

■ Nursing considerations
Assessment
• **History:** Allergy to ziprasidone, pregnancy, lactation, cardiac disease, hepatic or renal impairment, prolonged QTc interval
• **Physical:** T, weight; reflexes, orientation; P, ECG; bowel sounds, normal output, liver evaluation; normal urine output; urinalysis, LFTs, renal function tests

Interventions
⊗ *Warning* Ensure that patient is not pregnant before beginning therapy; advise patient to use contraceptive measures while using this drug.
⊗ **Black box warning** Increased risk of death if used in elderly patients with dementia-related psychosis; do not use drug in these patients; drug not approved for this use.
• Obtain baseline ECG to rule out prolonged QTc interval; monitor periodically throughout therapy.
• Monitor weight before beginning therapy and periodically during therapy. Weight gain is not usually a concern with this drug.
• Monitor patient regularly for signs and symptoms of diabetes mellitus.
• Alert patient that infants born to mothers who take this drug in the last trimester of pregnancy are at risk for abnormal muscle movements.
• Follow patients with renal or hepatic impairment carefully throughout therapy.
• Continue other measures used to deal with schizophrenia.

Teaching points
• This drug cannot be taken during pregnancy. If you think you are pregnant, or want to become pregnant, consult your health care provider.
• You may experience these side effects: Somnolence, drowsiness, dizziness, sedation (avoid driving a car, operating machinery, or performing tasks that require concentra-

tion); nausea, dyspepsia (eat frequent small meals); headache (analgesics may be available to help, consult your health care provider).
• Report lethargy, weakness, fever, sore throat, palpitations, return of symptoms, weight gain.

▽ ziv-aflibercept
See Appendix R, *Less commonly used drugs*.

▽ zoledronic acid
*(zoh leh **droh'** nik)*

Reclast, Zometa

PREGNANCY CATEGORY D

Drug classes
Bisphosphonate
Calcium regulator

Therapeutic actions
A bisphosphonic acid that inhibits bone resorption, possibly by inhibiting osteoclast activity and promoting osteoclast cell apoptosis; this action leads to a decrease in the release of calcium from bone and a decrease in serum calcium.

Indications
• IV treatment of the hypercalcemia of malignancy (*Zometa*)
• Treatment of Paget disease of bone in men and women (*Reclast*)
• Treatment of postmenopausal osteoporosis and osteoporosis in men (*Reclast*)
• Prevention of new clinical fractures in patients with low-trauma hip fractures (*Reclast*)
• Treatment of patients with multiple myelomas and patients with documented bone metastases from solid tumors in conjunction with standard antineoplastic therapy (*Zometa*)
• Treatment and prevention of glucocorticoid-induced osteoporosis (*Reclast*)
• Prevention of osteoporosis in postmenopausal women (*Reclast*)
• Unlabeled uses: Osteopenia in androgen-deprived prostate cancer patients or estrogen-deprived breast cancer patients; prevention of postrenal transplant bone loss

Z

Contraindications and cautions

- Contraindicated with allergy to any components of the drug or to bisphosphonates; severe renal impairment.
- Use cautiously with renal impairment (do not exceed single doses of 4 mg, and duration of infusion must not be less than 15 min), hepatic impairment, aspirin-sensitive asthmatic patients, pregnancy, or lactation.

Available forms

Injection—4 mg/5 mL (*Zometa*); 5 mg/100 mL (*Reclast*)

Dosages

Adults

Zometa: 4 mg IV as a single-dose infusion of not less than 15 min for hypercalcemia of malignancy with albumin-corrected serum calcium levels of 12 mg/dL or greater. Retreatment may be done with 4 mg IV if needed; a minimum of 7 days should elapse between doses with careful monitoring of serum creatinine levels. Patients with solid tumors should receive 4 mg IV every 3–4 wk to treat bone metastasis.

Reclast: 5 mg IV infused via vented infusion line over at least 15 min. Retreatment may be considered as needed once every 2 yr for osteoporosis.

Pediatric patients

Safety and efficacy not established.

Patients with renal impairment

Zometa: Mild to moderate renal impairment for patients with multiple myeloma and bone metastases from solid tumors (see chart for dosages).

CrCl (mL/min)	Dose (IV)
More than 60	4 mg
50–60	3.5 mg
40–49	3.3 mg
30–39	3 mg
Less than 30	Contraindicated

Reclast: If creatinine clearance 35 mL/min or greater, 5 mg over at least 15 min. Not recommended for patients with severe renal failure.

Pharmacokinetics

Route	Onset	Peak
IV	Slow	8 hr

Metabolism: Hepatic; $T_{1/2}$: 0.23 hr then 1.75 hr

Distribution: May cross placenta; may enter breast milk
Excretion: Urine

▼▼ IV FACTS

Preparation: Withdraw solution, equivalent to 4 mg *Zometa*, further dilute in 100 mL 0.9% sodium chloride, 5% dextrose injection. May be refrigerated and stored for up to 24 hr before the time of the end of the infusion. For *Reclast*, no additional preparation needed; use a vented infusion line.

Infusion: Infuse over no less than 15 min. Risk of acute infusion reaction for first 3 days; risk decreased with pre- and post-treatment with acetaminophen.

Incompatibilities: Do not mix with any other drug solution; always administer via a separate line. Physically incompatible with calcium-containing infusions.

Adverse effects

- **CNS:** Agitation, confusion, *insomnia*, anxiety
- **CV:** *Hypotension*
- **GI:** *Nausea, constipation,* vomiting, diarrhea, abdominal pain, anorexia
- **Hematologic:** Hypophosphatemia, hypokalemia, hypomagnesemia, hypocalcemia
- **Respiratory:** *Dyspnea,* coughing, pleural effusion
- **Other:** *Infections* (UTI, candidiasis), *fever,* progression of cancer, **osteonecrosis of the jaw,** renal impairment, fatigue

Interactions

✳ **Drug-drug** • Possible increased risk of hypocalcemia if taken with aminoglycosides, loop diuretics; if this combination is used, monitor serum calcium levels closely • Increased risk of nephrotoxicity if combined with other nephrotoxic drugs

■ Nursing considerations

Assessment

- **History:** Allergy to components of the drug or any bisphosphonate, hepatic or renal impairment, aspirin-sensitive asthma, pregnancy, lactation
- **Physical:** T, BP, R, orientation and affect, adventitious sounds, CBC and electrolytes, renal function tests

Interventions

- Do not confuse *Reclast* and *Zometa*; dosage varies.
- Arrange for the patient to have a dental examination and any needed preventive treatments before beginning therapy. Avoid any invasive dental work or surgery while on this drug to decrease risk of osteonecrosis of the jaw.
- Patients who receive zoledronic acid should also receive 500 mg of elemental calcium daily and a multivitamin containing 400 units of vitamin D daily.
- Make sure that patient is well hydrated before use; vigorous saline hydration to establish a urine output of about 2 L/day is suggested.
- Monitor urinary output and assess patient for hydration status continually.

⊗ *Warning* Monitor serum creatinine levels prior to each dose of zoledronic acid; follow dosage guidelines for any indication of renal toxicity.

⊗ *Warning* There is an increased risk of renal impairment and renal failure with drug administration. Check renal function regularly; use caution with other nephrotoxic drugs.

- Ensure that reconstituted solution is infused within 24 hr of reconstitution.
- For *Reclast,* make sure to use a vented infusion line.
- Ensure that drug infuses over not less than 15 min.
- Provide frequent small meals if GI upset occurs.
- Arrange for nutritional consult if nausea and vomiting are persistent.
- Monitor patient for any sign of infection and arrange for appropriate interventions.

Teaching points

- Arrange to have a dental examination and complete any needed treatment before starting this drug.
- This drug must be given by IV infusion; you will be closely monitored prior to and following the infusion.
- If you are returning for infusions every 3–4 weeks or once per year, mark a calendar with your return dates.
- It is important to maintain your fluid levels before using this drug; drink fluids as much as possible to ensure that you are hydrated.
- It is important to take vitamin D and calcium supplements to help prevent osteoporosis and reduce the risk of new fractures.

- Avoid invasive dental procedures and dental surgery.
- You may experience these side effects: Nausea, vomiting (eat frequent small meals); agitation, confusion, anxiety (consult your health care provider if this becomes a problem).
- Report difficulty breathing, muscle pain, tremors, pain at injection site.

▷ zolmitriptan
*(zohl mah **trip**' tan)*

Zomig ⊕, Zomig-ZMT

PREGNANCY CATEGORY C

Drug classes
Antimigraine drug
Serotonin selective agonist

Therapeutic actions
Binds to serotonin receptors to cause vascular constrictive effects on cranial blood vessels, causing the relief of migraine in select patients.

Indications
- Treatment of acute migraine attacks with or without aura
- Unlabeled use: Treatment of migraines in adolescents

Contraindications and cautions
- Contraindicated with allergy to zolmitriptan, active CAD, Prinzmetal angina, pregnancy.
- Use cautiously with the elderly and with lactation.

Available forms
Tablets ⊕—2.5, 5 mg; nasal spray—5 mg; orally disintegrating tablet—2.5, 5 mg

Dosages
Adults
Oral
For tablets or orally disintegrating tablets, 2.5 mg PO at onset of headache or with beginning of aura; may repeat dose if headache persists after 2 hr; do not exceed 10 mg in 24 hr.
Nasal spray
1 spray in nostril at onset of headache or beginning of aura; may repeat in 2 hr if needed. Maximum dose, 10 mg/24 hr (2 sprays).

Z

Pediatric patients
Safety and efficacy not established.

Patients with hepatic impairment
Use caution; keep doses at 2.5 mg or less. Significant increases in BP can occur.

Pharmacokinetics

Route	Onset	Peak
Oral	Varies	2–4 hr
Nasal	15 min	2 hr

Metabolism: Hepatic; $T_{1/2}$: 2.5–3.7 hr
Distribution: Crosses placenta; may enter breast milk
Excretion: Feces, urine

Adverse effects

- **CNS:** *Dizziness, vertigo,* headache, anxiety, malaise or fatigue, *weakness, myalgia*
- **CV:** *BP alterations, tightness or pressure in chest*
- **GI:** Abdominal discomfort, dysphagia
- **Other:** *Tingling, warm/hot sensations, burning sensation, feeling of heaviness, pressure sensation, numbness, feeling of tightness,* feeling strange, cold sensation

Interactions

✳ **Drug-drug** ⊗ *Warning* Risk of severe effects with an MAOI or within 2 wk of discontinuing an MAOI.

- Prolonged vasoactive reactions with ergot-containing drugs ● Increased risk of toxic effects with cimetidine, hormonal contraceptives ● A serotonin syndrome may occur when sibutramine is coadministered ● Increased risk of prolonged QT interval and potentially fatal arrhythmias if combined with other drugs that prolong QT interval

■ Nursing considerations

Assessment

- **History:** Allergy to zolmitriptan, active CAD, Prinzmetal angina, pregnancy, lactation
- **Physical:** Skin color and lesions; orientation, reflexes, peripheral sensation; P, BP; LFTs, renal function tests

Interventions

- Administer to relieve acute migraine, not as prophylactic measure. Ensure that patient does not cut, crush, or chew tablets.

- Establish safety measures if CNS or visual disturbances occur.
- Control environment as appropriate to help relieve migraine (eg, lighting, temperature).

⊗ *Warning* Monitor BP of patients with possible CAD; discontinue at any sign of angina or prolonged high BP.

Teaching points

- Take this drug exactly as prescribed, at the onset of headache or aura.
- Use drug right after removing from blister package. Do not break, crush, or chew tablet. Place orally disintegrating tablet on your tongue and let it dissolve. If using nasal spray, use one spray only; spray may be repeated after 2 hours if needed.
- This drug should not be taken during pregnancy; if you suspect that you are pregnant, contact your health care provider and stop using the drug.
- Continue measures that usually help you during a migraine (adjust lighting, noise).
- Contact your health care provider immediately if you experience chest pain or pressure that is severe or does not go away.
- You may experience these side effects: Dizziness, drowsiness (avoid driving or using dangerous machinery); numbness, tingling, feelings of tightness or pressure.
- Report feelings of heat, flushing, tiredness, nausea, swelling of lips or eyelids.

▽**zolpidem tartrate**
(zol' pih dem)

Ambien, Ambien CR⊞, Edluar⊞, Intermezzo, Tovalt ODT⊞, Zolpimist

PREGNANCY CATEGORY C

CONTROLLED SUBSTANCE C-IV

Drug class

Sedative-hypnotic (nonbarbiturate)

Therapeutic actions

Modulates GABA receptors to cause suppression of neurons, leading to sedation, anticonvulsant, anxiolytic, and relaxant properties.

Adverse effects in *italics* are most common; those in **bold** are life-threatening. ⊞ Do not crush.

Indications

- Short-term treatment of insomnia
- Treatment of insomnia in adults who experience difficulties with sleep onset and sleep maintenance (ER tablets)
- ■ NEW INDICATION: Treatment of insomnia when middle-of-the-night awakening is followed by difficulty returning to sleep when patient has at least 4 hr of bedtime remaining (*Intermezzo*)

Contraindications and cautions

- Contraindicated with hypersensitivity to zolpidem.
- Use cautiously with acute intermittent porphyria, impaired hepatic or renal function, addiction-prone patients, pregnancy, lactation.

Available forms

Tablets—5, 10 mg; ER tablets ⊕⊖—6.25, 12.5 mg; orally disintegrating tablets ⊕⊖—5, 10 mg; oral spray—5 mg; sublingual tablet—1.75, 3.5, 5, 10 mg

Dosages

Adults
10 mg PO at bedtime. Do not exceed 10 mg/day. ER tablets—12.5 mg/day PO. Oral spray—Two to three sprays in mouth, over tongue at bedtime. Or, 1.75 mg (women) or 3.5 mg (men) sublingually with middle-of-the-night awakening (*Intermezzo*); limit to 1.75 mg once per night if also on CNS depressants.

Pediatric patients
Safety and efficacy not established.

Geriatric patients
Increased chance of confusion, acute brain syndrome; initiate treatment with 5 mg PO or 6.25 mg/day PO ER tablets, or 1.75 mg sublingually (*Intermezzo*).

Pharmacokinetics

Route	Onset	Peak
Oral	45 min	1.6 hr

Metabolism: Hepatic; $T_{1/2}$: 2.6 hr
Distribution: Crosses placenta; may enter breast milk
Excretion: Urine

Adverse effects

- **CNS:** Seizures, hallucinations, ataxia, EEG changes, pyrexia, *morning drowsiness, hang-*over, *headache, dizziness,* vertigo, acute brain syndrome and confusion; paradoxical excitation, anxiety, depression, nightmares, dreaming, diplopia, blurred vision, *suppression of REM sleep,* REM rebound when drug is discontinued, complex sleep disorders
- **GI:** Esophagitis, vomiting, *nausea,* diarrhea, constipation
- **Hypersensitivity:** Generalized allergic reactions; pruritus, rash
- **Other:** Flulike symptoms, dry mouth, infection, **anaphylaxis, angioedema**

■ Nursing considerations
Assessment

- **History:** Hypersensitivity to zolpidem, acute intermittent porphyria, impaired hepatic or renal function, addiction-prone, lactation, pregnancy
- **Physical:** T; skin color, lesions; orientation, affect, reflexes, vision examination; P, BP; bowel sounds, normal output, liver evaluation; CBC with differential; LFTs, renal function tests

Interventions

⊗ **Warning** Limit amount of drug dispensed to patients who are depressed or suicidal.

⊗ **Warning** Withdraw drug gradually if patient has used drug long-term or if patient has developed tolerance. Supportive therapy similar to that for withdrawal from barbiturates may be necessary to prevent dangerous withdrawal symptoms.

- Place orally disintegrating tablet in patient's mouth; have patient swallow tablet with saliva. Do not allow patient to chew, break, or split tablet.
- Prime oral spray before first use by compressing the container five times. Teach the patient proper administration.
- Make sure patient places sublingual tablet under the tongue and allows it to dissolve. Sublingual tablets should not be swallowed whole.

Teaching points

- Take this drug exactly as prescribed. Do not exceed prescribed dosage. Long-term use is not recommended. Make sure you have at least 4 hours of bedtime left after taking the drug.
- If using oral spray, prime container before initial use by compressing the container five times. Hold container upright and aim it

Z

directly into your open mouth. Compress the container completely, spraying over your tongue and directly into your mouth. If drug is not used for 14 or more days, prime the container once before using.

- If using sublingual form for middle-of-the-night awakening, place tablet under your tongue and allow it to dissolve; do not swallow tablet whole. Make sure you have at least 4 hours of bedtime remaining.
- You may experience these side effects: Drowsiness, allergic reaction, swelling, dizziness, blurred vision (avoid driving or performing tasks requiring alertness or visual acuity); GI upset (eat frequent small meals), sleep disorders.
- Report rash, sore throat, fever, bruising, allergic reaction, swelling, complex sleep-related behaviors, thoughts of suicide.

▽ zonisamide
*(zoh **niss'** ah myde)*

Zonegran

PREGNANCY CATEGORY C

Drug class
Anticonvulsant

Therapeutic actions
Mechanism of action not fully understood; inhibits voltage-sensitive sodium and calcium channels, stabilizing the neuronal membrane and modulating calcium-dependent presynaptic release of excitatory amino acids; may also have dopaminergic effects.

Indications
- Adjuvant therapy in the treatment of partial seizures in adults with epilepsy

Contraindications and cautions
- Contraindicated with lactation, history of sulfonamide hypersensitivity.
- Use cautiously with impaired hepatic, renal, or cardiac function; pregnancy.

Available forms
Capsules—25, 50, 100 mg

Dosages
Adults
Initial dose, 100 mg PO daily as a single dose—not divided—subsequent doses can be divided; may increase by 100 mg/day every 2 wk to achieve control. Maximum dose, 600 mg/day.
Pediatric patients
Not recommended in patients younger than 16 yr.
Patients with renal impairment
Do not use in patients with a glomerular filtration rate of less than 50 mL/min.

Pharmacokinetics

Route	Onset	Peak
Oral	Rapid	2–6 hr

Metabolism: Hepatic; $T_{1/2}$: 49.7–130 hr
Distribution: Crosses placenta; enters breast milk
Excretion: Urine

Adverse effects
- **CNS:** *Dizziness,* insomnia, headache, *somnolence, ataxia,* diplopia, blurred vision, nystagmus, *decrease in mental functioning,* **suicidality**
- **Dermatologic:** *Rash,* **Stevens-Johnson syndrome**
- **GI:** *Nausea,* vomiting, *dry mouth, unusual taste in mouth, anorexia*
- **Other:** Bone marrow depression, *renal calculi,* **oligohidrosis and hyperthermia** (pediatric), metabolic acidosis

Interactions
✳ **Drug-drug** • Rapid elimination of zonisamide if taken with enzyme-inducing antiepileptics—carbamazepine, phenytoin, phenobarbital, primidone • Increased levels and potential for toxicity with carbamazepine if taken with zonisamide; adjust dosage and monitor patient carefully • Increased risk of metabolic acidosis if combined with carbonic anhydrase inhibitors; monitor patient closely.

■ Nursing considerations
Assessment
- **History:** Lactation; impaired hepatic, renal, or cardiac function; pregnancy
- **Physical:** Weight; T; skin color, lesions; orientation, affect, reflexes; P, BP, perfusion; bowel sounds, normal output; LFTs, renal function test, CBC

Interventions

⊗ *Warning* Monitor drug doses carefully when starting therapy and with each increase in dose; special care will need to be taken when changing the dose or frequency of any other antiepileptic.

⊗ *Warning* There is a risk of metabolic acidosis with drug administration. Measure serum bicarbonate level before and periodically during therapy. Alkali therapy is recommended if drug is needed and acidosis occurs.

⊗ **Black box warning** Patient may be at increased risk for suicidal ideation and suicidality; monitor accordingly.

⊗ *Warning* Taper drug slowly over a 2-wk period when discontinuing.

- Monitor patient for rash; potentially fatal Stevens-Johnson syndrome has occurred.
- Discontinue drug if patient develops acute renal failure or a clinically significant increase in creatinine or BUN level.
- Ensure that patient is well hydrated to prevent formation of renal calculi.
- Provide safety measures if CNS effects occur.

Teaching points

- Take this drug exactly as prescribed. Dosage may be increased slowly.
- Do not discontinue this drug abruptly or change dosage, except on the advice of your health care provider.
- You should wear a medical alert tag at all times so that any emergency medical personnel taking care of you will know that you have epilepsy and are taking antiepileptic medication.
- You may experience these side effects: Dizziness, drowsiness, decreased mental functioning (avoid driving a car or performing other tasks requiring alertness or visual acuity if this occurs); GI upset (taking the drug with food or milk and eating frequent small meals may help); headache (medication can be ordered); rash (skin care and lotions may be helpful).
- Report yellowing of skin, abdominal pain, changes in color of urine or stools, flank pain, painful urination, worsening rash, thoughts of suicide.

Z

Appendices

APPENDIX A

Alternative and complementary therapies

Many dietary supplements and "natural" remedies are used by the public for self-treatment. These substances, many derived from the folklore of various cultures, commonly contain ingredients that have been identified and that have known therapeutic activities. Some of these substances have unknown mechanisms of action but over the years have been reliably used to relieve specific symptoms. Many of these substances lack scientific studies and documentation, but it is important to be aware of what patients may use them for. There is an element of the placebo effect in using some of these substances. The power of believing that something will work and that there is some control over the problem is often beneficial in achieving relief from pain or suffering. Some of these substances may contain yet unidentified ingredients, which eventually may prove useful in the modern field of pharmacology. Because these products are not regulated or monitored, there is always a possibility of toxic effects. Some of these products may contain ingredients that interact with prescription drugs. A history of the use of these alternative therapies may explain unexpected reactions to some drugs. Drugs that the substance has been reported to interact with are in **bold.**

Substance	Reported uses and possible risks
acidophilus (probiotics)	Oral: prevention or treatment of uncomplicated diarrhea; restoration of intestinal flora Decreased effectiveness of **warfarin.**
alfalfa	Topical: healing ointment, relief of arthritis pain Oral: treatment of arthritis, hot flashes; strength giving; reduction of cholesterol level Increased risk of bleeding with **warfarin;** increased photosensitivity with **chlorpromazine;** increased risk of hypoglycemia with **anti-diabetic drugs;** loss of effectiveness with **hormonal contraceptives** or **hormone replacement**
allspice	Topical: anesthetic for teeth and gums; soothes sore joints and muscles Oral: treatment of indigestion, flatulence, diarrhea, fatigue Risk of seizures with excessive use; decreased **iron** absorption; can irritate mucosa; ingestion of extracts may be toxic, with CNS effects.
aloe leaves	Topical: treatment of burns, healing of wounds Oral: treatment of chronic constipation Caution: Oral use may cause serious hypokalemia; risk of spontaneous abortion if used in third trimester
androstenedione	Oral, spray: anabolic steroid to increase muscle mass and strength Caution: May increase risk of CV disease and certain cancers.
angelica	Oral: "cure all" for gynecologic problems, headaches, backaches, loss of appetite, and GI spasms; increases circulation in the periphery Risk of bleeding if combined with **anticoagulants.**
anise	Oral: relief of dry cough, treatment of flatulence and bloating May increase **iron** absorption and cause toxicity.
apple	Oral: control of blood glucose, constipation, cancer, heart problems May interfere with **antidiabetic drugs, fexofenadine.**

Substance	Reported uses and possible risks
arnica	Topical: relief of pain from muscle or soft tissue injury Oral: immune system stimulant May decrease effects of **antihypertensives** and increase effects of **anticoagulants** and **antiplatelet drugs;** very toxic to children.
ashwagandha	Oral: to improve mental and physical functioning; general tonic; to protect cells during cancer chemotherapy and radiation therapy May increase bleeding with **anticoagulants;** may interfere with **thyroid replacement** therapy. Discourage use during pregnancy and lactation.
astragalus	Oral: to increase stamina, energy; to improve immune function, resistance to disease; to treat upper respiratory tract infection, common cold May increase effects of **antihypertensives.** Caution against use during fever or acute infection.
barberry	Oral: antidiarrheal, antipyretic, cough suppressant Risk of spontaneous abortion if taken during pregnancy. May increase effects of **antihypertensives, antiarrhythmics.**
basil	Oral: analgesic, anti-inflammatory, hypoglycemic Risk of increased hypoglycemic effects of **antidiabetic drugs.**
bayberry	Topical: to promote wound healing Oral: stimulant, emetic, antidiarrheal May block effects of **antihypertensives.**
bee pollen	Oral: to treat allergies, asthma, impotence, prostatitis; suggested use to decrease cholesterol levels, premenstrual syndrome Risk of hyperglycemia; discourage use by diabetic patients or with **antidiabetic drugs.** May cause allergic reaction in patients allergic to bees.
betel palm	Oral: mild stimulant, digestive aid Increased risk of hypertensive crisis with **MAOIs;** blocks heart-rate reduction of **beta blockers, digoxin;** alters effects of **antiglaucoma drugs.**
bilberry	Oral: treatment of diabetes; cardiovascular problems; lowers cholesterol and triglycerides; treatment of diabetic retinopathy; treatment of cataracts, night blindness Increased risk of bleeding with **anticoagulants;** disulfiram-like reaction with **alcohol.**
birch bark	Topical: treatment of infected wounds, cuts Oral: as tea for relief of stomachache Topical form very toxic to children.
blackberry	Oral: as tea for generalized healing; treatment of diabetes Risk of interaction with **antidiabetic drugs.**

(continued)

Substance	Reported uses and possible risks
black cohosh root	Oral: treatment of PMS, menopausal disorders, rheumatoid arthritis Contains estrogen-like components. Caution against use with **hormone replacement therapy** or **hormonal contraceptives;** discourage use during pregnancy and lactation; may lower blood pressure with **sedatives, antihypertensives, anesthetics;** increased risk of fungal infection with **immunosuppressants.**
bromelain	Oral: treatment of inflammation, sports injuries, upper respiratory tract infection, PMS, and adjunctive therapy in cancer treatment May cause nausea, vomiting, diarrhea, menstrual disorders.
burdock	Oral: treatment of diabetes; atropine-like adverse effects, uterine stimulant May increase hypoglycemic effects of **antidiabetic drugs.**
capsicum	Topical: external analgesic Oral: treatment of bowel disorders, chronic laryngitis, peripheral vascular disease May increase bleeding with **warfarin, aspirin;** increases cough with **ACE inhibitors;** increases toxicity with **MAOIs;** increases sedation with **sedatives.**
catnip leaves	Oral: treatment of bronchitis, diarrhea
cat's claw	Oral: treatment of allergies, arthritis; adjunct in the treatment of cancers and AIDS Discourage use during pregnancy and lactation and use by transplant recipients; increased risk of bleeding episodes if taken with oral **anticoagulants;** increased hypotension with **antihypertensives.**
cayenne pepper	Topical: treatment of burns, wounds, relief of toothache
celery	Oral: lowers blood glucose, acts as a diuretic; may cause potassium depletion Advise caution when taken with **antidiabetic drugs.**
chamomile	Topical: treatment of wounds, ulcer, conjunctivitis Oral: treatment of migraines, gastric cramps, relief of anxiety, inflammatory diseases Contains coumarin–closely monitor patients taking **anticoagulants.** May cause depression; monitor patients on **antidepressants.** Cross-reaction with ragweed allergies may occur. Discourage use during pregnancy and lactation.
chaste-tree berry	Oral: progesterone-like effects; used to treat PMS and menopausal problems, and to stimulate lactation Advise caution when taken with **hormone replacement therapy** and **hormonal contraceptives.**
chicken soup	Oral: breaks up respiratory secretions, bronchodilator, relieves anxiety
chicory	Oral: treatment of digestive tract problems, gout; stimulates bile secretions

Substance	Reported uses and possible risks
Chinese angelica (dong quai)	Oral: general tonic; treatment of anemias, PMS, menopause, antihypertensive, laxative Use caution with the flu, hemorrhagic diseases. Monitor patients on **antihypertensives, vasodilators,** or **anticoagulants** for toxic effects. Advise caution when taken with **hormone replacement therapy.**
chondroitin	Oral: treatment of osteoarthritis and related disorders (usually combined with glucosamine) Risk of increased bleeding if combined with **anticoagulants.**
chong cao fungi	Oral: antioxidant; promotes stamina, sexual function Discourage use by children.
coleus forskohlii	Oral: treatment of asthma, hypertension, eczema Urge caution when taken with **antihypertensives** or **antihistamines;** severe additive effects can occur. Discourage use if patient has hypotension or peptic ulcer.
comfrey	Topical: treatment of wounds, cuts, ulcers Oral: gargle for tonsillitis Warn against using with **eucalyptus;** monitor liver function.
coriander	Oral: weight loss, lowers blood glucose Advise caution when taken with **antidiabetic drugs.**
creatine monohydrate	Oral: enhancement of athletic performance Warn against using with **insulin;** do not use with caffeine.
dandelion root	Oral: treatment of liver and kidney problems; decreases lactation (after delivery or with weaning); lowers blood glucose Advise caution when taken with **antidiabetic drugs, antihypertensives,** and **quinolone antibiotics.**
DHEA	Oral: slows aging, improves vigor ("Fountain of Youth"); androgenic side effects Risk of interactions with **alprazolam, calcium channel blockers,** and **antidiabetic drugs.** Screen patients older than 40 yr for hormonally sensitive cancers before use.
di huang	Oral: treatment of diabetes mellitus Risk of hypoglycemia with **antidiabetic drugs.**
dried root bark of lycium Chinese mill	Oral: lowers cholesterol, lowers blood glucose Advise caution with **antidiabetic drugs.**
echinacea (cone flower)	Oral: treatment of colds, flu; stimulates the immune system, attacks viruses; causes immunosuppression if used long-term May be liver toxic. Discourage use longer than 12 wk. Caution against taking with **liver-toxic drugs** or **immunosuppressants.** Discourage use with **antifungals;** serious liver injury could occur. Advise against use by patients with SLE, TB, AIDS.
elder bark and flowers	Topical: gargle for tonsillitis, pharyngitis Oral: treatment of fever, chills

(continued)

Substance	Reported uses and possible risks
ephedra	Oral: increases energy, relieves fatigue May cause serious complications, including death; increased risk of hypertension, stroke, MI; interacts with many drugs; **banned by the FDA.**
ergot	Oral: treatment of migraine headaches, treatment of menstrual problems, hemorrhage Monitor patient who takes ergot with **antihypertensives.**
eucalyptus	Topical: treatment of wounds Oral: decreases respiratory secretions; suppresses cough Warn against using with **comfrey;** very toxic in children.
evening primrose	Oral: treatment of PMS, menopause, rheumatoid arthritis, diabetic neuropathy Discourage use with **phenothiazines, antidepressants**—increases risk of seizures; discourage use by those with epilepsy, schizophrenia.
false unicorn root	Oral: treatment of menstrual and uterine problems Advise against use during pregnancy and lactation.
fennel	Oral: treatment of colic, gout, flatulence; enhances lactation Significantly decreases levels of **ciprofloxacin.**
fenugreek	Oral: lowers cholesterol level; reduces blood glucose; aids in healing Advise caution when taken with **antidiabetic drugs, anticoagulants.**
feverfew	Oral: treatment of arthritis, fever, migraine Advise caution when taken with **anticoagulants;** may increase bleeding. Discourage use before or immediately after surgery because of bleeding risk.
fish oil	Oral: treatment of coronary diseases, arthritis, colitis, depression, aggression, attention deficit disorder
gamboge	Oral: appetite suppressant, lowers cholesterol, promotes weight loss Oral use may be unsafe; discourage use.
garlic	Oral: treatment of colds; diuretic; prevention of CAD; intestinal antiseptic; lowers blood glucose; anticoagulant effects; decreases BP Advise caution if patient has diabetes or takes an **oral anticoagulant.** Known to affect blood clotting. Anemia reported with long-term use.
ginger	Oral: treatment of nausea, motion sickness, postoperative nausea (may increase risk of miscarriage) Affects blood clotting. Warn against use with **anticoagulants.**
ginkgobiloba	Oral: vascular dilation; increases blood flow to the brain, improving cognitive function; used in treating Alzheimer disease; antioxidant Can inhibit blood clotting. Seizures reported with high doses. Warn against use with **anticoagulants, aspirin,** or **NSAIDs.** Can interact with **phenytoin, carbamazepine, phenobarbital, TCAs, MAOIs,** and **antidiabetic drugs;** advise caution.

Substance	Reported uses and possible risks
ginseng	Oral: aphrodisiac, mood elevator, tonic; antihypertensive; decreases cholesterol levels; lowers blood glucose; adjunct in cancer chemotherapy and radiation therapy May cause irritability if combined with **caffeine.** Inhibits clotting. Warn against use with **anticoagulants, aspirin, NSAIDs.** Warn against use for longer than 3 mo. May cause headaches, manic episodes if used with **phenelzine, MAOIs.** Additive effects of **estrogens** and **corticosteroids.** May also interfere with cardiac effects of **digoxin.** Monitor patient closely if he takes these drugs or an **antidiabetic drug.**
glucosamine	Oral: treatment of osteoarthritis and joint diseases, usually combined with chondroitin Monitor glucose levels in diabetic patients.
goldenrod leaves	Oral: treatment of renal disease, rheumatism, sore throat, eczema May decrease effects of **diuretics** by increasing sodium retention. Advise caution if patient has a history of allergies.
goldenseal	Oral: lowers blood glucose, aids healing; treatment of bronchitis, colds, flulike symptoms, cystitis May cause false-negative test results in those who use such drugs as marijuana and cocaine. Large amounts may cause paralysis. Affects blood clotting; warn against use with **anticoagulants.** May interfere with **antihypertensives, acid blockers, barbiturates.** May increase effects of **sedatives.** Death can result from overdose.
gotu kola	Topical: chronic venous insufficiency Warn against using with **antidiabetic drugs, cholesterol-lowering drugs, sedatives.**
grape seed extract	Oral: treatment of allergies, asthma; improves circulation; decreases platelet aggregation Advise caution with **oral anticoagulants;** may increase bleeding.
green tea leaf	Oral: antioxidant, to prevent cancer and cardiovascular disease, to increase cognitive function (caffeine effects) Advise caution with **oral anticoagulants;** may increase bleeding. May increase BP. Caution against using with milk.
guarana	Oral: decreases appetite, promotes weight loss Advise caution; increases blood pressure, risk of CV events.
guayusa	Oral: lowers blood glucose; promotes weight loss Advise caution with **antihypertensives.** Decreases absorption of **iron.** May decrease clearance of **lithium.**
hawthorn	Oral: treatment of angina, arrhythmias, BP problems; decreases cholesterol Advise caution with **digoxin, ACE inhibitors, CNS depressants;** may potentiate effects.
hop	Oral: sedative; aids healing; alters blood glucose Discourage use with **CNS depressants, antipsychotics.**

(continued)

Substance	Reported uses and possible risks
horehound	Oral: expectorant; treatment of respiratory problems, GI disorders Use caution with **antidiabetic drugs, antihypertensives.**
horse chestnut seed	Oral: treatment of varicose veins, hemorrhoids, venous insufficiency Advise caution with oral **anticoagulants;** may increase bleeding.
hyssop	Topical: treatment of cold sores, genital herpes, burns, wounds Oral: treatment of coughs, colds, indigestion, and flatulence Warn against use by pregnant patients and those with seizures; toxic in children and pets.
jambul	Oral: treatment of diarrhea, dysentery; lowers blood glucose Use caution with **CNS depressants.**
Java plum	Oral: treatment of diabetes mellitus Advise caution with **antidiabetic drugs.**
jojoba	Topical: promotion of hair growth, relief of skin problems Toxic if ingested.
juniper berries	Oral: increases appetite, aids digestion; diuretic; urinary tract disinfectant; lowers blood glucose level Advise caution when taken with **antidiabetic drugs.** Not for use in pregnancy.
kava	Oral: treatment of nervous anxiety, stress, restlessness; tranquilizer Warn against use with **alprazolam;** may cause coma. Advise against use with Parkinson disease or history of stroke. Discourage use with **St. John's Wort, anxiolytics, alcohol.** Risk of serious liver toxicity.
kudzu	Oral: reduces cravings for **alcohol;** being researched for use with alcoholics Interacts with **anticoagulants, aspirin, antidiabetic drugs, CV drugs.**
lavender	Topical: astringent for minor cuts, burns Oral: treatment of insomnia, restlessness Advise caution with **CNS depressants.** Oil is potentially poisonous.
ledum tincture	Topical: treatment of insect bites, puncture wounds; dissolves some blood clots and bruises
licorice	Oral: prevents thirst, soothes coughs; treats "incurable" chronic fatigue syndrome; treatment of duodenal ulcer. Acts like aldosterone. Blocks **spironolactone** effects. Can lead to **digoxin** toxicity because of effects of lowering aldosterone. Advise extreme caution. Contraindicated with renal or liver disease, hypertension, CAD, pregnancy, lactation. Warn against taking with **thyroid drugs, antihypertensives, hormonal contraceptives.**
ma huang	Oral: treatment of colds, nasal congestion, asthma Contains ephedrine. Warn against use with **antihypertensives, antidiabetic drugs, MAOIs, digoxin.** Serious adverse effects could occur.
mandrake root	Oral: treatment of fertility problems

Substance	Reported uses and possible risks
marigold leaves and flowers	Oral: relief of muscle tension, increases wound healing Advise against use during pregnancy and breast-feeding.
melatonin	Oral: relief of jet lag, treatment of insomnia Advise caution with **antihypertensives, benzodiazepines, beta blockers, methamphetamine.**
milk thistle	Oral: treatment of hepatitis, cirrhosis, fatty liver caused by alcohol or drug use May affect metabolism and increase toxicity of **drugs using CP450, CYP3A4,** and **CYP2C9** systems.
milk vetch	Oral: improves resistance to disease; adjunct therapy in cancer chemotherapy and radiation therapy
mistletoe leaves	Oral: promotes weight loss; relief of signs and symptoms of diabetes Advise caution with **antihypertensives, CNS depressants, immunosuppressants.**
momordica charantia (Karela)	Oral: blocks intestinal absorption of glucose; lowers blood glucose; weight loss Advise caution when taken with **antidiabetic drugs.**
nettle	Topical: stimulation of hair growth, treatment of bleeding Oral: treatment of rheumatism, allergic rhinitis; antispasmodic; expectorant Advise against use during pregnancy and breast-feeding. Increases effects of **diuretics.**
nightshade leaves and roots	Oral: stimulates circulatory system; treatment of eye disorders
octacosanol	Oral: treatment of parkinsonism, enhancement of athletic performance Advise against use during pregnancy and lactation; avoid use with **carbidopa-levodopa.**
parsley seeds and leaves	Oral: treatment of jaundice, asthma, menstrual difficulties, urinary infections, conjunctivitis Risk of serotonin syndrome with **SSRIs, lithium, opioids;** increased hypotension with **antihypertensives.**
passionflower vine	Oral: sedative and hypnotic May increase sedation with other **CNS depressants, MAOIs.** Advise against drinking **alcohol** while taking this herb. Tell patient not to use with **anticoagulants.**
peppermint leaves	Oral: treatment of nervousness, insomnia, dizziness, cramps, coughs Topical: rubbed on forehead to relieve tension headaches
psyllium	Oral: treatment of constipation; lowers cholesterol Can cause severe gas and stomach pain; may interfere with nutrient absorption. Avoid use with **warfarin, digoxin, lithium**—absorption of drug may be blocked; take 2 hr before or after other oral medications. Do not combine with **laxatives.**

(continued)

Substance	Reported uses and possible risks
raspberry	Oral: healing of minor wounds; control and treatment of diabetes, GI disorders, upper respiratory disorders Advise caution with **antidiabetic drugs;** disulfiram-like reaction with **alcohol.**
red clover	Oral: estrogen replacement in menopause, suppresses whooping cough, asthma Risk of bleeding with **anticoagulants, antiplatelets;** discourage use in pregnancy.
red yeast rice	Oral: cholesterol-lowering agent Increased risk of rhabdomyolysis with **cyclosporine, fibric acid, niacin, lovastatin, grapefruit juice.**
rose hips	Oral: laxative, to boost the immune system and prevent illness Advise caution with **estrogens, iron, warfarin.**
rosemary	Topical: relief of rheumatism, sprains, wounds, bruises, eczema Oral: gastric stimulation, relief of flatulence, stimulation of bile release, relief of colic Disulfiram-like reaction with **alcohol.**
rue extract	Topical: relief of pain associated with sprains, groin pulls, whiplash Advise caution with **antihypertensive drugs, digoxin, warfarin.**
saffron	Oral: treatment of menstrual problems, abortifacient
sage	Oral: lowers BP; lowers blood glucose Advise caution with **antidiabetic drugs, anticonvulsants, alcohol.**
SAM-e (adomet)	Oral: promotion of general well-being and health May cause frequent GI complaints and headache. Risk of serotonin syndrome with **antidepressants.**
sarsaparilla	Oral: treatment of skin disorders, rheumatism Advise caution with **anticonvulsants.**
sassafras	Topical: treatment of local pain, skin eruptions Oral: enhancement of athletic performance, "cure" for syphilis Oil may be toxic to fetus, children, and adults when ingested. Interacts with many drugs.
saw palmetto	Oral: treatment of BPH Warn against use with estrogen replacement or hormonal contraceptives—may greatly increase adverse effects. May decrease iron absorption. Advise against use with **finasteride;** toxicity could occur.
schisandra	Oral: health tonic, liver protectant; adjunct in cancer chemotherapy and radiation therapy Warn against use during pregnancy; causes uterine stimulation. Advise caution with all **drugs metabolized in the liver.**
squaw vine	Oral: diuretic, tonic, aid in labor and childbirth, treatment of menstrual problems May cause liver toxicity; increased toxicity of **digoxin.** Disulfiram-like reaction with **alcohol.**

Substance	Reported uses and possible risks
St. John's Wort	Oral: treatment of depression, PMS symptoms; antiviral Topical: to treat puncture wounds, insect bites, crushed fingers or toes Discourage tyramine-containing foods; hypertensive crisis is possible. Thrombocytopenia has been reported. Can increase sensitivity to light; advise against taking with drugs that cause photosensitivity. Severe photosensitivity can occur in light-skinned people. Serious interactions have been reported with **SSRIs, MAOIs, kava, digoxin, theophylline, AIDS antiviral drugs, sympathomimetics, antineoplastics, hormonal contraceptives.** Advise against these combinations.
sweet violet flowers	Oral: treatment of respiratory disorders; emetic Increases effects of **laxatives.**
tarragon	Oral: weight loss; prevents cancer; lowers blood glucose Advise caution with **antidiabetic drugs.**
tea tree oil	Topical: antifungal, antibacterial; used to treat burns, insect bites, irritated skin, acne; used as a mouthwash
thyme	Topical: as liniment, gargle; to treat wounds Oral: antidiarrheal, relief of bronchitis, laryngitis May increase sensitivity to light; warn against combining with **photosensitivity-causing drugs.** Also warn against combining with **MAOIs** or **SSRIs;** may cause serious adverse effects.
turmeric	Oral: antioxidant, anti-inflammatory; used to treat arthritis May cause GI distress. Warn against use with known biliary obstruction. May cause increased bleeding with oral **anticoagulants, NSAIDs.** Advise caution with **immunosuppressants.**
valerian	Oral: sedative and hypnotic; reduces anxiety, relaxes muscles Can cause severe liver damage. Warn against use with **barbiturates, alcohol, CNS depressants, benzodiazepines,** or **antihistamines;** can cause serious sedation.
went rice	Oral: cholesterol- and triglyceride-lowering effects Warn against use in pregnancy, liver disease, alcoholism, or acute infection.
white willow bark	Oral: treatment of fevers Advise caution with **anticoagulants, NSAIDs, diuretics.**
xuan shen	Oral: lowers blood glucose; slows heart rate; treatment of HF Advise caution when taken with **antidiabetic drugs.**
yohimbe	Oral: treatment of ED Can affect BP; CNS stimulant; has cardiac effects. Manic episodes have been reported in psychiatric patients. Warn against use with **SSRIs,** tyramine-containing foods. Advise caution with **TCAs.**

APPENDIX B

Important dietary guidelines for patient teaching

Tyramine-rich foods (important to avoid with MAOIs, some antihypertensives)

Aged cheese	Bologna	Liver	Red wine	Smoked fish
Avocados	Caffeinated	Pepperoni	(Chianti)	Yeast
Bananas	beverages	Pickled fish	Ripe fruit	Yogurt
Beer	Chocolate		Salami	

Potassium-rich foods (important to eat with potassium-wasting diuretics)

Avocados	Dried fruit	Nuts	Prunes	Sunflower seeds
Bananas	Grapefruit	Oranges	Rhubarb	Tomatoes
Broccoli	Lima beans	Peaches	*Sanka* coffee	
Cantaloupe	Navy beans	Potatoes	Spinach	

Calcium-rich foods (important after menopause, in children, in hypocalcemic states)

Bok choy	Canned	Creamed soup	Dairy products	Oysters
Broccoli	sardines	(made with	Milk	Spinach
Canned salmon	Clams	milk)	Molasses	Tofu

Urine acidifiers (important in maintaining excretion of some drugs)

Cheese	Eggs	Grains	Poultry	Red meat
Cranberries	Fish	Plums	Prunes	

Urine alkalinizers (important in maintaining excretion of some drugs)

Apples	Berries	Citrus fruit	Milk	Vegetables

Iron-rich foods (important in maintaining RBCs)

Beets	Dried beans and	Dried fruit	Leafy green	Organ meats
Cereals	peas	Enriched grains	vegetables	(liver, heart,
				kidney)

Low-sodium foods (important in HF, hypertension, fluid overload)

Egg yolks	Honey	Macaroons	Puffed wheat	Sherbet
Fresh fruit	Jam and jelly	Potatoes	Pumpkin	Unsalted nuts
Fresh vegetables	Lean meat	Poultry	Red kidney	
Grits	Lima beans	Puffed rice	beans	

High-sodium foods (important to avoid in HF, hypertension, fluid overload)

Barbecue	Canned	Cured meat	Prepackaged	Snack foods
Beer	seafood	Fast food	dinners	Tomato
Butter	Canned soup	Microwave	Pretzels	ketchup
Buttermilk	Canned	dinners	Sauces	TV dinners
Cake, bread, and	spaghetti	Pickles	Sauerkraut	
other mixes	Cookies			

APPENDIX C

Drugs that interact with grapefruit juice

Grapefruit juice inhibits the CYP450 3A4 system in the liver, which can cause a decrease in the metabolism of many drugs. Decreasing the metabolism of the drug can lead to increased serum drug levels and toxicity. If any of these drugs is being given, the patient should avoid the use of grapefruit juice. If a patient has been stabilized on one of these drugs and suddenly begins to develop signs of drug toxicity, ask the patient specifically if he or she has been drinking grapefruit juice. If a patient is receiving one of these drugs, a key point of patient education should be to avoid the use of grapefruit juice. It takes approximately 48 hr for grapefruit juice to be cleared from the body.

albendazole	fentanyl	sirolimus
alfentanil	fexofenadine	sufentanil
amiodarone	fluoxetine	tacrolimus
amlodipine	fluvastatin	tadalafil
atorvastatin	fluvoxamine	tamoxifen
17 beta-estradiol	indinavir	temsirolimus
budesonide	itraconazole	testosterone
buspirone	losartan	theophylline
caffeine	lovastatin	triazolam
calcium channel blockers	methadone	troleandomycin
carbamazepine	methylprednisolone	verapamil
carvedilol	nelfinavir	vinblastine
cilostazol	nicardipine	vincristine
clarithromycin	nifedipine	warfarin
clomipramine	nimodipine	
cortisol	nisoldipine	
cyclophosphamide	progesterone	
cyclosporine A	quinidine	
dextromethorphan	ritonavir	
diltiazem	saquinavir	
erythromycin	scopolamine	
estrogens	sertraline	
etoposide	sildenafil	
felodipine	simvastatin	

APPENDIX D

Intramuscular and subcutaneous routes of administration

Choosing an IM injection site

When reviewing sites for IM injection, avoid any site that looks inflamed, edematous, or irritated. Also, avoid using a site that contains moles, birthmarks, scar tissue, or other lesions. Then select an appropriate site, such as one of those shown at right, and consider these guidelines:

- The dorsogluteal and ventrogluteal muscles are used most commonly for IM injections.
- The deltoid muscle may be used for injections of 2 mL or less.
- The vastus lateralis muscle is used most commonly in children.
- The rectus femoris may be used in infants.

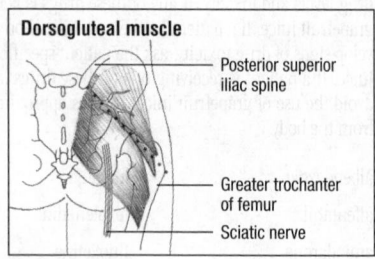

Dorsogluteal muscle

- Posterior superior iliac spine
- Greater trochanter of femur
- Sciatic nerve

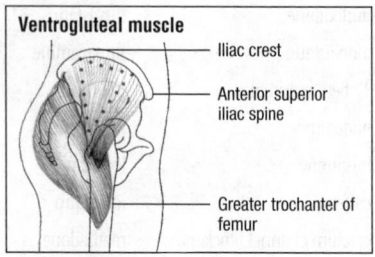

Ventrogluteal muscle

- Iliac crest
- Anterior superior iliac spine
- Greater trochanter of femur

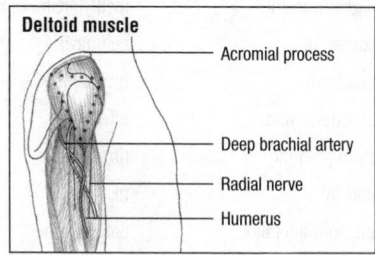

Deltoid muscle

- Acromial process
- Deep brachial artery
- Radial nerve
- Humerus

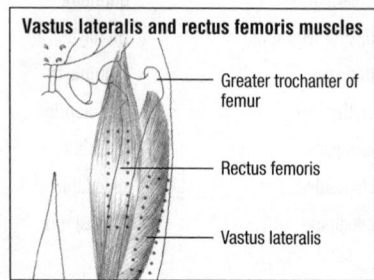

Vastus lateralis and rectus femoris muscles

- Greater trochanter of femur
- Rectus femoris
- Vastus lateralis

Selecting a subcutaneous injection site

To select an appropriate injection site, consider the available areas for subcutaneous injection. These areas offer sites on the abdomen, upper arms, thighs, shoulders, and lower back, as shown here. Also consider the patient's site rotation pattern and plan to use the next available injection site. This promotes drug absorption and helps prevent adverse reactions.

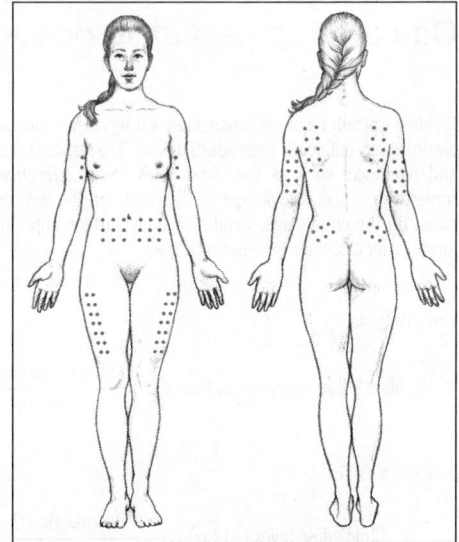

Injecting a subcutaneous drug

While pinching up the patient's skin with your nondominant hand, hold the syringe in your dominant hand and grip the needle sheath with the free fingers of your nondominant hand. Pull the sheath back to uncover the needle, but do not touch the needle. Position the needle with its bevel up.

Tell the patient he or she will feel a prick as you insert the needle. Do so quickly, in one motion, at a 45- or 90-degree angle, as shown at right. The needle length and the angle you use depend on the amount of subcutaneous tissue at the site. Some drugs, such as heparin, should always be injected at a 90-degree angle.

Release the skin to avoid injecting the drug into compressed tissue and irritating the nerves. Slowly inject the drug.

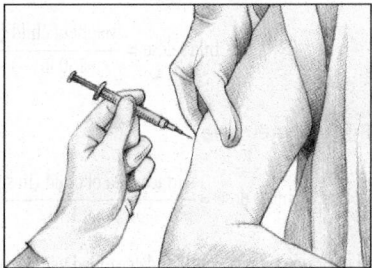

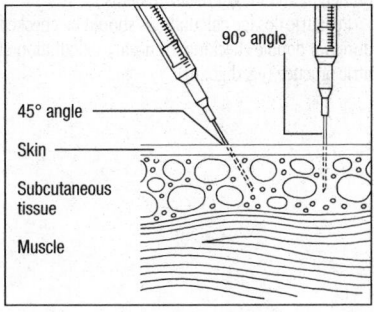

APPENDIX E

Calculating pediatric dosages

Children typically require different doses of drugs than adults because children's bodies often handle drugs very differently from adults' bodies. The standard drug dosages listed in package inserts and references such as the *Physician's Desk Reference* refer to the adult dosage. In some cases, a pediatric dosage is suggested, but in many cases it will need to be calculated based on the child's age, weight, or body surface area. The following are some standard formulas for calculating the pediatric dose.

Fried's rule

$$\text{Infant's dose (age younger than 1 yr)} = \frac{\text{infant's age (in mo)}}{150 \text{ mo}} \times \text{average adult dose}$$

Young's rule

$$\text{Child's dose (ages 1–12 yr)} = \frac{\text{child's age (in yr)}}{\text{child's age (in yr)} + 12} \times \text{average adult dose}$$

Clark's rule

$$\text{Child's dose} = \frac{\text{weight of child (lb)}}{150 \text{ lb}} \times \text{average adult dose}$$

Surface area rule

$$\text{Child's dose} = \frac{\text{surface area of child (in square meters)}}{1.73} \times \text{average adult dose}$$

The surface area of a child is determined using a nomogram that determines surface area based on height and weight measurements.

Pediatric dosage calculations should be checked by two people. Many institutions have procedures for double checking the dosage calculation of those drugs used most frequently in the pediatric practice (eg, digoxin).

Federal drug classifications

FDA pregnancy categories

The FDA has established five categories to indicate the potential for a systemically absorbed drug to cause birth defects. The key differentiation among the categories rests on the degree (reliability) of documentation and the risk-benefit ratio.

Category A: Adequate studies in pregnant women have not demonstrated a risk to the fetus in the first trimester of pregnancy, and there is no evidence of risk in later trimesters.

Category B: Animal studies have not demonstrated a risk to the fetus but there are no adequate studies in pregnant women. *Or,* animal studies have shown an adverse effect, but adequate studies in pregnant women have not demonstrated a risk to the fetus during the first trimester of pregnancy, and there is no evidence of risk in later trimesters.

Category C: Animal studies have shown an adverse effect on the fetus but there are no adequate studies in humans; the benefits from the use of the drug in pregnant women may be acceptable despite its potential risks. *Or,* there are no animal reproduction studies and no adequate studies in humans.

Category D: There is evidence of human fetal risk, but the potential benefits from the use of the drug in pregnant women may be acceptable despite its potential risks.

Category X: Studies in animals or humans demonstrate fetal abnormalities or adverse reaction; reports indicate evidence of fetal risk. The risk of use in a pregnant woman clearly outweighs any possible benefit.

Regardless of the designated pregnancy category or presumed safety, *no drug* should be administered during pregnancy unless it is clearly needed.

DEA schedules of controlled substances

The Controlled Substances Act of 1970 regulates the manufacturing, distribution, and dispensing of drugs that are known to have abuse potential. The DEA is responsible for the enforcement of these regulations. The controlled drugs are divided into five DEA schedules based on their potential for abuse and physical and psychological dependence.

Schedule I *(C-I):* High abuse potential and no accepted medical use (heroin, marijuana, LSD)

Schedule II *(C-II):* High abuse potential with severe dependence liability (narcotics, amphetamines, and barbiturates)

Schedule III *(C-III):* Less abuse potential than Schedule II drugs and moderate dependence liability (nonbarbiturate sedatives, nonamphetamine stimulants, limited amounts of certain narcotics)

Schedule IV *(C-IV):* Less abuse potential than Schedule III drugs and limited dependence liability (some sedatives, antianxiety agents, and nonnarcotic analgesics)

Schedule V *(C-V):* Limited abuse potential. Primarily small amounts of narcotics (codeine) used as antitussives or antidiarrheals. Under federal law, limited quantities of certain Schedule V drugs may be purchased without a prescription directly from a pharmacist. The purchaser must be at least 18 years of age and must furnish suitable identification. All such transactions must be recorded by the dispensing pharmacist.

Prescribing physicians and dispensing pharmacists must be registered with the DEA, which also provides forms for the transfer of Schedules I and II substances and establishes criteria for the inventory and prescribing of controlled substances. State and local laws are often more stringent than federal law. In any given situation, the more stringent law applies.

Cardiovascular guidelines

Classification of blood lipid levels

Serum level	Low*	Optimal*	Normal or desirable*	Borderline high*	High*	Very high*
Total cholesterol			Less than 200	200–239	240 or more	
LDL cholesterol		Less than 100	100–129	130–159	160–189	190 or more
HDL cholesterol	Less than 40				60 or more	
Triglycerides			Less than 150	150–199	200–499	500 or more

* In mg/dL.

LDL target goal is determined by the presence of other major cardiovascular risk factors (cigarette smoking, hypertension, low HDL, family history of premature CAD, men 45 years or older, women 55 years or older).

For 0–1 risk factor, goal for total cholesterol is 160 mg/dL; for 2 or more risk factors, goal is less than 130 mg/dL; for persons with congestive heart disease or diabetes, goal is less than 100 mg/dL.

From the Third Report of the National Cholesterol Education Program (NCEP) Expert Panel on Detection, Evaluation, and Treatment of High Blood Cholesterol in Adults (Adult Treatment Panel III). U.S. Department of Health and Human Services, National Institutes of Health, National Heart, Lung, and Blood Institute, 2004. Available at http://www.nhlbi.nih.gov/guidelines/cholesterol/atp3full.pdf.

Classification of blood pressure

Category	Systolic blood pressure (mm Hg)		Diastolic blood pressure (mm Hg)
Normal	Less than 120	and	Less than 80
Prehypertension	120–139	or	80–89
Hypertension, Stage 1	140–159	or	90–99
Hypertension, Stage 2	160 or more	or	100 or more

From the Seventh Report of the Joint National Committee on Prevention, Detection, Evaluation, and Treatment of High Blood Pressure (JNC 7). U.S. Department of Health and Human Services, National Institutes of Health, National Heart, Lung, and Blood Institute, 2003. Available at http://www.nhlbi.nih.gov/guidelines/hypertension/jnc7full.pdf.

Normal laboratory values

Test	Conventional units	Systems international units
albumin	3.5–5.0 g/dL	35–50 g/L
aminotransferases		
ALT	7–53 international units/L	0.12–0.88 μkat/L
AST	11–47 international units/L	0.8–0.78 μkat/L
ammonia	15–56 mcg/dL	9–33 μmol/L
amylase	25–115 international units/L	0.42–1.92 μkat/L
bilirubin		
total	0.3–1.1 mg/dL	5.13–18.80 μmol/L
direct	0–0.3 mg/dL	0–5.1 μmol/L
blood gases		
pH	7.35–7.45	7.35–7.45
PO_2	80–105 mm Hg	10.6–14 kPa
PCO_2	35–45 mm Hg	4.7–6 kPa
BUN	8–25 mg/dL	2.9–8.9 mmol/L
calcium		
total	8.6–10.3 mg/dL	2.15–2.58 mmol/L
ionized	4.5–5.1 mg/dL	1.13–1.28 mmol/L
chloride	97–110 mEq/L	97–110 mmol/L
coagulation studies		
bleeding time	2.5–9.5 min	150–570 sec
fibrinogen	150–360 mg/dL	1.5–3.6 g/L
PTT	21–32 sec	21–32 sec
prothrombin time	8.2–10.3 sec	8.2–10.3 sec
INR	0.9–1.13	0.9–1.13
thrombin time	11.3–18.5 sec	11.3–18.5 sec
creatinine	0.5–1.7 mg/dL	44–150 μmol/L
erythrocyte count		
male	$4.5–5.7 \times 10^6/mm^3$	$4.5–5.7 \times 10^{12}/L$
female	$3.9–5 \times 10^6/mm^3$	$3.9–5 \times 10^{12}/L$
glucose (fasting)	65–109 mg/dL	3.58–6.1 mmol/L
hematocrit		
male	41%–50%	138–172 g/L
female	35%–46%	120–156 g/L

Always check test results against the values considered normal by the laboratory doing the test.
Variations between laboratories are possible.

Test	Conventional units	Systems international units
hemoglobin		
male	13.8–17.2 g/dL	138–172 g/L
female	12–15.6 g/dL	120–156 g/L
hemoglobin A_{1c}	Less than 6% of total Hb	Less than 0.06 of total Hb
iron		
male	45–160 mcg/dL	8.1–31.3 μmol/L
female	30–160 mcg/dL	5.4–31.3 μmol/L
LDH	100–250 international units/L	1.67–4.17 μkat/L
leukocyte count		
total	3.8–9.8 × 10^3/μL	3.8–9.8 × 10^9/L
lymphocytes	1.2–3.3 × 10^3/μL	1.2–3.3 × 10^9/L
mononuclear cells	0.2–0.7 × 10^3/μL	0.2–0.7 × 10^9/L
granulocytes	1.8–6.6 × 10^3/μL	1.8–6.6 × 10^9/L
lipase	10–150 units/L	10–150 units/L
magnesium	1.3–2.2 mEq/L	0.65–1.10 mmol/L
phosphate	2.5–4.5 mg/dL	0.75–1.35 mmol/L
platelet count	140–440 × 10^3/μL	140–440 × 10^9/L
reticulocyte count		
adults	0.5%–1.5%	0.005%–0.015%
children	2.5%–6.5%	
potassium	3.3–4.9 mEq/L	3.3–4.9 mmol/L
sodium	135–145 mEq/L	135–145 mmol/L
uric acid	3–8 mg/dL	179–476 μmol/L

Always check test results against the values considered normal by the laboratory doing the test.
Variations between laboratories are possible.

APPENDIX I

Canadian drug information

Narcotics, controlled drugs, benzodiazepines, and other targeted substances

This table summarizes the requirements for prescribing, dispensing, and record-keeping for narcotics, controlled drugs, benzodiazepines, and other targeted substances. This information is not a comprehensive review; the reader is encouraged to seek additional and confirmatory information (eg, Controlled Drugs and Substances Act, Narcotic Control Regulations, parts G and J of the Food and Drug Regulations, Benzodiazepines, and Other Targeted Substances Regulations). *Reviewed 2011 by the Office of Controlled Substances, Health Canada.*

Classification and description	Legal requirements
Narcotic drugs*	
• 1 narcotic (eg, cocaine, codeine, hydromorphone, ketamine, morphine) • 1 narcotic + 1 active non-narcotic ingredient (eg, *Novahistex DH, Tylenol No. 4*) • All narcotics for parenteral use (eg, fentanyl, pethidine) • All products containing hydrocodone, oxycodone, methadone, or pentazocine • Dextropropoxyphene (eg, *Darvon-N, 642*) • Nabilone (ie, Cesamet)	• Written prescription required. • Verbal prescriptions not permitted. • Refills not permitted. • Written prescription may be prescribed to be dispensed in divided portions (part-fills). • For part-fills, copies of prescriptions should be made in reference to the original prescription. Indicate on the original prescription: the new prescription number, the date of the part-fill, the quantity dispensed, and the pharmacist's initials. • Transfers not permitted. • Record and retain all documents pertaining to all transactions for at least 2 years in a manner that permits an audit. • Sales reports required except for dextropropoxyphene, propoxyphene. • Report any loss or theft of narcotic drugs within 10 days after the discovery date to the Office of Controlled Substances at the address indicated on the forms.
Narcotic preparations*	
• Verbal prescription narcotics: 1 narcotic + 2 or more active non-narcotic ingredients in a recognized therapeutic dose (eg, *Fiorinal-C¼, Fiorinal-C½, Robitussin AC, 282, 292, Tylenol No. 2, Tylenol No. 3*) • Exempted codeine compounds: contain codeine up to 8 mg/solid dosage form or 20 mg/30 mL liquid + 2 or more active non-narcotic ingredients (eg, *Atasol-8*).	• Written or verbal prescriptions permitted. • Refills not permitted. • Written or verbal prescriptions may be prescribed to be dispensed in divided portions (part-fills). • For part-fills, copies of prescriptions should be made in reference to the original prescription. Indicate on the original prescription: the new prescription number, the date of the part-fill, the quantity dispensed, and the pharmacist's initials. • Transfers not permitted. • Exempted codeine compounds when dispensed pursuant to a prescription follow the same regulations as for verbal prescription narcotics.

*The products noted are examples only.

Classification and description	Legal requirements

Narcotic preparations* (continued)

- Record and retain all documents pertaining to all transactions for at least 2 years, in a manner that permits an audit.
- Sales reports not required.
- Report any loss or theft of narcotic drugs within 10 days after the discovery date to the Office of Controlled Substances at the address indicated on the forms.

Controlled drugs*

- Part I
  Amphetamines (eg, *Dexedrine, Adderall XR*)
  Methylphenidate (eg, *Biphentin, Concerta, Ritalin*)
  Pentobarbital
  Preparations: 1 controlled drug + 1 or more active noncontrolled ingredient(s) in a recognized therapeutic dose (eg, *Bellergal Spacetabs*)

- Written or verbal prescriptions permitted.
- Refills not permitted for verbal prescriptions.
- Refills permitted for written prescriptions if the prescriber has indicated in writing the number of refills and dates for, or intervals between, refills.
- Written or verbal prescriptions may be prescribed to be dispensed in divided portions (part-fills).
- For refills and part-fills, copies of prescriptions should be made in reference to the original prescription. Indicate on the original prescription: the new prescription number, the date of the repeat or part-fill, the quantity dispensed, and the pharmacist's initials.
- Transfers not permitted.
- Record and retain all documents pertaining to all transactions for a period of at least 2 years, in a manner that permits an audit.
- Sales reports required except for controlled drug preparations.
- Report any loss or theft of controlled drugs within 10 days after the discovery date to the Office of Controlled Substances at the address indicated on the forms.

- Part II
  Barbiturates (eg, phenobarbital)
  Butorphanol
  Nalbuphine (*Nubain* injection)
  Preparations: 1 controlled drug + 1 or more active noncontrolled ingredient(s) in a recognized therapeutic dose (eg, *Fiorinal*)
- Part III
  Anabolic steroids including:
  Testosterone (eg, *Androderm*)
  Testosterone cypionate (eg, *Depo-Testosterone*)
  Testosterone undecanoate (eg, *Andriol*)

- Written or verbal prescriptions permitted.
- Refills permitted for written or verbal prescriptions if the prescriber has authorized in writing or verbally (at the time of issuance) the number of refills and dates for, or intervals between, refills.
- Written or verbal prescriptions may be prescribed to be dispensed in divided portions (part-fills).
- For refills and part-fills, copies of prescriptions should be made in reference to the original prescription. Indicate on the original prescription: the new prescription number, the date of the repeat or part-fill, the quantity dispensed, and the pharmacist's initials.
- Transfers not permitted.
- Record and retain all documents pertaining to all transactions for a period of at least 2 years, in a manner that permits an audit.
- Sales reports not required.
- Report the loss or theft of controlled drugs within 10 days after the discovery date to the Office of Controlled Substances at the address indicated on the forms.

*The products noted are examples only.

Classification and description	Legal requirements

Benzodiazepines and other targeted substances*

Alprazolam
Bromazepam
Chlordiazepoxide
Clobazam
Diazepam
Ethchlorvynol
Lorazepam
Meprobamate
Oxazepam
Temazepam
Triazolam

- Written and verbal prescriptions permitted.
- Refills for written or verbal prescriptions permitted if indicated by prescriber and less than 1 yr has elapsed since the day the prescription was issued by the prescriber.
- Part-fills permitted as per prescriber's instructions.
- For refills or part-fills of prescriptions, record the following information: date of the repeat or part-fill, prescription number, quantity dispensed, and the pharmacist's initials.
- Transfer of prescriptions permitted except for a prescription that has been already transferred.
- Record and retain all documents pertaining to all transactions for a period of at least 2 years, in a manner that permits an audit.
- Sales reports not required.
- Report any loss or theft of benzodiazepines and other targeted substances within 10 days after the discovery date to the Office of Controlled Substances at the address indicated on the forms.

Adapted with permission from *Compendium of Pharmaceuticals and Specialties.* Ottawa, Canada: Canadian Pharmacists Association, 2013.

*The products noted are only examples.

Adverse reaction and medical device problem reporting

Consumers/patients and health professionals can report adverse reactions (also known as side effects) to health products, including prescription and non-prescription medications, biologics, natural health products and radiopharmaceuticals, to the Canada Vigilance Program: http://www.hc-sc.gc.ca/dhp-mps/medeff/vigilance-eng.php

The **Canada Vigilance Program** is Health Canada's post-market surveillance program that collects and assesses reports of suspected adverse reactions to health products marketed in Canada. Post-market surveillance enables Health Canada to monitor the safety profile of health products once they are marketed to ensure that the benefits of the products continue to outweigh the risks.

The Canada Vigilance Program has collected reports of suspected adverse reactions since 1965. Adverse reaction reports are submitted by health professionals and consumers on a voluntary basis either directly to Health Canada or via Market Authorization Holders. The following health products marketed in Canada are collected by the program: prescription and non-prescription medications, biologics, natural health products and radiopharmaceuticals. The information collected by the program can be accessed through the Canada Vigilance Online Database.

The Canada Vigilance Program is supported by seven Canada Vigilance Regional Offices who provide a regional point-of-contact for health professionals and consumers. Reports are collected by the regional offices before being forwarded to the Canada Vigilance National Office for further analysis.

The **Canada Vigilance Regional Offices** work collaboratively with the Canada Vigilance National Office to collect reports submitted by health professionals and consumers. (Market Authorization Holders send reports directly to the Canada Vigilance National Office). Each office has regional responsibility for collection of adverse reaction reports, which are then reviewed for completeness before being forwarded to the Canada Vigilance National Office for further analysis.

The regional offices also:
- increase health professional and consumer awareness of, and participation in the Canada Vigilance Program
- improve communication between the adverse reaction program and individuals who report adverse reactions
- provide guidance on adverse reaction reporting in order to maximize the quality of reports
- direct Canadians to Health Canada sources of new safety information regarding Canadian marketed health products.

Below is a list of the regional offices.

For all regional offices:
Telephone (automatic redirect):   1-866-234-2345
Facsimile (automatic redirect):   1-866-678-6789
Teletypewriter: 1-800-267-1245 (Health Canada)

British Columbia and Yukon
Canada Vigilance Regional Office-British
   Columbia and Yukon
Health Canada
400-4595 Canada Way,
Burnaby, British Columbia
V5G 1J9
E-mail: CanadaVigilance_BC@hc-sc.gc.ca

Alberta and Northwest Territories
Canada Vigilance Regional Office-Alberta and
   Northwest Territories
Health Canada
Suite 730, 9700 Jasper Avenue
Edmonton, Alberta
T5J 4C3
E-mail: CanadaVigilance_AB@hc-sc.gc.ca

Saskatchewan
Canada Vigilance Regional Office-Saskatchewan
Health Canada
4th floor, Room 412
101 - 22nd Street East
Saskatoon, Saskatchewan
S7K 0E1
E-mail: CanadaVigilance_SK@hc-sc.gc.ca

Manitoba
Canada Vigilance Regional Office-Manitoba
Health Canada
510 Lagimodière Boulevard
Winnipeg, Manitoba
R2J 3Y1
E-mail: CanadaVigilance_MB@hc-sc.gc.ca

Ontario and Nunavut
Canada Vigilance Regional Office-Ontario and
   Nunavut
Health Canada
2301 Midland Avenue
Toronto, Ontario
M1P 4R7
E-mail: CanadaVigilance_ON@hc-sc.gc.ca

Québec
Canada Vigilance Regional Office-Québec
Health Canada
Suite 202-40, 2nd Floor, East Tower
200 René-Lévesque Boulevard West
Montréal, Québec
H2Z 1X4
E-mail: CanadaVigilance_QC@hc-sc.gc.ca

**New Brunswick, Nova Scotia, Prince
   Edward Island and, Newfoundland and
   Labrador**
Canada Vigilance Regional Office-Atlantic
Health Canada
Suite 1625, 16th floor
1505 Barrington Street, Maritime Centre
Halifax, Nova Scotia
B3J 3Y6
E-mail: CanadaVigilance_ATL@hc-sc.gc.ca

If you are outside the country:
Canada Vigilance National Office
Marketed Health Products Safety and Effectiveness Information Division
Marketed Health Products Directorate
Health Products and Food Branch
Health Canada
Address Locator 0701E
Ottawa, Ontario
K1A 0K9
Canada
Email: CanadaVigilance@hc-sc.gc.ca

The Canada Vigilance Program provides a variety of tools for health professionals and consumers to report suspected adverse reactions. Reporting is simple and can be done online, by phone or by submitting the Canada Vigilance Reporting Form by fax or mail.

Source: Health Canada, 2011. Reproduced with permission from the Minister of Health, 2013.

APPENDIX J

Commonly used Canadian drugs

▷ cyproterone acetate

ANDROCUR, ANDROCUR DEPOT, AND OTHERS

Drug class and indications
Androgen receptor antagonist, antineoplastic, contraceptive

Treatment of prostate cancer, hypersexuality, hirsutism; hormone therapy for male-to-female transgender patients, hot flashes; part of combination oral contraceptives

Dosages and special alerts
25–50 mg PO bid. Up to 100 mg/day can be used for hypersexuality, hirsutism, hormone therapy for male-to-female transgender persons, hot flashes; 300 mg/day PO or IM for prostate cancer; 2 mg with 35 or 50 mcg/day PO ethinyl estradiol for contraception. Not for use in pregnancy. Monitor for liver toxicity; risk increases with higher doses. Risk of adrenal suppression, depression and mood changes, gynecomastia, and sexual dysfunction in males exists. Dosage should be tapered when discontinuing to allow adrenal function to return and to balance testosterone production.

▷ doxylamine succinate and pyridoxine hydrochloride

DICLECTIN

Drug class and indications
Antinausea drug, antihistamine, vitamin

Prevention of nausea and vomiting in pregnancy

Dosages and special alerts
Two DR tablets (10 mg doxylamine, 10 mg pyridoxine/tablet) PO at bedtime. One tablet in the morning and one tablet midday may be added if needed to control nausea and vomiting. Tablet must be swallowed whole; do not cut, crush, or chew tablet. Drug may cause drowsiness, vertigo, nervousness, disorientation. Warn patient to avoid driving or operating dangerous machinery until the effects of the drug are known. Do not combine with alcohol or other CNS depressants. Not for use in patients with epilepsy.

▷ flunarizine hydrochloride

Drug class and indications
Antimigraine drug

Prevention of migraine with or without aura

Dosages and special alerts
10 mg/day PO in the evening. 5 mg/day may be tried in patients who experience adverse effects. Not for treatment of acute migraine. Contraindicated for use in patients with history or depression and in patients with pre-existing extrapyramidal disorders. Not recommended for use in pregnancy.

Motor disturbances are very common, but these disturbances do not respond to antiparkinsonian drugs. Effects usually reverse with discontinuation of the drug. Sedation and drowsiness may occur. Warn patient to avoid driving or operating dangerous machinery until the effects of the drug are known.

▽ flupenthixol

FLUANXOL

Drug class and indications

Antipsychotic, thioxanthene derivative

Maintenance therapy for chronic schizophrenia in patients whose main manifestations do not include excitement, agitation, or hyperactivity

Dosages and special alerts

IM: 20 mg by deep IM injection; a second dose of 20–40 mg IM may be given in 4 to 10 days. If patient is controlled and tolerates the drug well, maintenance dose is 20–40 mg IM every 2–3 wk.

PO: 1 mg PO tid. May be increased to control symptoms to maintenance dose of 3–6 mg/day. Once stabilized, patients may be switched to IM coverage every 2–3 weeks. Contraindicated with CNS depression, blood dyscrasias, pheochromocytoma, liver damage, renal dysfunction. Do not use to treat severe agitation in psychiatric or psychoneurotic patients or to treat elderly patients with agitation. Use cautiously with pregnancy and lactation. Monitor for sedation and extrapyramidal responses. Warn patient to avoid driving or operating dangerous machinery until the effects of the drug are known.

▽ L-tryptophan

TRYPTAN AND OTHERS

Drug class and indications

Amino acid, sleep aid

To improve sleep and enhance mood

Dosages and special alerts

One or two 500-mg tablets PO at bedtime with food; may be increased to a maximum of 8–12 g per day. The amino acid is converted to serotonin in the brain to promote natural sleep and improve mood. No known contraindications exist. Few adverse effects reported.

▽ nitrazepam

MOGADON, NITRAZADON

Drug class and indications

Hypnotic, anticonvulsant, benzodiazepine

Symptomatic relief of transient and short-term insomnia characterized by difficulty falling asleep, frequent nocturnal awakenings, or early morning awakenings for a maximum of 7–10 days. May also be useful for the treatment of myoclonic seizures.

Dosages and special alerts
5–10 mg PO before bedtime for a maximum of 7–10 days. Elderly or debilitated patients should start at 2.5 mg/day and should not exceed 5 mg/day PO. *Children treated for myoclonic seizures (up to 30 kg):* 0.3–1 mg/kg/day PO divided into three doses. Contraindicated with myasthenia gravis, sleep apnea syndrome, known paradoxical reactions to alcohol or sedative medications, hypersensitivity to any benzodiazepine; use extreme caution with history of substance of alcohol abuse. Not recommended during pregnancy. Sedative effects, confusion, and drowsiness are common. Caution patient to avoid driving or operating hazardous machinery. Use of flumazenil (benzodiazepine antagonist) not recommended in patients with epilepsy who are treated with nitrazepam; this combination may precipitate seizures.

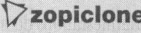

zopiclone

IMOVANE, RHOVANE

Drug class and indications
Sedative-hypnotic; cyclopyrrolone derivative
   Treatment of insomnia

Dosages and special alerts
5–7.5 mg PO taken at bedtime. Use cautiously with elderly or debilitated patients and patients with hepatic impairment or chronic respiratory insufficiency (reduce dosage to 3.75 mg PO at bedtime); history of depression; pregnancy, lactation; and history of substance abuse (may be habit-forming). Monitor for dizziness, sedation, anxiety, nervousness; warn patient to avoid driving or operating hazardous machinery until the effects of the drug are known. Dry mouth, metallic taste may occur; frequent mouth care and sucking sugarless candies may help. Be alert for sudden mood changes when drug is stopped.

APPENDIX K

Topical drugs

Topical drugs are agents that are intended for surface use, not ingestion or injection. They may be very toxic if absorbed into the system, but they serve several purposes when used topically.

Pregnancy Category C
Contraindications and cautions

Contraindicated with allergy to these drugs, open wounds, or abrasions.

Adverse effects

Local irritation (common), stinging, burning, dermatitis, toxic effects if absorbed systemically.

Teaching points

Apply sparingly to affected area as directed. Do not use with open wounds or broken skin. Avoid contact with eyes. Report any local irritation, allergic reaction, worsening of condition being treated.

Drug	Selected trade names	Instructions and preparations
Acne, rosacea, and melasma products		
adapalene	*Differin*	Do not use on cuts or any open area. Do not use in children younger than 12 yr. Avoid use on sunburned skin, in combination with other products, or exposure to sun. Apply a thin film to affected area after washing every night at bedtime. Drug is less drying than other products. Available as lotion, cream, gel; 0.1%, 0.3% concentrations.
alitretinoin	*Panretin*	Used for treatment of lesions of Kaposi sarcoma. 1% gel; apply as needed to cover lesions twice daily. Photosensitivity common. Inflammation, peeling, redness may occur. Pregnancy Category D.
azelaic acid	*Azelex* *Finacea*	Wash and dry skin. Massage a thin layer into affected area twice daily. Wash hands thoroughly after application. Improvement usually occurs within 4 wk. Initial irritation usually occurs but passes with time. Gel—15%.
clindamycin	*Clindesse* *Evoclin*	2% vaginal cream for the treatment of bacterial vaginitis; one applicatorful (100 mg) given vaginally at any time of the day. 1% foam used for the treatment of acne vulgaris; apply once daily to affected areas that have been washed and are fully dry.
clindamycin and benzoyl peroxide	*Acanya* *BenzaClin*	Apply gel to affected areas bid. Wash area and pat dry before application. Gel—1.2%, 2.5% (*Acanya*); 1%, 5% (*BenzaClin*).
clindamycin and tretinoin	*Veltin* *Ziana*	Rub pea-size amount over entire face once daily at bedtime. Not for use by patients with colitis. Avoid exposure to sunlight. Gel—0.025%, 1.2%.
dapsone	*Aczone Gel*	Apply thin layer of gel to affected areas bid. Closely follow Hgb, reticulocyte count in patients with G6PD deficiencies. Gel—5%.

(continued)

Drug	Selected trade names	Instructions and preparations
Acne, rosacea, and melasma products *(continued)*		
fluocinolone acetonide, hydroquinone, and tretinoin	*Tri-Luma*	Do not use during pregnancy. Apply to depigmented area of melasma once each evening, at least 30 min before bedtime after cleansing and patting dry; avoid occlusive dressings. Use a sunscreen and protective clothing if outside; skin dryness and peeling may occur. Cream—0.01% fluocinolone, 4% hydroquinone, 0.05% tretinoin.
ingenol mebutate	*Picato*	Apply 0.015% gel once daily to face and scalp for 3 days. Apply 0.05% gel once daily to trunk and extremities for 2 days.
metronidazole	*MetroCream MetroGel MetroLotion Noritate*	For treatment of rosacea. Apply cream to affected area bid. Cream—0.75%, 1%.
sodium sulfacetamide	*Klaron*	Apply a thin film bid to affected areas. Wash affected area with mild soap and water; pat dry. Avoid use in denuded or abraded areas.
tazarotene	*Fabior Tazorac*	Treatment of psoriasis. Avoid use in pregnancy. Apply thin film once daily in the evening. Do not use with irritants or products with high alcohol content. Drying causes photosensitivity. Cream, gel—0.05%, 1%.
tretinoin, 0.025% cream	*Avita*	Apply thin layer once daily. Discomfort, peeling, redness may occur for the first 2–4 wk. Worsened acne may occur in first few wk.
tretinoin, 0.05% cream	*Renova*	Used for removal of fine wrinkles. Apply thin coat in the evening.
tretinoin, gel	*Retin-A* Micro*	Apply to cover once daily after cleansing. Exacerbation of inflammation may occur at first. Therapeutic effects usually seen in first 2 wk.
Analgesics		
capsaicin	*Axsain Capsin Capzasin Icy Hot PM No Pain-HP Pain Doctor Qutenza Zostrix Zostrix-HP*	Apply not more than tid to qid. Applied locally, provides temporary relief from the pain of osteoarthritis, rheumatoid arthritis, neuralgias. Do not bandage tightly. Stop use and seek health care if condition worsens or persists after 14–28 days. *Qutenza*: Apply patch to relieve pain of postherpetic neuralgia.
Antibiotics		
ciprofloxacin and dexamethasone	*Ciprodex*	Apply drops to ears of child with acute otitis media who has tympanostomy tubes; apply to outer ear canal of patients with acute otitis externa. Use twice daily for 7 days.
ciprofloxacin and hydrocortisone	*Cipro-HC Otic Drops*	Apply drops to ears of child with acute otitis media who has tympanostomy tubes; apply to outer ear canal of patients with acute otitis externa. Use twice daily for 7 days.

Drug	Selected trade names	Instructions and preparations

Antibiotics (continued)

Drug	Selected trade names	Instructions and preparations
mupirocin	*Bactroban* *Centany*	Used to treat impetigo caused by *Staphylococcus aureus, Streptococcus,* and *Staphylococcus pyogenes* (2% ointment). Apply small amount to affected area tid; may be covered with a gauze dressing. Monitor for signs of superinfection; reevaluate if no clinical response in 3–5 days.
mupirocin calcium	*Bactroban Nasal*	Used to eradicate the nasal colonization of methicillin-resistant *S. aureus* (2.15% ointment, cream). Apply one-half of the ointment from single-use tube between nostrils and apply bid for 5 days.
retapamulin	*Altabax*	Used to treat impetigo. Apply thin layer of ointment to affected area bid for 5 days. May be used on patients 9 mo and older.

Anti–diaper-rash drug

Drug	Selected trade names	Instructions and preparations
miconazole, zinc oxide, petrolatum	*Vusion*	Apply gently to diaper area for 7 days. Verify *Candida* infection before beginning treatment. Combine with frequent diaper changes and gentle washing.

Antifungals

Drug	Selected trade names	Instructions and preparations
butenafine hydrochloride	*Mentax*	Used to treat intradigital pedia (athlete's foot), tinea corporis, ringworm, tinea cruris. Apply to affected area once a day for 4 wk.
butoconazole nitrate	*Gynazole-1*	Used to treat complicated and uncomplicated vulvovaginal candidiasis. Apply intravaginally as one dose (2% cream). Culture fungus; if no response, reculture. Ensure use of full course of therapy. May cause irritation, burning. May damage diaphragms and condoms.
ciclopirox	*Loprox* *Penlac Nail Lacquer*	Used to treat onychomycosis of fingernails and toenails in immunocompromised patients. Apply directly to affected fingernails or toenails.
clotrimazole	*Cruex* *Desenex* *Lotrimin* *Mycelex*	Clean area before applying. Gently massage into affected area up to twice daily. Use for up to 4 wk. Discontinue if irritation, worsening of condition occurs.
econazole nitrate	*Spectazole*	Apply locally once or twice daily. Clean area before applying. Treat for 2–4 wk. Discontinue if irritation, burning, or worsening of condition occurs. For athlete's foot, change socks and shoes at least once a day.
gentian violet		Do not apply to active lesions. Apply locally up to twice daily. May stain skin and clothing.
ketoconazole	*Extina* *Nizoral* *Xolegel*	Used to treat wide range of topical fungal infections from tinea to seborrheic dermatitis. Available as cream, foam, gel, shampoo. Apply as shampoo daily. Itching or stinging of the scalp may occur.
naftifine hydro-chloride	*Naftin*	Gently massage into affected area twice daily. Avoid occlusive dressings. Wash hands thoroughly after application. Do not use longer than 4 wk.

(continued)

Drug	Selected trade names	Instructions and preparations

Antifungals (continued)

oxiconazole	*Oxistat*	Apply every day up to twice daily. May be needed for up to 1 mo.
sertaconazole nitrate	*Ertaczo*	Apply to areas between toes affected by tinea pedis and to the surrounding healthy tissue bid for 4 wk.
terbinafine	*Lamisil*	Apply to area bid until clinical signs are improved, 1–4 wk. Do not use occlusive dressings. Report local irritation. Discontinue if local irritation occurs.
tolnaftate	*Absorbine Aftate Genaspor Quinsana Plus Tinactin*	Apply small amount bid for 2–3 wk; 4–6 wk may be needed if skin is very thick. Clean skin with soap and water before applying drug; dry thoroughly; wear loose, well-fitting shoes; change socks at least four times a day.

Antihistamine

azelastine hydrochloride	*Astelin Astepro*	Use two sprays per nostril bid. Avoid use of alcohol and OTC antihistamines; dizziness and sedation can occur.

Antipsoriatics

anthralin	*Balnetar Fototar Dritho-Cream HP Zithranol Zithranol RR*	Apply every day only to psoriatic lesions. Use protective dressing. Avoid contact with eyes. May stain fabrics, skin, hair, fingernails.
calcipotriene	*Dovonex*	Used as a synthetic vitamin D_2. Use only for disorder prescribed. Apply thin layer once or twice a day. Monitor serum calcium levels with extended use. May cause local irritation.
calcipotriene and betamethasone	*Taclonex Taclonex Scalp*	Apply to affected area once daily for up to 4 wk. Maximum, 100 g/wk. Limit treatment area to 30% of body surface. Do not use occlusive dressings on the area.

Antiseborrheics

selenium sulfide	*Selsun Blue*	Massage 5–10 mL into scalp; rest 2–3 min, rinse, repeat. May damage jewelry; remove jewelry before use. Discontinue use if local irritation occurs.

Antiseptics

benzalkonium chloride	*Benza Mycocide NS Zephiran*	Mix in solution as needed. Spray for preoperative use; store instruments in solution. Thoroughly rinse detergents and soaps from skin before use. Add antirust tablets for instruments stored in solution; dilute solution as indicated for use.
chlorhexidine gluconate	*BactoShield Dyna-Hex Exidine Hibistat*	Use for surgical scrub, preoperative skin prep, wound cleansing, preoperative bathing and showering. Scrub or rinse. Leave on for 15 sec; for surgical scrub, leave on for 3 min.

Drug	Selected trade names	Instructions and preparations

Antiseptics (continued)

Drug	Selected trade names	Instructions and preparations
hexachlorophene	*pHisoHex*	Use for surgical wash, scrub. Apply as wash; do not use with burns or on mucous membranes. Rinse thoroughly. Do not use routinely for bathing infants.
iodine		Wash affected area with solution. Solution is highly toxic; avoid occlusive dressings; stains skin and clothing.
povidone iodine	*ACU-dyne* *Betadine* *Betagen* *Etodine* *Iodex* *Minidyne* *Operand* *Polydine*	HIV may be inactivated in this solution. Apply as needed; treated areas may be bandaged. Causes less irritation than iodine and is less toxic.
sodium hypochlorite	*Dakin's solution*	Apply as antiseptic. *Caution:* Chemical burns can occur.

Antivirals

Drug	Selected trade names	Instructions and preparations
acyclovir	*Zovirax*	Apply cream five times/day for 4 days.
acyclovir and hydrocortisone	*Xerese*	Used to treat cold sores in patients 6 yr and older. Apply five times a day for 5 days. Use early in outbreak to reduce ulcerations and decrease healing time.
docosanol	*Abreva*	Used to treat oral and facial herpes simplex cold sores, fever blisters. Apply five times per day for 10 days. Caution patient not to overuse.
imiquimod	*Aldara*	Used to treat external genital warts and perianal warts. Apply a thin layer to warts and rub in three times per wk at bedtime for 16 wk; remove with soap and water after 6–10 hr. For typical nonhyperkeratotic actinic keratoses on face or scalp in immune-compromised patients, apply cream to affected area before bed twice weekly for 16 wk. For topical treatment of superficial basal cell carcinoma in immune-compromised patients, 10–40 mg applied to lesion five times weekly at bedtime for 6 wk.
	Zyclara	3.75% cream used to treat nonhyperkeratotic, nonhypertrophic, visible, or palpable acitinic keratose on the face or balding scalp of adults. Apply once daily to the affected area at bedtime for 2 wk. Treatment cycle is 2 wk of treatment followed by 2 wk of nontreatment. Once-a-day treatment for genital and perianal warts in patients 12 yr and older.
kunecatechins	*Veregen*	Used to treat external and perianal warts in immunocompetent patients older than 18 yr. Apply to each wart tid for up to 16 wk; do not cover treated area.
penciclovir	*Denavir*	Used to treat cold sores in healthy patients. Reserve use for herpes labialis on lips and face; avoid mucous membranes. Use at first sign of cold sore. Apply thin layer to affected area every 2 hr while awake for 4 days.

(continued)

Drug	Selected trade names	Instructions and preparations
Burn treatments		
mafenide	*Sulfamylon*	Apply to a clean, debrided wound, one or two times per day with a gloved hand. Cover burn at all times with drug, reapply as needed. Bathe patient in a whirlpool daily to aid debridement. Continue mafenide until healing occurs; monitor for infection and toxicity—acidosis. May cause marked discomfort on application.
silver sulfadiazine	*Silvadene* *SSD cream* *Thermazene*	Apply once or twice a day to a clean, debrided wound. Use a ⅟₁₆-inch thickness. Bathe patient in a whirlpool to aid debridement. Dressings are not necessary but may be used; reapply as needed. Monitor for fungal superinfections.
Corticosteroids		
alclometasone diproprionate	*Aclovate*	Available as ointment and cream in 0.05% concentration.
beclomethasone dipropionate	*Beconase AQ* *Qnasl*	Nasal spray for rhinitis.
betamethasone dipropionate		Available as ointment, cream, gel, lotion, aerosol in 0.05% concentration.
betamethasone dipropionate augmented	*Diprolene* *Diprolene AF*	Available as ointment, cream, lotion in 0.05% concentration.
betamethasone valerate	*Betaderm (CAN)* *Beta-Val* *Luxiq, Prevex B (CAN)*	Available as ointment, cream, and lotion in 0.1% concentration.
	Valisone	Available as foam in 0.12% concentration.
ciclesonide	*Alvesco*	Available as 80 mcg and 160 mcg/actuation, as nasal spray or solution for inhalation.
	Omnaris *Zetonna*	Available as nasal aerosol for seasonal and perennial allergic rhinitis.
clobetasol propionate	*Clobex*	Available as 0.05% spray.
	Cormax *Dermovate (CAN)* *Olux* *Temovate*	Available as ointment, cream, foam, and gel in 0.05% concentration.
clocortolone pivalate	*Cloderm*	Available as cream in 0.1% concentration.
desonide	*DesOwen*	Available as ointment, lotion, and cream in 0.05% concentration.
	Verdeso	Available as foam in 0.05% concentration.

Drug	Selected trade names	Instructions and preparations
Corticosteroids *(continued)*		
desoximetasone	*Topicort*	Available as ointment and cream in 0.25% concentration. Available as cream and gel in 0.05% concentration.
dexamethasone	*Aeroseb-Dex*	Available as aerosol in 0.01% and 0.04% concentrations.
diflorasone diacetate	*Florone* *Florone E* *Maxiflor* *Psorcon E*	Available as ointment and cream in 0.05% concentration.
fluocinolone acetonide	*Fluonid*	Available as solution in 0.01% concentration.
	Synalar	Available as ointment in 0.025% concentration, as cream in 0.01% and 0.025% concentrations, and as solution in 0.01% concentration.
fluocinonide	*Fluonex* *Lyderm Cream* *(CAN)*	Available as cream in 0.05% concentration.
	Lidex	Available as ointment, cream, solution, and gel in 0.05% concentration.
	Vanos	Available as cream in 0.1% concentration.
flurandrenolide		Available as ointment, cream, and lotion in 0.05% concentration and as tape containing 4 mcg/cm^2.
fluticasone fumarate	*Veramyst*	Available as nasal spray containing 55 mcg/spray.
fluticasone propionate	*Cutivate*	Available as cream in 0.05% concentration and ointment in 0.005% concentration.
halcinonide	*Halog*	Available as ointment, cream, and solution in 0.1% concentration.
halobetasol propionate	*Ultravate*	Available as ointment and cream in 0.05% concentration.
hydrocortisone	*Bactine Hydro-cortisone* *Cort-Dome* *Dermolate* *Dermtex HC*	Available as lotion in 0.25%, 0.5%, 1%, 2%, 2.5% concentrations.
	Cortizone-10 *Hycort* *Tegrin-HC*	Available as cream, lotion, ointment, and aerosol in 0.5% concentration.
	Hytone	Available as cream, ointment, and solution at 1% concentration.

(continued)

Drug	Selected trade names	Instructions and preparations

Corticosteroids (continued)

Drug	Selected trade names	Instructions and preparations
hydrocortisone acetate	Anusol-HC1	Available as cream in 1% concentration.
	Cortaid Lanacort-5	Available as ointment in 0.5% concentration.
	Cortaid with Aloe	Available as cream in 0.5% concentration.
	Gynecort Lanacort-5	Available as cream in 0.5% concentration.
hydrocortisone buteprate		Available as cream in 0.1% concentration.
hydrocortisone butyrate	Locoid	Available as ointment and cream in 0.1% concentration.
hydrocortisone valerate	Westcort	Available as ointment and cream in 0.2% concentration.
mometasone furoate	Asmanex Twisthaler	Available as powder for oral inhalation at 220 mcg/actuation; for patients 4 yr and older.
	Elocon	Available as ointment, cream, and lotion in 0.1% concentration.
	Nasonex	Available as nasal spray in 0.2% concentration.
prednicarbate	Dermatop	Available as preservative-free cream in 0.1% concentration.
triamcinolone acetonide	Triacet, Triderm	Available as cream in 0.1% concentration and as lotion in 0.025% and 0.1% concentrations.

Emollients

Drug	Selected trade names	Instructions and preparations
dexpanthenol	Panthoderm	Relieves itching and aids in healing for mild skin irritations. Apply once or twice daily.
urea	Aquacare Carmol 10 Carmol 20 Carmol 40 Gordon's Urea 40% Nutraplus Ureacin-10 Ureacin-20	Apply bid to qid to area affected; rub in completely. Also used to restore nails (Gordon's Urea 40%)—cover with plastic wrap; keep dry and remove in 3–7 days.
vitamins A and D		Relieves minor burns, chafing, skin irritations. Apply locally with gentle massage bid to qid. Consult physician if not improved within 7 days.
zinc oxide	Borofax Skin Protectant	Relieves burns, abrasions, diaper rash. Apply as needed.

Drug	Selected trade names	Instructions and preparations
Estrogen		
estradiol hemihydrate	*Vagifem*	For treatment of atrophic vaginitis. Use one tablet inserted vaginally every day for 2 wk; then one tablet inserted vaginally two times per week. Try to taper every 3–6 months.
Growth factor		
becaplermin	*Regranex*	Increases incidence of healing of diabetic foot ulcers as adjunctive therapy. Apply to diabetic foot ulcers daily; patient must have an adequate blood supply. Risk of cancer increases with prolonged use.
Hair removal product		
eflornithine	*Vaniqa*	Approved for use in women only. Apply to unwanted facial hair bid for up to 24 wk. Do not wash treated areas until at least 4 hr after treatment.
Hemostatics		
absorbable gelatin (also comes in powder form)	*Gelfoam*	To prepare paste, add 3–4 mL sterile saline to contents of jar. Apply sponge dry or saturated with saline. Smear or press paste to cut surface; when bleeding stops, remove excess. Apply sponge and leave in place; it will be absorbed. Assess continually for infection; agent may act as site of infection or abscess formation. Do not use with infection.
absorbable fibrin sealant	*TachoSil*	For use in cardiovascular surgery when control of bleeding by usual techniques is not effective. Apply yellow, active side of patch directly to bleeding area; number of patches needed depends on size of bleeding area. Do not apply intravascularly; do not use with known hypersensitivity to human blood products or horse protein.
human fibrin sealant	*Artiss* *Evicel* *Tisseel*	Spray or drip onto tissue in short bursts (0.1–0.2 mL) to produce a thin, even layer. If hemostasis is not complete, a second layer may be applied. Adjunct to decrease bleeding in vascular and liver surgery or used to adhere to autologous skin grafts for burns (*Artiss*). Adjunct to hemostasis in patients undergoing surgery when standard bleeding-control methods are ineffective (*Evicel*). Monitor patient for anaphylactic reaction.
microfibrillar collagen	*Hemopad*	Use dry. Apply directly to the source of bleeding; apply pressure. Time will vary from 3–5 min depending on the site. Discard any unused product; monitor for infection; do not use with infection. Remove any excess material once bleeding has been controlled.
thrombin	*Thrombinar* *Thrombostat*	Prepare in sterile distilled water or isotonic saline; 100–1,000 units/mL. Mix freely with blood on the surface of injury; contraindicated with any bovine allergies. Watch for any sign of severe allergic reaction in sensitive individuals.
thrombin, recombinant	*Recothrom*	Apply solution directly to bleeding site with absorbable gelatin sponge; amount needed varies with area to be treated. Reserve use for minor bleeding or oozing. Contraindicated with allergy to hamster or snake proteins.

(continued)

Drug	Selected trade names	Instructions and preparations
Immune modulator		
pimecrolimus	*Elidel*	Treatment of mild to moderate atopic dermatitis in non-immunocompromised patients older than 2 yr in whom conventional therapy is inappropriate or ineffective. Apply thin layer to affected area bid; discontinue if resolution of disease occurs.
Keratolytics		
podofilox	*Condylox*	Apply every 12 hr for 3 consecutive days. Allow to dry before using area. Dispose of used applicator. May cause burning and discomfort.
podophyllum resin	*Podocon-25* *Podofin*	Applied only by physician. Do not use if wart is inflamed or irritated. Very toxic; use minimum amount possible to avoid absorption.
Local anesthetic/analgesic		
lidocaine/ tetracaine	*Synera*	Dermal analgesia for superficial venous access and dermatological procedures. Apply one patch to intact skin 20–30 min before dermal procedure.
Lotions and solutions		
Burow's solution aluminum acetate	*Domeboro Powder*	Astringent wet dressing for relief of inflammatory conditions, insect bites, athlete's foot, bruises. Dissolve packet or tablet in pint of water, apply every 15–30 min for 4–8 hr; do not use occlusive dressing or in plastic containers.
calamine lotion		Relieves itching; pain of poison ivy, poison sumac, poison oak, insect bites, and minor skin irritations. Apply to affected area tid to qid.
hamamelis water	*A-E-R* *Witch Hazel*	Relieves itching and irritation of vaginal infection, hemorrhoids, postepisiotomy discomfort, posthemorrhoidectomy care. Apply locally up to six times per day.
Nasal corticosteroid		
fluticasone propionate	*Flonase*	Used as preventive treatment of asthma, not as primary treatment. May take several weeks to work. Clean nasal spray adapter weekly. *Adult:* Two sprays in each nostril daily. Approved for children 4–11 yr.
	Flovent Diskus *Flovent HFA*	Used as prophylactic treatment of asthma for patients age 4 and older who require a corticosteroid: 88–220 mcg bid using provided inhalation device or nasal inhalation.
Oral preparation		
amlexanox	*Aphthasol*	Apply solution or mucoadhesive disc to each aphthous ulcer qid—after meals, at bedtime, following oral hygiene—for 10 days; consult with dentist if ulcers are not healed within 10 days. May cause local pain.

Drug	Selected trade names	Instructions and preparations
Pediculicides and scabicides		
benzyl alcohol		5% lotion for treatment of head lice in patients 6 mo and older; not for use in infants. Apply to scalp or hair near scalp.
crotamiton	*Eurax*	For external use. Shake well, and massage into skin of entire body; repeat in 24 hr. Bathe or shower 48 hr after last use. Change bed linens and clothing the next day. Dry-clean contaminated clothing or wash in hot water.
ivermectin	*Sklice*	0.5% lotion for treatment of head lice in patients 6 mo and older; single 10-min application with no need for nit picking.
lindane		For external use; not for use in premature neonates. Apply thin layer to entire body; leave on 8–12 hr, then wash thoroughly. Shampoo 1–2 oz into dry hair and leave for 4 min. Reapply after 7 days if signs of live lice recur. Teach hygiene and prevention; treat all contacts. Inform parents that this is a readily communicable disease.
malathion	*Ovide Lotion*	Avoid use with open lesions. Apply to dry hair; leave on 8–12 hr. Repeat in 7–9 days. Change bed linens and clothing. Treat all contacts. Contains flammable alcohol.
permethrin	*Acticin* *Elimite* *Nix*	For external use, including prophylaxis during head lice epidemics. Thoroughly massage into skin (30 g/adult); wash off after 8–14 hr. Shampoo into freshly washed, rinsed, towel-dried hair. Leave on 10 min; rinse. Notify health care provider if rash, itching worsen.
spinosad	*Natroba*	Used to treat head lice in patients 4 yr and older (0.9% suspension). Apply to dry scalp and hair; leave on for 10 min, then rinse. May repeat every 7 days as needed.

APPENDIX L

Ophthalmic drugs

Ophthalmic drugs are intended for direct administration into the conjunctiva of the eye. These drugs are used to treat glaucoma (miotics constrict the pupil and decrease the resistance to aqueous flow), to aid in diagnosis of eye problems (mydriatics dilate the pupil for examination of the retina; cycloplegics paralyze the muscles that control the lens to aid refraction), to treat local ophthalmic infections or inflammation, and to provide relief from the signs and symptoms of allergic reactions.

Pregnancy Category C
Contraindicated in cases of allergy to these drugs. These drugs are seldom absorbed systemically, but caution should be taken with any patient who would have problems with the systemic effects of the drug if it were absorbed systemically.

Adverse effects
Local irritation, stinging, burning, blurring of vision (prolonged when using ointment), tearing; headache.

Dosage
1–2 drops to each eye bid to qid or 0.25–0.5 inch of ointment to each eye is the usual dosage.

Solution or drops
Wash hands thoroughly before administering; do not touch dropper to eye or to any other surface; have patient tilt head backward or lie down and stare upward; gently grasp lower eyelid and pull the eyelid away from the eyeball; instill drop(s) into pouch formed by eyelid; release lid slowly; have patient close eye and look downward; apply gentle pressure to the inside corner of the eye for 3–5 min to retard drainage; do not rub eyes; do not rinse eyedropper. Do not use eyedrops that have changed color; if more than one type of eyedrop is used, separate administration by 5 min.

Ointment
Wash hands thoroughly before administering; hold tube between hands for several minutes to warm the ointment; discard the first cm of ointment when opening the tube for the first time; tilt head backward or lie down and stare upward; gently pull out lower lid to form pouch; place 0.25–0.5 inch of ointment inside the lower lid; have patient close eyes for 1–2 min and roll eyeball in all directions; remove any excess ointment from around eye. If using more than one kind of ointment, wait 10 min before administration.

Teaching points
Teach patient the proper administration technique for the ophthalmic drug ordered; caution patients that transient stinging or burning may occur and that blurring vision may also occur—appropriate safety measures should be taken; sensitivity to sun will occur with mydriatic agents, which cause pupils to dilate; sunglasses may be needed. Report severe eye discomfort, palpitations, nausea, headache.

Drug	Trade names	Usage	Special considerations
alcaftadine	*Lastacaft*	Prevention of itching associated with allergic conjunctivitis	One drop in each eye daily. Remove contact lenses. Not for use to treat contact lens irritation.
apraclonidine	*Iopidine*	To control or prevent post-surgical elevations of IOP in patients after argon-laser eye surgery; short-term adjunct in patients on maximum tolerated therapy who need additional IOP reduction	Monitor for the possibility of vaso-vagal attack; do not give to patients with allergy to clonidine.
azelastine hydro-chloride	*Optivar*	Treatment of ocular itching associated with allergic conjunctivitis	Antihistamine, mast cell stabilizer. *3 yr and older:* 1 drop bid. Rapid onset, 8 hr duration.
azithromycin	*AzaSite*	Treatment of bacterial conjunctivitis	For patients 1 yr and older: One drop in affected eye bid, 8–12 hr apart for 2 days, then once a day for 5 days.
bepotastine besilate	*Bepreve*	Treatment of ocular itching associated with allergic rhinitis	Apply twice daily. Not for children younger than 2 yr.
besifloxacin	*Besivance*	Treatment of bacterial conjunctivitis (pinkeye)	1 drop in affected eye tid (6–8 hr apart); use for 7 days.
	Latisse	Treatment of hypertrichosis of the eyelashes	First- or second-line treatment; darkening of iris may occur; 1 drop daily in the evening.
bimatoprost	*Lumigan*	Treatment of open-angle glaucoma and ocular hypertension	First- or second-line treatment; darkening of iris may occur; 1 drop daily in the evening.
brimonidine tartrate	*Alphagan P*	Treatment of open-angle glaucoma and ocular hypertension	Selective alpha$_2$-antagonist; minimal effects on CV and pulmonary systems; may stain soft contact lenses. Do not use with MAOIs. 1 drop tid.
brimonidine and timolol	*Combigan*	Treatment of IOP	1 drop every 12 hr. Do not use with contact lenses.
brinzolamide	*Azopt*	Decrease IOP in open-angle glaucoma	May be given with other agents; 1 drop tid. Give 10 min apart from other agents.
bromfenac 0.09%	*Bromday* *Xibrom*	Treatment of postsurgical inflammation and reduction of ocular pain in patients who have undergone cataract extraction	1 drop in affected eye bid, beginning 24 hr after surgery and continuing for 2 wk. Once daily if using *Bromday*.

(continued)

Drug	Trade names	Usage	Special considerations
carbachol	*Miostat*	Direct-acting miotic; for treatment of glaucoma; for miosis during surgery	Surgical dose a one-use only portion; 1 or 2 drops up to tid as needed for glaucoma.
carteolol		Reduction of IOP in chronic open-angle glaucoma	1 drop in affected eye(s) bid. Monitor pressure closely.
ciprofloxacin	*Ciloxan*	Treatment of ocular infections and conjunctivitis	½ inch ribbon of ointment to eye sac tid for 2 days, then bid for 5 days, or 1–2 drops in eye sac every 2 hr while awake for 2 days, then every 4 hr while awake for 5 days.
cyclopentolate	*AK-Pentolate Cyclogyl Paremyd*	Mydriasis or cycloplegia in diagnostic procedures	Individuals with dark pigmented irides may require higher doses; compress lacrimal sac for 2–3 min after administration to decrease any systemic absorption.
cyclosporine emulsion 0.05%	*Restasis*	Increases tear production in patients whose tear production is presumed to be suppressed because of ocular inflammation associated with keratoconjunctivitis sicca	1 drop in each eye twice a day, approximately 12 hr apart; remove contact lenses before using.
dexamethasone intravitreal	*Ozurdex*	Extended-release intravitreal injection for treatment of macular edema following branch retinal artery occlusion or central retinal vein occlusion; treatment of noninfectious uveitis of the posterior segment of the eye	Monitor for infection, retinal detachment, and increased intraocular pressure after injection. Use cautiously with history of ocular herpes simplex.
diclofenac sodium	*Voltaren*	Photophobia; for use in patients undergoing incisional refractive surgery and for postoperative ocular inflammation	Apply 1 drop qid beginning 24 hr after cataract surgery; continue through the first 2 wk postoperatively. For postoperative ocular inflammation, 1–2 drops within the hour before corneal refractive surgery then 1–2 drops within 15 min after surgery, then qid for up to 3 days for ocular pain and photophobia.
difluprednate	*Durezol*	Anti-inflammatory and analgesic for treatment of postoperative ocular pain and inflammation; treatment of endogenous anterior uveitis	Apply 1 drop to affected eye qid beginning 24 hr after surgery and continuing for 2 wk.
dorzolamide	*Trusopt*	Treatment of elevated IOP in patients with ocular hypertension or open-angle glaucoma	A sulfonamide; monitor patients on parenteral sulfonamides for possible additive effects. Children: 1 drop in each eye tid.

Drug	Trade names	Usage	Special considerations
dorzolamide 2% and timolol 0.5%	*Cosopt*	Decrease IOP in open-angle glaucoma or ocular hypertension in patients who do not respond to beta blockers alone	Administer 1 drop in affected eye bid. Monitor for cardiac failure; if absorbed, may mask symptoms of hypoglycemia or thyrotoxicosis.
echothiophate		Treatment of open-angle glaucoma, accommodative estropia; irreversible cholinesterase inhibitor; long-acting.	Given only once or twice a day because of long action; tolerance may develop with prolonged use. Usually responds to a rest period.
emedastine	*Emadine*	Temporary relief of signs and symptoms of allergic conjunctivitis	For patients 3 yr and older: 1 drop in affected eye or eyes up to qid. Do not wear contact lenses if eyes are red; may cause headache, blurred vision.
epinastine hydrochloride	*Elestat*	Prevention of itching caused by allergic conjunctivitis	Remove contact lenses before applying. Instill 1 drop in each eye bid for entire time of exposure, even if itching subsides.
fluocinolone acetonide intravitreal implant	*Retisert*	Treatment of chronic noninfectious uveitis affecting the posterior segment of the eye	1 surgically implanted insert (releases 0.6 mcg per day for approximately 30 mo). May be replaced after 30 mo if needed.
fluorometholone	*Flarex Fluor-Op FML*	Topical corticosteroid used for treatment of inflammatory conditions of the eye	Improvement should occur within several days, discontinue if no improvement is seen. Monitor IOP if used longer than 10 days. Discontinue if swelling of the eye occurs. Take care not to discontinue therapy prematurely.
ganciclovir	*Zirgan*	Treatment of acute herpetic keratitis	1 drop to affected eye five times a day until ulcer heals; then 1 drop tid for 7 days.
gatifloxacin	*Zymar Zymaxid*	Treatment of bacterial conjunctivitis caused by susceptible strains of *Corynebacterium propinquum*, *Staphylococcus aureus*, *Staphylococcus epidermidis*, *Streptococcus mitis*, *Streptococcus pneumoniae*, *Haemophilus influenzae*	1 drop to affected eye every 2 hr while awake, up to eight times a day, on days 1 and 2; then 1 drop every 4 hr up to four times a day, while awake for 5 days. Contacts should not be worn during these infections; ensure that patient is not allergic to any quinolone antibiotic. Can cause blurred vision.
homatropine	*Homatropine HBr Isopto-Homatropine*	Long-acting mydriatic and cycloplegic used for refraction and treatment of inflammatory conditions of the uveal tract or preoperative and postoperative states when mydriasis is required	Individuals with dark pigmented irides may require larger doses; 5–10 min is usually required for refraction.

(continued)

Drug	Trade names	Usage	Special considerations
ketorolac	*Acuvail* (0.45%)	Treatment of pain and inflammation following cataract surgery	Apply to affected eye bid.
ketotifen	*Alaway* *Zaditor*	An antihistamine and mast cell stabilizer; provides temporary relief of itching due to allergic conjunctivitis	1 drop in affected eye every 8–12 hr. For patients 3 yr and older: Remove contact lenses before use—may be replaced within 10 min.
latanoprost	*Xalatan*	Treatment of open-angle glaucoma or ocular hypertension in patients intolerant or nonresponsive to other agents	Remove contact lenses before and for 15 min after use; allow at least 5 min between this and the use of any other agents; expect burning, blurred vision.
levobunolol	*AKBeta* *Betagan* *Liquifilm*	Lowering of IOP with chronic, open-angle glaucoma, ocular hypertension	1 or 2 drops bid. Do not combine with other beta blockers.
levofloxacin	*Quixin*	Treatment of bacterial conjunctivitis caused by susceptible bacteria	1 or 2 drops in affected eye every 2 hr while awake, up to eight times a day, on days 1 and 2; then every 4 hr while awake, up to four times per day for days 3 to 7.
lodoxamide tromethamine	*Alomide*	Treatment of vernal conjunctivitis and keratitis for patients older than 2 yr	Patients should not wear contact lenses while using this drug; discontinue if stinging and burning persist after instillation.
loteprednol etabonate	*Alrex* (0.2%)	Treatment of postoperative inflammation after ocular surgery	1 or 2 drops qid.
	Lotemax (0.5%)	Treatment of steroid-resistant ocular disease	1 or 2 drops qid beginning 24 hr after surgery and continuing for 2 wk. Shake vigorously before use. Discard after 14 days; prolonged use may cause nerve or eye damage.
loteprednol etabonate/ tobramycin	*Zylet*	Treatment of steroid-responsive inflammatory ocular conditions where there is a risk of superficial bacterial ocular infection	1 or 2 drops into conjunctival sac every 4–6 hr; during first 24–48 hr, dose may increase to every 1–2 hr.
metipranolol	*OptiPranolol*	Beta blocker; used in treating chronic open-angle glaucoma and ocular hypertension	Concomitant therapy may be needed; caution patient about possible vision changes.

Drug	Trade names	Usage	Special considerations
mitomycin-C	*Mitosol*	Adjunct to ab externo glaucoma surgery.	Apply fully saturated sponges to treatment area; leave on for 2 min. Requires bioltazard disposal. For topical use only; intraocular administration can result in corneal infarction, ciliary body atrophy.
moxifloxacin	*Moxeza* *Vigamox*	Treatment of bacterial conjunctivitis caused by susceptible strains of *Corynebacterium* species, *Micrococcus luteus*, *Staphylococcus*, *Staphylococcus aureus*, *Staphylococcus haemolyticus*, *Staphylococcus hominis*, *Staphylococcus warneri*, *Streptococcus pneumoniae*, *Streptococcus viridans* group, *Acinetobacter lwoffii*, *Haemophilus influenzae*, *Haemophilus parainfluenzae*, *Chlamydia trachomatis*	Contact lenses should not be worn during these infections; ensure that patient is not allergic to any quinolone antibiotic. Can cause blurred vision. *Moxeza:* For patients 4 mo and older: 1 drop to affected eye bid for 7 days. *Vigamox:* For patients 1 yr and older: 1 drop to affected eye tid for 7 days.
natamycin	*Natacyn*	Antibiotic used to treat fungal blepharitis, conjunctivitis, and keratitis; drug of choice for *Fusarium sotani* keratitis	Shake well before each use; store at room temperature; failure to improve in 7–10 days suggests a non-susceptible organism; reevaluate.
nedocromil sodium	*Alocril*	Treatment of itching of allergic conjunctivitis	Use at regular intervals through the entire allergic season: 1 or 2 drops in each eye bid.
olopatadine hydrochloride	*Pataday* *Patanol*	Mast cell stabilizer and antihistamine; provides fast onset of relief of itching due to conjunctivitis with prolonged action	For patients 3 yr and older: 0.1%, 1–2 drops bid at 6- to 8-hr intervals. 0.2%, 1 drop to affected eye once daily. Not for use with contact lenses; headache is a common adverse effect.
pemirolast potassium	*Alamast*	Prevention of itchy eyes due to allergic conjunctivitis	1 or 2 drops qid.
pilocarpine	*Adsorbocarpine* *Piloptic* *Pilostat*	Chronic and acute glaucoma; treatment of mydriasis caused by drugs; direct-acting miotic drug	Can be stored at room temperature for up to 8 wk, then discard. 1 or 2 drops up to six times per day may be needed, based on patient response.
polydimethylsiloxane	*AdatoSil 5000*	Treatment of retinal detachments where other therapy is not effective or is inappropriate; primary choice for retinal detachment due to AIDS-related CMV retinitis or viral infection	Monitor for cataracts; must be injected into aqueous humor.

(continued)

Drug	Trade names	Usage	Special considerations
rimexolone	*Vexol*	Corticosteroid; postoperative ocular surgery and for treatment of anterior uveitis	Monitor for signs of steroid absorption.
sulfacetamide	*Bleph-10*	Treatment of ocular infections	1–2 drops or 0.5 inch ointment to affected eye every 2–3 hr initially; gradually taper over 7–10 days.
tafluprost	*Zioptan*	Reduction of elevated IOP with open-angle glaucoma or ocular hypertension.	1 drop in affected eye(s) in the evening. Changes in eyelashes, iris color are possible.
timolol maleate	*Timoptic XE*	Treatment of elevated IOP in ocular hypertension or open-angle glaucoma	1 drop in affected eye once a day in the morning.
travoprost	*Travatan Z*	Treatment of open-angle glaucoma and ocular hypertension	1 drop in affected eye or eyes each evening; eye discomfort, pain, darkening of iris, growth of eyelashes common.
trifluridine	*Viroptic*	Antiviral; used to treat primary keratoconjunctivitis and recurrent epithelial keratitis due to herpes simplex virus types 1 and 2	Transient burning and stinging may occur; reconsider drug if improvement is not seen within 7 days. Do not administer for longer than 21 days at a time. Maximum, 9 drops/day to affected eye
tropicamide	*Mydral* *Mydriacyl* *Tropicacyl*	Mydriatic and cycloplegic; used for refraction	1 or 2 drops of 1% solution; repeat in 5 min. May repeat in 30 min for prolonged effects.

Laxatives

Laxative use has been replaced by the use of proper diet and exercise in many clinical situations. Most laxatives are available as OTC preparations and are often abused by people who become dependent on them for GI movement.

Indications
Short-term relief of constipation; to prevent straining; to evacuate the bowel for diagnostic procedures; to remove ingested poisons from the lower GI tract; as adjunct in anthelmintic therapy.

Pregnancy Category C
Contraindicated in cases of allergy to these drugs, third trimester of pregnancy, acute abdominal pain.

Adverse effects
Excessive bowel activity, perianal irritation, abdominal cramps, *weakness, dizziness,* cathartic dependence.

Teaching points
Use as a temporary measure. Swallow tablets whole. Do not take this drug within 1 hr of any other drugs. Report sweating, flushing, muscle cramps, excessive thirst.

Drug	Selected trade names	Type
bisacodyl	*Bisa-Lax* *Dulcolax*	Stimulant
cascara		Stimulant
castor oil		Stimulant
docusate	*Colace* *ex-lax Stool Softener* *Genasoft* *Phillips' Liqui-Gels*	Detergent, softener
glycerin	*Fleet Babylax* *Fleet Liquid Glycerin* *Suppository* *Sani-Supp*	Hyperosmolar agent
lactulose	*Cephulac* *Chronulac* *Constilac* *Constulose*	Hyperosmolar agent
lubiprostone	*Amitiza*	Chloride channel activator
magnesium citrate	*Citrate of Magnesia*	Saline
magnesium hydroxide	*Milk of Magnesia* *MOM* *Philip's MOM*	Saline
magnesium sulfate	*Epsom Salts*	Saline
mineral oil	*Kondremul Plain*	Emollient
polycarbophil	*Equalactin* *FiberCon* *Konsyl Fiber*	Bulk
polyethylene glycol	*MiraLax*	Bulk

Dosage	Onset	Special considerations
5–15 mg PO 2.5 g in water via enema	6–12 hr Rapid	Allergy to tartrazine in *Dulcolax* tablets; may discolor urine. Not for children younger than 6 yr.
325 mg–6 g PO	6–10 hr	Use caution in patients taking prescription drugs; may discolor urine; not for children younger than 18 yr.
15–60 mL PO	2–6 hr	May be very vigorous; may cause abdominal cramping.
50–300 mg PO	12–72 hr	Gentle; beneficial with anorectal conditions that are painful and with dry or hard feces.
Rectal suppository; 4 mL liquid by rectum (pediatric rectal liquid)	15–60 min	Insert suppository high into rectum, retain 15 min; insert liquid dispenser and apply gentle, steady pressure until all liquid is gone, then remove.
15–30 mL PO; up to 60 mL may be used	24–48 hr	Also used for treatment of portal system encephalopathy. May be more palatable mixed with fruit juice, water, or milk.
24 mcg PO bid with food and water	1–2 hr	May cause nausea, diarrhea; also approved for the treatment of IBS with constipation in women 18 yr and older. Take with food and water. Contains sorbitol.
1 glassful PO	0.5–3 hr	Reduce pediatric dosage by one-half.
30–60 mL PO at bedtime; 15–30 mL concentrate	0.5–3 hr	Take with liquids; flavored varieties vary.
5–10 mL PO	0.5–3 hr	Take mixed with full glass of water; reduce pediatric dose to 2.5–5 mL in one-half glass of water.
5–45 mL PO	6–8 hr	Reduce pediatric dose to 5–15 mL. May decrease absorption of fat-soluble vitamins. Use caution to avoid lipid pneumonia with aspiration. Not for children younger than 6 yr.
1–2 tablets up to four times a day as needed	12–72 hr	Good with IBS, diverticulitis. Abdominal fullness may occur. Smaller doses more frequently may alleviate discomfort. Taking with inadequate liquid may cause drug to expand in throat or esophagus, causing choking.
Dissolve 17 g in 8 oz water and drink every day for up to 2 wk	48–72 hr	Do not use with bowel obstruction; diarrhea common.

(continued)

Drug	Selected trade names	Type
polyethylene glycol-electrolyte solution	*CoLyte* *GoLYTELY* *NuLYTELY*	Bulk
polyethylene glycol, sodium sulfate, sodium chloride, potassium chloride, sodium ascorbate, ascorbic acid	*MoviPrep*	Osmotic
psyllium	*Fiberall* *Hydrocil Instant* *Metamucil*	Bulk
senna	*Agoral* *Black-Draught* *Fletcher's Castoria* *Senna-Gen* *Senokot*	Stimulant
sodium picosulfate, magnesium oxide, anhydrous citric acid	*Prepopik*	Stimulant Bulk

Dosage	Onset	Special considerations
4 L oral solution before GI examination	1 hr	Used as bowel evacuant before GI examinations. Do not use with GI obstruction, megacolon. GI discomfort common.
1 L PO followed by 16 oz of fluid the evening before colonoscopy and repeated the morning of colonoscopy; or 2 L followed by 32 oz of fluid the evening before colonoscopy	1 hr	Maintain hydration. Use caution in patients with history of seizures.
1 tsp or packet in cool water or juice, 1–3 times per day PO in children	12–72 hr	Safest and most physiologic. Ensure that patient has sufficient water to completely swallow dose. Taking with inadequate liquid may cause drug to expand in throat or esophagus, causing choking.
1–8 tablets per day PO at bedtime; suppository by rectum; syrup— 10–30 mL PO	6–10 hr	May be very aggressive; abdominal cramps and discomfort may occur.
Reconstitute one packet with cold water; patient should swallow immediately and follow with clear liquids; repeat (total of two doses). Take doses evening before and morning of colonoscopy.		Used for bowel cleansing before colonoscopy; risk of fluid and electrolyte abnormalities.

APPENDIX N

Combination products by therapeutic class

AMPHETAMINES

▽ dextroamphetamine and amphetamine

CONTROLLED SUBSTANCE C-II

Adderall●, Adderall XR

Tablets:

  1.25 mg (5-mg tablet), 2.5 mg (10-mg tablet), 5 mg (20-mg tablet), or 7.5 mg (30-mg tablet) each of dextroamphetamine sulfate and saccharate, amphetamine aspartate, and sulfate

ER capsules●:

  1.25 mg (5-mg capsule), 1.875 (7.5-mg tablet), 2.5 mg (10-mg capsule), 3.125 (12.5-mg tablet), 3.75 mg (15-mg capsule), 5 mg (20-mg capsule), 6.25 mg (25-mg capsule), or 7.5 mg (30-mg capsule) of each component

Usual adult and pediatric dosage: 5–60 mg PO per day in divided doses to control symptoms of narcolepsy or ADHD; ER capsules: 10–30 mg per day.

See also **dextroamphetamine.**

ANALGESICS

▽ acetaminophen and codeine

CONTROLLED SUBSTANCE C-III (TABLETS), C-IV (SOLUTION)

Tylenol with Codeine

Solution:

  12 mg codeine, 120 mg acetaminophen/5 mL

Tablets:

  No. 2: 15 mg codeine, 300 mg acetaminophen
  No. 3: 30 mg codeine, 300 mg acetaminophen
  No. 4: 60 mg codeine, 300 mg acetaminophen

Usual adult dosage: One or two tablets PO every 4–6 hr as needed or 15 mL every 4–6 hr.

See also **acetaminophen, codeine.**

▽ aspirin and codeine

CONTROLLED SUBSTANCE C-III

Empirin with Codeine

Tablets:

  No. 3: 30 mg codeine, 325 mg aspirin
  No. 4: 60 mg codeine, 325 mg aspirin

Usual adult dosage: One or two tablets PO every 4–6 hr as needed.

See also **aspirin, codeine.**

● Do not crush.

▽ codeine, aspirin, caffeine, and butalbital

CONTROLLED SUBSTANCE C-III

Fiorinal with Codeine

Capsules:
   30 mg codeine, 325 mg aspirin, 40 mg caffeine, 50 mg butalbital
Usual adult dosage: One or two capsules PO every 4 hr as needed for pain, up to 6 per day.
See also **codeine, aspirin, caffeine, butalbital.**

▽ diclofenac sodium and misoprostol

PREGNANCY CATEGORY X

Arthrotec

Tablets:
   '50': 50 mg diclofenac, 200 mcg misoprostol
   '75': 75 mg diclofenac, 200 mcg misoprostol
Usual adult dosage:
• *Osteoarthritis: Arthrotec* '50' PO tid; *Arthrotec* '50' or '75' PO bid.
• *Rheumatoid arthritis: Arthrotec* '50' PO tid or qid; *Arthrotec* '50' or '75' PO bid.
See also **diclofenac, misoprostol.**

▽ famotidine and ibuprofen

Duexis

Tablets:
   26.6 mg famotidine, 800 mg ibuprofen
Usual adult dosage: One tablet PO tid for arthritis pain.
See also **famotidine, ibuprofen.**

▽ hydrocodone and aspirin

CONTROLLED SUBSTANCE C-IV

Damason-P

Tablets:
   5 mg hydrocodone, 500 mg aspirin
Usual adult dosage: One tablet PO every 4–6 hr as needed.
See also **aspirin.**

▽ hydrocodone bitartrate and acetaminophen

CONTROLLED SUBSTANCE C-III

Anexsia, Co-Gesic, DuoCet, Hydrogesic, Lorcet Plus Tablets,
Lortab Tablets, Margesic H, Norco, Stagesic, Vicodin, Vicodin ES,
Vicodin HP, Zydone

Elixir:
   2.5 mg hydrocodone, 167 mg acetaminophen/5 mL

Capsules or tablets:
    2.5 mg hydrocodone, 500 mg acetaminophen
    5 mg hydrocodone, 500 mg acetaminophen
    5, 7.5, 10 mg hydrocodone, 400 mg acetaminophen
    7.5 mg hydrocodone, 500 mg acetaminophen
    7.5 mg hydrocodone, 650 mg acetaminophen
    10 mg hydrocodone, 650 mg acetaminophen
Norco tablets:
    5 mg hydrocodone, 325 mg acetaminophen
    7.5 mg hydrocodone, 325 mg acetaminophen
    10 mg hydrocodone, 325 mg acetaminophen
Usual adult dosage: Check brand-name products to determine specific dosage combinations available. One or two tablets or capsules PO every 4–6 hr, up to 8 per day.
See also **acetaminophen.**

▽ **hydrocodone and ibuprofen**

CONTROLLED SUBSTANCE C-III

Reprexain, Vicoprofen

Tablets:
    2.5 mg hydrocodone, 200 mg ibuprofen
    7.5 mg hydrocodone, 200 mg ibuprofen
    10 mg hydrocodone, 200 mg ibuprofen
Usual adult dosage: One tablet PO every 4–6 hr as needed.
See also **ibuprofen.**

▽ **methylsalicylate and menthol**

Salonpas

Dermal patch:
    10% methysalicylate, 3% menthol
Usual adult dosage: Apply one patch to clean, dry affected area; leave on for 8–12 hr. Remove patch and apply another as needed. For relief of pain from sprains, bruises, strains, backache.
See also **methylsalicylate.**

▽ **morphine and naltrexone**

CONTROLLED SUBSTANCE C-II

Embeda

ER capsules ⊡:
    20 mg morphine, 0.8 mg naltrexone
    30 mg morphine, 1.2 mg naltrexone
    50 mg morphine, 2 mg naltrexone
    60 mg morphine, 2.4 mg naltrexone
    80 mg morphine, 3.2 mg naltrexone
    100 mg morphine, 4 mg naltrexone
Usual adult dosage: One or two tablets PO daily when a continuous, around-the-clock analgesic is needed for a prolonged period; capsules may be opened and sprinkled over applesauce.
See also **morphine, naltrexone.**

⊡ Do not crush.

▷naproxen and esomeprazole

Vimovo

DR tablets:
  375 mg naproxen, 20 mg esomeprazole
  500 mg naproxen, 20 mg esomeprazole
Usual adult dosage: One tablet PO twice daily. Not recommended in moderate to severe renal insufficiency or severe hepatic insufficiency. Reduce dose with mild to moderate hepatic insufficiency.
See also **naproxen, esomeprazole.**

▷oxycodone and acetaminophen

CONTROLLED SUBSTANCE C-II

Percocet, Roxicet, Roxilox, Tylox

Roxilox, Tylox capsules:
  5 mg oxycodone, 500 mg acetaminophen
Tablets:
  2.5, 5 mg oxycodone, 325 mg acetaminophen
Roxicet solution:
  5 mg oxycodone, 325 mg acetaminophen/5 mL
Usual adult dosage: One or two tablets or capsules or 5 mL solution PO every 4–6 hr as needed.
See also **oxycodone, acetaminophen.**

▷oxycodone and aspirin

CONTROLLED SUBSTANCE C-II

Percodan, Roxiprin

Tablets:
  4.5 mg oxycodone, 325 mg aspirin
Usual adult dosage: One or two tablets PO every 6 hr as needed.
See also **oxycodone, aspirin.**

▷oxycodone and ibuprofen

CONTROLLED SUBSTANCE C-II

Tablets:
  5 mg oxycodone, 400 mg ibuprofen
Usual adult dosage: One tablet PO every 6 hr as needed for moderate to severe pain. Do not exceed four tablets in 24 hr or use for more than 7 days.
See also **ibuprofen, oxycodone.**

▷pentazocine and acetaminophen

CONTROLLED SUBSTANCE C-IV

Tablets:
  25 mg pentazocine, 650 mg acetaminophen

Usual adult dosage: One tablet PO every 4 hr, up to a maximum 6 tablets per day.
See also **pentazocine, acetaminophen.**

▷tramadol hydrochloride and acetaminophen

Ultracet

Tablets:
    37.5 mg tramadol, 325 mg acetaminophen
Usual adult dosage: Two tablets PO every 4–6 hr as needed. Do not exceed eight tablets per day. Reduce dosage with geriatric or renally impaired patients.
See also **tramadol, acetaminophen.**

ANTIACNE DRUGS

▷ethinyl estradiol and norethindrone

Estrostep Fe

Tablets:
    1 mg norethindrone, 20 mcg ethinyl estradiol
    1 mg norethindrone, 30 mcg ethinyl estradiol
    1 mg norethindrone, 35 mcg ethinyl estradiol
Usual adult dosage: One tablet PO each day (21 tablets contain active ingredients and seven are inert).
See also **norethindrone, estradiol.**

▷norgestimate and ethinyl estradiol

Ortho Tri-Cyclen

Tablets:
    0.18 mg norgestimate, 35 mcg ethinyl estradiol (7 tablets)
    0.215 mg norgestimate, 35 mcg ethinyl estradiol (7 tablets)
    0.25 mg norgestimate, 35 mcg ethinyl estradiol (7 tablets)
Usual adult dosage: For women older than 15 yr: One tablet PO per day.
Birth control agent used cyclically (21 tablets contain active ingredients, 7 are inert).
See also **estradiol.**

ANTIBACTERIALS

▷amoxicillin and clavulanic acid

Augmentin, Augmentin ES-600, Augmentin XR

Tablets:
    '250': 250 mg amoxicillin, 125 mg clavulanic acid
    '500': 500 mg amoxicillin, 125 mg clavulanic acid
    '875': 875 mg amoxicillin, 125 mg clavulanic acid
Powder for oral suspension:
    '125' powder: 125 mg amoxicillin, 31.25 mg clavulanic acid
    '250' powder: 250 mg amoxicillin, 62.5 mg clavulanic acid
    '400' powder: 400 mg amoxicillin, 57 mg clavulanic acid

Solution (*Augmentin ES-600*):

    600 mg amoxicillin, 42.9 mg clavulanic acid/5 mL

Chewable tablets:

    '125': 125 mg amoxicillin, 31.25 mg clavulanic acid

    '200': 200 mg amoxicillin, 28.5 mg clavulanic acid

    '400': 400 mg amoxicillin, 57 mg clavulanic acid

XR tablets:

    1,000 mg amoxicillin, 62.5 mg clavulanic acid

Usual adult dosage: One 250-mg tablet or one 500-mg tablet PO every 8 hr. For severe infections: 875-mg tablet PO every 12 hr. For those with difficulty swallowing, substitute the 125 mg/5 mL or 250 mg/5 mL for the 500-mg tablet or the 200 mg/5 mL or 400 mg/5 mL for the 875-mg tablet.

Usual pediatric dosage: In children weighing less than 40 kg: 20–40 mg amoxicillin/kg PO per day in divided doses every 8 hr (pediatric dosage is based on amoxicillin content) or every 12 hr; 90 mg/kg per day PO oral solution divided every 12 hr (*Augmentin ES-600*).

See also **amoxicillin.** Clavulanic acid protects amoxicillin from breakdown by bacterial beta-lactamase enzymes and is given only in combination with certain antibiotics that are broken down by beta-lactamase.

▷ co-trimoxazole (TMP-SMZ)

Bactrim, Bactrim DS, Septra, Septra DS, Sulfatrim Pediatric

Tablets:

    80 mg trimethoprim (TMP), 400 mg sulfamethoxazole (SMZ)

    160 mg TMP, 800 mg SMZ

Oral suspension:

    40 mg TMP, 200 mg SMZ per 5 mL

Usual adult dosage:

- *UTIs, shigellosis, acute otitis media:* 160 mg TMP and 800 mg SMZ PO every 12 hr. Treat for up to 14 days (UTI) or for 5 days (shigellosis).
- *Acute exacerbations of chronic bronchitis:* 160 mg TMP and 800 mg SMZ PO every 12 hr for 14 days.
- Pneumocystis jiroveci *pneumonitis*: 20 mg/kg TMP and 100 mg/kg SMZ every 24 hr PO in divided doses every 6 hr. Treat for 14 days.
- *Traveler's diarrhea:* 160 mg TMP and 800 mg SMZ PO every 12 hr for 5 days

Usual pediatric dosage:

- *UTIs, shigellosis, acute otitis media:* 8 mg/kg/day TMP and 40 mg/kg/day SMZ PO in two divided doses every 12 hr. Treat for 10–14 days (UTIs and acute otitis media) or for 5 days (shigellosis).
- P. jiroveci *pneumonitis:* 20 mg/kg TMP and 100 mg/kg SMZ every 24 hr PO in divided doses every 6 hr. Treat for 14 days.

Impaired renal function:

CrCl (mL/min)	Dosage
More than 30	Use standard dosage.
15–30	Use one-half of standard dosage.
Less than 15	Not recommended.

See also **sulfamethoxazole, trimethoprim.**

▷ erythromycin and sulfisoxazole

Granules for oral suspension:

    Erythromycin ethylsuccinate (equivalent of 200 mg erythromycin activity) and 600 mg sulfisoxazole per 5 mL when reconstituted according to manufacturer's directions

- Usual dosage for acute otitis media: 50 mg/kg per day erythromycin and 150 mg/kg per day sulfisoxazole PO in divided doses qid for 10 days.
- Administer without regard to meals; refrigerate after reconstitution; use within 14 days.

See also **erythromycin, sulfisoxazole.**

▷ imipenem and cilastatin
Primaxin

Powder for injection (IV):
  250 mg imipenem, 250 mg cilastatin
  500 mg imipenem, 500 mg cilastatin
Powder for injection (IM):
  500 mg imipenem, 500 mg cilastatin

- Follow manufacturer's instructions for reconstituting and diluting the drug.
- Administer each 250- to 500-mg dose by IV infusion over 20–30 min; infuse each 1-g dose over 40–60 min. Give 500–750 mg IM every 12 hr. Do not exceed 1,500 mg/day.
- Dosage recommendations based on imipenem. Initially based on type and severity of infection and later on severity of patient's illness, degree of susceptibility of the pathogens, and patient's age, weight, and creatinine clearance. Dosage for adults with normal renal function is 250 mg to 1 g IV every 6–8 hr, not to exceed 50 mg/kg/day or 4 g/day, whichever is less.
- Dosage for patients with renal impairment is based on creatinine clearance and weight. Consult manufacturer's guidelines.
- Imipenem inhibits cell wall synthesis in susceptible bacteria; cilastatin inhibits the renal enzyme that metabolizes imipenem; these drugs are available **only** in the combined form.

▷ piperacillin sodium and tazobactam sodium
Zosyn

Tazobactam is a beta-lactamase inhibitor used in combination with the broad-spectrum penicillin.
Powder for injection:
  2 g piperacillin, 0.25 g tazobactam
  3 g piperacillin, 0.375 g tazobactam
  4 g piperacillin, 0.5 g tazobactam
Usual adult dosage: 12 g/1.5 g IV given as 3.375 g every 6 hr.

- Recommended for appendicitis, peritonitis, postpartum endometritis and PID, community-acquired pneumonia, nosocomial pneumonia if agent is responsive in sensitivity testing.
- Reduced dosage required for renal impairment or dialysis.
- Administer by IV infusion over 30 min. Reconstitute with 5 mL of suitable diluent per 1 g piperacillin. Discard after 24 hr.

See also **piperacillin.**

▷ quinupristin and dalfopristin
Synercid

New class of drugs available **only** as this combination product.
Streptogramin antibiotics:
  500-mg/10-mL vial contains 150 mg quinupristin, 350 mg dalfopristin

- Treatment of life-threatening, susceptible infections associated with vancomycin-resistant *E. faecium* bacteremia (VREF), complicated skin infections due to *S. aureus, S. pyogenes.*
- Skin infections in patients older than 16 yr: 7.5 mg/kg IV every 12 hr for 7 days.
- VREF in patients older than 16 yr: 7.5 mg/kg IV every 8 hr.
- ⊗ **Warning** Dangerous when used with drugs that prolong the QTc interval.
- May cause pseudomembranous colitis.

▷ sulbactam and ampicillin

Unasyn

Powder for injection:
    1.5-g vial: 1 g ampicillin, 0.5 g sulbactam
    3-g vial: 2 g ampicillin, 1 g sulbactam
Usual adult dosage: 0.5–1 g sulbactam with 1–2 g ampicillin IM or IV every 6–8 hr.
Pediatric dosage:
    Less than 40 kg: 300 mg/kg per day IV in divided doses every 6 hr.
    40 kg or more: adult dosage, do not exceed 4 g per day.
See also **ampicillin.** Sulbactam inhibits many bacterial penicillinase enzymes, thus broadening the spectrum of ampicillin; sulbactam is also weakly antibacterial alone.

▷ ticarcillin and clavulanic acid

Timentin

Powder for injection, solution for injection:
    3.1-g vial (3 g ticarcillin, 0.1 g clavulanic acid)
Administer by IV infusion over 30 min.
- Dosage for 60-kg or more adults: 3.1 g (3 g ticarcillin, 0.1 g clavulanic acid) IV every 4–6 hr. Dosage for adults less than 60 kg: 200–300 mg ticarcillin/kg per day IV in divided doses every 4–6 hr.
- Urinary tract infections: 3.1 g (3 g ticarcillin, 0.1 g clavulanic acid) IV every 8 hr.
- Pediatric dosage in children 3 mo and older: 3.1 g (3 g ticarcillin, 0.1 g clavulanic acid) IV every 4–6 hr or 200–300 mg/kg per day IV in divided doses every 4–6 hr.
- Geriatric or renal-failure patients: For patients on hemodialysis, give 2 g IV every 12 hr, supplemented with 3.1 g after each dialysis. For patients with renal impairment, give initial loading dose of 3.1 g, then as follows:

CrCl (mL/min)	Dosage
More than 60	3.1 g IV every 4 hr
30–60	2 g IV every 4 hr
10–30	2 g IV every 8 hr
Less than 10	2 g IV every 12 hr
Less than 10 with hepatic disease	2 g IV every 24 hr

- Continue treatment for 2 days after signs and symptoms of infection have disappeared. Usual duration of therapy is 10–14 days.
See also **ticarcillin.** Clavulanic acid protects ticarcillin from breakdown by bacterial beta-lactamase enzymes and is given only in combination with certain antibiotics that are broken down by beta-lactamase.

ANTI–CORONARY ARTERY DISEASE DRUGS

▷ amlodipine besylate and atorvastatin calcium

Caduet

Tablets:

2.5 mg amlodipine with 10, 20, or 40 mg atorvastatin
5 mg amlodipine with 10, 20, 40, or 80 mg atorvastatin
10 mg amlodipine with 10, 20, 40, or 80 mg atorvastatin

Usual adult dosage: One tablet PO every day, taken in the evening. Dosage should be adjusted using the individual products; then switch to appropriate combination product.
See also **amlodipine, atorvastatin.**

ANTIDEPRESSANTS

▷ chlordiazepoxide and amitriptyline

CONTROLLED SUBSTANCE C-IV

Limbitrol, Limbitrol DS

Tablets:

5 mg chlordiazepoxide, 12.5 mg amitriptyline
10 mg chlordiazepoxide, 25 mg amitriptyline

Usual adult dosage: 10 mg chlordiazepoxide with 25 mg amitriptyline PO three or four times per day up to six times daily. For patients who do not tolerate higher doses, 5 mg chlordiazepoxide with 12.5 mg amitriptyline PO three or four times per day. Reduce dosage after initial response.
See also **amitriptyline, chlordiazepoxide.**

▷ olanzapine and fluoxetine

Symbyax

Capsules:

6 mg olanzapine, 25 mg fluoxetine
6 mg olanzapine, 50 mg fluoxetine
12 mg olanzapine, 25 mg fluoxetine
12 mg olanzapine, 50 mg fluoxetine

Usual adult dosage: One capsule PO daily in the evening.
See also **fluoxetine, olanzapine.**

▷ perphenazine and amitriptyline

Etrafon, Etrafon-A, Etrafon-Forte

Tablets:

2 mg perphenazine, 10 mg amitriptyline
2 mg perphenazine, 25 mg amitriptyline
4 mg perphenazine; 10 mg amitriptyline
4 mg perphenazine, 25 mg amitriptyline
4 mg perphenazine, 50 mg amitriptyline

Usual adult dosage: 2–4 mg perphenazine with 10–50 mg amitriptyline PO three or four times per day. Reduce dosage after initial response.
See also **amitriptyline, perphenazine.**

ANTIDIABETIC

▷ glyburide and metformin
Glucovance

Tablets:
   1.25 mg glyburide, 250 mg metformin
   2.5 mg glyburide, 500 mg metformin
   5 mg glyburide, 500 mg metformin
Usual adult dosage: One tablet daily PO with a meal, usually in the morning.
Not for initial therapy; drug should be adjusted using the individual products, switching to appropriate dosage of this combination product.
See also **glyburide, metformin.**

▷ linagliptin and metformin
Jentadueto

Tablets:
   2.5 mg linagliptin, 500 mg metformin
   2.5 mg linagliptin, 850 mg metformin
   2.5 mg linagliptin, 1 g metformin
Usual adult dosage: Base dosage on current use of individual drugs. Given twice a day with meals.
See also **linagliptin, metformin.**

▷ pioglitazone and glimepiride
Duetact

Tablets:
   30 mg pioglitazone with 2 or 4 mg glimepiride
Usual adult dosage: One tablet/day PO with first meal of the day.
See also **pioglitazone, glimepiride.**

▷ pioglitazone and metformin
ActoPlus Met⊕, ActoPlus Met XR⊕

Tablets:
   15 mg pioglitazone, 500 mg metformin
   15 mg pioglitazone, 850 mg metformin
ER tablets⊕:
   15 mg pioglitazone, 1,000 mg metformin
   30 mg pioglitazone, 1,000 mg metformin
Usual adult dosage: One tablet PO once or twice a day with meals based on patient response and glycemic control; ER tablets, once a day with evening meal.
See also **metformin, pioglitazone.**

▽repaglinide and metformin

PrandiMet

Tablets:
  1 mg repaglinide, 500 mg metformin
  2 mg repaglinide, 500 mg metformin
Usual adult dosage: 1 tablet PO bid to tid; titrate as needed for glycemic control.
See also **repaglinide, metformin.**

▽rosiglitazone and glimepiride

Avandaryl

Tablets:
  4 mg rosiglitazone, 1 mg glimepiride
  4 mg rosiglitazone, 2 mg glimepiride
  4 mg rosiglitazone, 4 mg glimepiride
  8 mg rosiglitazone, 2 mg glimepiride
  8 mg rosiglitazone, 4 mg glimepiride
Usual adult dosage: 4 mg rosiglitazone with 1 or 2 mg glimepiride PO once daily with first meal of the day. Titrate as needed for glycemic control. Available through limited-access program only.
See also **rosiglitazone, glimepiride.**

▽rosiglitazone and metformin

Avandamet

Tablets:
  1 mg rosiglitazone, 500 mg metformin
  2 mg rosiglitazone, 500 mg metformin
  2 mg rosiglitazone, 1 g metformin
  4 mg rosiglitazone, 500 mg metformin
  4 mg rosiglitazone, 1 g metformin
Usual adult dosage: 4 mg rosiglitazone with 500 mg metformin, PO once a day or in divided doses. Not for initial therapy; dosage should be adjusted using individual drugs alone and then switching to the appropriate dosage of the combination product. See package insert for details on adjusting dosage based on use of other agents and previous dosage levels. Available through limited-access program only.
See also **metformin, rosiglitazone.**

▽saxagliptin and metformin

Kombiglyze XR⊕

Tablets:
  5 mg saxagliptin, 500 mg metformin
  5 mg saxagliptin, 1,000 mg metformin
  2.5 mg saxagliptin, 1,000 mg metformin
Usual adult dosage: One tablet PO daily. Do not cut, crush, or allow patient to chew tablets.
See also **saxagliptin, metformin.**

▷ sitagliptin and metformin
Janumet, Janumet XR⬚

Tablets:
    50 mg sitagliptin, 500 or 1,000 mg metformin
ER Tablets:
    50 mg sitagliptin, 500 mg metformin
    50 mg sitagliptin, 1 g metformin
    100 mg sitagliptin, 1 g metformin
Usual adult dosage: One tablet PO bid with meals, or once a day with evening meal for ER tablet; maximum daily dosage 100 mg sitagliptin, 2,000 mg metformin. Do not cut, crush, or, chew ER tablet.
See also **sitagliptin, metformin.**

ANTIDIABETIC/LIPID-LOWERING DRUGS

▷ sitagliptin and simvastatin
Juvisync

Tablets:
    100 mg sitagliptin, 10 mg simvastatin
    100 mg sitagliptin, 20 mg simvastatin
    100 mg sitagliptin, 40 mg simvastatin
Usual adult dosage: Initially, 100 mg sitagliptin/40 mg simvastatin PO in the evening; adjust dosage based on patient response. Use in conjunction with diet and exercise program.
See also **sitagliptin, simvastatin.**

ANTIDIARRHEALS

▷ diphenoxylate hydrochloride and atropine sulfate
CONTROLLED SUBSTANCE C-V
Logen, Lomanate, Lomotil, Lonox

Tablets:
    2.5 mg diphenoxylate hydrochloride, 0.025 mg atropine sulfate
Liquid:
    2.5 mg diphenoxylate hydrochloride, 0.025 mg atropine sulfate/5 mL
• Individualized dosage.
Usual adult dosage: 5 mg PO qid.
• Pediatric initial dosage (use only liquid in children 2–12 yr): 0.3–0.4 mg/kg PO daily in four divided doses.

Age (yr)	Weight (kg)	Dose (mL)	Frequency
2	11–14	1.5–3	4 times daily
3	12–16	2–3	4 times daily
4	14–20	2–4	4 times daily
5	16–23	2.5–4.5	4 times daily
6–8	17–32	2.5–5	4 times daily
9–12	23–55	3.5–5	4 times daily

- Reduce dosage as soon as initial control of symptoms is achieved. Maintenance dosage may be as low as one-fourth of the initial dosage.

See also **atropine sulfate.**

ANTIHYPERTENSIVES

▽ aliskiren and amlodipine

Tekamlo

Tablets:
150 mg aliskiren, 5 mg amlodipine
150 mg aliskiren, 10 mg amlodipine
300 mg aliskiren, 5 mg amlodipine
300 mg aliskiren, 10 mg amlodipine

Usual adult dosage: One tablet PO daily; may give with other antihypertensives. Should give at about the same time each day.

See also **aliskiren, amlodipine.**

▽ aliskiren and amlodipine and hydrochlorothiazide

Amturnide

Tablets:
150 mg aliskiren, 5 mg amlodipine, 12.5 mg hydrochlorothiazide
300 mg aliskiren, 5 mg amlodipine, 12.5 mg hydrochlorothiazide
300 mg aliskiren, 5 mg amlodipine, 25 mg hydrochlorothiazide
300 mg aliskiren, 10 mg amlodipine, 12.5 mg hydrochlorothiazide
300 mg aliskiren, 10 mg amlodipine, 25 mg hydrochlorothiazide

Usual adult dosage: One tablet PO daily at about the same time each day.

See also **aliskiren, amlodipine, hydrochlorothiazide.**

▽ aliskiren and hydrochlorothiazide

Tekturna HCT

Tablets:
150 mg aliskiren, 12.5 mg hydrochlorothiazide
150 mg aliskiren, 25 mg hydrochlorothiazide
300 mg aliskiren, 12.5 mg hydrochlorothiazide
300 mg aliskiren, 25 mg hydrochlorothiazide

Usual adult dosage: One tablet PO daily.

May be given with other antihypertensives. Should be taken at about the same time each day.

See also **aliskiren, hydrochlorothiazide.**

▽ aliskiren and valsartan

Valturna

Tablets:
150 mg aliskiren, 160 mg valsartan
300 mg aliskiren, 320 mg valsartan

Usual adult dosage: One tablet PO daily.

Indicated when hypertension is not controlled by one drug alone.
See also **aliskiren, valsartan.**

▽ amlodipine and benazepril

Lotrel

Capsules:
    2.5 mg amlodipine, 10 mg benazepril
    5 mg amlodipine, 10 mg benazepril
    5 mg amlodipine, 20 mg benazepril
    5 mg amlodipine, 40 mg benazepril
    10 mg amlodipine, 20 mg benazepril
    10 mg amlodipine, 40 mg benazepril
Usual adult dosage: One tablet PO daily in the morning.
Monitor patient for hypotension and adverse effects closely over first 2 wk and regularly thereafter.
See also **amlodipine, benazepril.**

▽ amlodipine and olmesartan

Azor

Tablets:
    5 mg amlodipine, 20 mg olmesartan
    10 mg amlodipine, 20 mg olmesartan
    5 mg amlodipine, 40 mg olmesartan
    10 mg amlodipine, 40 mg olmesartan
Usual adult dosage: One tablet PO daily; titrate based on patient response.
See also **amlodipine, olmesartan.**

▽ amlodipine and valsartan

Exforge

Tablets:
    5 mg amlodipine, 160 mg valsartan
    5 mg amlodipine, 320 mg valsartan
    10 mg amlodipine, 160 mg valsartan
    10 mg amlodipine, 320 mg valsartan
Usual adult dosage: One tablet PO daily at about the same time each day.
Dosage based on patient response.
See also **amlodipine, valsartan.**

▽ amlodipine, valsartan, and hydrochlorothiazide

Exforge HCT

Tablets:
    5 mg amlodipine, 160 mg valsartan, 12.5 mg hydrochlorothiazide
    10 mg amlodipine, 160 mg valsartan, 12.5 mg hydrochlorothiazide
    5 mg amlodipine, 160 mg valsartan, 25 mg hydrochlorothiazide
    10 mg amlodipine, 320 mg valsartan, 25 mg hydrochlorothiazide
Usual adult dosage: One tablet PO daily; titrate based on patient response.
See also **amlodipine, hydrochlorothiazide, valsartan.**

▽ atenolol and chlorthalidone

Tenoretic

Tablets:
    50 mg atenolol, 25 mg chlorthalidone
    100 mg atenolol, 25 mg chlorthalidone
Usual adult dosage: One tablet PO daily in the morning.
Drug should be adjusted using the individual products, then switched to appropriate dosage.
See also **atenolol, chlorthalidone.**

▽ azilsartan and chlorthalidone

Edarbyclor

Tablets:
    40 mg azilsartan, 12.5 mg chlorthalidone
    40 mg azilsartan, 25 mg chlorthalidone
Usual adult dosage: 1 tablet PO daily. Not for use in pregnancy or renal failure. Monitor potassium level.
See also **azilsartan, chlorthalidone.**

▽ bisoprolol and hydrochlorothiazide

Ziac

Tablets:
    2.5 mg bisoprolol, 6.25 mg hydrochlorothiazide
    5 mg bisoprolol, 6.25 mg hydrochlorothiazide
    10 mg bisoprolol, 6.25 mg hydrochlorothiazide
Usual adult dosage: One tablet daily PO in morning. Initial dose is 2.5/6.25 mg tablet PO daily.
Dosage should be adjusted within 1 wk; optimal antihypertensive effect may require 2–3 wk.
See also **bisoprolol, hydrochlorothiazide.**

▽ candesartan and hydrochlorothiazide

Atacand HCT

Tablets:
    16 mg candesartan, 12.5 mg hydrochlorothiazide
    32 mg candesartan, 12.5 mg hydrochlorothiazide
Usual adult dosage: One tablet PO daily in the morning.
Drug should be adjusted using the individual products, then switched to appropriate dosage.
See also **candesartan, hydrochlorothiazide.**

▽ chlorthalidone and clonidine

Clorpres

Tablets:
    15 mg chlorthalidone, 0.1 mg clonidine hydrochloride
    15 mg chlorthalidone, 0.2 mg clonidine hydrochloride
    15 mg chlorthalidone, 0.3 mg clonidine hydrochloride
Usual adult dosage: One or two tablets per day PO in the morning; may be given once or twice daily.

Dosage should be adjusted with the individual products, switching to this combination product when patient's condition is stabilized on the dosage of each drug available in this combination. See also **clonidine.**

▷ **enalapril and hydrochlorothiazide**

Vaseretic

Tablets:
   5 mg enalapril maleate, 12.5 mg hydrochlorothiazide
   10 mg enalapril maleate, 25 mg hydrochlorothiazide
Usual adult dosage: One or two tablets per day PO in the morning.
Dosage should be adjusted with individual products, switching to combination product after patient's condition is stabilized on the dosage of each drug that is available in this combination.
See also **enalapril maleate, hydrochlorothiazide.**

▷ **eprosartan and hydrochlorothiazide**

Teveten HCT

Tablets:
   600 mg eprosartan, 12.5 mg hydrochlorothiazide
   600 mg eprosartan, 25 mg hydrochlorothiazide
Usual adult dosage: One tablet PO each day. Dosage should be established with each component alone before using the combination product; if BP is still not controlled, 300 mg eprosartan may be added each evening.
See also **eprosartan mesylate, hydrochlorothiazide.**

▷ **fosinopril and hydrochlorothiazide**

Monopril-HCT

Tablets:
   10 mg fosinopril, 12.5 mg hydrochlorothiazide
   20 mg fosinopril, 12.5 mg hydrochlorothiazide
Usual adult dosage: One tablet PO per day in the morning.
Drug should be adjusted using the individual products, switching to appropriate dosage of this combination product.
See also **fosinopril, hydrochlorothiazide.**

▷ **hydrochlorothiazide and benazepril**

Lotensin HCT

Tablets:
   6.25 mg hydrochlorothiazide, 5 mg benazepril
   12.5 mg hydrochlorothiazide, 10 mg benazepril
   12.5 mg hydrochlorothiazide, 20 mg benazepril
   25 mg hydrochlorothiazide, 20 mg benazepril
Usual adult dosage: One tablet per day PO in the morning.
Dosage should be adjusted with the individual products, switching to this combination product once the patient's condition is stabilized.
See also **benazepril, hydrochlorothiazide.**

▷ hydrochlorothiazide and captopril

Capozide

Tablets:
    15 mg hydrochlorothiazide, 25 mg captopril
    15 mg hydrochlorothiazide, 50 mg captopril
    25 mg hydrochlorothiazide, 25 mg captopril
    25 mg hydrochlorothiazide, 50 mg captopril
Usual adult dosage: One or two tablets PO daily, 1 hr before or 2 hr after meals.
Dosage should be adjusted with individual products, switching to this combination product when patient's condition is stabilized on the dosage of each drug available in this combination.
See also **captopril, hydrochlorothiazide.**

▷ hydrochlorothiazide and propranolol

Tablets:
    25 mg hydrochlorothiazide, 40 mg propranolol
    25 mg hydrochlorothiazide, 80 mg propranolol
Usual adult dosage: One or two tablets PO bid.
Dosage should be adjusted with individual products, switching to combination product when patient's condition is stabilized on the dosage of each drug available in this combination.
See also **hydrochlorothiazide, propranolol.**

▷ irbesartan and hydrochlorothiazide

Avalide

Tablets:
    150 mg irbesartan, 12.5 mg hydrochlorothiazide
    300 mg irbesartan, 12.5 mg hydrochlorothiazide
Usual adult dosage: One or two tablets per day PO.
Dosage should be adjusted with individual products, switching to combination product when patient's condition is stabilized.
See also **hydrochlorothiazide, irbesartan.**

▷ lisinopril and hydrochlorothiazide

Prinzide, Zestoretic

Tablets:
    10 mg lisinopril, 12.5 mg hydrochlorothiazide
    20 mg lisinopril, 12.5 mg hydrochlorothiazide
    20 mg lisinopril, 25 mg hydrochlorothiazide
Usual adult dosage: One tablet per day PO taken in the morning.
Dosage should be adjusted with individual products, switching to combination product when patient's condition is stabilized.
See also **hydrochlorothiazide, lisinopril.**

▽ losartan and hydrochlorothiazide

Hyzaar

Tablets:
    50 mg losartan, 12.5 mg hydrochlorothiazide
    100 mg losartan, 12.5 mg hydrochlorothiazide
    100 mg losartan, 25 mg hydrochlorothiazide
Usual adult dosage: One tablet per day PO in the morning.
- Not for initial therapy; start using each component and if desired effects are obtained, *Hyzaar* may be used.
- Used to reduce the incidence of CVA in hypertensive patients with left ventricular hypertrophy (not effective for this use in black patients).
See also **hydrochlorothiazide, losartan.**

▽ metoprolol and hydrochlorothiazide

Dutoprol⊛, Lopressor HCT

Tablets:
    50 mg metoprolol, 25 mg hydrochlorothiazide
    100 mg metoprolol, 25 mg hydrochlorothiazide
    100 mg metoprolol, 50 mg hydrochlorothiazide
ER Tablets:
    25 mg metoprolol, 12.5 mg hydrochlorothiazide
    50 mg metoprolol, 12.5 mg hydrochlorothiazide
    100 mg metoprolol, 12.5 mg hydrochlorothiazide
Usual adult dosage: One tablet PO per day.
Drug should be adjusted using the individual products, switching to appropriate dosage of this combination product. Do not cut, crush, or allow patient to chew ER tablets.
See also **hydrochlorothiazide, metoprolol.**

▽ moexipril and hydrochlorothiazide

Uniretic

Tablets:
    7.5 mg moexipril, 12.5 mg hydrochlorothiazide
    15 mg moexipril, 12.5 mg hydrochlorothiazide
    15 mg moexipril, 25 mg hydrochlorothiazide
Usual adult dosage: One or two tablets per day 1 hr before or 2 hr after a meal.
Not for initial therapy. Adjust dose to maintain appropriate BP.
See also **hydrochlorothiazide, moexipril.**

▽ nadolol and bendroflumethiazide

Corzide

Tablets:
    40 mg nadolol, 5 mg bendroflumethiazide
    80 mg nadolol, 5 mg bendroflumethiazide
Usual adult dosage: One tablet PO per day in the morning.
Drug should be adjusted using the individual products, switching to appropriate dosage of this combination product.
See also **bendroflumethiazide, nadolol.**

▷ olmesartan, amlodipine, and hydrochlorothiazide
Tribenzor

Tablets:
  20 mg olmesartan, 5 mg amlodipine, 12.5 mg hydrochlorothiazide
  40 mg olmesartan, 5 mg amlodipine, 12.5 mg hydrochlorothiazide
  40 mg olmesartan, 5 mg amlodipine, 25 mg hydrochlorothiazide
  40 mg olmesartan, 10 mg amlodipine, 12.5 mg hydrochlorothiazide
Usual adult dosage: One tablet PO daily. Not for initial therapy. For use in patients whose blood pressure is not controlled by any two of the drugs in the tablet.
See also **olmesartan, amlodipine, hydrochlorothiazide**

▷ olmesartan medoxomil and hydrochlorothiazide
Benicar HCT

Tablets:
  20 mg olmesartan, 12.5 mg hydrochlorothiazide
  40 mg olmesartan, 12.5 mg hydrochlorothiazide
  40 mg olmesartan, 25 mg hydrochlorothiazide
Usual adult dosage: One tablet PO per day in the morning.
Establish dosage with each drug individually, then switch to appropriate dosage of the combined product.
See also **hydrochlorothiazide, olmesartan.**

▷ quinapril and hydrochlorothiazide
Accuretic

Tablets:
  10 mg quinapril, 12.5 mg hydrochlorothiazide
  20 mg quinapril, 12.5 mg hydrochlorothiazide
  20 mg quinapril, 25 mg hydrochlorothiazide
Usual adult dosage: One tablet PO per day in the morning.
Drug should be adjusted using the individual products, switching to appropriate dosage of this combination product.
See also **hydrochlorothiazide, quinapril.**

▷ telmisartan and amlodipine
Twynsta

Tablets:
  40 mg telmisartan, 5 mg amlodipine
  40 mg telmisartan, 10 mg amlodipine
  80 mg telmisartan, 5 mg amlodipine
  80 mg telmisartan, 10 mg amlodipine
Usual adult dosage: One tablet PO daily.
May be used in combination with other drugs.
See also **amlodipine, telmisartan.**

▽ telmisartan and hydrochlorothiazide
Micardis HCT

Tablets:
  40 mg telmisartan, 12.5 mg hydrochlorothiazide
  80 mg telmisartan, 12.5 mg hydrochlorothiazide
  80 mg telmisartan, 25 mg hydrochlorothiazide
Usual adult dosage: One tablet PO per day; may be adjusted up to 160 mg telmisartan and 25 mg hydrochlorothiazide, based on patient's response.
See also **hydrochlorothiazide, telmisartan.**

▽ trandolapril and verapamil
Tarka

Tablets:
  1 mg trandolapril, 240 mg verapamil
  2 mg trandolapril, 180 mg verapamil
  2 mg trandolapril, 240 mg verapamil
  4 mg trandolapril, 240 mg verapamil
Usual adult dosage: One tablet PO per day, taken with food.
Dosage should be adjusted with the individual products, switching to this combination product when the patient's condition is stabilized on the dosage of each drug available in combination. Ensure that patient swallows tablet whole. Do not cut, crush, or chew.
See also **trandolapril, verapamil.**

▽ valsartan and hydrochlorothiazide
Diovan HCT

Tablets:
  80 mg valsartan, 12.5 mg hydrochlorothiazide
  160 mg valsartan, 12.5 mg hydrochlorothiazide
  160 mg valsartan, 25 mg hydrochlorothiazide
  320 mg valsartan, 12.5 mg hydrochlorothiazide
  320 mg valsartan, 25 mg hydrochlorothiazide
Usual adult dosage: One tablet per day PO.
Not for initial therapy; start using each component first.
See also **hydrochlorothiazide, valsartan.**

ANTIMIGRAINE DRUGS

▽ acetaminophen, caffeine, and isometheptene
MigraTen

Capsules:
  325 mg acetaminophen, 100 mg caffeine, 65 mg isometheptene
Usual adult dosage: Two capsules at onset of migraine; then one every hour until resolved. Maximum, 5 capsules in 12 hr. For tension headache, one to two capsules every 4 hr, up to 8 capsules per day.
See also **acetaminophen.**

▽ergotamine and caffeine

Cafergot, Migergot

Tablets:
    1 mg ergotamine tartrate, 100 mg caffeine
Usual adult oral dosage: Two tablets at first sign of attack. Follow with one tablet every 30 min, if needed. Maximum dose is six tablets per attack. Do not exceed 10 tablets per wk.
Do not combine this drug with ritonavir, nelfinavir, indinavir, erythromycin, clarithromycin, or troleandomycin—serious vasospasm events could occur.
See also **ergotamine.**

▽sumatriptan and naproxen sodium

Treximet

Tablets:
    85 mg sumatriptan, 500 mg naproxen
Usual adult dosage: One tablet PO at the onset of acute migraine; may repeat after at least 2 hour. Maximum dose, two tablets/24 hr.
See also **naproxen, sumatriptan.**

ANTIPARKINSONIANS

▽levodopa and carbidopa

Parcopa, Sinemet, Sinemet CR⊕

Tablets:
    100 mg levodopa, 10 mg carbidopa
    100 mg levodopa, 25 mg carbidopa
    250 mg levodopa, 25 mg carbidopa
Orally disintegrating tablets:
    100 mg levodopa, 10 mg carbidopa
    100 mg levodopa, 25 mg carbidopa
    250 mg levodopa, 25 mg carbidopa
Controlled release tablets⊕:
    100 mg levodopa, 25 mg carbidopa
    200 mg levodopa, 50 mg carbidopa
Usual adult dosage: Starting dose for patients not presently receiving levodopa: One tablet of 100 mg levodopa/10 mg carbidopa or 100 mg levodopa/25 mg carbidopa PO tid. For patients receiving levodopa: Start combination therapy with the morning dose at least 8 hr after the last dose of levodopa and choose a daily dosage of levodopa and carbidopa that will provide 25% of the previous levodopa daily dose. Dosage must be adjusted based on the patient's clinical response. See manufacturer's directions for adjusting the combination and single-agent drugs. *Orally disintegrating tablets:* Initially, one 100/25-mg tablet PO tid. Place tablet on top of the tongue where it will dissolve within seconds, then have the patient swallow the saliva; no additional liquid is required. Dosage may be increased by one tablet every day or every other day as needed to total daily dose of eight tablets (two tablets qid) as needed to control symptoms.
    Carbidopa is available alone only by a specific request to the manufacturer from physicians who have a patient who needs a different dosage of carbidopa than is provided by the fixed combination drug; carbidopa is a peripheral inhibitor of dopa decarboxylase, an enzyme that converts dopa to dopamine, which cannot penetrate the CNS. The addition of carbidopa to the levodopa regimen

reduces the dose of levodopa needed and decreases the incidence of certain adverse reactions to levodopa.

See also **carbidopa, levodopa.**

▷ levodopa, carbidopa, and entacapone

Stalevo 50, Stalevo 75, Stalevo 100, Stalevo 125, Stalevo 150, Stalevo 200

Tablets:
    50 mg levodopa, 12.5 mg carbidopa, 200 mg entacapone
    75 mg levodopa, 18.75 mg carbidopa, 200 mg entacapone
    100 mg levodopa, 25 mg carbidopa, 200 mg entacapone
    125 mg levodopa, 31.25 mg carbidopa, 200 mg entacapone
    150 mg levodopa, 37.5 mg carbidopa, 200 mg entacapone
    200 mg levodopa, 50 mg carbidopa, 200 mg entacapone
Usual adult dosage: One tablet every 3–8 hr, based on the patient's clinical response.
See also **carbidopa, entacapone, levodopa.**

ANTIPLATELETS

▷ aspirin and dipyridamole

Aggrenox

Capsules:
    25 mg aspirin, 200 mg dipyridamole
Usual adult dosage: One capsule PO bid to decrease risk of CVA in patients with known cerebrovascular disease.
See also **aspirin, dipyridamole.**

ANTIULCER DRUGS

▷ bismuth subsalicylate, metronidazole, and tetracycline

Helidac

Tablets:
    262.4 mg bismuth subsalicylate, 250 mg metronidazole, 500 mg tetracycline hydrochloride
Usual adult dosage: Two tablets bismuth subsalicylate, one tablet metronidazole, and one capsule tetracycline PO qid for 14 days along with a prescribed histamine-2 antagonist. Indicated for the treatment of active duodenal ulcers associated with *Helicobacter pylori* infection. Do not use in pregnant or breast-feeding women or in children.
See also **bismuth subsalicylate, metronidazole, tetracycline.**

▷ lansoprazole, amoxicillin, and clarithromycin

Prevpac

Daily administration pack:
    Two 30-mg lansoprazole capsules, four 500-mg amoxicillin capsules, and two 500-mg clarithromycin tablets.
Usual adult dosage: Divide pack equally to take twice daily, morning and evening for 10–14 days.

ANTIVIRALS

▷ abacavir and lamivudine

Epzicom

Tablets:
  600 mg abacavir with 300 mg lamivudine
Usual adult dosage: One tablet PO daily, taken without regard to food and in combination with other antiretroviral drugs for treatment of HIV infection.
See also **abacavir, lamivudine.**

▷ abacavir, zidovudine, and lamivudine

Trizivir

Tablets:
  300 mg abacavir, 300 mg zidovudine, 150 mg lamivudine
Usual adult dosage: One tablet PO bid for treatment of HIV infection.
Carefully monitor patient for hypersensitivity reactions; potential increased risk of heart attack.
See also **abacavir, lamivudine, zidovudine.**

▷ efavirenz, emtricitabine, and tenofovir

Atripla

Tablets:
  600 mg efavirenz, 200 mg emtricitabine, 300 mg tenofovir
Usual adult dosage: One tablet PO at bedtime on an empty stomach for treatment of HIV infection.
Pediatric patients 12 yr of age and older, weighing at least 40 kg: One tablet/day PO at bedtime.
Renal impairment: Not recommended for patients with moderate or severe renal impairment.
See also **efavirenz, emtricitabine, tenofovir.**

▷ elvitegravir, cobicistat, emtricitabine, and tenofovir

Stribild

Tablets:
  150 mg elvitegravir, 150 mg cobicistat, 200 mg emtricitabine, 300 mg tenofovir
Usual adult dosage: One tablet PO per day for patients who have never been treated for HIV infection. Elvitegravir is an HIV integrase strand transfer inhibitor only available in this combination form; cobicistat is a pharmacokinetic enhancer, delaying the metabolism of the other drugs to prolong effect.
See also **emtricitabine, tenofovir.**

▷ emtricitabine, rilpivirine, and tenofovir

Complera

Tablets:
  200 mg emtricitabine, 25 mg rilpivirine, 300 mg tenofovir

Usual adult dosage: One tablet PO per day for treatment of treatment-naïve patients with HIV infection. Administer with food.

See also **emtricitabine, rilpivirine, tenofovir.**

▷ emtricitabine and tenofovir disoproxil fumarate

Truvada

Tablets:
200 mg emtricitabine with 300 mg tenofovir

Usual dosage for patients 12 yr and older: One tablet PO daily, taken without regard to food in combination with other antiretroviral drugs for treatment of HIV infection and in combination with safe-sex practices as preexposure prophylaxis to reduce risk of sexually acquired HIV-1 infection in adults at high risk.

See also **emtricitabine, tenofovir.**

▷ lamivudine and zidovudine

Combivir

Tablets:
150 mg lamivudine, 300 mg zidovudine

Usual adult dose: One tablet PO bid for treatment of HIV infection.

Not recommended for children or adults weighing less than 30 kg. May be taken with food. Does not decrease risk of spreading infections; use caution.

See also **lamivudine, zidovudine.**

BENIGN PROSTATIC HYPERTROPHY DRUGS

▷ dutasteride and tamsulosin

Jalyn

Capsules:
0.5 mg dutasteride, 0.4 mg tamsulosin

Usual adult dosage: One capsule PO per day.

See also **dutasteride, tamsulosin.**

DIURETICS

▷ amiloride and hydrochlorothiazide

Moduretic

Tablets:
5 mg amiloride, 50 mg hydrochlorothiazide

Usual adult dosage: One or two tablets per day PO with meals.

See also **amiloride, hydrochlorothiazide.**

▷ hydrochlorothiazide and triamterene

Dyazide

Capsules:
25 mg hydrochlorothiazide, 37.5 mg triamterene

Usual adult dosage: One or two capsules PO per day or bid after meals.
See also **hydrochlorothiazide, triamterene.**

Maxzide, Maxzide-25

Tablets:
  25 mg hydrochlorothiazide, 37.5 mg triamterene
  50 mg hydrochlorothiazide, 75 mg triamterene
Usual adult dosage: One or two tablets PO per day.
See also **hydrochlorothiazide, triamterene**

▷ spironolactone and hydrochlorothiazide

Aldactazide

Tablets:
  25 mg spironolactone, 25 mg hydrochlorothiazide
Usual adult dosage: One to eight tablets PO daily.
Tablets:
  50 mg spironolactone, 50 mg hydrochlorothiazide
Usual adult dosage: One to four tablets PO daily.
See also **hydrochlorothiazide, spironolactone.**

HEART FAILURE DRUGS

▷ isosorbide dinitrate and hydralazine hydrochloride

BiDil

Tablets:
  20 mg isosorbide dinitrate, 37.5 mg hydralazine
Usual adult dosage: One tablet PO tid; may be increased to two tablets tid. For adjunct therapy in self-identified black patients to improve functional survival.
See also **isosorbide dinitrate, hydralazine.**

LIPID-LOWERING DRUGS

▷ ezetimibe and simvastatin

Vytorin

Tablets:
  10 mg ezetimibe; 10 mg simvastatin
  10 mg ezetimibe; 20 mg simvastatin
  10 mg ezetimibe; 40 mg simvastatin
  10 mg ezetimibe; 80 mg simvastatin
Usual adult dosage: One tablet PO daily, taken in evening in combination with cholesterol-lowering diet and exercise. Dosage of simvastatin in the combination may be adjusted based on patient response. If given with a bile sequestrant, must be given at least 2 hr before or 4 hr after the bile sequestrant.
See also **ezetimibe, simvastatin.**

niacin and lovastatin

Advicor

Tablets:

500 mg niacin, 20 mg lovastatin
750 mg niacin, 20 mg lovastatin
1,000 mg niacin, 20 mg lovastatin
1,000 mg niacin, 40 mg lovastatin

Usual adult dosage: One tablet daily PO at night with low-fast snack.
See also **lovastatin, niacin.**

simvastatin and niacin

Simcor

Tablets:

20 mg simvastatin, 500 mg niacin
20 mg simvastatin, 750 mg niacin
20 mg simvastatin, 1,000 mg niacin
40 mg simvastatin, 500 mg niacin
40 mg simvastatin, 1,000 mg niacin

Usual adult dosage: One tablet PO per day; titrate based on lipid levels. Maximum dose 2,000 mg niacin with 40 mg simvastatin per day.
See also **niacin, simvastatin.**

MENOPAUSE DRUGS

drospirenone and estradiol

Angeliq

Tablets:

0.25 mg drospirenone, 0.5 mg estradiol
0.5 mg drospirenone, 1 mg estradiol

Usual adult dosage: One tablet each day PO. Monitor potassium level closely.
See also **estradiol.**

drospirenone and ethinyl estradiol

YAZ

Tablets:

3 mg drospirenone, 0.02 mg ethinyl estradiol

Usual adult dosage: One tablet each day PO. Monitor potassium level closely.
Also approved to treat premenstrual dysphoric disorder, acne.

estradiol and norethindrone (transdermal)

CombiPatch

Patch:

0.05 mg per day estradiol, 0.14 mg per day norethindrone
0.05 mg per day estradiol, 0.25 mg per day norethindrone

Usual adult dosage: Change patch twice a week.
For relief of symptoms of menopause in women with intact uterus.
See also **estrogens.**

▽ estradiol and norethindrone (oral)
Activella

Tablets:
    0.5 mg estradiol, 0.1 mg norethindrone
    1 mg estradiol, 0.5 mg norethindrone
Usual adult dosage: One tablet each day.
For treatment of moderate to severe vasomotor symptoms, vulvar and vaginal atrophy, prevention
of postmenopausal osteoporosis in women with intact uterus.
See also **estrogens.**

▽ estradiol and norgestimate
Ortho-Prefest

Tablets:
    1 mg estradiol, 0.09 mg norgestimate
Usual adult dosage: One tablet per day PO (3 days of pink tablets: estradiol alone; followed by 3
days of white tablets: estradiol and norgestimate combination; continue cycle uninterrupted).
Treatment of moderate to severe symptoms of menopause and prevention of osteoporosis in women
with intact uterus.
See also **estradiol.**

▽ estrogens, conjugated, and medroxyprogesterone
Premphase

Tablets:
    0.625 mg conjugated estrogens, 5 mg medroxyprogesterone
Usual adult dosage: One tablet per day PO.
Treatment of moderate to severe symptoms of menopause and prevention of osteoporosis in women
with intact uterus.
See also **estrogen, medroxyprogesterone.**

▽ ethinyl estradiol and norethindrone acetate
femhrt

Tablets:
    2.5 mcg ethinyl estradiol, 0.5 mg norethindrone acetate
    5 mcg ethinyl estradiol, 1 mg norethindrone acetate
Usual adult dosage: One tablet per day PO.
Treatment of signs and symptoms of menopause and prevention of osteoporosis in women with
intact uterus.
See also **estradiol, norethindrone.**

medroxyprogesterone and conjugated estrogens

Prempro

Tablets:
0.3 mg conjugated estrogen, 1.5 mg medroxygesterone
0.45 mg conjugated estrogen, 1.5 mg medroxygesterone
0.625 mg conjugated estrogen, 2.5 mg medroxyprogesterone
0.625 mg conjugated estrogen, 5 mg medroxyprogesterone
Usual adult dosage: One tablet per day PO.
For relief of symptoms of menopause and prevention of osteoporosis in women with intact uterus.
See also **estrogen.**

OPIOID AGONISTS

buprenorphine and naloxone

CONTROLLED SUBSTANCE C-III

Suboxone

Sublingual tablets:
2 mg buprenorphine, 0.5 mg naloxone
8 mg buprenorphine, 2 mg naloxone
Usual adult dosage: One to two tablets sublingually once each day following induction with sublingual buprenorphine for treatment of opioid dependence.
See also **buprenorphine, naloxone.**

PSYCHIATRIC DRUGS

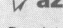dextromethorphan and quinidine

Nuedexta

Capsules:
20 mg dextromethorphan, 10 mg quinidine
Usual adult dosage: One capsule PO daily for 7 days; then one capsule PO every 12 hr for maintenance. To treat pseudobulbar affect associated with neurologic conditions.
See also **dextromethorphan, quinidine.**

RESPIRATORY DRUGS

azelastine and fluticasone

Dymista

Nasal spray:
137 mcg azelastine, 50 mcg fluticasone
Usual dosage for patients 12 yr and older: One spray in each nostril bid for relief of symptoms of seasonal allergic rhinitis.
See also **azelastine, fluticasone.**

▷budesonide and formoterol fumarate

Symbicort 80/4.5, Symbicort 160/4.5

Inhalation:
   80 mcg budesonide, 4.5 mcg formoterol fumarate
   160 mcg budesonide, 4.5 mcg formoterol fumarate
Usual dosage in patients 12 yr and older: Two inhalations bid, morning and evening.
Use for long-term maintenance of asthma, not for acute attacks.
See also **budesonide, formoterol.**

▷fluticasone and salmeterol

Advair Diskus, Advair HFA

Inhalation:
   100 mcg fluticasone, 50 mcg salmeterol
   250 mcg fluticasone, 50 mcg salmeterol
   500 mcg fluticasone, 50 mcg salmeterol
Usual dosage in patients 12 yr and older: One inhalation bid to manage asthma.
Usual dosage in patients 4–11 yr: One inhalation (100 mcg fluticasone, 50 mcg salmeterol) bid in the morning and evening about 12 hr apart.
See also **fluticasone, salmeterol.**

▷hydrocodone and pseudoephedrine

Rezira

Oral solution:
   5 mg hydrocodone, 60 mg pseudoephedrine per 5-mL solution
Usual adult dosage: 5 mL PO every 4–6 hr as needed; do not exceed four doses in 24 hr.
See also **hydrocodone, pseudoephedrine.**

▷hydrocodone and pseudoephedrine and chlorpheniramine

Zutripro

Oral solution:
   5 mg hydrocodone, 60 mg pseudoephedrine, 4 mg chlorpheniramine in 5-mL solution
Usual adult dosage: 5 mL PO every 4-6 hr as needed; do not exceed four doses in 24 hr.
See also **hydrocodone, pseudoephedrine, chlorpheniramine.**

▷ipratropium and albuterol

Combivent

Metered-dose inhaler:
   18 mcg ipratropium bromide, 90 mcg albuterol
Usual adult dosage: Two inhalations four times per day
Not for use during acute attack.
Use caution with known sensitivity to atropine, soy beans, soya lecithin, peanuts.
Treatment of bronchospasm with COPD in patients who require more than a single bronchodilator.
See also **albuterol, ipratropium.**

CRUSH Do not crush.

▽loratadine and pseudoephedrine

Claritin-D℞

ER tablets:
  5 mg loratadine, 120 mg pseudoephedrine
Usual adult dosage: One tablet PO every 12 hr.
See also **loratadine, pseudoephedrine.**

Claritin-D 24 Hour℞

ER tablets:
  10 mg loratadine, 240 mg pseudoephedrine
Usual adult dosage: One tablet PO every day.
See also **loratadine, pseudoephedrine.**

▽mometasone and formoterol

Dulera 100/5, Dulera 200/5

Metered aerosol inhaler:
  100 mcg mometasone, 5 mcg formoterol
  200 mcg mometasone, 5 mcg formoterol
Usual adult dosage: For maintenance treatment of asthma, 2 inhalations twice a day, AM and PM; rinse mouth after use. For adults only.
See also **mometasone, formoterol.**

TENSION HEADACHE DRUGS

▽butalbital, acetaminophen, and caffeine

Esgic-Plus

Capsules and tablets:
  50 mg butalbital, 500 mg acetaminophen, 40 mg caffeine
Usual adult dosage: One capsule or tablet PO every 4 hr as needed, up to six per day. May be habit-forming; avoid driving and dangerous tasks.
See also **acetaminophen, caffeine.**

WEIGHT-LOSS DRUGS

▽phentermine and topiramate

Qsymia

Capsules:
  3.75 mg phentermine, 23 mg topiramate
  7.5 mg phentermine, 46 mg topiramate
  11.25 mg phentermine, 69 mg topiramate
  15 mg phentermine, 92 mg topiramate
Usual adult dosage: One capsule daily in the morning with diet and exercise for help in weight loss with body mass index of 30 kg/m^2 or greater or 27 kg/m^2 with comorbidities. Risk of heart valve issues, surcidality. Hormonal contraceptines may be ineffective. Stop drug if loss of 5% body weight does not occur within 12 wk.
See also **topiramate.**

Frequently used combination products by trade name

Many products are available on the market in combination form. Many of these are OTC preparations. It is helpful to have a guide to the ingredients of these products when instructing patients or assessing for drug interactions. The following is a list of brand names, active ingredients, and common usages for various combination products. Nursing process information can be checked by looking up the active ingredients.

Trade name	Active ingredients	Common usage
Acanya	clindamycin, benzoyl peroxide	Anti-acne drug
Accuretic	quinapril, hydrochlorothiazide	Antihypertensive
Actifed Cold & Allergy	pseudoephedrine, triprolidine	Decongestant, antihistamine
ACTOplus Met	pioglitazone, metformin	Antidiabetic
ACTOplus Met XR	pioglitazone, metformin	Antidiabetic
Adderall	dextroamphetamine sulfate and saccharate, amphetamine aspartate and sulfate	Treatment of ADHD
Adderall XL	dextroamphetamine sulfate and saccharate, amphetamine aspartate and sulfate	Treatment of ADHD
Advair Diskus	fluticasone, salmeterol	Antiasthmatic
Advair HFA	fluticasone, salmeterol	Antiasthmatic
Advicor	niacin, lovastatin	Antihyperlipidemic
Advil Cold and Sinus	ibuprofen, pseudoephedrine	Decongestant, analgesic
Aggrenox	aspirin, dipyridamole	Stroke prevention
Aldactazide	spironolactone, hydrochlorothiazide	Diuretic
Alka-Seltzer Plus Cold & Cough	chlorpheniramine, dextromethorphan, phenylephrine	Decongestant, antihistamine, antitussive
Alka-Seltzer Plus Flu Medicine	dextromethorphan, chlorpheniramine, aspirin	Antitussive, analgesic, decongestant
Allegra-D	pseudoephedrine, fexofenadine	Decongestant, antihistamine
Allegra-D 24 hour	pseudoephedrine, fexofenadine	Decongestant, antihistamine
Allerest Maximum Strength	pseudoephedrine, chlorpheniramine	Decongestant, antihistamine

Trade name	Active ingredients	Common usage
Amturnide	aliskiren, amlodipine, hydrochlorothiazide	Antihypertensive
Anacin	aspirin, caffeine	Analgesic
Anexsia	hydrocodone, acetaminophen	Analgesic
Angeliq	drospirenone, estradiol	Menopause
Antrocol	atropine, phenobarbital	Sedative, GI anticholinergic
Apri	ethinyl estradiol, desogestrel	Hormonal contraceptive
Atacand HCT	candesartan, hydrochlorothiazide	Antihypertensive
Atripla	efavirenz, emtricitabine, tenofovir	Antiviral
Augmentin	amoxicillin, clavulanic acid	Antibiotic
Augmentin ES-600	amoxicillin, clavulanic acid	Antibiotic
Augmentin XR	amoxicillin, clavulanic acid	Antibiotic
Avalide	irbesartan, hydrochlorothiazide	Antihypertensive
Avandamet	rosiglitazone, metformin	Antidiabetic
Avandaryl	rosiglitazone, glimepiride	Antidiabetic
Aviane	estradiol, levonorgestrel	Hormonal contraceptive
Azdone	hydrocodone, aspirin	Analgesic
Azor	amlodipine, olmesartan	Antihypertensive
Bactrim	trimethoprim, sulfamethoxazole	Antibiotic
Bayer Plus Extra Strength	aspirin, calcium carbonate	Analgesic
Bayer Select Maximum Strength Backache	magnesium salicylate tetrahydrate,	Analgesic
Bayer Select Maximum Strength Night Time Pain Relief	acetaminophen, diphenhydramine	Analgesic
Benadryl Allergy & Sinus	diphenhydramine, pseudoephedrine, acetaminophen	Decongestant
Benicar HCT	olmesartan, hydrochlorothiazide	Antihypertensive
BenzaClin	clindamycin, benzoyl peroxide	Anti-acne drug
Beyaz	drosperinone, ethinyl estradiol, levomefolate	Hormonal contraceptive
BiDil	isosorbide dinitrate, hydralazine	Heart failure

(continued)

Trade name	Active ingredients	Common usage
Bromo Seltzer	acetaminophen, sodium bicarbonate, citric acid	Analgesic, antacid
Bronkaid Dual Action	theophylline, ephedrine, guaifenesin	Antiasthmatic
Bufferin	aspirin, magnesium carbonate, calcium carbonate, magnesium oxide	Analgesic, antacid
Caduet	amlodipine, atorvastatin	CAD prevention
Cafergot	ergotamine, caffeine	Antimigraine
Cheracol Plus	codeine, guaifenesin, alcohol	Antitussive, expectorant
Chlor-Trimeton Allergy-D 8-Hr	pseudoephedrine, chlorpheniramine	Antihistamine, decongestant
Chlor-Trimeton Allergy-D 12-H	pseudoephedrine, chlorpheniramine	Antihistamine, decongestant
Ciprodex	ciprofloxacin, dexamethasone	Antibiotic, corticosteroid
Claritin-D 12 Hour	loratadine, pseudoephedrine	Decongestant, antihistamine
Claritin-D 24 Hour	loratadine, pseudoephedrine	Decongestant, antihistamine
Clorpres	chlorthalidone, clonidine	Antihypertensive
Co-Gesic	hydrocodone, acetaminophen	Analgesic
CombiPatch	estrogen, norethindrone	Menopause drug
Combivent	ipratropium, albuterol	Antiasthmatic, COPD drug
Combivir	lamivudine, zidovudine	Antiviral
Complera	emtricitabine, rilpivirine, tenofovir	Antiviral
Coricidin "D" Cold, Flu & Sinus	chlorpheniramine, acetaminophen, pseudoephedrine	Antihistamine, decongestant, analgesic
Coricidin HBP Cold & Flu Tablets	chlorpheniramine, acetaminophen	Antihistamine, analgesic
Corzide	nadolol, bendroflumethiazide	Antihypertensive
Cryselle	ethinyl estradiol, norgestrel	Hormonal contraceptive
Cyclessa	desogestrel, ethinyl estradiol	Hormonal contraceptive
Cyclomydril	cyclopentolate, phenylephrine	Ophthalmic
Damason-P	hydrocodone, aspirin	Analgesic
Dermoplast	benzocaine, menthol, methylparaben	Local anesthetic

Trade name	Active ingredients	Common usage
Di Gel	magnesium hydroxide, aluminum hydroxide, magnesium carbonate, simethicone	Antacid, anti-gas
Dimetapp Cold & Cough	brompheniramine, phenylehrine, dextromethorphan	Antihistamine, decongestant
Dimetapp Cold & Allergy	phenylephrine, brompheniramine	Antihistamine, decongestant
Diovan HCT	valsartan, hydrochlorothiazide	Antihypertensive
Dristan Cold Multi-Symptom	phenylephrine, chlorpheniramine, acetaminophen	Antihistamine, decongestant
Drixoral Cold + Allergy Sinus	pseudoephedrine, dexbromphenir-amine, acetaminophen	Antihistamine, decongestant
Duetact	pioglitazone, glimepiride	Antidiabetic
Duexis	ibuprofen, famotidine	Analgesic, antiarthritis
Dulera 100/5, 200/5	mometasone, formoterol	Antiasthmatic
Duocet	hydrocodone, acetaminophen	Analgesic
Dutoprol	metoprolol, hydrochlorothiazide	Antihypertensive
Dyazide	triamterene, hydrochlorothiazide	Diuretic
Dymista	azelastine, fluticasone	antihistamine, corticosteroid
Embeda	morphine, naltrexone	Analgesic
Emoquette	desogestrel, ethinyl estradiol	Hormonal contraceptive
Empirin with Codeine	aspirin, codeine	Analgesic
Epzicom	abacavir, lamivudine	Antiviral
Esgic Plus	butalbital, acetaminophen, caffeine	Anti–tension headache
Estrostep FE	ethinyl estradiol, norethindrone	Hormonal contraceptive
Etrafon	perphenazine, amitriptyline	Antidepressant
Excedrin Extra Strength	aspirin, acetaminophen, caffeine	Analgesic
Excedrin P.M.	acetaminophen, dimenhydramine	Analgesic
Exforge	amlodipine, valsartan	Antihypertensive
Exforge HCT	amlodipine, valsartan, hydrochlorothiazide	Antihypertensive
Femcon Fe	ethinyl estradiol, norethindrone	Hormonal contraceptive
femhrt	ethinyl estradiol, norethindrone	Menopause drug

(continued)

Trade name	Active ingredients	Common usage
Fioricet	acetaminophen, butalbital, caffeine	Analgesic
Fiorinal	aspirin, butalbital, caffeine	Analgesic
Fiorinal with Codeine	aspirin, butalbital, caffeine, codeine	Analgesic
Fosamax Plus D	alendronate, cholecalciferol	Osteoporosis
Gaviscon	aluminum hydroxide, magnesium carbonate	Antacid
Gelusil	aluminum hydroxide, magnesium hydroxide, simethicone	Antacid
Glucovance	glyburide, metformin	Antidiabetic
Granulex	trypsin, Balsam Peru, castor oil	Topical enzyme
Haley's MO	mineral oil, magnesium hydroxide	Laxative
Helidac	bismuth subsalicylate, metronidazole, tetracycline	Antiulcer
Hydrogesic	hydrocodone, acetaminophen	Analgesic
Hyzaar	losartan, hydrochlorothiazide	Antihypertensive
Jalyn	dutasteride, tamsulosin	BPH drug
Janumet	sitagliptin, metformin	Antidiabetic
Janumet XR	sitagliptin, metformin	Antidiabetic
Jentadueto	linagliptin, metformin	Antidiabetic
Junel 21 Day 1/20	ethinyl estradiol, norethindrone	Hormonal contraceptive
Junel 21 Day 1.5/30	ethinyl estradiol, norethindrone	Hormonal contraceptive
Junel Fe 1/20	ethinyl estradiol, norethindrone	Hormonal contraceptive
Junel Fe 1.5/30	ethinyl estradiol, norethindrone	Hormonal contraceptive
Kariva	ethinyl estradiol, desogestrel	Hormonal contraceptive
Kombiglyze XR	saxagliptin, metformin	Antidiabetic
Kondremul Plain	mineral oil, Irish moss, glycerin, acacia	Laxative
Librax	chlordiazepoxide, clidinium	Anticholinergic, antispasmodic
Limbitrol DS 10-25	chlordiazepoxide, amitriptyline	Antidepressant
Logen	diphenoxylate, atropine	Antidiarrheal
Lomanate	diphenoxylate, atropine	Antidiarrheal

Trade name	Active ingredients	Common usage
Lomotil	diphenoxylate, atropine	Antidiarrheal
Lonox	diphenoxylate, atropine	Antidiarrheal
Lopressor HCT	metoprolol, hydrochlorothiazide	Antihypertensive
Lorcet Plus Tablets	hydrocodone, acetaminophen	Analgesic
Lortab Tablets	hydrocodone, acetaminophen	Analgesic
LoSeasonique	levonorgestrel, estradiol	Hormonal contraceptive
Lotensin HCT	hydrochlorothiazide, benazepril	Antihypertensive
Lotrel	amlodipine, benazepril	Antihypertensive
Low-Ogestrel	ethinyl estradiol, norgestrel	Hormonal contraceptive
Lufyllin GG	dyphylline, guaifenesin	Bronchodilator, expectorant
Lybrel	norgestrel, estradiol	Hormonal contraceptive
Malarone	atovaquone, proguanil	Antimalarial
Margesic H	hydrocodone, acetaminophen	Analgesic
Maxitrol	dexamethasone, neomycin, polymyxin B	Ophthalmic
Maxzide	triamterene, hydrochlorothiazide	Diuretic
Maxzide-25	hydrochlorothiazide, triamterene	Diuretic
Micardis HCT	telmisartan, hydrochlorothiazide	Antihypertensive
Microgestin Fe 1/20	ethinyl estradiol, norethindrone	Hormonal contraceptive
Microgestin Fe 1.5/30	ethinyl estradiol, norethindrone	Hormonal contraceptive
Midol Complete	acetaminophen, caffeine pyrilamine maleate	Analgesic, diuretic
Midol Teen	acetaminophen, pamabrom	Analgesic
Migergot	ergotamine, caffeine	Antimigraine
MigraTen	acetaminophen, caffeine	Antimigraine
Moduretic	amiloride, hydrochlorothiazide	Diuretic
MonoNessa	ethinyl estradiol, norgestimate	Hormonal contraceptive
Monopril-HCT	fosinopril, hydrochlorothiazide	Antihypertensive
Mucinex DM	guaifenesin, dextromethorphan	Expectorant, cough suppressant
Mycolog-II	triamcinolone, nystatin	Antifungal

(continued)

Trade name	Active ingredients	Common usage
Mylagen Gelcaps	magnesium carbonate	Antacid
Mylagen II Liquid	aluminum hydroxide, magnesium hydroxide, simethicone	Antacid
Mylanta	aluminum hydroxide, magnesium hydroxide, simethicone, sorbitol	Antacid
Mylanta Gelcaps	calcium carbonate, magnesium hydroxide	Antacid
Natazia	estradiol valerate, dienogest	Hormonal contraceptive
Necon 0.5/35	norethindrone, ethinyl estradiol	Hormonal contraceptive
Necon 1/35E	norethindrone, ethinyl estradiol	Hormonal contraceptive
Necon 1/50	mestranol, norethindrone	Hormonal contraceptive
Necon 7/7/7	ethinyl estradiol, norethindrone	Hormonal contraceptive
Necon 10/11	ethinyl estradiol, norethindrone	Hormonal contraceptive
Neosporin	polymyxin B, neomycin, bacitracin	Antibiotic
Nuedexta	dextromethorphan, quinidine	Psychiatric drug
NuvaRing	etonogestrel, ethinyl estradiol	Contraceptive ring
NyQuil Cold/Cough Relief	pseudoephedrine, chlorpheniramine, dextromethorphan	Antihistamine, decongestant, antitussive
Ogestrel	ethinyl estradiol, norgestrel	Hormonal contraceptive
Orsythia	levonorgestrel, ethinyl estradiol	Hormonal contraceptive
Ortho-Cyclen	ethinyl estradiol, norgestimate	Hormonal contraceptive
Ortho-Evra	norelgestromin, ethinyl estradiol	Contraceptive patch
Ortho-Novum 1/35	ethinyl estradiol, norethindrone	Hormonal contraceptive
Ortho-Novum 7/7/7	ethinyl estradiol, norethindrone	Hormonal contraceptive
Ortho-Prefest	estradiol, norgestimate	Menopause drug
Ortho Tri-Cyclen	norgestimate, ethinyl estradiol	Antiacne drug, hormonal contraceptive
Ortho Tri-Cyclen Lo	ethinyl estradiol, norgestimate	Hormonal contraceptive
Otocort	hydrocortisone, neomycin, polymyxin B	Antibiotic, steroid
Ovcon-50	ethinyl estradiol, norethindrone	Hormonal contraceptive
Pamprin Multi-Symptom	acetaminophen, pamabrom, pyrilamine	Analgesic

Trade name	Active ingredients	Common usage
Parcopa	levodopa, carbidopa	Antiparkinsonian
Pepcid Complete	famotidine, calcium carbonate, magnesium hydroxide	Antacid
Percocet	oxycodone, acetaminophen	Analgesic
Percodan	oxycodone, aspirin	Analgesic
Polysporin	polymyxin B, bacitracin	Antibiotic
Portia	levonorgestrel, ethinyl estradiol	Hormonal contraceptive
PrandiMet	repaglinide, metformin	Antidiabetic
Premphase	estrogen, medroxyprogesterone	Menopause drug
Prempro	conjugated estrogens, medroxyprogesterone	Menopause drug
Premsyn PMS	acetaminophen, pamabrom, pyrilamine	Analgesic
Prevpac	lansoprazole, amoxicillin, clarithromycin	Ulcer treatment
Primaxin	imipenem, cilastin	Antibiotic
Prinzide	lisinopril, hydrochlorothiazide	Antihypertensive
Qsymia	phentermine topiramate	Weight loss drug
Quasense	levonorgestrel, ethinyl estradiol	Hormonal contraceptive
Repan	acetaminophen, caffeine, butalbital	Analgesic
Rezira	hydrocodone, pseudoephedrine	Antitussive, decongestant
RID	pyrethrins, piperonyl butoxide	Pediculicide
Rifamate	isoniazid, rifampin	Antituberculotic
Riopan Plus	magaldrate, simethicone	Antacid
Robitussin Cold Multisymptom	phenylephrine, guaifenesin, alcohol, dextromethorphan	Antitussive, expectorant, decongestant
Robitussin Cold, Nighttime Multi-Symptom	acetaminophen, guaifenesin, alcohol, phenylephrine	Antitussive, expectorant, decongestant, analgesic
Robitussin Cold, Cough, and Chest Congestion DM	guaifenesin, dextromethorphan, alcohol	Antitussive, expectorant
Roxilox	oxycodone, acetaminophen	Analgesic
Roxiprin	oxycodone, aspirin	Analgesic

(continued)

Trade name	Active ingredients	Common usage
RuLox Plus	aluminum hydroxide, magnesium hydroxide	Antacid
Safyral	drospirenone, ethinyl estradiol, levomefolate	Hormonal contraceptive
Salonpas	methylsalicylate, menthol	Analgesic
Seasonale	levonorgestrel, ethinyl estradiol	Hormonal contraceptive
Seasonique	levonorgestrel, ethinyl estradiol	Hormonal contraceptive
Sedapap	acetaminophen, butalbital	Analgesic
Senokot-S	senna, docusate	Laxative
Septra DS	trimethoprim, sulfamethoxazole	Antibiotic
Simcor	simvastatin, niacin	Antihyperlipidemic
Sinemet	levodopa, carbidopa	Antiparkinsonian
Sinemet-CR	levodopa, carbidopa	Antiparkinsonian
Sine-Off Non-Drowsy	phenylephrine, acetaminophen	Decongestant, analgesic
Sinutab	pseudoephedrine, chlorphenir- amine, acetaminophen	Decongestant, analgesic, antihistamine
Sprintec	norgestimate, ethinyl estradiol	Oral contraceptive
Stagesic	hydrocodone, acetaminophen	Analgesic
Stalevo	levodopa, carbidopa, entacapone	Antiparkinsonian
Suboxone	buprenorphine, naloxone	Opioid agonist/antagonist
Sudafed Sinus 12-Hour Pressure and Pain	pseudoephedrine, naproxen	Decongestant, analgesic
Sulfatrim	trimethoprim, sulfamethoxazole	Antibiotic
Symbicort	budesonide, formoterol	Antiasthmatic
Synalgos DC	aspirin, caffeine, dihydrocodeine	Analgesic
Synercid	quinupristin, dalfopristin	Antibiotic
Tarka	trandolapril, verapamil	Antihypertensive
Tavist Allergy/Sinus Headache	clemastine, acetaminophen	Antihistamine, analgesic
Tekamlo	aliskiren, amlodipine	Antihypertensive
Tekturna HCT	aliskiren, hydrochlorothiazide	Antihypertensive
Tenoretic	atenolol, chlorthalidone	Antihypertensive

Trade name	Active ingredients	Common usage
Teveten HCT	eprosartan, hydrochlorothiazide	Antihypertensive
TheraFlu Flu & Sore Throat	phenylephrine, chlorpheniramine, acetaminophen	Antihistamine, decongestant
TMP-SMZ	trimethoprim, sulfamethoxazole	Antibiotic
Treximet	sumatriptan, naproxen	Antimigraine drug
Triad	acetaminophen, caffeine, butalbital	Analgesic
Triaminic Chest & Nasal Congestion	phenylephrine, guaifenesin	Antitussive, decongestant
Triaminic Cold & Cough	phenylephrine, dextromethorphan	Antihistamine, decongestant, antitussive
Tribenzor	olmesartan, amlodipine, hydrochlorothiazide	Antihypertensive
Tri-Legest FE	estradiol, norethindrone	Hormonal contraceptive
Trivora-28	ethinyl estradiol, levonorgestrel	Hormonal contraceptive
Trizivir	abacavir, zidovudine, lamivudine	Antiviral, AIDS drug
Truvada	emtricitabine, tenofovir	Antiviral
Twynsta	amlodipine, telmisartan	Antihypertensive
Tylenol Cold Multi-Symptom	acetaminophen, phenylephrine, dextromethorphan, guaifenesin	Antitussive, decongestant, expectorant, analgesic
Tylenol with Codeine	acetaminophen, codeine	Analgesic
Tylox	oxycodone, acetaminophen	Analgesic
Ultracet	tramadol, acetaminophen	Analgesic
Unasyn	ampicillin, sulbactam	Antibiotic
Uniretic	moexipril, hydrochlorothiazide	Antihypertensive
Valturna	aliskiren, valsartan	Antihypertensive
Vaseretic	enalapril, hydrochlorothiazide	Antihypertensive
Vicks Formula 44 Custom Care Chesty Cough Medicine	dextromethorphan, guaifenesin	Antitussive, expectorant
Vicks DayQuil Cold and Flu	dextromethorphan, phenylephrine, acetaminophen	Antitussive, decongestant
Vicks Formula 44 Custom Care Dry Cough Suppressant	dextromethorphan	Antitussive

(continued)

Trade name	Active ingredients	Common usage
Vicks NyQuil Cold & Flu Relief	dextromethorphan, doxylamine, acetaminophen	Antihistamine, antitussive, analgesic
Vicodin	hydrocodone, acetaminophen	Analgesic
Vicoprofen	hydrocodone, ibuprofen	Analgesic
Vimovo	naproxen, esomeprazole	Anti-inflammatory, acid reducer
Vytorin	ezetimibe, simvastatin	Lipid-lowering drug
Xerese	acyclovir, hydrocortisone	Antiviral
Yasmin	drospirenone, ethinyl estradiol	Hormonal contraceptive
YAZ	drospirenone, ethinyl estradiol	Menopause, PMDD
Zenchent	ethinyl estradiol, norethindrone	Hormonal contraceptive
Zestoretic	lisinopril, hydrochlorothiazide	Antihypertensive
Ziac	bisoprolol, hydrochlorothiazide	Antihypertensive
Zosyn	piperacillin, tazobactam	Antibiotic
Zovia 1/35E	ethinyl estradiol, ethynodiol di-acetate	Hormonal contraceptive
Zovia 1/50E	ethinyl estradiol, ethynodiol di-acetate	Hormonal contraceptive
Zutripro	hydrocodone, chlorpheniramine, pseudoephedrine	Antitussive antihistamine, decongestant
Zydone	hydrocodone, acetaminophen	Analgesic
Zyrtec-D	cetirizine, pseudoephedrine	Antihistamine, decongestant

Hormonal contraceptives

Usual dosage for oral contraceptives: Take one tablet PO daily for 21 days, beginning within 5 days of the first day of menstrual bleeding (day 1 of the cycle is the first day of menstrual bleeding). Inert tablets or no tablets are taken for the next 7 days. Then start a new course of 21 days. Sunday start: Take first tablet on first Sunday after menstruation begins.

Suggested measures for missed doses of oral contraceptives:

One tablet missed: Take tablet as soon as possible, or take two tablets the next day.

Two consecutive tablets missed: Take two tablets daily for the next 2 days, then resume the regular schedule.

Three consecutive tablets missed: If a Sunday starter, take 1 pill every day until Sunday; then discard pack and start new pack on that day. If a day 1 starter, discard rest of pack and start new pack that same day. Use an additional method of birth control until the start of the next menstrual period. Postcoital contraception ("morning after" pills): Safe and effective for emergency contraception. Dosing regimen starts within 72 hr of unprotected intercourse with a follow-up dose of the same number of pills 12 hr after the first dose.

Ovral: two white tablets

Nordette: four light orange tablets

Lo/Ovral: four white tablets

Triphasil: four yellow tablets

Plan B: 0.75 mg levonorgestrel; take one tablet within 72 hr of sexual intercourse, take the second tablet 12 hr later.

Plan B One-Step: 1.5 mg levonorgestrel; take one tablet within 72 hr of unprotected sexual intercourse. Available OTC for patients 17 yr and older.

Ella (ulipristal): 30 mg tablet; take within 5 days of unprotected sexual intercourse. A progesterone agonist/antagonist.

Oral contraceptives

Trade name	Combination
Monophasic	
Aviane, Lessina, Lutera, Orsythia, Sronyx	20 mcg ethinyl estradiol and 0.10 mg levonorgestrel
Altavera, Jolessa, Levora 0.15/30, Nordette, Portia	30 mcg ethinyl estradiol and 0.15 mg levonorgestrel
Apri, Desogen, Emoquette, Ortho-Cept, Reclipsen, Solia	30 mcg ethinyl estradiol and 0.15 mg desogestrel
Balziva, Femcon Fe chewable tablets, Ovcon-35, Zenchent	35 mcg ethinyl estradiol and 0.4 mg norethindrone
Beyaz	3 mg drospirenone, 20 mcg ethinyl estradiol, and 0.45 mg levomefolate; must monitor potassium levels.
Brevicon, Modicon, Necon 0.5/35, Zenchent	35 mcg ethinyl estradiol and 0.5 mg norethindrone

(continued)

Trade name	Combination
Monophasic (continued)	
Cryselle, Lo/Ovral, Low-Ogestrel	30 mcg ethinyl estradiol and 0.3 mg norgestrel
Gianvi, Loryna, Yaz	30 mg drospirenone, 20 mcg ethinyl estradiol
Kelnor 1/35, Zovia 1/35E	35 mcg ethinyl estradiol and 1 mg ethynodiol diacetate
Junel Fe 1/20, Junel 21 Day 1/20, Loestrin 21 1/20, Loestrin Fe 21 1/20, Loestrin 24 Fe, Microgestin Fe 1/20	20 mcg ethinyl estradiol and 1 mg norethindrone
Junel Fe 1.5/30, Junel 21 Day 1.5/30, Loestrin 21 1.5/30, Loestrin Fe 1.5/30, Microgestin Fe 1.5/30	30 mcg ethinyl estradiol and 1.5 mg norethindrone acetate
Lybrel	0.09 mg levonorgestrel and 20 mcg ethinyl estradiol in continual use to eliminate menstrual periods
MonoNessa, Ortho-Cyclen, Previfem, Sprintec	35 mcg ethinyl estradiol and 0.25 mg norgestimate
Necon 1/35, Norinyl 1+35, Ortho-Novum 1/35	35 mcg ethinyl estradiol and 1 mg norethindrone
Necon 1/50, Norinyl 1+50	50 mcg mestranol and 1 mg norethindrone
Ocella, Syeda, Yasmin, Zaran	3 mg drospirenone and 30 mcg ethinyl estradiol; must monitor potassium levels. Increased risk of thrombotic event.
Ogestrel, Ovral-28	50 mcg ethinyl estradiol and 0.5 mg norgestrel
Ovcon-50	50 mcg ethinyl estradiol and 1 mg norethindrone acetate
Quasense, Seasonale, Seasonique	0.15 levonorgestrel and 30 mcg ethinyl estradiol taken as 84 days active tablets, 7 days inactive
Safyral	3 mg drospirenone, 30 mcg ethinyl estradiol, 45 mcg levomefolate. Increased risk of thrombotic event.
Zovia 1/50E	50 mcg ethinyl estradiol and 1 mg ethynodiol diacetate
Biphasic	
Azurette, Kariva, Mircette	phase 1—21 tablets, 0.15 mg desogestrel, 20 mcg ethinyl estradiol phase 2—5 tablets: 10 mcg ethinyl estradiol
Lo Loestrin Fe	phase 1—24 tablets, 1 mg norethindrone, 10 mcg ethinyl estradiol phase 2—2 tablets, 10 mcg ethinyl estradiol

Trade name	Combination
Biphasic (continued)	
LoSeasonique	phase 1—84 tablets, 0.15 mg levonorgestrel, 20 mcg ethinyl estradiol
	phase 2—7 tablets, 10 mcg ethinyl estradiol
Seasonique	phase 1—84 tablets, 0.15 mg levonorgestrel, 30 mcg ethinyl estradiol
	phase 2—7 tablets, 10 mcg ethinyl estradiol
Necon 10/11	phase 1—10 tablets, 0.5 mg norethindrone and 35 mcg ethinyl estradiol;
	phase 2—11 tablets, 1 mg norethindrone and 35 mcg ethinyl estradiol
Triphasic	
Aranelle, Leena, Tri-Norinyl	phase 1—7 tablets, 0.5 mg norethindrone (progestin) and 35 mcg ethinyl estradiol (estrogen)
	phase 2—9 tablets, 1 mg norethindrone (progestin) and 35 mcg ethinyl estradiol (estrogen)
	phase 3—5 tablets, 0.5 mg norethindrone (progestin) and 35 mcg ethinyl estradiol (estrogen)
Caziant, Cesia, Cyclessa, Velivet	phase 1—7 tablets, 0.1 mg desogestrel and 25 mcg ethinyl estradiol
	phase 2—7 tablets, 0.125 mg desogestrel and 25 mcg ethinyl estradiol
	phase 3—7 tablets, 0.15 mg desogestrel and 25 mcg ethinyl estradiol
Enpresse, Triphasil	phase 1—6 tablets, 0.05 mg levonorgestrel (progestin) and 30 mcg ethinyl estradiol (estrogen)
	phase 2—5 tablets, 0.075 mg levonorgestrel (progestin) and 40 mcg ethinyl estradiol (estrogen)
	phase 3—10 tablets, 0.125 mg levonorgestrel (progestin) and 30 mcg ethinyl estradiol (estrogen)
Estrostep Fe, Tilia Fe, Tri-Legest Fe	phase 1—5 tablets, 1 mg norethindrone and 20 mcg ethinyl estradiol; with 75 mg ferrous fumarate
	phase 2—7 tablets, 1 mg norethindrone and 30 mcg ethinyl estradiol; with 75 mg ferrous fumarate
	phase 3—9 tablets, 1 mg norethindrone and 35 mcg ethinyl estradiol with 75 mg ferrous fumarate

(continued)

Trade name	Combination
Triphasic (continued)	
Ortho-Novum 7/7/7, Necon 7/7/7	phase 1—7 tablets, 0.5 mg norethindrone (progestin) and 35 mcg ethinyl estradiol (estrogen)
	phase 2—7 tablets, 0.75 mg norethindrone (progestin) and 35 mcg ethinyl estradiol (estrogen)
	phase 3—7 tablets, 1 mg norethindrone (progestin) and 35 mcg ethinyl estradiol (estrogen)
Ortho Tri-Cyclen, TriNessa, Tri-Previfem, Tri-Sprintec	phase 1—7 tablets, 0.18 mg norgestimate and 35 mcg ethinyl estradiol
	phase 2—7 tablets, 0.215 mg norgestimate and 35 mcg ethinyl estradiol
	phase 3—7 tablets, 0.25 mg norgestimate and 35 mcg ethinyl estradiol
Ortho Tri-Cyclen Lo	phase 1—7 tablets, 0.18 mg norgestimate and 25 mcg ethinyl estradiol
	phase 2—7 tablets, 0.215 mg norgestimate and 25 mcg ethinyl estradiol
	phase 3—7 tablets, 0.25 mg norgestimate and 25 mcg ethinyl estradiol
Tri-Legest	phase 1—5 tablets, 1 mg norethindrone, 20 mcg ethinyl estradiol
	phase 2—7 tablets, 1 mg norethindrone, 30 mcg ethinyl estradiol
	phase 3—9 tablets, 1 mg norethindrone, 35 mcg ethinyl estradiol
Trivora-28	phase 1—6 tablets, 0.5 mg levonorgestrel (progestin) and 30 mcg ethinyl estradiol (estrogen)
	phase 2—5 tablets, 0.075 mg levonorgestrel (progestin) and 40 mcg ethinyl estradiol (estrogen)
	phase 3—10 tablets, 0.125 mg levonorgestrel (progestin) and 30 mcg ethinyl estradiol (estrogen)
4-Phasic	
Natazia	phase 1—2 tablets, 3 mg estradiol valerate
	phase 2—5 tablets, 2 mg estradiol valerate and 2 mg dienogest
	phase 3—17 tablets, 2 mg estradiol valerate and 3 mg dienogest
	phase 4—2 tablets, 1 mg estradiol valerate

(continued)

Trade name	Combination
Progestin only	
Camila, Errin, Heather, Jolivette, Nora-BE, Ortho Micronor	0.35 mg norethindrone

Implantable system

Trade name	Combination
Implanon, Nexplanon	68 mg etonogestrel implanted subdermally in inner aspect of nondominant upper arm. Left in place for no longer than 3 yr and then must be removed. New implants may then be inserted.

Injectable contraceptives

Trade name	Combination
Depo-Provera	150, 400 mg/mL medroxyprogesterone Give 1-mL injection deep IM, repeated every 3 mo.
Depo-subQ Provera 104	104 mg medroxyprogesterone. Give 0.65 mL subcutaneously into the anterior thigh or abdomen.

Intrauterine systems

Trade name	Combination
Mirena	52 mg levonorgestrel inserted into the uterus for up to 5 yr. (Also approved to treat heavy menstrual bleeding in women using an intrauterine system for contraception.) Releases 20 mcg/day.

Transdermal system

Trade name	Combination
Ortho Evra	6 mg norelgestromin, 0.75 ethinyl estradiol in a patch form, which releases 150 mcg norelgestromin and 20 mcg ethinyl estradiol each 24 hr for 1 wk. Patch is applied on the same day of the wk for 3 consecutive wk, followed by a patch-free week. ⊗ ***Black box warning*** Higher risk of thromboembolic events and death if combined with smoking.

Vaginal ring

Trade name	Combination
NuvaRing	0.12 mg etonogestrel (progestin), 0.015 mg ethinyl estradiol (estrogen) per day; insert ring into vagina on or before the 5th day of menstrual period; remove after 3 wk. Insert new ring after 1-wk rest.

Commonly used biologics

▷ **diphtheria and tetanus toxoids, combined, adsorbed (DT, Td) (available in adult and pediatric preparations)**

Therapeutic actions
Contains reduced dose of inactivated diphtheria toxin and full dose of inactivated tetanus toxin to provide adequate immunization in adults without the severe sensitivity reactions caused when full pediatric doses of diphtheria toxoid are given to adults.

Indications
- Active immunization of adults and children 7 yr and older against diphtheria and tetanus. *Trivalent DTP* is preferred for use in most children; DT can be used for children 6 wk and older when pertussis vaccine is contraindicated.

Adverse effects
Fretfulness; drowsiness; anorexia; vomiting; transient fever; malaise; generalized aches and pains; edema of injection area with redness, swelling, induration, pain (may persist for a few days); hypersensitivity reactions.

Dosage
Two primary IM doses of 0.5 mL each given at 4- to 8-wk intervals, followed by a third 0.5-mL IM dose given in 6–12 mo. Routine booster of 0.5 mL IM every 10 yr for maintenance of immunity.

Nursing considerations
- Use caution in pregnant women. **Pregnancy Category C**—safety not established.
- Defer administration of routine immunizing or booster doses in case of acute infection.
- Arrange to interrupt immunosuppressive therapy if emergency booster doses of *Td* are required after injury.
- Not for treatment of acute tetanus or diphtheria infections.
- Administer by IM injection only; avoid subcutaneous or IV injection. Deltoid muscle is the preferred site. Do not administer into the same site more than once.
⊗ *Warning* Arrange for epinephrine 1:1,000 to be immediately available at time of injection in case of hypersensitivity reactions.
- Provide comfort measures to help patient cope with discomforts of injection: analgesics, warm soaks for injection site, small meals, environmental control—temperature, stimuli.
- Provide patient with written record of immunization and reminder of when booster injection is needed.

▷ **diphtheria and tetanus toxoids and acellular pertussis vaccine, adsorbed (DTaP, Tdap)**

Adacel, Boostrix, Daptacel, Infanrix, Tripedia

Therapeutic actions
Provides detoxified diphtheria and tetanus toxins and acellular pertussis vaccine to stimulate an immunologic response in children leading to an active immunity against these diseases.

Indications

- Primary immunization of children 6 wk and older–7 yr. Induction of immunity against diphtheria, tetanus, and pertussis. Immunization of adults against pertussis.

Adverse effects

Hypersensitivity reactions; erythema, induration, redness, pain, swelling of the injection area; nodule at the injection site, which may persist for several weeks; temperature elevations, malaise, chills, irritability, fretfulness, drowsiness, anorexia, vomiting, persistent crying; rarely—fatal reactions.

Dosage

- As primary immunization: 3 IM doses of 0.5 mL at 4- to 8-wk intervals. Start doses by 6–8 wk of age; finish by 7th birthday. Use the same vaccine for all three doses.
- Fourth dose: 0.5 mL IM at 15–20 mo, at least 6 mo after previous dose.
- Fifth dose: 0.5 mL IM at 4–6 yr or preferably before entry into school (*Infanrix, Tripedia, Daptacel*). If fourth dose was given after the 4-yr birthday, the preschool dose may be omitted.
- Booster injections: 10 yr and older (*Boostrix*) 0.5 mL IM; 11–64 yr (*Adacel*) 0.5 mL IM. Allow at least 5 yr between last of the series and booster dose.

Nursing considerations

- Do not use for treatment of acute tetanus, diphtheria, or whooping cough infections.
- Do not administer primary series to any person 7 yr or older.
- Do not attempt routine immunization with DTaP if the child has a personal history of CNS disease or convulsions.
- Do not administer DTaP after recent blood transfusions or receipt of immune globulin, in immunodeficiency disorders or with immunosuppressive therapy, or to patients with malignancy.
- Question the parent concerning occurrence of any signs or symptoms of adverse reactions after the previous dose before administering a repeat dose of the vaccine. If temperature higher than 39°C (103°F), convulsions with or without fever, alterations of consciousness, focal neurologic signs, screaming episodes, shock, collapse, somnolence, or encephalopathy has occurred, DTP is contraindicated and diphtheria and tetanus toxoids without pertussis should be used for immunization.
- Administer by IM injection only. Avoid subcutaneous or IV injection. Midlateral muscle of the thigh is the preferred site for infants; deltoid muscle is the preferred site for older children. Do not administer at same site more than once.
- ⊗ *Warning* Arrange for epinephrine 1:1,000 to be immediately available at time of injection in case of hypersensitivity reactions.
- DTaP products are not generically equivalent and are not interchangeable. Use vaccines from the same manufacturer for at least the first three doses.
- Provide comfort measures and teach parents to provide comfort measures to help the patient cope with the discomforts of the injection: analgesics, warm soaks for injection site, small meals, environmental control—temperature, stimuli.
- Provide parent with written record of immunization and reminder of when booster injection is needed.

▷ diphtheria and tetanus toxoids and acellular pertussis adsorbed, hepatitis B (recombinant), and inactivated poliovirus vaccine combined (DTaP-HePB-IPV)

Pediarix

Therapeutic actions

Contains diphtheria and tetanus toxoids, acellular pertussis vaccine, recombinant antigenic hepatitis B vaccine and inactivated poliovirus vaccine in one injection to stimulate active immunity against these diseases in children who have received all doses of the vaccine.

Indications

- Active immunization against diphtheria, tetanus, pertussis, hepatitis B virus, and poliomyelitis caused by poliovirus Types 1, 2, and 3 as a three-dose primary series in infants born to HBsAg-negative mothers.

Adverse effects

Hypersensitivity reactions: erythema, induration, redness, pain, swelling of the injection area; nodule at the injection site, which may persist for several weeks; temperature elevations, malaise, chills, irritability, fretfulness, drowsiness, anorexia, vomiting, persistent crying; rarely—fatal reactions.

Dosage

- Infants with hepatitis B surface antigen (HBsAG)–negative mothers, three 0.5-mL doses IM given at 6- to 8- (preferably 8-) wk intervals beginning at 2 mo.
- Children previously vaccinated with one dose of hepatitis B vaccine should receive the three-dose series.
- Children previously vaccinated with one or more doses of *Infanrix* or *IPV: Pediarix* may be used to complete the series.

Nursing considerations

- Administer only to children of HbsAg-negative mothers.
- Do not administer to children with immunodeficiency, immunosuppression, or malignancy.
- Do not administer to any person younger than 6 wk or older than 7 yr.
- Do not administer if patient is febrile.
- Administer by IM injection only; avoid subcutaneous or IV injection. Midlateral muscle of the thigh is the preferred site for infants; deltoid muscle is the preferred site for older children.
- Shake the vial vigorously to suspend the drug; do not use if particles are apparent; do not reenter the vial; discard any unused portion.
- Do not administer into the same site more than once.
- ⊗ *Warning* Arrange for epinephrine 1:1,000 to be immediately available at time of injection because of risk of hypersensitivity reactions.
- Provide comfort measures and teach parents to provide comfort measures to help the patient cope with the discomforts of the injection: analgesics, warm soaks for the injection site, small meals, environmental control—temperature, stimuli.
- Provide parents with written record of immunization and reminder of when booster injections are needed.
- Do not use this drug as a booster injection after the completion of the three-shot series; use appropriate single vaccines for boosters.

> ▷ **diphtheria and tetanus toxoids and acellular pertussis adsorbed and inactivated poliovirus vaccine (DTaP-IIPV)**
>
> Kinrix

Therapeutic actions

Contains diphtheria and tetanus toxoids, acellular pertussis, and inactivated poliovirus in one injection to stimulate active immunity against these diseases in children.

Indications

- Active immunization against diphtheria, tetanus, pertussis, and poliomyelitis as the fifth dose in the diphtheria, tetanus, acellular pertussis series and the fourth dose in the inactivated poliovirus series in children 4–6 yr whose previous immunizations have been with *Infanrix* or *Pediarix* for the first three doses and *Infanrix* for the fourth dose.

Adverse effects

Hypersensitivity reactions; local reactions at injection site, including warmth, redness, swelling, pain; headache; nausea; myalgia; fever; URI symptoms.

Dosage

One IM injection of 0.5 mL.

Nursing considerations

- Drug is contraindicated with severe allergic reaction to any other vaccine, encephalopathy, and progressive neurologic diseases.
- Ensure that patient has received other immunizations in the series before administration.
- Use cautiously in patients with latex allergy.
- Children at high risk for seizures should receive an antipyretic at time of administration.
- Do not administer if patient is febrile or shows signs of active infection.
- Do not mix in syringe with other vaccines; administer at different sites than other vaccines.
- Provide comfort measures and teach parents to provide comfort measures (analgesics, antipyretics, warm packs to injection site, small meals, environmental control of temperature and stimuli) to help patient cope with effects of the injection.
- Provide parents with a written record of the immunization.

▷**diphtheria and tetanus toxoids and acellular pertussis adsorbed, inactivated poliovirus vaccine, and *Haemophilus* b conjugate (tetanus toxoid conjugate) vaccine (DTaP-IPV/Hib)**

Pentacel

Therapeutic actions

Contains diphtheria and tetanus toxoids, acellular pertussis, inactivated poliovirus and *Haemophilus* b conjugate vaccine in one injection to stimulate active immunity against these diseases in children.

Indications

- Primary active immunization of children between 6 wk and 4 yr against diphtheria, tetanus, pertussis, poliomyelitis, and *H. influenza* b.

Adverse effects

Hypersensitivity reactions; local reactions at injection site, including warmth, redness, swelling, pain; headache; nausea; myalgia; fever; URI symptoms.

Dosage

Four-dose series of IM injections of 0.5 mL given at 2, 4, and 6 mo and at 15–18 mo.

Nursing considerations

- Contraindicated with severe allergic reaction to any other vaccine, encephalopathy, progressive neurologic diseases.
- Children at high risk for seizures should receive an antipyretic at time of administration.
- Do not administer if patient is febrile or shows signs of active infection.
- Do not mix in syringe with other vaccines; administer at different sites than other vaccines.

- Provide comfort measures and teach parents to provide comfort measures (analgesics, antipyretics, warm packs to injection site, small meals, environmental control of temperature and stimuli) to help patient cope with effects of the injection.
- Provide parents with a written record of the immunization and a date to return for the second dose in the series.

▽ *Haemophilus* b conjugate vaccine

ActHIB, Hiberix, Liquid PedvaxHIB

Therapeutic actions

Provides antigenic combination of *Haemophilus* b conjugate vaccine to stimulate an immunologic response in children, leading to an active immunity against these diseases.

Indications

- Active immunization of infants and children against *H. influenzae* b for primary immunization and routine recall; 2–71 mo (*PedvaxHIB*), 2–18 mo (*ActHIB* with DPT), or 15–18 mo (*ActHIB, Hiberix* with *Tripedia*).

Adverse effects

Hypersensitivity reactions; erythema, induration, redness, pain, swelling of the injection area; nodule at the injection site, which may persist for several weeks; temperature elevations, malaise, chills, irritability, fretfulness, drowsiness, anorexia, vomiting, persistent crying; rarely—fatal reactions.

Dosage

ActHIB: Reconstitute with DTP, *Tripedia*, or saline.
- *2–6 mo:* 3 IM injections of 0.5 mL at 2, 4, and 6 mo; 0.5 mL at 15–18 mo and DPT alone at 4–6 yr.
- *7–11 mo:* 2 IM injections of 0.5 mL at 8-wk intervals; booster dose at 15–18 mo.
- *12–14 mo:* 0.5 mL IM with a booster 2 mo later.
- *15–18 mo:* 0.5 mL IM, booster of *Tripedia* at 4–6 yr.

Hiberix
- *15 mo–4 yr:* Booster dose: 0.5 mL IM as a single dose.

PedvaxHIB
- *2–14 mo:* 2 IM injections of 0.5 mL at 2 mo of age and 2 mo later; 0.5-mL booster at 12 mo (if 2 doses complete before 12 mo, not less than 2 mo after last dose).
- *15–71 mo:* 0.5 mL IM, single injection.

Nursing considerations

- Do not administer to children with immunodeficiency, immunosuppression, or malignancy.
- Do not administer to adults.
- Do not administer in the presence of febrile illness.
- Administer by IM injection only. Avoid subcutaneous or IV injection. Midlateral muscle of the thigh is the preferred site for infants; deltoid muscle is the preferred site for older children. Do not administer at same site more than once.
- ⊗ *Warning* Arrange for epinephrine 1:1,000 to be immediately available at time of injection in case of hypersensitivity reaction.
- Provide comfort measures and teach parents to provide comfort measures to help patient cope with the discomforts of the injection: analgesics, warm soaks for injection site, small meals, environmental control—temperature, stimuli.
- Provide parents with written record of immunization and reminder of when booster injection is needed.
- Conjugate vaccines can be given simultaneously with other routine vaccines using separate sites and syringes.

▷ *Haemophilus* b conjugate vaccine with hepatitis B surface antigen (recombinant)

Comvax

Therapeutic actions

Provides antigenic hepatitis B vaccine to stimulate an immunologic response in children, leading to an active immunity against the disease.

Indications

• Active immunization against *Haemophilus* and hepatitis B in infants 6 wk to 15 mo born to HBsAg–negative mothers.

Adverse effects

Hypersensitivity reactions: erythema, induration, redness, pain, swelling of the injection area; nodule at the injection site, which may persist for several weeks; temperature elevations, malaise, chills, irritability, fretfulness, drowsiness, anorexia, vomiting, persistent crying; rarely—fatal reactions.

Dosage

• Infants with hepatitis B surface antigen (HBsAg)–negative mothers: Three 0.5-mL IM doses at 2, 4, and 12–15 mo.
• Children previously vaccinated with one or more doses of hepatitis B vaccine or *Haemophilus* b vaccine: 0.5-mL IM doses at 2, 4, and 12–15 mo.

Nursing considerations

• Administer only to children of HBsAg-negative mothers.
• Do not administer to children with immunodeficiency, immunosuppression, or malignancy.
• Do not administer to adults.
• Do not administer if patient has febrile illness.
• Administer by IM injection only. Avoid subcutaneous or IV injection. Midlateral muscle of the thigh is the preferred site for infants; deltoid muscle is the preferred site for older children.
• Do not administer into same site more than once.
⊗ *Warning* Arrange for epinephrine 1:1,000 to be immediately available at time of injection because of risk of hypersensitivity reactions.
• Provide comfort measures and teach parents to provide comfort measures to help patient cope with the discomforts of the injection: analgesics, warm soaks for injection site, small meals, environmental control—temperature, stimuli.
• Provide parents with written record of immunization and reminder of when booster injection is needed.
• Conjugate vaccines can be given simultaneously with other routine vaccines, using separate sites and syringes.

▷ hepatitis A vaccine, inactivated

Havrix, Vaqta

Therapeutic actions

Contains hepatitis A antigen that stimulates production of specific antibodies against hepatitis A virus (HAV), which protects against HAV infection. The immunity does not protect against hepatitis caused by other agents.

Indications

• Active immunization of adults and children 12 mo and older against disease caused by HAV in situations that warrant immunization (eg, travel, institutionalization); used with immune globulin for immediate and long-term protection against hepatitis. Administer at least 2 wk before expected exposure.

Adverse effects

Transient fever; edema of injection area with redness, swelling, induration, pain (may persist for a few days); upper respiratory illness, headache, rash.

Dosage

- Adults: *Havrix*—1 mL; same dose booster in 6–12 mo. *Vaqta*—1 mL IM; same dose booster in 6–18 mo.
- Pediatric patients 12 mo–18 yr: 0.5 mL IM with a repeat dose in 6–18 mo (*Vaqta*); IM; repeat dose in 6–12 mo (*Havrix)*.

Nursing considerations

- Use caution in pregnancy. **Pregnancy Category C**—safety not established.
- Defer administration in case of acute infection.
- Administer by IM injection only. Deltoid muscle is the preferred site; do not give in the gluteal site.
- ⊗ *Warning* Arrange for epinephrine 1:1,000 to be immediately available at time of injection in case of hypersensitivity reaction.
- Provide comfort measures to help patient cope with the discomforts of the injection (analgesics, warm soaks for injection site, small meals, environmental control of temperature and stimuli).
- Provide patient with written record of immunization and timing for booster immunization.

▷ hepatitis A inactivated and hepatitis B recombinant vaccine

Twinrix

Therapeutic actions

Provides inactivated hepatitis A antigens that stimulate production of specific antibodies against hepatitis A virus (HAV), which protect against hepatitis A, and inactivated human hepatitis B surface antigen particles, which stimulate active immunity and production of antibodies against hepatitis B surface antigens.

Indications

- Active immunization against disease caused by HAV and hepatitis B virus in persons 18 yr and older who want protection against or are at high risk of exposure to the viruses.

Adverse effects

Soreness, swelling, erythema, warmth, induration at injection site; malaise, fatigue, headache, nausea, vomiting, dizziness; myalgia, arthralgia, rash, low-grade fever; pharyngitis, rhinitis, cough; lymphadenopathy; hypotension; dysuria.

Dosage

- Three doses (1 mL by IM injection) given on a 0-, 1-, and 6-month schedule.
- Accelerated dosage: Four doses (1 mL by IM injection) on days 0, 7, 21, and 30, followed by booster dose at 12 mo.
- Safety for use in patients younger than 18 yr not established.

Nursing considerations

- Do not administer to any patient with a known hypersensitivity to hepatitis A vaccine or hepatitis B vaccine or any components used in the solution.

- Use cautiously with bleeding disorders, immunosuppression, pregnancy, and lactation. **Pregnancy Category C**—safety not established.
- Postpone injection in the presence of moderate to severe illness.
- Administer IM, preferably in the deltoid region. Do not administer in the gluteal region.
- Shake vial or syringe well before withdrawal; observe for any particulate matter or discoloration. Should appear as a white, homogenous, turbid suspension; discard if it appears otherwise.
- Administer drug as provided; do not dilute.
- Provide comfort measures—analgesics, antipyretics, care of injection site—to help patient cope with the effects of the injection.
- Provide patient with a written record of the immunization and the dates that repeat vaccinations and antibody tests are needed.

▷ hepatitis B immune globulin (HBIG)

HepaGam B, HyperHEP B S/D, Nabi-HB

Therapeutic actions

Globulin contains a high titer of antibody to hepatitis B surface antigen (HBsAg), providing a passive immunity to HBsAg.

Indications

- Postexposure prophylaxis following parenteral exposure (accidental "needle-stick"), direct mucous membrane contact (accidental splash), or oral ingestion (pipetting accident) involving HBsAg-positive materials such as blood, plasma, serum, or sexual exposure to an HbsAg-positive person.
- Prophylaxis in infants born to HBsAg-positive mothers.
- Adjunct to hepatitis B vaccine when rapid achievement of protective levels of antibodies is desirable.
- Prevention of hepatitis B recurrence after liver transplant in HBsAg-positive transplant recipients *(HepaGam B)*.

Adverse effects

Hypersensitivity reactions; tenderness, muscle stiffness at the injection site; urticaria, angioedema; fever, chills, nausea, vomiting, chest tightness.

Dosage

- Perinatal exposure: 0.5 mL IM within 12 hr of birth; repeat dose at 1 mo and 6 mo after initial dose.
- Percutaneous exposure: 0.06 mL/kg IM immediately (within 7 days) and repeat 28–30 days after exposure. Usual adult dose is 3–5 mL.
- Individuals at high risk of infection: 0.06 mL/kg IM at same time (but at a different site) as hepatitis B vaccine is given.
- *HepaGam B* after liver transplant: 20,000 international units IV at 2 mL/min. Give first dose with liver transplant and then daily on days 1–7, every 2 wk from day 14 through 12 wk, and monthly from month 4 onward.
- Sexual exposure: A single dose of 0.06 mL/kg IM within 14 days of last sexual contact.

Nursing considerations

- Do not administer to patients with history of allergic response to gamma globulin or with anti–immunoglobulin A antibodies.
- Use caution in pregnant women. **Pregnancy Category C**—safety not established. Use only if benefits outweigh potential unknown risks to the fetus.
- HBIG may be administered at the same time or up to 1 mo preceding hepatitis B vaccination without impairing the active immune response from the vaccination.

- Administer IM in the deltoid region or anterolateral aspect of upper thigh. May give IV liver transplantation.
- Administer the appropriate dose as soon after exposure as possible (within 7 days is preferable); repeat 28–30 days after exposure.

⊗ **Warning** Have epinephrine 1:1,000 immediately available at time of injection in case of anaphylactic reaction.

- Provide comfort measures to help patient deal with discomfort of drug therapy—analgesics, antipyretics, environmental control.

▽ hepatitis B vaccine

Engerix-B, Recombivax HB

Therapeutic actions

Provides inactivated human hepatitis B surface antigen particles to stimulate active immunity and production of antibodies against hepatitis B surface antigens using surface antigen produced by yeast.

Indications

- Immunization against infection caused by all known subtypes of hepatitis B virus, especially those at high risk for infection—health care personnel, military personnel identified to be at risk, prisoners, users of illicit drugs, populations with high incidence (Eskimos, Indochinese refugees, Haitian refugees), morticians and embalmers, persons at increased risk because of their sexual practices (repeated STDs, homosexually active males, prostitutes), patients in hemodialysis units, patients requiring frequent blood transfusions, residents of mental institutions, household contacts of people with persistent hepatitis B antigenemia.
- All infants, adolescents 11–12 yr, and older unvaccinated adolescents at high risk.

Adverse effects

Soreness, swelling, erythema, warmth, induration at injection site; malaise, fatigue, headache, nausea, vomiting, dizziness; myalgia, arthralgia, rash; low-grade fever, pharyngitis, rhinitis, cough; lymphadenopathy; hypotension; dysuria.

Dosage

- *Birth–10 yr:* Initial dose—0.5 mL IM, followed by 0.5 mL IM at 1 mo and 6 mo after initial dose.
- *11–19 yr:* 1 mL IM, followed by 1 mL IM at 1 mo and 6 mo after initial dose.
- *Adults:* Initial dose—1 mL IM, followed by 1 mL IM at 1 mo and 6 mo after initial dose, all types.
- *Dialysis or predialysis patients:* Initial dose—40 mcg (2 mL) IM; repeat dose at 1 mo, 2 mo, and 6 mo after initial dose (*Engerix-B*). Or, 40 mcg (1 mL) IM; repeat dose at 1 mo and 6 mo (*Recombivax HB*).
- Revaccination (a booster dose should be considered with anti-HBs levels less than 10 milliinternational units/mL 1–2 mo after third dose). *Children younger than 10 yr:* 10 mcg. *Adults and patients older than 10 yr:* 20 mcg. *Hemodialysis patients (when antibody testing indicates need):* two 20-mcg doses.

Nursing considerations

- Do not administer to any patient with known hypersensitivity to any component of the vaccine or allergy to yeast.
- Use caution in pregnant or nursing women. **Pregnancy Category C**—safety not established. Use only if clearly needed and benefits outweigh potential unknown effects.

- Use caution in any patient with active infection. Delay use of vaccine if possible. Use with caution in any patient with compromised cardiopulmonary status or patients in whom a febrile or systemic reaction could present a significant risk.
- Administer IM, preferably in the deltoid muscle in adults or the anterolateral thigh muscle in infants and small children. Do not administer IV or intradermally; subcutaneous route may be used in patients who are at high risk for hemorrhage following IM injection, but increased incidence of local effects has been noted.
- Shake vaccine container well before withdrawing solution; no dilution is needed. Use vaccine as supplied. Vaccine appears as a slightly opaque, white suspension. Refrigerate vials; do not freeze.

⊗ **Warning** Have epinephrine 1:1,000 immediately available at time of injection in case of severe anaphylactic reaction.

- Provide comfort measures—analgesics, antipyretics, care of injection site—to help patient cope with effects of the drug.
- Provide patient or parent with a written record of the immunization and dates that repeat injections and antibody tests are needed.

▷ human papillomavirus recombinant vaccine, bivalent types 16 and 18

Cervarix

Therapeutic actions

Human papillomavirus capsid proteins that generate the formation of immunoglobulin G–neutralizing antibodies directed against those strains of human papillomavirus.

Indications

- Prevention of diseases caused by oncogenic human papillomavirus types 16 and 18 in young girls and women ages 10–25 yr, including cervical cancer, cervical intraepithelial neoplasia grade 2 or worse, adenocarcinoma in situ, and cervical intraepithelial neoplasia grade 1.

Adverse effects

Injection site reactions (pain, redness, swelling), fatigue, headache, myalgia, GI symptoms, arthralgia, syncope.

Dosage

Three doses of 0.5 mL IM given at 0, 1, and 6 months.

Nursing considerations

- Do not administer to anyone with immunodeficiency/suppression or malignancy.
- Do not administer with antiviral medications or other immunizations or immune suppressants.
- Do not administer if patient has febrile illness or active infection.
- Do not administer to patient with known allergy to components of drug or to latex.
- Do not administer to women who are pregnant unless the benefit clearly outweighs the risk.

⊗ **Warning** Have epinephrine 1:1000 immediately available at time of injection in case of anaphylactic reaction.

- Observe patient for 15 minutes following vaccine administration; syncope is common and may occur with any dose of the series.
- Provide comfort measures (analgesics, rest, decongestants) to help patient cope with discomforts of immunization.
- Ensure that patient understands the importance of regular cervical cancer screening throughout life.
- Provide patient with written record of immunization; give patient a reminder for return dates to complete the series.

▷ human papillomavirus recombinant vaccine, quadrivalent

Gardasil

Therapeutic actions

Noninfectious, recombinant virus particles that stimulate antibody production to human papillomavirus types 6, 11, 16, and 18; providing humoral immunity to virus that cause such diseases as cervical cancer, genital warts, cervical adenocarcinoma in situ, cervical intraepithelial neoplasia, vulvar intraepithelial neoplasia, vaginal intraepithelial neoplasia, cervical intraepithelial neoplasia, anal intraepithelial neoplasia.

Indications

- Prevention of diseases caused by human papillomavirus types 6, 11, 16, and 18 in young girls and women ages 9–26 yr, including cervical cancer, precancerous genital lesions, genital warts, vaginal and vulvar cancer, and anal cancer.
- Prevention of genital warts caused by human papillomavirus types 6 and 11 in men and boys 9–26 yr.
- Prevention of anal cancer and precancerous lesions caused by human papillomavirus types 6, 11 in men and boys 9–26 yr.

Adverse effects

Injection site reactions (redness, warmth, swelling, bruising, pain), dizziness, diarrhea, nasal congestion, myalgia, arthralgia, fever, fainting, anaphylaxis (rare).

Dosage

- Three separate IM injections of 0.5 mL each, second dose 2 mo after the initial dose and last dose 6 mo after the first dose; for males and females 9–26 yr.

Nursing considerations

- Do not administer to anyone with immunodeficiency/suppression or malignancy.
- Do not administer with any antiviral drugs or with other immunizations or immune suppressants.
- Do not administer if patient has febrile illness or active infection.
- Do not administer to patient allergic to any component of the drug or with history of allergic reactions to yeast; do not repeat injections in patients who experience hypersensitivity reactions.
- Do not administer to women who are pregnant. **Pregnancy Category B.**
- Shake well before administering.
- Administer by IM injection in the deltoid or upper thigh. Do not use if drug is discolored or contains particulate matter.
- ⊗ **Warning** Have epinephrine 1:1,000 immediately available at time of injection in case of anaphylactic reaction.
- Have patient remain seated or lying down for 15 min after vaccination for safety; fainting, twitching, and seizurelike activity have occurred.
- Provide comfort measures (analgesics, rest, decongestants) to help the patient cope with discomforts of immunization.
- Ensure that patients understand the importance of regular cervical cancer screening throughout life.
- Provide patient with written record of immunization and reminders for second and third injections.

▷immune globulin intramuscular (IG; gamma globulin; IGIM)

GamaSTAN S/D

immune globulin intravenous (IGIV)

Carimune NF, Flebogamma 5%, Flebogamma 10%, Gammagard Liquid, Privigen

immune globulin subcutaneous (IGSC, SCIG)

Gamunex-C, Hizentra, Vivaglobin

Therapeutic actions

Contains human globulin (16.5% IM, 10% subcutaneously, 5% IV), which provides passive immunity through the presence of injected antibodies. IM gamma globulin involves a 2- to 5-day delay before adequate serum levels are obtained. IV gamma globulin provides immediate antibody levels. Mechanism of action in idiopathic thrombocytopenic purpura not determined.

Indications

- Prophylaxis after exposure to hepatitis A, measles (rubeola), varicella, rubella; IM route is preferred.
- Prophylaxis for patients with immunoglobulin deficiency—subcutaneously, IM; IV if immediate increase in antibodies is necessary.
- Idiopathic thrombocytopenic purpura. IV route has produced temporary increase in platelets in emergency situations (*Carimune NF*).
- Primary immune deficient diseases (*Vivaglobin*).
- Primary humoral immunodeficiencies (*Flebogamma, Gamunex-C*).
- Maintenance treatment of patients with primary immunodeficiencies (*Carimune NF*).
- Treatment of chronic inflammatory demyelinating polyneuropathy (*Gamunex-C*).
- Treatment of idiopathic thrombocytopenic purpura (*Gamunex-C*)

Adverse effects

Tenderness, muscle stiffness at injection site; urticaria, angioedema, nausea, vomiting, chills, fever, chest tightness; anaphylactic reactions, precipitous fall in blood pressure—more likely with IV administration. Risk of acute renal failure with IV products.

Dosage

- Hepatitis A: 0.02 mL/kg IM for household and institutional contacts. Persons traveling to areas where hepatitis A is common: 0.02 mL/kg IM if staying less than 2 mo; 0.06 mL/kg IM repeated every 5 mo for prolonged stay.
- Measles (rubeola): 0.25 mL/kg IM if exposed less than 6 days previously; immunocompromised child exposed to measles: 0.5 mL/kg to a maximum of 15 mL IM given immediately.
- Varicella: 0.6–1.2 mL/kg IM given promptly if zoster immune globulin is unavailable.
- Rubella: 0.55 mL/kg IM given to those pregnant women who have been exposed to rubella and will not consider a therapeutic abortion may decrease likelihood of infection and fetal damage.
- Immunoglobulin deficiency: Initial dosage of 1.3 mL/kg IM, followed in 3–4 wk by 0.66 mL/kg IM every 3–4 wk; some patients may require more frequent injections.
- *Carimune NF*: 0.4–0.8 g/kg by IV infusion every 3–4 wk.
- *Flebogamma*: 300–600 mg/kg IV every 3–4 wk.
- Patients with primary immune deficiency, idiopathic thrombocytopenic purpura, chronic inflammatory demyelinating polyneuropathy: 100–200 mg/kg subcutaneously every wk. Or, initially 1.37 × previous IGIV dose (grams)/number of weeks between IGIV doses (*Gamunex-C*). Adjust dosage based on patient's response.

Nursing considerations

⊗ **Black box warning** Risk of renal dysfunction, renal failure, or death exists. Monitor patient accordingly.

- Do not administer to patients with history of allergy to gamma globulin or antiimmunoglobulin A antibodies.
- Use IM gamma globulin with caution in patients with thrombocytopenia or any coagulation disorder that would contraindicate IM injections. Use only if benefits outweigh risks.
- Use with caution in pregnant women. **Pregnancy Category C**—safety not established.
- Administer vaccines 2 wk before or 3 mo after immune globulin administration because antibodies in the globulin preparation may interfere with the immune response to the vaccination.

⊗ **Warning** Have epinephrine 1:1,000 immediately available at time of injection in case of anaphylactic reaction, which is more likely with IV immune globulin, large IM doses, and repeated injections.

- Refrigerate drug; do not freeze. Discard partially used vials.
- Administer IM preparation by IM injection only; do not administer subcutaneously or intradermally.
- Check manufacturer's guidelines before using any immune globulin.
- Do not shake.
- Administer IV preparation with extreme caution, using separate IV line.
- Do not mix immune globulin with any other medications.
- Monitor patient's vital signs continuously and observe for any symptoms during IV administration. Adverse effects appear to be related to the rate of infusion.
- Teach patient doing home subcutaneous injections for primary immune deficiency the proper administration technique and disposal of needless and syringes. Proper storage is based on brand being used.
- Provide comfort measures or teach patient to provide comfort measures—analgesics, antipyretics, warm soaks to injection site—to help patient to cope with the discomforts of drug therapy.
- Provide patient with written record of injection and dates for follow-up injections as needed.

▽ influenza type A and B virus vaccine

Afluria, Agriflu, Fluarix, FluLaval, Fluvirin, Fluzone, Fluzone High Dose

Therapeutic actions

Inactivated influenza virus antigens stimulate an active immunity through the production of antibodies specific to the antigens used; the antigens used vary from yr to yr depending on which influenza virus strains are anticipated to be prevalent. The 2011–2012 version includes H1N1 (swine flu) and H3N2 strains.

Indications

- Prophylaxis for patients 6 mo and older, including those at high risk for developing complications from infection with influenza virus, including adults and children with chronic cardiovascular or pulmonary disorders, chronic metabolic disorders, renal impairment, anemia, immunosuppression, asthma; residents of long-term care facilities; medical personnel with extensive contact with high-risk patients, to prevent their transmitting the virus to these patients; children on long-term aspirin therapy who are at high risk of developing Reye syndrome; people who provide essential community services (to decrease the risk of disruption of services).
- Active immunization against influenza caused by influenza virus types A and B in children 6 mo and older (*Fluzone*), children 4 yr and older (*Fluvirin*), children 3–17 yr and adults (*Fluarix*), adults 18 yr and older (*FluLaval*), adults 65 yr and older at high risk for complications (*Fluzone High Dose*).
- Priority active immunization in patients at high risk for influenza complications when dosages are limited.

Adverse effects

Tenderness, redness, and induration at the injection site; fever, malaise, myalgia; allergic responses—flare, wheal, respiratory symptoms; Guillain-Barré syndrome.

Dosage

- *6–35 mo:* 0.25 mL IM, repeated in 4 wk (*Afluria, Fluzone*).
- *3 yr and older:* 0.5 mL IM (*Afluria, Fluzone, Fluarix*). Under 9 yr and receiving the vaccine for the first time or who received only one dose last year, give a repeat dose in 4 wk.
- *4 yr and older:* 0.5 mL IM (*Fluvirin*). Under 8 yr and receiving the vaccine for the first time or who received only one dose last year, give a repeat dose in 4 wk.
- *18 yr and older:* 0.5 mL IM; using the prefilled syringe, shake the syringe before use (*Agriflu, Afluria, Fluarix, FluLaval, Fluzone, Fluvirin*).
- *18–64 yr:* 0.1 mL intradermally (*Fluzone Intradermal*).
- *65 yr and older:* 0.5 mL IM (*Fluzone High Dose*).

Nursing considerations

- Do not administer to patients with sensitivities to eggs, chicken, chicken feathers, or chicken dander. If an allergic condition is suspected, administer a scratch test or an intradermal injection (0.05–0.1 mL) of vaccine diluted 1:100 in sterile saline. A wheal greater than 5 mm justifies withholding immunization.
- Do not administer to patient with a hypersensitivity to any component of the vaccine or history of Guillain-Barré syndrome.
- Do not administer to infants and children at the same time as diphtheria, tetanus toxoid, and pertussis vaccine (DTP) or within 14 days after measles virus vaccine.
- Delay administration in the presence of acute respiratory disease or other active infection or acute febrile illness.
- Use caution in pregnant women. **Pregnancy Category C**—safety not established. Delay use until the second or third trimester to minimize concern over possible teratogenicity.
- Monitor patient for enhanced drug effects and possible toxicity of theophylline, warfarin sodium for as long as 3 wk after vaccine injection.
- Administer IM only. The deltoid muscle is preferred for adults and older children, the anterolateral aspect of the thigh for infants and younger children.
- Consider the possible need for amantadine for therapeutic use for patients in high-risk groups who develop illness compatible with influenza during a period of known influenza A activity in the community.
- ⊗ *Warning* Have epinephrine 1:1,000 immediately available at time of injection in case of anaphylactic reaction.
- Provide comfort measures or teach patient to provide comfort measures—analgesics, antipyretics, warm soaks to injection site—to help patient cope with effects of the drug.
- Provide patient with written record of vaccination and dates of second injection as appropriate.
- Do not use vaccine supplies remaining from previous years for current year vaccination.

▽ **influenza virus vaccine, H5N1**

H5N1

Therapeutic actions

Contains inactivated type A influenza virus H5N1 (avian flu), which induces antibodies against this viral strain and blocks attachment of the virus to respiratory cells.

Indications

- Active immunization of persons 18–64 yr at increased risk of exposure to H5N1 influenza (avian flu) virus.

Adverse effects

Hypersensitivity reactions; injection site reactions, including warmth, redness, swelling, pain; headache; nausea; fever; symptoms of URI.

Dosage

- *Adults 18–64 yr:* 1 mL IM into deltoid muscle of upper arm, followed by 1 mL IM 21–35 days later.

Nursing considerations

- Virus is grown in chicken eggs; use caution in patients allergic to chickens.
- Use caution in pregnant women; vaccine is **Pregnancy Category C.** Use only if potential benefit outweighs risk to fetus.
- Do not mix in syringe with other vaccines or inject at same site as other vaccines.
- Provide comfort measures as needed, such as analgesics, antipyretics, and warm packs to injection site.
- Give patient a written record of the vaccination and a date to return for the second dose.

▷ influenza type A and B virus vaccine, live, intranasal
FluMist

Therapeutic actions

Contains attenuated virus reassortants of the three most commonly encountered viruses each year, as determined by the US Public Health Service; administered intranasally, these antigens produce a protective immunity against these strains.

Indications

- Active immunization for prevention of disease caused by influenza A and B viruses in healthy children, adolescents, and adults 2–49 yr.

Adverse effects

Irritability, *headache;* vomiting; sore throat, *runny nose,* nasal congestion, *cough;* fever, chills, muscle aches, decreased activity, tiredness.

Dosage

- *2–8 yr, not previously vaccinated:* Two doses (0.2 mL each) intranasally, given as one spray (0.1 mL) per nostril, at least 1 month apart.
- *2–8 yr, previously vaccinated*: One dose (0.2 mL) intranasally, given as one spray (0.1 mL) per each nostril.
- *9–49 yr:* One dose of one spray (0.1 mL) in each nostril each flu season.
- *2–8 yr not previously vaccinated with* flu vaccine: Two doses (0.2 mL [0.1 mL per nostril]), given at least 1 mo apart.
- *2–8 yr previously vaccinated with* flu vaccine: One dose (0.2 mL [0.1 mL per nostril]) per flu season.

Nursing considerations

- Do not administer to anyone with immunodeficiency, immunosuppression, or malignancy.
- Do not administer with any antiviral drugs or with other immunizations.
- Do not administer to a patient with febrile illness.
- Do not administer with aspirin or aspirin-related products in children; these products could mask Reye syndrome.
- Do not administer to women who are pregnant or nursing a baby. **Pregnancy Category C.**
- Administer this vaccine as one spray (0.1 mL) in each nostril for a total of 0.2 mL.

- Provide comfort measures and teach patients to provide comfort measures to help the patient cope with the discomforts of the immunization (analgesics, rest, decongestants).
- Caution patients that they may be able to transmit influenza after they have received the vaccine; they should avoid close contact with any people who may be immunocompromised.
- Provide parents with written record of immunization and reminder that the vaccine is needed every year just before flu season.

▽measles (rubeola) virus vaccine, live, attenuated

Attenuvax

Therapeutic actions

Attenuated measles virus produces a modified measles infection and stimulates an active immune reaction with antibodies to the measles virus.

Indications

- Immunization against measles (rubeola) immediately (within 72 hr) after exposure to natural measles; more effective if given before exposure—children 12 mo and older (immunization with trivalent MMR vaccine is the preferred product for routine vaccinations).
- Revaccination for children immunized before age 12 mo or vaccinated with inactivated vaccine alone.
- Prophylaxis for high school or college age persons in epidemic situations or for adults in isolated communities where measles is not endemic.

Adverse effects

Moderate fever, rash; high temperature (less common); febrile convulsions, Guillain-Barré syndrome, ocular palsies (less common); burning or stinging wheal or flare at injection site.

Dosage

Inject the total volume of the reconstituted vaccine or 0.5 mL of multi-dose vial subcutaneously into the outer aspect of the upper arm; dose is the same for all patients. Recommended age for primary vaccination is 12–15 mo.

Nursing considerations

- Do not administer to patients with a history of anaphylactic hypersensitivity to neomycin (contained in injection), to patients with immune deficiency conditions (immunosuppressive therapy with corticosteroids, antineoplastics; neoplasms; immunodeficiency states), to patients receiving immune serum globulin.
- Do not administer to pregnant women. **Pregnancy Category C**—advise patients to avoid pregnancy for 3 mo following vaccination. If measles exposure occurs during pregnancy, provide passive immunity with immune serum globulin.
- Use caution if administering to children with history of febrile convulsions, cerebral injury, or other conditions in which stress due to fever should be avoided.
- Use caution if administering to patient with a history of sensitivity to eggs, chicken, chicken feathers.
- Do not administer within 1 mo of immunization with other live virus vaccines; may be administered concurrently with monovalent or trivalent polio vaccine, rubella vaccine, mumps vaccine.
- Do not administer for at least 3 mo following blood or plasma transfusions or administration of serum immune globulin.
- Monitor for possible depression of tuberculin skin sensitivity; administer test before or simultaneously with vaccine.
- Administer with a sterile syringe free of preservatives, antiseptics, and detergents for each injection (these may inactivate the live virus vaccine). Use a 25-gauge, ⅝-inch needle.
- Refrigerate unreconstituted vial; protect from exposure to light. Use only the diluent supplied with the vaccine and reconstitute just before using. Discard reconstituted vaccine if not used within 8 hr.

⊗ *Warning* Have epinephrine 1:1,000 immediately available at time of injection in case of anaphylactic reaction.
- Provide comfort measures or teach patient or parent to provide comfort measures to help patient to cope with the discomforts of drug therapy: analgesics, antipyretics, warm soaks to injection site.
- Provide patient or parent with a written record of immunization.

▽ **measles, mumps, rubella vaccine, live (MMR)**
M-M-R II

Therapeutic actions
Attenuated measles, mumps, and rubella viruses produce a modified infection and stimulate an active immune reaction with antibodies to these viruses.

Indications
- Immunization against measles, mumps, rubella in children 12 mo and older adults.

Adverse effects
Moderate fever, rash, burning or stinging wheal or flare at injection site, high temperature; less common: febrile convulsions, Guillain-Barré syndrome, ocular palsies.

Dosage
0.5 mL reconstituted vaccine subcutaneously into the outer aspect of the upper arm. Dose is the same for all patients. Booster dose is recommended on entry into elementary school.

Nursing considerations
- Do not administer to patients with a history of anaphylactic hypersensitivity to neomycin (contained in injection), to patients with immune deficiency conditions (immunosuppressive therapy with corticosteroids, antineoplastics; neoplasms; immunodeficiency states), to patients receiving immune serum globulin.
- Do not administer to pregnant women. **Pregnancy Category C**—advise patients to avoid pregnancy for 3 mo following vaccination. If measles exposure occurs during pregnancy, provide passive immunity with immune serum globulin.
- Use caution if administering to children with history of febrile convulsions, cerebral injury, or other conditions in which stress due to fever should be avoided.
- Use caution if administering to patient with a history of sensitivity to eggs, chicken, chicken feathers.
- Do not administer within 1 mo of immunization with other live virus vaccines; may be administered concurrently with monovalent or trivalent polio vaccine, rubella vaccine, mumps vaccine.
- Do not administer for at least 3 mo following blood or plasma transfusions or administration of serum immune globulin.
- Monitor for possible depression of tuberculin skin sensitivity. Administer the test before or simultaneously with the vaccine.
- Administer with a sterile syringe free of preservatives, antiseptics, and detergents for each injection (these may inactivate the live virus vaccine). Use a 25-gauge, ⅝-inch needle.
- Refrigerate unreconstituted vial. Protect from exposure to light. Use only the diluent supplied with the vaccine and reconstitute just before using. Discard reconstituted vaccine if not used within 8 hr.
⊗ *Warning* Have epinephrine 1:1,000 immediately available at time of injection in case of anaphylactic reaction.
- Provide comfort measures or teach patient or parent to provide comfort measures to help patient cope with the discomforts of drug therapy (analgesics, antipyretics, warm soaks to injection site).
- Provide patient or parent with a written record of immunization.
- Trivalent measles, mumps, and rubella vaccine is the vaccination of choice for routine vaccinations. Another combination—rubella and mumps vaccine (*Biavax II*)—is used for specific situations.

▷ measles, mumps, rubella, and varicella virus vaccine, live

ProQuad

Therapeutic actions

Attenuated measles, mumps, rubella, and varicella viruses produce a modified infection and stimulate an active immune reaction with antibodies to these viruses.

Indications

- Active immunization of children ages 12 mo–12 yr, for the prevention of measles, mumps, rubella, and varicella virus infections.

Adverse effects

Irritability; diarrhea, fever, chills, muscle aches, injection site reactions; less common—fever, convulsions, ocular palsies.

Dosage

0.5 mL by subcutaneous injection; allow 1 mo to elapse between the administration of any vaccine containing measles antigens and the administration of *ProQuad;* if a second varicella vaccine is needed, allow 3 mo between administration of the two doses.

Nursing considerations

- Do not administer to anyone with immunodeficiency/suppression or malignancy.
- Do not administer with any antiviral medications or with other immunizations or immune suppressants.
- Do not administer in the presence of febrile illness or with active, untreated TB.
- Do not administer to a patient with known allergy to any component of the drug, gelatin, or neomycin.
- Defer vaccination for at least 3 mo after blood or plasma transfusion or administration of immunoglobulin.
- Do not administer with aspirin or aspirin-related products in children. These products could mask the presence of Reye syndrome; advise parents not to use aspirin for 6 wk following the vaccination.
- Do not administer to women who are pregnant or nursing. **Pregnancy Category C**—safety not established.
- Administer by subcutaneous injection only; inspect solution for particulate matter.
- Administer immediately after reconstituting with provided sterile water.
- ⊗ *Warning* Have epinephrine 1:1,000 immediately available at time of injection in case of anaphylactic reaction.
- Provide comfort measures or teach parents to provide comfort measures to help the patient cope with the discomforts of the immunization (analgesics, rest, decongestants).
- Provide parents with written record of immunization.

▷ Meningococcal groups C and Y, *Haemophilus* b tetanus toxoid conjugate vaccine

MenHibrix

Therapeutic actions

Capsular polysaccharides from *Neisseria meningitidis* serogroups C and Y and *Haemophilus influenzae* b, which will induce production of bactericidal antibodies to these serogroups of bacteria to provide active immunization.

Indications
• Active immunization to prevent invasive meningococcal disease caused by *N meningitidis* subgroups C and Y and *H. influenzae* type b in children 6-18 mo.

Adverse effects
Injection-site reactions (pain, redness, swelling), fever, chills, headache, malaise, fatigue, anorexia, Guillain-Barré syndrome.

Dosage
Four doses of 0.5 mL each, by IM injection at 2, 4, 6, and 12-15 mo. May give first dose as early as 6 wk; fourth dose may be as late as 18 mo.

Nursing considerations
• Do not mix in syringe with other vaccines.
• Do not administer to patient with known allergy to components of drug.
• Do not use in children younger than 6 wk or between 19 mo and 6 yr; safety not established.
• Weigh benefits versus risks in patients who experienced Guillain-Barré syndrome within 6 wk of any tetanus toxoid-containing vaccine; also weigh benefits/risks in premature infants (apnea has been reported).
• Maintain procedures to avoid falling injury and to restore cerebral perfusion if syncope occurs at time of injection.
• Provide comfort measures (analgesics, rest, decongestants) to help patient cope with discomforts of immunization.
• Provide parents or caregivers with written record of immunization and instructions on completing the series.

▽meningococcal vaccine

Menactra, Menomune A/C/Y/W-135, Menveo

Therapeutic actions
Capsular polysaccharides from *Neisseria meningitidis* serogroups A, C, Y, and W-135, which will induce production of bactericidal antibodies to these serogroups of bacteria to provide active immunization.

Indications
• Active immunization to prevent invasive meningococcal disease caused by *N. meningitidis* serogroups A, C, Y, and W-125; control of outbreaks of serogroup C disease (*Menomune*).

Adverse effects
Injection-site reactions (pain, redness, swelling), fever, chills, headache, malaise, fatigue, anorexia, Guillain-Barré syndrome.

Dosage
• *Menactra:* 9 mo–55 yr: 0.5 mL IM in the deltoid region as one dose.
• *Menomune:* 2–55 yr: 0.5 mL IM; may give booster in 3–5 yr.
• *Menveo:* 9 mo–55 yr: 0.5 mL IM as one dose. Children 2–5 yr may receive a second dose 2 mo after first dose.

Nursing considerations
• Do not administer to patient with immunodeficiency/suppression or malignancy.
• Do not administer with antivirals or other immunizations or immune suppressants.

- Do not administer if patient has febrile illness or active infection.
- Do not administer to patient with known allergy to components of drug or to latex.
- Do not administer to women who are pregnant unless the benefit clearly outweighs the risk.

⊗ *Warning* Have epinephrine 1:1,000 immediately available at time of injection in case of anaphylactic reaction.

- Provide comfort measures (analgesics, rest, decongestants) to help patient cope with discomforts of immunization.
- Provide patient with written record of immunization.

▷ pneumococcal vaccine, polyvalent
Pneumovax 23

Therapeutic actions
Polysaccharide capsules of the 23 most prevalent or invasive pneumococcal types stimulate active immunity through antipneumococcal antibody production against the capsule types contained in the vaccine.

Indications
- Immunization against pneumococcal pneumonia and bacteremia caused by the types of pneumococci included in the vaccine, specifically in children older than 2 yr and adults with chronic illnesses or who are immunocompromised and at increased risk for pneumococcal infections routine immunization of immunocompetent adults 65 yr and older.
- Prophylaxis in children 2 yr and older with asymptomatic or symptomatic HIV infections.
- Prophylaxis in community groups at high risk for pneumococcal infections—institutionalized persons, groups in an area of outbreak, patients at high risk of influenza complications, including pneumococcal infection.

Adverse effects
Erythema, induration, soreness at injection site; fever, myalgia; acute febrile reactions, rash, arthralgia (less common); paresthesias, acute radiculoneuropathy (rare); anaphylactic reaction.

Dosage
One 0.5-mL dose subcutaneously or IM. Not recommended for children younger than 2 yr.

Nursing considerations
- Do not administer to patients with hypersensitivity to any component of the vaccine or with previous immunization with any polyvalent pneumococcal vaccine.
- Administer at least 2 wk before initiation of cancer chemotherapy or other immunosuppressive therapy.
- Use caution if administering to patients who are nursing or pregnant. **Pregnancy Category C**—safety not established.
- Use caution if administering to patients with cardiac, pulmonary disorders; systemic reaction could pose a significant risk.
- May be administered concomitantly with influenza virus vaccine by separate injection in the other arm.
- Administer subcutaneously or IM only, preferably in the deltoid muscle or lateral mid-thigh; do not give IV.
- Refrigerate vials. Use directly as supplied; do not dilute (reconstitution is not necessary).

⊗ *Warning* Have epinephrine 1:1,000 immediately available at time of injection in case of anaphylactic reaction.

- Provide or teach patient to provide appropriate comfort measures—analgesics, antipyretics, warm soaks to injection site—to help patient to cope with effects of the drug therapy.

- Provide patient with written record of immunization and caution patient not to have another polyvalent pneumococcal vaccine injection.

▷ pneumococcal 13-valent conjugate vaccine (diphtheria CRM$_{197}$ protein)

Prevnar-13

Therapeutic actions

Stimulates active immunity against disease caused by *Streptococcus pneumoniae* by introduction of 13 capsular serotypes.

Indications

- Prevention of invasive *S. pneumoniae* disease in children 6 wk–5 yr (before 6th birthday); in patients 19 yr and older with weakened immune systems caused by advanced kidney disease, cancer, HIV; in adults so yr and older to prevent pneumonia and invasive disease caused by *S. Pneumoniae*.
- Active immunization of infants and toddlers against otitis media caused by vaccine serotypes.
- Prevention of otitis media caused by resistant strains.

Adverse effects

Fretfulness; drowsiness; anorexia; vomiting; transient fever; malaise; generalized aches and pains; edema of injection area with redness, swelling, induration, pain (may persist for a few days); hypersensitivity reactions.

Dosage

0.5 mg IM, preferably injected in the anterolateral aspect of the thigh in infants and the deltoid muscle of the upper arm in older children.

- Four-dose series administered 4–8 wk apart at 2, 4, and 6 mo; then at 12–15 mo.

Catch-up schedule for children 7 mo and older:

- 7–11 mo: three doses, first two doses at least 4 wk apart; third dose after first birthday.
- 12–23 mo: two doses at least 2 mo apart.
- 24 mo–5 yr: one dose (before 6th birthday).
- 19 yr and older with weakened immune system: one dose.
- 50 yr and older: one dose.

Nursing considerations

- Defer administration of routine immunizing or booster doses in case of acute infection or febrile illness.
- Not for treatment of acute pneumococcal infections.
- Shake vigorously before use. Do not use if a uniform suspension is not attained.
- Administer by IM injection only; avoid subcutaneous or IV injection. Do not inject vaccine in gluteal area.

⊗ **Warning** Arrange for epinephrine 1:1,000 to be immediately available at time of injection because of risk of hypersensitivity reactions.

- Provide comfort measures to help patient cope with the discomforts of the injection (analgesics, warm soaks for injection site, small meals, environmental control of temperature and stimuli).
- Provide parent with written record of immunization and reminder of when additional injections are needed.

▽poliovirus vaccine, inactivated (IPV, Salk)

IPOL

Therapeutic actions

Inactivated, attenuated sterile suspension of three types of poliovirus used to produce antibody response against poliomyelitis infection.

Indications

• Prevention of poliomyelitis caused by poliovirus types 1, 2, and 3 as routine immunization of infants, children, and adults.

Adverse effects

Local reaction at site of injection within 48 hr.

Dosage

• *Children:* 0.5 mL subcutaneously at 2 mo, 4 mo, and 6–18 mo. A booster dose is needed at time of entry into elementary school.
• *Adults:* Not usually needed in adults in the United States; if unimmunized adult is exposed, is traveling to a high-risk area, or is a household contact of children receiving IPV (inactivated poliovirus vaccine; Salk vaccine) immunization is recommended. 0.5 mL subcutaneously: two doses given at 1- to 2-mo intervals and a third dose given 6–12 mo later. Previously vaccinated adults at risk for exposure should receive a 0.5-mL dose of this drug.

Nursing considerations

• Do not administer to patients with known hypersensitivity to streptomycin or neomycin (each dose contains less than 25 mcg of each).
• Defer administration in the presence of persistent vomiting or diarrhea and in patients with acute illness or any advanced debilitating condition.
• Do not administer to any patient with immune deficiency conditions; do not administer shortly after immune serum globulin (ISG) unless necessary because of travel or exposure; if given with or shortly after ISG dose should be repeated after 3 mo.
• Use caution if administering to pregnant patients. **Pregnancy Category C**—safety not established; use only if clearly needed and benefits outweigh potential unknown effects on the fetus.
• Refrigerate vaccine. Do not freeze.
• Provide patient or parent with a written record of the vaccination and information on when additional doses are needed.

▽RH₀ (D) immune globulin

HyperRHO S/D Full Dose, RhoGAM, Ultra-Filtered Plus

RH₀ (D) immune globulin micro-dose

HyperRHO S/D Minidose, MICRhoGAM, Ultra-Filtered Plus

RH₀ (D) immune globulin IV (human) (RH₀ D IGIV)

Rhophylac, WinRho SDF

Therapeutic actions

Suppresses the immune response of nonsensitized Rh₀-negative individuals who receive Rh₀-positive blood as the result of a fetomaternal hemorrhage or a transfusion accident; raises platelet counts in Rh₀ D-positive, non-splenectomized adults with chronic immune thrombocytopenic purpura; each vial of Rh₀-immune globulin completely suppresses immunity to 15 mL of Rh-positive packed RBCs (about 30 mL whole blood); each vial of Rh₀ immune globulin micro-dose suppresses immunity to 2.5 mL Rh-positive packed RBCs.

Indications

- Prevention of sensitization to the Rh$_0$ factor.
- To prevent hemolytic disease of the newborn (erythroblastosis fetalis) in a subsequent pregnancy—mother must be Rh$_0$ negative; mother must not be previously sensitized to Rh$_0$ factor; infant must be Rh$_0$ positive and direct antiglobulin negative—used at full-term delivery, for incomplete pregnancy, for antepartum prophylaxis in case of abortion or ectopic pregnancy.
- To prevent Rh$_0$ sensitization in Rh$_0$-negative patients accidentally transfused with Rh$_0$-positive blood.
- To raise platelet count in Rh$_0$-positive adults with intact spleen and ITP.

Adverse effects

Pain and soreness at injection site.

Dosage

- *Postpartum prophylaxis:* One vial IM or IV (*WinRho SDF*) within 72 hr of delivery.
- *Antepartum prophylaxis:* One vial IM or IV (*WinRho SDF*) at 26–28 wk gestation and one vial within 72 hr after an Rh-incompatible delivery to prevent Rh isoimmunization during pregnancy.
- *Following amniocentesis, miscarriage, abortion, ectopic pregnancy at or beyond 13 wk gestation:* One vial IM or IV.
- *Transfusion accidents:* Multiply the volume in mL of Rh-positive whole blood administered by the Hct of the donor unit and divide this volume (in mL) by 15 to obtain the number of syringes to be administered. If results of calculation are a fraction, administer the next whole number of syringes (*Hyper Rh$_0$ S/D Full Dose*).
- *ITP:* 250 international units/kg IV at 2 mL/15–60 sec.
- *Spontaneous abortion, induced abortion, or termination of ectopic pregnancy up to and including 12 wk gestation (unless the father is Rh negative):* One vial micro-dose IM given as soon as possible after termination of pregnancy.

Nursing considerations

⊗ **Black box warning** There is risk of intravascular hemolysis and death when drug is used for ITP (*WinRho*). Monitor dipstick urinalysis at baseline, then at 2, 4, and 8 hr; ask patient to report back pain, chills, or discolored urine.

- Rh$_0$ globulin is not needed in Rh$_0$-negative mothers if the father can be determined to be Rh$_0$ negative.
- Do not administer to the Rh$_0$-positive postpartum infant, to an Rh$_0$-positive individual, to an Rh$_0$-negative individual previously sensitized to the Rh$_0$ antigen (if it is not known whether a woman is Rh$_0$ sensitized, administer the Rh$_0$ globulin).
- Before administration, determine the infant's blood type and arrange for a direct antiglobulin test using umbilical cord, venous, or capillary blood; confirm that the mother is Rh$_0$ negative.

⊗ **Warning** Do not administer *HyperRHO S/D, RhoGam* IV; administer IM within 72 hr after Rh$_0$-incompatible delivery, miscarriage, abortion, or transfusion.

- For IM use, prepare one vial dose by withdrawing entire contents of vial; inject entire contents.
- For IM use, prepare two or more vial doses using 5- to 10-mL syringes. Withdraw contents from the vials to be administered at one time and inject. Contents of the total number of vials may be injected as a divided dose at different injection sites at the same time, or the total dosage may be divided and injected at intervals, as long as the total dose is administered within 72 hr postpartum or after a transfusion accident.
- Refrigerate vials; do not freeze.
- Provide appropriate comfort measures if injection sites are painful.
- Reassure patient and explain what has been given and why; the patient needs to know what was given in the event of future pregnancies.

▽rotavirus vaccine, live, oral pentavalent

Rotarix, RotaTeq

Therapeutic actions

Live, reassortant rotaviruses that replicate in the small intestine and stimulate an active immunity to prevent rotavirus gastroenteritis.

Indications

• Prevention of rotavirus gastroenteritis in infants and children.

Adverse effects

Irritability; diarrhea, vomiting, fever, pneumonia, gastroenteritis, UTI.

Dosage

• Three ready-to-use liquid pouch doses (2 mL each) PO starting at age 6–12 wk, with subsequent doses at 4–10 wk intervals (third dose should not be given after age 32 wk) (*RotaTeq*).
• Two doses of 1 mL each PO beginning at age 6 wk. Allow 4 wk before the second dose. Series must be completed by age 24 wk (*Rotarix*).

Nursing considerations

• Do not administer to anyone with immunodeficiency, immunosuppression, or malignancy.
• Do not administer in the presence of febrile illness.
• Do not administer to a patient with a known allergy to any component of the drug.
• Do not administer to women who are pregnant or nursing. **Pregnancy Category C.**
• Do not have close contact with people with malignancies or who are immune compromised; live virus may shed.
• Provide comfort measures or teach parents to provide comfort measures to help patient cope with discomforts of immunization. Provide analgesics, fluids, and limited diet.
• Provide parents with written record of immunization.

▽typhoid vaccine

Typhim Vi, Vivotif Berna

Therapeutic actions

Contains live attenuated strains of typhoid bacteria; produces a humoral antibody response against the causative agent of typhoid fever. Precise mechanism of action is not understood.

Indications

• Active immunization against typhoid fever (*Typhim Vi, Vivotif Berna*).
• Immunization of adults and children against disease caused by *Salmonella typhi* (routine immunization is not recommended in the United States but is recommended for travelers, workers in microbiology fields, or those who may come into household contact with typhoid fever).

Adverse effects

Transient fever; edema of injection area with redness, swelling, induration, pain (may persist for a few days); headache, malaise.

Dosage

• Parenteral (*HP*). *Older than 10 yr:* 2 doses of 0.5 mL subcutaneously at intervals of 4 wk or longer. *10 yr or younger:* Two doses of 0.25 mL subcutaneously at 4-wk or longer intervals.

- Booster dose (given every 3 yr in cases of continued exposure). *Older than 10 yr:* 0.5 mL subcutaneously or 0.1 mL intradermally. *6 mo–10 yr:* 0.25 mL subcutaneously or 0.1 mL intradermally.
- Parenteral (*Typhim Vi*). *Children 2 yr and older:* 0.5 mL IM; booster dose every 2 yr: 0.5 mL IM.
- Oral (*Vivotif Berna*). *Patients older than 6 yr:* One capsule on days 1, 3, 5, and 7 taken 1 hr before a meal with a cold or lukewarm drink. There are no data on the need for a booster dose at this time; 4 capsules on alternating days—once every 5 yr is suggested.
- Complete vaccine regimen 1–2 wk before potential exposure.

Nursing considerations
- Use caution with pregnancy. **Pregnancy Category C**—safety not established.
- Defer administration in case of acute infection, GI illness, nausea, vomiting.
- Have patient swallow capsules whole; do not chew. All four doses must be taken to ensure antibody response.
- Administer *Typhim Vi* parenteral doses by IM injection; deltoid muscle is the preferred site.
- ⊗ **Warning** Arrange for epinephrine 1:1,000 to be immediately available at time of injection because of risk of hypersensitivity reactions.
- Provide comfort measures to help patient cope with the discomforts of the injection (analgesics, warm soaks for injection site, small meals, environmental control of temperature and stimuli).
- Provide patient with written record of immunization and information on booster immunization if appropriate.
- Vaccines must be kept refrigerated. Do not freeze injectable products.

▷ varicella virus vaccine, live
Varivax

Therapeutic actions
Contains live attenuated varicella virus obtained from human or guinea pig cell cultures. Varicella virus causes chickenpox in children and adults. Vaccine produces an active immunity to the virus; longevity of immunity is not known.

Indications
- Active immunization of adults and children 12 mo or older against chickenpox (varicella).

Adverse effects
Transient fever; edema of injection area with redness, swelling, induration, pain (may persist for a few days); upper respiratory illness, cough, rash.

Dosage
- *Adult and patients 13 yr and older:* 0.5 mL subcutaneously in the deltoid area followed by 0.5 mL 4–8 wk later.
- *Children 1–12 yr:* Single 0.5-mL dose subcutaneously.

Nursing considerations
- Use caution with allergy to neomycin or gelatin; use caution in pregnancy. **Pregnancy Category C**—safety not established.
- Defer administration in case of acute infection and for at least 5 mo after plasma transfusion or receipt of immune globulin, other immunizations.
- Do not administer salicylates for up to 6 wk after immunization; cases of Reye syndrome have been reported.
- Use reconstituted vaccine within 30 min. Only use diluent supplied.
- Administer by subcutaneous injection. Outer aspect of upper arm is preferred site.
- ⊗ **Warning** Arrange for epinephrine 1:1,000 to be immediately available at time of injection because of risk of hypersensitivity reactions.

- Provide comfort measures to help patient cope with the discomforts of the injection (analgesics, warm soaks for injection site, small meals, environmental control of temperature and stimuli).
- Provide patient with written record of immunization. It is not known whether booster immunization will be needed.

▽zoster vaccine, live
Zostavax

Therapeutic actions
Attenuated, live varicella-zoster virus causes a boost in the varicella-zoster virus immunity in older individuals; stimulating production of their own varicella-zoster virus antibodies. Herpes zoster, which causes shingles, is a reactivation of the varicella-zoster virus that causes chickenpox.

Indications
Prevention of herpes zoster (shingles) in patients older than 50 yr.

Adverse effects
Injection site reactions (redness, warmth, swelling, bruising, pain), headache, diarrhea, rhinitis, fever, flulike symptoms.

Dosage
One injection of the single-dose vaccine by subcutaneous injection in the upper arm. Vaccine should be frozen and reconstituted, using the supplied diluent, immediately after removal from the freezer; administer immediately after reconstituting.

Nursing considerations
- Do not administer to anyone with immunodeficiency/suppression or malignancy.
- Do not administer with any antiviral medications or with other immunizations or immune suppressants.
- Caution patient to avoid people who are immune suppressed after they receive the vaccine; the disease could be transmitted to them and they could become ill.
- Do not administer in the presence of febrile illness or with active, untreated tuberculosis.
- Do not administer to a patient with known allergy to any component of the drug, gelatin, or neomycin.
- Do not administer to women who are pregnant; recommend use of contraceptive measures at time of vaccination and for 3 mo after the injection. **Pregnancy Category C**—safety not established.
- Administer by subcutaneous injection only; inspect solution for particulate matter.
- Administer immediately after reconstituting with provided diluent.
- ⊗ *Warning* Have epinephrine 1:1,000 immediately available at time of injection in case of anaphylactic reaction.
- Provide comfort measures to help the patient cope with the discomforts of the immunization—analgesics, rest, decongestants.
- Provide patient with written record of immunization.

Other biologicals

Name	Indications	Instructions
Immune globulins		
anti-thymocyte globulin (*Thymoglobulin*)	Treatment of renal transplant acute rejection in conjunction with immunosuppression.	1.5 mg/kg/day for 7–14 days as 6-hr IV infusion for first dose and at least 4 hr each subsequent dose. Administer through on 0.22-micron filter. Store in refrigerator and use within 4 hr of reconstitution.
botulism immune globulin (*BabyBIG*)	Treatment of patients younger than 1 yr with infant botulism caused by toxin A or B.	1 mL/kg as a single IV infusion as soon as diagnosis has been made.
cytomegalovirus immune globulin IV (CMV-IGIV) (*CytoGam*)	Prophylaxis of CMV disease following renal, lung, liver, pancreas, and heart transplant.	15 mg/kg IV over 30 min, increase to 30 mg/kg IV for 30 min, then 60 mg/kg IV to a maximum of 150 mg/kg. Infuse at 72 hr, 2 wk, and then 4, 6, 8, 12, and 16 wk. Monitor for allergic reactions. Use within 6 hr of entering vial. Administer through an IV line with an in-line filter (15 micron).
lymphocyte, immune globulin (*Atgam*)	Management of allograft rejection in renal transplants; treatment of aplastic anemia.	10–30 mg/kg/day IV adult transplant; 5–25 mg/kg/day IV pediatric transplant, 10–20 mg/kg/day IV for 8–14 days for aplastic anemia. Stable for up to 12 hr after reconstitution. Administer a skin test prior to administration of first dose.
rabies immune globulin (*HyperRab S/D*, *Imogam Rabies-HT*)	Passive protection against rabies in nonimmunized patients with exposure to rabies.	20 international units/kg IM as single dose at same time as rabies vaccine. Infuse wound area if possible. Never give in same site as vaccine. Refrigerate vial.
vaccinia immune globulin IV (*VIGIV*)	Treatment or modification of vaccinia infections.	2 mL/kg (100 mg/kg) IV.
Antitoxins and antivenins		
antivenin (micrurus fulvius)	Neutralize the venom of coral snakes in the United States.	3–5 vials by slow IV injection. Give first 1 to 2 mL over 3–5 min and observe for allergic reaction. Flush with IV fluids after antivenin has been infused. May require up to 100 mL.
Black Widow spider species antivenin (*Antivenin Latrodectus mactans*)	Treatment of symptoms of Black Widow spider bites.	2.5 mL IM; may be given IV in 10–50 mL saline over 15 min. Ensure supportive therapy and use of muscle relaxants.
centruroides (*scorpion*) immune fab (*Anascorp*)	Treatment of scorpion stings.	Initially, 3 vials infused IV over 10 min; then one vial at a time at intervals of 30–60 min until clinically stable. Begin as soon as possible after sting. Severe hypersensitivity reactions and delayed serum sickness reaction possible (contains equine proteins).

Name	Indications	Instructions

Antitoxins and antivenins (continued)

Name	Indications	Instructions
crotalidae polyvalent immune fab (ovine) (*CroFab*)	Treatment of rattlesnake bites.	4–6 vials IV; may be repeated based on patient response. Dilute each vial with 10 mL sterile water, then with 250 mL 0.9% sodium chloride. Give each 250 mL over 60 min. Contains specific antibody fragments that bind to four different rattlesnake toxins. Removal of venom should be done at once. Monitor patient carefully for hypersensitivity reaction. Most effective if given within first 6 hr after snake bite.

Bacterial vaccines

Name	Indications	Instructions
BCG (*BCG Vaccine*)	Prevantion of TB in skin test—negative people at high risk for exposure; groups with high rates or TB; travel to areas with high rates of endemic TB.	0.2–0.3 mL percutaneous using a sterile multipuncture disc. Refrigerate, protect from light; keep the vaccination site clean until reaction disappears.

Viral vaccines

Name	Indications	Instructions
Japanese encephalitis vaccine (*JE-VAX*)	Active immunization in persons older than 1 yr who will reside or travel in areas where it is endemic or epidemic.	3 subcutaneous doses of 1 mL given at days 0, 7, and 30; children 1–3 yr: three subcutaneous doses of 0.5 mL. Refrigerate vial. Do not remove rubber stopper. Do not travel within 10 days of vaccination.
Japanese encephalitis vaccine, inactivated, adsorbed (*Ixiaro*)	Active immunization for prevention of disease caused by Japanese encephalitis virus (JEV) in patients 17 yr and older	2 doses of 0.5 mL each IM, given 28 days apart. Series should be completed at least 1 week before exposure to JEV. Contains protamine sulfate. Use only if clearly needed in pregnant or breast-feeding women.
rabies vaccine (*Imovax Rabies, RabAvert*)	Preexposure rabies immunization for patients in high-risk area; postexposure antirabies regimen in conjunction with rabies immunoglobulin.	Preexposure: 1 mL IM on days 0, 7, and 21 or 28. Postexposure: 1 mL IM on days 0, 3, 7, 14, and 28. Refrigerate. If titers are low, booster may be needed.
yellow fever vaccine (*YF-Vax*)	Immunization of persons 9 mo and older living in or traveling to endemic areas.	0.5 mL subcutaneously. Booster dose suggested every 10 yr. Use cautiously with allergy to chicken or egg products.

APPENDIX R

Less commonly used drugs

abatacept
Orencia

Drug class and indications
Immune modulator, antiarthritic

Reduction of the signs and symptoms, including major clinical response, slowing the progression of structural damage, and improving physical function in adult patients with moderately to severely active rheumatoid arthritis who have had an inadequate response to one or more disease-modifying antirheumatic drugs, as monotherapy or in combination with other drugs other than tumor necrosis factor (TNF) antagonists.

Reduction of signs and symptoms of moderately active polyarticular juvenile idiopathic arthritis in children 6 yr and older as monotherapy or in combination with methotrexate.

Dosages and special alerts
Adults: Less than 60 kg: 500 mg IV over 30 min, repeated at 2 and 4 wk, then every 4 wk. 60–100 kg: 750 mg IV over 30 min, repeated at 2 and 4 wk, then every 4 wk. More than 100 kg: 1 g IV over 30 min, repeated at 2 and 4 wk, then every 4 wk. Pediatric patients: Less than 75 kg: 10 mg/kg IV over 30 min repeated at 2 and 4 wk, then every 4 wk. Maximum dose: 1,000 mg. 75–100 kg: 750 mg IV over 30 min, repeated at 2 and 4 wk, then every 4 wk. More than 100 kg: 1,000 mg IV over 30 min, repeated at 2 and 4 wk, then every 4 wk. Risk of serious infection with TNF antagonists; do not give with live vaccines.

abiraterone acetate
Zytiga

Drug class and indications
CYP17 inhibitor; antineoplastic

In combination with prednisone treatment of patients with metastatic castration-resistant prostate cancer who have received prior chemotherapy containing docetaxel.

Dosages and special alerts
1,000 mg/day PO in combination with prednisone 5 mg PO bid; reduce dosage with hepatic impairment. Must be taken on an empty stomach, with no food for at least 1 hr before and 2 hr after dosing. Contraindicated in pregnancy and lactation. Risk of cardiac toxicity; monitor blood pressure and potassium levels carefully. Risk of hepatotoxicity. Risk of adrenal insufficiency; monitor closely and consider use of corticosteroids in stressful situations. Hot flashes, hypertension, edema, swelling, and discomfort are most common adverse effects.

acitretin
Soriatane

Drug class and indications
Antipsoriatic agent; retinoic acid

Treatment of severe psoriasis.

Dosages and special alerts
25–50 mg/day PO with the main meal. Numerous adverse effects. Stop drug when lesions resolve. Do not crush capsules. Do not allow patient to donate blood. Monitor vision periodically; protect patient from sun exposure. ⊗ *Black box warning* Pregnancy category X; do not give to pregnant women. Two forms of contraception required; signed Patient Agreement/Informed Consent required. Males should not father a child during or for 2–3 mo following treatment. Patients cannot donate blood during and for 3 yr following treatment.

DANGEROUS DRUG
adalimumab
Humira

Drug class and indications
Antiarthritic, monoclonal antibody

Reduction of the signs and symptoms of and inhibition of the progression of structural damage in adults with moderately to severely active rheumatoid arthritis and in children 4 yr and older with moderately to severely active polyarticular rheumatoid arthritis.

Reduction of the signs and symptoms of active arthritis in patients with psoriatic arthritis.

Reduction of the signs and symptoms of active ankylosing spondylitis.

Reduction of signs and symptoms of Crohn disease in adults.

Treatment of moderate to severe plaque psoriasis when other therapies are ineffective.

Dosages and special alerts

Adults: Maintenance therapy—40 mg subcutaneously every other wk, may be increased to 40 mg subcutaneously every wk in patients not on methotrexate. Pediatric patients ages 4–17 yr: Weighing 15 to less than 30 kg: 20 mg subcutaneously every other wk. Weighing 30 kg or more: 40 mg subcutaneously every other wk. Use cautiously with immunosuppressants; severe infection can occur. Avoid use in pregnancy. Monitor for CNS effects, demyelinating disease has been reported. ⊗ **Black box warning** High risk of infection, including from *Legionella* and *Listeria* organisms; monitor patient accordingly. ⊗ **Black box warning** Risk of potentially fatal hepatosplenic T-cell lymphoma; monitor patient accordingly.

adenosine
Adenocard, Adenoscan

Drug class and indications

Antiarrhythmic, diagnostic agent

Conversion to sinus rhythm of paroxysmal supraventricular tachycardias (*Adenocard*); with thallium, assessment of patients with suspected CAD (*Adenoscan*).

Dosages and special alerts

Conversion of arrhythmias in patients weighing more than 50 kg: 6 mg by rapid IV bolus; for repeat dose, use 12 mg by IV bolus within 1–2 min. May be repeated a second time. *Patients weighing less than 50 kg:* 0.05–0.1 mg/kg as rapid IV bolus, may give another bolus in 1–2 min, increased by 0.05–0.1 mg/kg. Maximum single dose, 0.3 mg/kg. *Cardiac assessment:* 140 mcg/kg/min IV, infused over 6 min. Inject thallium at 3 min. Maintain emergency equipment on standby, and monitor continually. Have methylxanthines available as antidote.

aflibercept
Eylea

Drug class and indications

Fusion protein; ophthalmic drug

Treatment of neovascular (wet) age-related macular degeneration.

Dosages and special alerts

2 mg (0.05 mL) by intravitreal injection every 4 wk for the first 3 mo; then once every 8 wk. Do not use for ocular or periocular infections, active intraocular inflammation. Risk of retinal detachment following injection; risk of increased intraocular pressure. Vitreous floaters, eye pain, cataract development, and conjunctival hemorrhage are common adverse reactions.

agalsidase beta
Fabrazyme

Drug class and indications

Enzyme

Treatment of Fabry disease.

Dosages and special alerts

1 mg/kg body weight IV every 2 wk; infused at a rate of no more than 0.25 mg/min. Infusion reactions are common; antipyretics and corticosteroids are given before the infusion; fever and chills may occur later. Continue regular regimen for treatment of Fabry disease.

DANGEROUS DRUG
aldesleukin
Proleukin

Drug class and indications

Antineoplastic

Metastatic renal cell carcinoma in adults.

Treatment of adult metastatic melanoma.

Dosages and special alerts

600,000 units/kg IV every 8 hr, given over 15 min as two 50-day cycles; total of 14 doses, followed by 9 days of rest, then 14 more doses; can be retreated after 7 wk if tumor shrinkage occurs. Monitor for capillary leak syndrome with third spacing of fluids and hypotension; GI bleeding has been reported.

alglucosidase alfa
Lumizyme, Myozyme

Drug class and indications
Enzyme, Pompe disease drug

To improve ventilator-free survival in patients with infantile-onset Pompe disease (*Myozyme*).

Treatment of patients 8 yr and older with late-onset Pompe disease without cardiac hypertrophy (*Lumizyme*).

Dosages and special alerts
20 mg/kg by IV infusion administered over 4 hr, every 2 wk. Because of a high risk of infusion reaction, infusion should be started as 1mg/kg/hr and then increased by 2 mg/kg/hr every 30 min, based on patient tolerance, to a maximum of 7 mg/kg/hr. Do not infuse in solution with any other drug. Monitor carefully for hypersensitivity reaction, cardiorespiratory failure.

⊗ **Black box warning** Risk of life-threatening allergic reactions; ensure medical support is readily available.

⊗ **Black box warning** *Lumizyme* is only available through *Lumizyme ACE* program because of risk of rapid disease progression.

DANGEROUS DRUG

alogliptin
Nesina (OTC)

Drug class and indications
Antidiabetic, DPP-4 inhibitor

Adjunct to diet and exercise to improve glycemic control in adults with type 2 diabetes

Dosages and special alerts
6.25 mg/day PO, increase based on patient response; max 25 mg/day PO. Monitor blood glucose levels and renal function; ensure continuation of diet and exercise program; may be used with other drugs for type 2 diabetes. Pregnancy Category B. Monitor drugs, herbs being used. Switch to insulin in times of extreme stress

alpha₁-proteinase inhibitor
Aralast NP, Prolastin, Prolastin C, Zemaira

Drug class and indications
Blood product
Aralast NP/Prolastin
Treatment of congenital alpha₁-antitrypsin deficiency, chronic treatment of adults with early evidence of panacinar emphysema.
Zemaira
Chronic augmentation and maintenance therapy in patients with alpha₁-proteinase inhibitor deficiency and clinical evidence of emphysema.

Dosages and special alerts
Aralast NP/Prolastin, Prolastin C
60 mg/kg IV once a wk to achieve functional levels of alpha₁-proteinase inhibitor in lower respiratory tract. Monitor for possible hepatitis related to the use of human blood products. Administer *Prolastin* C at 0.08 mL/kg/min IV once a week.
Zemaira
60 mg/kg IV weekly, infused over 15 min. Monitor for any sign of hypersensitivity reactions; drug should be discontinued if these occur. Warn the patient that product is made from human plasma and possible viral infection could occur—rash, drowsiness, chills, and joint pain should be reported immediately.

alpha₁-proteinase inhibitor (human)
Glassia

Drug class and indications
Alpha₁-proteinase inhibitor

Chronic augmentation therapy and maintenance therapy in adult patients with emphysema due to congenital deficiency of alpha₁-proteinase inhibitor.

Dosages and special alerts
60 mg/kg by IV infusion over 60–80 min once a wk. Do not mix with other drugs or diluting solutions. May contain large amounts of IgA; do not use in patients with known hypersensitivity to IgA. Human blood product; risk of transmitting

infectious agents. Transfusion reactions have been reported; reduce rate and monitor patient closely. Headache and dizziness are most common adverse reactions.

DANGEROUS DRUG
---

altretamine

Hexalen

Drug class and indications

Antineoplastic

Used as a single agent for the palliative treatment of patients with persistent or recurrent ovarian cancer following first-line treatment with cisplatin or alkylating agents.

Dosages and special alerts

260 mg/m^2/day PO given for 14 or 21 consecutive days of a 28-day cycle given as divided doses with meals and at bedtime. Consider an antiemetic or decreased dose if severe nausea or vomiting occur. ⊗ **Black box warning** Monitor blood counts and neurologic status frequently; risk of cytopenias, infections.

alvimopan

Entereg

Drug class and indications

Peripheral mu-opioid receptor antagonist

To accelerate upper and lower GI recovery following partial large- or small-bowel resection surgery with primary anastomosis.

Dosages and special alerts

12 mg PO given 30 min to 5 hr before surgery followed by 12 mg PO bid for up to 7 days to a maximum of 15 doses. For use in hospitalized patients only. Contraindicated in patients with more than 7 consecutive days of opioid therapy before treatment. Patients recently exposed to opioids will be more sensitive to drug effects and may experience nausea, vomiting, and diarrhea. Not recommended for patients with severe hepatic or renal disease. Risk of MI exists.

ambrisentan

Letairis

Drug class and indications

Endothelin receptor antagonist, antihypertensive

Treatment of pulmonary artery hypertension in patients with class II or III symptoms to improve exercise capacity and delay clinical worsening.

Dosages and special alerts

Initially, 5 mg/day PO; may be increased to 10 mg/day if needed and tolerated. Not recommended with moderate to severe hepatic impairment; risk of severe liver injury. Pregnancy category X; use of two forms of contraception advised. Available only through Letairis Access Program. ⊗ **Black box warning** Not for use in pregnancy.

amifostine

Ethyol

Drug class and indications

Cytoprotective drug

Reduction of renal toxicity associated with repeated administration of cisplatin in patients with advanced ovarian cancer; reduction of incidence of xerostomia in patients receiving radiation for head and neck cancers.

Unlabeled use: Protection of lung fibroblasts from effects of paclitaxel.

Dosages and special alerts

910 mg/m^2 IV daily as a 15-min infusion. Start within 30 min of starting chemotherapy. Monitor BP carefully; severe hypotension has been reported.

aminolevulinic acid hydrochloride

Levulan Kerastick

Drug class and indications

Photosensitizer

Treatment of nonkeratotic actinic keratoses of the face and scalp.

Dosages and special alerts

Must be applied in timing with blue light photodynamic illuminator; clean and dry area to be treated, break ampule, and apply solution with applicator provided. Light treatment must be done within the next 14–18 hr. One application of solution and one dose illumination per treatment site per 8-wk treatment session.

antihemophilic factor, recombinant

Advate, Xyntha

Drug class and indications
Antihemophilia drug

Prevention and control of bleeding episodes in hemophilia A; perioperative management of patients with hemophilia A.

Dosages and special alerts
Dosage is based on serum factor VIII level needed and body weight. See manufacturer's details. Antihemophilic factor required (international units) = body wt (kg) × desired factor VIII increase (% of normal) × 0.5.

antithrombin, recombinant

ATryn

Drug class and indications
Coagulation inhibitor

Prevention of perioperative and peripartum thromboembolic events in patients with hereditary antithrombin (AT) deficiency.

Dosages and special alerts
Loading dose given as a 15-min IV infusion based on AT level and body weight; maintenance dose given by continuous IV infusion to maintain AT activity levels between 80% and 120% of normal; perioperative: 100 − baseline AT ÷ 2.3 (for loading dose) or 10.2 (for maintenance) × body weight in kg; pregnant women: 100 − baseline AT ÷ 1.3 (loading dose) or 5.4 (maintenance) × body weight in kg. Contraindicated with allergy to goats or goat products; risk of hemorrhage and injection site reactions. Coagulation parameters must be followed closely.

DANGEROUS DRUG
antithrombin III

Thrombate III

Drug class and indications
Coagulation inhibitor

Treatment of patients with hereditary antithrombin III deficiency in connection with surgical or obstetric procedures or when they have thromboembolism.

Replacement therapy in congenital antithrombin III deficiency.

Dosages and special alerts
Dosage units = desired antithrombin level (%)—baseline ATIII level (%) × body weight (kg) divided by 1.4 every 2–8 days. Dosage varies greatly; frequent blood tests are needed

DANGEROUS DRUG
apixaban

Eliquis

Drug class and indications
Activated thrombin inhibitor, anticoagulant

Reduction of risk of stroke and systemic embolism in patients with nonvalvular atrial fibrillation

Dosages and special alerts
5 mg PO bid; patients over 80 yr, under 60 kg or with moderate renal impairment, 2.5 mg PO bid. Not for use with severe hepatic impairment, prosthetic heart valves. ⊗ **Black box warning** Increased risk of stroke and thrombotic events if discontinued in patient who are not continuing anticoagulation with other anticoagulants. Pregnancy Category B, but risk of bleeding at delivery, use not recommended. Not for use while breast feeding. Reduce dose with ketoconazole, itraconazole, ritonavir, clarithromycin; do not use with phenytoin, St Johns' Wort, rifampin, carbamazepine. Caution with any drug that alters bleeding. Serious to fatal bleeding possible. Warn patient not to stop drug suddenly; report any signs of bleeding.

apomorphine

Apokyn

Drug class and indications
Dopamine agonist, antiparkinsonism drug

Intermittent treatment of hypomobility, "off" episodes (drug wearing off) caused by advanced Parkinson disease.

Dosages and special alerts
2 mg by subcutaneous injection, increased slowly while monitoring BP to achieve control; maximum dose 6 mg. Give 300 mg trimethobenzamide PO tid from 3 days before starting apomorphine to completion of at least 2 mo

of therapy. Monitor patient for prolonged QT interval. GI effects common.

DANGEROUS DRUG

argatroban

Argatroban

Drug class and indications

Anticoagulant

Prophylaxis or treatment of thrombosis in heparin-induced thrombocytopenia; as an anticoagulant in patients at risk of heparin-induced thrombocytopenia undergoing percutaneous coronary intervention (PCI).

Dosages and special alerts

Dilute to concentration of 1 mg/mL; administer 2 mcg/kg/min as a continuous infusion. Monitor aPTT, usually achieves desired level within 1–3 hr; adjust dose of infusion to maintain a steady state aPPT that is 1.5–3 times the initial baseline value; do not exceed 10 mcg/kg/hr. Reduce initial dose to 0.5 mcg/kg/min with hepatic impairment. With PCI—25 mcg/kg/min with a bolus of 350 mcg/kg over 3–5 min. Excessive bleeding and hemorrhage may occur; monitor patient carefully for any sign of excess bleeding, decrease infusion rate or stop drug if excessive bleeding occurs.

DANGEROUS DRUG

arsenic trioxide

Trisenox

Drug class and indications

Antineoplastic

Induction and remission of acute promyelocytic leukemia in patients refractory to retinoid or anthracycline chemotherapy and whose leukemia is characterized by t(15;17) translocation or PML/RAR-alpha gene expression.

Dosages and special alerts

Induction: 0.15 mg/kg/day IV until bone marrow remission (maximum, 60 doses). Consolidation: 0.15 mg/kg/day IV starting 3–6 wk after completion of induction (maximum, 25 doses over 5 wk). Cardiac and CNS toxicity common; baseline and weekly ECG; biweekly electrolytes, CBC with differential and clotting profiles advised.

Avoid seafood and many alternative therapies (arsenic in many of these). Advise patient to avoid pregnancy, driving, or dangerous activities. ⊗ *Black box warning* Drug can be highly toxic and carcinogenic.

---

asparaginase *Erwinia chrysanthemi*

Erwinaze

Drug class and indications

Antineoplastic

Treatment of patients with acute lymphoblastic leukemia (ALL) who have developed hypersensitivity to *Escherichia coli*–derived asparaginase and pegaspargase used to treat ALL.

Dosages and special alerts

25,000 international units/m^2 IM three times a wk if substituting for pegaspargase; 25,000 international units/m^2 IM as substitute for each scheduled dose of *E. coli*–derived asparaginase. Contraindicated with history of serious pancreatitis, serious thrombosis, or serious hemorrhagic events with prior L-asparaginase therapy. Risk of serious hypersensitivity reactions; severe or hemmorhagic pancreatitis; glucose intolerance (monitor patient and treat hyperglycemia with insulin as needed); thrombosis or hemorrhage (discontinue therapy should either of these occur). GI complaints are common.

---

auranofin

Ridaura

Drug class and indications

Gold compound, antirheumatic

Management of adults with active classic or definite rheumatoid arthritis who have insufficient response to or intolerance to NSAIDs.

Dosages and special alerts

3 mg PO bid or 6 mg/day PO as a single dose; after 6 mo may be increased to 3 mg PO tid; do not exceed 9 mg/day. Monitor lung function, renal status, and blood counts. Protect patient from sunlight and UV exposure; systemic corticosteroids can be used for mild reactions. ⊗ *Black box warning* Discontinue drug at first sign of toxicity; severe bone marrow suppression, renal toxicity, and diarrhea are possible.

axitinib
Inlyta ⊞

Drug class and indications
Kinase inhibitor; antineoplastic

Treatment of advanced renal cell cancer after failure of one prior systemic therapy

Dosages and special alerts
Initially, 5 mg PO bid, spaced 12 hr apart, swallowed whole with a full glass of water. Thrombotic events, GI perforation and fistula, hypertensive crisis, hemorrhagic events, proteinuria, hepatotoxicity, reversible posterior leukoencephalopathy syndrome have occurred; monitor patient closely and be prepared to discontinue drug and provide supportive measures. Discontinue at least 24 hr before scheduled surgery. Pregnancy Category D: not for use in pregnancy. GI problems are very common.

DANGEROUS DRUG

azacitidine
Vidaza

Drug class and indications
Antineoplastic

Treatment of myelodysplastic syndrome including refractory anemias and chronic myelomonocytic leukemia.

Dosages and special alerts
75 mg/m^2/day by subcutaneous injection for 7 days every 4 wk; patients should receive at least four cycles. May be increased to 100 mg/m^2/day if no benefit after two cycles. Premedicate for nausea and vomiting. Monitor blood counts and adjust dosage as needed. Pregnancy should be avoided, and men taking this drug should not father children.

---

basiliximab
Simulect

Drug class and indications
Immunosuppressant, monoclonal antibody

Prophylaxis of acute rejection in renal transplant patients in combination with cyclosporine and corticosteroids.

Dosages and special alerts
Two doses of 20 mg IV with the first dose 2 hr before transplant, then 4 days after transplant. Drug must be given in combination with other immunosuppressant drugs. GI effects common.

DANGEROUS DRUG

BCG intravesical
TheraCys, Tice BCG

Drug class and indications
Antineoplastic

Treatment and prophylaxis for carcinoma in situ of the urinary bladder; prophylaxis of primary or recurrent Ta and T1 papillary tumors following transurethral resection; administered intravesically only.

Dosages and special alerts
Do not drink fluids for 4 hr before treatment; empty bladder before treatment. Instill 1 ampule, diluted as indicated in saline solution by catheter, allow to flow slowly. Have patient lie down for first hr, turning side to side, and then stay upright for 1 hr. Try to retain solution for 2 hr, and void retained solution trying not to splash liquid. Increase fluid intake for next few days. Monitor patient for local discomfort and reactions and for bone marrow depression and infection. ⊗ **Black box warning** Take precautions when handling drug; infection can occur.

---

bedaquiline
Sirturo ⊞

Drug class and indications
Antimycobacterial; antituberculosis drug

Treatment of adults with multidrug resistant pulmonary tuberculosis in combination with other antituberculosis drugs

Dosages and special alerts
400 mg/day PO for 2 wks, then 200 mg PO 3 x/wk for 22 weeks. ⊗ **Black box warning** Increased risk of death, reserve use for patients resistance to any other effective therapy. ⊗ **Black box warning** Increased QT interval and risk of serious to fatal arrhythmia; monitor patient, avoid use with other drugs that prolong QT interval. Pregnancy

Category B. Avoid use with rifampin, ketoconazole, lopinavir, ritonavir, drugs that prolong QT interval. Monitor heart rhythm; monitor LFTs. Nausea, arthralgia, headache are common.

belimumab

Benlysta

Drug class and indications

B-lymphocyte stimulator inhibitor; systemic lupus erythematosus drug (SLE)

Treatment of adult patients with active, autoantibody positive SLE who are receiving standard therapy; not for use with severe active lupus nephritis, severe active CNS lupus, or in combination with other biologics or IV cyclophosphamide.

Dosages and special alerts

10 mg/kg IV over 1 hr at 2-wk intervals for the first three doses, then at 4-wk intervals. Do not mix with other drugs or medical products; use a separate infusion line. Hypersensitivity reactions may occur; prophylaxis before each infusion is recommended. Increased risk of death, serious infections, depression, and suicidality. Nausea, diarrhea, fever, insomnia, URIs, and headache are most common adverse reactions. Do not give live vaccines to patient taking this drug.

DANGEROUS DRUG

bevacizumab

Avastin

Drug class and indications

Monoclonal antibody, antineoplastic

Used with 5-fluorouracil for first-line or second-line treatment of patients with metastatic carcinoma of the colon or rectum.

Used with paclitaxel and carboplatin for first-line treatment of unresectable, locally advanced recurrent or metastatic non-squamous, non–small-cell lung cancer.

Treatment of glioblastoma multiforme with progression following standard therapy.

Treatment of metastatic renal cell carcinoma with interferon-alfa.

Dosages and special alerts

For colon cancer, 5–10 mg/kg as an IV infusion every 14 days until disease progression is detected. First infusion over 90 min; second over 60 min; then infuse over 30 min. For lung cancer, 15 mg/kg as an IV infusion every 3 wk. For breast cancer: 10 mg/kg as an IV infusion every 14 days. Monitor blood counts and nutritional state. Patient may need treatment for constipation. May cause ovarian failure; discuss risk with patient. Increased risk of thrombotic events and osteonecrosis of the jaw in patients taking anticoagulants. ⊗ **Black box warning** High risk of serious to fatal GI perforations; risk of serious to fatal hemorrhage; reports of serious wound-healing complications. Monitor patient very closely.

DANGEROUS DRUG

bexarotene

Targretin

Drug class and indications

Antineoplastic

Treatment of the cutaneous manifestations of cutaneous T-cell lymphoma in patients refractory to at least one other systemic therapy.

Dosages and special alerts

300 mg/m^2 PO daily; may be increased to 400 mg/m^2 PO daily. Risk of serious pancreatitis, photosensitivity. ⊗ **Black box warning** Pregnancy Category X.

bicalutamide

Casodex

Drug class and indications

Antiandrogen

Treatment of advanced prostatic carcinoma in combination with LHRH analogue.

Dosages and special alerts

50 mg/day PO at the same time each day. Monitor liver function regularly. Administer only with LHRH analogue.

DANGEROUS DRUG

bivalirudin

Angiomax

Drug class and indications

Anticoagulant; thrombin inhibitor

Anticoagulation of patients undergoing percutaneous transluminal angioplasty who have unstable angina and who are receiving aspirin.

Treatment of patients with, or at risk for, heparin-induced thrombocytopenia and thrombosis syndromes who are undergoing percutaneous cardiac intervention.

Dosages and special alerts
0.75 mg/kg IV bolus, then 1.75 mg/kg/hr IV for duration of procedure; infusion can be continued for 4 hr after procedure. After 4 hr, IV infusion of 0.2 mg/kg/hr may be used for up to 20 hr, if needed. Reduce dosage with renal impairment. Give with aspirin. Monitor for excessive bleeding, which would indicate need to discontinue drug.

bosutinib
Bosulif ⓞⓝⓒ

Drug class and indications
Kinase inhibitor; antineoplastic

Treatment of adults with chronic-, accelerated-, or blast-phase Philadelphia chromosome-positive CML with resistance to or intolerance of prior therapy

Dosages and special alerts
500 mg/day PO with food. May increase to 600 mg/day with inadequate response; 200 mg/day PO with hepatic impairment. Risk of severe GI toxicity, bone marrow suppression, hepatotoxicity, fluid retention. Pregnancy Category D: not for use in pregnancy. GI problems, rash, fever, fatigue are common. Monitor patient for drug interactions with proton pump inhibitors, CY3PA inducers or inhibitors.

DANGEROUS DRUG
bortezomib
Velcade

Drug class and indications
Antineoplastic

Treatment of multiple myeloma or mantle cell lymphoma in patients who have received at least one prior therapy, or in those previously untreated.

Dosages and special alerts
1.3 mg/m² /dose IV twice weekly for 2 wk (days 1, 4, 8, and 11) followed by a 10-day rest (days

12–21); then repeat the cycle. Use lower dose with hepatic impairment. Monitor for peripheral neuropathies and thrombocytopenia; provide appropriate safety measures.

botulinum toxin type B (rimabotulinumtoxin B)
Myobloc

Drug class and indications
Skeletal muscle relaxant, direct acting

Reduction of the severity of abnormal head position and neck pain associated with cervical dystonia.

Dosages and special alerts
2,500–5,000 units IM, injected locally into affected muscles. Blocks cholinergic transmission between the nerve and muscle. Monitor for lack of muscle function, infection at injection site.
⊗ **Black box warning** Not for use in treatment of muscle spasms or cerebral palsy. Risk of botulinum toxicity if drug spreads from area of injection.

brentuximab vedotin
Adcetris

Drug class and indications
CD30-antibody drug conjugate; antineoplastic

Treatment of Hodgkin lymphoma after failure of autologous stem cell transplant or failure of at least two multidrug chemotherapy regimens

Treatment of systemic anaplastic large-cell lymphoma after failure of at least one prior multidrug chemotherapy regimen.

Dosages and special alerts
1.8 mg/kg IV over 30 min every 3 wk for maximum of 16 cycles or until disease progression or unacceptable toxicity. Infusion reaction possible; interrupt infusion and manage medically. Do not use with bleomycin; risk of pulmonary toxicity. Risk of peripheral neuropathy and neutropenia; monitor patient and adjust dosage as needed. Risk of tumor lysis syndrome, Stevens-Johnson syndrome. Do not use in pregnancy. Most common adverse effects include fatigue, nausea, URI, diarrhea, rash, vomiting, anemia, peripheral sensory neuropathy.
⊗ **Black box warning** Risk of progres-

sive multifocal leukoencephalopathy; report changes in mood, vision, coordination.

bumetanide

Burinex (CAN)

Drug class and indications
Loop diuretic

Treatment of edema associated with heart failure, hepatic and renal disease.

Unlabeled use: Treatment of adult nocturia; not effective in men with BPH.

Dosages and special alerts
0.5–2 mg/day PO as a single dose but may be repeated at 4- to 5-hr intervals if needed; maximum daily dose, 10 mg. Or 0.1 mg IV over 1–2 min or IM. May be repeated at 2- to 3-hr intervals if needed; maximum daily dose, 10 mg. Not for breast-feeding women. Provide supplemental potassium. Give early in the day so increased urination will not disrupt sleep. Dizziness, weakness, headache, hypotension, and hypokalemia are common adverse effects. ⊗ *Black box warning* Monitor patient closely for water and electrolyte depletion and hepatic dysfunction, especially with long-term use.

busPIRone

Apo-Buspirone (CAN)

Drug class and indications
Anxiolytic

Management of anxiety disorders or short-term relief of anxiety.

Unlabeled uses: PMS, traumatic brain injury.

Dosages and special alerts
Initially 7.5 mg PO bid. Increase at 2- to 3-day intervals by 5 mg/day to achieve desired effect. Usual range, 20–30 mg/day; do not exceed 60 mg/day. Advise patient to avoid alcohol, grapefruit juice, and OTC drugs. Usual adverse effects include mental changes, headache, insomnia, suicidality, dry mouth, GI upset, diarrhea, extrapyramidal effects. Suggest use of sugarless candies, analgesics for headache.

C1 esterase inhibitor (human)

Berinert, Cinryze

Drug class and indications
Proteinase inhibitor, blood product

Routine prophylaxis against angioedema attacks in adults and adolescents with hereditary angioedema.

Treatment of acute laryngeal attacks of hereditary angioedema (*Cinryze*).

Treatment of acute abdominal, facial, or laryngeal attacks of hereditary angioedema in adults and adolescents (*Berinert*).

Dosages and special alerts
Cinryze:

Berinert: 20 units/kg IV; do not use lower doses. 1,000 units IV every 3–4 days at rate of 1 mL/min. Monitor for immediate, potentially life-threatening hypersensitivity reactions (have epinephrine readily available). Associated risks include thrombotic events in patients with risk factors for thrombosis and potential for infectious agents in product because it is made from human plasma. Possible use for self-administration after training. Ensure proper disposal of needles, drug products.

cabazitaxel

Jevtana

Drug class and indications
Microtubular inhibitor, antineoplastic

In combination with oral prednisone for the treatment of patients with hormone-refractory metastatic prostate cancer previously treated with a docetaxel-containing regimen.

Dosages and special alerts
25 mg/m^2 as a 1-hr IV infusion every 3 wk. Pretreat with IV antihistamine, corticosteroid, and H$_2$ antagonist 30 min before each infusion; an antiemetic is also suggested. ⊗ *Black box warning* Severe hypersensitivity reactions have occurred; discontinue drug and support patient if these occur. Do not give to patient with a history of sensitivity reaction to this drug or to polysorbates. ⊗ *Black box warning* Severe neutropenia and deaths due to neutropenia have been reported; monitor neutrophil count and withhold

drug as appropriate. Patient may experience GI disturbances, renal failure, hepatic failure. Drug is pregnancy category D; not for use in pregnant women. Elderly patients are more likely to experience severe effects; monitor accordingly.

cabozantinib

Cometriq

Drug class and indications
Antineoplastic; kinase inhibitor
Treatment of patients with progressive, metastatic medullary thyroid cancer

Dosages and special alerts
140 mg/day PO. ⊗ **Black box warning** Risk of GI perforation, fistulas; severe to fatal hemorrhage has been reported Pregnancy Category D, not for use in pregnancy or while breast feeding. Avoid strong CYP3A4 inducers or inhibitors, including grapefruit juice. Monitor for thrombotic events, wound complications, hypertension, osteonecrosis of the jaw, hand-foot syndrome, proteinuria, reversible posterior leukoencephalopathy syndrome (RPLS). Common effects include hair color change, GI disturbances, fatigue, stomatitis.

canakinumab

Ilaris

Drug class and indications
Interleukin blocker
Treatment of cryopyrin-associated periodic syndrome in patients 4 yr and older, including familial cold autoinflammatory syndrome.
Treatment of Muckle-Wells syndrome.

Dosages and special alerts
40 kg and more: 150 mg by subcutaneous injection; 15–40 kg: 2 mg/kg by subcutaneous injection; children 15–40 kg with inadequate response: dose may be increased to 3 mg/kg. Injections are given every 8 wk. Patient may be at increased risk for infections. Do not give live vaccines to patient using this drug. URI symptoms are most common adverse effect.

carfilzomib

Kyprolis **ⓄⒷⒸ**

Drug class and indications
Proteasome inhibitor; antineoplastic
Treatment of multiple myeloma in patients who have received at least two prior therapies, including bortezomib and an immunomodulatory agent, and have demonstrated disease progression on or within 60 days of completing last therapy

Dosages and special alerts
Cycle 1: 20 mg/m^2/day IV over 2–10 min on 2 consecutive days each week for 3 weeks (days 1, 2, 8, 9, 15, 16) followed by a 12-day rest period. Cycle 2 and beyond: Increase to 27 mg/m^2/day IV over 2–10 min, following the same dosing days schedule. Premedicate with dexamethasone. Hydrate patient prior to and following treatment. Monitor patient closely and adjust dose based on toxicity. Risk of cardiac adverse reactions, pulmonary toxicity, pulmonary hypertension, tumor lysis syndrome, infusion reactions, thrombocytopenia, hepatic toxicity and failure. Pregnancy Category D; avoid pregnancy.

carglumic acid

Carbaglu

Drug class and indications
Carbamoyl phosphate synthetase 1 activator
Adjunctive therapy for the treatment of acute hyperammonemia due to the deficiency of hepatic *N*-acetylglutamate synthase; maintenance treatment of chronic hyperammonemia due to this deficiency.

Dosages and special alerts
100–250 mg/kg/day PO; adjust dosage based on patient response. Divide daily dose into two to four doses, and give before meals or feedings. Monitor ammonia levels regularly. Before treatment, protein is limited in the diet; once ammonia levels are stable, protein can be introduced. Patient may experience GI upset, fever, headache.

caspofungin acetate

Cancidas

Drug class and indications

Echinocandin, antifungal

Treatment of invasive aspergillosis in patients who are unresponsive to or who cannot tolerate standard therapy.

Treatment of esophageal candidiasis.

Treatment of candidemia and other *Candida* infections.

Empirical treatment when fungal infection is suspected in febrile and neutropenic patients.

Dosages and special alerts

Single loading dose of 70 mg IV, followed by daily IV infusion of 50 mg/day for at least 14 days. No loading dose is given for esophageal candidiasis. Monitor for IV complications. Use with cyclosporin is not recommended.

cellulose sodium phosphate (CSP)

Calcibind

Drug class and indications

Antilithic, resin exchange drug

Absorptive hypercalciuria type 1 (recurrent calcium oxalate or calcium phosphate stones).

Dosages and special alerts

15 g/day PO (5 g with each meal) in patients with urinary calcium exceeding 300 mg/day; reduce to 10 g/day PO (5 g with supper and 2.5 g with other meals) when urinary calcium falls to less than 150 mg/day. Caution patient to continue diet to moderate calcium oxalate intake; give supplemental magnesium gluconate while giving this drug; suspend powder in water, soft drink, or fruit juice and give 1 hr before the meal; urge patient to increase fluid intake.

certolizumab pegol

Cimzia

Drug class and indications

Tumor necrosis factor blocker, immune modulator

Reduction of the signs and symptoms of Crohn disease; maintenance of clinical response in adult patients with moderately to severely active disease who responded inadequately to conventional therapy.

Treatment of moderately to severely active rheumatoid arthritis in adults.

Dosages and special alerts

400 mg subcutaneously, repeated at wk 2 and 4; if clinical response occurs, maintenance dose of 400 mg subcutaneously every 4 wk.

⊗ **Black box warning** Associated risks include serious infections including infections caused by *Legionella* and *Listeria* bacteria; malignancies; and CNS demyelinating disorder. Prescreen for TB and hepatitis B and monitor patient closely.

cetrorelix acetate

Cetrotide

Drug class and indications

Fertility drug

Inhibition of premature LH surges in women undergoing controlled ovarian stimulation.

Dosages and special alerts

3 mg subcutaneously given with gonadotropins when serum estradiol levels show appropriate stimulation; if HCG is not given within 4 days, continue giving 0.25 mg/day subcutaneously until HCG is given or 0.25 mg subcutaneously morning or evening of stimulation day 5, or morning of stimulation day 6, continue daily until HCG is given. Patient or significant other should learn to give subcutaneous injections using the proper technique. Given only as part of overall fertility program.

DANGEROUS DRUG

cetuximab

Erbitux

Drug class and indications

Monoclonal antibody, antineoplastic

Monotherapy or in combination with irinotecan for the treatment of advanced epidermal growth factor receptor-expressing colorectal carcinoma.

With radiation for the treatment of locally or regionally advanced squamous cell carcinoma of the head and neck.

Monotherapy for recurrent or metastatic squamous cell cancer of the head and neck after failure of platinum therapy.

▪ **NEW INDICATION:** Treatment of recurrent regional disease or metastatic squamous cell carcinoma of the head and neck with platinum-based treatment as first-line therapy with 5-FU

Dosages and special alerts

400 mg/m^2 IV as a loading dose, infused over 120 min; weekly maintenance of 250 mg/m^2 IV infused over 60 min. Premedication with an antihistamine is recommended. Monitor for acute infusion reaction; interstitial pulmonary disease and dermatologic toxicity. ⊗ **Black box warning** Serious to fatal infusion reactions possible; discontinue with severe infusion reactions. ⊗ **Black box warning** Cardiopulmonary arrest has occurred in patients with head and neck cancers also receiving radiation and in patients with squamous cell cancer receiving platinum-based therapy; monitor electrolyte levels closely during and after infusion in those patients.

cevimeline hydrochloride

Evoxac

Drug class and indications

Parasympathomimetic

Treatment of symptoms of dry mouth in patients with Sjögren syndrome.

Dosages and special alerts

30 mg PO tid; administer with food if GI upset is severe; monitor swallowing; monitor patient for dehydration and provide supportive therapy.

chenodiol

Chenodal

Drug class and indications

Gallstone solubilizer

Treatment of select patients with radiolucent gallstones in well-opacifying gallbladders when elective surgery is contraindicated.

Dosages and special alerts

13–16 mg/kg/day in two doses, AM and PM. Start with 250 mg PO bid for 2 wk, then increase by 250 mg/day each wk. ⊗ **Black box warning** Hepatotoxicity is possible; drug not appropriate for many patients. Monitor liver function carefully. Discontinue if hepatitis occurs; caution patient to use barrier contraceptives and avoid pregnancy.

chlorproPAMIDE

Drug class and indications

Antidiabetic, sulfonylurea (first generation)

Adjunct to diet to lower blood glucose level in patients with type 2 diabetes mellitus.

Dosages and special alerts

250 mg/day PO. For maintenance therapy, 100–250 mg/day; do not exceed 750 mg/day. Not for pediatric use. May increase risk of CV events. Watch for possible hypoglycemia.

choline magnesium trisalicylate

Tricosal

Drug class and indications

NSAID, salicylate, antipyretic, analgesic

Treatment of osteoarthritis, rheumatoid arthritis; relief of moderate pain, fever.

Dosages and special alerts

Adults: For arthritis, 1.5–2.5 g/day PO in divided doses; do not exceed 4.5 g/day. For pain or fever, 2–3 g/day PO in divided doses.

Pediatric patients: Base dosage on patient's age; see manufacturer's guidelines. Usually 217.5–652.5 mg PO every 4 hr as needed.

GI effects common; give with meals to decrease them. Dizziness can also occur.

chorionic gonadotropin alfa (recombinant)

Ovidrel

Drug class and indications

Fertility drug

Induction of ovulation in infertile females who have been pretreated with FSH.

Induction of final follicular maturation and early luteinization in infertile women who have undergone pituitary desensitization and who have been appropriately pretreated with FSH.

Dosages and special alerts

250 mcg subcutaneously given 1 day following the last dose of a follicle-stimulating agent. Administer only when adequate follicular development has occurred. Do not administer if there is an excessive ovarian response. Inject into stomach area. Alert patient to risk of multiple births; patient should report shortness of breath, sudden abdominal pain, nausea, vomiting.

cidofovir
Vistide

Drug class and indications
Antiviral
Treatment of CMV retinitis in AIDS patients.

Dosages and special alerts

5 mg/kg IV infused over 1 hr once per wk for 2 wk; then 5 mg/kg IV every 2 wk. Probenecid must be given orally, 2 g PO before dose and 1 g at 2 and 8 hr after each dose. Maintain hydration. ⊗ *Black box warning* Monitor renal function closely; renal toxicity is common. Monitor neutrophils.

DANGEROUS DRUG
clofarabine
Clolar

Drug class and indications
Antimetabolite, antineoplastic
Treatment of patients ages 1–21 yr with ALL after at least two relapses from other regimens.

Dosages and special alerts

52 mg/m² by IV infusion over 2 hr daily for 5 consecutive days; repeat every 2–6 wk, based on recovery of baseline function. GI toxicity, bone marrow suppression, risk of infection are common.

coagulation factor VIIa (recombinant)
NovoSeven RT

Drug class and indications
Antihemophilic
Treatment of bleeding episodes in hemophilia A or B patients with inhibitors to factor VIII or factor IX.

Dosages and special alerts

70–90 mcg/kg as a slow IV bolus every 2 hr until hemostasis is achieved; continue dosing at 3- to 6-hr intervals after hemostasis in severe bleeds. Monitor for early signs of hypersensitivity reactions (hives, wheezing, hypotension, anaphylaxis).

collagenase clostridium histolyticum
Xiaflex

Drug class and indications
Proteinase enzyme
Treatment of adults with Dupuytren contraction with a palpable cord.

Dosages and special alerts

0.58 mg injected into the palpable cord; approximately 24 hr later, perform a finger extension procedure if the contraction still exists. May be repeated up to three times per cord at 4-wk intervals. Risk of tendon rupture and serious injury if injected into tendons, nerves, or other structures of the hand. Use with caution in patients taking anticoagulants. Patient may experience swelling and bruising at the injection site.

cosyntropin
Cortrosyn

Drug class and indications
Diagnostic agent
Diagnostic tests of adrenal function.

Dosages and special alerts

0.25–0.75 mg IV or IM or as an IV infusion of 0.04 mg/hr. Monitor for seizures, anaphylactoid reactions, excessive adrenal effects. Monitor plasma and urinary corticosteroid levels to determine adrenal function.

crofelemer
Fulyzaq ⓞⓝⓒ

Drug class and indications
Antidiarrheal
Relief of noninfectious diarrhea in adults with HIV/AIDS on antiretroviral therapy

Dosages and special alerts

125 mg/day PO, DR tablet. Swallow whole, not be to cut, crushed or chewed. Pregnancy Category C. Not for use while breast-feeding. Rule out infectious causes of diarrhea; ensure patient is on antiretroviral therapy. Cough, flatulence, bronchitis, URI common.

cromolyn sodium
Nalcrom (CAN), NasalCrom

Drug class and indications
Antiallergy drug

Prevention and treatment of allergic rhinitis, allergy eye disorders (ophthalmic).

Dosages and special alerts

1 spray in each nostril three to six times a day, as needed, or 1 to 2 drops in each eye four to six times a day as needed. Do not wear soft contact lenses if using ophthalmic preparation. Encourage continued use for optimal effects.

crizotinib
Xalkori

Drug class and indications
Tyrosine kinase inhibitor; antineoplastic

Treatment of locally advanced or metastatic non–small-cell lung cancer that is anaplastic lymphoma kinase–positive as detected by FDA approved *Vysis ALK Break Apart FISH Probe Kit*.

Dosages and special alerts

250 mg PO bid without regard to food. May reduce dosage to 200 mg PO bid based on patient safety and tolerability; 250 mg/day PO has been used in some cases. Ensure that patient has been tested for the appropriate sensitivity using the approved test. Not for use in pregnancy; fetal harm has occurred. Risk of serious to fatal pneumonitis; discontinue if this occurs. Risk of prolonged QT interval; monitor patient carefully. Liver toxicity can occur; monitor liver enzymes and reduce dosage or suspend dosing if enzyme elevations are high. Do not use with strong CYP3A inducers or inhibitors. Common adverse effects include nausea, vomiting, diarrhea or constipation (medication may be available to help); vision changes including blurry vision, light sensitivity, floaters, flashes of light. Advise patient

to use caution when driving or operating machinery if vision changes occur.

dalfampridine
Ampyra (BNC)

Drug class and indications
Potassium channel blocker

To improve walking in patients with multiple sclerosis (MS).

Dosages and special alerts

10 mg PO bid, approximately 12 hr apart; not for use with renal impairment. Tablet must be swallowed whole, not cut, crushed, or chewed; patient should not make up missed doses. Not for use in pregnancy or breast-feeding or in children. Patient may experience nausea, dizziness, headache, insomnia, balance disorder, relapse of MS. Risk of seizures, increased in patients with renal impairment; obtain baseline and periodic renal function tests; do not use in patients with history of seizures or moderate to severe renal impairment.

dapsone

Drug class and indications
Leprostatic

Treatment of Hansen disease.
Treatment of dermatitis herpetiformis.

Dosages and special alerts

50–100 mg/day PO (leprosy). 50 mg/day PO (dermatitis herpetiformis); 50–300 mg/day has been used. Children should not receive more than 100 mg/day. Monitor patients for bone marrow suppression and for the development of resistance if relapse occurs. Give with food to decrease GI upset. Drug will need to be used for prolonged time.

darunavir
Prezista

Drug class and indications
Antiviral, protesase inhibitor

Treatment of adults with advanced HIV disease with progression of disease following antiretroviral treatment; used with 100 mg ritonavir and combinations of other HIV drugs.

Dosages and special alerts

Treatment-experienced patients 600 mg PO bid with ritonavir 100 mg PO bid with food. Treatment-naïve patients: 800 mg PO daily with ritonavir 100 mg/day PO with food. Interacts with many other drugs; check drug regimen carefully before starting therapy. Monitor patient for rash, bone marrow suppression. Watch for increased bleeding in patients with hemophilia and glucose alterations in diabetics.

DANGEROUS DRUG

dasatinib

Sprycel

Drug class and indications

Kinase inhibitor, antineoplastic

Treatment of adults in all phases of CML (chronic, accelerated, or myeloid or lymphoid blast phase) with resistance or intolerance to prior treatment, given with imatinib.

Treatment of adults with Philadelphia chromosome–positive acute lymphoblastic leukemia (ALL) with resistance or tolerance to prior therapy and chronic phrase.

Dosages and special alerts

140 mg/day PO with or without food. Tablets should be swallowed whole, not cut, crushed, or chewed. Monitor patient for edema, excessive bleeding, bone marrow suppression. Increases risk of pulmonary artery hypertension; monitor according. Advise use of barrier contraceptives for both men and women using the drug.

DANGEROUS DRUG

DAUNOrubicin citrate

DaunoXome

Drug class and indications

Antineoplastic

First-line treatment of advanced HIV-associated Kaposi sarcoma.

Dosages and special alerts

40 mg/m^2 IV, infused over 1 hr; repeat every 2 wk. Decrease dose with renal or hepatic impairment. Monitor for extravasation; severe damage can occur. Do not use during pregnancy.
⊗ **Black box warning** Cardiac toxicity possible; monitor ECG and enzymes, and decrease dosage as needed.

DANGEROUS DRUG

decitabine

Dacogen

Drug class and indications

Antineoplastic antibiotic

Treatment of patients with myelodysplastic syndromes.

Dosages and special alerts

15 mg/m^2 IV, infused over 3 hr every 8 hr for 3 days. Repeat cycle every 6 wk for at least four cycles; may be continued as long as it benefits the patient. Premedicate patient with antiemetics. Monitor patient carefully for GI disturbances, bone marrow suppression.

---

deferasirox

Exjade

Drug class and indications

Chelate

Treatment of chronic iron overload due to blood transfusion (transfusional hemosiderosis) in patients 2 yr and older.

Dosages and special alerts

20 mg/kg/day PO. Therapy should be started when a patient has evidence of chronic iron overload as with transfusions of 100 mL/kg packed red cells. Maintenance: monthly serum ferritin levels should be drawn and dosage adjusted in steps of 5–10 mg/kg. If serum ferritin levels fall below 500 mcg/L, consider stopping therapy. Do not exceed 30 mg/kg/day. Monitor for changes in vision and hearing.
⊗ **Black box warning** May cause hepatic or renal impairment and GI hemorrhage, including fatal reactions. Monitor LFTs, renal function prior to, weekly for 2 wk, then monthly during therapy.

---

deferiprone

Ferriprox

Drug class and indications

Iron chelator

Treatment of transfusional iron overload due to thalassemia syndrome when standard chelation therapy is inadequate.

Dosages and special alerts

25–33 mg/kg PO tid for total daily dose of 75–99 mg/kg. Not for use in pregnant women because of possible harm to fetus; use of contraceptive measures is advised. Not for use in breast-feeding women; another method of feeding the baby should be found. Use cautiously with renal or hepatic impairment. GI upset, nausea, vomiting, joint pain, neutropenia are the most common adverse reactions. ⊗ *Black box warning* Can cause serious agranulocytosis with serious to fatal infections. Monitor neutrophil count and monitor patient for signs and symptoms of infection; interrupt therapy if infection or serious drop in neutrophil count occurs.

deferoxamine mesylate

Desferal

Drug class and indications

Chelate

Treatment of acute iron toxicity and chronic iron overload.

Dosages and special alerts

Acute toxicity: 1 g IM or IV, followed by 0.5 g every 4 hr for 2 doses, then every 4–12 hr based on patient response.
Chronic overload: 0.5–1 g IM qid; 2 g IV with each unit of blood or 20–40 mg/kg/day as a continuous subcutaneous infusion over 8–24 hr. IM preferred for acute intoxication; slow IV infusion for chronic overload. Monitor serum iron levels. Note that injection can be very painful.

degarelix

Degarelix for Injection, Firmagon

Drug class and indications

GnRH receptor antagonist, antineoplastic
Treatment of advanced prostate cancer.

Dosages and special alerts

Initially, 240 mg by subcutaneous injection, given as two separate 120-mg injections, followed by maintenance dose of 80 mg subcutaneously every 28 days. Pregnancy category X. Risk of prolonged QT interval. Injection site reactions, hot flashes, weight gain are common.

denileukin diftitox

Ontak

Drug class and indications

Biologic protein
Treatment of cutaneous T-cell lymphoma in patients whose cells express the CD25 component of the IL-2-receptor.

Dosages and special alerts

Adults: 9 or 18 mcg/kg/day IV over at least 30–60 min for 5 consecutive days every 21 days for eight cycles. Premedicate with antihistamine, acetaminophen. Monitor for capillary leak syndrome, serious infusion reactions, loss of visual acuity.
⊗ *Black box warning* Severe hypersensitivity reactions may occur; have life-support equipment available.

DANGEROUS DRUG

desirudin

Iprivask

Drug class and indications

Anticoagulant; thrombin inhibitor
Prevention of DVT in patients undergoing elective hip replacement.

Dosages and special alerts

15 mg every 12 hr by subcutaneous injection, initial dose given 5–15 min before surgery but after induction of anesthesia; give for 9–12 days. Administer by deep subcutaneous injection; alternate sites. Monitor blood clotting daily and protect from injury. ⊗ *Black box warning* Risk of epidural or spinal hematomas with long-term or permanent paralysis. Carefully weigh benefits and risks before using epidural or spinal anesthesia or spinal puncture.

DANGEROUS DRUG

dexmedetomidine hydrochloride

Precedex

Drug class and indications

Sedative, hypnotic
Sedation of initially intubated and mechanically ventilated patients during treatment in an ICU setting.

Dosages and special alerts

1 mcg/kg infused over 10 min, then 0.2–0.7 mcg/kg/hr using a controlled infusion device for up to 24 hr; drug is not indicated for use longer than 24 hr.

dexrazoxane

Totect

Drug class and indications

Lyopilizate

Treatment of extravasation resulting from IV anthracycline chemotherapy.

Dosages and special alerts

Given IV once daily for 3 days. *Day 1:* 1,000 mg/m^2; maximum dose, 2,000 mg. *Day 2:* 1,000 mg/m^2; maximum dose, 2,000 mg. *Day 3:* 500 mg/m^2; maximum dose, 1,000 mg. Infuse over 1–2 hr. Reduce dose by 50% in patients with creatinine clearance less than 40 mL/min. Monitor patient for bone marrow suppression, fever, and pain and burning at injection site. Do not give to pregnant women or nursing mothers.

dihydroergotamine mesylate

D.H.E. 45, Migranal

Drug class and indications

Ergot derivative, antimigraine drug

Acute treatment of migraine headaches with or without aura; acute treatment of cluster headache (parenteral).

Dosages and special alerts

1 mg IM, IV, or subcutaneously at first sign of headache; may repeat at 1-hr intervals for a total of 3 mg. Or one spray (0.5 mg) in each nostril followed by another spray in each nostril 15 min later for a total of 3 mg. Be aware of possible coronary artery vasoconstriction. Numbness, tingling are common. If patient has nausea or vomiting, give drug with an antiemetic. ⊗ *Warning* Serious to life-threatening peripheral ischemia possible when combined with potent CYP3A4 inhibitors; this combination is contraindicated.

dimercaprol

BAL in Oil

Drug class and indications

Antidote, chelate

Treatment of arsenic, gold, mercury poisoning.

Treatment of acute lead poisoning when used with calcium edetate disodium.

Treatment of acute mercury poisoning if used within the first 1–2 hr.

Dosages and special alerts

2.5–5 mg/kg IM qid for 2 days, taper to bid for 10 days. Can cause severe renal damage; alkalinize urine to increase chelated complex excretion. Use extreme caution with children.

dipyridamole

Dipridacot (CAN), Persantine

Drug class and indications

Antianginal, antiplatelet, diagnostic agent

With warfarin to prevent thromboembolism in patients with prosthetic heart valves; diagnostic aid to assess CAD in patients unable to exercise.

Dosages and special alerts

75–100 mg PO qid to prevent thromboembolism. For CAD, 0.142 mg/kg/min IV, infused over 4 min. Continually monitor patient receiving IV form. Give oral drug at least 1 hr before meals. Warn patient about possible lightheadedness.

dornase alfa

Pulmozyme

Drug class and indications

Cystic fibrosis drug

Management of respiratory symptoms of cystic fibrosis in conjunction with other drugs; treatment of advanced cystic fibrosis.

Dosages and special alerts

2.5 mg daily through a nebulizer; may increase to 2.5 mg bid in patients 5 yr or older. Store drug in the refrigerator. Make sure the patient knows how to use the nebulizer properly. Continue other treatments for cystic fibrosis.

doxercalciferol
Hectorol

Drug class and indications
Vitamin D analogue

Reduction of elevated intact parathyroid hormone (iPTH) levels in the management of secondary hyperparathyroidism in patients undergoing chronic renal dialysis; secondary hyperparathyroidism in patients with stage 3 or 4 chronic kidney disease who do not need dialysis.

Dosages and special alerts
With dialysis: 10 mcg three times per wk at dialysis. Maximum, 20 mcg three times per wk. Regulate dose by iPTH levels. Monitor carefully for hypercalcemia (arrhythmias, seizures, calcifications). Without dialysis: 1 mcg PO daily; adjust dosage based on PTH levels. Maximum dose, 3.5 mcg/day.

droperidol

Drug class and indications
Antiemetic

Dosages and special alerts
2.5 mg IM or IV. Use caution with renal or hepatic failure. Monitor patient for hypotension. Onset 3–10 min, recovery 2–4 hr; patient may have drowsiness, chills, or hallucinations during recovery. ⊗ *Black box warning* May prolong QT interval; monitor appropriately.

ecallantide
Kalbitor

Drug class and indications
Plasma kallikrein inhibitor

Treatment of acute attacks of hereditary angioedema in patients 16 yr and older.

Dosages and special alerts
30 mg by subcutaneous injection given as three 10-mg injections; may be repeated once in 24 hr. ⊗ *Black box warning* Risk of severe anaphylaxis; should only be given by health care provider familiar with anaphylaxis and with full medical support readily available. Patient may

also experience headache, nausea, diarrhea, injection-site reactions.

eculizumab
Soliris

Drug class and indications
Monoclonal antibody, complement inhibitor

Treatment of patients with paroxysmal nocturnal hemoglobinuria to reduce hemolysis.

Treatment of atypical hemolytic uremic syndrome.

Dosages and special alerts
Paroxysmal nocturnal hemoglobinemia: 600 mg IV over 35 min every 7 days for first 4 wk, followed by 900 mg IV as fifth dose 7 days later, and then 900 mg IV every 14 days.

Atypical hemolytic uremic syndrome: 900 mg IV weekly for first 4 wk, followed by 1,200 mg IV as fifth dose 1 wk later; then 1,200 mg IV every 2 wk.

⊗ *Black box warning* Patient must have had recent meningococcal vaccine before starting therapy; drug increases risk of infection. Monitor patient for early signs of meningococcal infection. Stopping drug can cause serious hemolysis; must monitor patient for 8 wk after stopping drug.

eltrombopag
Promacta

Drug class and indications
Thrombopoietin receptor agonist

Treatment of chronic immune idiopathic thrombocytopenic purpura in patients who have insufficient response to conventional therapies, including splenectomy.

Dosages and special alerts
50 mg PO once daily; may be increased to a maximum 75 mg/day. Patients of eastern Asian ancestry or with mild to moderate hepatic dysfunction should be started on 25 mg/day PO. May increase the risk of bone marrow–related malignancies; monitor CBC carefully. ⊗ *Black box warning* Risk of severe to fatal hepatotoxicity exists; monitor patient very closely and adjust dosage or discontinue drug if liver enzymes start to rise. Drug available only through limited distribution programs.

enzalutamide

Xtandi ඕ

Drug class and indications
Androgen receptor inhibitor; antineoplastic
Treatment of patients with metastatic, castration-resistant prostate cancer who have recently received docetaxel

Dosages and special alerts
160 mg/day PO once daily. Patient must swallow capsules whole. Pregnancy Category X: not for use in pregnancy. Interacts with many drugs; check drug regimen carefully before use. Pain, diarrhea, peripheral edema, dizziness, anxiety, hypertension, spinal cord compression have been reported.

DANGEROUS DRUG

epirubicin hydrochloride

Ellence

Drug class and indications
Antineoplastic, antibiotic
Adjunctive therapy in patients with evidence of axillary node tumor involvement after resection of primary breast cancer.

Dosages and special alerts
100–120 mg/m² IV given in repeated 3- to 4-wk cycles, all on day 1; given with cyclophosphamide and 5-fluorouracil. Premedicate with antiemetics and antibiotics; encourage patient to drink plenty of fluids. Alert patient that hair loss may occur. ⊗ *Black box warning* Cardiac toxicity can occur; obtain baseline ECG. Monitor for bone marrow suppression. Severe local cellulitis can occur with extravasation; discontinue immediately if burning or stinging occurs.

epoprostenol sodium (prostacyclin, PGX, PGI₂)

Flolan, Veletri

Drug class and indications
Prostaglandin

Treatment of primary pulmonary hypertension in patients unresponsive to standard therapy.

Dosages and special alerts
2 ng/kg/min with increases in increments of 2 ng/kg as tolerated using a portable infusion pump through a central venous catheter; 20–40 ng/kg/min common dosage after 6 mo of continuous therapy. Teach patient and significant other the proper maintenance and use of infusion pump; ensure that therapy is continuous. Headache, muscle aches, and pains are common.

ergotamine tartrate

Ergomar

Drug class and indications
Ergot derivative, antimigraine drug
Prevention or abortion of vascular headaches, such as migraine and cluster headaches.

Dosages and special alerts
One tablet (2 mg) under the tongue soon after the first symptoms, with subsequent doses at 30-min intervals. Do not exceed 3 tablets/day or 10 mg/week. Nausea and numbness and tingling are common. CV effects, including chest pain, may occur. Drug is Pregnancy Category X. ⊗ *Black box warning* Serious to life-threatening peripheral ischemia has occurred when administered with potent CYP3A4 inhibitors; this combination is contraindicate.

eribulin mesylate

Halaven

Drug class and indications
Microtubular inhibitor, antineoplastic
Treatment of patients with metastatic breast cancer who have previously received at least two chemotherapeutic regimens for the treatment of metastatic disease.

Dosages and special alerts
1.4 mg/m² IV over 2–5 min on days 1 and 8 of a 21-day cycle. Do not administer with dextrose-containing solutions. Reduce dosage in patients with hepatic or renal impairment. Not for use in pregnancy or breast-feeding.

Monitor patient for bone marrow suppression, which is common; adjust dosage as needed. Establish baseline ECG as QT-interval prolongation may occur; do not administer with other drugs that prolong QT interval. Watch for peripheral neuropathy; manage with dose delay or dosage adjustment. Alopecia may occur; GI upset is common.

DANGEROUS DRUG

erlotinib

Tarceva

Drug class and indications
Monoclonal antibody, antineoplastic

Treatment of patients with locally advanced or metastatic non–small-cell lung cancer after failure of at least one course of chemotherapy.

In combination with gemcitabine for first-line treatment of locally advanced, unresectable, or metastatic pancreatic cancer.

Dosages and special alerts
Non–small-cell lung cancer: 150 mg/day PO on an empty stomach. Monitor for potentially serious interstitial lung disease. GI effects are common.
Pancreatic cancer: 100 mg/day PO on an empty stomach with IV gemcitabine.
Risk of GI perforation, Stevens-Johnson syndrome, ocular disorders.

ethacrynic acid

Edecrin

Drug class and indications
Loop, high ceiling diuretic

Treatment of edema associated with HF, cirrhosis, renal disease; acute pulmonary edema; ascites associated with malignancy, idiopathic edema, lymphedema; short-term management of congenital heart disease in children.

Dosages and special alerts
50–200 mg/day PO, based on patient response. IV use in adults: 50 mg IV run slowly over several min to a maximum of 100 mg. Oral use in children, 25 mg/day, adjust in 25 mg increments as needed. Give oral dose with food or milk. Monitor weight and output regularly. Monitor potassium levels and provide replacement as needed.

everolimus

Afinitor, Zortress

Drug class and indications
Kinase inhibitor, antineoplastic

Treatment of advanced renal cell carcinoma after failure with sunitinib or sorafenib (*Afinitor*).

Treatment of subependymal giant-cell astrocytoma in patients who are not candidates for surgery (*Afinitor*).

Treatment of progressive neuroendocrine pancreatic tumors that cannot be removed surgically or that are metastatic (*Afinitor*).

Prevention of organ rejection in adults at low to moderate immunologic risk receiving a kidney transplant (*Zortress*).

■ **NEW INDICATION:** Treatment of patients 1 yr and older with tuberous sclerosis complect who have developed a brain tumor (*Afinitor Disperz*).

■ **NEW INDICATION:** Treatment of noncancerous kidney tumors (renal angiomyolipomas) not requiring immediate surgery in patients with tuberous sclerosis complex (*Afinitor*).

■ **NEW INDICATION:** Treatment of postmenopausal women with advanced hormone receptor–positive, HER2 -negative breast cancer with recurrence or progression after treatment with letrozole or anastrazole (*Afinitor*).

Dosages and special alerts
10 mg PO once daily with food. May be decreased to 5 mg/day to manage adverse effects or with moderate hepatic impairment. For renal transplant: 0.75 mg PO bid with cyclosporine starting as soon as possible after transplant (*Zortress*). Patients with tuberous sclerosis complex: 4.5 mg/m^2/day. Pregnancy Category D; fetal harm can occur. Risk of pneumonitis, serious to fatal infections, oral ulcerations, and elevations in blood glucose, lipid, and serum creatinine levels. Patients must be monitored very closely. Avoid use with strong CYP3A4 inhibitors; increase dose to a maximum 20 mg/day (*Afinitor*) if drug must be given with strong CYP3A4 inducers. Do not give live vaccines to patient taking this drug. ⊗ **Black box warning** *Zortress* only: Risk of serious infections, cancer development, including lymphoma and skin cancers; risk of nephrotoxicity with cyclosporine; risk of venous thrombosis and loss of kidney, usually

within 30 days. Increased mortality when used for heart transplant patients; not for use in heart transplant patients.

exemestane
Aromasin

Drug class and indications
Antineoplastic
Treatment of advanced breast cancer in postmenopausal women whose disease has progressed following tamoxifen therapy.

Dosages and special alerts
25 mg PO every day with meals. May be antagonized by estrogens. Avoid use during premenopause or with renal or hepatic impairment. Hot flashes, GI upset, anxiety, depression, headache are common.

factor XIII concentrate (human)
Corifact

Drug class and indications
Clotting factor
Routine prophylactic treatment of congenital factor XIII deficiency.

Dosages and special alerts
Individualize dosage based on patient weight, lab values, and clinical condition. Initially, 40 units/kg IV over not less than 4 mL/min; base subsequent dosing on patient response (see manufacturer's details). Do not mix with other drugs or medical products; use a separate infusion line. Hypersensitivity reactions may occur; discontinue drug and offer supportive care. Most common adverse effects include fever, chills, headache, arthralgia, increase in liver enzyme levels. Thrombotic events have occurred. Product is made from human blood, so may carry risk of transmission of blood-borne agents and Creutzfeldt-Jakob disease.

ferumoxytol
Feraheme

Drug class and indications
Iron replacement product

Treatment of iron deficiency anemia in adults with chronic renal failure.

Dosages and special alerts
510 mg IV, followed by 500 mg IV 3–8 days later depending on patient response. Infuse as undiluted injection at 30 mg/sec (1 mL/sec). May be readministered if indicated by persistent or recurrent anemia. Risk of iron overload; blood pressure changes are common. Monitor patient carefully for possible hypersensitivity reactions for 30 min after infusion. Drug is a superparamagnetic iron oxide that can alter MRI results and interpretation for up to 3 mo following administration; does not interfere with CAT scans or regular X-rays.

fibrinogen concentrate, human
RiaSTAP

Drug class and indications
Coagulation factor
Treatment of acute bleeding episodes in patients with congenital fibrinogen deficiency, including afibrinogenemia and hypofibrinogenemia.

Dosages and special alerts
70 mg/kg by slow IV injection, not to exceed 5 mL/min; dosage adjusted to a target fibrinogen level of 100 mg/dL. Risk of thrombotic events, severe hypersensitivity reactions. Drug is prepared from pooled human plasma; patient should be aware of potential infection risk.

floxuridine
FUDR

Drug class and indications
Antimetabolite, antineoplastic
Palliative management of GI adenocarcinoma metastatic to the liver that is incurable by surgery or other means.

Dosages and special alerts
0.1–0.6 mg/kg/day per intra-arterial infusion; continue until adverse effects occur, and resume when adverse effects resolve. Monitor bone marrow status; warn patient of possible severe GI effects.

fludrocortisone acetate
Florinef Acetate

Drug class and indications
Corticosteroid, hormone, mineralocorticoid
Partial replacement therapy in primary and secondary adrenocortical insufficiency.
Treatment of salt-losing adrenogenital syndrome with glucocorticoid therapy.

Dosages and special alerts
Adrenocortical insufficiency: 0.1 mg/day PO; may decrease to 0.05 mg/day PO if hypertension occurs. Salt-losing adrenogenital syndrome: 0.1–0.2 mg/day PO. Always use in conjunction with glucocorticoid therapy. Risk of increased fluid volume, headaches, tendon contractures. Discontinue at any sign of overdose (hypertension, edema, excessive weight gain, increased heart size). If infants or children are maintained on long-term therapy, monitor growth and development closely.

follitropin alfa
Gonal-F, Gonal-F REF Pen

Drug class and indications
Fertility drug
Induction of ovulation, stimulation, and development of multiple follicles for in vitro fertilization.
Also used to increase spermatogenesis in men with hypogonadism.

Dosages and special alerts
Ovulation induction: 75 international units/day subcutaneously, increase by 37.5 international units/day after 14 days; may increase again after 7 days; do not exceed 35 days of treatment.
Follicle development: 150 international units/day subcutaneously on days 2 or 3 and continue for 10 days. In patients whose endogenous gonadotropin levels are suppressed, initiate at 225 international units/day subcutaneously. Adjust dose after 5 days based on patient response; dosage should be adjusted no more than every 3–5 days and by no more than 75–150 international units at each adjustment. Maximum, 450 international units/day; then give 5,000–10,000 units HCG.
Spermatogenesis: 150 international units subcutaneously three times per wk in conjunction with HCG. May increase to 300 international units three times per wk, as needed. May administer up to 18 mo for adequate effect. Pregnancy category X. Explain risk of multiple births; risk of arterial thromboembolism.

follitropin beta
Follistim AQ, Puregon (CAN)

Drug class and indications
Fertility drug
Induction of ovulation, stimulation and development of multiple follicles for in vitro fertilization.

Dosages and special alerts
Ovulation induction: 75 international units/day subcutaneously, increase by 37.5 international units/day after 14 days; do not exceed 35 days of treatment.
Follicle development: 150–225 international units/day subcutaneously or IM for at least 4 days of treatment. Adjust dose based on ovarian response; then give 5,000–10,000 international units. HCG: maintenance dosage of 375–600 international units/day subcutaneously or IM may be necessary. Drug is Pregnancy Category X. Give subcutaneously in navel or abdomen. Warn patients of risk of multiple births.

fomepizole
Antizol

Drug class and indications
Antidote
Antidote for antifreeze (ethylene glycol) poisoning or for use in suspected poisoning.
Antidote for methanol poisoning.

Dosages and special alerts
15 mg/kg IV loading dose followed by doses of 10 mg/kg IV every 12 hr for 12 doses given as a slow IV infusion over 30 min. Start immediately after diagnosis is made. Headache, nausea, and dizziness are common. Consider hemodialysis as added therapy.

gadobutrol
Gadavist

Drug class and indications
Contrast agent

Diagnostic contrast agent in adults and children older than 2 yr to detect and visualize areas with disrupted blood-brain barrier or abnormal vascularity of the CNS

Dosages and special alerts

IV dosage is based on body weight, 0.1 mL/kg; given as an IV bolus injection at 2 mL/sec. Flush line with normal saline after injection. May cause fetal harm. Most common reactions are headache, nausea, feeling hot, injection-site reaction. Monitor patient for potentially serious hypersensitivity reactions. ⊗ *Black box warning* Increased risk of nephrogenic systemic fibrosis; contraindicated in patients with chronic, severe kidney disease or acute renal injury. Screen renal function before use.

galsulfase
Naglazyme

Drug class and indications
Enzyme

Treatment of patients with mucopolysaccharidosis VI to improve walking and stair climbing capacity.

Dosages and special alerts
1 mg/kg once weekly by IV infusion, diluted and infused over 4 hr. Patient should receive antihistamine with or without an antipyretic 30–60 min before the infusion begins.

ganirelix acetate

Drug class and indications
Fertility drug

Inhibition of premature LH surges in women undergoing controlled ovarian overstimulation as part of a fertility program.

Dosages and special alerts
250 mcg subcutaneously once daily starting on day 2 or 3 of the cycle. Drug is Pregnancy Category X. Teach patient to administer subcutaneous injections. Abdominal pain is a common adverse effect.

DANGEROUS DRUG

gefitinib
Iressa

Drug class and indications
Antineoplastic

Monotherapy for treatment of patients with locally advanced or metastatic non–small-cell lung cancer who have been receiving the drug and have been doing well. No longer available for initiating therapy.

Dosages and special alerts
250 mg/day PO with or without food. Monitor pulmonary function; potentially fatal interstitial lung disease possible. Eye pain and corneal erosion also reported.

glatiramer acetate
Copaxone

Drug class and indications
MS drug

Reduction of frequency of relapses in patients with relapsing or remitting MS.

Treatment of patients who have experienced a first clinical episode of MS and who have MRI features consistent with MS.

Dosages and special alerts
20 mg/day by subcutaneous injection; rotate injection sites. Photosensitivity may occur.

glucarpidase
Voraxaze

Drug class and indications
Carboxypeptidase enzyme

Treatment of toxic plasma methotrexate concentrations in patients with delayed methotrexate clearance due to impaired renal function

Dosages and special alerts
Single IV injection of 50 units/kg. Continue hydration and alkalinization of urine; do not administer leucovorin within 2 hr before or after glucarpidase. Serious allergic reactions have been reported; monitor patient closely during and directly after injection. Use in pregnancy

only if clearly needed. Paresthesia, flushing, nausea and vomiting, hypotension, and headache are common.

gold sodium thiomalate
Aurolate

Drug class and indications
Gold compound, antirheumatic

Treatment of select, early cases of adult and juvenile rheumatoid arthritis.

Dosages and special alerts
Weekly IM injections: 10 mg IM wk 1, 25 mg IM wk 2 and 3; then 25–50 mg/wk IM to a total dose of 1 g. Maintenance injections of 25–50 mg IM every other wk for 2–30 wk, may change to every third or fourth wk if response is adequate. Pediatric dosing: 10 mg IM test dose, then 1 mg/kg/wk IM; do not exceed 50 mg/dose. Injection reactions are common. Protect patient from sunlight and UV exposure; systemic corticosteroids can be used to manage mild reactions. ⊗ **Black box warning** Monitor lung, renal function and blood counts; discontinue at first sign of toxicity.

DANGEROUS DRUG
histrelin implant
Vantas

Drug class and indications
Gonadotrophic-releasing hormone used as antineoplastic.

Palliative treatment of advanced prostate cancer.

Dosages and special alerts
One implant inserted subcutaneously and left in for 12 mo. May be removed and a new implant inserted after 12 mo. Monitor for insertion site reactions. Patient may be at increased risk for CV events, including MI and stroke. Monitor accordingly. Contraindicated in pregnant and pediatric patients.

hyaluronic acid derivatives
Euflexxa, Hyalgan, Orthovisc, Supartz, Synvisc, Synvisc One

Drug class and indications
Glycosamine polysaccharide

Treatment of pain in osteoarthritis of the knee in patients who have failed to respond to other therapies.

Dosages and special alerts
2 mL by intra-articular injection in knee once weekly for a total of 3–5 injections. Use caution with latex allergies. Joint swelling may occur; avoid strenuous activities or prolonged weight bearing for 48 hr. Headache may occur.

hyaluronidase
Amphadase, Hylenex, Vitrase

Drug class and indications
Enzyme

Used to increase absorption and dispersion of injected drugs.

For hypodermoclysis.

Used as an adjunct in subcutaneous urography for improving the resorption of radiopaque agents.

Dosages and special alerts
Absorption of injected drugs: Adults: Add 150 units of hyaluronidase to the injection solution. Pediatric patients: Add 150 units of hyaluronidase to the injection solution, may be added to small amounts up to 200 mL. Do not administer with dopamine or alpha adrenergic drugs. Monitor the patient for local reactions.

Hypodermoclysis: Adults: 150 units injected under the skin, close to the clysis. Pediatric patients younger than 3 yr: limit single clysis to 200 mL; premature infants or during the neonatal period: do not exceed 25 mL/kg at a rate no greater than 2 mL/min. Use care to avoid overhydration by controlling rate and volume. Do not administer with dopamine or alpha adrenergic drugs. Monitor the patient for local reactions.

Adjunct to subcutaneous urography: 75 units injected subcutaneously over each scapula, followed by injection of the contrast media at the same sites.

hydroxocobalamin

Cyanokit

Drug class and indications

Antidote

Treatment of known or suspected cyanide poisoning.

Dosages and special alerts

5 g (2 vials) by IV infusion over 15 min; a second dose may be given if needed by IV infusion over 15–120 min, based on patient condition. Warn patient that urine will be red for up to 5 wk after treatment. Skin and mucous membranes may be red up to 2 wk after treatment; protect from sun exposure during this period.

hydroxyethyl starch in sodium chloride

Voluven

Drug class and indications

Colloid, plasma expander

Treatment and prophylaxis of hypovolemia.

Dosages and special alerts

Begin IV infusion slowly to monitor patient for anaphylactic reaction; base daily dosage and rate of infusion on patient's blood loss, hemodynamics, and hemodilution effects. Up to 50 mL/kg/day (3,500 mL for a 70-kg patient). For children, 7–25 mL/kg/day IV has been used. Monitor patient very closely, and adjust rate based on response. Watch for hypervolemia and anaphylactoid reactions.

DANGEROUS DRUG

ibritumomab

Zevalin

Drug class and indications

Monoclonal antibody, antineoplastic

Treatment of patients with relapsed or refractory low-grade follicular transformed B-cell non-Hodgkin lymphoma.

Treatment of patients with previously untreated follicular non-Hodgkin lymphoma who experience relapse to first-line therapy.

Dosages and special alerts

Single infusion of 250 mg/m² rituximab preceding a fixed dose of 5 mCi/kg ibritumomab as a 10-min IV push. Administer a second cycle 7–9 days later. Premedicate with acetaminophen and diphenhydramine before each rituximab infusion. ⊗ **Black box warning** Risk of serious infusion reactions, including fatalities; serious prolonged cytopenias; and cutaneous and mucocutaneous reactions. Monitor patient continuously.

icatibant

Firazyr

Drug class and indications

Peptidomimetic; bradykinin antagonist

Treatment of acute attacks of hereditary angioedema in adults

Dosages and special alerts

30 mg subcutaneously at first sign of an attack. May give additional dose at intervals of at least 6 hr if response is inadequate or symptoms recur. Use cautiously in patients with coronary artery disease, history of stroke. Injection-site reaction very common.

icosapent ethyl

Vascepa ⓞⓝⓒ

Drug class and indications

Ethyl ester; antihyperlipidemic

Adjunct to diet to reduce triglyceride levels in adults with severe (500 mg/dL or higher) hypertriglyceridemia

Dosages and special alerts

2 g PO bid with food. Patient should swallow capsules whole and not cut, crush, or chew them. Use caution with hepatic impairment; monitor LFTs carefully. Use caution with known hypersensitivity to fish or shellfish. May affect bleeding time; closely monitor patients taking drugs that affect coagulation. Arthralgia is common.

idursulfase

Elaprase

Drug class and indications

Enzyme, Hunter syndrome drug

Treatment of patients with Hunter syndrome (mucopolysaccharidosis II).

Dosages and special alerts
0.5 mg/kg IV every week, infused over 1–3 hr. First infusion should be at 8 mL/hour (must be diluted in 100 mL of 0.9% sodium chloride injection) for the first 15 min; then increase by 8 mL/hr at 15-min intervals if patient tolerates infusion; do not exceed 100 mL/hr. Drug improves walking capacity. ⊗ **Black box warning** Risk of serious anaphylactoid reactions; start therapy slowly, and monitor patient closely.

iloprost
Ventavis

Drug class and indications
Vasodilator

Treatment of pulmonary arterial hypertension in patients with New York Heart Association classes III to IV symptoms to improve composite endpoints.

Dosages and special alerts
2.5 mcg inhaled using the *ProDose* or *I-neb AAD system*. May be increased to 5 mcg; repeat inhalation 6–9 times/day while awake. Maximum dose 45 mcg/day. Monitor exercise and activity tolerances.

infliximab
Remicade

Drug class and indications
Monoclonal antibody

Used to reduce the signs and symptoms of moderate to severe Crohn disease in adults and children who do not respond adequately to conventional therapy.

Treatment of rheumatoid arthritis (RA) together with methotrexate as a first-line therapy.

Treatment of patients with fistulizing Crohn disease.

Used to reduce signs and symptoms, inhibit structural damage, and improve physical functioning of active arthritis in patients with psoriatic arthritis.

Used to reduce the signs and symptoms, and decrease the corticosteroid use in patients with moderately to severely active ulcerative colitis.

Treatment of moderately to severely active ulcerative colitis in children older than 6 yr who have inadequate response to conventional therapy.

Dosages and special alerts
5 mg/kg IV over 2 hr given once (Crohn disease). May repeat dose with fistulating or psoriatic arthritis disease at 2 wk and 6 wk after first dose, then every 8 wk with psoriatic arthritis or Crohn disease. 3 mg/kg IV followed by 3 mg/kg at 2 and 6 wk, then every 8 wk (RA). 5 mg/kg IV at 0, 2, and 6 wk for induction, followed by 5 mg/kg IV every 8 wk for maintenance (ulcerative colitis). Do not use in patients with allergy to mouse protein. Discontinue if lupus-like reaction occurs. ⊗ **Black box warning** There is an increased risk of malignancies and infections, including infections caused by *Legionella* and *Listeria* bacteria; monitor patient closely.

insoluble Prussian blue
Radiogardase

Drug class and indications
Ferric hexacyanoferrate

Treatment of patients with known or suspected contamination with radioactive cesium or radioactive or nonradioactive thallium to increase their rates of elimination.

Dosages and special alerts
Adults and children 12 yr and older: 3 g PO tid. Children 2–12 yr: 1 g PO tid. Prevent constipation; stool will be blue. If capsules cannot be swallowed, contents may be added to food and eaten. Alert patient that teeth and mouth may become blue. Protect others from contamination by flushing toilet several times with each use, washing hands carefully, and cleaning up any spilled urine, blood, or feces.

interferon alfacon-1
Infergen

Drug class and indications
Interferon, immune modulator

Treatment of chronic hepatitis C in patients 18 yr and older with compensated liver disease and HCV antibodies.

Dosages and special alerts

9 mcg by subcutaneous injection three times per wk for 24 wk; at least 48 hr should separate doses. Monitor for possible severe adverse reactions. Monitor for suicidal ideation and take appropriate precautions. Tell female patients to use contraceptives. Treat nausea and vomiting as needed. ⊗ *Black box warning* May cause or aggravate fatal or life-threatening neuropsychiatric, autoimmune, ischemic, and infectious disorders.

ipilimumab

Yervoy

Drug class and indications

Cytotoxic T-cell antigen 4–blocking antibody

Treatment of unresectable or metastatic melanoma

Dosages and special alerts

3 mg/kg IV over 90 min every 3 wk for a total of four doses. Suggest use of contraceptives. Patient should not breast-feed during therapy. Common adverse effects include fatigue, diarrhea, pruritus, rash, colitis. ⊗ *Black box warning* Can cause severe to fatal immune-mediated reactions involving many organs that may occur during treatment or weeks to months after treatment ends. Permanently discontinue drug and treat with high-dose systemic corticosteroids if signs and symptoms of immune reactions appear. Establish baseline LFT, thyroid function, skin condition, and endocrine and GI function; assess regularly for changes.

iron sucrose

Venofer

Drug class and indications

Iron salt

Treatment of iron deficiency anemia in patients undergoing chronic hemodialysis or peritoneal dialysis who are receiving supplemental erythropoietin therapy and non-dialysis dependent chronic renal failure patients with or without erythropoietin.

Dosages and special alerts

100 mg (5 mL) IV, one to three times per wk, during dialysis. Administer slowly, 1 mL over

2–5 min. Non-dialysis patients receive 1,000 mg IV over 14 days given as 200 mg IV on 5 different days. Serious to fatal hypersensitivity reactions have occurred. Administer test dose and monitor patient carefully during administration.

isocarboxazid

Marplan

Drug class and indications

MAOI

Treatment of depression (not a first choice for initial treatment).

Dosages and special alerts

Up to 40 mg PO daily. Dosage can usually be reduced after 3–4 wk because drug effects are cumulative. Not a first-line treatment for depression because of potential for serious adverse effects and food interactions. Might be useful in patients unable to tolerate newer and safer antidepressants. Patient must be given list of tyramine-containing foods. ⊗ *Black box warning* Increased risk of suicidality in children and adolescents; monitor accordingly.

ivacaftor

Kalydeco

Drug class and indications

Cystic fibrosis transmembrane conductance regulator (CFTR) potentiator

Treatment of cystic fibrosis in patients 6 yr and older with G55ID mutation in the CFTR gene

Dosages and special alerts

150 mg PO every 12 hr with fat-containing food; reduce dose with severe hepatic impairment, concurrent use of moderate or strong CYP3A inhibitors. Not for use with patients who do not express this mutation. Liver toxicity possible. URI, nasopharyngitis, abdominal pain with diarrhea and nausea, dizziness common. Patient should avoid grapefruit juice while taking this drug.

ivermectin
Stromectol

Drug class and indications
Anthelmintic
Treatment of intestinal strongyloidiasis.
Treatment of onchocerciasis.

Dosages and special alerts
Strongyloidiasis: 200 mcg/kg PO as a single dose.
Onchocerciasis: 150 mcg/kg PO as a single dose; may be repeated in 3–12 mo if needed. Give with a full glass of water. Nausea and vomiting very common. Instruct patient to use barrier contraceptives while on this drug.

ixabepilone
Ixempra

Drug class and indications
Antineoplastic, microtubule inhibitor
As monotherapy or with capecitabine for the treatment of metastatic or locally advanced breast cancer after failure of anthracycline and a taxane.

Dosages and special alerts
40 mg/m² IV infused over 3 hr every 3 wk. Premedicate with corticosteroids. Adjust dosage based on blood counts. ⊗ **Black box warning** Severe liver failure possible; monitor for bone marrow suppression, neuropathies, cardiac effects. Pregnancy Category D.

lanreotide acetate
Somatuline Depot

Drug class and indications
Hormone, growth hormone (GH) inhibitor
Long-term treatment of acromegaly in patients who have had inadequate response to or cannot be treated with surgery or radiation therapy.

Dosages and special alerts
Initially, 90 mg (range, 60–120 mg) subcutaneously every 4 wk for 3 mo; adjust dosage based on GH or insulin growth factor-1 level. Reduce dose with renal or hepatic impairment. Risk of gallstones, thyroid suppression, hypoglycemia,

hyperglycemia, bradycardia. Monitor GH and insulin growth factor-1 serum levels to establish dosage.

lanthanum carbonate
Fosrenol

Drug class and indications
Phosphate binder
Reduction of serum phosphate levels in patients with end stage renal disease.

Dosages and special alerts
750–1,500 mg/day PO in divided doses taken with meals. Titrate to achieve desired serum phosphate levels. Chew tablets thoroughly. GI upset may occur.

DANGEROUS DRUG
lapatinib
Tykerb

Drug class and indications
Kinase inhibitor, antineoplastic
With capecitabine, for treatment of patients with advanced or metastatic breast cancer whose tumors overexpress HER2 and who have received treatment including an anthracycline, a taxane, and trastuzumab.

In combination with letrozole for treatment of hormone-positive and HER2-positive advanced breast cancer in postmenopausal women for whom hormonal therapy is indicated.

Dosages and special alerts
1,250 mg (5 tablets) PO once daily 1 hr before or after meals on days 1–21. On days 1–14, given with capecitabine 2,000 mg/m²/day PO in two doses about 12 hr apart. Give in repeating 21-day cycle. Reduce lapatinib dosage to 750 mg/day PO with severe hepatic impairment. Stop drug if left ventricular ejection fraction (LVEF) is grade 2 or higher or it falls below lower limit of normal; may be restarted at 1,000 mg/day after at least 2 wk if LVEF returns to normal. Monitor heart function. Rash and GI upset common. Numerous drug interactions possible; avoid grapefruit juice. ⊗ **Black box warning** Severe to fatal hepatotoxicity has been reported; monitor patient accordingly.

laronidase
Aldurazyme

Drug class and indications
Enzyme

Treatment of patients with Hurler and Hurler-Scheie forms of mucopolysaccharidosis 1 and for patients with Scheie form who have moderate to severe symptoms.

Dosages and special alerts
0.58 mg/kg IV, infused over 3–4 hr, once each wk. Infusion reaction common, antipyretic and antihistamine given 60 min before infusion helps; regular follow-up essential; drug improves respiratory function and walking capacity. ⊗ *Black box warning* Life-threatening anaphylactic reactions have occurred; ensure appropriate medical support is available during infusion.

lenalidomide
Revlimid

Drug class and indications
Immune modulator, antianemic

Treatment of patients with transfusion-dependent anemia due to low or intermediate-1-risk myelodysplastic syndromes associated with a deletion of 5q cytogenetic abnormality with or without additional cytogenetic abnormalities.

Treatment of multiple myeloma, with dexamethasone, in patients who have received at least one other therapy.

Dosages and special alerts
Patients with anemia: 10 mg/day PO with water. Dosage may need to be lowered based on patient response and blood counts. Female patients must be tested to ensure that they are not pregnant and must agree to use two forms of contraception while using this drug. Male patients must agree to use contraceptive measures while using this drug.
Patients with multiple myeloma: 25 mg/day PO on days 1–21 of a 28-day cycle with dexamethasone 40 mg/day PO on days 1–4, 9–12, and 17–20 for first four cycles; for remaining cycles, given only on days 1–4.
Patients with renal impairment: Patient should be monitored closely and dosage adjusted down-

ward as needed. ⊗ *Black box warning* Increased risk of new secondary cancers, including acute leukemias, lymphomas, when used in patients with newly diagnosed multiple myeloma. Associated with serious birth defects; only dispensed through the Revassist Program and requires frequent pregnancy tests and signed agreement of understanding of risks; risk of PE, DVTs. Patient cannot donate blood or sperm.

DANGEROUS DRUG

lepirudin
Refludan

Drug class and indications
Anticoagulant

Treatment of heparin-induced thrombocytopenia associated with thromboembolic disease; a rare allergic reaction to heparin; directly inhibits thrombin.

Dosages and special alerts
0.4 mg/kg initial IV bolus followed by a continuous infusion of 0.15 mg/kg for 2–10 days. Monitor for bleeding from any sites; watch for hepatic injury. Reduce dosage with renal failure. Increased risk of bleeding if combined with chamomile, garlic, ginger, ginkgo biloba, or ginseng therapy.

levoleucovorin
Fusilev

Drug class and indications
Folate analogue, rescue drug

To diminish the toxicity and counteract the effects of impaired methotrexate elimination and of inadvertent overdosage of folic acid antagonists after high-dose methotrexate therapy in osteosarcoma.

■ NEW INDICATION: In combination with 5-FU for palliative treatment of patients with advanced metastatic colorectal cancer; dose is one-half the usual dose.

Dosages and special alerts
Serum methotrexate level of 10 micromolars at 24 hr, one micromolar at 48 hr, and less than 0.2 micromolar at 72 hr after methotrexate administration: 7.5 mg IV every 6 hr for 60 hr. (Ten doses starting at 24 hr after start of methotrexate.)

Serum methotrexate level remaining about 0.2 micromolar at 72 hr and more than 0.05 micromolar at 96 hr after methotrexate administration: Continue 7.5 mg IV every 6 hr until the methotrexate level is less than 0.05 micromolar.

Serum methotrexate level of 50 micromolars or more at 24 hr or 5 micromolars or more at 48 hr after administration, or a 100% or greater increase in serum creatinine level at 24 hr after methotrexate administration: 75 mg IV every 3 hr until methotrexate is less than 1 micromolar. Then 7.5 mg IV every 3 hr until methotrexate is less than 0.5 micromolar.

Inadvertent methotrexate overdose: 7.5 mg IV every 6 hr beginning within 24 hr of overdosage. Continue until methotrexate levels are within nontoxic range. Administer slowly because of high calcium levels in solution.

linaclotide

Linzess

Drug class and indications
Guanylate cyclase agonist; IBS drug
  Treatment of IBS with constipation; treatment of chronic idiopathic constipation

Dosages and special alerts
IBS: 290 mcg/day PO on an empty stomach at least 30 min before first meal of the day. Chronic idiopathic constipation: 145 mcg/day PO on an empty stomach at least 30 min before first meal of the day. Avoid use with mechanical obstruction of the GI tract. Diarrhea is commonly seen. May cause abdominal pain, abdominal distention, flatulence. ⊗ **Black box warning** Contraindicated for children younger than 6 yr and not recommended for children 6–17 yr; associated with death in young mice.

lincomycin hydrochloride

Lincocin

Drug class and indications
Lincosamide antibiotic
  Treatment of serious infections that are responsive to lincomycin, when less toxic antibiotics are not effective.

Dosages and special alerts
Adult: 600 mg IM every 12–24 hr, or 600 mg–1 g IV every 8–12 hr. Pediatric: 10 mg/kg IM every 12–24 hr, or 10–20 mg/kg/day IV in divided doses. ⊗ **Black box warning** Serious colitis can occur; have metronidazole or vancomycin and corticosteroids available; monitor for stomatitis. Evaluate patient for *Clostridium difficile* infection if diarrhea occurs.

lomitapide

Juxtapid

Drug class and indications
Antitriglyceride agent
  Adjunct to low fat diet and other lipid lowering treatments to reduce LDL, total cholesterol, apolipoprotein B and non-HDL cholesterol in patients with homozygous familial hypercholesterolemia

Dosages and special alerts
Initially 5 mg/d PO, increase to 10 mg/d after at least 2 wk, then at a minimum of 4 wk intervals to 20 mg, 40 mg then 60 mg/d. ⊗ **Black box warning** Increased elevations in transaminases, monitor closely and stop drug with significant liver toxicity; risk of hepatic steatosis and cirrhosis; available only through restricted access program. Pregnancy category X, ensure patient is not pregnant and agrees to use of barrier contraceptives; not for use while breast-feeding; GI effects can be severe and limit absorption of oral drugs. Strong CYP3A4 inhibitors contraindicated with use; avoid grapefruit juice, warfarin, limit dose of simvastatin, lovastatin; separate bile acid sequestrants by at least 4 hr

lutropin

Luveris

Drug class and indications
Luteinizing hormone, fertility drug
  Used in combination with *Gonal-f* to stimulate follicle development in hypogonadotropic hypogonadal women as part of a fertility regimen.

Dosages and special alerts

75 international units subcutaneously daily with 75–150 international units *Gonal-f* for up to 14 days per cycle. Monitor for ovarian overstimulation; there is a risk for multiple births.

mecasermin

Increlex

Drug class and indications

Insulin-like growth factor-1

Long-term treatment of growth failure in children with severe primary insulin growth factor-1 deficiency or with growth hormone gene deletion who have developed neutralizing antibodies to growth hormone.

Dosages and special alerts

Dosage is based on individual response and glucose levels. Initially, 0.04–0.08 mg/kg (40–80 mcg/kg) bid by subcutaneous injection; may be increased by 0.04 mg/kg per dose to a maximum dose of 0.12 mg/kg bid. Hypoglycemia is common, monitor patient and ensure that patient eats after administration; tonsillar hypertrophy is common.

mesna

Mesnex

Drug class and indications

Cytoprotective drug

Prophylaxis to reduce the incidence of ifosfamide-induced hemorrhagic cystitis.

Unlabeled use: Reduction of the incidence of cyclophosphamide-induced hemorrhagic cystitis.

Dosages and special alerts

20% ifosfamide dose IV at the time of ifosfamide injection and at 4 and 8 hr after that. Timing needs to be exact. Monitor for any signs of bladder hemorrhage.

methazolamide

Neptazane

Drug classes and indications

Glaucoma drug, carbonic anhydrase inhibitor

Adjunct treatment of chronic open angle glaucoma, secondary glaucoma.

Preoperative use in acute angle-closure glaucoma where delay in surgery is desired to lower IOP.

Lowering of IOP in conditions where lowering pressure would be beneficial (*Neptazane*).

Dosages and special alerts

50–100 mg PO bid or tid as needed to achieve best results. Administer with food if GI upset is a problem. Arrange for regular evaluation of IOP.

methoxsalen

8-MOP, Oxsoralen, Oxsoralen-Ultra, Uvadex

Drug class and indications

Psoralen

Symptomatic treatment of severe disabling psoriasis refractory to other forms of therapy; repigmentation of vitiliginous skin.

Treatment of cutaneous cell lymphoma.

Unlabeled use: With ultraviolet A radiation (UVAR), treatment of mycosis fungoides.

Orphan drug use: With UVAR photophoresis to treat diffuse systemic sclerosis; prevention of acute rejection of cardiac allografts.

Dosages and special alerts

Oral: Dosage varies with weight; dosing must be timed to coincide with UV light exposure. Do not expose patient to additional UV light. GI effects are very common. ⊗ ***Black box warning*** Methoxsalen and UV radiation should only be used by health care providers with special competence in the diagnosis and treatment of psoriasis and vitiligo. Reserve use for severe, disabling, recalcitrant psoriasis.

methsuximide

Celontin

Drug class and indications

Antiepileptic, succinimide

Control of absence seizures when refractory to other drugs.

Dosages and special alerts

300 mg/day PO for the first wk; may increase to a maximum of 1.2 g/day as needed. Reduce dosage slowly, do not stop suddenly. Discontinue

drug if rash, altered blood count, unusual depression, or aggression occurs. May be used with other antiepileptic drugs. Increased risk of suicidality.

methylnaltrexone bromide
Relistor

Drug class and indications
Opioid receptor antagonist, laxative

Treatment of opioid-induced constipation in patients with advanced illness receiving palliative care when response to laxative therapy has not been sufficient.

Dosages and special alerts
Dosage depends on weight. 38–less than 62 kg: 8 mg by subcutaneous injection every other day. 62–114 kg: 12 mg by subcutaneous injection every other day. If weight falls outside the above limits: 0.15 mg/kg per dose by subcutaneous injection every other day. Reduce dose by one-half with severe renal impairment. Monitor for severe diarrhea.

metyrosine
Demser

Drug class and indications
Enzyme inhibitor

Preoperative preparation for surgery for pheochromocytoma.

Management of pheochromocytoma when surgery is contraindicated.

Chronic treatment of malignant pheochromocytoma.

Dosages and special alerts
250–500 mg PO qid. Preoperative: 2–3 g/day PO for 5–7 days. Maximum, 4 g/day. Ensure a liberal intake of fluids. Severe diarrhea may occur; use antidiarrheals if needed.

midodrine
ProAmatine

Drug class and indications
Alpha agonist, antihypotensive

Treatment of symptomatic orthostatic hypotension in patients whose lives are impaired by this disorder and who have not responded to other therapy.

Dosages and special alerts
10 mg PO tid during daytime hours when upright; reduce dose to 2.5 mg PO tid with renal impairment. Risk of bradycardia, paresthesia, pruritus, dysuria, chills. Patient should empty bladder before taking drug. Patient should report changes in vision, pounding headache, very slow heart rate. ⊗ **Black box warning** Can cause marked elevation in supine blood pressure. Use should be reserved for patients whose lives are considerably impaired despite standard treatment.

miglustat
Zavesca

Drug class and indications
Enzyme inhibitor

Treatment of adult patients with mild to moderate type I Gaucher disease for whom enzyme replacement is not a therapeutic option.

Dosages and special alerts
100 mg PO tid at regular intervals. Monitor for diarrhea, weight loss, and tremor; dosage may need to be reduced. Drug is Pregnancy Category X and it may also alter men's fertility. Caution patient about tremor development.

milnacipran
Savella

Drug class and indications
Selective serotonin and norepinephrine reuptake inhibitor

Management of fibromyalgia in adults.

Dosages and special alerts
Initially, 12.5 mg/day PO; increase over 1 wk to recommended dose of 50 mg PO bid. Doses up to 200 mg/day have been used. ⊗ **Black box warning** Increased risk of suicidality; monitor patient accordingly. Avoid use with MAO inhibitors and in patients with uncontrolled narrow-angle glaucoma. Serotonin syndrome has been reported. Headache, nausea,

constipation, dizziness, insomnia, dry mouth, and palpitations are common.

DANGEROUS DRUG

mitotane

Lysodren

Drug class and indications

Antineoplastic

Treatment of inoperable hormone-secreting or hormone-non-secreting adrenal cortical carcinomas.

Dosages and special alerts

2–6 g/day PO in divided doses tid to qid, slowly increased to 9–10 g/day; if no benefits are seen by 3 mo, consider another form of treatment. Birth defects have been reported with use; suggest use of contraceptives. ⊗ **Black box warning** Discontinue temporarily in times of severe stress; adrenal hormone replacement may be needed in times of stress.

nefazodone

Drug class and indications

Antidepressant

Treatment of depression.

Dosages and special alerts

200 mg/day PO in divided doses, may be increased at 1-wk intervals to 300–600 mg/day. Limit available doses for severely depressed patients, and take suicide precautions. Use caution to assure at least 14 days between MAOI and nefazodone use and at least 7 days between stopping nefazodone and starting MAOIs. ⊗ **Black box warning** Watch for signs of hepatic impairment, and stop drug immediately if they occur. Increased risk of suicidality, suicidal ideation.

DANGEROUS DRUG

nelarabine

Arranon

Drug class and indications

Antimitotic drug, antineoplastic

Treatment of patients with T-cell acute lymphoblastic leukemia and T-cell lymphoblastic lymphoma whose disease has not responded to or has relapsed following treatment with at least two chemotherapy regimens.

Dosages and special alerts

Adults: 1,500 mg/m^2 IV over 2 hr on days 1, 3, and 5; repeat every 21 days. Pediatric patients: 650 mg/m^2 IV over 1 hr daily for 5 consecutive days; repeat every 21 days. Bone marrow suppression common. ⊗ **Black box warning** Watch for neurologic toxicity, including neuropathies and demyelination disorders.

nesiritide

Natrecor

Drug class and indications

Human B-type natriuretic peptide, vasodilator

Treatment of patients with acutely decompensated HF with dyspnea at rest or with minimal activity.

Dosages and special alerts

2 mcg/kg IV bolus followed by a continuous infusion of 0.01 mcg/kg/min for no longer than 48 hr. Monitor patient continuously. Discontinue if serious hypotension occurs, which could worsen condition. Maintain hydration. Replace any reconstituted solution every 24 hr.

nilotinib

Tasigna

Drug class and indications

Kinase inhibitor, antineoplastic

Initial treatment of chronic phase and accelerated phase Philadelphia chromosome–positive CML in adults resistant to or intolerant of prior therapy that included imatinib or for treatment at first diagnosis.

Dosages and special alerts

400 mg PO bid, about 12 hr apart, without food. Dosage may need adjustment based on myelosuppression during therapy. Watch for bone marrow suppression and possible liver toxicity. ⊗ **Black box warning** Risk of prolonged QT interval and sudden death. Obtain baseline and periodic ECG; monitor electrolytes levels.

nimodipine

Drug class and indications
Calcium channel blocker

Improvement of neurologic deficits due to spasm following a subarachnoid hemorrhage (SAH) from ruptured congenital intracranial aneurysm.

Dosages and special alerts
60 mg PO every 4 hr, beginning within 96 hr of SAH for 21 consecutive days. Monitor for cardiac effects (arrhythmias, hypotension). If patient is unable to take oral medications, remove contents of capsule using a needle and empty contents into nasogastric tube; flush with 30 mL normal saline. ⊗ **Black box warning** Do not administer by parenteral routes. Death and serious, life-threatening adverse reactions have occurred when capsule contents have been injected parenterally.

nitazoxanide

Alinia

Drug class and indications
Antiprotozoal

Treatment of diarrhea caused by *Cryptosporidium parvum* in patients 1 yr and older.

Treatment of *Giardia lamblia* in pediatric patients 1–11 yr.

Dosages and special alerts
Patients 12–47 mo: 5 mL (100 mg nitazoxanide) PO every 12 hr for 3 days. Patients 4–11 yr: 10 mL (200 mg nitazoxanide) PO every 12 hr for 3 days. Patients 12 yr and older: 500 mg (tablet or suspension) PO every 12 hr for 3 days taken with food. Obtain stool for ova and parasite testing before beginning therapy. To reconstitute, tap bottle until all powder flows freely; add about 24 mL of water to bottle and shake vigorously to suspend powder; add remaining 24 mL of water and shake vigorously again. Use cautiously with diabetic patients; suspension contains sucrose. Give drug with food. Advise parents to use good hand-washing technique and to dispose of diapers properly, when appropriate.

ofatumumab

Arzerra

Drug class and indications
Cytotoxic monoclonal antibody, antineoplastic

Treatment of chronic lymphocytic leukemia refractory to standard therapy.

Dosages and special alerts
12 doses given by IV infusion using the following schedule: 300 mg, followed in 1 wk by 2,000 mg/wk for seven doses, followed 4 wk later by 2,000 mg every 4 wk for four doses. Premedicate patient with acetaminophen, antihistamines, and IV corticosteroids. Infusion reaction is common; bone marrow suppression and infections, including progressive multifocal leukoencephalopathy and activation of hepatitis B, can occur; rash and GI effects are most common.

olsalazine sodium

Dipentum

Drug class and indications
Anti-inflammatory

Maintenance of remission of ulcerative colitis in patients intolerant to sulfasalazine.

Dosages and special alerts
1 g/day PO, divided into two doses. Give with meals. Monitor patient for renal impairment. Abdominal pain common.

omacetaxine mepesuccinate

Synribo⦿

Drug class and indications
Protein synthesis inhibitor; antineoplastic

Treatment of adults with chronic- or accelerated-phase chronic myeloid leukemia with resistance to or intolerance of two or more tyrosine kinase inhibitors

Dosages and special alerts
Induction: 1.25 mg/m^2 subcutaneously bid for 14 consecutive days of a 28-day cycle. Maintenance: 0.25 mg/m^2 subcutaneously bid for 7 consecutive days of a 28-day cycle. Adjust dosage

based on toxicity. Pregnancy Category D; use of barrier contraceptives is advised. Myelosuppression, bleeding, hyperglycemia can occur; monitor patient accordingly. Nausea, vomiting, diarrhea, fever, injection-site reactions, bone marrow depression are common.

omalizumab

Xolair

Drug class and indications

Monoclonal antibody, antiasthmatic

To decrease asthma exacerbation in patients 12 yr and older with moderate to severe persistent asthma who have a positive skin test to a perennial airborne allergen, who are not controlled by inhaled corticosteroids.

Dosages and special alerts

150–375 mg by subcutaneous injection every 2–4 wk, based on body weight and pretreatment immunoglobulin E levels. Discontinue and arrange for appropriate therapy at first sign of severe allergic reaction. Solution is thick; complete injection may take 5–10 sec. Do not use during pregnancy or lactation. ⊗ **Black box warning** Anaphylaxis with bronchospasm, hypotension, syncope, urticaria, and edema may occur. Monitor patient after administration; have medical support readily available.

oprelvekin

Neumega

Drug class and indications

Interleukin

Prevention of severe thrombocytopenia and reduction of platelet transfusions following myelosuppressive chemotherapy in patients with nonmyeloid malignancies at high risk to develop severe thrombocytopenia.

Dosages and special alerts

50 mcg/kg/day subcutaneously starting 1 day after chemotherapy and continuing for 14–21 days or until platelet count is at least 50,000 cells/mm^3. Protect patient from exposure to infection; urge the use of contraceptives. ⊗ **Black box warning** Drug may cause severe allergic reaction, including anaphylaxis.

DANGEROUS DRUG

oxaliplatin

Eloxatin

Drug class and indications

Antineoplastic

Treatment of patients with metastatic carcinoma of the colon or rectum whose disease has progressed during or within 6 mo of completion of first-line therapy with 5-fluorouracil (5-FU)/leucovorin (LV) and irinotecan; first-line therapy for advanced colorectal cancer with 5-FU and LV.

Dosages and special alerts

85 mg/m^2 IV infusion in 250–500 mL D$_5$W with leucovorin 200 mg/m^2 in D$_5$W both given over 2 hr followed by 5-FU 400 mg/m^2 IV bolus over 2–4 min, followed by 5-FU 600 mg/m^2 IV infusion in 500 mL D$_5$W as a 22-hr continuous infusion on day 1, then leucovorin 200 mg/m^2 IV infusion over 2 hr followed by 5-FU 400 mg/m^2 bolus given over 2–4 min, followed by 5-FU 600 mg/m^2 IV infusion in 500 mL D$_5$W as a 22-hr continuous infusion on day 2; repeat cycle every 2 wk. Premedicate with antiemetics and dexamethasone. ⊗ **Black box warning** Monitor for potentially dangerous anaphylactic reactions; reactions may occur within minutes of administration.

palifermin

Kepivance

Drug class and indications

Keratinocyte growth factor

To decrease the incidence and duration of severe oral mucositis in patients with hematologic malignancies receiving myelotoxic chemotherapy requiring hematopoietic stem cell support.

Dosages and special alerts

60 mcg/kg/day by IV bolus infusion for 3 consecutive days before and 3 consecutive days after chemotherapy regimen. Monitor for rash and mouth changes such as taste alteration.

DANGEROUS DRUG

panitumumab
Vectibix

Drug class and indications
Monoclonal antibody, antineoplastic

Treatment of epidermal growth factor receptor–expressing metastatic colorectal carcinoma with disease progressing with or after chemotherapy regimens containing fluoropyrimidine, cisplatin, and irinotecan.

Dosages and special alerts
6 mg/kg IV over 60 min every 14 days; doses larger than 1,000 mg should be given over 90 min. Dosage should be adjusted in patients experiencing infusion reactions or severe adverse reactions. ⊗ *Black box warning* Monitor patient for possibly severe infusion reactions, dermatologic toxicity, pulmonary fibrosis.

paricalcitol
Zemplar

Drug class and indications
Vitamin

Prevention and treatment of secondary hyperparathyroidism associated with chronic renal failure.

Dosages and special alerts
0.04–0.1 mcg/kg injected during dialysis, not more often than every other day. Patients not on dialysis: 1–2 mcg/day PO or 2–4 mcg PO three times a wk, based on parathyroid levels. Monitor for hypercalcemia, treat appropriately. Ensure adherence to dietary regimen and use of calcium supplements.

pazopanib
Votrient

Drug class and indications
Kinase inhibitor, antineoplastic

Treatment of advanced renal cell carcinoma.

▪▸**NEW INDICATION:** Treatment of advanced soft-tissue sarcoma in patients who have previously received chemotherapy.

Dosages and special alerts
800 mg/day PO without food (at least 1 hr before or 2 hr after meals). Not for use with severe hepatic impairment; limit to 200 mg/day with moderate hepatic impairment. Prolongs QT interval. Fatal hemorrhagic events have been reported. Arterial thrombotic events, some fatal; GI perforations and fistulas; hypertension; hypothyroidism; and proteinuria have occurred. Pregnancy Category D; advise use of contraceptives. Diarrhea, depigmentation of hair, and GI effects are common. Patient must be monitored very carefully. ⊗ *Black box warning* Serious to fatal hepatotoxicity has occurred; monitor patient closely.

pegaptanib
Macugen

Drug class and indications
Monoclonal antibody

Treatment of neovascular (wet) age-related macular degeneration.

Dosages and special alerts
0.3 mg once every 6 wk by intravitreous injection into the affected eye. Monitor for vision changes, eye infection, retinal detachment, and traumatic cataract.

DANGEROUS DRUG

pegaspargase
Oncaspar

Drug class and indications
Antineoplastic

Treatment of ALL in patients hypersensitive to native forms of L-asparaginase or as a component of a multi-drug regimen.

Dosages and special alerts
2,500 international units/m^2 IM or IV every 14 days. Associated with pancreatitis, bone marrow depression, and renal toxicity. Monitor patient closely. Save IV use for extreme situations. IM use is preferred.

peginterferon alfa-2a
Pegasys

Drug class and indications
Interferon

Treatment of adults with hepatitis C who have compensated liver disease and who have not been treated with interferon alfa.

Dosages and special alerts
180 mcg subcutaneously once each wk for 48 wk. Adjust dosage with low neutrophil counts, low platelet counts, and for patients on dialysis or who have impaired liver function. Interstitial pneumonitis has been reported; monitor lung function closely. Cardiac dysfunction and hepatic impairment can occur. Protect patient from exposure to infection. ⊗ **Black box warning** Fatal to life-threatening neuropsychiatric, autoimmune, ischemic, and infectious diseases have occurred; monitor patient accordingly.

peginterferon alfa-2b
Peg-Intron, Sylatron

Drug class and indications
Interferon

Treatment of patients older than 3 yr with chronic hepatitis C who have not received alpha interferon and who have compensated liver function; given with ribavirin.

Treatment of chronic hepatitis C in patients 18 yr and older with compensated liver disease previously untreated with interferon alfa as monotherapy.

▪ NEW INDICATION: Treatment of genotype 1 chronic hepatitis C infections in combination with hepatitis C virus protease inhibitors.

Unlabeled use: Renal carcinoma.

Dosages and special alerts
1.5 mcg/kg (60 mcg/m^2/wk for children) subcutaneously once per wk for 1 yr; flulike symptoms common. Monitor bone marrow and liver function. ⊗ **Black box warning** Fatal to life-threatening neuropsychiatric, autoimmune, ischemic, and infectious diseases have occurred; monitor patient accordingly.

pegloticase
Krystexxa

Drug class and indications
PEGylated uric-acid specific enzyme

Treatment of chronic gout in adult patients refractory to conventional therapy.

Dosages and special alerts
8 mg by IV infusion over no less than 120 min every 2 wk; do not give as IV push or bolus. Monitor serum uric-acid levels carefully. Premedicate with antihistamines and corticosteroids. Contraindicated with G6PD deficiencies. ⊗ **Black box warning** Administer in setting prepared to support patient if anaphylaxis occurs. Gout flare may occur during treatment; alert patient. Infusion reactions are common as well as GI symptoms. Use in pregnancy only if benefits outweigh risks; do not use in breast-feeding women.

pegvisomant
Somavert

Drug class and indications
Human growth hormone analogue

Treatment of acromegaly in patients who have had no adequate response to surgery or radiation and other standard therapies or patients for whom these therapies are not appropriate.

Dosages and special alerts
40 mg by subcutaneous injection as a loading dose; then 10 mg/day by subcutaneous injection. Local reactions to the injection are common; rotate sites regularly and monitor for infection. Monitor liver function and blood glucose levels regularly.

DANGEROUS DRUG

pemetrexed
Alimta

Drug class and indications
Antifolate antineoplastic given with cisplatin

Treatment of patients with malignant mesothelioma whose disease is unresectable or who are not candidates for surgery.

Treatment of locally advanced or metastatic non–small-cell lung cancer as a single agent after prior chemotherapy or with cisplatin for first-line treatment.

Dosages and special alerts

500 mg/m^2 IV infused over 10 min on day 1, followed by 75 mg/m^2 cisplatin (treatment of mesothelioma only) IV over 2 hr; repeat cycle every 21 days. Pretreat with corticosteroid, folic acid, and vitamin B$_{12}$. Monitor for bone marrow suppression and GI effects.

penicillamine

Cuprimine, Depen

Drug classes and indications

Chelate, antirheumatic

Treatment of severe, active rheumatoid arthritis when other therapies fail, Wilson disease, cystinuria when other measures fail.

Dosages and special alerts

125–250 mg/day PO; may be increased to 1 g/day if needed. Serious bone marrow suppression, myasthenic syndrome, polymyositis can occur; discontinue if drug fever occurs; Monitor patient closely; push fluids with cystinuria.

pentetate calcium trisodium (Ca-DTPA)

pentetate zinc trisodium (Zn-DTPA)

Drug class and indications

Chelate

Treatment of patients with known or suspected internal contamination with plutonium, americium, or curium, to increase rates of elimination.

Dosages and special alerts

1 g Ca-DTPA IV followed in 24 hr by 1 g Zn-DTPA IV using a slow IV push over 3–4 min. Pediatric patients: 14 mg/kg/day IV (not to exceed 1 g/dose), first using Ca-DTPA, then switching to Zn-DTPA 24 hr after initial dose. Use precautions for handling wastes to avoid contamination of others. Nursing mothers should express breast milk and dispose of it properly. Encourage hydration to improve elimination of the radioactive materials.

pentosan polysulfate sodium

Elmiron

Drug class and indications

Bladder protectant

Relief of bladder pain associated with interstitial cystitis.

Dosages and special alerts

100 mg PO tid on an empty stomach. May cause loss of hair (head should be covered at extremes of temperature); increased bleeding (is a low–molecular-weight heparin).

DANGEROUS DRUG

pentostatin (2' deoxycoformycin [DCF])

Nipent

Drug class and indications

Antineoplastic; antibiotic

Treatment of adults with alpha interferon refractory hairy cell leukemia, chronic lymphocytic leukemia, cutaneous T-cell lymphoma, peripheral T-cell lymphoma.

Dosages and special alerts

4 mg/m^2 IV every other wk, decrease to 2 mg/m^2 with renal impairment. Hydrate patient before each dose and monitor closely.
⊗ **Black box warning** Associated with fatal pulmonary toxicity and bone marrow depression.

pertuzumab

Perjeta

Drug class and indications

HER2/neu receptor antagonist; antineoplastic

Treatment of patients with HER2-positive metastatic breast cancer who have not received prior anti-HER2 therapy or chemotherapy for metastatic disease, in combination with trastuzumab and docetaxel

Dosages and special alerts

Initially, 840 mg IV over 60 min; then 420 mg IV over 30–60 min every 3 weeks. Ensure patient is HER2 positive. Infusion reactions possible.

Monitor patient closely; slow or interrupt infusion and provide supportive treatment if infusion reaction occurs. Left ventricular dysfunction has been reported; monitor patient closely. Not for use while breast-feeding. Must be given with trastuzumab and docetaxel; most common adverse effects with this combination are diarrhea, nausea, alopecia, rash, peripheral neuropathy. and bone marrow suppression. ⊗ **Black box warning** Can cause embryo-fetal death and/or birth defects. Not for use in pregnancy; use of contraceptives is advised.

pilocarpine hydrochloride
Salagen

Drug class and indications
Parasympathomimetic; mouth and throat product

Treatment of symptoms of xerostomia from salivary gland dysfunction caused by radiation therapy for cancers of the head and neck.

Dosages and special alerts
5–10 mg PO tid. Can cause blurred vision, parasympathomimetic effects. Monitor susceptible patients carefully.

pimozide
Orap

Drug class and indications
Antipsychotic; diphenylbutylpiperidine

Suppression of severely compromising motor or phonic tics in patients with Tourette syndrome who have not responded to other therapy.

Dosages and special alerts
1–2 mg/day PO in divided doses; up to a maximum of 10 mg/day. Monitor for prolonged QTc interval. Has been associated with severe cardiac complications; may cause dizziness, sedation, Parkinson-like symptoms.

plerixafor
Mozobil

Drug class and indications
Hematopoietic stem cell mobilizer

Mobilization of hematopoietic stem cells to the peripheral blood for collection and subsequent autologous transplantation in patients with non-Hodgkin lymphoma and multiple myeloma in combination with a granulocyte-colony stimulating factor (G-CSF).

Dosages and special alerts
Start therapy after patient has received G-CSF once daily for 4 days; 0.24 mg/kg by subcutaneous injection, repeated for up to 4 consecutive days. Administer approximately 11 hours before apheresis. In severe renal impairment, reduce dose to 0.16 mg/kg. May mobilize leukemic cells; do not use in leukemia. Monitor blood counts and watch for potential splenic rupture. Headache, dizziness, nausea, vomiting, and injection site reactions are common.

polidocanol
Asclera

Drug class and indications
Sclerosing agent

Treatment of uncomplicated spider veins, and reticular veins in the lower extremities. No experience in treating varicose veins over 3 mm in diameter.

Dosages and special alerts
IV injections at the site of the varicose vein; dosage varies with size and extent of varicosity. Usual dose, 0.1–0.3 mL per varicose vein; maximum volume per session, 10 mL. Must be administered by health care professional familiar with this therapy. Patient may experience mild local reactions at injection sites.

poly-L-lactic acid
Sculptra

Drug classes and indications
Polymer, cosmetic device

Restoration and correction of the signs of lipoatrophy in patients with HIV syndrome.

Dosages and special alerts
0.1–0.2 mL injected intradermally at each injection site. Up to 20 injections per cheek may be needed; re-treat periodically. Do not use if any sign of skin infection is present. Apply ice packs to area immediately after

injection and for first 24 hr; massage injection sites daily.

DANGEROUS DRUG

porfimer sodium
Photofrin

Drug class and indications
Antineoplastic

Photodynamic therapy for palliation of patients with completely or partially obstructing esophageal cancer or transitional cancer who cannot be treated with laser alone, transitional cell carcinoma in situ of urinary bladder, endobronchial non–small-cell lung cancer.

Dosages and special alerts
2 mg/kg IV given as a slow injection over 3–5 min; must be followed in 40–50 hr and again in 96–120 hr by laser therapy. Monitor for pleural effusion and respiratory complications. Avoid any contact with the drug. Protect patient from exposure to light for 30 days after treatment.

---

pralatrexate
Folotyn

Drug class and indications
Folate analogue metabolic inhibitor, antineoplastic

Treatment of relapsed or refractory peripheral T-cell lymphoma.

Dosages and special alerts
30 mg/m^2 as an IV push over 3–5 min once weekly for 6 wk in a 7-wk cycle. Patient should also receive vitamin B$_{12}$, 1 mg IM every 8–10 wk, and folic acid, 1–1.25 mg/day PO. Pregnancy Category X. Bone marrow suppression is common. Mucositis can be severe; dosage may need to be modified.

---

praziquantel
Biltricide

Drug class and indications
Anthelmintic

Treatment of *Schistosoma* infections, liver flukes.

Orphan drug use: treatment of neurocysticercosis.

Dosages and special alerts
3 doses of 20–25 mg/kg PO as a one-day treatment; allow 4–6 hr between doses. Administer with food. Do not cut, crush, or chew tablets; swallow whole. GI upset is common.

DANGEROUS DRUG

procarbazine hydrochloride
Matulane

Drug class and indications
Antineoplastic

Used in combination with other antineoplastics for treatment of stages III and IV Hodgkin lymphoma (part of MOPP chemotherapy regimen).

Dosages and special alerts
2–4 mg/kg/day PO for the first wk, and then 4–6 mg/kg/day PO. Maintenance dosage: 1–2 mg/kg/day. Monitor bone marrow and adjust dosage accordingly. Stress need for barrier contraceptives. Advise patient to avoid alcohol and foods high in tyramine.

---

propantheline bromide

Drug class and indications
Anticholinergic, antimuscarinic, parasympatholytic, antispasmodic

Adjunct therapy in the treatment of peptic ulcer.

Unlabeled uses: antisecretory and antispasmodic.

Dosages and special alerts
7.5–15 mg PO 30 min before meals and at bedtime. Pediatric patients: 1.5 mg/kg/day PO in divided doses tid to qid as an antisecretory or 2–3 mg/kg/day PO in divided doses every 4–6 hr and at bedtime as an antispasmodic. Not approved for peptic ulcer. Monitor patient's hydration. Control environment to prevent hyperpyrexia. Encourage patient to void before each dose because urine retention can occur.

DANGEROUS DRUG

protein C concentrate (human)
Ceprotin

Drug class and indications
Blood product, anticoagulant

Replacement therapy for patients with severe congenital protein C deficiency to prevent and treat venous thrombosis and purpura fulminans.

Dosages and special alerts
Initially, 100–120 international units/kg by IV injection. Then 60–80 international units/kg IV every 6 hr for three more doses. Maintenance dose, 45–60 international units/kg IV every 6–12 hr based on patient response. Monitor patient closely for possibly severe allergic reaction. Risk of disease transmission in blood products.

quinine sulfate
Qualaquin

Drug class and indications
Cinchonan, antimalarial

Treatment of uncomplicated *Plasmodium falciparum* malaria.

Dosages and special alerts
648 mg (two capsules) PO every 8 hr for 7 days. Not for use in children. Reduce dosage with severe renal impairment. Cinchonism causes vision changes, dizziness, sweating, tinnitus, headache, progressing to GI problems. Use caution with prolonged QT interval. Not for treating nocturnal leg cramps. ⊗ **Black box warning** Risk of serious to life-threatening blood-related reactions; use with caution.

ranibizumab
Lucentis

Drug class and indications
Monoclonal antibody, ophthalmic agent

Treatment of patients with neovascular (wet) age-related macular degeneration.

Treatment of macular edema following retinal vein occlusion.

Dosages and special alerts
0.5 mg (0.05 mL) by intravitreal injection once every mo; may be changed to once every 3 mo after the first four injections if monthly injections are not feasible. Monitor patient carefully for detached retina, increased IOP. Patient should be anesthesized before injection and should receive antibiotic treatment.

rasburicase
Elitek

Drug class and indications
Enzyme

Initial management of plasma uric acid levels in patients with leukemia, lymphoma, and solid tumor malignancies who are receiving anti-cancer therapy expected to result in tumor lysis and subsequent elevation of plasma uric acid.

Dosages and special alerts
0.15 or 0.2 mg/kg IV as a single daily infusion over 30 min for 5 days. Chemotherapy should be started 4–24 hr after the first dose. Blood drawn to monitor uric acid levels must be collected in pre-chilled, heparinized vials and kept in an ice-water bath. Analysis must be done within 4 hr. ⊗ **Black box warning** May cause severe hypersensitivity reactions, including anaplylaxis. Do not administer to patients with G6PD deficiency. Immediately discontinue if patient develops hemolysis, do not restart.

regorafenib
Stivarga ⓄⓃⒸ

Drug class and indications
Kinase inhibitor; antineoplastic

Treatment of metastatic colorectal cancer in patients previously treated with fluoropyrimidine-, oxaliplatin-, and irinotecan-based chemotherapy, an anti-VEGF therapy and, if KRAS wild type, an anti-EGFR therapy

Dosages and special alerts
160 mg PO once daily for first 21 days of a 28-day cycle, taken with a low-fat breakfast. Cardiac ischemia, GI perforation and fistula, hypertensive crisis, hemorrhagic events, hepatotoxicity, reversible posterior leukoencephalopathy syndrome, and wound-healing

problems have occurred; monitor patient closely and be prepared to discontinue drug and provide supportive measures. Discontinue at least 24 hours before scheduled surgery. Pregnancy Category D: not for use in pregnancy. Anorexia, diarrhea, weight loss, hand-foot syndrome, mucositis, asthenia/fatigue are common. ⊗ **Black box warning** Severe to fatal hepatotoxicity has been reported; monitor liver function before and during treatment; reduce dose or discontinue at first sign of hepatotoxicity.

rifabutin

Mycobutin

Drug class and indications

Antibiotic

Prevention and treatment of disseminated *Mycobacterium avium* complex disease in patients with advanced HIV infection.

Dosages and special alerts

Adults: 300 mg PO daily. Children: 5 mg/kg/day. GI effects, bone marrow depression common. Body fluids turn a reddish-orange; contact lenses may be stained. Do not use with active TB.

rilonacept

Arcalyst

Drug class and indications

Interleukin blocker, anti-inflammatory drug

Treatment of cryopyrin-associated periodic syndromes, including familial cold autoinflammatory syndrome and Muckle-Wells syndrome in adults and children 12 yr and older.

Dosages and special alerts

Adults: Loading dose of 320 mg given as two 160–mg (2-mL) subcutaneous injections given at different sites; then once-weekly subcutaneous injections of 160 mg (2 mL). Pediatric patients 12–17 yr: Loading dose of 4.4 mg/kg up to a maximum of 320 mg subcutaneously. May be given in divided doses if necessary; then once-weekly injections of 2.2 mg/kg up to a maximum 160 mg. Monitor lipid levels. Risk of severe infection exists.

riluzole

Rilutek

Drug class and indications

Amyotrophic lateral sclerosis (ALS) drug

Treatment of ALS; extends survival time or time to tracheostomy.

Orphan drug use: Treatment of Huntington disease.

Dosages and special alerts

50 mg PO every 12 hr. Slows disease but does not cure it. Take on an empty stomach at the same time each day. Protect drug from light. Commonly causes nausea and vomiting.

DANGEROUS DRUG

rituximab

Rituxan

Drug class and indications

Antineoplastic, monoclonal antibody

First-line treatment or maintenance treatment of relapsed or refractory, low-grade or follicular CD20-positive non-Hodgkin B-cell lymphoma.

With methotrexate, to reduce signs and symptoms of moderately to severely active rheumatoid arthritis in patients with inadequate response to tumor necrosis factor antagonists.

With corticosteroids to treat Wegener granulomatosis, microscopic polyangiitis.

With fludarabine and cyclophosphamide for the treatment of CD20-positive chronic lymphocytic leukemia (CLL).

Dosages and special alerts

Lymphoma in adults: 375 mg/m² IV, once weekly for four or eight doses.

Arthritis: Two 1,000-mg infusions separated by 2 wk, given with methotrexate.

CLL: 375 mg/m² IV the day before fludarabine and cyclophosphamide; then 500 mg/m² on day 1 of cycles 2–6 (every 28 days).

Premedicate patient with acetaminophen and diphenhydramine to decrease fever, chills associated with infusion. Protect patient from exposure to infection. Monitor for reactivation of hepatitis B; discontinue use if viral hepatitis occurs. ⊗ **Black box warning** Fatal infusion reactions, severe cutaneous reactions, and tumor lysis syndrome are possible.

romidepsin

Istodax

Drug class and indications

Histone deacetylase inhibitor, antineoplastic

Treatment of patients with cutaneous or peripheral T-cell lymphoma who have received at least one prior systemic therapy.

Dosages and special alerts

14 mg/m^2 IV over a 4-hr period on days 1, 8, and 15 of a 28-day cycle. Repeat every 28 days if patient tolerates drug and benefits from it effects. Pregnancy Category D. Associated with ECG changes, including prolonged QT interval. Binds to estrogen receptors and may cause fetal harm. May negate effects of hormonal contraceptives; use of barrier contraceptives is advised. May cause GI upset and bone marrow depression.

romiplostim

Nplate

Drug class and indications

Thrombopoietin receptor agonist

Treatment of thrombocytopenia in patients with chronic immune thrombocytopenic purpura who have insufficient response to corticosteroids, immunoglobulins, or splenectomy.

Dosages and special alerts

1 mcg/kg by subcutaneous injection once a wk; adjust dosage in increments of 1 mcg/kg to achieve platelet count of 50 × 10^9. Maximum weekly dose is 10 mcg/kg. Risk of thrombosis, reticulin deposition in the bone marrow, and hematologic malignancies. Patient must be enrolled in the *Nplate NEXUS* program; drug must be administered by a health care provider enrolled in the program. Not for use in pregnant or nursing women.

rosiglitazone

Avandia

Drug class and indications

Antidiabetic; thiazolidinedione

As an adjunct to diet and exercise to improve glycemic control in adults who are already on rosiglitazone and tolerating it well or cannot achieve glycemic control with other antidiabetics and have decided not to take pioglitazone. Available by limited-access program only.

Dosages and special alerts

4 mg PO daily, not to exceed 8 mg/day. Patients must enroll in limited-access program; drug not available in pharmacies. Risk of liver injury, hypoglycemia, hyperglycemia, fatigue. ⊗ **Black box warning** Increased risk of heart failure and myocardial infarction; do not use in patients with known heart disease or symptomatic heart failure; monitor patients accordingly.

rufinamide

Banzel

Drug class and indications

Antiepileptic, sodium channel blocker

Adjunctive treatment of seizures associated with Lennox-Gastaut syndrome in adults and children 4 yr and older.

Dosages and special alerts

Adults: Initially, 400–800 mg/day PO in two equally divided doses. Increase to a target 3,200 mg/day PO in two equally divided doses. Pediatric patients age 4 and older: Initially, 10 mg/kg/day PO in two equally divided doses to a target of 45 mg/kg/day or 3,200 mg/day, whichever is less. Monitor for suicidal ideation and mood changes. Hormonal contraceptives may not be effective if combined with this drug.

ruxolitinib

Jakafi

Drug class and indications

Kinase inhibitor

Treatment of intermediate or high-risk myelofibrosis, including primary myelofibrosis, post–polycythemia vera myelofibrosis and post–essential thrombocythemia myelofibrosis.

Dosages and special alerts

20 mg PO bid. Monitor platelet count closely; adjust dosage based on platelet levels. Maximum dosage, 25 mg bid. Decrease dosage to 10 mg PO bid with renal or hepatic impairment. Discontinue after 6 mo if no spleen reduction

or symptom improvement. Risk of serious infections; monitor patient accordingly and treat appropriately. Not for use in breast-feeding women. Headache, bruising, anemia, and dizziness are most common adverse effects.

sacrosidase

Sucraid

Drug class and indications
Enzyme
Oral replacement of genetically determined sucrase deficiency.

Dosages and special alerts
15 kg or less: 1 mL or 22 drops per meal or snack. Dilute dose with 2–4 ounces of water, milik, or infant formula. More than 15 kg: 2 mL or 44 drops per meal or snack. Do not use in patients with known allergy to yeast. Refrigerate bottle; discard 4 wk after opening.

sapropterin dihydrochloride

Kuvan

Drug class and indications
Coenzyme factor, phenylalanine reducer
With diet, to reduce blood phenylalanine level in patients with hyperphenylalaninemia caused by tetrahydrobiopterin-responsive phenylketonuria.

Dosages and special alerts
4 yr and older: Starting dose 10 mg/kg/day PO once daily. May be adjusted to 5–20 mg/kg/day based on blood phenylalanine level. Dissolve tablets in water or apple juice and have patient drink within 15 min. Monitor phenylalanine level and adjust dosage as needed. Must be used with dietary restrictions.

secretin

ChiRhoStim

Drug class and indications
Diagnostic agent
Stimulation of pancreatic secretions to aid in the diagnosis of pancreatic exocrine dysfunction.
Stimulation of gastrin secretion to aid in the diagnosis of gastrinoma.

Dosages and special alerts
0.2–0.4 mcg/kg IV over 1 min.

sevelamer hydrochloride

Renagel

Drug class and indications
Calcium-phosphate binder
Reduction of serum phosphorus levels in hemodialysis patients in end-stage renal disease.

Dosages and special alerts
800–1,600 mg with each meal based on serum phosphorus levels; may be increased by 400–800 mg per meal to achieve desired serum phosphorus level. Does not cause increase in calcium levels.

sipuleucel-T

Provenge

Drug class and indications
Cellular immunotherapy
Treatment of asymptomatic or minimally symptomatic metastatic castrate-resistant (hormone refractory) prostate cancer.

Dosages and special alerts
Administer IV over 60 min; do not use a cell filter. Administer three doses at approximately 2-wk intervals. Premedicate with oral acetaminophen and an antihistamine. Risk of acute infusion reactions; closely monitor patient during administration. Universal precautions are required. Patient may experience chills, fever, headache, nausea, joint pain.

sirolimus

Rapamune

Drug class and indications
Immunosuppressant
Prophylaxis for organ rejection in renal transplants in conjunction with adrenal corticosteroids and cyclosporine.

Dosages and special alerts
Dosage based on weight. Less than 40 kg: Loading dose of 3 mg/m^2 then 1 mg/m^2/day PO.

40 kg or more: Loading dose of 6 mg PO as soon after transplant as possible, and then daily dose of 2 mg PO in combination with cyclosporine and corticosteroids. Monitor liver and renal function closely; changes could indicate need to change dose or discontinue drug. ⊗ **Black box warning** Drug is associated with these risks: Increased susceptibility to infections, graft loss and hepatic artery thrombosis with liver transplant, bronchial anastomotic dehiscence in lung transplants.

sodium ferric gluconate complex

Ferrlecit

Drug class and indications
Iron product

Treatment of iron deficiency in patients undergoing chronic hemodialysis who are also receiving erythropoietin therapy.

Dosages and special alerts
Test dose: 2 mL diluted in 50 mL 0.9% sodium chloride for injection, given IV over 60 min. Adults: 10 mL diluted in 100 mL 0.9% sodium chloride for injection given IV over 60 min. Most patients will initially require 8 doses given at sequential dialysis sessions, then periodic use based on hematocrit. Flushing and hypertension are common effects.

sodium phenylacetate/ sodium benzoate

Ammonul

Drug class and indications
Urea substitute, ammonia reducer

Adjunctive therapy in the treatment of hyperammonemia and associated encephalopathy in patients with deficiencies in enzymes associated with the urea cycle.

Dosages and special alerts
0–20 kg: 2.5 mL/kg; more than 20 kg: 55 mL/m². Given IV through a central line with arginine. Patients not responsive will require hemodialysis.

DANGEROUS DRUG

sorafenib tosylate

Nexavar

Drug class and indications
Kinase inhibitor, antineoplastic

Treatment of patients with advanced renal cell carcinoma, hepatocellular carcinoma.

Dosages and special alerts
Adults: 400 mg PO bid on an empty stomach (1 hr before or 2 hr after eating). Swallow tablets whole. Patients with cutaneous toxicity: Temporarily stop drug, or reduce dose to 400 mg/day PO and monitor patient closely. Not recommended for pediatric patients.
Monitor for skin reactions, hand-foot syndrome, hypertension.

streptomycin sulfate

Drug class and indications
Antibiotic

Treatment of tularemia, plague, subacute bacterial endocarditis (if less toxic agents are not appropriate).

Fourth drug in the treatment of TB.

Dosages and special alerts
Adults: 15 mg/kg/day IM, or 25–30 mg/kg IM 2 or 3 times a wk. Pediatric patients: 20–40 mg/kg/day IM or 25–30 mg/kg/IM 2 or 3 times a wk.
Tularemia: 1–2 g/day IM for 7–14 days.
Plague: 2 g/day IM in two divided doses for at least 10 days.
Tinnitus, dizziness, ringing in the ears, hearing loss are common. Monitor patient for renal toxicity, injection site infections.

DANGEROUS DRUG

streptozocin

Zanosar

Drug classes and indications
Alkylating drug, antineoplastic

Treatment of metastatic islet cell carcinoma of the pancreas.

Dosages and special alerts

500 mg/m^2 IV for 5 consecutive days every 6 wk, or 1,000 mg/m^2 IV once per wk for 2 wk, and then increase to 1,500 mg/m^2 IV each wk. Bone marrow suppression likely; monitor counts carefully and reduce dosage as needed. ⊗ **Black box warning** Monitor for renal and liver toxicity. Special handling of toxic drug required.

DANGEROUS DRUG

sunitinib

Sutent

Drug class and indications

Kinase inhibitor, antineoplastic

Treatment of GI stromal tumor if patient is intolerant to or tumor progresses after imatinib therapy.

Treatment of advanced renal cell carcinoma.

Treatment of progressive neuroendocrine cancerous pancreatic tumors that cannot be treated surgically or that have metastasized.

Dosages and special alerts

Advanced renal cell carcinoma: 50 mg/day PO for 4 wk, followed by 2 wk of rest; repeat cycle. Advanced pancreatic neuroendocrine tumors: 37.5 mg/day PO. Monitor patient carefully for GI disturbances, bone marrow suppression; dosage adjustment may be needed. ⊗ **Black box warning** Risk of serious to fatal hepatotoxicity. Monitor LFTs closely.

talc, USP

Sterile Talc Powder

Drug class and indications

Sclerosing drug

To decrease the recurrence of malignant pleural effusion.

Dosages and special alerts

5 g in 50–100 mL sodium chloride injection injected into a chest tube after pleural fluid has been drained. Clamp chest tube and have patient change positions for 2 hr; unclamp chest tube and continue external suction. Acute respiratory distress syndrome, PE, MI, local reactions are common. Monitor patient closely.

taliglucerase alfa

Elelyso

Drug class and indications

Lysosomal glucocerebroside-specific enzyme

Long-term enzyme replacement treatment for adults with confirmed diagnosis of Type 1 Gaucher disease

Dosages and special alerts

60 units/kg IV over 60–120 min every other week. Anaphylaxis and allergic and infusion reactions have been reported; stopping infusion at first sign of reaction, or use of antihistamines and antipyretics is advised. Pregnancy Category B. URI, pharyngitis, throat infections, flulike syndrome are common.

teduglutide

Gattex

Drug class and indications

Glucagon-like peptide-2

Treatment of adults with short bowel syndrome who are dependent on parenteral support

Dosages and special alerts

0.05 mg/kg subcutaneously. Pregnancy Category B; risk of accelerated neoplastic growth, full colonoscopy removing any polyps must be done before treatment and at least q5yr afte; may interfer with absorption of oral drugs, monitor closely and adjust doses as needed; GI obstruction, biliary and pancreatic disease may occur; fluid overload may occur; rotate injection sites; abdominal pain, headache, nausea, vomiting, URI may occur.

telbivudine

Tyzeka

Drug class and indications

Nucleoside, antiviral

Treatment of chronic hepatitis B in adult patients with evidence of viral replication and either evidence of persistent elevations in serum aminotransferases (ALT or AST) or histologically active disease.

Dosages and special alerts
Adults older than 16 yr: 600 mg/day PO with or without food. Pediatric patients: Safety and efficacy not established. Patients with renal impairment: For creatinine clearance greater than 50 mL/min, no adjustment needed; for clearance of 30–49 mL/min, 600 mg PO every 48 hr; for clearance less than 30 mL/min, 600 mg PO every 72 hr; for end-stage renal disease, 600 mg PO every 96 hr. ⊗ *Black box warning* Monitor patient for myopathy, severe hepatic failure with steatosis, exacerbation of hepatitis B with discontinuation of drug.

DANGEROUS DRUG
temozolomide
Temodar

Drug class and indications
Antineoplastic

Treatment of refractory astrocytoma in patients at first relapse with disease progression on a drug regimen including a nitrosourea and procarbazine; treatment of advanced metastatic melanoma.

Treatment of adult patients with newly diagnosed glioblastoma multiforme with radiation therapy and then as maintenance therapy.

Dosages and special alerts
Anaplastic astrocytoma: Dose is based on body surface area. Taken for 5 consecutive days for a 28-day treatment cycle. Adjusted dose is based on neutrophil and platelet counts. Monitor bone marrow function closely. Especially toxic in women and the elderly.
Glioblastoma: 75 mg/m^2/day PO or IV for 42 days with focal radiation therapy, then 6 cycles: cycle 1—150 mg/m^2/day PO or IV for 5 days, 23 days rest; cycles 2–6—200 mg/m^2/day PO or IV for 5 days, 23 days rest.

DANGEROUS DRUG
temsirolimus
Torisel

Drug class and indications
Kinase inhibitor, antineoplastic
Treatment of advanced renal cell carcinoma.

Dosages and special alerts
30 min after giving prophylactic diphenhydramine 25–50 mg IV, give 25 mg IV infused over 30–60 min once per wk until disease progresses or unacceptable toxicity occurs. Monitor lung function, blood glucose level, bowel sounds, renal function. Assess patient for slowed healing. Do not give with vaccines. Do not give to pregnant women. Avoid giving with grapefruit juice, St. John's Wort, numerous drugs.

---

teriflunomide
Aubagio ⒩

Drug class and indications
Pyrimidine synthesis inhibitor; MS drug
Treatment of patients with the relapsing form of MS

Dosages and special alerts
7–14 mg PO once daily without regard to food. Monitor patient for potential leukopenia, renal impairment, severe skin reactions, peripheral neuropathy, and changes in blood pressure. Known to react with many drugs; monitor drug history. Most common adverse effects include alopecia, nausea, diarrhea, and paresthesia.
⊗ *Black box warning* Risk of severe to fatal liver toxicity; monitor liver function before treatment, then monthly for 6 months; discontinue at any sign of liver injury.
⊗ *Black box warning* Pregnancy Category X: not for use in pregnancy.

---

teriparatide
Forteo

Drug class and indications
Parathyroid hormone, calcium regulator
Treatment of postmenopausal women with osteoporosis and high risk of fracture.

Treatment of men and women with osteoporosis associated with sustained systemic glucocorticoid therapy at high risk for fracture.

To increase bone mass in men with primary or hypogonadal osteoporosis at high risk for fracture.

Dosages and special alerts

20 mcg/day subcutaneously in thigh or abdominal wall; use for more than 2 yr is not recommended. ⊗ *Black box warning* Increased risk of osteosarcoma in rats; should not be use in patients with increased risk of osteosarcoma (Paget disease, unexplained elevations in alkaline phosphatase level, open epiphyses, prior external beam or implant radiation therapy involving the skeleton). Not recommended for treatment of bone disease other than osteoporosis. May cause orthostatic hypotension; may increase risk of renal stones. Not for use by nursing mothers. Arthralgia, pain, and nausea are common.

tesamorelin
Egrifta

Drug class and indications

Growth hormone releasing factor analogue
    Reduction of excess abdominal fat in HIV-infected patients with lipodystrophy related to use of antivirals.

Dosages and special alerts

2 mg/day subcutaneously. Not for use in pregnancy or breast-feeding. Monitor patient for fluid retention, glucose intolerance, and injection-site reactions. Encourage patient to rotate injection sites.

thalidomide
Thalomid

Drug class and indications

Immune modulator
    Treatment of erythema nodosum leprosum—painful inflammatory condition related to an immune reaction to dead bacteria following treatment of leprosy; newly diagnosed multiple myeloma; brain tumors; Crohn disease; HIV-wasting syndrome; graft-host reaction in bone marrow transplant.

Dosages and special alerts

100–300 mg/day PO. Taken once daily with water at bedtime for at least 2 wk. Taper off in decrements of 50 mg every 2–4 wk. ⊗ *Black box warning* Associated with severe birth defects; women must have a pregnancy test and sign consent to use birth control

to avoid pregnancy while on this drug (STEPS program).

tiludronate disodium
Skelid

Drug class and indications

Bisphosphonate
    Treatment of Paget disease in patients with alkaline phosphatase at least two times the upper limit of normal who are asymptomatic and at risk for future complications.

Dosages and special alerts

400 mg/day PO for 3 mo taken with 6–8 oz of plain water at least 2 hr before any other food or beverage. Monitor serum calcium closely; patient should increase intake of vitamin D and calcium; allow a 3-mo rest period if re-treatment is needed.

tiopronin
Thiola

Drug class and indications

Thiol compound
    Prevention of cystine kidney stone formation in patients with severe homozygous cystinuria with urine cystine levels exceeding 500 mg/day who are resistant to other therapy.

Dosages and special alerts

800 mg/day PO; increase to 1,000 mg/day in divided doses; take on an empty stomach. Children 9 yr and older: 15 mg/kg/day PO; adjust dose based on urinary cystine level. Monitor cystine levels at 1 mo and then every 3 mo. Patient should drink fluids liberally to 3 L/day.

tofacitinib
Xeljanz ⓞⓡⓒ

Drug class and indications

Kinase inhibitor; antirheumatic

Treatment of adults with moderately to severely active rheumatoid arthritis who have inadequate response to or are intolerant of methotrexate, as monotherapy or in combination with methotrexate or other nonbiologic disease-modifying antirheumatic drugs

Dosages and special alerts
Initially, 5 mg PO bid without regard to food. Not recommended with severe hepatic impairment; reduce dose to 5 mg/day PO with moderate or severe renal impairment or moderate hepatic impairment. Risk of GI perforation, immune suppression; monitor patient accordingly. URIs, headache, diarrhea, nasopharyngitis very common. Pregnancy Category C. Do not give vaccines; many drug interactions possible. ⊗ **Black box warning** Risk of serious to fatal infections, including TB. Screen patient for TB before use; do not give to patient with signs of active infection. Lymphoma and other malignancies can occur.

TOLAZamide

Drug class and indications
Antidiabetic, first-generation sulfonylurea
Adjunct to diet and exercise to control blood glucose in patients with type 2 diabetes.
With insulin to control blood glucose levels and decrease the insulin dose in select patients with type 1 diabetes.

Dosages and special alerts
If fasting blood glucose is less than 200 mg/dL, 100 mg/day PO in the morning before breakfast. If fasting blood glucose is greater than 200 mg/dL, 250 mg/day PO. Do not exceed 1 g/day. Use caution with geriatric patients, who may be more sensitive to glucose-lowering effects. Adjust dosage based on patient response; switch to insulin in times of high stress. Be aware that patient may be at increased risk for CV events.

TOLBUTamide
Apo-Tolbutaminde (CAN), Orinase

Drug class and indications
Antidiabetic, first-generation sulfonylurea, diagnostic agent
Adjunct to diet and exercise to control blood glucose level in patients with type 2 diabetes.
With insulin to control blood glucose levels and decrease insulin dose in select patients with type 1 diabetes.

To aid in diagnosis of pancreatic islet cell adenoma

Dosages and special alerts
1–2 g/day PO in the morning before breakfast; maintenance dose of 0.25–3 g/day PO based on patient response. Do not exceed 3 g/day. As a diagnostic agent: 20 mL IV infused over 2–3 min. Use caution with geriatric patients, who may be more sensitive to glucose-lowering effects; switch to insulin in times of high stress. Be aware that patient may be at increased risk for CV events.

tolvaptan
Samsca

Drug class and indications
Selective vasopressin receptor antagonist
Treatment of clinically significant hypervolemic or euvolemic hyponatremia, including patients with heart failure, cirrhosis, and SIADH.

Dosages and special alerts
15 mg PO once daily; may increase after at least 24 hr, based on patient response, to a maximum of 60 mg/day. ⊗ **Black box warning** Therapy should be initiated in a hospital setting, with close supervision of sodium and volume. Not for use when rapid correction of hyponatremia is needed. May cause fetal harm; do not give to nursing women. Dry mouth, constipation, increased blood glucose level, and polyuria are common.

DANGEROUS DRUG
topotecan hydrochloride
Hycamtin

Drug class and indications
Antineoplastic
Treatment of metastatic ovarian cancer after failure of traditional chemotherapy.
Treatment of small-cell lung cancer after failure of first-line treatment.
With cisplatin, for treatment of stage V recurrent or persistent carcinoma of the cervix when not amenable to surgery or radiation.

Dosages and special alerts

1.5 mg/m^2 IV over 30 min daily for 5 days, starting on day 1 of a 21-day course; minimum of 4 courses recommended (lung cancer, ovarian cancer).

0.75 mg/m^2 by IV infusion over 30 min on days 1, 2, 3 followed by cisplatin on day 1; repeat every 21 days (cervical cancer).

Provide analgesics. Suggest use of wig or head covering. Protect patient from exposure to infection. Barrier contraceptives should be urged. ⊗ **Black box warning** Monitor bone marrow carefully.

DANGEROUS DRUG

tositumomab and iodine I-131 tositumomab

Bexxar

Drug class and indications

Antineoplastic, monoclonal antibody

Treatment of CD20-positive, follicular non-Hodgkin lymphoma in patients whose disease is refractory to rituximab and who have relapsed following chemotherapy.

Dosages and special alerts

Two-step treatment: 450 mg tositumomab IV in 50 mL 0.9% sodium chloride over 60 min, 5 mCi I-131 with 35 mg tositumomab in 30 mL sodium chloride IV over 20 min; then repeat as a therapeutic step, adjusting I-131 based on patient response. Drug is Pregnancy Category X. ⊗ **Black box warning** Risk of severe and prolonged cytopenia; hypersensitivity reactions including anaphylaxis have occurred.

tranexamic acid

Lysteda

Drug class and indications

Antifibrinolytic

Treatment of cyclic heavy menstrual bleeding.

Dosages and special alerts

1,300 mg PO tid for a maximum of 5 days during monthly menstruation. Reduce dosage with renal impairment. Increased risk of clots, stroke, and MI if combined with hormonal

contraceptives, antihemophilic agents, or oral tretinoin. Visual changes or severe allergic reaction should lead to immediate discontinuation of drug. Cerebral infarct and cerebral edema have occurred. Most common adverse effects include pain, sinus and nasal symptoms, anemia, and fatigue.

trazodone hydrochloride

Apo-Trazodone (CAN), NuTrazadone (CAN), Oleptro ⊕

Drug class and indications

Antidepressant

Treatment of depression in inpatients and outpatients and for depressed patients with or without anxiety.

Dosages and special alerts

150 mg/day PO in divided doses; may be increased to maximum of 400 mg/day PO in divided doses. ER tablets (*Oleptro*)— 150 mg/day PO, up to a maximum 375 mg/day, once daily. For severe depression, maximum dosage 600 mg/day PO; adjust to a lower dosage as soon as possible. Geriatric patients should start at 75 mg/day PO in divided doses with close monitoring. Do not cut, crush, or allow patient to chew ER tablet. ⊗ **Black box warning** Limit quantities of drug in depressed and suicidal patients. Monitor patient for low BP. Discontinue drug if priapism occurs. Risk of suicidality is increased, especially in children, adolescents, and young adults.

trientine hydrochloride

Syprine

Drug class and indications

Chelate

Treatment of patients with Wilson disease who are intolerant of penicillamine.

Dosages and special alerts

Adults: 750–1,250 mg/day PO in divided doses, maximum 2 g/day. Children: 500–750 mg/day PO; maximum, 1,500 mg/day. Interruption of therapy can lead to severe hypersensitivity reactions when drug is restarted. If iron supplements are taken, separate by at least 2 hr.

urofollitropin

Bravelle

Drug class and indications

Fertility drug

Sequentially with HCG to induce ovulation in patients who have previously received pituitary suppression.

Stimulation of multiple follicle development in ovulatory patients.

Dosages and special alerts

Patients who have received gonadotropin-releasing hormone agonist or antagonist suppression: 150 units daily subcutaneously or IM for the first 5 days of treatment. Subsequent dosing should be adjusted according to individual patient response, should not be made more frequently than once every 2 days, and should not exceed more than 75–150 units per adjustment. The maximum daily dose is 450 units; treatment beyond 12 days is not recommended. If patient response is appropriate, give HCG 5,000 to 10,000 units 1 day following the last dose of *Bravelle*. Monitor patient for ovarian overstimulation; warn patient of risk of multiple births.

ustekinumab

Stelara

Drug class and indications

Monoclonal antibody

Treatment of mild to moderate plaque psoriasis in adults who are candidates for phototherapy or systemic therapy.

Dosages and special alerts

100 kg or less: 45 mg subcutaneously, followed by 45 mg in 4 wk and then every 12 wk; more than 100 kg: 90 mg subcutaneously, followed by 90 mg in 4 wk and then every 12 wk. Risk of serious infections and malignancy. Do not use during active infection; if infection occurs, stop treatment. Most common adverse effects are headache, fatigue, and URI symptoms.

velaglucerase alfa

VPRIV

Drug class and indications

Lysosomal enzyme

Long-term replacement therapy for children and adults with type 1 Gaucher disease.

Dosages and special alerts

60 units/kg as a 60-min IV infusion every other wk. Most common reactions are infusion-related; monitor patient closely during administration. Patient may also experience headache, joint pain, dizziness, abdominal pain, fatigue.

vemurafenib

Zelboraf OTC

Drug class and indications

Kinase inhibitor; antineoplastic

Treatment of patients with unresectable or metastatic melanoma with BRAF mutation as detected by the approved BRAF test

Dosages and special alerts

960 mg PO bid, approximately 12 hr apart. Tablets must be swallowed whole; cannot be cut, crushed, or chewed. BRAF confirmation test is required before use to ensure appropriate selection of drug. Serious hypersensitivity reactions and severe dermatologic reactions have occurred; discontinue at first sign of such reactions. Drug can prolong QT interval; monitor ECG and electrolytes before and periodically during therapy. Liver injury is possible; monitor liver enzymes before and periodically during therapy. Use ophthalmic exams to detect possible eye damage. Patient should avoid sun exposure because of risk of photosensitivity. Patient should be screened for potential new melanomas and cutaneous squamous cell carcinomas. Avoid use in pregnancy.

verteporfin

Visudyne

Drug class and indications

Ophthalmic drug

Treatment of age-related macular degeneration, pathologic myopia, ocular histoplasmosis.

Dosages and special alerts

6 mg/m^2 diluted in D$_5$W to total 30 mL IV into a free-flowing IV over 10 min at 3 mL/min using an inline filter and syringe pump. Laser light therapy should begin within 15 min of starting IV; may be repeated in 3 mo if needed. Protect patient from exposure to bright light for at least 5 days after treatment. Avoid use with hepatic impairment or sensitivity to eggs.

vigabatrin
Sabril

Drug class and indications

Antiepileptic, GABAase inhibitor

Monotherapy for children 1 mo–2 yr with infantile spasms.

Adjunctive therapy for adults with complex partial seizures not controlled by other therapy.

Dosages and special alerts

Children 1 mo–2 yr: 50 mg/kg/day PO bid oral solution to a maximum of 150 mg/kg/day PO bid. Adults: 500 mg PO bid to a maximum of 1.5 g PO bid with other antiepileptics. ⊗ **Black box warning** Risk of vision loss; limit dosage and duration of therapy and monitor patient's vision. Stop drug if vision changes occur. Risk of suicidal ideation; monitor patient accordingly. Causes anemia, somnolence, peripheral neuropathy, weight gain, edema. Taper dosage when discontinuing.

vismodegib
Erivedge

Drug class and indications

Hedgehog pathway inhibitor; antineoplastic

Treatment of metastatic or locally advanced basal cell carcinoma in patients who are not candidates for surgery or radiation

Dosages and special alerts

150 mg/day PO. Muscle spasms, alopecia, weight loss, fatigue, nausea, vomiting, diarrhea are common. Advise patients that they cannot donate blood during and for 7 months following treatment. ⊗ **Black box warning** Can cause embryo-fetal death or severe birth defects. Ensure patient is not pregnant prior to therapy. Advise use of contraceptives. Male

patients should not father a child while on taking drug.

DANGEROUS DRUG

vorinostat
Zolinza

Drug class and indications

Histone deacetylase inhibitor, antineoplastic

Treatment of cutaneous manifestations in patients with cutaneous T-cell lymphoma who have progressive, persistent, or recurrent disease on or following two systemic therapies.

Dosages and special alerts

400 mg PO once daily with food; continue until there is evidence of progression of disease or unacceptable toxicity. ⊗ **Black box warning** Monitor patient for increased bleeding, excessive nausea and vomiting, thromboembolic events. Encourage 2 L/day of fluid intake to prevent dehydration.

ziconotide
Prialt

Drug class and indications

N-type calcium channel blocker, analgesic

Management of severe chronic pain in patients who need intrathecal therapy and are intolerant or unresponsive to traditional therapy.

Dosages and special alerts

Initially 2.4 mcg/day by continuous intrathecal pump; may be titrated to a maximum 19.2 mcg/day (0.8 mcg/hr). Monitor for development of meningitis, psychotic behaviors, and neurologic impairment.

ziv-aflibercept
Zaltrap

Drug class and indications

Ligand binding factor; antineoplastic

In combination with 5-FU, leucovorin, and irinotecan for the treatment of adults with metastatic colorectal cancer that is resistant to or has progressed following an oxaliplatin-containing regimen

Dosages and special alerts

4 mg/kg IV over 1 hr every 2 wk; do not give as an IV bolus or push. Monitor patients for hypertension, thromboembolic events, fistula formation, proteinuria, bone marrow suppression, diarrhea, dehydration, and headache. Not for use while breast-feeding.

⊗ **Black box warning** Risk of serious to fatal hemorrhage (do not administer to patients with hemorrhage), GI perforation (do not administer with history of GI perforation), impaired wound healing (suspend use at least 4 wk before elective surgery and do not restart for at least 4 wk after surgery and after the surgical wound has healed).

Appendix S

Drugs commonly used to treat specific disorders

The list below includes 50 specific disorders and the medications most commonly prescribed to treat them.

Alzheimer disease
Cholinergics
- donepezil (*Aricept*)
- galantamine (*Razadyne*)
- rivastigmine (*Exelon*)

NMDA receptor antagonist
- memantine (*Namenda*)

Angina
Nitrates
- *isosorbide dinitrate (Isordil)*
- *isosorbide mononitrate (Imdur)*
- *nitroglycerin (Nitro-Bid, Nitrostat, others)*

Beta blockers
- metoprolol (*Toprol*)
- nadolol (*Corgard*)
- propranolol (*Inderal*)

Calcium channel blockers
- amlodipine (*Norvasc*)
- diltiazem (*Cardizem*)
- nicardipine (*Cardene*)
- nifedipine (*Adalat*)
- verapamil (*Calan*)

Piperazine-acetamide
- ranolazine (*Ranexa*)

Anxiety disorder
Benzodiazepines
- alprazolam (*Xanax*)
- chlordiazepoxide
- clonazepam (*Klonopin*)
- clorazepate (*Tranxene*)
- diazepam (*Valium*)
- lorazepam (*Ativan*)
- oxazepam (*Serax*)

Barbiturates
- mephobarbital (*Mebaral*)

Others
- buspirone (*BuSpar*)
- meprobamate (*Miltown*)

Arthritis, rheumatoid
Pain relief
- aspirin (generic)
- capsaicin (*Zostrix*)
- celecoxib (*Celebrex*)
- diclofenac (*Cataflam*)

Immune modulators
- abatacept (*Orencia*)
- adalimumab (*Humira*)
- anakinra (*Kineret*)
- auranofin (*Ridaura*)
- aurothioglucose (*Solganal*)
- azathioprine (*Imuran*)
- certolizumab (*Cimzia*)
- cyclosporine (*Sandimmune*)
- etanercept (*Enbrel*)
- hydoxychloroquine (*Plaquenil*)
- infliximab (*Remicade*)
- leflunomide (*Arava*)
- methotrexate (generic)
- pencillamine (*Caprimine*)
- prednisone (*Delasone*)
- rituximab (*Rituxan*)

Asthma
Xanthines
- aminophylline (*Truphylline*)
- diphylline (*Dilor*)
- theophylline (*SloBid*, others)

Sympathomimetics
- albuterol (*Proventil*)
- ephedrine (generic)
- epinephrine (*SusPhrine*)
- formoterol (*Foradil*)
- isoetharine (generic)
- isoproterenol (*Isuprel*)
- levalbuterol (*Xopenex*)
- metaproterenol (*Alupent*)
- pirbuterol (*Maxair*)
- salmeterol (*Serevent*)
- terbutaline (*Brethaire*)

Inhaled steroids
- beclomethasone (*Beclovent*)
- budesonide (*Pulmicort*)
- ciclesonide (*Alvesco*)
- fluticasone (*Flovent*)
- triamcinolone (*Azmacort*)

Leukotriene receptor antagonists
- montelukast (*Singulair*)
- zafirlukast (*Accolate*)
- zileuton (*Zyflo*)

Attention deficit hyperactivity disorder

Stimulants
- dexmethylphenidate (*Focalin*)
- dextroamphetamine (*Dexedrine*)
- lisdexamfetamine (*Vyvanse*)
- methylphenidate (*Concerta, Ritalin*)
- mixed amphetamines (*Adderall*)

Nonstimulants
- atomoxetine (*Strattera*)
- guanfacine (*Intuniv*)

Benign prostatic hyperplasia

Alpha₁ blockers
- afluzosin (*UroXatral*)
- doxazosin (*Cardura*)
- tamsulosin (*Flomax*)
- terazosin (*Hytrin*)

Androgen inhibitors
- dutasteride (*Avodart*)
- finasteride (*Proscar*)

Cancer, breast

Antineoplastics
- anastrozole (*Arimidex*)
- capecitabine (*Xeloda*)
- cyclophosphamide (*Cytoxan*)
- docetaxel (*Taxotere*)
- doxorubicin (*Adriamycin*)
- epirubicin (*Ellence*)
- eribulin (*Halaven*)
- exemestane (*Aromasin*)
- fluorouracil (*Efudex, Fluoroplex*)
- fulvestrant (*Faslodex*)
- gemcitabine (*Gemzar*)
- ixabepilone (*Ixempra*)
- lapatinib (*Tykerb*)
- letrozole (*Femara*)
- methotrexate (*Abitrexate, Folex, Folex PFS*)
- paclitaxel (*Abraxane, Taxol*)
- tamoxifen (*Nolvadex*)
- toremifene (*Fareston*)

Cancer, colon

Antineoplastics
- bevacizumab (*Avastin*)
- capecitabine (*Xeloda*)
- cetuximab (*Erbitux*)
- irinotecan (*Camptosar*)
- leucovorin (*Wellcovorin*)
- oxaliplatin (*Eloxatin*)
- panitumumab (*Vectibix*)

Cancer, lung

Antineoplastics
- bevacizumab (*Avastin*)
- carboplatin (*Paraplatin*)
- cisplatin (*Platinol-AQ*)
- docetaxel (*Taxotere*)
- erlotinib (*Tarceva*)
- etoposide (*VePesid*)
- gemcitabine (*Gemzar*)
- irinotecan (*Camptosar*)
- paclitaxel (*Taxol*)
- pemetrexed (*Alimta*)
- vinorelbine (*Navelbine*)

Cancer, prostate

LH-RH agonists
- degarelix (*Firmagon*)
- goserelin (*Zoladex*)
- histrelin (*Vantas*)
- leuprolide (*Lupron*)
- triptorelin (*Trelstar*)

Antiandrogens
- bicalutamide (*Casodex*)
- flutamide (generic)
- nilutamide (*Nilandron*)

Antineoplastics
- abiraterone (*Zytiga*)
- cabazitaxel (*Jevtana*)

Immunotherapy
- sipuleucel-T (*Provenge*)

Chronic obstructive pulmonary disease

Xanthines
- aminophylline (*Truphylline*)
- diphylline (*Dilor*)
- theophylline (*SloBid*, others)

Sympathomimetics
- arformoterol (*Brovana*)
- indacaterol (*Arcapta*)

Anticholinergics
- aclidinium
- ipratropium (*Atrovent*)
- tiotropium (*Spiriva*)

Phosphodiesterase inhibitor
- roflumilast (*Daliresp*)

Constipation
Chemical stimulants
- bisacodyl (*Dulcolax*)
- cascara (generic)
- castor oil (*Neolid*)
- senna (*Senokot*)

Bulk stimulants
- lactulose (*Chronulac*)
- magnesium citrate (*Citrate of Magnesia*)
- magnesium hydroxide (*Milk of Magnesia*)
- magnesium sulfate (*Epsom Salts*)
- polycarbophil (*FiberCon*)
- polyethylene glycol (*Miralax*)
- polyethylene glycol electrolyte solution (*GoLYTELY*, others)
- psyllium (*Metamucil*)

Lubricants
- docusate (*Colace*)
- glycerin (*Sani-Supp*)
- mineral oil (*Agoral Plain*)

Crohn disease
Salicylates
- mesalamine (*Apriso, Asacol*)
- sulfasalazine (*Azulfidine*)

Antibiotics
- ciprofloxacin (*Cipro*)
- metronidazole (*Flagyl*)

Corticosteroids
- budesonide (*Entocort EC*)
- prednisone (*Sterapred*)

Immune modulators
- azathioprine (*Imuran*)
- mercaptopurine (*Purinethol*)

Monoclonal antibodies
- adalimumab (*Humira*)
- infliximab (*Remicade*)

Cystic fibrosis
Bronchodilators
- albuterol (*Proventil*)
- salmeterol (*Serevent*)

Mucolytic
- acetylcysteine (*Mucomyst*)

Digestive enzyme
- pancrelipase (*Creon, Pancrease*)

Others
- Donase alfa: dornase (*Pulmozyme*)

Depression
Tricyclic antidepressants
- amitriptyline (generic)
- amoxapine (*Ascendin*)
- clomipramine (*Anafranil*)
- desipramine (*Norpramin*)
- doxepin (*Sinequan*)
- imipramine (*Tofranil*)
- maprotiline (generic)
- nortriptyline (*Aventyl*)
- protriptyline (*Vivactil*)
- trimipramine (*Surmontil*)

Monoamine oxidase inhibitors
- isocarboxazid (*Marplan*)
- phenelzine (*Nardil*)
- tranylcypromine (*Parnate*)

Selective serotonin reuptake inhibitors
- citalopram (*Celexa*)
- escitalopram (*Lexapro*)
- fluoxetine (*Prozac*)
- fluvoxamine (*Luvox*)
- paroxetine (*Paxil*)
- sertraline (*Zoloft*)
- vilazodone (*Viibyrd*)

Others
- bupropion (*Wellbutrin*)
- desvenlafaxine (*Pristiq*)
- duloxetine (*Cymbalta*)
- mirtazipine (*Remeron*)
- nefazodone (generic)
- selegiline (*Emsam*)
- trazodone (*Desyrel*)
- venlafaxine (*Effexor*)

Diabetes mellitus
Insulin
- insulin (*Humulin*, others)

Sulfonylureas
- chlorpropamide (*Diabinese*)
- glimepiride (*Amaryl*)
- glipizide (*Glucotrol*)
- glyburide (*DiaBeta*)
- tolazamide (*Tolinase*)
- tolbutamide (*Orinase*)

Alpha-glucosidase inhibitors
- acarbose (*Precose*)
- miglitol (*Glyset*)

Biguanide
- metformin (*Glucophage*)

DPP4 inhibitors
- alogliptin
- linagliptin (*Tradjenta*)
- saxagliptin (*Onglyza*)
- sitagliptin (*Januvia*)

Human amylin
- pramlintide (*Symlin*)

Incretin mimetics
- exenatide (*Baraclude*)
- liraglutide (*Victoza*)

Meglitinides
- nateglinide (*Starlix*)
- repaglinide (*Prandin*)

Thiazolidinediones
- pioglitazone (*Actos*)
- rosiglitazone (*Avandia*)

Diarrhea
Antidiarrheals
- bismuth subsalicylate (*Pepto-Bismol*)
- loperamide (*Imodium*)
- opium derivatives (*Paregoric*)

Erectile dysfunction
Prostaglandin
- alprostadil (*Caverject*)

Phosphodiesterase inhibitors
- avanafil (*Stendra*)
- sildenafil (*Viagra*)
- tadalafil (*Cialis*)
- vardenafil (*Levitra*)

Gastroesophageal reflux disease
Antacids
- aluminum salts (*AlternGel*)
- calcium salts (*Tums*)
- magaldrate (*Riopan*)
- magnesium salts (*Milk of Magnesia*)
- sodium bicarbonate (*Bells/ans*)

Histamine-2 antagonists
- cimetidine (*Tagamet*)
- famotidine (*Pepcid*)
- nizatidine (*Axid*)
- ranitidine (*Zantac*)

Proton pump inhibitors
- dexlansoprazole (*Kapidex*)
- esomeprazole (*Nexium*)
- lansoprazole (*Prevacid*)
- omeprazole (*Prilosec*)
- pantoprazole (*Protonix*)
- rabeprazole (*Aciphex*)

Glaucoma
Ophthalmic agents
- acetazolamide (*Diamox*)
- apraclonidine (*Topidine*)
- betaxolol (*Betoptic*)
- bimatoprost (*Lumigan*)
- brimonidine (*Alphagan*)
- carbachol (generic)
- carteolol (*Ocupress*)
- dipivefrin (*Propine*)
- dorzolamide (*Trusopt*)
- echothiophate (*Phospholine*)
- latanoprost (*Xalatan*)
- levobunolol (*Betagan*)
- metipranolol (*Optipranolol*)
- pilocarpine (*Isopto Carpine*)
- timolol (*Timoptic*)
- travoprost (*Travatan*)

Heart failure
Cardiac glycoside
- digoxin (*Lanoxin*)

Phosphodiesterase inhibitors
- inamrinone (*Inocor*)
- milrinone (*Primacor*)

Nitrates
- isosorbide dinitrate (*Isordil*)
- isosorbide mononitrate (*Imdur*)
- nitroglycerin (*Nitro-Bid, Nitrostat, others*)

Beta-adrenergic blockers
- metoprolol (*Toprol*)
- nadolol (*Corgard*)
- propranolol (*Inderal*)

Angiotensin converting enzyme inhibitors
- benazepril (*Lotensin*)
- captopril (*Capoten*)
- enalapril (*Vasotec*)
- fosinopril (*Monopril*)
- lisinopril (*Zestril*)
- moexipril (*Univasc*)
- perindopril (*Aceon*)
- quinapril (*Accupril*)
- ramipril (*Altace*)
- trandolapril (*Mavik*)

Diuretics
- bumetanide (*Bumex*)
- furosemide (*Lasix*)
- torsemide (*Demadex*)

Natriuretic peptide
- nesiritide (*Natrecor*)

Hepatitis
Hepatitis B
Antivirals
- adefovir (*Hepsera*)

- entecavir (*Baraclude*)
- telbivudine (*Tyzeka*)

Hepatitis C
- boceprevir (*Victrelis*)
- telaprevir (*Incivek*)

HIV/AIDS
Non-nucleoside reverse transcriptase inhibitors
- delaviridine (*Rescriptor*)
- effavirenz (*Sustiva*)
- etravirine (*Intelance*)
- nevirapine (*Viramune*)
- rilpivirine (*Edurant*)

Nucleoside reverse transcriptase inhibitors
- abacavir (*Ziagen*)
- didanosine (*Videx*)
- emtricitabine (*Emtriva*)
- lamivudine (*Epivir*)
- stavudine (*Zerit XR*)
- tenofovir (*Viread*)
- zidovudine (*Retrovir*)

Protease inhibitors
- atazanavir (*Reyataz*)
- darunavir (*Prezista*)
- fosamprenavir (*Lexiva*)
- indinavir (*Crixivan*)
- lopinavir (*Kaletra*)
- nelfinavir (*Viracept*)
- ritonavir (*Norvir*)
- saquinavir (*Fortovase*)
- tipranavir (*Aptivus*)

Fusion inhibitor
- enfuvirtide (*Fuzeon*)

CCR5 coreceptor antagonist
- maraviroc (*Selzentry*)

Integrase inhibitor
- raltegravir (*Isentress*)

Hyperlipidemia
Bile acid sequestrants
- cholestyramine (*Questran*)
- colesevelam (generic)
- colestipol (*Colestid*)

Statins
- atorvastatin (*Lipitor*)
- fluvastatin (*Lescol*)
- lovastatin (*Mevacor*)
- pitavastatin (*Livalo*)
- pravastatin (*Pravachol*)
- rosuvastatin (*Crestor*)
- simvastatin (*Zocor*)

Cholesterol absorption inhibitor
- ezetimibe (*Zetia*)

Fibrates
- fenofibrate (*Tricor*)
- fenofibric acid (*Trilipix*)
- gemfibrozil (*Lopid*)

Vitamin B
- niacin (*Niaspan*)

Other
- omega-3-acid ethyl esters (*Lovaza*)

Hypertension
Angiotensin converting enzyme inhibitors
- benazepril (*Lotensin*)
- captopril (*Capoten*)
- enalapril (*Vasotec*)
- fosinopril (*Monopril*)
- lisinopril (*Zestril*)
- moexipril (*Univasc*)
- perindopril (*Aceon*)
- quinapril (*Accupril*)
- ramipril (*Altace*)
- trandolapril (*Mavik*)

Angiotensin II receptor blockers
- azilsartan (*Edarbi*)
- candesartan (*Atacand*)
- eprosartan (*Teveten*)
- irbesartan (*Avapro*)
- losartan (*Cozaar*)
- olmesartan (*Benicar*)
- telmisartan (*Micardis*)
- valsartan (*Diovan*)

Calcium channel blockers
- amlodipine (*Norvasc*)
- clevidipine (*Cleviprex*)
- diltiazem (*Cardizem*)
- felodipine (*Plendil*)
- isradipine (*DynaCirc*)
- nicardipine (*Cardene*)
- nifedipine (*Procardia XL*)
- nisoldipine (*Sular*)
- verapamil (*Calan SR*)

Renin inhibitor
- aliskiren (*Tekturna*)

Thiazide diuretics
- chlorothiazide (*Diuril*)
- hydrochlorothiazide (*HydroDIURIL*)

Adrenergic blockers
- acebutolol (*Sectral*)
- atenolol (*Tenormin*)
- betaxolol (*Kerlone*)
- bisoprolol (*Zebeta*)

- carteolol (*Cartrol*)
- metoprolol (*Lopressor*)
- nadolol (*Corgard*)
- nebivolol (*Bystolic*)
- propranolol (*Inderal*)
- timolol (*Blocadren*)

Infertility
Hormones
- cetrorelix (*Cetrotide*)
- chorionic gonadotropin (*Chorex*)
- chorionic gonadotropin alpha (*Ovidrel*)
- clomiphene (*Clomid*)
- follitropin alfa (*Gonal-F*)
- follitropin beta (*Follistim*)
- ganirelix (*Antagon*)
- lutropin alfa (*Luveris*)
- menotropins (*Pergonal*)
- urofollitropin (*Bravelle*)

Influenza
Antivirals
- amantadine (*Symmetrel*)
- oseltamavir (*Tamiflu*)
- ribavirin (*Rebetron*)
- rimantadine (*Flumadine*)
- zanamivir (*Relenza*)

Insomnia
Benzodiazepines
- estazolam (*ProSom*)
- flurazepam (*Dalmane*)
- quazepam (*Doral*)
- temazepam (*Restoril*)
- triazolam (*Halcion*)
Other
- diphenhydramine (*Benadryl*)
- eszopiclone (*Lunesta*)
- ramelteon (*Rozerem*)
- zaleplon (*Sonata*)
- zolpidem (*Ambien*)

Irritable bladder syndrome
Anticholinerics
- darifenacin (*Enablex*)
- fesoterodine (*Toviaz*)
- flavoxate (*Urispas*)
- oxybutynin (*Ditropan, Gelnique, Oxytol*)
- solifenacin (*VESIcare*)
- tolterodine (*Detrol*)
- trospium (*Santura*)

Menopause
Estrogens
- estradiol (*Estrace*)
- estrogens, conjugated (*Premarin*)
- estrogens, esterified (*Menest*)
- estropipate (*Ortho-Est*)
Progestins
- drospirenone (*Yasmin* with ethinyl estradiol)
Estrogen receptor modulator
- raloxifene (*Evista*)

Migraine headache
Ergots
- dihydroergotamine (*Migranal*)
- ergotamine
Triptans
- almotriptan (*Axert*)
- eletriptan (*Relpax*)
- frovatriptan (*Frova*)
- naratriptan (*Amerge*)
- rizatriptan (*Maxalt*)
- sumatriptan (*Imitrex*)

Myocardial infarction
Platelet inhibitors
- abciximab (*ReoPro*)
- aspirin (generic)
- clopidogrel (*Plavix*)
- eptifibatide (*Integrilin*)
- prasugrel (*Effient*)
- ticagrelor (*Brilinta*)
- ticlodipine (*Ticlid*)
- tirofiban (*Aggrastat*)
Anticoagulants
- dalteparin (*Fragmin*)
- enoxaparin (*Lovenox*)
- heparin (generic)
Pain relief
- morphine (generic)
Nitrates
- isosorbide dinitrate (*Isordil*)
- isosorbide mononitrate (*Imdur*)
- nitroglycerin (*Nitro-Bid, Nitrostat,* others)
Beta adrenergic blockers
- metoprolol (*Toprol*)
- nadolol (*Corgard*)
- propranolol (*Inderal*)
Calcium channel blockers
- amlodipine (*Norvasc*)
- diltiazem (*Cardizem*)
- nicardipine (*Cardene*)

- nifedipine (*Adalat*)
- verapamil (*Calan*)

Nausea and vomiting
Phenothiazines
- chlorpromazine (*Thorazine*)
- prochlorperazine (generic)
- promethazine (*Phenergan*)
- perphenazine (*Trilafon*)
Nonphenothiazines
- metoclopramide (*Reglan*)
Anticholinergics/antihistamines
- buclizine (*Bucladin*)
- cyclizine (*Marezine*)
- meclizine (*Antivert*)
5HT3 receptor blockers
- dolasetron (*Anzemet*)
- granisetron (*Kytril*)
- ondansetron (*Zofran*)
- palonosetron (*Aloxi*)
Substance P/neurokinin 1 receptor antagonist
- aprepitant (*Emend*)
Other
- dronabinol (*Marinol*)
- hydroxyzine (*Vistaril*)
- nabilone (*Cesamet)*
- trimethobenzamide (*Tigan*)

Obsessive compulsive disorder
Tricyclic antidepressants
- clomipramine (*Anafranil*)
Selective serotonin reuptake inhibitors
- citalopram (*Celexa*)
- fluoxetine (*Prozac*)
- fluvoxamine (*Luvox*)
- paroxetine (*Paxil*)
- sertraline (*Zoloft*)

Osteoporosis
Bisphosphonates
- alendronate (*Fosamax*)
- etidronate (*Didronel*)
- ibandronate (*Boniva*)
- pamidronate (*Aredia*)
- risedronate (*Actonel*)
- tiludronate (*Skelid*)
- zolendronic acid (*Reclast, Zometa*)
Calcitonin
- calcitonin, salmon (*Fortical, Miacalcin*)
Parathyroid hormone
- teriparatide (*Forteo*)

Estrogen modulator
- raloxifene (*Evista*)

Otitis media
Analgesics
- acetaminophen (*Tylenol*)
- ibuprofen (*Advil, Motrin*)
- benzocaine, topical (*Cyclex*)
Antibiotics
- amoxicillin (*Amoxil*)
- amoxicillin/clavulanate (*Augmentin*)
- cefdinir (*Omnicef*)
- ofloxacin (*Floxin*)

Parkinson disease
Dopaminergics
- amanatadine (*Symmetrel*)
- apomorphine (*Apokyn*)
- bromocriptine (*Parlodel*)
- carbidopa/levodopa (*Sinemet*)
- levodopa (*Dopar*)
- pramipexole (*Mirapex*)
- rasagiline (*Azilect*)
- ropinirole (*Requip*)
- rotigone (*Neupro*)
Anticholinergics
- benzotropine (*Cogentin*)
- diphenhydramine (*Benadryl*)
- trihexyphenidyl (*Artanei*)
Adjuncts
- entacapone (*Comtan*)
- selegiline (*Carbex, Eldepryl*)
- tolcapone (*Tasmar*)

Peptic ulcers
Histamine-2 antagonists
- cimetidine (*Tagamet*)
- famotidine (*Pepcid*)
- ranitidine (*Zantac*)
Proton pump inhibitors
- dexlansoprazole (*Kapidex*)
- esomeprazole (*Nexium*)
- lansoprazole (*Prevacid*)
- omeprazole (*Prilosec*)
- pantoprazole (*Protonix*)
- rabeprazole (*Aciphex*)
GI protectant
- sucralfate (*Carafate*)
Prostaglandin
- misoprostol (*Cyotec*)

Post-traumatic stress disorder
Selected serotonin reuptake inhibitors
- citalopram (*Celexa*)
- escitalopram (*Lexapro*)
- fluoxetine (*Prozac*)
- paroxetine (*Paxil*)
- sertraline (*Zoloft*)
- venlafaxine (*Effexor*)

Tricyclic antidepessant
- amitriptyline (*Elavil*)

Antipsychotics
- aripiprazole (*Abilify*)
- olanzapine (*Zyprexa*)
- quetiapine (*Seroquel*)
- risperidone (*Risperdol*)
- ziprasidone (*Geodon*)

Pulmonary artery hypertension
Endothelin receptor antagonist
- ambrisentan (*Letairis*)
- bosentan (*Tracleer*)
- treprostinil (*Remodulin*)

Phosphodiesterase inhibitors
- sildenafil (*Viagra*)
- tadalafil (*Adcirca*)

Prostaglandin
- epoprostenol (*Flolan*)

Prostacyclin
- iloprost (*Ventavis*)

Renal failure
Angiotensin converting enzyme inhibitors
- benazepril (*Lotensin*)
- captopril (*Capoten*)
- enalapril (*Vasotec*)
- fosinopril (*Monopril*)
- lisinopril (*Zestril*)
- moexipril (*Univasc*)
- perindopril (*Aceon*)
- quinapril (*Accupril*)
- ramipril (*Altace*)
- trandolapril (*Mavik*)

Angiotensin II receptor blockers
- azilsartan (*Edarbi*)
- candesartan (*Atacand*)
- eprosartan (*Teveten*)
- irbesartan (*Avapro*)
- losartan (*Cozaar*)
- olmesartan (*Benicar*)
- telmisartan (*Micardis*)
- valsartan (*Diovan*)

Diuretics
- bumetanide (*Bumex*)
- furosemide (*Lasix*)

Erythropoietins
- darbapoetin (*Aranesp*)
- epoetin alfa (*Procrit*)
- methoxy polyethylene glycol-epoetin beta (*Mircera*)

Vitamins
- doxercalciferol (*Hectoral*)
- paricalcitol (*Zemplar*)

Iron
- ferumoxytol (*Feraheme*)
- iron sucrose (*Venofer*)
- sodium ferric gluconate complex (*Ferrlacit*)

Phosphate binder
- lanthanum (*Fosrenol*)

Rhinitis (allergic/seasonal)
Topical nasal decongestants
- ephedrine (*Pretz-D*)
- oxymetazoline (*Afrinz*)
- phenylephrine (*Coricidin*)
- tetrahydrozoline (*Tyzine*)
- xylometazoline (*Otrivin*)

Nasal steroids
- beclomethasone (*Beclovent*)
- budesonide (*Pulmicort*)
- dexamethasone (*Decadron*)
- flunisolide (*AeroBid*)
- fluticasone (*Flovent*)
- triamcinolone (*Azamacort*)

Antihistamines
- brompheniramine (*Bidhist*)
- buclizine (*Bucladin-S*)
- carbinoxamine (*Histex*)
- chlorpheniramine (*Aller-Chlor*, others)
- clemastine (*Tavist*)
- cyclizine (*Marezine*)
- cyproheptadine (generic)
- dexchlorpheniramine (generic)
- dimenhydrinate (*Dimentabs*)
- diphenhydramine (*Benadryl*)
- hydroxyzine (*Vistaril*)
- phenindamine (*Nolahist*)
- promethazine (*Phergan*)
- tripolidine (*Zymine*)

Nonsedating nasal spray–only antihistamines
- azelastine (*Astelin*)
- cetirizine (*Zyrtec*)
- desloratadine (*Clarinex*)

- fexofenadine (*Allegra*)
- levocetirizine (*Xytal*)
- loratadine (*Claritin*)

Oral decongestant
- pseudoephedrine (*Sudafed*)

Schizophrenia
Typical antipsychotics
- chlorpromazine (*Thorazine*)
- fluphenazine (*Prolixin*)
- haloperidol (*Haldol*)
- loxapine (*Loxitane*)
- perphenazine (*Trilafon*)
- pimozide (*Orap*)
- prochlorperazine (generic)
- thioridazine (generic)
- thiothixene (*Navane*)
- trifluoperazine (generic)

Atypical antipsychotics
- aripiprazole (*Abilify*)
- clozapine (*Clozaril*)
- iloperidone (*Fanapt*)
- lurasidone (*Latuda*)
- olanzapine (*Zyprexa*)
- paliperidone (*Invega*)
- quetiapine (*Seroquel*)
- risperidone (*Risperdal*)
- ziprasidone (*Geodon*)

Seizure disorder
Hydantoins
- ethotoin (*Peganone*)
- fosphenytoin (*Cerebyx*)
- phenytoin (*Dilantin*)

Barbiturates
- mephobarbital (*Mebaral*)
- phenobarbital (*Solfoton*)
- primidone (*Mysoline*)

Benzodiazepines
- clobazam (*Onfi*)
- clonazepam (*Klonopin*)
- diazepam (*Valium*)

Succinimides
- ethosuximide (*Zarontin*)
- methsuximide (*Celontin*)

GABA modulators
- acetazolamide (*Diamox*)
- valproic acid (*Depakene*)
- zonisamide (*Zonegran*)

Drugs for partial seizures
- carbamazepine (*Tegretol*)
- clorazepate (*Tranxene*)
- felbamate (*Felbatol*)

- gabapentin (*Neurontin*)
- lacosamide (Vimpat*)
- lamotrigine (*Lamictal*)
- levetiracetam (*Keppra*)
- oxcarbazepine (*Trileptal*)
- pregabalin (*Lyrica*)
- rufinamide (*Banzel*)
- tiagabine (*Gabitril*)
- topiramate (*Topamax*)

Shock
Vasopressors
- dobutamine (*Dobutrex*)
- dopamine (*Intropin*)
- ephedrine (generic)
- epinephrine (*Adrenalin*)
- isoproterenol (*Isuprel*)
- norepinephrine (*Levophed*)

Thromboembolic disorders
Heparins
- dalteparin (*Fragmin*)
- enoxaparin (*Lovenox*)
- heparin
- tinzaparin (*Innohep*)

Oral anticoagulants
- dabigatran (*Pradaxa*)
- rivaroxaban (*Xarelto*)
- warfarin (*Coumadin*)

Thyroid dysfunction
Replacement
- levothyroxine (*Synthroid, Levoxyl,* others)
- liothyronine (*Cytomel*)
- liotrix (*Thyrolar*)
- thyroid, dessicated (*Armour Thyroid*)

Antithyroid
- methimazole (*Tapazole*)
- propylthiouracil
- sodium iodide/potassium iodide (*Thyroblock*)

Tuberculosis
First line
Antimycobacterial antibiotics
- ethambutol (*Myambutol*)
- isoniazid (*Nydrazid*)
- pyrazinamide (generic)
- rifampin (*Rifadin*)
- rifapentine (*Priftin*)
- streptomycin (generic)

Second line
- capreomycin (*Capastat*)
- cycloserine (*Seromycin*)
- ethionamide (*Treactor*)
- rifabutin (*Mycobutin*)

Urinary tract infection
Anti-infectives
- cinoxacin (*Cinobac*)
- co-trimoxazole (*Bactrim, Septra*)

- fosfomycin (*Monurol*)
- methenamine (*Hiprex*)
- methylene blue (*Urolene Blue*)
- nitrofurantoin (*Furadantin*)
- norfloxaxin (*Noraxin*)

Appendix T

Quick guide to reputable Internet sites

Agency for Healthcare Research and Quality (AHRQ)
www.ahrq.gov

American Diabetes Association
www.diabetes.org

American Heart Association
www.americanheart.org

Centers for Disease Control and Prevention (CDC)
www.cdc.gov

Drugs @ FDA
www.accessdata.fda.gov/scripts/cder/
drugsatfda

Food and Drug Administration (FDA)
www.fda.gov

Healthfinder
www.healthfinder.gov

Institute for Safe Medication Practices
www.ismp.org

The Joint Commission (TJC)
www.jointcommission.org

Medwatch
www.fda.gov/Safety/Medwatch

National Cancer Institute (Cancer Net)
www.cancer.gov

National Center for Complementary and Alternative Medicine
www.nccam.nih.gov

National Heart Lung and Blood Institute
www.nhlbi.nih.gov

National Institute for Occupational Safety and Health
www.cdc.gov/niosh

National Institutes of Health
www.nih.gov

National Library of Medicine
www.nlm.nih.gov

Bibliography

Aschenbrenner, D., & Venable, S. (2011). *Drug therapy in nursing* (4th ed.). Philadelphia, PA: Lippincott Williams & Wilkins.

Brunton, L., Chabner, B., & Khollman, B. (2010). *Goodman and Gilman's the pharmacological basis of therapeutics* (12th ed.). New York, NY: McGraw-Hill.

Carpenito-Moyet, L. J. (2012). *Nursing diagnosis: Application to clinical practice* (14th ed.). Philadelphia, PA: Lippincott Williams & Wilkins.

Drug evaluations subscription. (2012). Chicago, IL: American Medical Association.

Drug facts and comparisons. (2013). St. Louis, MO: Facts and Comparisons.

Drug facts update: Physicians on-line. (2012). Multimedia.

Fetrow, C. W., & Avila, J. (2003). *Professional handbook of complementary and alternative medicines* (3rd ed.). Springhouse, PA: Lippincott Williams & Wilkins.

Griffiths, M. C. (Ed.). (2012). *USAN and the USP 2012 dictionary of drug names.* Rockville, MD: United States Pharmacopeial Convention.

Handbook of adverse drug interactions. (2012). New Rochelle, NY: The Medical Letter.

ISMP medication safety alert! (2012). Huntingdon Valley, PA: Institute for Safe Medication Practices.

Karch, A. M. (2013). *Focus on nursing pharmacology* (6th ed.). Philadelphia, PA: Lippincott Williams & Wilkins.

The medical letter on drugs and therapeutics. (2013). New Rochelle, NY: Medical Letter.

PDR for nonprescriptive drugs. (2013). Oradell, NJ: Medical Economics.

PDR for ophthalmic medications. (2012). Oradell, NJ: Medical Economics.

Physicians' desk reference (67th ed.). (2013). Oradell, NJ: Medical Economics.

Smeltzer, S. C., & Bare, B. G. (2009). *Brunner and Suddarth's textbook of medical-surgical nursing* (12th ed.). Philadelphia, PA: Lippincott Williams & Wilkins.

Tatro, D. S. (Ed.). (2012). *Drug interaction facts.* St. Louis, MO: Facts and Comparisons.

Index

Generic names and alternative therapies are boldface in main entries. *Brand names* of drugs are in italics, followed by the generic name in parentheses. Brand names of Canadian drugs are followed by (CAN). Chemical or nonofficial names appear in regular typeface. **DRUG CLASSES** appear in bold capital letters with the drugs that fall in that class listed as official names under the CLASS HEADING.

ANTINEOPLASTICS *(continued)*
medroxyprogesterone: 728
megestrol: 731
melphalan: 734
mercaptopurine: 742
methotrexate: 756
mitomycin: 796
mitotane: 1379
mitoxantrone: 798
nelarabine: 1379
nilotinib: 1379
ofatumumab: 1380
omacetaxine: 1380
oxaliplatin: 1381
paclitaxel: 896
panitumumab: 1382
pegaspargase: 1382
pemetrexed: 1383
pentostatin: 1384
pertuzumab: 1384
porfimer: 1386
pralatrexate: 1386
procarbazine: 1386
regorafenib: 1387
rituximab: 1388
romidepsin: 1389
sorafenib: 1391
streptozocin: 1391
sunitinib: 1392
tamoxifen: 1090
temozolomide: 1393
temsirolimus: 1393
thioguanine: 1120
thiotepa: 1121
tolvaptan: 1395
topotecan: 1395
toremifene: 1150
tositumomab: 1396
trastuzumab: 1158
tretinoin: 1161
triptorelin: 1175
vinblastine: 1196
vincristine: 1198
vinorelbine: 1200
vemurafenib: 1397
vismodegib: 1398

ANTINEOPLASTICS *(continued)*
vorinostat: 1398
ziv-aflibercept: 1398
ANTIPARKINSONIANS
amantadine: 105
apomorphine: 1350
atropine: 159
benztropine: 181
bromocriptine: 199
diphenhydramine: 391
entacapone: 436
levodopa: 676
pramipexole: 956
rasagiline: 1010
ropinirole: 1032
rotigotine: 1036
selegiline: 1050
tolcapone: 1144
trihexyphenidyl: 1169
ANTIPEPTIC ULCER DRUG
sucralfate: 1077
ANTIPLATELETS
abciximab: 68
anagrelide: 132
aspirin: 148
cilostazol: 281
clopidogrel: 308
dipyridamole: 1363
eptifibatide: 449
prasugrel: 959
ticagrelor: 1127
ticlopidine: 1128
tirofiban: 1138
ANTIPROTOZOALS
atovaquone: 158
metronidazole: 775
nitazoxanide: 1380
pentamidine: 917
tinidazole: 1133
ANTIPSORIATICS
acitretin: 1346
ANTIPSORIATICS, TOPICAL
anthralin: 1252
calcipotriene: 1252

auranofin: 1351
Aurolate (gold sodium): 1370
Author's acknowledgments: xvii
Avalide (irbesartan, hydrochlorothiazide): 1288, 1303
avanafil: 162
Avandamet (rosiglitazone, metformin): 1282, 1303
Avandaryl (rosiglitazone, glimepiride): 1282, 1303
Avandia (rosiglitazone): 1389, C26
Avapro (irbesartan): 635, C14
Avastin (bevacizumab): 1353
Avelox (moxifloxacin): 807, C20
Avelox ABC Pack (moxifloxacin): 807
Avelox IV (moxifloxacin): 807
Aventyl (nortriptyline): 857
Aviane (estradiol, levonorgestrel): 1303, 1313
Avinza (morphine): 804
Avita (tretinoin): 1161, 1250
Avodart (dutasteride): 420, C9
Avonex (interferon beta-1a): 628
Axert (almotriptan): 95
Axid (nizatidine): 849
Axid AR (nizatidine): 849
Axid Pulvules (nizatidine): 849
Axiron (testosterone): 1109
axitinib: 1352
Axsain (capsaicin): 1250
Aygestin (norethindrone): 852
azacitidine: 1352
Azactam (aztreonam): 168
Azasan (azathioprine): 163
AzaSite (azithromycin): 166, 1261
azathioprine: 163
Azdone (hydrocodone, aspirin): 1303
azelaic acid: 1249
azelastine hydrochloride: 1252, 1261
Azelex (azelaic acid): 1249
azidothymidine (zidovudine): 1209
Azilect (rasagiline): 1010, C25
azilsartan medoxomil: 165
azithromycin: 166, 1261, C5
Azopt (brinzolamide): 1261
Azor (amlodipine, olmesartan): 1285, 1303
AZO-Standard (phenazopyridine): 927

AZT (zidovudine): 1209
aztreonam: 168
Azulfidine (sulfasalazine): 1081
Azulfidine EN-Tabs (sulfasalazine): 1081
Azurette (desogestrel, ethinyl estradiol): 1314

B

B-LYMPHOCYTE STIMULANT INHIBITOR
   belimumab: 1353
BabyBIG (botulism immune globulin): 1344
Baciguent (CAN) (bacitracin): 170
Baci-IM (bacitracin): 170
Baciject (CAN) (bacitracin): 170
bacitracin: 170
baclofen: 171
BactoShield (chlorhexidine): 1252
Bactrim (co-trimoxazole): 1277, 1303
Bactrim DS (co-trimoxazole): 1277, C27
Bactroban (mupirocin): 1251
Bactroban Nasal (mupirocin): 1251
BAL in Oil (dimercaprol): 1363
Balminil DM (CAN) (dextromethorphan): 372
Balnetar (anthralin): 1252
balsalazide disodium: 173
Balziva (estradiol, norethindrone): 1313
Banflex (orphenadrine): 875
Banophen (diphenhydramine): 391
Banzel (rufinamide): 1389
Baraclude (entecavir): 438
barberry: 1223
BARBITURATES (see also page 32)
   pentobarbital: 921
   phenobarbital: 931
   secobarbital: 1048
Baridium (phenazopyridine): 927
basil: 1223
basiliximab: 1352
bayberry: 1223
Bayer (aspirin): 148
Bayer Advanced Aspirin (aspirin): 148
Bayer Plus Extra Strength (aspirin, calcium carbonate): 1303

Qutenza (capsaicin): 1250
QVAR (beclomethasone): 174

R

rabeprazole sodium: 1000, C25
rabies immune globulin: 1344
rabies vaccine: 1345
Rabivert (rabies vaccine): 1345
Radiogardase (insoluble Prussian blue): 1372
raloxifene hydrochloride: 1001, C25
raltegravir: 1002
ramelteon: 1003
ramipril: 1005
Ranexa (ranolazine): 1008, C25
ranibizumab: 1387
Raniclor (cefaclor): 237
ranitidine: 1007, C25
ranolazine: 1008, C25
Rapaflo (silodosin): 1055
Rapamune (sirolimus): 1390
rasagiline: 1010, C25
rasburicase: 1387
raspberry: 1230
ratio-Acyclovir (CAN) (acyclovir): 81
ratio-Alendronate (CAN) (alendronate): 88
ratio-Amiodarone (CAN) (amiodarone): 117
ratio-Atenolol (CAN) (atenolol): 153
ratio-Baclofen (CAN) (baclofen): 171
ratio-Beclomethasone AQ (CAN)
    (beclomethasone): 174
ratio-Carvedilol (CAN) (carvedilol): 235
ratio-Ciprofloxacin (CAN) (ciprofloxacin): 285
ratio-Citalopram (CAN) (citalopram): 289
ratio-Clonazepam (CAN) (clonazepam): 303
ratio-Cyclobenzaprine (CAN)
    (cyclobenzaprine): 324
ratio-Desipramine (CAN) (desipramine): 352
ratio-Dexamethasone (CAN) (dexamethasone):
    359
ratio-Diltiazem (CAN) (diltiazem): 386
ratio-Fenofibrate MC (CAN) (fenofibrate): 499
ratio-Flunisolide (CAN) (flunisolide): 522
ratio-Fluoxetine (CAN) (fluoxetine): 525
ratio-Fluvoxamine (CAN) (fluvoxamine): 535
ratio-Gabapentin (CAN) (gabapentin): 553
ratio-Glimepiride (CAN) (glimepiride): 565

ratio-Glyburide (CAN) (glyburide): 569
ratio-Ipratropium (CAN) (ipratropium): 634
ratio-Ipratropium UDV (CAN) (ipratropium):
    634
ratio-Lactulose (CAN) (lactulose): 659
ratio-Lamotrigine (CAN) (lamotrigine): 662
ratio-Lovastatin (CAN) (lovastatin): 711
ratio-Meloxicam (CAN) (meloxicam): 733
ratio-Metformin (CAN) (metformin): 749
ratio-Methotrexate (CAN) (methotrexate): 756
ratio-Minocycline (CAN) (minocycline): 788
ratio-Morphine SR (CAN) (morphine): 804
ratio-Nortriptyline (CAN) (nortriptyline): 857
ratio-Nystatin (CAN) (nystatin): 859
ratio-Paroxetine (CAN) (paroxetine): 906
ratio-Pentoxifylline (CAN) (pentoxifylline):
    923
ratio-Pioglitazone (CAN) (pioglitazone): 943
ratio-Pravastatin (CAN) (pravastatin): 961
ratio-Prednisolone (CAN) (prednisolone): 964
ratio-Ranitidine (CAN) (ranitidine): 1007
ratio-Sertraline (CAN) (sertraline): 1051
ratio-Simvastatin (CAN) (simvastatin): 1057
ratio-Sotalol (CAN) (sotalol): 1071
ratio-Sumatriptan (CAN) (sumatriptan): 1084
ratio-Temazepam (CAN) (temazepam): 1100
ratio-Terazosin (CAN) (terazosin): 1105
ratio-Topiramate (CAN) (topiramate): 1148
ratio-Valproic (CAN) (valproic acid): 1183
Razadyne (galantamine): 554
Razadyne ER (galantamine): 554
Reactine (CAN) (cetirizine): 261
Rebetol (ribavirin): 1013
Rebif (interferon beta-1a): 628
Reclast (zoledronic acid): 1213
Reclipsen (estradiol, desogestrel): 1313
recombinant human deoxyribonuclease
    (dornase): 1363
recombinant human erythropoietin (epoetin):
    446
recombinant human interleukin (oprelvekin):
    1381
recombinant tissue-type plasminogen activator
    (alteplase): 102
Recombinate (antihemophilic factor): 137
Recombivax-HB (hepatitis B vaccine): 1326

S

S_2 (epinephrine): 441
Sabril (vigabatrin): 1398
sacrosidase: 1390
Safyral (drospirenone, ethinyl estradiol, levonorgestrel): 1310, 1314
saffron: 1230
sage: 1230
Saint John's wort: 1231
Saizen (somatropin): 1068
Salagen (pilocarpine hydrochloride): 1385
Salazopyrin EN-Tabs (CAN) (sulfasalazine): 1081
Salflex (salsalate): 1039
SALICYLATES
  aspirin: 148
  choline magnesium trisalicylate: 1358
  salsalate: 1039
  salicylsalicylic acid (salsalate): 1039
SALIVA SUBSTITUTE
  saliva substitute: 1037
saliva substitute: 1037
Salivart (saliva substitute): 1037
Salk (poliovirus vaccine): 1339
salmeterol: 1038
Salmonine (calcitonin, salmon): 215
Salofalk (CAN) (mesalamine): 745
Salonpas (methylsalicylate, menthol): 1274, 1310
salsalate: 1039
Salsitab (salsalate): 1039
SAM-e: 1230
Samsca (tolvaptan): 1395
Sanctura (trospium): 1177
Sanctura XR (trospium): 1177
Sancuso (granisetron): 576
Sandimmune (cyclosporine): 328
Sandostatin (octreotide): 860
Sandostatin LAR Depot (octreotide): 860
Sandoz-Mirtazapine (CAN) (mirtazapine): 793
Sani-Supp (glycerin): 1268
Saphris (asenapine): 146
sapropterin: 1390
saquinavir mesylate: 1041
Sarafem (fluoxetine): 525, C12

Sarafem Pulvules (fluoxetine): 525
sargramostim: 1042
sarsaparilla: 1230
sassafras: 1230
Savella (milnacipran): 1378
saw palmetto: 1230
saxagliptin: 1044
schisandra: 1230
SCIG (immune globulin, subcutaneous): 1329
SCLEROSING AGENT
  polidocanol: 1385
  talc, USP: 1392
Scopolamine Hbr (scopolamine): 1046
scopolamine hydrobromide: 1046
Scot-tussin Expectorant (guaifenesin): 577
Sculptra (poly-L-lactic acid): 1385
Seasonale (ethinyl estradiol, levonorgestrel): 1310, 1314
Seasonique (ethinyl estradiol, levonorgestrel): 1310, 1314, 1315
secobarbital sodium: 1048
Seconal Sodium (secobarbital): 1048
secretin: 1390
Sectral (acebutolol): 72
Sedapap (acetaminophen, butalbital): 1310
SEDATIVES AND HYPNOTICS
  chloral hydrate: 264
  dexmedetomidine: 1362
  diphenhydramine: 391
  estazolam: 461
  eszopiclone: 472
  flurazepam: 530
  fospropofol: 547
  lorazepam: 706
  nitrazepam (CAN): 1247
  pentobarbital: 921
  phenobarbital: 931
  promethazine: 977
  quazepam: 993
  ramelteon: 1003
  secobarbital: 1048
  temazepam: 1100
  triazolam: 1168
  zaleplon: 1207
  zolpidem: 1216
  zopiclone (CAN): 1248